Anderson's
PATHOLOGY

VOLUME ONE

Anderson's
PATHOLOGY

Edited by

JOHN M. KISSANE, M.D.

Professor of Pathology and of Pathology in Pediatrics,
Washington University School of Medicine;
Pathologist, Barnes and Affiliated Hospitals,
St. Louis Children's Hospital, St. Louis, Missouri

NINTH EDITION

with **2269** illustrations and **8** color plates

The C. V. Mosby Company

ST. LOUIS • BALTIMORE • PHILADELPHIA • TORONTO   1990

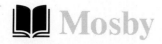

Editor: George Stamathis
Developmental Editor: Elaine Steinborn
Assistant Editor: Jo Salway
Project Manager: Kathleen L. Teal
Production Editor: Carl Masthay
Book and Cover Design: Gail Morey Hudson
Production: Ginny Douglas, Teresa Breckwoldt

Two volumes

NINTH EDITION

The C.V. Mosby Company
11830 Westline Industrial Drive, St. Louis, Missouri 63146

Library of Congress Cataloging in Publication Data

Pathology (Saint Louis, Mo.)
    Anderson's pathology.—9th ed. / edited by John M. Kissane.
        p.   cm.
    Includes bibliographies and index.
    ISBN 0-8016-2772-9 (set)
    1. Pathology.   I. Kissane, John M., 1928-   . II. Anderson,
W.A.D. (William Arnold Douglas), 1910-1986. III. Title. IV. Title:
Pathology.
    [DNLM: 1. Pathology.   QZ 4 P2984]
RB111.P3   1990
616.07—dc19
DNLM/DLC   89-3072
for Library of Congress   CIP

C/VH/VH   9 8 7 6 5 4 3 2 1

Contributors

ARTHUR C. ALLEN, M.D.

Professor of Pathology, State University of New York,
Downstate Medical Center; Consultant Pathologist,
The Brooklyn Hospital–Caledonian Hospital,
Brooklyn, New York

ROBERT E. ANDERSON, M.D.

Frederick H. Harvey Professor and Chairman,
Department of Pathology, The University of New Mexico,
Albuquerque, New Mexico

FREDERIC B. ASKIN, M.D.

Professor of Pathology
University of North Carolina School of Medicine;
Director of Surgical Pathology,
North Carolina Memorial Hospital,
Chapel Hill, North Carolina

SAROJA BHARATI, MD.

Professor of Pathology, Department of Pathology,
Rush Medical School, Rush–Presbyterian–
St. Luke's Medical Center, Chicago;
Director, Congenital Heart and Conduction System Center,
Heart Institute for Children of Christ Hospital,
Palos Heights, Illinois

CHAPMAN H. BINFORD, M.D.

Formerly Chief, Special Mycobacterial Diseases Branch,
Geographic Pathology Division,
Armed Forces Institute of Pathology,
Washington, D.C.

FRANCIS W. CHANDLER, D.V.M., Ph.D.

Professor of Pathology, Department of Pathology,
Medical College of Georgia,
Augusta, Georgia

JOSÉ COSTA, M.D.

Professor of Pathology, Director, Institute of Pathology,
University of Lausanne,
Lausanne, Switzerland

JOHN REDFERND CRAIG, M.D., Ph.D.

Associate Clinical Professor, Department of Pathology,
University of Southern California School of Medicine,
Los Angeles;
Chief Pathologist, Department of Pathology,
St. Luke Medical Center, Pasadena;
St. Jude Hospital and Rehabilitation Center,
Fullerton, California

CHARLES J. DAVIS, Jr., M.D.

Associate Chairman, Department of Genitourinary
Pathology, Armed Forces Institute of Pathology,
Professor of Pathology,
Uniformed Services University of Health Sciences,
Washington, D.C.

KATHERINE De SCHRYVER-KECSKEMÉTI, M.D.

Professor of Pathology, Director, Anatomic and
Surgical Pathology, Case Western Reserve University,
Cleveland, Ohio

MICHAEL D. FALLON, M.D.

Associate Professor of Pathology and Cell Biology,
Department of Pathology,
Thomas Jefferson Medical College;
Attending Pathologist, Division of Surgical Pathology;
Director of the Division of Orthopaedic Pathology,
Department of Pathology,
Thomas Jefferson University Hospital,
Philadelphia, Pennsylvania

ROBERT E. FECHNER, M.D.

Royster Professor of Pathology and Director,
Division of Surgical Pathology,
University of Virginia Health Sciences Center,
Charlottesville, Virginia

GERALD FINE, M.D.

Formerly Chief, Division of Anatomic Pathology,
Henry Ford Hospital, Detroit;
Consulting Pathologist, Holy Cross Hospital, Detroit;
St. Joseph's Hospital,
Mt. Clemens, Michigan

KAARLE O. FRANSSILA, M.D. Ph.D.

Chief of Pathology Laboratory, Department of Radiotherapy
and Oncology, Helsinki University Central Hospital,
Helsinki, Finland

VICTOR E. GOULD, M.D.

Professor and Associate Chairman of Pathology,
Rush Medical College, Chicago, Illinois

ROGERS C. GRIFFITH, M.D.

Assistant Professor of Pathology, Brown University,
Providence, Rhode Island

JOHN G. GRUHN, M.D.

Associate Professor of Pathology, Rush Medical College,
Chicago, Illinois

DONALD B. HACKEL, M.D.

Professor of Pathology, Department of Pathology,
Duke University Medical Center,
Durham, North Carolina

REID R. HEFFNER, Jr., M.D.

Professor of Pathology, Department of Pathology,
State University of New York,
Buffalo, New York

GORDON R. HENNIGAR, M.D.

Professor of Pathology, Department of Pathology and
Laboratory Medicine, Medical University of South Carolina,
Charleston, South Carolina

CHARLES S. HIRSCH, M.D.

Chief Medical Examiner, Suffolk County, New York;
Professor of Forensic Pathology,
SUNY Medical School at Stony Brook,
Stony Brook, New York

PHILIP M. IANNACCONE, M.D., D.Phil. (Oxon)

Associate Professor of Pathology,
Northwestern University, Chicago;
Associate Staff Attending, Pathology,
Northwestern Memorial Hospital,
Chicago, Illinois

CHRISTINE G. JANNEY, M.D.

Assistant Professor of Pathology,
St. Louis University School of Medicine,
St. Louis, Missouri

HAN-SEOB KIM, M.D.

Associate Professor of Pathology,
Baylor College of Medicine;
Attending Pathologist, The Methodist Hospital,
Harris County Hospital District, Houston, Texas

JOHN M. KISSANE, M.D.

Professor of Pathology and Pathology in Pediatrics,
Washington University School of Medicine; Pathologist,
Barnes and Affiliated Hospitals, St. Louis Children's
Hospital at Washington University Medical Center,
St. Louis, Missouri

FREDERICK T. KRAUS, M.D.

Professor of Pathology (Visiting Staff),
Washington University School of Medicine;
Director of Laboratory Medicine,
St. John's Mercy Medical Center,
St. Louis, Missouri

CHARLES KUHN III, M.D.

Professor of Pathology, Brown University,
Providence, Rhode Island;
Pathologist in Chief, Memorial Hospital of Rhode Island,
Pawtucket, Rhode Island

MICHAEL KYRIAKOS, M.D.

Professor of Pathology, Washington University School of
Medicine; Surgical Pathologist, Barnes Hospital;
Consultant to St. Louis Children's Hospital at
Washington University Medical Center and to
Shriner's Hospital for Crippled Children,
St. Louis, Missouri

PAUL E. LACY, M.D.

Mallinckrodt Professor and Chairman, Department of
Pathology, Washington University School of Medicine,
St. Louis, Missouri

RUSSELL M. LEBOVITZ, M.D., Ph.D.

Assistant Professor of Pathology, Baylor College of Medicine,
Houston, Texas

MAURICE LEV, M.D.

Professor of Pathology, Department of Pathology,
Rush Medical School, Rush–Presbyterian–
St. Luke's Medical Center, Chicago;
Associate Director, Congenital Heart and Conduction
System Center, Heart Institute for
Children of Christ Hospital,
Palos Heights, Illinois

MICHAEL W. LIEBERMAN, M.D. Ph.D.

Professor and The W.L. Moody, Jr., Chairman,
Department of Pathology, Baylor College of Medicine,
Houston, Texas

CHAN K. MA, M.D.

Staff Pathologist, Department of Pathology,
Henry Ford Hospital,
Detroit, Michigan

JOSEPH A. MADRI, M.D., Ph.D.

Department of Pathology,
Yale University School of Medicine,
New Haven, Connecticut

MANUEL A. MARCIAL, M.D.

Associate Professor and Chairman,
Department of Pathology and Laboratory Medicine,
Universidad Central del Caribe, Escuela de Medicina,
Bayamón, Puerto Rico

RAÚL A. MARCIAL-ROJAS, M.D., J.D.

Professor and Dean, Universidad Central del Caribe,
Escuela de Medicina,
Bayamón, Puerto Rico

ROBERT W. McDIVITT, M.D.

Director, Division of Anatomic Pathology,
Department of Anatomic Pathology,
Washington University School of Medicine;
Chief of Anatomic Pathology,
Department of Anatomic Pathology, Barnes Hospital;
Consultant St. Louis Children's Hospital at Washington
University Medical Center, St. Louis, Missouri

WAYNE M. MEYERS, M.D., Ph.D.

Chief, Division of Microbiology,
Armed Forces Institute of Pathology,
Washington, D.C.

F. KASH MOSTOFI, M.D.

Chairman, Department of Genitourinary Pathology,
Armed Forces Institute of Pathology, Washington, D.C.;
Professor of Pathology,
Uniformed Services University of Health Sciences,
Bethesda, Maryland;
Associate Professor of Pathology,
Johns Hopkins University School of Medicine,
Clinical Professor of Pathology,
University of Maryland Medical School,
Baltimore, Maryland;
Clinical Professor of Pathology,
Georgetown University School of Medicine,
Washington, D.C.

JAMES S. NELSON, M.D.

Clinical Professor of Pathology, Department of Pathology,
University of Michigan, Ann Arbor, Michigan;
Division Head, Neuropathology, Department of Pathology,
Henry Ford Hospital, Detroit, Michigan

JAMES E. OERTEL, M.D.

Chairman, Department of Endocrine Pathology,
Armed Forces Institute of Pathology,
Washington, D.C.

JEFFREY M. OGORZALEK, M.D.

Major, US Air Force, Medical Corps;
Pathologist, Department of Endocrine Pathology,
Armed Forces Institute of Pathology,
Washington, D.C.

ALAN S. RABSON, M.D.

Director, Division of Cancer Biology and Diagnosis,
National Cancer Institute,
Bethesda, Maryland

KEITH A. REIMER, M.D., Ph.D.

Professor of Pathology, Department of Pathology,
Duke University Medical Center,
Durham, North Carolina

JUAN ROSAI, M.D.

Professor and Director of Anatomic Pathology,
Department of Pathology,
Yale University School of Medicine,
New Haven, Connecticut

DANTE G. SCARPELLI, M.D., Ph.D.

Ernest J. and Hattie H. Magerstadt Professor and Chairman,
Department of Pathology,
Northwestern University Medical School;
Chief of Service, Northwestern Memorial Hospital,
Chicago, Illinois

HARRY A. SCHWAMM, M.D.

Chairman, Department of Pathology,
The Graduate Hospital;
Clinical Professor of Orthopaedic Surgery (Pathology),
Department of Orthopaedic Surgery;
Clinical Professor of Pathology, Department of Pathology,
University of Pennsylvania School of Medicine,
Philadelphia, Pennsylvania

STEWART SELL, M.D.

Professor, Department of Pathology and Laboratory Medicine,
University of Texas Health Science Center at Houston,
Houston, Texas

GEORGE F. SCHREINER, M.D. Ph.D.

Assistant Professor of Medicine and Pathology,
Department of Medicine, Pathology,
Washington University School of Medicine;
Assistant Physician, Department of Medicine,
Barnes Hospital,
St. Louis, Missouri

HERSCHEL SIDRANSKY, M.D.

Professor and Chairman, Department of Pathology,
The George Washington University Medical Center,
Washington, D.C.

RUTH SILBERBERG, M.D.

Visiting Scientist,
Hadassah Hebrew University School of Medicine,
Jerusalem, Israel

MORTON E. SMITH, M.D.

Professor of Ophthalmology and Pathology,
Washington University School of Medicine,
St. Louis, Missouri

JACK L. TITUS, M.D., Ph.D.

Director, Jesse E. Edwards Registry of Cardiovascular
Disease, United Hospital;
Clinical Professor of Pathology, University of Minnesota,
St. Paul, Minnesota;
Formerly Professor and The W.L. Moody, Jr., Chairman,
Department of Pathology, Baylor College of Medicine;
Chief, Pathology Service, The Methodist Hospital;
Pathologist-in-Chief, Harris County Hospital District,
Houston, Texas

CHARLES A. WALDRON, D.D.S., M.S.D.

Professor Emeritus and Consultant, Oral Pathology,
Emory University School of Postgraduate Dentistry,
Atlanta, Georgia

DAVID H. WALKER, M.D.

Professor and Chairman, Department of Pathology,
The University of Texas Medical Branch at Galveston,
Galveston, Texas

NANCY E. WARNER, M.D.

Hastings Professor of Pathology,
University of Southern California School of Medicine,
Los Angeles, California

JOHN C. WATTS, M.D.

Attending Pathologist, Department of Anatomic Pathology,
William Beaumont Hospital, Royal Oak, Michigan;
Clinical Associate Professor of Pathology,
Wayne State University School of Medicine,
Detroit, Michigan

ROSS E. ZUMWALT, M.D.

Associate Professor, Department of Pathology,
University of New Mexico School of Medicine;
Assistant Chief Medical Investigator–State of New Mexico,
Office of the Medical Investigator,
Albuquerque, New Mexico

Preface to the Ninth Edition

My first responsibility, and it is a sad one, as editor of this ninth edition of *Anderson's Pathology,* is to mourn the loss of Dr. W.A.D. Anderson, creator and through nearly four decades guiding spirit of this book, which bears his name. He was an Emeritus Professor of Pathology and former Chairman of the Department of Pathology at the University of Miami School of Medicine in Miami, Florida. When he died on January 20, 1986, many of us lost a friend, and Pathology lost a scholarly spokesman. We will all miss him.

This edition continues the tradition of prior editions' concern. In the introductory chapters, mechanisms of human disease are addressed; these are followed by chapters that consider diseases of the several organ systems. Consideration of diseases of the various organ systems is deliberately made thorough so that the book can remain a useful and reliable source of information not only for medical students and trainees in pathology, but also for those training and practicing in other disciplines.

The eighth edition witnessed the emergence of acquired immunodeficiency syndrome (AIDS) as a major public health problem in industrialized societies as well as, by virtue of its protean clinical and morphologic manifestations, an important diagnostic consideration in specific patients. In preparing for this ninth edition, I considered allocating a separate chapter to AIDS. Eventually I decided to leave the consideration of AIDS within the several chapters addressing various organ systems, both for its basic aspects and for the descriptions of specific clinicopathologic features. Somewhat similar considerations related to the treatment of transplantation pathology, and the same decision was reached. These decisions remain very much open and may be amended in future revisions.

This edition of *Pathology* includes more than the usual number of chapters by new contributors. I welcome each of them and at the same time express my gratitude to their predecessors who have participated so importantly in the success this book has enjoyed throughout its long life.

John M. Kissane

Preface to First Edition

Pathology should form the basis of every physician's thinking about his patients. The study of the nature of disease, which constitutes pathology in the broad sense, has many facets. Any science or technique which contributes to our knowledge of the nature and constitution of disease belongs in the broad realm of pathology. Different aspects of a disease may be stressed by the geneticist, the cytologist, the biochemist, the clinical diagnostician, etc., and it is the difficult function of the pathologist to attempt to bring about a synthesis, and to present disease in as whole or as true an aspect as can be done with present knowledge. Pathologists often have been accused, and sometimes justly, of stressing the morphologic changes in disease to the neglect of functional effects. Nevertheless, pathologic anatomy and histology remain as an essential foundation of knowledge about disease, without which basis the concepts of many diseases are easily distorted.

In this volume is brought together the specialized knowledge of a number of pathologists in particular aspects or fields of pathology. A time-tested order of presentation is maintained, both because it has been found logical and effective in teaching medical students and because it facilitates study and reference by graduates. Although presented in an order and form to serve as a textbook, it is intended also to have sufficient comprehensiveness and completeness to be useful to the practicing or graduate physician. It is hoped that this book will be both a foundation and a useful tool for those who deal with the problems of disease.

For obvious reasons, the nature and effects of radiation have been given unusual relative prominence. The changing order of things, with increase of rapid, worldwide travel and communication, necessitates increased attention to certain viral, protozoal, parasitic, and other conditions often dismissed as "tropical," to bring them nearer their true relative importance. Also, given more than usual attention are diseases of the skin, of the organs of special senses, of the nervous system, and of the skeletal system. These are fields which often have not been given sufficient consideration in accordance with their true relative importance among diseases.

The Editor is highly appreciative of the spirit of the various contributors to this book. They are busy people, who, at the sacrifice of other duties and of leisure, freely cooperated in its production, uncomplainingly tolerated delays and difficulties, and were understanding in their willingness to work together for the good of the book as a whole. Particular thanks are due the directors of the Army Institute of Pathology and the American Registry of Pathology, for making available many illustrations. Dr. G.L. Duff, Strathcona Professor of Pathology, McGill University, Dr. H.A. Edmondson, Department of Pathology of the University of Southern California School of Medicine, Dr. J.S. Hirschboeck, Dean, and Dr. Harry Beckman, Professor of Pharmacology, Marquette University School of Medicine, all generously gave advice and assistance with certain parts.

To the members of the Department of Pathology and Bacteriology at Marquette University, the Editor wishes to express gratitude, both for tolerance and for assistance. Especially valuable has been the help of Dr. R.S. Haukohl, Dr. J.F. Kuzma, Dr. S.B. Pessin, and Dr. H. Everett. A large burden was assumed by the Editor's secretaries, Miss Charlotte Skacel and Miss Ann Cassady. Miss Patricia Blakeslee also assisted at various stages and with the index. To all of these the Editor's thanks, and also to the many others who at some time assisted by helpful and kindly acts, or by words of encouragement or interest.

W.A.D. Anderson

Contents

VOLUME ONE

1   Cell injury and errors of metabolism, 1
Dante G. Scarpelli
Philip M. Iannaccone

2   Inflammation and healing, 67
Joseph A. Madri

3   Injuries caused by physical agents, 111
Charles S. Hirsch
Ross E. Zumwalt

4   Drug and chemical injury—environmental pathology, 146
Gordon R. Hennigar

5   Radiation injury, 247
Robert E. Anderson

6   Bacterial diseases, 289
John M. Kissane

7   Leprosy, 333
Wayne M. Meyers
Chapman H. Binford

8   Rickettsial and chlamydial diseases, 348
David H. Walker

9   Viral diseases, 362
José Costa
Alan S. Rabson

10   Mycotic, actinomycotic, and algal infections, 391
Francis W. Chandler
John C. Watts

11   Protozoal and helminthic diseases, 433
Manuel A. Marcial
Raúl A. Marcial-Rojas

12   Immunopathology (hypersensitivity diseases), 487
Stewart Sell

13   Malnutrition and deficiency diseases, 546
Herschel Sidransky

14   Neoplasia, 566
Michael W. Lieberman
Russell M. Lebovitz

15   Heart, 615
Donald B. Hackel
Keith A. Reimer

16   Congenital heart disease, 730
Maurice Lev
Saroja Bharati

17   Blood vessels and lymphatics, 752
Jack L. Titus
Han-Seob Kim

18   The urinary system, 804
George F. Schreiner
John M. Kissane

19   Male reproductive system and prostate, 871
F. Kash Mostofi
Charles J. Davis, Jr.

20   Lung and mediastinum, 920
Charles Kuhn III
Frederic B. Askin

21   Ophthalmic pathology, 1047
Morton E. Smith

VOLUME TWO

22   Upper respiratory tract and ear, 1077
Robert E. Fechner

23   Face, lips, tongue, teeth, oral soft tissues, jaws, salivary glands, and neck, 1095
Charles A. Waldron

24   Alimentary tract, 1153
Gerald Fine
Chan K. Ma

25   Liver, 1199
John Redfernd Craig

26 Gallbladder and biliary ducts, 1321

Katherine De Schryver-Kecskeméti

27 Pancreas and diabetes mellitus, 1347

John M. Kissane
Paul E. Lacy

28 Hematopoietic system: bone marrow and blood, spleen, and lymph nodes, 1373

Rogers C. Griffith
Christine G. Janney

29 Thymus gland, 1493

Rogers C. Griffith

30 Pituitary gland, 1517

Nancy E. Warner

31 Thyroid gland, 1544

Kaarle O. Franssila

32 Parathyroid glands, 1570

James E. Oertel
Jeffrey M. Ogorzalek

33 The adrenal glands, 1580

John G. Gruhn
Victor E. Gould

34 Female genitalia, 1620

Frederick T. Kraus

35 Breast, 1726

Robert W. McDivitt

36 Skin, 1751

Arthur C. Allen

37 Tumors and tumorlike conditions of the soft tissue, 1838

Michael Kyriakos

38 Metabolic and other nontumorous disorders of bone, 1929

Michael D. Fallon
Harry A. Schwamm

39 Tumors and tumorlike conditions of bone, 2018

Juan Rosai

40 Diseases of joints, 2065

Ruth Silberberg

41 Diseases of skeletal muscle, 2105

Reid R. Heffner, Jr.

42 Pathology of the nervous system, 2123

James S. Nelson

Color Plates

1 Acute hemorrhagic myocardial infarct with complete occlusion; infarct with central necrosis and peripheral organization; old infarct with aneurysm and thrombus, 640

2 Congenital aganglionic megacolon; multifocal epidermoid carcinoma of esophagus; familial multiple polyposis of colon; multiple chronic gastric (peptic) ulcers; carcinomatous ulcer of stomach; carcinoma of stomach, linitis plastica type; multiple carcinoid tumors of ileum, 1156

3 Needle biopsy in epidemic hepatitis; centrilobular bile stasis in patient taking oral contraceptive; acute pericholangitis and cholestasis in needle biopsy; hyaline necrosis in alcoholic, 1220

4 Submassive hepatic necrosis from viral hepatitis; large, deep yellow fatty liver, cause unknown; granular to nodular liver of advanced Laënnec's cirrhosis; small liver with bulging nodules in patient with postnecrotic cirrhosis; suppurative cholangitis with multiple abscesses secondary to carcinomatous obstruction of common duct, 1220

5 Hepatic cirrhosis; arteriovenous fistulas in diabetic cirrhosis; Kayser-Fleischer ring in Wilson's disease; jaundice and biliary cirrhosis after ligation of common bile duct, 1220

6 Cystic disease, fibroadenoma, scirrhous carcinoma, and medullary carcinoma, 1732

7 Beta$_2$-microglobulin amyloidosis of bone in chronic renal failure: whole mount of fracture by two different stains; polarized light shows amyloid; immunoperoxidase shows beta$_2$-microglobulin, 1988

8 Ochronosis of knee joint and of intervertebral discs; purulent arthritis developing in course of staphylococcic osteomyelitis, with purulent exudate in both joint capsule and bone marrow; osteoarthrosis of femoral head, with ulceration of articular cartilage and marginal lipping, 2084

1 Cell Injury and Errors of Metabolism

DANTE G. SCARPELLI
PHILIP M. IANNACCONE

Fundamental knowledge of the morphologic and functional reactions of cells and tissues to various injurious agents and genetic defects is critical for the understanding of disease processes. In recent years, the march of biologic science has allowed the study of cellular processes at the molecular level. Thus, as we near the twenty-first century, pathology (the study of disease) has undergone a metamorphosis from a visual science, in which descriptive morphology was the centerpiece, to one where diseases are defined and interpreted in molecular terms. The foregoing, correlated with morphologic and functional alterations of cells and tissues, form the content of this chapter.

Cells are complex units driven by vital processes whose function depends on the fine integration of numerous extracellular and intracellular events. Injury occurs when adverse chemical, physical, or biologic elements in the environment alter these processes such that cells lose their capacity to generate energy, mediate transport of small molecules of biologic importance such as electrolytes, glucose, and amino acids, and finally synthesize vital macromolecules and assemble cell membranes. A few of the more common elements in the environment that are known to cause cell injury in humans are classified and listed below:

Chemical
  Industrial chemicals
  Therapeutic drugs
  Ethanol
  Tobacco smoke
  Aflatoxins and other toxic natural products
Physical
  Ultraviolet and ionizing radiation
  Mechanical trauma
  Heat and cold
Biologic
  Bacteria
  Fungi
  Viruses
  Metazoan parasites

Diseases attributable to errors of gene function are included because they are both a form of cell injury and, as they are expressed, ultimately a cause of cell injury.

MAJOR FUNCTIONS OF NORMAL CELLS

Since deterioration of cell function is the hallmark of cell injury, it seems appropriate to consider major functions of cells as an introduction to general cellular pathology. Although this is necessarily brief, it is intended to review some of the cellular and molecular mechanisms involved in cell structure and function. Inasmuch as the fine structure of cells is now the routine content of beginning courses in biology, it is not dealt with in any detail; instead, function is considered from the point of view of more recent developments in cell and molecular biology.

Energy production

The generation of energy in the form of adenosine triphosphate (ATP) is derived largely from the oxidative metabolism of glucose, fatty acids, and amino acids. The various enzymes and cofactors involved in these reactions are localized in mitochondria and their adjacent cytosol. Glucose converted to pyruvate by glycolysis in the cytosol, and fatty acids oxidized in mitochondria are broken down to the two-carbon acetyl group, which interacts with coenzyme A (CoA) to form acetyl CoA. CoA facilitates the entry of acetyl groups into the citric acid cycle localized in the matrix and inner membrane of mitochondria for further metabolism, the generation of high-energy electrons, and their capture by NAD^+ and FAD to form NADH and $FADH_2$. The conversion of this energy to the storable form (ATP) is accomplished by electron transport along the respiratory chain and ATP synthetase embedded in the inner mitochondrial membrane culminating in the phosphorylation of ADP to ATP and the formation of water according to the reaction $2H^+ + \frac{1}{2}O_2 \rightarrow H_2O$, the end product of respiratory oxidative metabolism. The foregoing is made possible by the specific orientation of respiratory and electron transport enzymes in the inner membrane, as well as its impermeability to the H^+ and OH^- ions produced during oxidative metabolism. It turns out that the active sites of the enzymes that discharge H^+ during dehydrogenation of substrates are placed in the membrane such that these ions are released on one side of the membrane while OH^- ions are discharged on the other side as a result of the orientation of cytochrome oxidase, the terminal enzyme in the respiratory chain. The vectorial separation of H^+ and OH^- creates an electrochemical gradient across the inner mitochondrial membrane. As a result of the gradient, protons (H^+) flow from the intermembrane space across the inner mitochondrial membrane and drive the generation of ATP from ADP and inorganic phosphate (P_i) as they interact with ATP synthetase. This enzyme extracts H^+ and OH^- asymmetrically from ADP and HPO_4^{-2} in directions opposite to those during dehydrogenation and electron transport noted previously.[107] As is probably evident to the reader, the reaction responsible for the conversion and conservation of energy by the formation of ATP is the reverse of that for its release by dephosphorylation. It is not surprising then that ATP synthetase can also function in reverse to hydrolyze ATP and actively pump H^+ ions. The reactions involved in ATP formation and hydrolysis respectively are shown below.

ATP formation from glucose oxidation

Glycolysis (cytosol)

$$Glucose + 2P_i + 2ADP + 2NAD^+ \longrightarrow$$
$$2\ Pyruvate + 2NADH + 2H^+ + 2ATP + 2H_2O$$

Oxidation of NADH

$$2NADH + 2H^+ + O_2 + 4P_i + 4ADP \longrightarrow$$
$$2NAD^+ + 4ATP + 6H_2O$$

Citric acid cycle (mitochondria)

$$2\ Pyruvate + 5O_2 + 30ADP + 30P_i \longrightarrow$$
$$6CO_2 + \underline{30ATP} + 34H_2O$$

TOTAL ATP FORMED 36ATP

Free energy of hydrolysis of ATP

$$ATP + H_2O \longrightarrow ADP + P_i + H^+$$
$$\Delta G = -7.3\ kcal/mol$$

Under cellular conditions ΔG is higher at about -12 kcal/mol.

The foregoing aspects of energy production are presented to emphasize its high efficiency, the importance of the vectorial movement of ions, and its dependence on the organization and orientation of the multiple membrane-bound enzymes involved in the extraction of protons and electron transport. These points assume greater significance when we consider the loss of oxidative metabolism and energy generation that accompany the extensive structural alterations encountered in injured cells.

Synthesis of proteins and macromolecules

A typical mammalian cell synthesizes more than 10,000 different proteins, many of which are enzymes, as well as numerous species of structural proteins, lipoproteins, glycoproteins, and complex polysaccharide-protein molecules called "proteoglycans." These macromolecules are the means by which the "cryptic" functions encoded in DNA are expressed and activated. They serve to impart the many functions to cells that allow them not only to maintain and renew themselves, but also to recognize and signal other cells and organize into multicellular aggregates called "tissues," which provide a greater functional complexity and diversity than they can achieve as single cells. Protein synthesis is localized in the cytosolic, endoplasmic reticular, and to a lesser extent mitochondrial compartment. Protein synthesis is a complex process that begins with RNA polymerase copying a specific sequence of DNA into messenger RNA (mRNA), a process known as "transcription." The polymerase binds to the promoter that signals the site on the DNA molecule from which RNA synthesis must begin to encode for the synthesis of a specific protein; mRNA synthesis ceases when the polymerase encounters a second site on the DNA, which signals that the appropriate mRNA has been produced and the molecule is released.[17,69]

A family of more than 20 different RNA molecules called "transfer RNAs" (tRNA), including at least one tRNA for each amino acid, are responsible for specifically binding amino acids, a reaction catalyzed by enzymes named aminoacyl-tRNA synthetases, again one for each amino acid. The amino acyl-tRNAs thus formed serve to bring each specific amino acid to its appropriate place in the protein molecule being synthesized by recognizing its appropriate codon in the mRNA molecule and pairing with complementary nucleotides at their anticodon tips.[133] Amino acids are added to the carboxyl terminal end of the growing chain of peptides. These events occur on ribosomes, large multienzyme complexes consisting of protein and RNA.[110] Ribosomes are composed of a small and large subunit and have two grooves, one that fits onto an mRNA molecule and the other accommodating the growing polypeptide chain. In addition, there are two binding sites for tRNAs, one for the molecule that is contributing its amino acid to the protein being synthesized, the other for binding the tRNA carrying the next amino acid to be inserted.

Initiation of protein synthesis involves binding of the small ribosomal subunit to mRNA that has previously bound an initiator rRNA molecule that recognizes its AUG starter codon.[80] Once the initiation reaction is complete, the various factors involved are discharged from the small subunit and the large ribosomal subunit is bound and all is ready for protein synthesis to begin. It is noteworthy that initiation factors not only initiate the process of synthesis, but can also regulate its overall rate presumably by their phosphorylation by protein kinases in one system and perhaps by other cellular mechanisms that modulate the function of proteins.[113] The conversion of information in a molecule of mRNA by its interaction with ribosomes and to RNAs culminating in the synthesis of a specific cellular protein is known as "translation."

Ribosomes exist as free 30 nm particles or as multiple ribosomes bound to a single mRNA molecule giving rise to polymorphous complex structures called polyribosomes in the cytosol, or as highly ordered parallel tubular arrays composed of membrane-bound ribosomes termed "rough-surfaced endoplasmic reticulum" (RER).[2] Proteins synthesized by the first of the two varieties of ribosomal profiles are released directly into the cytosol where they function as soluble proteins. Those that are targeted for a specific intracellular site are guided there by a specific carrier molecules as apparently is the case for some molecular components of mitochondria. In the case of RER organized into tubular structures (cisternae) with ribosomes attached to their outer surface, the proteins once synthesized are extruded across the RER membrane into the cisternal lumen. Although the problem of directed intracellular transport is at least partially solved, there still remains the need to assist proteins to reach their ultimate correct destination. This is accomplished by a system of coated vesicles that enclose proteins, especially those destined for insertion into or on a cell membrane. Transportation to specific locations is guided by so-called specific "docking" proteins that recognize complementary acceptor proteins at the various sites. The RER serves as the site for the synthesis of proteins and macromolecules for most of the cell's organelles, which undergo the addition of O-linked oligosaccharides, a reaction known as "glycosylation."[93] This occurs as soon as the growing polypeptide chain enters the cisternal lumen and is completed before it is released. Soluble proteins not destined for transport to membranous cell structures are not glycosylated.

The Golgi apparatus, with its parallel arrays of stacked cisternae and vacuoles, plays a major role in the biology of cell proteins and macromolecules. This is so because all such molecules destined for either membranous sites or export pass through this complex cell organelle and are chemically modified by it. These modifications include alterations of the O-linked oligosaccharide residues just mentioned, as well as a variety of other reactions such as glycosylation, sulfation, the addition of fatty acids, and proteolysis because these are required to allow proteins to achieve their full functional capacity.[49] In the case of proteins that are exported, the Golgi apparatus packages the product into secretory vacuoles that ultimately fuse with the plasma membrane during their secretion.

Transport, endocytosis and exocytosis

The plasma membrane serves both as an effective barrier that maintains the essential differences between the cell interior and its external environment and as a highly competent monitor regulating the entry and exit of specific molecules. In certain types of specialized cells it mediates the ingestion of large particles. The various properties of the plasma membrane are the result of transport enzymes specific for the uptake and output of ions, sugars, and amino acids and other small molecules, numerous different and specific receptors that recognize various molecules, and the ability to undergo gross conformational changes as a result of membrane fluidity and flow. The plasma membrane consists of a lipid bilayer[57] rich in cholesterol, four phospholipids with head groups of different sizes and charges, and glycolipids. The fluidity of the membrane is a function of its composition, that is, the amount of cholesterol and the types and amounts of constitutive fatty acids.[18,123] Since the majority of phospholipids are neutral at a physiologic pH, they readily accommodate intramembrane and transmembrane proteins embedded in the membrane bilayer. Membrane proteins have hydrophilic and hydrophobic domains; the former are localized at the external and internal surfaces of the membrane that are exposed to water, whereas the latter lie within the lipid-rich interior of the bilayer.[90] The latter interactions serve to firmly hold membrane proteins in the bilayer, and so they can be considered as integral constituents, whereas proteins that are inserted more superficially are not so anchored and are referred to as superficial proteins.[140]

The transport of ions involves membrane proteins, the best studied of which is the Na^+-K^+ pump, energized by ATP, where Na^+ is pumped out while K^+ ions are transported into the cell.[40] The vectorial movements of both ions in opposite directions are believed to occur in tandem; first Na^+ is bound on the cytoplasmic face of the carrier protein complex followed by hydrolysis of ATP and phosphorylation of the protein, which causes a conformational change and release of Na^+ to the cell exterior. This is then followed by binding of K^+ at the external surface of the protein and its subsequent dephosphylation and release of K^+ into the cytoplasm. For each molecule of ATP hydrolyzed $3Na^+$ and $2K^+$ ions are translocated. The Na^+-K^+ pump serves to control cell volume by regulating levels of these ions inside cells.[141] Other Na^+-carrier protein systems not driven by ATP are involved in the transport of other vital small molecules such as glucose and other sugars and amino acids in which these are taken into the cell driven by the chemical gradient of Na^+ uptake.[40] A third means by which ion transport occurs in excitable cells such as nerve and muscle involves so-called channels formed by parallel transmembrane proteins that "open" and "close" either by changes in membrane potential or by binding of a specific substance to a membrane receptor.[147] The latter is exemplified by the binding of acetylcholine at the activated neuromuscular junction causing the loss of K^+ and the uptake of Na$^+$, ultimately resulting in muscular contraction.

The uptake of macromolecules such as large proteins, polysaccharides and nucleic acids, small bits of plasma membrane, and in specialized cells large particles across the cell membrane is accomplished by the formation and fusion of membrane-bounded vesicles a process called "endocytosis."[139] In the case of the uptake of macromolecules, the plasma membrane invaginates and pinches off small vesicles enclosing a bit of the extracellular fluid, a process termed "pinocytosis" ('cell drinking'). Cells are continuously ingesting materials at different rates depending on the cell type. Although most pinocytic vesicles move inward into the cytoplasm and fuse with primary lysosomes (organelles that contain hydrolytic enzymes), some bypass lysosomes and transport their contents through the cytoplasm to the cell periphery, fuse with the plasma membrane, and discharge their contents to the outside, a process called "exocytosis."[115] An excellent example of this is afforded by endothelial cells, which directly transport material from the blood into the extracellular fluid. A special class of endocytotic vesicles that bear mention are the "coated" variety, so called because they are composed of specific fibrous proteins that form a basketlike network.[55] These vesicles are capable of internalizing large numbers of specific macromolecules with only a minimum of extracellular fluid. This is accomplished by the presence of specific receptors in the vesicle membrane that bind and thus concentrate certain macromolecules. Cases in point are the insulin and low-density lipoprotein (LDL) molecules and their respective receptors. In these two examples there are special features of both that merit mention. Binding of insulin to its receptor mediates the entry of glucose into the cell; subsequent proteolysis of the insulin-receptor complex limits the action of the hormone and simultaneously regulates the number of receptor molecules on the cell surface.[117] Binding of LDL to its receptor and their endocytosis and delivery to lysosomes supplies the cell with cholesterol, after hydrolysis of the cholesterol ester moiety of LDL and, in contrast to the fate of insulin receptor, recycles the LDL receptor to the plasma membrane into which it is reinserted.

The cellular uptake of large particles including bacteria, is a subset of endocytosis, referred to as phagocytosis,[139] and a property largely of specialized cells such as polymorphonuclear (PMN) leukocytes and macrophages. These are major components of the host cellular defense mechanisms against infection by microorganisms, as well as for the removal of senescent and dead cells and internalized foreign materials such as mineral dusts and pigments. In this instance endocytosis involves the formation of a very large invagination of the plasma membrane and subsequently a corresponding-ly large vacuole or phagosome. This then fuses with primary lysosomes, which release their complement of hydrolytic enzymes and digest its contents. Phagocytosis is not a random process but one that is mediated by specific receptors on PMNs and macrophages.[149] Some of these receptors recognize antibody molecules, and in individuals with specific immunity, avidly bind, internalize, and destroy microorganisms that have previously bound the specific antibody. The foregoing represents the major humoral protective mechanism against infection. Although intracellular digestion is a very efficient process, the cell not infrequently ingests materials that cannot be totally degraded; these remain in secondary lysosomes for the lifetime of the cell and are called "residual bodies."

Exocytosis is the reverse of endocytosis and involves the formation of intracellular vacuoles containing specific macromolecules. These migrate to the cell periphery, fuse with the plasma membrane, and release their contents into the extracellular fluid or, in the case of exocrine gland cells, into ductules. This is the means by which cells secrete macromolecules. Some are released continuously, whereas others are packaged into secretory vesicles, stored, and released after an extracellular signal.[96] A specific signal triggers the secretion of a particular substance, or in the case of certain cells a group of macromolecules packaged into single vesicles. Macromolecules synthesized in the RER move to the Golgi apparatus via transport vesicles that bud off the cisternae and transfer their content to so-called condensing vesicles. Here they are progressively concentrated and end up as mature dense secretory granules on the luminal face of the Golgi appartus.

Digestion and detoxication

Controlled intracellular digestion is a vital property of all mammalian cells and is mediated by lysosomes, organelles that contain a spectrum of acid hydrolases capable of degrading proteins, carbohydrates, lipids, and nucleic acids.[33] Because of their important role, lysosomes are an integral part of the pathways involved in the uptake of materials, are formed by budding from the Golgi membranes facing the apical surface of the cells, and are strategically localized to degrade ingestive substances. Special features of this organelle that allow lysosomes to function optimally as the principal sites of intracellular digestion are localization of an ATPase-driven membrane transport protein that accumulates H$^+$ within them to create an acid milieu and a selective membrane that, together with that of the phagosome, allows free passage of the products of digestion while sequestering hydrolases from the cytosol. The logistics of incorporating the 40 or so appropriate hydrolytic enzymes into lysosomes during their formation is presumably accomplished by receptors (docking proteins) localized in their membranes that bind specific transport vesicles bearing the enzymes. Studies of fibroblasts from patients with a genetic defect affecting their lysosomes have served to identify a critical aspect of docking, that is, that lysosomal membrane receptors recognize and internalize only enzymes that contain a mannose phosphate–containing oligosaccharide moiety. Two additional features of this signal-targeting system that enhance its function are that the mannose-6-phosphate–containing oligosaccharide is an uncommon one in the cell's economy and that once the enzymes are delivered to the lysosome the marker sugar is rapidly cleaved and removed.[109] These features not only assure delivery to a specific organelle, but also serve to prevent inappropriate signals, as during events such as membrane recycling.

The recognition and metabolic biotransformation of xenobiotic compounds that leads to their rapid elimination is a property common to all body cells that endows the organism with the capacity to detoxify potentially toxic substances, an advantage for survival in a noxious environment. In vertebrates, the liver and to a lesser degree the kidney and the lung are the organs involved in the detoxication of drugs and other foreign compounds by oxidation, reduction, hydrolysis, and conjugation. Oxidative metabolism, which includes hydroxylation, demethylation, dealkylation, deamination, sulfoxide formation, oxidation, and N-oxidation among others, is localized in the smooth endoplasmic reticulum (SER) and mediated by the NADPH–cytochrome P-450 drug-metabolizing enzyme system. The system requires the electron donor NADPH, and the flavoprotein cytochrome P-450 serves to bind a drug to form a complex after its acceptance of electrons from NADPH and with O_2 to form two active oxygen molecules, one of which reacts with the drug and the second to react with $2H^+$ ions to form water. The ferric iron moiety in cytochrome P-450 is reduced to ferrous iron upon interaction with NADPH and returns to the ferric state when the electrons are donated to form H_2O; the drug-

metabolizing enzyme system and its various reactions are shown below (Fig. 1-1).

Two features of this system that significantly enhance its effectiveness are its stimulation after exposure of the organism to a drug or foreign compound and its capacity to metabolize a wide variety of chemicals. Increased activity of the cytochrome P-450 system is the result of higher levels of the enzyme than in the basal or unexposed state and is accomplished by synthesis of new molecules of hemoprotein and the SER membrane in which it is localized. Xenobiotic compounds such as phenobarbital, 3,4-benzo[a]pyrene, and polychlorinated biphenyls, are particularly potent inducers of augmented synthesis of the cytochrome P-450 drug-metabolizing enzyme system. Although not all the details of induction are completely understood, specific cytoplasmic receptors that recognize each class of compound bind them, enter the cell nucleus, and interact with DNA thereby activating specific genes. This leads to synthesis of the mRNAs, which code for the proteins that constitute and assemble the various components of the enzyme system. The trait of induction is inherited as an autosome dominant and varies significantly among different species. Activity of the enzyme system can be inhibited by certain chemicals and starvation. The capability of the enzyme system to metabolically degrade a surprisingly broad spectrum of different foreign compounds is achieved by the presence of a variety of isozyme forms of cytochrome P-450 that possess different catalytic properties. In contrast to the foregoing, the second major mechanism for the detoxication of drugs or their metabolites involves nonhemoprotein enzymes, some of which are localized in SER membranes and others in the soluble fraction. These enzymes catalyze drugs to react with a variety of small molecules. These include glucuronic acid, glutathione, sulfate, and methyl and acetyl groups, which form water-soluble compounds, which are readily excreted in the urine. These evolutionary developments have served to ensure the protection and survival of organisms constantly

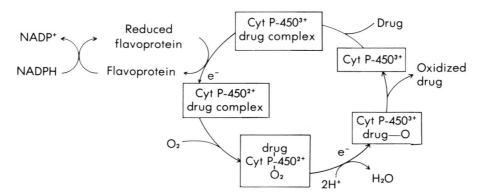

Fig. 1-1. Microsomal drug-oxidizing enzyme system. (Modified from Hildebrandt, A., and Estabrook, R.W.: Arch. Biochem. Biophys. **143**:66, 1971.)

exposed to toxic substances. Before this section is concluded, however, it should be pointed out that there are two edges to every sword and that drug metabolism is not always protective to the host. During the metabolic degradation of some chemicals, it turns out that there are formed certain intermediates that are highly reactive, interact with critical cell macromolecules, and not infrequently are toxic to the organism.

Intracellular storage

The most readily apparent storage of materials in the cytoplasm of normal cells involves glycogen and neutral lipids, substances that can be rapidly degraded and metabolized as sources of energy. Although many different types of cells can accumulate either or both substances to varying degrees, the liver is a major store of glycogen and, to a much lesser degree, neutral lipids. The amounts of each vary considerably during the course of each day with the highest amounts present after a meal and the lowest just before the next. Both substances accumulate in the SER; glycogen is distributed as characteristic deposits consisting of either the more common rosette-like clusters of dense particles, the alpha form, or the smaller aggregates of roughly spherical granules, the beta form. In the case of neutral fat, its accumulation early is in the SER when it appears as dense microdroplets; as these increase in number, they coalesce into large, dense homogeneous spherical deposits in vacuoles. In fat deposits in the body where the largest amounts of fat are stored in fat cells, virtually the entire cytoplasm of these cells is occupied by a single macrodrop of neutral lipids. This fat is mobilized when other more readily available sources of substrate from which energy is derived are depleted, as in sustained dieting and malnutrition. Other examples of intracellular storage involve endocrine and exocrine glandular cells, mucin-secreting cells, and various leukocytes in which the various secretory products are stored in cytoplasmic granules, which are secreted by exocytosis into the blood, a ductal system, or the extracellular fluid in response to specific molecular signals. A second form of storage that is not morphologically apparent but is both important and dynamic includes the so-called metabolic pools of various molecules and macromolecules whose size at a given steady state represents the difference between the rates of their formation and utilization respectively. Examples abound in which the size a metabolic pool for a specific molecule varies widely depending on rate changes. There are also instances in which the same molecule may be simultaneously localized in several different cell compartments, each representing a pool of dissimilar size.

Cell movement

Cell locomotion is a basic property of cells that plays important roles in the formation of tissues and organs during embryonic development, chemotaxis, phagocytosis, and wound healing among other important events in the life of an organism. Cell movement depends on complex and dynamic assemblies of actin filaments in the cytoplasm immediately beneath the plasma membrane coupled with interaction with other components of the cytoskeleton.[54,66] Although the mechanical details of cell movement are elusive, information gained from microcinematographic analysis of single cells in vitro and from the behavior of isolated components of the cytoskeleton and its associated proteins alone and in various mixtures under different conditions have led to hypothetical explanations that await biophysical and biochemical confirmation. Studies of cells lying on a plastic surface or collagen substrate in culture indicate that locomotion may be accomplished by focal forward extension of the cytoplasm (leading edge) in the direction of movement followed by its adhesion to the surface. This, in turn, is followed by a contraction of the trailing edge of the cytoplasm; the cell is pulled forward in a unidirectional movement. Movement in vertebrate cells is quite slow and difficult to analyze, as contrasted to primitive eucaryotes, such as amebas, wherein movement is rapid and can be observed directly. In these cells the cytoplasm in the advancing extension undergoes noticeable changes in viscosity, or a so-called gel-sol transition, where the peripheral zone of the extension is gel-like, as contrasted to its central portion, which is quite fluid and is seen to stream or flow forward in the direction of the extension.[155] Current dogma, based on experimental observations, suggests that these phase changes in the peripheral and central zones of the cytoplasmic extension may be related to the formation, cross-linking, and breakdown of actin filaments and bundles. For example, a solution of actin filaments cross-linked into bundles by the small protein fimbrin are converted to a gel when the long flexible proteins actinin or filamin are added to bind adjacent actin filaments into three-dimensional networks. Gel-to-sol transition is further modulated by a family of Ca^{++}-dependent proteins, so-called actin-fragmenting proteins, one of which has been named "gelsolin,"[167] that in the presence of high levels of Ca^{++} ions bind to actin filaments so avidly that they insert themselves between their component subunits and cause their disassembly and solation of the gel to a less viscous state. Contraction of cytoplasm is believed to be attributable to the interaction of nonmuscle myosin with the actin molecules in the gel phase in the presence of a high level of Ca^{++} ions. Ca^{++} ions, together with actin-fragmenting proteins, break down the actin networks characteristic of cytoplasmic gels; concerted movement is accomplished by the attachment of aggregates of myosin molecules to adjacent and parallel actin filaments, which in turn pull one filament against the other causing a net shortening in length. Reduced to its simplest terms, cell movement appears to be closely linked to gel-sol transitions of actin filaments as they interact with various small proteins capable of either cross-linking them into bundles or networks, or disassembling them into subunits, and also interact with myosin, which imparts the force of contraction.[150] There is a growing awareness that there are interactions of actin and myosin with various other components of the cytoskeleton that are probably involved in cell motion, but these are not yet fully elucidated.

Cell recognition, communication, and excitation

The growth, formation, and organization of individual cells into tissues, organs, and an entire organism such that it functions as an integrated whole is dependent on their ability to recognize and communicate with each other. Cell-cell recognition and communication are accomplished by a variety of strategies ranging from binding between cell surface molecules and direct transfer of informational molecules afforded by close physical contact between cells to indirect mechanisms mediated by chemical signals secreted by distant cells into the blood and extracellular fluid compartment. Our current state of knowledge indicates that the model of endocrine glands signaling remote cells by the hormones they secrete is reiterated at all levels of organization including single cells. Many if not all cell functions are triggered and modulated by specific chemical signals be they ions, small proteins, or complex macromolecules. The simplest and most effective strategy by which signals can be sent to cells is by having them as molecular components of the environment with which the cell is in immediate contact as is the case of the extracellular matrix. A variety of specific constituent molecules and macromolecules, expecially collagen,[64,65] have been identified in the extracellular matrix and impart signals important in cell-cell interaction (adhesion), histogenesis, growth, and differentiation. The specificity of such signals is assured by the presence of complementary proteins on and in the surface membrane of the cell that serve as receptors that bind to specific signal molecules. Such interactions mediate orientational and positional signals critical to the formation of functional tissue structures, or they can trigger intracellular events if the receptor protein is a transmembrane one.

In addition to interaction with molecules in the extracellular matrix, cells also recognize signals from other cells in their proximity. These signals play an important role not only in cell-cell recognition by which cells are organized into tissues, but also in their specialized functions. Two cases in point are cardiac muscle cells, which interact with each other to form a syncytium allowing for the transmission of electrical activity throughout the organ during contraction and ensuring its coordinated contraction, and the intestinal lumen, which is lined by a highly folded layer of single cells and is surrounded by alternating circular and longitudinal layers of smooth muscle cells, an organizational plan that optimizes both the absorption of nutrients and the unidirectional movement of its luminal content. Recognition of cells for cells of the same tissue is a well-established phenomenon of high specificity that can identify and sort out its counterparts from a mixture of cells from different tissues rapidly and with surprising accuracy.[158] Although such mutual adhesion of like cells is a key in tissue formation, it is not yet clear whether it is attributable to an extracellular aggregation factor or to the recognition of complementary cell surface molecules, or both. Although these signals serve to bring similar component cells of a tissue together, they are not sufficient by themselves to assure the appropriate orientation and polarity necessary for their function.

Cell orientation and polarity are achieved by specialized contact sites of the lateral plasma membranes of adjacent cells linking them to one another and of the basal plasma membrane linked to the basal lamina, a component of the extracellular matrix. These contact sites or cell junctions include adhering, impermeable, and communicating varieties, which serve mechanical, barrier, and transport functions respectively. Variations in the structure of the latter two expands their functions beyond that of cell-cell attachment. The tight junctions present at the apical lateral aspect of cells are highly impermeable and prevent the passage of molecules between adjacent cells.[145] Contrast this with the so-called gap junction, which is permeable, allows the passage of small molecules between adjacent cells, and thus allows for their communication.[45] The passage of ions, amino acids, sugars, vitamins, and nucleotides through gap junctions between cells links adjacent cells both electrically and metabolically. For example, the passage of Ca^{++} ions from one cell to another can in certain circumstances serve as a chemical signal triggering a set of cytoplasmic events. The channels of gap junctions are apparently regulated so that the movement of materials between adjacent cells can be controlled. However, it is not clear at present how this control is mediated.

Recognition between cells separated by some distance is important not only in their migration to specific remote sites during embryogenesis, but also in critical physiologic events such as the direction of leukocytes from the vascular compartment to sites of infection or tissue injury during the inflammatory process. Cell recognition across distances is mediated by at least two strategies. The first consists in the secretion of chemical signals that attract cells (chemotaxis); these are potent signals that are effective despite their high dilution in the extracellular fluid compartment.[129] The second means by which cells are guided from one site to another involves the creation of a pathway through the extracellular matrix by chemical marking by a previous migration of cells, called "contact guidance," presumably by secretion of cell-specific adhesion molecules, which serve to direct subsequent cells.[100] In the examples cited above, the migration of nerve cells along specific pathways is mediated by both nerve growth factor, a chemotactic polypeptide,[15] and contact guidance, whereas chemotaxis of leukocytes to a site of infection or tissue injury is accomplished solely by means of a family of well-characterized small peptides.[72] These are generated locally at the affected tissue site, taken up by the leukocytes, and rapidly destroyed and so their effect is localized and limited. There are two other types of signal molecules that bear mention, hormones secreted into the blood by specialized tissues that affect target cells at distant sites and neurotransmitters that act over very short distances on postsynaptic cells. Lipid-soluble hormones cross the plasma membrane by diffusion and bind to specific cytoplasmic receptors, which carry them into the nucleus where they activate the transcription of specific genes.[118,166] Water-soluble hormones, on the other hand, unable to cross the lipid barrier of the plasma membrane, bind to specific cell surface receptors, which are rapidly endocytosed.[84] Once internalized, they trigger a plasma membrane bound enzyme adenyl cyclase, which generates cyclic AMP (cAMP), which in turn serves as a second signal or messenger, which ultimately mediates a variety of intracellular events.[152] Since one receptor protein molecule leads to the generation of many cAMP molecules, amplification of the signal is achieved.

Excitation of certain specialized cells, such as neurons and muscle, involves their reception, conduction, and transmission of electrical signals. These involve the generation of a voltage difference or membrane potential across the plasma membrane by the to-and-fro movement of Na^+, K^+, Cl^-, and Ca^{++} ions. These ions pass across the lipid bilayer via protein channels, which open and close to regulate their passage. The reciprocal differences in Na^+- and K^+-ion content of these cells, like others, is dependent on the ATPase-driven pump mentioned previously in the section on transport and serves as a source of free energy to drive these ions across the plasma membrane. Since propagation of the membrane potential (action potential) involves a focal change in selective membrane permeability,[8] only a very small flow of ions into the cell is sufficient to generate it. This involves the opening of Na^+ channels[148]; as the positively charged ions enter the cells, the plasma membrane is further depolarized causing more Na^+ channels to open. Na^+ channels remain open for about 0.5 msec, close, and become inactivated,[71] unable to open again until a few milliseconds have elapsed. The action potential of a neuron is propagated along the plasma membrane of the axonal process, which allows for rapid communication across a long distance.

Transmission of the electrical impulse from a nerve to its target cell is accomplished by a miniaturized version of the chemical signaling model described previously. This is accomplished at locations called "synaptic junctions" where the end of the axon interfaces with the target or postsynaptic cell. This specialized axonal structure consists of its plasma membrane lying on the basal lamina of the target cell so that the plasma membranes of the two cells are separated by a minute space of a fraction of a micrometer called the "synaptic cleft."[70] Acetylcholine, the signal molecule packaged in numerous small vesicles, is stored in the cytoplasm of the axon just beneath its plasma membrane. When the action potential has reached the synapse, it opens Ca^{++} channels and allows Ca^{++} ions to enter the axon terminal and trigger fusion of the vesicles with the plasma membrane of the axon releasing their content of acetylcholine into the synaptic cleft.[27,86] The acetylcholine binds to its specific receptor on the plasma membrane of the target cell, in this case, a muscle cell, and the chemical signal is transduced into an electrical one. The foregoing involves the focal increased permeability of the muscle cell membrane to Na^+, K^+, and Ca^{++} and its depolarization, and an action potential is propagated.[87] The acetylcholine is rapidly hydrolyzed by acetylcholine esterase assuring that the signal is not a prolonged one. Although we have presented this topic as primarily one that is involved in cell excitation, we should point out in closing that the complex electrical events in the nervous system and the tissues it innervates are exquisitely modulated by synapses that are excitatory, as well as those that are inhibitory, both mediated by the events just described.

Reproduction

The mechanisms involved in the replication of DNA are central to the continuity and transfer of genetic information, and they must allow for the duplication of new DNA to occur rapidly and accurately. The rate of polymerization of DNA achieved by a multienzyme system in mammalian cells adds about 50 nucleotides per second to the preexisting chain as contrasted to about a tenfold increased rate for the synthetic system in bacterial cells. The fidelity of the copied strand in the mammalian cell is assured by the obligatory requirement of DNA polymerase such that the proximate nucleotide in the primer strand be base-paired *before* it can add a new nucleotide to its 3'-OH end.[13,39] This "proofreading" strategy is *so* efficient that an error of only about one nucleotide is made in about 10^9 base-pair replications. It guards against errors of mispairing of nucleotides as a result of isomeric forms, which spontaneously occur in ratios of about one to 10^4 nucleotides. The rare imino isomer of cytosine is a case in point, wherein it base-pairs with adenine rather than with guanosine as its normal isomeric form does.

Disposition of the two strands of DNA as a double helix and the very high stability of hydrogen bonding between base pairs pose several sizable problems that arise during replication that nature appears to have solved rather nicely. The first deals with the need to open the helix, separate the DNA strands, and straighten them out so that DNA polymerase can add the complementary nucleotides. Destabilization of the DNA helix, enhancing its opening and allowing straightening of the strands, is accomplished by single-strand DNA-binding (SSB) proteins,[23] which bind to the DNA in such a fashion that the bases are exposed for pairing. Straightening of the DNA strand is optimized by the fact that SSB protein monomers tend to bind cooperatively with others already bound to form long clusters along the strand. Unwinding of the helix involves an ATP-dependent enzyme (helicase) that opens the helix ahead of the replication sites on the separated strands.[1] A second problem is the prevention of tangling of the DNA helix resulting from the strain caused by its clockwise winding ahead of the newly synthesized strands. The helix winds about one turn for every new 10 base pairs formed, which in the case of mammalian cells means five rotations per second. Two enzymes, topoisomerases I and II cause single- and double-strand nicks respectively by virtue of their activity as nucleases, the first enzyme allowing the helix to move about the phosphodiester bond opposite the nick, thereby releasing the strain and preventing tangling, the second allowing complete separation of DNA helices when an entire chromosome has been replicated to prevent tangling.[48]

DNA synthesis occurs in S phase of the now well-known cell cycle; once the S phase is completed, the cell is prepared to enter the G_2 phase and then undergo division at M (mitosis). The rate at which various cells of the body divide differs considerably from one cell type to another[19] and is attributable largely to the length of time they remain in the G_1 phase; once cells have passed through G_1,[121] they all traverse through the rest of the cycle at a relatively constant rate. In rapidly dividing intestinal epithelial cells, for example, the G_1 period is measured in hours as contrasted to the much more slow-growing liver cells, which remain in G_1 for many months. Studies have identified a point late in G_1 that must be passed by a cell before it can proceed through the remainder of the cycle and divide. This is referred to as the restriction, or R, point[116] and has been the focus of much attention, since it appears to be a crucial factor in the regulation of cell division. Despite many efforts, clarification of the nature of the restriction point and the mechanism or mechanisms involved in its release remain elusive. At present it is postulated that release from R depends on the accumulation of an unstable protein that, upon reaching a sufficient concentration, allows the cell to enter S phase and begin to synthesize DNA.[127] Because the protein is postulated to be unstable and short lived, its synthesis would necessarily have to occur very late in G_1 and be very rapid.

In addition to intracellular control of cell growth and division, several extracellular regulatory factors such as endocrine hormones, specific small peptide growth factors, matrices that surround cells, and perhaps even cell-cell contact have been identified. These include endocrine secretions that stimulate cell growth such as somatotropin and thyroxin and several other potent non-endocrine growth factors that have been identified, purified, and characterized and also prompt the growth of a variety of epithelial and connective tissue cell types. Although in the main these are quite cell specific, some of them can also stimulate growth of other cell types, though in some instances less so than its primary specific cell target. These growth factors may be synthesized by cells at some distance from their targets. For example, epithelial growth factor (EGF), which originates in cells of the submaxillary gland, can stimulate a wide variety of epithelial cells, many of which are located great distances away. Other growth factors are produced by nearby cells, and still others by the target cell itself, so-called paracrine and autocrine growth factors respectively. If results obtained with cells in culture are also applicable to cells in tissues, the proliferation of some cells may require several growth factors acting in concert.

The role of extracellular matrices in cell replication is well documented not only in early development where it appears to be particularly crucial, but also in more well-differentiated cells. As judged from observations in cultured cells, an important aspect of matrix-cell interaction that influences cell division is the adhesion of cells to the matrix because this provides the stability required for the cell movements involved in cell division. Recent evidence suggests that in addition to cell stabilization there may also be important signals involved in matrix-cell interaction that are positional in nature and thus modulate cell division. Cell-cell interaction can also influence cell division by signals that identify cell loss as occurs in a wound where cell replication is stimulated at the edges of the wound and cells migrate progressively into the tissue defect to fill it.[41] However, it should be noted that in liver stimulated to regeneration by partial hepatectomy the replication of hepatocytes appears to be stimulated not only by the physical loss of cell mass, but also at least in part by the production of a potent polypeptide growth factor specific for liver cell proliferation called "hepatopoietin."[105] Finally, the role of cell-cell interaction in the regulation of cell replication must be considered in the context of the active transfer of signal molecules from one cell to the other across gap junctions mentioned previously in the section dealing with cell communication.

CELL CONTROL MECHANISMS AND HOMEOSTASIS

Cells exist in an *external milieu* that requires virtually continuous work against chemical gradients with the expenditure of energy so that they can maintain close regulation of their internal environment. Thus cell control systems are of vital importance for optimal function and survival of cells.

Points of control of cell metabolism exist throughout the various compartments of the cell and at different levels of structural organization. These range from the interaction of free molecules in the cell sap, which apparently do not require spatial or oriented relationships, to highly ordered arrays of macromolecules embedded in cell membranes, where function and structures are intimately interrelated. In the case of unbound catalytic molecules such as those involved in glycolysis, organization and coordination of multisequential reactions are afforded solely by their *chemical* specificity for a particular substrate. Thus the product of one reaction can continue along a particular metabolic pathway by virtue of its specificity for the next enzyme in the sequence. Contrast this with the citric acid cycle enzymes, many of which are physically embedded in the inner membrane of mitochondria facilitating enzyme substrate interaction and electron transport. Control can also be accomplished by regulation of the *amounts* of enzymes and other macromolecules synthesized by cells.[162] The means by which control is effected by this strategy is so obvious that it need not be discussed further.

Regulation of metabolism by the synthesis of various molecular forms (isoenzymes) of the same enzyme is a more complex mechanism. An excellent example is the stimulation of glycolysis in mammalian liver by insulin, in which a special isoenzyme of pyruvate kinase, called "liver pyruvate kinase," is synthesized. This enzyme possesses catalytic and regulatory properties that are better able to meet the increased demand for glycolysis imposed by a high-carbohydrate diet than is another form of pyruvate kinase also present in liver, muscle, brain, heart, and other tissues that is less responsive to insulin.[154] This means of control is necessarily slow because it involves protein synthesis and of course because it precludes fine adjustments of metabolism. Another example of hormone-mediated control of metabolism involves the stimulation of glycogenolysis by epinephrine in which the hormone simultaneously exerts different effects, that is, inhibition of glycogen synthetase and activation of gluconeogenesis. Such regulation is modulated by a variety of environmental factors, notable among which is the concentration of specific substrates and certain hormones. On the other hand, modulation of the activity of enzyme molecules offers both a rapid response and a fine degree of regulation, which allow cells to effect smooth metabolic control.

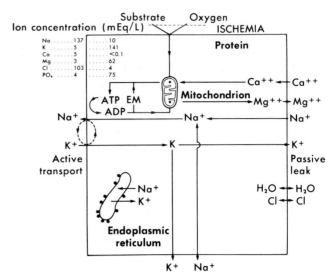

Fig. 1-2. Diagram of various factors responsible for control of cell volume. High intracellular concentration of protein requires continuous active pumping of ions (largely sodium and potassium ions) and passive outward diffusion of water to counteract the tendency for water to enter cells because intracellular osmolality is higher than that in the extracellular space. Control is mediated by vectorial transport enzymes associated with cell membranes, particularly the plasma membrane, that are driven by dephosphorylation of high-energy compounds such as adenosine triphosphate (ATP). *Upper left,* Extracellular and intracellular concentrations of various ions in "normal" cells are shown; maintenance of the intracellular concentration of various ions requires expenditure of considerable work against a chemical gradient. Energy in the form of ATP is supplied by aerobic glycolysis and mitochondrial phosphorylation (oxidative phosphorylation). The latter reaction or reactions are highly sensitive to alterations of substrate and oxygen concentration and are interrupted by ischemia. When the pump is effective, it pumps sodium ions at a rate to balance their entry into the cell by passive leak, which in turn regulates inward passive diffusion of water and thus the cell volume. Notice that active transport of sodium and potassium ions also occurs in intracellular membrane systems such as endoplasmic reticulum. *EM,* Embden-Meyerhof pathway. (From Scarpelli, D., and Trump, B.F.: Cell injury, Bethesda, MD., 1974, Universities Associated for Research and Education in Pathology, Inc.)

Such modulation can be achieved by conformational changes in the enzyme protein molecule, termed "allosteric regulation,"[108] in which the enzyme-substrate affinity is altered. Slight changes in the enzyme-substrate affinity can result in significant alterations in the rate of catalysis.[4,135]

At the highest level of organization, metabolic control depends on the functional integrity of the various membranes, organelles, and compartments of the cell,[138] such as the plasma membrane, endoplasmic reticulum, Golgi complex, mitochondria, lysosomes, peroxisomes, nuclear membrane, chromatin, nucleoplasm, and nucleolus. These components regulate the types and amounts of substances that enter their metabolic interactions (synthetic or catabolic), intracellular incorporation, transport, concentration and storage of synthesized products (secretory granules), and export; and all of these functions are controlled by expression of the various genes in the nucleus that direct the synthesis of the myriad proteins necessary to support them. Membrane-bound and free cytoplasmic receptors capable of recognizing a variety of hormones, growth factors, and other molecules by specific high-affinity binding represent a major mechanism by which cell functions, including transduction of extracellular signals and cell-cell interaction are regulated and integrated. The foregoing brief summary emphasizes the extent to which normal control of cell metabolism and function are closely dependent on molecular, supramolecular, and anatomic levels of cell structure.

A cell's capacity rapidly and effectively to regulate its internal environment and function in order to adapt to a variety of external environments is a property that has obvious selective advantages. The fine regulation of cell volume depends on the continuous function of active transport systems for a variety of ions. The ionic composition and protein concentration of the cell interior differ greatly from those of the extracellular fluid. These differences would lead to a passive diffusion of water into the cell, which would be considerable if unopposed by active transport of sodium ions into the extracellular fluid and the intracellular uptake of potassium ions by the adenosine triphosphatase (ATPase)–sodium–potassium pump in the plasma membrane (Fig. 1-2). Only by continuous chemical work and expenditure of energy is the cell prevented from reaching the Gibbs-Donnan equilibrium in which ingress of water into the cell would lead to massive swelling and its eventual death.

Cell injury and death

The brilliant intuitive insight of Rudolph Virchow, a German pathologist whose treatise *Cellular Pathology*, published in 1855, revolutionized the scientific basis of medicine, is revealed in the following excerpt from his writings: "All diseases are in the last analysis reducible to disturbances, either active or passive, of large groups of living units whose functional capacity is altered in accordance with the state of their molecular composition and is thus dependent on physical and chemical changes of their contents."[160] This statement presaged by some 50 years the wealth of scientific developments in the biology of medicine that began in the early 1900s and continues at an ever-increasing pace today. With our current state of knowledge concerning the biology of disease, terms such as "degeneration" to denote progressive deterioration of cells or "infiltration" to describe intracellular or extracellular accumulations of normal or abnormal substances are of little more than

historical interest and should not be used. The various responses of cells to stress and injury are being increasingly described in the more precise and quantitative terms of cell and molecular biology.

Cellular reactions to stress vary depending on the type, duration, and severity of injury induced (Fig. 1-3). The response can range from a minimal and reversible disturbance of cell volume to massive irreversible swelling with a concomitant loss of cell function, followed by death.[159] When injury develops rapidly, it is conventionally referred to as "acute." The factor or factors that ultimately determine whether a cell will survive or succumb after injury remain to be unequivocally established. Irreversibility is probably attributable to the effect of the loss of several vital functions coupled with increased degradation of intracellular components. Recent studies indicate that in the early stages of cell injury there are significant losses of phospholipids from cell membranes. This leads to functional alterations of the cell, presumably resulting from activation of intracellular phospholipases.[20] Clearly the impaired capacity to generate adenosine triphosphate (ATP) and synthesize protein is insufficient to cause death of liver cells. Experimental studies have shown that hepatocytes faced with such dire events are capable of downmodulating their functional demands, thereby decreasing their requirement for ATP generation to the extent that they can survive short periods of stress. If stress is sufficiently prolonged, cells will certainly die; perhaps this occurs when the synthesis of a certain vital molecule or molecules is sufficiently compromised that the renewal of cell substance is critically impaired. The factors responsible for the point beyond which survival is no longer possible, aptly referred to as the "point of no return," have not been identified because we still do not know precisely what vital func-

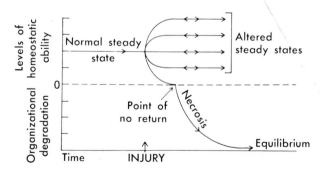

Fig. 1-3. In the "normal" steady state a cell is able to maintain a homeostasis (internal milieu) that allows optimum function. When injury occurs, the cell alters its steady state and function; if injury is sufficiently intense and protracted, it is unable to maintain its homeostasis at a level sufficient for function compatible with life, and cell death results. (From Scarpelli, D., and Trump, B.F.: Cell injury, Bethesda, Md., 1974, Universities Associated for Research and Education in Pathology, Inc.)

tions must be compromised before a cell dies. In less intense and prolonged forms of stress, termed "chronic," cells are able to adapt to environmental abnormalities to the extent that they are capable of augmented rather than diminished function (see Fig. 1-3). Cases in point are (1) the increase in cell mass (hypertrophy) of muscle cells after increased demands for work, as occurs in the heart after pathologic stress or in peripheral striated muscle of athletes as a consequence of increased physiologic stress, and (2) the enlargement of hepatocytes, accompanied by an increase in smooth-surfaced endoplasmic reticulum membranes and the associated drug-metabolizing enzyme systems, after exposure to foreign and potentially toxic compounds such as phenobarbital and other drugs.

The response of cells to an adverse environment is conditioned by numerous intracellular and extracellular factors. These can be classified into four broad categories: (1) extracellular and intracellular milieu, (2) pattern and degree of metabolic activity, (3) level of cell differentiation, and (4) type, amount, and expression of information contained in the genome. A brief discussion of each of these follows.

Several experimental models have demonstrated that manipulation of either the intracellular or extracellular milieu can to some degree protect cells from the deleterious effects of injury. Perfusion of isolated rat heart with a high concentration of glucose in the oxygenated perfusate sharply diminishes ischemic injury of myocardium induced subsequently by 30 minutes of perfusion with perfusate charged with nitrogen. Protection is characterized by a return of nearly normal cardiac function as well as ultrastructural integrity of myocardial cells after reperfusion with perfusate containing oxygen. Presumably protection is afforded by the glycolytic pathway's ability to generate sufficient ATP to maintain myocardial cells until they are again supplied with oxygen.[163]

The pattern and degree of metabolic activity of a cell also determine to some extent its reponse to certain types of injury. For example, the high sensitivity of cardiac muscle cells to ischemia is largely attributable to their almost total dependence on aerobic metabolism for a continuous supply of high levels of ATP required for their contractile and other functions. When ATP generation is totally interrupted for as short a period as 20 to 30 minutes, injury is irreversible and cardiac cell death ensues. Cells such as hepatocytes and fibroblasts appear to be somewhat more resistant to ischemic injury, since they apparently do not require such steady and high levels of ATP to survive. As mentioned previously, such cells can apparently modulate their energy requirements for extended periods and thus adapt to an adversely altered environment and survive.

Increased resistance of the relatively undifferentiated neuronal cell layers of the developing infant brain to hypoxic injury, as contrasted to the increased susceptibility of fully differentiated neurons in the brain of growing and adult animals, including humans, is an example of the altered response to injury that differentiation confers on cells. The increased sensitivity of differentiated cells is probably related to their more complex metabolic machinery and greater dependence on oxidative metabolism than is true for less differentiated cells.

The role of the genome in determining how and to what extent a cell population will respond to an injurious agent is an area in which there is a rapidly growing fund of information. For example, the inability of individuals with xeroderma pigmentosum to repair injury to DNA of squamous epithelium of skin after exposure to ultraviolet radiation is apparently caused by a genetically determined lack of the necessary repair enzymes[22] and is probably closely related to the high incidence of skin cancer in such persons in young adulthood. In this case, the absence, abnormality, or inexpression of a specific bit of genetic information has made exposure to sunlight a serious hazard.

Studies of acute injury caused by a variety of noxious agents on both isolated cells and tissue have shown a striking similarity in the types and sequence of morphologic changes, regardless of the nature of the injurious agent. Some of the most impressive findings have resulted from time-lapse cinematographic phase-contrast microscopy of cells in culture[9] because these have emphasized the rapidity, variety, and extent of cytologic changes incident to injury. The initial event, occurring almost immediately after exposure of a cell to a noxious environment, is a loss of cell volume control, which is rapidly followed by a decrease in the optical density of the cytoplasm because of intracellular swelling (hydropic change) and eventual accumulation of lipid droplets (fatty change). If the noxious agent is particularly toxic and the exposure is sufficiently prolonged to be lethal, additional alterations are seen: violent movements of the plasma membrane followed by the development of bizarre pseudopods and blebs of the plasma membrane, nuclear swelling, condensation of nuclear chromatin (pyknosis), dissolution of the nucleus (karyolysis), and finally lysis of the cell (cytolysis).

Cell death, autolysis, and necrosis

Cell death is that state in which cells are incapable of *any function*, including energy generation, homeostatic control, motility, uptake of materials, synthesis, export, cell communication and excitability, and reproduction. Within minutes after cell death, hydrolytic enzymes are released from lysosomes in the cytoplasm and activated by the increasingly acid pH arising from lactic acidosis caused by diminished or absent oxidative metabolism. Hydrolytic enzymes rapidly degrade intracellular materials including organelles and other cell membrane

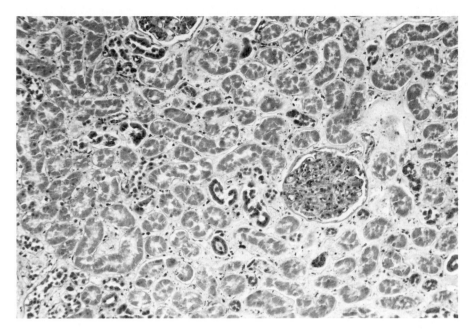

Fig. 1-4. Autolysis of kidney removed from body 72 hours after death. Epithelial cells lining the renal tubules are no longer attached to basement membrane (desquamated) and are devoid of nuclei. Absence of inflammatory cells indicates that cell death and necrosis did not occur during life of the patient.

systems; this process of self-digestion is referred to as *autolysis.* As autolysis proceeds, the cell cytoplasm becomes homogeneous in appearance and intensely eosinophilic. Eventually cellular details are lost and cell debris remains. The onset of autolysis is rapid in cells with a high content of hydrolytic enzymes such as those of the pancreas and gastric mucosa; intermediate in the heart, liver, and kidney; and slow in fibroblasts, which have relatively few lysosomes and a corresponding low level of hydrolytic enzymes. When focal death and autolysis of a tissue occur in a living body, the process is referred to as *necrosis;* since the focus rapidly incites activation of body cellular defenses, it is quickly surrounded by inflammatory cells. Autolysis of normal tissues in a dead body, termed postmortem change, can be distinguished from autolysis in the living body by the fact that the former is diffuse rather than focal and does not invoke an inflammatory reaction (Fig. 1-4). When sufficiently advanced, both autolysis and necrosis result in softening and eventual liquefaction of tissues.

Types of necrosis. Based on the gross appearance of tissues obtained from autopsy or surgery, three different major types of necrosis have been described. Each type also has characteristic microscopic features. In *coagulation necrosis* the tissue has an opaque appearance likened to that of boiled meat and is somewhat drier than surrounding normal tissue (Fig. 1-5). This type of necrosis in humans is most frequently caused by irreversible focal injury after sudden cessation of blood flow (ischemia) in organs such as the heart, kidney, or spleen. Less common causes are potent bacterial toxins

and phenol, mercurials, and other corrosive chemicals. Foci of coagulation necrosis vary in their gross appearance depending on their age. Areas of fresh coagulation necrosis are pale, firm, and slightly swollen; as it progresses, the tissue becomes more yellowish as a result of increasing numbers of inflammatory cells and softer as a result of autolysis. Foci of early coagulation necrosis contain cells that are slightly more eosinophilic than normal with little or no alteration of cellular detail. As the necrosis progresses, eosinophilia becomes intense and cells swell and undergo the changes described previously. Eventually the focus becomes infiltrated with inflammatory cells, which help to digest the dead cells, leaving residual cellular debris.

Caseation necrosis (Fig. 1-6) is a variant of coagulation necrosis encountered when cell death is attributable to certain microorganisms such as *Mycobacterium tuberculosis.* Grossly, such foci are yellowish white and sharply circumscribed from the surrounding normal tissues. The necrotic tissue is soft, granular, and friable, reminiscent of dry cheese (hence the name). The necrosis is in part attributable to the severe histotoxic effects of high-molecular-weight lipoidal substances present in tubercle bacilli. Because of limited growth of capillary-sized blood vessels from the surrounding normal tissues into the area of necrosis, intense scarring around such foci, and inhibition of intracellular hydrolytic enzymes by certain chemical components of mycobacteria, the caseous material remains in situ in tissues for long periods.

Liquefaction necrosis (Fig. 1-7) is the focal degrada-

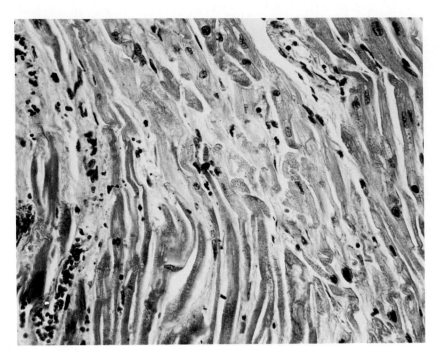

Fig. 1-5. Coagulation necrosis of cardiac muscle. Contrast deeply staining necrotic muscle fibers devoid of nuclei at lower left with more normal-appearing muscle fibers at upper right.

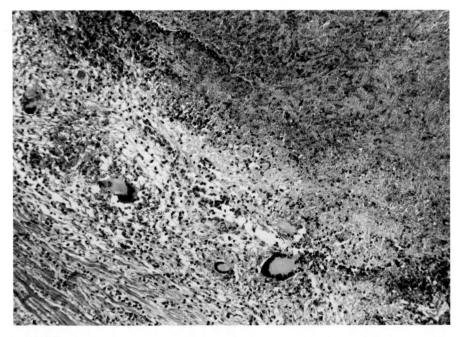

Fig. 1-6. Caseation necrosis in patient with widespread pulmonary tuberculosis; area of necrosis appears at the right with an adjacent zone of inflammation including multinucleated giant cells.

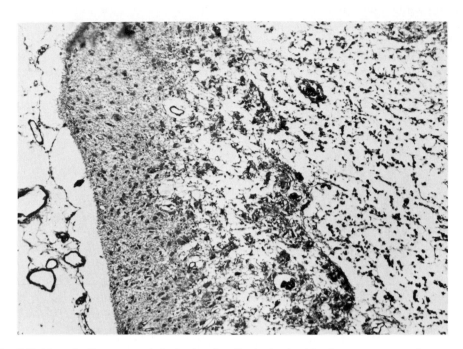

Fig. 1-7. Liquefaction necrosis in brain of patient who had had numerous cerebrovascular accidents. Liquefaction necrosis, present at right, consists of cellular debris and numerous glial cells; the cyst is limited by a thin rim of brain substance at left.

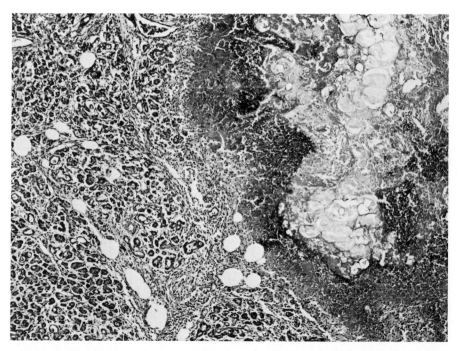

Fig. 1-8. Fat necrosis of pancreas. Necrotic area, visible at right, consists of accumulations of pale amorphous material (sodium, magnesium, and calcium salts of fatty acids).

tion of tissue that rapidly undergoes softening and liquefaction. It is most frequently encountered in the central nervous system after ischemic injury resulting from primary occlusion of an artery, or after massive cerebral trauma. Grossly, the necrotic area is soft and the center is liquefied. As time passes, a cystic space whose walls are defined by nonnecrotic tissue develops. Histologically, the cystic space contains necrotic cell debris, among which can be seen free glial cells containing phagocytized material, and the cyst wall is lined by a network of proliferating capillaries and numerous glial cells.

Fat necrosis (Fig. 1-8) is encountered in adipose tissue contiguous to the pancreas and more rarely at distant sites, as a result of leakage of lipase after acute injury to pancreatic acinar tissue, most commonly from obstruction of pancreatic ducts. Grossly, fat necrosis appears as firm, yellow-white deposits in peripancreatic and mesenteric adipose tissue. When the extent of pancreatic injury is severe, fat necrosis may be widespread, affecting extra-abdominal adipose tissue such as that in the anterior mediastinum and bone marrow. The necrotic foci consist of necrotic fat cells in which the triglycerides have been hydrolyzed by pancreatic lipase into fatty acids and glycerol. The fatty acids are subsequently converted into soaps (saponification) by reaction with calcium, magnesium, and sodium ions. As the concentration of calcium and magnesium soaps increases, the deposits become firmer and chalky white. Histologically, necrotic fat cells are distinguishable as pale outlines, and their cytoplasm is filled with an amorphous-appearing, faintly basophilic material (soap).

Some details of cell injury caused by chemical, physical, and biologic agents

Although the basic pattern of cellular response tends to be similar for injury caused by different types of noxious agents, there are significant variations, especially in the early stages of injury. These appear to be related to the nature of the injurious agent, including the mechanism by which it exerts its effects, its severity, and its duration. In this discussion we consider the sequential biochemical and other functional and structural changes that occur in injury caused by several types of agents.

Chemical agents
Carbon tetrachloride

Toxic injury of the liver is a common outcome of ethanol abuse; exposure to certain industrial chemicals or, to a lesser extent, to therapeutic drugs or naturally occurring toxicants such as the aflatoxins may also be the cause. This discussion focuses on cell injury by carbon tetrachloride and ethanol, the former because it has been well studied and is a classic example of an industrial toxicant and the latter because of its obvious clinical and social significance.

Injury of liver cells by carbon tetrachloride (CCl_4) is a much-studied model system of toxic insult that has served to establish some of the salient mechanisms involved in toxic chemical injury. Cell damage by CCl_4 is the result of its metabolic conversion by the NADPH-cytochrome P-450 drug-metabolizing enzyme system to highly reactive chemical species. In contrast to the usual reaction in which ferric (Fe^{+++}) iron in cytochrome P-450 is reduced to ferrous (Fe^{++}) iron by addition of an electron to the cytochrome when a foreign chemical substrate binds to it, in the case of CCl_4 the electron is not accepted by Fe^{+++}, but rather by CCl_4; this leads to its reductive cleavage of the carbon-chlorine bond as follows:

$$CCl_4 + e \rightarrow CCl_3^{\cdot} + Cl \cdot$$

The products formed have unpaired electrons and are highly reactive free radicals as shown below for one of these, the chloromethyl ($CCl_3^{\cdot}$) radical. $CCl_3^{\cdot}$, like other free radicals, react with molecules in the immediate vicinity of their formation, most notably unsaturated lipids of intracellular membranes, by abstracting a hydrogen atom through the following reactions:

$$-CH_2-\overset{H}{\underset{}{C}}=\overset{H}{\underset{}{C}}- + CCl_3^{\cdot} \rightarrow -CH_2-\overset{\cdot}{C}=\overset{H}{C}- + CCl_3H$$
$$-CH_2-\overset{\cdot}{C}=\overset{H}{C}- + CCl_3^{\cdot} \rightarrow -CH_2-CH=\overset{H}{C}\cdot + CCl_3H$$

In each instance reaction with a free radical leads to the formation of still another free radical. These organic free radicals react rapidly with molecular oxygen to form lipid peroxides such as

$$-\overset{H}{\underset{H}{C}}-\overset{H}{\underset{H}{C}}-\overset{O}{\overset{\|}{C}}-$$

These are highly unstable and break down to aldehydes, malonaldehyde, ketones, and other products that are also highly reactive and react with nearby methylene bridges leading to formation of additional unstable molecules. The foregoing is responsible for the fact that free-radical formation is autocatalytic and progresses from a focus leading to widespread membrane damage. Proteins are spared, especially those with sulfhydryl (—SH) moieties, and hydrogen atoms are abstracted through the following reactions:

$$CCl_3^{\cdot} + HS-R \rightarrow \cdot S-R + CCl_3H$$
$$CCl_3^{\cdot} + \cdot S-R \rightarrow Cl_3C\mathbf{:}S-R$$

For example, the function of enzymes depending on glutathione and other —SH-containing compounds as cofactors would be seriously compromised by their progressive alkylation.

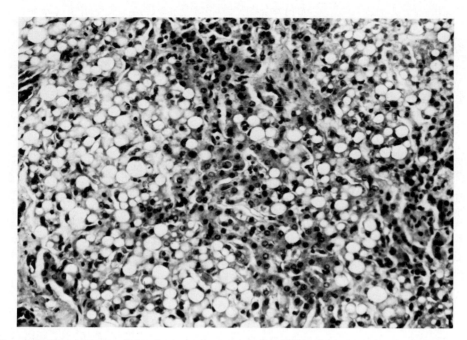

Fig. 1-9. Fatty liver in a patient after a protracted alcohol debauch. Hepatocytes are vacuolated; these represent accumulations of neutral lipids that have been removed by lipid solvents during tissue processing.

The earliest change that has been detected in rat liver cells is a functional one that occurs 30 minutes after the intragastric administration of a single dose of 0.25 ml of CCl_4. It consists in a rapid decrease in synthesis of the export protein albumin, as well as cytochrome c.[143,144] The liver grossly and histologically appears entirely normal; ultrastructural studies, however, indicate a slight dilatation of the cisternae of the endoplasmic reticulum (ER), suggestive of very early swelling, and dissociation of ribosomes from the ER membrane. Ultracentrifugal analysis of ribosomes from experimental animals supports the morphologic findings and demonstrates a progressive loss of 200S polysome aggregates and a concomitant increase in 54S subunits, indicating that disaggregation has occurred. The diminution of protein synthesis after CCl_4 intoxication appears to be linked to disaggregation of polysomes and probably represents a physical disruption of its obligatory association with mRNA. Significantly, in this early phase of CCl_4-induced injury, mitochondria appear morphologically intact and are capable of normal oxidative phosphorylation and fatty acid oxidation among their many other functions.

Within a few hours after administration of CCl_4, neutral lipids (triglycerides) begin to accumulate in the cytoplasm, making their first appearance as osmiophilic droplets in the ER cisternae. These coalesce to form larger droplets, which ultimately fill the entire cytoplasm. Approximately 10 to 12 hours after CCl_4 administration, the liver is grossly enlarged and pale because

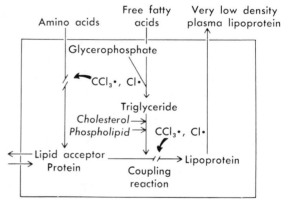

Formation of plasma lipoproteins by the hepatocyte showing sites of CCl_4 effect

Fig. 1-10. Diagram of lipid metabolism involved in development of fatty liver. (From Scarpelli, D., and Trump, B.F.: Cell injury, Bethesda, Md., 1974, Universities Associated for Research and Education in Pathology, Inc.)

of accumulated fat (Fig. 1-9). This experimental model, which reproducibly leads to the development of fatty liver, has been of signal importance in elucidating one of the major pathogenetic mechanisms responsible for this condition.[102] Impairment of protein synthesis leads to a rapid diminution of lipoprotein secretion by the liver because the synthesis of the protein (lipid acceptor protein) necessary for the coupling of triglyceride to phospholipids to form lipoprotein has been interrupted (Fig. 1-10). This results in the accumulation of lipid in

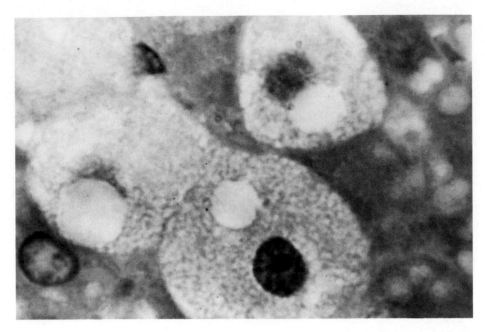

Fig. 1-11. Liver cells 8 hours after administration of CCl_4. Hepatocytes are large and swollen with a finely granular cytoplasm; clear vacuoles probably represent early accumulation of neutral lipids (triglycerides). Nuclei appear unaltered.

the form of triglycerides, since these can be secreted into the blood from the liver only as lipoproteins. Lipid can also accumulate in the liver by other mechanisms, as by increased mobilization of free fatty acids from depot fat, as occurs in early starvation and after the excessive ingestion of ethanol such that the capacity for its metabolism and secretion by liver is exceeded, or by concomitant stimulation of synthesis and decreased oxidation of fatty acids as occurs in toxic injury by ethanol. Mitochondrial injury after CCl_4 intoxication occurs somewhat later than that of ER and appears first as a loosening of the coupling between oxygen consumption and the esterification of adenosine diphosphate (ADP) to form ATP, which may progress to total uncoupling. The cells then undergo progressive swelling, which begins in the early phases of injury and becomes more severe as they lose their capacity to oppose the passive inward diffusion of sodium and calcium ions and water because of decreased function of the plasma membrane. The swollen cells have a pale, almost clear-appearing cytoplasm and are referred to as balloon cells (Fig. 1-11). In the late stages of injury, dense basophilic granules appear in the cytoplasm becoming progressively larger with time. These granules represent focal aggregates of precipitated calcium salts in the matrix of swollen mitochondria, the result of massive unregulated influx of calcium ions in dying and dead liver cells.

Nuclear and nucleolar injury also occurs; however, the sequence of injury is difficult to describe because structure-function relationships for these organelles are still poorly understood. Clumping and margination of nuclear chromatin may be related to sharp alterations of electrolytes and pH resulting from injury and are accompanied by impaired DNA and RNA synthesis. Thus impaired transcription is superimposed on the previously described defects of translation. Dead hepatocytes appear in increasing numbers, undergo necrosis, and are characterized by a flocculent eosinophilic cytoplasm and a dense basophilic nucleus that becomes progressively shrunken (pyknosis), fragmented, and ultimately totally digested (karyolysis). Digestion of necrotic liver cells is attributable to activation of proteolytic enzymes by the lactic acidosis after the loss of oxidative metabolism. These and other metabolic alterations that characterize toxic cell injury by CCl_4 are summarized schematically in Fig. 1-12. Notice how these various events are linked both chemically and temporally.

Ethanol

Ethanol is a less potent toxicant than carbon tetrachloride (CCl_4) though a single bout of excessive ingestion can induce significant functional disturbances of the liver, which subside rapidly with abstinence. Chronic ethanol abuse leads to severe hepatotoxicity and liver cell death. Although ethanol is a normal metabolite of the mammalian organism, formed both from the reduction of acetaldehyde in tissues and in the gut by bacteria, a high level of ethanol is toxic to cells. Recent evidence indicates that unmetabolized ethanol can inhibit amino acid uptake by liver cells.[126] Since ethanol is metabolized rapidly after its ingestion, attention has been focused on the cellular effects of its metabolism. Ethanol is metabolized largely in the liver by

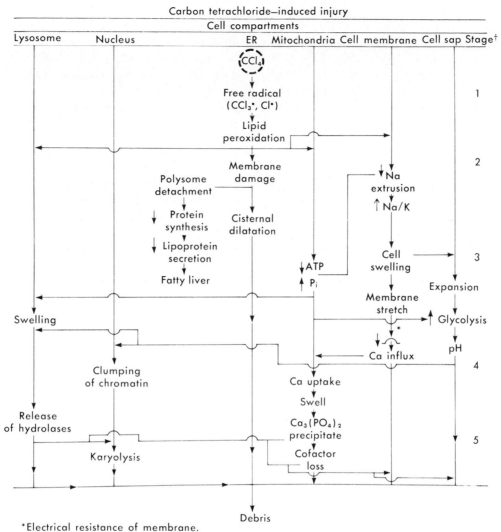

Carbon tetrachloride–induced injury

Fig. 1-12. Flow sheet of sequential events during acute CCl₄ intoxication. (From Scarpelli,. D., and Trump, B.F.: Cell injury, Bethesda, Md., 1974, Universities Associated for Research and Education in Pathology, Inc.)

three pathways. The first and primary one involves alcohol dehydrogenase; the second, catalase; and the third, the drug-metabolizing enzyme system. All of these lead to the formation of acetaldehyde, which in turn is rapidly oxidized to acetate by acetaldehyde dehydrogenase. The overall result of sustained ethanol metabolism, which involves NAD^+-linked oxidation in two major steps, its oxidation to acetaldehyde and subsequently to acetate and acetyl coenzyme A (CoA), is to produce an excess of intracellular NADH and a concomitant decrease in the ratio of NAD^+ to NADH. The sustained increase in NADH leads to enhanced reduction of pyruvate to lactate, decreased gluconeogenesis, and a higher concentration of α-glycerophosphate, which in turn lead to increased esterification of fatty acids to triglycerides. It also causes inhibition of mitochondrial β-oxidation of fatty acids and an increased synthesis of fatty acids by the coupling of ethanol oxi-

dation with the oxalocetate-malate cycle and the production of NADPH necessary for lipogenesis. These changes together are responsible for the accumulation of triglyceride in liver cells, a cardinal though not exclusive sign of alcohol-induced liver cell injury.

Chronic excessive ingestion of ethanol leads to enhanced synthesis of drug-metabolizing enzymes. Such adapted hepatocytes have an increased capacity for the metabolism of ethanol and as a consequence produce excessive amounts of acetaldehyde. On the other hand, chronic ingestion of ethanol significantly impairs the capacity of liver mitochrondria to oxidize acetaldehyde,[63] so that the net effect is an increased level of the metabolite in the liver and other tissues and in the blood. As a class, aldehydes are highly reactive compounds capable of a variety of chemical reactions, including oxidation, reduction, addition, substitution, and polymerization. In tissue, acetaldehyde reacts with the active hydrogen atoms of the amines of protein to form cross-linking methylene bridges. It is also capable of reacting with other chemical groups of living matter such as amide, peptide, hydroxyl, carboxyl, imine, thiol, disulfide, and indole. It is not surprising, then, that acetaldehyde has been suggested as the toxic metabolite involved in ethanol toxicity. Studies have shown that chronic ingestion of ethanol adversely affects mitochondria by inducing decreased fluidity of their inner membranes, changes in the temperature dependence of respiration and ATPase activity,[128] and impaired mitochondrial protein synthesis.[14] In addition to the implication of acetaldehyde in ethanol toxicity, there is increasing evidence that free radicals causing lipid peroxidation of cell membranes may also be involved. Some of these effects are no doubt responsible for the toxic injury and cell death in the liver and in some cases other organs, such as the heart and brain, in chronic alcoholic patients. Whatever the mechanisms responsible for ethanol toxicity, it should be clear that continued abuse of ethanol leads to serious disease and eventual death.

Physical agents
Ischemic injury

Injury resulting from ischemia differs considerably from that caused by chemical toxicants in both the initial focus of dysfunction and the general sequence of events, especially in the early phases of injury. Ischemic injury and subsequent cell death are all too frequently encountered in clinical medicine. They occur when the vascular supply of an organ is interrupted by spontaneous formation of an occluding blood clot or thrombus, a process discussed in Chapter 3. Ischemic injury has been studied most profitably in two experimental models, the heart and the kidney, in which the blood supply has been suddenly interrupted by ligation of the coronary arteries or the renal artery respectively. The heart is the simpler of the two models because of its less complex blood supply, and it has been studied much more extensively. Experimental ischemia of the heart induced by arterial ligation is characterized initially by several functional changes that are followed by morphologic ones.[82,83] The earliest gross change occurs within a few beats after ligation; the ischemic focus of myocardium becomes pale and ceases to contract, and so the focus bulges passively with each contraction. The rapid and focal loss of contractility is attributable to depletion of the small pool of ATP that normally energizes the shuttling of Ca^{++} from the cisternae of the sarcoplasmic reticulum (SR) into the sarcoplasm where it binds actin and myosin; this contractility causes conformational changes resulting both in contraction and dephosphorylation of ATP. The actin-myosin intermolecular relationships return to those of the relaxed state, ADP is rephosphorylated, and Ca^{++} ions are actively pumped into the SR where they remain sequestered until the next cycle of contraction. Mitochondrial phosphorylation continues to diminish rapidly, leading to depletion of creatine phosphate and ATP. This in turn stimulates phosphorylase and phosphofructokinase activity and an increase in anaerobic glycolysis. However, since no new substrate is available, this regulatory mechanism for the generation of ATP in the face of a low oxygen tension ceases in a few minutes when myocardial stores of glycogen are depleted and low ATP levels and acidosis inhibit anaerobic glycolysis. As ATP levels fall, the sodium-potassium pump and sodium-calcium exchange cease to function, and the active transport of K^+ and Ca^{++} is interrupted. At this point, the electrical potential of the cells decreases as Na^+, Cl^-, K^+, and water freely cross the sarcolemmal membrane, and edema ensues. The sarcoplasmic reticulum and mitochondria also fail to control their transport of ions and water, and they swell (Fig. 1-13). ATP deprivation also leads to the development of severe focal contractures of heart muscle fibers characterized by the formation of "rigor" bands of actin and myosin. If ATP depletion is severe and sustained, the permeability of the sarcolemma increases to the point that large protein molecules, including enzymes, and other cellular components leak into the extracellular space and the cells are irreversibly injured. In cardiac muscle, irreversible damage develops after 30 to 40 minutes of sustained ischemia. In contrast to toxic injury of liver, the initial salient effects of ischemic injury seem to involve energy production and ion transport by cell membranes (Fig. 1-14). As the duration of ischemic injury increases, the sequence of events tends to resemble that seen in toxic injury of liver—failure of protein synthesis, alterations of membrane structure, activation of lysosomes, and ultimately death and self-digestion.

An understanding of the events that follow the return of blood flow to ischemic myocardium is important because of the dire consequences. At the interface between ischemic and normally perfused heart muscle, return of blood to irreversibly injured myocardium induces a sudden contraction of muscle cells with a clumping of sarcomeres followed by an explosive swelling of the cells, sarcolemmal rupture, and a rapid intracellular influx of Ca^{++} and water leading to rapid cell death. As one would expect, these changes are accompanied by a massive loss of myoglobin and intracellular proteins including creatine kinase and other enzymes. Knowledge of these effects, coupled with the demonstration that the viability of heart muscle cells can be maintained for several hours in the absence of blood flow if high intracellular levels of ATP are preserved, has led to the methodology routinely employed in open-heart surgery. Hypothermia and stilling of the heart (cardioplegia) are used to drastically diminish energy requirements of the heart and thus conserve cel-

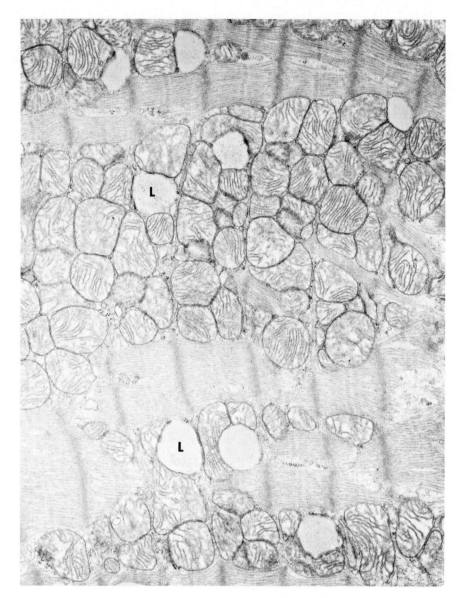

Fig. 1-13. Ischemic injury of myocardium in a patient who died of irreversible shock. Mitochondria are swollen, and numerous droplets of neutral lipid *(L)* are present. (From Scarpelli, D., and Trump, B.F.: Cell injury, Bethesda, Md., 1974, Universities Associated for Research and Education in Pathology, Inc.)

lular ATP levels. The protective effects of hypothermia and cardioplegia are additive, and the early recovery of heart function appears directly related to the cellular ATP levels remaining at the end of the ischemic interval.

Before concluding this discussion, it is noteworthy that the mechanism or mechanisms involved in reperfusion injury are a matter of some controversy. Some believe that the damage of the plasma membrane responsible for these lethal intracellular events occurred before reperfusion and involves constitutive alterations. This is consonant with the finding that sustained ischemia causes rapid degradation of membrane phospholipids. Other workers maintain that membrane damage is attributable to the production of oxygen free-radical species such as superoxide (O_2^-), hydrogen peroxide (H_2O_2), and the hydroxyl (OH·) radical formed during reperfusion from the reaction of purines with O_2 catalyzed by the enzyme xanthine oxidase. More recent work has identified some pronounced alterations of the cytoskeletal framework of ischemic myocardial cells, which adds still another facet to this already complex problem.

Disturbances in intracellular ion homeostasis

There are major differences in the early phases of cell injury depending on the nature of the insult and the target cell affected. In contrast, the later phases, in

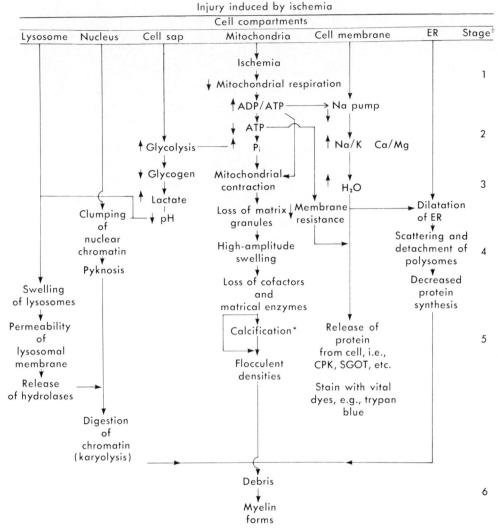

*Calcification does not generally occur in the centers of infarcts unless reflow of blood is permitted.

‡Numbers at the right correspond to the temporal sequence of events.

Fig. 1-14. Flow sheet of sequential events in ischemic injury. *ER,* Endoplasmic reticulum. (From Scarpelli, D., and Trump, B.F.: Cell injury, Bethesda, Md., 1974, Universities Associated for Research and Education in Pathology, Inc.)

which the biochemical and structural events are similar regardless of the toxicant and cell involved, have been referred to as the final common pathway. One common thread in cell injury and death is the major disturbances in intracellular ion homeostasis that have been identified in cells lethally injured by a toxicant or by sustained ischemia. Recent evidence indicates that an abnormality in intracellular levels of Ca^{++} may be a central event in coagulation necrosis. This is based on the demonstration that cultured hepatocytes remain viable in the presence of a variety of potent chemical toxins as long as they are kept in calcium-free medium and that cell death rapidly follows exposure to Ca^{++}.[132] The lethal event has been postulated to be the massive influx of Ca^{++} across the damaged plasma membrane, rather than the preexisting membrane damage. Other studies of freshly isolated hepatocytes, however, indicate that uncontrolled fluxes of other ions such as Na^{+} and K^{+} may be involved.[142] Although it has been known for many years that abnormally high accumulations of Ca^{++} and other ions are present in severely injured and dead cells, only recently have studies focused on the kinetics of their intracellular accumulation and the biochemical effects that follow.

Ionizing radiation

Exposure to ionizing radiation is a fact of life that has become increasingly important in the latter half of the twentieth century. In addition to natural sources of ionizing radiation in the environment over which we have little control, such as cosmic radiation, terrestrial radiation, and natural radioisotopes in our bodies, we are

Table 1-1. Various types of ionizing radiation of importance to medicine

Type	Mass	Charge	Description	Tissue penetration
X rays	None	None	Electromagnetic and	High (ft)
Gamma (γ) rays	None	None	nonparticulate	High (ft)
Beta (β) particles	1/1836	Either + or −	Charged electrons	Low (mm-cm)
Alpha (α) particles	4	+2	Ionized helium atoms	Very low (<mm)
Protons	1	+1	Hydrogen nuclei	Intermediate between α and β
Neutrons	1	None	Neutrons	High (ft)

exposed to radiation from a variety of man-made sources, which we can control; these include diagnostic radiology, therapeutic, industrial, and fallout radiation. The physician may encounter injury from excessive exposure to ionizing radiation as a complication of intensive radiation therapy for the treatment of cancer or more rarely from industrial accidents in facilities that produce fissionable materials or generate electrical power by atomic energy. The recent disaster at Chernobyl in the Soviet Union emphasizes the magnitude of the problem.

Ionizing radiations are classified according to their physical properties into two general categories; radiations that are electromagnetic, nonparticulate, and devoid of mass and charge and those that are particulate, have mass, and may be charged as shown in Table 1-1. The physician should be aware of the general characteristics and source of x rays, gamma rays, and beta particles and to a lesser extent of alpha particles, protons, and neutrons. This section deals with the physical and chemical events that occur in irradiated cells and ultimately lead to their injury.

The effects of ionizing radiation on cells begin with the absorption of energy by cell substance. This leads to the formation of ions when the energy is sufficient to expel external electrons from constituent atoms, causing them to become positively charged. The ejected electrons may interact with a nearby atom so that it becomes negatively charged, and thus an ion pair is formed. When x rays or gamma rays are the source of radiation, the expelled electrons are so highly energized that they give rise to multiple ion pairs before their energy is sufficiently reduced to make them incapable of displacing electrons. Alpha and beta particles may also dislodge electrons if their energy is sufficient; such electrons become secondary ionizing particles. Chemical bonds in molecules are broken when the absorbed energy is greater than that of the bond. Thus, in brief, the interaction of ionizing radiation with cell matter leads to excitation of atoms to form ions,[97] resulting in a series of localized physicochemical perturbations in the cell.

Studies of the radiochemistry of water have been of salient importance in elucidating the reactions that probably occur in irradiated cells. Cell substance is a dilute complex mixture of proteins, carbohydrates, and lipids, present either in aqueous solution or in suspension. Water, the major component of cell substance, absorbs energy from ionizing radiation to a greater extent than do solute molecules, which are more infrequent. The interaction of ionizing radiation with water leads to the formation of ionizing water molecules, H_2O^+ and H_2^-, which dissociate to form the free radicals H· and OH·; subsequently these react with each other, with water molecules, with their own reaction products, and finally with other substances in the cell, including organic molecules.[28] Interactions of free radicals with each other, their reaction products, and cell macromolecules are largely dependent on their volume concentration, that is, how closely together the free radicals are formed.[25] As the energy transfer from ionizing radiation to surrounding matter in a given volume increases, the number of free radicals formed and the ensuing interactions also increase. Various types of ionizing radiation differ in the amounts of energy they lose as they pass through matter; this property is referred to as linear energy transfer (LET). Highly penetrating gamma rays, for example, have a low LET; they lose their energy over a long distance and thus generate a very low ion concentration. Conversely, radiations with low penetration such as alpha particles have a high LET and generate a high ion concentration. X rays and beta particles have intermediate LET values and generate moderate ion concentrations. H_2O^+ and H_2O^- are unstable ions that dissociate in about 10^{-16} second; the resultant free radicals react with nearby molecules in about 10^{-5} second.[7] These various reactions are summarized in Table 1-2.

Irradiation of deaerated solutions of simple organic molecules leads to their decomposition, a reaction that may also occur in irradiated cells. The decomposition of the amino acid glycine in irradiated water, for example, is as follows:

$$OH· + {}^+NH_3CH_2COO^- \rightarrow OHCH_2COO^- + NH_3^+$$
$$NH_3^+ + H_2O \rightarrow NH_4^+ + OH·$$

Irradiation of proteins, including enzymes, leads to their denaturation through attack on their peptide link-

Table 1-2. Summary of various reactions that occur during the irradiation of water molecules

Initial reactions	$H_2O \longrightarrow H_2O^+ + e^-$
	$H_2O^+ \longrightarrow H^+ + OH\cdot$
	$e^- + H_2O \longrightarrow H_2O^-$
	$H_2O^- \longrightarrow H\cdot + OH^-$
Reactions of free radicals	$H\cdot + OH\cdot \longrightarrow H_2O$
	$H\cdot + H\cdot \longrightarrow H_2$
	$OH\cdot + OH\cdot \longrightarrow H_2O_2$
Reactions with reaction products	$H_2O_2 + OH\cdot \longrightarrow HO_2\cdot + H_2O$
	$HO_2\cdot + HO_2\cdot \longrightarrow H_2O_2 + O_2$
	$HO_2\cdot + OH\cdot \longrightarrow H_2O_2 + O_2$
Reactions with organic molecules	$HO_2\cdot + RH \longrightarrow R\cdot + H_2O_2$
	$RH + HO_2\cdot \longrightarrow RO\cdot + H_2O$

ages and oxidation of sulfhydryl groups to disulfide bonds; the latter reaction appears to be enhanced by the presence of oxygen dissolved in the water. Ionizing radiation rapidly depolymerizes DNA and decreases its viscosity; in addition, chemical changes occur because of the rupture of glycoside and phosphate ester linkages and the ring opening of heterocyclic bases.[134]

High doses of ionizing radiation rapidly induce cell injury characterized by swelling and vacuolization of the cytoplasm, rupture of the nucleus and nucleolus, pyknosis, karyorrhexis (nuclear fragmentation), karyolysis, and cytolysis. These changes are of course identical to those seen in any acutely injured cell and must be considered nonspecific reactions to injury. Elegant experiments with amphibian eggs have shown that injection of minute amounts of cytoplasm from previously irradiated cells into nonirradiated ones promptly induces nuclear injury. These experiments also demonstrated that nuclei freed of cytoplasm by microdissection are very radioresistant, withstanding doses levels of x irradiation as high as 30,000 roentgens (R), whereas nuclei surrounded by cytoplasm in cells are injured by a dose of only 3000 R, a finding indicating that toxic substances that promote radiation injury may arise in irradiated cytoplasm.[37] These experiments also point out that at least part of the injury induced by irradiation must be indirect in nature; that is, the injury must be mediated through chemical alterations of the cytoplasm that secondarily affect the nucleus. In view of the extremely short half-life of ions and free radicals and the short life of hydrogen peroxide at body temperature, it is doubtful that these can be implicated in injury induced by injection of cytoplasm from irradiated cells into normal cells. Radiobiologists have also postulated that cell injury can be caused by a "direct" effect of ionizing radiation in which the radiation effect is localized totally to the smallest structural unit in the cell. Considering the diffuse nature of the physical interaction of ionizing radiation with matter and the complex-

ity of biologic organization of cells, it seems fruitless to attempt to explain the mechanism or mechanisms of injury induced by ionizing radiation in this manner.

The most thoroughly studied effects of ionizing radiations on cells are those that are localized in the nucleus and more especially the chromosomes. This is so because it became apparent to the early workers in radiobiology that these organelles were altered by very small doses of radiation and that the changes were readily detectable by light microscopy. All phases of the cell cycle can be affected by ionizing radiation, depending on the intensity and duration of exposure. Sensitivity of the cell appears to be greatest in G_2, that phase of the cycle just preceding mitosis (M); irradiation during this phase leads to a temporary block and retards the onset of cell division. Irradiation during mitosis induces chromosome aberrations, which differ depending on when exposure occurred. Exposure during or after metaphase and before S phase when DNA is synthesized induces lesions of the whole chromosome that become apparent at the first mitotic division *after* exposure. These lesions consist of breaks in the continuity of chromosomes, which may remain broken (deletion) or may be rejoined (repair). The rejoining may be such that no visible lesion is apparent, or it may be grossly abnormal if different broken ends are rejoined, leading to a so-called exchange. If, on the other hand, exposure to irradiation occurs late in the S phase, or early in G_2, after the chromosomes have doubled, the lesions involve one of a pair of chromatids of the replicated chromosomes. Chromatid lesions range from simple breaks to complex rejoining of various fragments, which may be symmetric or asymmetric. Chromosome lesions may lead to mutations because of structural changes in the purine and pyrimidine bases. These may result from the formation of hydrogen bonds between two bases after ionization or from the deletion of bases as a result of their interaction with free radicals. When such "errors" are replicated, the functional disturbance, often a negative one such as the deletion of an enzyme, is perpetuated in the daughter cells. If the mutation involves the deletion of a critical function or functions, it may be lethal. One of the most dreaded complications of mutation is the transformation of a previously normal cell to a malignant one. Radiation-induced damage of chromosomes becomes especially apparent morphologically during the metaphase, anaphase, and telophase stages of mitosis when their movements in the cytoplasm are more pronounced. Lesions at these latter stages consist of so-called lagging chromosomes where whole or fragments of chromosomes bridge the gap between the two separated masses of chromosomes. These are believed to be attributable to an increased stickiness of the chromosomes, a view consonant with the fact mentioned earlier that DNA is depolymerized by ionizing radiation. Aberrant movement of chromosomes may also be attri-

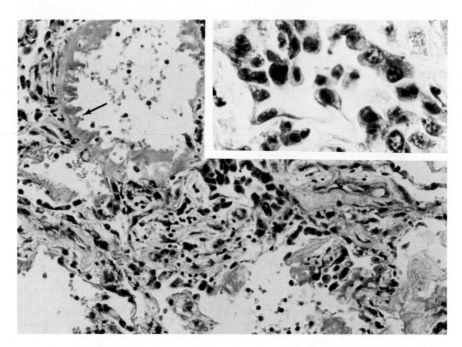

Fig. 1-15. Radiation-induced giant cells in the lung of patient who received radiation therapy for disseminated cancer. Notice fibrin deposits resulting from increased vascular permeability *(arrow)* and the cluster of large deeply staining cells *(center)*, which are much larger than other cells in the lung. *Inset,* At higher magnification these appear to be giant cells with large basophilic nuclei probably derived from pneumocytes.

butable to radiation-induced injury to the microtubules of the mitotic spindle, especially at the centromeres where they are attached to the chromosomes. This injury probably involves denaturation of tubulin, the major protein component of microtubules. Exposure of cells to ionizing radiation in the G_1 phase immediately after mitosis or in the S phase leads to a temporary inhibition of DNA synthesis. Such cells eventually enter the S phase and synthesize DNA even when they are exposed to high doses of radiation. Thus cell injury after irradiation is manifest at one or more of the following levels of biologic organization; structural damage to its DNA; breaks in the continuity of the chromosome, the organelle responsible for replication and transmission of genetic material; and finally denaturation of the proteins of the spindle, the organelle involved in distribution of genetic material to daughter cells.

As a result of inhibition of mitosis and DNA synthesis and premature cell death after irradiation of a cell population, there is a rapid decline in the number of cells that are in mitosis at any given time. The extent and duration of the overall effect are dependent on the dose of irradiation. A classic series of experiments[122] for studying the ability of single HeLa cells in culture to replicate and form clones after exposure to x irradiation as a biologic index of radiation effect showed that mammalian cells respond in one of three ways. Irradiated single cells that cannot proliferate give rise to colonies

that survive as single cells, or undergo a limited number of mitotic divisions (abortive colonies) and develop into cells that eventually become giant cells (Fig. 1-15). These reactions appear to be dose related. The average number of cells in an abortive colony varies inversely with the dose; the number of giant cells appears to vary directly with the dose. In abortive colonies the mitotic rate is reduced in direct proportion to the dose. Such studies have important clinical relevance because they form a basis for rational approaches to dosimetry in radiotherapy.

Biologic agent—virus

Viruses are a class of infectious particles that are obligate intracellular parasites. They consist of a core of either DNA or RNA surrounded by a protein coat that both protects the core and facilitates its entry into a host cell. In view of the large number of viruses and the numerous variations encountered in their interactions with susceptible cells, this section is limited to a general discussion of virus–host cell interactions and a presentation of a few examples in detail.

The interaction of virus with host cells can be modulated by numerous factors such as immune competence, tolerance, genetic variation in host susceptibility, and age and body temperature of the host. Viruses can rapidly produce irreversible and lethal injury in highly susceptible cells in an immunosuppressed host.

On the other hand, if a symbiotic equilibrium is reached between the virus and host cell, persistent inapparent infection may result. In the latter instance, cell injury does not develop and virus persists. This occurs when immune tolerance is present, as in the case of the common "fever blister" caused by the DNA virus herpes labialis. The virus remains latent or occult in apparently healthy ganglion cells until it is activated to replicate,[56] giving rise to lethal cell injury of epithelial cells of the lip characterized by the blisters.

The earliest stage of interaction between virus and a sensitive host cell begins with primary attachment of viral particles to the cell surface.[29,92] The initial binding involves ionic, van der Waals' forces and hydrogen bonds. Adsorption becomes stable when sufficient complementarity exists between specific-receptor molecules on the protein coat of the virus and the cell surface. Such virus-specific receptors have been identified and studied with appropriate host cells for the myxoviruses, rhabdoviruses, poliovirus, and more recently the herpesviruses.

Once stable adsorption has occurred, the virus is internalized by phagocytosis. The cell membrane adjacent to the virus flows around it, the invaginated membrane separates from the plasma membrane, and the vesicle moves into the cytoplasm of the virus particle. There follows a series of complex reactions that ultimately uncoats the virus or virion and releases viral nucleic acid into cytoplasm. The complexity of the uncoating phenomenon appears to depend on the number of coats possessed by the virus. In the case of vaccinia, a disease from a poxvirus that contains several coats, uncoating has been studied in detail from both a biochemical and a morphologic point of view. Within 20 minutes after phagocytosis the large (250×300 nm), brick-shaped virons begin to break down. This begins with dissolution of phospholipid of the outer coat and vacuolar membrane; since it occurs almost immediately after ingestion, it probably involves already existing hydrolytic enzymes of the host cell. The nucleoprotein core is freed from the outer coat, and approximately 1 hour later its protein coat begins to undergo digestion. This lag period is apparently the time required for synthesis of a specific proteolytic enzyme. This enzyme seems to be coded for the host cell genome, but its expression is continuously repressed and is redepressed only by the presence of specific viral protein made available by digestion of the core outer coat. The viral DNA that is liberated into the cytoplasm collects in pools, and information encoded in it is transcribed and translated. The truly parasitic nature of viruses becomes evident as the synthesis of vital macromolecules by the host cell is progressively inhibited while the synthetic machinery of the cell is utilized to form viral DNA and proteins (Fig. 1-16).[44] In vaccinia infection the rate and extent of

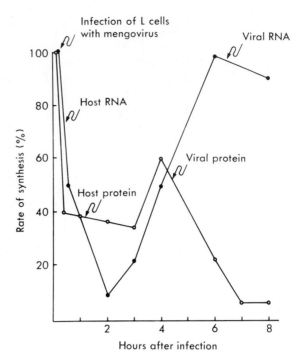

Fig. 1-16. Effect of virus on synthesis of RNA and protein by infected host cells. Synthesis of host cell RNA and protein is greatly inhibited almost immediately after infection. Return of synthesis of these macromolecules represents synthesis of viral RNA and protein by parasitized host cells. (Modified from Franklin, R.M., and Baltimore, D.: Cold Spring Harbor Symp. Quant. Biol. **27:**175, 1962.)

inhibition of protein synthesis are more pronounced than those observed with actinomycin D, a potent antibiotic that interferes with transcription. Since inhibition of host protein synthesis after infection by mengovirus reaches a level of about 10% of normal in 2 hours after infection, inhibition is mediated either by inactivation of host messenger RNA, which normally has a half-life of about 3 hours, or by prevention of its translation. Inhibition of host protein synthesis has also been documented for poliovirus.

The rate of host DNA synthesis decreases to approximately one third of normal within the first hour after infection by vaccinia virus because of virus-induced changes in host DNA, which impair its function as a template, after which viral DNA synthesis proceeds at a rate several times greater than that of the host cell. Such synthesis is mediated in the cytoplasm by a new virus-induced DNA polymerase synthesized by a specific messenger RNA copied from viral DNA released from the virion. Other examples of intracellular alterations induced by virus infection include disruption of the vimentin–intermediate filament components of the cytoskeleton by reovirus and diminished synthesis of growth hormone by involvement of the anterior pituitary by lymphocytic choriomeningitis virus in mice.

Although the foregoing events ensure replication of virus at the expense of synthesis of host macromolecules, they do not necessarily injure the cell. This is precisely what one would expect from a nearly perfectly adapted parasite. The means by which cell injury, or a cytopathic effect,[119] is produced by virus is not altogether understood. Although viral infections significantly inhibit synthesis of vital host macromolecules, this influence is usually short lived, and so interference with the normal turnover of macromolecules necessary for cell survival is an unlikely explanation. Two facts tend to support this finding: first, the amount of viral components synthesized is approximately 15% of total host cell material and so a critical paucity of precursor molecules for synthesis of host molecules probably does not develop; second, in some virus infections, such as vaccinia and poliomyelitis, increased synthesis of host membrane phospholipids and lipids has been observed. During the course of virus replication, inclusion bodies (intracellular accumulations of virus particles) (Fig. 1-17) may reach such proportions that they make up a large percentage of the host cell volume and could conceivably interfere with normal function of cell organelles and intracellular transport to cause cell injury. Several observations indicate that viral coat protein, especially that synthesized in the late stages of viral replication, may exert a toxic effect on host cells by increasing the permeability of lysosomal and plasma membranes through mechanisms that remain obscure. For example, it has been observed that high concentrations of vaccinia virus can rapidly injure host cells in culture. Furthermore, intravenous injections of concentrated vaccinia virus or mumps virus into mice cause death within 24 hours, without evidence of viral multiplication or at most with synthesis of incomplete viral particles, which in the case of vaccinia virus consist largely of the outer protein coat. Increased permeability of cell membranes develops, leading to cell injury and death.

In addition to a direct cytopathic effect, viruses can also cause cell injury indirectly through mediation of the host immune response by the following mechanisms: (1) coating, or insertion, of viral antigen into the plasma membrane of infected host cells such that the host now recognizes these cells as nonself, or foreign, or (2) damage of host cells by cytoxic lymphokines or monokines released by T-lymphocytes and macrophages in the inflammatory response mounted by the host to virus, the so-called bystander effect. In each instance, the immune response of the host leads to injury of its own cells, a perverse twist of a defense mechanism. Some cases in point include hepatitis B virus, which during persistent and protracted infection cause cell damage by the first mechanism, and Theiler's, Chandipura, and vesicular stomatitis viruses, which cause demyelinatin of the central nervous system me-

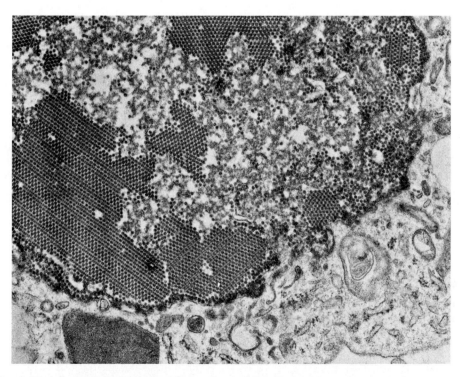

Fig. 1-17. Intranuclear inclusion of virus in a glial cell of patient with progressive multifocal leukoencephalopathy. Virions are in a tightly packed crystalline arrangement. (Courtesy of Dr. Itaru Watanabe, Kansas City, Mo.)

diated, in part, by the second mechanism, and by additional mechanism or mechanisms that remain to be elucidated.

In addition to necrosis, viruses can induce fusion of an infected cell with its neighbors, ultimately leading to the formation of multinucleated giant cells, or polykaryocytes. This can be considered a nonlethal expression of cell injury. The giant cells induced in lymphoid tissue by measles virus and in other tissues by herpesvirus and Sendai virus, a parainfluenza virus that causes respiratory disease in humans, are cases in point.

Experimental evidence indicates that polykaryocytosis and cell proliferation are phenomena mediated in large part by basic alterations in the structure and function of the plasma membrane, an organelle that appears to be significantly involved in both lethal and nonlethal effects of virus on host cells. Augmented cell replication is another nonlethal effect of certain viruses; the pocks induced by variola (smallpox) and vaccinia (cowpox) viruses growing on the chorioallantoic membranes of chick embryos in the laboratory and on the skin of human hosts are the result of numerous focal nodular aggregations of proliferated cells. Cell proliferation is a salient feature of certain groups of DNA and RNA viruses that cause neoplasms in animals and humans and that are appropriately classified as oncogenic, or tumor, viruses.

Cellular reactions to sustained sublethal injury

As pointed out previously, a fundamental property of cells is their capacity to adapt to an adverse environment, especially when the environmental alterations develop slowly and are not of sufficient intensity to be lethal, at least at their onset. Such adaptations are mediated through feedback control mechanisms that initiate and modulate structural and functional alterations to allow cell survival under adverse conditions. Cellular adaptations are a common and integral part of many disease states. In some instances it is difficult to ascertain what is a pathologic response and what represents an extreme adaptation to an excessive functional demand. It should be recalled that in the early stages of a successful adaptive response cells may be capable of enhanced function.

Cellular accumulations

When injury is sublethal and sustained, cells and tissues tend to accumulate substances in abnormal quantities, a phenomenon referred to as "infiltration" in the older literature. Most commonly such accumulations consist of molecules that are normally present, such as triglycerides, glycogen, calcium, uric acid, melanin, and bilirubin. In the preceding section on acute cell injury, a few examples of these were described. More uncommonly the accumulated substances are abnormal,

as in amyloidosis, or more rarely in diseases attributable to defective genes in which abnormal metabolites accumulate because of faulty synthetic or degradative pathways, to be discussed in a later section of this chapter. In addition, exogenous materials such as mineral dusts, pigments, and certain heavy metals may accumulate in the cytoplasm of cells after their introduction into the body by inhalation, ingestion, or injection.

The basic processes of ingestion, digestion, and storage of materials by cells discussed in some detail earlier[34,35] involves their complex interactions of cell membranes and their fusion with lysosomes. Ingestion involves the inward flow of plasma membrane, which eventually encloses either fluid (pinocytosis) or particulate material (heterophagocytosis) that is internalized in the cytoplasm though still enclosed in a membrane-limited vacuole. As the vacuole (phagosome) moves inward, its membrane fuses with that of a preexisting lysosome whereupon hydrolytic enzymes are released into the phagosome, interacting with and digesting the enclosed material (Fig. 1-18). Because of the rapidity of pinocytosis, phagocytosis, phagosome movement, and fusion with lysosomes, certain types of cells may ingest and digest prodigious amounts of material. When the material is ingested in amounts so large that they exceed the capacity of lysosomes to digest them, or if the material is degraded slowly or not at all, it tends to accumulate in the cytoplasm, a condition referred to as "lysosomal overloading."

Lysosomal overloading may occur rapidly if not all the ingested material is subject to attack by digestive enzymes or more slowly, sometimes a matter of years, if only a small proportion of ingested material is undigested. Digestion of biologic material leads to the formation of soluble substances such as small peptides, amino acids, and sugars, which are reutilized by the cell. Accumulation of material may cause the organs involved to become enlarged and firm; in the case of pigments the tissues may be strikingly colored. When the storage of material is excessive, cells may be mechanically compromised and their functions may be impaired to the point that cell death occurs. Lysosomal overloading can also result from material originating within the cell (Fig. 1-19), for example, the indigestible material resulting from focal cytoplasmic degradation, a process referred to as autophagy ("self-eating"). Autophagy is probably a normal cellular event responsible for the turnover of cell organelles and membranes, a sober reminder that "living" is dying.

Glycogen, complex lipids, and carbohydrates

Pathologic accumulations of glycogen occur in the tissues of patients with diabetes mellitus in whom the normal cellular uptake of glucose is impaired. Excessive storage of glycogen is also found in genetic diseases in which there is absence of one or another of the en-

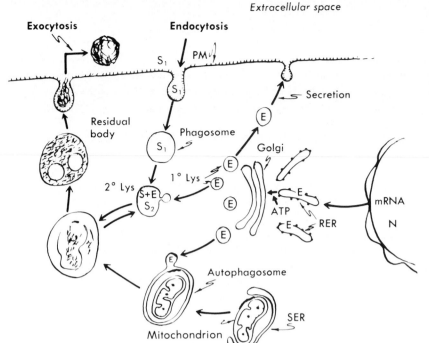

Fig. 1-18. Diagram of the lysosome system. Notice the interrelationships of endocytosis, phagosomes, primary lysosomes, secretion granules, autophagosomes, and residual bodies. *E*, Acid hydrolase; *Lys,* lysosome; *mRNA,* messenger RNA; *N,* nucleus; *PM,* plasma membrane; *RER,* rough endoplasmic reticulum; *S₁,* substrate; *S₂,* partially digested substrate; *SER,* smooth endoplasmic reticulum. (From Scarpelli, D., and Trump, B.F.: Cell injury, Bethesda, Md., 1974, Universities Associated for Research and Education in Pathology, Inc.)

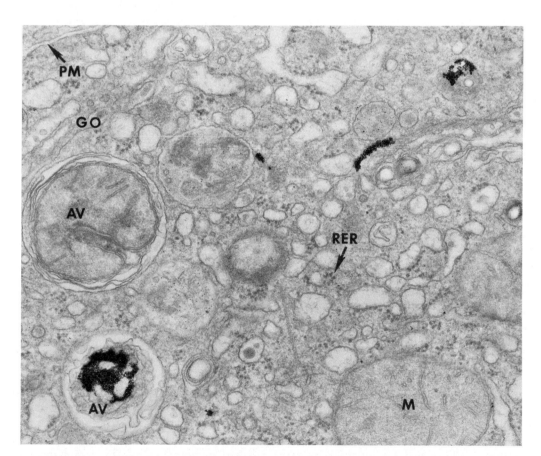

Fig. 1-19. Autophagy induced experimentally in rat liver by administration of catabolic hormone glucagon. Dense deposits represent sites of acid phosphatase activity in membranes of the Golgi apparatus at upper right. Mitochondrion is enclosed in a newly formed autophagic vacuole at middle left. Beneath it a second autophagic vacuole containing membrane arrays and exhibiting acid phosphatase activity may be seen. *AV,* Autophagic vacuoles; *GO,* Golgi apparatus; *M,* mitochondrion; *PM,* plasma membrane; *RER,* rough-surfaced endoplasmic reticulum. (From Scarpelli, D., and Trump, B.F.: Cell injury, Bethesda, Md., 1974, Universities Associated for Research and Education in Pathology, Inc.)

zymes that constitute the Embden-Meyerhof glycolytic pathway, or when an abnormally structured glycogen that cannot be degraded by glycolytic enzymes is synthesized. Intracellular accumulations of glycogen impart a vacuolated appearance to the cytoplasm. Since accumulations of glycogen morphologically resemble those of water (hydropic swelling) and fat (triglyceride under the light microscope), one of the following tests is necessary to establish that the deposit is glycogen: (1) application of the periodic acid–Schiff test in which glycogen is stained a reddish purple (tissues previously digested with diastase serve as negative controls) or (2) quantitative analysis of the glycogen content of affected tissues. Massive intracellular deposits of glycogen occurring in glycogen storage disease cause affected organs such as the liver, kidney, or heart to be greatly enlarged and their function to be ultimately compromised.

In diabetes mellitus, glycogen deposits are encountered in epithelium of the distal segment of the proximal convoluted renal tubules and the descending loop of Henle, hepatocytes, beta cells of pancreatic islets, and cardiac muscle. Accumulation in the kidney occurs when the degree of glycosuria leads to levels of glucose in the glomerular filtrate that exceed the rate at which glucose is reabsorbed by epithelial cells of the renal tubules (tubular mass).

Excessive intracellular deposits of glycogen lipids, glycolipids, mucolipids, and mucopolysaccharides develop in patients with genetic disorders characterized by lysosomes with specific enzyme deficiencies that render them incapable of hydrolyzing them. Abnormal metabolites accumulate in neurons of the central nervous system, as well as parenchymal cells of the liver, kidney, and heart, and cells of the reticuloendothelial system such that massive enlargement of the spleen and to a lesser degree the lymph nodes and liver occurs. As in the other storage diseases attributable to gene defects, involvement may become so severe that it is incompatible with life. These and similar diseases are considered in greater detail in a subsequent section dealing with inborn errors of metabolism.

Pigments

Pigments are colored substances present in the majority of living forms, including humans, and are widely distributed in our environment both as pollutants and as artifacts of cultural practices such as smoking tobacco and tattooing the skin. Pigments are generally classified into two broad categories: (1) endogenous pigments, which are normal constituents of cells and tissues, for example, tyrosine- and tryptophan-derived pigments, such as melanin, argentaffin substances, and adrenochromes; hemoproteins, which include porphyrins, hemoglobin, and hemosiderin (ferritin); and lipid-rich pigments such as lipofuscin and ceroid; and (2) exogenous pigments introduced into the body from without, such as anthracotic pigments, mineral dusts containing silica and oxides of iron, ingested iron, lead, and silver salts, and the various pigments that are used in tattoos of the skin.

Melanin. Melanin is a brown-black pigment synthesized by melanocytes from tyrosine. In humans, as in lower animals (the ink of cuttlefish and the cutaneous pigment cells of some animals), melanin serves a protective function. The skin of individuals adapted to long exposure to sunlight contains much more melanin than does the skin of those living in northern latitudes where such exposure is much less. This is believed to be an important factor in the widely differing incidences of skin cancer in these two population groups; skin cancer, which is virtually unknown among blacks, is a very common neoplasm in fair-skinned whites. Measurements of sheets of stratum corneum for their effectiveness in screening out ultraviolet light have shown that such material derived from blacks is much more effective than that from less-pigmented people.[156] Ultraviolet radiation, which stimulates the synthesis of melanin, is also highly absorbed by the pigment as part of the protective mechanism. In addition, since melanin's properties indicate that it is a stable free radical and that its free-radical content increases after exposure to ultraviolet radiation, it may protect by capturing injurious free radicals formed by the action of ultraviolet rays on skin.[30,104]

Melanin is formed by the oxidation of tyrosine to dihydroxyphenylalanine (dopa), a reaction catalyzed by tyrosinase, a copper-containing enzyme. Dopa is further oxidized to indole-5,6-quinone (dopachrome), which in turn is converted by oxidation-reduction to 5,6-dihydroxyindole, which is polymerized to a highly insoluble substance.

A generalized increase in skin melanin commonly occurs with continued exposure to sunlight; more rarely it is seen in persons with Addison's disease, an adrenocortical insufficiency resulting from destruction of the adrenal cortex. The mechanism by which melanogenesis is stimulated in such cases is an interesting facet of comparative endocrinology. In the lower animals, melanin formation is under control of a polypeptide hormone called melanin-stimulating hormone (MSH), which is localized in the pars intermedia of the pituitary. Its existence has not been unequivocally established in humans, in whom melanogenesis appears to be stimulated by adrenocorticotropic hormone (ACTH). The loss of adrenocortical hormones in Addison's disease leads to a loss of feedback control of ACTH secretion and so it continues to be secreted at high levels. The melanin-stimulating properties of ACTH are no doubt related to the fact that a segment of the molecule bears a strong chemical homology to MSH through an identical amino acid sequence.

Increased melanogenesis is also seen in patients with proliferative lesions of melanocytes. The benign form includes the commonly occurring "pigmented moles" (nevi). The malignant equivalent, malignant melanoma, is a highly malignant neoplasm that invades normal tissues early and widely and that almost invariably terminates in death. Such tumors are highly pigmented because of the synthesis of excessive amounts of melanin, which may accumulate in serum and urine, making them gray to black. An interesting although less common variant is the so-called amelanotic melanoma, in which the neoplastic melanocytes have lost their capacity to produce melanin pigment because of the deletion of one or more of the enzymes necessary for its synthesis.

Albinism is an inherited disorder of melanin metabolism in which there is a decrease or absence of the pigment in the skin and choroid of the eye. It occurs in both lower animals and mammals, including humans. Careful histologic and ultrastructural studies of the skin of albinos have definitely established that, although melanocytes are present and show an essentially normal structure and complement of cell organelles, including premelanosomes, the latter are devoid of melanin. The condition may be diffuse, involving all the skin, the eyes, and the hair, or it may be localized to a certain site or sites (piebalding). Such curious distributions are attributable to the fact that the genetic defect is limited to only a specific group or groups of precursor melanocytes that migrate during embryonic development from the neural crest to peripheral sites where albinism is localized. Patients with oculocutaneous albinism have poor vision and severe photophobia. The hair is blond, often with a slight reddish cast, and the skin is exquisitely sensitive to sunlight, becoming rapidly erythematous on exposure. Chronic exposure invariably leads to the development of precancerous lesions of the skin that ultimately evolve into squamous and basal cell cancers.

A melanin-like pigment is produced in large amounts in alkaptonuria, a rare metabolic disorder involving abnormal metabolism of homogentisic acid, an intermediate product formed in the metabolism of phenylalanine and tyrosine. The metabolic block is caused by the lack of homogentisic acid oxidase, an enzyme that converts homogentisic acid to methylacetoacetic acid. The black pigment, a polymer derived from homogentisic acid, accumulates in the skin and connective tissues, especially cartilage of the nose, ears, ribs, joints, and the tendons of the hands; such pigmentation is referred to as ochronosis. The pigment also appears in perspiration and is excreted in the urine.

Pigments derived from hemoproteins. Hemoproteins constitute some of the most important normal endogenous pigments because they include hemoglobin, the cytochromes, and a variety of enzymes. Central to an understanding of disorders involving these pigments is a knowledge of the uptake, metabolism, excretion, and storage of iron. A normal adult male requires approximately 1 mg of iron per day to balance the average net loss each day through bile, sweat, minute episodic blood loss in the gut, and cell turnover in the gastrointestinal tract and skin. During periods of rapid body growth (infancy and puberty), menstrual years of women, and the last two trimesters of pregnancy, daily iron requirements are increased. Iron in food, which is in the ferric state, is reduced to the ferrous form by reducing substances present in food and is absorbed across the duodenal and jejunal mucosa. The sites of absorption merit mention because of their important function of closely regulating the uptake of iron into the body. Clinical and experimental studies indicate that some of the iron entering the mucosal cell may be complexed to transferrin, a β-globulin, which is the major iron transport protein and transferred directly and rapidly (within 8 hours after ingestion) into the plasma. The remainder of iron is oxidized back to the ferric form and unites with a β-globulin called apoferritin to form ferritin, a compound containing about 17% to 23% iron. Ferritin is then slowly absorbed into the blood, taking several days; since it is in equilibrium with ferrous iron in the cell, its slow removal tends to maintain ferrous iron at a high saturated level. Such intracellular levels of ferrous iron inhibit further uptake of iron from the lumen of the intestine and enhance the movement of ferritin from the cell into the blood. Iron absorption is also regulated by the level of plasma iron, being increased when plasma iron is low, as in individuals with sustained blood loss or anemia. A variety of dietary factors affect iron absorption; alcohol, ascorbic acid, and fructose tend to enhance absorption, whereas phytates (plant salts), phosphates, fats, and calcium impair it. Conditions such as achlorhydria (very low levels of gastric acid) and the altered gastric mucosa associated with it also tend to diminish absorption.

Tissue iron. Iron enters the plasma from tissue stores, from the intestinal mucosa, and from reticuloendothelial cells, which remove and destroy effete and damaged red cells. Plasma iron then enters the bone marrow where it is used for synthesis of hemoglobin. Iron is stored in tissues in essentially two forms: ferritin, which is not apparent with light microscopy but is visualized with electron microscopy as a tetrad aggregation of intensely electron-dense particles, and hemosiderin, which is composed of large, irregular aggregates of ferritin that are insoluble and appear as coarse, brown cytoplasmic granules. The granules can be demonstrated to contain ferric iron because they form a deep blue product, ferric ferrocyanide, on reaction of tissue with an acid solution of potassium ferrocyanide (Prussian blue reaction). The equilibrium between storage and plasma iron depends on the degree of transfer-

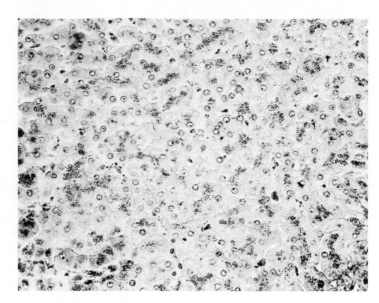

Fig. 1-20. Hemosiderosis of liver in patient with severe hemolytic anemia who required numerous blood transfusions. Notice fine granular deposits of hemosiderin in cytoplasm of hepatocytes.

rin saturation by iron. Low plasma iron levels and reduced saturation shift the equilibrium so that iron is mobilized from stores to the plasma; when the converse is true, iron moves from plasma to tissue stores.

HEMOSIDERIN AND HEMOSIDEROSIS. Local accumulations of hemosiderin (hemosiderosis) occur regularly around areas of bruising and hemorrhage and in lungs and spleen subjected to the protracted congestion that accompanies recurrent heart failure. In each instance the pigment is localized in cells of the reticuloendothelial system. In the lungs hemosiderin-laden macrophages are appropriately referred to as "heart failure cells." The pigment imparts a deep brown color to tissues and organs when it is present in high concentrations. The generalized form of this condition, also referred to as secondary hemochromatosis, is most commonly encountered in patients who have received repeated blood transfusions or more rarely after prolonged parenteral administration of iron; it can also occur in patients with chronic ineffective erythropoiesis (such as thalassemia major), presumably from increased absorption of dietary iron across the duodenal mucosa. Alcohol ingestion when carried to extremes can lead to hemosiderosis (Fig. 1-20) because of the augmentation of iron uptake by alcohol; wines, which are rich in iron, place the alcoholic in double jeopardy. In the South African Bantu there is an added interesting facet in that the alcoholic beverages are conventionally prepared in iron pots, which probably serve as an abundant source of additional dietary iron (estimated to be as high as 100 mg per day). Although iron deposition in hemosiderosis is initially limited to the reticuloendothelial system, with time the parenchymal cells of the liver, kidney,

and heart are also affected and the condition becomes clinically and pathologically indistinguishable from primary hemochromatosis.

PRIMARY HEMOCHROMATOSIS. The rare disease hemochromatosis is genetically determined by a locus on chromosome 6 with variable penetrance, the full clinical disorder having an autosomal recessive inheritance. A linkage to HLA types A3, B7, and B14 has been found in kindreds. Primary hemochromatosis is a disorder of iron metabolism that appears in middle life (80% of cases appear after 40 years of age). It is characterized clinically by the triad of pigment cirrhosis of liver, diabetes mellitus, and slate gray to bronze-colored pigmentation of the skin, which interestingly enough is caused by increased melanin deposition rather than iron. In some instances heart failure is added to the triad, attributable presumably to injury of heart muscle cells resulting from intracellular accumulation of iron. Primary hemochromatosis is more common in men; women presumably are protected by their periodic loss of blood by menstruation, and therefore the disease is usually manifest during the postmenopausal years. The average woman may lose between 10 and 35 g of iron through menstruation, pregnancy, and lactation during her lifetime. Approximately 50% of women with the disease have a history of scant or absent menses. The protective effect of menstruation on the development of this genetic disease is an excellent example of sex-determined modification of gene expression. Since normal function of the X chromosome is responsible for normal menses, its abnormal function, as would be expected, allows the autosomal dominant gene defect to be expressed.

Liver, pancreas, spleen, heart, and in fact all other tissues contain increased amounts of iron and are brown to chocolate brown in color. Affected organs are enlarged and firm. The liver is cirrhotic with numerous nodules measuring from several millimeters to 1 cm in diameter and may contain more than 50 g of iron. Granular deposits of hemosiderin are present in the cytoplasm of affected cells: in the liver, granules are present in both hepatocytes and Kupffer cells. The basic metabolic defect in this disease is still not clear; however, results of careful clinical studies indicate an increased uptake of iron by the duodenal mucosa and an absence of iron-binding protein gastroferrin, which has been found in gastric juice.[32] This protein has been implicated in the regulation of iron absorption from the gut. The latter defect may have a genetic basis and may ultimately fit into the complex pathogenetic mechanism responsible for this disease.

Iron accumulation in tissues is common in chronic alcoholics, but alcohol consumption may occasionally help to unmask a genetic predisposition to primary hemochromatosis. In general, iron accumulation in alcoholism remains confined to the reticuloendothelial system and hepatic scarring is more prominent than tissue accumulation of iron, whereas in primary hemochromatosis the reverse is true. Occasionally, however, a precise diagnosis is difficult.

Hematin. Hematin is a brown-black pigment derived from hemoglobin. Although its precise composition has not yet been determined, it is known to contain heme iron in the ferric form. The pigment is associated most commonly with a severe hemolytic crisis after transfusion of incompatible blood or chronic parasitization of red blood cells by malarial protozoa. It is usually found in the cytoplasm of reticuloendothelial cells. This pigment is not stained by the Prussian blue reaction despite the presence of ferric iron; this anomaly is believed to be attributable to the presence of an as yet unknown material, perhaps a protein that has formed a complex with the iron so that it is unable to react.

Bilirubin. Bilirubin is a non–iron containing yellow pigment derived from the porphyrin ring of the heme moiety of hemoglobin as a result of red cell destruction by cells of the reticuloendothelial system. Bilirubin is essentially water insoluble and is kept in solution in blood plasma by binding to albumin. Since it is formed normally as a result of the turnover of red cells, there is an efficient pathway in the body for its metabolic conversion and ultimate excretion.

Circulating bilirubin in plasma (normal levels range between 0.1 and 0.8 mg/dl) is removed from albumin at the surface of the hepatocyte and subsequently bound by two cytoplasmic proteins, ligandin and a fatty acid–binding protein. The amount of ligandin is increased by administration of phenobarbital. In the hepatocyte, bilirubin is conjugated to glucuronic acid to form the water-soluble diglucuronide. This reaction is catalyzed by glucuronyl transferase, an enzyme that is localized in the smooth endoplasmic reticulum and is one of a group of enzymes capable of modifying foreign toxic compounds by conjugation. All these enzymes, interestingly enough, are also induced by phenobarbital. Thus the liver handles bilirubin as a potentially toxic compound. In this regard, it is significant to note that phenobarbital is used to treat patients with low levels of glucuronyl transferase attributable to a defective gene (Gilbert's disease and the Crigler-Najjar type of congenital jaundice). If, however, the defect is so severe that the enzyme is totally absent, such treatment is fruitless. Conjugated bilirubin is excreted through the biliary tract into the intestine as bile, a micellar complex of cholesterol, phospholipid, bilirubin diglucuronide, and bile salts. In the small intestine, bilirubin is changed to urobilinogen, a small amount of which is reabsorbed into the portal circulation. Most of it is excreted by the kidneys or is reduced to stercobilin in the large bowel and excreted as a brown pigment in the feces.

Jaundice is a condition in which the level of bilirubin in plasma is greater than 2 mg/dl and the skin and scleras are yellow. Clinically, jaundice is classified into three major types: hemolytic, obstructive, and hepatocellular.

Hemolytic jaundice results from an excessive breakdown of the red blood cell membrane in a variety of conditions, which include a genetic membrane defect, an immune reaction, a severe infection, circulating intravascular toxic substances causing red cell destruction (snake venoms), or transfusion of incompatible blood. Because of the amount and rapid rate of formation of bilirubin in hemolytic crises, the liver's capacity to conjugate it is exceeded, and the level of unconjugated bilirubin rises in the plasma. However, since the liver's capacity is much greater than is normally required, even massive red cell destruction does not lead to bilirubin levels in plasma higher than 5 mg/dl. Since unconjugated bilirubin is not water soluble, its concentration in plasma cannot be measured by chemical means until alcohol is added; alcohol, a lipid solvent that allows the bilirubin to react with diazotized sulfanilic acid to form the red compound azobilirubin, which is then measured. This is the indirect van den Bergh test, which should be distinguished from the direct van den Bergh test in which water-soluble conjugate reacts directly with the reagent. As one would expect, in patients with hemolytic jaundice the level of unconjugated bilirubin is elevated and bilirubinuria is not present.

Obstructive jaundice results from an obstruction of the passage of conjugated bilirubin from hepatocytes to the intestine. Clinically, this is broadly classified on the basis of the location of obstruction as (1) extrahepatic caused by obstruction of the common bile duct by gallstones, carcinomas of the pancreas and the common duct, and extrinsic masses, or (2) intrahepatic because of obstruction of normal bile flow through the bile canaliculi, most commonly caused by adverse reactions to drugs such as chlorpromazine and other phenothiazine derivatives, estrogenic hormones, and the anesthetic halothane. Ultrastructural studies have demonstrated dilatation of bile canaliculi with a sharp diminution of microvilli on the secretory surface. In obstructive jaundice, bilirubin in the plasma is predominantly the conjugated diglucuronide and results in a direct van den Bergh reaction.

Hepatocellular jaundice results from failure both of hepatocytes to conjugate bilirubin and of bilirubin to pass through the liver into the intestine. Failure to conjugate may involve a primary defect in the hepatocyte because of the absence or very low levels of glucuronyl transferase, the enzyme responsible for catalyzing the reaction of uridinediphosphoglucuronic acid with bilirubin to form the diglucuronide. Jaundice in a newborn infant, after postnatal physiologic hemolysis of red blood cells, is attributable to functional immaturity of the infant, who has had little or no need for conjugation of foreign compounds during its intrauterine existence. Enzyme levels rise a few days after birth, and the jaundice begins to subside. In severe cases of jaundice, as in prematurity, Rh incompatibility, or infection, very high levels of bilirubin can exert a toxic effect on neurons in the basal ganglia (kernicterus). This occurs because the blood-brain barrier in newborn infants, unlike that in adults, is permeable to bilirubin. Such injury can lead to mental retardation, motor dysfunction, and muscle atrophy. Low to absent levels of glucuronyl transferase resulting from a gene defect are a much rarer occurrence. The obstructive element in hepatocellular jaundice is characterized by intrahepatic cholestasis with fine structural alterations of bile canaliculi and ductules described earlier. The dual features of impaired cell function and obstruction are reflected in the fact that high levels of both indirect- and direct-reacting bilirubin are present in the plasma.

The organs of patients with jaundice are deeply stained, being yellow early and becoming dark green in more protracted cases. Bilirubin is present in cells as dark mahogany brown to green droplets; in liver, bile fills the sinusoids, canaliculi, and ductules.

Because of its lipid solubility and structure, bilirubin has the potential for inducing cell injury, a fact that has been documented clinically especially in the case of kernicterus. However, the precise mechanism or mechanisms by which cytotoxicity occurs have not been elucidated. In the body, albumin has a significant protective effect by binding free bilirubin, a fact amply supported by experimental studies in which it was shown that albumin-bound bilirubin is nontoxic to tissue-culture cells and that albumin is capable of extracting significant amounts of cell-bound bilirubin from such cells.[26] Free bilirubin exerts two effects—uncoupling of oxidative phosphorylation and a loss of cell pro-

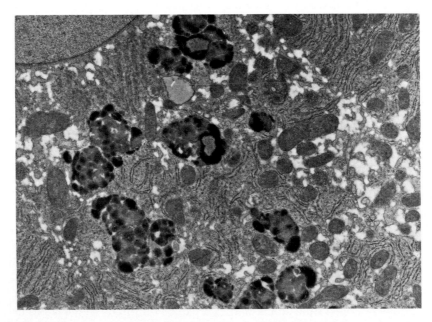

Fig. 1-21. Lipofuscin granules in liver biopsy specimens from patient with a history of drug abuse and acute hepatitis. Lipofuscin granules are the result of protracted autophagy and are synonymous with residual bodies. (Courtesy Dr. Itaru Watanabe, Kansas City, Mo.)

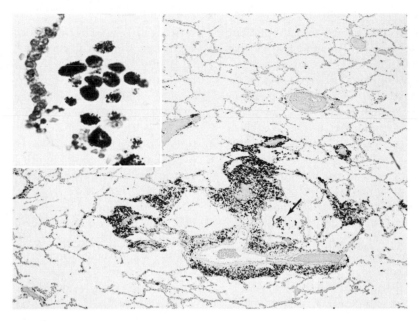

Fig. 1-22. Anthracosis of lung in a patient who had been a city dweller all his life. Particles of inhaled carbon are phagocytized by macrophages in perivascular connective tissue and desquamated pneumocytes *(arrow). Inset,* These are shown at higher magnification; carbon particles fill the entire cytoplasm and obscure nuclear detail.

teins—suggestive of a primary effect on the inner membrane of mitochondria and other cell membranes, including the plasma membrane. Clearly, that one does not encounter overt evidence of significant cell injury in most cases of jaundice is probably the result of the protective effects of serum albumin and conjugation.

Lipofuscin. Lipofuscin is an insoluble lipid pigment present in cells of elderly persons and those with malnutrition or a chronic wasting disease. It is a brown intracellular pigment found in hepatocytes, cardiocytes, and neurons (Fig. 1-21). It represents the accumulation of indigestible membrane material in lysosomes after autophagy. Ingested material may accumulate when the rate of autophagy exceeds the capacity for digestion or when it has been chemically altered, as by lipid peroxidation, which would render it resistant to enzymatic degradation. Organs containing large amounts of lipofuscin are deep brown; in the heart this is referred to as brown atrophy. This condition appears to correlate directly with age[151]; however, since such pigment can also accumulate rapidly with extensive tissue wasting, it seems prudent not to attribute its presence strictly to aging.

Mineral dusts. The presence of considerable amounts of inhaled pigmented particulate materials in the lungs of the majority of persons, especially those in urban centers, attests to the state of the environment. The most common condition, anthracosis, is seen in the lungs of almost every adult and is most noticeable in smokers. Black pigment is localized subpleurally in irregular patches, in the hilar lymph nodes, and around bronchi and intrapulmonic vasculature. Microscopically, the pigment consists of coal-like dust in lymph nodes and alveolar macrophages and around capillaries and larger vessels (Fig. 1-22). Such material is apparently bland, since it does not appear to incite either inflammation or scarring. However, it may be accompanied by toxic substances, including polycyclic hydrocarbons, which are cytoxic and account for the deleterious effects of cigarette smoking.

Pneumoconiosis of coal workers is a serious condition encountered in anthracite coal miners. It develops over a period of years and leads to excessive deposition of black pigment in the lung. The impairment of respiratory function after the development of emphysema indicates that the dusts causing pneumoconiosis may not be identical to the common dusts responsible for anthracosis. This is a major health problem today, and much effort is being directed to elucidating the cause and understanding the pathogenetic mechanism or mechanisms responsible for this disease (see p. 1000).

Silica. Silicosis, also encountered in coal miners, is caused by fine (10 μm or smaller) silica dust particles, which after inhalation are phagocytized and carried through lymphatics to lymphoid tissues in the lung and hilar lymph nodes. Fibrosis develops in areas of tissue injury and inflammation wherever the silica particles reside. The fibrosis is quite extensive, leading to crippling pulmonary insufficiency and right-sided heart failure. The persistence of fibrosis even when the patient has left the dust-laden environment responsible for this disease indicates that the silica already present perpetuates the development of fibrosis. The current popular theory concerning pathogenesis involves the ingestion of silica by macrophages, which lead to their cytolysis and release of a fibroblast-stimulating factor. The silica is reingested by macrophages and the cycle is repeated again and again. The sustained stimulation of fibroblasts leads to augmented synthesis and deposition of collagen, and the formation of dense silicotic nodules and diffuse scarring. A second hypothesis holds that an immunologic mechanism based on abnormal and increased serum immunoglobulins capable of reacting with nuclear antigens may be responsible.

Heavy metals. Long-term use of silver and gold salts for therapeutic purposes leads to their deposition in the basement membranes of skin and other tissues, causing pigmentation. At one time when silver nitrate was widely used as a disinfectant, argyria, a slate gray pigmentation of skin, was not uncommon.

Long-standing exposure to lead, usually through ingestion, gives rise to a line of black pigment on teeth at the gum line, presumably because of the formation of lead sulfide attributable to the presence of hydrogen sulfide–forming bacteria.

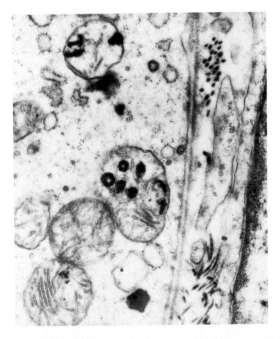

Fig. 1-23. Accumulation of calcium salt (hydroxyapatite) in mitochondria of an epithelial cell of proximal convoluted tubule in kidney of rat in which hypercalcemia was induced by high doses of vitamin D. Dense circular structures represent deposits of calcium phosphate. *Left,* Linear deposits are aligned along a crista. (From Scarpelli, D., and Trump, B.F.: Cell injury, Bethesda, Md., 1974, Universities Associated for Research and Education in Pathology, Inc.)

Calcium

Abnormal deposits of calcium in injured and dead tissue are a common finding in human pathologic conditions (Fig. 1-23). Earlier, we dealt with one important mechanism for the accumulation of calcium in injured tissues: rapid influx across damaged plasma membranes and calcium uptake by injured mitochondria. Another mechanism explaining the predilection of calcium salts to localize on the walls of alveoli in lungs, basilar cytoplasm, and basement membrane of renal tubules and gastric epithelium is the secretion of acid at each of these sites, leading to local increases in hydroxyl ions, which subsequently result in precipitation of calcium ions that form calcium hydroxide ($Ca[OH]_2$) and the mixed salt hydroxyapatite ($3\ Ca_3[PO_4]_2 \cdot Ca[OH]_2$).

Pathologic calcification is classified into two types: dystrophic and metastatic. "Dystrophic" denotes the calcification of severely injured and dead tissues. It is frequently localized in necrotic tissues. The mechanism for calcification in such instances is unclear, but it is suggested that denatured proteins preferentially bind phosphate ions, which in turn react with calcium ions to form a precipitate of calcium phosphate. "Metastatic calcification" is a term used for a condition in which mineral deposits appear in undamaged normal tissues, most commonly because of persistent hypercalcemia such as that encountered in hyperparathyroidism, hypervitaminosis D, or the rapid and extensive demineralization of bone that results from the spread of cancer to bone (Fig. 1-24). Experimental studies of hypervitaminosis D in rats indicate that excessive levels of calcium accumulate in kidney only after the oxidative phosphorylative capacity of kidney mitochondria is impaired and furthermore that pathologic calcification can be accelerated by the administration of 2,4-dinitrophenol, a potent uncoupler of phosphorylation. These findings indicate that even in so-called metastatic calcification, cell injury may precede the morphologic appearance of calcium.[131]

Urate

In mammals the purine moieties of nucleic acids and nucleotides are catabolized and appear in urine as uric acid or allantoin. In humans and other primates, uric acid is the major end product of purine catabolism because of the absence of urate oxidase (uricase). Other mammals have urate oxidase in the liver and excrete allantoin as the end product. Dalmatian dogs, though possessing urate oxidase, excrete uric acid because of a defect in the renal tubular reabsorption of uric acid.

In humans, uric acid is present as the monosodium salt in plasma at pH 7.4. The solubility of monosodium urate in body fluid is approximately 6.4 mg/dl. The serum urate concentration is in general quite stable, the average being approximately 5 mg/dl in postpubertal males and 4.1 mg/dl in postpubertal females. Al-

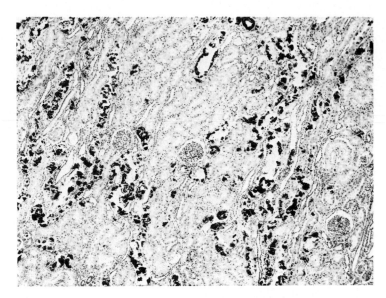

Fig. 1-24. Calcification in kidney of a patient with breast cancer that has metastasized widely to the bony skeleton. Hypercalcemia resulting from lytic bone lesions led to numerous deposits of calcium salts in epithelial cells of renal tubules.

though the intake of foods rich in nucleoprotein, such as liver, thymus, pancreas, and certain fish, tends to increase the serum urate concentration whereas the restriction of such foods tends to reduce it, the influence of exogenous purine on the serum urate concentration is considered minor. There is a complex interrelated balance among the production of purine nucleotides, catabolism of purine-containing compounds to produce free purine, oxidation of purine to uric acid by xanthine oxidase, tubular reabsorption of urate, and finally tubular secretion of urate. Disturbances of this balance can result in hyperuricemia and deposition of sodium urate crystals in the tissues, leading to painful acute arthritis, chronic gouty arthritis, tophus formation, and nephritis.[91] Hyperuricemia is the cardinal biochemical feature of the group of clinical disorders collectively referred to as gout. Ninety-five percent of the cases occur in males.

In primary gout, hyperuricemia is attributable to gene defects leading to repeated overproduction of uric acid through increased purine biosynthesis[89] or undersecretion of uric acid by the proximal renal tubules,[125] or in some cases both. Some of these are associated with specific genetic metabolic diseases, such as type I glycogen storage disease and the Lesch-Nyhan syndrome.[99]

In secondary gout, hyperuricemia occurs as a complication of other diseases, of the administration of certain drugs, and in some instances of both. In leukemia and lymphoma, particularly after their treatment with cytotoxic antineoplastic agents, accelerated catabolism of nucleic acids after cell death results in overproduction of uric acid. Hyperuricemia is a common feature of eclampsia. Although hyperuricemia in this condition is

attributable to the frequent occurrence of tissue injury and necrosis, there are probably other mechanisms involved, especially the secretion of uric acid by the kidney. Indeed, uric acid secretion is often impaired in diseased kidneys regardless of cause. The mechanism of uric acid secretion by renal tubules is a sensitive one. It is impaired by a variety of disease states and therapeutic agents, such as the accumulation of the keto acids acetoacetate and β-hydroxybutyrate in diabetic ketoacidosis and starvation[53]; the lactic acidemia that accompanies excessive ethanol ingestion[101]; and the thiazide diuretics used in the treatment of edema in cardiac and renal failure. In some cases of secondary gout, particularly those induced by the use of diuretics, there may be a preexisting genetically determined disposition toward hyperuricemia.

Persistent hyperuricemia results in the deposition of urate in tissues, cell injury, and an inflammatory reaction. Microcrystals of monosodium urate are phagocytized by leukocytes and eventually enter lysosomes. This is followed by increased permeability of the lysosomal membrane, which leads to leakage of hydrolytic enzymes.[137,164] Since urate crystals are not degradable by lysosomal enzymes, they remain in the face of the digestion of dead cells and cellular debris. Labilization of lysosomes may play an important pathogenetic role in chronic gout, particularly in the severe damage that occurs in the joint space and articular surfaces of joints. The crystals of monosodium urate initiate an inflammatory reaction by virtue of their physical presence in the interstitial fluid and tissues. Urate crystals activate Hageman factor,[88] which in turn leads to activation of the kallikreinogen-kininogen system and ultimately increased capillary permeability. Urate crystals cause the

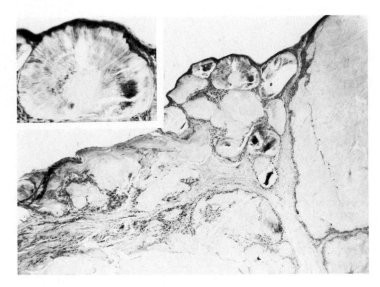

Fig. 1-25. Deposits of urate crystals in connective tissue of skin in patient with gout. Large nodular deposits are surrounded by thin strands of connective tissue with inflammatory foci. *Inset,* Higher magnification of a deposit shows radial arrays of urate crystals.

emigration of inflammatory cells to crystalline deposits in tissues and tissue spaces by activating the complement system. The combination of these events precipitates the clinically well-known severe inflammatory reaction seen in acute bouts of gout. These are characterized by the development of hot, swollen, and very painful joints, especially those of the great toe. The most effective drug for treatment of an acute attack of gout is the plant alkaloid colchicine, which is a potent stabilizer of the lysosomal membrane and, furthermore, inhibits leukocyte motility and function by interfering with microtubules in the cytoplasm.

Continued deposition of urate results in the formation of characteristic tophi; these are firm, nodular, subcutaneous deposits of urate crystals surrounded by foreign body giant cells and fibrosis (Fig. 1-25). When such deposits are preserved by fixation of tissue in absolute alcohol, urate crystals can be demonstrated as brilliantly double refractile crystals by polarized light (birefringence). They can also be demonstrated by a silver-containing stain as brown-black crystals. Urate deposition tends to occur in relatively avascular tissues, such as cartilage, epiphyseal bone, and periarticular structures. In chronic gouty arthritis, both cartilage and subchondral bone are destroyed. Proliferation of fibrous tissue and marginal bone tissue leads finally to crippling immobilization of the joint. Urate deposits also occur in the kidney, leading to severe renal damage. Crystals of monosodium urate monohydrate are needle shaped and are arranged radially in small, sheaflike clusters. Calcific material may be deposited in the matrix, rendering such deposits radiopaque. The tissues in which urate deposits commonly occur are those rich in mucopolysaccharides. Some authorities have suggested that the

release of lysosomal enzymes from leukocytes may alter protein-mucopolysaccharide conjugates in connective tissues so that urates are preferentially deposited in this matrix.

Amyloid

Amyloidosis is associated with advanced aging and with a variety of chronic diseases, especially those accompanied by chronic infection and inflammation, disturbances of immune and autoimmune reactions, excessive tissue breakdown and wasting, and certain neoplasms.[114] These include chronic tuberculosis, osteomyelitis, lupus erythematosus, rheumatoid arthritis, Hodgkin's disease, multiple myeloma, and medullary carcinoma of the thyroid. More rarely amyloidosis is encountered as a primary disease that in some cases appears to have a genetic background and is familial. The most common form of this disease is the secondary type, which is systemic with involvement of multiple organs including the kidney, liver, spleen, adrenals, pancreas, and lymph nodes. Occasionally more widespread involvement including the heart, gastrointestinal tract, and blood vessels is encountered. Amyloid accumulation may in some cases be limited to one organ such as the heart, tongue, brain, or, in association with diabetes mellitus, the islets of Langerhans in the pancreas.

Amyloid is an amorphous, insoluble, pink-staining material deposited between cells; involved organs are pale and enlarged and have the consistency of hard rubber. More rarely, the kidney may be smaller than normal because of atrophy resulting from vascular narrowing by intramural deposits of amyloid. In the kidney, amyloid is present as homogeneous eosinophilic depos-

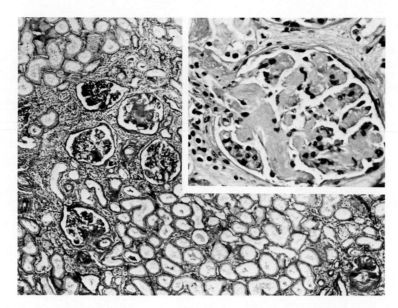

Fig. 1-26. Amyloidosis of kidney in a patient with severe long-standing infection of bone (osteomyelitis) occurring after trauma. Amyloid deposits obliterate normal structure of glomeruli. *Inset,* High magnification of glomerulus shows amyloid deposited along the course of capillaries. There is a reduction in the number of nuclei and patency of capillary lumens.

its in the mesangium of the glomerulus, the basement membrane of interstitial arteries and arterioles, and, in advanced cases, the basement membrane and peritubular tissue of renal tubules (Fig. 1-26). In the liver, deposits begin in the space of Disse between the endothelium of the sinusoids and the hepatocytes and ultimately extend to involve the entire liver lobule. Deposits in spleen are localized either to the splenic follicles where amyloid accumulates between and around individual or small groups of lymphoid cells or to the pulp where it is deposited along the basement membrane of the sinuses and between the connective tissue cells and fibers that surround them. In other organs the same general pattern of extracellular deposits pertains. As the condition worsens, the deposits enlarge to the point that entrapped cells become atrophic and ultimately die. When cell loss is excessive and the vascular supply to an organ is severely diminished, its function is compromised. Thus renal or cardiac failure is not uncommon in patients with advanced amyloidosis. Amyloid can be further identified in tissue sections by its staining reaction with the metachromatic dyes crystal violet and toluidine blue, which impart a rose-pink coloration to the deposits, and its avid binding of Congo red dye, which stains it orange and has an intense green birefringence when viewed with polarized light. Congo red has been used clinically for the diagnosis of amyloidosis in living patients by virtue of its rapid disappearance from the blood after injection, presumably because it is bound by amyloid deposits. High-resolution electron microscopy has established that the homogeneous-appearing deposits in tissues actually consist of a meshwork of nonbranching fibrils each measuring 7.5 nm in diameter; each fiber in turn appears to be composed of a pentagonal array of protofibrils that measure 2.5 to 3.5 nm in diameter and are twisted in a plaitlike fashion so that they impart periodicity to the fibril.[136] A second component contained in such deposits consists of short, ringlike structures with a pentagonal profile (P component),[10] which appears to be identical to a 9.5S α-glycoprotein normally present in serum. P component constitutes about 10% of the protein in all amyloid proteins and is periodic acid–Schiff positive. The third component, a glycosaminoglycan usually heparan sulfate, is responsible for the intense staining of these deposits by iodine.

After its initial description in 1842 by Rokitansky and subsequent studies by Virchow[160] that led to its naming a few years later, the nature of amyloid until recent years was a matter of considerable controversy. On the basis of its mahogany-brown staining reaction with an aqueous solution of iodine and violet coloration after subsequent exposure to dilute sulfuric acid (Fig. 1-27), Virchow was convinced that such deposits consist of a starchlike carbohydrate, hence its name.

The clinical association of amyloid with diseases characterized by chronic antigenic stimulation, plasma cell proliferation, and frequently the presence of abnormal immunoglobulins in the blood and urine has long indicated that the condition may be related to a protracted immune response that has gone awry.[10] Amyloid is frequently encountered in horses that have been used for

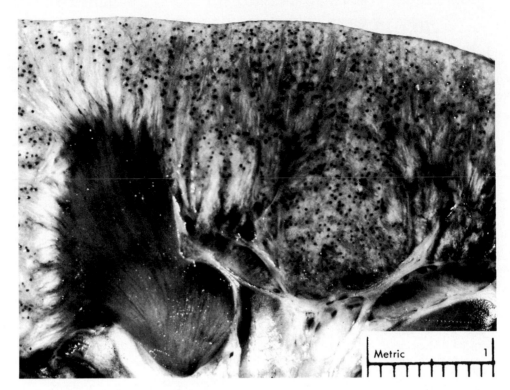

Fig. 1-27. Amyloidosis of kidney, showing glomeruli deeply stained with Lugol's solution. (Courtesy Dr. Joseph H. Davis, Miami, Fla. From Rezek, P.R., and Millard, M.: Autopsy pathology, Springfield, Ill., 1963, Charles C Thomas, Publisher.)

20 years or so for the commercial production of antitoxin by the pharmaceutical industry. Although an immune mechanism for the formation of some cases of amyloid was supported by experimental studies showing that splenectomy prevented the development of amyloid in mice after the injection of casein[120] and that it could be induced in normal syngeneic hosts by transfer of splenic cells from animals with amyloidosis,[61] it remained largely a point of speculation rather than fact. A major feature of amyloid that proved to be a hurdle to its definitive chemical characterization was its insolubility. The finding that amyloid could be readily solubilized in a 6 M solution of guanidine hydrochloride allowed a detailed analysis of its amino acid sequence. Solubilized amyloid fibrils have an amino acid sequence identical to that found in the amino terminal variable segment of the light chains of immunoglobulin, usually of the λ type.[52] The current view is that amyloid is a fibrillar protein with a β-pleated structure and a molecular weight ranging from 5000 to 18,000 daltons.[50] A feature of plasma cell myeloma that has been of assistance in furthering our knowledge of the nature of amyloid is the synthesis and secretion of immunoglobulins and their light-chain subunits (Bence Jones proteins) by this tumor. On proteolytic digestion the fraction of Bence Jones protein that contains the variable portion of the light-chain molecule forms fibrils with properties similar to those of amyloid.[50]

On the basis of detailed studies of the sequence of amino acids in solubilized amyloid "protein," it has become clear that amyloid is a heterogeneous spectrum of proteins.[51] At least the following five clearly distinct types have been identified:

1. *AL type.* Its major protein component is derived from immunoglobulin.
2. *AA type.* This type is encountered in patients with recurrent and protracted inflammatory diseases such as rheumatoid arthritis, tuberculosis, malaria, familial Mediterranean fever, and a variety of malignancies including those of the kidney, Hodgkin's disease, and multiple myeloma. Its major protein component is that of the amino terminal, two thirds of acute phase protein, and differs from that of the AL type.
3. *AE type.* The major protein is a polypeptide with an amino acid sequence identical to part of the hormone thyrocalcitonin and believed to represent calcitonin precursor protein.
4. *A type.* The major protein in this type of amyloid is prealbumin (transthyretin), a protein that migrates ahead of albumin in electrophoresis, binds vitamin and thyroid hormones, and carries them in the blood. This type of amyloid accumulates in the heart of patients in the eighth and ninth decades of life, giving rise to so-called senile amyloid heart disease.

5. *AP type.* Its protein component present in all types of amyloid is derived from a normal serum protein called serum amyloid p (SAP) substance.

Since amyloid can arise from a variety of different proteins that are converted to β-pleated fibrils, the catalog of amyloid proteins may increase as more cases of this disease complex are chemically studied. Although the pathogenesis of amyloid is far from understood, it appears that one facet involves the proteolytic alteration of protein to β-pleated fibrils.

Hypertrophy

A variety of somatic cells respond to an increased demand for work by undergoing an increase in size or hypertrophic growth; among them are the cells of the heart and kidneys, which are particularly responsive and have served as excellent experimental models for the study of this condition. Any sustained abnormality of the heart such as a malfunctioning valve or increased resistance of the peripheral arterial system will lead to its enlargement. Experimental studies indicate that initially the enlargement is caused by dilatation of the cardiac chambers but that this is relatively short lived and is followed by augmented synthesis of cardiac muscle proteins and subsequent physical enlargement of the muscle fibers, enabling them to perform more work. The synthetic events are apparently triggered by the stretch of muscle fibers induced by cardiac dilatation. When muscle fibers are stretched, the uptake of amino acids increases within a matter of minutes, mediated by an augmentation of transport enzymes localized in the plasma membrane.[98] Shortly after this, protein and lipid synthesis is increased and new cytoplasmic components of the muscle cell, such as mitochondria, sarcoplasmic reticulum, and myofibrils, are formed.[124]

In cardiac hypertrophy in humans, the nucleus is also hypertrophic, and there appears to be augmented synthesis of DNA. Thus, even though differentiated heart muscle cells are unable to undergo mitosis, they are capable of increased DNA synthesis when appropriately stimulated. Although the basis for the inability of cardiac muscle cells to progress through the cell cycle to mitosis is not known, it is postulated that this is attributable to a block that prevents them from entering G_2 (Fig. 1-28). The role if any that redundant genetic material plays in the hypertrophic response is not clear. Cardiac hypertrophy is limited by the vascular supply for the delivery of substrates required for increased synthetic metabolism. Since the interstitial capillary bed does not proliferate significantly in hypertrophy, especially when it is in response to an increased work demand imposed as a consequence of a cardiovascular pathologic condition, the hypertrophic muscle fibers eventually outstrip the capillaries' capacity to supply them adequately and their growth stops. Furthermore, since hypertrophic muscle fibers have increased oxygen consumption, a marginal vascular supply dooms them to a tenuous and often short-lived existence.

Hypertrophy of the kidney after removal of the contralateral kidney deserves mention because in this situation the adaptive response to increased demand for work involves not only an increase in the size of cells of the renal tubules but also an increase in the number of cells.[103] The proliferative phase of the response consists in a brief burst of mitosis leading to about a 7% increase in the number of epithelial cells. However, since this accounts for only 25% of the increase in kidney cell mass, it represents only a minor part of the response. The major contribution to renal enlargement is hypertrophy (Fig. 1-29). The hyperplastic phase begins within an hour or so after removal of the contralateral kidney, the initial event being an increased synthesis of RNA followed rapidly by an increase in protein synthesis that plateaus at 3 hours and is sustained at this level. Synthesis of DNA does not begin until about 9 to 10 hours after nephrectomy (Fig. 1-30). Although the factors that initiate and control compensatory renal growth are not clearly defined, the nutritional state and age of the animal appear to be important. Other examples of cell hypertrophy that bear mention are the enlargement of liver cells caused by proliferation of SER in response to exposure to foreign compounds, and the enlargement of smooth muscle cells of the urinary bladder caused by the obstruction of urinary flow.

In addition to the foregoing examples of pathologic stimuli for cell hypertrophy, there are periodically increased demands on tissues and organs that are part of

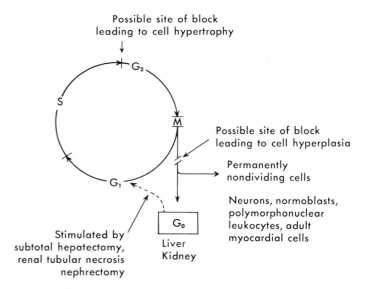

Fig. 1-28. Cell cycle showing possible sites of blocks in G_2, the "gap" or period between completion of DNA synthesis and initiation of mitosis (M). Blocks in this phase lead to hypertrophy. Blocks after mitosis prevent cells from entering G_0, which leads to hyperplasia. (From Scarpelli, D., and Trump, B.F.: Cell injury, Bethesda, Md., 1974, Universities Associated for Research and Education in Pathology, Inc.)

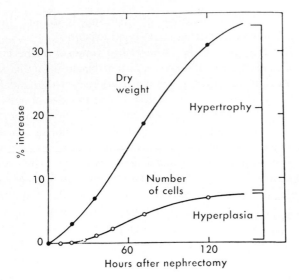

Fig. 1-29. Compensatory renal enlargement after unilateral nephrectomy is caused by hypertrophy and hyperplasia; this graph shows relative contributions of both cellular reactions. (From Johnson, H.A., and Vera-Roman, J.M.: Am. J. Pathol. **49:**1, 1966.)

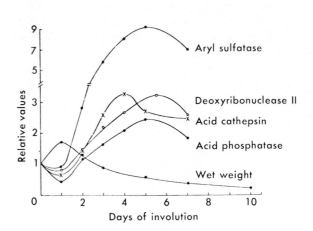

Fig. 1-31. Activity of various hydrolytic enzymes during atrophy of mammary gland after cessation of weaning. (From Woessner, F.J., Jr. In Dingle, J.T., and Fell, H.B., editors: Lysosomes in biology and medicine, vol. 1, Amsterdam, 1969, Elsevier/North-Holland Biomedical Press.)

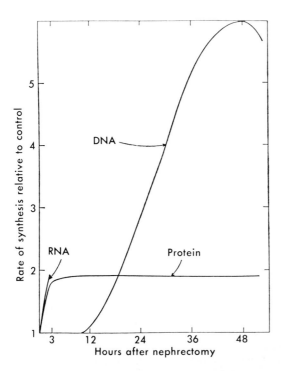

Fig. 1-30. Sequence and rate of metabolic alterations in RNA, DNA, and protein synthesis during compensatory renal enlargement after unilateral nephrectomy. (From Johnson, H.A., and Vera-Roman, J.M.: Am. J. Pathol. **49:**1, 1966.)

normal living and therefore must be considered as physiologic. A case in point is the augmented growth of the uterus and mammary glands in response to pregnancy. Numerous studies have established that the growth of these organs is triggered and maintained by hormones. In the uterus, smooth muscle cells bind estrogen, a receptor in the cytosol that transports the hormone into the nucleus where it interacts with nuclear DNA, ultimately activating specific genes responsible for the synthesis of smooth muscle proteins as well as other cytoplasmic components. The uterine muscle mass increases manyfold so that the organ is eventually transformed into a large, saclike structure with a thick muscular wall capable of the contractions necessary to expel the fetus at the time of birth. The mammary glands also grow during pregnancy as a result of high levels of estrogen, progesterone, and prolactin. These hormones stimulate both proliferative and hypertrophic growth of the terminal ends of the mammary ducts. In addition, prolactin induces the synthesis of milk proteins. The synthesis and secretion of milk continue as long as suckling is permitted; if milk is not removed, the mammary glands become greatly distended and milk production rapidly ceases.

Atrophy

In both instances just mentioned, regression of augmented physiologic growth occurs when the need for increased function is over. The degree of involution is remarkable; the term uterus with a weight of 1000 g and a wall 5 cm thick returns to its nongravid state of

100 g and a muscular wall only 0.4 cm thick in a period of 5 to 6 weeks. Changes of a similar magnitude occur in the mammary glands. Regression is characterized by macrophages that infiltrate the tissues and ingest and digest some of the augmented cell mass, an increased rate of focal self-digestion by muscle cells (autophagy),[3] and a rapid diminution of cell growth caused by an absence of the stimulating hormones as well as a decrease in the local blood supply. There is an increase in the activity of various hydrolytic enzymes in involution of the mammary gland after weaning (Fig. 1-31).[68] Secondary sex characteristics diminish as a consequence of aging or surgical ablation of the gonads. Regression of a tissue or organ because of a decrease in the size and number of cells is commonly referred to as atrophy. Atrophy also occurs in other organs such as skeletal muscle, the heart, and the central nervous system as an adaptation to a decrease in work load, use, nutrition, denervation, or blood supply. Experimental studies of muscle atrophy after denervation illustrate that a sharp lowering of oxygen consumption, amino acid uptake, and protein synthesis occurs within 15 to 24 hours. This is ultimately reflected in decreased synthesis of sarcoplasmic components such as mitochondria and myofibrillar proteins. Muscle fibers decrease in size and within several weeks are reduced to thin, ribbonlike cells. In such cells there seems to be an increased turnover of proteins. Thus denervation atrophy appears to be the net result of diminished synthesis amplified by increased breakdown of muscle protein. Since denervation of a muscle also quickly leads to a diminution of its blood supply, it is difficult to separate general effects from local cellular ones. This model is of interest to students of aging because it closely resembles the pattern of muscle atrophy in animals of advanced age.

In heart muscle and liver cells of animals that have lost considerable body weight as a result of either extended malnutrition or a debilitating chronic disease, the cytoplasm contains numerous, refractile, yellow-brown granules that are highly insoluble pigments termed "lipofuscin," or "aging pigments," the latter because they are seen with greater frequency in old individuals.[151] Ultrastructural and biochemical studies indicate that the pigment granules may represent cytoplasmic foci of self-digestion, or autophagy. Focal autophagy is a common cellular reaction to sublethal injury and is a major mechanism for decremental modulation of cell size in response to an adverse environment.[3] Autophagic vacuoles arise in the cytoplasm apparently around a focus that is to be digested; these then fuse with primary lysosomes. Such vacuoles frequently contain mitochondria and endoplasmic reticulum and presumably are responsible for their removal by virtue of a full complement of acid hydrolases. Lipofuscin pigment is believed to arise from the presence of lipid debris that has been rendered indigestible by previous oxidation as the consequence of an injurious insult. In individuals with debilitating diseases, such pigment arises in part as a result of the rapid tissue breakdown that accompanies wasting.

Hyperplasia

As mentioned previously, organ growth can also be the result of an increase in the number of cells, a process called "hyperplasia." In the context of this discussion, hyperplasia as a response to injury occurs when the injury has been sufficiently severe and prolonged to have caused cell death. The loss of cells in epithelial surfaces and in liver and kidney triggers DNA synthesis, which is followed by mitosis. The transduction of cell loss into augmented cell growth is a complex multistep process. For example, in the case of the liver, it appears to involve the production of a specific growth factor that stimulates remaining hepatocytes through a receptor-mediated series of intracellular events to synthesize new cell components and ultimately divide to produce more liver cells. Regeneration of the renal tubules after injury with mercuric chloride has shown that the proliferative response leads to an increase in the rate of DNA synthesis reflected by a shortening of the synthetic (S) phase of the cell cycle of tubular epithelial cells from the normal 12 hours to 9 hours. Increased mitoses become apparent about 20 hours after the administration of mercuric chloride and reach a peak on the third day. Proliferating epithelial cells rapidly reline the renal tubules and largely complete this stage by the fifth day. By the ninth day the mitotic index has returned to its normal preinjury level. The glomerular filtration rate drops to a low level by the fifth day and returns to normal by the ninth day. Tubular reabsorption does not return to normal levels until the twentieth day after the initial injury, indicating that considerable differentiation of the epithelial cells must occur before they are capable of effective transport.

The liver has an even greater capacity for regeneration than the kidney does and because of the greater homogeneity of its cell population has been the model of choice for studies of hyperplastic growth. Surgical removal of 75% of the liver mass leads to mitosis of hepatocytes, which peaks at about 25 to 30 hours and begins a gradual decline at 44 hours. This is followed by a second and small wave of mitosis that reaches a maximum at 56 hours and ceases at 65 hours. DNA synthesis begins 12 hours after hepatectomy and peaks at 27 hours. The mass of liver excised is totally restored by the twelfth day. In contrast to the kidney, the liver rapidly regains its normal capacity for function, indicating that newly formed hepatocytes may not have to undergo an extensive period of differentiation to carry on the numerous synthetic, catabolic, and transport functions characteristic of the liver in adults. The extent to which liver cells respond to the perturbation of hepatectomy can be emphasized if one recalls that in the normal liver in an adult less than 1% of the liver is synthesizing DNA at any one time, whereas at the peak of regeneration about 10% of the cells are in the S phase of the mitotic cycle. Epithelial cells of the kidney tubules and hepatocytes are examples of differentiated cells that are in the G_0, or resting, phase of the mitotic cycle but are capable of reentering the mitotic cycle when stimulated appropriately (Fig. 1-28).

Thus far we have limited our discussion of hyperplasia to instances of repair and regeneration. Neoplasia is a major condition in which hyperplastic growth plays a central role. Hyperplasia associated with neoplasia differs from that just described in that growth-regulatory mechanisms are lost because of a change in cellular heredity. The growth advantage of neoplastic cells operates to the disadvantage of the host because it is often accompanied by either loss or abnormality of cell function and in the case of malignant tumors leads ultimately to death.

GENETIC DISORDERS

It is axiomatic that the genetic constitution of an organism establishes the way in which that organism interacts with its environment. The more inflexible the adaptive response potential of an organism, the more restricted is the habitat the organism can occupy. Individuals within a group of organisms can be segregated by their genetic constitution, and therefore "normal" must be defined in terms of population dynamics within a group. Disease state then may be defined in terms of the inability of an individual organism to interact with its environment in a homeostatic manner common to the group. Although this process can be treated formally with both linear and nonlinear mathematics, it is perhaps more useful here to take a descriptive approach and explore what specific elements of the human genome have, by mutation, caused disequilibrium of homeostasis.

Genetically determined disease is related to cell injury to the extent that disequilibrium results from disorder within the cell. The rich and complex manner in which higher orders of existing organisms interact with their environment offer many opportunities for mistakes (mutations) in requisite biochemical processes. Frequently these mistakes have disastrous consequences to the individual. Most often, though, the genetic change that mutation (and recombination) causes is neutral to the species in which it occurs. Much of the DNA that composes our genome is not directly relevant to any of those functions that might be regarded as essential to individual survival in a changing ecosystem. In that sense reproduction provides no more than a mechanism to perpetuate base sequences of DNA in time.

However, it must be remembered that mutation as a process still remains an important source of variation in the biosphere in general. Mutation provides the variation upon which selection can act to allow organisms to grow into new niches or to allow species to survive catastrophic changes in habitat.

Although variation is crucial in the sense of geologic time, it can be devastating to the individual and can preclude reproduction. Variation is not always a threat to individuals, however. Consider antibody responses, which clearly represent a cell-based adaptive response to a threatening environment. The ability of individuals to respond to a truly impressive array of structures (both living and nonliving) that pose a danger is the result of antibody diversity. Antibody diversity is now known to primarily be the result of genetic recombination.

Diversity in proteins, both desirable and undesirable, can result from changes in primary amino acid sequence from altered base sequence in a gene. Proteins may also be altered posttranslationally in such a way that structure and hence function deviate from normal in a population. Those proteins that regulate posttranslational modification can indirectly cause an altered protein species if they themselves are changed in some way. Protein variation also occurs as a result of posttranscriptional modification of RNA before transport to the cytoplasm, a "normal" process. Introns must be removed from the RNA molecule, and the message then results from splicing RNA exons together. In several well-documented cases there are several different ways to do this within a given gene. Regulation of this process offers yet another opportunity for variability in proteins, hence another mechanism of adaptive response and another risk of accident.

The genome with all of its alterability remains basically a conservative entity and a great deal of energy seems to be expended to maintain its basic parameters. For example, specific enzymatic mechanisms exist for DNA repair. Although a great deal is known about DNA repair, the process is complex beyond current understanding. DNA repair serves to ensure that the most injurious of alterations in the genome are survivable by the individual. DNA repair attempts to force the genome back to its original state.

The processes that are essential to normal homeostasis are mediated through the action of specific proteins, glycoproteins, sterols, lipids, and other cellular macromolecules. The study of alterations in these molecules offers the opportunity to establish the relationship of genome, gene product, and biochemistry of normal homeostatic physiology.

Given some thought, one could construct a valid list

of ways in which heritable changes in genes would result in inherited diseases. Such a list might include immunologic disorders, steroidogenic disorders, sterologenic disorders, receptor-based disorders, and disorders of metabolite accumulation (such as gout, Lesch-Nyhan disease, and glycogen storage disease).

It is important also to consider maternal effects in the genetic development of offspring. Although mammals surely do not suffer the extreme sensitivity to maternal genome that is apparent in *Drosophila* (perhaps another indication of our developmental adaptability), we know that maternal effects influence the fetal environment and can adversely affect pregnancy outcome.

The seriousness of a class of disease is frequently judged on the basis of the impact that class of disease has on the human population. Impact can be a function of the numbers of people affected or the seriousness of the disease in individuals. A disease without serious long-term consequence that affects all human beings obviously has a high impact on humans. On the other hand, a disease that does not affect large numbers of humans but has devastating consequences in the individuals who suffer it is also a high-impact process. Genetic disorders have high impact in both ways. Some genetic disorders affect relatively large numbers of individuals, whereas others have very dire consequences for the few individuals who are affected.

Historical aspects

The success of a theory is frequently determined by the length of its survival. One of the longest-lived theories in biology attempted to explain why characteristics of living things could be passed from generation to generation. Hippocrates, in the fourth century BC, taught that procreative semen was derived from every part of the body. This theory, called "pangenesis," survived for over 2000 years and was even invoked by Darwin. In the nineteenth century it became the dominant theory of inherited disorders. It is, of course, absolutely wrong. The germ plasm theory of Weismann formally set the modern concept of inheritance by arguing that specialized cells are responsible for passing genetic determinants to offspring. Experimental proof of this idea came from the landmark studies of Boveri who established that specialized cells fated to become germ cells in *Ascaris* embryos are set aside early in development.

Rudolf Virchow established the concept of pathologic process as based in the physiology of the cell. Virchow observed that irrespective of the multiplicity of sizes and shapes of various cells their nuclei all looked basically the same, an observation suggesting to him that something very important must occur in this structure. Theodore Boveri, some 40 years later, began a series of experiments to show that the nucleus was a singularly important organelle and that it contained chromosomes

that were central to the function of the nucleus. In experiments with sea urchin eggs he showed that mitotic divisions occasionally resulted in unequal chromosome numbers in daughter cells but that most usually the chromosomes were segregated in equal numbers to both daughter cells. He showed that when unequal chromosome numbers occurred they would most often result in the death of the cell. Only rare cells would survive with inappropriate chromosome numbers. At the turn of the century, with the rediscovery of Mendel's principles of inheritance, the contention that chromosomes were the unit of inheritance was generally held. The isolation of DNA in purified form and the proof of its role as the chemical basis of inheritance was the result of experiments begun in the 1930s by Avery and completed in the 1940s by Avery, MacLeod, and McCarty. Their experiments proved that the DNA was the molecular species responsible for transmission of the so-called transforming principle in pneumococci.[5] These results demonstrated that the DNA was the most likely candidate for the transmission of inherited factors. Transformation of pneumococcal phenotypes was permanent and represented a heritable trait. Thus by the early 1950s it was known that chromosomes were the segregating units of inheritance and that DNA was the chemical basis of the transmission of inherited factors.

The correct chromosome number in humans was not established until 1956 by Tio and Levan[157] and independently by Charles Ford.[42] The number 46 was a matter of some debate until methods of preparation of metaphase chromosomes for high-resolution observation were established, most notably by Ford. Modern technique can distinguish 23 pairs of chromosomes with great precision.

Genetic disorders can be classified into two broad areas: cytogenetic disorders (those involving abnormalities of chromosomes) and errors in mechanisms of cellular homeostasis.

Cytogenetic disorders

The constructs established by the experiments described in the preceding section opened an era of study of cytogenetic disorders. Cytogenetic disorders can be classified into two groups: those caused by aberrant chromosome number and those caused by aberrant chromosome structure.

The number of chromosomes in an individual is established from some mitotic population within the individual, most frequently dividing blood cells. The correct chromosome number is not determined from a single cell but rather from a population of cells. The modal chromosome number in such a population study is taken to be the chromosome number of the individual. Generally, in a euploid individual (one with a nor-

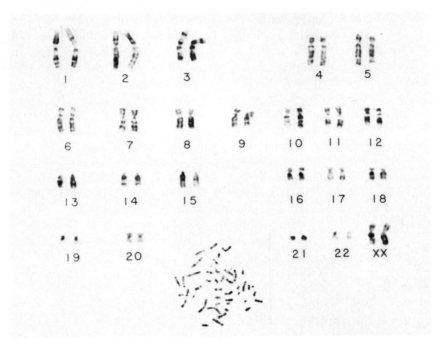

Fig. 1-32. Normal diploid female human karotype, Giemsa banded (A8097 human embryo fibroblasts). *Inset,* Metaphase cell from which the karyotype was obtained. (Courtesy Prof. W. Fahl, University of Wisconsin, McArdle Laboratory for Cancer Research, Madison, Wisc.)

mal chromosome constitution) the population of mitotic cells shows little variation with only one or two cells deviating from the mode. However, in an aneuploid individual many cells deviate from the population norm. The deviation may be in a population of like cells, all with the same inappropriate chromosome number, or the cells may have divergent chromosome numbers. In some conditions the distribution of chromosome number shows bimodality, with essentially two populations of cells with respect to chromosome number. These individuals are mosaics whose chromosome constitution defines a mixture of cells, some with the correct chromosome constitution and some with an incorrect chromosome constitution.

Precise identification of chromosome identity requires preparations that result in distinct stained bands on the chromosome (Fig. 1-32). Such procedures generally include some form of peptidase treatment of the spread metaphase chromosomes. These bands are not necessarily correlated with specific genetic features of the chromosomes. The bands are, however, consistent morphologic landmarks on each of the chromosomes, which are numbered from the longest to the shortest. In humans there are 22 chromosome pairs, plus the sex chromosome pair.

The karyotype of an individual is defined with a shorthand statement that begins with the modal number, cytologic sex, and a list of structural alterations followed by additions or deletions, indicated by "+" or "−" respectively. The short arm is designated "p" and the long arm is designated "q."

There are several limitations in the study of metaphase chromosomes. First, the size of the chromosome is at or near the limits of optical resolution of the light microscope, and so oil-immersion lens with high numerical aperture are required to adequately visualize chromosomes. Secondly, banding patterns, though reproducible, often cannot locate precise regions of chromosomes, particularly on smaller chromosomes. High-resolution banding techniques are available, but these are very tedious and demanding procedures. As a result, the loss or duplication of small parts of chromosomes may go undetected.

Numeric abnormalities of autosomes

Aneuploidy. Gain of a whole chromosome is called "primary trisomy," whereas such loss is called "monosomy." The loss of a whole chromosome or even a significant part of a chromosome is most often lethal to the cell in which it occurs. As a consequence, incorrect chromosome number (aneuploidy) in a zygote almost always results in the loss of the conceptus early in embryonic development. Several conditions do occur, however, as the result of fetal survival with abnormal chromosome number.

One in every 500 newborns has an autosomal chromosome abnormality always associated with congenital abnormalities. These individuals, though, represent a small subset of fetuses with chromosome abnormalities that are probably responsible for the loss of 10% to 20% of all conceptions during pregnancy. Aneuploidy in surviving fetuses results in gene-dosage effects only. There are no widespread effects on gene expression. The DNA in trisomic individuals is apparently unaffected at both the structural and the biochemical level. Moreover, only the genes on the duplicated chromosome show abnormal product quantity. There is no evidence for altered gene products in these individuals; thus there are no biochemical abnormalities. Even so, profound structural abnormalities exist in these individuals as a result of having the incorrect number of normal genes.[38,161]

It is generally held that a 50% increase or decrease in the amount of a given gene product is sufficient change to cause abnormal function. Where would such abnormal function manifest itself? Epstein has classified possible sites of action in order to suggest possible mechanisms of action of abnormal product quantity. Molecular abnormalities may include alterations in the concentration of rate-limiting enzymes, the concentrations of regulatory molecules, alterations in structural macromolecules, changes in the levels of cell surface recognition molecules (several of these are known to influence three-dimensional morphogenesis), or alterations in the quantity of organizing molecules important in pattern formation.

In human populations, only trisomic aneuploidies (those with one extra copy of one chromosome) have been identified in late-gestation fetuses. Fetuses trisomic for all autosomal chromosomes except 1, 5, 6, 11, 12, and 19 have been described. The trisomies are, for the most part, incompatible with postnatal life and often with intrauterine life as the result of very severe developmental defects.

Trisomy 16 is the most common trisomy seen in fetuses but has never been described in an individual surviving birth. Only trisomy 13, 18, and 21 are sufficiently compatible with life to allow postnatal survival. Several cases of trisomy 14 are now in the literature, but these are very rare. Death occurs rapidly after birth, and these individuals have severe cardiac anomalies. Of all aneuploidies, only trisomy 21 individuals can survive as nonmosaics with all their cells containing the extra chromosome 21. The trisomic conditions are invariably associated with growth retardation and mental retardation. The conditions are very frequently associated with fetal anatomic anomalies or defects (usually cardiovascular in nature). Growth retardation occurs during fetal development as well, with a resulting increase in variability of anatomic structures, frequent supernumerary structures, and frequent missing structures. The trisomic individuals express great phenotypic diversity as a group. As a result, it is difficult to correctly establish which chromosome is trisomic by phenotype alone.[38,73,85,95]

Trisomy 21. The most significant of the trisomies from the standpoint of impact in human populations is trisomy 21, or Down's syndrome. This condition represents the most common chromosome abnormality in newborns. It is the most frequent genetic cause of mental retardation and the most frequent identifiable cause of congenital heart disease.

Down's syndrome occurs with a frequency of about 1 in every 2000 live births. The frequency of the condition increases with increasing maternal age over 30 years. The effect of maternal age on the frequency of Down's syndrome is most striking over 40 years. The role of paternal age is much less clearly established though some authors contend that increasing paternal age also correlates with increasing incidence of the condition. Of course, the frequency of cytogenetic abnormalities in gametes of both parents will increase with the age of the individual, but the probability of an abnormal sperm successfully participating in fertilization is very much lower than that of an abnormal ovum.

Patients with trisomy 21 have a characteristic face (round with oblique palpebral fissures), bilateral clinodactyly (medial curvature of the fifth digit), and a simian crease. Patients are growth retarded and have cardiac anomalies and gastrointestinal tract anomalies. They are mentally retarded and suffer seizures. These patients also have immune defects and an increased susceptibility to leukemia as well as greatly enhanced probability of developing Alzheimer's disease (presenile dementia) as young adults in the third decade. Essentially nothing is known about how one extra chromosome 21 could have such profound effects.

Human gene mapping techniques have been used to establish which genes are actually on this chromosome. The known loci include superoxide dismutase, α- and β-interferon receptor, and several other biochemical markers. These have been unequivocally established to be enhanced by 50% at the product level, in accordance with the gene dosage prediction. If, however, biologic effects related to some of these loci are established, threefold to tenfold differences are found. Thus a relatively small gene-dosage change can have a much more pronounced functional effect.

Edward's syndrome. Trisomy 18, called Edward's syndrome, causes severe mental retardation, seizures, severe cardiac anomalies, and a typical facial structure including lowset ears. These individuals display specific neuromuscular phenotypes particularly in forearm development. Many of these variations turn out to be atavistic, and some of them appear briefly in normal human embryology. These alterations, which also occur to a certain extent with trisomies 13 and 21, in aggregate support the contention that aneuploidy is associated with growth retardation at various stages of embryonic development. In some cases specific neuromuscular phenotypes have proved useful for the accurate diagnosis in suspected cases. For example, flexion deformities of the wrist and digits occur in most individuals with trisomy 18.[36]

Research approaches. New animal models of trisomies and monosomies are available now to allow the study of mechanisms of action of aneuploidy in disease state. Monosomies of autosomes are uniformly fatal in early embryonic development. Conceptuses with anomalies of these sorts result when an aneuploid gamete is fertilized by, or fertilizes, a normal haploid gamete. The most frequent cause of aneuploidy in a gamete is meiotic nondisjunction. This results from the failure of homologous pairs of chromosomes to segregate during the first and second meiotic division in oogenesis or spermatogenesis. Both monosomy and trisomy can occur after fertilization as well. If the nondysjunctional event occurs after the initiation of cleavage in the embryo, mosaicism is the likely outcome. Only some of the cells of the fetus or newborn then will display aneuploidy.[38,47,60]

Numeric abnormalities of sex chromosomes

Abnormalities in the number of the sex chromosomes are recognized. An additional X chromosome produces individuals with Klinefelter's syndrome (sex chromosome constitution XXY or XXXY; occasionally higher numbers of X chromosomes occur). This condition is characterized by mental retardation in some cases. These individuals suffer testicular dysgenesis resulting in sterility.

Monosomic X individuals (Turner's syndrome) have sex chromosome constitutions of XO. Those that survive to term have streak ovaries and poorly developed secondary sexual characteristics. They have widely spaced nipples and a webbed neck and are growth retarded. These individuals are phenotypically female but do not reproduce. They have a short stature, numerous congenital malformations, and mild mental retardation. In some individuals, mosaicism ameliorates the symptoms. Two things are evident in these individuals: (1) absence of one sex chromosome does not allow normal development and (2) monosomic X individuals can be viable. These findings indicate that normal development requires some X chromosome–coded function or functions but that the organism requires only one active X chromosome for viability.

Structural abnormalities

Increasing sophistication in banding techniques is resulting in the discovery of more and more structural alterations in chromosomes of individuals. The majority of these structural aberrations are related to cancer. Morphologic (structural) alterations include translocations, inversions, and deletions; see Fig. 1-33 and the following list:

Structural alteration in chromosomes
 Translocations
  Balanced
  Unbalanced
  Centric fusions (robertsonian)
 Inversions
  Paracentric
  Pericentric
 Deletions
  Interstitial
  Terminal
 Ring chromosomes
 Fragile sites

Translocations are the result of movement of one portion of a chromosome to another nonhomologous chromosome. They may be balanced, with no loss or gain of genetic material, or unbalanced where some material is lost or gained. Translocations may be inherited. One of the most famous of these is the Philadelphia translocation first described by Nowell and Hungerford.[111] Most of the neoplastic cells of almost all individuals with chronic myelocytic leukemia display this translocation. Robertsonian translocations occur when two acrocentric chromosomes are joined together at the centromere. It is now clear that translocations can modify the behavior of genes at the site of the translocation. Translocations generate small fragments of chromosomes that are not likely to appear in all daughter cells after mitosis, unless the genes present on the fragments are required for each cell's survival, in which case there is selection for the presence of the fragment. A fragment that includes a centromere can segregate itself during mitosis.

Another form of structural abnormality in chromosomes is an inversion, in which a portion of the chromosome breaks out and then reinserts itself in the opposite orientation. This process has the effect of reversing the order of the gene sequence in a local area of a given chromosome. Inversions may be paracentric, on one side of the centromere, or pericentric, spanning the centromere.

Finally, deletions may remove portions of the chromosome and yet allow survival of the cell. Such alterations are often associated with specific cancers. An example of this is the association of the deletion of the short arm of chromosome 3, which is present in many individuals with small cell carcinoma of the lung.

Deletion of the short arm of chromosome 5 is associated with cri-du-chat syndrome. The peculiar cry of these children to which the disease owes its name appears because of structural anomalies within the larynx. This condition is always accompanied by mental retardation and growth failures. It is frequently associated with abnormal facial appearance including low-set ears and oblique palpebral fissures. Patients usually die at a very early age.

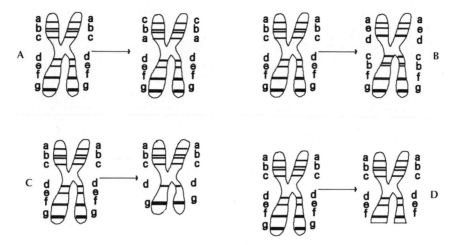

Fig. 1-33. Diagram of various forms of structural aberration of chromosomes. **A,** Paracentric inversion. **B,** Pericentric inversion. **C,** Interstitial deletion. **D,** Terminal deletion. *Stripes,* Hypothetical bands from Giemsa preparation of the spread chromosome. *Letters,* Hypothetical genetic loci.

Fragile chromosome sites

The study of fragile sites began with the observation that a consistent 25% excess of males was present in institutional populations of retarded individuals. In 1969 a marker X chromosome (bearing a rare fragile site) was observed in some of these individuals and pedigrees quickly confirmed a syndrome of X chromosome–linked mental retardation. Affected males may have severe retardation and there is an associated physiognomy—a long face, large ears, and macroorchidism. These individuals have a large head circumference and numerous connective tissue abnormalities. The fragile X syndrome may not present a cytogenetic disorder but rather may be an inherited monogenic disorder in which the fragile site is nothing more than a coincident marker. Alternatively, the fragile site may be intimately involved in the disease.[21,106,112]

Fragile sites on chromosomes were defined by Sutherland as a site on a chromosome evident as a nonstaining gap of variable length. Usually such sites are present on both sister chromatids. The location and size of such gaps is precisely the same in all the cells of a given individual. The sites are inherited in a mendelian codominant manner. The presence of such sites is identified by the production (under appropriate in vitro conditions) of acentric fragments, deleted chromosomes, and multiradial figures. Fragile sites of this type are referred to as rare fragile sites and have been described on chromosomes 2, 3, 6, 7, 8, 9, 10, 11, 12, 16, 17, 20, and X. There are 21 known rare fragile sites in all. Another type of fragile site, the common fragile site, though nonrandom in distribution, occur in virtually all individuals. They are not known to be inherited and are not associated with any disease. It is not known whether either type of fragile site is fragile in vivo or if they simply represent an in vitro manifestation of specific structural alterations in the chromosome.

These sites appear in culture media low in thymidylate. This stress increases uracil incorporation in DNA during replication. The fragile site may be a DNA sequence particularly prone to uracil misincorporation because of the presence of the uracil bases, which, by themselves, disrupt the cytogenetic appearance. Alternatively, the fragile site may be a DNA sequence that slows the replication fork, resulting in incomplete replication when DNA precursors are limited. The suspicion that a given individual has a rare fragile site–based disorder must be pursued with a special culture medium, since the fragile sites are not apparent under the usual culture conditions employed for cytogenetic analysis. The clinician must alert the cytogenetist of the possibility of fragile sites.

Pedigree analysis

Analysis of pedigree is an important tool available to the clinician for the study of inherited disorders. The family data are presented in a diagrammatic form in which individuals are depicted as symbols of geometric shape. Most usually, a square will be used to indicate a male and a circle is used to indicate a female. The relationships between these individuals are depicted by lines connecting them. Marriage or, more specifically, mating is indicated by a straight line connecting the two involved individuals. Succeeding generations are depicted by vertical lines connecting offspring with their parents so that each generation is on the same horizontal level. The index case, or the case that promoted investigation of the family, is known as the "propositus," or the "proband," and is usually indicated with an arrow. Affected individuals are depicted by filling in the

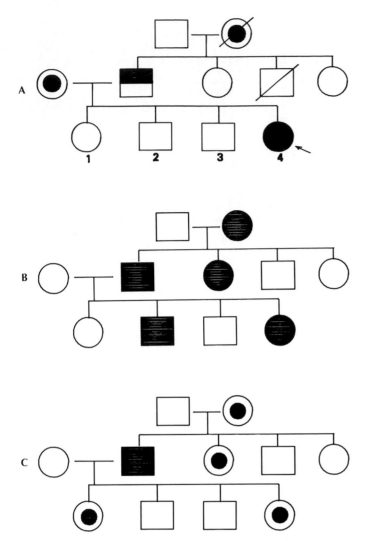

Fig. 1-34. Hypothetical pedigree analysis of the major patterns of inheritance of genetic disorders. **A,** Autosomal recessive pattern. **B,** Autosomal dominant pattern. **C,** X chromosome–linked recessive pattern. *Squares,* males; *circles,* females; *partially filled shapes,* incomplete expression of the phenotype or carrier state; *slash,* deceased members of the family; *numbers under symbols,* order of birth; *arrow,* proband.

symbol, either fully for complete expression of the phenotype, or partially to indicate incomplete expression of the phenotype. Incomplete expression of the phenotype occurs either as a result of heterozygosity in recessive conditions or incomplete expressivity in homozygous recessive individuals or in dominant conditions. Incomplete expression is different from incomplete penetrance. Incomplete penetrance occurs when less than the expected number of affected individuals is observed. Individuals who have died are depicted with a slash drawn through the symbol, and the order of birth is shown by placement of a small number under the symbol for that individual (Fig. 1-34).

Autosomal inheritance
Autosomal dominant conditions

Autosomal dominant conditions (Fig. 1-34, *B*) show a transmission pattern from either sex to either sex. Males and females are equally at risk, and there is a 50% chance of each child of an affected individual having the disease. The probability of expression of the phenotype is based on the potential of all offspring of all affected individuals to express the phenotype. Therefore it is not necessarily true that a 50% incidence of the phenotype occurs in every set of offspring in all afflicted families.

This group of conditions includes Marfan's syndrome, which is a highly complex connective tissue disorder characterized by skeletal abnormalities, subluxation of the lens of the eye, and dissecting aortic aneurysms. These individuals also have floppy cardiac valves. The disease is caused by a wide variety of structural alterations in collagen. The net result of these defects is that given individuals will have less or weakened collagen throughout their body.

Another autosomal dominant condition is multiple neurofibromatosis (von Recklinghausen's disease). These people suffer multiple neurofibromas over most of their body and have characteristic *café-au-lait* spots distributed within various skin dermatomes. These individuals probably inherit an alteration expressed within neural sheath cells that render them highly susceptible to transformation. An early event, necessary but not sufficient for transformation of this cell population, occurs as a germ line mutation.

Familial hypercholesterolemia is a disease with an autosomal dominant pattern of inheritance in which there is an alteration in a structural protein. Affected individuals have serious heart disease and stroke. The patients generally die between the third and sixth decade of life. Rare homozygotes have extremely high blood cholesterol levels. Death in these people occurs before 30 years of age from myocardial infarction. Frequently fatal heart attacks occur earlier. Gene mapping by somatic cell hybridization (see p. 60) has shown a synteny of the loci (that is, both loci are on the same chromosome, in this case chromosome 19) for low-density lipoprotein (LDL) and the gene coding for the low-density lipoprotein receptor (LDLR). Family studies show an association of the disease with the same chromosome. The proximity of the two loci, the association of elevated LDL and cholesterol in the disease, and the association of the disease with the same chromosome indicated that an abnormal LDLR caused familial hypercholesterolemia.

Low-density lipoproteins (LDL) form a complex spherical structure that carries large numbers of cholesterol molecules through the circulatory system. LDL interaction with LDLR on the cell surface results in internalization of cholesterol through coated pits. Mutant LDLR fail to internalize lipoproteins into the cell, leading to an elevation in circulating lipids but a decrease in intracellular cholesterol concentration. As the intracellular cholesterol levels fall, 3-hydroxy-3-methylglutamyl coenzyme A (HMG CoA) reductase activity increases. This enzyme, which is rate limiting in the endogenous synthesis of cholesterol, is normally inhibited by intracellular cholesterol. Therefore the inability to internalize cholesterol results in increased intracellular cholesterol synthesis. The excess cholesterol is transported out of the cell adding to the circulating pool of cholesterol. Therapeutic intervention has been attempted by lowering of LDL levels in the circulation by removal of bile acids from the intestinal tract with special resins. Inhibitors of HMG CoA reductase are being developed in an attempt to reduce intracellular cholesterol production. Since circulating LDL and cholesterol levels are a principal risk factor in myocardial infarction, it is hoped that this form of intervention will lessen the risk of premature death from heart attack in this disorder.[12,43]

Autosomal recessive conditions

In autosomal recessive conditions, the affected offspring of normal parents occur in equal proportions of males and females (Fig. 1-34, *A*). Rarer recessive conditions are frequently associated with consanguinity in the parents. Recessive mutations are in general loss-of-function mutations, or null mutations. The diseases that result are attributable to the loss of a specific enzyme that because of its role in key metabolic processes results in a disease condition. This category of genetic disorder is by far the most important in terms of impact. Certainly, this group represents the most numerous group of individual diseases and the most numbers of affected individuals. In addition, some of the most devastating of the genetic disorders such as the glycogen storage diseases are in this category.

The concept that one gene contains the information necessary for one protein was first suggested by Beadle and Tatum. The relationship of this concept to inborn errors of metabolism provides a framework for the consideration of these disorders. This framework indicates that all biochemical processes may be under genetic control, these processes are resolvable into individual stepwise reactions, each biochemical reaction is under the control of a different single gene, and a single gene mutation can alter the ability to perform a single reaction. These concepts were generated at a time when the physical constitution of the gene was not even firmly established as DNA. The current dramatic advances in molecular genetics were not even imagined. Functional units of transcriptions, regulatory elements (both upstream and downstream), genes that contain multiple open reading frames, and modification of RNA (RNA splicing) are but a few of many aspects of the "gene" that belie the simplicity of the one gene–one protein concept. Interestingly, Beadle and Tatum deduced a paradigm that implies linearity. That is, their theory suggested that genetic events proceeded one after another, as if on a string, and correlated on a one-to-one basis with proteins. This linearity was sought experimentally and, of course, found in the form of the base sequence of DNA. But DNA structure and function actually imply a dynamic system that has nonlinear features. It is certain that advances in nonlinear analysis will enhance our understanding of the complex ways in which genes are interpreted by transcriptional mechanisms.

Errors of metabolism

The concept of inborn errors of metabolism originates in Garrod's lectures and in his monograph entitled *Inborn Errors of Metabolism*, published early in this century, in which he described the familial distribution of alcaptonuria. He observed that parents were often normal and many families had consanguinous marriages. Mendel's laws had recently been rediscovered, and it was clear that in Mendel's construct alcaptonuria acted as a recessive heritable trait. These patients were found by observation of the constant urinary excretion of homogentisic acid. Homogentisic acid is an oxidation product of tyrosine, normally converted to fumaric acid and acetoacetic acid by homogentisic acid oxidase, which alcaptonuries lack. The metabolite homogentisic acid forms a black pigment, "ochronotic pigment," in the presence of oxygen and results in black urine.

Garrod also studied and published reports describing albinism, cystinuria, and pentosuria. He correctly concluded that diseases of this sort could be caused by failure of a single metabolic step because of an inherited error. He further concluded that the accumulation of a given metabolite suggested that the metabolite was normal.

The key forms of inborn errors of metabolism are the absence of an end product as in albinism, the accumulation of intermediate compounds as in alcaptonuria, galactosemia, or glycogen storage diseases, the increased use of a minor pathway with detrimental consequences such as phenylketonuria, and the loss of feedback control as in Lesch-Nyhan syndrome.

Albinism. Albinism is the hypomelanotic syndrome that results from failure to produce mature melanin-containing melanosomes within pigment cells, the melanocytes. One rare form of this disease affects only the eyes and is called the ocular form. The other form, oculocutaneous albinism, affects both the skin and the eyes. These individuals may lack tyrosinase and are thus incapable of converting L-tyrosine into dihydroxyphenylalanine (dopa). Dopa is subsequently converted to a quinone and then to melanin. Oculocutaneous albinism may also be tyrosinase positive, occurring in individuals who have normal tyrosinase levels. The disease state in these people is attributable to a defect in the uptake of tyrosine. Both forms of oculocutaneous albinism involve a high risk of ultraviolet-induced squamous cell carcinoma of the skin.

Lysosomal storage diseases. Lysosomal storage diseases result from the abnormal accumulation of cytoplasmic materials or metabolites in secondary lysosomes. The secondary lysosomes are formed by fusion of primary lysosomes and autosomal vacuoles. The primary lysosomes contain a variety of enzymes, including hydrolases, that are responsible for the catalysis of cytoplasmic materials and metabolites. These substances are digested when the organelles fuse. If an enzyme is absent or nonfunctional, the metabolite or material whose production the enzyme catalyzes will accumulate.

Genetically determined lysosomal storage diseases result from the lack of synthesis of a particular enzyme, the synthesis of abnormal enzyme (either abnormal stability, transport, or structure), the inability to transport normal enzyme into the lysosome, the synthesis of enzyme that is unstable or inactive when inside the lysosomal compartments, and the absence or inactivity of activator enzymes responsible for converting inactive forms of metabolic enzyme into an active form.[94]

Four general categories of inborn errors of metabolism can be classified as lysosomal storage diseases: sphingolipidoses, mucopolysaccharidoses, mucolipidoses, and some glycogen storage diseases (Table 1-3).

Sphingolipidoses. The most common disease of this storage category is Tay-Sachs disease, in which large amounts of G_{M2} ganglioside accumulates in ganglion cells. The accumulation of this product results in swelling of the cells, which ultimately causes their death. This disease has a high incidence among Jews of eastern European extraction. The ganglion cells of the macula are involved in the process, and this causes a characteristic cherry-red spot evident on funduscopic examination of the eye. Homozygous offspring of carriers are afflicted with a progressive neurologic disorder associated with blindness and a prominent startle reflex. Death ensues before the end of the third year from infection after loss of mental function, seizures, and severe spasticity.

Gangliosides are complex sphingolipids that accumulate as the result of a deficiency in hexaminidase A in the primary lysosomes of affected neurons. Accumulation of this material results in a characteristic onion-skin appearance of neurons and ganglion cells as membranous cytoplasmic bodies comprising secondary lysosomes stuffed with uncatalyzed sphingolipid accumulate in these cells.

The absence of a compartmentalized enzyme that results in the accumulation of sphingolipid can cause diseases distant from the usual sites of sphingolipid manufacture and utilization. Lysosomal compartmentalization of certain enzymes can confer organotropy on deficiencies of these enzymes. An example of this phenomenon is Gaucher's disease in which glucocerebroside accumulates because of a deficiency of β-galactosidase. β-Galactosidase is normally present within the primary lysosome of cells of the reticuloendothelial system (RE cells). In this location, the enzyme participates in the catalysis of glucocerebroside. Accumulation of this material in the secondary lysosomes of RE cells causes hypersplenism and an enlarged liver. The enlargements are so striking that clinically they can recall malignant tumors, and, indeed, originally this condition was believed to be a cancer. The ceramide lipid can be seen in peculiar tubule-like inclusions in affected cells. The most devastating form of the disease is the infantile form. These patients die before 2 years of age and have severe failure to thrive (that is, they do not gain weight). They invariably suffer seizures.

Mucopolysaccharidoses. The mucopolysaccharides, or glycosaminoglycans, are extremely complex molecules that form the ground substance of connective tissue in higher organisms. It is chemically similar to a jelly-like substance surrounding unicellular organisms. These intercellular substances are remarkably constant throughout the animal kingdom. For the most part, patients with these diseases accumulate dermatan sulfate and heparan sulfate because of a deficiency of one or more of the degradative enzymes responsible for catabolism of these ground substances.

Deficiency in iduronidase causes three separate clinical conditions with strikingly different clinical patterns. These are attributable to variation in the severity of the deficiency; however, the patterns are constant within a given family. The enzyme defect results in the accumulation of nondegradable mucopolysaccharides in the brain, heart, bones, liver, and spleen.[75] Pathologic appearance varies with the organ. For example, the liver displays many large clear nearly empty lysosomes giving the microscopic section of this tissue a characteristic "Swiss-cheese" appearance. In the cerebral cortex on the other hand, lysosomes are filled with lamina of material creating structures aptly known as "zebra bodies" (Fig. 1-35). In Hurler's syndrome (mucopolysaccharidosis type I, or MPS I), the most severe form, dementia occurs after normal mental development up to about 20 months of age. Death results between 6 and 10 years of age. Scheie's disease is a much more mild form of iduronidase deficiency with normal mental development. There is an intermediate form known a Hurler-Scheie disease, in which mental retardation usually occurs but death is generally forestalled until the third

Table 1-3. Storage disease

Disease	Inheritance pattern	Defect
LYSOSOMAL STORAGE DISEASES		
Sphingolipidoses		
Tay-Sachs disease	AR	Hexosaminidase A
Fabry's disease	X	α-Galactosidase
Gaucher's disease	AR	β-Galactosidase
Krabbe's disease	AR	β-Galactosidase
Niemann-Pick disease	AR	Sphingomyelinase
Mucopolysaccharidoses		
Type I (Hurler's, Scheie's, and Hurler-Scheie)	AR	α-L-Iduronidase
Type II (Hunter's)	X	L-Iduronosulfate sulfatase
Type III	AR	Heparan sulfatase, *N*-acetyl-α-D-glucosaminidase
Type IV	AR	*N*-Acetyl hexosaminidase-6-sulfate sulfatase
Mucolipidoses		
Type I (sialidosis)	AR	Neuraminidase
Type II	AR	Hydrolases
Type III	AR	Hydrolases
Type IV	AR	Unknown
Glycogen storage disease II, GSD II (Pompe's disease)	AR	α-Glucosidases
GLYCOGEN STORAGE DISEASES		
Hypoglycemic		
GSD O	AR	Glycogen synthetase
GSD Ia	AR	Glucose-6-phosphatase
GSD Ib	AR	G-6-Pase translocase
Accumulation		
GSD IIa	AR	Structural abnormality of α-glucosidase
GSD IIb	AR	Reduced amount of normal α-glucosidase
GSD IIIa	AR	Amylo-1,6-glucosidase "debrancher"
GSD IIIb	AR	Amylo-1,6-glycosidase "debrancher"
GSD IV	AR	Amylo-1,4→1,6-transglucosidase "brancher"
GSD V	AR	Muscle phosphorylase
GSD VI	AR	Hepatic phosphorylase
GSD VII	AR	Phosphofructokinase
GSD VIII	AR	Inactive hepatic phosphorylase
GSD IXa	AR	Endogenous kinase
GSD IXb	X	Endogenous kinase
GSD IXc	AR	Hepatic and muscle phosphorylase kinase
GSD X	AR	cAMP-dependent kinase
GSD XI	AR	Unknown

AR, Autosomal recessive; *X,* X-linked recessive.

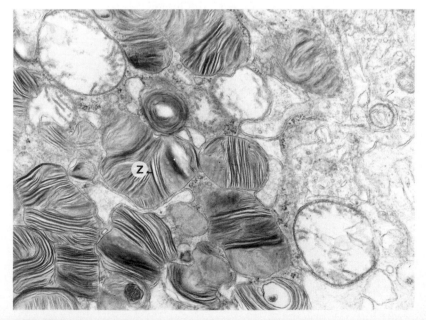

Fig. 1-35. Ultrastructural photomicrograph of a brain specimen from a patient with mucopolysaccharidosis type I. The abnormal accumulation of material within lysosomes create characteristic structures known as "zebra bodies," *Z.* (26,200×; courtesy Prof. G. Hug, University of Cincinnati.)

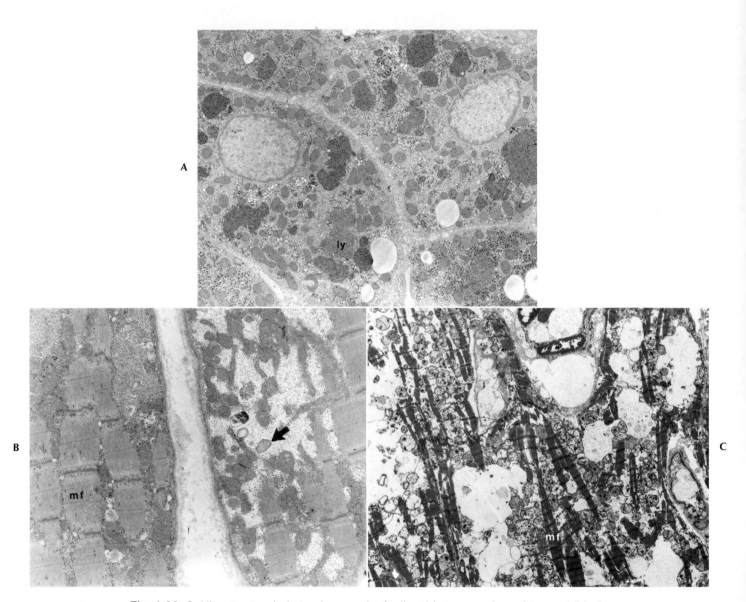

Fig. 1-36. A, Ultrastructural photomicrograph of a liver biopsy specimen from a child with Pompe's disease (GSD IIa). Glycogen *(small dark dots)* accumulation is apparent in both the cytoplasm and in abnormal lysosomes, *ly*. The role of such accumulations in disruption of hepatocyte function is currently under investigation. (3550×.) **B,** Ultrastructural photomicrograph of a skeletal muscle biopsy specimen from the same child (GSD IIa). Cytoplasmic accumulation of glycogen has caused a great deal of disruption of muscle fibers (as in *mf*). Glycogen accumulation can also be seen within lysosomes, *arrow*. Such morphologic distortion will prevent normal contraction of such cells. It is less clear that simply removing the glycogen in some way will restore normal function. (7700×.) **C,** Ultrastructural photomicrograph of a left ventricular specimen from the same child (GSD IIa). The large spaces are autolytic changes in the autopsy material. Profound disruption of the normal myofibril structure, *mf,* is evident as a result of large amounts of glycogen *(small dark dots)* within the cells. (2150×.) (**A** to **C** courtesy Prof. G. Hug, University of Cincinnati.)

decade. These diseases are important because they provide an example of defects in one enzyme controlled at multiple allelic sites resulting in several diseases. These diseases provide an example of the oversimplification of the one gene–one protein–one disease concept. Most probably, there are at least two sets of alleles involved in the synthesis of iduronidase, and homozygosity at both will result in the most severe deficiency of the enzyme activity.

Mucopolysaccharidosis type II (Hunter's syndrome, MPS II) involves a different degradative enzyme and displays an X-chromosome-linked recessive pattern of inheritance. The enzyme defect in this disorder is L-iduronosulfate sulfatase. It has proved possible in some cases to arrest the progress of the disorder by the subcutaneous transplantation of normal fibroblasts. Normal enzyme levels were achieved in serum and leukocytes after this procedure.

Many of the lysosomal storage diseases affect skeletal muscle cells. As stated above, the affected cell is the one that accumulates the material. The storage diseases may be caused by direct cell injury as a result of metabolite accumulation caused by a deficiency of a specific enzyme. Damage to skeletal muscle cells as a result of deficient lysosomal enzymes may be caused by many materials. At this time, however, there is no definitive evidence that proves metabolite accumulation within the cells causes the cell to malfunction.

Acid maltase deficiency (glycogenosis II, GSD II) includes two syndromes that occur in different age groups. All are caused by a deficiency of the enzyme α-1,4-glucosidase. Since this results in the accumulation of glucogen, these diseases may also be considered glycogen storage diseases. The infantile form is known as Pompe's disease (or GSD IIa), and there is an adult onset form. In Pompe's disease, glycogen accumulates in all skeletal muscle fibers both free in the cytoplasmic compartment of the cells and in lysosomes. Glycogen accumulation also occurs in other organs as well, such as the heart, liver, kidney, brain, and spinal cord. The effect of the accumulated glycogen is predictable. Affected infants have severe hypotonia, progressive weakness, and cardiomegaly. The babies usually die before the end of their second year from congestive heart failure. The adult onset form shows involvement within individual muscles. In these patients weakness resembles a mild form of muscular dystrophy, which may be nonprogressive. The less severe forms of the disease often show residual acid maltase activity within muscle cells, and the only organ involved is skeletal muscle. GSD II is an example of a storage disease that may be considered both a glycogen storage disease, because of the metabolite which accumulates, and a lysosomal storage disease because the metabolite can accumulate in lysosomes (Fig. 1-36).

Fabry's disease, caused by a deficiency of α-galactosidase, results in the accumulation of ceramide trihexoside in skin, skeletal muscle, smooth muscle, kidney, heart, and the central nervous system. The two clinical forms (type I, type II) of this disease that are currently recognized show a X-linked recessive pattern of inheritance. Kidney involvement, particularly in the glomeruli, results in kidney failure. Skeletal muscles are involved in type I but not in type II.[16,75,78,94]

Mucolipidoses. There are four types of mucolipidoses, types I, II, III, and IV (ML I, ML II, ML III, and ML IV). Type II is also known as I-cell disease and causes a Hurler-like clinical syndrome.[6] This disease, however, can be diagnosed early in infancy (Fig. 1-37). The lysosomal defect in these diseases is the result of the absence of certain recognition markers (because of a deficiency in a phosphotransferase) that are necessary for the correct transport of lysosomal acid hydrolases into the lysosomes. The lysosomes then are deficient in or completely lack many of the lysosomal enzymes normally present. In addition to the Hurler-like appearance, these individuals have very severe retardation of ossification. Type III is also known as pseudo-Hurler polydystrophy. Genetic evidence indicates that the phosphotransferase may be oligomeric. The enzyme deficiency responsible for type IV mucolipidosis has not been clearly established. Dense lamellar bodies accumulate in nearly all muscle fibers. The disease appears early in infancy and causes spasticity and corneal clouding. Many cell types are involved including endothelium, Schwann cells, and eccrine secretory cells.

Glycogen storage diseases. Glycogen storage diseases (GSD) are a series of diseases involving enzymes that regulate glycogen. This set of disorders as a group is not rare. These diseases present with an impressive array of clinical manifestations recently reviewed by Hug.[76] These clinical manifestations include hepatomegaly, cardiac dysfunction, muscular hypotonia, ascites, splenomegaly, and degenerative brain disease. When the enzyme responsible for the disease is normally found in the lysosome, the disease may also be considered a lysosomal storage disease.

Hug has defined glycogen storage disease as an abnormal concentration or structure of glycogen in any tissue of the body because of a metabolic inborn error. These diseases are classified by assignment of a different roman numeral to each particular enzyme deficiency. Letters are assigned to clinical or pathologic variants of a given enzyme deficiency. This classification is much more understandable when the normal pathways of glycogenesis and metabolism are considered (Fig. 1-38). Glycogen molecules are elongated by the addition of glucose from uridinediphosphoglucose in 1,4 linkages. This elongation is catalyzed by glycogen synthetase. After the chaiin attains a given length, the chain branches by transferring the glucose to 1,6 regu-

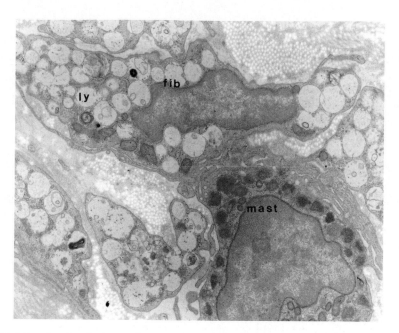

Fig. 1-37. Ultrastructural photomicrograph of a skin biopsy from a patient with I-cell disease. Several fibroblasts, *fib,* and a mast cell, *mast,* are visible. Abnormal lysosomes, *ly,* are present within the fibroblasts. (10,000×.) (Courtesy Prof. G. Hug, University of Cincinnati.)

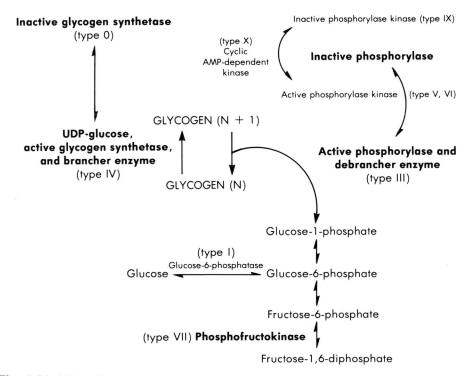

Fig. 1-38. Major biosynthetic and catabolic pathways of glycogen. *Brackets,* Type of glycogen storage disease (GSD) caused by the deficiency of that particular enzyme. (Redrawn from Hug, G.: Glycogen storage disease, Pract. Pediatr. **6:**1, 1984.)

lated by amylo-1,4→1,6-transglucosidase, or brancher enzyme.

Glycogen metabolism is a cyclic AMP–dependent process. cAMP-dependent kinase causes the phosphorylation of phosphorylase kinase phosphatase, activating it, and glycogen synthetase, inactivating it. Phosphorylase kinase phosphatase degrades 1,4-linked glucose but cannot degrade the 1,6-linked branch points. Amylo-1,6-glucosidase, or debrancher enzyme, removes the branch point as free glucose. Thus the action of kinase phosphatase phosphorylase and debranching enzyme alternate as the glycogen molecule is degraded to glucose and glucose-1-phosphate.

The ultrastructural appearance of glycogen often forms an important part of the scheme used to establish the correct diagnosis of GSD. Glycogen is normally present in the intracellular compartment as small electron-dense spherical particles about 20 nm in diameter. These are known as beta particles. Alpha particles are present normally within hepatocytes and appear as electron-dense rosettes, typically 200 nm in diameter. Glycogen can attain a molecular weight of millions of daltons, and these particles represent the aggregation of many molecules.

Hypoglycemic disorders. Both GSD type 0, which is a deficiency of glycogen synthetase, and GSD types Ia and Ib, which show defects in glucose-6-phosphatase, result in hypoglycemia. The enzyme defects are most profound in liver and muscle. In GSD Ib the levels of glucose-6-phosphatase activity are normal, but a translocase, necessary for the glucose-6-phosphatase to reach its substrate, is absent. Thus the *effective* activity of glucose-6-phosphatase is deficient. GSD 0 causes hypoglycemia after fasting and, if untreated, may result in convulsions and mental retardation. GSD Ia and Ib are associated with enlarged liver and kidneys, glucagon nonresponsive hypoglycemia, and a "doll-face" appearance.

Disorders with abnormal metabolite accumulation. GSD IIa and IIb are attributable to defects in α-glucosidase, a lysosomal enzyme. In GSD IIa the normal amount of this enzyme is present, but the structure is altered at the molecular level in a way that makes it ineffective. In GSD IIb the structure of the enzyme is normal, but the amount is greatly reduced. GSD IIa is the classical infantile form of the disease and causes excessive glycogen in all tissues. The infant is normal at birth, but noticeable hypotonia develops within a few months followed by pronounced cardiomegaly, hepatomegaly, and death in infancy. GSD IIb is the adult form of this disease and causes glycogen accumulation in liver, muscle, and skin. This form of the disease is much less severe and is compatible with a normal life span. The principal clinical manifestation is muscle weakness.

GSD IIIa and IIIb are caused by a deficiency in amylo-1,6-glucosidase, or debrancher enzyme. GSD IIIa affects only the liver, whereas IIIb is a generalized defect. Patients with this disorder have pronounced hepatomegaly but only moderate cardiomegaly. Frequently there is no demonstrable hypotonia though muscle involvement can be demonstrated histologically. Mental development is normal in almost all patients, and the prognosis is good.

GSD IV is a deficiency of amylo-1,4→1,6-transglucosidase, or brancher enzyme. The inability to correctly branch the growing glycogen molecule causes the accumulation of structurally abnormal molecules though they remain appropriate in number. The defect results in hepatosplenomegaly, ascites, cirrhosis, and liver failure. Death occurs in early childhood, unless liver transplantation is performed.

GSD V is caused by the congenital absence of skeletal muscle phosphorylase. Inability to utilize glycogen causes weakness and painful contracture of muscles after exercise. These patients have normal mental development. GSD VI is a deficiency in liver phosphorylase causing pronounced hepatomegaly as the principal clinical manifestation.

GSD VII results from a deficiency of phosphofructokinase in skeletal muscle and erythrocytes. The principal clinical manifestation is temporary weakness and exercise intolerance. The disease may be disabling but not fatal.

GSD VIII is demonstrated by the presence of cerebral glycogen accumulation in the form of giant alpha particles particularly within the axons and synapses. Skeletal muscle is unaffected, and these patients have hepatomegaly. Ataxia and nystagmus are among neurologic symptoms that result from this disorder. Neurologic deterioration will progress to spasticity. Up to now the enzyme defect responsible is unknown. The phosphorylase-activating system is intact though most of the phosphorylase is in the inactive form. In vitro homogenates of liver from these patients will activate endogenous phosphorylase if ATP and $MgCl_2$ are added. This activation indicates that a defect in regulation of the endogenous activation system may be involved in the disease. GSD VIII results in death at an early age.

There are three forms of GSD IX: a, b, and c. These disorders are attributable to deficient phophorylase kinase activity, and so endogenous activation of phosphorylase does not occur. This results in increased liver glycogen concentration but no functional alteration. In type IXc, glycogen accumulates in skeletal muscle as well as liver though clinical symptoms are minimal.

GSD X is attributable to ineffective cAMP-dependent kinase in liver and muscle. The phosphorylase therefore, though present in normal amounts, is completely inactive. The phosphorylase kinase has a much

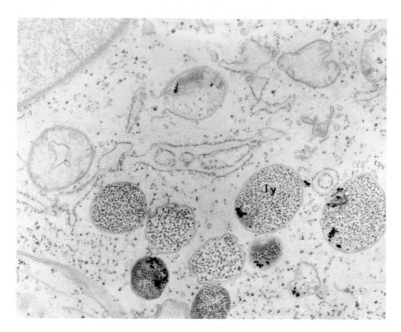

Fig. 1-39. Ultrastructural photomicrograph of a human muscle cell grown in tissue culture. The original material was obtained from a muscle biopsy of a patient with GSD IIa. Abnormal lysosomes, *ly,* are evident with accumulations of glycogen. The black dots within the lysosomes are colloidal gold, proving uptake from extracellular pools. This was an attempt to target enzyme to the correct compartment of the cells. The explant and culture experiments were performed by Prof. S.T. Iannaccone, University of Cincinnati. (16,500×; courtesy Prof. G. Hug, University of Cincinnati.)

lower than normal activity because of the deficiency of cAMP kinase activity. Hepatomegaly appears to be the only clinical manifestation of this disorder.

Patients with GSD XI may have hyperlipidemia, galactosuria, glucosuria, growth retardation, and vitamin D–resistant rickets. Up to now there is no known enzyme defect to account for this form of glycogen storage disease.

Prenatal diagnosis of GSD II, III, and IV is possible by enzyme analysis of cultured amniotic cells and ultrastructural analysis of uncultured amniotic cells. Material for enzyme studies and ultrastructural examination may also be obtained from chorionic villus biopsy during the first trimester of pregnancy. Thus genetic counseling can be offered to parents who have previously given birth to children with GSD. This is most important for fatal diseases such as GSD IIa. All the glycogen storage diseases, except for GSD IXb, are autosomal recessive conditions. Therefore, on average, one in four offspring of heterozygous carrier parents will be expected to have the disease.

Treatment has been attempted in three ways. One is by providing the patients with special diets. This approach has met with limited succcess in some of the diseases. The second is by liver transplantation, which has proved successful in those conditions where in-

volvement is limited to the liver. The third is by administration of the enzyme that is deficient or nonfunctional in the patients. The enzymes have been administered orally, intravenously, or by bone marrow transplant. Enzymes have been prepared from both fungal and human sources for intravenous administration. These procedures have met with limited success. Oral administration for example has been shown to remove glycogen from the liver but hasn't prevented progression of the disease. It is clear now that the enzyme must be in the correct compartment of the cell to be of any use (Fig. 1-39). It is less clear that even if this were achieved and the metabolite accumulation were reversed the disease process would stop. There may be other unsuspected problems associated with the genetic defect.[24,62,74-78,153]

Sex-linked conditions

In sex-linked conditions, the male with the disorder transmits the gene from an affected X chromosome to daughters who can then pass the gene to daughters or to males. The males manifest the disorder, since they have a single X chromosome. Females can also show the sex-linked disorder but much less frequently because of the low probability of homozygosity. Holandric inheritance patterns are those that display direct father-to-son transmission of a condition (that is, those that are Y linked). There are no known Y-transmitted disorders. Indeed, the only known structural genes on the Y chromosomes are those that direct testicular differentiation of the indifferent fetal gonad. Although XO embryos can survive to birth, the complete absence of X chromosomes is incompatible with life. These features indicate that there are no vital genes on the Y chromosome and that its function in Mammalia is solely to establish maleness in these Y-male heterogametic species.

Therefore a sex-linked disorder really means an X-linked disorder. There are two peculiarities of the sex chromosomes relevant to X-linked disorders. The first is that the male X chromosome is maternally derived. The second is that one X chromosome of the two present in females is inactivated early in embryonic life. In 1961, Mary Lyon first proposed X-chromosome inactivation as a gene-compensation mechanism. The presence of both a maternal and a paternal genome are required at fertilization to allow embryonic development in mammals.[46] The fact that females then will have an extra chromosome would lead to the problems previously discussed for aneuploidy if there were no mechanism for gene dose compensation. The process of X-chromosome inactivation serves the purpose of maintaining the appropriate number of active X-linked genes. As a result, mammalian females are a mosaic of cells, some with the maternal X chromosome active and some with paternal X chromosome active.[31]

The Lyon hypothesis now embodies several key precepts. One entire X chromosome of the two present in females is inactivated and remains heritably present as the Barr body. The inactivation is all or nothing; that is, the X chromosome in each cell is fully inactivated. The inactivation is normally irreversible in somatic cells and is heritable. That is, the maternal or the paternal X chromosome, once inactive, will also be inactive in daughter cells after division. The inactivation occurs early in embryogenesis some time around implantation, and in eutherian mammals it is a random process among the early embryonic cells that will form the fetus. Primordial germ cells in females have two active X chromosomes. This could be the result of reactivation of one previously inactivated X chromosome or the result of some sequestered cell that was fated to develop into primordial germ cells but escaped X-chromosome inactivation. It is now established, at least in the mouse, that there is no sequestered population of germ cells and that the X chromosome must reactivate in the primordial germ cell population. This is an important aspect of mammalian development that varies in other animals.

The consequences of these features of sex chromosomes in man are that the sex-linked affected phenotype appears in male offspring of heterozygous females; among male offspring of heterozygous females, 50% should have the affected phenotype; and affected male offspring will not transmit the trait to male children but will transmit the trait to all female children. Complete expression of a recessive X-linked trait in female offspring is possible only in offspring of a carrier female and affected males. Partial phenotypic expression (low expressivity) can occur as a result of inactivation of the mutant X chromosome in some cells with the expression of the normal allele in those cells. In some conditions, however, mosaicism does not fully compensate for the cells with the abnormal phenotype.

For example, in glucose-6-phosphate dehydrogenase deficiency, affected individuals suffer from hemolytic anemia. In females with two populations of red blood cells, one with the affected X chromosome and one with a normal X chromosome, the anemia is less severe than in affected males with only one population of red blood cells. Thus mosaicism ameliorates the phenotype.

Most X-linked disorders are recessive and include hemophilia, Hunter's syndrome (previously discussed), and Lesch-Nyhan syndrome. Lesch-Nyhan syndrome is an unusual disorder characterized by hyperuricemia, mental retardation, and behavioral anomalies including self-mutilation of fingertips and lips. The accumulation of uric acid results in goutlike symptoms in affected males. The syndrome is caused by a deficiency in hypoxanthine-guanine phosphoribosyl transferase (HGPRT). HGPRT is an enzyme in the purine salvage pathway that obviates the complete de novo synthesis of purines required for DNA synthesis. When cells are grown in medium containing hypoxanthine, aminopterine, and thymidine, only cells that have HGPRT will survive. Aminopterine blocks normal de novo synthesis, and without HGPRT the cell cannot utilize hypoxanthine or thymidine for purine production and the cell dies. In vivo the intermediate metabolite uric acid accumulates.

The X-linked recessive disorder ichthyosis is a scaling disorder that has been shown to be attributable to a deficiency of cholesterol sulfatase. During normal differentiation of squamous cells in the epidermis, maturation of the squamous cells serves two purposes. One is to establish an effective permeability barrier and the other is to ensure correct regulation of the thickness of that barrier. The permeability barrier is established by the synthesis of neutral lipids and cholesterol. These sterols are deposited extracellularly but can also be present in specialized organelles within the squamous cells. Interestingly the synthesis of cholesterol in squamous cells is not regulated by circulating LDL as it is in other tissues. Cholesterol is converted to cholesterol sulfate in a reaction catalyzed by sulfotransferase; the back reaction is catalyzed by cholesterol sulfatase. The process of desquamation (the second role of squamous maturation in the skin) appears to be regulated by the ratio of cholesterol to cholesterol sulfate. Therefore, in X-linked recessive ichthyosis, the deficiency in cholesterol sulfatase results in an inappropriate, nonregulatable ratio of cholesterol to cholesterol sulfate and desquamation is abnormal. The scaling disorder results.[165]

Duchenne muscular dystrophy (DMD) is an X chromosome–linked disorder that illustrates an important point about the utilization of a full array of molecular techniques in biomedical research. DMD causes progressive muscle wasting and affects about one in 3000 males. There are affected females, and this is known to be attributable to the translocation of a portion of the X chromosome to autosomal chromosomes. Molecular analysis of these translocations has led to the precise localization of the gene responsible for DMD. Interstitial deletions in this area of the X chromosome have been described in patients with DMD. Since such cytogenetic abnormalities are undoubtedly responsible for the disease, the deletion area was cloned and sequenced. The sequence data ultimately led to the discovery of dystrophin, a protein component of intracellular membranes in skeletal muscle important to muscle function. Defects in this protein may be responsible for DMD. This form of "reverse genetics" will play an increasing important role in establishing the mechanisms of genetic disorders.

Somatic cell genetics

The field of somatic cell genetics embodies genetic analysis in vitro as opposed to sexual genetic analysis. Obviously the practical approach to mendelian genetics without the necessity of breeding is very important in the advance of knowledge in human populations where sexual genetical information is largely fortuitous and requires generations to obtain. Principally the analysis of genetic problems in vitro is accomplished by cell fusion, whereby genomes from cells of differing sources are combined. This approach allows analysis in a manner analogous to breeding experiments. Cell fusion produces hybrid cells with combined genomic and cytoplasmic contents. The analysis must proceed with cells that have actually fused, and under the best of experimental conditions this can be accomplished in only a small fraction of the two types of cells originally mixed. Selective growth conditions are required to eliminate the parental cells that have not been induced to fuse. Hybrid cells containing both genomes are then selected because the parental cells of the fusion are killed in the growth medium. One such selective system takes advantage of the consequences of HGPRT deficiency. The growth medium contains hypoxanthine, aminopterine, and thymidine. In this case, one of the cell types to be fused lacks HGPRT and is incapable of purine salvage synthesis, aminopterine blocks the uptake of thymidine, and the HGPRT-deficient cells are incapable of

synthesizing DNA and cannot divide. Selection of the other parental cell type in the fusion can be accomplished in a variety of ways. The result is that only those cells that contain both genomes and can compliment each other to survive the selective medium are capable of division. These cells form clonal colonies in the culture flask and can be harvested and propagated for analysis.

Human chromosome mapping

If one of the cell types used in cell fusion is human in origin whereas the other cell type is from a rodent, the cells will lose human chromosomes preferentially with time in culture. New clones that have relatively few, indeed usually one, human chromosome can be established. This allows specific enzymes or phenotypes to be assigned to specific chromosomes. If, in a series of such hybrids, there is a chromosome that is always present when the enzyme activity or the phenotype is expressed and is never present when the enzyme activity or phenotype is not expressed, then the locus for the gene or genes responsible must be on that chromosome. HGPRT was proved to be on the X chromosome with this technique. The genes for the low-density lipoprotein receptor and for LDL synthesis were assigned to human chromosome 19 in this way. Family studies have previously shown an association between the disease familial hypercholesterolemia (see p. 50) and chromosome 19.[43]

If the human chromosomes are fragmented by irradiation of the human cells before fusion, it is possible to map human chromosomes regionally. This is done by determination of how frequently two enzyme activities or two phenotypes are lost together when one phenotype is at a known location in the human genome (several human loci have been previously mapped by tedious family studies). If in a small fragment of human chromosome the two phenotypes are always present together and always lost together, the genes for these phenotypes must be close to each other. One can quantitate the distance between them by varying the amount of radiation used initially and thereby varying the size of the fragments. The probability of cosegregation with increasing radiation dose then is a measure of the distance between the genes.[58,59]

Genetic analysis of malignancy

Cancer cells may be defined operationally as cells that have the ability to grow progressively in an appropriate host, eventually killing the host. If cancer cells are fused with normal cells, the resulting hybrid cells are nonmalignant for a time in culture. This condition indicates that the cancer cells may have been malignant because they lacked something that normal cells have. Thus fusion supplies the missing element or elements from the normal genome. As the hybrid cells are grown in culture in successive generations, chromosomes that are not essential for the cells' survival are lost. Eventually a stage is reached at which the cells are once again malignant, having lost the gene or genes responsible for the expression of the suppressing product. Such cancer-suppressor genes are now being actively sought, with accumulating evidence that at least one such gene is on human chromosome 1.

Xeroderma pigmentosum

The foregoing analysis of malignancy provides an example of complementation of one genome by another. Similar genetic analyses have been applied to other disorders as well.

Xeroderma pigmentosum is an autosomal recessive condition characterized by a predilection to form skin cancers on sun-exposed areas of the body. All affected individuals will have skin cancer by their third decade of life. Fibroblasts from these people have been shown to be defective in their ability to repair damaged DNA. Ultraviolet radiation induces dimerization of thymidine bases in DNA molecules. These thymidine dimers may cause misreading during DNA transcription or during DNA replication. They may cause polymerases to stop. These dimers are normally repaired by excision, base replacement, and ligation. Xeroderma fibroblasts are incapable of repairing the lesions.

If more than one gene is required to cause the correct repair of such DNA lesions, a deficit of any of these genes would result in repair deficiency. Fusion of these cells with normal cells results in normal DNA repair as the defective gene or genes are complimented by the normal genome. In a group of individuals with this disorder, different ones will have defects in different genes. If cells from individuals with xeroderma are fused with xeroderma cells from other individuals, DNA repair will be normal if the defect was in a gene different in the two individuals. However, DNA repair will be defective if the lesion is in the same gene in both individuals. If such cell fusion analysis is applied to a large number of individuals with this disorder, each individual can be assigned to a group according to whether their cells complement the deficiency in some other individuals. These groups are called complementation groups, and their number equals the lowest number of genes that can be responsible for the disorder or the phenotype. Complementation analysis has been done for xeroderma pigmentosum, and so far five complementation groups have been identified, meaning that in man at least five genes are involved in this type of DNA repair.

Maternal effects

The mother can greatly influence the pregnancy outcome as a result of her role in establishing and maintaining the fetal environment throughout gestation.

There are two fundamental ways in which this occurs. One is genetically, in which the genetic disorder occurs in the mother and results in a uterine environment that damages the offspring. For example, mothers with phenylketonuria expose their fetuses to high levels of phenylalanine, which results in damage to the developing brain of the fetus. Birth defects among offspring of diabetic mothers is a serious unresolved problem. Recently, Freinkel has established that glucose loading at specific stages of fetal development will cause dysmorphogenesis. Thus a metabolic defect in the mother produces a damaging environment to the fetus.

The other way maternal effects influence fetal environment is by exposure to toxic substances through maternal serum. These substances may be acquired accidentally, or they may be self-inflicted. Maternal smoking, for example, is associated with lowered implantation rates. The spontaneous abortion rate and the incidence of idiopathic, prenatal mortality as well as babies small for gestational age are higher in smoking mothers than in nonsmoking mothers. Late effects in offspring of smoking mothers have also been well documented, including sudden infant death syndrome (SIDS) and decreased intellectual functioning. We have established that mutagens (similar to those present in cigarette smoke) can cause gross dysmorphogenesis, growth retardation, and increased perinatal mortality when administered in the preimplantation period. This period has traditionally been regarded as refractory to the effects of chemical exposure. We now know that this is not the case, and mothers should not wait until pregnancy is clinically defined to refine the environment in which the conceptus must develop.[11,81]

Therapeutic approaches

Several novel approaches to the treatment of genetic disorders are being developed. Familial hypercholesterolemia is an example. As we have seen, this disease is caused by the underproduction of functional low-density lipoprotein receptor (LDLR) as a result of a mutant gene. Elevated circulating levels of low-density lipoprotein (LDL) and cholesterol result, but since the cholesterol cannot get into the cell, HMG-CoA reductase remains active and endogenous cholesterol synthesis proceeds. LDL can be removed from the circulation of these individuals by removal of bile acids from the intestinal tract with special resins. Simultaneously, inactivation of HMG-CoA reductase activity can prevent endogenous cholesterol synthesis and also stimulate the production of LDLR. This approach is being tested now in the hope that significant reduction of the circulating LDL and cholesterol levels will reduce the risk of fatal myocardial infarction in these persons. The rational approach to therapy in this instance required a thorough fundamental understanding of the mechanisms of cholesterol transport and biochemistry of its synthesis as well as genetic regulation of the receptor expression. These were all learned as a result of intensive investigation at the cellular level.

The elucidation of enzyme deficiencies responsible for glycogen storage diseases led to an attempt to replace these enzymes in affected individuals. Although success has been achieved in getting the enzyme into the correct cells, it has not been thus far possible to get the enzymes into the correct *compartment* of the cell. Nevertheless, limited success in some instances has been achieved in MPS II by transplantation of normal fibroblasts capable of production of missing enzymes. Recently, lysosomal placement of normal enzyme has been achieved in cultured human skeletal muscle from patients with GSD II. Limited success in eliminating the enzyme deficiency in infants with GSD II has been achieved though survival has not yet been extended. Ultimately, gene replacement therapy with appropriate regulatory elements will be required to cure genetic disorders.

Molecular approaches to therapy are now beginning to be undertaken. In the fatal disease β^0 thalassemia no adult hemoglobin is produced. This inevitably leads to the death of affected individuals in young adulthood. Since the gene for β-globin in humans has been cloned, it should in principal be possible to replace the defective gene in these individuals. This has been attempted by transfection of the globin gene into stem cells of the bone marrow of a few patients with this disease along with the TK (thymidine kinase) promoter of HSV (herpes simplex virus). It was hoped that this recombinant gene would have a selective advantage in the bone marrow stem population after transplantation of genetically engineered cells into patients. This should lead to appropriate expression of globin in red blood cells. Until recently this has been a highly controversial approach to the disease, but one hopes as our knowledge increases and the rhetoric wanes people with devastating diseases like β^0 thalassemia can turn to gene manipulation with hope.

Zygotic gene replacement therapy represents another possible approach to some genetic disorders in the future. Mammalian embryos can be given exogenous DNA microsurgically and develop normally with the exogenous gene incorporated into the host genome. In many instances, the gene will be temporally and spatially expressed in an appropriate manner. The way in which this technology might be applied to genetic disorders in the future is a matter of pure speculation, but we can expect that the information gathered by the production of transgenic animals will prove invaluable for the appropriate use of recombinant-DNA therapies.

REFERENCES

1. Abdel-Monem, M., and Hoffmann-Berling, H.: DNA unwinding enzymes, Trends Biochem. Sci. **5**:128, 1980.
2. Adelman, M., Sabatini, D., and Blobel, G.: Ribosome-membrane interaction, J. Cell Biol. **56**:206, 1973.
3. Arstila, A.U., and Trump, B.F.: Studies on cellular autophagocytosis: the formation of autophagic vacuoles in the liver after glucagon administration, Am. J. Pathol. **53**:687, 1968.
4. Atkinson, D.E.: Regulation of enzyme activity, Annu. Rev. Biochem. **35**:85, 1966.
5. Avery, O.T., MacLeod, C.M., and McCarty, M.: Studies on the chemical nature of the substance inducing transformation of pneumococcal types: induction of transformation by a desoxyribonucleic acid fraction isolated from pneumococcus type III, J. Exp. Med. **79**:137, 1944.
6. Babcock, D.S., Bove, K.E., Hug, G., Dignan, P.S.J., Soukup, S., and Warren, N.S.: Fetal mucolipidosis II (I-cell disease): radiologic and pathologic correlation, Pediatr. Radiol. **16**:32, 1986.
7. Bacq, Z.M., and Alexander, P.: Fundamentals of radiobiology, New York, 1955, Academic Press, Inc.
8. Baker, P.F., Hodgkin, A.L., and Shaw, T.I.: The effects of changes in internal ionic concentrations on the electrical properties of perfused giant axons, J. Physiol. **164**:355, 1962.
9. Bessis, M.: Studies on cell agony and death: an attempt at classification. In De Reuck, A.V.S., and Knight, J., editors: Cellular injury, Boston, 1964, Little, Brown & Co.
10. Bladen, H.A., Nylen, M.U., and Glenner, G.G.: The ultrastructure of human amyloid as revealed by the negative staining technique, J. Ultrastruct. Res. **14**:449, 1966.
11. Bossert, N.L., and Iannaccone, P.M.: Midgestational abnormalities associated with in vitro preimplantation N-methyl-N-nitrosourea exposure with subsequent transfer to surrogate mothers, Proc. Natl. Acad. Sci. USA **82**:8757, 1985.
12. Brown, M.S., and Goldstein, J.L.: How LDL receptors influence cholesterol and atherosclerosis, Sci. Am. **251**:58, 1984.
13. Brutlag, D., and Kornberg, A.: Enzymatic synthesis of deoxyribonucleic acid: a proofreading function for the 3′ to 5′ exonuclease activity in DNA polymerases, J. Biol. Chem. **247**:241, 1972.
14. Burke, J.P., and Rubin, E.: The effects of ethanol and acetaldehyde on the products of protein synthesis by liver and mitochondria, Lab. Invest. **41**:393, 1979.
15. Campenot, R.B.: Local control of neurite development by nerve growth factor, Proc. Natl. Acad. Sci. USA **74**:4516, 1977.
16. Carpenter, S., and Karpati, G.: Lysosomal storage in human skeletal muscle, Hum. Pathol. **17**:683, 1986.
17. Chamberlin, M.J.: RNA polymerase: an overview. In Losick, R., and Chamberlin, M., editors: RNA polymerase, Cold Spring Harbor, N.Y., 1976, Cold Spring Harbor Laboratory.
18. Chapman, D.: Lipid dynamics in cell membranes. In Weissmann, G., and Claiborne, R., editors: Cell membranes: biochemistry, cell biology and pathology, New York, 1975, HP Publishing Co., Inc.
19. Cheng, H., and LeBlond, C.P.: Origin, differentiation and renewal of the four main epithelial cell types in the mouse small intestine, Am. J. Anat. **141**:461, 1974.
20. Chien, K.R., Abrams, J., Serroni, A., Martin, J.T., and Farber, J.L.: Accelerated phospholipid turnover and associated membrane dysfunction in irreversible ischemic liver cell injury, J. Biol. Chem. **253**:4809, 1978.
21. Chudley, A.E., and Hagerman, R.J.: Fragile X syndrome, J. Pediatr. **110**:821, 1987.
22. Cleaver, J.E.: DNA repair and radiation sensitivity in human (xeroderma pigmentosum) cells, Int. J. Radiat. Biol. **18**:557, 1970.
23. Coleman, J.E., and Oakley, J.L.: Physical chemical studies of the structure and function of DNA binding (helix-destabilizing) proteins, CRC Crit. Rev. Biochem. **7**:247, 1979.

24. Collins, J.E., and Leonard, J.V.: Hepatic glycogen storage disease, Br. J. Hosp. Med. **38**:168, 1987.
25. Cormack, D.V., and Johns, H.E.: Electron energies and ion densities in water irradiated with 200 keV, 1 MeV and 25 MeV radiation, Br. J. Radiol. **25**:369, 1952.
26. Cowger, M.L.: Mechanism of bilirubin toxicity on tissue culture cells: factors that affect toxicity, reversibility by albumin, and comparison with other respiratory poisons and surfactants, Biochem. Med. **5**:1, 1971.
27. Dale, H.H., Feldberg, W., and Vogt, M.: Release of acetylcholine at voluntary motor nerve endings, J. Physiol. **86**:353, 1936.
28. Dale, W.M., Davies, J.V., and Gilbert, C.W.: The kinetics and specificities of deamination of nitrogenous compounds by X-radiation, Biochem. J. **45**:93, 1949.
29. Dales, S.: Penetration of animal viruses into cells, Prog. Med. Virol. **7**:1, 1965.
30. Daniels, F., Jr.: Physiological effects of sunlight, J. Invest. Dermatol. **32**:147, 1959.
31. Davies, K.E.: Molecular genetics of the human X chromosome, J. Med. Genet. **22**:243, 1985.
32. Davis, P.S., Luke, C.G., and Deller, D.J.: Reduction of gastric iron-binding protein in haemochromatosis: a previously unrecognized metabolic defect, Lancet **2**:1431, 1966.
33. de Duve, C.: Exploring cells with a centrifuge, Science **189**:186, 1975.
34. de Duve, C., and Wattiaux, R.: Functions of lysosomes, Annu. Rev. Physiol. **28**:435, 1966.
35. Dingle, J.T., and Fell, H., editors: Lysosomes in biology and pathology (in two parts), Amsterdam, 1969, North Holland Publishing Co.
36. Dunlap, S.S., and Rosenbaum, K.N.: Comparative anatomical analysis of human trisomies 13, 18, and 21. I. The forelimb, Teratology **33**:159, 1986.
37. Duryee, W.R.: The nature of radiation injury to amphibian cell nuclei, J. Natl. Cancer Inst. **10**:735, 1949.
38. Epstein, C.J.: Developmental genetics, Experientia **42**:1117, 1986.
39. Fersht, A.R.: Enzymatic editing mechanism in protein synthesis and DNA replication, Trends Biochem. Sci. **5**:262, 1980.
40. Finean, J.B., Coleman, R., and Michell, R.H.: Membranes and their cellular functions, ed. 2, London, 1978, Blackwell.
41. Folkman, J., and Moscona, A.: Role of cell shape in growth control, Nature **273**:345, 1978.
42. Ford, C.E., and Hamerton, J.L.: The chromosomes of man, Nature [Lond.] **178**:1020, 1956.
43. Francke, U., Brown, M.S., and Goldstein, J.L.: Assignment of the human gene for the low density lipoprotein receptor to chromosome 19: synteny of a receptor, a ligand, and a genetic disease, Proc. Natl. Acad. Sci. USA **81**:2826, 1984.
44. Franklin, R.M., and Baltimore, D.: Patterns of macromolecular synthesis in normal and virus-infected mammalian cells, Cold Spring Harbor Symp. Quant. Biol. **27**:175, 1962.
45. Furshpan, E.J., and Potter, D.D.: Low-resistance junctions between cells in embryos and tissue culture, Curr. Top. Dev. Biol. **3**:95, 1968.
46. Gartler, S.M., and Riggs, A.O.: Mammalian X chromosome inactivation, Annu. Rev. Genet. **17**:155, 1983.
47. Gearhart, H.D., Davisson, M.T., and Granite, M.L.: Autosomal aneuploidy in mice: generation and developmental consequences, Brain Res. Bull. **16**:789, 1986.
48. Gellert, M.: DNA topoisomerases, Annu. Rev. Biochem. **50**:879, 1981.
49. Gibson, R., Kornfeld, S., and Schlesinger, S.: A role for oligosaccharides in glycoprotein biosynthesis, Trends Biochem. Sci. **5**:290, 1980.
50. Glenner, G.G.: The creation of "amyloid" fibrils from Bence Jones proteins in vitro, Science **174**:712, 1971.
51. Glenner, G.G.: Amyloid deposits and amyloidosis: the β-fibrilloses, N. Engl. J. Med. **302**:1283, 1980.
52. Glenner, G.G., Ein, D., and Terry, W.D.: The immunoglobulin origin of amyloid, Am. J. Med. **52**:141, 1972.
53. Goldfinger, S., Klinenberg, J.R., and Seegmiller, J.E.: Renal retention of uric acid induced by infusion of beta-hydroxybutyrate and acetoacetate, N. Engl. J. Med. **272**:351, 1965.
54. Goldman, R., Pollard, T., and Rosenbaum, J., editors: Cell motility, Cold Spring Harbor, New York, 1976, Cold Spring Harbor Laboratories.
55. Goldstein, J.L., Anderson, R.G.W., and Brown, M.S.: Coated pits, coated vesicles, and receptor-mediated endocytosis, Nature **279**:679, 1979.
56. Good, R.A., and Campbell, B.: The precipitation of latent herpes simplex and encephalitis by anaphylactic shock, Proc. Soc. Exp. Biol. Med. **68**:82, 1948.
57. Gorter, E., and Grendel, F.: On bimolecular layers of lipoids on the chromocytes of the blood, J. Exp. Med. **41**:439, 1925.
58. Goss, S.J.: Gene mapping by cell fusion, Int. Rev. Cytol. **8**:127, 1978.
59. Goss, S.J., and Harris, H.: Gene transfer by means of cell fusion I, II, J. Cell Sci. **25**:17, 1977.
60. Granite, M.L.: The neurobiologic consequences of autosomal trisomy in mice and men, Br. Res. Bull. **16**:767, 1986.
61. Hardt, F.: Transfer amyloidosis. I. Studies on the transfer of various lymphoid cells from amyloidotic mice to syngeneic non-amyloidotic recipients. II. Induction of amyloidosis in mice with spleen, thymus and lymph node tissue from casein-sensitized donors, Am. J. Pathol. **65**:411, 1971.
62. Harris, R.E., Hannon, D., Vogler, C., and Hug, G.: Bone marrow transplantation type IIa glycogen storage disease, Birth Defects **22**:119, 1986.
63. Hasumura, Y., Teschke, R., and Lieber, C.S.: Characteristics of acetaldehyde oxidation in rat liver mitochondria, J. Biol. Chem. **251**:4908, 1976.
64. Hay, E.D.: Extracellular matrix, J. Cell Biol. **91**:205s, 1981.
65. Hay, E.D., editor: Cell biology of extracellular matrix, New York, 1982, Plenum Press.
66. Heath, J.P., and Dunn, G.A.: Cell to substratum contacts of chick fibroblasts and their relation to the microfilament system: a correlated interference-reflexion and high-voltage electron-microscope study, J. Cell Sci. **29**:197, 1978.
67. Hecht, F., Hecht, B.K., Morgan, R., Sandberg, A.A., and Link, M.P.: Chromosome clues to acute leukemia in Down's syndrome, Cancer Genet. Cytogenet. **21**:93, 1986.
68. Helminen, H.J., Ericsson, J.L.E., and Orrenius, S.: Studies on mammary gland involution. IV. Histochemical and biochemical observations on alterations in lysosomes and lysosomal enzymes, J. Ultrastruct. Res. **25**:240, 1968.
69. Hershey, J.W.B.: The translational machinery. In Prescott, D.M., and Goldstein, L., editors: A comprehensive treatise, vol. 4, New York, 1980, Academic Press, Inc.
70. Heuser, J.E., and Reese, T.: Structure of the synapse. In Kandel, E.R., editor: Handbook of physiology: the nervous system, vol. 1, Cellular biology of neurons, Baltimore, 1977, Williams & Wilkins Co.
71. Hodgkin, A.L., and Huxley, A.F.: The dual effect of membrane potential on sodium conductance in the giant axon of *Loligo*, J. Physiol. **116**:497, 1952.
72. Houck, J.C., editor: Chemical messengers of the inflammatory process, New York, 1979, Elsevier/North-Holland Inc.
73. Huang, C., Chiang, J., Yeh, G., Chou, P., Shiau, H., Lai, Y., and Li, S.: Cyclopia with trisomy 13, Aust. NZ Obstet. Gynaecol. **27**:251, 1987.
74. Hug, G.: Pre- and postnatal diagnosis of glycogen storage disease, J. Inherited Metab. Dis. **1**:327, 1978.
75. Hug, G.: Pre- and postnatal pathology, enzyme treatment and unresolved issues in five lysosomal disorders, Pharmacol. Rev. **30**:565, 1979.
76. Hug, G.: Glycogen storage disease, Pract. Pediatr. **6**:1, 1984.
77. Hug, G., and Schubert, W.K.: Lysosomes in type II glycogenosis, J. Cell Biol. **35**:C1, 1967.

78. Hug, G., Soukup, S., Chuck, G., and Ryan, M.: Antenatal diagnosis of mucopolysaccharidosis type I (Hurler's disease) is not possible by electronmicroscopy of uncultured amniotic fluid cells, J. Med. Genet. **21**:359, 1984.

79. Hug, G., Soukup, S., Ryan, M., and Chuck, G.: Rapid prenatal diagnosis of glycogen-storage disease type II by electron microscopy of uncultured amniotic-fluid cells, N. Engl. J. Med. **310**:1018, 1984.

80. Hunt, T.: The initiation of protein synthesis, Trends Biochem. Sci. **5**:178, 1980.

81. Iannaccone, P.M., Bossert, N.L., and Connelly, C.S.: Disruption of embryonic and fetal development due to preimplantation chemical insults: a critical review, Am. J. Obstet. Gynecol. **157**:476, 1987.

82. Jennings, R.B., Sommers, H.B., Herdson, P.B., and Kaltenbach, J.P.: Ischemic injury of myocardium, Ann. NY Acad. Sci. **156**:61, 1969.

83. Jennings, R.B., and Reimer, K.A.: Lethal myocardial ischemic injury, Am. J. Pathol. **102**:241, 1981.

84. Kahn, C.R.: Membrane receptors for hormones and neurotransmitters, J. Cell Biol. **70**:261, 1976.

85. Kaplan, L.C., Wayne, A., Crowell, S., and Latt, S.: Trisomy 14 mosaicism in a liveborn male: clinical report and review of the literature, Am. J. Med. Genet. **23**:925, 1986.

86. Katz, B.: The release of neural transmitter substances, Liverpool, 1969, Liverpool University Press.

87. Katz, B., and Miledi, R.: The timing of calcium action during neuromuscular transmission, J. Physiol. **189**:535, 1967.

88. Killenmeyer, R.W.: Hageman factor and acute gouty arthritis, Arthritis Rheum. **11**:452, 1968.

89. Kelley, W.N., and Wyngaarden, J.B.: Enzymology of gout, Adv. Enzymol. **41**:1, 1974.

90. Kimelberg, H.K.: The influence of membrane fluidity on the activity of membrane-bound enzymes. In Poste, G., and Nicolson, G.L., editors: Dynamic aspects of cell surface organization, cell surface reviews, vol. 3, Amsterdam, 1977, Elsevier Publishing Co.

91. Klinenberg, J.R., editor: Proceedings of the second conference on gout and purine metabolism, Arthritis Rheum. **18**(suppl. 6), 1975.

92. Kohn, A., and Fuchs, P.: Initial effects of viral infection in bacterial and animal host cells, Adv. Virus Res. **18**:159, 1973.

93. Kornfeld, R., and Kornfeld, S.: Comparative aspects of glycoprotein structure, Annu. Rev. Biochem. **45**:217, 1976.

94. Kornfeld, S.: Trafficking of lysosomal enzymes in normal and disease states, J. Clin. Invest. **77**:1, 1986.

95. Kuhn, E.M., Sarto, G.E., Bates, B., and Therman, E.: Gene-rich chromosome regions and autosomal trisomy, Hum. Genet. **77**:214, 1987.

96. Lawson, D., Fewtrell, C., and Raff, M.: Localized mast cell degranulation induced by concanavalin A–sepharose beads: implications for the Ca^{++} hypothesis of stimulus-secretion coupling, J. Cell Biol. **79**:394, 1978.

97. Lea, D.E.: Actions of radiations on living cells, Cambridge, 1946, Cambridge University Press.

98. Lesch, M., Gorlin, F., and Sonnenblick, E.H.: Myocardial amino acid transport in the isolated rabbit right ventricular papillary muscle: general characteristics and effects of passive stretch, Circ. Res. **27**:445, 1970.

99. Lesch, M., and Nyhan, W.L.: A familial disorder of uric acid metabolism and central nervous system function, Am. J. Med. **36**:561, 1964.

100. Letourneau, P.C.: Cell-to-substratum adhesion and guidance of axonal elongation, Dev. Biol. **44**:92, 1975.

101. Lieber, C.S., Jones, D.P., Losowsky, M.S., and Davidson, C.S.: Interrelation of uric acid and ethanol metabolism in man, J. Clin. Invest. **41**:1863, 1962.

102. Lombardi, B.: Considerations on the pathogenesis of fatty liver, Lab. Invest. **15**:1, 1966.

103. Malt, R.A.: Compensatory growth of the kidney, N. Engl. J. Med. **280**:1446, 1969.

104. Mason, H.S., Ingram, D.J.E., and Allen, B.: Free radical property of melanins, Arch. Biochem. Biophys. **86**:226, 1960.

105. Michalopoulos, G., Houck, K.A., Dolan, M.L., and Luetteke, N.C.: Control of hepatocyte replication by two serum factors, Cancer Res. **44**:4414, 1984.

106. Michels, V.V.: Fragile sites on human chromosomes: description and clinical significance, Mayo Clin. Proc. **60**:690, 1985.

107. Mitchell, P.: A chemiosmotic hypothesis for the mechanism of oxidative and photosynthetic phosphorylation, Nature **191**:144, 1961.

108. Monod, J., Changeux, J.P., and Jacob, F.: Allosteric proteins and cellular control systems, J. Mol. Biol. **6**:306, 1963.

109. Neufeld, E.F., and Ashwell, G.: Carbohydrate recognition systems for receptor-mediated pinocytosis. In Lennarz, W.J., editor: The biochemistry of glycoproteins and proteoglycans, New York, 1980, Plenum Press.

110. Nomura, M., Tissières, A, and Lengyel, P., editors: Ribosomes, Cold Spring Harbor, New York, 1974, Cold Spring Harbor Laboratory.

111. Nowell, P.L., and Hungerford, D.A.: The etiology of leukemia: some comments on current studies, Semin. Hematol. **3**:114, 1966.

112. Nussbaum, R.L., and Ledbetter, D.H.: Fragile X syndrome: a unique mutation in man, Annu. Rev. Genet. **20**:109, 1986.

113. Ochoa, S., and de Haro, C.: Regulation of protein synthesis in eukaryotes, Annu. Rev. Biochem. **48**:549, 1979.

114. Osserman, E.F.: Plasma-cell myeloma. II. Clinical aspects, N. Engl. J. Med. **261**:952, 1959.

115. Palade, G.: Intracellular aspects of the process of protein synthesis, Science **189**:347, 1975.

116. Pardee, A.B.: A restriction point for control of normal animal cell proliferation, Proc. Natl. Acad. Sci. USA **71**:1286, 1974.

117. Pastan, I.H., and Willingham, M.C.: Receptor-mediated endocytosis of hormones in cultured cells, Annu. Rev. Physiol. **43**:239, 1981.

118. Payvar, F., Wrange, O., Carlstedt-Duke, J., Okret, S., Gustafsson, J.A., and Yamamoto, K.R.: Purified glucocorticoid receptors bind selectively in vitro to a cloned DNA fragment whose transcription is regulated by glucocorticoids in vivo, Proc. Natl. Acad. Sci. USA **78**:6628, 1981.

119. Pereira, H.G.: The cytopathic effect of animal viruses, Adv. Virus Res. **8**:245, 1961.

120. Pirani, C.L., Catchpole, H.R., and Moore, O.: Prevention of casein-induced amyloidosis by splenectomy, Fed. Proc. **18**:500, 1959.

121. Potten, C.S., Schofield, R., and Lajtha, L.G.: A comparison of cell replacement in bone marrow, testis, and three regions of surface epithelium, Biochim. Biophys. Acta **560**:281, 1979.

122. Puck, T.T., and Marcus, P.I.: Action of x-rays on mammalian cells, J. Exp. Med. **103**:653, 1956.

123. Quinn, A.J., and Chapman, D.: The dynamics of membrane structure, CRC Crit. Rev. Biochem. **8**:1, 1980.

124. Rabinowitz, M., Aschenbrenner, V., Albin, R., Gross, N.J., Zak, R., and Nair, K.G.: Synthesis and turnover of heart mitochondria in normal hypertrophied and hypoxic rat. In Alpert, N.R., editor: Cardiac hypertrophy, New York, 1971, Academic Press, Inc.

125. Rieselbach, R.W., Sorenson, L.B., Shelp, W.D., et al.: Diminished renal urate secretion per nephron as a basis for primary gout, Ann. Intern. Med. **73**:359, 1970.

126. Rosa, J., and Rubin, E.: Effects of ethanol on amino acid uptake by rat liver cells, Lab. Invest. **43**:366, 1980.

127. Rossow, P.W., Riddle, V.G.H., and Pardee, A.B.: Synthesis of labile, serum-dependent protein in early G_1 controls animal growth, Proc. Natl. Acad. Sci. USA **76**:4446, 1979.

128. Rottenberg, H., Robertson, D.E., and Rubin, E.: The effect of ethanol on the temperture dependence of respiration and ATPase activities of rat liver mitochondria, Lab. Invest. **42**:318, 1980.

129. Samuelsson, B., Granström, E., Green, K., Hamberg, M., and Hammarström, S.: Prostaglandins, Annu. Rev. Biochem. **44**:669, 1975.

130. Sapienza, C., Peterson, A.C., Rossant, J., and Balling, R.: Degree of methylation of transgenes is dependent on gamete of origin, Nature **328**:251, 1987.

131. Scarpelli, D.G.: Experimental nephrocalcinosis: a biochemical and morphologic study, Lab. Invest. **14**:123, 1965.

132. Schanne, F.A.X., Kane, A.B., Young, E.E., and Farber, J.L.: Calcium dependence of toxic cell death: a final common pathway, Science **206**:700, 1979.

133. Schimmel, P.R., and Söll, D.: Aminoacyl tRNA synthetases: general features and recognition of transfer RNAs, Annu. Rev. Biochem. **48**:601, 1979.

134. Scholes, G., and Weiss, J.: Chemical action of x-rays on nucleic acids and related substances in aqueous systems. II. The mechanism of the action of x-rays on nucleic acids in aqueous systems, Biochem. J. **56**:65, 1954.

135. Scrutton, M.C., and Utter, M.F.: Regulation of glycolysis and gluconeogenesis in animal tissues, Annu. Rev. Biochem. **37**:249, 1968.

136. Shirahama, T., and Cohen, A.S.: High resolution electron microscopic analysis of the amyloid fibril, J. Cell Biol. **33**:679, 1967.

137. Shirahama, T., and Cohen, A.S.: Ultrastructural evidence for leakage of lysosomal contents after phagocytosis of monosodium urate crystals, Am. J. Pathol. **76**:501, 1974.

138. Siekevitz, P.: On the meaning of intracellular structure for metabolic regulation. In Wolstenholme, G.E.W., and O'Connor, C.A., editors: Regulation of cell metabolism, London, 1959, J. & A. Churchill.

139. Silverstein, S.C., Steinman, R.M., and Cohn, Z.A.: Endocytosis, Annu. Rev. Biochem. **46**:669, 1977.

140. Singer, S.J., and Nicolson, G.L.: The fluid mosaic model of the structure of cell membranes, Science **175**:720, 1972.

141. Skou, J.C., and Norby, J.G., editors: Na$^+$-K$^+$ ATP-ase: structure and kinetics, New York, 1979, Academic Press, Inc.

142. Smith, M.T., Thor, H., and Orrenius, S.: Toxic injury to isolated hepatocytes is not dependent on extracellular calcium, Science **213**:1257, 1981.

143. Smuckler, E.A., and Benditt, E.P.: Studies on CCl$_4$ intoxication. III. A subcellular defect in protein synthesis, Biochemistry **4**:671, 1965.

144. Smuckler, E.A., Iseri, O.A., and Benditt, E.P.: A defect in protein synthesis induced by carbon tetrachloride, J. Exp. Med. **116**:55, 1962.

145. Staehelin, L.A., and Hull, B.E.: Junctions between living cells, Sci. Am. **238**(5):141, 1978.

146. Stein, Z.A.: A woman's age: childbearing and child rearing, Am. J. Epidemiol. **121**:327, 1985.

147. Stevens, C.F.: The neuron, Sci. Am. **24**(3):54, 1979.

148. Stevens, C.F.: Ionic channels in neuromembranes: methods for studying their properties. In Koester, J., and Byrne, J.H., editors: Molluscan nerve cells: from biophysics to behavior, Cold Spring Harbor, N.Y., 1980, Cold Spring Harbor Laboratory.

149. Stossel, T.P.: Phagocytosis, N. Engl. J. Med. **290**:717, 774, 833, 1974.

150. Stossel, T.P., and Hartwig, J.H.: Interactions of actin, myosin, and a new actin-binding protein of rabbit pulmonary macrophages: role in cytoplasmic movement and phagocytosis, J. Cell Biol. **68**:602, 1976.

151. Strehler, B.L., and Mildvan, A.S.: Rate and magnitude of age pigment accumulation in the human myocardium, J. Gerontol. **14**:430, 1959.

152. Sutherland, E.W.: Studies on the mechanism of hormone action. Science **177**:401, 1972.

153. Tager, J.M., Elferink, R.P.J.O., Reuser, A., Kroos, M., Ginsel, L.A., Fransen, J.A.M., and Klumperman, J.: α-Glucosidase deficiency (Pompe's disease), Enzyme **38**:280, 1987.

154. Tanaka, T., Harano, Y., Sue, F., et al.: Crystallization, characterization and metabolic regulation of two types of pyruvate kinase from rat tissues, J. Biochem. (Tokyo) **62**:71, 1967.

155. Taylor, D.L., and Condeelis, J.S.: Cytoplasmic structure and contractility in amoeboid cells, Int. Rev. Cytol. **56**:57, 1979.

156. Thomson, M.L.: Relative efficiency of pigment and horny layer thickness in protecting the skin of Europeans and Africans against solar ultraviolet radiation, J. Physiol. **127**:236, 1955.

157. Tijo, J.H., and Levan, A.: The chromosome number of man, Hereditas **42**:1, 1956.

158. Townes, P., and Holtfreter, J.: Directed movements and selective adhesion of embryonic amphibian cells, J. Exp. Zool. **128**:53, 1955.

159. Trump, B.F., Croker, B.P., Jr., and Mergner, W.J.: The role of energy metabolism, ion, and water shifts in the pathogenesis of cell injury. In Richter, G.W., and Scarpelli, D.G., editors: Cell membranes: biological and pathological aspects, Baltimore, 1971, The Williams & Wilkins Co.

160. Virchow, R.: Die Cellularpathologie in ihrer Begründung auf physiologische und pathologische Gewebelehre, Berlin, 1958, A. Hirschwald.

161. Warburton, D.: Chromosomal causes of fetal death, Clin. Obstet. Gynecol. **30**:268, 1987.

162. Weber, G., Singhal, R.L., and Srivastava, S.K.: Regulation of biosynthesis of hepatic gluconeogenetic enzymes. In Weber, G., editor: Advances in enzyme regulation, vol. 3, Oxford, 1965, Pergamon Press, Inc.

163. Weissler, A.M., Kruger, F.A., Baba, N., et al.: Role of anaerobic metabolism in the preservation of functional capacity and structure of anoxic myocardium, J. Clin. Invest. **47**:403, 1968.

164. Weissman, G.: Crystals, lysosomes and gout, Adv. Intern. Med. **19**:239, 1974.

165. Williams, M.L., Feingold, K.R., Grubauer, G., and Elias, P.M.: Ichthyosis induced by cholesterol-lowering drugs, Arch. Dermatol. **123**:1535, 1987.

166. Yamamoto, K.R., and Alberts, B.M.: Steroid receptors: elements for modulation of eukaryotic transcription, Annu. Rev. Biochem. **45**:721, 1976.

167. Yin, H.L., and Stossel, T.P.: Control of cytoplasmic actin gelsol transformation by gelsolin: a calcium-dependent regulatory protein, Nature **281**:583, 1979.

2 Inflammation and Healing

JOSEPH A. MADRI

INFLAMMATION

Inflammation is the characteristic response of mammalian tissue to injury. Whenever tissue is injured, there follows at the site of injury a series of events that tend to destroy or limit the spread of the injurious agent. The early events in this so-called *inflammatory response* are mainly vascular and are usually succeeded by repair and healing of the injured tissue. The inflammatory response might therefore be taken to include the subsequent healing and repair processes, but in this chapter I will consider inflammation and healing as separate events while remembering that inflammation and subsequent repair do merge and overlap and that a clear-cut chronologic distinction is impossible.

The agents that injure tissues and therefore evoke the inflammatory response include bacteria and other types of microorganisms and nonliving agents such as trauma, heat, cold, radiant and electrical energy, and chemicals. Because of the diversity of the causative factors, inflammation is one of the most common and important conditions with which the physician has to deal.

Historical perspective

Inflammation, the response of any vascularized tissue to injury, has been written about and studied for at least 4000 years. The roman Celsus described the four cardinal signs of inflammation: *rubor* 'redness,' *calor* 'heat,' *dolor* 'pain,' and *tumor* 'swelling.' Before the writings of Hunter in the late 1700s which describe the inflammatory response as salutary this response was believed to be attributable to an unhealthful breakdown of the blood elements, which prompted phlebotomy as a treatment. It wasn't until the 1800s that the importance of the microvasculature became evident. In several classic experiments Cohnheim elegantly demonstrated and documented the microcirculation using living whole mounts of frog tongue and mesentery. Furthermore, when he injured the microvascular beds he noticed dramatic changes in blood flow, permeability, and inflammatory cell movements into tissues. These findings were the first correlation between the signs of inflammation first written about by the ancients and the changes in the microcirculation of the affected areas. Thus, although at first glance it may appear that western medical science has made great strides in advancing our understanding of the inflammatory process, a brief look back indicates that we have just begun a long, complex investigation of a process of major importance to our health.[12,13]

Definition and signs of inflammation

A definition of inflammation is complicated because the local vascular and tissue reactions may be accompanied by systemic effects that include malaise, fever, leukocytosis, metabolic disturbances, and shock.

According to its duration, inflammation is described as acute or chronic. Sometimes the acute process subsides but the stimulus persists sufficiently to evoke a subsequent chronic inflammation. In other cases, with a stimulus that typically induces chronic inflammation, the tissue response may be acute for the first day or so. The tissue response differs considerably in acute and chronic inflammation. However, when inflammation or the inflammatory response is mentioned in this chapter without qualification, it is acute inflammation that is being discussed.

Main events in an acute inflammatory process—a vascular reaction

The following account of acute inflammation describes the main events composing the inflammatory process, discusses the mechanism of these events, and indicates how the events are responsible for the clinical signs of inflammation.

The early features of the inflammatory response result from reactions of the small blood vessels in the injured tissue. Some of the features are demonstrated by the events induced by firm stroking of the skin on the inner aspect of the forearm. The line of the stroke is accurately marked by a red line that appears in 3 to 18 seconds and reaches a peak in 30 to 50 seconds. When the stroking is heavy or repeated several times in succession, the red line becomes bordered by a spreading flush that appears in the first minute and intensifies into a bright red flare. Finally, the red line becomes replaced by a pale wheal, which begins 1 to 3 minutes

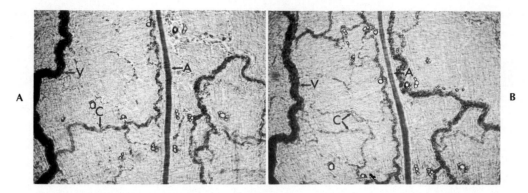

Fig. 2-1. A, Arteriole, *A,* capillary, *C,* and venule, *V,* in periphery of uninjured rabbit ear chamber. **B,** Same area shown in **A** 24 hours after injury. Notice engorgement of additional capillaries, *C.* (65×; from Allison, F., Jr., Smith, M.R., and Wood, W.B., Jr.: J. Exp. Med. **102:**655, 1955.)

after the stroking and becomes maximal in 3 to 5 minutes. Next, the wheal and then the flare become pale, but it is 1 or several hours before the wheal subsides.

The red line results from local vasodilatation of capillaries and small venules, the flare is caused by dilatation of the neighboring arterioles, and the wheal represents local edema. The local *vasodilatation* and the *flare* and *wheal* constitute what Lewis[6] termed the "triple response."

One can obtain similar effects by pricking or scratching, by freezing or burning, or by inducing electrical or chemical injury. With cold, electrical, or chemical injury, the triple response is often accompanied by itching or pain. These simple experiments therefore elicit the four classic signs of inflammation—redness, swelling, heat, and pain. They also demonstrate that the same events are evoked by various kinds of stimuli and that the events themselves are predominantly vascular in nature.

Microscopic observations

When the early vascular events in injured tissue are observed microscopically, it becomes apparent that the responses of the vessels[2,3] are far more complex than might be believed from macroscopic observation.

The events can be demonstrated in the vessels of the exposed frog tongue or mesenteric loops of rats. Both tissues are thin enough to be examined in the living state with the light microscope and were used by Cohnheim in his pioneering classic studies on inflammation.[7,10] The connective tissue beds of rabbit ears have also proved to be a valuable experimental model. Special chambers (called ear chambers) are inserted into rabbit ears to allow one to see the vascular bed with great clarity and watch what happens when it is injured. A typical view of the microvessels obtained in this way is shown in Fig. 2-1, *A.*

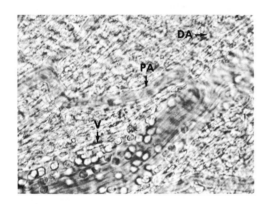

Fig. 2-2. Vascular shunt in which blood flow bypasses lesion located at upper right. Blood is flowing from proximal arteriole, *PA,* to venule, *V,* and bypassing distal arteriole, *DA.* Sticking of leukocytes is pronounced in venule. (250×; from Allison, F., Jr., Smith, M.R., and Wood, W.B., Jr.: J. Exp. Med. **102:**655, 1955.)

Immediately after injury, regardless of the stimulus, there is transient vasoconstriction of the arterioles. With mild injury, blood flow may be reestablished in a few seconds. With strong thermal injury, however, the vasoconstriction lasts about 5 minutes. Then follows a progressive dilatation of the blood vessels, which involves mainly the arterioles but also, to less extent, the venules and capillaries. Within 30 minutes, the arteriolar dilatation is evident, and blood flow through the injured tissues is greater than before injury. The arteriolar dilatation continues to increase, so that by 24 hours after injury the blood vessels of the area are engorged, and the capillaries and veins in which there was previously little or no blood flow now carry a rapid stream (Figs. 2-1 and 2-2). Arteriolar pulsation becomes so strong that it is transmitted to the capillaries and venules, and the whole area visibly pulsates.

Two further events are important in the development of the inflammatory response. The first is the exudation of plasma from blood vessels in the injured tissues. This exudation is accompanied by a decrease in blood flow. As the bloodstream slows, the formed elements become redistributed in the local circulation as a preliminary to the second important event—the emigration of neutrophilic leukocytes into the injured tissues.

Exudation of plasma. From microscopic examination, the tissues in and adjacent to the injured areas appear increasingly dense from the accumulation of edema fluid, which indicates the escape of plasma through the wall of the peripheral vascular bed. Immediately adjacent to the site of injury, edema begins to develop in the first 10 to 15 minutes. Farther afield, where the intensity of the stimulus is less, edema appears more slowly. Edema causes swelling of inflamed tissue. Edema is also recognizable in blisters, such as occur in second-degree burns, and exudation also results in the accumulation of fluid in cavities lined by inflamed serosal membranes (for example, pleurisy with effusion).

Edema fluid in inflamed tissue is characterized by high protein content (1 to 6 g/dl) and ready coagulability (because of the content of fibrinogen and other clotting factors). In contrast to exudate, the term *transudate* refers to fluid that leaks out of vessels in noninflammatory conditions such as congestive cardiac failure. Transudates have a protein content less than 1 g/dl and less tendency to coagulate. The protein is mainly albumin.

The local exudation of plasma in inflammation can be demonstrated by intravenous administration of a marker dye to animals fitted with ear chambers. Using mercuric sulfide as a marker Arnold noted this in 1875.[7,10] Such dyes become bound to plasma albumin, so that their accumulation provides an indicator of the exudation of plasma protein. By this technique,[14] dye is observed to begin escaping in ear chambers as early as 3 minutes after injury. Coloration of the lesions by dye reaches a peak 3 hours after injury. As vascular stasis spreads from the center to the periphery of the lesions and adjacent tissues, the vessels exhibiting stasis cease to exude dye. Finally, as stasis becomes more prominent, hemorrhage occurs adjacent to the obstructed vessels.

Changes in formed elements of blood. In the early stages of the inflammatory response, blood flow through the dilated vessels becomes accelerated, so that the movement of the individual blood cells is too rapid to be followed by the eye. But after some hours, the rate decreases and flow may even cease. The early acceleration is readily explained by the dilatation of the arteriolar bed, which results in an increase in hydrostatic pressure at the proximal end of the capillaries and hence an increased gradient of hydrostatic pressure in

the capillary bed. The subsequent slowing of blood flow has been attributed to an increase in blood viscosity. It has been hypothesized that the escape of plasma into the tissues has the effect of increasing the concentration of red cells in the circulating blood that enters the venules. The consequent rise in the viscosity of the blood increases the resistance to flow in the venules with a corresponding rise in hydrostatic pressure in the capillary bed. The later effect assists the expulsion of more plasma and therefore further increases viscosity, the slowing of venular blood flow, and the ensuing cycle of events that terminate in stasis.

While stasis is developing, the distribution of the red and white cells change within the affected vessels (Fig. 2-3). As blood flow slows in the dilated vessels, the axial column of blood cells becomes relatively wider and the plasmatic zone much narrower—as might be expected from the loss of plasma by exudation. The redistribution of the blood cells is followed by striking behavior on the part of the neutrophilic leukocytes.

Emigration of neutrophilic leukocytes. The peripheral leukocytes begin to stick to the vascular endothelium. At first they stick momentarily and then move on with the flow of the blood. But the duration of sticking gradually increases, and finally some of the neutrophils remain adherent to the endothelium.

In rabbit ear chambers, neutrophils begin adhering to the endothelium within a few minutes, the response becoming quite distinct in 15 to 30 minutes (Fig. 2-2).

Ear chamber studies after thermal injury have revealed that vasodilatation is the rule, though not a necessary precursor for the adherence of neutrophils. Another part is the frequent sticking of white cells to one another. Furthermore, when leukocytes sticking to endothelium become dislodged, the displaced cells do not attach themselves to uninjured endothelium farther along the same vessel.

Soon after the onset of sticking of neutrophils to endothelium, the cells begin to migrate through the vascular wall into the adjacent tissues. The adherent cells first move over the endothelium (Fig. 2-4). When a suitable site is found, the process of emigration commences, with each cell taking several minutes to migrate through the wall of a blood vessel. After a cell has passed through the vessel wall, a defect seems to exist in the vessel wall and additional cells often flow the same route.

Initially, emigration of neutrophils is more evident in vessels nearer the lesion than in those farther removed. But, as stasis develops adjacent to the lesion, emigration becomes more noticeable in vessels farther afield.

Hemorrhage. Hemorrhage often occurs in severe inflammation. In the ear chamber, thermal burns cause noticeable hemorrhage 3 to 6 hours after injury, particularly adjacent to vessels that are dilated and exhibiting

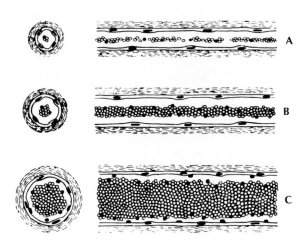

Fig. 2-3. Progressive changes in caliber of blood vessels and character of blood flow in an area of inflammation. **A,** Normal venule with its axial stream of cells. White cells *(closed circles)* tend to lie centrally among column of red cells *(open circles),* surrounded by wide plasmatic zone. **B,** Early stage of inflammation showing vascular dilatation and broader axial stream of cells. Leukocytes are now more peripheral in column, but plasmatic zone is still conspicuous. **C,** Later stage of inflammation showing still further vascular dilatation. Central column of cells is now much broader and plasmatic zone correspondingly reduced. Peripherally placed white cells are now close or even adhering to endothelium. (From Wright, G.P.: An introduction of pathology, ed. 3, London, 1958, Longmans, Green & Co. Ltd.)

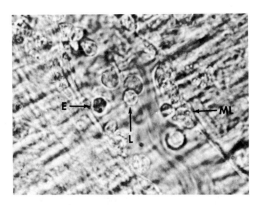

Fig. 2-4. Leukocytes migrating on endothelial surface before emigrating through wall of blood vessel. Motile cells, *ML,* have lost their usual globular shape, *L.* One erythrocyte, *E,* is adhering to endothelium. (250×; from Allison, F., Jr., Smith, M.R., and Wood, W.B., Jr.: J. Exp. Med. **102:**655, 1955.)

stasis. Red cells escape through the vessel wall by a seemingly passive process termed "diapedesis." Often they become trapped in the endothelial defects left by emigrating leukocytes, and one or several erythrocytes "trickle" through the wall of the vessel.

• • •

In summary, acute inflammation is characterized by three main vascular events: (1) vasodilatation and changes in blood flow, (2) exudation of plasma, and (3) emigration of neutrophilic leukocytes. These events will now be considered in some detail.

Vasodilatation and changes in blood flow

In the triple response, vasodilatation involves first the postcapillary venules and capillaries at the site of injury and then the adjacent arterioles.

The mechanism responsible for the local dilatation of capillaries and venules are examined by Lewis[6] in a series of experiments whose simplicity is a lesson in experimental technique. The response can be compared on both forearms of the same subject, with one arm having its circulation occluded by an inflated sphygmomanometer cuff above the elbow. Firm stroking of the skin of both forearms results in vasodilatation of each. Vasodilatation on the unobstructed arm lasts about 10 minutes. On the arm with the cuff, the vasodilatation lasts as long as the arterial obstruction is continued, with the longest test period being 25 minutes. As soon as the sphygmomanometer cuff is released, the erythema behaves like that on the unobstructed arm and fades during the ensuing 10 minutes. With heating at 43° to 44° C, the duration of the initial erythema can be similarly prolonged by arterial obstruction.

Lewis interpreted these results to indicate that injury leads to the local release of a substance responsible for the dilatation of the capillaries and venules. When blood is circulating freely in the vessels of the injured tissues, the vasodilator substance is removed by the flowing blood in about 10 minutes. But when the arterial circulation is obstructed, the liberated substance is retained locally as long as the circulation is occluded. Lewis obtained strong support for these conclusions by obtaining similar results when low doses of histamine were pricked into the skin. Not only did histamine induce a typical triple response, but the fading of the initial erythema was also delayed by arterial obstruction as with injury by stroking.

There are other substances, apart from histamine, that play a role in mediating vasodilatation. Kinins,[25,29,32,33] in particular, have attracted attention because (1) kinin-forming enzymes appear to be associated with physiologic vasodilatation and (2) kinins accumulate in inflammatory exudates.[28] Since kinins are vasodilators under physiologic conditions, they may well play a similar role in pathologic conditions such as inflammation. These and other substances are discussed below.

Exudation of plasma

Under physiologic conditions the endothelium of the capillaries and proximal portion of the venules permits free movement of water and small molecules to and fro across the endothelium but normally restricts the passage of plasma protein. According to Starling's theory, fluid equilibrium across this endothelial barrier is maintained by the hydrostatic pressure of the capillary blood being balanced by the equal and opposite restraint of the osmotic pressure of the plasma proteins. In inflammation, there is a net movement of fluid into the tissues that has been estimated to be five to seven times greater than that from a normal vessel with similar levels of hydrostatic pressure and plasma protein. The fluid exudate of inflammation characteristically contains 1 to 6 g of plasma protein per 100 ml. The protein content of the exudate may even reach that of plasma itself.

Demonstration of permeability responses in inflammation. A simple method of identifying and quantifying increased vascular permeability depends on the use of vital dyes. When circulating in the blood, such dyes accumulate in skin sites that have been damaged by injury. Vital dyes all form complexes with plasma albumin and other plasma proteins, so that their local accumulation in tissues indicates a movement of plasma protein across vascular endothelium.

For experimental injury, one can assess a permeability response by measuring the amount of dye that exudes into the injured tissue (Fig. 2-5).[82] When factors believed to increase permeability are tested by injection into skin, the exuded dye forms a round blue lesion at the injection site, with the mean diameter of the lesion being proportional to the dose of factor injected.

One performs the dye technique by giving a standard dose of dye intravenously to experimental animals from which the fur on the back of the trunk has been removed. Experimental injury (such as by heating) can be obtained by application of a heated metal disk to the skin, as described in the legend for Fig. 2-5. Dye accumulates locally in a few minutes after injury, but the coloration then remains unchanged for some hours, and so subsequent fluctuations in the permeability of the local vascular bed cannot be discerned. This disadvantage is easily overcome by withholding of the intravenous injection of dye until the animal bears several sites heated at intervals beforehand to give lesions of different ages. Intravenous dye will now exude only into sites where vascular permeability is still increased. The technique therefore allows us to map the life history or time course of the permeability response.

Permeability factors. Much effort has gone into identifying substances produced at sites of injury that might

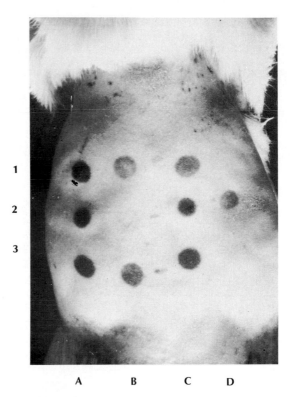

Fig. 2-5. Method of demonstrating increased vascular permeability. Metal disk (8.5 mm in diameter) heated to 54° C was applied for 5 seconds to depilated skin of back of trunk of guinea pig previously given Evans blue dye intravenously. Dye exudes into injured sites, and intensity of permeability response can be assessed by estimation of amount of dye extracted from each lesion. (From Wilhelm, D.L., and Mason, B.: Br. J. Exp. Pathol. **45**:487, 1960.)

be responsible for the characteristic increase of vascular permeability. Since histamine and other factors did not provide all the answers to the problem, the continuing search has resulted in an ever-growing list of so-called permeability factors that were isolated from normal and inflamed tissues. These substances fall into four main groups:

1. Pharmacologically active amines, such as histamine and 5-hydroxytryptamine
2. Polypeptides such as bradykinin, together with various proteolytic enzymes whose activity probably results in the production of these polypeptides; such enzymes include kallikrein, plasmin, and possibly trypsin
3. Prostaglandins, particularly E_1 and E_2 and leukotrienes
4. Derivatives of the third and fifth components of complement such as the anaphylatoxins

Histamine. Histamine is still the first substance considered in any discussion of the natural mediators of inflammation. Histamine is widespread in the tissues

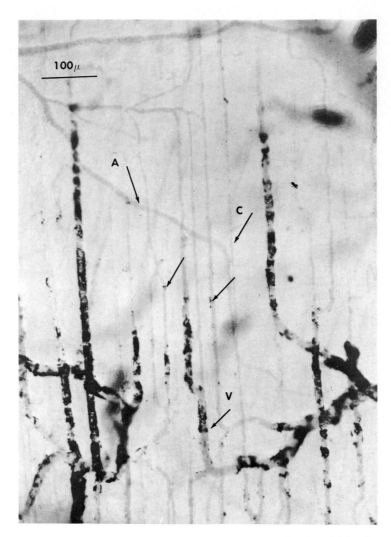

Fig. 2-6. From preparation of rat cremaster muscle 1 hour after local injection of histamine and intravenous injection of colloidal carbon. This field shows arteriole, *A*, branching into capillaries, *C*, with later draining into venules, *V*. Histamine-induced leaks are marked by deposits of carbon. Notice that there are no deposits at arterial end of capillaries, that occasional small deposits appear along venous end, and that heavy deposits occur only in venules *(arrows)*. (140×; from Majno, G.: Mechanism of abnormal vascular permeability in acute inflammation. In Thomas, L., Uhr, J.W., and Grant, L., editors: International symposium on injury, inflammation and immunity, Baltimore, 1964, The Williams & Wilkins Co.; copyrighted by Miles Laboratories, Inc.)

and is associated particularly with the granules of mast cells.[27,31]

Tissue histamine is probably obtained from three main sources[23,24]: (1) decarboxylation of histidine in the tissues, (2) decarboxylation of histidine by bacteria in the bowel, and (3) the diet. Although the actual mechanism of the release of histamine is unclear, this agent is readily released as a result of various kinds of tissue injury, including anaphylaxis. Histamine causes dilatation of capillaries and increases the permeability of venules to plasma protein.

Claims that histamine is a natural permeability factor in injury are based on three main pieces of evidence:

1. Lewis's work[6] on the triple response
2. Its widespread distribution, ready release, and high activity as a permeability factor, particularly in guinea pigs, rabbits, and humans
3. Suppression of the permeability response in mild inflammation by histamine antagonists[11,36] (Fig. 2-5)
4. In several recent studies investigators have demonstrated histamine receptors on endothelial cells of a variety of vascular beds[18]

5-Hydroxytryptamine. 5-Hydroxytryptamine (5-HT, serotonin) was found to be a potent permeability factor in rats.[11] Rats have long been popular for experimental work on inflammation, but the low activity of histamine as a permeability factor in this species provided at least one good reason for doubting the overall importance of histamine in inflammation. When 5-HT was demonstrated to have high activity in both rats and mice, it seemed possible that a family of amines might be involved rather than histamine itself.

As with histamine, 5-HT is widely distributed in the body tissues, with the highest concentrations occurring in the intestine, blood, spleen, and nervous system. In rats its activity as a permeability factor is exceeded only by bradykinin. Furthermore, there is evidence consistent with the presence of 5-hydroxytryptamine receptors on endothelial cells of various microvascular beds.[19]

Recent studies with the electron microscope have revealed that the increased permeability of injured small blood vessels is associated with intercellular changes in and contraction of vascular endothelium.[17,22]

In addition to dyes, circulating colloidal carbon also allows identification of vessels having increased permeability by becoming deposited in the walls of the involved vessels. In animals given india ink intravenously, deposits of carbon quickly fill venules and capillaries in the injured tissues (Fig. 2-6). After treatment of cremaster muscle of the rats with histamine or 5-HT, the labeling is confined to venules 7 to 100 μm in diameter, with the heaviest labeling in venules 20 to 30 μm in diameter. The capillaries do not exhibit labeling. Electron microscopic examination of the labeled venules reveals that the endothelial cells become separated by gaps 0.1 to 1 μm in width (Fig. 2-7), which appear as early as 1 minute after histamine or 5-HT is applied. The affected endothelial cells appear to be partially disconnected along their intercellular junctions, whereas the basement membrane remains intact and serves as an additional barrier.

The gaps between the endothelial cells provide a ready passage for the escape of plasma through the vessel wall to the basement membrane. The plasma passes on, but if the circulating blood contains a "marker" substance such as colloidal carbon, particles of the marker are restrained by the basement membrane. The mechanism responsible for the separation of the endothelial cells remain to be identified, but progress has been made in the identification of several cytoskeletal elements (including actin, myosin, tropomyosin, alpha-actinin, and vinculin) in various endothelial cells that may participate in receptor-mediated contraction.[17,18]

Kinins and proteolytic enzymes. The generation of biologically active peptides from larger inactive precursor proteins by specific proteolytic enzymes is a biologic principle that is encountered frequently in living systems. This biochemical mechanism recurs repeatedly throughout all stages of the inflammatory reaction. An extremely active peptide generated by proteolytic cleavage of a plasma protein is the nonapeptide bradykinin. Bradykinin is generated by the action of a class of proteolytic enzymes called the kallikreins. These act on larger proteins, generating either the nonapeptide bradykinin or the decapeptide kallidin, which is simply bradykinin containing an extra lysine residue.

Kallidin

H.Lys.Arg.Pro.Pro.Gly.Phe.Ser.Pro.Phe.Arg.OH

Bradykinin

All kallikreins are proteolytic and esterolytic enzymes, and most share with trypsin the ability to hydrolyze certain peptide bonds. Kallikreins are widely distributed in the body and fall into two groups: (1) tissue kallikreins, which occur particularly in glandular organs (such as the salivary glands, the pancreas, and the sweat and lacrimal glands), as well as in the kidney and intestinal mucosa, and (2) plasma kallikrein. Although closely related, the tissue kallikreins appear to be distinct. They are produced in the various tissues as the active enzyme or the inert precursor.

Kinins[25,29,32,33] are formed from high–molecular weight glycoproteins termed "kininogens." Kinins have an extremely short half-life in circulating blood, being hydrolyzed by kininases to inactive peptides. The interrelation of the kinin system can therefore be summarized as follows:

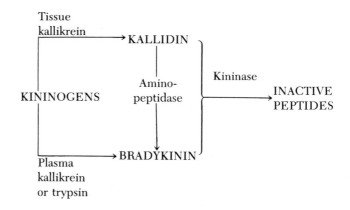

Bradykinin, kallidin, and other kinins have high activity as permeability factors,[34] their high potency being apparent whatever the species of test animal. The technique of vascular labeling with colloidal carbon given intravenously (Fig. 2-6) and subsequent examination by electron microscopy indicates that the effects of bradykinin (Fig. 2-7) parallel those of histamine and 5-HT in causing interendothelial gaps in venules.[20]

Leukotrienes. The leukotrienes are complex lipid molecules that are derived enzymatically from the breakdown of phospholipid molecules of cell membranes. Leukotrienes were originally described as being derived from leukocytes (hence the name), but it now appears that leukotrienes of different types can be gen-

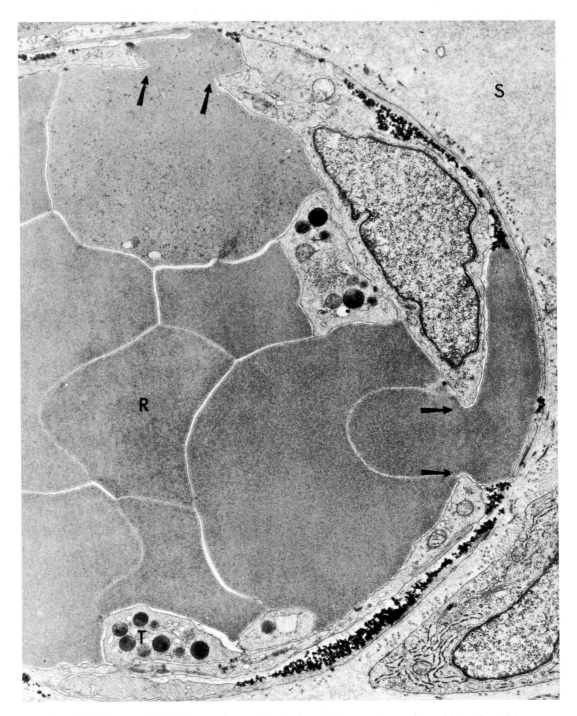

Fig. 2-7. Interendothelial gaps in venules induced by agents such as histamine, 5-hy-droxytryptamine, or bradykinin. Electron micrograph of venule in rat striated muscle 6 minutes after treatment with bradykinin. Lumen is packed with red blood cells, *R*. Three gaps have formed in venular wall by separation of endothelial cells: one at top *(between arrows)* plugged by reticulocyte; one at right *(between arrows)* plugged by red blood cell; one at bottom plugged by thrombocyte, *T*. Dark granules in venular wall represent carbon particles, which had been administered intravenously just before local injection of bradykinin. Basement membrane, which is holding back components of blood that have passed through endothelial gaps, is visible as faint gray line just outside endothelium. *S*, Extracellular space. (19,400×; courtesy Prof. Guido Majno; from Wilhelm, D.L.: Rev. Can. Biol. **30:**153, 1971.)

erated from macrophages, tissue mast cells, and other connective tissue cells as well.[70] Leukotrienes are generated first by the action of phospholipases on membrane phospholipids that release arachidonic acid, which is in turn converted by a series of enzymes to many complex forms, among them prostaglandins, thromboxanes, and the family of molecules called leukotrienes. Some of the leukotrienes are extremely potent bronchoconstricting and vasoconstricting agents, and some have actions similar to histamine but are far more powerful. When applied to appropriate vascular beds, some of the leukotrienes (LTC$_4$) cause transient vasoconstriction that is followed by a sharp increase in the leakiness of the venules of the treated vessels. The leukotrienes seem to act directly on the vessel wall, rather than acting through the liberation of histamine. Another leukotriene, LTE$_4$ has been found to induce gaps between endothelial cells of postcapillary venules by causing contraction of the endothelial cells.[55] Another class of leukotrienes, distinct from those that act on blood vessels, appears to act directly on leukocytes, causing effects that mimic those found in inflammatory reactions. This particular class of leukotrienes promotes adhesion of leukocytes to the walls of venules and their subsequent extravasation into the tissue spaces. These leukotrienes are also chemotactic for neutrophils, eosin-

ophils, and monocytes. Finally, such leukotrienes stimulate leukocytes to release lysosomal enzymes, consistent with the idea that these leukotrienes play an important role in activating many of the cellular reactions found in acute inflammation. Leukotrienes are now known to be the biologically active agents that were once referred to as the slow-reacting substances of anaphylaxis (SRS-A).[47-49]

Pattern and mechanism of increased vascular permeability. The permeability responses in various examples of experimental injury fall into three main categories, according to their onset after injury: (1) immediate, (2) delayed, and (3) early. For each category the response may have a shorter or longer duration, so that there is a total of six main types of response (Fig. 2-8).

Immediate responses (Fig. 2-8, curves A and B) are exhibited in thermal injury and injury from ultraviolet light, as well as in anaphylaxis in both guinea pigs and rats. The provocative stimuli are usually mild or short lived, though for injury to occur from ultraviolet light the stimulus needs to be quite strong. The permeability response is transient, with peak effects being reached in 5 minutes and normal permeability usually restored in 10 to 15 minutes. The same type of response is also obtained with histamine, 5-HT, and bradykinin.

The immediate response is usually mediated in injury

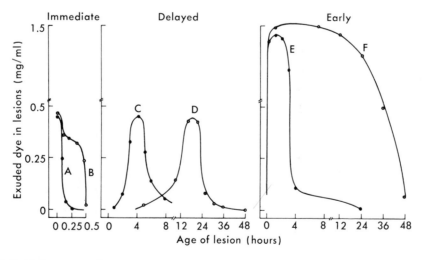

Fig. 2-8. Main types of vascular permeability responses induced in skin of guinea pig. Animals had previously received Evans blue dye, and exudation was induced by thermal injury of varying intensity, by ultraviolet injury, and by intracutaneous injection of the histamine liberator, compound 48/80. Immediate responses *(left side):* curve *A* (heating at 54° C for 5 seconds); curve *B* (intracutaneous injection of compound 48/80). Delayed responses *(center):* curve *C* (heating at 54° C for 20 seconds); curve *D* (ultraviolet radiation for 20 seconds). Early responses *(right side):* curve *E* (heating at 58° C for 20 seconds); curve *F* (heating at 60° C for 60 seconds). (From Wilhelm, E.L.: Pattern and mechanism of increased vascular permeability in inflammation. In Zweifach, B.W., Grant, L., and McCluskey, R.T., editors: The inflammatory process, vol. 2, ed. 2, New York, 1973, Academic Press, Inc.)

by histamine or 5-HT released from the injured cells. This response is readily suppressed by antihistamines or antagonists of 5-HT. As might be expected, the lesion (for example, in mild thermal injury of skin) is the interendothelial gap in venules (Figs. 2-6 and 2-7).

Some immediate responses are slightly prolonged as illustrated by curve *B* in Fig. 2-8.

Delayed responses have a comparatively late onset, being preceded by a latent interval of normal low permeability. Peak effects occur at about 4 hours (Fig. 2-8, curve *C*) or 24 hours (Fig. 2-8, curve *D*).

A typical delayed response of short duration can be elicited by thermal injury in guinea pig skin. This pattern is often combined with a preceding early response to give a diphasic effect. For thermal injury, the initial responses depend to some extent on the animal species. The same pattern of increased permeability is also induced by bacterial infection[15] and the alpha toxin of *Clostridium welchii*,[21] one of the organisms that causes gas gangrene.

Delayed responses of prolonged duration are observed in mild ultraviolet light or chemical injury, in delayed hypersensitivity, and in skin sites injected with various bacterial toxins. Carbon labeling indicates that both venules and capillaries are affected. Electron microscopically, the venules show intercellular gaps in the endothelium of small and medium-sized vessels, whereas the smaller capillaries contain thrombi that plug their lumens and often show damage and disruption of the endothelium.[16] This type of response is also usually part of a diphasic effect.

The results indicate that such responses may involve pharmacologic mediation affecting venules, as well as direct damage of vascular endothelium, particularly of capillaries.

Early responses seem to represent the effects of relatively strong stimuli[35] such as surgical incision, heating (for example, at 60° C), or the application of organic solvents such as xylol, benzene, or chloroform. A strong permeability response may begin within a few minutes of injury and reach a peak in 15 to 30 minutes, or in about 60 minutes with weaker stimuli (Fig. 2-8). Early responses may last 1 to several hours or may be greatly prolonged as in the case of severe burns. As might be expected, endothelial disruption is a prominent feature. Carbon labeling indicates that venules, capillaries, and even arterioles are involved. Electron microscopically, there is injury to endothelium and pericytes, as well as fragmentation and sloughing of endothelial cells. Leaking vessels, particularly capillaries, often are occluded by thrombi consisting of platelets and fibrin.

Summary. The permeability effects in acute inflammation may include six types of response. Under particular circumstances, each of the six types may occur alone as a monophasic permeability response, but an immediate response or a short-term early response may be succeeded after a latent interval by a delayed response to give a diphasic response.

As for the mechanisms involved, immediate responses are usually mediated by amines such as histamine and 5-HT. Electron microscopic evidence indicates that pharmacologic mediation may be mainly responsible for lesions in the faster type of delayed response but is accompanied by endothelial damage in the slower type. Kinins have been proposed as the natural mediators of delayed responses, but there is no convincing evidence for this proposal. Endothelial damage is prominent in lesions of early responses.

Emigration of neutrophilic leukocytes

The emigration of neutrophilic leukocytes through the wall of blood vessels into the adjacent tissues represents the main cellular phase of acute inflammation.[26]

Reference has already been made to the evidence from studies of transparent preparations and rabbit ear chambers that neutrophils bind to the endothelium of venules and, to a lesser extent, of capillaries before migrating through the vascular wall (Fig. 2-9). *Adherence* and *emigration* of neutrophils is now discussed in the light of additional information obtained with the electron microscope.

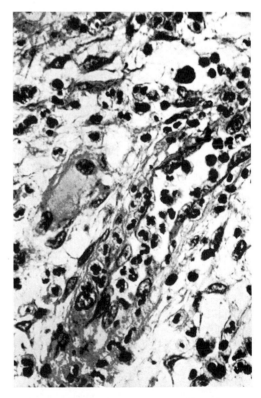

Fig. 2-9. Emigration of leukocytes of nasal polyp. Neutrophilic leukocytes are present in lumen of vessel in center, but number of neutrophils are emigrating through vessel wall or have reached tissues immediately around vessel. (640×.)

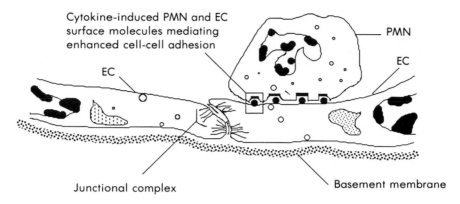

Fig. 2-10. Adhesion of a polymorphonuclear leukocyte to a microvascular endothelial cell after cytokine activation.

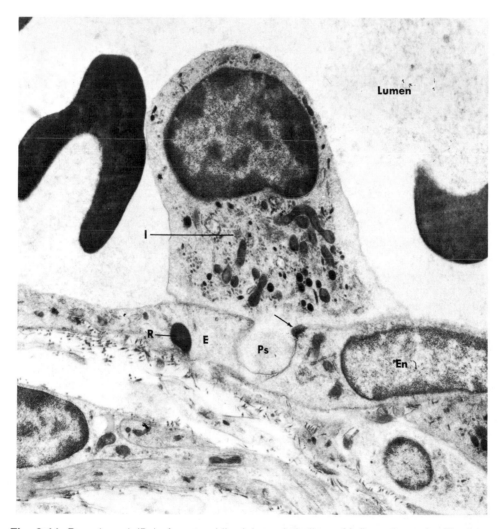

Fig. 2-11. Pseudopod *(Ps)* of neutrophils, *I,* in endothelium of inflamed venule. Electron-dense material *(arrow)* may be part of attachment belt. *R,* Part of red blood cell within cytoplasm of endothelial cell, *E. En,* Nucleus of endothelial cell. (11,700×; from Marchesi, V.T., and Florey, H.W.: Q. J. Exp. Physiol. **45:**343, 1960.)

Sticking of neutrophils. With the light microscope, neutrophils are seen to adhere to the walls of *venules.* The cells behave as though attached to a sticky surface, along which they are slowly pushed by the bloodstream.

As leukocytes come into contact with the endothelium of venules in injured tissue, the cells adhere to the endothelium, and the margin of the cell in contact with the endothelium becomes flattened. Some of these neutrophils appear to move on the inner surface of the endothelium by ameboid motion. The phenomenon of leukocytic adhesion seems to be attributable to soluble factor–induced changes in the cell surfaces of the leukocyte and the endothelial cell (Fig. 2-10). The biochemical mechanisms are currently only incompletely understood.[39,50,51]

Escape of neutrophils. Once a neutrophil becomes closely apposed to the endothelium of venules, it extrudes a pseudopod preparatory to migrating (Fig. 2-11). If extrusion occurs at or near a cell junction, the neutrophil forces its way through the junction down to the basement membrane of the endothelium (Fig. 2-12 and 2-13). Serial sections of neutrophils in different stages of emigration indicate that the pseudopod separates the intercellular junctions between the endothelial cells. The advancing pseudopod is then followed by the main body of the cell. How the pseudopod separates the junction is not understood, but it may be the result of physical force or be associated with enzymatic activity.

Neutrophils that manage to emigrate between the endothelial cells come against a second barrier—the basement membrane[59]—which, with the periendothelial cells and connective tissue, collectively forms the periendothelial sheath. This barrier hinders the continued migration of the neutrophil so that its pseudopod usually changes course to take up a position between an endothelial cell and its basement membrane. Eventually, the neutrophil penetrates the periendothelial sheath and emerges into the connective tissue around the venule (Fig. 2-13). Penetration of the wall takes about 3 to 9 minutes. Once clear of the wall, the neutrophils move in the perivascular tissues at rates of up to 20 μm per minute. Eosinophils and monocytes migrate through the venular wall in the same manner as neutrophils.

The migration of neutrophils does not appear to leave a breach in the endothelium. The edges of the adjacent endothelial cells that are separated keep in contact with the emigrating cell and apparently come together again after the leukocyte has escaped through the endothelium.[46,59] Nevertheless, the escape of a neutrophil is sometimes followed by a trickle of erythrocytes from the same site in the endothelium. This process, diapedesis of the red cells, appears to be passive.

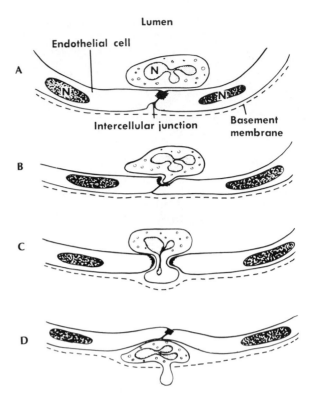

Fig. 2-12. Progressive stages in migration of neutrophil, *N*, through venule in acute inflammation. Cell penetrates intercellular junction and separates endothelial cells. (From Marchesi, V.T., and Gowans, J.L.: Proc. R. Soc. Lond. [Biol.] **159**:283, 1964.)

Sequential accumulation of cells in inflamed tissues. Practically any type of tissue injury evokes an initial accumulation of neutrophilic leukocytes. If the lesion persists for some time, these polymorphonuclear cells often become replaced by mononuclear cells (monocytes, macrophages, and their derivatives), as well as by lymphocytes. Such a transition is typically illustrated by the cellular accumulation in lobar pneumonia: the initial dense accumulation of neutrophils exhibits an increasing proportion of mononuclear phagocytes. Although not invariable, such a transition is common, whatever the type of infection or cause of injury, but differs in time of onset, rate of development, and the proportion of mononuclear cells in the inflamed tissue. If some infections, either acute (such as typhoid fever) or chronic (tuberculosis), the cellular reaction is characteristically "mononuclear"—but even in these cases there is an initial transient infiltration by neutrophils, which quickly gives way to a substantial and persistent accumulation of mononuclear cells.

Since the initial cellular reaction is similar whatever the type of injury, how does the cell type change from predominantly neutrophils to mononuclear cells? Current hypotheses include changes in the surface proteins

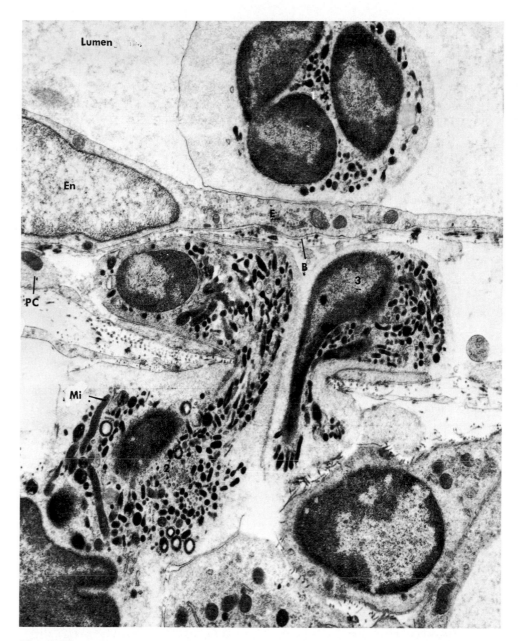

Fig. 2-13. *1,* Neutrophil adherent to endothelium, *E. 2* and *3,* Neutrophils streaming through periendothelial sheath into adjacent connective tissue. *En,* Nucleus of endothelial cell. *B,* Basement membrane of endothelium. *Pc,* Periendothelial cell. *Mi,* Mitochondria. (14,000×; from Marchesi, V.T., and Florey, H.W.: Q. J. Exp. Physiol. **45:**343, 1960.)

of the activated endothelial cells or monocytes, leading to increased adhesion and emigration.[61]

Chemotaxis and leukocytic emigration. When grains of starch are injected into the tail of a tadpole, leukocytes adhere to the vascular endothelium, emigrate through the vessel wall, and move toward the starch grains.[42] Such a directional response is referred to as *chemotaxis*[60]—the phenomenon being defined as a response in which the direction of locomotion of a cell or organism is determined by a substance in its environ-

ment. Chemotaxis ensures that, rather than wandering at random, the leukocytes move toward the site of injury and therefore concentrate in the infected or injured tissues.

Work on chemotaxis has been stimulated by a technique developed by Boyden.[40] A Perspex chamber is separated into two compartments by a Millipore filter membrane through which leukocytes can pass only by active migration. Blood cells are allowed to settle on one side of the membrane, and a solution of a substance to be tested for chemotactic activity is placed in the chamber on the other side of the membrane. After incubation for suitable periods, the membrane is removed and the cells that have migrated through it are counted microscopically.

In a medium containing normal rabbit serum, Boyden observed that human albumin was strongly chemotactic in the presence of its own antiserum. The chemotactic substance appeared to be a heat-stable product released into the solution in the chamber, although not produced when the rabbit serum was "inactivated" by being heated at 56° C for 30 minutes.

Boyden's results recalled an earlier finding that immune precipitates were capable of inducing the chemotaxis of neutrophils in vitro in the presence of fresh plasma. The incubation of serum with minced liver or a suspension of neutrophils also produces a chemotactic factor.[53] The clue to the problem appears to be the presence of *fresh* plasma because the results become inconsistent with aged plasma and negative when the plasma is replaced by serum, whether fresh or aged.

The nature of the chemotactic factors in fresh plasma is now beginning to emerge. The key factors appear to be various components of complement, since chemotactic activity is not obtained when complement fixation is prevented by the heating of serum, by removal of divalent cations, or by the use of antibodies that fix complement poorly. Three factors derived from complement and chemotactic for neutrophils have been identified—a trimolecular complex of components C5, C6, and C7 of complement, and two factors with low molecular weight (C3a and C5a), which correspond respectively to cleavage products of C3 and C5.[69] However, chemotaxis for neutrophils has also been demonstrated for kallikrein, products of virus-infected cells, and bacterial products of both high and low molecular weight.[72] The exhibition of chemotaxis by rabbit neutrophils involves the activation of an esterase with serine in its active site.[38] Such activation has been demonstrated for C$\overline{567}$, C5a, C3a, and a chemotactic factor from culture filtrates of *Escherichia coli*. In detail, the inert proesterase exists in or on the leukocyte, being activated to the esterase by any of the chemotactic factors just mentioned. In addition to activation of proesterase, chemotaxis requires metabolic energy provided mainly or wholly by anaerobic glycolysis and also requires the presence of Ca^{++} and Mg^{++} in the external medium. The process of chemotaxis possibly involves the contractile mechanism of the cell.[38]

Experiments with these chemotactic factors associated with complement indicate that neutrophils may move toward regions of greatest concentration of the chemotactic factors. On the other hand, the addition of activated C$\overline{567}$ complex to the cells themselves prevents their migration through the filter membrane. It

may be that chemotactic factors induce neutrophil migration toward the source of activated factor. Once the cells have accumulated, however, they may be unable to move away from the higher concentration of chemotactic factors.[77]

Eosinophilic granulocytes are particularly associated with immunologic lesions and parasitic infestations. Eosinophils seem particularly involved in immunologic responses when antigen is persistently present as in chronic infections or is subsequently reintroduced into the body.[67] They are chemotactically attracted to specific memory cells that contain components of both the priming antigen and the challenge antigen, being later engulfed by macrophages before the formation of plasma cells. A factor chemotactic for eosinophils has been isolated from human lung sensitized with IgE antibody.[56]

Factors inducing the accumulation of eosinophils in tissues harboring parasites have received little attention. One such factor has been recovered, however, from *Ascaris suum,* as well as the wall and fluid of hydatid cysts. The factor is a lecithin plasmalogen.[37]

The numerical paucity of *basophilic granulocytes* in human blood is matched by our lack of knowledge of their function. Nothing is known of factors chemotactic for basophils, though these cells seem implicated in certain types of immediate and delayed hypersensitivity.[79]

Factor chemotactic for *monocytes* overlap with those for neutrophils and include cleavage products of C3 and C5, other serum factors that are distinct from C$\overline{567}$, and soluble bacterial products.[71] *Lymphocytes* do not respond chemotactically to substances that induce directional movement in other varieties of leukocytes. Nevertheless, a substance that can influence the movement of lymphocytes in vitro has been identified among the products released by lymphocytes stimulated with antigen.[83]

In addition to this older data there has been a dramatic advancement in our understanding of the cellular biology of the complex endothelial cell-leukocyte-lymphocyte interactions that modulate cell traffic during the inflammatory response. Data have been accrued supporting the concept that specific, inducible cell surface receptors are utilized by neutrophils to modulate their interactions with endothelial cells during the acute phases of the inflammatory response.[39,50,51] These receptors are believed to be similar to those involved in lymphocyte homing to specific vascular beds.[58] The discovery of these inducible cell surface molecules as well as other adhesion proteins such as LFA-1 and MAC-1, belonging to the "integrin" gene family, will be potentially very helpful in advancing our understanding of this dynamic, complex cell-gating process.[41,50,54] Similarly, endothelial cells "activated" by soluble factors present in areas of inflammation, such as interferon-gamma, interleukin-1, and tumor necrosis factor, have been found to increase the expression of endothelial cell surface proteins, some of which enhance leukocyte and lymphocyte binding.[43] Furthermore, investigators have demonstrated distinct but overlapping endothelial cell responses (enhanced expression of Ia molecules, pro-coagulant activity and surface molecules which elicit increased leukocyte binding) to selected factors (interferon-gamma, interleukin-1, and tumor necrosis factor), indicating that the "activation" of endothelial cells may be "factor specific" and that the mixture of the various cytokines present during an inflammatory response may, in part, dictate the cellular response.[44,45,62,63]

Leukocytes in inflammation

Neutrophils. Neutrophils have a diameter ranging from 10 to 15 μm.[52] Phase-contrast microscopy reveals the cells to be actively motile and constantly changing in shape, with the leading margin having the form of a ruffled border or pseudopod. The cytoplasm contains 50 to 200 granules, which vary in size and shape according to species, but lack other organized structures. The granules contain various proteases, carbohydrases, lipases, and miscellaneous enzymes such as nucleotidase, peroxidase, oxidases, esterases, arylsulfatase, and acid and alkaline phosphatases. Nonenzymatic components of the granules include sulfated and nonsulfated mucopolysaccharides, as well as cationic proteins.

In the adult mammal, neutrophils arise in the bone marrow from the population of stem cells. Mature neutrophils from the bone marrow are released into the bloodstream, in which about half the neutrophils form a circulating pool and the other half provide a reserve pool in blood vessels at sites of slow or stagnant circulation. The latter cells are concentrated on the endothelial surface of the corresponding vasculature. Neutrophils in the peripheral blood leave the circulation in a random one-way migration into the tissues after a mean half-life in the circulation of 6 to 7 hours. In the tissues the cells die of senility or are excreted in the stool and respiratory tract secretions. Alternatively, they may be lyzed during combat with infecting microorganisms or in dealing with other forms of tissue injury.

The neutrophil utilizes glucose as a source of energy and has a reserve supply of glycogen in its cytoplasm.[52] But even under aerobic conditions, neutrophils derive 90% of their energy supply from glycolysis. They also exhibit an active turnover of various types of lipids, though practically no metabolism of deoxyribonucleic acid, in keeping with the inability of the mature cell for mitosis.

The function of neutrophils is associated mainly with the initial phagocytosis of microorganisms and other foreign material introduced into the tissues. To meet this function, the neutrophil adheres to vascular endothelium and exhibits locomotion on endothelium or in the tissues, emigration through the vascular wall, chemotaxis, phagocytosis, degranulation, and digestion or egestion of the foreign material. The importance of neutrophils in the defense of the host against microbial invaders is illustrated by the high incidence of infection in persons with agranulocytosis. In other examples of lowered host resistance (such as after massive x radiation or excessive levels of certain adrenal corticosteroids), there is a decrease in the availability or functional capacity of neutrophils.[52] In these latter circumstances, however, host resistance is also decreased by the concurrent impairment of antibody formation. Unusual forms of neutrophilic granulocytes in certain congenital disorders also leave the individual highly vulnerable to infection.

Neutrophils also engulf antigen-antibody complexes, as well as nonmicrobial material introduced into the tissues. Undigested materials are engulfed by neutrophils or by mononuclear phagocytes. Besides this role of scavenger, neutrophils also seem to play a key role in various types of immunologic injury. Many examples are known in which the leukocytes contribute to the breakdown of the host's own tissue.

Deleterious effects of neutrophils seem particularly directed at the internal elastic lamina of arteries and the basement membrane of smaller vessels and glomeruli.[77] The accumulation of neutrophils on or near these membranes is succeeded by damage and lysis of the membrane. Up to now, this field of study has been confined to the Arthus and Shwartzman reactions, acute experimental glomerulonephritis, and the arteries in serum sickness. But as the scope of investigation is widened, it seems that a similar picture will be revealed in various acute clinical conditions with an immunologic basis.

Eosinophils. Larger than the neutrophil though less numerous, the eosinophil has much in common with the neutrophil, both structurally and functionally.[4] Both types of cell are produced in the bone marrow, have a short life in the blood stream, and pass into the tissues. Both exhibit locomotion and phagocytosis, and both carry cytoplasmic granules that are disrupted during the phagocytosis of particulate material. Even many of their enzymes are similar, though the granules of eosinophils have a higher content of peroxidase and contain an unidentified crystalline structure but no lysozyme.

The function of eosinophils remains unknown. In health they are present in large numbers in the skin, lungs, and bowel. It may be relevant that these parts of the body have contact either with the outside world or with substances from the exterior. The blood and tissue levels of eosinophils are elevated in allergies, parasitic infestations, skin diseases, and some types of malignant lymphoma. However, the long-recognized association of eosinophilia with parasitic infestation may be part of an immunologic phenomenon. This possibility is suggested by the finding that, in infestation of the rat by the nematode *Trichinella spiralis*, the eosinophil response is sharply decreased by procedures that deplete or inactivate the pool of circulating lymphocytes.[75]

The distribution of these cells is strikingly affected by hormonal secretion, particularly of the adrenal cortex. High levels of cortisone lead to decreased numbers or even disappearance of eosinophils from the blood.

Basophils. In humans, basophils comprise about 1% of circulating leukocytes. Their large basophilic granules contain heparin and histamine, which are released when the cells degranulate. Reference has already been made to the apparent involvement of basophils in both immediate and delayed types of hypersensitivity. Human homocytotropic antibody (IgE) is bound specifically to basophils and sensitizes them for antigen-induced release of histamine. Basophils therefore seem likely to participate in atopic allergic disease.[79] Furthermore, several varieties of delayed hypersensitivity are characterized in both humans and animals by intense infiltration of tissue by basophils (so-called cutaneous basophil hypersensitivity). Such reactions are particularly prominent in the guinea pig but also occur in humans. Lymphocytes play an essential role in such reactions.[79] The morphologic and pharmacologic similarities of basophils with tissue mast cells and the predominance of one or the other type of cell in various species indicate that basophils and mast cells may well have allied functions.

Lymphocytes. In histologic sections, lymphocytes are rather smaller than neutrophils and consist almost entirely of nucleus, with little or no cytoplasm (Fig. 2-14). The living cell, however, has a distinct and more abundant cytoplasm. Lymphocytes comprise the major variety of cells in normal lymph nodes, white pulp of the spleen, and the lymphoid tissue of the alimentary tract and lungs. They also comprise 15% to 30% of the leukocytes in peripheral blood, being more numerous in children than in adults, and are the predominant type of cell in lymph that has passed through lymph nodes. Their number in blood increases little or not at all in acute infections, though their number may increase relatively during convalescence or in chronic infections such as tuberculosis. In the tissues, lymphocytes are particularly numerous in chronic inflammation (for example, renal interstitial tissue in chronic pyelonephritis). They are prominent as a perivascular infiltration in the brain in syphilis and various types of viral encephalitis (Fig. 2-15) and at the periphery of tuberculous lesions. Periportal infiltration by lymphocytes is common in cirrhosis of the liver, and cells often occur at the periphery of neoplasms. They form a feature of the tissue reaction in delayed hypersensitivity and transplanted organs.

Monocytes. In most species, monocytes seldom comprise more than 8% to 10% of the circulating leukocytes. These cells in the blood belong to a system of mononuclear phagocytes, which are widely distributed

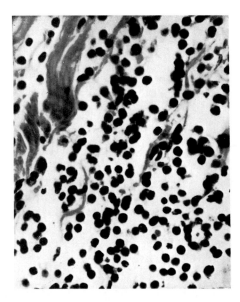

Fig. 2-14. Lymphocytes infiltrating connective tissue. In tissue preparations, cells exhibit little cytoplasm. (510×.)

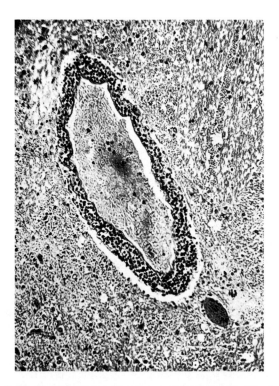

Fig. 2-15. Lymphocytes forming perivascular "cuff" of cells in brain in lethargic encephalitis. (130×.)

in the body, being found in bone marrow, blood, liver, lymphoid tissue, lungs, connective tissue, and serous cavities. Important because of their phagocytic ability, the cells share a common morphology, origin, function, and other properties that have prompted their designation collectively as the "mononuclear phagocyte system," which includes the following elements[57]:

Promonocyte (bone marrow)
↓
Monocyte (blood)
↓
Macrophage (tissues)
 Histiocyte (connective tissue)
 Kupffer cell (liver)
 Alveolar macrophage (lung)
 Free and fixed macrophage and sinusoidal lining cell (spleen)
 Free and fixed macrophage (lymph node)
 Macrophage and sinusoidal lining cell (bone marrow)
 Peritoneal macrophage (serous cavity)
 Osteoclast (bone tissue)
 Microglia? (nervous system)

Accordingly, "the monocytes of the peripheral blood form a population of young cells on the way from their place of origin, the bone marrow, to their ultimate location, the tissues.[69]

Circulating monocytes[10] arise in the bone marrow by division of promonocytes, which in turn are derived from an unidentified precursor stem cell.[68] Under normal conditions the tissue macrophages have a relatively long life, with the normal turnover of Kupffer cells taking about 60 days; of alveolar macrophages, about 50 days; and of peritoneal macrophages, about 30 to 40 days.

Reference has already been made to the emigration of monocytes through postcapillary venules in inflammation to the concurrence of their emigration with that of neutrophils.

Phagocytosis. Many cells possess the ability to ingest material by engulfment.[73] The ingested matter is usually particulate, such as bacteria, protozoal parasites or other microorganisms, tissue cells (usually necrotic), dust, pigment, and other foreign material. When engulfment involves such particulate matter, the process is termed *phagocytosis.*

Phagocytes comprise two main classes of cells: those that are capable of migrating to the site where their phagocytic ability is required (such as neutrophilic and eosinophilic leukocytes and circulating mononuclear phagocytes) and those that are fixed in tissues during all or most of their life and therefore depend on chance encounter with foreign materials (such as Kupffer cells in liver and lining sinusoid of lymph node).

In the act of phagocytosis, small particles such as a grain of charcoal may be ingested in an instant. In the rapid engulfment of a small particle viewed with a light microscope, the particle appears to pass directly through the cell membrane. But electron microscopy indicates that this is not the case; firm contact is first established between cell membrane and particle. The area of contact is then extended by invagination of the cell membrane until the apposing membrane surfaces meet and fuse (Fig. 2-16). Larger objects such as tissue cells, clumps of bacteria, or a single large bacterium (such as *Bacillus megaterium*) are ingested by a more active response. Fig. 2-16 illustrates the sequence of events in the phagocytosis of *B. megaterium* by a neutrophilic leukocyte; the leukocyte flows slowly about the bacillus until ingestion has been completed. This process is similar for neutrophils (microphages), monocytes, and tissue macrophages.

The process of phagocytosis involves two stages:
1. The attachment stage, in which the particle becomes bound to the surface of the phagocyte
2. The ingestion stage, involving invagination of the surface membrane and the surrounding of the particle

The fate of ingested particulate matter is closely related to the process of degranulation and the discharge of granule contents into the newly formed digestive pouch (Fig. 2-16) or phagosome. The nature of the surface of the object to be ingested (whether bacterium, cell, or foreign body) determines whether there can be firm fixation to the neutrophil surface as the necessary prelude to phagocytosis. Since both bacteria and neutrophils usually have a net surface charge that is negative and therefore repellent, some form of physical or chemical bond must be established between particle and cell membrane. Opsonins (such as plasma fibronectin) are factors that act on the surface of many bacteria, presumably by adsorption, and render them susceptible to phagocytosis. In the absence of opsonins (as in serum), ingestion of most microorganisms by neutrophils proceeds slowly or not at all. Besides the coating of bacteria with a film of opsonin, the beneficial effects of serum on phagocytosis also include colloid osmotic effects and the binding or inactivation of toxins.

The physical nature of the environment also influences phagocytosis by neutrophils. Even encapsulated unopsonized microorganisms are engulfed, provided that the cells can trap the bacteria "in corners" or between cells. This phenomenon of "surface phagocytosis" may have considerable importance in the tissues.[74]

Phagocytosis is accompanied by degranulation of the neutrophils (Fig. 2-16), resulting in the liberation of digestive enzymes and antibacterial substances. The degranulation seems to result from contact of the membranes of the cytoplasmic granules with the membranes of the "phagocytic pouch" surrounding the ingested particle. The hydrolases released by the granules are discharged into the pouch, and so the cell's cytoplasm

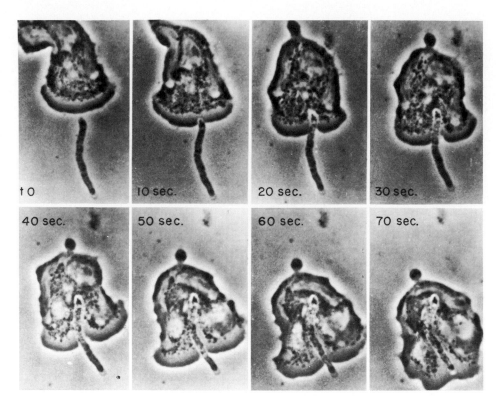

Fig. 2-16. Timed sequences from motion picture of human neutrophil engulfing *Bacillus megaterium*. Notice invagination of cell membrane and formation of digestive pouch. There is overall reduction in cytoplasmic content of granules by the time ingestion has been completed. (Phase contrast; approximately 1400×; from Hirsch, J.G.: J. Exp. Med. **116:**827, 1962.)

is protected from its own ferments. The antibacterial substances released include lysosome, hydrogen peroxide, basic peptides (leukins), and a basic protein (phagocytin) that kills a wide range of organisms without lyzing them.[52]

Lymph flow in inflammation

The fluid exudate that accumulates in inflamed tissues is mainly drained away by the lymphatics.[1] The regional lymph nodes are admirably constructed as a filtering mechanism,[76] with the efficiency of filtration being improved when the rate of flow of incoming lymph is decreased. This factor assumes considerable importance in the management of inflamed tissues by rest and immobilization.[132]

Cardinal signs of inflammation

Thus the cardinal signs of inflammation (redness, swelling, heat, and pain) can now be partially explained.

The *redness* is caused by vasodilatation. The *swelling* results mainly from the accumulation of fluid exudate consequent to increased vascular permeability, with smaller contributions from the cellular infiltration of the affected tissues and the engorgement of their blood vessels.

The sensation of *heat* is attributable to the rapid inflow of relatively warm blood through dilated vessels in the inflamed area, the incoming blood from the deep tissues being warmer than that in the superficial tissues and skin.

Various factors contribute to the *pain*. Distension of tissue, particularly when there is little room for expansion, results in the all too familiar throbbing pain of an infected nail bed of the finger or toe. But other factors such as kinins, histamine, and metabolites, which are liberated or activated by injured cells, probably also play a role in causing the pain felt in acutely inflamed lesions.

Varieties of acute inflammation
Factors in variation of inflammatory response

Inflammation is referred to as *acute* when it lasts days or 2 to 3 weeks and as *chronic* when more prolonged. The typical case of acute inflammation is characterized by vasodilatation, exudation of plasma, and emigration of neutrophilic leukocytes into the injured tissues. But not all examples of acute inflammation exhibit neutrophilic infiltration, and conversely neutrophils may be associated with prolonged and therefore chronic inflammation. Typhoid fever represents an acute inflammatory process in which the cellular response in the submucous lymphoid tissue of the small bowel is typically mononuclear, and chronic osteomyelitis is an example of prolonged chronic inflammation in which the cellular response is mainly neutrophilic. Between acute and chronic inflammation is a wide range of overlapping processes.

The main events in acute inflammation are vascular in origin and remarkably consistent for a wide range of stimuli. Nevertheless, the response exhibits considerable differences that depend, first, on factors related to the injury or infection and, second, on the condition of the host and nature of the tissue involved.[9] For example, skin reacts to the virus of herpes simplex by forming a vesicle (or blister), to staphylococci with an abscess (such as a boil), and to streptococci with a diffuse brawny red swelling known as erysipelas. Furthermore, there is a remarkable difference in the way the lung reacts to pneumococci in lobar pneumonia and to mycobacteria in chronic tuberculosis.

The site of an inflammation also modifies the inflammatory response—the lung with its loose texture would be expected to exhibit a response differing from that in dense compact tissue such as bone. But, in general, the picture of inflammation in an organ depends largely on the predominance of one of three processes: exudation, proliferation of tissue cells, or necrosis caused by the injurious agent. Although these three processes are combined in varying proportions, all are usually present to a greater or lesser extent. They may be combined in various proportions to produce recognizable types of inflamation that are influenced by the character and site of the tissue involved in the inflammatory process.

Exudation. The term *exudation* is preferably limited to the escape of plasma rather than emigrating leukocytes, but both can be conveniently included in the present context. The exudate is described as *serous* when it resembles serum (that is, consists of water, solutes, and plasma protein but with scanty fibrin and neutrophils). Serous exudates are found in tuberculous pleurisy.

A *fibrinous* exudate has a high content of fibrin. It is common on the pleura when pneumonia extends to the pleural surface and on the pericardium in pneumococcal or rheumatic pericarditis. Fibrinous inflammation frequently involves serous membranes and the meninges (Fig. 2-17). The exudate has a gray, lusterless appearance and can be readily peeled off with forceps or by rubbing with a finger.

The terms *purulent* and *suppurative* refer to the presence of pus. It seems noteworthy that pus consists of both dead and still viable neutrophils, with a contri-

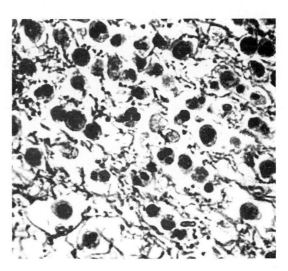

Fig. 2-17. Fibrinocellular exudate in pneumococcal meningitis. Neutrophils and macrophages lie in mesh of fibrin. (760×.)

bution of necrotic cells and tissue, as well as exuded plasma. Initially thick and creamy, pus becomes thinner in consistency after the proteolysis that results from the activity of proteolytic enzymes released from dying and dead neutrophils.

In severe inflammation there is often sufficient vascular damage to cause hemorrhage, the inflammation then being referred to as *hemorrhagic*. Some degree of hemorrhage is common in severe or advanced inflammation such as acute appendicitis.

Proliferation. Cell proliferation is usually inconspicuous in acute inflammation caused by bacteria, but a notable exception is typhoid fever, in which there is considerable multiplication of large mononuclear cells in the intestinal lymphoid tissue. Viral infections have a characteristic ability to stimulate cell division, and so the early stages of a number of viral diseases show cellular proliferation. This is particularly true for epidermis, with proliferation occurring in the early stages of herpes simplex, chickenpox, smallpox, and vaccinia. Another example of proliferation in inflammation is the formation of "crescents" resulting from proliferation of glomerular capsular epithelium in glomerulonephritis.

Proliferation is also a common feature of chronic inflammation, with cellular multiplication particularly involving macrophages and fibroblasts and endothelial cells.

Necrosis. Although necrosis often involves individual cells in inflammation, it sometimes dominates the picture, as in gas gangrene. In this condition the tissues may be discolored and foul, with microscopic evidence of nuclear fragmentation. Leukocytes are scarce. Necrosis results from the action of toxins of the responsible organisms that belong to the genus *Clostridium*.

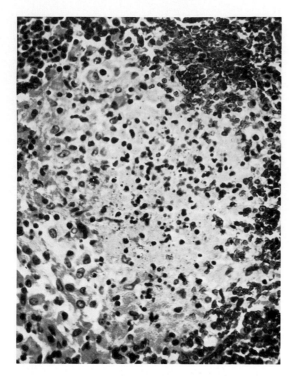

Fig. 2-18. Necrosis in inflammation. Necrotic area is in center of tubercle. Such necrosis is referred to as caseation and contains nuclear remnants and debris. Pale cells at periphery of necrosis are macrophages (so-called epithelioid cells), with lymphocytes still farther afield, particularly in upper and lower right-hand corners. (760×.)

Some microorganisms are associated with necrotizing inflammation in the mouth and throat. In other instances, necrosis may result from vascular obstruction caused by bacterial infection. Such obstruction is a common cause of acute appendicitis progressing to gangrenous appendicitis and rupture of the appendix. Necrosis is often prominent in chronic inflammation, a common example being the caseous necrosis (caseation) that characteristically occurs in tuberculous lesions (Fig. 2-18).

Pseudomembranous inflammation

Pseudomembranous inflammation is a response of mucous surfaces (as in the pharynx, larynx, trachea, bronchi, and bowel) to necrotizing agents such as the toxin of diphtheria bacilli or irritant gases. The surface epithelium is destroyed, a condition that allows the irritant to penetrate the underlying tissues, where it increases the permeability of the blood vessels. Plasma therefore exudes onto the eroded surface, coagulates, and encloses the necrotic epithelium in its fibrinous meshes. This coagulum of necrotic tissue constitutes the false membrane that gives this type of inflammation its name.

Such inflammation in the trachea is typical of diphtheria. At this site, the formation of a false membrane carries a particular risk of respiratory obstruction and hence the need for relief by tracheotomy. With the

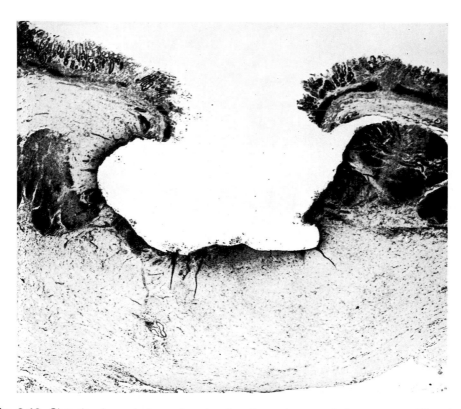

Fig. 2-19. Chronic ulcer of stomach extending through muscularis mucosae. Fibrosis of submucosa and base of ulcer provides evidence of long-continued process. (8×.)

present-day programs of immunization against diphtheria, the condition has become uncommon except where immunization is not the rule.

Ulceration

The term *ulceration* means a circumscribed loss of substances from the surface of an organ, usually accompanied by inflammation of the adjacent tissue (Fig. 2-19). Ulceration results from necrosis occurring as the sequel to cell destruction by toxins and poisons or from interference with blood supply. The necrotic tissue becomes loosened and finally separated from the adjacent viable tissue.

Frequent sites of ulceration are the stomach and first part of the duodenum. Intestinal ulcers are a common feature of typhoid fever, intestinal tuberculosis, and both bacillary and amebic dysentery. On the legs, ulcers are associated with varicose veins. Ulcers are among the most common and important inflammatory lesions.

Abscess formation

An abscess is a localized collection of pus in a tissue, organ, or confined space. Common sites of abscess formation include the dermis of skin, the lung, brain, kidney, and liver, or a cyst. Abscesses are often caused by strong irritants that remain localized rather than spreading diffusely. Examples are the ingress of staphylococci through hair follicles to cause a boil or the embolism of infected thrombi in pyemia.

The established focus of infection incites an outpouring of large numbers of neutrophilic leukocytes (Fig. 2-20). These become concentrated in the infected area and liberate proteases that digest damage and dead tissues and so convert it into the semiliquid material known as pus.

An abscess therefore consists of a collection of pus surrounded by inflamed tissue heavily infiltrated with neutrophils. As long as the irritant (such as staphylococcus) persists, more leukocytes are attracted, more tissue is liquified, and further pus is formed. Proteolysis results in the splitting of larger molecules into smaller ones, with a consequent increase in osmotic pressure, which attracts more water from the surrounding tissues. The increasing pressure in the abscess often causes the pus to "track" or burrow through adjacent tissues along lines of least resistance, such as intermuscular septa. Eventually, the pus reaches a surface, where it is discharged. Tracking and erosion cause considerable damage, which the surgeon tries to prevent by opening the abscess to establish drainage of the pus.

Suppuration (formation of visible pus) involves the destruction of tissue. It is therefore an irreversible process that cannot be restored to normal by resolution but rather results in healing with scarring. The healing process is described later in this chapter.

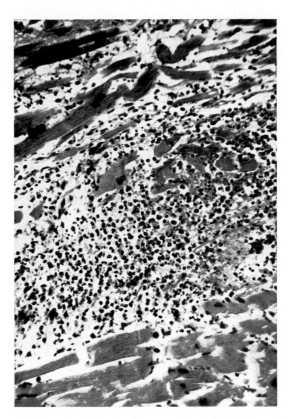

Fig. 2-20. Small abscess of myocardium. Collection of neutrophils has replaced muscle fibers. Fragments of dead muscle are present near periphery of abscess. (370×.)

Sometimes the irritant is overcome by natural defenses before pus reaches a surface. Under these circumstances pus may be absorbed. If too abundant, however, it may persist as a collection of sterile fluid (a cyst) or become dehydrated and circumscribed by a fibrous tissue capsule.

Cellulitis (diffuse inflammation)

By contrast with the circumscription of an abscess, other inflammatory lesions may be diffuse (Fig. 2-21). The diffuseness results when the irritant, such as bacteria causing infection, is equipped with factors that aid the spread of the infection. For example, the rapid spread of infection by hemolytic streptococci is largely attributable to their production of hyaluronidase, or "spreading factor," which breaks down hyaluronic acid in the ground substance of connective tissue.

Inflammation in hypersensitivity

An important part of our defense mechanism involves the production of antibodies against antigens such as bacterial toxins. But the union of antigen with antibody is not always advantageous to the host. Sometimes the outcome is unfavorable, with a result worse than the effects of the antigen itself. When such conditions are

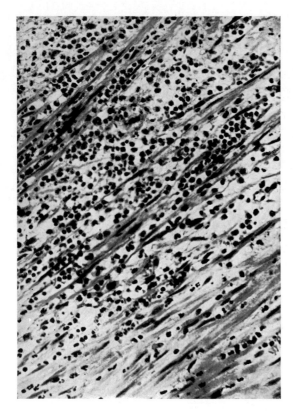

Fig. 2-21. Acute inflammation of appendix. Muscle fibers are separated by inflammatory exudate in which many neutrophils are recognizable. Lesion is example of diffuse type of inflammation. (270×.)

acquired and have a specific immunologic basis, they constitute examples of hypersensitivity. The current usage of the term *hypersensitivity* is synonymous with *allergy*. Allergic reactions are, then, defined according to common usage as those immunologic reactions that damage the tissues or disrupt the physiology of the vertebrate host. Although we carefully distinguish in words and in fact between allergy and immunity, the same mechanisms operate in both; the fundamental difference in any individual reaction is who or what is the primary target of the given immunologic mechanism— whether the invading organism and its products are affected in the case of immunity or the host itself in the case of allergy.

Disorders that come within the category of hypersensitivity include a wide range of conditions that may be conveniently divided into immediate type and delayed type of hypersensitivity, on the basis of rapidity of onset and duration. Immediate-type reactions begin seconds or minutes after contact of antigen with antibody, though the effects may take minutes or even hours to become apparent. Delayed-type reactions are slower in onset and take at least some hours, usually 24 to 48 hours, to become obvious. They run a prolonged

course, which is often associated with chronic disease.

Although the division of hypersensitivity into immediate type and delayed type is based simply on the time course of the disorder, such a division corresponds to important differences in the underlying mechanisms. Of these, the most fundamental is the dependence of immediate-type hypersensitivity on the presence of circulating antibody. Delayed-type hypersensitivity undoubtedly involves the immune mechanism, but the presence of circulating antibody is not essential for the exhibition of the disorder, though often accompanying it. Delayed-type hypersensitivity is mediated by sensitized lymphoid cells and is transferable by means of such cells, though not by serum. Hypersensitivity reactions that may evoke damage of tissues have been classified into four types.[78]

1. *Type I* (anaphylactic) reactions result from the interaction of antigen with antibody "fixed" on tissue cells, particularly mast cells. In humans, atopic or reaginic antibodies (IgE) are mainly responsible. Challenge by antigen locally or systemically results in an acute release of short-lived factors, such as histamine, 5-hydroxytryptamine, kinins, and "slow-reacting substance" (SRS), having both local and systemic effects.[81]

2. *Type II* (cytotoxic) reactions are initiated by heterologous or autologous antibodies that provoke complement-dependent lysis of target cells or a local inflammatory response (transient or persistent) in the target tissue.[81] The antibody is usually IgG or IgM. One example of a type II hypersensitivity reaction is Goodpasture's syndrome. In this disease the patient develops antibodies that are cross-reactive with basement membrane components. When these antibodies bind to the basement membranes of the kidney, lung choroid plexus, and so on, they elicit complement activation and evoke an inflammatory response leading to tissue destruction.

3. *Type III* (damage by immune complexes) reactions involve aggregation of antigen-antibody under two sets of circumstances: first, in the bloodstream when relatively large amounts of antigen persist until corresponding antibody is formed and then combine with that antibody; second, when antibody is circulating in the blood and antigen is introduced locally in the tissues in high concentration.[78] The first situation results in "serum sickness," and the second in an *Arthus reaction*. The antibodies are IgG or gamma globulin.

Another example of a type III hypersensitivity reaction is the immune complex–mediated glomerulonephritis observed in systemic lupus erythematosus. In this autoimmune disease the patient develops circulating antigen-antibody complexes, which deposit in various tissues and elicit complement activation and tissue destruction.

4. *Type IV* (delayed hypersensitivity) reactions are

cell mediated and include bacterial or tuberculin type of hypersensitivity and contact dermatitis.

Types I, II, and III therefore represent varieties of immediate types of hypersensitivity, whereas type IV corresponds to the delayed type.

Hypersensitivity constitutes another form of injury that evokes the nonspecific inflammatory response. The picture varies, however, according to whether the inflammation is provoked by antigen-antibody reactions without the presence of additional agents, as in the Arthus and Shwartzman reactions,[81] or results from an agent that is also the provocative antigen, as in many bacterial infections.

When hypersensitivity provides the only factor responsible for inflammation, the tissue reaction is a rapid development of edema resulting from increased vascular permeability and an accumulation of neutrophils, macrophages, and often eosinophils. Vascular lesions may be prominent and particularly include arteriolar necrosis and extensive thrombosis. In addition to its acute exudative onset, hypersensitivity differs qualitatively from other varieties of inflammation in provoking rapid proliferation of macrophages and plasma cells.

A good example of the tissue reaction in delayed-type hypersensitivity is the response to the intradermal injection of old tuberculin in a person previously infected with tubercle bacilli. In contrast to the edema and comparatively sparse cellular infiltration of the immediate type of reaction, the delayed type of reaction histologically shows a dense accumulation of cells, mainly lymphocytes and macrophages. The reaction of delayed-type hypersensitivity to chronic granulomatous inflammation, necrosis, and immunity (as in tuberculosis) is a complex subject that warrants further reading.[81,84]

Systemic effects of acute inflammation

The present account of the acute inflammatory response has purposely been concentrated on the local responses at the site of injury. This approach, however, should not be taken to indicate that systemic responses have little magnitude or importance. On the contrary, as noted early in this chapter, the systemic effects are both complex and comprehensive. They include malaise, fever, leukocytosis, fibrinolysis, metabolic disturbances, shock, and endocrine and immunologic responses.

Functions of inflammatory response

The exudation of plasma and the accumulation of neutrophilic leukocytes in foci of inflammation provide important protective mechanisms in the defense of the host. The outpouring of plasma dilutes bacterial toxins or other noxious factors, whereas the protein content of the plasma includes specific and nonspecific antibodies that antagonize the toxins as well as the kinin, clotting,

and complement-amplification systems. The benefits of the fluid phase of the response overlap with those of the emigrated neutrophils. These leukocytes compose the first wave of phagocytes that arrive to deal with invading bacteria, but their role as phagocytes is considerably facilitated by the presence of antibodies in the fluid exudate. In addition, the fibrin mesh that is formed from the exuded fibrinogen probably provides an important framework on which the neutrophils move about in the tissues.

The role of inflammation is not as obvious in nonbacterial inflammation. The increased vascularity ensures that both sites involved by infection and those of noninfective injury have a blood supply adequate for the local metabolic demands. In addition, the close relation of repair to inflammation indicates that the latter process may act as a stimulus for subsequent healing and regeneration.

Nevertheless, inflammation in certain circumstances may have disadvantages.[12] Phagocytosed bacteria may survive within phagocytes and even be protected against antibodies or antibiotics. Or again, the "successful" outcome of the inflammatory response may extract a high price in terms of functional loss in organs such as the eye.

In the final summing up, however, the definite advantages of inflammation seem amply illustrated by the harmful effects that follow experimental suppression of vasodilatation in bacterial infection. After the experimental inoculation of bacteria in skin, the number of bacteria capable of establishing infection is considerably greater in sites treated with a vasoconstrictor, such as epinephrine, than in control sites with a normally responsive vasculature.[8]

Chronic inflammation

Textbook accounts of acute and chronic inflammation often separate the two conditions by a description of healing and regeneration. An understanding of the histologic picture of chronic inflammation is certainly assisted by a knowledge of the processes involved in repair, but the separation from acute inflammation leaves the impression that these two varieties of inflammation are distinct from each other, though sharing the term "inflammation" in their names. This is not the case. In general, the term *acute*, as applied to inflammation, refers to a response with a rapid onset and relatively short duration characterized by particular vascular phenomena. The common sequel is resolution of the inflammatory exudate and restoration of normal structure and function. In some cases, however, the acute events lose their intensity, and so the process continues as a smoldering chronic condition. In other cases the initial infection may be attributable to an organism of low pathogenicity, which therefore evokes a less intense response from the outset. Such is the case with *Mycobacterium tuberculosis*. Even so, the experimental introduction of this organism into the tissues evokes an initial response of acute inflammation for the first 24 hours; then there is a rapid change to the picture of chronic inflammation.

Besides infection by bacteria and other microorganisms of low-grade pathogenicity, causes of chronic inflammation include physical agents of mild intensity or chemical agents of low concentration. Examples of such agents are particles of sand entering the tissues through an abrasion or laceration, and talc powder from a surgeon's glove contaminating an operative incision. The pneumoconioses are a group of diseases of the lung in which chronic inflammatory lesions result from the inhalation of dust containing silica or other irritants. Sometimes the agent is a chemical factor of plant or occupational origin to which a low-grade sensitivity has developed, usually after continued exposure, as in some types of contact or occupational dermatitis.

Other circumstances favoring the development of chronic inflammation include minor trauma or infection involving tissues that are handicapped by restricted blood supply attributable to disease or by poor venous return as in varicose veins of the legs. In such cases an injury or infection that normally would evoke no more than transient acute inflammation is followed by a persistent chronic inflammation.

As long as irritation persists, the lesion should be considered inflammatory. Once the irritation abates or is removed, the process becomes reparative. The ensuing process of repair commonly takes the form of fibrosis with the formation of "scar tissue," adhesions, and fibrous bands. Such lesions are relatively common as the outcome of chronic inflammation of serous membranes but should not be labeled "chronic peritonitis" or "chronic pericarditis." The chronic inflammation has subsided and the condition is one of peritoneal or pericardial adhesion or fibrosis, respectively.

Features of chronic inflammation

Inflammation is said to be chronic when its duration is relatively prolonged—often for months or years. Its prolonged course is provoked by persistence of the causative factor in the tissues, whether the factor be an infection or an inanimate foreign body. The tissues are infiltrated by several cell types: mononuclear phagocytes, lymphoid cells, fibroblasts, and endothelial cells. In addition, there may be granulocytic leukocytes, particularly eosinophils.[66] Mononuclear phagocytes are represented by macrophages, epithelioid cells, or multinucleated giant cells. Lymphoid cells are present as lymphocytes, plasma cells, or immunoblasts. Fibroblasts produce collagen and ground substance and proliferate to form more fibroblasts. Endothelial cells migrate and proliferate forming a rich neovascular network necessary for the maintenance of the inflammatory response. At varying stages during the course of the lesion, lymphocytes, fibroblasts, or granulocytes may predominate, but the most important unit of chronic inflammation is almost always the macrophage and its derivatives, the epithelioid cell and the giant cell.[66]

Necrosis is also common in chronic inflammatory lesions. Quite often, there are episodes of necrosis that stimulate the formation of granulation tissue and hence of fibrous tissue, even to such extent that fibrosis becomes a feature of older lesions. The overall participation of the "dividing" tissue cells and their efforts in producing new tissue have resulted in chronic inflammation being described as *proliferative*, in contrast to the *exudative* features of acute inflammation.

The accumulation of macrophages, lymphocytes, and plasma cells may be diffuse or focal. Although the histologic picture can be variable, a distinctive pattern often occurs in conditions such as tuberculosis, leprosy, syphilis, sarcoidosis, brucellosis, rheumatic fever, and certain mycoses. A proliferative type of reaction, which is focal in distribution, results in a lesion that is often described as a "granuloma." When the condition is caused by infection, the lesion is referred to as an "infective granuloma." The term *granuloma* is alleged to have two origins: (1) it goes back to the time when the

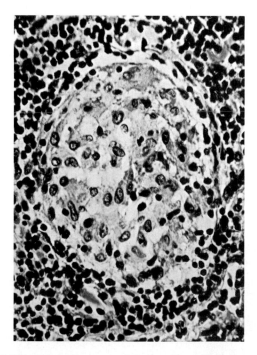

Fig. 2-22. Macrophages of tubercle, which is circumscribed ovoid focus in center. Peripheral cells are mostly lymphocytes. Fig. 2-18 illustrates caseous necrosis subsequently developing at center of tubercle. (510×.)

nodular foci were considered to be neoplastic, hence the name "granule-*oma*," and (2) the term refers to the tumorlike nodules of proliferating granulation tissue.

Granulomatous inflammation. The development of granulomatous inflammation is well illustrated by the tissue response to the primary lodgment of tubercle bacilli in the lungs of guinea pigs or rabbits. When the bacilli are injected intravenously, those that lodge in the pulmonary capillaries evoke a transient neutrophil response. After 12 hours, however, the immigrant neutrophils are overshadowed by incoming macrophages that predominate throughout the remaining life of the lesion. When the tubercle bacilli are inspired into the pulmonary alveoli, macrophages predominant from the outset. In either case the macrophages proceed to engulf the tubercle bacilli and, by the second or third day, they form clusters of elongated cells that are closely packed at the center of the lesion (Fig. 2-22). In these macrophage clusters, adjacent cells often fuse to form multinucleated giant cells, containing up to 50 to 100 nuclei; these are the so-called Langhans' giant cells (Fig. 2-23) that are common in tuberculosis.

Beyond 10 to 12 days, the central macrophages begin to undergo a characteristic necrosis termed *caseation* (Fig. 2-18), a term that refers to the caseous or cheeselike appearance and consistency of the necrotic tissue. The development of such necrosis in tuberculosis appears to be related to the onset of tissue hypersensitivity resulting from an immunologic response to the mi-

crobial invader. By 2 or 3 weeks, each lesion usually exhibits a central area of necrosis surrounded by macrophages and often one or several multinucleated giant cells. Surrounding the macrophages is a zone of lymphocytes (Figs. 2-18 and 2-22). The periphery of the granulomatous focus is bounded by fibroblasts and fibrous tissue. In tuberculosis each such lesion is about 1 mm in diameter and is known as a "tubercle." The focal lesions gradually coalesce, while much of the remaining tissue becomes infiltrated by mononuclear cells (lymphocytes, plasma cells, and macrophages) and exhibits progressive fibrosis. But even at an advanced stage of the disease, the microscopic picture usually shows some evidence of the focal lesions.

Granulomatous inflammation is evoked by various infections, particularly by tuberculosis, leprosy, syphilis, and actinomycosis, and less commonly by brucellosis and various mycoses. In other cases the condition is associated with diseases having an allergic (or hypersensitive) background, such as rheumatic fever and rheumatoid disease. Still other examples are provided by beryllium poisoning and by the presence of foreign bodies such as talc, grit, sutures, or splinters of wood. Finally, the condition named "sarcoidosis" includes several conditions that share the feature of granulomatous lesions resembling tubercles, but with minimal or no necrosis (Fig. 2-24).

It should be emphasized that the histologic picture of granulomatous inflammation is both variable and nonspecific. In some cases a causative organism is estab-

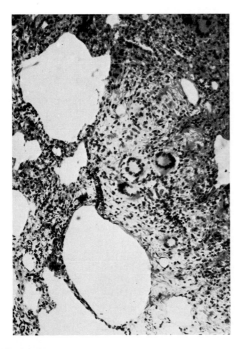

Fig. 2-23. Multinucleated giant cells of Langhans type in lipid pneumonia. (110×.)

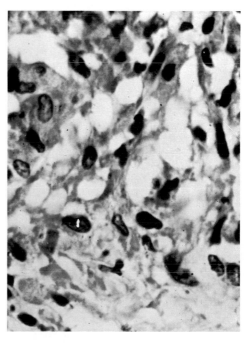

Fig. 2-24. Macrophages, more highly magnified than in Fig. 2-22, in sarcoidosis. (1130×.)

lished, in others the lesion probably results from hypersensitivity associated with infection, and in still others there is no suggestion of an association with infection. Some of the diseases have widespread systemic manifestations, whereas for others the clinical features remain almost entirely local. The focal proliferative lesions may predominate or may be infrequent—for example, the tubercle is common in tuberculosis, whereas the gumma is much less common in syphilis. Under various conditions of dosage, virulence, and host resistance, some of the organisms responsible for granulomatous inflammation produce tissue responses that are nongranulomatous. The tubercle bacillus, for example, usually evokes the formation of a tubercle, but occasionally it incites a distinctively exudative inflammation.

The giant cells also exhibit considerable variation in incidence and morphology. In tuberculosis they are relatively large and contain many rounded nuclei, arranged either peripherally or at one or both poles. Their cytoplasm is acidophilic and finely granular and contains fine filaments. In sarcoidosis the giant cells sometimes contain cytoplasmic inclusions, whereas in "foreign body" reactions the giant cells tend to be variable in size and morphology (Fig. 2-25).

Two points warrant reiteration:

1. The histologic picture in granulomatous inflammation is seldom specific, though the Aschoff nodule in rheumatic heart disease may be one excep-

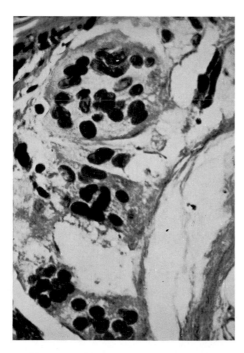

Fig. 2-25. Three multinucleated giant cells of "foreign body" type in response to keratin that was retained in hair follicle. (450×.)

tion to this rule. In general, however, the microscopic appearances are inconclusive.

2. There is a strong tendency for granulomatous inflammation to be associated with hypersensitivity. This association is established for some conditions and seems probable in others. Such a relation may appear less likely for reactions to foreign bodies, but so many foreign bodies are chemical in nature, endogenous or plant in origin, that an associated delayed type of hypersensitivity cannot be entirely excluded.

Macrophages. The circulating monocyte is the main precursor of the mononuclear macrophage in inflamed tissues. However, the infiltration of inflamed tissues by macrophages may be transient or persistent, according to the cause of the lesion. In acute inflammation, macrophages disappear in a few days because of death of the cells, their removal by lymphatics, or migration elsewhere. In chronic inflammation the persistence of macrophages may result from their local proliferation, from longevity of the cells in the tissues, or from their continuing mobilization from the bone marrow. There is, in fact, evidence for all three possibilities.[66]

Functionally, the macrophage has a high capacity for phagocytosis and a highly developed system for digesting engulfed material. These features are best illustrated in infections by large facultative bacteria such as *Mycobacterium tuberculosis* or by fungi, or in lesions provoked by the introduction of foreign bodies. Compared with the neutrophil as a phagocyte, the macrophage has a longer life, greater hardiness, and different functions.[65]

Epithelioid cells provide a major feature of various examples of granulomatous inflammation, such as tuberculosis (Fig. 2-22), leprosy, and sarcoidosis (Fig. 2-24). They are relatively large cells (Fig. 2-22), polygonal or somewhat elongate, with a pale nucleus and the cell membranes of adjacent cells in apposition. Epithelioid cells are derived from macrophages by natural maturation, provided that (1) the macrophage survives and remains in situ for long enough, (2) it is not required to undertake phagocytosis, or (3) if it does so, the particle is completely degraded or eliminated. Macrophages that ingest poorly degradable material (such as mycobacteria) do not mature into epithelioid cells.[65]

Epithelioid cells in the mouse normally live for 1 to 4 weeks and are nonphagocytic but retain high pinocytic activity. Epithelioid cells divide to produce small round cells that develop, in turn, into typical macrophages that are phagocytic but that mature into epithelioid cells when appropriate conditions prevail.[65]

Giant cells are large multinucleate cells formed by fusion of macrophages (Fig. 2-26). They are common granulomatous inflammation, particularly when the lesions are caused by the following:

1. Infection such as tuberculosis, syphilis, and fungal infections
2. Insoluble exogeneous substances such as talc, ligatures, and other foreign bodies
3. Insoluble endogenous substances such as fat, keratin, and sodium biurate crystals

The morphology of giant cells is variable. Nuclei arranged peripherally in the cell are characteristic of the so-called Langhans' giant cell (Fig. 2-23), which is common in tuberculosis, whereas nuclei positioned centrally in the cell are more common in giant cells in foreign-body reactions (Fig. 2-25). All the nuclei of these multinucleated cells exhibit synchronous synthesis of DNA.[64]

Lymphocytes and plasma cells. The occurrence of lymphocytes and plasma cells (Fig. 2-27) in chronic inflammation, particularly in granulomatous lesions, and their role in antibody formation raise the question of the part that immune mechanisms play in chronic inflammation, especially where the lesions are granulomatous.

The possible importance of such immunologic mechanisms is highlighted by the number of diseases exhibiting granulomatous inflammation for which an associated delayed type of hypersensitivity provides the basis for a diagnostic skin test. The list of conditions includes infection by the following:

1. Bacteria—tuberculosis, leprosy, syphilis, and brucellosis

2. Viruses—lymphogranuloma inguinale and cat-scratch fever
3. Fungi—dermatomycosis, coccidioidomycosis, and histoplasmosis
4. Metazoa—hydatid disease
5. Protozoa—leishmaniasis

Eosinophils. Eosinophils are common in chronic inflammatory lesions, particularly when the disease is associated with hypersensitivity or attributable to parasitic infestation. Reference has already been made in this chapter to the decrease of the eosinophil response that occurs in trichinosis when there is depletion or inactivation of the pool of lymphocytes normally recirculating in the body.[75]

Fibroblasts are prominent in chronic inflammation when organization is in process (as at the periphery of a tubercle) or when the reaction is fibrogenic (as in silicosis).[65] Fibroblasts arise by proliferation of other local fibroblasts and synthesize collagen.

Over the past several years the complex modulation of the fibroblast by immune and other mesenchymal cells during the inflammatory process has been partially elucidated.[85] A variety of lymphokines and monokines have been found to profoundly affect fibroblast proliferation, migration, and extracellular matrix synthesis and degradation. Cytokines have been isolated, and they have inhibitory as well as stimulatory activities, indicating that there may be immune-modulated down-regulation of the fibroblastic response as well as up-

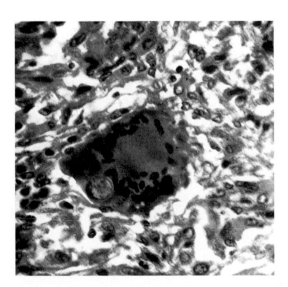

Fig. 2-26. Phagocytosis of pathogenic fungus. *Coccidioides immitis,* by multinucleated giant cell in human lung. Doubly contoured organism is seen at lower left-hand side of giant cell. (420×.)

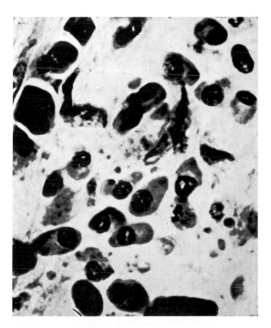

Fig. 2-27. Plasma cells have eccentric nucleus with chromatin arranged peripherally to give "cartwheel" or "clock-face" appearance. Large cells are macrophages. (1070×.)

regulation of this mesenchymal cell population during the inflammatory response.[133]

Causes of chronicity of inflammation

Experimental work with various irritants labeled with radioactive isotopes indicates that persistence of a granulomatous reaction is accompanied by the intracellular presence of irritant. Disappearance of irritant results in disappearance of the reaction.[65] Persistence of irritant within cells may result from survival of viable microorganisms or from failure of macrophages to degrade dead organisms to diffusible breakdown products.

The development of hypersensitivity is frequently put forward as a cause of chronicity. An excess of antibody over antigen in the formation of immune complexes certainly provokes a granulomatous reaction rather than an acute inflammation, but the reaction is nevertheless exhibited by thymectomized animals. Recurrent reactions of immediate-type hypersensitivity (for example, to circulating antigen-antibody complexes as in allergic vasculitis) may provoke chronic inflammation, but the evidence also indicates that delayed-type hypersensitivity may accompany chronic inflammation and may also cause it.[65]

HEALING

The resolution of inflammation involves the removal of exudate and dead cells by enzymatic dissolution and phagocytosis. These events are followed by healing: the replacement of the killed or damaged tissue by cells derived from the parenchymal or connective tissue elements of the injured tissue. When healing is accomplished mainly by proliferation of the parenchymal ele-

ments, the process is termed *regeneration* and often results in complete restoration of the original tissue. When the main contribution is made by the nonspecialized elements of connective tissue, fibrosis or scarring results, and the process is called *repair*. The same principles are involved in the restoration of destroyed tissue whether the process involves mainly regeneration or repair.

Regeneration

The cells of the body can be divided into three groups according to their capacity to regenerate[92,111]:

1. *Labile cells* continue to multiply throughout life, even under normal physiologic conditions. They include the epithelial cells of the skin and mucous membranes and the cells of the bone marrow and lymph nodes.
2. *Stable cells* have a decrease or loss of ability for physiologic regeneration in adolescence but retain the ability to proliferate throughout adult life. They include parenchymatous cells of the liver, pancreas, kidney, adrenal, and thyroid.
3. *Permanent cells* lose their ability to proliferate around the time of birth. The most important example is the neuron of the central nervous system.

Regeneration of labile cells

The process of regeneration is basically similar whatever the tissue involved. The events are well illustrated after the curettage of a longitudinal strip 2 mm wide from the mucosal epithelium of the trachea. The rings of tracheal cartilage prevent distortion of the injured

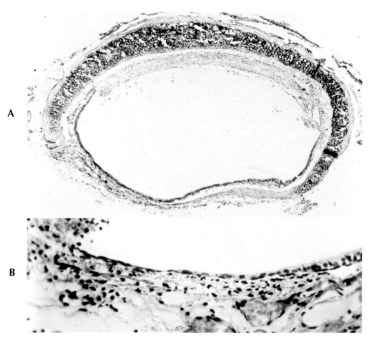

Fig. 2-28. A, Regeneration of tracheal mucosa in rat. Two fifths of mucosa has been removed by curettage. Six hours after curettage, migration of epithelial cells has commenced at margins of residual mucosa. **B,** Higher magnification of migrating epithelial cells illustrated in **A.** (**A,** 35×; **B,** 150×; from Wilhelm, D.L.: J. Pathol. Bacteriol. **65:**543, 1953.)

tissue and hence make it easy to follow the regeneration of the thin layer of specialized cells in the mucosa.

Regeneration proceeds in four stages[134]: (1) thrombosis and inflammation, (2) regeneration of epithelium over the denuded surface, (3) multiplication of the new cells, and (4) differentiation of the new epithelium.

In *thrombosis and inflammation* the denuded surface is quickly covered by fibrin clot (Figs. 2-28, *A*, and 2-29) with entangled blood cells, while the adjacent underlying tissues exhibit an acute inflammatory response that reaches a peak in 24 to 36 hours and then subsides over the next few days.

Regeneration of epithelium over the denuded surface occurs by the migration of cells from the margin of the wound. The tracheal mucosa consists of a pseudostratified ciliated epithelium with intervening goblet cells and a basal layer of germinal cells that proliferate, migrating toward the surface as they mature.

In regeneration the resurfacing of the denuded area is performed by the epithelial cells at the wound margin (Fig. 2-28). These cells lose their cilia and then migrate laterally as a sheet of cells that are noticeably thinned as though each were covering as great an area as possible. Some cells still exhibit cilia as they begin to migrate, but not for long. Such migration begins as early as 1 hour after injury and is usually well established in 6 hours. The migrating cells cover distances of about 200 μm in the first 8 hours and 400 to 1200 μm in 24 hours, with the migrating cells at both edges of a longitudinal curettage together covering the 2 mm defects within 48 hours (Fig. 2-30, *A*). Cells from the curetted necks of submucosal glands make smaller contributions to the sheet of spreading cells.

When the lesions are about 24 hours old, the original mucosal cells just lateral to the initial margin of the wound exhibit a sudden wave of mitotic activity. The proliferation begins six to eight cells behind the margin of curettage and involves both ciliated columnar cells

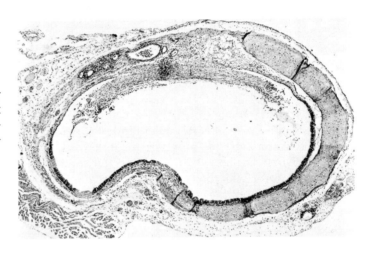

Fig. 2-29. Regeneration of tracheal mucosa 18 hours after curettage. Advancing epithelium is undermining fibrin clot on curetted surface. Peritracheal tissues exhibit inflammatory edema and infiltration by neutrophils. (35×; from Wilhelm, D.L.: J. Pathol. Bacteriol. **65:**543, 1953.)

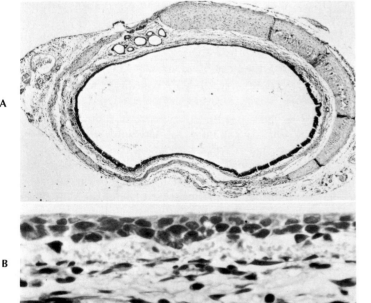

Fig. 2-30. A, Regeneration of tracheal mucosa 48 hours after curettage. Curetted surface is reepithelialized by shallow epithelium. **B,** Higher magnification of new epithelium illustrated in **A.** New epithelium is simple and stratified. (**A,** 35×; **B,** 625×; from Wilhelm, D.L.: J. Pathol. Bacteriol. **65:**543, 1953.)

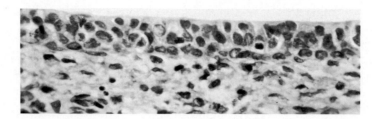

Fig. 2-31. Regeneration of tracheal mucosa 96 hours after curettage. New epithelium shows evidence of redifferentiation. (550×; from Wilhelm, D.L.: J. Pathol. Bacteriol. **65:**543, 1953.)

and basal cells. This mitotic activity provides a population of cells to replace those lost by migration and ensures a continuing supply of cells for migration. Mitosis involves most of the original mucosa. Another factor of importance in regeneration is the requirement of an appropriate surface on which the spreading cells can migrate. Recent data indicates that the composition and organization of the underlying connective tissue, in part, may determine the attachment, spreading, migration, and proliferation rates of the overlying migrating epithelial cells as well as their differentiation state.[129,130] If the injury is slight and the underlying basement membrane is intact, reconstitution by the epithelium is rapid. If the basement membrane is destroyed, the migrating epithelial cells synthesize a new basal lamina as they migrate. Inhibition of this matrix synthesis results in inhibition of migration and repair.[129] The advancing cells undermine the superficial blood clot, presumably by fibrinolytic activity, and continue migrating until the defect is covered. With migration complete, the retromarginal mitosis ceases abruptly. The migrating cells are therefore derived mainly from the original mucosal cells, though lesser numbers arise by mitosis of the spreading cells themselves.

Multiplication of the new cells follows as soon as the defect has been covered by the new epithelium. A fresh wave of mitotic activity appears in the regenerated mucosa. This second wave is strictly confined to the new mucosal epithelium, occupies the next 24 to 48 hours, and results in the new mucosa's becoming multilayered, the cells at this stage being simple and stratified in type.

Differentiation of the new epithelium begins by the time the whole process is 4 days old. The new cells are rearranged into a superficial layer of cuboid cells and a basal layer of flattened germinal cells (Fig. 2-31). In 5 to 7 days, differentiation is advanced, with the cuboid cells already becoming columnar and some containing droplets of mucin. Differentiation into goblet cells takes 12 to 14 days. Cilia begin to form during the second week, but more so in the third week. The final restoration of normal tissue may take up to 6 weeks (Fig. 2-32).

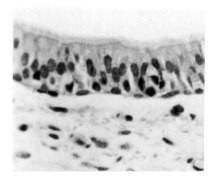

Fig. 2-32. Regenerated tracheal mucosa 6 weeks after curettage. Normal mucosal epithelium with mitosis in basal cell. (550×; from Wilhelm, D.L.: J. Pathol. Bacteriol. **65:**543, 1953.)

The same sequence of events is evident in regeneration of columnar cell epithelium of other organs and of *squamous cell epithelium* of the epidermis and cornea. In the skin there is no regeneration of specialized structures such as sweat glands, sebaceous glands, or hair follicles unless viable remnants of these structures persist in the dermis.

With *burns*, the severity of destruction is closely related to the depth of the tissue affected. Burns are described as *first degree* (epidermal) when the superficial epidermis is involved but its continuity is maintained; as *second degree* (dermal) when the epidermis is virtually destroyed so that the underlying dermis with its sweat glands, nerve endings, and bulbs of hair follicles is exposed; and as *third degree* (full thickness) when all epithelial structures in the dermis have been destroyed. In second-degree burns the epidermis is largely reformed from surviving cells of the dermal appendages. Without this possibility in third-degree burns, reepithelialization can occur only from the edges, and the depth of the burn results in substantial scarring and the dermal appendages are not reconstituted, illustrating the importance of the surrounding connective tissues in maintaining specialized structures and functions of epithelial cells.

Regeneration of stable cells

The liver has remarkable powers of regeneration that have been repeatedly described after surgical resection or exposure to chemical poisons causing hepatic necrosis. Regeneration after the resection of healthy liver was originally demonstrated in rabbits by Ponfick[122,123] in the 1890s. In a series of animals of comparable body weight, he estimated the proportional weight of the liver lobes to that of the whole liver and therefore could calculate the proportion that was surgically excised.

The liver has a striking regenerative capacity. Successful regeneration can occur even when nearly 90% of the organ is removed. A residuum of 10% of the liver might be expected to be too little for postoperative survival, but it proved adequate for Ponfick's rabbits, as well as for rats and dogs in later studies by other workers.

A wide range of chemical poisons and biochemical and metabolic disorders, as well as certain viral infections, all produce liver necrosis that may be focal, zonal, or diffuse in distribution. For example, the hepatic necrosis induced by exposure to carbon tetrachloride chiefly involves the parenchyma around the central veins.[93] The necrotic cells are removed by lysis and phagocytosis, but the supporting mesenchymal stroma survives. Proliferation soon occurs in the surviving liver cells throughout each lobule, and new cells migrate into the centrilobular zones, being guided by the persistent reticulin framework, which normally supports the columns of hepatocytes. Remarkably satisfactory regeneration is achieved within 2 weeks. But if necrosis is again induced before regeneration is complete, or the lesion results in damage of the supporting stroma, "regeneration nodules" of liver tissue are formed without restoration of normal hepatic architecture.

In the liver, just as in the trachea, lung, and skin, maintenance of the connective tissue skeleton is necessary for regeneration to occur. If necrosis after injury destroys the complex connective tissue structure of the lobule, hepatocytes will still undergo proliferation but the normal lobular architecture will not be maintained. The repair process progresses with the formation of nodules of hepatocytes having no organized portal, trabecular, or central venous architecture or organization, but with Ito cell proliferation with the formation of broad fibrous bands of connective tissue.[98-100,113]

Regeneration of permanent cells

Permanent cells occur predominantly in the central nervous system. At birth the nervous system already has its full complement of neurons, which lack a capacity for regeneration. For peripheral nerves, however, limited regeneration can occur, though it is confined to the axons (the cytoplasmic extensions of the neurons).

Regeneration of peripheral nerves. The divided ends of a sectioned nerve[137] become united by proliferating Schwann cells and fibroblasts, which arise from the cut end, though mainly from the distal stump. On about the third day, the myelin sheath and axon of the remaining intact nerve degenerate back as far as the next node of Ranvier of the proximal surviving axon. From the peripheral end of the viable axon appear numerous new sprouts: 25 to 50 such fibrils emerge from the central stump, but most become lost in the "union scar" joining the cut ends of the fiber.

Meanwhile, in the peripheral stump, there is breakdown and phagocytosis of the axon and myelin, as well as proliferation of the surviving Schwann cells. About 50 days after injury, the peripheral stump consists of tubes filled with elongated Schwann cells. Of the fibrils emerging from the proximal stump, one or more enter the old neural tube; one of the entering fibrils in turn grows in diameter, becomes medullated, and develops into the new functional axon. After crushing or division and suture of a nerve, function is restored after an initial lag of 20 to 40 days, the rate of advance being 2 to 3 mm per day.

The success of regeneration depends on the width of the union scar and the alignment of the cut ends; the nature of any intervening tissue; and suturing of the cut ends. Suturing is well worthwhile, even some time after a nerve is sectioned, though the results are unsatisfactory if suture is delayed more than 6 months.

Regeneration of muscle. Regeneration of striated muscle[96] resembles that of peripheral nerve in that each fiber must be regarded as a unit that can be regenerated only when there is survival of a reasonable part of the unit. When muscle fibers are divided, the subsequent retraction of the cut ends seriously handicaps regeneration. But after crushing, the ends of injured fibers are held together by the connective tissue stroma. The injured site is first filled with fibrinous exudate containing neutrophils and macrophages. The damaged portions of the fibers are soon removed, with short lengths of sarcolemmal tubes filled with histiocytes being left. At about 3 days, outgrowths of sarcoplasm extend from the fiber stumps along these tubes. These outgrowths contain numerous nuclei and have a characteristic pointed tip. The regenerating strands meet, overlap, and anastomose, though complete restoration of muscle architecture is slow and individual fibers may be disoriented for up to 3 months. When the sheath of the fibers is destroyed, the outgrowth of sarcoplasm may be obstructed by connective tissue and therefore forms a multinucleated mass.

With muscle damage from ischemia or bacterial toxins, new endomysial tubes are formed on the scaffolding of the dead fibers and provide the channels that guide the new fibers. Regeneration is independent of an intact nerve supply.

Smooth muscle (as of the ureter, bladder, and bowel) has similar, though lesser, capacity for regeneration than striated muscle does.

• • •

This discussion of regeneration has been purposely restricted to only a few tissues and organs because the process basically consists in (1) cell migration, with proliferation of the original cells to maintain a population of cells available for migration, and (2) proliferation of the migrated cells constituting the regenerated tissue and their subsequent differentiation and maturation. These processes are modified for the various parenchymal cells, according to their morphologic features and functional requirements.

Repair

Repair refers to the replacement of tissue defects by fibrous tissue, whereas *regeneration* should be restricted to the replacement of a single type of parenchymatous cell by proliferating survivors of the same kind. Both terms come under the more general one of *healing*.

The most common example of healing is the healing of wounds. Before considering the healing process, however, it is helpful to discuss two aspects of the process: the formation of granulation tissue and the contraction of wounds.

Formation of granulation tissue

Much of our information on the formation of granulation tissue comes from the work of E.R. and E.L. Clark,[94,95] who microscopically observed the events provoked by injury of the tail of the tadpole, and from Sandison,[127] who studied repair in mammalian tissues in the rabbit ear chamber. After insertion of an ear chamber, the central table of the chamber is soon covered by blood clot containing strands of fibrin, erythrocytes, and a few leukocytes. During the next day or two, the fibrin becomes more evident, the red cells less so, and the central table covered by a light brown granular mass. Concurrent with these preliminary changes, *macrophages* appear on the table, invade the blood clot, and begin to ingest and digest cellular debris, fragments of fibrin, and red cells. Some of the macrophages fuse to form giant cells. The digestion of the fibrin clot is also facilitated by extracellular enzymes derived from the macrophages, as well as from disintegrated neutrophils.

The advancing macrophages are soon followed by *capillaries* that arise from blood vessels at the periphery of the table where preexisting tissue adjoins the blood clot. The young capillaries usually reach the edge of the table by the seventh day after insertion of the chamber and continue to advance at a rate of 0.1 to 0.6 mm daily. The new capillaries are formed by migration and mitosis of endothelial cells of adjacent preexisting blood vessels in a manner analogous to that for regeneration of mucosal epithelium. Endothelial cells at the line of severance of blood vessels migrate forward beyond the cut vessel to form a small sprout with a fine terminal prolongation. This new capillary is initially solid (Fig. 2-33), but within a few hours it develops a lumen and carries blood. The tips of proliferating vessels have blunt, plump, or even bulbous ends, into the lumen of which are forced red cells, platelets, and a few white cells. However, the fluid exhibits no movement other than oscillations imparted by the heartbeat and respiration. The new capillaries gradually proliferate into the areas of the blood clot cleared by the scavenging macrophages and sometimes join one another or anastomose to form capillary loops.[77] The outcome is an advancing margin of delicate vascular arches through which blood flows (Fig. 2-34). The newly formed capillaries are abnormally premeable at or near the advancing tip, the interendothelial junctions being tenuous and exhibiting distinct gaps. The newly formed vessels also bleed readily, their fragility possibly being attributable to the morphologic features underlying their abnormal permeability.[128]

The new blood vessels initially consist of endothelial cells alone. Within a few days they develop into arterioles, true capillaries, or venules, possibly according to intravascular pressure and the amount of blood flow.[4] During the next weeks the new vessels continue to differentiate until after some months the field on the table of an ear chamber exhibits a whole range of vascular elements—artery, arterioles, true capillaries, venules, and vein.[94,95] While the vascular bed is differentiating, there is a constant remodeling of the vasculature. This remodeling particularly involves obliteration of many of the initial capillaries, consequent to absence of blood flow through these vessels. The process begins by a decrease in diameter and then a loss of lumen. The solid cord so produced breaks in two, and the ends retract to the level of the next patent vessel.[127]

Vasomotor nerves appear on the arterioles as early as 2 to 3 days after the formation of endothelial tubes. The development of muscle cells in the vascular wall imparts tone, but contraction is not evident until the cells are reached by vasomotor twigs.[4]

Lymphatics proliferate in much the same manner as blood vessels, though the growth of lymphatic vessels is slower and less labile.[4]

Fibrous tissue. At the stage when the formed elements of the initial blood clot have been removed from an ear chamber, the cells and proliferating elements are supported by an amorphous gelatinous matrix ("ground substance"). This matrix has a relatively high content of mucopolysaccharide, the concentration of which begins

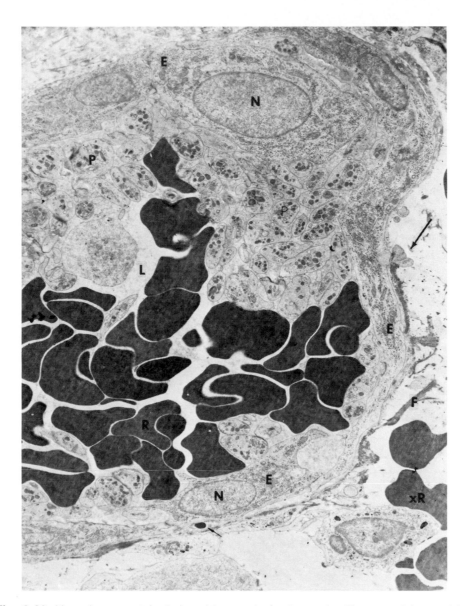

Fig. 2-33. Vascular sprout in 3-day-old wound of rat muscle. The sprout has a blunt extremity, and lumen, *L,* is filled with platelets, *P,* and red blood cells, *R. Lower right,* Extravasated red cells, *xR.* Notice cytoplasmic extrusion *(right arrow)* of endothelial cell, *E.* Shreds of fibrin, *F,* coat the adventitial aspect of vessel. *Bottom arrow,* Portion of red cell in cleft in vascular wall. *N,* Nucleus of endothelial cell. (Karnovsky stain; 3800×; from Schoefl, G.I.: Virchows Arch. [Pathol. Anat.] **337:**97, 1963.)

to decrease when the first young fibrils of collagen are produced by fibroblasts. The fibroblasts probably arise from fibrocytes or some less differentiated precursor in the tissues around the table of the chamber, particularly the loose connective tissue. Fibroblasts enter the clot just after the macrophages and at about the same time as the blood vessels, advancing at a rate of about 0.2 mm a day. Their number is constantly increased by further cells from the surrounding tissue, as well as by mitotic division of fibroblasts already on the scene. Col-

lagen fibers become identifiable by about the sixth day. At first they are radially disposed and lie in a single plane, but other layers of fibers subsequently appear, roughly at right angles to the first. The direction of the fibers seems to be determined by lines of tension during the laying down of the fibers.

The outcome of these processes is the formation of vascular young connective tissue containing a variable number of inflammatory cells. This so-called *granulation tissue* (Fig. 2-35) derives its name from its appear-

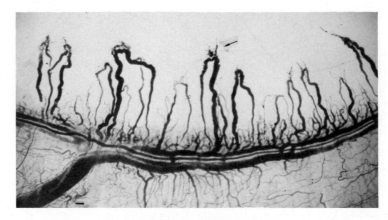

Fig. 2-34. Cornea of rat, 5 days after silver nitrate injury. Arcades of new blood vessels appear in healing wound. Abnormal permeability of new vessels is indicated by escape of circulating colloidal carbon into the perivascular tissue *(arrows)*. (22×; from Schoefl, G.I.: Virchows Arch. [Pathol. Anat.] **337:**97, 1963.)

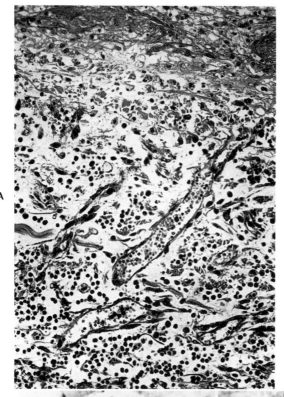

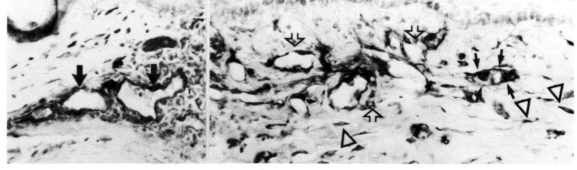

Fig. 2-35. A, Granulation tissue in pericarditis. Newly formed blood vessels are supported by loosely arranged connective tissue, in interstices of which lie inflammatory cells. Fibrinous exudate *(at top)* obscures outline of serosal pericardium. (170×.) **B,** Immunoperoxidase staining of murine corneal neovascularization using antibodies raised against laminin. *Left,* Proximal area of neovascularization near the preexisting limbal vessels *(large arrows)* and newly formed vessels stain with laminin antibodies. *Right,* High-power photomicrograph of the distal area of neovascularization illustrating the distal tips of the newly forming vessels *(small arrows)* stained with laminin antibodies. All the segments of the newly formed vessels as well as single putative endothelial cells in this area *(arrowheads)* stain positively. (400×.)

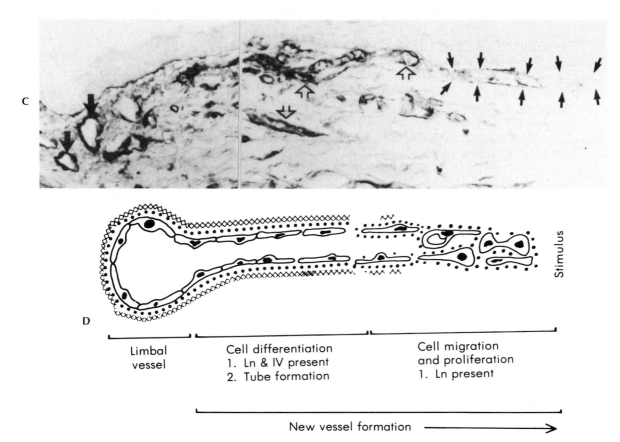

Limbal
vessel

Cell differentiation
1. Ln & IV present
2. Tube formation

Cell migration
and proliferation
1. Ln present

New vessel formation ⟶

Fig. 2-35, cont'd. C, Immunoperoxidase staining of murine corneal neovascularization using antibodies raised against type IV collagen. *Left,* Proximal area of neovascularization near the preexisting limbal vessels *(large arrows)* and newly formed vessels stain with type IV collagen antibodies. *Right,* High-power photomicrograph of the distal area of neovascularization illustrating the distal tips of the newly forming vessels *(small arrows)* stained with type IV collagen antibodies. There is an absence of staining for type IV collagen at the distal tips of the newly forming vessels, whereas irregular, patchy staining is observed a short distance behind the tips *(small arrows).* Neovasculature farther behind this area stains more intensely and uniformly for type IV collagen *(large open arrows).* In contrast to the staining pattern noted in **B** individual cells in the stroma in proximity to the vessel tips are negative for type IV collagen staining. (400×.) **D,** Schema of the angiogenic response noted in the murine cornea. After stimulation, the endothelial cells lining the limbal vessels degrade their investing basement membrane and migrate into the stroma toward the injury site in response to a variety of factors. After the initial migratory response, the endothelial cells undergo a proliferative response. Migration and proliferation occur at or near the distal tip of the neovascular response, whereas endothelial cells farther back, near the limbal vessels, exhibit a lower proliferative rate and organize into tubelike structures with definite lumens and cell-cell and cell-matrix interactions. Endothelial cells in the more distal area secrete laminin but do not form a morphologically identifiable basement membrane. Endothelial cells farther back secrete both laminin and type IV collagen and form morphologically identifiable basement membranes. The temporally staggered appearance of laminin and type IV collagen correlates with the rates of endothelial cell proliferation noted in situ during angiogenesis and the in vitro effects of these basement membrane components. *Dots,* Laminin (Ln); *cross-hatching,* type IV collagen (IV).

ance, as in the base of a large open wound. The new tissue has a slightly granular surface with each "granule" corresponding to a vascular arcade of new capillaries, elevating their thin covering of young collagen slightly above the adjacent unsupported matrix. The term *granulation tissue* refers to the consequent impression of granularity of the surface.

Since these now classical descriptions of the angiogenic process observed to occur after wounding, there has been a remarkable advance in our understanding of this dynamic, complex process, which plays a central, if not pivotal, role in not only repair but also in neoplasia and atherosclerosis.[90,104,105,131] The phenomenon of angiogenesis can be arbitrarily broken down into several processes: endothelial cell activation; migration; proliferation, differentiation—tube formation; stabilization; and regression.[107,114,115,124] Recently there have been identified several endothelial cell growth factors that share some common properties (heparin binding) as well as having differences (pI, molecular weight).[103,112] From these and other studies it has become clear that angiogenesis can be triggered by any one of several stimuli (cytokines, tumor factors, clotting proteins, and so on) all leading to a similar end point—neovascularization.[88,104,107,119,125] In addition to the various soluble factors that are capable of modulating the angiogenic response, investigators have noted that the surrounding extracellular matrix and that newly synthesized by the local endothelial cell population dramatically affect the behavior of microvascular endothelial cells.[106,114-116,124] Selected matrix components appear to function as solid-phase autocrine and paracrine effectors of the angiogenic response. Specifically, laminin, which is detected early in the angiogenic response, is associated with a highly proliferative and migratory phenotype; whereas type IV collagen is noted later in areas exhibiting lower migratory and proliferative rates where tube formation is occurring.[106,119] Fig. 2-35, *B* to *D*, illustrates this staggered appearance of basement membrane components in experimentally induced murine corneal neovascularization.

Thus the angiogenic response observed during healing and repair appears to be modulated by a complex number of positive and negative stimuli including soluble and solid-phase factors, vasomotor control, and shear forces.

Chemical estimations of the constituents of healing wounds reveal two phases of activity: (1) an initial phase, during which there is accumulation of proteins and an increase in content of hexosamine, the latter possibly corresponding to the entry of glycoproteins with the inflammatory exudate, succeeded by (2) a collagen phase. The level of hexosamine in the healing tissue decreases with the progression of fibroplasia.[101,102] The amount of collagen formed, assessed by the wound

is content of hydroxyproline, increases as the argyrophilic reticulin fibers disappear. This corresponds to a lateral growth of collagen fibrils as well as to an increase in the number of fibrils. For some weeks the amount of collagen and collagen cross-linking parallel the increasing tensile strength of the healing tissue.

Repair with organization

The process whereby coagulated blood becomes replaced by granulation tissue is known as *organization*. The same process occurs in four main sets of circumstances:

1. *Repair.* This was just described.
2. *Inflammation.* Acute inflammation generally resolves, leaving little or no evidence of the episode. Occasionally, however, resolution is incomplete or delayed, whereupon fibrinous exudate in particular becomes invaded by proliferating fibroblasts and blood vessels, with the enhanced vascular supply being required to meet the heightened metabolic needs of the granulation tissue. This process of organization may complicate unresolved pneumonia, being associated with persistence of fibrin in lobar pneumonia and with mixed bacterial infections in bronchopneumonia. It also occurs in rheumatic pneumonia, bronchiectasis, and lung abscess. Organization also complicates inflammatory lesions of serous membranes, such as fibrinous pericarditis (Fig. 2-35), empyema of the pleural cavity, and inflammation of the peritoneal cavity. The process results in adhesions, bands, and scarring.
3. *Thrombosis.* Thrombi that persist at their site of formation are often invaded by granulation tissue and converted into fibrous tissue.
4. *Infarction.* A slow ingrowth of granulation tissue frequently occurs at the periphery of infarcts exhibiting coagulative necrosis, such as that in the kidney, spleen, myocardium, and lung. The infarct is eventually converted into a fibrous scar.

In addition to playing a major role in the repair process, angiogenesis is a prerequisite for metastatic growth of tumors.[103,104] To increase in size, tumors necessarily have to evoke a local angiogenic response. The presence of these new vessels provides the tumor mass with the nutrients needs for continued growth as well as a potential portal to the vascular system that can be instrumental for distant metastatic spread. These observations have led investigators to study the possibilities of inhibiting tumor-induced angiogenesis. Normally during the healing process there is a significant regression of the neovasculature (Fig. 2-36). Folkman and his colleagues have taken several approaches to this problem including the use of heparin antagonists such as protamine and cartilage extracts to downregulate and

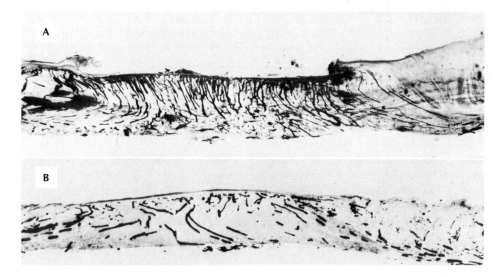

Fig. 2-36. Vasculature of wounds healing by second intention. Full thickness of disk of skin was excised from back of trunk of rats, and regenerated blood vessels were demonstrated by intra-arterial injection with opaque colloidal medium. **A,** Numerous new blood vessels supplying wound that has been filled by granulation tissue. **B,** Decreased vasculature in wound healed in rat 2 months after injury.

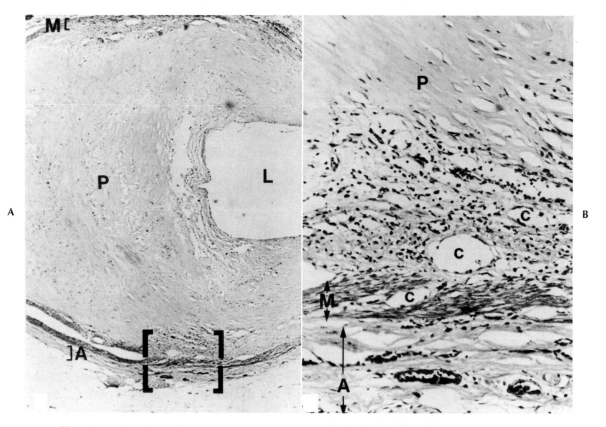

Fig. 2-37. Neovascularization in an atherosclerotic plaque. **A,** Low-power micrograph (100×) of an atherosclerotic coronary artery. Atheromatous material *(P)* is noted above the tunica media *(M)* of the vessel, compromising the lumen *(L).* Adventitial tissue with noticeable vascularization *(A)* surrounding the vessel is also seen. **B,** High-power micrograph (200×) of the bracketed area in **A** illustrating neovascularization of the atherosclerotic plaque *(P)* by vessels *(c)* originating in the adventitia *(A)* and coursing through and disrupting the media *(m).*

inhibit the angiogenic response.[88,104,109] Another approach used by Folkman centers around the discovery that certain steroids (so-called angiostatic steriods) when given in combination with heparin or specific heparin fragments have the ability to inhibit angiogenesis and cause newly formed capillary regression by induction of capillary basement membrane dissolution.[97,108] Additional work in these areas is needed to assess this approach in the treatment of cancer and other diseases in which angiogenesis plays a significant role. One such area in which angiogenesis appears to play a significant role in the development of disease is atherosclerosis. Although known and observed for over 50 years, neovascularization of atherosclerotic plaques has taken on renewed importance.[90,131] It has been postulated that the neovasculature, observed in the vessel walls of atherosclerotic plagues (Fig. 2-37) may be susceptible to hemorrhage, leading to medial hemorrhage, which may result in occlusion or dissection of the affected vessel. In addition, it has been postulated that the presence of increased vasculature in regions of atherosclerotic injury might lead to higher local tissue concentrations of circulating vasoconstrictors, evoking arterial spasm.[90] Thus angiogenesis may play a significant role in the pathogenesis and complications of atherosclerosis and its control may develop into an important therapeutic approach.

Contraction of wounds

The rapidity of the healing of wounds depends to considerable extent on the contraction that begins a few days after injury and continues for several weeks. The magnitude of such contraction is not always appreciated. In rats the scar occupies about 20% to 30% of the area of the original wound, and in rabbits the process is even more successful. But until quite recently, the mechanisms of wound contraction remained uncertain. Dehydration was claimed to contribute, though the main factor was alleged to be contraction of the mature reparative collagen.[13] Nevertheless, the theory of contraction of collagen was acknowledged to be inconsistent with the fact that contraction proceeds at a stage when the collagen content of granulation tissue is negligible. An even greater difficulty is the fact that formation of collagen is decreased in scorbutic animals though wound contraction in such animals proceeds as in normal controls.

The observation that contraction occurs when granulation tissue is being formed prompted various workers to regard granulation tissue as an *organ of contraction*,[87,91] a proposal that gained support from the observation that comparable contraction occurs in scorbutic animals.[86] The puzzle concerning the element responsible for contraction seems resolved by work in Majno's laboratory.[110,126] In wounds of the rat's skin, fibroblasts increase in number from the third day onward. Be-

tween 7 and 21 days, according to the type of lesion, many of the fibroblasts in granulation tissue develop three morphologic modifications: (1) bundles of fibrils in the cytoplasm, resembling those of smooth muscle cells, as well as opaque areas among the bundles or beneath the plasmalemma, resembling "attachment sites" of smooth muscle; (2) nuclear indentations, comparable to those on nuclear membranes of contracted muscle cells; and (3) differentiation of the cell's surface to provide numerous intercellular connections resembling desmosomes. The morphologic similarity of these modified fibroblasts to smooth muscle cells is supported by other observations. The cytoplasm of the modified cells exhibits immunofluorescent labeling with human anti-smooth muscle serum, and strips of granulation tissue respond to various drugs in vitro similarly to smooth muscle. Furthermore, the extraction of granulation tissue yields quantities of actomyosin (with the same adenosine triphosphate activity) similar to those obtained from nonstriated muscle of the pregnant rat uterus. The overall results therefore indicate that modified fibroblasts ("myofibroblasts") are responsible for the process of contraction of granulation tissue in healing wounds.[110] Similar myofibroblasts have been identified in granulation tissue from human lesions.[126]

The phenomenon of wound contracture is also evident in parenchymal organs such as the lung and liver and "myofibroblast-like" cells have been identified in both organs during the repair process.[89,113,117,118,120] In the liver the vitamin A storage cell (the Ito cell) has been identified as a mesenchymal cell that proliferates and produces connective tissue components during fibrosis and also displays the phenotype of a myofibroblast (including desmin positivity and abundant microfilaments and attachment sites).[89,98-100,117,118,120]

Healing by first intention

When the surgeon sutures a clean incision, healing takes place with minimum loss of tissue and without significant bacterial infection. This is referred to as *healing by first intention* or *primary union* (Fig. 2-37). The space between the opposing surfaces of the incised skin becomes filled with blood from *hemorrhage* of severed vessels; the blood then coagulates to form a clot that seals the incision against dehydration and infection.

Acute inflammation quickly ensues, and within 24 hours the margins of the incision are infiltrated by neutrophils and monocytes, and swollen by fluid exudate. Autolytic enzymes liberated by dead tissue cells, proteolytic enzymes from neutrophils, and phagocytic activity by monocytes and tissue macrophages combine to clear away the necrotic tissue, debris, and red blood cells. The ingested hemoglobin becomes converted into hemosiderin and hematoidin.

The early events in healing by first intention include an important contribution by the *epidermis*.[121] At both margins of the incision, the epidermis responds within hours by becoming thickened and migrating from the margins of the wound down into the upper part of the incisional gap and uniting in the upper dermis. The advancing epidermis cleaves the overlying necrotic epithelium and associated necrotic dermis from underlying viable dermis (Fig. 2-37), so that the scab over the migrated epidermis finally contains dry blood clot, fragments of dead epidermis, and fibers of collagen and elastin. Throughout the invasion by the epidermis, the migrating cells are nondividing. Mitotic activity is confined to basal cells adjacent to the margins of the wound.

With well-approximated wounds, a continuous layer of epidermis usually forms in 48 hours (Fig. 2-37). During the next day or so, the new epidermis may further invade the dermal breach to form a downward-pointing spur (Fig. 2-38). Thereafter, the new epidermis takes on the morphologic features of the adjacent uninjured epidermis, and the epidermal spurs are remodeled from early in the second week onward.

Organization proceeds meanwhile in the incisional deficit of the dermis, protected by the overlying new epidermis. By about the third day, the dermal lesion contains fibroblasts and capillary buds emigrating from the edges of the wound. Reticulin is demonstrable by the second or third day, and new collagen by the fifth day. During the fourth week (and even earlier in the tissue adjacent to the margins of the wound site), the cellular and vascular elements are decreasing in both number and concentration.

Response to sutures. Healing by first intention of a wound more than minimal in size requires that the wound be sutured. However, the suture material itself evokes a complex and often prolonged reaction.[121] During the initial 3 days, the epidermis and the epithelium of dermal appendages react to the presence of the foreign material by advancing along the suture track to form an incomplete tube of epithelium two to three cells thick around the whole length of the suture (Fig. 2-38). Between the epithelial tube and the suture lie fibrin, neutrophils, and erythocytes. Externally, the epithelium initially lies on the collagen of the dermis, though in a day or two, mononuclear cells come to surround the epithelial tube. Deep to the advancing margin of downgrowing epithelium, the suture is encased by (1) leukocytes and nuclear debris, (2) foreign-body granulation tissue containing macrophages and giant cells, and (3) young collagen.

Removal of sutures at about the tenth day usually re-

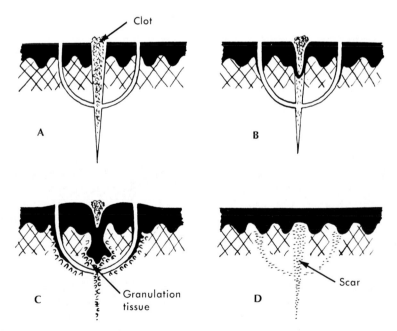

Fig. 2-38. Healing of incised wound that has been sutured. Track alone of suture is illustrated. **A,** Wound rapidly fills with blood clot. **B,** Soon afterwards, epidermis *(black)* migrates both into wound and around suture track. **C,** Epithelial tongues or spurs are formed, and granulation tissue begins to be formed. For convenience, zone of necrotic tissue flanking incision is not illustrated but is nevertheless present and becomes separated from underlying viable dermis by invading epithelial cells from the epidermis. These epithelial cells are represented in **B** and **C** by the centrally placed spur. **D,** Suture has been removed and scar tissue marks sites of incision and of suture track. Epithelial tongues and spurs have degenerated. (From Walter, J.B., and Israel, M.S.: General pathology, ed. 3, Edinburgh, 1970, J. & A. Churchill.)

sults in part or much of the epithelial tube being left in the suture tract. The epithelium so isolated in the dermis provokes a strong foreign-body reaction. However, the epithelium is resorbed during the next week and the breach in the epidermis is healed by regeneration (Fig. 2-38).

In summary, the insertion of sutures itself entails incisional damage. To this damage is added a brisk granulomatous reaction evoked by both the suture material and the downgrowing epithelium, which arises particularly from dermal appendages injured by suturing. The tissue reaction is equally severe for monofilament nylon as for polyfilament Mersilk of equivalent caliber. The earlier the sutures are removed, the less will be the granulomatous response. However, the use of adhesive tape avoids even the lesser granulomatous response obtained by early removal of sutures.[121]

Healing by second intention

Not all wounds can or should be sutured. In either case the edges gape and the open wound has a red base and margins that become swollen from inflammatory edema. The floor of the wound exudes a yellowish pink fluid that contains protein, including fibrinogen, and therefore coagulates over the wound.

The relatively wide separation of the wound edges means that healing has to progress from the base upward. Nevertheless, the basic events in healing by second intention resemble those for first intention. Acute inflammation and clearing of debris are accompanied chronologically by downgrowth of epidermis to form a layer of epithelium that separates viable preexisting col-

lagen of the dermis from injured necrotic collagen at the wound's margin (Fig. 2-39).

Meanwhile, the base of the coagulum becomes replaced by granulation tissue, produced by fibroblasts and vascular sprouts from the adjacent viable dermis (Fig. 2-36, A). The surface of the young granulation tissue is deep red, granular, and fragile. Concurrent with the development of the granulation tissue, there is contraction of the wound induced by myofibroblasts. The advancing sheets of epidermis finally cover the granulation tissue so that the scab is separated and cast off. Progressive contraction decreases the size of the wound, and the new epidermis is elevated by the increasing amount of granulation tissue (Fig. 2-39). The scar is at first pink but becomes pale and whitish because of a decrease in vasculature over the succeeding months (Fig. 2-36).

The *presence of infection* is an important factor in handicapping the healing of wounds. The increased amount of exudate enlarges the wound, bacterial toxins provoke necrosis and suppuration, and the fibrinolytic enzymes in pus destroy the framework of fibrin, which is so important for the ingrowth of fibroblasts and capillaries. Finally, bacterial toxins may induce thrombosis of blood vessels and therefore interfere with the blood supply of healing tissue.

Metaplasia

Metaplasia ("transformation") is usually defined as the transformation of fully differentiated cells on one kind into differentiated cells of another kind in response to abnormal stimuli. This definition is misleading, how-

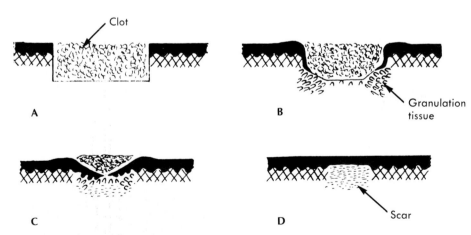

Fig. 2-39. Healing of excised wound by second intention. **A,** Blood clot rapidly fills the wound. **B,** Epidermal cells migrate into the wound as a tongue of cells, separating blood clot and zone of necrotic tissue from underlying viable dermis. **C,** In center of wound, clot becomes organized and rising body of granulation tissue elevates tongues of epithelium until they meet and reform the surface. **D,** Most or all of the clot is cast off without being organized. Contraction of wound results in relatively small scar. (From Walter, J.B., and Israel, M.S.: General pathology, ed. 3, Edinburgh, 1970, J. & A. Churchill.)

ever, because the change in form of the mature cells results from a *change in the usual line of differentiation*, not a transformation of the fully differentiated cell. For example, the progeny of the germinal cells of tracheal mucosa normally differentiate into ciliated columnar and goblet cells, but in rats deficient in vitamin A the proliferating cells abandon their usual line of differentiation for one that results in squamous cells.[134] The term *metaplasia* therefore refers to a change in the line of differentiation of proliferating cells, such that the type of fully differentiated cell usual for a tissue becomes replaced by a different variety of differentiated cell. Since metaplasia is confined to proliferating cells, the condition is associated mainly with regeneration or neoplasia. It particularly involves epithelium or connective tissue.[136]

Metaplasia in epithelium

Under various circumstances, columnar cell and transitional cell epithelia are transformed into squamous cell epithelium resembling epidermis, the process being referred to as *squamous* or *epidermoid metaplasia*. Squamous metaplasia of a transitional cell epithelium, such as the mucosa of the urinary tract, represents little substantial change in character of the epithelium. On the other hand, squamous metaplasia of the pseudostratified ciliated columnar cells lining the respiratory tract (Fig. 2-40) results in an epithelium that is entirely different morphologically and has lost important features of the normal mucosa that make it such an effective guardian against the entry of inhaled bacteria and foreign material. Such metaplasia is common in the presence of chronic bronchitis and bronchiectasis and in smokers. Squamous metaplasia is reasonably common in the ducts of the salivary glands (Fig. 2-41) and pancreas, in the mucosa of prolapsed bowel, in endometrial polyps, in hyperplasia of the prostate, and in

chronic inflammation of the epididymis and thyroid gland.

The same process of squamous metaplasia is common in neoplasms, particularly in adenocarcinoma of the lung, uterus, breast, and gallbladder, as well as in pleomorphic salivary adenoma. It occurs occasionally in carcinoma of the stomach, large bowel, pancreas, and prostate and in transitional cell cancers of the urinary tract.

Metaplasia in connective tissues

The extraosseous formation of bone or cartilage has been frequently observed in scars, chronic inflammatory and degenerative lesions, sclerotic arteries, and muscle. Ossification sometimes occurs in scars from operative incisions, particularly of the upper abdomen, in or near the linea alba. In degenerative necrotic lesions, ossification is preceded by the deposition of calcium. Myositis ossificans is frequently related to previous injury, with ensuring fibrosis and vascularization of the injured muscle.

The most surprising example of osseous metaplasia is that associated with the mucosa of the urinary tract. The process occurs in connective tissues closely related to the transitional cell epithelium of the mucosa of the bladder, ureter, or renal pelvis, being possibly related to the phosphatase activity of regenerating epithelium of the urinary tract.

Bony or cartilaginous metaplasia is not unusual in the connective tissue stroma of neoplasms and has been described in carcinoma of the stomach, bowel, gallbladder, salivary gland, and prostate. Less commonly, mus-

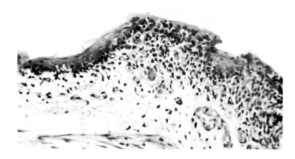

Fig. 2-40. Early squamous metaplasia of ciliated columnar epithelium of tracheal mucosa from 35-day-old rat fed diet deficient in vitamin A. Metaplasia begins in small foci that extend and coalesce until whole circumference of tracheal mucosa is involved. (185×; from Wilhelm, D.L.: J. Pathol. Bacteriol. **67**:361, 1954.)

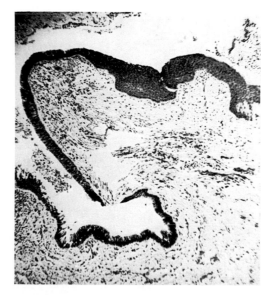

Fig. 2-41. Metaplasia of epithelial lining of salivary duct. Columnar epithelium *(bottom left)* has been replaced by squamous epithelium *(upper right)*. (50×.)

cle may exhibit metaplasia, in which nonstriated muscle becomes striated.[136]

• • •

Metaplasia therefore represents a change in the direction of cellular differentiation, resulting in the development of mature cells having a character different from that usually occurring in a particular tissue. On the other hand, when tissue occurs in an unusual site as the result of alleged "primary displacement" or developmental abnormality, the foreign tissue is termed a *heterotopia* (for example, the presence of gastric mucosa in a congenital Meckel's diverticulum of the terminal ileum).

In conclusion, attention should be drawn to the disadvantages that may follow the development of metaplasia. The replacement of the usual cell by another type of cell often results in decreased function of the affected organ or in impairment of mechanisms that are important in defense against infection (as in the respiratory tract).

ACKNOWLEDGMENT

I am indebted to the previous authors of this chapter, D.L. Wilhelm and Vincent T. Marchesi, for providing me with an excellent foundation to build upon.

REFERENCES
General

1. Casley-Smith, J.R.: An electron microscopic study of injured and abnormally permeable lymphatics, Ann. NY Acad. Sci. **116**:803, 1964.
2. Chambers, R., and Zweifach, B.W.: Capillary endothelial cement in relation to permeability, J. Cell. Physiol. **15**:255, 1940.
3. Chambers, R., and Zweifach, B.W.: Topography and junction of mesenteric capillary circulation, Am. J. Anat. **75**:173, 1944.
4. Florey, H.W., editor: General pathology, ed. 4, London, 1970, Lloyd-Luke (Medical Books), Ltd.
5. Hunter, J.: A treatise on the blood, inflammation and gunshot wounds, vol. 1, London, 1974, G. Nicoll.
6. Lewis, T.: The blood vessels of the human skin and their responses, London, 1927, Shaw & Sons, Ltd.
7. Macleod, A.G., Aspects of acute inflammation. In Thomas, B.A., editor: Scope Monograph, Kalamazoo, 1969, The Upjohn Co.
8. Miles, A.A.: Ann. NY Acad. Sci. **66**:356, 1956.
9. Robbins, D.L.: Pathologic basis of disease, Philadelphia, 1974, W.B. Saunders Co.
10. Ryan, G.B., and Majno, G.: Inflammation. In Thomas, B.A., editor: Scope Monograph, Kalamazoo, 1977, The Upjohn Co.
11. Spector, W.G., and Willoughby, D.A.: The inflammatory response, Bacteriol. Rev. **27**:117, 1963.
12. Thomas, L.: Inflammation as a disease mechanism. In Zweifach, B.W., Grant, L., and McCluskey, R.T., editors: The inflammatory process, ed. 2, vol. 3, New York, 1974, Academic Press, Inc.
13. Walter, J.B., and Israel, M.S.: General pathology, ed. 4, Edinburgh, 1974, Churchill Livingstone.

Inflammation—plasma components

14. Allison, F., Jr., and Lancaster, M.G.: Studies on the pathogenesis of acute inflammation. II. The relationship of fibrinogen and fibrin to the leucocyte sticking reaction in ear chambers of rabbits injured by heat, Br. J. Exp. Pathol. **40**:324, 1959.
15. Burke, J.F., and Miles, A.A.: The sequence of vascular events in early infective inflammation, J. Pathol. Bacteriol. **76**:1, 1958.

16. Cotran, R.S., Suter, E.R., and Majno, G.: The use of colloidal carbon as a tracer for vascular injury: a review, Vasc. Dis. **4**:107, 1967.
17. Crone, C.: Modulation of solute permeability in microvascular endothelium, Fed. Proc. **45**:77-83, 1986.
18. Duling, B.R., Hogan, R.D., Langille, B.L., Lelkes, P., Segal, S.S., Vatner, S.F., Weigelt, H., and Young, M.A.: Vasomotor control: functional hyperemia and beyond, Fed. Proc. **46**:251-263, 1987.
19. Grega, G.J., and Adamski, S.W.: Patterns of constriction produced by vasoactive agents, Fed. Proc. **46**:270-275, 1987.
20. Majno, G.: Mechanism of abnormal vascular permeability in acute inflammation. In Thomas, L., Uhr, J.W., and Grant, L., editors: International symposium on injury, inflammation and immunity, Baltimore, 1964, The Williams & Wilkins Co.
21. Miles, A.A.: Large molecular substances as mediators of the inflammatory reaction, Ann. NY Acad. Sci. **116**:855, 1964.
22. Miller, F.N., and Sims, D.E.: Contractile elements in the regulation of macromolecular permeability, Fed. Proc. **45**:84-88, 1986.
23. Paton, W.D.M.: Histamine release by compounds of simple chemical structure, Pharmacol. Rev. **9**:269, 1957.
24. Paton, W.D.M.: The release of histamine, Prog. Allergy **5**:79, 1958.
25. Pierce, J.V.: Fed. Proc. **27**:52, 1968.
26. Pullinger, B.D., and Florey, H.W.: Some observations on structure and functions of lymphatics: Their behavior in local edema, Br. J. Exp. Pathol. **16**:49, 1935.
27. Riley, J.F., and West, G.B.: Tissue mast cells: studies with histamine-liberator of low toxicity (compound 48/80), J. Pathol. Bacteriol. **69**:269, 1955.
28. Rocha e Silva, M.: The physiological significance of bradykinin, Ann. NY Acad. Sci. **104**:190, 1963.
29. Schachter, M.: Kallikreins and kinins, Physiol. Rev. **49**:509, 1969.
30. Simionescu, N., Heltianu, C., Antohe, F., and Simionescu, M.: Endothelial cell receptors for histamine, Ann. NY Acad. Sci. **401**:132-149, 1982.
31. Uvnas, B.: Mechanism of histamine release in mast cells, Ann. NY Acad. Sci. **103**:278, 1963.
32. Webster, M.E.: Fed. Proc. **27**:84, 1968.
33. Webster, M.E.: Kinin system. In Movat, H.Z., editor: Cellular and humoral mechanisms in anaphylaxis and allergy, New York, 1969, S. Karger AG.
34. Wilhelm, D.L.: Pattern and mechanism of increased vascular permeability in inflammation. In Zweifach, B.W., Grant, L., and McClusky, R.T., editors: The inflammatory process, ed. 2, vol. 2, New York, 1973, Academic Press, Inc.
35. Wilhelm, D.L., Bertelli, G., and Hoceck, J.C., editors: Symposium on inflammation, biochemistry, and drug interaction, Amsterdam, 1969, Excerpta Medica Foundation.
36. Wilhelm, D.L., and Mason, B.: Vascular permeability changes in inflammation: the role of endogenous permeability factors in mild thermal injury, Br. J. Exp. Pathol. **45**:487, 1960.

Inflammation—blood cells and endothelial cells

37. Archer, G.T., Robson, J., and Thompson, A.R.: Proc. Aust. Biochem. Soc, **8**:96, 1975.
38. Becker, E.L.: Enzyme activation and the mechanism of neutrophil chemotaxis, Antibiot. Chemother. **19**:409, 1974.
39. Bevilacqua, M.P., Wheeler, M.E., Pober, J.S., Fiers, W., Mendrick, D.L., Cotran, R.S., and Gimbrone, M.A.: Endothelial-dependent mechanisms of leukocyte adhesion: Regulation by interleukin-1 and tumor necrosis factor. In Movat, H.Z., editor: Leukocyte emigration and its sequelae, pp. 79-93, Basel, 1987, S. Karger AG.
40. Boyden, S.: The chemotactic effect of mixtures of antibody and antigen on polymorphonuclear leucocytes, J. Exp. Med. **115**:453, 1962.
41. Butcher, E.C., Lewinsohn, D., Duijestijn, A., Bargatze, R., Wu, N., and Jalkanen, S.: Interactions between endothelial cells and leukocytes, J. Cell. Biochem. **30**:121-131, 1986.
42. Clark, E.R., and Clark, E.L.: Anat. Rec. **24**:127, 1922.
43. Duijestijn, A., Kerkhove, M., Bargatze, R., and Butcher, E.C.:

Lymphoid tissue and inflammation-specific endothelial cell differentiation defined by monoclonal antibodies, J. Immunol. **138**:713-719, 1987.

44. Collins, T., Korman, A.J., Wake, C.T., Boss, J.M., Kappes, D.J., Fiers, W., Ault, K.A., Gimbrone, M.A., Strominger, J.L., and Pober, J.S.: Immune interferon activates multiple class II major histocompatibility complex genes and associated invariant chain gene in human umbilical endothelial cells and dermal fibroblasts, Proc. Natl. Acad. Sci. (USA) **81**:4917-4921, 1984.

45. Collins, T., Lapierre, L.A., Fiers, W., Strominger, J.L., and Pober, J.S.: Recombinant human tumor necrosis factor increases mRNA levels and surface expression of HLA-A,B antigens in vascular endothelial cells and dermal fibroblasts in vitro, Proc. Natl. Acad. Sci. (USA) **83**:446-450, 1986.

46. Florey, H.W., and Grant, L.H. Leucocyte migration from small blood vessels stimulated with ultraviolet light: an electron-microscope study, J. Pathol. Bacteriol. **82**:13, 1961.

47. Goetzl, E.J.: Leukocyte recognition and metabolism of leukotrienes, Fed. Proc. **42**:3128-3132, 1983.

48. Goetzl, E.J.: Leukocyte receptors for lipid and peptide mediators, Fed. Proc. **46**:190-191, 1987.

49. Goldman, D.W., Gifford, L.A., Marotti, T., Koo, C.H., and Goetzl, E.J.: Molecular and cellular properties of human polymorphonuclear leukocyte receptors for leukotriene B$_4$, Fed. Proc. **46**:200-203, 1987.

50. Harlan, J.M., Schwartz, B.R., Wallis, W.J., and Pohlman, T.H.: The role of neutrophil membrane proteins in neutrophil emigration, In Movat H.Z., editor: Leukocyte emigration and its sequelae, pp. 94-104, Basel, 1987. S. Karger AG.

51. Haskard, D.O., Cavender, D., and Ziff, M.: Mechanisms of lymphocyte adhesion to endothelial cells. In Movat, H.Z., editor: Leukocyte emigration and its sequelae, pp. 119-122, Basel, 1987, S. Karger AG.

52. Hirsch, J.G.: Neutrophilic leukocytes. In Zweifach, B.W., Grant, G., and McCluskey, R.T., editors: The inflammatory process, ed. 2, vol. 1, New York, 1973, Academic Press, Inc.

53. Hurley, J.V.: Incubation of serum with tissue extracts as a cause of chemotaxis of granulocytes, Nature (Lond.) **198**:1212, 1963.

54. Hynes, R.O.: Integrins: A family of cell surface receptors, Cell **48**:549-554, 1987.

55. Joris, I, Majno, G., Corey, E.J., and Lewis, R.A.: The mechanism of vascular leakage induced by leukotriene E$_4$: endothelial contraction, Am. J. Pathol. **126**:19-24, 1987.

56. Kay, A.B., and Austen, K.F.: The IgE-mediated release of an eosinophil leukocyte chemotactic factor from human lung, J. Immunol. **107**:899, 1971.

57. Langevoort, H.Z., et al.: Classification of mononuclear phagocytic cells. In van Furth, R., editor: Mononuclear phagocytes, Oxford, 1970, Blackwell Scientific Publications, Ltd.

58. Lewinsohn, D.M., Bargatze, R.F., and Butcher, E.C.: Leukocyte-endothelial cell rocognition: evidence of a common molecular mechanism shared by neutrophils, lymphocytes and other leukocytes, J. Immunol. **138**:4313-4321, June 15, 1987.

59. Marchesi, V.T., and Florey, H.W.: Electron micrographic observations on the emigration of leucocytes, Q. J. Exp. Physiol. Rev. **26**:319, 1946.

60. McCutcheon, M.: Chemotaxis in leukocytes, Physiol. Rev. **26**:319, 1946.

61. Pawlowski, N.A., Abraham, E.L., Pontier, S., Scott, W.A., and Cohn, Z.A.: Human monocyte–endothelial cell interaction in vitro, Proc. Natl. Acad. Sci. (USA) **82**:8208-8212, 1985.

62. Pober, J.S., Bevilacqua, M.P., Mendrick, M.L., Lapierre, L.A., Fiers, W., and Gimbrone, M.A.: Two distinct monokines, interleukin-1 and tumor necrosis factor, each independently induce biosynthesis and transient expression of the same antigen on the surface of cultured human vascular endothelial cells, J. Immunol. **136**:1680-1687, 1986.

63. Pober, J.S., Gimbrone, M.A., Lapierre, L.A., Mendrick, M.L., Fiers, W., Rothelein, R., and Springer, T.A.: Overlapping patterns of activation of human endothelial cells by interleukin-1, tumor necrosis factor, and immune interferon, J. Immunol. **137**:1893-1896, 1986.

64. Ryan, G.B., and Spector, W.G.: Natural selection of long-lived macrophages in experimental granulomata, Proc. R. Soc. Lond. (Biol.) **175**:269, 1970.

65. Spector, W.G.: Chronic inflammation. In Zweifach, B.W., Grant, L., and McCluskey, R.T., editors: The inflammatory process, ed. 2, vol. 3, New York, 1974, Academic Press, Inc.

66. Spector, W.G., and Willoughby, D.A.: Recruitment of macrophages in granuloma. In van Arman, C.G., editor: White cells in inflammation, Springfield, Ill., 1974, Charles C Thomas, Publisher.

67. Speirs, R.S., and Speirs, E.S.: Eosinophils in granulomatous inflammation. In van Arman, C.G., editor: White cells in inflammation, Springfield, Ill., 1974, Charles C Thomas, Publisher.

68. Steinman, R.M., and Cohn, Z.A.: Metabolism and physiology of mononuclear phagocytes. In Zweifach, B.W., Grant, L., and McCluskey, R.T., editors: The inflammatory process, ed. 2, vol. 1, New York, 1974, Academic Press, Inc.

69. van Furth, R., editor: Mononuclear phagocytes, Oxford, 1970, Blackwell Scientific Publications, Ltd.

70. Vane, J., and Botting, R.: Inflammation and the mechanism of action of anti-inflammatory drugs. FASEB J. **1**:89-96, 1987.

71. Ward, P.A.: Chemotaxis of mononuclear cells, J. Exp. Med. **128**:1201, 1968.

72. Ward, P.A.: Mechanisms of phagocytosis. In Lepow, I.H., and Ward, P.A., editors: Inflammation: mechanisms and control, New York, 1972, Academic Press, Inc.

Inflammation—phagocytosis

73. Elsbach, P.: Phagocytosis. In Zweifach, B.W., Grant, L., and McCluskey, R.T., editors: The inflammatory process, ed. 2, vol. 1, New York, 1974, Academic Press, Inc.

74. Wood, W.B., Jr.: Phagocytoses with particular reference to encapsulated bacteria, Bacteriol. Rev. **24**:41, 1960.

Inflammation—hypersensitivity

75. Basten, A., and Beeson, P.B.: Mechanism of eosinophilia. II. Role of the lymphocyte, J. Exp. Med. **131**:1288, 1970.

76. Burnet, M.: Self and non-self, Cambridge, Eng., 1969, Cambridge University Press.

77. Cochrane, C.G.: Immunologic tissue injury mediated by neutrophilic leukocytes, Adv. Immunol. **9**:97, 1968.

78. Coombs, R.R.A., and Gell, P.G.H.: Classification of hypersensitivity. In Fell, P.G.H., and Coombs, R.R.A., editors: Clinical aspects of immunology, ed. 2, Oxford, 1968, Blackwell Scientific Publications, Ltd.

79. Dvorak, H.F., and Dvorak, A.M.: Basophils, mast cells, and cellular immunity in animals and man, Hum. Pathol. **3**:454, 1972.

80. Ford, W.L., and Gowans, J.L.: The traffic of lymphocytes, Semin. Hematol. **6**:67, 1969.

81. Humphrey, J.H., and White, R.G.: Immunology for students of medicine, ed. 3, Oxford, 1970, Blackwell Scientific Publications, Ltd.

82. Lykke, A.W.J., and Cumings, R.: Increased vascular permeability in the primary cutaneous allograft response in the rat, Experientia **24**:1287, 1969.

83. McGregor, D.D., and Mackaness, G.B.: Life history and function of lymphocytes. In Zweifach, B.W., Grant, L., and McCluskey, R.T., editors: The inflammatory process, ed. 2, vol. 3, New York, 1974, Academic Press, Inc.

84. Waksman, B.M.: In Wolstenholme, G.E.W., and O'Connor, M., editors: Cellular aspects of immunity, Ciba Foundation Symposium, Boston, 1960, Little, Brown & Co.

85. Fibrosis, Ciba Foundation Symposium 114, London, 1985, Pitman.

Healing and repair

86. Abercrombie, M., Flint, M.H., and James D.L.: J. Embryol. Exp. Morphol. **4**:167, 1956.

87. Abercrombie, M., James, D.L., and Newcombe, J.F.: Wound contraction in rabbit skin, studied by splinting the wound margins, J. Anat. **94**:170, 1960.

88. Azizkhan, R.G., Azizkhan, J.C., Zetter, B.R., and Folkman, J.: Mast cell heparin stimulates migration of capillary endothelial cells in vitro, J. Exp. Med. **152**:931-944, 1980.

89. Ballardini, G., Esposti, S.D., Bianchi, F.B., DeGiorgi, L.B., Faccani, A., Biolchini, L., Busachi, C.A., and Pisi, E.: Correlation between Ito cells and fibrogenesis in an experimental model of hepatic fibrosis: a sequential stereological study, Liver 3:58-63, 1983.

90. Barger, C.A., Beeuwkes, R., Lainey, L.L., and Silverman, K.J.: Hypothesis: vasa vasorum and neovascularization of human coronary arteries a possible role in the pathophysiology of atherosclerosis, New Eng. J. Med. 310:175-177, 1984.

91. Billingham, R.E., and Russell, P.S.: Studies on wound healing, with special reference to the phenomenon of contracture in experimental wounds in rabbits' skin, Ann. Surg. 144:961, 1951.

92. Bizzozero, G.: Accrescimento e rigenerazione nell' organismo, Arch. Sci. Med. (Torino) 18:245, 1894.

93. Cameron, G.R., and Karunaratne, W.A.E.: Massive necrosis ("toxic infarction") of liver following intra-portal administration of poisons, J. Pathol. Bacteriol. 44:297, 1937.

94. Clark, E.R., and Clark, E.L.: Microscopic observations on growth of blood capillaries in living mammal, Am. J. Anat. 64:251, 1939.

95. Clark, E.R., et al.: General observations on ingrowth of new blood vessels into standardized chambers in rabbit's ear, and subsequent changes in newly grown vessels over period of months, Anat. Rec. 50:129, 1931.

96. Clark, W.E.L.: Experimental study of regeneration of mammalian striped muscle, J. Anat. 80:24, 1946.

97. Crum, R., Szabo, S., and Folkman, J.: A new class of steroids inhibits angiogenesis in the presence of heparin or a heparin fragment, Science 230:1375-1378, 1985.

98. Davis, B., and Madri, J.A.: Type I and III procollagen propeptides during hepatic fibrogenesis: an immunohistochemical and ELISA serum study in the CCL₄ rat model, Am. J. Pathol. 126:137-147, 1986.

99. Davis, B., and Madri, J.A.: An immunohistochemical and serum ELISA study of type I and III procollagen amino propeptides in chronic liver disease. Am. J. Pathol. 128:265-275, 1987.

100. Davis, B., Pratt, B.M., and Madri, J.A.: Hepatic Ito cell culture: modulation of collagen phenotype and cellular retinol binding protein and extracellular collagen matrix, J. Biol. Chem. 262:10280-10286, 1987.

101. Dunphy, J.E.: On the nature and care of wounds, Ann. R. Coll. Surg. Eng. 26:69, 1960.

102. Edwards, L.C., and Dunphy, J.D.: Wound healing (in two parts), N. Engl. J. Med. 259:224, 275, 1958.

103. Fett, J.W., Strydom, D.J., Lobb, R.R., Alderman, E.M., Bethune, J.L., Riordan, J.F., and Vallee, B.L.: Isolation and characterization of angiogenin, an angiogenic protein from human carcinoma cells, Biochemistry 24:5480-5486, 1985.

104. Folkman, J., and Cotran, R.: Relation of vascular proliferation to tumor growth, Int. Rev. Exp. Pathol. 16:208-248, New York, 1976, Academic Press, Inc.

105. Folkman, J., and Cotran, R.: Relation of vascular proliferation to tumor growth, Intl. Rev. Exp. Pathol. 16:208-248, New York, 1976, Academic Press, Inc.

106. Form, D.M., Pratt, B.M., and Madri, J.A.: Endothelial cell proliferation during angiogenesis: in vitro modulation by basement membrane components, Lab. Invest. 55:521-530, 1986.

107. Furcht, L.T.: Critical factors controlling angiogenesis: cell products, cell matrix and growth factors, Lab. Invest. 55:505-509, 1986.

108. Ingber, D.E., Madri, J.A., and Folkman, J.: A possible mechanism for inhibition of angiogenesis by angiostatic steroids: induction of capillary basement membrane dissolution, Endocrinol. 119:1768-1775, 1986.

109. Langer, R., Conn, H., Vacanti, J., Haudenschild, C., and Folkman, J.: Control of tumor growth in animals by infusion of an angiogenesis inhibitor, Proc. Natl. Acad. Aci. (USA) 77:4331-4335, 1980.

110. Gabbiani, G., et al.: Granulation tissue as a contractile organ: a study of structure and function, J. Exp. Med. 135:719, 1972.

111. Leblond, C.P., and Walker, B.E.: Renewal of cell populations, Physiol. Rev. 36:255, 1956.

112. Lobb, R., Sasse, J., Sullivan, R., Shing, Y., D'Amore, P., Jacobs, J., and Klagsbrun, M.: Purification and characterization of heparin-binding endothelial cell growth factors, J. Biol. Chem. 261:1924-1928, 1986.

113. Madri, J.A., and Furthmayr, H.: Collagen polymorphism in the lung: an immunochemical study of pulmonary fibrosis, Hum. Pathol. 11:353-366, 1980.

114. Madri, J.A., and Pratt, B.M.: Endothelial cell–matrix interactions: in vitro models of angiogenesis, J. Histochem. Cytochem. 34:85-91, 1986.

115. Madri, J.A., and Pratt, B.M.: Angiogenesis. In Clark, R.F., and Henson, P., editors: The molecular and cellular biology of wound healing, New York, 1987, Plenum Press.

116. Madri, J.A., Pratt, B.M., and Yannariello-Brown, J.: Endothelial cell extracellular matrix interactions: matrix as a modulator of cell function. In Simionescu, N., and Simionescu, M., editors: Endothelial cell biology in health and disease, New York, 1988, Plenum Press.

117. Mak, K.M., Leo, M.A., and Lieber, C.S.: Alcoholic liver injury in baboons: transformation of lipocytes to transitional cells, Gastroenterology 87:188-200, 1984.

118. Minato, Y., Hasumura, Y., and Takeuchi, J.: The role of fat-storing cells in Disse space fibrogenesis in alcoholic liver disease, Hepatology 3:559-566, 1983.

119. Nicosia, R.F., and Madri, J.A.: The microvascular extracellular matrix: developmental changes during angiogenesis in the aortic ring–plasma clot model, Am. J. Pathol. 128:78-90, 1987.

120. Ogawa, K., Suzuki, J., Mulai, H., and Mori, M.,: Sequential changes of extracellular matrix and proliferation of Ito cells with enhanced expression of desmin and actin in focal hepatic injury, Am. J. Pathol. 125:611-619, 1986.

121. Ordman, L.J., and Gillman, T.: Studies in the healing of cutaneous wounds (in three parts), Arch. Surg. 93:857, 883, 911, 1966.

122. Ponfick, E.: Verh. Dtsch. Ges. Chir. 19:28, 1890.

123. Ponfick, E.: Experimentelle Beiträge zur Pathologie der Leber, Virchows Arch. (Pathol. Anat.) 138(suppl.):81, 1895.

124. Pratt, B.M., Form, D., and Madri, J.A.: Endothelial cell–extracellular matrix interactions. In Fleischmajer, R., Olsen, B.R., and Kuhn, K., editors: Biology, chemistry and pathology of collagen, Ann. NY Acad. Sci. 460:129-139, 1986.

125. Roberts, A.B., Sporn, M.B., Assoian, R.K., Smith, J.M., Roche, N.S., Wakefield, L.M., Heine, U.I., Liotta, L.A., Falanga, V., Kehrl, J.H., and Fauci, A.S.: Transforming growth factor type β: rapid induction of fibrosis and angiogenesis in vivo and stimulation of collagen formation in vitro, Proc. Natl. Acad. Sci. (USA) 83:4167-4172, 1986.

126. Ryan, G.B., et al.: Myofibroblasts in human granulation tissue, Hum. Pathol. 5:55, 1974.

127. Sandison, J.: Observations on growth of blood vessels as seen in transparent chamber introduced into rabbit's ear, Am. J. Anat. 41:475, 1928.

128. Schoefl, G.I.: Studies on inflammation. III. Growing capillaries: their structure and permeability, Virchows Arch. (Pathol. Anat.) 337:97, 1962.

129. Stenn, K.S., Madri, J.A., and Roll, F.J.: Migrating epidermis produces AB₂ collagen and requires continual collagen synthesis for movement, Nature 277:229-232, 1979.

130. Stenn, K.S., Madri, J.A., Tinghitella, T., and Terranova, V.: Multiple mechanisms of dissociated epidermal cell spreading, J. Cell Biol. 96:63-67, 1983.

131. Train, J.S., Mitty, H.A., Effremidis, S.C., and Rabinowitz, J.G.: Visualization of a fine periluminal vascular network following transluminal angioplasty: possible demonstration of the vasa vasorum, Radiology 143:399-403, 1982.

132. Trueta, R.J.: The principles and practice of war surgery, ed. 3, London, 1946, Hamish Hamilton, Ltd.

133. Wahl, S.M.: Host immune factors regulating fibrosis. In Fibrosis, Ciba Foundation Symposium 114, pp. 175-195, London, 1985, Pitman.

134. Wilhelm, D.L.: Regeneration of tracheal epithelium, J. Pathol. Bacteriol. 65:543, 1953.

135. Wilhelm, D.L.: Regeneration of tracheal epithelium in vitamin-A–deficient rats, J. Pathol. Bacteriol. 67:361, 1954.

136. Willis, R.A.: In King, E.S.J., Lowe, T.E., and Cox, L.B., editors: Studies in pathology, Melbourne, 1950, Melbourne University Press.

137. Young, J.Z.: Functional repair of nervous tissue, Physiol. Rev. 22:318, 1942.

3 Injuries Caused by Physical Agents

CHARLES S. HIRSCH
ROSS E. ZUMWALT

Physical injuries include those caused by mechanical trauma, increases or decreases of atmospheric pressure, sound waves, heat (local and systemic), cold (local and systemic), and electricity. In terms of morbidity and mortality, mechanical trauma is more important by an order of magnitude than all other modalities of physical injury combined. Therefore more than half of this chapter is devoted to mechanical trauma.

MECHANICAL TRAUMA

Force or mechanical energy is that which changes the state of rest or uniform motion of matter. When force applied to any part of the body results in a harmful disturbance in function or structure, a mechanical injury is said to have been sustained.

The most common manifestation of such an injury is a disruption in the continuity of tissue, or a wound. The force responsible for wound production is usually liberated incident to a collision between the body and some external mass and may be derived from the motion of the body itself, from the motion of the other participant in the collision, or from both.

Wounding by mechanical trauma is governed by (1) the amount of force transmitted to the tissues, (2) the rate of application of force to the tissues, (3) the surface area involved in energy transfer, and (4) the characteristics of the target area.

Physical principles
Amount of force

The kinetic energy or wound-producing capacity that an object has in consequence of its motion is determined by its weight and velocity. In the case of simple forward motion, this force may be computed by the formula $MV^2/2g$, in which M = weight, V = velocity, and g = the acceleration of gravity. It is important to note that the kinetic energy of a moving object increases arithmetically in relation to its weight and geometrically in relation to its velocity. If two objects, one weighing twice as much as the other, are traveling at the same velocity, the kinetic energy of the former will be twice that of the latter; however, if they weigh the same but

one is traveling twice as fast as the other, the energy will be four times as great. Wounding by bullets provides an important application of this principle to an understanding of the resulting injuries. Bullets fired from military and hunting rifles commonly have muzzle velocities three to four times as great as those fired from handguns. Consequently, such high-velocity bullets have kinetic energies 9 to 16 times greater than their low-velocity counterparts.

One should not infer that the kinetic energy and the wound-producing factor of a mass in motion are necessarily identical. Only that part of the total energy of motion actually utilized in changing the state of rest or uniform motion of the tissues is capable of contributing to injury production. Unexpended force, possessed by the source of energy after the impulse of collision, is still capable of doing work and has not contributed to injury production. Force of impact utilized to induce uniform motion of the tissues or to displace or deform the object that has struck the tissue is likewise noninjurious, since it has been expended for work other than disturbing the uniform state of rest or motion of the tissues.

In addition to the kinetic energy of forward motion, an object may possess energy by reason of the fact that it is rotating on its own axis. Such energy frequently is possessed by a flying missile and adds to the wound-producing capacity of bullets. The extra energy possessed by a spinning object may be calculated from the formula $IW^2/2g$, in which I = the rotary inertia or $Mr^2/2g$ (r = radius of cross section and M = weight), W = the angular velocity in radians per second or $2\pi \times$ number of rotations/second, and g = the acceleration of gravity.

Rate of energy transfer

The duration of impulse or period of energy transfer is an important factor in determining how much of the force of an impact will be expended in the causation of uniform or noninjurious motion and how much in the causation of nonuniform or potentially injurious movement of the tissues. Athletes are aware of the desirability of prolonging the duration of impulse. To diminish the amount of force likely to be expended in the production of nonuniform or disruptive movement of tissues, the tumbler rolls with his fall, the ballplayer moves his gloved hand with the caught ball, and the fighter endeavors to move with his opponent's blow. Protracted deceleration probably accounts in large measure for the occasional and seemingly miraculous survival of people who have fallen from great heights.

Surface area

Another important factor in determining the wound-producing capacity of an impact is the size of the surface area to which the force is applied. The larger the area through which a given amount of impact force is transmitted, the less will be its intensity. Thus an impulse of a certain number of foot-pounds might cause uniform tissue displacement without injury when acting over a large area and yet be capable of causing severe disruption of tissue when acting through an area comparable to the edge or point of a knife.

Target area

Many other factors may modify the disruptive effects of impacts even when they are similar in respect to the amount of energy expended, the duration of impulse, and the area of collision contact. Among these is the extent to which the force may be intensified by lever action or by hydrostatic effect. A small force applied near the end of a liver will be greatly intensified as the fulcrum is approached. This phenomenon is particularly important in relation to the production of fractures of long bones. Similarly, a relatively small compression of a large hollow viscus may displace a sufficient volume of fluid to rupture the wall of a less voluminous communicating structure. Differences in the elasticity, plasticity, or inertia of tissues are of great importance in respect to whether a given force will produce disruptive change. Liver is ordinarily more friable and more readily disrupted by distortion than lung or muscle is. A hyperplastic and friable spleen may be torn to pieces by an impact that would be harmless to a normal spleen. The capillary fragility of persons with certain vitamin deficiencies is often greater than that of the normal person.

The foregoing discussion of the mechanics of injury production by the energy of motion has concerned disruption of tissue or wound production. Although a wound is the most common manifestation of injury caused by the energy of motion, it is by no means the only one. Force has been defined as that which changes the state of rest or uniform motion of matter. The application of force to the surface of the body may alter subsurface relationships sufficiently to cause severe functional disturbance even though no cutaneous

wound is produced. In fact, many victims of fatal blunt trauma have no externally visible wound. This pertains especially to persons with head injuries whose scalp is shielded by thick hair or a hat and to persons who sustain chest and abdominal impacts over a broad area.

Also, the application of pressure in many situations may cause harmful interference with the function of the compressed or displaced tissue even though the force is insufficient to produce a wound. Mechanical obstruction of the air passages for more than a few minutes is likely to cause death from systemic anoxia. A tight tourniquet applied for 30 minutes may result in ischemic necrosis of a limb. Furthermore, as in many other areas of pathology, traumatically induced functional disturbances can be profound, or even lethal, yet not structurally demonstrable. For example, the term *instantaneous physiologic death* can be used to describe the rapidly fatal outcome of a blunt impact to the chest that fails to mark the skin, causes no fractures of the sternum or ribs, and does not produce a cardiac contusion.[2] Such deaths probably result from ventricular fibrillation, a structurally traceless lethal mechanism.

Local effects of mechanical violence
Wounds

As previously indicated, a wound is a mechanically produced interruption in the continuity of tissue. There are several anatomic types of such disruptive lesions, for which distinctive terms are used.

Abrasion. An abrasion (scratch or scrape) represents the tearing away of epidermal cells by friction or crushing. Such a defect may or may not penetrate to the corium. Although an abrasion may provide a portal of entry for infection, such a wound is ordinarily of little pathologic significance beyond the fact that it provides objective evidence that force has been applied to the surface of the body. The direction of motion responsible for an abrasion can frequently be recognized by the manner in which the partially detached sheets of epidermis have been rolled on themselves at the distal end of the defect (Fig. 3-1). In some instances the nature of the abrading object can be recognized by the distribution and configuration of the epidermal defects.

Laceration. The word "laceration" is commonly *misused* as a synonym for a cut (or incised wound). A laceration is a split or tear and represents the effect of excessive stretching of tissue. Although any tissue may be disrupted in this manner, such injuries most commonly involve the integument, particularly where it is stretched over bone, as in the hands or over the skull. Lacerations of skin caused by the unidirectional displacement and stretching that occur incident to the impact of an obliquely directed force are likely to be linear or curve, whereas those produced by the multidirectional radial displacement of a crushing impact oriented

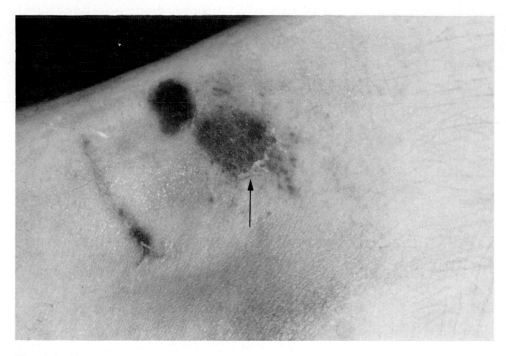

Fig. 3-1. Abrasion of left medial malleolus of a pedestrian who was "knocked out of his shoes" when struck by auto. Force acting on ankle as it exited the shoe was directed distally and nearly parallel to the surface. Heaping of epidermis *(arrow)* on lower margin of injury reflects direction and orientation of abrading force.

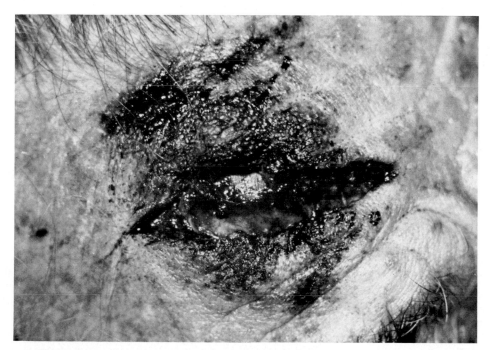

Fig. 3-2. Abraded laceration of forehead caused by impact of circumscribed object with force directed perpendicular to the skin. Abrasion resulted from crushing of epidermis, and laceration was caused by stretching of skin over subjacent bone.

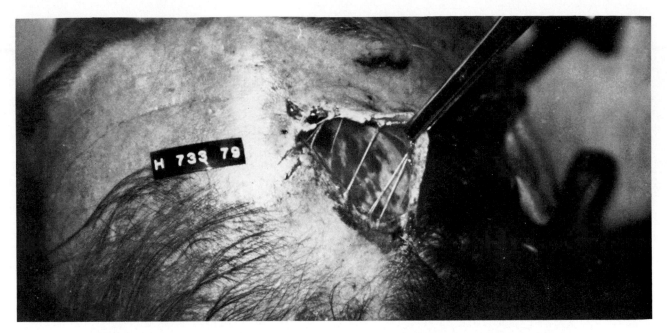

Fig. 3-3. Linear laceration of forehead with undermining of distal margin. Strands of tissue bridging defect indicate that injury is a laceration rather than an incised wound, because a cutting instrument cannot leave intact tissue above its deepest penetration.

at a right angle to the skin may be linear or stellate. The latter commonly have crushed, abraded margins; such an injury is an *abraded laceration* (Fig. 3-2). Linear lacerations may be so cleanly disrupted as to resemble an incised wound. In such a circumstance it may be necessary to identify the attenuated strands of tissue that bridge the margins of the defect in order to recognize it as a laceration (Fig. 3-3). In the case of curved or angular lacerations of the skin, the apex of the angle or the convexity of the curve will face the direction from which the force was applied.

The force of an external impact may lacerate internal structures without damage to the skin or subcutaneous tissue (Fig. 3-4). Thus ligaments, muscles, or blood vessels are frequently lacerated by excessive stretching with or without superficial injury. Compression of fluid or gas in hollow viscera may cause laceration and perforation of their walls (Fig. 3-5). Soft tissues adjacent to the site of a fracture are usually lacerated by the broken ends of the bone.

Contusion. A contusion or bruise is an injury in which the force of an impact is transmitted through the skin to the underlying tissues with sufficient intensity to disrupt the walls of small blood vessels and to cause interstitial bleeding without disruption of the epidermis (Fig. 3-6).

Usually the interstitial bleeding is so superficial as to be almost immediately visible through the skin. However, a bruise may be so deep that either hours elapse before the extravasated blood becomes superficial

enough to be visible or it is never seen from the surface. An external impact may cause extensive bruising of internal viscera without damage to the skin or subcutaneous tissue.

Individuals vary enormously in their susceptibility to mechanical disruption of small blood vessels. Persons with certain dietary deficiencies or blood dyscrasias are likely to sustain remarkably extensive contusions as a result of relatively mild impacts.

Incision. An *incised wound* (or cut) is one produced by the pressure and friction against skin or other tissues by an instrument having a sharp edge. By definition an incised wound is longer than it is deep. *Stab wounds* are deeper than they are long. In these types of injury the tissues are uniformly displaced to either side of the cutting edge with the result that the primary damage is limited largely to the immediate vicinity of the defect.

Penetrating injury. The impact of an appropriately shaped resistant object against the skin may produce a defect so deep and of such relatively small diameter that its outstanding characteristic is penetration. Slender sharp objects and flying missiles are the most common causes of such injuries. Although the majority of penetrating wounds involve the skin and subcutaneous tissue, the broken end of a bone often causes penetrating injury without involving the integument.

Fracture. Any force that tends to change the state of uniform motion or rest of the body is likely to disrupt its least plastic tissue, the bony skeleton. A fracture is a mechanically produced disruption in the continuity of

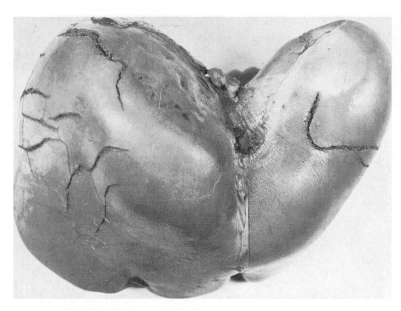

Fig. 3-4. Multiple lacerations of liver caused by lateral compression of thorax. There were no external wounds or fractures. Death resulted from hemoperitoneum.

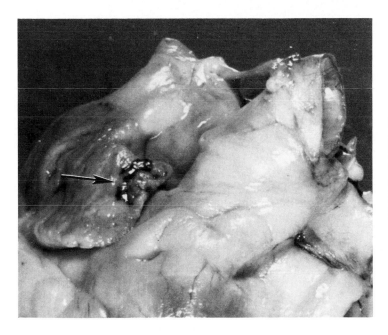

Fig. 3-5. "Blowout" laceration of right atrial appendage *(arrow),* the sole cardiac injury in young woman who fell from a height and landed on her chest. Compression of right atrium during diastole caused hydrostatic transmission of pressure into atrial appendage with laceration of its tip. Death resulted from hemopericardium with tamponade.

bone. Such osseous defects vary from a simple linear break, caused by excessive bending, to an explosive comminution caused by the impact of a high-velocity projectile. Of particular importance in the mechanics of fracture production is the transmission of force from the site of external application and its intensification at a distant point through lever action. One should not assume that the stress responsible for a fracture is necessarily of unusual magnitude or of external origin. A relatively minor stress may cause *pathologic fractures* of diseased bones.

Traffic injuries

Because traffic injuries are so common and exemplify the physical principles involved in blunt wound production, they deserve separate consideration.[48]

Injuries to vehicle occupants. The most straightforward situation with respect to the fate of vehicle occupants is a head-on crash without ejection. Such a collision with another vehicle or fixed object (such as a bridge abutment) causes the car to decelerate rapidly or come to a dead stop. The occupants are, of course, moving at the same speed and in the same direction as

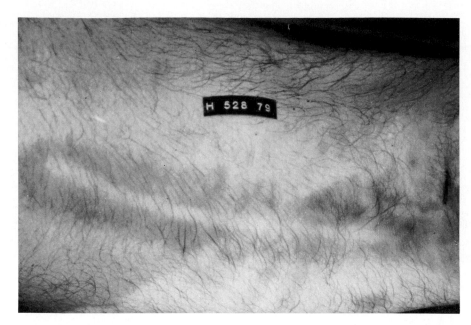

Fig. 3-6. Contusions caused by one impact with cylindrical object on posterior thigh. Linear pale mark indicates point of impact, which was subjected to uniform compressive stress. Adjacent, parallel, linear contusions correspond to areas of maximal shearing stress along edges of striking object.

the vehicle at the instant of its crash. However, because they are not riveted to the vehicular frame, they do not decelerate and stop with it. Instead, they continue on their forward course as masses in motion until they meet an opposing force. The latter force is exerted by their impact against the vehicle interior. To recapitulate, the first collision involves the vehicle and some other object; the second collision involves the occupant and the interior of the vehicle, and this is the injury-producing energy transfer. Other types of vehicular crash (such as side impacts) add a complicating factor in that the initial collision changes the vehicle's direction as well as its speed. In these more complex situations, the occupants move toward the point of vehicular crash en route to their decelerating impact with the car's interior.

The extent and severity of resulting injuries are determined by the initial velocity of the occupant, the rate of the occupant's deceleration, the nature and distribution of the opposing force that causes occupant deceleration, and the part of the body involved in energy transfer. As with other modalities of mechanical violence, rapid energy transfer and concentration of force over a small area produce more injurious, nonuniform displacement of tissues than does slowly applied, widely distributed force. All types of occupant safety systems, whether some form of restraining belt or an air bag, a collapsible steering column, padded interior panels, or recessed knobs and buttons, are designed to prolong the energy transfer of deceleration, to distribute the decelerating force over the broadest or sturdiest

possible area of the occupant's body, and to prevent unrestrained movement (and ejection) of the occupant after the vehicular crash.

Injuries to the head and neck commonly result from impacts against the windshield, side windows, or upper part of the vehicular frame. Trunk injuries are caused by decelerating impacts against the steering wheel (Fig. 3-7) or column, dashboard, or back of the front seat in the case of rear-seat passengers. Injuries of the lower limbs are frequently produced by impacts against the dashboard, foot compression against the floor, or entanglement of the feet in pedals or beneath the seats. Arm fractures can be produced when an occupant braces for a front-end collision by gripping the steering wheel or the dashboard.

Improperly worn safety belts can cause or contribute to patterns of injury.[18,60] Lap belts should be worn over the pelvic area so that the sturdy iliac crests absorb the stress of deceleration. If they are worn loosely or high, the force thereby transmitted to the abdomen can injure virtually any structure between the diaphragm and pelvis (Fig. 3-8). Likewise, an improperly worn shoulder strap, resting against the side of the neck rather than the upper chest, can cause severe cervical injury.

Occupant ejection from the vehicle allows for second or additional impacts with the road and other objects, greatly increasing the likelihood of serious injury or death. A crash that causes such severe deformity of the vehicle interior that the occupants are crushed is a nonsurvivable accident.

Injuries to pedestrians. Pedestrian fatalities are of

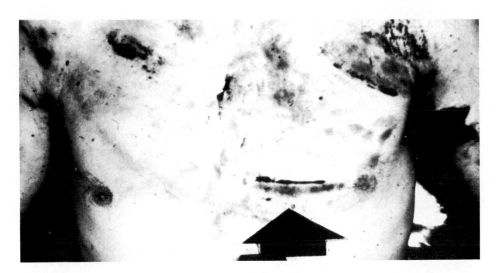

Fig. 3-7. Multiple contusions and abrasions on chest of driver killed in head-on collision. Curved abrasion *(arrow)* resulted from impact against steering wheel. (Courtesy Office of the Chief Medical Examiner, Baltimore, Md.)

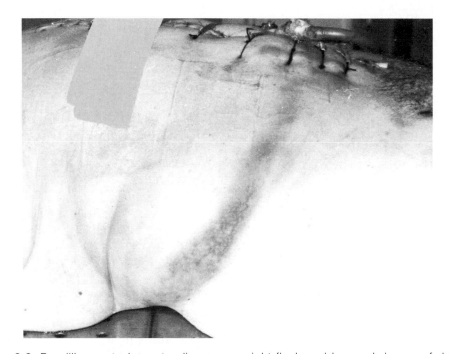

Fig. 3-8. Bandlike contusion extending across right flank and lower abdomen of driver who sustained mesenteric and small intestinal lacerations in a head-on collision. Patterned bruise and visceral injuries probably resulted from force applied to trunk by way of improperly worn lap belt.

three general types, with an approximately equal incidence. One third are children who carelessly dart into the path of a moving vehicle; one third are elderly persons who may have defective vision or hearing, which usually is coupled with diminished agility; and one third are healthy adults who commonly are under the influence of ethanol. Pedestrians sustain injuries when they are run over, "run under," or violently slammed aside.

A person is run over in one of two circumstances; either he is lying in the path of a moving vehicle or his center of gravity lies below the point of impact with the vehicle. The latter situation arises with children and crouching adults or when the involved vehicle is a bus or truck whose front end is high and broad. Tire tread marks on the victim's skin or clothing can be conspicuous or subtle, but the injured area almost invariably shows underlying avulsions of subcutaneous fat and severe crushing. An exception to the foregoing sometimes occurs when the victim is lying on a surface that yields, such as soft dirt or grass.

It is far more common for pedestrians to be *run under* than *run over*.[48] This occurs when an upright adult is struck by a moving vehicle below his center of gravity. Compound ("bumper") fractures of the lower legs are the classic stigmas of such impacts, but the thighs, hips, and low back are other common areas of initial impact.[57] As a result of the primary impact, the pedestrian's legs are thrown forward and elevated. His next impact usually occurs when he strikes the automobile hood or roof, after which he bounces to the pavement. The point or points of secondary impact with the vehicle are determined by the victim's height and weight and the speed and configuration of the moving vehicle. If the auto is moving rapidly, it may pass completely beneath the victim, who is tossed high into the air and comes down on the road. The majority of pedestrian fatalities result from head injuries.

Victims who walk or run into the side of a moving vehicle usually are hurled aside. They may impact against a wide variety of nearby objects before hitting the ground and generally sustain head injuries.

Injuries to cyclists. Cyclists sustain injuries when they are struck by motor vehicles, when they drive into a vehicle or some other object, or when they lose their balance and fall. The cyclist who is hit by a moving vehicle is the mechanical equivalent of a "sitting pedestrian," and the principles governing injury in this circumstance are similar to those mentioned previously. The cyclist who hits another object is the mechanical equivalent of an unrestrained, open-vehicle occupant who is "launched" when he continues in forward motion after his cycle is stopped by its decelerating impact. As with pedestrians, the vulnerability of cyclists allows for multiple severe injuries of more than one body area, though craniocerebral trauma is the leading cause of cyclist fatalities.

Common medicolegal problems associated with traffic injuries

Toxicology. Blood ethanol determinations should be done on all teenage and adult victims of traffic accidents who survive their injuries for less than 24 hours. Tests for carboxyhemoglobin are indicated when vehicles catch fire or when there is a possibility that the car had a defective exhaust system or extensive rusting of its undersurface. On the latter basis, we have seen fatal asphyxia by carbon monoxide in occupants of a car parked in an open area with its engine running.

The slightest suspicion of drug involvement in any victim of a fatal traffic incident should prompt the pathologist to save at least 50 ml of blood and urine, all available bile, stomach content, and generous samples of liver, kidney, and brain. Toxicologists have adequate means to dispose of samples they do not need, but none can retrieve a specimen that went down the drain or into an incinerator. Nothing frustrates the toxicologist more than a 5 to 10 ml sample of blood accompanied by an all-encompassing request that it be analyzed for "drugs."

Identity of driver. When all vehicle occupants are ejected, important medicolegal questions may arise concerning the identity of the driver. Patterns of injury may provide the answer, and comparison of the victims' blood groups with the location of blood stains in the car may be helpful. Hair samples should be plucked from any hairbearing area that is injured. The victims' clothing should be preserved carefully for evidentiary evaluation by trained personnel. In this regard, smooth-soled shoes should be examined, since they may show patterned imprints imparted by forces transmitted through the brake or accelerator pedals or the floor mats.

Hit-skip (hit and run) pedestrians. Samples of blood and hair should be saved as mentioned previously. In addition, fragments of metal, glass, or paint are usually present on the victim's clothing and may be on or in the victim's body. Reconstruction of the accident situa-

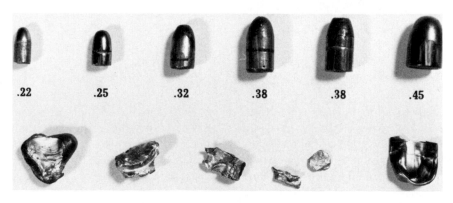

Fig. 3-9. *Top row,* Bullets of commonly available calibers for handguns. *Bottom row,* Deformed bullets, misshapen bullet fragments, and a deformed partial jacket (see text).

tion may hinge on correlation of the victim's impact areas with damage to the suspected vehicle. It should be standard practice to measure the height or impact areas on the lower limbs above the level of the heels. The presence of cataracts or optic atrophy occasionally helps to explain why an elderly pedestrian walked into the path of an oncoming vehicle, thereby exonerating an innocent driver.

Firearm injuries

Guns and bullets. Pulling the trigger or a loaded gun causes the firing pin to strike the cartridge base, detonating the primer. The latter event causes ignition of gunpowder in the cartridge. Gunpowder combustion produces rapidly expanding gas, the pressure of which propels the bullet.

A bullet's diameter, or caliber, can be expressed in hundredths of an inch or in millimeters. Fig. 3-9 shows representative handgun bullets of commonly available

calibers. The .25- and .45-caliber bullets have full copper jackets, and the .38-caliber bullet on the right has a partial copper jacket. The .22-caliber bullet has been coated with a thin film of copper ("copper wash"), which is not a discrete jacket. The specimens arranged on the bottom row of Fig. 3-9 are bullets that have been deformed and fragmented as a result of their passage through a hard object such as bone. A misshapen partial jacket, which has been separated from the bullet core after contact with a hard object, is shown at the far right of the bottom row. Deformed bullets and fragments such as these present irregular surfaces to the tissues in their path. Consequently, they are likely to expend all of their energy in wound production. From the standpoint of "wounding efficiency," the residual kinetic energy possessed by a bullet as it exits from the victim is wasted because it has not been utilized in injury production.

During the manufacture of handgun and rifle barrels,

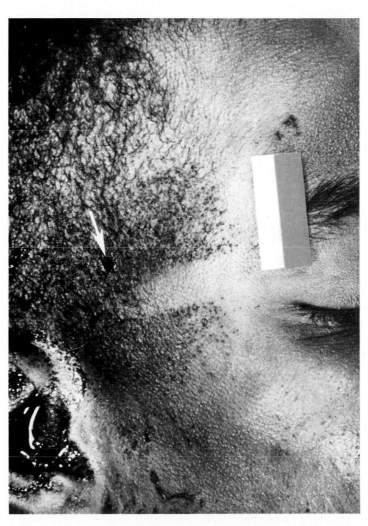

Fig. 3-10. Entrance gunshot wound of right temple *(arrow)* with surrounding dense zone of fouling. Skin adjacent to lateral aspect of eyebrow has been shielded by frame of decedent's eyeglasses. (Courtesy Office of the Chief Medical Examiner, Baltimore, Md.)

a rifling tool cuts a series of spiral grooves in their interiors. The elevated surfaces between the grooves are called "lands." Because the interior diameter of the barrel is slightly smaller than the bullets intended for use in the gun, the fired bullet entering the breech end of the barrel is gripped by the lands, which impart a spin to it as it passes through the barrel. This spin about its long axis produces the bullet's gyroscopic stability while it is in flight.

In addition to the bullet, a variety of particulate matter emerges from the muzzle of a fired gun. The smallest particles are the residue of completely burned gunpowder and take the form of a black, dustlike material. These particles are so light that they generally travel only 6 to 8 inches from the gun muzzle. As a result, targets shot at ranges closer than 6 to 8 inches usually show a zone of black *fouling* or *smudging* surrounding the bullet perforation (Fig. 3-10). Larger particles emerging with or behind the bullet consist of partially burned or unburned gunpowder, metal shavings, and

other debris or lubricant from the barrel interior or bullet surface. Since these particles are larger and heavier than the dustlike residue of completely burned powder, they travel farther. In flight they take the form of tiny individual missiles, each creating a punctate impression on or in the target. Collectively, these individual marks are referred to as *stippling* or *tattooing* (Fig. 3-11). Most handguns produce stippling up to ranges of 1½ to 3 feet.

Cutaneous entrance wounds. In reference to muzzle-target distance, we use the following classification for handgun and rifle wounds.[72] *Contact* shots are those in which the muzzle of the gun touches the target. When the muzzle is pressed firmly against the skin so that all of the powder residue is blasted *into* the tissue, the wound is classified as *tight contact* (Fig. 3-12). If the seal between muzzle and skin is imperfect, a *loose contact* wound results in which powder residue is deposited *on* the cutaneous surface as well as being blasted *into* the wound track (Fig. 3-13). In either instance the

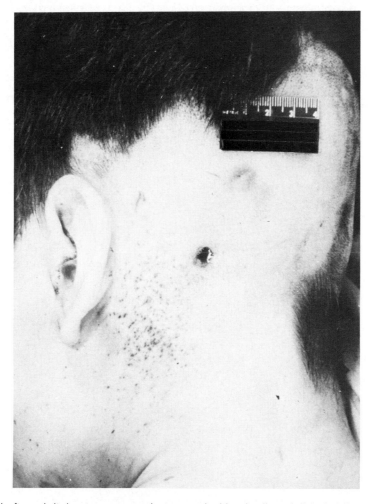

Fig. 3-11. Left occipital entrance gunshot wound with stippling visible in left mastoid area and on decedent's left cheek. The scalp, exposed by postmortem shaving, shows no stippling because it was shielded by hair. Fouling is absent. (Courtesy Office of the Chief Medical Examiner, Baltimore, Md.)

expanding gas that follows the bullet augments the severity of the injury. When the muzzle does not touch the target but is sufficiently close to produce fouling, the wound is *close range*. Wounds having stippling but no fouling are *intermediate range*, and those beyond the range of stippling are *distant*. In reference to cutaneous wounds, the foregoing criteria are inappropriate when the skin is not the primary target. Passage of a bullet through thick hair, clothing, or some other object before it strikes the skin may filter some or all of the powder residue, shielding the skin from fouling and stippling (Figs. 3-10 and 3-11).

The appearance of a contact-range gunshot wound is determined by the amount of gunpowder in the car-

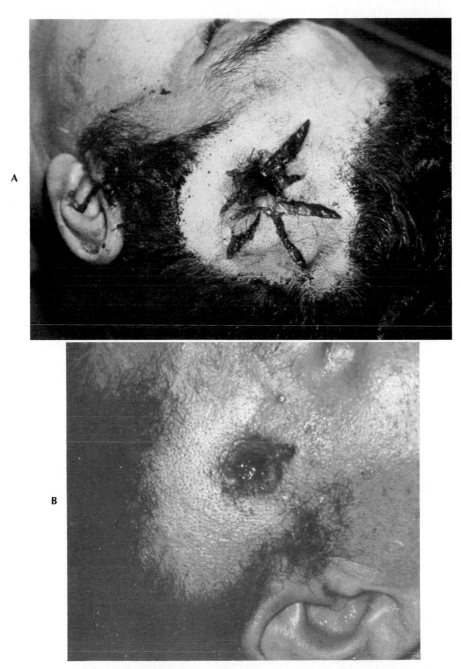

Fig. 3-12. Typical, tight contact-range gunshot wounds with no escape of powder residue onto cutaneous surface adjacent to perforations. Expanding gas blasted into wound in **A** caused extensive lacerations, whereas in **B,** gas elevated scalp and pressed it against gun, producing "muzzle stamp" abrasion that includes impression of the gun site in 3 o'clock position. In **B,** quantity of gas was insufficient to lacerate skin. Internally both wounds contain abundant powder residue.

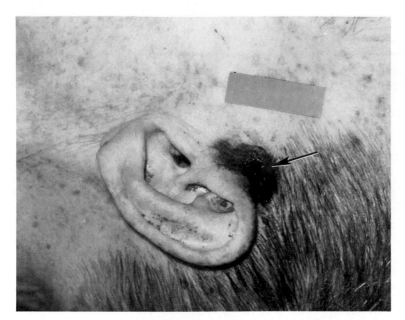

Fig. 3-13. Loose contact-range gunshot wound with imperfect seal between muzzle and skin, allowing escape of gas and powder residue onto cutaneous surface adjacent to perforation. Arrow indicates centrally located perforation. Internally, tracks of such wounds contain powder residue.

Fig. 3-14. Schema of mechanism whereby spinning bullets cause abraded defects when they perforate an elastic structure such as skin. Bullet striking at a right angle, **A,** creates a uniform margin of abrasion, whereas bullet approaching at an acute angle, **B,** leaves asymmetric abrasion that is widest on the side from which the bullet approached.

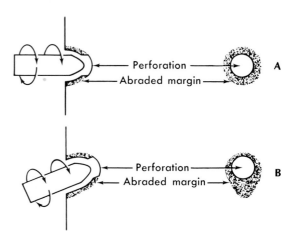

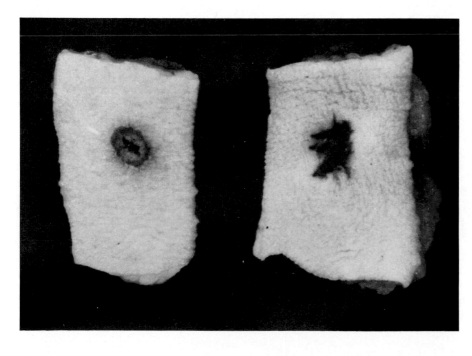

Fig. 3-15. Cutaneous entrance *(left)* and exit wounds made by same bullet. Symmetric, uniform margin of abrasion surrounding entrance perforation indicates that bullet approached at a nearly right angle. Exit wound is a lacerated, nonabraded perforation.

tridge (load), the characteristics of the firearm, the firmness of the seal between muzzle and skin, and the part of the body that is shot. If sufficient expanding gas is blasted into an area with underlying firm bony support (such as the head), the skin is torn loose from its attachment and lacerated (Fig. 3-12, *A*). Such wounds are commonplace with contact-range wounds produced by handguns of .32 caliber or greater. Smaller-caliber handgun ammunition often does not produce sufficient gas to lacerate the skin. Instead it may elevate the skin from its support and press it back against the face of the gun, imparting a "muzzle stamp" to the skin surrounding the gunshot perforation (Fig. 3-12, *B*). If the arrangement of the tissues is such that the explosive force can be decompressed *internally,* as is likely with contact wounds of the chest or abdomen, the external characteristics of the cutaneous wound may resemble those of a distant wound.

Typical distant cutaneous entrance wounds are abraded perforations whose central defect is slightly smaller than the bullet diameter. This characteristic appearance is the combined result of the bullet's forward motion and the skin's elasticity. In the process of perforating the skin, the bullet initially indents and stretches it. The epidermis in contact with the margin of the moving bullet is scraped away, creating a rim of abrasion about the perforation. The outer circumference of the abrasion collar may be soiled by lubricant

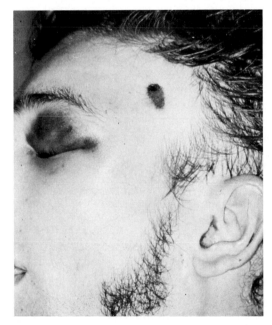

Fig. 3-16. Entrance gunshot wound of left side of forehead. Bullet approached victim at acute angle from his lower left, creating asymmetric margin of abrasion that is widest at lower left side of perforation. Ecchymosis and swelling of his left upper eyelid were produced by fracture of orbital roof as a result of gunshot wound rather than by direct facial trauma.

or dirt ("gray ring"), which must not be misinterpreted as fouling. Bullets striking the skin at right angles usually produce a uniform margin of abrasion (Figs. 3-14 and 3-15), whereas those that strike at an angle of less than 90 degrees leave asymmetric abrasions whose widest margin indicates the direction from which the bullet approached the skin (Figs. 3-14 and 3-16).

Atypical entrance gunshot wounds are those having unusual configurations, which commonly include lacerated margins and alteration of the typical abrasion collar described previously. Such anomalies occur in a variety of circumstances. Alterations of a bullet's normal gyroscopic spin and exaggerations of its yaw may be produced by defective guns or faulty ammunition, ricochet off a solid object, or passage of a bullet through some other target before it strikes the skin. In the last instance, if the primary target is close to the victim or is a personal item, such as spectacles or jewelry, fragments of the article may act as secondary missiles, which complicate the bullet perforation. In like fashion, primary perforation of a victim's hand or arm may render a wound of reentrance on his trunk or face decidedly atypical (Fig. 3-17). Finally, when the skin of the target area has a texture or contour different from that of ordinary skin, its wound (of entrance or exit) may have a totally different appearance. Examples of such areas include the eyelids, nose, lips, external ears, penis, scrotum, and fingertips.

Rifle wounds usually differ from those inflicted by handguns because the former typically are caused by bullets with much greater kinetic energy. Commonly available handguns loaded with standard ammunition generally fire bullets with an initial muzzle velocity of 600 to 1000 feet per second, whereas rifle bullets frequently are in the range of 2000 to 3000 feet per second. Since a bullet's kinetic energy varies with the square of its velocity, a tripling of velocity increases its energy by a factor of 9.

Contact-range wounding with military and powerful civilian rifles causes massively destructive or explosive injuries. Distant wounding with these weapons will, in many instances, produce cutaneous wounds of entrance and exit that are atypical and larger than those inflicted by handguns (Fig. 3-18). Although distant rifle wounds may resemble handgun injuries externally, they generally inflict far more visceral trauma than handgun bullets do (Fig. 3-19). Small-caliber, low-velocity civilian rifle wounds may be similar to those produced by handguns.

Cutaneous exit wounds. When a bullet leaves the body, it is traveling at a slower speed and is frequently deformed. It normally produces an irregularly lacerated wound with everted edges (Fig. 3-15). A slowly moving bullet may leave only a small, easily overlooked slit in the skin. The surface of an exit wound lacks the mar-

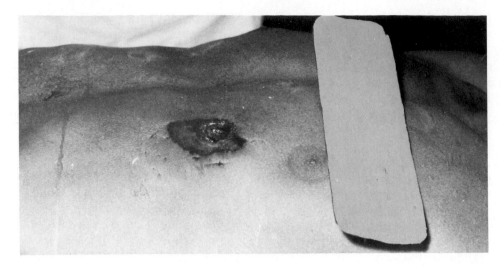

Fig. 3-17. Gunshot wound of reentrance in left inframammary area. Before striking decedent's chest, bullet perforated his right hand, passing from dorsum to palm, with exit defect on thenar eminence. At instant of wounding, palmar surface of his hand was resting against the chest. Oval abrasion, asymmetrically surrounding perforation, reflects configuration of his thenar eminence.

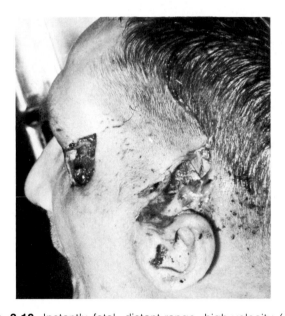

Fig. 3-18. Instantly fatal, distant-range, high-velocity (.30-caliber rifle) bullet wound of head. Entrance defect is adjacent to lateral aspect of left eyebrow, and exit defect is located above superior attachment of auricle. Skin between entrance and exit wounds has been torn loose from its attachments and shows tiny, stretch type of lacerations. (Dark spots on and behind ear are dry blood rather than stippling.) Subjacent skull was shattered, and multiple bone fragments ("secondary missiles") penetrated brain.

ginal epidermal abrasion that characterizes an entrance wound unless the skin was somehow supported at the moment it was perforated by the exiting missile. Support of this type can be provided by elastic bands of undergarments, belts, articles in pockets, or a firm external surface, such as a wall or the floor, against which the cutaneous surface was resting when perforated. With high-velocity bullets, the exit wound is usually larger than the entrance wound.

Internal injuries produced by gunfire have peculiar and important characteristics caused principally by the velocity of the wounding missile and the nature of the target area. Tissues in direct contact with the bullet are crushed and devitalized as they are perforated. Such crushing results in a permanent cavity or wound track. Radial or centrifugal displacement of force from the path of the bullet causes temporary cavitation of tissue and generates potentially damaging, stretching stress at a considerable distance from the bullet track (Figs. 3-19 and 3-20).[15] Any fragmentation of the projectile can augment wound production by providing points of weakness where the stretching effect is focused rather than being uniformly absorbed by the tissue.[17] Rigid tissues and structures are more susceptible to injury by stretching than soft, elastic tissues such as muscle. One of the more commonly encountered manifestations of radially transmitted forces from bullets is comminution of the orbital plates, which occurs frequently in association with transcerebral passage of projectiles (Fig. 3-16). Bullet perforations in bones are characteristically conical, with the entrance defect being smaller than the corresponding exit (Fig. 3-21).

Medicolegal evidence in death by gunfire. Fre-

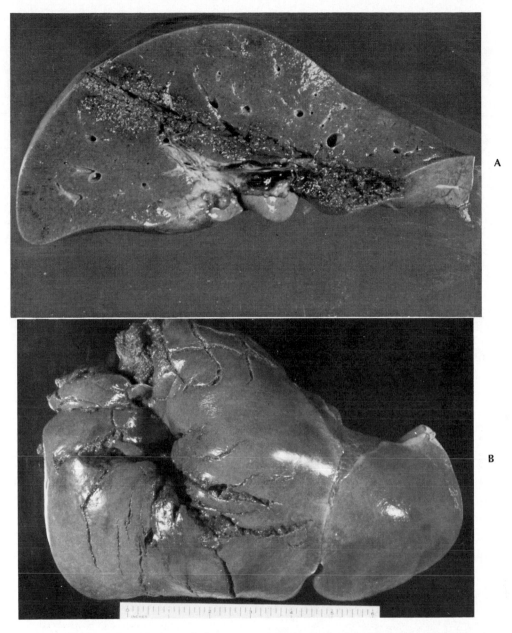

Fig. 3-19. A, Wound track through liver caused by low-velocity, .38-caliber bullet fired from revolver. Zone of tissue damage is larger than diameter of bullet, but the injury is far less destructive than that shown in **B. B,** Injury caused by high-velocity, .30-caliber rifle bullet. Extensive splits of Glisson's capsule reflect radial transmission of energy. Striking contrast between the two specimens exemplifies the dominance of velocity over weight in determining wounding potential, because the .38-caliber handgun bullet was slightly heavier than the .30-caliber rifle bullet.

quently, the only opportunity to acquire reliable evidence as to the circumstances in which the injury occurred or to establish the identifying characteristics of the responsible weapon is provided by the autopsy. Such evidence may be readily lost or destroyed unless it is looked for and preserved. Loss or destruction of such medical and paramedical evidence can be disastrous. Thus failure to recognize powder residue in the interior of a wound may lead to the exclusion of suicide and give support to the erroneous suspicion that murder has been committed. Failure to distinguish an entrance wound from an exit wound may seriously distort the official investigation of a homicidal incident.

General considerations. A detailed examination and description of all skin wounds, all associated holes in the clothing, and such changes in either as might have

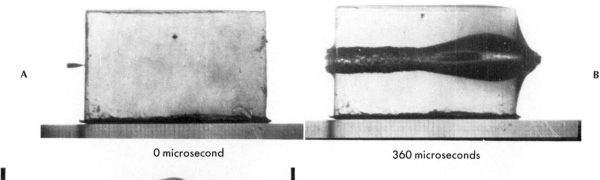

A

0 microsecond

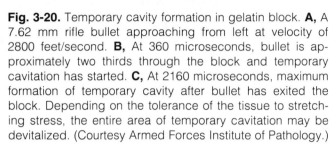

B

360 microseconds

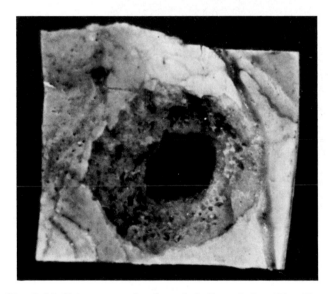

C

2160 microseconds

Fig. 3-20. Temporary cavity formation in gelatin block. **A,** A 7.62 mm rifle bullet approaching from left at velocity of 2800 feet/second. **B,** At 360 microseconds, bullet is approximately two thirds through the block and temporary cavitation has started. **C,** At 2160 microseconds, maximum formation of temporary cavity after bullet has exited the block. Depending on the tolerance of the tissue to stretching stress, the entire area of temporary cavitation may be devitalized. (Courtesy Armed Forces Institute of Pathology.)

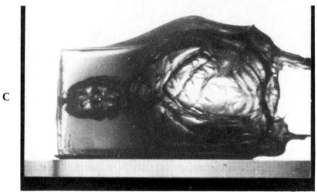

Fig. 3-21. Entrance perforation of skull made by .38-caliber bullet, viewed from the inner table, showing bone beveling in direction of flight and exemplifying principle that fractures dissipate forces acting on bone. In entrance wound of skull, bullet first strikes and fractures outer table. Force is dissipated as it is transmitted through bony trabeculas and therefore is exerted over larger area on inner table, causing larger perforation of the latter. Beveling is reversed in exit wounds, with the larger defect on outer table of skull. Most bones develop morphologically similar defects when perforated by bullets.

resulted from powder residue should be routine practice in all cases of death by gunfire. It is common for a bullet that has passed through the body to be found in the clothing. The dimensions and precise location of each wound, each hole in clothing, and each area of fouling or stippling should be recorded with their locations related to standard anatomic landmarks as well as to the standing height of the victim. Color photographs are an indispensable supplement to the descriptive text.

Bullets or fragments of bullets. Any bullet or fragment of a bullet (sufficiently large to be recovered) in the body should be retrieved, even though no reason for preserving the bullet is anticipated at the time of operation or autopsy. Each bullet should be placed in its own properly labeled container and saved. In cases where more than one bullet or fragment of bullet are recovered, each should be identified in relation to the entrance wound with which it is associated.

Although the need for exercising care in the handling of projectiles and projectile fragments recovered from a victim should be common knowledge, many surgeons and some pathologists still make the mistake of extracting and handling such objects in the unprotected jaws of metal instruments or of scratching identifying initials across rifling marks on the sides of the bullet. Fig. 3-22 shows two bullets, each of which has been inscribed with the victim's initials, J.D.H. The specimen on the left is improperly marked because the initials obliterate some of the rifling striations. The correctly initialed specimen on the right has been marked on its base.

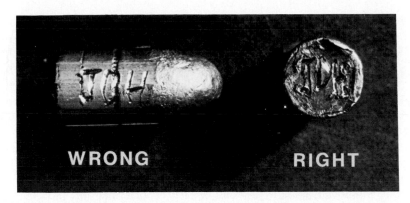

Fig. 3-22. Two nonjacketed .38-caliber bullets, each bearing initials J.D.H. Specimen on left is marked improperly because initials obscure rifling striations ("autograph" of gun from which it was fired). Specimen on right has been properly marked on its base.

Because bullets often migrate or travel considerable distances from their entrance sites, autopsies of persons who have died from gunfire should be performed in locales where x-ray facilities are available. In the case of a perforating wound, where the bullet has emerged from the victim and has been lost, it may be extremely important to collect bullet fragments that have been sheared off in passing through a bone or deposited along the track of the wound. X-ray examination is often essential to locate such metallic debris. Subsequent identification of the chemical composition of the fragment or fragments may establish that it could or could not represent a certain type or branch of ammunition.

Direction of fire. In a case of death by gunfire, it is necessary to verify the direction from which the bullet came. If there is only one surface wound (that is, entrance defect) and the bullet is still in the victim, the problem is simplified. With low-power handguns, the bullet is frequently palpable beneath the skin of the side of the body opposite to the site of entrance. Skin offers greater resistance to perforation than any tissue other than bone or tooth.

If more than one hole is present in the skin, entrance must be distinguished from exit. The gross appearances of typical and atypical entrance and exit wounds have been described already; Adelson[1] has reported the histopathologic characteristics of cutaneous gunshot wounds. Also, one should be aware that bullet defects in clothing are frequently easier to orient as entrance or exit wounds than are the corresponding perforations of the victim's skin.

If bullet wounds in the skin (entrance or exit) have been altered or destroyed as a result of putrefaction or other postmortem change or surgery, it may still be possible to recognize the direction in which the bullet was traveling by the manner in which bones have been fractured. In passing through a bone, a bullet characteristically produces a larger defect at the site of exit

than at the site of entrance (Fig. 3-21). It also displaces fragments of bone in the direction of its flight.

Range of fire. The evidence needed to establish the distance between the gun and the target when the shot was fired has been mentioned in connection with entrance wounds. Gray-black powder residue beneath the periosteum of the outer table of the skull or on the underlying dural margins is often seen with contact gunshot wounds of the head. Blotting of the wound with paper towels may help demonstrate powder soiling by removing excess blood. Removal of blood by this means must be done with care because contact or near-contact wounds produced by some ammunition may result in minimal surface fouling that is easily overlooked. The potential importance of such evidence for reconstructing the fatal incident is so great that the decedent should be examined by the pathologist before clothing has been removed and before the skin has been washed. If the clothing is dark, it may need to be photographed with infrared technique or tested chemically to disclose the presence or absence of combustion residues. When gunshot wounds are sustained through clothing, range of fire determinations rests on an evaluation of the garments rather than the person's skin. The effectiveness with which clothing shields the skin from powder residue is determined by the range of fire, characteristics of the gunpowder, number of layers of cloth perforated, and tightness of weave of the fabric.

Contact wounds in areas with underlying skeletal muscle (such as the chest) commonly show a zone of pink discoloration in muscle surrounding the wound-track. This is attributable to an uptake of carbon monoxide by myoglobin and probably also to a staining of muscle by nitrites in powder residue. The pink discoloration fades when the muscle is exposed to air.

Number and sequence of shots fired. The number of entrance wounds may not coincide with the number of bullets that have been fired into the body. Since the *number* of shots fired is often a matter of critical medicolegal importance, the causes of such "discrepancies" deserve investigation. The most common circumstance in which there may be a disparity between the number of bullets fired and the number of entrance wounds occurs when a bullet passes through an arm or hand before entering the trunk or head (Fig. 3-17). In such circumstances it is obvious that a single bullet can produce two or more entrances. Another type of discrepancy arises when a bullet strikes a compact bone and splits into two or more pieces. In such circumstances there may be more than one exit wound for a single hole of entrance. In rare instances, two bullets enter the same cutaneous perforation. This can occur with tandem or "piggyback" bullets or in contact-range wounding when the muzzle of the gun is pressed against a previous site of entrance. Bullets can be coughed up, expectorated, vomited, or defected when their tracks terminate in an air passage or the gastrointestinal tract, explaining the occasional situation in which there is an entrance wound without a corresponding exit defect and no bullet in the body.

Time and degree of disability after gunshot injury. Great caution should be exercised in estimating the immediate disabling effects of a bullet wound. Through-and-through wounds of the heart commonly fail to cause immediate disability. Only when there is massive destruction of the motor area of the central nervous system or of the brainstem or cervical cord, or when the heart or aorta has been extensively damaged can it be said "with reasonable medical certainty" that the injury was immediately and totally disabling.

Shotgun wounds. Shotguns are smooth-bore weapons that fire a charge composed of one or more projectiles plus wadding. The single-projectile shotgun ammunition, called a rifled slug, is encountered rarely in human wounding and will not be considered further. Pellets in shotgun shells vary in size from 0.36 inch (000 buckshot) to 0.05 inch (number 12 shot). In our jurisdiction, the most frequently encountered sizes of shot in civilian wounding are from 0.10 to 0.15 inch in diameter, and average loads contain 100 to 250 such pellets. Police "riot guns" usually are loaded with large-sized buckshot.

Shotgun *gauge* formerly was defined as the number of spherical lead balls, each of the same diameter as the bore, required to weigh 1 pound. In actual measure a 12-gauge shotgun has a bore diameter of 0.729 inch and a 16-gauge bore is 0.662 inch in diameter. Bore diameter also can be expressed in thousandths of an inch—for example, .410 ("four-ten").

Choke refers to constriction of the muzzle end of the barrel and is designed to reduce pellet dispersion. The amount of choke varies from "full" to none. It is measured functionally by the percentage of shot falling in a 30-inch circle when the weapon is fired at a distance of 40 yards and ranges from 65% to 75% for full choke to 25% to 35% in the case of an unchoked cylinder bore. Choke either is added to the barrel during the manufacturing process or can be controlled with a variable choke adapter.

Contact-range shotgun wounds of the trunk are round or oval, smoothly marginated defects that may or may not contain an abundance of powder residue. Contact wounds in the interior of the mouth or against the scalp frequently produce explosive semidecapitation. The appearance of shotgun wounds beyond contact range is determined by the muzzle-target distance, barrel choke and length, shot size, and presence or absence of clothing or other intermediate objects in the path of the charge. Consequently, an estimate of range of fire in a given case is made with considerable latitude unless appropriate experimental test firings have been done. Generally speaking, at ranges beyond 3 to 6 feet the charge begins to separate, producing a skin defect with ragged margins, often referred to as a "rat hole." Next, a few pellets create individual satellite perforations adjacent to the major defect. As the distance lengthens, the main defect becomes smaller, more satellite perforations appear, and the spread of satellite perforations increases. Beyond approximately 5 yards, the wound pattern consists mainly of individual perforations with or without wad injuries in the form of circular, nonpenetrating abrasions.

Passage of the shotgun charge through clothing or any intermediate object, no matter how flimsy, accelerates the pellet spread and renders the skin pattern inappropriate for estimating range of fire. An x-ray film of the victim showing the spread of pellets cannot be utilized to estimate range of fire because the final distribution of pellets may be identical in contact and distant wounds.

Shotgun pellets usually do not exit from the body except for the following situations: contact wounds of the head that cause virtual explosions; tangentially oriented wounds, either close or distant, where part or all of the charge follows a short track through the body; wounding of a thin part of the body, such as the neck or a limb; and wounding by large-sized buckshot.

Local sequelae of mechanical injury

The mechanical disruption of living tissue is attended and followed by various local disturbances, the nature of which depends in part on the site and severity of the disruptive lesion and in part on the organism's capacity to react.

Hemorrhage. Hemorrhage is an immediate and inevitable sequel to mechanical disruption of living vascularized tissue. Blood continues to flow from the damaged vessels until prevented from doing so by thrombosis, vasoconstriction, or equalization of intravascular and extravascular pressures (through a drop in the former or a rise in the latter).

In the case of damage to the small vessels (capillaries, arterioles, venules), vasoconstriction is a more important mechanism than thrombosis in the induction of hemostasis. This is also true when vessels, whether large or small, are lacerated or crushed. When a vessel is incised or injured in such a manner that the disturbance is limited to the site of the defect, hemostasis is more dependent on the occurrence of thrombosis.

In noncommunicating injuries such as may occur with fracture or other forms of internal laceration, the opposition offered by the surrounding intact tissue to the accumulating mass of extravascular blood is an important mechanism of hemostasis. When injury has caused a state of shock, the fall in systemic blood pressure contributes to other factors in preventing further loss of blood.

Mechanical disturbances resulting from an extravascular accumulation of blood may be caused by distension, compression, or obstruction. Pain is an outstanding manifestation of distension of tissue by hemorrhage. It may be the first evidence of the accumulation of a relatively small amount of blood beneath the periosteum or immediately below the peritoneum. The most important compressive effects of extravasated blood are those seen in relation to intracranial and intrapericardial hemorrhage. The rapid accumulation of as little as 50 ml in the former situation or 150 ml in the latter may be fatal by its compressive effect. The importance of the rate of hemorrhage in determining such a mechanical effect is revealed by the fact that a considerably larger amount of blood can be tolerated in either situation if it has accumulated slowly. In the case of a slowly developing subdural hemorrhage, more than 100 ml may accumulate before signs of increased intracranial pressure become apparent. If the pericardium is distended slowly, a liter or more of fluid may be tolerated without the occurrence of fatal cardiac tamponade.

One of the best examples of obstructive disturbance caused by extravasated blood may occur when blood is aspirated into the lower air passages. The foam created by mixing blood and air in such a situation may be sufficiently obstructive to cause asphyxiation, though the lungs need not be heavier than normal.

The preceding paragraphs have been concerned with early mechanical disturbances caused by the extravascular accumulation of blood. The possibility of late mechanical disturbances attributable to secondary edema incident to the presence of blood in tissue spaces should not be ignored. One of the best examples of this phenomenon is the progressive expansion of a subdural hematoma. Although the space originally consumed by such a hemorrhage may fail to cause a significant amount of cerebral compression, the subsequent imbibition of fluid by the hematoma or secondary spontaneous bleeding from capillaries contained in newly formed granulation tissue sometimes gives rise to a progressively incapacitating or even fatal rise in intracranial pressure.

Pigmentary changes are a striking feature of the deterioration of blood at the site of hemorrhage. As the oxyhemoglobin is reduced, the color of the injured tissue changes from red through purple to blue. In the case of small extravasations, either the erythrocytes are ingested by phagocytes and transported from the site of injury or the products of their disintegraton in situ are carried away by the lymph so rapidly that secondary pigmentary changes are inconspicuous. If the mass of extravasated blood is large or its disposal is delayed by inadequate lymph flow, the iron is separated from the globin after hemolysis in situ and the pigment is subsequently converted to bilirubin and biliverdin, with chromatic changes ranging through brown, green, and yellow. In addition to these color changes, two types of crystalline derivatives of hemoglobin may be identified on microscopic examination: hematoidin and hemosiderin. (For further discussion of hemoglobin pigments, see p. 1380.)

Chronologic changes in the gross and microscopic appearances of contusions can provide the basis for important medicolegal interpretations. However, caution is in order when making such interpretations because of variability in temporal evolution of the gross appearances of bruises and of the histopathologic inflammatory responses. Such variability is governed by the vascularity of the injured locus, the quantity of blood accumulating in the tissues, the integrity of the overlying skin, and the factors that combine to define the host response to injury.

Aseptic inflammation. Unless immediately fatal, a mechanical injury of living tissue is almost invariably followed by a series of local reactive changes producing the phenomenon of aseptic inflammation. The extent to which the inflammatory reaction progresses or eventually disturbs the tissue usually depends on the severity and location of the injury that elicited it. The inflammatory cycle in such instances is probably set in motion and maintained by a variety of chemical and physical alterations. (Inflammation and wound healing are discussed in detail in Chapter 2.)

Other local circulatory disturbances. Attention has already been directed to the circulatory disturbances that may be induced by an expanding hematoma and to those that occur incident to vascular participation in the phenomenon of inflammation. Various other factors may contribute to local disturbances in circulation after a mechanical injury.

One of these is the occurrence of regional vascular

spasm of sufficient extent and severity that the original injury is enlarged by the occurrence of secondary ischemic necrosis. Generalized ischemia of a limb may result from reactive spasm of large and apparently unwounded arteries after the occurrence of an injury whose disruptive effects were local. Nonthrombotic ischemia apparently from vasospasm is sometimes responsible for the progressive enlargement, by infarction, of relatively small primary injuries of the brain or kidney.

Similar enlargement of the original scope of injury may result from the propagation of a thrombus from the site of a disruptive vascular injury or from stasis and thrombosis caused by posttraumatic vascular compression by edema or interstitial hemorrhage. In the case of disabling injuries, the inactivity imposed by disability is an additional cause of stasis and may be responsible for thrombosis in the region of injury or in the lower extremities.

Intravascular stasis may be sufficient to cause thrombosis independent of preceding injury to the affected vessel. Although it is unlikely that thrombosis will occur in a normal vessel, the lining of a vessel does not remain normal for long after the blood within it has ceased to flow. Degeneration of the lining endothelium and edema of the intima occur concomitantly with stasis. Platelets adhere to the damaged lining. In larger vessels, clot formation begins at the periphery of the stream and progresses toward the center until the obstruction is complete. In small vessels, much or most of the fluid elements of the blood diffuse through the vascular wall, leaving the distended lumen occluded by a solid, sausagelike mass of closely packed erythrocytes.

Local infection. Any injury that disturbs the continuity of the protective and especially adapted layer of cells that stands between the organism and its external environment, whether it be the integument or the mucous membrane lining an internal passage, may create a portal of entry for infection. The infective agent may be carried into the tissues on the surface of the instrument that was responsible for the wound, or it may subsequently gain access to the tissues because of the existence of a wound.

Under nonsurgical conditions, any instrument responsible for the production of a mechanical injury is likely to be contaminated with pathogenic organisms. Soil is an important source of such contamination, and *Clostridium tetani* and *Clostridium welchii* are among the more important pathogenic inhabitants of soil. Streptococci, staphylococci, *Proteus vulgaris*, *Pseudomonas aeruginosa*, and *Escherichia coli* are commonly present on the skin. Pathogenic organisms that may be present on mucous membranes of the body include streptococci, pneumococci, meningococci, *Haemophilus influenzae*, *Klebsiella pneumoniae*, *E. coli*, *Corynebacterium diphtheriae*, and *C. welchii*.

The creation of an external portal of entry is by no means the only mechanism by which mechanical violence may render the site of an injury vulnerable to infection. Even though primary wound infection does not take place, a locus of diminished resistance may be established. Delayed infection of the injured tissue by way of the bloodstream may occur because of the creation of conditions favorable to bacterial growth at the wound site.

Systemic effects of mechanical injury

Almost immediately incapacitating systemic anoxia may be the direct consequence of an injury if its primary effect is such as to interfere with respiration or systemic circulation. Certain types of disruptive injury of the brain or heart may thus be the direct and immediate cause of fatal systemic disturbance. One should not conclude, however, that wounds of these structures are invariably fatal. As long as the brainstem escapes damage, extensive and disruptive cerebral injury may be survived. Through-and-through stab or bullet wounds of the heart are sometimes survived, and even those that eventually cause death may not be immediately incapacitating.

It is a fact, however, that even though the function of the damaged tissue is not normally concerned with such basic physiologic processes as respiration, circulation, nutrition, or elimination, such an injury may be responsible for systemic disturbances by any of several mechanisms.

Although the cause and nature of such disturbances are described in detail in various other places in this book, it is not unduly repetitive to bring them to the reader's attention at this time.

Primary shock

A mechanical injury to any part of the body may elicit a reflex vasodilatation and a fall in blood pressure of sufficient severity to cause collapse, loss of consciousness, and in some instances death. This type of posttraumatic circulatory disturbance constitutes the syndrome of primary or neurogenic shock. Pressure on the carotid sinuses, a blow to the epigastrium or a testicle, puncture of the pleura, a dilatation of the rectum may lead to sufficient fall in blood pressure to result in unconsciousness and occasionally in death. The reduction in blood pressure in such circumstances is caused by vasodilatation rather than by heart failure or a reduction in blood volume.

Secondary shock

Secondary shock is the state of circulatory failure that results from an excessive reduction in blood volume. It occurs whenever the amount of blood or plasma that has escaped from damaged vessels exceeds the limits of physiologic compensation. The vascular damage responsible for the escape of blood or plasma may be local and attributable to the direct effects of trauma or may be generalized and attributable to infection or some other systemic complication of what was originally a local injury.

Vasoconstriction is the initial homeostatic reaction to reduced blood volume. This may or may not be sufficient to maintain blood pressure, depending on the amount of blood lost. The secondary compensation is a movement of extravascular fluid into the vascular system, with hemodilution that may or may not be compensated by the mobilization of the erythrocyte reserves from the bone marrow and spleen. In its initial stages, shock is reversible. Severe and uncompensated shock may become irreversible as a result of widespread hypoxic parenchymatous injury. If bleeding or plasma loss continues, compensation fails and the volume of circulating blood decreases. When the pressure falls below a certain critical level, the vasomotor centers become anoxic and the resulting vasodilatation leads to rapid circulatory collapse and death.

The amount of hemorrhage necessary to produce circulatory collapse is governed by the rate of blood loss, the person's general cardiovascular condition, and the presence or absence of other factors, such as alcohol or drug intoxication, that may predispose to hypotension. In otherwise healthy persons, rapid loss of one third of the blood volume causes hemorrhagic shock, and death ensues when half of the blood volume is lost rapidly. Slow bleeding permits the occurrence of previously mentioned physiologic compensations and allows larger volumes of blood to be lost without causing shock or death.

In cases of death from acute massive hemorrhage, the most significant postmortem changes are gross rather than microscopic and consist in generalized pallor of tissue, collapse of the great veins, and a flabby, shrunken, gray spleen.

Shock kidney

Irreversible renal injury leading to anuria and death as a complication of secondary shock first attracted general attention during World War II. It did so because of the frequency with which persons who had sustained severe crushing injuries as a result of being caught in buildings demolished by air raids subsequently became anuric and died of renal insufficiency. Examination disclosed segmental obstruction of the renal tubules by pigmented casts, which were particularly conspicuous in the lower portions of the nephrons. It was first believed that the extensive crushing of skeletal muscle was responsible for the renal lesion. Subsequent stud-

ies, however, indicated that the essential damage to the kidney in such circumstances was probably attributable primarily to the renal ischemia that occurs during and may be prolonged beyond the posttraumatic episode of systemic hypotension. Any injury that is followed by secondary shock is capable of causing renal damage if the state of shock is sufficiently severe or protracted. If the original injury is associated with extensive muscle injury or intravascular hemolysis, the renal casts tend to be conspicuous by reason of their brown pigment. The injury is not confined to the lower reaches of the nephrons, and the casts represent the result rather than the cause of renal injury (pp. 809 and 832).

Shock lung

The term "shock lung" is probably a misnomer because shock alone fails to explain the pathogenesis of a variety of nonspecific pulmonary abnormalities that occur in injured persons. Lung injury from shock can be regarded as one of the local and systemic causes of the adult respiratory distress syndrome. In addition to chest wall and lung injuries, such patients may have aspiration of gastric content with pneumonia or lung abscess, bronchopneumonia, septicemia, fat embolism, large or small thromboemboli, embolism of cellular aggregates in massive blood transfusions, cardiac failure, fluid overloads, retained secretions, abdominal distension, atelectasis, and all the complications of prolonged mechanical ventilation.

Pulmonary pathologic changes are understandably variable and include alveolar and interstitial edema, thickening and fibrosis of alveolar septa, interstitial lymphocytic infiltrates, and alveolar hyaline membranes in various stages of organization. Obliterative changes in the pulmonary microvasculature, attributable to fibrin and platelet thromboemboli, commonly complicate disseminated intravascular coagulation and multiple transfusions. Bacterial, fungal, and viral pulmonary infections are common complications of trauma associated with coma, burns, debility, or inactivity.

General adaptation syndrome

The frequent occurrence of a posttraumatic neuroendocrine disturbance in the form of an evanescent hyperglycemia has long been recognized. That the neuroendocrine reaction to an injury may be such as to modify significantly the injury's total effect on the organism was not fully appreciated before the investigations of Selye.[55]

It is postulated that a wide variety of damaging stimuli may cause the pituitary gland to discharge an excessive amount of corticotropic hormone, which in turn leads to an outpouring of cortical hormones from the adrenal glands. Pathologic evidence of this effect on the adrenal glands is partial or complete depletion of lipid from the cortical cells within the first few days after an injury. That the reaction is part of a defense mechanism can be inferred from the fact that cortical hormone may cause a rapid release of antibodies from lymphoid tissue. The pathologic evidence of this effect is the rapid involution of thymus and lymphoid tissue.

Embolism

Fat droplets of sufficient size to obstruct capillaries may be found in the blood after almost any kind of disruptive injury involving adipose tissue and particularly after fractures of long bones. Unless the number and size of the emboli are such that fat-distended arterioles and capillaries are seen in every low-power field of lung, their lethality is doubtful. Usually when droplets and cylinders of fat are numerous in the pulmonary capillaries, emboli will also be found in the brain and kidneys (Fig. 3-23). Scully[54] found that only when the cerebral vessels are obstructed are fat emboli capable of causing death. In massive fat embolism, clinical features of the fat embolism syndrome, respiratory distress, and petechiae are present within 3 days of the injury.[67]

Controversy exists regarding the origin of the fat. Originally it was believed that fat released from the damaged adipose tissue (or bone marrow) at the site of injury was forced or aspirated into the central ends of the lacerated value. That this does happen is indicated by the occasional finding of organized masses of myeloid tissue in the pulmonary vessels of persons who have died after fractures. However, the amount of fat found in the pulmonary vascular bed in some instances is far in excess of what might plausibly be derived from the site of injury.

Lehman and Moore[29] were among the first researchers to suggest that the phenomenon of posttraumatic fat embolism was the result of a change in the droplet size of the endogenous plasma lipids. Support for this point of view has been provided by the work of LeQuire and associates,[32] who found that the cholesterol content of the embolic fat was much higher than that of adipose tissue. More recent investigations have demonstrated posttraumatic alterations in lipid metabolism and mobilization. Elevated plasma levels of free fatty acids (FFA) and macroglobules and prolonged shifts in lipoprotein composition distinguish those patients at risk for developing fat embolism.[51,62] Pulmonary fat embolism occurring independent of mechanical violence may be encountered in association with such diverse conditions as diabetes mellitus, extensive cutaneous burns, and decompression sickness.[56]

A detached blood clot is another type of embolism frequently caused by mechanical injury. Venous thrombosis may occur as a direct result of trauma to a vein or as a result of stasis caused by edema or inactivity. Thus the thrombus may form at the site of injury or at some remote place in the body. The spontaneous detachment of such a thrombus frequently results in fatal pulmonary embolism.

A third type of embolism that may be caused by me-

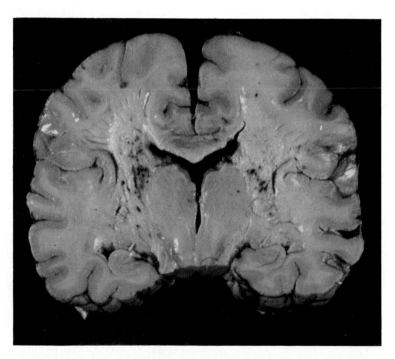

Fig. 3-23. Cerebral fat embolism. Small hemorrhagic infarcts caused by fat emboli produce gross appearance of white matter petechiae.

chanical injury results from the entrance of air into the circulating blood. The most common portals of entry for fatal air embolism are the dilated veins of the gravid uterus. Large amounts of air may be sucked into the uterine veins during orogenital sex[8] or an attempt to empty the uterus by instrumentation or by irrigation. Air embolism may result from tubal insufflation, from the insufflation of a nongravid uterus, from the injection of air into the peritoneal cavity, or from incision or laceration of veins anywhere in the body. Iatrogenic air embolism may occur with disconnection of intravenous catheters or intraoperatively, particularly in procedures of the posterior cranial fossae. Small amounts of air may enter the veins and be carried to the lung without causing significant disturbance. If the amount of air is large, however, the right side of the heart and the pulmonary arteries become occluded by foam, and death results from acute circulatory failure. As a result of penetrating injuries of the lungs, air may be carried to the left side of the heart and thence to the systemic circulation, where it causes death as the result of cerebral or coronary air embolism.[27] The autopsy diagnosis of fatal air embolism can be substantiated by a postmortem x-ray film or opening the heart under water.

INJURIES CAUSED BY CHANGES IN ATMOSPHERIC PRESSURE

The biologic consequences of changes in atmospheric pressure are dependent on two physical properties of gases:

1. The volume of gas contained in an elastic membrane increases in size as the surrounding barometric pressure is reduced.
2. The solubility of a gas in a liquid solvent (such as blood) is proportional to the partial pressure of that gas in the ambient atmosphere.

These two characteristics of gases in general are responsible for the signs and symptoms created by *trapped* and *evolved* gases that are observed with sudden changes in barometric pressure.

Gases may be trapped in body cavities that are usually in free communication with the ambient atmosphere if ready passage of air into and out of the cavity is blocked. Thus, in the presence of acute upper respiratory tract inflammation with resultant edema and swelling of the mucous membrane, the sinus orifices and eustachian tubes may be blocked or narrowed so that equalization of pressures within the paranasal air sinuses or middle ear cavities and the outside atmosphere is delayed or prevented. The clinical consequences may be severe.

Sufficient decrease in atmospheric pressure leads to expansion of gastric and intestinal gases with resultant abdominal distension. Expansion progresses until deflation occurs as a result of gaseous eructations or the passage of flatus or both.

Injuries associated with changes in atmospheric pressure may be seen in underwater use of a caisson, in high-altitude climbing or flight, or most commonly in diving with *s*elf-*c*ontained *u*nderwater *b*reating *a*pparatus (scuba). The three characteristics of an episode of abnormal atmospheric pressure that determine its injurious effects on humans are as follows:

1. Direction and magnitude of change
2. Rate of change
3. Duration of change

Decreased atmospheric pressure

The human organism tolerates an increase in atmospheric pressure better than a decrease of equal magnitude. Thus the atmospheric pressure of the human environment can be tripled without harm, and yet a lowering of the pressure by as little as 50% incident to elevation to an altitude of 20,000 feet results in severe systemic hypoxia and may cause death.

Rapid accentuation of hypoxia as a result of diminished barometric pressure is followed by strong peripheral vasoconstriction with consequent shifting of a large portion of the blood volume to the pulmonary circuit. This hemodynamic disturbance leads to pulmonary arterial hypertension associated with anoxic damage to pulmonary capillary endothelium and alveolar pneumocytes. The result of the combined action of these two responses to the abnormal physical environment is the so-called high-altitude pulmonary edema and high-altitude cerebral edema.[22,47] The pulmonary edema fluid is characterized by high molecular weight proteins, erythrocytes, and alveolar macrophages without significant neutrophil accumulation and is a result of loss of integrity of the endothelial-epithelial barrier with a transient leak in the pulmonary circulation.[52]

Acute high-altitude pulmonary edema usually occurs between 3 and 48 hours after exposure to altitudes above 3000 meters, especially if severe physical exertion has taken place in the unaccustomed environment. This illness poses a particular hazard to those who climb or ski at high altitudes. Therefore most instances occur in athletic young adults who are otherwise healthy. The condition is also a threat to those who live and work permanently at high altitudes, especially if they are faced with repeated reentry into the hypoxic environment after trips to lower altitudes. Fatalities can be indistinguishable clinically from fulminant pneumonia. At autopsy the lungs are congested and have interstitial and alveolar edema. Hyaline membranes may be present.[21]

In addition to decreased barometric pressure and decreased partial oxygen pressure encountered at high altitudes, there is often a simultaneous exposure to decreased environmental temperature and increased ultraviolet irradiation. A further source of physiologic stress is the decreasing humidity of air at high altitudes. This factor in concert with the hyperventilation that accompanies even moderate physical exertion can lead to rapid dehydration with resultant extreme thirst. The combination of hyperventilation and profuse diaphoresis can bring about a moderate degree of hypokalemic alkalosis. These multiple physical and biochemical assaults may give rise to acute mountain sickness, a syndrome characterized by headache, palpitations, nausea, anorexia, weakness, and insomnia.

Exposure to increasing altitudes activates various adaptive mechanisms that permit the body to tolerate the changes. The types and degrees of adaptation depend on many factors, including duration of exposure, level of physical activity, age, and general physical condition. Persons with limited cardiorespiratory reserve may experience dyspnea, nausea, and insomnia at altitudes as low as 1500 meters above sea level.

Increased atmospheric pressure

Injuries associated with increased atmospheric pressure usually occur during the return from elevated to normal barometric pressure. The rate at which the atmospheric pressure changes—more particularly, the rate at which it is decreased—is an exceedingly important factor in injury production. Unless barometric pressure is lowered slowly to normal, decompression sickness (also known as dysbarism, caisson disease, the bends, the staggers, or the chokes) may occur. A very rapid change from normal to subnormal pressure, as may occur during rapid ascent in supersonic aircraft, may also cause decompression sickness.

An increase in atmospheric pressure results in a net flow of nitrogen, which makes up four fifths of the inspired air, from the alveoli through the blood in which the gas dissolves, to tissue. When the return to normal pressure is slow, the loss of gas from tissue is analogous to gas uptake. However, if the return to normal pressure is rapid, gas bubbles form in tissue and blood because nitrogen evolves faster than it can be transported to the lungs and expired.[59]

Some degree of microscopic bubble formation probably occurs whenever the tissue partial pressure of nitrogen even moderately exceeds that in the surrounding atmosphere. However, symptom-producing bubbles (decompression sickness) will not occur until the partial pressure of nitrogen is more than twice that of the surrounding atmosphere.[43] (At the ocean's surface a diver and his viscera are under a pressure of 1 atmosphere [760 mm Hg], and 1 additional atmosphere of pressure is added for each 33 feet he descends.[58])

The nature and severity of decompression sickness are determined by the rate and location of nitrogen release. Disability and death may supervene within minutes or hours after decompression. Pulmonary and central nervous system involvement dominate in the causation of sudden fatalities. Subacute or chronic effects of decompression are characterized by lower limb, bladder, and rectal paralysis from demyelination of the dorsal and lateral columns of the inferior thoracic spinal cord rather than the upper cord or brain.[19] In divers and tunnelers with a history of the bends and persistent joint symptoms, foci of aseptic necrosis have usually developed in bones. Venous gas embolism with resultant vascular obstruction is the most likely basis for the localized areas of osseous destruction. Because of the solubility of nitrogen in fat, obesity predisposes to the development of decompression sickness.[66]

With the acute decompression seen in rapid ascent of a scuba diver who fails to exhale, mediastinal interstitial emphysema, subcutaneous emphysema, pneumothorax, and *arterial* air embolism may follow rupture of distended pulmonary alveoli from expanding intrapulmonary air. The air embolism is the most serious consequence because of the possibility of cerebrovascular involvement with the production of such phenomena as hemiplegia, confusion, blindness, unconsciousness, and death.[30] Inasmuch as the incident occurs in an aquatic environment, the victim may drown. It is of interest that this series of catastrophic events can occur during rapid ascent in water from a depth of only 10 feet.

Rapid descent in an aircraft or rapid ascent during a scuba dive can lead to sinus barotrauma, so-called *aerosinusitis* and *aero–otitis media* with rupture of the tympanum. As the air in the intracranial spaces expands during ascent (1 volume of air at sea level becomes 2 volumes at 18,000 feet and 4 volumes at 33,000 feet), it passes easily through the natural ostia of the sinuses to equilibrate with the ambient barometic pressure. During *descent*, air must enter the sinuses through the ostia to equalize the intrasinus pressure with the *increasing* atmospheric tension. When sinus ostia and nasal mucosa are normal, the air exchange occurs efficiently and promptly. (Similar dynamic changes occur in all the hollow body structures that communicate with the exterior.)

However, if a sinus ostium is obstructed by tenacious mucus (a "mucus plug"), edematous mucosa, or a bony structural deformity, the defect may act as a cork during descent, effectively occluding the orifice, which is now under negative pressure. The negative pressure in the sealed-off sinus cavity is resolved by the sinus's filling with fluid transudate or blood. Indeed, if the pressure changes are especially rapid or severe, the mucous membrane may be stripped from the sinus wall with formation of a hematoma. The frontal sinus is most vulnerable to barotrauma because of the long, narrow bony nasofrontal defect with its dependent position on the floor of the sinus and the lack of accessory ostia.[65]

Although most cases of sinus barotrauma occur with compression (rapid descent in an aircraft or in diving), a considerable pressure disequilibrium can occur during *ascent* if the same type of interference exists with the passage of air *out* of the sinus.[24]

Explosions

The term *blast injury* designates the disruptive effects of the sudden changes in pressure that result from an explosion. If the force of the explosion is transmitted through the air, the term *air blast* is employed; if through water, *immersion blast*, and if through more or less rigid structures, *solid blast*.[11]

The shock wave of an air blast is a sound wave of very high pressure that emanates radially from an explosive source at the speed of sound. The air pressure is highest in the region of the explosion and falls rapidly, almost exponentially, as the distance from the blast increases. The amount of injury inflicted depends on the peak pressure and to a lesser degree on the duration of the shock wave.[45] In the case of an air blast the compression tends to be unilateral, and its principal effect is on the side of the body that faces the explosion. Here, much of the energy is reflected, but at least part is transmitted through the tissues and strikes the subjacent organs during the succeeding millisecond or less. Solid organs are virtually incompressible and consequently undergo little or no internal displacement. They vibrate as a whole and so escape serious injury. However, organs that contain air or gas respond differently because they *are* compressible and contain gas-liquid interfaces. Compression generates displacement, and whenever tissues of different density exist side by side, the amount of displacement varies from point to point, causing distension and tearing. An air blast also gives rise to surface phenomena such as epithelial shredding. Lesions tend to be most severe at tissue junctions. When loose, poorly supported tissues attached to dense unyielding tissues are displaced beyond their elastic limits, they are lacerated or otherwise damaged. Differences in fixation, cohesion, compressibility, and inertia on the part of the various components of the body result in nonuniform response to the displacing force and in widespread disruptive change. Thus the walls or compartments of hollow viscera are particularly susceptible to blast injury.

The lungs are especially vulnerable to blast injury. Alveolar septa are torn, permitting neighboring alveoli to coalesce, with ensuing emphysema. Alveolar parenchyma shears away from vascular structures, and alveolar epithelium is shredded. At the same time, bronchiolar epithelium is stripped from its basement membrane. These lesions lead to destruction of the fluid-air barrier. Blood and edema fluid escape into the alveoli, and air is forced into pulmonary vessels as a result of the for-mation of alveolar-venous fistulas. Cerebral air embolism attributable to the aspiration of air by disrupted pulmonary veins may be an important component of such an injury. Visible damage ranges from petechiae to massive hemorrhages and extensive areas of hemorrhagic edema. The hemorrhages tend to be more severe in the pulmonary parenchyma underlying the intercostal spaces, with the lung tissue beneath the protecting ribs being comparatively only slightly damaged. At autopsy, the pleural surfaces show alternating light and dark bands, the former corresponding to the ribs ("rib markings") and the latter to the intercostal spaces. Diffuse injuries of both the thoracic and the abdominal viscera may occur and may be sustained with little or no external evidence of trauma. Hemorrhage may occur in the gastric wall and elsewhere. The greater the degree of distension of the viscus when the shock waves strike, the more severe the injury.[14]

Since a blast wave is a sound wave of high intensity, it is obvious that the ear, built specifically for the reception of sound, is likely to be damaged by explosions. The pressure pulse approaching the human ear is concentrated as it passes down the external auditory canal so that the pressure on the tympanic membrane is approximately 20% higher than that just outside the ear. Injuries to the ears range from hyperemia and punctate bruising of the intact tympanic membrane to laceration of the membrane and damage to the cochlea. Membrane laceration usually occurs when the pressure rises to 15 psi and typically is associated with bleeding into the middle ear.[23]

In the case of an immersion blast, a shock wave is propagated at approximately the speed of sound in water (1450 m/second). Since water is much less compressible than air, corresponding pressures are much higher in a water shock wave than in those produced in air. Injury can occur from the shock wave or from the subsidiary pulse when the shock wave is reflected, for example, from the surface or from the bottom. The sequel of the pressure pulse injury is hemorrhage and laceration of air-containing organs. Lung damage of the type already described under air blast is a constant feature in deaths. Small perforations of the gut, especially of the cecum, may occur, and there may be subperitoneal contusions.[45]

In the case of solid blast, the disruptive force of the explosion is transmitted to the body through those parts that are in contact with an agitated rigid structure, such as the deck of a ship or the wall of an air raid shelter. Most solid blast injuries involve fractures of the lower extremities with considerable soft-tissue damage.[6]

One should bear in mind that proximity to either air or immersion blast may result in virtual destruction of the body by the extreme air or water turbulence induced by the blast. Flying missiles may add an infinite variety of wounds to those induced by turbulence and compression. These lesions are called *secondary blast* injuries; they result from missiles energized by blast pressure and winds and are distinguished from the *primary blast* injuries caused by the blast per se. In civilian explosions, including terrorist bombings, most deaths are caused by injuries from high-velocity fragments and falling debris (secondary blast injuries).[37]

Blast injuries sustained incident to atomic bomb explosion may be complicated by exposure to excessive heat and ionizing radiation. The cutaneous burns incurred in this manner are often unique by reason of the extremely high intensity and short duration of the hyperthermic episode. The injurious effects of ionizing radiation frequently require weeks to years for the development of signs and symptoms (p. 265).

INJURIES CAUSED BY SOUND WAVES
Noise

Permanent hearing loss resulting from excessive exposure to noise has long been recognized as an occupational hazard in industry. Such hearing defects develop with chronic exposure when the "work noise" exceeds the critical level of 80 to 90 decibels (dB).[53] It is less well known that many noise levels encountered in the community exceed standards found injurious in industry. For example, animals exposed to live rock music for 2½ hours in a discotheque had loss of sensory cells in the organ of Corti. The average sound pressure level measured in the discotheque was 107 dB.[7]

Chemical and structural changes in the spiral ganglion and hair cells have been demonstrated during exposure to sound, and exposure to sound levels of the degree produced by home food blenders causes noticeable changes in the hair cells, which characteristically show cytoplasmic vacuolization and swelling with compression of their nuclei and changes in their shape.[16]

In human autopsy studies no clear histologic picture has been identified in which morbid anatomic changes can be correlated with clinical hearing loss. Postmortem changes in the organ of Corti are the rule and complicate attempts to find such relationships.

Studies of persons subjected to high noise levels have revealed that long-term exposure to acoustic insult first affects hearing in the range between 3000 and 6000 hertz (Hz, cycles per second), whereas hearing for frequencies below 3000 Hz and above 8000 Hz remains essentially normal for long periods of time. High-frequency receptors deteriorate with age, and the burden of extra noise increases the wear.[49]

Ultrasound

Ultrasonic vibrations are those above limits of hearing of the human ear. Although ultrasound can be generated at frequencies exceeding 1000 megahertz (MHz),

in current medical practice the useful range is generally from 900 kilohertz (kHz) to 6 MHz. The medical literature has been almost unanimous in suggesting that there is little or no danger associated with diagnostic or therapeutic exposure of current levels.[5] Reports that diagnostic levels of ultrasound produced chromosomal damage in vitro and retarded rapidly growing tissue have not been confirmed in human cells.[33,36]

High-frequency ultrasound producing intensities many times that used in diagnostic or therapeutic procedures may cause biologic changes by increasing tissue temperature or producing tissue microcavitation. Wittenzellner[69] carried out self-experiments by irradiating both thighs in the frequency range of 20 to 800 kHz. Postirradiation changes in the skin receiving 800 kHz for 25 minutes included an acute inflammatory infiltrate and intraepidermal vesicles. Twenty-five years later the irradiated skin showed no significant signs.

Recently, shock waves have been employed as a treatment for renal calculus disease. These generated shock waves differ from ultrasound in having a positive-pressure front of multiple frequencies with a steep onset rather than a sinusoid waveform.[10] Although theoretically designed to be propagated through the body without energy loss or damage to body tissue, morphologic and functional renal changes attributed to kidney contusion resulting in edema and extravasation of urine and blood into the interstitial, subcapsular, and perirenal spaces have been described.[26]

INJURIES FROM HEAT AND COLD

Despite humans' ability to survive wide variations in environmental temperature, internal temperature must be maintained within a narrow range to avoid thermal injury. Cellular injury or death occurs if tissue temperature is maintained at a level more than 5° C above or more than 15° C below that which is normal for the blood. The severity of injury caused at any given temperature tends to be proportional to the duration of the hypothermal or hyperthermal episode. The somatic function of circulation is more susceptible to irreversible disturbance by dysthermia than are the individual cells of the body, and hence somatic death may result from a systemic alteration in temperature that would not cause cellular death if it were localized.

The skin is the principal site of heat loss during exposure to a cold environment or of heat gain during exposure to a hot environment. The respiratory membranes are rarely injured by heat or cold—and then only when the alteration of air temperature is so extreme that the skin is burned or frozen.[40,41]

Local hypothermia

Chilling of tissue retards the metabolic activity of the cells and may cause irreversible cellular change attributable to intracellular ice formation. This is not to imply, however, that hypothermal injury is dependent on the occurrence of congelation. The most important injurious effects of chilling are alterations in the walls and contents of the small blood vessels. A brief period of severe tissue hypothermia or a protracted period of mild tissue hypothermia may injure capillary endothelium sufficiently to cause transudation of fluid and edema. Superficially, such edema may lead to extensive vesication. The threshold for edema formation incident to chilling varies greatly among individuals.

If chilling is rapid and severe, the tissue may be rendered ischemic so quickly that evidence of vascular injury does not become apparent until the temperature rises and circulation is reestablished. Intense hyperemia is usually the immediate response to restitution of circulation after hypothermia. The hyperemia is followed by edema as soon as sufficient time has elapsed for plasma to diffuse through the cells of the injured vessels.

During a protracted episode of nonfreezing hypothermia such as that causing immersion or trench foot or after a brief episode of freezing hypothermia such as that causing frostbite, the local vascular injury may be so severe that the capillaries and even the larger vessels become plugged by tightly packed masses of erythrocytes. The nature and severity of the subsequent changes are determined by the extent and permanence of the ensuing ischemia. If the vascular occlusion is extensive, complete infarction in the form of moist or dry gangrene takes place. If the necrotic tissue becomes moist and dark colored, one can infer that infarction was preceded or accompanied by some degree of vascular patency. If the necrotis tissue becomes dry and mummified, one can infer that vascular occlusion was complete from the beginning.

Most if not all of the residual injury from protracted nonfreezing hypothermia can be attributed to the ischemia that results from the vascular occlusion. Atrophic and degenerative changes are seen in the epidermis, sweat glands, nerves, subcutaneous fat, and skeletal muscle, with proliferation of fibrous connective tissue in all situations.

Systemic hypothermia

If the area exposed to cold is relatively small, a severe local injury may be sustained without significant lowering of the blood temperature. If the area of exposure is large, the body temperature may be lowered sufficiently to cause death from circulatory failure even though no local injury has been sustained. Circulation fails when the temperature of the blood is reduced to approximately 20° C. Immersion in cold water or exposure to a rapidly moving current of cold air may lower the body temperature to a fatal level in a remarkably short time. However, prolonged exposure to cool temperatures may also result in hypothermia, particu-

larly in susceptible elderly persons with impaired homeostatic reactions or with chronic disease. The full extent of the problem of hypothermia in the elderly is not recognized because of the limited awareness of the hazard of mildly cold temperatures to the elderly and the focus on the medical complications of the hospitalized victim of the exposure.[42] There are no histologic or anatomic changes that can be regarded as pathognomonic of death from systemic hypothermia. However, autopsy examinations of some persons who have died after accidental hypothermia have demonstrated widespread thromboses and visceral infarction along with acute, necrotizing pancreatitis (Fig. 3-24).

Circulatory stasis and ischemia are probably responsible for the vascular phenomena and for the acute pancreatitis that has been observed in experimental and clinical situations. In accidental hypothermia the pancreatitis usually occurs when exposure to cold is prolonged, with coma preceding death.[46,50]

Local hyperthermia

Humans are far more susceptible to injury from an increase in tissue temperature than from a corresponding decrease.

Cutaneous burns

An elevation of tissue temperature by even a few degrees above that which is normal for the blood may be injurious. At any given temperature the nature and extent of the resulting injury are determined by the duration of the hyperthermal episode. During episodes of low intensity (40° to 45° C), injury is the result of accelerated metabolism of the hyperthermal tissue, and ordinarily many hours are required before irreversible changes have occurred. The higher the temperature, the shorter is the time required to cause cell death.[38,39] Transepidermal necrosis occurs if the epidermal temperature is brought to and maintained at 70° C or higher for a second or less, whereas transepidermal temperature elevation to 50° C for periods as long as 10 minutes may or may not destroy the epidermis.

The earliest evidence of hyperthermal injury is functional rather than structural. Capillaries and small blood vessels become dilated as the tissue temperature is raised, the permeability of the capillary walls is increased, and the fluid components of the blood leave the vessel and enter the interstitial spaces, with resulting edema. When thermal edema occurs in the superficial portion of the skin, the fluid may collect beneath the epidermis, with resulting vesiculation.

The earliest cytologic evidence of hyperthermal injury is a redistribution of the fluid and solid components of the nuclei, followed by nuclear swelling attributable to the imbibition of fluid, rupture of the nuclear membranes, and finally pyknosis. Since the rise in tissue temperature incident to exposure of the sur-

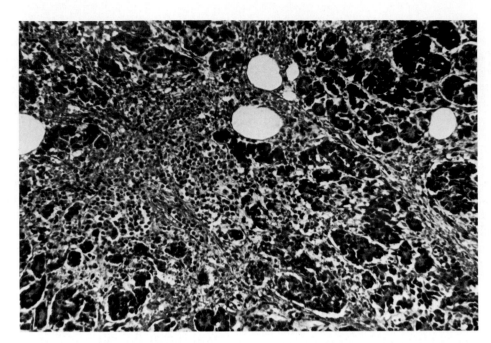

Fig. 3-24. Pancreas from 85-year-old man who died approximately 24 hours after being found in a snowbank and who suffered from exposure. Parenchyma is abundantly infiltrated with acute inflammatory cells. (150×.)

face of the skin to excessive heat is greatest at the surface and becomes progressively less as the distance from the surface is increased, it is apparent that any given burn will include a wide range of thermal effects. The cytoplasm of thermally injured cells becomes at first granular and later homogeneously coagulated. The collagen tends to lose its fibrillar character and to take on the appearance of a more or less homogeneous gel. The pH of the thermally denatured cells falls, as indicated by their increased affinity for basic stains.

Cutaneous burns may be designated as either first, second, or third degree or now more commonly as partial thickness or full thickness. Partial-thickness burns result in no permanent damage to the dermis and include both first- and second-degree burns from the older classification (Figs. 3-25 and 3-26). If vesication occurs with partial-thickness burns, regeneration of epithelium is generally rapid and is derived in part from the margin of the burned area and in part from the underlying hair follicles. Full-thickness burns are those in which there has been sufficient damage to the dermis to interfere with epithelial regeneration.

The irreversibly injured dermis must be disposed of before a new layer of epithelium can be regenerated. The organization and repair of the damaged dermis are accomplished by growth of new fibrous connective tissue and often result in extensive scar formation.

The flash burn resulting from exposure to the tremendous caloric flux of the first 0.6 second of the fire-

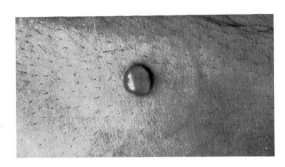

Fig. 3-25. Experimentally produced partial-thickness (second-degree) burn of human skin caused by maintaining surface temperature at 45° C for 3 hours. There is transepidermal necrosis with vesication. Irreversible dermal injury was minimal, and epidermal regeneration was complete in 10 days.

ball of the atomic bomb explosion differs from the ordinary relatively low temperature burn in several respects.[34,44] Despite carbonization of the epidermis and subjacent dermis, the zone of injury may be shallow and sharply demarcated.

Vascular reaction with hyperemia and edema is inevitable if the tissue hyperthermia has been sufficient to be injurious, and this reaction frequently occurs before the duration or the intensity of the exposure has been great enough to cause other perceptible evidence of injury.

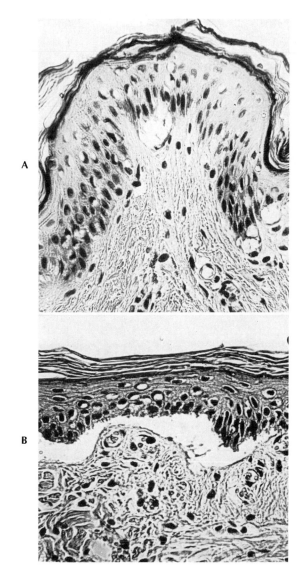

Fig. 3-26. Partial-thickness cutaneous burns. **A,** Mild burn (first degree). Although epidermis is damaged, it is not completely destroyed. Many nuclei are swollen and show eccentric displacement of chromatin. Minute vesicles have formed at junction of dermis and epidermis. **B,** More severe burn (second degree). Vesication is complete. Entire thickness of epidermis is necrotic and detached from relatively uninjured dermis. (400×.).

In the case of exposure to intense heat, the superficial vessels may become so rapidly fixed in a state of contraction that neither edema nor hyperemia is visible from the surface. In such an event, the reactive vascular changes will occur at a lower level but with no less severity. One of the most important systemic effects of extensive cutaneous burning is secondary shock brought on by hemoconcentration from loss of plasma at the site of injury.

Thermally denatured tissue elicits an aseptic inflammatory reaction, represents a foreign body, and must undergo lysis and organization or be sloughed off as a sequestrum. Before organization or sequestration, it provides a favorable medium for bacterial growth and predisposes the adjacent tissue to infection.

The use of topical antibacterial agents in current burn therapy show bacterial growth and usually prevent infection by the common bacteria that colonize burn wounds. However, the later appearance of resistant microorganisms, bacterial, fungal, and viral, often causes invasive infection and systemic sepsis, which combined remain the leading immediate cause of death among hospitalized burn patients.[35]

Systemic disturbances caused by cutaneous burns. Burning of the surface of the body may result in a wide variety of secondary disturbances. Such an injury may precipitate the development of primary or neurogenic shock with rapid peripheral circulatory collapse leading to syncope or death. The progressive loss of plasma from the burned surface or into the damaged tissue beneath it may result in hemoconcentration and secondary shock.

Patients with third-degree burns experience an average water loss of 0.35 ml/cm^2 of burned area per day during the first week.[13] It is a reasonable inference that the hemoconcentration, low blood pressure, and systemic anoxia of secondary shock predispose not only to phlebothrombosis, particularly in immobilized limbs, but also to the occurrence of the degenerative changes so commonly observed in the kidneys, liver, and adrenal glands of burned persons.

Although the precise cause of the ulcers that sometimes develop in the proximal portion of the small intestine of severely burned persons is not known, local mesenteric thrombosis and mucosal infarction would appear to constitute a plausible explanation.

Erythrocytes break down rapidly in vitro at temperatures over 50° C and in vivo at temperatures over 42.5° C, and intravascular hemolysis usually takes place if the hyperthermal episode has been of sufficient intensity or duration to destroy the epidermis. Free plasma hemoglobin is excreted rapidly by the kidneys, where it may be precipitated in the lower segments of the nephrons to form obstructive casts similar to those formed as a result of a mismatched transfusion.

The combined effects of these pigmented casts and the irreversible tubular damage caused by prolonged shock result in the renal failure so often associated with severe burns.

Since most cutaneous burns are associated with fire, the possibility of inhalation injury must be considered in most burn victims. Many homes and other buildings are built and furnished with synthetic materials that give off copious smoke and toxic gases when burned. In addition to carbon monoxide, victims of cutaneous burns may be exposed to such toxic gases as cyanide, hydrogen chloride, and acrolein. Upper airway occlusion may result from thermal damage or edema secondary to burns from soluble toxic gases. Lower airway obstruction may occur as the result of sloughing of mucosa, bronchospasm, or peribronchial edema. At the alveolar level, inactivation of surfactant with subsequent atelectasis and an increase in pulmonary capillary permeability further impair ventilation-perfusion abilities.[12,68]

Systemic hyperthermia

The temperature of the body may be raised to an injurious level either by the inflow of heat from without or by the body's failure to eliminate the heat developed by metabolic processes. A general rise in the temperature of the circulating blood to a level higher than 42.5° C leads to profound functional disturbances, including the following:

1. Generalized vasodilatation with resulting reduction in effective blood volume as a consequence of the disparity between the newly expanded capacity of the circulatory apparatus and the unchanged quantity of the fluid (blood) available to fill it
2. Rapid pulse and dilatation of the heart with impairment of cardiac efficiency
3. Stimulation of the respiratory centers, manifested first by tachypnea, later by irregularity, and finally by suspension of respiratory activity

It is difficult to determine which of these several physiologic effects of systemic hyperthermia may contribute most to somatic deterioration and death. It is of interest in this connection that a heart-lung preparation fails when the temperature of the perfusate reaches approximately 42.5° C.

Heatstroke is the result of uncontrolled overproduction of body heat or impairment of the body's ability to lose heat; it occurs most frequently in susceptible persons exposed to unusually hot conditions. Heat is dissipated principally by evaporative cooling through sweating and by cutaneous vasodilatation with increased cardiac output. The more labile thermoregulatory mechanism of small children and, particularly, the elderly renders them vulnerable to heatstroke; heatstroke rates are 10 to 12 times higher in persons older than 65 years than in younger adults. Other factors that predispose persons to heatstroke include alcoholism, any skin disease or injury that impairs or prevents sweating, cardiovascular disease, general debility, coexistence of a febrile disorder, dehydration, obesity, anticholinergic drugs, and some medications that are used to treat psychiatric disorders (such as chlorpromazine, fluphenazine, promazine, and haloperidol). Environmental risk factors include hot temperature, high humidity, and the entire complex of living conditions in poorly insulated urban housing, especially the multistory buildings of slums.[25]

Heatstroke also can occur in healthy persons who exert themselves with such intensity that the heat produced by skeletal muscles cannot be dissipated quickly enough to cool the body. This exertional heatstroke occurs in unacclimated athletes, such as football players during spring training, or in military recruits who undergo basic training in summer. Athletes wearing heavy equipment or impervious plastic sweatsuits increase their risk. Autopsy findings in heatstroke deaths are nonspecific and are governed by the survival interval, treatment, and previous condition of the victim.

Delayed systemic disturbances from systemic hyperthermia include widely distributed degenerative changes in the parenchymatous viscera and particularly in the brain.[4]

ELECTRICAL INJURY

Electrical injury does not occur unless some part of the body completes the circuit betwen two conductors. An electrician supported by an insulated boom may safely handle a high-tension conductor because he is isolated from the ground.

The path of a current through the body tends to follow the most direct route between the contact points. The current may cause injury or death by altering the function of a vital organ (for example, throwing the heart into ventricular fibrillation or paralyzing the respiratory center), by stimulating strong (and occasionally tetanic) muscular contractions, or by creating large quantities of heat (electrothermal effect).

When conditions (contacts) are appropriate for the flow of current through the body (or tissues), the occurrence and nature of the harmful effects created by its passage depend on the following:

1. The kind of current (direct or alternating)
2. The amount of current (amperage)
3. The electromotive force (voltage)
4. The amount of resistance offered by the tissues in the path of the current
5. The actual path of the current between the sites of contact
6. The duration of current flow
7. The surface area of contact

An alternating current is more effective in the production of physiologic disturbances than a direct current is, and some alternating frequencies are more disturbing than others. The 60-cycle alternating current commonly available for domestic and industrial use lies in the frequency range that is particularly disturbing to the respiratory centers of the brain and to the heart where it can induce fibrillation by interacting with the vulnerable phase of the cardiac cycle. Increasing the duration of current flow increases the risk of disrupting the vulnerable phase. One of the major dangers of alternating current is its tetanizing effect, so that a person becomes "locked" to the contact until the circuit is broken. Since the amount of current necessary to cause tetany may be less than that necessary to cause fibrillation, he may succumb to a current that would otherwise not be lethal.

The amount of current that will flow through the body when it becomes part of a circuit is determined by the formula $C = V/R$, in which C is the current in amperes, V is potential in volts, and R is the resistance in ohms with which the body opposes the flow of the current. Thus the higher the voltage or the lower the resistance, the greater the flow of current. The usual currents available for domestic use have a fixed potential of either 110 volts or 220 volts. Therefore the resistance R is the major variable in determining the flow of current in an electrical accident in the home. The resistance of the human body may be reduced to less than 40 ohms under particularly favorable conditions (large areas of electrode contact against a moist skin surface). Since a 60-cycle alternating current as small as 100 milliamperes, applied at the body surface and passing through the trunk, can be sufficient to cause ventricular fibrillation, household currents with a potential of 110 volts greatly exceed the threshold for fatal electrocution.

Currents applied to the body surface tend to disperse over multiple pathways as they pass through the trunk. Therefore the amount of current passing through the heart will be considerably less than the amount of current on the surface of the body. The result is that currents far lower than 100 milliamperes, currents in the microampere range, can cause fibrillation if directly applied at the heart. Persons susceptible to such "microshocks" are those with indwelling catheters, particularly cardiac catheters hooked to monitors where there is a potential of leakage of current along the catheter.[28,31]

That the path taken by the current is of critical importance in determining whether a fatal shock will occur is indicated by the fact that, in electroshock therapy, transcranial current flow as great as 1 ampere may be survived without injury.

In general, the severity of the disturbance caused by the flow of a given amount of current between similar external contacts is proportional to the duration of flow. Certainly the generation of heat bears a linear relationship to time. Physiologic disturbances that are evanescent after a momentary shock may be rendered irreversible by a longer period of electrical exposure.

Electrical burns

The amount and place of heat formation incident to the flow of a given amount of electricity through the body are determined by the resistance that the tissue offers to the current. Most of the resistance offered by the human body to an electrical current is that of the skin and the interface between skin and external conductor. Thus electrothermal burns are ordinarily limited to the skin and the immediately subjacent tissue.

Thin skin is less resistant to the flow of electricity than thick skin is, and moist skin offers less resistance than dry skin does. Heavily callused dry skin may provide a resistance-protection of several hundred thousand ohms. Because of this fact, persons with callused hands often handle with impunity live wires that would be exceedingly dangerous if brought into contact with a less-resistant portion of the body surface.

If the contact between the skin and an external conductor is large, the generation of heat in terms of calories per square centimeter of surface per second may be too low to produce a burn, and yet the amperage may be more than enough to paralyze respiration or circulation. On the other hand, if the skin contact is a small one such as may occur by touching the end of a live wire, the amount of heat generated in a few cubic millimeters of epidermis may be sufficient to produce a burn even though the total amperage has been insufficient to cause a significant degree of physiologic disturbance. The significance of the surface area of contact is best exemplified by what is observed in low-voltage incidents. A child sucking on a live cord may sustain deep labial burns without suffering systemic effects because contact is limited to the mouth, whereas a person lying in a bathtub who touches an ungrounded electrical element of identical voltage may well be killed immediately without the production of any localized injuries.

In a study of 108 electrocutions by low voltage (less than 1000 volts), electrical burns were absent in over 40% of the cases.[70] In the absence of electrical burns the determination of a fatal electrical shock may depend on the circumstances of the death and an "autopsy" of the electrical source.

Typical low-voltage cutaneous electrical burns are small, circumscribed, indurated lesions that have a central, depressed, gray or black focus of charring surrounded by a zone of grayish white discoloration (Fig. 3-27). The latter change represents coagulation necrosis of the skin and often is surrounded by a narrow areola of erythema. Microscopically there is an abrupt transition from normal to burned skin. The burn commonly shows microvesicles in the epidermis, separation of the lower epidermis, and transcutaneous coagulation extending into the dermis. Epidermal nuclei are pyknotic, elongated, and aligned in a parallel or palisading fashion, often referred to as "nuclear streaming" (Fig. 3-28). High-voltage burns usually have large areas of contact and generate sufficient heat to produce extensive, deep charring that may amputate extremities (Fig. 3-29). Ignition of clothing is a frequent concomitant of contact with high-voltage electrical current and results in the superimposition of ordinary burning on electrical injury.

Arcing of the current may produce pitlike defects on

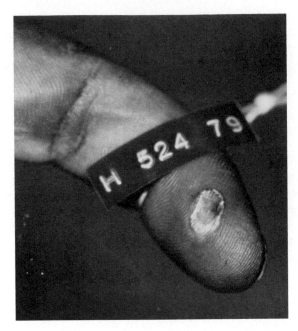

Fig. 3-27. Typical low-voltage electrical burn of index finger.

the surface of hair or epidermis that are rarely, if ever, produced by other forms of heat. Metallic constituents of the external conductor may be deposited in or on the surface of an electrical burn, and their presence may help to establish the kind of electrode with which the skin was in contact. In the case of alternating current, such metallic deposits may be present at both sites of contact. With direct current the deposits will occur only at the site of contact with the negative electrode.

In persons who survive high-voltage electrical injury, the size of the primary burn does not change, but a surrounding zone of secondary ischemic necrosis may enlarge progressively in the days or weeks after the incident. Such ischemic progression results primarily from thrombosis of arterioles and arteries whose intima was damaged when they served as conduits for the transmission of electricity. These arterial sequelae may necessitate repeated débridement or amputations before the circulatory state is stabilized.

Electrothermal injuries should not be confused with the burns caused by contact with an object that has been rendered hot by a short circuit. If a short circuit

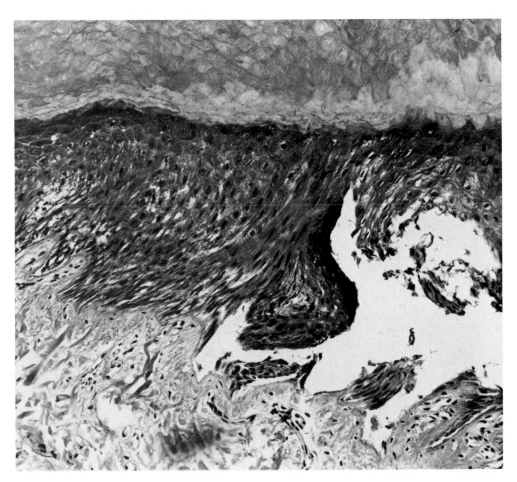

Fig. 3-28. Low-voltage electrical burn of hand. Epidermal separation *(right)* and nuclear streaming *(left)*.

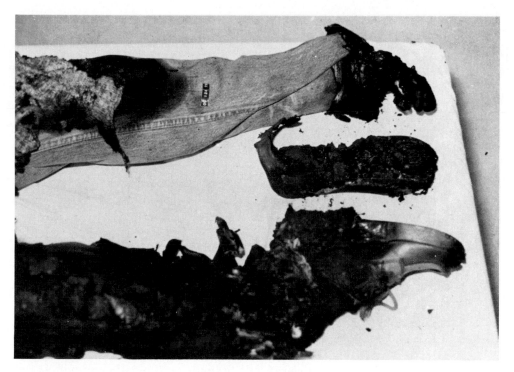

Fig. 3-29. High-voltage electrical burns of lower extremities in young woman who came into contact with downed 13,000-volt power line. There is extensive charring, with partial amputation of left foot and heat fractures of right tibia and fibula. Shoes and clothing were ignited, with superimposed thermal trauma.

occurs through a metallic conductor, the flow of current through it may be so great that even with a potential of 110 volts its temperature is raised almost immediately to the melting point. Contact with such a superheated conductor will cause severe and instantaneous burning even though no electricity flows through the skin. When a current of 110 volts flows through the skin, the resistance is ordinarily so great that there is insufficient amperage for rapid elaboration of heat. Rarely does a current of 110 volts produce a large electrothermal injury of the skin unless the contact is maintained for a considerable period of time.

Apart from injuries caused by heat production and the explosive effects of currents of extremely high voltage, there are no tissue changes that can be regarded as consistently pathognomonic of electricity. Attention has already been directed to the facts that an electrical current flowing through the brainstem may cause death by inhibition of the respiratory centers and that electricity flowing through the heart may cause death by central circulatory failure. Victims of fatal accidental electrocution resulting from a transthoracic current pathway have spoken rationally and continued breathing up to 15 seconds after contact with the electrical circuit was broken. This is typical of ventricular fibrillation or asystole from any cause such as coronary arteriosclerosis. During this interval, they complained of such symptoms as "tightness" in the chest, difficulty in breathing, a sensation of "strangulation," and a feeling of the heart pounding fiercely against the chest wall.[63]

Whether death results from ventricular fibrillation or from respiratory paralysis is immaterial from the standpoint of the production of characteristic gross or microscopic alterations in the viscera. In neither instance are there internal organic lesions that indicate the cause or mechanism of death. In both circumstances, somatic death is likely to be preceded by a brief period of intense systemic anoxemia, which may lead to the occurrence of petechiae in the serous membranes and central nervous system.

Myoglobinuria of the type that occurs after muscle injury from crushing force or excessive exercise is occasionally encountered in survivors of electric shock. It is a consequence of tissue damage caused by heat generation and coagulation necrosis, both of which are functions of current intensity (amperage), duration and pathway of current flow, tissue resistance, and grounding of the victim.

The myoglobinuria is usually associated with renal tubular necrosis with resulting oliguria or even anuria. The extremely high voltage and amperage characteristics of lightening (see the following) render the survivor of a lightning stroke a likely candidate for this life-threatening, posttraumatic sequel.[71]

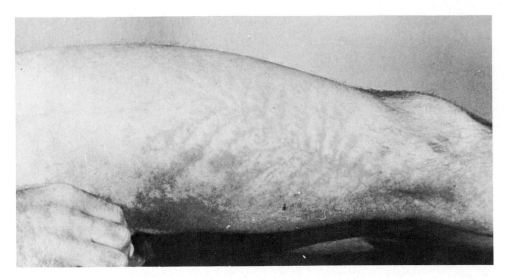

Fig. 3-30. Arborescent pattern of injury marking site of passage of lightning on surface of skin.

Lightning

When a bolt of lightning approaches the earth or a grounded conductor, it tends to break up into many paths of varying intensity. In such circumstances a person struck by lightning may become the conductor of a current so small that his injury is superficial and inconsequential or so large as to be fatal with or without extensive burning. In some instances the current produces an arborescent cutaneous hyperemia that resembles a fern (Fig. 3-30). That some of the electrical energy of a bolt of lightning has produced a superficial injury does not preclude the simultaneous passage of a fatal current through the body with severe burning at the sites of entrance, exit, or both.

In addition to skin burns of varying degrees of severity, victims of lightning may suffer fractures and ruptures of blood vessels and abdominal viscera. The enormous energy (as much as 10^9 volts) of a lightning bolt may cause injury by direct effect of the current or by the expanded (and returning) air resulting in blastlike injuries.[9] Current passing through the body may cause either ventricular fibrillation or respiratory paralysis. Instances of fetal electrocution with maternal survival have been reported in which the path of electrical current passed through the gravid uterus after a lightning strike.[20,64]

In addition to thermal injuries, persons surviving lightning strikes may develop diverse serious complications such as myoglobinuria, cardiac arrhythmias and infarction, peripheral nerve lesions, and tympanic membrane rupture.[3]

A broad variety of ocular injuries can develop in survivors of lightning strikes. These include cataracts, corneal ulcers (occasionally going on to perforation), irido-cyclitis, hyphema, and vitreous hemorrhage. In rare instances, choroidal ruptures, chorioretinitis, macular tears, retinal detachments, and even optic nerve injury have been recorded.[61]

REFERENCES

1. Adelson, L.: A microscopic study of dermal gunshot wounds, Am. J. Clin. Pathol. **35**:393, 1961.
2. Adelson, L., and Hirsch, C.S.: Sudden and unexpected death from natural causes in adults. In Spitz, W.U., and Fisher, R.S., editors: Medicolegal investigation of death, ed. 2, Springfield, Ill., 1980, Charles C Thomas, Publisher.
3. Amy, B.W., McManus, W.F., Goodwin, C.W., Jr., and Pruitt, B.A.: Lightning injury with survival in five patients, JAMA **253**:243, 1985.
4. Anderson, R.J., Reed, G., and Knochel, J.: Heatstroke, Adv. Int. Med. **28**:115, 1983.
5. Baker, M.L., and Dalrymple, G.V.: Biological effects of diagnostic ultrasound: a review, Radiology **126**:479, 1978.
6. Barr, J.S., Draeger, R.H., and Sager, W.W.: Solid blast personnel injury: a clinical study, Milit. Surg. **98**:1, 1946.
7. Bohne, B.A., Ward, P.H., and Fernandez, C.: Rock music and inner ear damage, Am. Fam. Physician **15**:117, 1979.
8. Bray, P., Myers, R.A.M., and Cowley, R.A.: Orogenital sex as a cause of nonfatal air embolism in pregnancy, Obstet. Gynecol. **61**:653, 1983.
9. Brown, K.L.: Electrical injuries, J. Trauma **4**:608, 1964.
10. Chaussey, C., Schüller, J., Schmiedt, E., Brandi, H., Jocham, D., and Liedl, B.: Extracorporeal shock-wave lithotripsy (ESWL) for treatment of urolithiasis, Urology **23**(special issue):59, 1984.
11. Cohen, J., and Biskind, G.R.: Pathologic aspects of atmospheric blast injuries in man, Arch. Pathol. **42**:12, 1946.
12. Cohen, M.A., and Guzzardi, L.J.: Inhalation of products of combustion, Ann. Intern Med. **12**:628, 1983.
13. Davies, J.W.L., Lamke, L.O., and Liljedahl, S.O.: A guide to the rate of non-renal water loss from patients with burns, Br. J. Plast. Surg. **27**:325, 1974.
14. Decandole, C.A.: Blast injury, Can. Med. Assoc. J. **96**:207, 1967.
15. Department of the Army: Wound ballistics, Washington, D.C., 1962, Superintendent of Documents.
16. Doughterty, J.D., and Welsh, O.L.: Community noise and hearing loss, N. Engl. Med. J. **275**:759, 1966.

17. Fackler, M.L.: Wound ballistics, a review of common misconceptions, JAMA **259**:2730, 1988.
18. Fletcher, B.D., and Brogdon, B.G.: Seat-belt fractures of the spine and sternum, JAMA **200**:167, 1967.
19. Fryer, D.I.: Pathological findings in fatal sub-atmospheric decompression sickness, Med. Sci. Law **2**:110, 1962.
20. Guha-Ray, D.K.: Fetal death at term due to lightning, Am. J. Obstet. Gynecol. **134**:103, 1979.
21. Health, D., and Williams, D.R.: Man at high altitude, Edinburgh, 1977, Churchill Livingstone.
22. Heath, D., and Williams, D.R.: The lung at high altitude, Invest. Cell Pathol. **2**:147, 1979.
23. Hill, J.F.: Blast injury with particular reference to recent terrorist bombing incidents, Ann. R. Coll. Surg. Engl. **61**:4, 1979.
24. Idicula, J.: Perplexing case of maxillary sinus barotrauma, Aerospace Med. **43**:891, 1972.
25. Jones, T.S., Liang, A.P., Kilbourne, E.M., Griffin, M.R., Patriarca, P.A., Wassilak, S.C., Mullan, R.J., Herrick, R.F., Donnell, H.D., Jr., Choi, K, and Thacker, S.B.: Morbidity and mortality associated with the July 1980 heat wave in St. Louis and Kansas City, Mo., JAMA **247**:3327, 1982.
26. Kaude, J.V., Williams, C.M., Millner, M.R., Scott, K.N., and Finlayson, B.: Renal morphology and function immediately after extracorporeal shock-wave lithotripsy, AJR **1450**:305, 1985.
27. King, M.W., Aitchison, J.M., and Nel, J.P.: Fatal air embolism following penetrating lung trauma: an autopsy study, J. Trauma **24**:753, 1984.
28. Leeming, M.N.: Protection of the electrically susceptible patient, Anesthesiology **38**:370, 1973.
29. Lehman, E.P., and Moore, R.M.: Fat embolism including experimental production without trauma, Arch. Surg. **14**:621, 1927.
30. Leitch, D.R., and Green, R.D.: Pulmonary barotrauma in divers and the treatment of cerebral arterial gas embolism, Aviat. Space Environ. Med. **57**:931, 1986.
31. Leonard, P.F.: Characteristics of electrical hazards, anesthesia and analgesia, Curr. Res. **51**:798, 1972.
32. LeQuire, V.S., Shapiro, J.L., Lequire, C.B., Cobb, C.A., Jr., and Fleet, W.F., Jr.: A study of the pathogenesis of fat embolism based on human necropsy material and animal experiments, Am. J. Pathol. **35**:999, 1959.
33. Liebeskind, D., Bases, R., Elequin, F., Neubort, S., Leifer, R., Goldberg, R., and Koenigsberg, M.: Diagnostic ultrasound: effects on the DNA and growth patterns of animal cells, Radiology **131**:177, 1979.
34. Leibow, A.A., Warren, S., and DeCoursey, E.: Pathology of atomic bomb casualties, Am. J. Pathol. **25**:853, 1949.
35. Luterman, A., Dacso, C.C., and Curreri, P.W.: Infections in burn patients, Am. J. Med. **81**(suppl. 1A):45, 1986.
36. Lyon, M.F., and Simpson, G.M.: An investigation into the possible genetic hazards of ultrasound, Br. J. Radiol. **47**:712, 1974.
37. Marshall, T.K.: Explosion injuries in forensic medicine. In Tedeschi, C.G., Eckert, W.G., and Tedeschi, L.G., editors: Forensic medicine, Philadelphia, 1977, W.B. Saunders Co.
38. Moritz, A.R.: Studies of thermal injury: pathology and pathogenesis of cutaneous burns: experimental study, Am. J. Pathol. **23**:915, 1947.
39. Moritz, A.R., and Henriques, F.C., Jr.: Studies of thermal injury: relative importance of time and surface temperature in causation of cutaneous burns, Am. J. Pathol. **23**:695, 1947.
40. Moritz, A.R., Henriques, F.C., Jr., and McLean, R.: Effects of inhaled heat on air passages and lungs, Am. J. Pathol. **21**:311, 1945.
41. Moritz, A.R., and Weisiger, J.R.: Effects of cold air on air passages and lungs: experimental investigation, Arch. Intern. Med. **75**:233, 1945.
42. Moss, J.: Accidental severe hypothermia, Surg. Gynecol. Obstet. **162**:501, 1986.
43. Neuman, T.S., Spragg, R.G., Wagner, P.D., and Moser, K.M.: Cardiopulmonary consequences of decompression stress, Respir. Physiol. **41**:143, 1980.
44. Pearse, H.E., and Kingsley, H.D.: Thermal burns from atomic bombs, Surg. Gynecol. Obstet. **98**:385, 1954.
45. Rawlins, J.S.P.: Physical and pathophysiological effects of blast, Injury **9**:313, 1978.
46. Read, A.E., Emslie-Smith, D., Gough, K.R., and Holmes, R.: Pancreatitis and accidental hypothermia, Lancet **2**:1219, 1961.
47. Roy, S.B., Guleria, J.S., Khanna, P.K., et al.: Haemodynamic studies in high altitude pulmonary oedema, Br. Heart J. **31**:52, 1969.
48. Ryan, G.A.: Injuries in traffic accidents, N. Engl. J. Med. **276**:1066, 1967.
49. Sataloff, J., Vassalo, J., and Menduke, H.: Occupational healing loss and high frequency thresholds, Arch. Environ. Health **14**:832, 1967.
50. Savides, E.P., and Huffband, B.I.: Hypothermia, thrombosis and acute pancreatitis, Br. Med. J. **1**:614, 1974.
51. Schnaid, E., Lamprey, J.M., Viljoen, M.J., Joffe, B.I., Seftel, H.C.: The early biochemical and hormonal profile of patients with long bone fractures at risk of fat embolism syndrome, J. Trauma **27**:309, 1987.
52. Schoene, R.B., Hackett, P.H., Henderson, W.R., Sage, E.H., Chow, M., Roach, R.C., Mills, W.J., Jr., and Martin, T.R.: High altitude pulmonary edema: characteristics of lung lavage fluid, JAMA **256**:63, 1986.
53. Schwetz, F.: The critical intensity for occupation noise, Acta Otolaryngol. **89**:358, 1980.
54. Scully, R.E.: Fat embolism in Korean battle casualties: its incidence, clinical significance and pathologic aspects, Am. J. Pathol. **32**:379, 1956.
55. Selye, H.: Stress and disease, Science **122**:625, 1955.
56. Sevitt, S.: Fat embolism, London, 1962, Butterworth & Co.
57. Spitz, W.U.: Essential postmortem findings in the traffic accident victim, Arch. Pathol. **90**:451, 1970.
58. Strauss, R.H., and Prockop, L.D.: Decompression sickness among scuba divers, JAMA **223**:637, 1973.
59. Strauss, R.H., and Yount, D.E.: Decompression sickness, Am. Sci. **65**:598, 1977.
60. Sube, J., Ziperman, H.H., and McIver, W.J.: Seat belt trauma to the abdomen, Am. J. Surg. **133**:346, 1967.
61. Taussig, H.B.: "Death" from lightning—and the possibility of living again, Ann. Intern. Med. **68**:1345, 1968.
62. Treiman, N., Waisbrod, V., and Waisbrod, H.: Lipoprotein electrophoresis in fat embolism, Injury **13**:108, 1981.
63. Walter, C.W.: Is death from accidental electric shock instantaneous? JAMA **221**:922, 1972.
64. Weinstein, L.: Lightning: a rare cause of intrauterine death with maternal survival, South. Med. J. **72**:103, 1979.
65. Weissman, B., Green, R.S., and Roberts, P.T.: Frontal sinus barotrauma, Laryngoscope **82**:2160, 1972.
66. Whitcraft, D.D., III, and Karas, S.: Air embolism and decompression sickness in scuba divers, JACEP **5**:355, 1976.
67. Williams, A.G., Mettler, F.A., Jr., Christie, J.H., and Gordon, R.E.: Fat embolism syndrome, Clin. Nucl. Med. **7**:497, 1986.
68. Witten, M.G., Quan, S.F., Sobonya, R.E., and Lemen, R.J.: New developments in the pathogenesis if smoke inhalation induced pulmonary edema, West. J. Med. **148**:33, 1988.
69. Wittenzellner, R.: Tissue damaging effects of ultrasound, Ultrasonics **14**:281, 1976.
70. Wright, R.K., and Davis, J.H.: The investigation of electrical deaths: a report of 220 fatalities, J. Forensic Sci. **25**:514, 1980.
71. Yost, J.W., and Olmes, F.F.: Myoglobinuria following lightning stroke, JAMA **228**:1147, 1974.
72. Zumwalt, R.E., and Hirsch, C.S.: Medicolegal interpretation of gunshot wounds, Am. J. Emerg. Med. **5**:133, 1987.

4 Drug and Chemical Injury— Environmental Pathology

GORDON R. HENNIGAR

DRUG INJURY AND IATROGENIC DISEASES
Adverse medicinal drug reactions

An adverse drug reaction (ADR) is defined as any response to a drug that is noxious and unintended and that occurs at dosage used in humans for prophylaxis, diagnosis, or therapy, excluding failure to accomplish the intended purpose.

Incidence

It is frequently stated that 5% of patients are admitted to the hospital as a result of drug reactions. One study suggested that, during their hospital stay, 20% of all patients had suffered from the complications of diagnostic or therapeutic procedures utilizing drugs. Adverse effects from drug therapy may account for 1 in 40 consultations in general practice. They are obviously important in terms of morbidity and may affect the physician-patient relationship and cause noncompliance in the future. One group is heard to cry, "Bad prescriptions kill thousands a year," and to assert that 30,000 Americans die as a direct result of the drugs their physicians prescribe. A second group holds an altogether different view and considers the seriousness of drug toxicity to be overemphasized; they are quick to point out that a drug-related fatality of 2.4:1000 patients admitted to the hospital medical services represents a small risk and that drugs, compared with many daily hazards to which we all are exposed, are in general remarkably benign. A third group considers the debate useless on the grounds that valid data on the prevalence and incidence of adverse drug reactions are unavailable.

Considering the number of prescription and over-the-counter preparations (approximately 1500 generic types) that are dispensed to the public, the number of toxic and allergic reactions is small. Physicians, and the public as well, should not be concerned about all adverse reactions but rather about the number of *unwarranted* adverse reactions. A patient who appears to be dying of advanced congestive failure and is not responding to conventional doses of digitalis may be given larger doses of this drug in a desperate attempt that is recognized as heroic. Signs of digitalis intoxication may supervene, and if the patient dies, he may well be classified as having a toxic drug reaction contributing to his death. But the use of additional digitalis in this instance was a well-considered and warranted intervention. The death may be classified for statistical purposes as drug related, but this statistic has no bearing on the quality of medical practice. This kind of warranted drug reaction is part of the risk any physician and patient must assume when treatment, whether medical or surgical, is instituted. The crucial parameter is the one that will indicate whether the quality of drug use is good or bad, and this will be governed by the number of unwarranted adverse reactions noted.

Consider the instance in which diarrhea develops in a patient receiving clindamycin. The pathologist interprets biopsy results as indicative of early ulcerative colitis when actually the patient has a clindamycin-associated lesion. A state of toxic megacolon develops and the patient dies. The cause of death is recorded as complications of *Clostridium difficile* toxic colitis associated with the administration of clindamycin. In this instance the compound is blamed for the death, though the clinician and pathologist using their gross and microscopic findings should not have rendered the diagnosis of ulcerative colitis in the first place. Ulcerative colitis is a diffuse disease, whereas antibiotic-associated colitis is focal, becoming diffuse only in fatal or nearly fatal incidences.

Causative components of adverse drug reactions

Drugs as toxins. The term *toxin* is frequently used loosely to encompass all injurious substances, whatever the means by which injury is induced. We use it here in a more restricted sense to refer to chemical agents producing a predictable, dose-related injury to cells and organs, thus excluding a large group of ADRs related to immunologic responses.

Although most toxic ADRs result from overdose or

prolonged high-dose therapy, in some instances an ADR may occur from normal dosage. This may be the result of (1) preexisting kidney or liver disease, with limited ability to excrete or detoxify the drug, producing high concentrations in tissues or circulation in the face of normal dosage; (2) interaction with other drugs, producing synergistic effects; or (3) quantitative alterations in pharmacokinetics, that is, absorption, distribution, and elimination.

Toxic reactions in cells and organs are predictable and dose related, occur within a specific time after administration of the drug, and can be consistently reproduced in animals. All these characteristics are also true of the desired pharmacologic effect; thus toxic ADRs may simply be a magnification of the pharmacologic effect or may include new, unrelated responses (Table 4-1).

The dose-responding curves for the two may overlap, as in the case of digoxin: a dose of digoxin sufficient to ensure fully therapeutic levels for 100% of patients will also cause troublesome vomiting. All drugs must be tested in animals before they are administered to man in clinical trials. Additional animal tests are subsequently required before a drug is approved for general use. Although species-specific toxicities are not unknown, these animal tests have been useful in defining the toxic potentials of drugs. In particular, attempts to assess the immunoallergic and oncogenic potential of drugs and chemicals in animals has been problematic.

Over the last two decades, a wide variety of studies in laboratory animals and man have made it abundantly clear that in many instances of chemically induced tissue injury the damage is caused by a metabolite of the chemical, rather than by the parent compound itself. Drugs and other environmental chemicals of toxicologic interest are generally highly lipophilic in nature and are not readily excreted by renal mechanisms. Clearance of lipophilic chemicals occurs by metabolic transformation to more water-soluble derivatives, which in turn are subject to renal or fecal elimination. The enzymes that are responsible for this metabolic clearance are located in the endoplasmic reticulum of the liver and other tissues and catalyze a wide variety of oxidation, reduction, and conjugative reactions.

On occasion, during the course of the metabolic transformation of a lipophilic chemical, there arise reaction intermediates that are chemically more reactive than the parent compound yet have sufficient stability to diffuse away from the active site of the enzyme that formed it. Such reactive metabolites may have several fates. Many of the reactive metabolites are electrophilic in nature and react spontaneously with cellular nucleophils. If the nucleophil is reduced glutathione or hydroxyl ion, the reactivity will be decreased and the potential for injury to the cell is usually lessened.

Table 4-1. Comparison of immunologic and "toxic" medicinal drug reactions

Immunologic	Toxic
Usually more than one exposure	Frequently only one exposure
Not necessarily dose related	Cellular severity of reaction related to amount of dose or cumulative dosage
Withdrawal of drug leads, in most cases, to prompt recovery	Permanent damage to cells and tissues depends on organ site and total amount of drug administered
Hypersensitivity or immunologic reactions variable and not target organ specific	Target organ specific

However, if the nucleophil is DNA or protein, the subsequent loss of structure and function of the cell macromolecule may result in severe toxicity such as the genesis of neoplasia (DNA as target) or cell death (vital protein as target). Other reactive metabolites are free radical in nature or have the capacity to generate free radicals on interaction with tissue molecular oxygen. Free radicals may attack the lipids of cellular membranes, resulting in the loss of fluidity of the membrane or inactivation of membrane enzymes responsible for maintaining ionic gradients across the membrane. Toxic oxygen species such as superoxide, hydroxyl radical, and singlet oxygen have also recently been implicated as possible causative agents in a variety of pathophysiologic states.

Appreciation of the central role played by reactive metabolites in tissue injury has allowed a rational explanation of several previously puzzling characteristics of ADRs, such as the pronounced differences observed in a patient's susceptibility, the target-tissue specificity of environmental chemicals, and the difficulty often experienced in reproducing in experimental animals the lesions seen in man, and vice versa. It is now well known that lipophilic compounds typically are simultaneously metabolized by several different detoxification enzymes such that the initial single chemical species is transformed into many metabolites. It is also well established that large interindividual differences occur between patients in the rates at which many of these pathways operate and that these rates are further influenced by factors such as age, sex, and pathophysiology, as well as by simultaneous or immediately prior exposure to other drugs and environmental chemicals. Since reactive metabolites may be formed in comparatively minor pathways, relatively small changes in the activity of the toxic pathway may lead to a large change in the amount of reactive metabolite formed and a correspondingly large tissue injury. Alternatively, an increase in the severity of the tissue lesion may occur if the activity of the enzyme pathways responsible for the nontoxic clearance of the chemical should be decreased by, for example, competition for the enzyme surface by a second drug or other ingested chemical.

Similar considerations apply to target-tissue specificity; since the ultimate toxic agent is the metabolite of the chemical, the target tissue for a chemical toxin is the tissue that forms the reactive metabolite at a rate greater than its capacity to detoxify it. The difficulty in extrapolation from man to animals and vice versa is also explicable in that the common laboratory animals—rat, mice, hamsters, and rabbits—all metabolize environmental chemicals at rates four or more times greater than that in man. This increased activity is seen in both the toxic and the nontoxic pathways of clearance. However, the relative activities of the various pathways may be very different from that of patients, with the result that susceptibility to the chemically induced lesion in a laboratory species may be very different, either greater or smaller, depending on the compound and on the species chosen for examinations.[30]

Drugs as antigens. Drugs, chemical structures with potent pharmacologic activity, are foreign to the body's immunologic system. They are also, in general, treated by the body as undesirable substances and are excreted as soon as possible. There is hardly a drug that is excreted in the form in which it is taken; this implies that the drug is chemically transformed by metabolic processes, with the ultimate effect of facilitating excretion. Hepatic microsomal enzymes are capable of hydroxylating, conjugating, reducing, or oxidizing drugs to make them more polar. Metabolites that are more polar than the original compound are more water soluble and are therefore easier to excrete via the urine or feces.

The possibility of a drug metabolite becoming immunologically significant rests with its ability to react with proteins or other macromolecule structures, since drug molecules, for the most part, are of low molecular weight and are by themselves unable to act as complete antigens.

The exact mechanism of covalent binding of the drug or its metabolite to an immunogenic carrier is not fully understood. Rarely, crescentic glomerulonephritis (rapidly progressive glomerulonephritis) may accompany acute interstitial nephritis because of both being mediated by circulating immune complex disease (Arthus phenomenon) after administration of penicillin. It has been estimated that approximately 10 per 100,000 injections of penicillin elicit a hypersensitivity response by the recipients. Skin eruptions—exanthema positive, erythema multiforme, toxic epidermal necrolysis (Lyell's syndrome), and purpura—constitute 69% of penicillin reactions. Next in incidence is immune complex disease, 20%, and anaphylactic shock, 10%. Occasionally unexpected death may be attributed to penicillin-induced anaphylactic shock. In forensic cases, particularly, it is essential to look for IgE and IgG antibodies to penicillin in the plasma in suspected cases of sudden death in which penicillin or its analogs may be suspected.

A supply of susceptible carrier molecules is essential for antigen formation. The proteins synthesized locally within the liver are ideally suited to combine with newly formed reactive drug metabolites. It is known that very few individuals develop altered immune (hypersensitivity) reactions to drugs, though reactive metabolic products are formed; this implies that factors *unique to the host* play a considerable part in the development of the allergic state.

Under appropriate conditions, then, altered immune responses of the humoral or cellular type may occur, characterized by the appearance of specific circulating antibody or skin sensitivity or both. However, attempts to demonstrate such evidence of sensitization may be unsuccessful in many patients with drug-induced hypersensitivities. For instance, the finding of so-called markers of autoimmunity, such as lupus erythematosus cell phenomenon, antinuclear factor, antimitochondrial antibody, rheumatoid factor, and positive Coombs' test results, indicates an altered immunologic response but may not be accompanied by *direct evidence* of humoral or cell-mediated drug sensitization and should not imply that such a reaction is responsible for the accompanying lesions.

Drugs are not generally reactive enough to form the irreversible complexes with proteins that are necessary for sensitization, but the metabolic or oxidative products of many common drugs are sufficiently reactive to form stable immunogenic complexes. Some of the minor metabolites, formed in minute quantities, can be responsible for the most severe reactions. The major metabolite responsible for sensitization with penicillin, for example, has been identified as the minor benzylpenicilloyl group, which combines irreversibly with proteins. With quinine or quinidine, it has been suggested that sensitization results from the drugs being metabolized to a more reactive molecule; antibodies from 20% of sensitized patients do not react with quinine and quinidine isomers but with quininone, an oxidative derivative of both drugs. Thus it is apparent that metabolic products of drugs, rather than native drugs, are frequently responsible for sensitization, even though the antibodies elicited by the metabolite, as a rule, react with the native drug.

In contrast to direct toxic action, altered immune responses are not necessarily dose related. Withdrawal of the drug leads in most instances to prompt recovery, and the hypersensitivity or immunologic reaction is variable and not target organ specific. Not infrequently, the clinical manifestations may be any one or more of the following: blood eosinophilia, mucocutaneous lesions, fleeting joint pains, hepatosplenomegaly, generalized lymphadenopathy, and (most important) fever.

A definitive diagnosis of an allergic drug reaction is often impossible to make. One frequently ends up with a diagnosis of "probable" or "possible," rather than "definitive." In attempting to demonstrate a causal relationship between the observed clinical manifestations and the drug, the investigator must recognize that the signs and symptoms that develop are those that are usually associated with the natural history of disease or that can be accounted for by a complication of the disease process. This was recently well illustrated when jaundice developed in a patient who had for several months been taking the phenothiazine chlorpromazine. A liver biopsy was performed. Within the bile canaliculi were observed bile "thrombi," accompanied by eosinophils and lymphocytes in the portal tracts. A diagnosis of chlorpromazine cholestatic hepatitis was made, and the drug was stopped. The direct-reacting serum bilirubin level continued to rise, and it was discovered that the patient had a small bile duct carcinoma at the bifurcation of the common bile duct!

Eosinophils are frequently suggestive of a drug reaction, but there are many other causes of tissue eosinophilia. One of the earliest signs of an ADR is the development of mild fever, but of course this is very nonspecific. However, careful and frequent scrutiny of the temperature chart should be routine during any drug treatment, especially with multiple drugs or if the drugs are known to be potential antigens. For example, one of the main causes of postsurgical fever, 4 to 7 days after an operation, is a hypersensitivity reaction to the anesthetic halothane. Therefore, if the surgeon is not satisfied that the fever is related directly to the surgical procedure, the anesthetic should be suspect.

The syndrome of fever, arthritis and myalgia, eosinophilia, lymphadenopathy, and hepatosplenomegaly is not uncommon in patients admitted to the hospital. Frequently the referring physician is thinking of diagnoses such as sarcoidosis, tuberculosis, and malignant lymphoma. A careful history, however, may reveal that the patient has been taking one or more medicinal compounds, and within a few days after withdrawal of these drugs, the fever subsides. Such a patient was a 45-year-old woman who was quite ill when admitted to the hospital, with fever, malaise, recent weight loss, and a mild leukocytosis. A bone marrow biopsy revealed the presence of several noncaseating granulomas, and similar granulomas were found during a liver biopsy. When attempts to identify organisms within the granulomas failed, it was decided that the granulomas could be drug induced. A survey of the woman's drug regimen

revealed that she had been, and was at the time of her hospital admission, taking some 18 different medicinal compounds for such varied problems as headache, pain, cardiac arrhythmia, and edema. All drugs except the antiarrhythmic were discontinued for 3 days. The patient's fever disappeared, her leukocyte count reverted to normal, and she was talking about leaving the hospital.

A classification of the mechanisms of immunologically induced adverse tissue reactions to drugs is as follows:

1. Anaphylactic (IgE-mediated) response
2. Circulating antigen-antibody complexes (the antigen being the drug or metabolite)
3. Cell-mediated response
4. Autoimmune response
   a. Lupus erythematosus phenomenon (antinuclear antibodies)
   b. Cytotoxic (for example, hemolytic anemia, agranulocytosis, thrombocytopenia)

It should be appreciated that *more than one* of these mechanisms may be operative in any immunologic reaction to a drug or its metabolite (Table 4-2). An additional immune mechanism is that of *neutralization*. Antibodies to drugs may neutralize the therapeutic effect. These antibodies may bring about resistance to antibiotics, cancer chemotherapeutic drugs, blood-clotting factors, and antibiotics.

Several drugs may initiate the systemic lupus erythematosus syndrome. Some of these drugs are hydralazine, procainamide, isonicotinic acid, and penicillamine. The laboratory and clinical features are identical to systemic lupus erythematosus but an observation of interest is that all these signs and symptoms disappear when the administration of the drug is stopped. Of great interest is the fact that antinuclear antibodies are demonstrated, an indication that the syndrome may be an immune-complex or autoimmune reaction to altered nuclear components. Withholding of the drug results in reversibility of the clinical and laboratory features.

Genetically related adverse drug reactions (pharmacogenetics)

Genetic factors may predispose an individual to ADRs, and in some cases there may be inheritance of abnormal receptors and enzymes. Examples include drug-induced hemolysis in glucose-6-phosphate dehydrogenase deficiency, prolonged paralysis after administration of succinylcholine to patients with atypical pseudocholinesterase, susceptibility to malignant hyperthermia during anesthesia, drug-induced exacerbation of porphyria, and the link between ABO blood group and thromboembolic disease caused by oral contraceptives. Polymorphic hydroxylation and acetylation of drugs may also predispose individuals to toxicity. Thus drug-induced lupus erythematosus, hemolysis, and peripheral neuropathy are related to polymorphic acetylation of procainamide and sulfasalazine, as well as isoniazid. There is an association between the HLA-DR antigen phenotype and adverse reactions to gold and penicillamine.

In the context of ADRs, the term *idiosyncrasy* has been used extensively as a label for bizarre responses that were assumed to result from some qualitative abnormality in the patient. Until recently, drug idiosyncrasies were a catchall classification for ADRs that could not be classified under any other heading. This situation is now changing slowly as the mechanisms of ADRs have become clearer and it has become apparent that the majority have a genetic basis.

Age and sex. The incidence of ADRs is greatest in the very young and the very old. The newborn are particularly vulnerable, especially if they are premature, and the responsiveness of the tissues to a given drug concentration may not be the same as in adults. Very young children are said to be particularly sensitive to narcotics, anticholinergics, diazepam, salicylates, and agents that cause methemoglobinemia (fetal hemoglobin is more easily oxidized to methemoglobin than is the adult form). In addition, the metabolism and renal excretion of drugs may be abnormally slow in neonates and infants, resulting in exaggerated and prolonged effects. Thus the maternal use of diazepam is associated with apneic spells, hypotonia, poor feeding, and hypothermia lasting for several days in the newborn—the "floppy baby syndrome."

The elderly are also vulnerable to ADRs. Not only are the functional reserves of many organs reduced and compensatory mechanisms impaired, but the capac'ty to metabolize and eliminate drugs is also reduced. Central nervous system (CNS) depressants are a particular problem for the elderly, in whom they readily cause confusion, disorientation, dementia, depression, incontinence, ataxia, and falls resulting in fractures. In most surveys the incidence of ADRs has been higher in women than in men, possibly because women take more drugs and make up a higher proportion of the vulnerable geriatric population.

Renal disease. ADRs are more common in patients with renal disease. Contributory factors include decreased renal clearance of drugs and their metabolites, increased receptor responsiveness, decreased plasma protein binding, changes in drug distribution, impaired drug metabolism, and the effects of acid-base and electrolyte disturbances. Many drugs are excreted in the urine largely unchanged, and the half-life increases disproportionately as the creatinine clearance falls below 20 to 30 ml/minute. Drug metabolites that normally have little or no activity may accumulate to a remarkable degree and cause toxicity. Use of nephrotoxic combinations such as gentamicin plus cephalothin should obviously be avoided, and preexisting renal disease may potentiate the nephrotoxicity of drugs such as tetracycline, sulfamethoxazole (Septra), phenylbutazone, and aspirin.

Morphologic aspects

Immunologic reactions. Generalized necrotizing vasculitis, especially polyarteritis, is one of the most common allergic drug reactions. For years the sulfonamides were the most common cause of this reaction, but more recently penicillin has assumed this role. The reaction is similar to the Arthus phenomenon and to polyarteritis nodosa, with complement and IgG demonstrable in the inflammatory necrotizing lesions of small vessels. The cellular reactions in drug-induced states show wide variability (see Table 4-2).

Immunologic reactions to drugs are frequently characterized by disproportionate numbers of eosinophils and "immunoblasts." These cells are prominent in other conditions as well, but when they are seen in tissue sections, it is important to entertain the diagnosis of allergic drug reaction. Immunoblastic lymphadenopathy, which occurs occasionally in patients taking phenytoin (Dilantin) and other drugs, has been mistaken for malignant lymphoma.

Noncaseous granulomatous inflammation is also seen occasionally as a marker of allergic drug reaction, particularly in the skin, liver, and bone marrow.

Toxic reactions. The tissue(s) or organ(s) involved and the nature of the reactions in a toxic response depend on the chemical and pharmacologic nature of the drug. There is thus a bewildering array of such reactions. The brain, kidneys, lungs, heart, liver, or gastrointestinal tract may be most seriously involved, and the lesion may be acute, inflammatory, necrotizing, fibrotic, metabolic, neoblastic, or thrombotic, to mention a few. A drug such as acetaminophen may appear to selectively involve a single organ—the liver—whereas the toxic manifestations of phenytoin include acute epithelial necrolysis of the skin, megaloblastic anemia, hepatitis, teratogenesis, and gingival hyperplasia, in addition to immunologic responses such as vasculitis, immunoblastic lymphadenopathy, and granulomatous reactions.

Table 4-3 presents a list of reactions in the liver, believed to be toxic, to illustrate the large variety of such reactions. The toxic reactions to each of the drugs listed may be more complex than is implied by this table, and the prototype drug listed is not the only one that can produce each of these lesions. Several reactions that appear to be allergic, such as granulomatous inflammation, chronic active hepatitis, and necrotizing vasculitis, are not included.

Medicinal hazards of therapy
Antibiotics

Tetracycline. The tetracyclines, when administered intravenously, particularly in the presence of renal dys-

Table 4-2. Classification of altered immune reactions to medicinal drugs

Type	Antibody	Disease state	Cellular reaction	Drugs*
Anaphylactic	Essentially IgE	Acute anaphylactic shock; status asthmaticus; laryngeal edema	Basophil and mast cell degeneration; eosinophils	Penicillins and cephalosporins; iodinated contrast media; vaccines and antisera
Cytotoxic	IgG or IgM	Hemolytic reactions; autoimmune reactions (e.g., lupus erythematosus phenomenon)	Lysed red cells; lymphocytes, plasma cells, and macrophages; vasculitis	Penicillins; sulfonylureas; phenothiazines; hydralazine and procainamide; rifampin
Acute immune complex disease (antigen-antibody complement)	IgG	Serum sickness	Eosinophils, lymphocytes, plasma cells, macrophages; acute vasculitis	Antisera; penicillins
		Membranous glomerulonephritis	No inflammatory cells	Gold salts; penicillamine; cimetidine; aspirin; phenytoin
Cell-mediated reactions	Sensitized T lymphocytes	Contact dermatitis	Lymphocytes; edema and necrosis of epidermal cells	Ethylene diamine; antibiotics (e.g., neomycin); benzocaine; procaine
		Organic and systemic granulomas	Focal collection of macrophages	Nonsteroid analgesics (e.g., phenylbutazone)

*Commonly implicated as prototypes of hypersensitivity reactions.

function, may lead to fat accumulation in the liver cells. This may be accompanied by acute tubular necrosis, characterized by swelling, hydropic change, and fatty accumulations within the cells of the proximal convoluted tubules. Other changes such as focal hemorrhagic pancreatitis and ulceration of the esophagus, stomach, and proximal portion of the small intestine have been noted.

Both in humans and in some laboratory animals, fatty degeneration (steatosis) of the liver is produced by the intravenous injection of tetracycline. Grossly, the liver is of normal size or slightly enlarged. Sectioning reveals it to be bulging, yellow, and greasy. This is not associated with inflammation or necrosis. Studies with tritium-labeled tetracycline show that this antibiotic accumulates in the spleen, lymph nodes, and skeleton, with the highest concentration in the liver. It is quickly excreted into the bile and within the liver acinus or lobule, where there tends to be a centrilobular localization. Microscopically, tetracycline localizes within mitochondria as demonstrated by fluorescence. The degree of involvement seems to depend on the dosage. At the cellular level, in contrast to the alcoholic type of fatty liver, the nuclei are in the center of the cell rather than "squeezed over" to the margin by a single large globule of intracellular fat (Fig. 4-1). The appearance is reminiscent of the liver in "obstetric yellow atrophy," or fatty liver of pregnancy. In that condition the fatty accumulation in the liver cell assumes the same cytologic configuration as in tetracycline toxicity, but, in addition, inflammatory changes and necrosis are frequently seen, whereas they are rare in tetracycline toxicity. There is no direct evidence that the liver of a

Table 4-3. Toxic hepatic injury

Lesion	Prototype
Fatty infiltration (steatosis)	Tetracycline
Hepatic cell necrosis	Acetaminophen
Cholangionecrosis	Chlorpromazine
Cirrhosis	Methotrexate
Cholestasis	Methyltestosterone
Cholestatic hepatitis	Chlorpropamide
Vascular thrombosis	Oral contraceptives
Peliosis hepatis	Methyltestosterone
Hyperplasia and adenoma	Oral contraceptives
Malignant neoplasia	Thorotrast

From Hennigar, G.R.: Adverse drug reactions. In Hill, R.B., and Terzian, J.A., editors: Environmental pathology: an evolving field, New York, 1982, Alan R. Liss, Inc.

pregnant woman is especially susceptible to tetracycline hepatotoxicity. Ultrastructurally, evidence of tetracycline toxicity is manifested by the finding of cytoplasmic collections of lipid closely associated with lipofuscins (Fig. 4-1, *A*). All of this swims in a sea of glycogen.

The centrilobular localization is not surprising, since these cells contain the highest levels of esterase and β-hydroxybutyric dehydrogenase. Such enzyme localization points to the central part of the liver as the location where most of the lipids are metabolized, and interference with such metabolism would allow changes to be visible initially in this portion of the lobule. Physiologically, intracellular lipids are believed to be in the form of laminar micelles, which in turn are incorporated into the membranous structures of the cell and are not identifiable as lipid by light microscopy. The stability of this

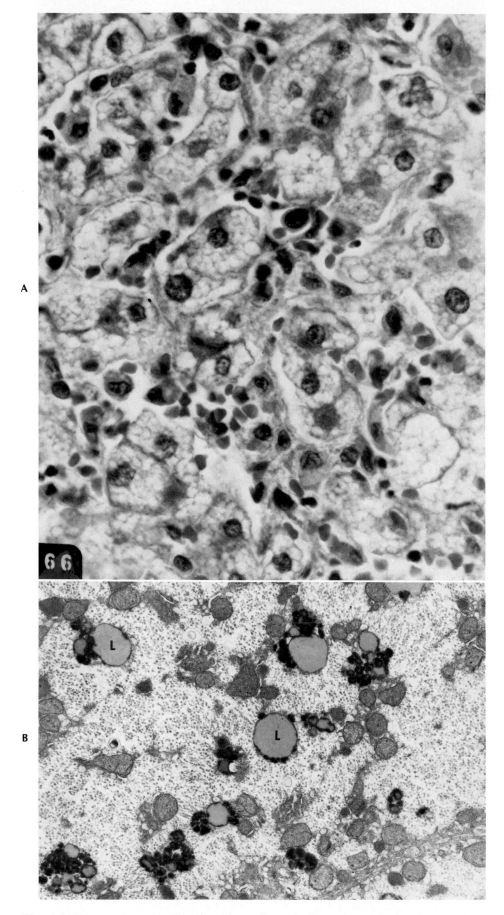

Fig. 4-1. Effects of tetracycline therapy on liver. **A,** There is steatosis of liver cells with centrally placed nuclei. Cytoplasm has a foamy, vacuolated appearance. Oil Red O stain for neutral fat was positive. **B,** Lipid droplets, *L,* are closely associated with lipofuscins (dark pigment). (**A,** Hematoxylin and eosin; 400×.)

lipid dispersion depends on protein and abundant phospholipid as an emulsifier or stabilizer. When there is a deficiency of these substances as well as choline and inositol, a low oxygen supply, or an excess of cholesterol, one may expect to find interference with this form of cellular lipid dispersion. The exact mechanism whereby tetracycline interferes with one or more of these factors is not clear. It is known, however, that the tetracyclines inhibit protein synthesis, so that an antianabolic effect is produced. If there is interference with the normal membrane localization of intracellular lipids, globules of fat that can be stained by the usual fat-staining methods appear. The fatty change in the liver in tetracycline toxicity is reversible.

The formation of lipoprotein-tetracycline complexes in the blood of patients may partially explain why tetracyclines sometimes have anticoagulant properties. They apparently impair the conversion of prothrombin to thrombin and the generation of thromboplastin. Both of these reactions require phospholipid for activation. The bleeding phenomenon noted clinically may be related in part to this property, but the hypoprothrombinemia that is observed probably also constitutes an important factor.

Renal tubular necrosis, when it occurs, is caused largely by the toxic degradation products of tetracycline metabolism, the most important of which is anhydrotetracycline. This substance has been responsible for producing the renal Fanconi syndrome (glucoaminophosphate diabetes). The syndrome, when related to tetracycline administration, is reversible.

All compounds of tetracycline may cause tooth discoloration, with oxytetracycline being the most innocuous. The mechanism of discoloration is that tetracyclines form chelation complexes with calcium at a physiologic pH and become incorporated into bone and teeth. Since teeth do not undergo a constant remodeling as does bone, they can be stained only during their calcification stage. Both deciduous and permanent teeth can be stained. Tetracycline passes the placental barrier and therefore stains teeth in the process of calcification in utero.

Amphotericin B. Amphotericin B is produced by the streptomycete *Streptomyces nodosus*. It is available in either the crystalline or the colloidal form. The crystalline form is useful only through oral administration and has been effective, for the most part, in the treatment of infections caused by *Candida albicans*. Very few signs or symptoms of toxicity are noted with oral administration. Colloidal amphotericin B that is solubilized with desoxycholate is used either intravenously or intrathecally. Signs of toxicity are associated mainly with these routes of administration. The toxic manifestations of intravenous administration consist of phlebitis, hypokalemia, abnormal renal function, and anemia, whereas those of intrathecal administration are pain at the site of injection or along the lumbar nerve roots, headache, paresthesias, nerve palsies, difficulty in voiding, and chemical meningitis.

The colloidal form of amphotericin B has been successful in the treatment of a wide spectrum of mycotic diseases. The two major toxic problems are related to abnormal renal function and anemia. Morphologically, in both humans and dogs, numerous renal lesions have been noted after amphotericin treatment. These predominantly involve the proximal and distal convoluted tubules and consist of hydropic degeneration or necrosis with tubulorrhexis and amorphous material containing calcium and phosphate in the lumen and interstitium. The effects of amphotericin B on the tubules are probably the result of vasospasm of the afferent arterioles leading to acute hypoxic nephrosis or tubular necrosis with renal shutdown. The glomerular lesions have included basement membrane thickening with increased lobulation and ischemic glomerular loops and infraglomerular epithelial reflux.

These renal changes are believed to be reversible, except for the nephrocalcinosis. The anemia is independent of the azotemia and occurs after a relatively small amount of the drug has been administered. The anemia is usually not incapacitating and is of the normocytic normochromic type. There is usually no reticulocytosis. Bone marrow examinations have shown no consistent histologic findings. There is, however, suppression of erythropoiesis without correlation between the total dose and duration of the drug and the degree of the anemia. In vitro studies using exceedingly high levels of amphotericin have shown damage to tissue culture cells and human red blood cells.

Clindamycin. Clindamycin (Cleocin) is an effective antibiotic against gram-positive bacteria. Recommended and particularly excessive doses may result in diarrhea, abdominal pain, and a shocklike state. These findings are highly suggestive of clindamycin-induced pseudomembranous colitis. Grossly, the initial lesion is white or gray plaques that extend from the ileocecal valve to the rectum (Fig. 4-2, *A*). More advanced lesions of antibiotic-associated colitis involve the mucosa, being manifested as a diffuse necrosis of the superficial layers of epithelium. The result is a sheetlike, gray, diffuse pseudomembrane. The underlying mucosa is red-brown, granular, and superficially denuded (Fig. 4-2, *B*).

Histologically, the earliest focal lesions are characterized by necrosis of the surface epithelium with exudation of mucus, fibrin, leukocytes, and necrotic glandular epithelium (Fig. 4-2, *C*). Advanced lesions appear as a diffuse pseudomembrane (Fig. 4-2, *C*). Superficially, the underlying mucosa is denuded and replaced by necrotic debris, inflammatory cells, fibrin, and "streamers" of mucus emanating from the overdistended, ruptured mucous glands (Fig. 4-2, *D* and *E*). The ap-

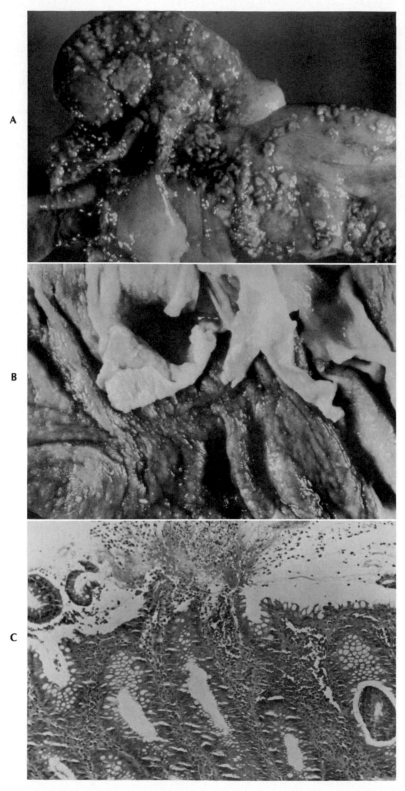

Fig. 4-2. Clindamycin colitis. **A,** Focal plaques of fibrin, mucus, and necrotic debris. **B,** Diffuse pseudomembrane reflected to demonstrate underlying red-brown, granular, superficially denuded mucosa. **C,** Early lesion showing focal necrosis of superficial epithelium and mucosa with outpouring of mucus, fibrin, and nuclear fragments.

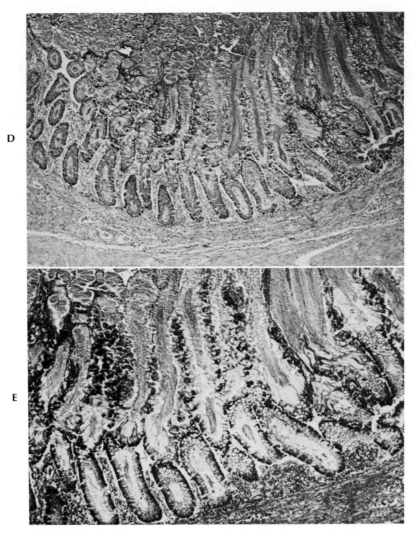

Fig. 4-2, cont'd. D, Necrosis and inflammatory infiltrate extends through mucosa and minimally involves submucosa. Muscularis is spared. Notice necrotic glands, hyperactive goblet cells, and "streamers" of mucus. The luminal side of lesions is composed of necrotic debris. **E,** Higher magnification of micrograph in **D.**

pearance is reminiscent of lava spewing from an activated volcanic crater. The underlying muscularis is not involved by the inflammatory process.

The microscopic appearance of early antibiotic-associated colitis has been confused with that of idiopathic ulcerative colitis. This confusion has led to continued use of clindamycin with fatal outcome. Interestingly, *C. difficile* toxin leads to aggravation of idiopathic ulcerative colitis. The necrosis of the mucosa is attributable to toxins of the *Clostridium* class, most notably *C. difficile* and in some cases *C. perfringens*. Antibiotic-associated colitis has also followed the administration of ampicillin and tetracycline. Recently, rifampin and metronidazole, an effective combination against *Bacteroides*, and other antibiotics have been documented as causes of the condition. Some years ago, vigorous anti-

biotic therapy before intestinal surgery was routine. Pseudomembranous enterocolitis developed in these patients and was attributed to antibiotic-resistant staphylococcal toxins. It should be noted that this is different from the current antibiotic-associated colitis that is confined to the colon, since the staphylococcal cases involved the small intestine as well. During the past several decades, stool cultures have failed to reveal the presence of staphylococci in cases of antibiotic-associated pseudomembranous colitis. The toxins of *C. difficile* can be identified by a tissue culture cell assay technique, both during life and at autopsy.

Chloramphenicol. The most serious complication after the administration of chloramphenicol is the development of aplastic anemia. Since there is no hemolysis, as one would expect to find as a manifestation of an autoimmune reaction, the development of the anemia probably represents specific idiosyncrasy of the individual. The reaction is not necessarily related to dosage but is more common with prolonged use.

Selective depression of bone marrow does occur in mild cases of toxicity, but this usually involves the granulocytes or platelets and spares erythropoiesis. Evidence for the direct toxic reaction is the observation of greatly vacuolated nucleated red cells in the marrow. The toxic action of chloramphenicol is believed to be attributable to the nitrobenzene ring within its structure. It is not clear why aplasia occurs in some patients after the administration of small doses, whereas other patients can receive very high doses without apparent permanent effect on the marrow.

Chloramphenicol is normally detoxified by conjugation with glucuronic acid in the liver and is excreted in the urine as inert nitro compounds. The idiosyncrasy may be related to the inability to metabolize chloramphenicol or may be the result of some other genetically determined defect in the marrow cells themselves. The possibility exists, as it does with virtually all drugs, that some form of hypersensitivity mechanism is at work. At autopsy the marrow has a pale or fatty appearance. There is no lymphadenopathy or splenomegaly. Microscopically, in patients with aplasia, the bone marrow takes on the appearance of vascularized adipose tissue. Hemosiderosis throughout the reticuloendothelial system is observed in patients who have received several blood transfusions. Focal myocardial hemorrhages sometimes occur. As is the case with many antibiotics, infections by opportunistic fungi is common.

Newborn infants are devoid of an effective glucuronic acid conjugation mechanism for degradation and detoxification of the antibiotic. Consequently, when such infants are given chloramphenicol in doses of 75 or more mg/kg body weight per day, the drug may accumulate, resulting in the "gray syndrome" with hyperthermia, acidity, gray color, shock, and collapse. This mechanism is also applicable to the neonatal hyperbilirubinemia occurring after the administration of streptomycin.

Penicillins. For many years the short-acting sulfonamides were the outstanding culprit that brought about hypersensitivity angiitis and polyarteritis nodosa, but penicillin has now assumed this role. Medium-sized and small vessels, as well as capillaries, may be the target of penicillin hypersensitivity. The metabolite benzylpenicilloyl serves as the antigen or hapten for the induction of humoral and cell-mediated responses. The semisynthetic penicillins such as methicillin, ampicillin, oxacillin, and carbenicillin have been clearly pinpointed as etiologic agents of acute interstitial nephritis of hypersensitivity etiology. The cephalosporins (prototype cephalothin), which have a cross-sensitivity with the penicillins, and the aminoglycosides (prototypes streptomycin, kanamycin, and gentamicin) also cause this hypersensitivity nephritis. Drug-induced acute interstitial nephritis is characterized by acute renal failure accompanied by pronounced hematuria, proteinuria, and the presence of tubular epithelial cells and eosinophils in the urine. Concomitantly, clinical manifestations of allergy, such as fever, skin rash, and joint pains, and blood eosinophilia are observed. It is estimated that acute interstitial nephritis may cause between 7% and 10% of cases of clinically obscure acute renal failure. Unexpected death, occurring within minutes after parenteral injection of penicillin, has been recorded numerous times. The mechanism is anaphylactic shock manifested by pulmonary arteriolar and bronchiolar spasm, leading to acute dilatation of the right side of the heart with pooling of blood in the vena caval system. Pulmonary alveolar congestion and edema are consistent findings (Fig. 4-3). Petechial hemorrhages of the conjunctiva and serosal surfaces of visceral organs are noted. Patients may complain of chest pain, which is followed by dyspnea, cyanosis, generalized convulsions, and frothing at the mouth. The manifestations are reminiscent of those seen after fatal bee sting, accidental parenteral injection or overdosage in clinical hyposensitization procedures, and anaphylaxis in experimental animals.

A syndrome characterized by transient eosinophilic pulmonary infiltrates and vasculitis may be the result of acute immune complex disease occurring after penicillin therapy. The syndrome is almost identical to that seen in patients who manifest hypersensitivity reactions to infection with the *Ascaris* parasite. In this instance the condition is referred to as Löffler's syndrome.

Cephalosporins. Cephalothin, a prototype of the cephalosporins, may produce immune hemolytic anemia. This effect is shared with the penicillins, with which there is cross-sensitivity. Antibiotic-associated colitis may follow the administration of cephalothin or penicillin, or both. Cephalothin therapy occasionally leads to a "toxic effect" on the proximal convoluted tubular epithelial cells, which may result in necrosis and subsequent acute renal failure. The hypersensitivity reaction in the kidney to cephalothin is characterized by the appearance of acute interstitial nephritis (see discussion of penicillins).

Aminoglycosides. Gentamicin and polymyxin B, like neomycin and kanamycin, are aminoglycosides that cause hydropic degeneration of the proximal convoluted tubules. On occasion, tubular necrosis supervenes. Gentamicin is concentrated in the renal cortex and excreted slowly. It is the most nephrotoxic of the aminoglycosides, causing nephrotoxicity in 2% to 14% of patients treated. The incidence is lowest in those who do not have preexisting renal disease. The evidence points to a direct cellular toxic damage to the proximal tubular

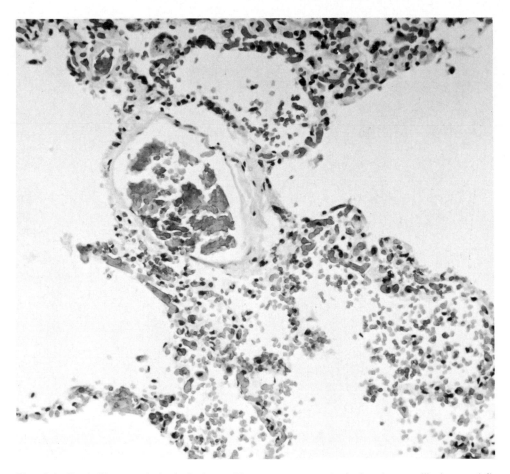

Fig. 4-3. Penicillin anaphylaxis in lung. There are congested alveolar capillaries and fibrinogen in vessel.

epithelium and is characterized by a granular type of necrosis, with the lumens being filled by an amorphous eosinophilic material. The basement membranes are intact. Electron microscopic examination shows a group of changes that are associated with toxic damage to the cell, including numerous phagosomes with myeloid bodies and swelling of the mitochondria (Fig. 4-4). There is an initial loss of brush-border microvilli, which is noted as the earliest lesion. Cellular necrosis follows, and the exact pathogenesis of cell death is not established. Recently, it has been demonstrated that inhibitors of the binding of aminoglycosides to brush-border membranes will negate the nephrotoxicity in rats. The newer aminoglycoside antibiotics tobramycin and amikacin produce renal lesions similar to those caused by gentamicin but are less nephrotoxic.

Neomycin and kanamycin. Orally administered neomycin in doses of 3 to 12 g/day produces moderate malabsorption of a variety of substances, including fat, protein and amino acids, cholesterol, glucose, sodium, calcium, vitamin B_{12}, iron, and penicillin. A lesser degree of malabsorption may occur after the administration of tetracycline, kanamycin, polymyxin, or bacitracin.

Neomycin has a cholesterol-lowering effect. The morphologic changes consist in shortening of the finger-like villi of the small intestine, accompanied by an infiltration of the lamina propria by round cells and macrophages. The latter frequently contain cellular debris and bacteria-like structures. Dense bodies that may represent aggregated neomycin are seen within the crypt cells. Since there is evidence that cholesterol synthesis takes place within intestinal crypt cells, these changes may explain the sharp cholesterol-lowering effect of neomycin. In addition to the disturbances in the structure and villi of the mucosa of the small intestine, there is evidence of defective reabsorption by the proximal convoluted tubules of the kidney after neomycin administration. Amino acid levels may be greatly increased in the urine, as well as the feces, because of this dual toxicity to the intestinal villi and the tubular epithelium (Fig. 4-5).

Kanamycin belongs to the same group as neomycin but is far less toxic. Acute swelling and hydropic degen-

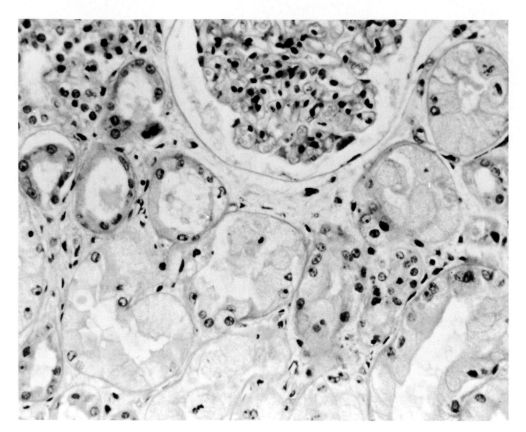

Fig. 4-4. Neomycin-kanamycin nephrosis in kidney. Cells of proximal convoluted tubules are swollen and hydropic with nuclei in various stages of degeneration.

eration of the proximal convoluted tubules may occur after dosage with either drug (Fig. 4-5).

Streptomycin. An effect on the eighth nerve, leading to vestibular impairment and sometimes hearing loss, is one of the toxicologic manifestations of streptomycin therapy. Streptomycin, like kanamycin, is autotoxic and is capable of bringing about swelling and hydropic degeneration of the proximal convoluted tubules, accompanied by mild proteinuria. The tubular changes are reversible when treatment is discontinued. This compound has been reported to cause polyarteritis nodosa. It is the least nephrotoxic of all the aminoglycosides.

From the above account, it is clear that the aminoglycosides are a group of compounds that are directly toxic to the plasma membrane and intracellular structures. The proximal convoluted tubule is the primary target cell of aminoglycoside toxicity. Organ cells, such as those in the mucosa of the small intestine and the sensory hair cells in the organ of Corti and the vestibular apparatus, are subject to toxic degenerative changes. The reasons for the localization of toxic damage in these organs is unexplained. In contrast to the toxic effects of the wide variety of aminoglycosides, altered immune responses are exceedingly rare.

Analgesics and antipyretics

Salicylates. Aspirin and methyl salicylate (wintergreen oil) are salicylates that together constitute the most common cause of accidental poisoning in children. Death has occurred in infants, children, and adults after an intake of 2 to 5 g of aspirin.

In acute salicylate poisoning the primary effect of salicylate overdosage is direct stimulation of the respiratory center. This provokes a respiratory alkalosis that at first is compensated by increased renal excretion of bicarbonate and retention of hydrogen ions. Disturbance of the intermediate metabolism of carbohydrate and fat leads to a superimposed metabolic acidosis, possibly from the accumulation of lactate and pyruvate. Hypokalemia then develops, partly because of the loss of potassium in the urine in the early stages, but probably mainly because the alkalosis causes a shift of potassium into the cells. Hypokalemia is known to impair renal excretion of bicarbonate and may increase renal excretion of hydrogen ions, with both factors tending to increase the alkalosis.

Aspirin and other nonsteroidal anti-inflammatory agents may be responsible for chronic oozing of blood from the gastric mucosa, leading to a hypochromic mi-

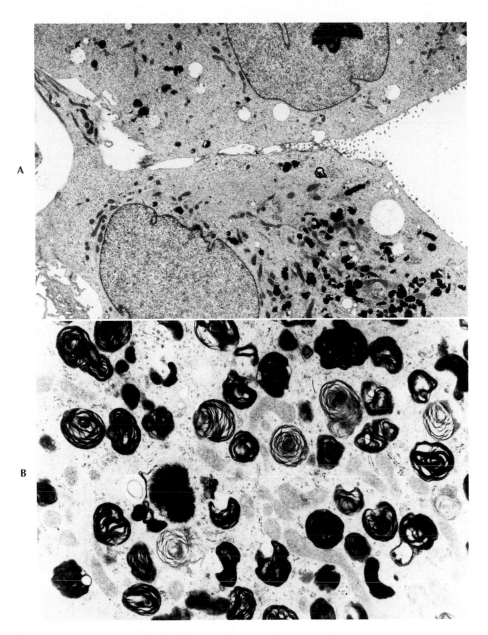

Fig. 4-5. A, Ultrastructural profile of human proximal tubule cells cultured in vitro in serum-free media and exposed for 3 days to 250 μg/ml streptomycin. The cytoplasm contains numerous electron-dense spheroid bodies, termed "myeloid bodies." **B,** A higher magnification of the cytoplasmic inclusions demonstrating the concentric swirls of electron-dense material. These bodies are distinct from lipofuscin pigment or residual phagolysosomes. They show in vitro aminoglycoside nephrotoxicity, among other conditions, and are proposed lysosomal in origin. Notice the interspersed, lighter staining mitochondria, which are morphologically normal. (**A,** 2360×; **B,** 11,800×; both from Sens, M.A., et al.: Ann. Clin. Lab. Sci. **18:**204, 1988; by permission of the Institute for Clinical Science.)

crocytic anemia. Not uncommonly, excessive aspirin ingestion will reveal itself to the endoscopist as a series of petechial hemorrhages that not infrequently are accompanied by an acute bleeding ulcer. In fatal cases of overdosage in children or adults, the gross anatomic finding is hemorrhagic gastroenteritis, sometimes with superficial ulceration. One may find necrosis of the germinal centers of the lymphoid tissue of the body, which is probably caused by lympholysis as a result of sudden sharp elevations in the serum corticosteroid level. The elevation is a manifestation of the "stress reaction" that acetylsalicylic acid readily produces in human and experimental animals. Acute ulceration of the stomach may be attributed in part to this phenomenon. The hemorrhagic gastrointestinal mucosa and the petechial hemorrhages in the meninges and serosal surfaces of the viscus may be attributed to the anticoagulant property of acetylsalicylic acid. This drug interferes with the production of factor IV by the platelets. Factor IV neutralizes heparin, and so a deficiency would lead to an increased serum heparin level. Salicylate depression of the formation of prothrombin by the liver accentuates the hemorrhagic diathesis. Aspirin added to platelet-rich plasma inhibits "second-phase" platelet aggregation, as well as release of platelet adenosine diphosphate (ADP), serotonin, and platelet factor IV after the addition of collagen, ADP, or epinephrine. The effect of aspirin on platelet function tests is not clear. In fact, the mechanism by which aspirin acts on platelets is incompletely understood. There remains enormous interest in the possibility of preventing thrombosis by inhibition of the platelet-release reaction.

The probable cause of death in most cases of fatal salicylate intoxication may be attributed to the metabolic and electrolyte disturbances. The shock resulting from loss of gastrointestinal fluids is also an important factor. Salicylates given to hypersensitive patients with bronchial asthma may precipitate serious systemic reactions within 30 minutes. The acute fatal event may be manifested by an uncontrollable attack of bronchial asthma. There is a high incidence of chronic peptic ulcer in patients who abuse analgesics.

Of the salicylic acid group of compounds, methyl salicylate is the most potent toxin. One teaspoon of methyl salicylate equals 12 ordinary aspirin tablets in contents of salicylate. Metabolic acidosis is a more prominent feature of poisoning by the methyl ester than with other common derivatives of salicylic acid.

Aminophenols. Acetaminophen (Tylenol) is a metabolite of phenacetin and acetanilid. It is an analgesic that has certain advantages over salicylates (aspirin). It does not initiate or aggravage hyperacidic states and gastroduodenitis. Chronic ethanol abusers frequently have chronic gastroduodenitis and varying degrees of malabsorption; acetaminophen is therefore a preferred compound for these individuals. A further advantage of acetaminophen is that it does not give rise to hypersensitivity reactions. On the other hand, acetaminophen is a dangerous drug when consumed in excess of therapeutic doses. It is rapidly and almost completely absorbed from the gastrointestinal tract. It is metabolized in the liver, and about 3% is excreted in the urine unchanged; the remainder is composed of 60% glucuronide conjugates, 30% sulfate conjugates, and 5% cystine conjugates. Acetaminophen is a hepatotoxin, and this action is mediated through the formation of active toxic metabolites that are normally detoxified in the liver by conjugation with glutathione. Overdosage of acetaminophen leads to depletion of liver cell glutathione and subsequent failure of the glutathione protective mechanism. The toxic metabolites then bind to macromolecules of hepatocellular protein. Through a mechanism that is not clear, there is a loss of vital cellular function, which leads to death of the hepatocytes. The central portion of the hepatic lobule is specifically involved (Fig. 4-6). The necrosis is characteristically of the coagulative type and is not preceded by the centrilobular fatty change that is characteristic of hepatocellular toxins in general. Early damage to the centrilobular hepatocytes is evidenced by the loss of glycogen from the cytoplasm of these cells. The functional and morphologic effects of long-standing acetaminophen therapy (greater than 2 g/day) have not been documented.

Phenacetin (acetophenetidin) also belongs to the group of aminophenol analgesics. It is rapidly absorbed after oral administration, reaching a maximum concentration in the blood at the end of 2 hours. One hour after administration to humans, the greater part of phenacetin has been converted to N-acetyl-p-aminophenol (acetaminophen), which is assumed to be the active ingredient and analgesic agent. A small part, less than 1%, is converted to p-phenitidin. Elimination is rapid, and only 0.2% is excreted in the urine as unconverted phenacetin. The greater part is eliminated in the urine within the first 22 hours as N-acetyl-p-aminophenol after conjugation in the liver with glucuronic acid, approximately 3% as free N-acetyl-p-aminophenol and less than 1% as p-phenetidin. Phenacetin is generally used in drug combinations with other antipyretics such as acetanilid and acetylsalicylic acid, as well as with barbiturates and caffeine. In the United States there is only the occasional over-the-counter preparation containing phenacetin. Although phenacetin is characterized by low toxicity in humans, during the past 25 years there have been an increasing number of reports of syndromes caused by persistent intake of prolonged high doses. Most of these reports have been from Switzerland, Australia, and the Scandinavian countries, where the consumption of phenacetin has increased multifold, and from areas where there has been severe abuse of phenacetin-containing compounds. The effect of such abuse is described mainly as an effect on the blood (hemolytic anemia, methemoglobinemia) and kidneys (chronic interstitial nephritis, papillitis necroticans).

The pathogenesis of chronic interstitial nephritis, with or without papillitis necroticans, after chronic analgesic abuse has not been clarified. Experimental studies indicate that the initial damage may be located in the medulla with subsequent cortical changes. Papillitis necroticans is believed to develop during the course of tubular epithelial necrosis caused by acetaminophen (phenacetin metabolite) and aspirin, both of which at-

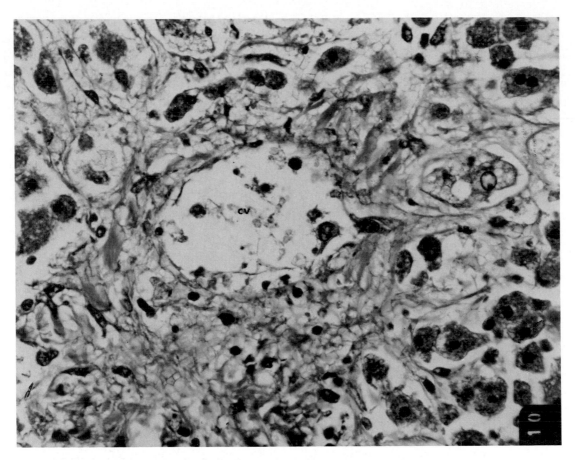

Fig. 4-6. Acetaminophen hepatotoxicity. Hepatocytolysis is visible around the central vein *(cv)*. Collagen-reticulin remains. Coagulative hepatocellular necrosis is displayed by the cells with intact cellular outlines and shrunken, pyknotic nuclei. An identical microscopic picture follows hepatic injury by acute ischemia, severe shock, or heatstroke.

tain a high concentration in the papillae. However, another theory invokes an ischemic mechanism as the cause of papillitis necroticans. Aspirin inhibits prostaglandin PGE_2 synthesis, resulting in a reduction of medullary blood flow. The observation in experimental animals that phenacetin and aspirin, when administered together, cause papillitis necroticans is in contrast to a diminished incidence when the drugs are used separately. This synergistic effect has not been explained. Compared with the general population, phenacetin abusers in Scandinavia and Australia are more prone to transitional cell carcinoma of the renal pelvis and bladder. This experience has rarely been documented in the United States and Canada.

Acute hemolytic anemia may follow short- or long-term intake of small therapeutic doses of phenacetin. It is likely that acute hemolytic anemia more often represents a hypersensitivity reaction, with the phenacetin playing the role of hapten. The more prolonged chronic type of anemia, after continuous high levels of phenacetin intake, probably represents a direct toxic effect on the erythropoietic tissues, leading to disturbance in hemoglobin synthesis with the accumulation of abnormal blood pigments (methemoglobin and sulfhemoglobin). In such instances, Heinz bodies are often demonstrable after careful staining, the results of direct and indirect Coombs' tests are negative, and the reticulocyte count is elevated, while white cell and platelet counts are normal. Moderate elevations of serum iron and serum bilirubin levels and splenomegaly may occur. Examination of the bone marrow reveals increased erythropoiesis and an increased deposition of iron.

The occurrence of unknown primary aromatic amines in the urine of patients receiving acetophenetidin (phenacetin) and acetaminophen (Tylenol) is recorded. Humans excrete only traces in their urine. It is of interest that the extent of excretion of these diazotizable amines parallels the ability of acetophenetidin to cause methemoglobinemia. There is also an indication of a direct relationship between the extent of the excretion of the diazotizable amines (2-hydroxyphenetidin sulfate and 2-hydroxyphenetidin glucuronide) and the concentration of methemoglobin. A stimulating observation is a significant reduction in erythrocyte survival after the administration of acetophenetidin to persons who have phenacetin-induced kidney damage. When similar dosage of phenacetin is given to patients with renal insufficiency of other origin, no decrease in the red blood cell life span is observed.

The individual variation in drug metabolism as a cause of drug toxicity is well known. Individual variation in the metabolism of phenacetin is obviously another example. Phenacetin-induced kidney damage in two or more members of the same family has been reported on several occasions. Time may clarify whether persons who show adverse hematologic reaction to phenacetin are candidates for interstitial nephritis.

Other nonsteroidal anti-inflammatory drugs. Ibuprofen, a propionic acid derivative excreted primarily by the kidneys, is indicated for the treatment of a variety of painful conditions, including those that are immune mediated, such as disseminated lupus erythematosus, rheumatoid arthritis, and autoimmune disease. Paradoxically, adverse reactions include hemolytic anemia, lupus-like syndrome, thrombocytopenic thrombotic purpura, and glomerular-tubular disease. Ibuprofen as a compound that is associated with renal dysfunction has received increasing attention in recent years. The primary renal target is the entire nephron, interstitium, and renal papillae. The blood vessels escape involvement. The most common glomerular lesion is mesangiopathic glomerulonephritis with IgM and C′3 deposition in the mesangium. Minimal thickening of the basement membrane with IgG and C′3 subepithelial complexes may occur alone or accompany the above-mentioned mesangial findings. Minimal change disease has also been incriminated as an adverse reaction to ibuprofen "toxicity." This is a rare lesion to be recognized as drug induced. Numerous medicinal drugs have been recognized as agents giving rise to acute tubulointerstitial nephritis. This type of nephritis is invariably characterized by a prominent interstitial lymphocytic response, eosinophilic leukocytes, and plasma cells. The tubular destruction is a direct response of the cytotoxic effects of the lymphocytes on the epithelium. The identification of immune complexes in the cells and the basement membranes of the tubules is infrequently demonstrated. Papillary necrosis after Ibuprofen administration has been recorded.

There has been considerable discussion concerning the role of increased renal prostaglandin E concentration after ibuprofen administration. Prostaglandins are vasodilators that play a role in regulating renal blood flow, particularly in the presence of renal arterial and arteriolar vasoconstriction. The impairment of glomerular blood flow may account, in part, for tubular dysfunction after nonsteroidal anti-inflammatory drug usage. Invariably, ibuprofen-associated renal dysfunction is reversible after discontinuance of the drug and the beginning of steroid therapy. The rapid response to steroids is strong circumstantial evidence that the glomerular and tubulointerstitial lesions are immune mediated.

Corticosteroids

The role of corticosteroids as anti-inflammatory and immunosuppressive agents is established. Only some of the mechanisms involved in cortisone action at the cellular level are understood. The compounds inhibit the release of lysosomes (neutrophilic granules) from the polymorphonuclear leukocytes. Cortisone and its analogs are capable of slowing down the proliferation of many types of cells (fibroblasts, histiocytes, and lymphocytes). The "lytic" effect on lymphocytes, particularly thymic-dependent lymphocytes, is of interest. With high concentrations, nuclear fragmentation of the lymphocytes is profound. Large lymphocytes and cells of the germinal centers of lymph follicles become pyknotic and karyorrhectic under the influence of these compounds. On the other hand, plasma cells are unaffected by adrenal hormones.

Cortisone may be considered an immunosuppressive drug by virtue of its ability to inhibit nucleoprotein synthesis and mitosis of lymphocytes. This effect on small lymphocytes is more readily demonstrable in animals than in humans, in whom there is some resistance to depletion by corticosteroids. The question of whether a steroid-induced mechanism affects the processing of antigen and transfer to lymphocytes has not been solved. Cortisone may inhibit or enhance an animal's ability to produce circulating antibodies, depending on the dose and time of administration. The maximum effect for suppression is obtained when treatment is started approximately 12 hours before the antigen administration. Steroid suppression of antibody synthesis in humans requires a great deal of new investigation. By virtue of its effect on cellular immunity, cortisone prolongs the survival of normal tissue allografts in many animals. It has been used to suppress tumor immunity and to increase the survival of tumor allografts and xenografts. Administration of steroids may facilitate metastases from tumors.

In graft rejection the union and interaction of antigen and antibody elicit a violent acute inflammatory reaction. There is a strong possibility that corticosteroids may enhance the likelihood of graft acceptance by suppressing inflammation and thereby improving the host environment for the graft. On the other hand, prolonged and continued use of steroids after the cessation of "graft rejection inflammation" may prove to be deleterious.

As opposed to the anti-inflammatory action, it should be kept in mind that patients with chronic recurring disease states (such as rheumatoid arthritis and lupus erythematosus) who are receiving continuous cortisone therapy may have reactivation of tuberculous foci or may die as a result of other disseminated bacterial or fungal infections. Under such circumstances, fever, leukocytosis, and constitutional signs and symptoms are masked by the steroid therapy. Necropsies on such patients may reveal adrenal atrophy of the zona fasciculata and reticularis with preservation of the glomerulosa zone. The beta cells of the pancreatic islets reveal glycogen infiltration, Crooke's changes develop in the mucoid cells of the pituitary gland, and fatty infiltration of the liver is observed.

Widespread necrosis of muscle fibers in experimental animals after the administration of large amounts of ACTH or cortisone has been demonstrated. Similar lesions in humans with Cushing's syndrome or after corticosteroid therapy are debatable.

It is well known that changes in carbohydrate metabolism are produced by steroids derived from the adrenal cortex. The term *steroid diabetes* therefore has usually been applied to the syndrome resulting from the administration of steroids. The diabetogenic action of adrenal corticosteroids was first suspected in 1925, when it was reported that patients with adrenocortical insufficiency exhibited pronounced sensitivity to insulin. After adrenalectomy there is a noticeable improvement in the diabetic state and a diminished insulin requirement. It is well known that patients with Cushing's syndrome have an abnormal glucose tolerance and that diabetic patients with Addison's disease require higher doses of insulin after cortisone treatment.

However, not all adrenal corticosteroids are diabetogenic. It seems that the steroids principally concerned with this action are those with an 11-oxy group. These glucocorticoids have an opposing action to insulin in the regulation of carbohydrate, protein, and lipid metabolism in that they stimulate glucose production, protein breakdown, and fatty acid mobilization. Some of the most potent and frequently administered drugs (such as cortisol and prednisone) belong to this type.

The mechanism of action of the 11-oxy steroids on metabolic processes is still insufficiently understood. They do not destroy insulin or accelerate insulin breakdown. The glucocorticoids enhance glucose production primarily by increasing hepatic glucose production. The catabolic action on proteins contributes by increasing the level of plasma amino acids, some of which are converted into glucose. The administration of 11-oxy steroids increases fatty acid release from tissue stores, and there is evidence that the intermediate metabolism of lipids is modified by steroid therapy, resulting in an increased production of glucose. From these facts it would appear that glucocorticoids interfere with the normal disposal of glucose, while at the same time the glucose concentration is increased by gluconeogenesis, mainly from amino acids.

Clinical observations lead us to believe that latent diabetes may become manifest and the severity of existing diabetes may be increased after the administration of these drugs. Whether treatment with corticosteroids induces diabetes in previously nondiabetic patients is not clear. There is no definite evidence that these drugs can induce diabetes in normal persons without a hereditary predisposition.

Early in the administration of steroids to rabbits, the pancreas shows glycogen accumulation in the small duct cells. After prolonged administration, the beta cells of the islets, as well as the ductules, contain increasing amounts of glycogen. The beta cells become degranulated, and proliferating ductules become filled with inspissated secretion. This results in leakage of pancreatic enzymes from increased hydrostatic pressure in the ductal lumens with separation of acinar cells, bringing about focal pancreatitis. Similar changes have been described in humans with chronically elevated corticosteroid levels.

In partially depancreatized dogs, permanent diabetes may result after termination of steroid treatment. Whether these findings can be extrapolated to humans receiving steroids is problematic.

The pathognomonic diabetic lesions of nodular glomerulosclerosis in the kidney and hyalinization of the islets have not been observed in patients treated with steroids in the absence of known hereditary diabetes. Likewise, the findings of these lesions in patients with Cushing's syndrome (endogenous steroid production), if they occur, are rare.

In recent years there has accumulated an impressive body of circumstantial evidence indicating that primary adult aseptic bone necrosis may be linked in some way to the use of corticosteroid drugs. The bones usually involved are the head of the femur and humerus, and in some cases concomitant involvement of the hip and shoulder joints has occurred. The osteolytic and necrotic process involves the trabeculas of the epiphyses and causes extreme joint pain (Fig. 4-7, *A*). There are disturbing indications that cessation of corticosteroid therapy once joint necrosis has begun may be of no benefit in altering the course of joint disorganization. The pathogenic mechanisms whereby corticosteroids predispose individuals to bone necrosis are not known. The possibility that the corticosteroids may produce a vasculitis in small vessels supplying the hip and shoulder joints has not been borne out by histologic examination of surgically removed specimens.

Suggestions that aseptic bone necrosis may result from fat embolism are intriguing. Patients with alcoholic (nutritional) fatty livers have been observed to have an increased incidence of the disease, and fatty metamorphosis in the normal liver after corticosteroid administration has been observed. Some workers have speculated that corticosteroid-induced fatty livers may be the source of embolus-sized fat globules that occlude the terminal interosseous capillaries and produce microinfarcts (Fig. 4-7, *B*).

Sclerosing retroperitonitis and sclerosing mediastinitis after the use of the corticosteroid dexamethasone

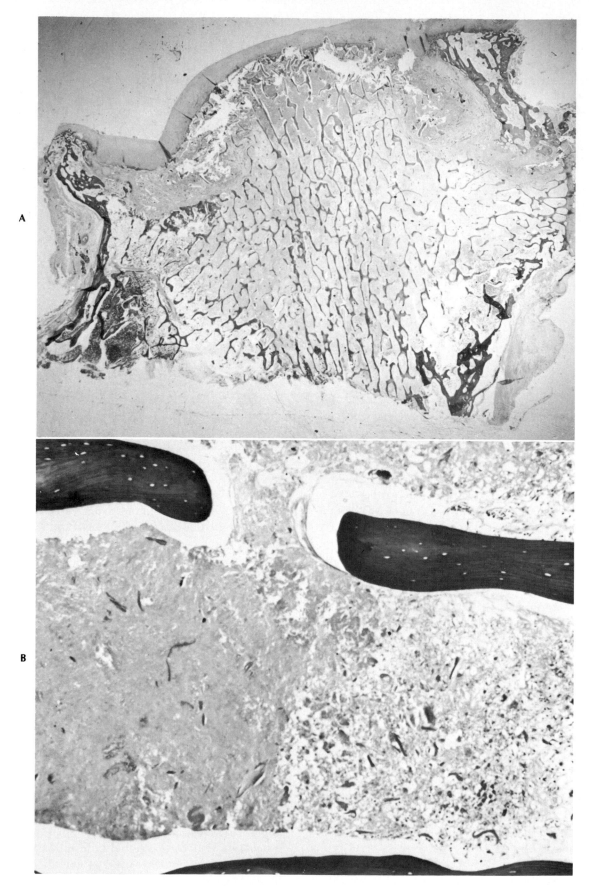

Fig. 4-7. Cortisone therapy. **A,** Aseptic necrosis of head of femur. Notice cyst formation beneath articular cartilage and necrosis of adjacent bony trabeculas and marrow. **B,** Same specimen shown in **A.** "Infarctlike" area of necrosis may be seen on left. Necrotic bone spicules are in evidence.

have frequently been reported. Similar reactions after the ingestion of halogen compounds (such as bromides or iodides) have been described. Administration of the corticosteroid prednisone to patients with rheumatic fever or leukemia has also resulted in the development of these lesions.

One of the best-known functions of the corticosteroids is their ability to retard the inflammatory process. Phagocytic activity is depressed, capillary permeability is decreased, the number of leukocytes and monocytes is reduced, and the exudate is less rich in fibrin. The inhibitory effect of the corticosteroids on the accumulation of ground substance and fibroblastic proliferation results in a diminution of the formation of granulation tissue. Once granulation tissue and fibrosis have appeared, the corticosteroids have no retarding influence on further development, nor will they lyse existing granulation of fibrous tissue elements.

Androgenic-anabolic steroids

Methyltestosterone. Methyltestosterone norethandrolone may, in the upper limits of dosage, give rise to one or more of the following adverse cellular reactions in the liver: (1) cholestatic hepatitis, (2) peliosis hepatis, and (3) biliary cirrhosis, indistinguishable from the entity described as primary biliary cirrhosis. The mechanism of action whereby the compound causes the characteristic destruction of the bile ductules and elicts a profound plasma cell response is not clear. In drug-induced hepatitis and biliary cirrhosis the patient's serum may contain macroglobulins, circulating antinuclear antibodies, and antibodies to bile ductules. The presence of nonspecific antimitochondrial antibodies may be observed. These immunologic findings tempt the observer to speculate that the drug or its metabolite acting on liver or bile duct protein has given rise to prolonged antigenic stimulation. This mechanism, referred to as autoimmunity, is veiled in mystery. With the passage of time many cases that are now referred to as primary biliary cirrhosis may be discovered to have resulted from medicinal drug therapy.

Oral contraceptives (the "pill")

Histologic changes in both arteries and veins of women receiving antiovulants have been described. The change may occur over a period of a week to months after initiation of the medication. Most individuals in whom vascular changes have developed received a combination type of preparation of estrogens and progestins. There is no absolute evidence that the type of oral contraceptive taken is responsible for the appearance of the vascular lesions.

Irey, Manion, and Taylor[84] have drawn attention to the involvement of pulmonary, systemic, and portal circulations. Arteries and veins of large, medium, and small caliber show changes throughout the vessel wall, frequently accompanied by thrombosis. Most spectacular are the intimal fibrosis and profound endothelial proliferation frequently found in small pulmonary arteries. This latter finding is interpreted by Irey and associates as a primary effect of the drugs on the vascular wall and can be distinguished from the secondary intimal changes occurring after thromboembolism in persons not taking the "pill."

Endothelial hyperplasia has been noted in blood vessels in the endometrium of women taking oral contraceptives. Other evidence of the hyperplastic effect of steroids is the hyperplasia of endocervical glandular epithelium and increased cellularity in uterine leiomyomas noted in women using oral contraceptives.

Substantiation of a direct cause-and-effect association between the administration of oral contraceptives and the development of vascular thrombosis and thromboembolism is fraught with conflicting statistical evidence. The increasing number of cases of the Budd-Chiari syndrome (hepatic vein thrombosis) that occur in women taking the "pill" may point to its implication in thrombus formation (Fig. 4-8). Despite an increasing number of reports in the literature suggesting the cause-and-effect relationship between oral contraceptives and cerebral artery occlusion, this relationship requires further scrutiny. Evidence strongly suggests that some type of thromboembolic disorder is associated with the use of oral contraceptives, particularly in the group of women with no known medical condition predisposing to thrombosis. The evidence is strongest for venous thrombosis (superficial and deep).

How oral contraceptives would contribute to the factors that could bring about thrombosis seems to be entirely obscure, and the many in vitro coagulation studies have not shed much light on the problem. In evaluating the thromboembolic phenomena, one must also take into consideration that thrombosis may strike the young and healthy without previous warning.

The ovaries of women taking oral contraceptives are devoid of corpora lutea with a paucity of developing graafian follicles. Follicular cysts are not uncommon. There are conflicting reports as to the presence or absence of stromal hyperplasia and fibrosis of the tunica albuginea. It is possible that FSH and LH activity may persist despite inhibition of ovulation. The gonadotropic function of the pituitary gland under such circumstances is in need of clarification. It has been suggested that the Stein-Leventhal syndrome may develop after prolonged usage of ovulation inhibitors. If and when ovarian fibrosis occurs, it is believed to be reversible in most instances. The role of these hormones as possible inducers of malignant neoplasia in humans will be established or refuted after a longer time interval of usage has been established.

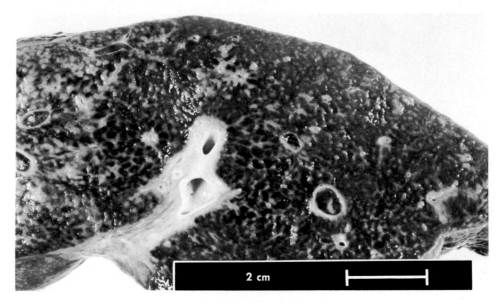

Fig. 4-8. The "pill" and Budd-Chiari syndrome. Large hepatic veins are filled with thrombus, and there is pronounced centrilobular congestion.

The incidence of jaundice in women using oral contraceptive tablets has been estimated to be 1 in 10,000. This event may occur during the first cycle of therapy or appear after several months. The laboratory findings reveal elevations in direct-reacting (conjugated) bilirubin and alkaline phosphatase and, frequently, a moderate rise in aspartate aminotransferase (AST, SGOT) and alanine aminotransferase (ALT, SGPT). There is invariably an increase in BSP retention. No abnormal levels in the flocculation tests have been observed. These findings are consistent with the morphologic features observed in liver biopsy specimens. The architectural pattern is normal and not associated with hepatocellular necrosis. A pronounced portal triad inflammatory reaction is usually present, and no bile duct hyperplasia is observed.

On the other hand, the microscopic picture is characterized by slightly swollen liver cells accompanied by pronounced intracanalicular bile stasis confined to the centrilobular area. Occasionally a mild portal inflammatory reaction composed of lymphocytes, plasma cells, and eosinophils is noted. The clinical, biochemical, and histologic findings are strikingly similar to those in intrahepatic cholestasis of pregnancy, indicating that hormonal effect may be the common denominator. Whether the estrogen or progesterone component of the oral contraceptive is the culprit is not clear. Likewise, the mechanism of interference with intracellular bile metabolism in these cases has not been elucidated by histochemical, light microscopic, and electron microscopic methods. In patients manifesting inflammatory reaction with a pronounced eosinophil infiltrate, the possibility of anaphylactic (immediate) type

of hypersensitivity may be considered. In the majority of cases the contraceptive steroids probably exert a toxic effect on the hepatocytes. Generally, when the patient discontinues the "pill," there is complete reversal of the cholestatic state within 1 week to 2 months. A clinicopathologic picture similar to that induced by the oral contraceptives may be observed after the administration of methyltestosterone and norethandrolone.

Experiments in laboratory rodents indicate that estrogenic compounds may be responsible for the development of focal nodular hyperplasia and liver cell adenomas. Adenomas of the liver are more often found in younger women in contrast to their infrequent appearance in older women and men. It is now clear that the appearance and regression of hepatic cell adenomas show a cause-and-effect relationship in young women taking the "pill." That focal nodular hyperplasia is caused by estrogenic and progestin components of the "pill" is not proved at this time. Whereas significant epidemiologic data point to the involvement of androgenic steroids in the development of hepatocellular carcinoma, this does not appear true of estrogenic stimulation in the form of Premarin or oral contraceptive steroids. In recent years it has been customary to associate development of intralobular vascular dilatation (peliosis hepatis) with the administration of androgenic anabolic steroids; it now seems clear that estrogen likewise can be realistically implicated. Since the induction of hepatogenic tumors seems to be related to the dosage and length of time of hormonal contraceptive use, a reduction of the tumor risk is likely if the organism is less exposed to these preparations. The initiation, cellular multiplication, and resolution of hepatic cell adenoma are clearly dose dependent.

Benign cholestatic jaundice associated with oral contraceptive use is similar to that of pregnancy. Some women apparently cannot metabolize increased secretions of estrogen and progesterone during pregnancy. Conjugated bilirubin and alkaline phosphatase accumulate in the bloodstream, and jaundice develops. However, the hepatic parenchymal cells remain normal, results of flocculation tests are normal, and serum transaminase levels are normal or slightly increased. Liver biopsy shows cholestasis in the liver cells and the bile canaliculi. There usually is a slight to moderate lymphocytic and eosinophilic cell response in the portal triads. Epidemiologic studies strongly suggest the increased incidence of inflammatory gallbladder disease after prolonged use of oral contraceptives.

Estrogens

Estrogen preparations came into use in the United States in the 1930s and were looked on by many menopausal women as the long-awaited "fountain of youth." Having drunk from the fountain, many of these women have had their enthusiasm dampened by the possibility of promotion of carcinoma of the endometrium. In predisposed women, the unopposed action of estrogenic substances, exogenous or endogenous, results in adenomatous hyperplasia, atypical hyperplasia, and adenocarcinoma of the endometrium. In menopausal and postmenopausal women, conjugated estrogenic preparations are effective in modifying menopausal symptoms including vasomotor instability (hot flashes, hot flushes), atrophy of the reproductive tract, and immediate postmenopausal osteoporosis.

Characteristic vaginal or cervical neoplasms designated as clear cell carcinoma may develop in women who have been exposed to diethylstilbestrol (DES) in utero. More commonly observed changes are cervical erosion, transverse ridges of the uterine cervix and upper vagina that may constitute the cervical or vaginal hood, a pseudopolypoid appearance of the uterine cervix, the so-called cockscomb cervix, and the changes that are designated as adenosis. The cellular detection of vaginal adenosis consists in the demonstration of columnar cells resembling those of the endocervix and metaplastic squamous cells. Cytologic examination of young girls or women with vaginal adenosis does not demonstrate sufficient atypicalities to suggest adenosis as a premalignant lesion. From 1948 to 1970, DES was used for threatened abortion. It was estimated that 10,000 to 16,000 females born between 1960 and 1970 are now at risk. In 85% of cases of vaginal and clear cell adenocarcinoma there is a history of maternal estrogen ingestion before the fourth month of pregnancy. Some 30% of young women whose mothers had estrogen during pregnancy have some vaginal lesion—partial strictures, firm ridges, or histologically confirmed adenosis. The investigation of these lesions and the relationship to adenocarcinoma of the vagina is a matter of urgency (see also p. 1641).

Tranquilizers

Chlorpromazine (Thorazine) is a phenothiazine that may produce intrahepatic cholestasis with or without accompanying changes of hepatitis. Various reports estimate that the incidence of cholestatic jaundice in patients receiving chlorpromazine ranges from less than 0.2% to 4%. The basic disorder of centrilobular cholestasis is postulated to be a disturbance of the biliary secretion of the micelles of bile salts, mixed with other biliary solids. Bile canaliculi and ductules are dilated and contain precipitated bile, referred to as bile plugs or thrombi. Bile canalicular microvilli are absent, distorted, or bleblike. The Golgi apparatus is enlarged, and conspicuous hypertrophic smooth endoplasmic reticulum is observed.

Chlorpromazine and other amine salts cause precipitation of bile salts, thus interfering with micelle formation and bile secretion. The cholestasis may persist for weeks or months. This may depend, in part, on the fact that retained bile salts interfere with the transformation of cholesterol to bile salts because of reduced hydroxylation. Subsequently, secretion of bile salt micelles is blocked, and this further leads to centrilobular cholestasis, creating a vicious circle. Severe and prolonged intrahepatic cholestasis results in more pronounced cellular changes and the appearance of inflammation. The hepatocytes become swollen, vacuolated, and feathery, as observed with the light microscope. Some liver cells have disappeared, and focal inflammatory exudate is seen in the vicinity of cellular disruption. Kupffer cells become prominent because of "stuffing" with bile pigment. This reactive cholestatic hepatitis is accompanied by cellular inflammation in the portal tracts. The cellular response is frequently composed of lymphocytes, plasma cells, and varying numbers of eosinophilic granulocytes. The observation of numerous eosinophilic leukocytes in the portal areas reveals a possible hypersensitivity mechanism. This is particularly significant when coupled with the clinical triad of blood eosinophilia, allergic rashes, and joint pains.

It appears that prolonged intraductal cholestasis itself may initiate the presence of lymphocytes in the portal areas, as well as ductular proliferation. The histopathologic distinction from mild viral hepatitis, with or without jaundice, may be impossible without relying on clinical information (such as epidemiologic history) or the results of a diagnostic virologic procedure. Although mild portal fibrosis may develop, clinical cirrhosis probably does not appear. From the laboratory standpoint, there is a serum increase in direct-reacting and indirect-reacting bilirubin. A rise in blood cholesterol, bile acids, and alpha and beta lipoproteins, as well as the activity of alkaline phosphatase enzymes, is the rule. Some believe that the drug or its metabolites acting in the role of hapten bring about the formation of antibodies, which are then believed to remain attached to the hepatocytes. On further administration of the drug, an antigen-antibody reaction occurs on the surface of the cells, leading to cytotoxic damage. Interestingly, a prolonged increase in the serum alkaline phosphatase level may be the only laboratory indication of hepatotoxicity.

Morphologic evidence of myocardial damage characterized by myofibrillar degeneration and some instances of necrosis has been found after chlorpromazine therapy. Focal interstitial myocarditis in association with chlorpromazine therapy is also documented.

Phenothiazines, notably chlorpromazine, may cause gynecomastia and galactorrhea. Several other medicinal compounds are likewise responsible for these findings, that is, spironolactone, reserpine, isoniazid, and those used in carcinoma of the prostate and in prolonged digitalis therapy and estrogen administration.

Antihypertensive drugs

Methyldopa (Aldomet) evokes an acute hypersensitivity reaction in approximately 3% of patients. Manifestations of this include acute colitis and granulocytopenia with thrombocytopenia. An autoimmune hemolytic anemia may occur. This is accompanied by the presence of antinuclear antibodies and lupus erythematosus phenomena, positive results of a rheumatoid arthritis test, and a not-infrequent elevation of the serum immunoglobin levels. Hypersensitivity myocarditis, rich in eosinophils, has been documented. Of the drugs that have been implicated as causing hypersensitivity myocarditis with sudden unexpected death, methyldopa leads the field. In recent years, this drug has been replaced by other antihypertensive medicinals, such as β-adrenergic receptor blockers, calcium-channel blockers, and angiotensin-converting enzyme inhibitors. Sulfonamide and sulfonamide derivatives have been closely linked to the development of hypersensitivity myocarditis. Unexpected fatal hypersensitivity myocarditis is uncommonly observed in hospital and forensic deaths. It is noteworthy that in numerous instances of death from methyldopa myocarditis the patient was also receiving hydrochlorothiazide. Penicillin and its synthetic counterparts are notorious for giving rise to both reversible and irreversible hypersensitivity myocarditis. One of the most notable adverse tissue reactions to methyldopa is acute diffuse and spotty hepatitis that is indistinguishable clinically and histologically from the usual viral hepatitis. Most of these reactions are mild and reversible. Occasionally, however, an autoimmune phenomenon appears to supervene so that chronic active hepatitis is observed. In this situation various degrees of hepatocellular necrosis may occur, and the eventu-

ality is a mixed macronodular and micronodular cirrhosis. Granulomatous hepatitis characterized by fever, eosinophilia, and a slight elevation of serum alkaline phosphatase levels may be detected. The granulomas in this instance are similar to those of other drug-induced granulomatous hepatitis in that they are noncaseous and may be situated in both the portal and the lobular areas of the liver. On discontinuation of the drug, the lesions rapidly disappear, leaving no residua.

Hydralazine (Apresoline) is a monoamine oxidase (MAO) inhibitor. The mechanism of its hypotensive action is intensification of beta-sympathomimetic effects rather than sympathoplegic. Hydralazine is not a powerful hypotensive agent. In some instances, indiscriminate administration of this compound gives rise to an end-stage chronic interstitial pulmonary fibrosis similar to that produced by the ganglion-blocking agents. The pathogenesis of the lesion is still unsettled. It is probable that the fibrosis is the terminal event in a series of episodes of hypersensitivity alveolitis with necrosis of bronchioloalveolar epithelium and intra-alveolar capillary thrombosis of the septa. In approximately 10% of patients receiving hydralazine, symptoms of peripheral neuritis that are responsive to pyridoxine develop.

Hydralazine is known to cause a clinical syndrome identical to that of classic systemic lupus erythematosus. The manifestations are protean and include arthritis, fever, skin rashes, and myalgia. The LE phenomenon is observed in the blood. The pathologic findings are the same as those of classic systemic lupus erythematosus in which there has been no history of causative medication. One difference, however, is the reversibility of the hydralazine syndrome when the inciting drug is discontinued.

Propranolol, a prototype of the β-adrenergic receptor blockers, has unquestionably been associated with the development of sclerosing peritonitis in man and animals. The exact cause, as with methysergide, is not clear. Whether the mechanism encompasses some altered immune response or is the result of the drug on the vasculature leading to vasoconstriction is not clear.

Epidemiologic studies have implicated reserpine (*Rauwolfia* alkaloids) in the development of human mammary carcinoma. Whether the mechanism is mediated by causing elevation of the serum prolactin level is not certain.

Sympathomimetic amines
Amphetamines

The amphetamines have medical applications in patients with severe hypotension and poisoning by central nervous system depressants. Under the Controlled Substances Act, the amphetamines fit into Schedule II. That is, they are looked upon as drugs with a high potential for abuse with severe liability to cause psychic or physical dependence. Of the entire group of sympathomimetic amines, the amphetamines and methamphetamines stand out as being most conspicuous in drug abuse. Toxic doses of amphetamines and methamphetamines when consumed by persons with hypertension or elevated ethanol levels are extremely dangerous. Within the framework of this background of drug abuse, amphetamine has been shown to initiate necrotizing angiitis with subsequent brain hematomas and subarachnoid hemorrhage, leading to permanent paralysis, coma, and in some instances death. The histologic appearance of this angiitis are reminiscent of the lesion seen in classical periarteritis nodosa.

Diuretics

Among the most effective of the diuretic drugs are the thiazides, with chlorothiazide serving as a prototype of the group. Pharmacologic adverse reactions include hypokalemia, hyperuricemia, and hyperglycemia. Toxic and hypersensitivity responses are manifested by skin rashes, agranulocytosis, and acute pancreatitis. Acute diffuse and spotty hepatitis and cholestatic hepatitis are uncommonly observed.

Furosemide possesses a structural configuration similar to that of chlorothiazide; therefore it is no surprise to learn that it likewise causes acute pancreatitis. At postmortem examination, inspissated mucus secretion is observed in the ductular lumens.

Hypersensitivity reaction to diuretics, if indeed they do occur, are of minimal importance. The potassium-sparing diuretic spironolactone may induce gynecomastia in males. There is no hard evidence incriminating spironolactone as a tumor-inducing agent.

Antithyroid drugs

Thiouracil and iodine compounds are frequently noted as a cause of hypersensitivity vasculitis (angiitis). As with many other drugs, notably penicillin, sulfonamides, and phenylbutazone, an acute or chronic vasculitis may emerge after therapy. If, after removal of the compound, the vasculitis persists for a long period of time, the drug should not be implicated as the source of the antigenic stimulus. Experimental findings do not point to any evidence that a brief exposure to an antigen can produce a chronic vasculitis in which fresh (acute) lesions appear many months after the immunologic stimulus is removed. Although not clear cut, it is feasible that a medicinal drug may bring about an autoimmune vasculitis of protracted nature.

Antidiabetic drugs—oral hypoglycemic agents

Prominent among the oral hypoglycemic compounds in general use are tolbutamide (Orinase), chlorpropamide (Diabinese), and phenformin (DPI). Of these, chlorpropamide evokes reactions with frequency of approximately 5%. The reactions are mainly cholestatic hepatitis similar to the changes occurring after hyper-

sensitivity reactions to the tranquilizers. Phenformin therapy has been associated with irreversible lactic acidosis in individuals with histories of renal disease and infection.

Patients receiving sulfonylurea therapy respond with some interesting islet cell changes. The maturity-onset diabetic subject usually has an increase in the number and size of the islets. Cytologically, the most striking finding is hyperplasia and new formation of the islets of Langerhans with a reduction in the percentage of beta cells and an increase in alpha cells. A further observation in this group of patients is the appearance of islet cell adenomas. Morphologic changes in the islets in patients treated with sulfonylureas are in need of further observation.

H₂ receptor antagonists

Cimetidine (Tagamet) is a potent antagonist of the H_2 receptors that exist in many cell types. Cimetidine is used to inhibit gastric acid secretion in diseases such as duodenal ulcer (short-term and maintenance therapy), Zollinger-Ellison syndrome, and other gastric hypersecretory states. The incidence of serious adverse tissue reactions to cimetidine is far less than 1%. A bothersome complication of the therapy is the appearance of gynecomastia, which is usually florid and which disappears after cessation of therapy in most cases. The gynecomastia is commonly bilateral, and the causative mechanism is unknown. In rare cases, renal adverse tissue reactions may occur in the form of acute interstitial nephritis. The renal biopsy reveals interstitial foci of lymphocytes, plasma cells, and abundant eosinophils. Destruction of the tubular basement membranes may occur as part of this hypersensitivity reaction. No chronic renal disease has resulted from the acute insult. Acute diffuse hepatitis is an additional hypersensitivity reaction to cimetidine. No instances of "chronic active" hepatitis or cirrhosis have been documented. Currently there is no convincing evidence that cimetidine is carcinogenic.

Antitubercular drugs

Isoniazid and rifampin are agents widely used in the prophylaxis and treatment of tuberculosis. Para-aminosalicylic acid is not as widely used, and it is associated with a greater incidence of hepatitis and hepatic necrosis than the other antitubercular agents are (Fig. 4-9).

Isoniazid. Isoniazid (INH, Rimifon) is metabolized by the liver by an acetylation pathway, producing innocuous metabolites. As a result of arylating and acrylating pathways, however, a metabolite known as acetylhydrazine is formed. It is this metabolite that probably brings about damage of the hepatocytes in the small percentage (1% to 2%) of people who are genetically predisposed to this damage. It may be postulated that, after the damage, a hypersensitivity state ensues that is re-

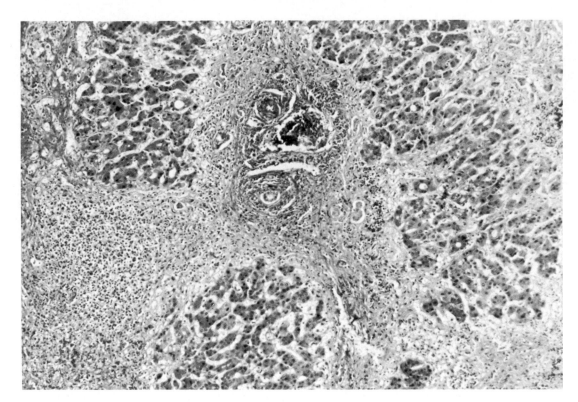

Fig. 4-9. INH hepatitis. Cells of peripheral lobules have disappeared and are replaced by condensed reticulum and lymphocytes. This may be impossible to distinguish from viral hepatitis.

sponsible for the hepatitis and, in rare instances, necrosis of the liver. Fifty percent of whites are slow acetylaters, and this group is prone to the development of autoimmune reactions characterized by the LE phenomenon. After cessation of the drug, all the clinical and serologic features of this phenomenon usually disappear rapidly, but in a few instances the time interval is prolonged over months. Whether it is advantageous to be a slow or a fast acetylater is controversial.

Isoniazid is similar to methyldopa, chlorpromazine, and halothane in that an increasing number of reports point to the occurrence of chronic active hepatitis, in some instances leading to cirrhosis. It is noteworthy that the morphologic changes induced by isoniazid may be identical to those of viral acute spotty hepatitis, as well as virus-initiated chronic active hepatitis and massive necrosis. Any drug- or virus-induced chronic active hepatitis may lead to cirrhosis. In INH-associated chronic active hepatitis the portal areas may contain numerous plasma cells, particularly in patients showing the concomitant LE phenomenon. The onset of clinical signs and symptoms of INH hepatitis usually occurs in the first 2 months of prophylactic or preventive therapy. Onset after 8 to 10 weeks is usually more severe. The hepatitis is also more severe in the older age groups and in black women, again suggestive of a genetic influence. Isoniazid, on infrequent occasions, may

be accountable for the appearance of numerous granulomatous lesions scattered throughout the left and right ventricular myocardium but particularly concentrated in the former. The majority of other drug-induced lesions are reversible when the drug is discontinued, and there are reports in the literature of cardiac cardiomyopathy with focal fibrosis after drug-induced hypersensitivity myocarditis.

Rifampin. Rifampin (Rifadin, Rimactane), a semisynthetic antibiotic that is derived from *Streptomyces mediterranei* and is similar to isoniazid, may cause transient abnormalities in liver function test results and, rarely, fatal hepatitis. It reduces or abolishes the tuberculin reaction in guinea pigs infected with tubercle bacilli. Likewise, in humans there is a strong suggestion that rifampin may suppress cell-mediated immunity as manifested by delayed cutaneous hypersensitivity to purified protein derivative of *Mycobacterium tuberculosis*. It also inhibits in vitro lymphoblast transformation in both phytohemagglutinin and purified protein derivative. Rifampin or its metabolite desacetylrifampicin may elicit a type II cytotoxic allergic reaction, based on the observation that in some cases antigen-antibody complexes are formed in the serum and attach to the cell surface of the erythrocyte, resulting in lysis. In patients demonstrating this hemolytic reaction, indirect Coombs' test results are positive in the presence of the drug. As in isoniazid therapy, acute spotty hepatitis with portal inflammatory infiltrate, rich in eosinophils, lymphocytes, and a few macrophages, and accompanied by focal intralobular necrosis, may be observed. In combined tuberculostatic therapy with rifampin and isoniazid, liver injuries are more severe than in monotherapy with either isoniazid or rifampin. Rifampin may interfere with bilirubin metabolism by impairment of transport of the unconjugated form from the sinusoid through the hepatocyte plasma membranes or by inhibiting the excretion of conjugated bilirubin. Interference with bile flow as manifested by rifampin has been attributed to a variety of mechanisms. These include disturbance of bile flow because of a lack of cellular ATP, injury to the hepatocellular membranes, impairment of bile salt–dependent flow by blocking the synthesis of bile acids or their transcanalicular transport, impairment of bile salt–independent flow by inhibition of sodium and potassium ATPase, intereference with the formation of normal micelles in the bile, and excessive reabsorption of water and electrolytes by the lining cells of the ductules.

Rifampin, being an enzyme inductor, results in a high level of the cytotoxic metabolite isoniazid acetylhydrazine. Although its exact mechanism of action has not been defined, rifampin is known to inhibit DNA-directed RNA synthesis, probably by interfering with the activity of RNA polymerase. Unlike isoniazid, rifampin is a powerful stimulator of the activity of drug-metabolizing enzymes of the human liver microsomes. Acute interstitial nephritis characterized by oliguria and rising BUN levels has been attributed to rifampin as an altered immune response to the drug or its metabolites. On cessation of the drug, the signs and symptoms disappear rapidly, and there is no evidence that irreversible damage to the interstitium of the kidney or the tubules has occurred.

Anesthetics

Halothane. There is little question that halothane is capable of causing a variety of morphologic types of hepatitis, including (1) acute diffuse and spotty hepatitis, (2) persistent hepatitis, (3) chronic active hepatitis, and (4) acute and subacute massive necrosis. The majority of hepatic reactions to halothane are either acute diffuse spotty hepatitis or persistent hepatitis. Massive necrosis is rare. These reactions depend on the appearance of the altered immune response in the patient, who has almost invariably received more than one dose of this quite safe anesthetic. Clinical and laboratory evidence of the altered immune reaction includes blood eosinophilia, low-grade fever, arthralgia, and rash. Recrudescence of halothane hypersensitivity follows rechallenge with the drug. The appearance of antimitochondrial antibodies and positive results of a lymphocyte transformation test have been observed in a significant number of cases. The exact location of halothane's effect on the hepatocyte remains unclear. Centrilobular fat accumulation, which commonly occurs in other direct toxic reactions, may be observed. The toxic reaction may bring about denatured proteins, to which the body now reacts unfavorably, and brings about many of the well-known altered immune reactions. Both the toxic reactions (if indeed they exist) and the hypersensitivity reactions are probably mediated at the hepatocyte cell membrane level. Histologically, the hepatic lesions are indistinguishable from those occurring in the many morphologic variations of viral hepatitis. Not infrequently, a plethora of eosinophils and noncaseous granuloma formations in the portal tracts and the lobules is the morphologic indicator of the hypersensitivity mechanism. The ultrastructural changes after halothane administration are nonspecific and include swelling of the mitochondria with crystalline inclusions and abnormal cristae and pronounced dilatation of both smooth and rough endoplasmic reticulum.

Methoxyflurane. Methoxyflurane, an excellent, non-explosive, fluorinated anesthetic agent, has occasionally been reported to produce liver injury. It may give rise to hepatitis identical to that caused by halothane, probably through the same mechanisms of action. Cross-sensitivity between the two agents has been observed. In addition to liver involvement, nephrotoxicity aimed primarily at the proximal convoluted tubules may develop. The degree of tubular dysfunction can be correlated with the dose of the anesthetic agent and its metabolites, inorganic fluoride and oxalic acid. Metabolically, methoxyflurane is readily defluorinated. The acute polyuria resulting from methoxyflurane administration is attributed to the effect of inorganic fluoride on the tubule. The amount of oxalic acid found in the kidney is probably not a significant factor in the development of the tubular lesion. In human cases of nephrotoxicity, light microscopic examination of the proximal convoluted tubules is unimpressive. It is characterized by some dilatation of the tubular lumen and flattening of the epithelium. Ultrastructurally, the mitochondria are swollen with disruption of their cristae, and they contain dense bodies (probably fluoride proteinate). The mechanism may be similar to the disturbance in oxidative phosphorylation observed in lead poisoning.

Anticonvulsants

Phenytoin. Of the anticonvulsants, phenytoin (Dilantin) appears to be the major compound eliciting adverse tissue reactions. Direct dose-related cytotoxicity has not been ascribed to phenytoin, nor has any toxic metabolite been identified. On the other hand, the altered hypersensitivity or altered immunologic responses of a human organism to phenytoin though uncommon, are protean. Foremost among these are the dermatologic reactions, which consist mainly in erythema multiforme and toxic epidermal necrolysis. Both of these are severe adverse reactions to the drug, and the mortality of toxic epidermal necrolysis has been reported to be approximately 25%. The histologic features of the epidermal form of erythema multiforme and toxic epidermal necrolysis reveal many similarities. There is eosinophilic necrosis of keratinocytes and hydropic degeneration of basal cells. Cleft formation at the dermal-epidermal junction follows necrosis of the basal cells. Pericapillary minimal infiltrates with lymphocytes are the rule. Occasionally thrombosis of the capillaries is observed. It is assumed that these two phenytoin-induced skin disorders are mediated through an immunologic cytotoxic mechanism.

Less frequently, hypersensitivity reactions are directed toward the kidney as acute interstitial nephritis accompanied by renal failure and peripheral eosinophilia. Renal dysfunction is promptly reversed after discontinuation of phenytoin administration. An interesting observation is the presentation of phenytoin-induced lymphadenopathy as clinical malignant lymphoma. The haptenic action of phenytoin may elicit any of the common immunologic responses known to exist. Circulating antibodies to phenytoin have been demonstrated. A lymph node may show a distortion of the architecture with lymphocyte hyperplasia, eosinophils, plasma cells, and necrosis. Large so-called histiocytic or reticulin cells are in evidence (Fig. 4-10). In other instances the enlarged lymph nodes may be characterized by the presence of numerous immunoblasts and endothelial proliferation of small blood vessels. This is referred to as angioimmunoblastic lymphadenopathy, and in some instances, it proceeds to the more serious condition of immunoblastic sarcoma. Finally, noncaseous granulomas, frequently accompanied by numerous eosinophils, may be noted.

Phenytoin is one of the drugs that has been identified as causing systemic hypersensitivity necrotizing angiitis. Disseminated granulomatous angiitis, in the absence of necrosis, may be reversible after withdrawal of phenytoin and the introduction of steroid therapy. In fatal cases of phenytoin allergic reactions, morphologic reflections of several of the basic altered immune responses may be present. On occasion, phenytoin may fire off an autoimmune response characterized by the LE phenomenon in the blood, hemolytic anemia, positive results of the indirect Coombs' test, antinuclear antibodies, and skin lesions, all of which are reminiscent of clinical disseminated lupus erythematosus. Withdrawal of the drug results in disappearance of the clinical and serologic manifestations. Phenytoin may invoke

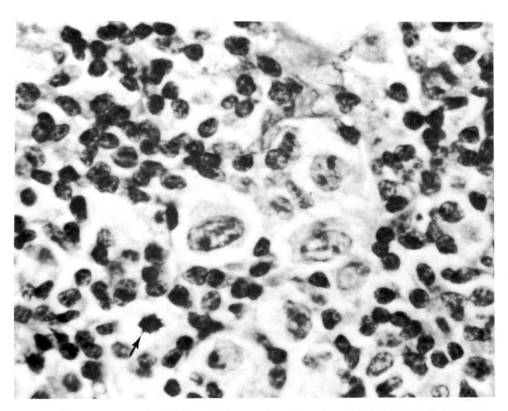

Fig. 4-10. Phenytoin (Dilantin) lymphadenopathy. Distortion of the normal cellular topography with replacement by numerous large cells (histiocytes, immunoblasts) with prominent nucleoli and mitoses (arrow) may lead to misdiagnosis of malignant lymphoma.

a microscopic appearance suggestive of Hodgkin's disease (Fig. 4-10). However, the Reed-Sternberg cells characteristic of Hodgkin's disease are not identified and, unlike Hodgkin's disease, the lymphadenopathy recedes after discontinuation of the drug. Nevertheless, an increasing number of reports suggest that long-term administration of phenytoin may give rise to Hodgkin's disease or non-Hodgkin's malignant lymphoma. Hepatic injury associated with phenytoin therapy reflects literally all the histologic features seen in viral hepatitis. The most common acute reaction is hepatocellular degeneration or necrosis, or both, with panlobular

"spotty" reaction. Hepatocellular and cholestatic injury may be displayed. Rarely, submassive and massive necrosis supervenes. Granulomatous hepatitis, with or without vasculitis, is one of the forms of hepatic injury. Phenytoin can cause megaloblastic anemia associated with low folate levels in the serum, red blood cells, and cerebrospinal fluid. There is a disturbance of cell utilization of folate by an as yet undetermined mechanism.

Gingival hyperplasia may promptly appear after phenytoin therapy is begun. After painless enlargement of the interdental papillae, the gingival surface becomes pebbled and lobulated (Fig. 4-11, A). Microscopically,

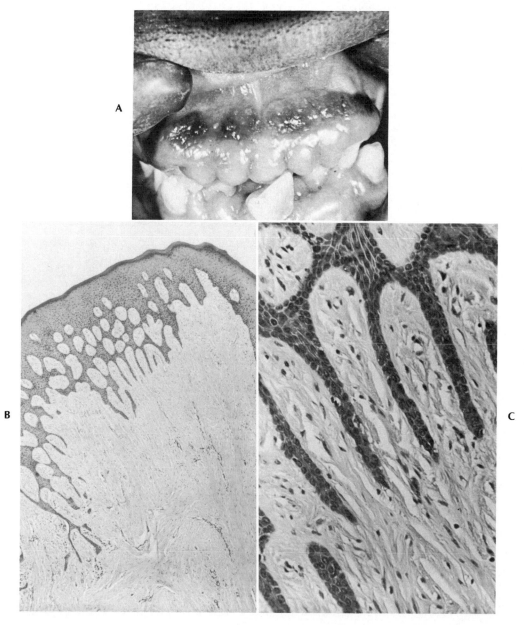

Fig. 4-11. A, Phenytoin (Dilantin) gingival hypertrophy. Prominent interdental papillae obscure teeth. **B** and **C,** Phenytoin gingival hypertrophy and hyperplasia characterized by penetrating rete pegs and fibrosis of submucosa. Relatively avascular connective tissue proliferation.

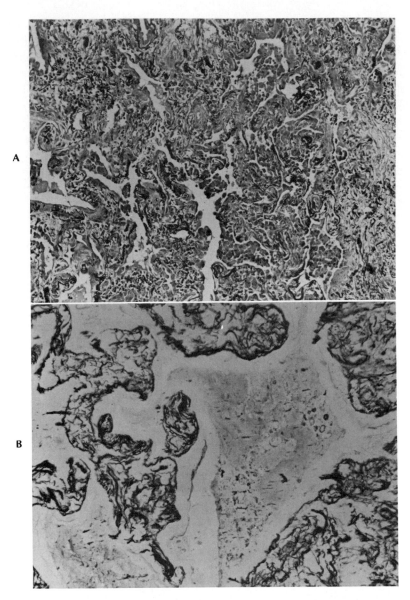

Fig. 4-12. A, Nitrofurantoin. Broad alveolar walls filled with lymphocytes, macrophages, and collagen severely constrict air spaces, which contain fibrin, desquamated macrophages, and pneumocytes. **B,** Reticulin stain emphasizes widened alveolar walls. Fibrin and cellular debris occupy terminal air spaces. (**A,** Hematoxylin and eosin, 250×; **B,** reticulin stain; 330×.)

the squamous epithelium projects down into the avascular hyperplastic connective tissue as prominent rete pegs (Fig. 4-11, *B* and *C*). Careful oral hygiene slows the hyperplastic process, but recurrence is common. Some anticonvulsants, including phenytoin, when administered to the mother during the first trimester of pregnancy, may result in congenital anomalies. These include cleft lip and palate and the fetal hydantoin syndrome. The latter shares with the fetal alcohol syndrome several anomalies, including ptosis, epicanthal folds, and flat nasal bridge.

Anti-infective agents

Nitrofurantoin. Nitrofurantoin (Furadantin, Macrodantin) is a synthetic antimicrobial agent used to treat urinary infections. It is primarily excreted by the kidney. This drug is a cause of acute pulmonary eosinophilia (Löffler's syndrome), which is characterized by blood eosinophilia and a variety of radiographic findings that were segmental fan-shaped infiltrations or, less commonly, a diffuse, small, nodular pattern. Microscopically, the alveolar walls are widened and the air spaces are filled with a fibrinous, nonhemorrhagic exudate containing macrophages, lymphocytes, and plasma cells. However, the preponderant cell in the inflammatory picture is the eosinophilic polymorphonuclear leukocyte. If the condition is recognized early and administration of the drug is discontinued, recovery is complete. If, however, the pulmonary damage is allowed to progress, a chronic eosinophilic pneumonia and a nonreversible, diffuse interstitial fibrosis may develop (Fig. 4-12). Nitrofurantoin-induced acute spotty and diffuse hepatitis has occurred concomitantly with eosinophilic pneumonia. Thus the single compound is focused on two target organs, and a patient with either organ involved should be tested for dysfunction of the other. In some instances, persistent therapy will bring about chronic active hepatitis.

Nitrofurantoin has been implicated in producing the clinical syndrome of lupus nephritis and the full-blown picture identical to disseminated lupus erythematosus. In the presence of chronic renal impairment, nitrofurantoin therapy may lead to peripheral axon degeneration, with resultant numbness and tingling of the extremities. Remyelination resulting from revision of the Schwann cells takes place after cessation of therapy.

Antiarrhythmics

Digitalis. Mixtures of steroid glycosides, all having the same effects on the heart, are present in at least 39 genera of the plant kingdom. The genus *Digitalis* is the common commercial source of the crude product, digitalis, as well as for the specific glycosides digoxin and digitoxin. Although the cardiac glycosides, in therapeutic doses, are valuable in the treatment of several heart diseases, in higher doses these agents are potent cardiac poisons. The immediate danger with digitalis poisoning is the production of fatal ventricular fibrillation.

Prolonged sublethal concentrations of the glycosides produce myocardial lesions, which have been described in humans and experimental animals. The histologic findings are focal necrosis, cellular infiltration, interstitial edema, fibrosis, and hyaline degeneration, these changes being especially prominent in the subendocardial region of the myocardium. Affected cardiac cells commonly show a loss of striations, fibrillar fraying, and pyknosis of nuclei. The coronary vessels remain patent. In dogs, ultrastructural changes become obvious in some cells within 2 hours after a toxic infusion of digoxin. These early changes consist in a degeneration of myofibrillar banding patterns and contracture band formation, intracellular edema, and clumping and margination of nuclear chromatin. The cardiac glycosides probably exert their beneficial effect on cardiac contractility by "facilitating" the handling of calcium by the sarcoplasmic reticulum, whereas the arrhythmic toxic effect is attributable to their inhibitory effect on sarcolemmal Na^+,K^+-activated ATPase (the sodium pump). The latter action produces potassium depletion, a situation frequently correlated with edema and myofibrillar degeneration. A severe interference with the normal cycle of intracellular flux of calcium between the sarcoplasmic reticulum and the myofilaments may also account for some of the lesions.

Gazes and associates[143] have drawn attention to profound venous engorgement of the small intestine with areas of mucosal hemorrhage in patients receiving high or toxic doses of digitalis (Fig. 4-13). This finding appeared particularly significant in patients who showed no evidence of congestive failure. The syndrome can be suspected when abdominal pain develops in a patient

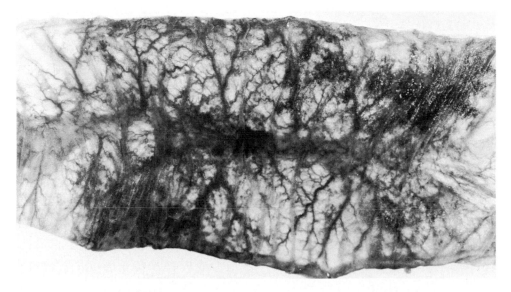

Fig. 4-13. Digitalization effect. Transilluminated segment of small intestine showing profound venous engorgement with areas of mucosal hemorrhage. (From Gazes, P.C., et al.: Circulation **23:**358, 1961; by permission of the American Heart Association, Inc.)

receiving large amounts of digitalis; unnecessary surgery thus may be avoided. Gazes and associates speculate that hepatic vein or sinusoid sphincter constriction with resultant portal splanchnic venous congestion is a possible mechanism by which digitalization produces this syndrome.

Digitalis therapy is occasionally associated with gynecomastia, the mechanism of which is not well understood. However, it may be attributed to the basic steroid structure of the digitalis glycosides. There is no accepted evidence of a relationship between digitalis therapy and breast cancer.

Quinidine. The antiarrhythmic quinidine in high therapeutic doses may be the cause of toxic myocarditis, characterized by myocytolysis and myocyte necrosis. The inflammatory response is characterized by lymphocyte infiltration, and evidence of a hypersensitivity reaction, such as eosinophils, plasma cells, giant cells, and granulomas, is absent.

Quinidine has been indicated in instances of mild granulomatous hepatitis characterized by a Kupffer cell hyperplasia and eosinophilia involving focal areas of lobules and portal tracts. The portal infiltrate is rich in eosinophils and plasma cells. Uncommonly, small noncaseating granulomas with giant cells are observed. As with most drugs that generate a granulomatous hepatitis, the lesions and abnormal liver function tests subside rather abruptly upon removal of the therapeutic drug involved.

Amiodarone. Amiodarone effect may be characterized by toxic macrovesicular fatty change in the hepatocytes resembling alcoholic hepatitis. Mallory bodies and polymorphonuclear leukocytes may be part of the acute inflammatory response. The administration of amiodarone may precipitate diffuse interstitial pneumonia. In such instances, the alveolar walls are widened by endothelial hyperplasia of capillaries, edema, and a mononuclear inflammatory response. Nuclear fragments and polymorphonuclear leukocytes are observed in the alveolar walls. Regenerating type II pneumocytes line the alveoli.

Oxygen

Respiratory therapy, using increased partial pressures of oxygen at sea level, as well as under hyperbaric conditions, is a vital constituent of modern medicine. Higher than normal atmospheric oxygen tensions at ambient as well as hyperbaric pressures are employed therapeutically in humans primarily in hypoxic states. However, oxygen must be employed with an understanding of its potential adverse effects. In humans these are primarily changes in the eyes of premature infants and in the lungs; however, experimental studies reveal that all organ systems, including the brain, heart, kidney, and liver, are at risk.

Biochemical data have shown that excessive oxygen inhibits many enzymes, including those involved in the Embden-Meyerhof pathway, the conversion of pyruvate to acetyl CoA, the tricarboxylic acid cycle, electron transport, synthesis of neurotransmitters, proteolysis, and membrane transport. Enzymes with essential sulfhydryl (SH) groups seem to be especially vulnerable. The biochemical mechanisms of oxygen toxicity are related to the metabolism of oxygen through free radical and hydroperoxide intermediates, a process that normally occurs in the cells and is accelerated on exposure to high oxygen tensions. This hypothesis is summarized in Fig. 4-14, *F*. The intermediate reactions in oxygen metabolism, through unknown mechanisms, induce lipid peroxidation. Lipid peroxides may disrupt membranes directly, oxidize SH groups, and shift the redox state of glutathione toward oxidation. The last results in the oxidation of pyridine nucleotides, which impairs energy production, leading, as does enzyme inhibition or disruption of membranes, to cell injury and eventual cell death. Hyperoxia may also directly inhibit RNA, DNA, and protein synthesis by free radical and hydroperoxide intermediates.

Pulmonary oxygen toxicity in the mature human lung is one of the many causes of diffuse alveolar damage (DAD), which begins with an exudative phase characterized by necrosis of epithelial and endothelial components of the alveolar wall, associated with pulmonary edema, congestion, fibrin deposition, and hemorrhage. The fibrin-rich inflammatory exudate leads to the formation of fibrin caps and, later, hyaline membranes (Fig. 4-14, *A*). The exudative changes are rapidly followed by proliferative alterations consisting in interstitial fibrosis, hyperplasia of the alveolar type II cells (granular pneumocytes), and organization and collagenosis (Fig. 4-14, *B*). Studies in a variety of experimental animals, as well as in humans, have shown that the exudative changes begin within 2 to 3 days of exposure to approximately 1 atmosphere absolute (ATA) of oxygen, and the proliferative changes are observed shortly thereafter. In human cases, interstitial fibrosis may appear after 3 days of oxygen therapy and become diffuse and severe by 1 to 2 weeks. Ultrastructural studies reveal that the initial changes in the lung consist of focal interstitial edema followed by swelling of endothelial and epithelial cells. After this, both endothelial and type I epithelial alveolar cells (membranous) become necrotic. The endothelial cells are more vulnerable than the alveolar pneumocytes. The sequence of events is summarized in Fig. 4-14, *C* to *E*.

With regard to the immature human lung, oxygen has been considered in the pathogenesis of the pathologic changes (hyaline membrane disease) associated with the idiopathic respiratory distress syndrome (IRDS) of premature infants. The IRDS begins before

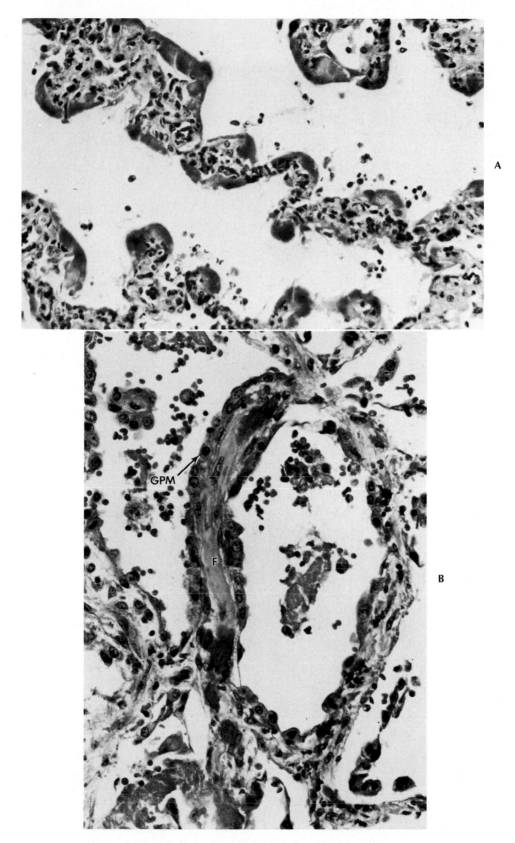

Fig. 4-14. A, Oxygen toxicity—early lesion. Fibrin "caps" adhere to surface of alveolar lining of epithelial cells. Alveolar capillaries show acute inflammatory reaction. **B,** Later lesion consists of thickened alveolar walls with fibrosis *(F)* and proliferative changes manifested by granular pneumocyte metaplasia *(GPM).* (**A,** 250×; **B,** hematoxylin and eosin, 300×; **C** to **E,** 2400×; **A, C,** and **E,** courtesy Dr. Robert M. Rosenbaum, Bronx, N.Y.; **B** and **F,** from Balentine, J.D.: Pathology of oxygen toxicity, New York, 1982, Academic Press, Inc.)   *Continued.*

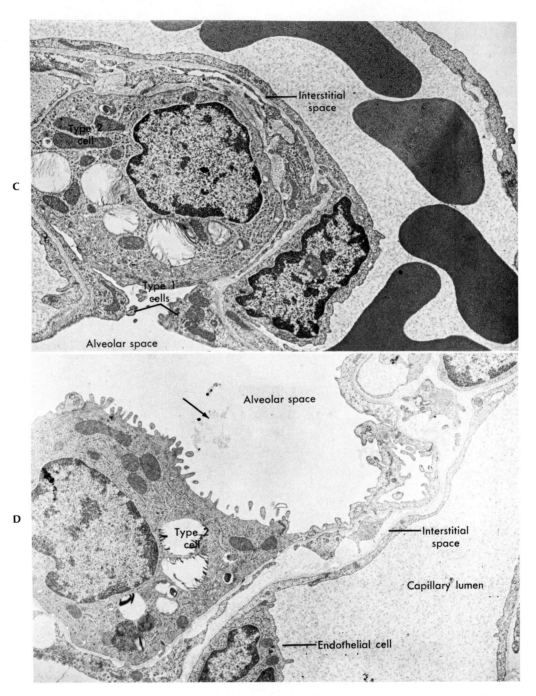

Fig. 4-14, cont'd. C, Normal rat lung—a type 2 cell is shown sunk beneath infolding of type 1 cells lining the alveolar space. Interstitital space is normal, is reduced in width, and contains some collagen bundles and fibroblasts. Fragments of fibroblasts appear in this section. **D,** Oxygen exposure (900 mm Hg), 24 hours—type 2 cell shown here is typically last affected by oxygen and remains so in a reversible lesion. Interstitital space is beginning to expand because of accumulation of edema fluid. Endothelial cell shows increased numbers of pinocytic vesicles but, as shown here, tight junctions remain intact. To right of type 2 cells (notice junction between the two) is a type 1 cell. This cell type responds to increased oxygen tension by surface blebbing and infolding before its death. The picture seen here continues to become more severe over the next 12 hours. *Arrow,* Tubular myelin fragments, possibly representing type 2 cell secretory material.

Continued.

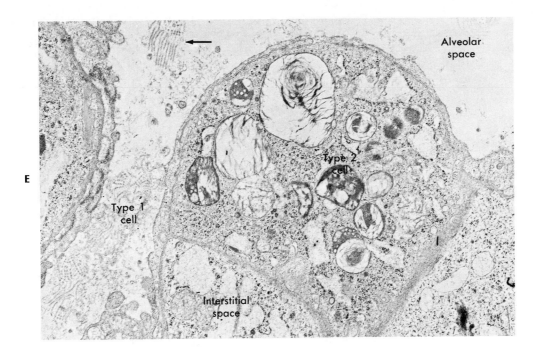

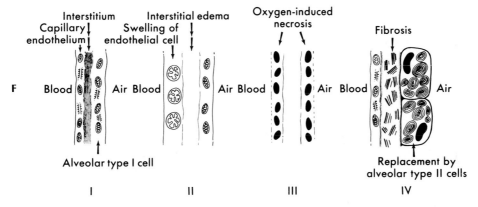

Fig. 4-14, cont'd. E, Oxygen exposure (900 mm Hg), 48 hours—this is an irreversible lesion caused by oxygen. Type 2 cell is relatively intact, but it contains numerous multivesicular bodies, many of which are closely associated with lamellar bodies. Under conditions of toxic Po_2 exposure these cells often hypersecrete. In alveolar space, numerous tubular myelin figures *(arrow)* offer additional evidence of such hypersecretion. In addition, alveolar space contains flocculent protein attributable presumably to capillary leakage. Remnants of endothelial cell on far left also have associated regions of fibrin accumulation. Several type 1 cells surround the central type 2 cell and, though they appear intact, show surface discontinuities and infolding indicative of early degenerative changes. The interstitial space is completely disrupted and contains cellular debris. **F,** Diagram of the changes occurring in experimentally induced hyperoxic DAD, progressing from the exudative *(II, III)* to the proliferative *(IV)*. The drawings represent a composite interpretation concerning the essential events in pulmonary oxygen toxicity. Initially *(II),* there is swelling of the interstitial space and capillary endothelium, emphasizing that the initial changes are related to the endothelial component of the air-blood barrier. Both membranous epithelial and capillary endothelial necrosis *(III)* ensue, however. The granular pneumocyte is a reserved repair cell and is relatively resistant to oxygen toxicity. The proliferative or reparative phase *(IV)* consists in interstitial fibrosis and replacement of the alveolar epithelium by alveolar type 2 cells (granular pneumocytes).

oxygen therapy, however, and it is clearly associated with biochemical immaturity of surfactant and morphologic immaturity of the lung. The IRDS is a disease entity related solely to factors involving the epithelial component of the air-blood barrier. Atelectasis is a prominent feature of the IRDS. Bronchopulmonary dysplasia is a chronic lung disease characterized by diffuse alveolar damage and obliterative bronchiolitis, attributed to prolonged oxygen therapy for the IRDS.

Acute central nervous system oxygen toxicity is manifested by grand mal epileptic convulsions in humans. In experimental adult animals, repeated exposure to hyperbaric oxygen results in paralysis and selective necrosis of neurons and gray matter. Prolonged exposure of neonatal animals to oxygen at or near 1 ATA inhibits RNA, DNA, and protein synthesis in the brain. Recent reports suggest that certain types of neuropathologic lesions (such as periventricular leukomalacia and pontosubicular necrosis) occurring in the brains of premature human infants suffering from hypoxia may be the result of oxygen therapy.

It has been established in humans and experimental animals that, during hyperoxic exposure, immature developing retinal vessels become necrotic and obliterated. This is followed by a proliferative reparative response resulting in the growth of new blood vessels, mesenchymal and glial cells from the inner retina extending into the vitreous. As the growth of this regenerative tissue progresses, the retina is detached, leading to blindness. The retinal response to hyperoxic exposure that occurs in premature infants is known as retrolental fibroplasia and was formerly referred to as the retinopathy of prematurity.

Antineoplastic and immunosuppressive agents

Alkylating agents. The more commonly used alkylating agents include the nitrogen mustards, chlorambucil, cyclophosphamide (Cytoxan), busulfan (Myleran), triethylenethiophosphoramide (thio-TEPA), triethylenemelamine (TEM), and mitomycin C. Although they differ in action, all have the capacity of replacing hydrogen atom with alkyl radicals (aliphatic hydrocarbons deprived of an H atom). They inhibit DNA synthesis, but the effect on RNA synthesis is less pronounced. The alkylating agents readily penetrate the cell walls and interfere with many enzymatic reactions, inhibit phosphorylation of ATP, glycolysis, respiration, protein synthesis, and mitosis, and, in addition to producing mutations, cause breaks in chromosomes and irregular accumulation of chromatin in proliferating cells (Fig. 4-15). A striking clinical improvement in patients with Burkitt's lymphoma and some forms of large cell non-Hodgkin's lymphoma may follow a single dose of cyclophosphamide.

The alkylating agents can initiate and enhance malignant tumor growth and suppress immune responses. The latter effect is characteristic of many antitumor agents. Of the group of alkylating agents, cyclophosphamide is the most widely used for immune response suppression. In experimental animals, particularly guinea pigs, suppression of antibody production is most evident if the agent is administered just before and immediately after introduction of the antigen. There is extensive lysis of small and large lymphocytes, but the cells of the reticuloendothelial system are not particularly affected.

Alkylating agents and antifolates cause epithelial atypias of the urogenital tract. The extent of the atypia correlates with the total dosage and duration of therapy. The epithelial abnormalities may persist for a long period after cessation of therapy. Cyclophosphamide, busulfan, thio-TEPA, and chlorambucil cause epithelial atypia and cytomegaly in a variety of epithelial surfaces, but particularly in the lungs, urinary tract, and cervix (Fig. 4-15, A). Type 2 alveolar cells develop strongly acidophilic cytoplasm, which is increased in amount (Fig. 4-15, B). The nuclei are arrested during the process of DNA synthesis and are converted to grotesque, shapeless masses of condensed chromatin. Mitoses are absent (Fig. 4-15, A). Ultrastructurally, an interesting observation is the finding of abundant intranuclear tubular structures in type 2 alveolar pneumocytes. This is probably the result of interaction of the drug with perichromatin (Fig. 4-15, C). Severe lung damage by the alkylating agent leads to diffuse interstitial fibrosis, with all the gross and microscopic characteristics of the "honey-comb" lung. Recent observations raise the possibility that the alkylating agents may actually generate the development of malignancies.

Bleomycin, unlike other antibiotic members of its class, seldom causes stem cell suppression of bone marrow elements. Like busulfan, it causes degeneration and necrosis of type 1 pulmonary alveolar and endothelial cells, with subsequent exudative alveolitis and eventual alveolar fibrosis. Regeneration by type 2 pneumocytes is reminiscent of that seen in the lung affected by busulfan (Fig. 4-15, A and B). Bleomycin does not affect as wide a variety of epithelial tissues as busulfan. For example, the uroepithelium is not affected.

Cyclophosphamide gives rise to acute myocardial changes, particularly if high dose levels are attained. The cardiac damage occurs in a matter of 2 to 5 days. The gross and microscopic features of the myocardial damage are shared by cyclophosphamide, the anthracycline antibiotics (see the following discussion), and the sympathetic catecholamines (norepinephrine). The endocardium, myocardium, and epicardium of the left ventricle, interventricular septum, and papillary muscles reveal toxic myocarditis as shown by the presence of myocytolysis and myocyte necrosis. Focal necrosis or

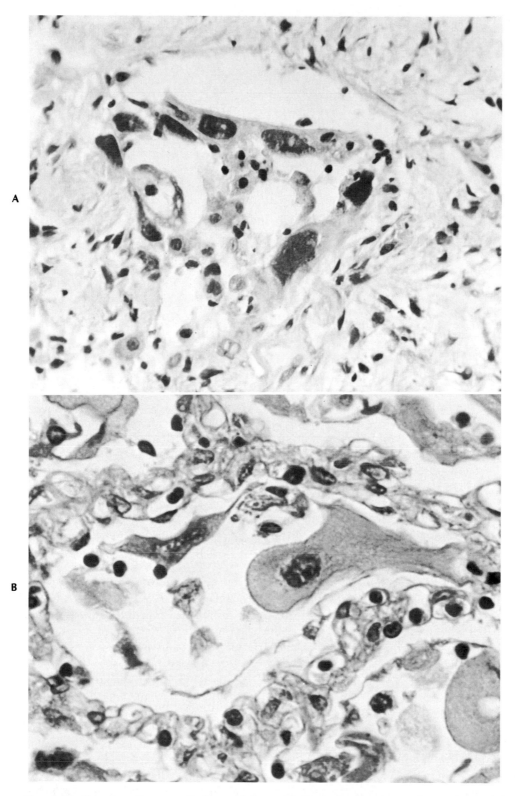

Fig. 4-15. Busulfan therapy. **A,** Bronchiolar epithelium showing hyperchromatic nuclei composed of condensed chromatin leading to bizarre nuclear contours. Nuclear fragments in evidence. **B,** This cytologic picture is reminiscent of radiation effect. Several large bronchioloalveolar cells have desquamated into air sac. Nuclear membrane of largest cell is fragmented.   *Continued.*

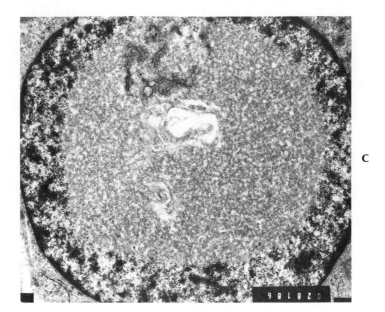

Fig. 4-15, cont'd. C, Type 2 pneumocyte from busulfan lung. Large numbers of curves, interwoven tubular structures, devoid of chromatinic DNA, fill the nucleus (**C** 32,500×; from Györkey, F., Györkey, P., and Sinkovics, J.G.: Ultrastruc. Pathol. **1:** 217, 1980.)

mini-infarcts are observed throughout the myocardium of the left side. The mini-infarcts result from capillary microthrombosis. Examination of the left ventricle also reveals small, focal subendocardial and intramyocardial hemorrhages. Ultrastructural studies of the lesions reveal endothelial damage with prominent thick and thin filaments in both the myocyte and the endothelial cell nuclei.

Small muscular arteries, capillaries, and venules reveal necrosis, hemorrhages, and fibrin deposition. As a result of high-dose cyclophosphamide therapy, the gross appearances of the urinary bladder reveal acute changes consisting of a diffusely hemorrhagic and focally ulcerated mucosa. As pointed out by Slavin, the mucosa is thrown up into multiple coarse folds. In the very high dose, patients' damage has been discovered to involve the entire wall of the urinary bladder. Extensive fibrosis of the wall of the bladder observed in children does not appear to be present in the adults.

Nitrogen mustard was one of the early antitumor agents to be given extensive clinical trial, specifically for the treatment of Hodgkin's disease. It quickly became apparent to pathologists that the cellular effects of the compound were bizarre and profound. The familiar and classic histologic features of Hodgkin's granuloma (Reed-Sternberg cells with "owl's-eye," reticulum cells, eosinophils, and lymphocyte hyperplasia) were converted to a bizarre conglomeration of cells with large, hyperchromatic pyknotic nuclei and increased chromatin content. In other words, the cellular pattern became more pleomorphic and malignant in cytologic appearance. These changes are reminiscent of cellular radia-

tion effect. With the development of additional alkylating agents, cellular changes similar to those observed after nitrogen mustard therapy appeared. The pathologist interpreting a "treated node" may be misled if he or she is unaware of this fact. The histologic appearance of a Hodgkin's granuloma may be converted into a false appearance of Hodgkin's sarcoma (reticulum cell sarcoma), a lesion of more serious prognostic import.

The role of nitrogen mustard therapy as a cause of the elaboration and deposition of amyloid in patients with malignant lymphoma is a controversial issue. Certainly, in untreated persons with malignant lymphoma, particularly Hodgkin's disease, generalized amyloidosis has been observed. In mice receiving casein injections with nitrogen mustard, there appears to be an acceleration in the deposition of amyloid. Whether the latter result can be extrapolated to humans is problematic.

Cyclosporin. Cyclosporin is a potent immunosuppressive drug that selectively inhibits T-cell function, permitting the survival of allografts without myelosuppression. Its advantage is that it lessens the numerous adverse effects of long-term steroid therapy. On the other hand, the benefits of its ability to suppress the immune response is clouded by its nephrotoxicity effects. These effects are those of a direct toxic reaction on the tubular epithelium, particularly the proximal and straight tubules. Characteristic, but not pathognomonic, degenerative changes are vacuolization and the presence of giant mitochondria. These are common in experimental animals but unusual in human tissue. In the final analysis it is not certain how the kidney handles the drug. Until a completely satisfactory animal model is developed, clarification will probably not be forthcoming. When cyclosporin A is prescribed during the rejection episodes, the pathologist frequently observes varying degrees of severity of acute tubulointerstitial nephritis, characterized by the presence of lymphocytes, tubular degeneration, and focal necrosis. It is of interest that in patients treated with steroids and other immunosuppressive agents, the lymphocytes, numerous plasma cells, and eosinophils characterize the inflammatory response. Successful cyclosporin A therapy alone reveals solely an interstitial lymphocyte population. Lymphocytes are found within the tubular cell cytoplasm demonstrating cytotoxic action. A great difficulty confronting the morphologist is the interpretation of the patient's kidney that is in the stage of chronic rejection. In this instance, one finds endothelial and intimal hyperplasia of the small arteries, interstitial fibrosis, tubular dilatation, and atrophy of the tubules. At the same time, one still has to consider the probability that these histologic characteristics may be shared by the cyclosporin tubular toxicity and chronic rejection.

Anthracycline antibiotics. Two important members of the anthracycline antibiotics group are daunorubicin (daunomycin) and doxorubicin (adriamycin), antineoplastic antibiotics that are effective in the treatment of acute leukemias in humans. The cardiotoxic effects of long-term therapy with daunorubicin and doxorubicin comprise a variety of histopathologic lesions consisting of myocytes characterized by the development of myeloid bodies, which is frequently observed in toxic cell damage. There is myofibril loss within the myocyte; the nucleus is frequently intact, and the mitochondria contain their compact cristae. With a high cumulative dose, one may observe myocyte necrosis, which progresses to interstitial fibrosis. Inflammatory cells are not a feature of chronic anthracycline cardiotoxicity. Reactive vascular lesions have not been described after therapeutic doses. The earliest lesions are to be found predominantly in the subendocardium and the ventricular trabeculas.

Antimetabolites. The antimetabolites include compounds that are folic acid and purine antagonists. Methotrexate (Amethopterin) acts by inhibition of folic acid reductase. The inhibition of dihydrofolate reductase blocks the conversion of folic acid to tetrahydrofolic acid, which is essential for the synthesis of DNA, RNA, and purine-containing coenzymes. The folic acid antagonists exert profound mitotic arrest. 6-Mercaptopurine acts by inhibition of de novo purine synthesis. Azathioprine (Imuran) is 6-mercaptopurine modified by the addition of an imidazole ring. This compound enjoys current clinical popularity. The synthesis of IgG is inhibited more readily by 6-mercaptopurine than is the synthesis of IgM. Both 6-mercaptopurine and azathioprine may prolong allograft survival and "stunt" the delayed hypersensitivity reaction.

Prolonged administration of azathioprine in renal transplant recipients has led to the appearance of large cell non-Hodgkin's lymphoma involving several organs of the body, including the lungs and meninges. The appearance of peliosis hepatis ("livid spots") in these patients is well documented (Fig. 4-16). Peliosis hepatis gives rise to hepatic dysfunction and, if extensive, even to portal hypertension and ascites. Bone marrow depression, usually leukopenia, has been the most common manifestation of azathioprine therapy.

Methotrexate is a derivative of aminopterin and circulates in the blood bound to plasma albumin. Approximately 80% is excreted unchanged in the urine within 12 hours after administration. Its use in patients with any degree of renal impairment is contraindicated, and this precludes its employment as an immunosuppressant in kidney transplant procedures. Most cancer chemotherapists agree that it is essential to administer doses that produce some degree of measurable host effect (toxicity) to achieve maximum response. The major toxic manifestations of methotrexate relate to cells with a high mitotic index, such as those found in the bone marrow, intestinal crypts, and hair follicles. Anemia, granulocytopenia, and thrombocytopenia may occur after long-term administration.

The extreme responsiveness of erythropoiesis to methotrexate probably depends on the observation that the turnover of erythroid precursors is more rapid than that of granulocytic elements. Bone marrow megaloblastosis of the red blood cell series may appear in patients receiving methotrexate. When given to patients with certain deficiency states, antimetabolites bring about selective decrease of DNA biosynthesis. Hence, the morphologic change may be attributed to continued protein and RNA synthesis in the face of arrested DNA synthesis. Methotrexate causes a decrease in the mitotic activity of immature proliferating granulocytes, which results in granulocytopenia. The danger of the development of severe infections and septicemia is obvious. By a similar mechanism, thrombocytopenia may develop, giving rise to severe hemorrhages. Ulcerations of the buccal mucosa and gastrointestinal tract are common signs of methotrexate toxicity.

One of the dangers of prolonged methotrexate therapy for psoriasis is the appearance of liver damage, predominantly a cirrhosis that is mixed macronodular and micronodular with the septal bands of connective tissue being frequently narrow. Fat is usually seen scattered through the regenerative nodules. Fatty changes in the hepatocytes are probably the initial microscopic lesions seen in prolonged methotrexate therapy. Hepatocytes undergoing cytolysis and necrosis are observed after prolonged therapy. These fatty and degenerative changes with septal fibrosis may precede the development of cirrhosis by years after administration of the drug. Almost uniformly in methotrexate toxicity of the

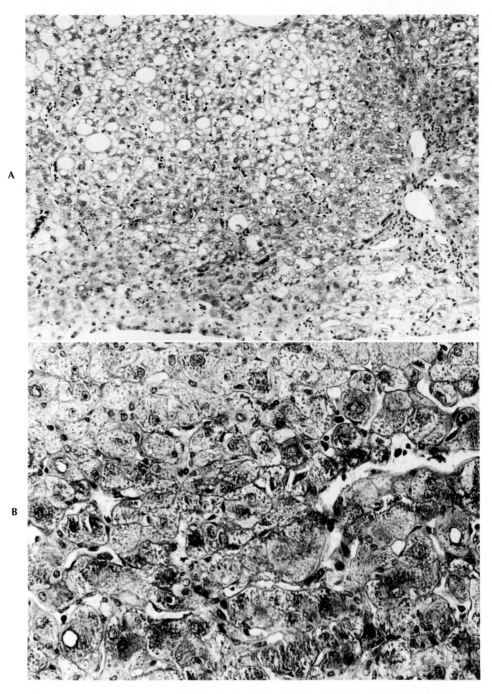

Fig. 4-16. A, The cytoplasm of numerous hepatocytes is replaced by fat. In the lower right hand corner notice swollen hepatocytes. **B,** Notice the variation in the staining characteristics of the hepatocytes. Some are swollen, whereas others fuse to present a syncytial appearance. There is considerable variation in the size, shape, and staining characteristics of the cells. Many nuclei are enlarged, irregular, and without discernible nucleoli and obviously contain increased masses of stagnant chromatin (inhibition of DNA turnover).

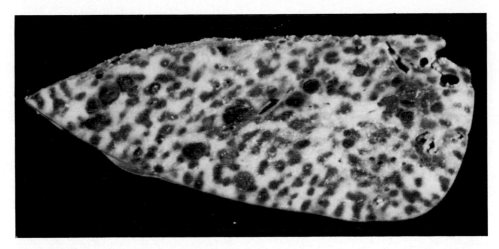

Fig. 4-17. Azathioprine. Peliosis hepatis. Livid spots characterized by dilated sinusoids and vascular channels.

liver, one observes nuclear vacuoles of varied dimensions located in the hepatocytes. These vacuoles do not stain for glycogen using the PAS reagent-diastase method. However, one may observe defects in the nuclear membrane, and this may be followed by glycogenic infiltration of the nucleus from the cytoplasm and therefore show PAS positivity (Fig. 4-17, A). The nuclei of methotrexate hepatotoxicity are consistently in the state of flux or unrest characterized by diploidy. Hyperchromatic collections of chromatin material without accompanied nucleoli are observed (Fig. 4-17, B). It is unusual to find any sustained elevation of serum transaminase, alkaline phosphatase, or serum bilirubin levels. These data indicate that liver biopsies may be mandatory every 12 to 24 months for patients undergoing prolonged therapy for severe psoriasis. The incidence of cirrhosis is calculated to be between 4% and 7%. The consensus is that the cirrhosis might well be accelerated if there is concomitant chronic ethanol toxicity. Chronic active hepatitis followed by cirrhosis has been observed after prolonged methotrexate therapy. There is no evidence that methotrexate predisposes patients directly to the development of hepatocellular carcinoma.

The severity of liver damage is related to the duration of therapy. Methotrexate may be responsible for diffuse interstitial pneumonia (DIP), which may progress to extensive interstitial fibrosis. Occasionally, widespread noncaseating granulomas may be induced by methotrexate; these are characterized by focal collections of macrophages, frequently accompanied by eosinophils and plasma cells.

The lung may also be the target for an adverse methotrexate reaction. At any time during the course of methotrexate therapy, an altered immune reaction may occur. This is manifested by alveolar lining cell damage, alveolitis characterized by cell infiltrate rich in eosino-phils, plasma cells and lymphocytes, and, to a lesser extent, macrophages. In occasional cases, noncaseating granulomas are observed. In prolonged methotrexate therapy after damage to the alveoli, a chronic alveolitis appears and irreversible fibrosis is established. Evidence of a direct toxic reaction is substantiated by the demonstration of cytoplasmic aggregates in type 2 alveolar lining cells. These aggregates are Mallory bodies, confirmed by light microscopy, cytochemistry, and ultrastructure. The extrahepatic nature and location of these bodies have been well described by Kuhn.

The folic acid antagonists affect both cellular and humoral immunity, but greater influence is on the cellular type. The antineoplastic agents affect the cell at various stages of the mitotic cycle. Methotrexate and cytosine arabinoside attack cell division during the DNA synthesis stage of the mitotic cycle. They are not aggressive when in contact with nonproliferating cells. The periwinkle alkaloids, vincristine and vinblastine, are also active only against proliferating cells in metaphase. The alkylating agents can inhibit cells exposed during any stage of their mitotic cycle.

The majority of cytotoxic drugs bring about an elevation in the levels of serum hepatic cell enzymes, as well as alkaline phosphatase enzymes, accompanied by increased bromosulfophthalein retention and a rise in the serum bilirubin level. Findings reminiscent of viral hepatitis can be produced by many of these cytotoxic drugs, including 6-mercaptopurine and 5-fluorodeoxyuridine.

Azathioprine is therapeutically employed for the treatment of acute myeloid leukemia and immunosuppressive therapy, commonly in patients undergoing transplantation of organs. Among the adverse tissue reactions is the development of cholestatic hepatitis, which is possibly the result of a direct toxic action of the compound. Tumors, in particular large cell (histiocytic non-Hodgkin's) malignant lymphoma and Kaposi's sarcoma, are frequently observed. Other malignancies, involving the bladder, breast, and endometrium, are also being found. Bone marrow suppression as a result of direct toxic action is to be expected, accompanying higher doses. Hypersensitivity reactions such as fever, skin rashes, and abdominal pain occasionally occur. In recent years, development of acute pancreatitis associated with long-term azathioprine therapy has been documented. The long-term therapy has usually been in patients being treated for rheumatoid arthritis, systemic lupus erythematosus, or Crohn's disease.

Other agents

Methysergide. Used in the therapy for migraine, methysergide (Sansert) possesses antiserotonin activity and is a powerful vasoconstrictor agent. The basic structure of the compound is similar to that of the ergot alkaloids, such as ergotamine tartrate. In addition to endomyocardial fibrosis, both methysergide and ergotamine tartrate bring about mitral, aortic, and tricuspid fibrosis resulting in valvular incompetence. The patchy endocardial fibrosis is reminiscent of that observed in carcinoid disease in which serotonin levels are elevated. The fibrous plaque covers, if it does not invade, the leaflets, and so the underlying valve architecture is normal, but it may extend to the chordae tendineae and papillary muscles. The major difference between the drug-induced cardiac changes and the carcinoid syndrome is the preponderance of right ventricular involvement in the latter, compared with a predominantly left-sided disease in methysergide. The drug may give rise to brawny edema and inflammatory fibrosis affecting retroperitoneal and pleuropulmonary tissues, endocardium, and large vessels. The mechanism of action has some similarities to serotonin activity but is not clearly understood.

The drug-induced fibrosis is microscopically identical to that found in the idiopathic forms. There is a distinct possibility that vasoconstriction and vasculitis may play some part in the causation of these drug-induced localized collagenoses. In most instances the disease process is reversible after discontinuation of the compound. Histologically, accompanying the fibrosis, the cellular component of the inflammatory reaction is composed primarily of lymphocytes in clumps and with the formation of germinal centers, frequently surrounded by plasma cells. As in the idiopathic variety, eosinophils may be prominent. Since the disease process is usually well advanced before clinical discovery, the nature of the earliest inflammatory lesion has not been delineated.

Thorotrast. Thorotrast is a colloidal solution containing 20% thorium (^{232}Th) dioxide and 20% dextran with 0.15% methyl-*p*-hydrobenzoate as a preservative. It was first used clinically in 1928. During the period from 1930 to 1945, it was used primarily in diagnostic radiology for visualization of the liver, spleen, and cerebral arteries. It was not until 1947 that this chemically inert and presumed innocuous compound was found to give rise to neoplasia. ^{232}Th, present in Thorotrast, is the parent of a series of radioactive daughter elements, including two long-lived daughters, mesothorium (^{228}Ra, radon) and radiothorium (^{228}Th). The unstable thorium nucleus goes through a chain of reactions, giving off alpha and beta particles and gamma rays until it reaches the stable element lead (^{208}Pb). ^{232}Th has a half-life of 1.4×10^{10} years and a biologic half-life of more than 400 years. Estimates by different investigators of the percentage of injected amounts of thorium retained in the organs of greatest Thorotrast deposition are as follows: liver, 71% to 73%; spleen, 7% to 17%; and bone marrow, 6% to 10%. More than 90% of ^{232}Th introduced into the body is deposited in the reticuloendothelial system.

The number and variety of malignant tumors that have been described and attributed to Thorotrast in humans are protean. Hemangioendothelioma of the liver was the neoplasm first associated with Thorotrast, and for some years it was believed to be the prevalent type (Fig. 4-18). Recently an increasing number of reports of hepatocarcinoma and cholangiocarcinoma have appeared. The time interval from the introduction of the compound to appearance of the tumor is greater than 20 years. Sarcomas and carcinomas may occur at injection sites and in body cavities into which Thorotrast has been instilled. Leukemia and carcinoma of the maxillary sinus have occurred after the introduction of Thorotrast into the body. Both Thorotrast sarcomas and carcinomas have been produced in experimental animals. There is a remarkable resemblance between the angiosarcoma produced by Thorotrast and that occurring after use of polyvinyl chloride in plastic workers. In each instance the earliest lesion appears to be sinusoid dilatation and hyperplasia of the endothelial and Kupffer cells.

Potassium chloride. The need for potassium chloride as replacement therapy in patients receiving thiazide type of drugs has resulted in the development of focal ulceration of the distal portion of the jejunum and of the ileum. Thiazide drugs deplete the body stores of potassium chloride, and the unpalatability of potassium chloride necessitated incorporation of the drug in an enteric-coated tablet or capsule form. Experiments on monkeys have shown that neither the coatings nor the thiazide itself is responsible for the development of the ulcer. The ileum and distal portion of the jejunum are highly susceptible to chemical trauma, since they lack mucous glands for protection. Chronic stenosing ulcers appear to be the result of repeated chemical irritation by localized potassium chloride released in the small

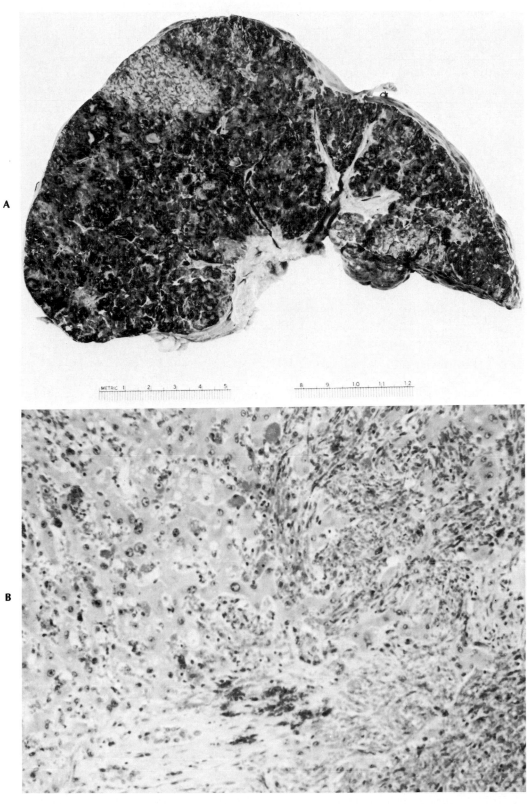

Fig. 4-18. Thorotrast. Hemangioendothelial sarcoma of liver. **A,** Light areas represent liver uninvolved by tumor. **B,** Liver biopsy. Aggregates (dark granules) of Thorotrast are embedded in connective tissue. Spindle areas are composed of neoplastic endothelial cells.   *Continued.*

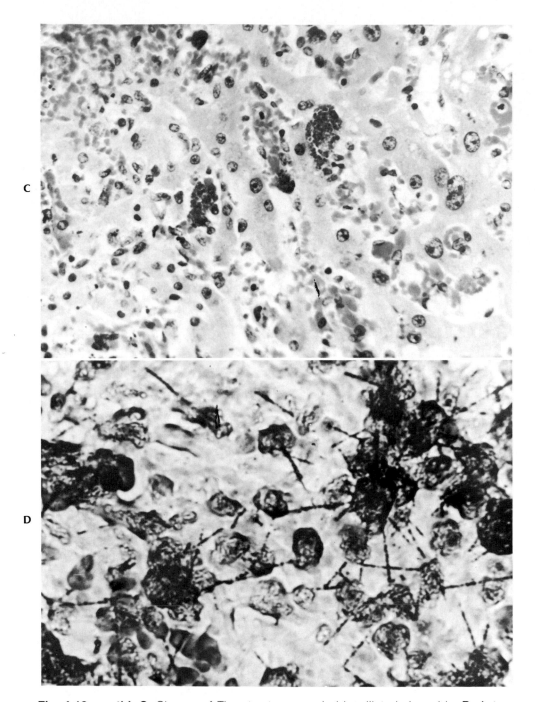

Fig. 4-18, cont'd. C, Clumps of Thorotrast surrounded by dilated sinusoids. **D,** Autoradiograph. Alpha-particle tracks "shoot out" from Thorotrast-laden Kupffer cells. Thorotrast was introduced 20 years earlier for demonstration of suspected amebic abscess of liver.

bowel (Fig. 4-19). A segment of previous irritation, spasm, and ulceration could block subsequent tablets, which would prevent healing and perpetuate the ulcerogenic process. Ulcers can apparently develop after an intake of very few tablets, but the individual susceptibility to the potassium-induced ulcers is not understood.

Grossly, the ulcers are acute or chronic and may be punctate or anular. They have a "punched-out" appearance. Proximal dilatation of the bowel occurs as a result of obstruction, in which case there is a tendency to perforation. Microscopically, the pathologic changes are confined to the mucosal and submucosal layers. There is an abrupt interruption of the normal mucosa, and the submucosa shows varying degrees of acute and chronic inflammatory infiltrate composed of neutrophils, eosin-

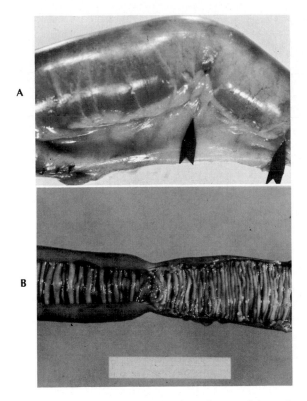

ophils, and plasma cells. Extension of the inflammatory process through the muscle of the small bowel is not frequently seen. Occasionally the mucosa may regenerate and regain an intact appearance. This is accompanied by disappearance of the inflammatory infiltrate in the submucosa with replacement fibrosis leading to a circumferential "napkin ring–like" stricture.

Milk and alkali. After the prolonged ingestion of milk and absorbable alkali in the treatment of peptic ulcer, the milk-alkali syndrome, characterized by hypercalcemia followed by calcium deposition in the kidneys, resulting in renal insufficiency, may occur. This renal calcification predisposes the patient to repeated attacks of acute pyelonephritis, resulting in a scarred, nonfunctional kidney. The syndrome must be distinguished from the calcification of hypervitaminosis D and primary pulmonary alveolar calcinosis. Other causes of hypercalcemia, such as hyperparathyroidism with the common complication of renal calcification, also may be complicated by peptic ulcer, thereby confusing the issue.

The association of pulmonary alveolar microlithiasis with the milk-alkali syndrome has been observed. In one case we observed, the alveoli were dilated throughout the lung and literally filled with calcified, desquamated bronchioloalveolar epithelial cells and macrophages. The conversion of the clumps of cells to microliths by their mineralization with calcium phosphate was extensive throughout all lobules (Fig. 4-20).

Fig. 4-19. Potassium chloride ulcer in small intestine. **A,** Constricted areas *(arrows)*. **B,** Focal, superficial ulcer and anular constriction of bowel. (Courtesy Dr. H. Rawling Pratt-Thomas, Medical University of South Carolina, Charleston, S.C.)

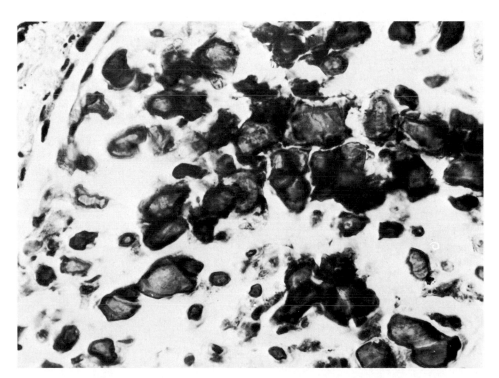

Fig. 4-20. Milk-alkali syndrome. Pulmonary alveolar microlithiasis associated with milk-alkali syndrome. Calcified desquamated alveolar cells occupy alveolar sac. (Hematoxylin and eosin; 350×.)

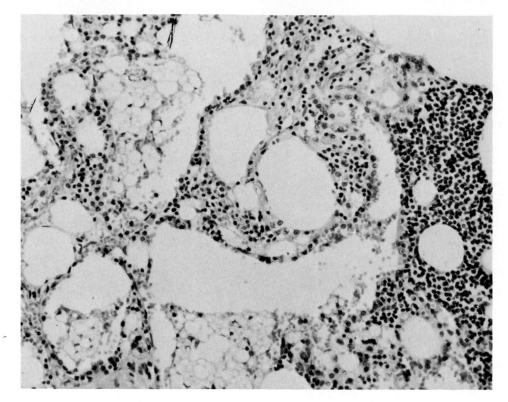

Fig. 4-21. Mineral oil pneumonitis. Small vacuoles coalesce to form larger ones. Inflammatory response is predominantly lymphocytic.

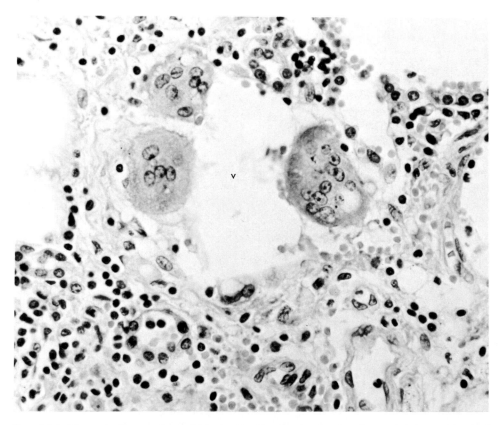

Fig. 4-22. Mineral oil granuloma in lung. Foreign-body giant cells containing mineral oil surround large vacuole *(v)*. Lymphocytes and plasma cells are prominent.

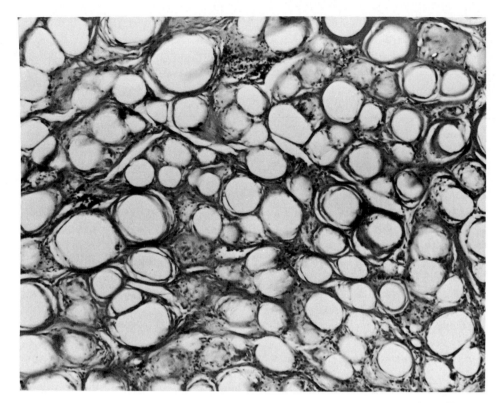

Fig. 4-23. Lung of patient who used mineral oil as laxative for 30 years. X-ray film suggested malignancy of right lower lobe. Large vacuoles of mineral oil are demarcated by bands of fibrous tissue.

The septa, though fibrosed in part, were free of mineral deposits. Cut sections of the lungs had the appearance and feel of grains of sand.

Mineral oil. At necropsy, the pathologist may find numerous lipogranulomas caused by mineral oil in such organs as the spleen, lymph nodes, and portal tracts of the liver. The source of the mineral oil in such cases is frequently foods, such as bread, that are prepared on stainless steel tables that are rubbed down daily with mineral oil. In many food-processing plants, rust is kept off the machinery by applying this substance. Thus, over many years, a considerable amount of mineral oil may be ingested in contaminated foods. Furthermore, mineral oil has been a common form of self-medication for such conditions as peptic ulcer, diarrhea, and constipation.

Since this petrolatum oil does not elicit the cough reflex, the oily substances may reach the dependent portions of the lungs. Unlike fish and animal oils, which contain varied amounts of unsaturated fatty acids that produce an acute hemorrhagic or necrotizing reaction, mineral oil produces a mild foreign body type of reaction. It elicits macrophages, which then phagocytose the foreign material (Fig. 4-21). Giant cells are abundant, depending on the amount and duration of the oil dosage (Fig. 4-22). Over a long period of time, the small globules of mineral oil coalesce to form large vacuoles, and the process is accompanied by a chronic in-

flammatory reaction rich in lymphocytes and plasma cells. The eventuality is a diffuse lobar interstitial pneumonia and fibrosis or a localized reaction referred to as a paraffinoma (Fig. 4-23). These lesions radiologically have simulated pneumonia and localized or diffuse tumor (p. 985).

Skin cancer caused by mineral oil was first noted during the latter part of the nineteenth century among mule spinners in the cotton industry. Between 1920 and 1943, no fewer than 1400 cases of skin cancer attributable to industrial exposure to mineral oil were reported. Of these, the scrotum was affected in 885 patients, nearly all of whom were cotton workers. Only 50 of the patients worked in the engineering industry. Mineral oils comprise three types of compounds—paraffins, naphthenic compounds, and aromatic compounds. It is believed that most of the carcinogenicity of cutting oils is attributable to compounds in the aromatic fraction, particularly the polycyclic aromatics containing four to six condensed benzene rings.

TOXICOLOGIC ASPECTS OF FORENSIC PATHOLOGY
Alcohols and glycols

Alcohol continues to be the most frequently abused chemical compound among adults in the United States. More socioeconomic problems are created by alcohol abuse than all other medicinal and illicit drugs combined. Alcoholism is the nation's leading public health problem. In a significant proportion of sudden unexpected deaths among adults, alcohol has been implicated as either a direct or a contributory cause. This statement holds true not only for natural deaths but also for those classified as homicide, accident, or suicide. What may be interpreted at first glance as sudden unexpected death in a chronic alcoholic on a spree may prove to be otherwise, such as asphyxia by aspiration of a meat bolus. In such cases there is a rapid onset of dyspnea, gasping for breath, and choking. This series of events has been referred to as "café coronary," a term that is misleading and should be discarded. A postmortem examination reveals that large chunks of food, undigested and unchewed, are present in the larynx. This is invariably accompanied by high blood-alcohol levels. It is mandatory that the student of chronic alcoholism realize that an alcoholic undergoing sudden or rapid death may have a background of numerous diseases that develop as a result of many years of recurrent alcohol-poisoning episodes.

Pathophysiologic effects of alcohol include interference with normal metabolic effects (hypoglycemia, acidosis) and suppression of phagocytosis and of normal immunologic responses. Common findings at autopsy are subdural hematoma and hemorrhage resulting from ruptured viscera, fatty and cirrhotic liver changes, acute hemorrhagic pancreatitis, anemia, and miscellaneous infections, notably Friedländer's pneumonia. Toxicologic studies may reveal that contaminants in alcoholic beverages may have contributed to the patient's demise; among these are lead, propyl alcohol, ethylene glycol, methanol, and cobalt. At autopsy the finding in alcoholics of dangerous levels of barbituric acid derivatives, and in recent years such compounds as amphetamines and tranquilizers, is not unusual. Well over 95% of the deaths attributed to alcohol may be classified as accidental and resulted from overdose unrelated to suicidal intent.

Acute subdural hematomas are not uncommon in alcoholics. There are innumerable documented cases of "jail death" in which alcoholics are moved to the jail cell and told to "sleep it off." Some hours later they are discovered dead, and autopsy reveals an acute subdural hematoma that has caused fatal supratentorial pressure on the brainstem. Interestingly, the blood-alcohol level may be very low as a result of the metabolic oxidation that occurred while the deceased was in the jail cell. However, the pathologist can closely estimate the alcohol level at the time of injury by analyzing the blood in the subdural hematoma for alcohol content. This portion of blood has not been recirculated through the liver for its metabolism and therefore reflects a more accurate blood-alcohol level at the time of injury. The hopeless alcohol addict may envision himself or herself as an inspired bartender and may devise a fatal concoction by adding such toxic substances as antifreeze, ethylene glycol, and rubbing alcohol (isopropyl alcohol) to the alcoholic drink. The addition of a touch of Sterno and paint thinner may prove to be the "straw that broke the camel's back."

Ethanol

A not uncommon set of circumstances associated with acute ethanol (alcohol) intoxication is that of a person who, after a heavy bout of drinking, retires and is found dead in bed the next morning with a blood-alcohol level that is well below the lethal level (Table 4-4). At autopsy, various changes may be found in the liver ranging from a large fatty liver to various stages of Laënnec's (alcoholic or nutritional) cirrhosis. The mechanism of death with central nervous system depression is not clearly understood. In other instances, unexpected deaths occur in chronic alcoholics, and the pathologist finds only a large fatty liver at autopsy. Again, the level of blood alcohol may be less than the levels associated with acute fatal poisoning.

Incidents of alcoholics who have consumed over a pint a day for several weeks without eating are commonly encountered. In these cases clinical manifestations are vomiting, jaundice, fever, and leukocytosis, with pneumonia and delirium tremens frequently complicating the picture. Death occurs in approximately 66% of the cases with this clinical setting. The pathologist usually finds evidence of hepatocellular necrosis and bile stasis superimposed on a fatty or cirrhotic liver, but occasionally the morphologic features of complicating acute viral hepatitis are observed. Indeed, the alcoholic liver may well have an increased susceptibility to acute and chronic viral hepatitis. Acute alcoholic hepatitis is an appropriate morphologic designation when focal scattered necrotic liver cells are observed among the fat cells. When the alcohol intake has been excessive (over a pint a day) for a long period of time in the presence of dietary lack, one not infrequently observes intracytoplasmic hyaline bodies that first appear in a perinuclear location and are known as Mallory's alcoholic hyaline bodies. When they are found abundantly in fatty livers, they are characteristic of an acute and severe alcoholic insult. The hyaline bodies may be observed in smaller numbers in conditions other than acute toxic alcoholic damage, namely, morbid obesity (twice normal weight) and acute viral hepatitis. Individuals with large fatty livers may suffer fat embolism after injury to the liver. Examination of the brain will reveal the telltale petechial hemorrhages caused by the embolic fatty material. Microscopically, the liver cells are so engorged with fat that the cell boundaries may rupture and form microcysts.

Some cases of sudden or unexpected death in acute

Table 4-4. Levels of common and uncommon chemicals and drugs found in body tissue at necropsy of accidental, suicidal, and homicidal poisoning victims (all values in mg/dl)

Chemical	Blood	Urine	Brain	Liver	Kidney	Other
COMMON						
Acetaminophen	150	—	—	—	—	—
Alcohols	84	—	—	—	—	—
Butanol						
Ethanol	360-544	—	—	—	—	—
Methanol	20-630	—	—	10-180	20-230	—
Propanol	150-200	—	—	—	—	—
Amphetamine	0.05-4.1	2.5-70	0.28-0.3	0.43-7.4	0.32-5.2	—
Aromatics	0.5-33	—	—	0.7-125	1.4-3	—
Barbiturates	2.9-6.8	0.7-9.8	17.2	10.6-58	21	—
Amobarbital						
Amobarbital and secobarbital (Tuinal)	0.6-8.5	0.3-12.1	—	3.8-26	—	—
Barbital	10-38	114	6.3	10-93	—	—
Barbiturates and alcohol (20-260 mg/dl)	0.8-5.3	0.1-17	3.4-4.8	3-16	1.7	—
Butabarbital	3-8.8	—	—	5.1-25	—	—
Pentobarbital	0.5-11.2	1.4-18	1.2	2.3-55	1.8	—
Phenobarbital	8-15	—	—	8.9-26.6	—	—
Carbon monoxide	10%, may be significant; 20%, chronic; 40%+, acute					
Cyanide	0.11-5.3	0.005-0.11	0.06-1.6	0.07-2.3	0.02-8.4	—
Glutethimide (Doriden)	1-9.7	2.8	1.1	6.3-14.1	0.4-1.6	—
Meprobamate	1.4-34.6	—	140	5.8-41.2	50	—
Morphine	0.02-0.23	1.4-8.1	0.002-0.75	0.04-1.8	0.02-0.15	Bile, 0.2-5.7
Nicotine	1.1-6.3	1.7-5.8	—	10-500	0.3-5.3	—
Propoxyphene (Darvon)	0.1-1.7	0.25-3.5	0.88-4	0.73-11.9	0.1-6.4	—
UNCOMMON						
Acetone	55	90	—	—	—	—
Amitriptyline (Elavil)	0.27-0.47	0.04-0.79	2.6-1.8	1.3-32	1.2-31	—
Arsenic	0.06-0.93	—	0.02-0.4	0.2-120	0.02-70	Bile, 14.1; stomach contents, 30.6
Benzene	0.09	0.06	3.9	1.6	1.8	—
Boron	8-296	—	—	—	—	—
Bromide	200	—	—	—	—	—
Brompheniramine	0.02	0.51	0.10	0.2	—	—
Caffeine	7.9-15.9	11.4-54.2	7.5-10.8	9.2-32.9	10.4-23	—
Chloral hydrate (trichloroethanol)	10-64	59	—	0.9-17	—	—
Chlordiazepoxide (Librium)	2	—	—	2	—	—
Chloroform	1-4.8	0-6	5.5-31	0.6-13	1.6-2.7	—
Chlorpromazine	0.3-3.5	—	—	5.4-211	—	—
Codeine	0.1-0.88	2.9-22.9	0	0.06-4.49	0.23-3.63	—
Desipramine	0.3	—	—	—	—	—
Diazepam (Valium)	2	—	—	—	—	—
2,4-Dichlorophenoxyacetic acid (2,4-D)	66.9-82.6	26.4	1.3	2.1-18.3	6.3	—

Data from Sunshine, I., editor: Handbook of analytical toxicology, Akron, Ohio, 1969, The Chemical Rubber Co.

Continued.

Table 4-4. Levels of common and uncommon chemicals and drugs found in body tissue at necropsy of accidental, suicidal, and homicidal poisoning victims (all values in mg/dl)—cont'd

Chemical	Blood	Urine	Brain	Liver	Kidney	Other
Dieldrin	5 (IV)	—	—	—	—	—
Ethchlorvynol (Placidyl)	15	3.1-5.4	1.3-5.7	1.8-7.2	1.8-6.3	Adipose, 6-104
Ethylene glycol	200-400	200-1130	30-390	20-1510	20-1130	—
Fluoride	0.2-0.3	—	—	—	—	—
Hydroxychloroquine (Plaquenil)	4.8-6.1	97	—	7.1	—	—
Imipramine (Tofranil)	0.28-0.7	0.69-6.4	3-7.4	8.6-25	3.8-5.6	—
Iron	1.9-5	—	—	—	—	—
Lead	0.11-0.35	—	—	—	—	—
Mebutamate	1	—	—	—	—	—
Meperidine	3	177	7	11	11.4	—
Mercury	—	—	0	0.9	1.2	—
Methamphetamine	4	—	—	—	—	—
Methapyrilene	0.4-3	—	—	2.5-16	0.6	—
Methaqualone	3	—	—	—	—	—
Methyprylon (Noludar)	8.9-10	—	—	22	1.1	—
Nortriptyline	0.1-3	2.5-12	—	0.78-22	0.7-9.4	—
Paraldehyde	11.5-48	13	15-37	20-60	50-260	—
Pentachlorophenol	4.6-17.3	2.8-5.2	1.4-3.5	5.9-22.5	4.1-12.3	—
Phenytoin	10	—	7.8	27	11	—
Quinine	1.2	—	—	—	—	—
Strychnine	0.05-0.61	0.1-3.3	0.05-2.6	0.5-25.7	0.007-10.6	—
Thioridazine	2-8	—	—	2.5-51.3	—	—
Trichloroethane	0.15-72	0.1-0.3	0.32-59	0.49-22	0.26-12	—
Trichloroethylene	0.3-11	0.2-7.3	0.7-27	0.5-25	1.1-11.2	—

alcohol poisoning have been attributed to alcoholic myocardiosis (alcoholic myopathy). It has been presumed that the mechanism of death in these cases is cardiac arrhythmia. An association between alcohol use and cardiac arrhythmias, particularly atrial fibrillation, has long been suspected, but the specific etiologic role of alcohol is difficult to establish. In an emergency room setting, one encounters patients who drink heavily and habitually, and examination shows that many have arrhythmias that return rather rapidly to sinus rhythm. Regan and Haider[193] point to this situation as a rather typical weekend or holiday presentation and refer to it as "holiday heart syndrome." They define this as an acute disturbance of cardiac rhythm or conduction, or both, that follows heavy ethanol consumption in a person without other clinical evidence of heart disease and that disappears, without evident residua, with abstinence.

Clinically, electrocardiographic changes indicate myocardial dysfunction in alcoholics, but the morphologist has not been able to characterize any pathognomonic lesions by light and electron microscopy. Of the morphologic observations on the myocardium of the chronic alcoholic, probably the most significant is the presence of myocytes containing numbers of irregularly deposited intramyocardial lipid droplets, which are composed of triglycerides. The action of alcohol on the myocytes results in the loss of some Krebs' cycle enzymes and electrolytes from the cell, thereby interfering with the utilization of fatty acids for energy production and leading to the accumulation of triglycerides. If, indeed, toxic alcoholic cardiomyopathy exists as a separate entity, its morphologic manifestations are shared in patients who demonstrate nutritional cardiomyopathy such as thiamine deficiency (beriberi heart disease).

Ferrans has clearly demonstrated that significant coronary occlusion (over 50%) is not a factor in producing myocyte and fibrotic changes in the musculature of the cardiac chambers of ethanol toxicity. An unusual finding is that of acute alcoholic rhabdomyolysis. This consists in acute necrosis of muscle fibers with the liberation of myoglobin in the plasma. Renal dysfunction, including renal failure, may follow the shocklike state and the plugging of the tubules with myoglobin.

Ethanol is a drug that has been classified as a food yielding 7 "empty" calories per gram. In excess amounts it behaves as a toxin. It supports growth, has a protein-sparing effect, is well absorbed from the gastrointestinal tract even in patients with malabsorption, and increases the smooth endoplasmic reticulum of the hepatocyte and the rate of hepatic drug metabolism, including its own oxidation. In general the fundamental cytologic differences between patients with alcoholic hepatitis who live and those who die lie in the amount of hepatic cell necrosis and the individual capability for hepatocellular regeneration. In acute alcoholic hepatitis, one observes, in addition to steatotic hepatic cells, the presence of nonfatty "balloon cells." The balloon cells contain deformed mitochondria, some being of giant configuration whereas others appear shrunken and are closely approximated into groups. The cristae frequently have a grotesque and bizarre pattern. Among the numerous nonspecific mitochondrial alterations, the most conspicuous are crystal-like inclusions resembling myelin degeneration. The smooth endoplasmic reticulum is diffusely hypertrophied and vacuolated. The changes in the endoplasmic reticulum reflect the fact that ethanol can influence microsomal drug metabolism in humans. Alcoholics metabolize tolbutamide more rapidly than do nonalcoholics, and this should be considered when alcoholics are given tolbutamide for the treatment of diabetes. People who ingest alcohol chron-

ically have an increased level of the hepatic enzyme that metabolizes pentobarbital, whereas the activity of this enzyme system is inhibited by the in vitro addition of alcohol to the incubation mixture. These observations may explain the increased tolerance of alcoholics to barbiturates and other sedatives when sober and the enhanced sensitivity of these individuals to sedatives when inebriated. The ergastoplasm is vacuolated, and dispersion of the ribosomes is observed.

It is my opinion that a major contribution if not the sole one to the formation of Mallory bodies is the fusion and disintegration of abnormal mitochondria. It has been observed for some time that a characteristic of alcoholic hepatocyte toxicity is mitochondrial damage with the appearance of crystalline inclusions and a considerable increase in the size of the mitochondrial structure (Fig. 4-24). Light microscopy reveals the clumping of large mitochondria in a paranuclear location and later the formation of characteristic "ropelike" Mallory bodies. The giant mitochondrial forms and altered endoplasmic reticulum probably form the morphologic basis for the alcoholic hyaline bodies of Mallory.

The oral and intravenous administration (respectively 25% and 20% ml of absolute alcohol in 100 ml of water) of lethal and sublethal doses of alcohol (respectively 12 and 8 ml of absolute alcohol per kilogram) to unanesthetized dogs produces changes in the lymphatic tissues.

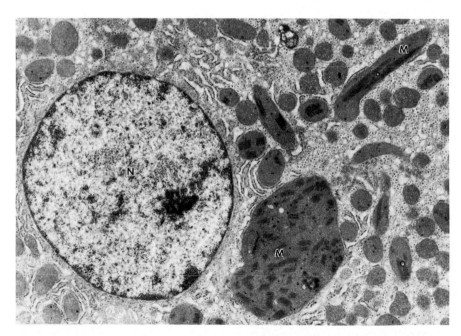

Fig. 4-24. Mitochondrial changes in ethanol toxicity. Notice the megamitochondrion *(M),* which is approximately a third the size of the nucleus *(N).* It is surrounded by bizarre mitochondria with similar crystalline protein inclusions.

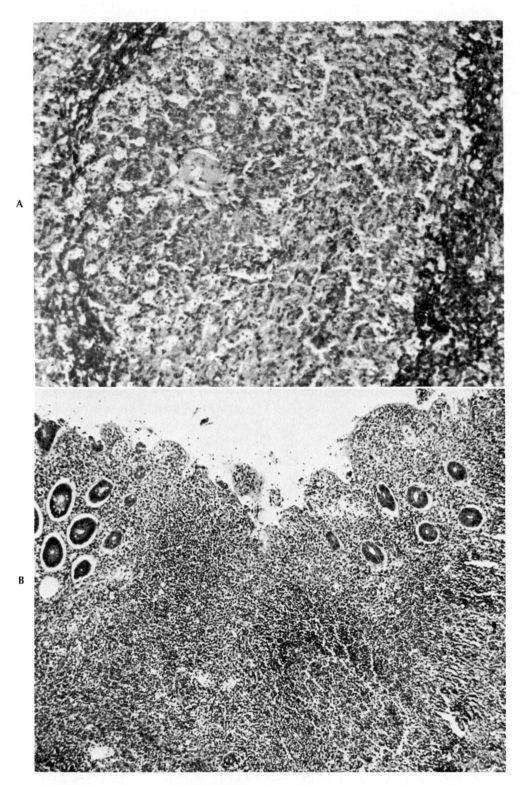

Fig. 4-25. A, Spleen of dog after sublethal dose of ethanol. Germinal follicles of all lymphatic tissues show necrosis of germinal follicles with presence of "nuclear dust" (lympholysis), which probably represents cortisone effect. Similar lesions are seen in humans after fatal salicylate poisoning and burns. **B,** Sublethal oral dose of ethanol in dog stomach. Superficial ulceration and gastritis 4 days after dosage.

These changes consist in necrosis of germinal follicles throughout the entire lymphatic system (Fig. 4-25, *A*). Hemorrhagic gastritis and superficial ulceration, particularly of the distal part of the stomach, were noted after oral administration (Fig. 4-25, *B*). Occasionally, loss of lipid in the deeper layers of the adrenal zona fasciculata was observed. Continuous intravenous infusion of epinephrine or norepinephrine to alcoholized dogs did not appear to intensify this reaction. These changes did not occur in adrenalectomized dogs. The lympholysis and germinal center necrosis were probably a reflection of adrenal stimulation with acutely elevated serum corticosteroid level.

It is of interest that these changes, particularly those in the mitochondria, probably occur only in persons who have a very excessive alcohol intake in the presence of adequate food consumption or in persons who consume lesser quantities of alcohol in the absence of adequate diet. In addition to the effect on the liver cell, ethanol may have a direct "toxic" effect on the bone marrow. This is reflected in the observation of vacuolation of primitive erythroblasts. The action appears independent of nutritional deficiencies of other toxins.

An excellent treatise on alcohol and the cell has been presented by Rubin, who points out that "the mechanism by which alcohol injures tissue is not fully understood." Hepatocyte disruption is occasioned by the metabolism of excessive intake of ethanol. During the oxidation of ethanol to acetaldehyde, NAD is reduced to NADH, thereby greatly increasing the reducing power of the cell. However, although certain metabolic abnormalities may be attributed to this change in the NAD/NADH ratio, no tissue injury has been directly shown to be caused by it. Moreover, other organs that also exhibit alcohol-induced injury, such as the heart and the pancreas, do not metabolize ethanol to any appreciable extent.

The occurrence of pancreatitis and pancreatic lithiasis in alcoholics is well known. Whether this can be accounted for by duct and ductule blockage by inspissated pancreatic secretion during a period of dehydration is unresolved. On the other hand, there may be a direct "toxic" effect on the pancreatic acinar cell (see discussion of methyl alcohol). Although alcohol administration regularly induces mild hyperlipemia, pronounced hyperlipemia develops in some persons at intoxicating levels. The explanation for this unusual response to alcohol is not clear. It is possible that pancreatitis is incriminated, or possibly the low plasma lipoprotein lipase, which often is decreased in patients with liver disease, is at fault. Zieve[200] reported hyperlipemia in association with jaundice, fatty liver, and hemolytic anemia, and this association of signs and symptoms is now known as Zieve's syndrome.

The congeners (which include fusel oil, aldehydes, furfural, esters, solids, tannins, and many uncharacterized compounds) are necessary for the taste, bouquet, and color of whiskey. Some workers believe that their presence in large amounts enhances the possibility of toxic reactions. The evidence indicates that small quantities of congeners in proper balance, such as found in some types of blended whiskies, may lessen undesirable physiologic effects through interaction with ethanol and other constituents of the beverage. A consideration of these factors points to the desirability of further biochemical and toxicologic investigations, with emphasis on the fundamental mechanisms.

Methanol (methyl alcohol)

In Atlanta, Georgia, in 1951, more than 300 patients who had ingested bootleg whiskey containing 35% methanol were treated at the Grady Memorial Hospital. They presented the classic symptoms of wood alcohol poisoning—visual disturbances from mild blurring to total blindness, severe abdominal pain, nausea, headache, and central nervous system manifestations ranging from dizziness and convulsions to coma. Many patients manifested severe acidosis as evidenced by reduction in plasma carbon dioxide–combining power. The mechanism of the acidosis is incompletely understood, although it is well known that the breakdown of methyl to formic acid and possibly formaldehyde may have some role in bringing it about. Some patients had initial serum amylase levels exceeding 300 units, and at autopsy the lesions varied from scattered areas of pancreatic acinar destruction with edema of the stroma to a pronounced hemorrhagic necrosis that was easily visualized in the gross examination. The mildest and possibly earliest changes were degranulation and increased basophilism of the acinar cells with pooling of secretion in the ducts accompanied by edema of the connective tissue of the lobules. More conspicuous changes consisted in necrosis of both arterial and venous walls with extravasation of blood through the parenchyma. Histologic examination of the eyes from fatal cases showed retinal ganglion cell degeneration with sparing of the optic nerve and tract.

Methanol is easily absorbed through the skin, respiratory tract, or gastrointestinal tract, and human poisoning is possible by any of these routes. According to several authorities, 200 parts of methanol per million parts of air is the maximum limit of safety in industry. In the Atlanta incident the smallest amount that produced a fatal result was about 15 ml of 40% methanol. The highest dose recorded in a survivor was 500 ml of the same concentration. This unusual variation in susceptibility constitutes one of the unusual features of this type of poisoning and has not been fully explained. The oxidation rate of methanol in the body is less than one fifth that of ethanol, hence its long persistence. A small proportion is excreted unchanged in the urine, but a much larger amount is lost in expired air. As stated previously, methanol poisoning is attributed partially to the acidosis caused by formic acid and partially to the local toxic effects of formaldehyde, both compounds resulting from metabolism of methanol. Both methanol and ethanol are converted by the enzymes alcohol dehydrogenase and aldehyde dehydrogenase. The consequence is that high doses of ethanol compete with methanol, delaying and reducing its toxification. Ethanol inhibits the bioactivation—in this case a toxification—of methanol.

Isopropanol (isopropyl alcohol)

Fatal isopropanol poisoning is much less common than that from methanol. Isopropyl alcohol has many important uses in industries, where it has been substituted for ethanol in several processes. At a concentration of 70%, it is readily available to the public as "rubbing alcohol." Adelson[179] points out that no specific organic lesions are found in persons who die within a few hours after ingestion of isopropanol. Death, which occurs rapidly after absorption, is the result of profound depression of the central nervous system with ultimate respiratory paralysis. In this respect isopropanol acts in the same manner as other respiratory depressants (ethanol, anesthetics, and barbiturates). The acute tubular nephrosis in cases of fatal poisoning probably is attributable to the circulatory effect of existing shock in the victims. Since 15% of isopropyl alcohol is metabolized to acetone, the patient in coma could be subject to an erroneous diagnosis of diabetic coma, except that glycosuria is absent.

Gadsden and associates[186] reported 50 cases of isopropanol intoxication after ingestion of what has been referred to as "scrap iron." The drink is made by using cracked corn, yeast, and sugar. The mixture is fermented for 48 hours, with Clorox used as a catalyst. Isopropanol and mothballs (naphthalene) are added at the end of the fermentation period. After distillation, the drink tastes like the galvanized steel drum in which it was made, hence the name "scrap iron." Gadsden and associates conclude that this drink is for high voltage and not vintage.

Glycols

Ethylene glycol, a hygroscopic secondary alcohol, is best known as a constituent of antifreeze. In the body it is metabolized to oxalic acid. The importance of this chemical in accidental and sometimes suicidal death cannot be overemphasized. It appears as an intentional contaminant in moonshine whiskey. Fatal accidental ingestion of numerous compounds containing oxalic acid and ethylene glycol has been recorded. Household cleaners such as brass polish and ink spot and iron stain removers are sometimes the culprits. Glycols are excellent industrial solvents; in the navy they are used for cleaning torpedoes and are known under names such as "torpedo juice," "pink lady," or "hen wine." These chemicals also are used by shoemakers, bookbinders, and straw hat manufacturers.

Shortly after the ingestion of as little as 100 ml of ethylene glycol, evidence of drunkenness ensues, followed rapidly by headache, convulsions, coma, and death. If the individual survives for 1 to 3 days, the initial central nervous system depressant effect lightens and cardiopulmonary manifestations appear with the development of pulmonary edema. By the second day there is evidence of azotemia and uremia. Depending on the dosage and the initiation of therapy, shock may appear at any time during the first 24 hours. At necropsy the kidneys are swollen and tense, and on cut section the pale cortex stands out in contrast to the dark color because of vascular stasis that occupies the medullary zone. If shock has been severe and prolonged, cortical necrosis may be evident. Microscopically, the cellular features of acute tubular nephrosis or necrosis accompanied by jamming of the lumens of the tubules by sheaf-shaped, semiopaque calcium oxylate crystals are observed (Fig. 4-26). The crystals are strongly birefringent. Lesser numbers of calcium oxalate crystals are to be found in the distal nephron. Tubulovenous anastomoses and red blood cell casts are part of the histologic picture. Other findings are chemical meningitis and pericapillary calcification of the meninges. Oxalate crystals may be demonstrated within the intrameningeal and intracerebral blood vessels and, less frequently, localized within the white matter of the brain. Gross hydropic degeneration of the hepatocytes of the centrilobular region is usual.

Diethylene glycol, also an occasional constituent of antifreeze and a one-time vehicle for drugs, is twice as toxic as ethylene glycol. It is not metabolized to oxalic acid, and crystals of calcium oxalate are not to be found in the tissues. Like ethylene glycol, the diethylene compound may bring about centrilobular hydropic or "ballooning" hepatocyte changes. Necrosis of the liver has been documented. Renal cortical necrosis is prone to develop and is probably more closely related to the tubular hypoxia of shock than to toxic nephropathy. In the majority of cases, remarkable swelling and hydropic degeneration occur in the proximal convoluted tubules. Ethylene glycol dinitrate produces methemoglobin formation, which may be a direct cause of the renal injury found after ingestion of this compound. Propylene glycol, however, induces hemolysis and tubular necrosis.

Among the various ethylene glycol derivatives of low molecular weight (such as diethylene glycol, dipropylene glycol, and dioxane), the presence of an ether linkage appears to cause a more intense renal damage.

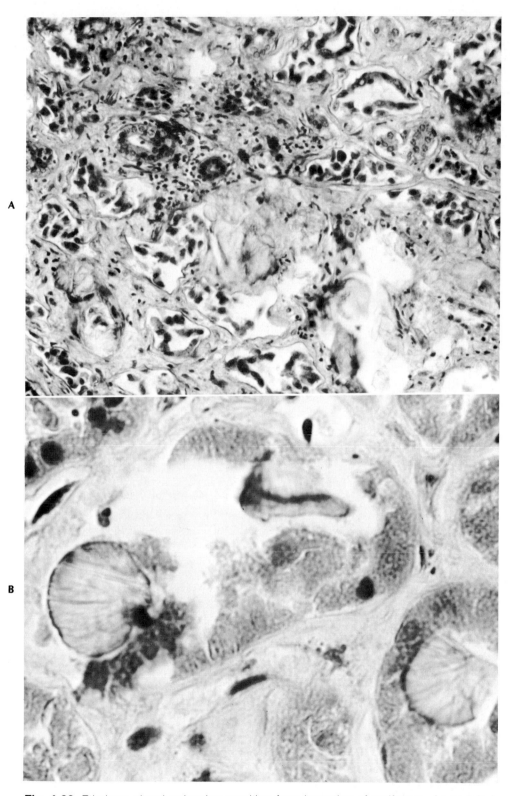

Fig. 4-26. Ethylene glycol poisoning resulting from ingestion of antifreeze. Acute tubular necrosis with "stuffing" of tubular lumens by calcium oxalate crystals. Focal chronic interstitial nephritis is evident. **A,** Characteristic calcium oxalate crystals. **B,** Nuclei at upper left pyknotic. Remainder of tubules reveal loss of nuclear staining, swelling, and necrosis of tubular cells.

Dioxane

Dioxane is a powerful dehydrating agent often used as a substitute for alcohol in tissue preparation and stains. In poorly ventilated areas, dangerous concentrations may develop in the air. Dioxane, like other nephrotoxins, causes cytoplasmic vacuolation, rarefaction, and loss of the brush border. Like mercuric chloride, this agent induces proliferation of the smooth endoplasmic reticulum; in contrast to mercuric chloride, it does not cause dissociation of polysomes. Mitochondria are severely damaged and undergo swelling, and amorphous intramatrical deposits develop. With established necrosis, spicular crystals, believed to be calcium salts, appear on the cristae and eventually fill up most of the mitochondrion.

Metals and metallic salts
Mercury

Mercury and its compounds enter the body by absorption through the skin, by ingestion, and by inhalation. However, the chemical form of mercury has a significant effect on its disposition. Practically, there are three general forms of mercury: elemental mercury (Hg^0); inorganic mercury—mercurous (Hg^{+1}) and mercuric (Hg^{+2}); and organic mercury, which is usually limited to methyl, ethyl, and phenyl mercury salts and the family of alkoxyalkyl mercury diuretics.

Inhalation is the most important route of absorption from the industrial point of view and is responsible for many cases of mercury poisoning. Elemental mercury and monoalkyl mercurials (such as methyl mercury) are important in this route of entry because both have high vapor pressures and high lipid solubility. Oral intake of mercury does occur but usually only in cases of suicide or as a result of accidental contamination of food and drink with mercury compounds. Elemental mercury is very poorly absorbed from the gastrointestinal tract (<0.01%), and organic mercury compounds are much better absorbed than inorganic compounds. Systemic absorption of all alkyl mercury compounds probably is substantial because there are cases of poisoning from the dermal application of methyl mercury ointments.

The distribution of mercury varies considerably depending on the chemical form and, to a lesser extent, on the route of administration. Mercurous compounds and metallic mercury are oxidized to mercuric mercury, whereas the organic mercury compounds are variably metabolized to the mercuric form. The mercuric salts form soluble compounds with proteins, sodium chloride, blood, and tissue fluid alkalis. The accumulation of mercury is independent of the mode of administration—mercury entering the body as a vapor behaves no differently from mercury injected into the body. However, the chemical form of administration significantly affects the disposition. For example, whereas both mercuric mercury and organic mercury (methyl mercury) are distributed preferentially to the kidneys, the amount of mercury in other tissues is much higher with methyl mercury. Mercuric chloride has a more toxic effect on parenchymal cells than the organic mercurials such as methyl mercury chloride and methyl mercury dicyanamide. Organic mercury is more firmly bound to the tissues than is inorganic mercury and possesses greater power of penetration of the blood-brain barrier. Mercury, regardless of form, moves readily across the placenta and may be concentrated in fetal tissue. The concentration of mercury in the blood has been used as a biologic indicator of exposure. In general, the distribution within the blood depends on the chemical form; organic mercury is carried mainly by erythrocytes and inorganic mercury by the plasma.

Absorbed mercury leaves the blood rapidly, with the greater part excreted in the urine and feces; some, however, is also excreted in bile, sweat, saliva, and milk. The relative contribution of urine and feces to the total elimination of mercury also depends on the chemical form of mercury present. With prolonged administration of metallic and mercuric mercury, urinary excretion somewhat exceeds the fecal route; however, methyl mercury is excreted mainly by the fecal route. After any short exposure in both animals and humans, excretion is normally greater in feces than in urine. The mechanism of renal excretion is poorly understood, but glomerular filtration is not believed to play a major role. There is also urinary reabsorption in the renal proximal tubules primarily, with some by distal tubules. During exposure of short duration, excretion is rapid; hence the tissue concentration is lowered within a week after cessation of exposure. After prolonged exposure, mercury accumulates in the brain, and the gradual buildup in the kidneys results in slow excretion. After termination of the exposure, the amount in the urine is approximately proportional to the mercury content of the kidneys. With prolonged low exposure, excretion approximately equals absorption so that the tissue levels of mercury remain the same. Interestingly, the administration of mercury, zinc, or cadmium stimulates the synthesis in the kidney of metallothionein, a low–molecular weight protein rich in sulfhydryl groups, with a high affinity by mercury for the sulfhydryl moiety. The renal concentration of metallothionein is increased as much as sixfold by administration of inorganic mercury, which may serve a protective role for the kidney by sequestering mercury, since the minimal concentration of mercury in kidney associated with toxic effects is considerably greater with long-term administration than with acute administration.

A significant local inflammatory reaction to metallic mercury and its compounds in the body tissues depends on the presence of, or the oxidation of such compounds to, the mercuric ion. The mercuric ion, when present in large amounts, will cause protein precipitation. Mercury also inhibits multiple enzyme systems such as oxidative mitochondrial phosphorylation and cytochrome c oxidase. Mercury decreases the activity of the liver microsomal detoxification systems and thus indirectly potentiates the harmful effects of other toxicants. It has been found that mercury combines with both sulfhydryl and phosphoryl groups in the cell membrane, particularly the former. The exact mechanism entailed in the diuretic action of mercuric chloride and organic mercurial compounds is not completely understood, but the result is a diminution in the reabsorption of sodium and chloride by the kidney tubules, particularly the straight portion of the loop of Henle.

The toxic effects of mercury involve numerous organs and systems, but the major target organs are the central nervous system and the kidney. Although the kidney contains the highest concentration of mercury regardless of the chemical form absorbed, it is the primary target organ only for inorganic mercury. In acute mercury poisoning, mercuric chloride is usually identified as causing the massive damage to proximal convoluted tubules that results in acute renal failure. The ingestion of this material is usually associated with suicide or accidental death. Autopsy findings reveal enlarged kidneys with pale and swollen cortices and dark and congested pyramids. When death does not ensue until a

period of 3 or 4 days has passed, the proximal convoluted tubules undergo extensive cellular necrosis, with the lumens becoming filled with eosinophilic granular cytoplasmic debris (Fig. 4-27). The basement membrane of the nephron is intact. The ascending limbs, distal convoluted tubules, and collecting tubules contain casts, and there is only slight epithelial loss in the distal convoluted tubules. At approximately 8 days the necrotic debris has disappeared from the tubular lumens. The proximal convoluted tubules are dilated, and the epithelium shows signs of regeneration as evidenced by the presence of mitotic figures (Fig. 4-28, A). By approximately 14 days the epithelium of the proximal convoluted tubules has returned to the normal configuration. Healing of the lesion is characterized by reabsorption of the interstitial edema fluid and repair of the tubular epithelium along the intact basement membrane, thereby reestablishing tubular integrity.

This is in contrast to pure ischemic changes in which the basement membrane is fragmented and ruptured, with complete disintegration of the tubular structure and leakage of the tubular contents into the renal interstitium. The latter lesion is referred to as tubulorrhexis. In severe acute tubular nephrosis or necrosis resulting from inorganic mercurial salt ingestion, ischemia, as well as direct toxic action of the insulting agent, may

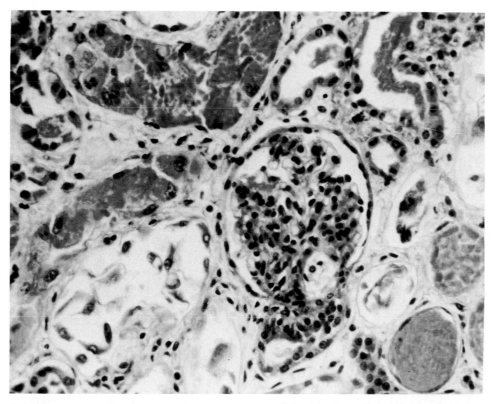

Fig. 4-27. Mercury poisoning. Death occurred 4 days after ingestion of several table-spoonfuls of bichloride of mercury. Coagulative necrosis of proximal convoluted tubules is characteristic.

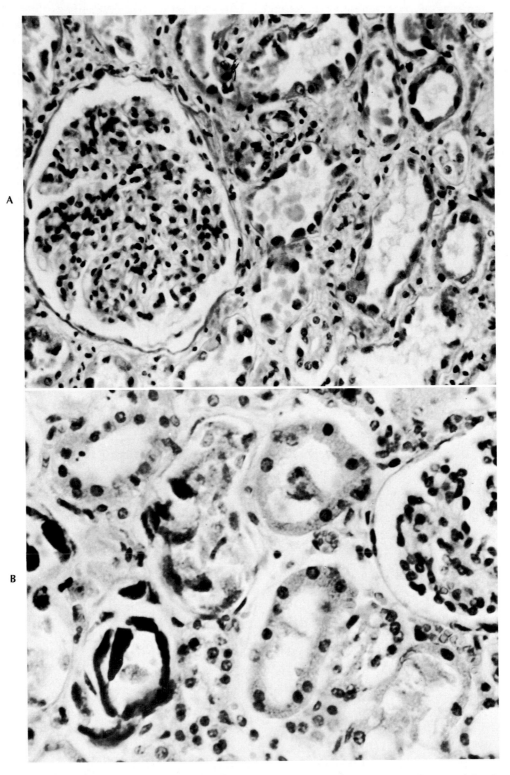

Fig. 4-28. A, Mercury poisoning. Death occurred 7 days after ingestion of mercurial salts. Attempts at regeneration of proximal tubular epithelial cells are observed. However, regeneration was not sufficient to prevent death from renal insufficiency. **B,** Calcification of renal tubules.

have its effect on the tubules. For example, in cases of severe mercury poisoning, there is considerable ulceration of the colonic mucosa, with severe diarrhea and fluid loss leading to hypovolemic shock with its accompanying peripheral circulatory failure. This set of circumstances results in tubular damage as a result of the ischemia of hypovolemic shock, as well as the direct toxic action of the mercury. Calcification, particularly of the proximal convoluted tubules, may occur in a matter of a few days (Fig. 4-28, *B*). Ultrastructural observations indicate that initially the intracellular calcification may be in the mitochondria.

It is known that detectable glomerular damage does not take place in acute poisoning, but in clinical cases of chronic industrial exposure there is documentation of thickening of the glomerular basement membrane leading to proteinuria. With severe damage, the nephrotic syndrome may appear characterized by all the features of membranous glomerulonephritis with subepithelial electron-dense deposits, reminiscent of an immune complex deposition. An additional mechanism in the development of proteinuria in such cases is tubular damage leading to inability of the tubule to resorb protein, which results in minor degrees of the nephrotic syndrome. Chronic poisoning usually develops in workers in the mercury industry who handle mainly mercuric oxide and calomel (mercurous chloride).

Electron microscopic examination of tubular epithelium of the pars recta of the rat kidney after subcutaneous injection of 4 to 16 mg of mercuric chloride per kilogram of body weight reveals tubular necrosis. The following changes are observed: fragmentation and disruption of the plasma membrane and its appendages, vesiculation and disruption of endoplasmic reticulum, dissociation of polysomes and loss of ribosomes, vesiculation of Golgi apparatus, mitochondrial swelling with loss of mitochondrium-dense granules, and condensation of the nuclear chromatin.

In acute mercury poisoning the brain is characterized by necrosis of gray matter, hyalinization of vessels, proliferation of capillaries, and astrocytic proliferation (Fig. 4-29). As stated previously, exposure to both elemental mercury vapor and short-chain alkyl mercury compounds exerts a pronounced effect on the central nervous system. There are similarities and striking differences between these two forms. Mercury vapor effects are neuropsychiatric in nature and occur at relatively low levels. Symptoms include excessive shyness, insomnia, and emotional instability with depression and irritability.

Intention tremors occur with both forms of mercury toxicity. In contrast to mercury vapor toxicity, methyl mercury effects are largely sensorimotor in nature and include paresthesias, constriction of the visual field, loss of hearing, loss of sense of smell and taste, incoordina-

tion, paralysis, and abnormal reflexes. In addition, spontaneous fits of laughing and crying and intellectual deterioration occur only in methyl mercury poisoning. Morphologically, in both forms of poisoning degenerative changes are widespread and include degeneration of both the plasma membrane and the myelin sheath. In addition, microscopic examination reveals both cerebral and cerebellum atrophy, with involvement of the granular layer of the cerebellum being particularly prominent. The Purkinje cells are intact. Spongy degeneration of the white matter in the visual cortex and other cortical regions are observed.

In addition to its role as a cytoplasmic toxin, mercury may assume the role of a hapten by virtue of its ability to denature protein. Uncommonly, mercurial diuretics have been implicated in the pathogenesis of the clinical nephrotic syndrome. In these instances there is a chronic transmembranous glomerulonephritis with dense deposits (presumably immune complexes) located between the visceral epithelial cells and the basement membrane of the glomeruli. Immunostaining has in some instances demonstrated immunoglobulin deposits at these sites. Other heavy metals such as gold have been implicated in the production of transmembranous glomerulonephritis, resulting in the nephrotic syndrome.

Our knowledge of inorganic and organic mercury poisoning of the central nervous system is almost entirely confined to the effects of these compounds on the brain. Although there is clinical evidence of involvement of peripheral nerves, morphologic changes in the human have not been well documented. The clinical features of inorganic mercury poisoning are well known. The phrase "mad as a hatter" arises from the use of mercury in the preparation of felt hats. This clinical syndrome, as popularized by Lewis Carroll, is a classic combination of emotional liability, depression, outbursts of anger, and insomnia. Neuropathologic findings on these cases is not well established. On the other hand, organic material especially in the form of short-change alkyl mercury exposure, is probably the best explored aspect of mercury toxicity. Acute and subacute methyl mercury poisoning in adults and chronic exposure in children may result in widespread spongy disruption of the cerebral cerebellum cortex with neuronal loss and gliosis. Prenatal exposure may result in a similar picture. Choi recorded in utero exposure as being teratogenic, leading to microcephaly, abnormal gyration patterns, gray matter heterotopias, and disruption of cortical architecture. Chronic instances of methyl mercury poisoning are reflected by gross atrophy of the calcarine cortex and cerebellum. In the calcarine cortex there is considerable neuronal loss and gliosis; lesser affected areas include pre- and postcentral gyri and temporal cortex. The outer cortical lay-

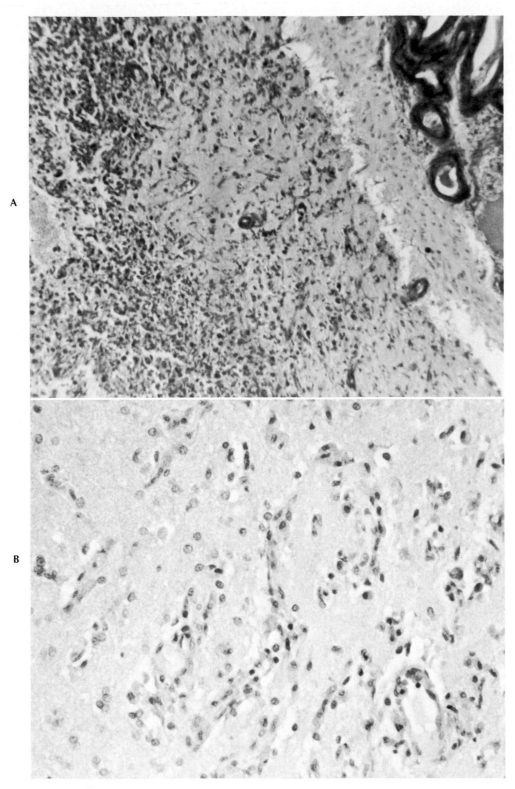

Fig. 4-29. Acute mercury poisoning (10 days' duration). **A,** Necrosis of occipital cortex and "fibrinoid necrosis of pia vessels." **B,** Capillary proliferation and necrosis. (Courtesy Dr. W.D. Hiers, Spartanburg, S.C.)

Fig. 4-29, cont'd. C, Astrocytic proliferation.

ers and depths of sulci appear most effective. In the cerebellum, internal granular cell neurons are lost along with small numbers of Purkinje cells. The route of administration seems unimportant as both ingestion and intravenous administration as well as other routes result in identical morphologic presentations. Short-change alkyl mercury compounds easily across the blood-brain barrier. They react nonspecifically with sulfhydryl groups. In particular, they may affect ribosomal proteins, resulting in ribosomal structural abnormalities detectable on electron microscopy.

Lead

The lead content of some exterior paints and a few interior paints, as well as that of glazing putty, offers a very serious and potential hazard for the development of lead poisoning in children. It is estimated that some 5% to 10% of children between 1 and 6 years of age have abnormally high blood levels of lead and so in the United States the projected figure may be as high as 200,000. The habit of eating nonfood objects such as peeling paint and slivers of glazed putty from window frames is known as pica (a reference to the omnivorous magpie). During the past 30 years there has been an increasing effort on the part of public health authorities to urge paint and putty manufacturers to discontinue the use of lead, substituting compounds such as tita-

nium dioxide as an opacifier. In fact, lead has been banned from use by manufacturers of paint. The occupational exposure by those working in the smelting of lead are subject to the inhaling of the metal fumes and deposits of lead oxide dust in the immediate environment. Also endangered are those who manufacture and recycle automobile batteries. Lead is a common heavy metal used in the construction of battery grids. Consumers of moonshine liquor also risk lead intoxication because metallic lead may be used in the construction of the still.

The diagnosis of lead poisoning encompasses such findings as high blood content of lead, increased free erythrocyte protoporphyrin (FEP) content, decreased erythrocyte δ-aminolevulinate dehydrase (ALAD) activity, convulsions, intestinal cramps, vomiting, anemia, and basophilic stippling of red blood cells (Fig. 4-30).

Lead inhibits several enzymes, notably ALAD, ferrochelatase, and nucleotidase. Inhibition of the first two enzymes blocks synthesis of hemoglobin. Inhibition of the nucleotidase is the probable cause for basophilic stippling and an associated increase in red cell fragility. Both effects contribute to iron-deficient microcytic hypochromic anemia. Lead and lead salts are absorbed by the gastrointestinal tract and fumes by the lung. Lead is deposited in the bones, nails, teeth, and hair. It frequently will be stored in these locations until dehydra-

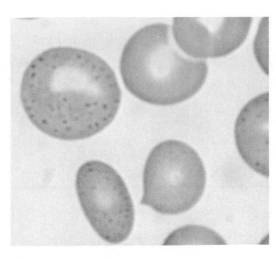

Fig. 4-30. Lead poisoning. Basophilic stippling of red blood cells.

tion, acidosis, and hyperthermia or increased body temperature occur. These factors mobilize the lead from bones into the bloodstream and are then deposited in the cells of the nervous system, kidney, liver, and bone marrow, resulting in clinical and laboratory manifestations of lead toxicity.

Feeding lead to rats for several weeks causes swelling of kidney mitochondria in vivo and inhibition of the phosphorylating system in vitro. Dense particles are found in both mitochondria and lysosomes of dogs fed lead at high levels for long periods of time. In part, they are composed of magnesium, calcium, and protein (Fig. 4-31, A). Electron-dense, lead-containing intranuclear inclusions are a common finding. The nuclear inclusions also contain other metals and are bound to a highly anionic protein. In humans and experimental animals they appear to be present only in acute lead intoxication and are acid fast when stained with carbol fuchsin (Fig. 4-31, B). Many of the morphologic and functional sequelae of lead poisoning are believed to be secondary results of a primary inhibition of mitochondrial activity by lead. Clinically, the lead tubular damage of the proximal convoluted tubule leads to the impaired reabsorption of amino acids, glucose, and phosphorus. The result is aminoaciduria, glycosuria, and hyperphosphaturia, referred to as "Fanconi's syndrome."

In acute cases of lead poisoning, the brain is extremely edematous and, microscopically, necrosis of the cerebral and cerebellar white matter may occur, followed by diffuse astrocytic proliferation (Fig. 4-32). This is probably attributable in part to the role of lead as a mitochondrial poison. Similar to mercurial encephalopathy, there is endothelial proliferation of small capillaries of the white matter and thickening of small in-

tercerebral arteries. Characteristically, protein droplets accumulate in perivascular spaces (Fig. 4-33). However, in severe lead encephalopathy (above 120 μg of Pb per ml) the neurotoxicity manifests itself as a peripheral motor neuropathy primarily involving the perineal and radial nerves, resulting in foot and wrist drop. Lead toxicity may also be responsible for recurrent episodes of gastrointestinal pain brought about by neuropathy. Experimentally, toxic levels of lead acetate may bring about liver necrosis in rats that are fed a diet containing 40% fat. Lipotropic agents, such as the sulfur-containing amino acid methionine, prevent this necrosis. In humans, necrosis of the liver is not observed in acute and chronic lead poisoning.

Cytochrome P-450 serum levels are diminished, suggestive of some hepatocyte dysfunction. The kidney lesions are restricted to the proximal convoluted tubule, where there is some interference with function, resulting in aminoaciduria. Changes in the mitochondria of the proximal convoluted tubules are observed. In children with chronic lead poisoning, lesions of the myocardium, consisting of edema and fibroblastic activation in the interstitial tissue accompanied by a lymphocytic inflammatory infiltrate, have been described. Similar lesions have not been described in chronic lead poisoning in adults. However, lead has been implicated as an etiologic factor in the production of premature atherosclerosis and of nephrosclerosis with hypertension and cardiac hypertrophy. Experimentally, such factors as vitamin D administration, ultraviolet radiation, increasing body temperatures, and acidosis have been shown to mobilize lead salts from the bony skeleton, thereby increasing the serum levels. The gingival dental margin is pigmented as a result of the deposition of lead sulfite, the so-called lead line of the gums.

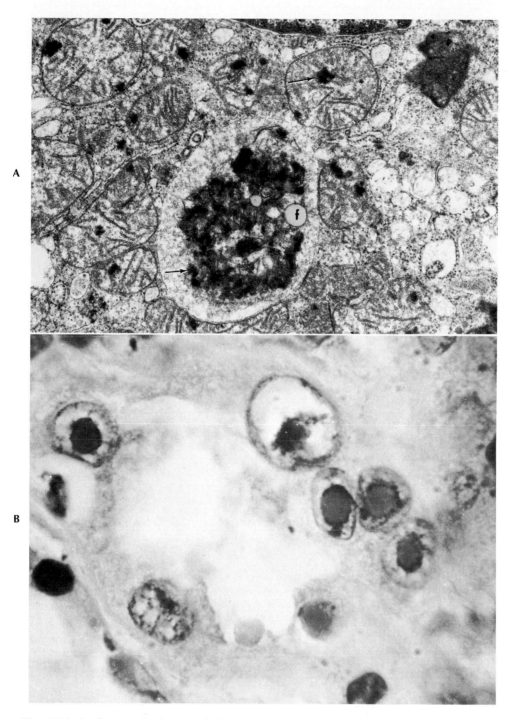

Fig. 4-31. A, Center of micrograph is occupied by large phagolysosome containing mitochondrial fragments, lipofuscin pigment, and fat *(f)*. Dense particles are observed in the mitochondria and phagolysosome *(arrows).* **B,** Lead poisoning. Intranuclear inclusions in cells of proximal convoluted tubules. (37,500×; courtesy William B. Greene, Medical University of South Carolina, Charleston, S.C.)

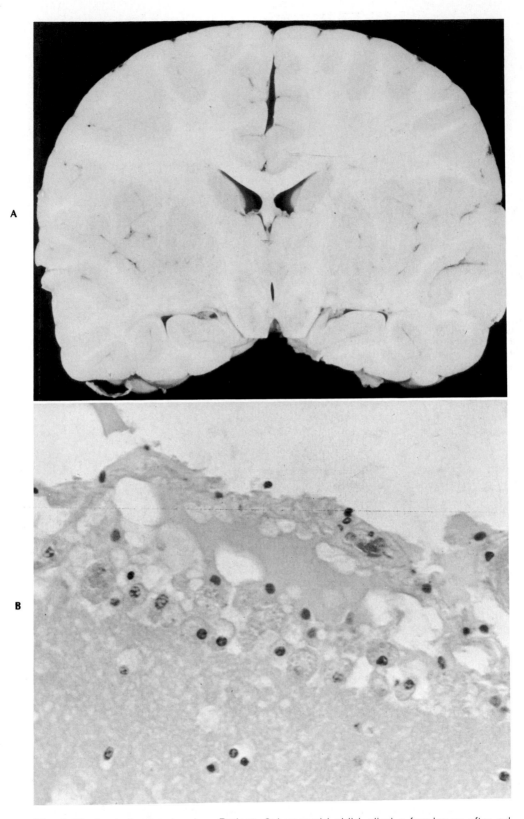

Fig. 4-32. Acute lead poisoning. Patient, 2½-year-old child, died a few hours after admission with diagnosis of brain tumor. **A,** Brain noticeably swollen. Samples of gray and white matter yielded toxic content of lead. **B,** Subpial vesicles filled with proteinaceous fluid and macrophages. (Courtesy Dr. Stanley M. Aronson, Brown University, Providence, R.I.)

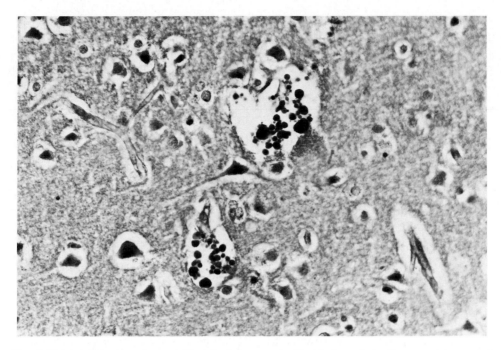

Fig. 4-33. Adult male, a "moonshiner" who was admitted to hospital with convulsions and died from pneumonia. Lead serum level was 140 μg/dl (normal 0 to 50). Notice protein globules, prominent astrocyte *(center),* and perinuclear and perivascular edema. (Phosphotungstic acid and hematoxylin stains; 270×.)

Arsenic

Arsenic is a metalloid, exhibiting variable valences −3, +3, +5; it is capable of forming both cationic and anionic salts. It is ubiquitous in distribution in soil, occurring mainly in the pentavalent state, whereas arsenic added to the environment is trivalent. Arsenic trioxide (As_2O_3) is used as the initial reactant in the manufacture of most arsenic compounds. Major uses of white arsenic and other arsenic compounds are as active ingredients of rodenticides, insecticides, fungicides, wood preservatives, soil sterilants, defoliants, feed additives, and weed killers. They are also used in the textile, tanning, and glass industries, as well as in the manufacture of pigments and in antifouling paints. Arsenic has been used therapeutically for 2000 years.

Compounds of arsenic may be absorbed after ingestion or by inhalation. It is generally true that trivalent forms of arsenic are more toxic than pentavalent forms and that most poisoning results from inorganic arsenicals. Arsenate in all its valent forms is most prevalent in nature and probably does not accumulate in the body, being rapidly excreted by the kidneys. Arsenites, however, bind easily to tissue proteins and accumulate primarily in liver, muscles, hair, nails, and skin. Acute arsenic poisoning has its major manifestation in the stomach, nervous system, and vascular endothelium. Symptoms include nausea; vomiting; diarrhea; acute and severe irritation of the nose, throat, and conjunc-tiva; severe abdominal pain; and inflammation. Total toxic effects may be produced by the gaseous form of arseniureted hydrogen (arsine, AsH_3). A 30-minute exposure to 250 ppm in air is lethal to humans and animals, the maximum concentration inhalable for 1 hour without toxicity being 5 to 20 ppm. The intensity of the acute toxic reaction depends to a great extent on the physical state of the subject and quantity of the arsenic ingested or inhaled. Shock may cause early death, in which case no striking anatomic changes are evident.

In suspected acute poisoning, obtaining an alkaline reaction with litmus on the vomitus may be helpful. Most common poisons are acid in reaction.

In acute as well as chronic poisoning, significant amounts of arsenic may be identified in clippings of hair, fingernails, and toenails. Contamination of fingernails from vomitus or other external sources must always be kept in mind. Arsenic binds rapidly and firmly with sulfhydryl (SH) groups in nails, hair, and skin. In fact, this ability to combine with SH groups probably explains the lethal action of high concentrations of arsenic by inhibition of respiratory SH enzymes. At necropsy, particles of yellow sulfide of arsenous oxide may be seen attached to the stomach mucosa. These crystals are readily identifiable on chemical and microscopic examination. In patients surviving a few days, there will be congestion, edema, and hemorrhage in the gastric mucosa and degenerative changes in the heart, liver, and kidneys. There may also be purpuric hemorrhages in various tissues, a striking feature being the discovery of extensive subendocardial splashes of hemorrhage in the left ventricle.

Chronic arsenic poisoning from repeated exposure results in a highly suggestive group of signs and symptoms: loss of weight, nausea, alternating constipation and diarrhea, paresthesia and numbness (frequently in a symmetric stocking-glove distribution), and muscle weakness of the limbs caused by peripheral neuritis. In addition, perforation of the nasal septum, ulceration of the alimentary tract, and tremors may occur. Dermatologic manifestations are protean: loss of hair, increased melanin pigmentation, maculopapular rash, "arsenical dermatitis," and hyperkeratosis of the palms and soles. Reported hepatic damage includes noncirrhotic portal hypertension, cirrhosis, and hemangiosarcoma of the liver. Arsenicals are readily excreted in the sweat, but the main route of elimination is the urine. Moderate anemia resulting from hemolysis and erythropoietic depression may be manifest. Basophilic stippling also occurs frequently. The diagnosis is substantiated by examination of the urine (over 0.2 mg of arsenic per liter is significant), sweat, hair, or nails.

Arsenous acid (arsenous oxide, white arsenic) is the substance most commonly employed in homicidal arsenical poisoning. It is manufactured as a gritty white material in the form of powder or cakes. It is quite insoluble in cold water. It dissolves in hot water, but three fourths of the particles settle out as the water cools. Solubility in caustic soda is easily accomplished. Exhumed bodies testify to the preservative action of arsenic on body tissues. As is the case with fluoride, gross and microscopic examinations are facilitated by prior tissue exposure.

Involvement of arsenic in carcinogenesis is not unequivocally established, since the epidemiologic and experimental findings are in contradiction. Epidemiologic evidence indicates that industrial and agricultural exposure to arsenic is implicated in cancer of the skin and respiratory tract. The persons at greatest risk are smelter workers, though there is some evidence that women residing near such operations incur a greater incidence of respiratory cancer. Also, studies have implicated arsenic ingestion as goitrogenic, and this possible effect has been confirmed in animals. Epithelial carcinomas of the skin develop with chronic arsenicalism, with latent periods of 3 to 40 or more years. Sound experimental evidence for the carcinogenic activity of inorganic arsenic compounds appears to be nonexistent.

Ferrous sulfate

Accidental ferrous sulfate intoxication is a relatively common and frequently fatal poisoning in childhood. The usual range is between 1 and 2 years of age. Approximately 2000 cases of acute poisoning occur an-

nually, with only acute intoxications from aspirin, other unknown medications, and phenobarbital occurring more frequently.

After ingestion of ferrous sulfate in toxic doses, there are five clinical phases of subsequent toxicity. The first phase, lasting 30 minutes to 2 hours, is characterized by lethargy, restlessness, hematemesis, abdominal pain, and bloody diarrhea. The direct corrosive effect of iron initiates necrosis of the gastrointestinal mucosa and may result in severe hemorrhagic necrosis and subsequent shock. Shock may also in part be attributed to vasodepressor activity of ferritin resulting from rapid iron absorption through the intact mucosa. "Shock lesions" (centrilobular necrosis of liver cells, acute tubular nephrosis, and brain and pulmonary congestion and edema) are observed. Experimentally, ferrous sulfate–induced liver damage is reminiscent of that seen in humans. At the lethal dose level, severe hepatic necrosis develops by 8 hours. Ultrastructural studies demonstrate mitochondrial damage in parenchymal cells within 2 hours after ingestion. Within 4 hours there is extensive mitochondrial alteration with the accumulation of iron particles between the cristae. As is common after the ingestion of numerous hepatocellular toxins, there is hypertrophy of the smooth endoplasmic reticulum.

The second phase represents apparent recovery, which progresses into the third phase 2 to 12 hours after the first phase. The third phase is heralded by the appearance of shock, cyanosis, fever, and acidoses. The last results from conversion of ferric$^{(+3)}$ to ferrous$^{(+2)}$ ions with concomitant release of hydrogen ions, as well as accumulation of lactic and citric acids. Signs of pneumonitis and convulsions may occur. The fourth phase occurs 2 to 4 days after ingestion and is characterized by the development of hepatic necrosis, again attributable to direct toxic action of iron on mitochondria. Recovery is generally rapid if survival is 3 to 4 days. The fifth phase, 2 to 4 weeks after ingestion, is characterized by gastrointestinal obstruction resulting from gastric or pyloric scarring.

Pertinent autopsy findings are confined to the gastroduodenal mucosa and liver. The mucosa is brown from staining with iron chloride and reveals focal or diffuse superficial necrosis with petechial hemorrhages. Stainable iron is easily identifiable in the mucosal lamina propria and connective tissue of the submucosa. This probably represents diffusion. Iron is readily demonstrated in the endothelium of the submucosal veins and lymphatics, as well as the intrahepatic portal vein branches and Kupffer cells. Staining of the reticulin fibers in the portal areas is eaily visualized. The periportal hepatocytes are swollen and contain stainable finely dispersed fat, and loss of glycogen and necrosis may be evident.

Whereas acute overload studies strongly suggest the

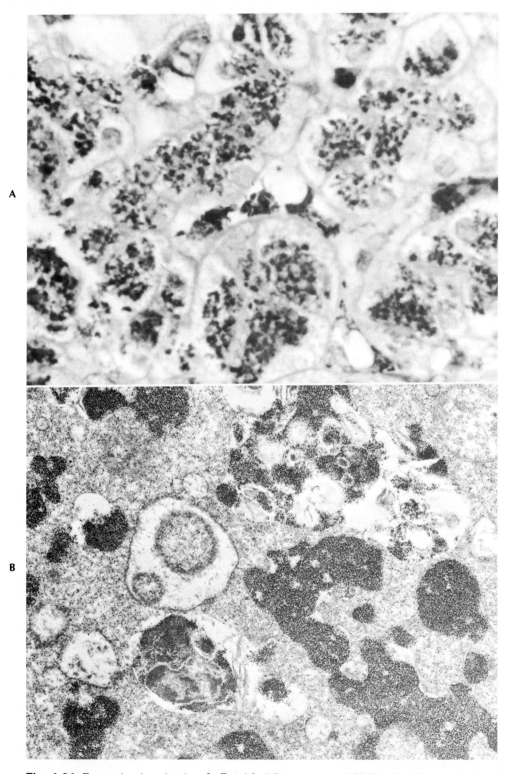

Fig. 4-34. Excessive iron intake. **A,** Food faddist consumed 5000 mixed iron and vitamin pills per annum for several years. Enlarged liver was an incidental finding on routine physical examination. Hepatocytes are loaded with hemosiderin. **B,** Normal amount of glycogen and dense intracellular aggregates of hemosiderin. No mitochondrial damage is noted. (34,000×.)

toxic role of iron for mitochondria, there may not be an analogous situation in chronic iron overload. Fig. 4-34, A, demonstrates hemosiderin-laden hepatocytes prepared from a man who ingested 5000 mixed vitamin and iron pills per annum for several years. He was in "good health," a nutritional faddist, and hepatosplenomegaly was discovered on a routine physical examination. Light and electron microscope examination revealed iron impregnation of collagen and reticulin fibers. The hepatocytes contained large aggregates of membrane-bound hemosiderin and intact mitochondria (Fig. 4-34, B).

Chronic excessive intake of iron may lead to hemosiderosis or hemochromatosis. Hemosiderosis refers to generalized increased iron content in body tissues, particularly the liver and reticuloendothelial system. Hemochromatosis indicates histologic hemosiderosis with diffuse fibrosis of the affected organ.

Cobalt

Cobalt is an essential micronutrient for mammals, but its function is unknown except as a component of vitamin B_{12}. Cobalt salts are generally well absorbed in normal dietary amounts, but larger doses are more poorly absorbed. It is not sequestered easily, since it is stored in intestinal mucosa and lost through desquamation of the epithelium. Cobalt salts are retained primarily in the heart, liver, bone marrow, pancreas, kidneys, and spleen. Excretion is mainly urinary. Poisoning can occur from inhalation of cobalt alloy vapors in industrial settings and from the therapeutic use of cobalt-containing compounds in treatment of anemia and radioactive cobalt in cancer treatment.

Polycythemia characteristically occurs with ingestion of excessive amounts of cobalt. Acute toxicity after ingestion has been reported to lead to vomiting, paralysis, lowering of blood pressure, liver and adrenal hemorrhages, alveolar thickening, and renal and pancreatic degeneration. Inhalation causes acute lung inflammation, edema, and hemorrhages; massive pericardial effusions; and peritoneal effusions.

Before the banning of cobalt in proprietary preparations, it was not uncommon to see diffuse thyroid hyperplasia primarily in children treated for anemia with Roncovite, an enteric-coated, ferrous-cobaltous chloride preparation. This goitrogenic compound did not give rise to thyrotoxicosis. Experimentally, the role of cobalt in stimulating erythrocytosis is well known.

A decade ago, beer manufacturers in the United States and Belgium added excessive amounts of cobalt acetate to their products so that the froth would stick to the sides of the glass to produce a good "head." However, the levels of ingestion were lower than doses tolerated in other conditions, such as those for treatment of anemia. Many of the beer drinkers were in a state of thiamine and nutritional deficiency, and it has been shown that thiamine and protein deficiencies enhance the cardiotoxicity of cobalt. In addition, ethanol sensitizes animals to cobalt toxicity. The situation is comparable to so-called alcoholic cardiomyopathy, making it impossible to characterize the entities of cobalt and alcoholic myocardiosis.

Grossly, the hearts of persons who have died of what has been referred to as beer drinkers' heart disease have shown cardiac dilatation and hypertrophy. Signs and symptoms were those of congestive heart failure. Histologically, in cases in which cobalt was a suspected factor in the death of the patient, the myocardium revealed vacuole formation and accumulation of sudanophilic material that appeared as fine droplets in all parts of the sarcoplasm. A slight and fine focal fibrosis was observed that is interpreted as a condensation fibrosis occurring after myocytolysis. Although pyknotic nuclei may be observed, there is no extensive overt necrosis.

Experimentally, structural changes in animal myofibrils and mitochondria have been produced by cobalt administration alone. Cobalt ions are known to depress oxygen uptake in heart mitochondria by inhibiting the enzymes α-ketoglutarate dehydrogenase and pyruvate dehydrogenase.

Mild cobalt toxicity has been reported to cause hyperglycemia in dogs and rats because of transient and reversible damage to alpha cells of the pancreas.

Although no evidence for carcinogenicity of dietary cobalt is known, it has been shown experimentally that oxides and sulfides of cobalt cause cancer in animals. Tumors reported include fibrosarcomas, liposarcomas, and tumors in the thyroid gland and at injection sites.

Cadmium

Cadmium is utilized in the manufacture of alkaline storage batteries, alloys, and electroplating of other metals. Instances of inhalation of cadmium oxide fumes during the course of welding steel parts that have been plated with a cadmium anticorrosive agent has been observed.

Acute inhalation of relatively large concentrations of cadmium vapors produces acute cadmium pneumonia approximately 8 to 10 hours after inhalation of the vapors. Histologically, the lung is characterized by diffuse alveolar damage, with striking congestion and edema of the alveolar capillaries. Death occurs in approximately 16% of those exposed to high concentration of the vapors. Chronic inhalation of smaller amounts of cadmium vapors can result in interstitial fibrosis of the lungs. This eventuates in the honeycomb lung that is the result of repeated attacks of acute bronchiolitis and interstitial pneumonia with reparative scarring (Fig. 4-35).

There are several reports of an increased incidence of emphysema in persons exposed to low concentrations of cadmium fumes over a long period of time. The maximum permissible level of cadmium vapors in the air,

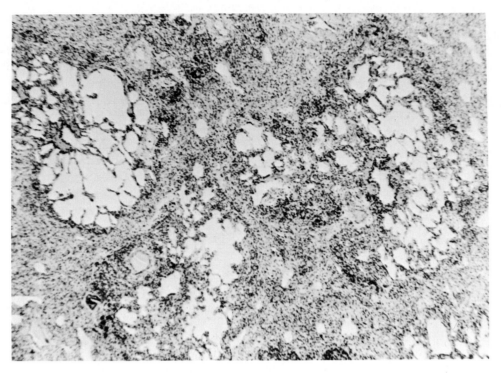

Fig. 4-35. Cadmium inhalation—dog lung. Interstitial fibrosis, lymphocyte infiltration, and expanded alveolar sacs. (Courtesy Dr. Charles B. Carrington, Stanford University, Stanford, Calif.)

in both England and the United States, is 100 μg/cubic meter. According to Nandi and associates,[225] the cadmium contained in cigarettes is transmitted to the lungs during smoking. One pack of 20 cigarettes contains 30 μg of cadmium. One must conclude therefore that cadmium accumulates in the tissues of heavy smokers and could theoretically cause lung, liver, and kidney disease. However, if *all* the cadmium in two packs of cigarettes were inhaled, this would still be less cadmium than would be inspired in 2 hours of normal breathing at maximum safe levels of atmospheric cadmium. There is no unchallenged evidence that cigarette smoking causes emphysema. There is no question, on the other hand, that cigarette smoking results in acute and chronic bronchitis and worsens the state of emphysema. Emphysema may develop in cadmium workers in the alkaline battery industry as a result of exposure to low concentrations of cadmium fumes over a long period of time. To properly assess the significance of the relationship of cadmium to the development of emphysema, further epidemiologic and other studies are required. At the present time there is no information available as to the type and degree of emphysema seen at autopsy in such persons.

It is now certain that cadmium accumulates in the kidney with age and, if exposure is excessive and prolonged, will induce a progressive form of chronic renal disease characterized by interstitial fibrosis and tubular atrophy. Unlike the heavy-metal tubular dysfunctions brought about by damage to the proximal tubular cells, cadmium does not manifest tubular damage acutely but in a chronic sequence. A growing documentation of evidence that points to the tubular cell damage is in proportion to the increasing concentration of calcium bound to metallothioneine. Bonding of calcium and tissues and transport has been shown to be related to the presence of the low-molecular-weight protein metallothioneine. There is a selective uptake by the proximal convoluted tubules of metallothioneine-bound cadmium. The toxic effects after a long-time exposure to the toxic levels of this union of cadmium with the protein metallothioneine is characterized by probable damage to the plasma cell membrane resulting in the eventuality of necrosis of the tubular cells. The effects of cadmium on proximal renal tubular function are characterized by increased calcium in the urine, proteinuria (primarily β_2-microglobulin), aminoaciduria, glycosuria, and decreased renal tubular reabsorption of phosphate. As stated by Goyer, the most important measure of excessive cadmium exposure is increased cadmium excretion in the urine, and this finding reflects the concentration. Studies of workers with cadmium exposure suggest that the "critical level" is a urine concentration of 10 to 15 mg, which means per gram of urinary creatine. At this level, proximal tubular reabsorption dysfunction will probably raise its ugly head.

Nickel

Nickel and its compounds have been implicated in producing a contact type of dermatitis, carcinoma of the lung and nasal passages, and various soft-tissue malignancies in experimental animals. Nickel dermatitis has been noted to be a rather common occurrence. Nickel workers in Great Britain, Germany, Norway, Russia, Japan, and Canada have been noted to have an increased incidence of respiratory cancer, particularly of the nasal passages.

Experimental studies with nickel carbonyl, $Ni(CO)_4$, have produced carcinomas in rats by inhalation of the vapor and by parenteral administration. It is interesting to note that even with intravenous administration of nickel carbonyl the lungs are the target of the acute reaction. There is also an increased mitotic index of the bronchiolar and alveolar epithelial cells. To a lesser extent the liver shows loss of glycogen, the kidney shows sporadic vacuolization of the proximal convoluted tubules without necrosis, and the adrenal glands reveal intense congestion of the cortical sinusoids. When viewed by electron microscopy, the proliferative reaction of the alveolar epithelium appears to involve both the granular and membranous pneumocytes. Discharge of cytoplasmic inclusions and granular pneumocytes is noted. The membranous pneumocytes develop large nucleoli, nuclei, and cytoplasm and have a distinct increase in cytoplasmic organelles, including free ribosomes, endoplasmic reticulum, and Golgi zones.

There are a few studies concerning the long-range effects of continued oral ingestion of nickel in mammals. Dogs fed nickel sulfate orally for a period of 2 years show a remarkable reaction in the lungs. Grossly there are pale subpleural collections of cholesterol macrophages that are associated with the peripheral chronic bronchiolitis observed (Figs. 4-36 and 4-37). This may be the result of irritative qualities of the nickel ion being secreted by the bronchial mucosa. Whereas nickel carbonyl has been implicated in the production of respiratory neoplasia, it is not known if nickel salts (sulfate, chloride) consumed orally over a long period of time cause tissue damage or serve as carcinogens.

Thallium

The etiologic agent of thallotoxicosis is a heavy metal. Thallium sulfate or acetate appears in rat poisons and common insecticides. Because it is one of the most toxic metals, it has been used as a homicidal poison and for suicidal purposes. As a medicinal agent, the compound has enjoyed its greatest popularity through the years in the topical treatment of ringworm. It also has been used as a depilatory agent. In fact, some cases of accidental poisoning have occurred when the use of the agent in this manner resulted in rapid absorption. The metal is dispersed widely throughout all the body tissues and is excreted slowly. It interferes with the telogen phase of hair follicle growth, and because of its delayed excretion, alopecia may occur approximately 2

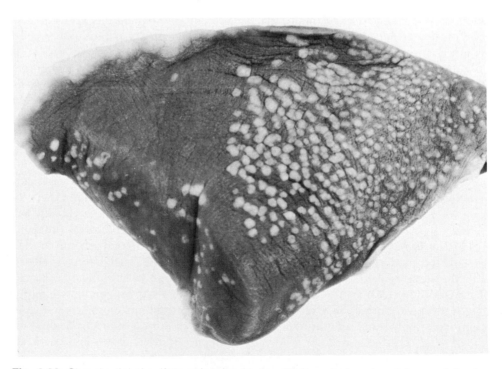

Fig. 4-36. Chronic nickel sulfate poisoning in dog. White subpleural nodules contain cholesterol macrophages. Edge of lung is pale after air trapping attributable to chronic bronchiolitis with mucus plugging.

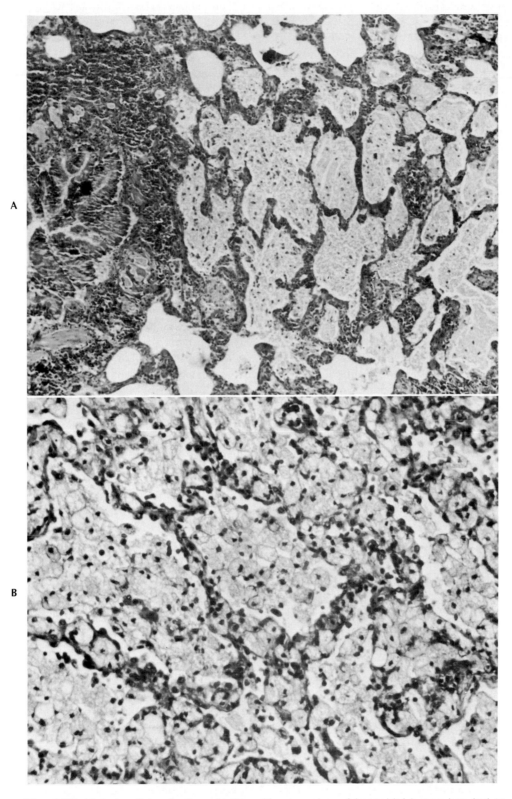

Fig. 4-37. Nickel sulfate. **A,** Bronchiolitis with narrowing of bronchial lumen has led to accumulation of cholesterol macrophages in alveolar sacs—often called "golden pneumonia." **B,** Higher magnification of section shown in **A.**

weeks after ingestion. Interestingly, axillary and facial hair and the inner one third of the eyebrows are spared, a feature of diagnostic importance.

Children are particularly susceptible to the effects of thallium compounds, with ingestion of 10 mg being responsible for fatal outcome. The lethal dose of thallium acetate in adults is approximately 1 g. Acute poisoning appears 12 to 36 hours after ingestion of a toxic amount. The signs and symptoms are abdominal pain, vomiting, and varied neurologic findings such as ataxia and other manifestations of toxic encephalopathy. Morphologically, neurons, nerve fibers, and glial elements throughout the central nervous system reveal various degenerative and even necrotic changes. More than 40 products containing 1% to 3% thallium salts are available in retail stores in the United States today. Reed and associates[242] point out that the ingestion of 1 ounce of a pesticide containing 1% thallium could be fatal to a small child. The actual mode of toxicity remains unclear.

Uranium

After the administration of uranyl nitrate to rats, renal tubular lesions become manifest. There is loss of the brush borders, dispersion of mitochondrial matrix, fragmentation and vesiculation of endoplasmic reticulum, and disruption of cytoplasmic membrane with whorl formation. The earliest observable changes after the administration of this compound appear to be clumping and margination of chromatin accompanied by nuclear shrinkage. This observation may indicate that uranyl nitrate attacks the nucleus before attacking cytoplasmic organelles, the intactness of which is responsible for the resorptive mechanism.

Platinum

For many years chemical injury from platinum was confined to the syndrome of platinosis, characterized by excessive histamine release and the concomitant hypersensitivity manifestations, in industrial platinum workers. In 1969, however, the compound *cis*-dichlorodiamine-platinum (II) was shown to be active against a transplantable rodent tumor. After extensive clinical evaluation, this compound was marketed as cisplatin in 1979. It is active against squamous cell carcinoma, lymphosarcoma, pancreatic carcinoma, and fibrosarcoma. It is particularly effective against metastatic ovarian tumors when combined with doxorubicin and cyclophosphamide and against metastatic testicular tumors when combined with vinblastine and bleomycin.

After intravenous administration, the first side effects noted in most patients are severe nausea and vomiting, occurring within a period of a few minutes to a few hours. This common reaction is so severe and long lasting that some patients refuse a second course of treatment. The mechanism of this effect is unknown.

The principal dose-limiting toxic action of cisplatin is nephrotoxicity; histologically similar renal lesions have been observed in rats, dogs, and humans after administration of the drug. The earliest marker of proximal tubular damage is an increased rate of excretion of β_2 microglobulins; this is followed by increases in BUN and serum creatinine levels, as well as hyperuricemia. The damage is considered mild when BUN and serum creatinine values are 25 to 35 mg/dl and 1.5 to 2 mg/dl respectively and severe when the BUN value increases to greater than 50 mg/dl or the serum creatinine level reaches more than 2.5 mg/dl, or both.

Histologically, the proximal tubular necrosis resembles that observed after administration of certain other heavy metals. Necrosis and desquamation of tubular epithelium are accompanied by the presence of intraluminal granular material and cellular debris. Cisplatin inactivates mitochondrial ATPase activity, thus inhibiting the energy-dependent functions of the tubular cells. Coadministration of cisplatin with large fluid volumes and mannitol to promote diuresis can ameliorate renal toxicity to some extent, but once incurred, damage is frequently irreversible.

Ototoxicity is observed in almost 30% of patients treated with a single dose of cisplatin at 50 mg/m². This is manifested by tinnitus or hearing loss in the high-frequency range, or both, and is more severe in children than in adults. Additional toxic effects of cisplatin include leukopenia, thrombocytopenia, a normocytic anemia, and marrow hypoplasia. Noted less often is neurotoxicity, characterized by peripheral neuropathies. Anaphylaxis-like reactions have also been reported.

Catecholamines

The vasopressor amines are commonly used to treat clinical states of shock and myocardial infarction. As early as 1906, experiments using multiple intravenous injections in rabbits were found to result in the appearance of hyaline necrosis with granular change, loss of muscle striation, and mononuclear leukocyte infiltration of the cardiac muscle fibers. The myocardial damage was not the result of arterial lesions, since no vascular change was demonstrated. Healing was characterized by interstitial edema and fibrosis of the myocardium.

Since that time, experimental cardiac lesions have been produced with epinephrine, isoproterenol, norepinephrine, and ephedrine. The most severe lesions are produced by isoproterenol, and the severity of the lesions can be correlated with increasing dosage. In cats, electrical stimulation of the midbrain reticular formation, the stellate ganglion, or the lateral hypothalamus can produce demonstrable myofibrillar degeneration. The degeneration is attributable to the rising

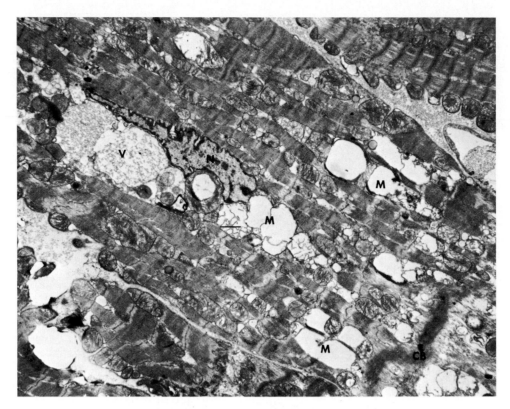

Fig. 4-38. Experimental isoproterenol hydrochloride in dog myocardium. After administration of 8 μg/kg body weight/minute for 2 hours, alterations include swelling of many mitochondria *(M)* with cristolysis and myofibrillar disruption with formation of contracture bands *(CB)*. Clumping and margination of nuclear chromatin *(N)* and vacuolization *(V)* of extracellular space. (4000×; courtesy Dr. David W. Hiott, Walterboro, S.C.)

concentration of catecholamines that have been induced by stimulation of the central nervous system pathways. The buildup and release of catecholamine in granular vesicles in close apposition to the sympathetic nervous system have been well demonstrated by Reichenbach and Benditt[253] after midbrain stimulation and the administration of isoproterenol. Histologically, by the end of the first day after the administration of norepinephrine or isoproterenol, the myocardial fibers are the "seat" of cytoplasmic banding, pyknosis of myocardial nuclei, loss of myocardial nuclear staining, and mononuclear proliferation (Fig. 4-38). At this stage there is disorganization of the cardiac myofibrils, and by the end of 3 days mineralization of mitochondria is evident. After 9 days, myocytolysis and fibrosis appear.

Factors capable of potentiating catecholamine induction of myofibrillar degeneration include sodium excess, deoxycorticosterone acetate (Doca) administration to animals deficient in dietary potassium, and low potassium content of the myocardial cells. Myofibrillar degeneration has been reported in patients dying of pheochromocytoma. Histologic findings in these patients were cytoplasmic band formation and mononuclear cell infiltration. Myofibrillar degeneration is not associated solely with endogenous or exogenous catecholamine states. On the other hand, it does explain the focal subendocardial patches of necrosis sometimes found after a variety of intracranial spontaneous and traumatic hemorrhages. It would seem logical that the cytotoxic effects of catecholamine may be the mechanism responsible for cardiac injury in many exogenous and endogenous disease states. From the standpoint of the pathologist, the recent enlightening literature concerning catecholamine damage may go a long way toward explaining early myofibrillar degeneration that was previously attributed to agonal or postmortem alterations. In addition, some cases of idiopathic myocardial fibrosis may in the future be discovered to be attributable to catecholamine myofibril toxicity.

Barbiturates

The barbiturates are similar in action to alcohol in that they are central nervous system depressants. The severity of the depression depends on the barbiturate used, mode of administration, degree of tolerance, presence or absence of other drugs in the body, and state of excitability of the individual. The potentially fatal oral doses of barbiturates are 5 g (long-acting) or 3 g

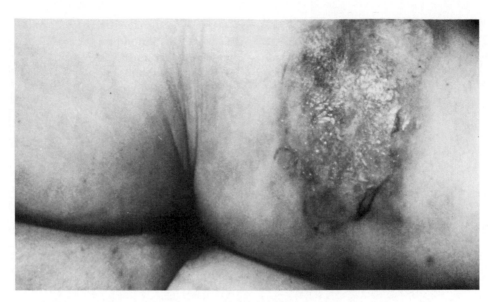

Fig. 4-39. Acute barbiturate intoxication. Patient died in coma 10 days after ingestion of pills. Irregularly outlined lesion of thigh is characterized by vesicles and excoriated epidermis with a dark coloration at periphery. (Courtesy Dr. Sandra E. Conradi, Medical University of South Carolina, Charleston, S.C.)

(short-acting). Potentially fatal blood levels are 8 mg/dl of a long-acting or 3.5 mg/dl of a short-acting barbiturate, indicating that short-acting barbiturates are more toxic. However, it is generally accepted that considerable individual variation exists. Recovery after the ingestion of 33 g of phenobarbital has been observed.

Barbiturates (goof balls, redbirds, yellow jackets, blue heavens), like innumerable other drugs, may play the role of a hapten and give rise to a wide spectrum of hypersensitivity tissue reactions. Notable among these is the development of polyarteritis nodosa lesions indistinguishable from the acute lesions of the spontaneous disease. Barbiturates are a leading cause of dermatitis medicamentosa, challenging penicillin for first place. Furthermore, the compounds may cause severe skin reactions such as those seen in exfoliative dermatitis and the Stevens-Johnson syndrome. Clinicians and pathologists are familiar with the large bullous lesions of the skin that develop in approximately 6% to 9% of patients with acute barbiturate intoxication. They are often referred to as the barbiturate blister (Fig. 4-39). Clinically, they are adequately characteristic to be valuable in the differential diagnosis of coma. The lesions are probably caused by a pressure phenomenon and are not the result of a specific toxic effect. In support of this is the common finding of the lesions on the inner aspects of the knees and ankles. The presence of lesions in other sites may be explained if the precise position of the patient when found is known.

Microscopically, the lesions are characterized by intraepidermal and subepidermal vesicles and bullae. Necrosis of eccrine sweat gland epithelia is a common ob-servation. The absence of abundant lymphocytes, plasma cells, macrophages, vasculitis, and granulomas leads the morphologist away from considering hypersensitivity-immunologic reactions as causative mechanisms for the production of the skin lesions. Clear-cut zones of hemorrhagic infarction are found in the subcutaneous fat. The barbiturates, like chloral hydrate, DDT isomers, and alcohol, generate hyperplasia of the smooth endoplasmic reticulum in the hepatocyte. This is the morphologic reflection of "enzyme induction," resulting in accelerated enzymatic action in the liver microsomes. This mechanism explains the depression of anticoagulant response in patients receiving both barbiturate derivatives and bishydroxycoumarin (dicumarol). The increased enzyme activity stimulated by barbiturates and chloral hydrate rapidly metabolizes the coumarin drug. In contrast, phenylbutazone and thyroxine inhibit the breakdown of coumarin, leading to an accentuated prolongation of the prothrombin time. Failure to recognize these effects may result in serious hemorrhagic complications.

Barbiturates should be administered with caution to patients who have hepatocellular damage such as fatty liver, alcoholic hepatitis, viral hepatitis, or severe generalized circulatory failure. The alcoholic with cirrhosis may show a prolonged peak of blood barbiturate after therapeutic dosage. The investigation of apparently natural deaths that actually resulted from alcohol-barbiturate intake is of immense importance to the medical examiner, the coroner, and the public. The *manner* of death determined from such investigations appears on the death certificate as accident, suicide, or undetermined. At the same time the probable *cause* of death may be clearly attributed to alcohol-barbiturate intake. The finding of a suicide note aids the investigator. On the other hand, a history of alcoholic and barbiturate intake is of little help in the determination of whether fatal consumption was intentional or accidental. What appears on the death certificate is important, since relatives are frequently emotionally upset when proved suicide occurs and rightfully resent a designation of suicide on suspicious grounds only. An understanding of the additive effect of alcohol and barbiturate is essential in determining the probable cause of death in such cases.

Currently, barbiturates are being used increasingly for nonmedicinal purposes and have outstripped alcohol in popularity in many age and socioeconomic groups. The question of accuracy of postmortem blood examinations is often raised. In a refrigerated room the blood-alcohol level remains stable for several days, but it is not known whether this is true of barbiturate. As mentioned previously, an estimation of the amount of barbiturate consumed, from postmortem chemical examination of the blood, depends on such factors as the varying speed of action of the compound and individual variation in metabolism, physical activity, and functional integrity of the liver cells. Obviously, in many accidental deaths caused by alcohol-barbiturate poisoning, some degree of liver damage exists. In his series of barbiturate suicides, Teare notes that "over 90% of cases were dead on arrival at the hospital—suggesting that death was rapid, though of course, many suicides choose circumstances and places for their final act where they are unlikely to be disturbed."[263] It is noteworthy that decomposition will raise the postmortem blood level of alcohol, whereas the opposite is true for barbiturates. In the analysis of suspected alcohol-barbiturate deaths, it is mandatory to observe the stomach contents, when present, and to submit a specimen for barbiturate content. Sometimes the contents are "loaded" with barbiturate but no barbiturate is found in the blood. A finding of this nature may be attributed to death from acute coma and aspiration after alcohol intake before sufficient time had elapsed for barbiturate absorption.

Narcotics

Complications of intravenous administration of narcotics (heroin and morphine) by addicts are arteritis and thrombosis of pulmonary arteries, arterioles, and capillaries ("mainline lesions") with the result of pulmonary hypertension and cor pulmonale. Addicts injecting a mixture known as "blue velvet" (concentrated paregoric and a tripelennamine hydrochloride tablet) and "red devil" (contents of a Seconal capsule) have shown these lesions. The offending agent was found to be the talc contained in the tripelennamine hydrochloride tablet

and the starch granules in the Seconal capsule. Kranier, Berman, and Wishnick[264] reported a similar case in a meperidine (Demerol) addict, in whom granulomatous lesions were found in the lungs. Again, the offending agent was talc, which was used as a filler in the Demerol oral tablet. Both starch and talc have been shown experimentally to produce these lesions. Multiple scars on the skin may be observed. Frequently the addict does not heed the principles of asepsis, and so pitted scars result from healed abscesses at the site of injection. Recent lesions have an ecchymotic appearance.

Homicidal death may follow the forced administration of a "hot shot," consisting of a narcotic plus strychnine. Accidental or homicidal death may result from the addict's administering a purer blend than he or she has been accustomed to receiving. Therefore the addict accidentally takes an overdose of the narcotic, not knowing of the increased potency at the same dose level. Heroin "cut" with lactose can be detected by tasting the sweet flavor. Quinine reestablishes the bitter taste of the narcotic. Some addicts have died as a result of hypersensitivity reaction to quinine.

Morphine may play a role in the death of patients receiving oxygen therapy. Because of its depressant action, morphine predisposes such patients to oxygen toxicity. Likewise, this characteristic of morphine makes it contraindicated in alcohol poisoning. Since morphine is detoxified by the liver, patients with hepatocellular damage should not receive the morphine group of narcotics. Morphine causes vasoconstriction of the bronchial smooth musculature. The administration of morphine to a person in a state of status asthmaticus (bronchiolar spasm, mucus plugging, and air trapping with oxygen retention) may rapidly bring on death. The postmortem appearance in cases of morphine poisoning is not particularly striking. Frequently the appearance is that of asphyxia. Cyanosis, congestion of the viscera, and abundant, dark, fluid blood may be observed. If an addict has taken morphine and quinine, the latter may be identified in the urine. This finding, particularly with the fluorescent demonstration of quinine sulfate in a fresh skin puncture wound, is significant. Sulfuric acid is applied to the skin, and it rapidly penetrates the dermis to combine with quinine, forming quinine sulfur, which is fluorescent under Wood's light. Congested lungs are commonly "beefy red" in fatal cases, probably attributable, in part, to the alveolar capillary damage from quinine.

The student should keep in mind that morphine may influence laboratory tests. Elevation of serum amylase levels after constriction of the sphincter of Oddi, leading to increased intraductular pressure, may occur after morphine administration. The increased intraluminal pressure "drives" amylase into the periacinar venular network. Morphine can cause BSP retention; elevation of transaminase levels in certain patients can precipitate attacks of acute intermittent porphyria.

Other agents
Cocaine

Cocaine toxicity affects various body organs, but in the last few years it is becoming more fully appreciated that abuse of the drug induces heart disease. The likelihood of the clinical association of cocaine toxicity to histologic myofibrillar changes is indeed strong. Epidemiologic studies and to a lesser extent morphologic observations support the concept that cocaine is probably responsible for a variety of coronary artery and myocardial insults. These include sudden death syndrome, ischemic heart disease, chronic heart failure, and contraction-band necrosis. Various hypotheses supporting the pathogenesis of myofibrillar fragmentation and contraction-band necrosis of the myocytes have been proposed. These hypotheses include the following: (1) coronary artery changes such as intimal hyperplasia and contraction-band necrosis of the media may result in the sudden death syndrome or ischemic cardiomegaly and, (2) increased localization of catecholamine concentration, especially norepinephrine, binds beta-adrenergic receptors and elevates intracytosolic calcium. A popular concept is that the elevation of intracellular calcium produces hypercontraction as a result of which the myofilaments will "ratchet" past each other and end up as an amorphous mass, incapable of contracting again. This phenomenon has been nicely demonstrated in experimental animals by Karch.

Carbon monoxide

The incidence of carbon monoxide intoxication is increasing at a faster rate than population growth and hence is of even greater significance than in the past. Although the popularity of carbon monoxide as a suicide agent has been superseded by the barbiturates, this form of intoxication has taken on greater significance in view of space and underwater conquests where confinement in enclosed space is necessary.

The medicolegal aspects of carbon monoxide intoxication are of great importance when related to the public interest and safety. Dangerous levels of carbon monoxide may accumulate when almost any heating device is defective from incomplete combustion of any carbon fuel. If negligence on the part of manufacturer leads to illness or death from carbon monoxide intoxication, the medicolegal importance of suits and compensation insurance becomes obvious. The proper investigation of a case of suspected suicide carries with it great responsibility. At first glance it is often impossible to determine whether the death of a victim of carbon monoxide poisoning is attributable to suicide, accident, or homicide. An exhaustive history at the scene by persons acting in the public interest (medical examiners, coroners, law enforcement officers, pathologists) is mandatory. The importance of the classification of death as homicide or accident is obvious. On the other hand, to glibly designate a death as suicide from carbon monoxide intoxication may lead to considerable psychologic trauma to the victim's family and friends.

From the purely medical standpoint, it should be appreciated that carbon monoxide intoxication may be responsible for coma. If recognition is not prompt and therapy is not quickly instituted, irreparable damage to the brain may ensue with eventual death. In the investigation of medical coma, blood is usually drawn and a reserve sample is placed in the refrigerator. This sample may be used to detect the stable carboxyhemoglobin hours or days after the specimen has been drawn. In interpreting the level of carbon monoxide, one must take many factors into consideration. Many smokers and some industrial workers normally carry a level of 10% carbon monoxide saturation in the blood. The functional integrity of the cardiovascular and pulmonary systems, the rate of blood flow in the vascular system, the number of red blood cells and total amount of hemoglobin available, and the age, physical activity at the time of exposure, and metabolic rate of the individual will affect the response to a given level of carbon monoxide. It is apparent that survival depends on the amount and length of exposure, as well as all of those factors that normally govern the optimum exchange of oxygen between the red blood cells and the parenchymal cells of the body. The presence of drugs such as alcohol and barbiturates in depressant doses will enhance the effects of carbon monoxide.

Means of detection include sampling of carbon monoxide by air-sampling devices and the rapid detection of carboxyhemoglobin in the blood. Recording spectrophotometry allows the rapid identification of carbon monoxide using as little as two drops of blood. Gas chromatographic demonstration of small quantities of carbon monoxide is used in practically all toxicology laboratories. An exact determination of blood carbon monoxide can be made by infrared spectrophotometry.

Carbon monoxide is odorless and tasteless. It unites with hemoglobin to form a compound, carboxyhemoglobin, which is over 200% more stable than oxyhemoglobin. Carbon monoxide displaces normal oxyhemoglobin and interferes with the exchange of oxygen between the red blood cells and the extravascular tissue. In fatal cases there is a cherry-red livor of the skin from the color of the carboxyhemoglobin that is present in the superficial capillaries. One can observe the blanching or lack of cherry-red color over the pressure areas because of mechanical obliteration of the skin capillaries. In cases of death not related to carbon monoxide poisoning, there is a blue discoloration of the skin (livor mortis) after somatic death. In this instance the blue color is caused by reduced hemoglobin. A cherry

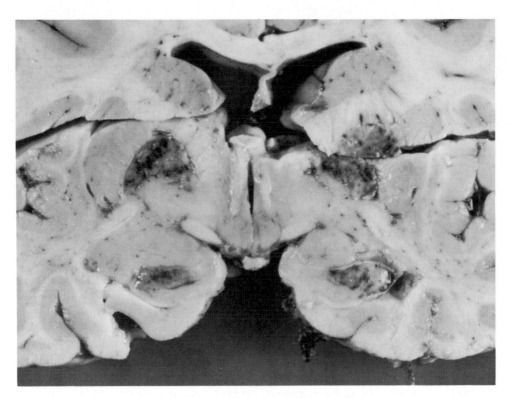

Fig. 4-40. Carbon monoxide poisoning. Patient, 15-year-old girl, was found comatose in automobile with motor running. She remained in coma for 5 days. Distribution of hemorrhagic necrosis is typical. Cross section of cerebral hemisphere at level of lenticular nuclei shows bilateral hemorrhage and necrosis of globus pallidus and hippocampus. (Courtesy Dr. Stanley M. Aronson, Brown University, Providence, R.I.)

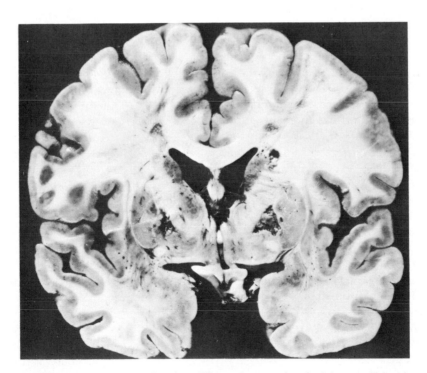

Fig. 4-41. Carbon monoxide poisoning. Bilateral necrosis of globus pallidus in patient who died 41 days after exposure. Also, necrosis of centrum semiovale, which may be caused by secondary vascular changes. Cystic transformation is evident. (From Finck, P.A.: Milit. Med. **131:**1513, 1966; AFIP.)

livor also may be caused by fluoroacetate or cyanide poisoning or by freezing. Fluoroacetate and cyanide are cellular toxins that paralyze the metabolism of the cells so that utilization of the freed oxygen from oxyhemoglobin cannot be incorporated into the cytoplasm.

In the acute, rapidly fatal type of carbon monoxide poisoning, anatomic findings may be limited to the observation of small petechial hemorrhages of serosal surfaces and white matter of the cerebral hemispheres. However, if the individual survives 4 to 5 days or more, gross lesions become evident and are characterized by striking hemorrhagic necrosis of the basal ganglia and lamellar necrosis of the cortical gray matter (Fig. 4-40). If there is longer survival, cystic areas develop in these regions (Fig. 4-41). The subendocardial layer of the myocardium is characterized by minute foci of necrosis. The findings in the brain and heart are not pathognomonic for carbon monoxide poisoning and may be seen in other conditions in which acute severe hypoxia develops.

Carbon tetrachloride

Shortly after the ingestion of as little as 5 ml to as much as 100 ml of carbon tetrachloride (a halogenated hydrocarbon) and depending on the resistance of the individual (high-fat diet increases the susceptibility to the toxicity), swelling and hydropic degeneration of the centrilobular hepatic cells develop. These changes progress to a diffuse fatty degeneration and necrosis in the centrilobular parenchyma with collapse of the reticulum network, followed shortly by hemorrhage and leukocytic infiltration. The relative specificity of this agent for the centrilobular areas appears to be related not to ischemia but to a direct effect of the agent on the cells in the centrilobular area. Autoradiographic studies have shown a rapid uptake of carbon tetrachloride by the cytoplasm and nuclei of the cells of the centrilobular areas (Fig. 4-42). There is moderate uptake in the midzonal areas and very little uptake in the periportal areas. Autoradiographic evidence shows that radioactive ^{14}C in carbon tetrachloride remains in the centrilobular areas as long as 2 days after ingestion. Regeneration of liver parenchyma begins on approximately the third day and is often completed by 2½ weeks.

The initial intracellular structure to be involved is the endoplasmic reticulum, which is damaged within 30 minutes of the administration of carbon tetrachloride, whereas the mitochondria survive unaltered for several hours. Experimentally, protein synthesis is reduced within 2 hours of poisoning. Fatty acids are mobilized from peripheral fat depots to the liver. In the liver cell they are oxidized to triglyceride. The latter is conjugated with globulin to form lipoproteins, which are secreted. This mechanism is believed to be responsible for the formation of plasma lipoproteins. If protein synthesis (carrier protein) is blocked, lipoprotein is not formed and fat accumulates in the liver cell. This explains the steatosis resulting from the inhibition of protein synthesis by carbon tetrachloride. At the same time, it must be realized that diminution of protein synthesis plays no major role in the pathogenesis of liver cell necrosis. Ultrastructurally an early observation is the direct "toxic" attack on the endoplasmic reticulum, leading to the detachment of ribosomes.

Renal lesions in acute carbon tetrachloride poisoning consist of acute tubular nephrosis or necrosis. Microscopically, tubulovenous communications and calcified necrotic tubular cells, the latter reminiscent of acute mercurial nephrosis, are observed.

Benzene

Benzene, an aromatic hydrocarbon, should be distinguished from benzine, which is a composite of aliphatic hydrocarbons. As a solvent, benzene is used widely in industrial processes, being the starting point for syntheses of a constituent of fuels. It is also used to extract the last water of hydration in the preparation of absolute alcohol. Also, benzene is to be distinguished from benzidine and its salts. Occupational workers exposed to benzidine include biochemists; dye, plastic, and rubber workers; and wood chemists. Of special interest is the exposure of medical personnel to benzidine using the compound to test for occult blood. Benzidine is classified as one of the industrial agents associated with cancer as a federally regulated carcinogen.

Chronic manifestations of benzene exposure include various disarrangements of the cellular bone marrow. Industrial workers exposed to chronic benzene intoxication may develop hypoplasia or aplasia of the bone marrow and pancytopenia. Long-standing anemia may set the stage for the development of acute myeloblastic leukemia, or erythroleukemia. The association of prolonged exposure to benzene with chronic myelocytic and lymphocytic leukemia is not certain at this time.

Boric acid

Boric acid (a boron compound) is a white crystalline powder used as a weak antiseptic, a food preservative, and a buffering and fungistatic agent in talcum powder. Fatalities have resulted from the accidental ingestion of boron or in some cases from the therapeutic use of the compound. Accidental ingestion has involved children almost entirely. Many of the accidents have resulted from boric acid powder being mistaken for an infant formula, from borate powders or solutions being left in places accessible to small children, and from the ingestion of sodium perborate as a mouthwash. In some instances the application of boric acid to large areas of denuded burned skin or excoriated dermatitis has resulted in boric acid poisoning.

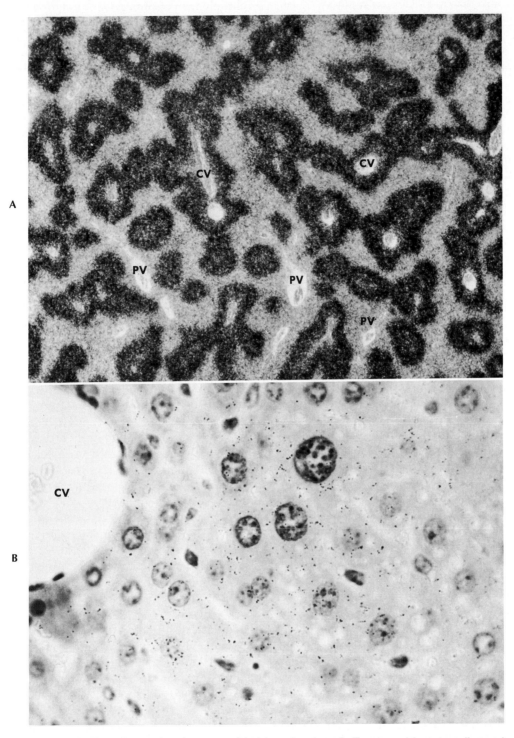

Fig. 4-42. Experimental carbon tetrachloride poisoning. **A,** Topographic autoradiography 1 hour after injection of ^{14}C-CCl_4. Localization of radioactive material concentrated around centrilobular veins *(CV)*, with periportal veins *(PV)* spared. **B,** Higher resolution showing ^{14}C-CCl_4 "grains." (Courtesy Dr. Augustine Roque, Carteret Hospital, Morehead City, N.C.)

A lethal dose of boric acid is estimated to be between 5 and 15 g. After ingestion a gastroenteritis develops and results in severe diarrhea. Autopsy findings are cerebral edema, petechial hemorrhages in the white matter of the brain, and acute tubular nephrosis or necrosis of the proximal convoluted tubules of the kidney. In the majority of cases a hemorrhagic cystitis is found. The skin manifestations in children are fairly constant and typical. Erythema is usually intense and may cover the entire body. The subject presents a characteristic "boiled lobster" appearance.

Hexachlorophene

Hexachlorophene is a chlorinated bisphenol. Hexachlorophene liquid soap is bactericidal and to some extent fungicidal. It has wide topical application, and many surgical and germicidal soaps contain this compound in a concentration of approximately 3%. Bathing of infants with detergents containing hexachlorophene has been shown to reduce greatly the incidence of staphylococcal infection. However, frequent bathing of premature infants may lead to a pronounced disturbance of myelin in the white matter of the reticular formation of the medulla, resulting in fatal respiratory distress. Premature infants under the weight of 1400 g are particularly susceptible. Hexachlorophene, when applied to large exposed areas of the skin that are the site of burns or skin diseases allowing rapid absorption, may also lead to splitting of the myelin and demyelination of the white matter of the cerebral hemispheres, brainstem, and medulla. The central nervous system damage in adults, however, is for the most part reversible.

Elemental phosphorus

The majority of cases of phosphorus poisoning in the United States in recent years have been attributable to the ingestion of certain rat poisons or roach pastes. In the past, yellow phosphorus matches were the primary source for such intoxication.

Phosphorus is a general protoplasmic poison, but it exerts its most profound effects on the liver and kidneys. After ingestion of as little as 15 mg of yellow phosphorus, immediate, mostly nonspecific gastrointestinal symptoms attributable to the local effect of this poison are usually noted. Clinical and pathologic evidence of hepatic damage usually is noted after a variable interval. Electron microscopic studies show that after the initial ingestion a decrease in the hepatocyte cytoplasmic basophilia, reflecting alterations of the ergastoplasm, is observable within 12 hours and that mitochondrial swelling is detectable by 24 hours. Abnormal accumulations of hemosiderin granules in the hepatocytes have been observed in experimental phosphorus poisoning. Steatosis of the hepatic cells usually begins approximately 15 hours after experimental injection of phosphorus. Uncoupling of oxidative phosphorylation is one reflection of enzymatic derangement in phosphorus poisoning. Perilobular necrosis is characteristic of phosphorus intoxication. Liver enlargement with extensive fatty degeneration, principally periportal, possibly with a mild inflammatory infiltrate in the portal triads, is usually found at autopsy. Only rarely is massive necrosis observed.

The liver lesions of Reye's syndrome may morphologically resemble phosphorus poisoning. In these fatty livers, necrosis when present is frequently situated in the periphery of the lobule.

Plant poisons

"Bush tea." The pyrrolizidine chemical series constitutes a group of some 50 alkaloids, many of which are known to be highly toxic to man and animals. These poisonous substances occur in all parts of the world. At least 2000 common plants contain pyrrolizidine.

Bras and associates[275] incriminated the pyrrolizidine alkaloid fulvine as being the hepatotoxic agent responsible for the occurrence of veno-occlusive disease of the liver among the natives of Jamaica. Many people in the West Indies are addicted to the ingestion of "bush teas." These aqueous infusions of plant material are imbibed in the belief that they are herbal remedies for a wide variety of common complaints. *Crotalaria fulva* (which contains the pyrrolizidine alkaloid fulvine) is used for one "bush tea." The consumption of an extract of *C. fulva* is not definitely linked with the high incidence of liver disease in the Caribbean ("veno-occlusive disease of the liver"). The disease, unlike Chiari's syndrome, does not affect the larger hepatic veins. The toxin exerts a dual attack on the liver—on the centrilobular hepatocytes, causing necrosis, and on the hepatic veins, leading to endothelial damage and thrombosis (Fig. 4-43).

Mushrooms. Mushroom poisoning is primarily caused by *Amanita phalloides* and *A. muscaria*. Of the 80 species of mushrooms known to be toxic for many individuals, only one, *A. phalloides*, affects the liver. Two types of toxins isolated from *A. phalloides* are phallin, a thermolabile glucoside with hemolytic properties, and *Amanita* toxin, a thermostable mixture of cyclic polypeptides. The former is readily destroyed by cooking and ingestion and probably plays little role in human poisoning.

On the other hand, the *Amanita* toxin causes a choleralike gastroenteritis, followed in several days by tender hepatomegaly and jaundice. In fatal cases death occurs within 10 days. There is a 50% mortality. At autopsy the liver is small because of the massive hemorrhagic hepatocellular necrosis. Persistent, peripherally located fatty liver cells are observed. An acute inflammatory exudate is found throughout the organ. In

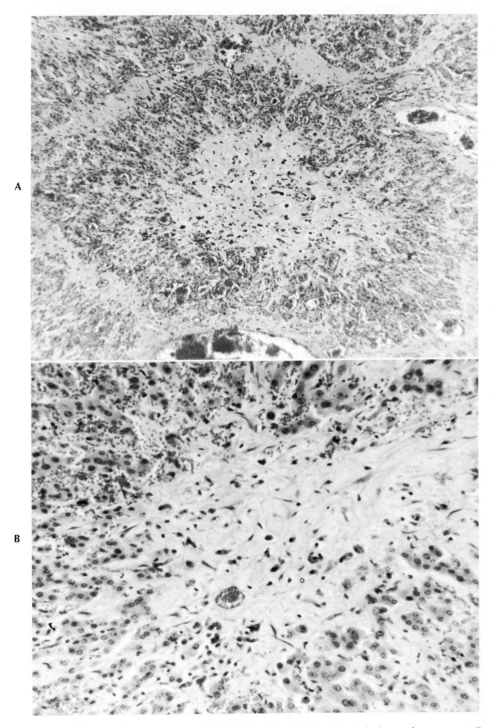

Fig. 4-43. "Bush tea" poisoning. Liver of pig after intraperitoneal dose of monocrotaline. Hepatic lobule with centrilobular disappearance of hepatic parenchymal cells and condensation of connective tissue supporting framework.

nonfatal cases, periportal hepatic fibrosis may be noted. Amanitine combines with and inhibits RNA polymerase and therefore blocks the synthesis of messenger RNA. The morphologic findings in other organs—kidney, brain, and heart—are of lesser severity and consist mainly in fatty changes and hydropic degeneration in the proximal convoluted tubules of the kidney, nonspecific neuronal reactions widely scattered throughout the brain, and fatty myocardial fibrils. The alkaloid muscarine is the toxin derived from *A. muscaria* and exhibits cholinergic effects.

ENVIRONMENTAL PATHOLOGY
Insecticides and pesticides
Organophosphates

Organophosphates, a large class of compounds, were originally prepared as nerve gases for warfare. Fortunately they were not released in this role, and it was discovered that they could be used in agriculture. The most widely used are parathion and malathion. Their action is based on the inhibition of cholinesterase. This leads to accumulation of acetylcholine, consequent blockade of the intercostal muscles, and respiratory failure resulting in brain anoxia. Although all the compounds are anticholinesterases, only a small group leads to the development of demyelination of peripheral nerves. The mechanism of the demyelination is unknown. At necropsy, no specific pathologic changes are noted.

There have been two instances of widespread poisoning of humans. One occurred in the 1930s in the United States, when a contaminated cargo of ginger, which was used primarily for preparing illicit alcoholic drinks in prohibition days, left several thousand people with nerve damage to the lower limbs. The resultant irregular motion of the victims became known as "ginger Jake paralysis." Another episode occurred in Morocco in the 1950s, when contaminated motor oil was sold for cooking purposes. In many parts of the world, parathion is sold over the counter as a pesticide. In Puerto Rico, for example, parathion poisoning leads acute alcoholism as a cause of accidental death.

Organic chlorinated hydrocarbons

DDT is an abbreviation of the earlier chemical name p,p′-dichlorodiphenyltrichloroethane. The present designation is 1,1,1-trichloro-2,2-bis(p-chlorophenyl) ethane. DDT is the most widely used insecticide, but since 1962 the volume has decreased because of the following factors: (1) increased insect resistance, (2) storage in plants and animals, which has led to environmental contamination, and (3) lack of understanding of its mode of action after deposition in the adipose tissue of humans. Disturbing also has been the observation of its possible role as a carcinogen, teratogen, and antifer-

tility agent, as demonstrated in experimental animals.

Vertebrate animals receiving fatal doses of DDT manifest a myriad of neurologic signs and symptoms including tremors, hyperexcitability, ataxia, and paralysis. The severity of the reaction is in proportion to the dose administered. the clinical response of acute poisoning in humans is similar to that in animals. At necropsy, no dramatic evidence of neurologic damage is appreciated. Minimal adrenolytic changes are evident in the inner fasciculata and reticularis zones. Ultrastructurally, the hepatocytes show hypertrophy of the smooth endoplasmic reticulum, probably representing an intracellular adaptive change (Fig. 4-44). It thus appears that DDT and its analogs are capable of increasing microsomal activity. In chronic DDT poisoning, animals respond with a variety of changes. Fatty degeneration occurs in the myocardium and in the centrilobular portions of the liver and the proximal convoluted tubules of the kidney. Pyknosis and shrinkage of neurons, including those of the cerebral cortex, dentate nucleus, and spinal cord, are observed.

In humans, chronic or recurrent deposition of DDT in adipose tissue, brain, liver, and adrenal zona fasciculata leads to no cellular changes observable by light microscopy. A remarkable change in the adrenal zona fasciculata and zona reticularis after the administration of DDT to dogs is of interest. After a total cumulative dose of approximately 1800 mg/kg body weight, the adrenal gland undergoes considerable atrophy, leaving little more than a fairly intact zona glomerulosa and medulla (Fig. 4-45). There is pronounced mitochondrial enlargement (Fig. 4-46). Correspondingly, serum corticosteroid levels fall. Regeneration occurs in approximately 90 days after withdrawal of the compound. Unfortunately, this antisteroid effect is seen to a strong degree only in dogs and should be considered a species-specific phenomenon.

Isomers of DDT, o,p′-DDD and m,p′-DDD, have been used to treat humans with Cushing's syndrome and functioning adrenocortical carcinoma. The compounds are especially useful as palliative agents if surgical procedures are not indicated.

Polychlorinated biphenyls

Polychlorinated biphenyls (PCBs) are a group of chlorinated aromatic compounds that are structurally similar to DDT but are more resistant to environmental degradation. DDT contains between its two phenyl rings an ethane portion, which serves as the site of its oxidative breakdown in the environment, whereas PCBs contain no ethane structure and are thus more stable in the ecosystem.

PCBs were introduced into commerce in 1929 and have been used as plasticizers, extenders for pesticides, heat exchangers, dielectric fluids, and nonflammable

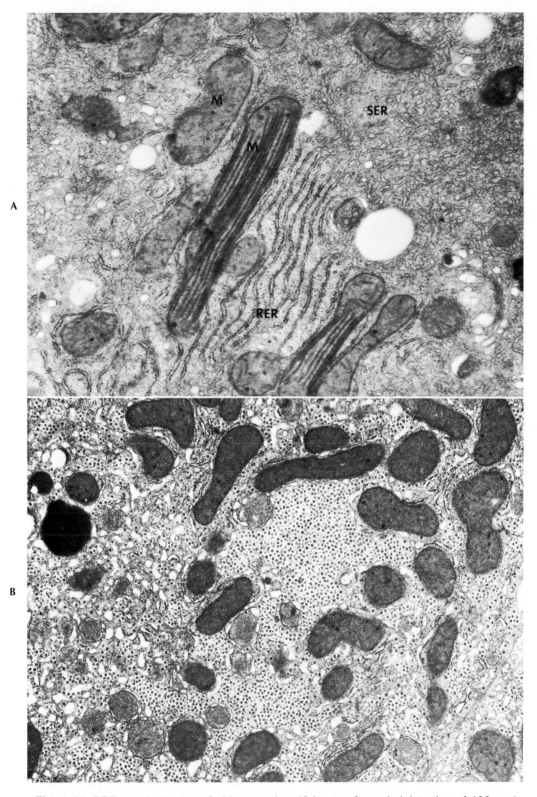

Fig. 4-44. DDT toxicity in dog. **A,** Liver section 48 hours after administration of 100 mg/kg body weight. Proliferation of smooth endoplasmic reticulum *(SER)* from rough endoplasmic reticulum *(RER)* may be seen. *M,* Mitochondria. **B,** Animal was sacrificed 56 hours after 200 mg/kg body weight was administered. Proliferation and dilatation of smooth endoplasmic reticulum in hepatocyte. Cell is rich in glycogen, and mitochondria are not abnormal. Dark globules at top left corner are fat. (**A,** 50,000×; **B,** 35,000×.)

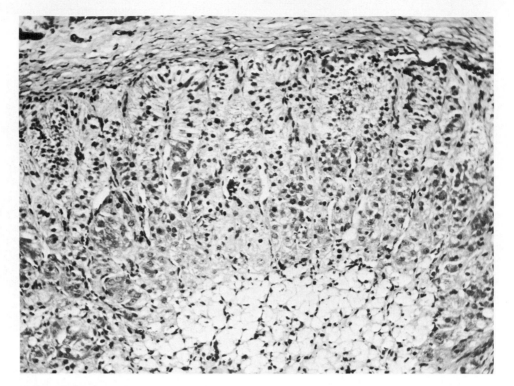

Fig. 4-45. DDT toxicity. Adrenal gland of dog that received 1800 mg/kg body weight over 3-week period. Capsule is thickened because of loss of underlying zona fasciculata cells. Zona glomerulosa is remarkably preserved (normally, 12 to 15 cell layers thick). Zona fasciculata adjacent to zona reticularis has undergone atrophy and replacement by adipose-appearing tissue. Remainder of zona fasciculata reveals granular cells in various stages of degeneration. Minor changes with these characteristics are found in humans with Cushing's syndrome who have been treated with o-p'-DDD.

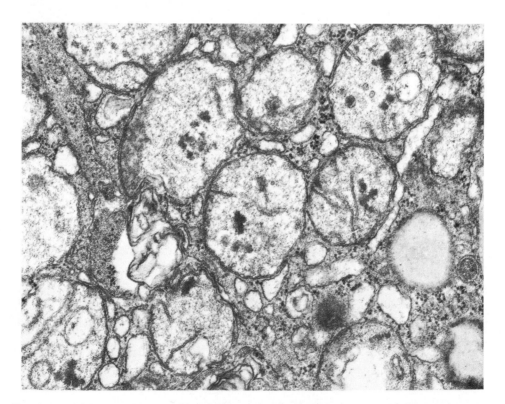

Fig. 4-46. DDT toxicity. Zona fasciculata cells in adrenal gland of dog 56 hours after administration of 200 mg/kg body weight. Mitochondria are swollen. Loss of cristae and normal contour and precipitation of electron-dense material in mitochondrial matrix. (40,000×.)

hydraulic and lubricating fluids and as an ingredient in caulking compounds, adhesive paints, printing inks, and carbonless duplicating paper. It is estimated that 25,000 tons of PCBs are lost into the environment each year. Recent studies strongly suggest that DDT vapor can be converted to PCBs by ultraviolet sunlight in the lower atmosphere.

Toxic findings in animals reveal liver lesions (fatty infiltration, centrilobular atrophy, necrosis, hyaline bodies), kidney and intestinal damage (especially in birds), hydropericardium and ascites (birds), immunosuppressive effects (chickens), and detrimental reproductive effects (rats). Toxic effects in exposed PCB workers are chiefly chloracne with dermal cysts and comedos developing after a latent period of about 7 months after the time of most recent exposure and lasting for periods ranging from several months to 4 years after removal from the source of exposure. The main sources in the human diet are believed to be fish, shellfish, and poultry.

Carbamates

Carbamates are derivatives of carbamic acid. Physostigmine (eserine) was identified from the beans of a poisonous plant, *Physostigma venenosum*, and neostigmine (Prostigmin) is a synthetic analog medically. The best known of the carbamate insecticides is carbaryl (arylam, Sevin). As with the organophosphates, the mode of action is cholinesterase inhibition. On the other hand, none of the carbamates causes demyelination.

Insects do not utilize cholinesterase in their neuromuscular junctions, and their vital cholinesterase is all central and protected by a barrier system that hinders penetration by ionized molecules. All the medicinal carbamates are ionized or ionizable and therefore have little effect on insects.

Fluorine compounds

The fluoro-organic compound known as fluoroacetate is an insecticide but is most widely used as a rodenticide. It is sold under the name "1080." Lethal doses cause symptoms in 20 to 60 minutes, at which time convulsions herald rapidly approaching death. Elevated citrate levels are found, particularly in the heart and kidney. Fluoroacetate is metabolically converted to fluorocitric acid, which is an acetate-activating enzyme. In the presence of this enzyme, there is formation of the coenzyme A derivative fluoroacetyl CoA followed by condensation with oxaloacetate to give fluorocitrate. It is possible that death results from "jamming" of the Krebs citric acid cycle, with resulting disruption of energy-producing reactions.

Sodium fluoride has long been used as a bait for cockroaches and ants. The findings in acute fluoride poisoning in humans and animals are analogous. Acute gastrointestinal disturbances develop, rapidly followed by respiratory or cardiac failure. Two teaspoons of fluoride may kill a human in 2 hours. Rapid absorption with high concentration of fluoride ion throughout the body is the rule. At the same time, rapid deposition in the skeleton and excretion in the urine occur. Depending on the circumstances, a patient surviving toxic levels for 4 or more hours may be expected to live. Fluoride is a powerful metabolic inhibitor. It forms complexes with and inhibits a large number of metal-containing enzymes. The magnesium-containing enzymes, especially acid phosphatase and ATPase, are inhibited. Other metal-containing enzymes such as succinic dehydrogenase, cytochrome oxidase, peroxidase, and catalase are likewise affected. Considering this wide spectrum of enzyme paralysis, it is not difficult to understand why the finger cannot be pointed at a specific mechanism responsible for the death of the organism. Superimposed on the enzyme effects is the old knowledge of the calcium-precipitating role of fluoride. Indeed, the myocardial effects of fluoride resemble those brought about by excess of calcium ion. It is probable, then, that calcium fluoride becomes deposited on the cell membrane, yielding a local excess of calcium. At necropsy the epithelial mucosa of the stomach and small intestine is desquamated, and widespread superficial ulceration is demonstrated. Rigor mortis appears rapidly, and preservation of the tissues is prolonged. A usual finding is unclotted blood, probably the result of calcium binding by fluoride. The microscopic examination of the myocardium, liver, and nephrons reveals no specific pathologic change.

Chronic fluorosis was first described as an industrial disease. A "poker back" hypermineralization of the skeleton and broad ligaments developed in cryolite powder workers. Exostoses evolved from both long and flat bones. Lipping of the vertebral bodies led to nerve root compression, with weakness and atrophy of leg muscles. Microscopically, distorted architecture of bony trabeculas, accompanied by poorly developed haversian canals, is suggestive of chronic fluorosis. Fluorine, unlike iodine, is not taken up preferentially by the thyroid gland, nor is there substitution of iodine by fluorine in the gland. These facts contradict an old concept that repeated large doses of fluorine could lead to the development of colloid goiter. Fluorine, at the recommended concentration level in fluoridated water supplies, has no proved deleterious effect on growth of teeth and bones in children. However, excessive fluoride intake may lead to brown staining and mottled tooth enamel. Mottled enamel develops during tooth formation, before eruption. The report of Dean[285] that caries resistance may be facilitated by fluoridation of drinking water (1 to 3 ppm) has been a notable advance in this area.

Herbicides

Paraquat dichloride, diquat dibromide, and morfamquat dichloride are weed killers. Paraquat is the one most commonly used. Animals may be poisoned by paraquat given parenterally, orally, or by aerosol spray. If death supervenes shortly after the initial dose, the lungs are the seat of severe pulmonary congestion and edema. If death occurs several days after dosage, proliferative alveolitis, hyaline membranes, and terminal bronchiolitis are observed. With longer survival, pulmonary fibrosis and subsequent cor pulmonale occur.

Paraquat toxicity in humans may occur after the oral ingestion of only a few milliliters of the compound. Absorption from the skin is also a method of introduction. Depending on the dosage, symptoms may appear within a few days or weeks. By the same token, death may occur within the first 24 hours or 3 to 4 weeks after imbibition of the paraquat solution. With smaller doses, gingival and oropharyngeal pseudomembranous ulcers (diphtheria-like membranes) are the initial signs. X-ray examination of the chest shows the basilar linear infiltration, which becomes progressively diffuse with time. Grossly, the lungs are dark and rubbery and have a "meaty" consistency during the first 5 days. What appears to be cystic change is the result of hemorrhage into the terminal air spaces (Fig. 4-47). The histologic findings in the first 6 days consist in hemorrhagic edema with bleeding into the air spaces. In the first few days, hyaline membranes are in evidence. From 6 to 30 days there is progressive buildup of a fibrous alveolitis leading eventually to interstitial fibrosis and the classic "honeycomb lung." During the later stages, bronchioloalveolar hyperplasia with squamous metaplasia is a prominent feature of honeycomb lung. Changes in hepatocytes and interlobular bile ducts vary with the amount of paraquat ingested and the survival time. Centrilobular necrosis, fatty changes in the lobular hepatocytes, acute cholangitis, and necrosis of the interlobular bile ducts have all been described as morphologic reflections of paraquat injury. With few exceptions, such as allopurinol and methotrexate, one does not associate these changes of acute cholangitis or bile duct injury with medicinal drugs. On the contrary, intrahepatic cholestasis is the most common morphologic adverse reaction to therapeutic compounds. Proximal renal tubular dysfunction as manifested by glycosuria and aminoaciduria, as well as acute tubular necrosis, has been recorded after paraquat ingestion. It is probable that the toxicity mediated by paraquat induces the production of a superoxide ion (through electron transfer) that, via an intermediate, reacts with lipids to form fatty acid hydroperoxides, which in turn interfere with pulmonary surfactant function. The formation of the toxic superoxide radical is more rapid under higher oxygen tension, which may explain why the lung is the preferential site of paraquat toxicity.

Diquat does not produce the same pulmonary changes as paraquat but results in gastrointestinal erosion. In severe toxicity, acute tubular necrosis of the kidneys and centrilobular hepatic necrosis may occur. Morfamquat primarily affects the kidneys, leading to necrosis of the proximal convoluted tubules. The mechanism of the toxic damage resulting from paraquat is the subject of disagreement among investigators.

Air pollutants

As long-term exposure to increasing levels of air pollution is experienced by larger segments of the population, the results in terms of human pathology will become increasingly obvious. The role of air pollution in the development of emphysema and other chronic respiratory conditions is generally recognized. Epidemiologic data indicate that the same causal relationship exists in conditions affecting the cardiovascular system. In the United States alone, approximately 150 million tons of air pollutants are emitted each year, with 60% of this amount resulting from vehicular emissions, including automobiles, trucks, and buses; 31% from industrial processes; 6% from the heating of homes and offices; and 3% from the burning of trash and refuse. Although the sources are varied, approximately 85% of all air pollution results from the burning of fossil fuels. Industrial pollutants are as varied as the types of industries, and many may be harmful to animal and plant life. The damage from acid emissions such as HCl, H_2SO_4, HNO_3, or HF can be readily recognized, but the relationship between some other emissions and human pathologic conditions is not yet clearly established.

Of increasing concern is the widespread and often indiscriminate use of toxic chemical compounds, especially pesticides and herbicides. Compounds such as DDT have reportedly caused massive bird kills and adversely affected reproduction in songbirds. Although specific human effects have not been noted as a result of minimal exposures, the compound is being found in increasing concentrations in human tissues. The main cause of concern with DDT and all the chlorinated hydrocarbons is that they remain in the environment for an indefinite period of time without loss of potency. We have no idea what the results of long-term exposure will be.

Ozone is a form of oxygen. Under ordinary circumstances it is a colorless or pale blue gas with a characteristic pungent odor. In high concentrations it is extremely flammable, and in liquid form it becomes a dangerous explosive. There are two general sources of exposure to ozone: (1) the discharge of high-voltage electrical equipment, welding operations, and ultraviolet spectrographic equipment and (2) emanations from ozone generators used in industrial processes (such as those involved in the production of ozone for use as a disinfecting germicide or for controlling growth of

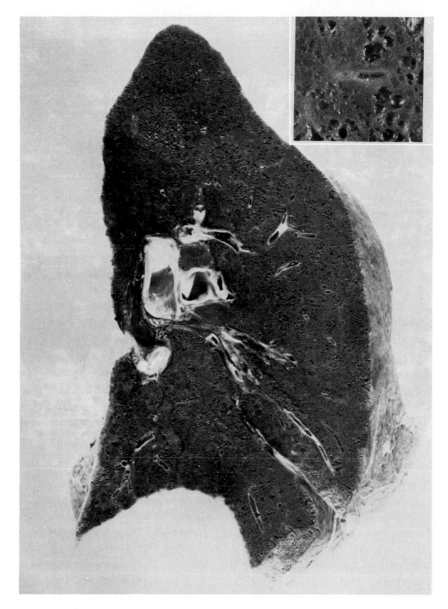

Fig. 4-47. Fatal paraquat poisoning. Lung is greatly congested, rubbery, and nonaerated. *Inset* shows what appear to be cysts but proved to be distended terminal airways filled with blood. Patient was admitted with acute glossitis and pharyngitis 5 days after ingestion of paraquat and died on the sixth hospital day as a result of respiratory, hepatic, and renal failure. (Courtesy Dr. Sandra E. Conradi, Medical University of South Carolina, Charleston, S.C.)

fungi, molds, and bacteria in food processing.

As pointed out by Deichmann and Gerarde, "The danger of undesirable health effects far outweigh any benefits presumed to be derived from the industrial or institutional use of ozone for the control of odors or bacteria in air."[292] Ozone, like many other chemical agents, including phosgene, chlorine, irritating smoke gases, ammonia, nitrogen dioxide, and cadmium fumes, may damage the alveolar capillaries, rendering them exceptionally permeable. Continued exposure to the irritating gases will lead to permanent damage

manifested by alveolar septal derangement, desquamative bronchioloalveolitis, and eventual interstitial fibrosis.

A classic example of such a mechanism occurs in silo-filler's disease. In this condition the culprits are nitric oxide and nitrogen dioxide. Nitric acid is used extensively in industry for copper, brass, and silver dipping, the preparation of nitrocellulose, collodion, and methyl nitrate, and the production of sulfuric, chromic, and picric acids. It is used as an oxidizer in rocket fuel. Nitrous fumes are expelled from silos filled with cattle for-

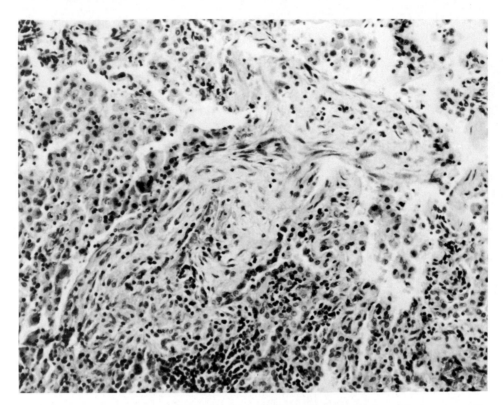

Fig. 4-48. Silo-filler's disease of lung. Bronchiolitis obliterans attributable to connective tissue proliferation. Lymphocytes and desquamative granulocytes complete microscopic picture.

age collected during times of partial drought. Under these circumstances the forage (corn) is often harvested before it is fully grown, and the young plants contain a high nitrate content. Later, during storage, anaerobic fermentation of potassium nitrate liberates nitrates, which, as the temperature rises with fermentation, liberate various oxides of nitrogen. The reaction to high concentrations of nitrogen dioxide is profound. Desquamation of bronchial and bronchioalveolar epithelium is prompt. The alveolar capillaries become rapidly dilated, and edema fluid flows into the alveoli. Within a matter of days, a well-developed bronchiolitis obliterans, accompanied by interstitial lymphocytic infiltration and slight fibrosis of the alveolar septa, appears (Fig. 4-48). If the pathologic process has been one primarily of edema with very little alveolar septal destruction, reversible changes may be expected within a period of 6 months. Severe cases result in the persistence of interstitial fibrosis, and centrilobular emphysema follows the bronchiolitic destruction.

Occupational chest diseases

As a result of acute or chronic occupational exposure to harmful aerosols or gases, any one or several of the following diseases may develop in the lower respiratory tract: pneumoconiosis, pneumonitis, pulmonary edema, bronchitis, bronchial constriction, pleural in-

flammation, or cancer. To a considerable degree, whether an aerosol will produce disease, or where the disease will be initiated in the respiratory tract, may be governed largely by the size of the suspended particles. Particles less than 7 μm are generally considered respirable. Small particles are deposited in the air spaces to a greater degree than a dust with a significantly larger average particle size. Larger particles tend to be trapped on the tracheobronchial mucous membrane by a combination of inertial and gravitational deposition. Deposition in the air spaces, on the other hand, occurs largely by diffusion—a process that is caused by collisions of gas molecules with the particles. It is dependent on the near absence of air flow that is the rule in the alveoli.

Dust particles that are deposited on the tracheobronchial mucous membrane are transported toward the pharynx by the mucociliary mechanism. The motive force is supplied by cilia that beat 20 times per second with a rapid, whiplike cephalad stroke requiring one third of the cycle, followed by a slower recovery stroke occupying the remaining time of the cycle. In the trachea the mucous film or blanket, normally about 5 μm thick, is thereby propelled proximally with its embedded macrophages and dust particles at a rate of about 1 cm per minute. It is apparent that at this rate the tracheobronchial tree is capable of cleansing itself within 24 hours of particles that have been deposited on its surface.

There is also an alveolar clearance mechanism. This consists of a film of fluid about 0.2 μm thick that moves from the most peripheral alveoli toward the terminal bronchiole where it merges with the mucous blanket and becomes its nethermost layer. Because the respiratory bronchiole has a surface area that is only ⅟₅₀₀ of the surface area of the structures draining into it, the respiratory bronchiole becomes the locus where stagnation of the alveolar clearance mechanism first becomes manifest. In effect, the respiratory bronchiole is the narrow end of a large funnel. Thus, when the clearance mechanism is overwhelmed by excessive dust deposition, dust macules form in the lungs. In the center of each macule is a respiratory bronchiole, the evaginating alveoli of which are filled with dust and dust-filled macrophages. As the exposure continues and more dust accumulates, alveoli situated peripheral to the respiratory bronchiole become filled and the macule thereby becomes larger and tends to fuse with adjacent macules.

Pneumoconiosis

Pneumoconiosis is defined as an accumulation of dust in the lungs and the tissue reaction to its presence. Pneumoconiosis occurs most often in people who have resided many years in highly industrialized smoky cities. The lungs of these people often accumulate enough soot and fly ash to give the lungs a mottled black appearance. These people have pneumoconiosis, but they are in no manner handicapped by it. There is no demonstrable departure from health because of the presence of this dust. Their pneumoconiosis is merely a condition, *not* a disease.

The pneumoconiosis-producing dusts have been divided into two main categories: those that are fibrogenic and those that are nonfibrogenic. The latter are also called nuisance dusts. A nonfibrogenic dust is defined as one whose tissue reaction has the following three characteristics: (1) the alveolar architecture remains intact, (2) the stromal proliferation is minimal and consists of reticulin fibers, and (3) the reaction is potentially reversible. In contrast, a fibrogenic dust is one that provokes a tissue reaction having the following features: (1) the alveolar architecture is destroyed, (2) the stromal proliferation is significant and tends to be collagenous, and (3) the reaction is irreversible.

Nonfibrogenic dusts. Examples of nonfibrogenic dusts include soot, kaolin, stannic oxide, barium sulfate, aluminum oxide, iron oxide, and coal, as well as many other dusts. These dusts, when deposited in the air spaces, evoke a macrophage reaction associated with very little stromal proliferation. The latter consists of delicate reticulin fibers that course between the dust-filled macrophages. The air spaces containing the dust generally are atelectatic, thereby sequestering the dust-containing cells. Because tin oxide, iron oxide, and barium sulfate dusts are radiopaque, the chest x-ray films of the workers who have inhaled these dusts may demonstrate alarming shadows even though there are no symptoms of disease.

Coal workers' pneumoconiosis. Coal workers' pneumoconiosis can be presumed to be present in all coal miners who have inhaled the dust. However, it has been found that only 10% of working coal miners have x-ray evidence of pneumoconiosis.

Simple coal workers' pneumoconiosis consists of coal dust macules scattered throughout the lungs. In the center of each macule is a respiratory bronchiole. This bronchiole is often greatly enlarged, a condition termed "focal emphysema." Focal emphysema is not productive of symptoms and must not be confused with the centrilobular emphysema (see Chapter 20) caused by cigarette smoking that affects many coal miners. Simple pneumoconiosis is asymptomatic and causes no disability, though it has been associated with a slight reduction in lung function values in some miners.

Complicated coal workers' pneumoconiosis, or progressive massive fibrosis (PMF), is characterized by black, dense, stony-hard masses in an anthracotic lung. The masses may be so small as to cast a shadow on the x-ray film only 1 cm in diameter, or they may be so large as to involve a major portion of one or both lungs and undergo cavitation. Only 3% of working coal miners have PMF (one third of the 10% that have x-ray evidence of pneumoconiosis). Many coal miners who have x-ray evidence of PMF are not incapacitated.

It has been possible to produce PMF experimentally in sensitized guinea pigs that have a large lung burden of coal dust by means of various kinds of living acid-fast bacilli, dead acid-fast organisms, and even tuberculin alone injected intratracheally. It is probable that an immunologically determined alteration in tissue reactivity is a requisite to the conversion of simple pneumoconiosis to PMF.

The development of PMF in coal miners may be associated with severe sclerosis of pulmonary vessels, resulting in pulmonary hypertension and cor pulmonale. The latter is a common immediate cause of death in cases of PMF in which the disease is far advanced.

Fibrogenic dusts

Silicosis. Silicosis has been recognized for centuries as a debilitating and often fatal disease. However, in more recent times, studies have demonstrated that, except for exposure to extremely heavy dosage of very fine dust of crystalline silica, the debility and fatal outcome of silicosis are usually attributable to an associated complicating tuberculosis. Of the crystalline forms of silica (SiO_2), quartz dust is the most common cause of silicosis. Silica particles ingested by macrophages cause death of the latter by dissolution of lysosomal membranes, thereby spilling autolytic enzymes into the ma-

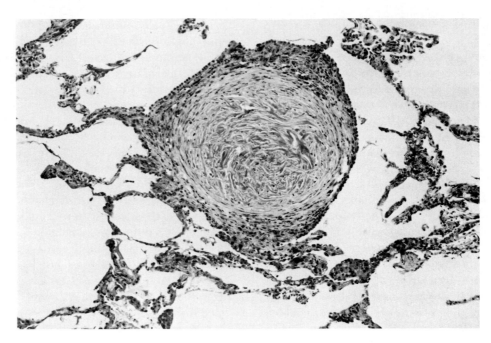

Fig. 4-49. Silicotic nodule, composed of acellular, hyaline collagenous tissue. Focal septal thickening and emphysema in area of nodule are frequent findings. (250×.)

crophagic cytoplasm. An unidentified substance from the dead macrophages stimulates the production of fibrous tissue.

As with nonfibrogenic dusts, the respiratory bronchiole with its evaginating alveoli is the locus of silica dust accumulation and therefore the site of the initial lesion. Within a very few days after the dust accumulation, the macrophages become associated with fibroblasts and reticulin fibers. This inflammatory tissue occludes the lumens of the respiratory bronchiole and the evaginating alveoli; thus the tissue is solidified. A silicotic nodule is formed by a cluster of involved respiratory bronchioles situated circumferentially around a central blood vessel that becomes obliterated as the nodule matures. Maturation of the inflammatory tissue in the nodule to the acellular, hyaline collagenous tissue characteristic of the mature silicotic nodule requires many months or even years (Fig. 4-49).

The number and size of the nodules in the lungs of an individual depend on the amount of silica dust deposited in the lung tissue over a lifetime. They may vary from very few widely scattered nodules no larger than 1 to 2 mm to hundreds of nodules, still widely separated but usually not more than 4 to 5 mm in diameter. Except for some paracicatricial types of emphysema, the alveolar tissue around and between silicotic nodules is normal. This is simple silicosis.

Simple silicosis, like the simple pneumoconiosis of coal miners, is asymptomatic. It is the abundance of normal lung tissue between the nodules in simple silicosis that is responsible for its asymptomatic character.

Although not handicapped for reasons still unknown, the worker with simple silicosis is highly susceptible to tuberculosis. The resultant silicotuberculosis is much more serious than tuberculosis alone and is more difficult to treat. Fifty years ago it was estimated that 75% of the deaths among silicotic workers were attributable to an associated tuberculosis. With the great reduction in the incidence of tuberculosis, this cause of death among silicotic workers has likewise decreased.

Another form of silicosis, diatomaceous-earth pneumoconiosis, is caused by a dust created when natural diatomaceous earth is heated to a high temperature in the presence of lime (flux-calcined) and a significant portion of the amorphous silica becomes crystalline. Usually this dust exposure is associated with exposure to the unaltered natural diatomaceous earth as well, the net result of this being a mixed-dust pneumoconiosis. Many of the airspaces not destroyed by scars are plugged with macrophages containing amorphous silica. Natural diatomaceous earth, without quartz admixture, does not cause silicosis. Amorphous silica, if it is prepared by precipitation from aqueous sodium silicate solution with acid, likewise does not cause silicosis. However, amorphous silica, prepared by heating silica above its boiling point, producing silica fumes, or by burning organic silicates, is fibrogenic and capable of causing pulmonary fibrosis. This fibrosis may be diffuse and interstitial in character rather than nodular.

Acute silicosis is caused by the inhalation of very high concentrations of extremely fine crystalline silica (less than 1 μm in diameter). The tissue reaction is different from that usually seen. Although silicotic nodules form, they are few and remain cellular in character, as well as microscopic in size. There is a diffuse alveolar lipoproteinosis that is the predominant aspect of the reaction and that, by extensive plugging of the air spaces, has been responsible for the early deaths of the afflicted workers.

Whether silicosis is responsible for an increased incidence of lung cancer is a question that is raised occasionally. Epidemiologic studies that have taken the tobacco-smoking history into account indicated that there was no increased risk of lung cancer production in silicotic lungs. Because silicotic nodules are scars, and cancers are known to arise in tuberculous and other scars of lungs, it would be logical to expect some lung cancers to arise in silicotic nodules. This expectation is nullified by the fact that, unlike other scars, silicotic nodules do not contain epithelial parenchymal remnants from which cancers might arise (see also p. 997).

Asbestos-related diseases. The mechanism by which asbestos dust induces tissue damage is not known at present, nor is there an explanation for the difference in biologic activity of the different kinds of asbestos. This biologic activity includes pulmonary and pleural inflammation as well as neoplastic involvement of the lungs, pleura, and peritoneum. The different kinds of asbestos include chrysotile, amosite, crocidolite, and anthophyllite. Of these, chrysotile, which is mined in Canada, constitutes more than 95% of the asbestos used in America. Amosite and crocidolite are imports from South Africa and have limited use. Anthophyllite is extensively mined in Finland and the Soviet Union but is not used in America. Another type of asbestos, tremolite, is not used as such, but it is associated with most talc deposits and may constitute as much as 25% of the weight of commercial talc.

Inasmuch as serpentine rock, the mother ore of chrysotile, as well as other mineral fiber–containing rocks are common geologic outcroppings, they are subject to erosion by streams and winds. As a result of this erosion, mineral fibers are ubiquitous in ambient air. However, because of a greatly increased industrial consumption of asbestos and other mineral fibers over the past 50 years, the ambient air of cities has a significantly greater mineral fiber content than that of rural communities. This is consonant with the discovery that the lungs of all adult city dwellers contain mineral fibers ranging from 140,000 to almost 7 million per gram of dry lung tissue. Of these fibers, about 6%, on the average, have been identified morphologically as chrysotile. The presence of mineral fibers in the lungs is not always accompanied by demonstrable pulmonary disease. This indicates that there may be a level of pulmonary asbestos deposition below which no demonstrable disease occurs.

The initial reaction to asbestos dust, similar to that of other dusts, involves the respiratory bronchioles and their evaginating alveoli. As with silicosis, there is a rapid proliferation of reticulin upon the alveolar surfaces that obliterates these alveoli. However, in contrast to silicosis, the bronchiole and alveolar ducts remain patent. Months and years later the reticulin is converted to collagen. With increased deposition of asbestos, the involvement extends peripherally, thereby causing confluence of neighboring lesions. In this process, some alveoli remain patent but their walls are thickened. There is thickening of the walls of respiratory bronchioles and alveolar ducts caused in part by the fibrous obliteration of their evaginating alveoli and in part by newly deposited fibrous tissue. The result is a relatively diffuse but nonuniform fibrosis that is most severe in the basal portions of the lower lobes and is more pronounced around bronchi and vessels and in the central portions of the primary lobule than in the peripheral portions.

Some alveolar septa are devoid of patent capillaries because of the fibrosis, and some that remain patent are covered by inflammatory tissue. The net result in advanced asbestosis is that some alveoli that are capable of being ventilated are poorly perfused or unperfused. Because of the fibrosis, some perfused alveoli are not ventilated. The interposition of inflammatory tissue between the capillary and the alveolar wall causes impairment in gaseous diffusion. All these deficiencies contribute to the dyspnea seen in advanced asbestosis. The collagenization and subsequent contraction of the scar tissue increase the stiffness of the lungs, decrease their compliance, restrict the respiratory excursions, and increase the cost of respiration in terms of the effort and work involved.

Some of the asbestos fibers become incorporated in the inflammatory tissue and are thereby sequestered. Other asbestos fibers remain in the air spaces and become covered by an iron-containing protein. Because of the characteristic high iron component, these coated fibers are called "ferruginous bodies." The ferruginous bodies are red-brown or golden structures, often segmented and clubbed, and straight or curved. Their length and thickness are variable, dependent on the length and diameter of the central fiber. Because inhaled fibers composed of materials other than asbestos may also be converted into ferruginous bodies, the latter are not specific for asbestos. Only if the central fiber of a ferruginous body is composed of asbestos may the latter be termed an "asbestos body."

The nature of the pulmonary fibrosis caused by the inhalation of asbestos dust is not distinctive or diagnostic of asbestosis. It is usually most severe in the basal portions of the lung. However, fibrosis and the presence of ferruginous bodies would constitute a fairly secure base upon which the diagnosis of asbestosis can rest.

Excessive lung carcinomas among asbestos workers occur in those most heavily exposed to dust; that is, asbestotic lung cancer occurs in association with severe asbestosis. The implication of this finding is that there is a dose-effect relationship between asbestos dust exposure and lung cancer development, so that there is a level of asbestos dust exposure below which lung cancer is not likely to develop. Support for this conclusion is found in the published statistics from a large English asbestos factory in which the lung cancer incidence prior to 1932 was about 10 times that of the general population. After the institution of "good-housekeeping" measures in the factory, another survey indicated that the risk of developing lung cancer in that factory was no higher than in the general population.

In a study of asbestos-insulation workers it was found that, among the nonsmokers, the risk of lung cancer was relatively slight. But compared with a cigarette smoker not exposed to asbestos, the risk of lung cancer in a cigarette-smoking asbestos insulation worker was eight times greater, and about 90 times greater than that of a nonsmoking worker not exposed to asbestos.

Many asbestos-related lung cancers are bronchogenic in character—squamous, or undifferentiated carcinomas—but some are adenocarcinomas of peripheral origin. Although much of the inhaled dust inclusive of asbestos is cleared from the lungs via the bronchial mucosa, it is difficult to explain the genesis of bronchogenic cancers on the basis of asbestos dust alone. The adenocarcinomas of peripheral origin are more readily explained inasmuch as all experimentally produced asbestotic lung cancers originated peripherally within asbestotic scars.

Mesotheliomas of the pleura and of the peritoneum have been reported not only in people occupationally exposed to asbestos dust, but also in people exposed to this dust nonoccupationally. Among the latter are the wives of workers who washed work clothes heavily impregnated with very fine asbestos fibers that tended to remain suspended in air indefinitely. Another type of nonoccupational exposure included in these reports was living within one-half mile of a factory or shipyard fabricating or applying asbestos.

A satisfactory explanation for the occurrence of peritoneal mesotheliomas does not exist. This occurrence is particularly perplexing in those workers who have no asbestotic involvement of the lungs. Even more puzzling is the occurrence of mesotheliomas in Karain, Nevşehir Province, Turkey, where mesothelioma deaths are endemic and asbestos exposure is nonexistent. Here exposure to alluminum silicate fibers of volcanic origin and classified as zeolite minerals is suspected as the cause.

The ability to cause mesothelioma is not shared equally by all types of asbestos. In South Africa, the excess of mesotheliomas was almost limited to the crocidolite-producing area. Very few mesotheliomas were reported from areas where amosite was mined and none from chrysotile mines. Among 380 deaths of New York asbestos-insulation workers who had been exposed to various types of asbestos dusts, 6% were attributed to mesothelioma. Of 436 British asbestos workers, also exposed to more than one kind of asbestos, 5% had died of mesotheliomas. On the other hand, of 2413 deaths among Canadian chrysotile mine and mill workers, only three, or 0.1%, died of mesothelioma.

Talcosis is a pneumonconiosis that closely resembles asbestosis. This resemblance is probably related to the tremolite asbestos content of the dust to which talc miners are exposed. As in exposure to other forms of asbestos dust, talc miners suffer from an increased incidence of lung cancer. However, mesotheliomas have not been reported associated with talc-dust exposure.

Another type of pneumoconiosis, though rarely encountered and inadequately studied, has been reported among some workers exposed to dust from hard metals such as tungsten carbide. Cobalt has been incriminated as the responsible agent in these cases. The disease takes the form of a diffuse pulmonary fibrosis with granulomatous features.

Pneumonitis

The occupationally induced pneumonitides are of two types: hypersensitivity and toxic. The hypersensitivity type is caused exclusively by certain dusts, whereas the toxic type may be caused by dust, vapor, or gas—any inhaled material that is chemically irritating to the lung parenchyma.

A dust-related hypersensitivity pneumonitis differs from a pneumoconiosis in that although the inflammation in the former is unquestionably caused by the inhaled dust there is no demonstrable dust accumulation. Most of the dusts causing these pneumonitides are organic in character, consisting of the spores of fungi, but one dust is inorganic—beryllium.

The inhalation of beryllium, either as a metallic dust or as a dust of its chemical compounds, may result in serious disease, berylliosis. There is, however, one notable exception. Miners exposed to beryl ore dust (beryllium aluminum silicate) have not been affected by this disease.

Berylliosis may occur as an acute pneumonitis in which alveoli are filled with fluid containing macrophages and few lymphocytes. Alveolar walls are swollen and infiltrated by lymphocytes, monocytes, and scattered plasma cells. With persistence of the inflammation, fibroblastic proliferation and multiplication of reticulin fibers upon the alveolar walls usher in the subacute stage of the disease. The chronic form of berylliosis is characterized by a granulomatous inflammation that so closely resembles sarcoidosis in all its histologic aspects that it is often difficult to differentiate these two diseases microscopically. As is true for sarcoidosis, the inflammatory stroma of berylliosis retains its reticulin character over periods of months and years. It is this delay in collagenization of the stroma that allows for successful therapy with steroid drugs.

Because lung cancers have been readily produced experimentally with beryllium compounds by intratracheal injection in rats and, after many years of inhalation, also in monkeys, beryllium-caused cancers have been anticipated in people exposed to these materials. However, no evidence of cancer production by occupational exposure to beryllium or its compounds has been forthcoming.

The other hypersensitivity pneumonitides of occupational origin are caused by aerosolized components of different kinds of fungi that are characteristic of particular occupational settings. The thermophilic organisms that grow on bagasse and cause bagassosis, or the organism growing on moldy hay, causing farmer's lung, the mold growing on the bark of maples, causing maple bark–stripper's disease, and the spores of mushrooms causing mushroom-grower's disease are but a few examples. The diseases named are pathologically identical, having similar pathogenic backgrounds and histopathologic features.

The pneumonitis is both proliferative and exudative. There is thickening of septal walls by fibroblastic proliferation associated with multiplication of reticulin fibers and infiltration of these tissues by lymphocytes and plasma cells. In addition, there is also a granulomatous component in the inflammation. This takes the form of scattered foci of foreign body giant cells surrounded by reticulin fibers, lymphocytes, monocytes, plasma cells, and fibroblasts.

The irritants responsible for the production of the chemical or toxic pneumonitides or pneumonias of occupational origin are generally agents that would cause death from pulmonary edema at higher dose levels. As a matter of fact, the first reaction to a sublethal dose of such inhaled irritant is the development of pulmonary edema. If the victim does not "drown" in his alveolar fluid and survives 24 hours or longer, exudation of leukocytes occurs in the air spaces. The chemical pneumonia may be complicated by infection and conversion to a bacterial pneumonia.

Manganese oxide has been reported to cause chemical pneumonia in workers inhaling this dust. Mercury vapor and nickel carbonyl vapor have caused chemical pneumonia and pneumonitis among workmen, ranging from the acute form to the chronic variety and pulmonary fibrosis. More frequent causes of chemical pneumonias are gases in common industrial use such as nitrogen dioxide, sulfur dioxide, chlorine, and ammonia. Nitrogen oxides are also produced by decomposition of silage and are responsible for the acute edema or chronic pneumonitis and bronchiolitis termed "silo-filler's disease."

Pulmonary edema

As indicated in the previous column, all inhaled irritants that cause chemical pneumonia initially traumatize the alveolar capillary endothelium and produce pulmonary edema. If the dose level of the inhaled irritant is sufficiently high, the amount of capillary endothelial damage may be so extensive that death occurs before much cellular exudation can take place. Because there is usually a latent period of some hours after exposure before the pulmonary edema becomes clinically manifest, an erroneous concept of the mechanism of the edema is often held, that is, that the inhaled irritant is continuing its pathogenic action over this period of time. Actually, the damaging action of the irritant upon the capillary endothelium is completed within minutes of the inhalation and leakage of fluid into the air spaces occurs promptly. If a major portion of the alveolar capillary bed has been injured, the development of pulmonary edema can be explosive. With only a minor portion of the capillary bed affected, hours may be required to fill a sufficient amount of lung tissue with fluid to become clinically apparent.

To the irritants that cause pulmonary edema by virtue of causing chemical pneumonia, cadmium oxide fumes (CdO) and phosgene ($COCl_2$) should be added as potent producers of pulmonary edema in occupational settings. Workers welding cadmium-coated steel under conditions of inadequate ventilation are often victims of pulmonary edema. Phosgene is manufactured as an intermediate for the production of other chemicals. It is a hermitized process, situated outside of buildings. However, accidents such as leakages do occasionally occur.

Irritant gases can be divided into two general categories: those with a high solubility in water and those with a low solubility in aqueous solutions. Gases in the first category are considered upper respiratory irritants because in the concentrations usually encountered and from which people can escape the lungs are generally not involved. These gases are removed from the airstream before reaching the air spaces by the moisture of the tracheobronchial mucosa. Included in this category are sulfur dioxide, chlorine, and ammonia. Nitrogen dioxide and phosgene belong in the class of gases with low solubility in water. They are deep lung irritants and are known to produce pulmonary edema even in low concentrations. It is to be noted that gases that are upper respiratory irritants may also cause severe pulmonary damage and death if they are inhaled at high dose levels.

Bronchitis

Chemically active gases that have a high solubility in water, inclusive of sulfur dioxide, chlorine, and ammonia, tend to cause acute bronchitis if inhaled in sufficiently high concentrations.

Industrial bronchitis

Occupationally caused chronic bronchitis has been a somewhat controversial subject because in the United Kingdom, where this illness was most intensively studied, it was difficult to determine whether an increased risk of this disease was caused by occupational factors or the more evident causes so prevalent in the general population. There now appears to be adequate evidence that soft-coal miners, foundry men, and byssinotic workers described below do have an increased risk of developing chronic bronchitis even after allowances are made for genetic factors and cigarette smoking. Evidence for an increased risk of chronic bronchitis in other dusty occupations is lacking.

Bronchial constriction

Byssinosis is an occupational bronchial constriction affecting cotton-mill workers as well as those working with flax and hemp. In the former, it is caused by the inhalation of cotton dust. Some of the workers develop a hypersensitivity to an as yet unknown but heat-labile component of bracts of cotton. Subsequent inhalation of this dust results in the local release of histamine followed by the development of bronchial constriction with a feeling of chest tightness. Investigators who have studied cotton-mill workers believe that some of the workers, after many years of exposure to cotton dust, develop chronic obstructive lung disease and cor pulmonale. It has been difficult to sort out the other more common causes of chronic obstructive lung disease in cotton-mill workers to be certain that the obstructive changes were indeed caused by the inhalation of cotton dust. Before the development of chronic obstructive lung disease, no morphologic changes in the bronchi or lung tissue that could be identified with the clinical symptoms of byssinosis are known.

Toluene 2,4-diisocyanate (TDI, $CH_3C_6H_3[NCO]_2$) is also known to sensitize workers. As with byssinosis, the sensitization that occurs has not been shown to have an immunologic basis. Exposure of sensitized workers to this vapor results in bronchial constriction and attendant symptoms. No morphologic changes have been documented as a result of such exposure, though concentrations of 1 to 2 ppm cause tracheobronchitis in rats and a concentration of 12 ppm is lethal to this animal. Related diisocyanates may have similar effects.

Pleural fibrosis

Except for the development of pleural hyaline plaques from exposure to asbestos dust, the role played by inhaled dust in the pathogenesis of pleural inflammation is uncertain. The inconstancy of pleural inflammation in the presence of substantial subpleural dust deposition raises the question of requisite factors additional to the inhaled dust for the production of pleural fibrosis. The occurrence of parietal pleural hyaline plaques in the absence of asbestos dust exposure would seem to support the assumption that factors other than dust also participate in the production of the pleural fibrosis encountered in some pneumoconiotic lungs.

Emphysema

Sporadic case reports have claimed that debilitating emphysema developed after a massive one-time exposure to nitrogen dioxide, phosgene, or cadmium oxide fumes. Emphysema has also been claimed to be the result of exposure to such dusts as coal, asbestos, silica, and cement. These claims rest upon very insecure bases. Most of the reports and claims neglected to consider cigarette smoking, recognized as the most common cause of emphysema, in the evaluation of causative factors. Nevertheless, it has been possible to produce emphysema in rats by long-term exposure to low concentrations of nitrogen dioxide (also present but in relatively high concentrations in cigarette smoke).

Oncogenesis

Two kinds of occupational cancers involving thoracic tissues are recognized today. The more common one is lung cancer and the other, mesothelioma. The most widespread occupational lung cancer is caused by excessive exposure to asbestos dust. The asbestotic lung cancer and the asbestos-related mesothelioma have already been discussed.

Other occupationally caused lung cancers include those caused by exposures in the refining of nickel and in the production of chromates and exposures to coke-oven emissions, inorganic arsenic compounds, and radioactive material in mines.

Nickel. The specific dusts involved as possible carcinogens include the subsulfide and oxide of nickel as well as the metal itself. However, nickel furnace workers are also exposed to polycyclic hydrocarbons, which may be factors in the cancer production. Lung cancer rates among nickel workers have been reported to be as much as 10 times greater than expected but are generally much lower.

Inasmuch as nickel carbonyl vapor exposure has produced lung cancers in rats, this material has been suspected of being responsible for human lung cancer production. Because the increase in risk of lung cancer production in a Wales nickel refinery disappeared despite the continued use of nickel carbonyl, it now appears unlikely that this chemical was the only or the main factor in the lung cancer production.

Coke-oven emissions. Coke-oven emissions contain particulate polycyclic organic matter (POM) and workers exposed to them suffer an increased risk of developing lung cancer. Which of the many components of POM is responsible for this increased risk is not known, although benzo[*a*]pyrene (BAP) is often selected.

Chromates. The number of deaths from respiratory tract cancers in chromate-producing plants between 1940 and 1948 in the United States was 29 times the expected number according to a 1953 report, but in a 1966 study the number had dropped ninefold. The lung cancers occurred in workers exposed mainly to hexavalent chromium, particularly lead and zinc chromate. The carcinogenicity of chromates has been confirmed experimentally by the production of lung cancer in rats that had pellets of calcium as well as zinc chromate in cholesterol embedded in their bronchi.

Radioactive materials. Uranium mines in Colorado and fluorspar mines in Nova Scotia contain radioactive materials consisting of radon gas and its radioactive decomposition products—the radon daughters. The radon daughters differ from each other physically. Some consist of submicronic solid particles. An investigation of 249 deaths among white underground uranium miners disclosed a lung cancer incidence that was four times the expected one.

Oncogenic bioassays

Because of the extensive use of bioassays performed in rodents to determine the human neoplastic potential of drugs and chemicals, a few comments might be useful in placing the results of such testing in perspective. First the terminology must be considered. The official term employed in reference to these tests is "carcinogenicity bioassays," and a positive result brands a compound "carcinogen." However, the results may be interpreted as positive even if only benign tumors are produced. Such a subtlety may be of concern only to a pathologist, but the more appropriate terms would be "oncogenicity" and "oncogene."

These tests employ the "maximum tolerated dose" (MTD) as the highest of two or three dose levels of administered for 2 (or more) years to rats and mice. This dose is variously defined, but the attempt is to expose the rodents to the maximum dose that will not affect their survival over the chronic course of drug or chemical exposure. Such doses have been shown to overload various physiologic mechanisms and produce metabolites, distribution patterns, and elimination pathways that are not represented in the human exposure.

These high doses are utilized in an attempt to negate various statistical concerns in an attempt to represent the human population by a relatively small number of test animals (50/sex/group/species). Similar concerns support the 2-year or longer exposure of the test animals. However, this necessitates the determination of treatment-induced tumors against the considerable background of spontaneous tumors that occur naturally in aged rats and mice. Consequently, statistical analysis becomes a significant factor in the evaluation of oncogenicity and the results are often difficult to interpret biologically. For example, a new cholesterol-lowering agent was recently approved by the Food and Drug Administration despite statistically significant increases in hepatocellular carcinomas and adenomas, as well as pulmonary adenomas in mice and a positive dose-response relationship for "hepatocellular carcinogenicity" in male rats. Indeed, "the implication of findings are unclear."

The lack of validation of the bioassay protocol and the variability of tumor incidences between different control groups constitute additional concerns. The inability of the rat to allow prediction of oncogenicity for the mouse and vice versa makes human extrapolation of rodent bioassay results very tenuous.

REFERENCES
General

1. Ahlstedt, S., and Kristofferson, A.: Immune mechanisms for induction of penicillin allergy, Prog. Allergy **30:**67, 1982.
2. Baselt, R.C.: Disposition of toxic drugs and chemicals in man, Canton, Ohio, 1978, Biomedical Publications.
3. Baselt, R.C., and Cravey, R.H.: A compendium of therapeutic and toxic concentrations of toxicologically significant drugs in human biofluids, J. Anal. Toxicol. **1:**81, 1977.
4. Biava, C.: Fine structure of hepatocellular and canalicular bile pigment, Lab. Invest. **13:**1099, 1964.
5. Browning, E.: Toxicity of industrial metals, ed. 2, New York, 1969, Appleton-Century-Crofts.
6. Camps, F., editor: Gradwohl's legal medicine, ed. 2, Baltimore, 1968, The Williams & Wilkins Co.
7. Davies, D.M.: Textbook of adverse drug reactions, ed. 2, New York, 1981, Oxford Medical Publications.
8. Deichmann, W.B., and Gerarde, H.W.: Toxicology of drugs and chemicals, ed. 4, New York, 1969, Academic Press, Inc.
9. Gonzales, T.A., et al.: Legal medicine: pathology and toxicology, ed. 2, New York, 1954, Appleton-Century-Crofts.
10. Grundmann, E.: Drug-induced pathology, Current Topics in Pathology, vol. 69, New York, 1980, Springer-Verlag.
11. Hennigar, G.R.: Iatrogenic drug toxicity in the pathologist and the environment. In Scarpelli, D.G., Craighead, J.E., and Kaufman, N., editors: International Academy of Pathology, Monographs in Pathology, no. 26, Chap. 4, Baltimore, 1985, The Williams & Wilkins Co.
12. Herrold, K.M., Rabson, A.S., and Smith, R.: Liver in generalized hypersensitivity, Arch. Pathol. **66:**306, 1958.
13. Inglefinger, F.J.: Counting adverse drug reactions that count, N. Engl. J. Med **294:**1003, 1976.
14. Irey, N.S.: Tissue reactions to drugs, Am. J. Pathol. **82:**617, 1976.
15. Landsteiner, K., and Jacobs, J.: Studies on the sensitization of animals with simple chemical compounds, J. Exp. Med. **61:**643, 1935.
16. McLean, A.E.M., and Judah, E.: Cellular necrosis in the liver induced and modified by drugs, Int. Rev. Exp. Pathol. **4:**127, 1965.
17. McMaster, K.R., III, and Hennigar, G.R.: Drug-induced granulomatous hepatitis, Lab. Invest. **44:**61, 1981.
18. Meyler, L.: In Dukes, M.N.G., editor: Meyler's side effects of drugs, ed. 9, Princeton, N.J., 1980, Excerpta Medica.
19. Meyler, L., and Peck, H.M.: Drug-induced diseases, vol. 4, Amsterdam, 1972, Excerpta Medica Foundation.

20. Meyler, L., and Peck, H.M.: In Bristow, M.R., editor: Meyler and Peck's drug-induced diseases, vol. 5, New York, 1980, Elsevier/North-Holland Biomedical Press.
21. Moser, R.H.: Disease of medical progress: a study of iatrogenic disease, ed. 3, Springfield, Ill., 1969, Charles C Thomas, Publisher.
22. Parker, C.W.: Mechanisms of drug allergy, N. Engl. J. Med. **292**:511, 1975.
23. Popper, H., and Schaffner, F.: Pathophysiology of cholestasis, Hum. Pathol. **1**:1, 1970.
24. Riddell, R.H.: Pathology of drug-induced and toxic diseases, New York, 1982, Churchill Livingstone.
25. Schimmel, M.E.: The hazards of hospitalization, Ann. Intern. Med. **60**:100, 1964.
26. Sell, S.: Immunology, immunopathology and immunity, ed. 4, New York, 1987, Elsevier Science Pub. Co., Inc.
27. Spain, D.M.: The complications of modern medical practices, New York, 1963, Grune & Stratton, Inc.

Drug injury and iatrogenic diseases
Drug-induced systemic lupus erythematosus

28. Dammin, G.J., Nora, J.R., and Reardan, J.B.: Hydralazine reactions: case with lupus erythematosus, J. Lab. Clin. Med. **46**:806, 1955.
29. Fakhro, A.M., Ritchie, R.F., and Lown, B.: Lupus-like syndrome induced by procainamide, Am. J. Cardiol. **20**:367, 1967.
30. Jollow, D.J.: Personal communication, Department of Pharmacology, Medical University of South Carolina, Charleston, S.C., 1988.
31. Ladd, A.T.: Procainamide-induced lupus erythematosus, N. Engl. J. Med. **267**:1357, 1962.
32. Lee, S.L., Rivero, I., and Siegel, M.: Activation of systemic lupus erythematosus by drugs, Arch. Intern. Med. **117**:620, 1966.
33. Shulman, L.E., and Harvey, A.M.: Nature of drug-induced systemic lupus erythematosus, Arthritis Rheum. **3**:464, 1960.
34. Siegel, M., Lee, S.L., and Peress, N.S.: Epidemiology of drug-induced systemic lupus erythematosus, Arthritis Rheum. **10**:407, 1967.

Medicinal hazards of therapy
Antimicrobial agents

35. Andres, G.A., and McCluskey, R.T.: Tubular and interstitial renal disease due to immunologic mechanisms, Kidney Int. **7**:271, 1975.
36. Andres, G.A., Brentjens, J., Kohli, R., Anthone, R., Anthone, S., Baliah, T., Montes, M., Mookerjee, B.K., Prezyna, A., Sepúlveda, M., Venuto, R., and Elwood, C.: Histology of human tubulo-interstitial nephritis associated with antibodies to renal basement membranes, Kidney Int. **13**:480, 1978.
37. Bartlett, J.G., Chang, T.W., Gurwith, M., Grobach, S.L., and Onderdonk, A.B.: Antibiotic-associated pseudomembranous colitis due to toxin-producing clostridia, N. Engl. J. Med. **298**:531, 1978.
38. George, R.H., Symonds, J.M., Dimock, F., Brown, J.D., Arabi, Y., Shinagawa, N., Keighley, M.R., Alexander-Williams, J., and Burdon, D.W.: Identification of *Clostridium difficile* as a cause of pseudomembranous colitis, Br. Med. J. **1**:695, 1978.
39. Heptinstall, R.H.: Interstitial nephritis: a brief review, Am. J. Pathol. **83**:214, 1976.
40. Linton, A.L., Clark, W.F., Driedger, A.A., Turnbull, D.I., and Lindsay, R.M.: Acute intersitial nephritis due to drugs: a review of the literature with a report of nine cases, Ann. Intern. Med. **93**:735, 1980.
41. Mayaud, C., Kanfer, A., Kourilsky, O., et al: Interstitial nephritis after methicillin, N. Engl. J. Med **292**:1132, 1975. (Letter.)
42. Medline, A., Shin, D.H., and Medline, N.M.: Pseudomembranous colitis associated with antibiotics, Hum. Pathol. **7**:693, 1976.
43. Méry, J., and Morel-Maroger, L.: Acute interstitial nephritis: a hypersensitivity reaction to drugs. In Giovannetti, S., and Bonomini, V., editors: Proc. Sixth International Congress of Nephrology, Florence, June 8-12, 1975, Basel, 1976, S. Karger AG., p. 524.

44. Ooi, B.S., Jao, W., First, M.R., Mancilla, R., and Pollak, V.E.: Acute interstitial nephritis: a clinical and pathologic study based on renal disease, Am. J. Med. **59**:614, 1975.
45. Pittman, F.E.: Antibiotic-associated colitis: an update, Adverse Drug Reaction Bull. **75**:268, 1979.
46. Price, A.B., and Davies, D.R.: Pseudomembranous colitis, J. Clin. Pathol. **30**:1, 1977.

TETRACYCLINE

47. André, T.: Studies on the distribution of tritium-labelled dehydrostreptomycin and tetracycline in the body, Acta Radiol. **142**(suppl):1, 1957.
48. Davis, J.S.: Drug-induced diseases, vol. 3, New York, 1968, Excerpta Medica Foundation.
49. Davis, J.S., and Kaufman, R.H.: Tetracycline toxicity, Am. J. Obstet. Gynecol. **95**:523, 1966.
50. Dowling, H.F., and Lepper, M.H.: Hepatic reactions to tetracycline, JAMA **188**:307, 1964.
51. Gale, E.F., and Folkes, J.P.: The assimilation of amino-acids by bacteria, Biochem. J. **53**:493, 1953.
52. Schultz, J.C., Adamson, J.S., Workman, W.W., and Norman, T.D.: Fatal liver disease after intravenous administration of tetracycline in high dosage, N. Engl. J. Med. **269**:999, 1963.
53. Sheehan, H.L.: The pathology of acute yellow atrophy and delayed chloroform poisoning, J. Obstet. Gynecol. Br. Emp. **47**:49, 1940.

AMPHOTERICIN B

54. Hill, G.J., II: Amphotericin nephrotoxicity, Ann. Intern. Med. **61**:349, 1964.
55. Kinsky, S.C., Avruch, J., Permutt, M., and Rogers, H.B.: Amphotericin and erythrocytes, Biochem. Biophys. Res. Commun. **9**:503, 1962.
56. Perlman, D., Giuffre, N.A., and Brindle, S.A.: Amphotericin and tissue culture cells, Proc. Soc. Exp. Biol. Med. **106**:880, 1961.
57. Sens, M.A., Hennigar, G.R., Hazen-Martin, D.J., Blackburn, J.G., and Sens, D.A.: Cultured human proximal tubule cells as a model for aminoglycoside nephrotoxicity, Ann. Clin. Lab. Sci. **18**:204, 1988.
58. Utz, J.P.: Amphotericin B toxicity, Ann. Intern. Med. **61**:334, 1964.

AMINOGLYCOSIDES: STREPTOMYCIN, NEOMYCIN, CHLORAMPHENICOL, GENTAMICIN

59. Dobbins, W.O., III, Herrero, B.A., and Mansbach, C.M.: Morphologic alterations associated with neomycin-induced malabsorption, Am. J. Med Sci. **255**:63, 1968.
60. Hottendorf, G.H.: Aminoglycoside nephrotoxicity, Toxicol. Pathol. **14**:66, 1986.
61. Kosek, J.C., Mazze, R.I., and Cousins, M.J.: Nephrotoxicity of gentamicin, Lab. Med. **30**:48, 1974.
62. McCurdy, P.R.: Action of chloramphenicol, Blood **21**:363, 1963.
63. Schentag, J.J., Lasezkay, G., Plaut, M.E., Jusko, W.J., and Cumbo, T.J.: Gentamicin tissue accumulation and nephrotoxic reactions, JAMA **240**:2067, 1978.

Analgesics and antipyretics; nonsteroidal anti-inflammatory drugs
SALICYLATES

64. Done, A.K.: Salicylamide toxicity, Pediatrics **23**:774, 1959.
65. Eichenholz A., Mulhausen, R.O., and Redleaf, P.S.: Salicylate effect on respiratory center, Metabolism **12**:164, 1963.
66. Lawson, A.A.H., et al.: Acute salicylate intoxication in adults, Q. J. Med. **38**:31, 1969.
67. Maher, J.F., and Schreiner, G.E.: Death in acute salicylate poisoning, Trans. Am. Soc. Artif. Intern. Organs **11**:349, 1965.
68. Smith, M.J.H., and Smith, P.K.: The salicylates, New York, 1966, Interscience Publishers, Inc.
69. Tobin, J.A., and Hennigar, G.R.: Salicylate intoxication, V. Med. Monthly **79**:486, 1952.

ACETAMINOPHEN

70. Jollow, D.J., Mitchell, J.R., Potter, W.Z., et al.: Acetaminophen-induced hepatic necrosis. IV. Protective role of glutathione, J. Pharm. Exp. Ther. **187**:211, 1973.

AMINOPHENOLS

71. Black, M.: Acetaminophen hepatotoxicity, Gastroenterology **78**:382, 1980.
72. Brodie, B.B., and Axelrod, J.: Fate of phenacetin in man, Pharmacol. Exp. Ther. **97**:58, 1949.
73. Burry, A.F.: Pathology of analgesic nephropathy: Australian experience, Kidney Int. **13**:34, 1978.
74. Gloor, F.J.: Changing concepts in pathogenesis and morphology of analgesic nephropathy as seen in Europe, Kidney Int. **13**:27, 1978.
75. Gonwa, T.A., Corbett, W.T., Schey, H.M., and Buckalew, V.M., Jr.: Analgesic-associated nephropathy in transitional cell carcinoma of the urinary tract, Ann. Intern. Med. **93**:249, 1980.
76. Grimlund, K.: Kidney damage in members of same family, Acta Med. Scand. **174**(suppl. 405):3, 1963.
77. Kincaid-Smith, P.: Analgesic nephropathy: a common form of renal disease in Australia, Med. J. Aust. **2**:1131, 1969.
78. MacGibbon, B.H., Loughridge, L.W., Hourihane, D.O., and Boyd, D.W.: Autoimmune haemolytic anaemia, with acute renal failure due to phenacetin and *p*-aminosalicylic acid, Lancet **1**:7, 1960.
79. Marsco, W.A., Gikas, P.W., Azziz-Baumgartner, R., Hyzy, R., Eldredge, C.J., and Stross, J.: Ibuprofen-associated renal dysfunction, Arch. Intern. Med. **147**:2107, 1987.
80. Mitchell, J.R., and Jollow, D.J.: Metabolic activation of drugs to toxic substances, Gastroenterology **68**:392, 1975.
81. Nissen, N.I., and Friis, T.: Phenacetin anuria and interstitial nephritis, Acta Med. Scand. **171**:125, 1962.

Androgenic-anabolic steroids

82. Antunes, C.M.F., Strolley, P.D., Rosenshein, N.B., Davies, J.L., Tonascia, J.A., Brown, C., Burnett, L., Rutledge, A., Pokempier, M., and García, R.: Endometrial cancer and estrogen use: report of a large case-control study, N. Engl. J. Med. **300**:9, 1979.
83. Glover, G.A., and Wilkerson, J.A.: Biliary cirrhosis following the administration of methyltestosterone, JAMA **204**:168, 1968.

Oral contraceptive (the "pill")

84. Irey, N.S., Manion, W.C., and Taylor, H.B.: Vascular lesions in women taking oral contraceptives, Arch. Pathol. **89**:1, 1970.
85. Mann, J.I., Vessey, M.P., Thorogood, M., and Doll, R.: Myocardial infarction in young women with special reference to oral contraceptive practice, Br. Med. J. **2**:241, 1975.
86. Tausk, M.: Drug-induced diseases, vol. 3, New York, 1968, Excerpta Medica Foundation.

Estrogens

87. Herbst, A.L., Kurman, R.J., and Scully, R.E.: Vaginal and cervical abnormalities after exposure to stilbestrol in utero, Obstet. Gynecol. **40**:287, 1972.
88. Herbst, A.L., and Scully, R.E.: Adenocarcinoma of vagina in adolescence, Cancer **25**:745, 1970.
89. Ng, A.B.P., Reagan, J.W., Hawliczek, S., and Wentz, W.B.: Cellular detection of vaginal adenosis, Obstet. Gynecol. **46**:323, 1975.

Tranquilizers

90. Alexander, C.S., and Nino, A.: Cardiovascular complications—phenothiazines, Am. Heart J. **78**:757, 1969.
91. Campbell, J.E.: Myocardial lesions—chlorpromazine, Am. J. Clin. Pathol. **34**:133, 1960.
92. Margolis, I.B., and Gross, C.G.: Gynecomastia during phenothiazine therapy, JAMA **199**:942, 1967.
93. Walker, C.O., and Combes, B.: Biliary cirrhosis induced by chlorpromazine, Gastroenterology **51**:631, 1966.

Antihypertensive drugs

94. Alarcón-Segovia, D., Fishbein, E., and Betancourt, V.M.: Antibodies to nucleoprotein and to hydrazide-altered soluble nucleoprotein in TB patients receiving isoniazid, Clin. Exp. Immunol. **5**:429, 1969.
95. Fenoglio, J.J., McAllister, H.A., and Mullick, F.G.: Drug related myocarditis, Hum. Pathol. **12**:900, 1981.

96. Graham, C.F., Gallagher, K., and Jones, J.K.: Acute colitis with methyldopa, N. Engl. J. Med. **304**:1044, 1981.
97. Maddrey, W.C., and Boitnott, J.K.: Severe hepatitis from methyldopa, Gastroenterology **68**:351, 1975.
98. Maddrey, W.C., and Boitnott, J.K.: Drug-induced chronic liver disease, Gastroenterology **72**:1348, 1977.
99. Seeverens, H., DeBruin, C.D., and Jordans, J.G.: Myocarditis and methyldopa, Acta Med. Scand. **211**:233, 1982.

Sympathomimetic amines
Amphetamines

100. Citron, B.P., Halpern, M., McCarron, M., Lundberg, G.D., McCormick, R., Pincus, I.J., Tatter, D., and Haverback, B.J.: Necrotizing angiitis associated with drug abuse, N. Engl. J. Med. **283**:1003, 1970.

Antithyroid drugs

101. Griswold, W.R., Mendoza, S.A., and Johnson, W.: Vasculitis associated with propylthiouracil: evidence for immune complex pathogenesis and response to therapy, West. J. Med. **128**:543, 1978.
102. Houston, B.D., Crouch, M.E., and Brick, J.E.: Apparent vasculitis associated with propylthiouracil use, Arthritis Rheum. **22**:925, 1979.

Antidiabetic drugs

103. Balodimos, M.C., Marble, A., Rippey, J.H., et al.: Pathologic findings after sulfonylurea, Diabetes **17**:503, 1968.
104. Bloodworth, J.M.B., Jr.: Morphologic changes associated with sulfonylurea, Metabolism **12**:287, 1963.
105. Sackner, M.A., and Balian, L.: Sulfonylurea-induced hypoglycemia, Am. J. Med. **28**:135, 1960.

H₂ receptor antagonists

106. Freston, J.W.: Cimetidine. II. Adverse reactions and patterns of use, Ann. Intern. Med. **97**:728, 1982.
107. McGowan, W.R., and Vermillion, S.E.: Acute interstitial nephritis related to cimetidine therapy, Gastroenterology **79**:746, 1980.
108. Sawyer, D., Conner, C.S., and Scalley, R.: Cimetidine: adverse reaction and acute toxicity, Am. J. Hosp. Pharm. **38**:188, 1981.

Antitubercular drugs

109. Bellamy, W.E., Jr., Mauck, H.P., Jr., Henningar, G.R., and Wigod, M.: Jaundice associated with the administration of sodium *p*-aminosalicylic acid, Ann. Intern. Med. **44**:764, 1956.
110. Elmendorf, D.F., Jr., et al.: INH toxicity, Am. Rev. Tuberc. **65**:429, 1952.
111. Lichenstein, M.R., and Cannemeyer, W.: PAS hypersensitivity, JAMA **152**:606, 1953.
112. Paine, D.: Fatal hepatic necrosis associated with aminosalicylic acid, JAMA **167**:285, 1958.
113. Reynolds, E.: INH jaundice, Tubercle **43**:375, 1962.
114. Warring, F.C., Jr., and Howlett, K.S.: Allergic reactions to PAS, Am. Rev. Tuberc. **65**:235, 1952.

Anesthetics
HALOTHANE

115. Paronetto, F., and Popper, H.: Lymphocyte-stimulation test, N. Engl. J. Med. **283**:277, 1970.
116. Peters, R.L., Edmondson, H.A., Reynolds, T.B., and Meister, J.C.: Hepatic necrosis associated with halothane, Am. J. Med. **47**:748, 1969.
117. Touloukian, J., and Kaplowitz, N.: Halothane-induced hepatic disease, Semin. Liver Dis. **1**:134, 1981.

METHOXYFLURANE

118. Cousins, M.J., Mazze, R.I., Kosek, J.C., et al.: Etiology of methoxyflurane nephrotoxicity, J. Pharmacol. Exp. Ther. **190**:530, 1975.
119. Frascino, J.A., Venemee, P., and Rosen, P.P.: Renal oxalosis and azotemia after methoxyflurane, N. Engl. J. Med. **283**:676, 1970.
120. Powell, H.C., Garrett, R.S., Bernstein, L., et al.: Methoxyflurane nephropathy, Hum. Pathol. **5**:359, 1974.

Anticonvulsants

121. Carrington, C.B., Addington, W.W., Goff, H.M., Madoff, I.M., Marks, A., Schwaber, J.R., and Gaensler, E.A.: Eosinophilic pneumonia, N. Engl. J. Med. **280**:787, 1969.
122. Crofton, J.W., Livingstone, J.L., Oswald, N.C., and Roberts, A.T.M.: Pulmonary eosinophilia, Thorax **7**:1, 1952.
123. Gaffy, C.M., Chun, B., Harvey, J.C., and Manz, H.J.: Phenytoin-induced systemic granulomatous vasculitis, Arch. Pathol. Lab. Med. **110**:131, 1986.
124. Gams, R.A., Neal, J.A., and Conrad, F.G.: Hydantoin-induced pseudo-pseudolymphoma, Ann. Intern. Med. **69**:557, 1968.
125. Gately, L.E., III, and Lam, M.A.: Phenytoin-induced toxic epidermal necrolysis, Ann. Intern. Med. **91**:59, 1979.
126. Hansen, J.W., Jones, K.L., and Smith, D.W.: Fetal alcohol syndrome, JAMA **235**:1458, 1976.
127. Hepner, G.W., et al.: Inhibition of intestinal ATPase by diphenylhydantoin and acetazolamide, Clin. Res. **18**:382, 1970.
128. Kleckner, H.B., Yakulis, V., and Heller, P.: Severe hypersensitivity to diphenylhydantoin with circulating antibodies to the drug, Ann. Intern. Med. **83**:522, 1975.
129. Larmas, L.: A comparative enzyme histochemical study of hydantoin-induced hyperplastic and normal human gingiva, Proc. Finn. Dent. Soc. **73**(suppl. 1): 1, 1977.
130. Li, F.P., Williard, D.R., Goodman, R., and Vawter, G.: Malignant lymphoma after diphenylhydantoin (Dilantin) therapy, Cancer **36**:1359, 1975.
131. McMaster, K.R., III, and Hennigar, G.R.: Drug-induced granulomatous hepatitis, Lab. Invest. **44**:61, 1981.
132. Meadow, S.R.: Harelip and cleft palate, Lancet **2**:1296, 1968.
133. Meynell, M.J.: Megaloblastic anemia in anticonvulsant therapy, Lancet **1**:487, 1966.
134. Monson, R.R., Rosenberg, L., Hartz, S.C., Shapiro, S., Heinonen, O.P., and Slone, D.: Congenital malformations and teratogenesis, N. Engl. J. Med. **289**:1049, 1973.
135. Mullick, F.G., and Ishak, D.G.: Hepatic injury associated with diphenylhydantoin therapy: a clinicopathologic study of 20 cases, Am. J. Clin. Pathol. **74**:442, 1980.
136. Rausing, A.: Hydantoin-induced lymphadenopathies and lymphomas, Rec. Res. Cancer Res. **64**:263, 1978.
137. Reynolds, E.H.: Diphenylhydantoin hematologic aspects of toxicity. In Woodbury, D.M., Penry, J.K., and Schmidt, R.P., editors: Antiepileptic drugs, New York, 1972, Raven Press.
138. Saltzstein, S.L., and Ackerman, L.V.: Dilantin-induced lymphadenopathy, Cancer **12**:164, 1959.
139. Sheth, K.J., Casper, J.T., and Good, T.A.: Interstitial nephritis due to phenytoin hypersensitivity, J. Pediatr. **91**:438, 1977.
140. Smith, D.W.: Fetal alcohol syndrome. In Shaffer, A.J., consulting editor: Recognizable patterns of human malformation, ed. 2, Philadelphia, 1976, W.B. Saunders Co.
141. Yermakov, V.M., Hitti, I.F., and Sutton, A.L.: Necrotizing vasculitis associated with diphenylhydantoin: two fatal cases, Hum. Pathol. **14**:182, 1983.

Digitalis

142. Dearing, W.H., Barnes, A.R., and Essex, H.E.: Experimental myocardial damage, Am. Heart J. **25**:648, 1943.
143. Gazes, P.C., Holmes, C.R., Moseley, V., and Pratt-Thomas, H.R.: Acute hemorrhage and necrosis of the intestines associated with digitalization, Circulation **23**:358, 1961.
144. Hiott, D.W.: Early ultrastructural changes in heart muscle produced by digoxin and emetine, Fed. Proc. **27**:347, 1968.
145. Molnar, Z., Larsen, K., and Spargo, B.: Cardiac changes in potassium-depleted rat, Arch. Pathol. **74**:339, 1962.
146. Reichenbach, D.D., and Benditt, E.P.: Catecholamines and cardiomyopathy: the pathogenesis and potential importance of myofibrillar degeneration, Hum. Pathol. **1**:125, 1970.
147. Walton, R.P., and Gazes, P.C.: Cardiac glycosides II: pharmacology and clinical use. In DiPalma, J.P., editor: Drill's pharmacology in medicine, ed. 3, New York, 1965, McGraw-Hill Book Co.
148. Wenzel, D.G.: Myocardial lesions, J. Pharm. Sci. **56**:1209, 1967.

Oxygen

149. Balentine, J.D.: Pathology of oxygen toxicity, New York, 1982, Academic Press, Inc.
150. Chance, B., and Boveris, A.: Hyperoxia and hydroperoxide metabolism. In Robin, E.D., editor: Extrapulmonary manifestations of respiratory disease, New York, 1978, Marcel Dekker, Inc.
151. Yamamoto, E., Wittner, M., and Rosenbaum, R.M.: Resistance and susceptibility to oxygen toxicity by cell types of the gas-blood barrier of the rat lung, Am. J. Pathol. **59**:409, 1970.

Antineoplastic and immunosuppressive drugs

152. Billingham, M.E.: Morphologic changes in drug-induced heart disease. In Bristow, M.R., editor: Meyler and Peck's drug-induced diseases. Vol. 5. Drug-induced heart disease, New York, 1980, Elsevier/North-Holland Biomedical Press.
153. Buja, L.M., and Ferrans, V.J.: Myocardial injury produced by antineoplastic drugs: pathophysiology and morphology of myocardial cell alterations, In Fleckenstein, A., and Rona, G., editors: Recent advances in the studies on cardiac structure and metabolism, vol. 6, Baltimore, 1975, University Park Press.
154. Buja, I.M., Ferrans, V.J., Mayer, R.J., Roberts, W.C., and Henderson, E.S.: Cardiac ultrastructural changes induced by daunorubicin therapy, Cancer **32**:771, 1973.
155. Bulkley, B.H., and Roberts, W.C.: The heart in systemic lupus erythematosus and the changes induced in it by corticosteroid therapy, Am. J. Med. **58**:243, 1975.
156. Castlemen, B., Schull, R.E., and McNeely, B.U.: Case records of the Massachusetts General Hospital. Case 6, N. Engl. J. Med. **290**:390, 1974.
157. Györkey, F., Györkey, B., and Sinkovics, J.G.: Origin and significance of intranuclear tubular inclusions in type II pulmonary alveolar epithelial cells of patients with bleomycin and busulfan toxicity, Ultrastruc. Pathol. **1**:211, 1980.
158. Jones, A.W.: Bleomycin lung damage: the pathology and nature of the lesion, Br. J. Dis. Chest **72**:321, 1978.
159. Kirschner, R.H., and Esterly, J.R.: Pulmonary lesions associated with busulfan therapy of chronic myelogenous leukemia, Cancer **27**:1074, 1971.
160. Kraus, H., Schuhman, R., Ganal, M., and Geier, G.: Cytologic findings in vaginal smears from patients under treatment with cyclophosphamide, Acta Cytol. **21**:726, 1977.
161. Mallory, A., and Kern, F., Jr.: Drug-induced pancreatitis: a critical review, Gastroenterology **78**:813, 1980.
162. Reimer, R.R., Hoover, R., Fraumeni, J.F., Jr., and Young, R.C.: Acute leukemia after alkylating-agent therapy of ovarian cancer, N. Engl. J. Med. **297**:177, 1977.
163. Seiber, S.M., and Adamson, R.H.: Toxicity of antineoplastic agents in man: chromosomal aberrations, antifertility effects, congenital malformations and carcinogenic potential, Adv. Cancer Res. **22**:57, 1975.
164. Slavin, R.E., Millan, J.C., and Mullins, G.M.: Pathology of high dose intermittent cyclophosphamide therapy, Hum. Pathol. **6**:693, 1975.
165. Weiss, B.R., and Muggia, F.M.: Cytotoxic drug-induced pulmonary disease: update 1980, Am. J. Med. **68**:259, 1980.
166. Williams, G.M., Burdick, J.F., and Solez, K.: Kidney transplant rejection, New York, 1986, Marcel Dekker, Inc.

Antimetabolites

167. Kuhn, C., III, and Kuo, T.-T.: Cytoplasmic hyalin in asbestosis: a reaction of injured alveolar epithelium, Arch. Pathol. **95**:190, 1973.

Other agents

168. Hache, L., Utz, D.C., and Woolner, L.B.: Methysergide and idiopathic fibrous retroperitonitis, Surg. Gynecol. Obstet. **115**:737, 1962.
169. Hursh, J.B., et al.: Thorotrast excretion, Acta Radiol. (Stockholm) **47**:481, 1957.
170. Karch, S.B., and Billingham, M.E.: The pathology of the heart in near drowning, Arch. Pathol. Lab. Med. **109**:171, 1985, *and* The pathology and etiology of cocaine-induced heart disease, Arch. Pathol. Lab. Med. **112**:225, 1988.

171. Looney, W.B.: Thorotrast: late clinical findings, Am. J. Roentgenol. **83**:163, 1960.
172. Mason, J.W., Billingham, M.E., and Friedman, J.P.: Methysergide-induced heart disease: a case of multivalvular and myocardial fibrosis, Circulation **56**:889, 1977.
173. Reeves, D.L., and Stuck, R.M.: Thorotrast: clinical and experimental, Medicine **17**:37, 1938.

POTASSIUM CHLORIDE, MILK AND ALKALI, MINERAL OIL

174. Baker, D.R., Schrader, W.H., and Hitchcock, C.R.: Small-bowel ulceration apparently associated with thiazide and potassium therapy, JAMA **190**:586, 1964.
175. Bingham, E., Horton, A.W., and Tye, R.: Cancer from mineral oil, Arch. Environ. Health **10**:449, 1965.
176. Diener, R.M., Shoffstall, D.H., and Earl, A.E.: Experimental potassium-induced ulcer in monkeys, Toxicol. Appl. Pharmacol. **7**:746, 1965.
177. Pinkerton, H.: Reaction to oils and fats in lung, Arch. Pathol. **5**:380, 1928.
178. Portnoy, L.M., Amadeo, B., and Hennigar, G.R.: Pulmonary alveolar microlithasis, Am. J. Clin. Pathol. **41**:194, 1964.

Toxicologic aspects of forensic pathology
Alcohols and glycols

179. Adelson, L.: Fatal intoxication with isopropyl alcohol (rubbing alcohol), Am. J. Clin. Pathol. **38**:144, 1962.
180. Bennett, I.L., Jr., Nation, T.C., and Olley, J.F.: Pancreatitis—methyl alcohol, J. Lab. Clin. Med. **40**:405, 1952.
181. Biava, C.: Mallory alcoholic hyalin, Lab. Invest. **13**:301, 1964.
182. Factor, S.M.: Intramyocardial small-vessel disease in chronic alcoholism, Am. Heart J. **92**:561, 1976.
183. Ferrans, V.J., Hibbs, R.G., Weilbaecher, D.G., et al.: Alcoholic cardiomyopathy: a histochemical study, Am. Heart J. **69**:748, 1965.
184. Ferrans, V.J., et al.: Cardiac morphologic changes produced by ethanol. In Rothschild, M.A., Oratz, M., and Schreiver, S.S., editors: Alcohol and abnormal protein biosynthesis: biochemical and clinical, New York, 1975, Pergamon Press.
185. Flax, M.H., and Tisdale, W.A.: Electron microscopy of alcoholic hyalin, Am. J. Pathol. **44**:441, 1964.
186. Gadsden, R.H., Mellette, R.R., and Miller, W.C., Jr.: Scrap-iron intoxication, JAMA **168**:1220, 1958.
187. Lieber, C.S.: Hepatic and metabolic effects of alcohol, Gastroenterology **50**:119, 1966.
188. MacDonald, R.A., and Baumslag, N.: Iron in alcoholic beverages, Am. J. Med. Sci. **247**:649, 1964.
189. Makar, A.B., Tephly, T.R., and Mannering, G.J.: Ethanol inhibition of bile activation and toxification by methanol, Mol. Pharmacol. **4**:471, 1968.
190. McCord, W.M., Switzer, P.K., and Brill, H.H., Jr.: Isopropyl alcohol intoxication, South. Med. J. **41**:639, 1948.
191. McKennis, H., Jr., and Haag, H.B.: On the congeners of whiskey, J. Am. Geriatr. Soc. **7**:848, 1959.
192. Popper, H., Rubin, E., Cardiol, D., et al.: Drug-induced liver disease, Arch. Intern. Med. **115**:128, 1965.
193. Regan, T.J., and Haider, B.: Pathophysiologic effects of ethanol on cardiac tissue. In Bristow, M.R., editor: Meyler and Peck's drug-induced diseases, vol. 5, New York, 1980, Elsevier/North-Holland Biomedical Press.
194. Reppart, J.T., Peters, R.L., Edmondson, A.A., et al.: Alcoholic hyalin bodies, Lab. Invest. **12**:1138, 1963.
195. Rubin, E., and Lieber, C.S.: Early fine structural changes in the human liver induced by alcohol, Gastroenterology **52**:1, 1967.
196. Rubin, E., and Lieber, C.S.: Induction and inhibition of hepatic microsomal enzymes by ethanol, Science **162**:690, 1968.
197. Rubin, E.: Alcohol and the cell, Ann. NY Acad. Sci., vol. 492, 1987.
198. Svoboda, J.D., and Manning, R.T.: Mitochondrial alterations, Am. J. Pathol. **44**:645, 1964.
199. Wendt, V.E., Wu, C., Balcon, R., et al.: Hemodynamic and metabolic effects of chronic alcoholism in man, Am. J. Cardiol. **15**:175, 1965.
200. Zieve, L.: Jaundice, hyperlipemia and hemolytic anemia: a heretofore unrecognized syndrome associated with alcoholic fatty liver and cirrhosis, Ann. Intern. Med. **48**:471, 1958.

Metals and metallic salts
Mercury

201. Becker, C.G., Becker, E.L., Maher, J.F., Schreiner, G.E.: Nephrotic syndrome, Arch. Intern. Med. **110**:178, 1962.
202. Brown, J.R., and Kulkarni, M.V.: Toxicity and metabolism of mercury: a review, Med. Serv. J. Canada **23**:786, 1967.
203. Cameron, J.S., and Trounce, J.R.: Membranous glomerulonephritis and the nephrotic syndrome, Guy's Hosp. Rep. **114**:101, 1965.
204. Choi, B.H., Lapham, L.W., Amin-Zaki, L., and Saleem, T.: Abnormal migration, deranged cerebral cortical organization, and diffuse white matter astrocytosis of human fetal brain: a major effect of methylmercury poisoning in-utero, J. Neuropathol. Exp. Neurol. **37**:719, 1978.
205. Gage, J.C.: Distribution and excretion of inhaled mercury vapor, Br. J. Ind. Med. **18**:287, 1961.
206. Gritzka, T.L., and Trump, B.F.: Renal tubular lesions caused by mercuric chloride, Am. J. Pathol. **52**:1225, 1968.

Lead

207. Aronson, S.M.: Lead encephalopathy. In Carter, C.H., editor: Medical aspects of mental retardation, Springfield, Ill., 1965, Charles C Thomas, Publisher.
208. Blackman, S.S., Jr.: Inclusions in lead poisoning, Bull. Johns Hopkins Hosp. **58**:384, 1936.
209. Blackman, S.S., Jr.: Lead encephalitis, Bull. Johns Hopkins Hosp. **61**:1, 1937.
210. Chiodi, H., and Cardeza, A.F.: Experimental hepatic lesions caused by lead, Arch. Pathol. **48**:395, 1949.
211. Cramer, K., et al.: Variation in morphology and function of kidney in humans with increased length of exposure to lead, Br. J. Ind. Med. **31**:113, 1974.
212. Goyer, R.A.: The renal tubule in lead poisoning, Lab. Invest. **19**:71, 1968.
213. Goyer, R.A., and Krall, A.: Ultrastructural transformation in mitochondria isolated from kidneys of normal and lead-intoxicated rats, J. Cell. Biol. **41**:393, 1969.
214. Goyer, R.A., Krall, R.A., and Kimball, J.P.: The renal tubule in lead poisoning, Lab. Invest. **19**:78, 1968.
215. Goyer, R.A., and Rhyne, B.C.: A general review of pathology of lead, Int. Rev. Exp. Pathol. **12**:1, 1973.
216. Landing, B.H., and Nakai, H.: Histochemistry of lead inclusions, Am. J. Clin. Pathol. **31**:499, 1959.
217. Moore, J.F., Goyer, R.A., and Wilson, M.: Lead inclusion bodies, Lab. Invest. **29**:488, 1973.
218. Paglia, D.E., Valentine, W.N., and Dahlgren, J.C.: Inhibition of pyrimidine 5-nucleotidase in workers chronically exposed to lead, J. Clin. Invest. **56**:1164, 1975.
219. Piomelli, S., Davidow, B., Guinee, V.F., Young, P., and Gay, G.: Free erthrocyte protoporphyrin (FEP) in blood as an indicator of lead intoxication, Pediatrics **51**:254, 1973.

Arsenic, cobalt, cadmium

220. Axelson, O.: Arsenic compounds and cancer, J. Toxicol. Environ. Health **6**:1229, 1980.
221. Goyer, R.A.: In Porter, G.A., editor: Cadmium nephropathology in nephrotoxic mechanisms of drugs and environmental toxins, New York, 1982, Plenum Medical Book Co.
222. Grice, H.C., Munro, I.C., and Wiberg, G.S.: Experimentally induced cobalt cardiomyopathies: comparison with beer drinker's cardiomyopathy, Clin. Toxicol. **2**:273, 1969.
223. Ivankovic, S., Eisenbrand, G., and Preussmann, R.: Lung carcinoma induction in BD rats after a single intratracheal instillation of an arsenic-containing pesticide mixture formerly used in vineyards, Int. J. Cancer **24**:786, 1979.
224. Lander, H., Hodge, P.R., and Crisp, C.S.: Arsenic in the hair and nails, J. Forensic Med. **12**:52, 1965.
225. Nandi, M., Slone, D., Jick, H., et al.: Cadmium content of cigarettes, Lancet **2**:1329, 1969.
226. Newman, J.A., Archer, V.E., Saccomanno, G., et al.: Histologic types of bronchogenic carcinoma among members of copper-mining and smelting communities, Ann. NY Acad. Sci. **271**:260, 1976.
227. Pryce, D.M., and Ross, C.F.: Ross's post-mortem appearances, ed. 6, London, 1963, Oxford University Press.

228. Rona, G., and Chappel, C.I.: Pathogenesis and pathology of cobalt cardiomyopathy: recent advances in studies on cardiac structure and metabolism. In the series Cardiomyopathies, vol. 2, Baltimore, 1973, University Park Press.

229. Sandusky, G.E., Henk, W.G., and Roberts, E.D.: Histochemistry and ultrastructure of the heart in experimental cobalt cardiomyopathy in the dog, Toxicol. Appl. Pharmacol. 61:89, 1981.

230. Schroeder, H.A., Nason, A.P., and Tipton, I.H.: Essential trace metals in man: cobalt, J. Chronic Dis. 20:869, 1967.

231. Szuler, I.M., Williams, C.N., Hindmarsh, J.T., and Park-Dincsoy, H.: Massive variceal hemorrhage secondary to presinusoidal portal hypertension due to arsenic poisoning, Can. Med. Assoc. J. 120:168, 1979.

232. Venugopal, B., and Luckey, T.D.: Metal toxicity in mammals, vol. 2, New York, 1977, Plenum Press.

233. Webb, J.L.: Enzyme and metabolic inhibitors, vol. 3, New York, 1966, Academic Press, Inc.

234. Wiberg, G.S., et al.: Factors affecting cardiotoxic potential of cobalt, Clin. Toxicol. 2:257, 1969.

Nickel, thallium, uranium, platinum, and other group VIIIb transition complexes

235. Bencosme, S.A., Stone, R.S., Latta, H., and Madden, S.C.: Acute tubular and glomerular lesions in rat kidneys after uranium injury, AMA Arch. Pathol. 69:470, 1960.

236. Committee On Medical and Biologic Effects of Environmental Pollutants, Division of Medical Sciences, National Research Council: Nickel, Washington, 1975, National Academy of Sciences.

237. Gale, G.R.: Platinum compounds. In Sartorelli, A.C., and Johns, D.G., editors: Handbuch der experimentellen Pharmakologie. Vol. 38. Antineoplastic and immunosuppressive agents, Berlin, 1975, Springer-Verlag.

238. Hackett, R.L., and Sunderman, F.W., Jr.: Acute pathologic reactions to administration of nickel carbonyl, Arch. Environ. Health 14:604, 1967.

239. Hackett, R.L., and Sunderman, F.W., Jr.: Nickel carbonyl and nickel compounds, Arch. Environ. Health 16:349, 1968.

240. Hardaker, W.T., Stone, R.A., and McCoy, R.: Platinum nephrotoxicity, Cancer 34:1030, 1974.

241. Prestayko, A.W., Crooke, S.T., and Carter, S.K.: Cisplatin: current status and new developments, New York, 1980, Academic Press, Inc.

242. Reed, D., Crawley, J., Faro, S.N., Pieper, S.J., and Kurland, L.T.: Thallitoxicosis, JAMA 183:516, 1963.

243. Rosenberg, B., Van Camp, L., and Krigas, T.: Inhibition of cell division in *Escherichia coli* by electrolysis products from platinum electrode, Nature 205:698, 1965.

244. Stone, R.S., Bencosme, S.A., Latta, H., and Madden, S.C.: Renal tubular fine structure studied during reaction to acute uranium injury, AMA Arch. Pathol. 71:160, 1961.

245. Watt, T.L., and Baumann, R.R.: Nickel dermatitis, Arch. Dermatol. 98:155, 1968.

Catecholamines

246. Bloom, S., and Cancill, P.A.: Myocytolysis and mitochondrial calcification in rat myocardium after low doses of isoproterenol, Am. J. Pathol. 54:373, 1969.

247. Ferrans, V.J., Hibbs, R.G., Black, W.C., et al.: Isoproterenol-induced myocardial necrosis, Am. Heart J. 68:71, 1964.

248. Greenhoot, J.H., and Reichenbach, D.D.: Cardiac injury and subarachnoid hemorrhage, Neurosurgery 30:521, 1969.

249. Hiott, D.W.: Heart muscle—experimental use of isoproterenol, Arch. Int. Pharmacodyn. Ther. 180:206, 1969.

250. Kline, I.K.: Myocardial alterations associated with pheochromocytomas, Am. J. Pathol. 38:539, 1961.

251. Lillehei, R.C., Lillehei, C.W., Grismer, J.T., et al.: Plasma catecholamines in open heart surgery, Surg. Forum 14:269, 1963.

252. Pearce, R.M.: Epinephrine myocarditis, J. Exp. Med. 8:400, 1906.

253. Reichenbach, D.D., and Benditt, E.P.: Catecholamines and cardiomyopathy, Hum. Pathol. 1:125, 1970.

254. Sode, J., Getzen, L.C., and Osborne, D.P.: Cardiac arrhythmias and cardiomyopathy associated with pheochromocytomas, Am. J. Surg. 114:927, 1967.

255. Wiswell, J.G., and Crazo, R.M.: Cardiomyopathy and pheochromocytoma, Trans. Am. Clin. Climatol. Assoc. 80:185, 1969.

Barbiturates

256. Beveridge, G.W., and Lawson, A.A.: Bullous lesions in acute barbiturate intoxication, Br. Med. J. 1:835, 1965.

257. Cucinell, S.A., Odessky, L., Weiss, M., et al.: The effect of chloral hydrate on bishydroxycoumarin metabolism, JAMA 197:366, 1966.

258. Dayton, P.G., et al.: Barbiturates and prothrombin response, J. Clin. Invest. 40:1797, 1961.

259. Matte, M.L., Winer, L.H., and Wright, E.T.: Dermatitis medicamentosa, Arch. Dermatol. 82:56, 1960.

260. Meyler, L., et al.: Barbiturates—arteritis, Acta Med. Scand. 167:95, 1960.

261. Rostenberg, A., Jr., and Fagelson, H.J.: Life threatening drug eruptions, JAMA 194:660, 1965.

262. Sorensen, B.F.: Barbiturate blister, Dan. Med. Bull. 10:130, 1963.

263. Teare, R.D.: Alcohol-barbiturate deaths. In Meyler, L., and Peck, H.M., editors: Drug-induced diseases, Amsterdam, 1965, Excerpta Medica Foundation.

Narcotics

264. Kranier, L., Berman, E., and Wishnick, S.C.: Parenteral talcum granulomatosis: complication in narcotic addicts, Lab. Invest. 11:671, 1962.

265. Puro, H.E., Wolf, P.L., Skirgaudas, J., et al.: Experimental production of human "blue velvet" and "red devil" lesions, JAMA 197:1100, 1966.

Other agents
Carbon monoxide

266. Finck, P.A.: Exposure to carbon monoxide: review of the literature and 567 autopsies, Milit. Med. 131:1513, 1966.

Carbon tetrachloride

267. Judah, J.D.: Mechanisms in acute carbon tetrachloride poisoning, NZ Med. J. 67(suppl.):73, 1968.

268. Magee, P.N.: Toxic liver necrosis, Lab. Invest. 15:111, 1966.

269. Recknagel, R.O.: Carbon tetrachloride effect on ribosomes, Pharmacol. Rev. 19:145, 1967.

270. Smuckler, E.A., Iseri, O.A., and Benditt, E.P.: Carbon tetrachloride poisoning and protein synthesis, J. Exp. Med. 116:55, 1962.

Boric acid

271. Fisher, R.S., Freimuth, H.C., O'Connor, K.A., and Johns, V.: Boron absorption from borated talc, JAMA 157:503, 1955.

272. Goldbloom, R.B., and Goldbloom, A.: Boric acid poisoning, J. Pediatr. 43:631, 1953.

Hexachlorophene

273. Shuman, R.M., Leech, R.W., and Alvord, E.C., Jr.: Neurotoxicity of hexachlorophene in humans. II, Arch. Neurol. 32:320, 1975.

Plant poisons
"BUSH TEA"

274. Allen, J.R., Carstens, L.A., and Katagiri, G.J.: Hepatic veins of monkeys with veno-occlusive disease: sequential ultrastructural changes, Arch. Pathol. 87:279, 1969.

275. Bras, G., Jelliffe, D.B., and Stuart, K.L.: Veno-occlusive disease of liver in Jamaica, Arch. Pathol. 57:285, 1954.

MUSHROOMS

276. Abul-Haj, S.K., Ewald, R.A., and Kazyak, L.: Fatal mushroom poisoning, N. Engl. J. Med. 269:223, 1963.

277. Dubash, J., and Teare, D.: Poisoning by *Amanita phalloides*, Br. Med. J. 1:45, 1946.

278. Grossman, C.M., and Malbin, B.: Mushroom poisoning: a review of the literature and report of two cases caused by a previously described species, Ann. Intern Med. **40:**249, 1954.
279. Himsworth, H.P.: Mushroom poisoning—hepatic fibrosis. In Himsworth, H.P., editor: Lectures on the liver and its diseases, Cambridge, Mass., 1947, Harvard University Press.

Environmental pathology
Insecticides and pesticides

280. Nichols, J., and Hennigar, G.R.: Studies on DDD, 2,2-bis(parachlorphenyl)-1,1,1-dichloroethane, Exp. Med. Surg. **15:**310, 1957.
281. Temple, T.E., Jr., Jones, D.J., Jr., Liddle, G.W., and Dexter, R.N.: Treatment of Cushing's disease, N. Engl. J. Med. **281:**801, 1969.

Polychlorinated biphenyls

282. Greene, W.B., et al.: PCB-DDT toxicity on mouse liver cells: an electron microscopic study. In Deichmann, W.B., editor: Pesticides and the environment: a continuing controversy, vol. II, New York, 1973, Intercontinental Medical Book Corp., Publisher.
283. Moilanen, K.W., and Crosby, D.G.: DDT: an unrecognized source of polychlorinated biphenyls, Science **180:**578, 1973.

Fluorine compounds

284. David, W.A.L., and Gardiner, B.O.A.: Fluoracetamide as a systemic insecticide, Nature **181:**1810, 1958.
285. Dean, H.T.: Endemic fluorosis and its relation to dental caries, Public Health Rep. **53:**1443, 1938.
286. Hodge, H.C.: Highlights of fluoride toxicology, J. Occup. Med. **10:**273, 1968.

287. Hodge, H.C., and Smith, F.A.: Fluorides and man, Annu. Rev. Pharmacol. **8:**395, 1968.
288. Loewi, O.: On the mechanism of the positive inotropic action of fluoride, oleate, and calcium on the frog's heart, J. Pharmacol. Exp. Ther. **114:**90, 1955.

Herbicides

289. Conning, D.M., Fletcher, K., and Swan, A.A.B.: Paraquat and related bipyridyls, Br. Med. Bull. **25:**245, 1969.
290. Parkinson, C.: The changing pattern of paraquat poisoning in man, Histopathology **4:**171, 1980.
291. Vaziri, N.E., Ness, R.L., Fairshter, R.D., Smith, W.R., and Rosen, S.M.: Nephrotoxicity of paraquat in man, Arch. Intern. Med. **139:**172, 1979.

Air pollutants

292. Deichmann, W.B., and Gerarde, H.W.: Toxicology of drugs and chemicals, ed. 4, New York, 1969, Academic Press, Inc.

Occupational chest diseases

293. Morgan, W.K.C., and Seaton, A.: Occupational lung diseases, Philadelphia, 1975, W.B. Saunders Co.

Oncogenesis

294. Hottendorf, G.H., and Pachter, I.J.: An analysis of the carcinogenesis testing experience of the National Cancer Institute, Toxicol. Pathol. **10:**22, 1982.
295. Hottendorf, G.H.: Risk assessment problems in chemical oncogenesis, Prog. Drug Res. **31:**257, 1987.

5 Radiation Injury

ROBERT E. ANDERSON

Under appropriate circumstances, all forms of radiation are potentially injurious to living organisms. The purpose of this chapter is to describe some of the injurious consequences that follow irradiation of cells and organs emphasizing injury to human tissues. For the latter, much of the background information was drawn from the accidental and therapeutic exposure of human populations to ionizing radiation.

Basic to an understanding of radiation-induced tissue injury is an appreciation of the physics of radiation and the effects of radiation on individual cells and their subcellular components. A discussion of these general concepts will be followed by a description of the morphologic and clinical features of radiation injury involving cells and tissues in vivo with particular reference to the acute and delayed effects of whole-body or partial-body exposure of humans.

This chapter is written with the understanding that radiation will continue to increase in importance in the diagnosis and treatment of disease. For this reason, considerable emphasis is placed on the biologic basis for the use of radiation in the treatment of persons with malignant tumors and on the consequences to the host of radioisotopes administered therapeutically or diagnostically.

RADIATION SPECTRUM

Radiation involves the emission, propagation, and absorption of radiant energy. This form of energy may be characterized in terms of the mode by which the energy is emitted, propagated, and absorbed. With respect to propagation, radiation classically has been classified as electromagnetic or particulate.

Electromagnetic radiation

Electromagnetic radiation can be conceived as bundles of energy. This form of energy is propagated by means of wave motion and is subclassified on the basis of the length and frequency of the waves. The penetrating power varies greatly depending on the wavelength. By definition, electromagnetic radiation travels at the speed of light in a vacuum.

As shown in Fig. 5-1, electromagnetic radiation forms a continuous spectrum covering a wide range of wavelengths and frequencies. Microwaves and radio waves exhibit long wavelengths (up to several miles), but the number of waves emitted per unit of time is small. At the other end of the spectrum are cosmic, gamma, and roentgen (x) rays, which exhibit short wavelengths and high frequencies. Intermediate between these extremes are ultraviolet, visible light, and infrared rays.

Those forms of electromagnetic radiation, characterized by short wavelengths and high frequencies, carry sufficient energy to cause ionization in the materials that absorb them. In other words, they produce ions (atoms or molecules that possess an electrical charge) on

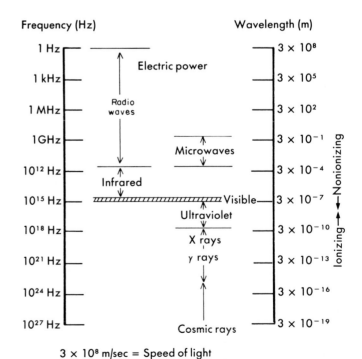

Fig. 5-1. Physical characteristics of ionizing and nonionizing radiation of electromagnetic spectrum. (From Human health and the environment—some research needs, DHEW Pub. no. NIH 77-1277, U.S. Department of Health, Education and Welfare, 1977.)

passage through matter. For this reason, these highly energetic forms of radiation are called "ionizing."

In terms of physical characteristics, gamma rays and x rays are for all intents and purposes identical. By convention, however, a distinction is made between the electromagnetic radiation produced artificially by a roentgen-ray tube (x rays) and that emitted spontaneously by a radioactive substance (gamma rays). Gamma rays have defined energies characteristic of the atomic nucleus responsible for their emission, whereas the energies of x rays involved depend on the energy characteristics of the source. Both x rays and gamma rays ionize matter indirectly by the ejection of high-speed electrons from the molecules that form the absorbing material.

Particulate radiation

Radiation caused by the movement of subatomic particles is known as "particulate radiation." This form of radiation may be generated either (1) directly by accelerating electrons, deuterons, protons, or other subatomic particles to high speeds in a man-made device such as a cyclotron or a linear accelerator, or (2) indirectly by the decay of naturally occurring or artificially produced radioactive substances.

Particulate radiation may be subclassified on the basis of the type of particles involved. The biologically important particles are alpha and beta particles, protons, neutrons, deuterons, and mesons. These particles differ primarily in terms of mass, charge, and angular momentum. Alpha and beta particles are emitted by the nuclei of certain radioactive nuclides, such as radium, thorium, and actinium. Alpha particles are helium nuclei and thus possess a mass of 4 and a positive charge. Beta particles are high-speed positrons or electrons and have an extremely small mass (1/1836) and may be either positively or negatively charged. These particles travel at speeds less than that of light, and like other moving bodies, their energy depends on their rest mass and their velocity. The energies of these particles are measured in electron volts or, more commonly, in million electron volts (MeV).

Protons and neutrons are constituents of the nuclei of atoms and each has a mass of 1. Protons possess a positive charge equal to that of an electron, but opposite in sign. Neutrons have no charge and therefore ionize indirectly by imparting their energy to protons. Deuterons represent nuclei of deuterium, a stable isotope of hydrogen. Recently, accelerators have been developed to utilize one type of meson, in the treatment of malignant tumors.

RADIOACTIVE SUBSTANCES

A substance is said to be radioactive when it possesses an unstable nucleus that spontaneously decays with the release of energy. This decay may involve nat-urally occurring atoms, such as radium or thorium, or atoms rendered radioactive by artificial means. Both natural and artificially produced radioactive substances are termed *radioisotopes*. These radioactive atoms, or nuclides, give off radiation as a result of the disintegration or decay of individual atoms. During radioactive decay, unstable daughter nuclei are often formed, and in turn they undergo disintegration.

Types of decay

There are three common modes of decay: alpha emission, beta emission, and electron capture. Many nuclei with high atomic numbers decay by emission of alpha particles and thus are known as alpha (α) emitters. During decay, energy is released. This is transmitted as the kinetic energy of the alpha particles. Alpha particles from a specific nuclide are ejected with discrete energies. Additional energy may also be released as gamma radiation. The total energy released during the radioactive decay of a nucleus is termed the *transition energy*. For example, radium, with an atomic number of 88 and a mass number of 226, decays to radon ($^{222}_{86}$Rn) as follows:

$$^{222}_{86}\text{Ra} \longrightarrow\ ^{222}_{86}\text{Rn} + ^4_2\text{He} + \text{gamma radiation}$$

Beta (β) emitters are the most numerous of the radioactive isotopes. β^- decay, or negatron decay, involves the transformation of a neutron into a proton. Energy is released as the kinetic energy of a neutrino (ν), energetic electrons (beta particles), and gamma rays. Neutrinos are uncharged particles with zero rest mass. β^+ decay, or positron decay, is somewhat more complicated but involves the transformation of a proton to a neutron followed by a variable series of steps that include the release of a neutrino and a positron. β^+ decay may also be accompanied by electron capture.

Beta decay leaves the nucleus lacking an electron. These holes or vacancies in electron shells are promptly filled by electrons cascading from energy levels farther away from the nucleus. As these vacancies are filled, energy is released, usually in the form of electromagnetic radiation. The movement of an electron, usually from the innermost shell to the nucleus, with the release of a neutrino, is known as "electron capture."

Gamma rays are often emitted during the transition from the excited state to a stable energy level. However, no radioactive substance decays solely by gamma emission. Gamma transition is always preceded by either electron capture or emission of an alpha or a beta particle.

Measurement of decay

The rate of decay of a radioactive substance is referred to as the activity of the sample and the unit of measurement is the curie (Ci).

1 Ci = 3.7 × 10^{10} disintegrations per second
1 mCi = 3.7 × 10^{7} disintegrations per second
1 μCi = 3.7 × 10^{4} disintegrations per second

The specific activity of a radioactive sample refers to the activity per unit mass.

The radioactive decay of substance is expressed as follows:

$$\frac{N}{N_0} = e^{-\lambda t}$$

N_0 is the initial number of radioactive atoms at zero time. N is the number of radioactive atoms left after a defined period of time (t). Lambda (λ) is the decay constant and represents the fraction of the radioactive nuclei that decays in unit time. This constant is characteristic of each radionuclide.

The character of the preceding equation implies that radioactive substances take an infinitely long time to decay totally. For this reason, it is customary to express the activity in terms of half-life ($t_{1/2}$) or the time necessary to reduce the activity to one half of the initial value. The half-life periods of the known radioactive isotopes range from a fraction of a second to many centuries.

It is important to note that the curie is not a measure of energy. In characterizing a radionuclide in terms of disintegrations per second, no indication is given as to the character of the radiation emitted of the energy involved.

Biologic effects

In addition to the specific activity and the physical characteristics of the radiation emitted, the biologic consequences of exposure to a radionuclide depend on at least two other factors: (1) the distribution of the isotope within the host and the rate of excretion and (2) the half-life of the substance involved. The internal deposition of radium in humans illustrates the importance of these factors. Radium has a very long half-life (1638 years), is concentrated in the skeleton, and, together with its poorly soluble decay products, subjects the involved tissues to a continuous bombardment of alpha and beta particles and gamma rays throughout the life span of the host. Thus as little as 0.1 to 0.3 μCi of radium deposited in the human body is dangerous to the health of the recipient.

RADIATION UNITS

Several units are employed to measure amounts of ionizing radiation. The oldest, the roentgen, is used for x and gamma (γ) rays as the unit of the charge produced as these rays ionize a given volume of air. Thus the roentgen is a unit of exposure and not absorption (see next paragraph). Furthermore, to encompass intensity, a time frame must also be indicated (for example, roentgens per minute).

To represent particulate radiation in terms that can be related to x and gamma rays, two other units—the rad and the gray—have been devised. These units are based on absorbed dose. One rad is the dose of radiation that will result in the absorption of 100 ergs of energy per gram of the absorbing substance. The energy absorbed by 1 gram of most tissues on exposure to 1 γ of roentgen rays is about 93 ergs or almost the same as 1 rad. Therefore, in many discussions involving radiobiology, rads and roentgens are employed almost interchangeably. As with roentgens, the rad is a measure of quantity, and to convey intensity, an indication of time in the form of dose rate must also be introduced.

Recently there has been a move toward the use of Système Internationale (SI) units in radiobiology and nuclear medicine. SI units are based on fundamental units of mass (kilograms), length (meters), and time (seconds). SI units have not yet achieved widespread use in the United States but probably will do so during the next several years. Therefore familiarity with both SI and traditional units is necessary.

The gray (Gy) is the accepted SI unit to measure absorbed dose. One gray is defined as that dose of any form of radiation resulting in the absorption of 1 joule of energy per kilogram of the absorbing material. Thus 1 gray corresponds to 100 rad.

One rad of particulate radiation generally causes more damage to a biologic system than 1 rad of x rays or gamma rays. For this reason, the rem was introduced as a means to normalize these differences in biologic effects produced by different types of radiation. One rem can be defined loosely as that dose of any type of radiation that produces a biologic effect equivalent to 1 rad of x or gamma rays. In situations where the rem is an inconveniently large unit of measure, the millirem (mrem), which is 1/1000 of a rem, is employed. The sievert is the accepted SI unit of dose equivalence. One sievert is that dose producing a biologic effect equivalent to 1 gray of x or gamma rays. One sievert thus corresponds to 100 rem.

The traditional unit to measure the activity of a radioactive substance is the curie. The corresponding SI unit is the becquerel. One becquerel (Bq) corresponds to a decay rate of one disintegration per second. Since 1 curie equals 3.7 × 10^{10} disintegrations per second, 1 curie is equivalent to 3.7 × 10^{10} becquerels.

ENVIRONMENTAL RADIATION

Life on earth has evolved in the presence of ionizing radiation. This natural, or background, radiation is derived from three major sources: cosmic rays from the sun and outer space, radium and other radioactive elements contained in the earth's crust, and potassium 40 and other naturally occurring radionuclides that are normally present in the body. Cosmic radiation varies with altitude, and residents of Albuquerque, New Mexico, for example, receive approximately twice the dose as the inhabitants of Boston, Massachusetts, receive. Airline personnel and astronauts are also exposed to above-average doses of cosmic rays. Similarly, the radiation emitted by the earth's crust varies greatly by geographic region depending on variations in the content of radioactive materials in the soil and subterranean rock. Terrestrial radiation is of particular importance to miners who may be exposed to radioactive components of the earth's crust in aerosol form in the atmosphere of mines. Inhalation of these substances, when they are of appropriate size and shape, results in their deposition in the terminal air passages of the lungs where they may emit radioactivity for a prolonged time, much to the detriment of the host.

In addition to natural radiation, humans are exposed to radiation from man-made sources. The largest component of man-made radiation comes from exposures associated with medical diagnosis and treatment. Lesser contributions come from "technologically enhanced" sources (such as the use of radionuclide-containing minerals in phosphate fertilizers and building materials), fallout from atomic weapons, nuclear power production, and consumer products (color television sets, smoke detectors, luminescent instrument and clock dials, and so on).

Table 5-1 shows the estimated annual exposure to various types of man-made and natural radiation. Table 5-2 shows how these doses compare with other whole-body exposures, the latter in tenfold increments. Only somatic effects are included in this table, since the dose levels at which an increased incidence of genetic abnormalities may be expected in humans are still uncertain.

CELLULAR AND MOLECULAR RADIATION BIOLOGY

Much of our understanding of the effects of ionizing radiation in humans comes from studies that involve the exposure of cells grown in tissue culture. Such cells can be analyzed for evidence of (1) overt injury such as cell death or loss of the ability to undergo cell division and (2) occult injury such as nonlethal alterations of plasma membranes, enzymes, and even specific molecules. In this section a portion of these data are discussed with particular reference to the mechanisms by which radiation injures and kills cells.

Reproductive death

After irradiation of a population of cells, a variable number become pyknotic, undergo lysis, or otherwise exhibit evidence of cell death. The residual cells remain viable and are indistinguishable morphologically from their nonirradiated counterparts. However, despite this absence of recognizable morphologic alterations, many of the irradiated cells have lost their capacity to divide

Table 5-1. Sources and average amounts of radiation exposure from the environment

Category	Source	Average annual dose(mrem)*
Natural	Cosmic radiation	44
	Terrestrial radiation	40
	Internally deposited radioactive isotopes	18
	Subtotal	—
		102
Man-made	Medical diagnosis and treatment	73
	Technologically enhanced sources	4
	Global fallout	4
	Nuclear power	0.003
	Occupational	0.8
	Miscellaneous	2
	Subtotal	84
	TOTAL	186

From Advisory Committee on the Biological Effects of Ionizing Radiation: The effects on populations of exposure to low levels of ionizing radiation (BEIR Report), Washington, D.C., 1980, National Academy of Sciences, National Research Council; Klement et al.: Estimates of ionizing radiation doses in the United States, 1960-2000, U.S. Environmental Protection Agency, 1972; and Interagency Task Force on the Health Effects of Ionizing Radiation: Report of the Work Group on Exposure Reduction, Dept. HEW, June 1979.

*Data for 1970 in the United States. Notice that dose rates for cosmic and terrestrial radiation vary greatly with altitude and geographic region. Also, estimates for nuclear power may be high because of improved technology.

and are therefore sterile. Loss of a cell's ability to divide in unlimited fashion is referred to as reproductive death, and this loss in reproductive capacity constitutes one of the most important effects of radiation on mammalian cells. On occasion, irradiated cells may continue to divide and grow but fail to separate. The result is the formation of multinucleated giant cells, which represents one of the morphologic hallmarks of radiation injury.

To document reproductive death, one needs to quantitate the loss of the ability of irradiated cells to proliferate indefinitely. This may be accomplished in vivo or in vitro. The ability of hematopoietic stem cells to form macroscopic colonies in the spleen after intravenous transfer to lethally irradiated mice of the same inbred strain is a frequently employed in vivo method to quantitate the reproductive capacity of stem cells. Since each colony is derived from a single stem cell that has divided innumerable times, irradiation of the bone marrow cells before transfer permits the development of a dose-response curve, which inversely relates radiation dose to the capacity of the irradiated cells to repro-

Table 5-2. Biologic significance of a single whole-body exposure to various doses of ionizing radiation in man

Dose (roentgens)	Biologic response
0.01	No detectable somatic effects. (this dose is 200 times the daily natural background)
0.1	No detectable somatic effects
1	No detectable somatic effects
10	Detectable morphologic and functional alterations in specific subpopulations of lymphocytes; probable chromosomal abnormalities
100	Mild radiation sickness in some persons with nausea and vomiting; decrease in mitotic index of bone marrow and transient leukopenia
1,000	Extensive damage to bone marrow with leukopenia, thrombocytopenia, and anemia; necrosis of gastrointestinal mucosa; severe radiation sickness; death within 30 days
10,000	Immediate disorientation or coma; death within hours
100,000	Acute death of most types of mammalian cells
1,000,000	Death of some bacteria
10,000,000	Death of all living organisms; some denaturation of proteins

Modified from Warren, S.: The pathology of ionizing radiation, Springfield, Ill., 1961, Charles C Thomas, Publisher.

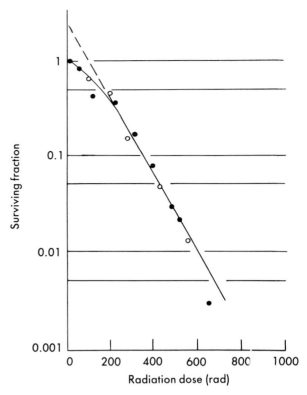

Fig. 5-2. Survival of reproductive capacity of normal mouse bone marrow stem cells as function of radiation dose. Open and closed circles represent two experiments. (From Till, J.E., and McCullock, E.A.: Radiat. Res.**14**:213, 1961.)

duce in their new environment. Results from such an experiment are shown in Fig. 5-2.

Alternatively, the irradiated cells may be grown in tissue culture and colony formation determined in vitro. In this setting, it is also known that each colony arises from a single viable cell whereas nonreproductive cells will not form colonies. Abortive colonies, containing subnormal numbers of cells, are not included in the calculation of the survival curves. Results from an experiment that employs this type of approach are shown in Fig. 5-3. Survival curves determined in vitro closely approximate those obtained in vivo for the same cell population.

The sequence of events that leads to reproductive death is not totally understood. There is general agreement that the initial event is the absorption of energy by cells with the subsequent disruption of individual molecules or sequences of molecules. Damage of this type is believed to be initiated randomly in cells as a result of a series of ionizations and excitations, which are known to occur along the tracks of charged particles moving with a high velocity. The mechanisms by which radiation-induced alterations of individual molecules in cells are translated into a loss of sustained reproductive capacity are poorly understood. Two broad theories have been postulated and are referred to as the "target theory" and the "indirect-effects theory."

Target theory

The target theory predicts that a biologic unit (such as a cell, a cell membrane, or a specific molecule) will undergo lethal damage after a minimum number of radiation "hits," or absorption events. Fig. 5-4 shows a hypothetical dose-response curve to illustrate this theory. Notice that the dose-response curve of Fig. 5-4, *A*, becomes a straight line in Fig. 5-4, *B*, when the surviving fraction is plotted on a logarithmic scale against the dose on a linear scale. Thus the number of surviving cells is an exponential function of dose. Even at low dose levels, there is a corresponding decrease in the number of survivors with each incremental increase in radiation dose. This type of dose-response curve is referred to as a "single-hit" curve because only one "hit" (ionization) is required for the inactivation of a de-

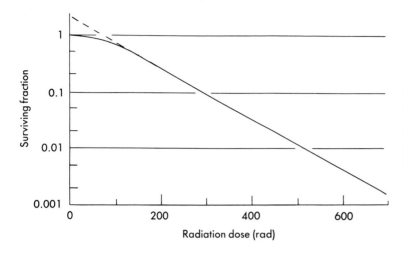

Fig. 5-3. Survival of reproductive capacity of HeLa cells as function of radiation dose. (From Puck, T.T., and Marcus, P.I. Reproduced from The Journal of Experimental Medicine, 1956, vol. 103, pp. 653-666, by copyright permission of The Rockefeller University Press.)

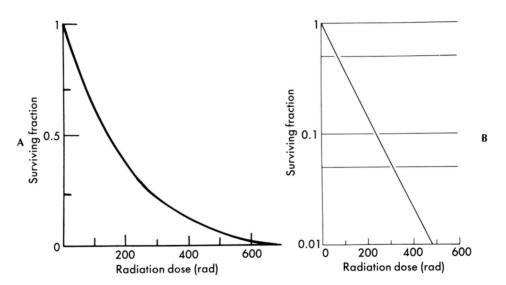

Fig. 5-4. A, Idealized dose-response curve in which fraction of surviving cells is plotted as function of radiation dose. Notice absence of shoulder. **B,** Semilog plot of curve from **A.** Dose is linearly related to logarithm of surviving fraction.

finable number of cells. This theory, which experimentally applies best to densely ionizing particles (see p. 254), predicts that cell death will be unaffected by the time over which the dose of radiation is administered (the dose rate) or whether it is administered on one or several occasions (fractionated).

Indirect-effects theory

Fig. 5-5 shows a second type of dose-response curve, which is not exponential at low dose levels. The nonlinear region in Fig. 5-5, *B,* is referred to as the shoulder or the threshold region of the curve. At least two explanations exist for this threshold effect: (1) each target must sustain more than one "hit" or related deleterious event in order to be inactivated, and, at low dose levels, the probability of two or more such random events

occurring to one cell, or perhaps even to a specific region of the cell, approaches zero; and (2) the damage sustained by individual cells at low dose levels is minimal and therefore susceptible to repair by intracellular enzymes.

Except for the shoulder region, Figs. 5-4, *B,* and 5-5, *B,* are identical. Therefore, in order to describe and compare survival curves, two pieces of information are generally included:

1. The slope of the linear portion of the curve or, more commonly, the dose that results in a 37% survival; this value is referred to as the D_{37}, the mean lethal dose, or the D_0; it is important to emphasize that these calculations must be made on the straight portion of the curve.

2. The intercept of the straight portion of the curve

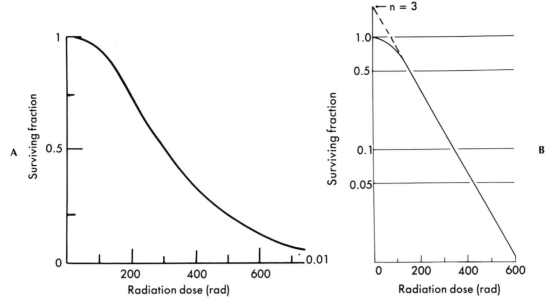

Fig. 5-5. A, Idealized dose-response curve in which fraction of surviving cells is plotted as function of radiation dose. Notice presence of shoulder. **B,** Semilog plot of curve from **A.** Dose is not linearly related to logarithm of surviving fraction, particularly at low dose levels.

extrapolated to zero dose (the dotted line in Fig. 5-5, *B*) gives a number known as the extrapolation number and in the example given is 3.

Dose-survival experiments utilizing the approaches outlined above have established D_{37} values of 80 to 200 rad for most mammalian cells exposed in vitro to x or gamma rays. These figures stand in contrast to similar data for microorganisms, such as *Escherichia coli*, yeasts, and viruses, which often exhibit D_{37} values in excess of several thousand rad.

Radiation-induced formation of free radicals has been suggested as a mechanism to explain the indirect inactivation of target molecules. Free radicals are known to be produced by ionizing radiation. Since water is an important constituent of all cells, it is postulated that many of these indirect effects are related to the interaction of radiation with water. In this situation, hydrogen and hydroxyl free radicals are formed. Free radicals are extremely strong oxidizing or reducing agents. As such they can (1) react with water to form peroxides; (2) form cross-linkages with critical molecules such as DNA and RNA, which may result in inactivation of the parent molecule; or (3) attach directly to key structures, such as plasma membranes, to render them incapable of discharging their normal functions.

Factors affecting radiation response

In biologic systems, several factors are known to affect the degree of radiation injury. The relative contribution of these factors depends on the system involved and a variety of other factors, especially the character of the radiation and the presence or absence of agents known to protect against the effects of radiation. Consideration will now be given to some of these factors.

The important factors that influence the radiosensitivity of mammalian cells can be divided into three general groups: physical, chemical, and biologic. These factors are considered separately though their contributions usually overlap in both the experimental and the therapeutic settings.

Physical factors

The most important physical factors that affect the magnitude of a biologic response to radiation are the character of the radiation, the total amount administered, and the time within which this dose is given. The term *relative biologic effectiveness* (RBE) is used to compare the effectiveness (in terms of absorbed dose) of two forms of radiation in producing the same biologic effect. The generally accepted reference standard for this type of comparison is x rays generated at 150 to 300 kiloelectron volts (keV) with a standard filter to remove extraneous energies. Fast neutrons are more effective than x rays in producing most of the late somatic effects associated with radiation injury. Therefore, with these effects, fast neutrons have an RBE of greater than 1.

The RBE of a particle is determined primarily by how it distributes energy along its track. This sequence of events is known as *linear energy transfer* (LET), which is a measure of the average rate at which an ionizing particle loses energy along its path. LET therefore depends on the mass, the charge, and the velocity of the particle. A particle with a relatively large mass and charge but a low velocity will in general exhibit a higher LET than a small noncharged particle with a high velocity. Heavy particles, such as atomic nuclei, which are given velocity (or accelerated) by a machine (a generator) constructed for this purpose, produce dense paths of ionization over short tracks and are referred to as *densely ionizing particles*. X and gamma rays, as well as energetic electrons produced by an accelerator, are referred to as *sparsely ionizing* because they lose small amounts of energy to the absorbing substance over a long path until finally all the energy is spent and they come to a halt.

Dose rate also influences cell survival, especially for low-LET radiations. With low-LET radiations, a greater total dose is required to produce a given effect when the radiation is (1) delivered in multiple small doses known as fractions or (2) given continuously over a prolonged period of time. The basis of these observations is believed to relate to the repair of sublethal radiation damage that occurs during the actual time of exposure at low dose rates or between exposures with fractionalization.

Chemical factors

Chemical factors may either exert a protective effect or potentiate the effects of ionizing radiation. Perhaps the most important substance in this regard is molecular oxygen. Bubbling oxygen into a cell suspension immediately before exposure potentiates cell killing, whereas reduction of the oxygen tension has a protective effect. This effect, known as the oxygen effect, is especially pronounced with low-LET radiations such as x and gamma rays. The involved mechanisms have not been completely defined but probably relate to the observation that oxygen increases the production of free radicals by radiation. The oxygen effect is especially important in the treatment of malignant tumors with ionizing radiation. Most tumors exhibit considerable variability in oxygen tension, presumably because of the nonuniform distribution of blood vessels within the neoplasm. When the discrepancy between local requirements and the available oxygen becomes critical, necrosis results. Adjacent to areas of necrosis are hypoxic but still viable tumor cells. Such hypoxic foci are less sensitive to many types of ionizing radiation than are the surrounding, well-oxygenated tissues, and they may give rise to local recurrence of tumor after radiotherapy. As a consequence of these observations, considerable effort has been devoted to attempts to increase the oxygen tension in tumors before radiotherapy.

Another group of agents that have been used chemically to increase the radiosensitivity of cells is the halogenated pyrimidines. These analogs of DNA bases can increase severalfold the radiosensitivity of cells in culture. The mechanism involved is not known.

Another class of chemical agents serves to protect against radiation-induced cell injury. The best-known examples of these radioprotective agents are the sulfhydryl amines such as cysteine and cystamine. Several hypotheses exist to explain the mechanisms of action of these compounds. One well-accepted theory postulates that sulfhydryl groups compete effectively with biologically important compounds, such as DNA, for free radicals formed by the interaction of radiation and water. Oxidation of the sulfhydryl amines to relatively stable compounds may serve to protect more complex molecules known to be critical to the viability of the cell.

Biologic factors

Although exceedingly complex and poorly understood, a variety of biologic factors are known to influence the response of individual cells to radiation. Two of the most important factors are the repair of nonlethal injury and the timing of the radiation exposure with respect to the cell cycle. The radiosensitivity of synchronized cell populations grown in tissue culture relates to the time in generation cycle when irradiation occurs. For most tissue culture lines, cells are most sensitive to radiation during G_2 and mitosis, less sensitive in G_1, and least sensitive toward the end of the S period.

Repair of sublethal radiation injury appears to begin immediately after the damage is incurred. Under optimal conditions, such repair proceeds rapidly. It is important to note that repair is much more effective after low-LET radiations (x rays, gamma rays) than with high-LET radiations (alpha particles). The point is illustrated in the hypothetical dose-response curves shown in Figs. 5-4, *B*, and 5-5, *B*. Fig. 5-5, *B*, with a well-defined shoulder, represents the situation that would be encountered experimentally utilizing low-LET radiations. The breadth of the shoulder is believed to reflect roughly the magnitude of repair. In contrast to Fig. 5-5, *B*, the dose-response curve of Fig. 5-4, *B*, demonstrates no shoulder and would be typical of high-LET radiation. From this and related evidence it appears that cells exposed to high-LET radiation either die or escape unscathed. In either case, there is no sublethal damage to repair. Repair is discussed in greater detail when radiation-induced injury to DNA is considered.

Radiation effects involving macromolecules

In the past several years a significant body of information has been developed with respect to the effects of radiation upon DNA, RNA, and several specific proteins. Much of this work points to DNA as the "target" of greatest radiobiologic importance. For example, in experiments utilizing microbeams of radiation, a cell was more likely to be killed if the nucleus rather than the cytoplasm was irradiated. In addition, the sensitivity of cells from different species to reproductive death is directly proportional to their DNA content. Finally, as will be seen subsequently, DNA alterations are implicated in many of the delayed effects of radiation exposure.

Both in vitro and in vivo, the effects of radiation on DNA are dependent on the dose, the quality or type of particle involved, and the stage of the cell cycle during which the irradiation occurs. In vitro, the irradiation of DNA results in (1) breaking of hydrogen bonds, (2) base damage, (3) disruption of the sugar-phosphate backbone of the molecule, (4) impairment of the ability of DNA to act as a template for the synthesis of a new DNA strand, and (5) formation of cross-linkages between adjacent strands or closely apposed regions of the same strand. The latter two observations have received particular attention recently.

In vitro and in vivo experiments show that radiation can result in breaks of one or both DNA strands. The effect may result directly from a strategically located ionization or indirectly by means of the activation of a specific nuclease. The majority of single-stranded breaks are believed to be rapidly repaired, with the intact strand serving as a template to direct the rejoining process. The intact strand apparently holds the broken strand in place while repair occurs and may also provide a coding function for the involved enzymes. The rejoining process proceeds exceedingly rapidly. In contradistinction to single-strand breaks, the majority of double-strain breaks are believed to be irreparable. The total loss of local structure, and the formation of DNA fragments that quickly become separated, are believed to produce a situation in which restoration of normal structure is extremely unlikely.

The exposure of rapidly dividing mammalian cells to intermediate doses of radiation generally results in a phenomenon known as "division delay." Typically, irradiated cells immediately cease cell division for a period of time proportional to the dose. After this delay, the cells resume their normal growth patterns for one or more generations. Cell death, when it occurs, usually takes place during the first postirradiation division though damaged cells occasionally undergo several divisions before death. Less commonly, radiation can induce DNA synthesis outside the period of normal synthesis in the cell cycle. This phenomenon, which involves all phases of the cell cycle, is referred to as *unscheduled* DNA synthesis. Unscheduled synthesis can also be induced by ultraviolet rays and alkylating agents. The biologic implications of unscheduled syn-

thesis are not entirely known, but the phenomenon is probably related to the repair process.

Experiments designed to evaluate the effects of radiation on RNA have in general been concerned with RNA synthesis in toto and have not included species analysis (messenger RNA, ribosomal RNA). In addition, RNA synthesis is dependent on DNA integrity, and the relative contribution of these two effects upon radiation-induced cell injury has been difficult to differentiate experimentally. Despite these technical problems, however, RNA synthesis is believed to be less radiosensitive than DNA synthesis.

Large doses of radiation are required to destroy the function of most proteins. Several enzymes have been carefully investigated in this regard. The apparent radioresistance of most proteins may be attributable to their relatively small size, particularly in comparison with such molecules as DNA and RNA.

GENERAL MORPHOLOGIC FEATURES OF RADIATION INJURY

Before beginning a discussion of the effects of radiation on select cell types and tissues, it is important to emphasize that none of the morphologic events that result from radiation injury is unique. Each of the alterations encountered in irradiated cells may be found in association with other forms of injury, such as that caused by ischemia, heat, cold, microbiologic agents, or toxic substances. In fact, the effects of some alkylating agents so closely mimic those associated with ionizing radiation that they are often referred to as radiomimetic drugs.

Cells injured by radiation show changes in both the nucleus and the cytoplasm. As noted previously, the nucleus of most cells appears to be more radiosensitive than the cytoplasm. At low dose levels, the nuclear chromatin becomes somewhat clumped, and the nucleus appears swollen and presumably is edematous. At moderate and high dose levels, the nucleus is often pyknotic and may show karyorrhexis. Swelling and focal loss of the nuclear membrane and fragmentation of the chromatin may be observed by electron microscopy. The cytoplasmic changes after irradiation include edema, vacuolization, and alterations in the various components of the plasma membrane. Variable degrees of disintegration of the endoplasmic reticulum are also apparent. Mitochondria have been noted to be enlarged, and distorted forms are readily apparent; but these changes may be secondary to metabolic and membrane alterations, since several studies have shown that mitochondria themselves are relatively radioresistant.

Although all mammalian cells are affected by ionizing radiation, moderate variability exists among different cell types and tissues with respect to their susceptibility to a specific effect such as cell death. In general, rapidly dividing cells are more radiosensitive than slowly dividing cells. This difference presumably has to do with radiation-induced inhibition of DNA synthesis and interference with normal cell division. The morphologic consequences of these changes are a variety of chromosomal abnormalities including translocations, breaks, deletions, and the formation of fragments and rings. Such alterations are best appreciated by chromosome analysis. However, abnormal mitotic figures may be seen in tissue sections, often in association with the multinucleated giant cells that reflect the failure of dividing cells to separate physically. The relationship between radiosensitivity and mitotic activity was first appreciated in 1906 by Bergonié and Tribondeau, and their names have been applied to what has become a key concept in radiobiology. They stated that:

X-rays are more effective on cells which have greater reproductive activity; the effectiveness is greater on those cells that have a longer dividing future ahead, on those cells the morphology and the function of which are least fixed. From this law, it is easy to understand that roentgen radiation destroys tumors without destroying healthy tissues.*

These relationships, semiquantitated for normal cells and tumors in Table 5-3, have been paraphrased as follows: radiosensitive tissues are those with the greatest mitotic activity and the least degree of differentiation.

Vascular changes are known to be an extremely important consequence of the irradiation of several tissues and may be responsible for many of the acute and delayed effects of such exposure. Vascular abnormalities are seen after irradiation of both normal and neoplastic tissues. As shown in Table 5-3, endothelial cells are not especially radiosensitive, but with time degenerative vascular abnormalities are almost always seen in association with an irradiated neoplasm. Furthermore, degenerative vascular changes are not confined to the tumor but also involve the adjacent normal parenchyma of the affected organ and other tissues that may be interposed between the source of the radiation and the tumor.

Vascular dilatation is responsible for the erythema of the skin that is frequently noted in the immediate post-irradiation period. Similar dilatation of the blood vessels probably occurs in a variety of other sites and may account for the transient increase in function documented in some organs after exposure. Somewhat later, and generally in association with high dose levels, regressive changes appear, including swelling and vacuolization of the endothelium, focal necrosis of the vessel wall sometimes with hemorrhage, or, on occasion, rup-

ture. Months or years after exposure various degenerative abnormalities are apparent. They include (1) fibrous and hyaline sclerosis of the subintimal region and media of small arteries and arterioles, which results in focal narrowing, (2) endothelial cell proliferation, which may partially obliterate the lumen, and (3) decreased numbers of capillaries with considerable ectasia of those that persist.

From the above description, it is not difficult to visualize some of the alterations that might be expected in a structure irradiated several years previously. Grossly, the organ will be smaller than normal because of necrosis and loss of radiosensitive parenchymal cells and subsequent ischemia of less radiosensitive cells by a compromised circulation. Microscopically, atrophic or absent parenchymal cells will have been replaced by dense hyalinized connective tissue, which may contain pleomorphic, often very large fibroblasts. Multinucleated giant cells may be present except in organs populated by fixed postmitotic cells. Small arteries and arterioles will be lined by increased numbers of unusually prominent endothelial cells. Focally, the walls of these vessels will be thick and sclerotic and the lumen small or obliterated.

The functional consequences of these morphologic abnormalities are significant. Loss of parenchymal cells may result in impairment of function. Diffusion across thickened capillary walls may be impeded. Structures may be distorted or compressed by the dense fibrous connective tissue referred to above. For example, obstruction of the ureter is not an uncommon complication of pelvic irradiation administered to eradicate or impede the growth of a malignant tumor of the urinary bladder. Surgical procedures are generally more difficult in areas that have been irradiated months or years previously. Increased amounts of dense connective tissue make dissection of vital structures more difficult than usual. Postoperatively, hypoperfusion of the area by abnormal blood vessels predisposes to poor wound healing and increases the likelihood of the breakdown of anastomotic sites. Impaired circulation also compromises local defense mechanisms needed to deal with untoward complications such as infection. Poor wound healing and an increased incidence of infection in a previously irradiated person are not confined to the postoperative state but may be associated with any form of trauma.

RADIATION INJURY IN HUMANS
General effects

Radiation effects can be divided into two general categories: somatic effects and genetic effects. Somatic effects are those manifested by the recipient. In contrast, genetic effects do not show up directly in the irradiated organism but rather in its progeny. Somatic effects may

---

*From Bergonié, J., and Tribondeau, L.: Compt. Rend. Acad. Sci. **143:**983, 1906.

Table 5-3. Relative radiosensitivity of normal cells and certain tumors

Radiosensitivity	Normal cells	Tumors
Very high	Lymphocytes Hematopoietic stem cells Crypt cells of intestinal epithelium Spermatogonia Ovarian follicular cells	Most forms of lymphoma; leukemia Seminoma, dysgerminoma Granulosa cell tumor Retinoblastoma

High	Glandular epithelium of breast
	Urinary bladder epithelium
	Esophageal epithelium
	Gastric mucosa
	Mucous membranes of mouth and pharynx
	Epidermal epithelium
	  (including hair follicles and sebaceous glands)
	Epithelium of optic lens
		Transitional cell carcinoma of bladder
		Adenocarcinoma of stomach
		Epidermoid carcinoma of skin, oropharynx,
		  esophagus, cervix
		Small cell carcinoma of lung

Intermediate	Endothelium
	Growing bone and cartilage
	Fibroblasts
	Glial cells
	Pulmonary epithelium
	Renal epithelium
	Hepatic epithelium
	Pancreatic epithelium
	Thyroid epithelium
	Adrenal epithelium
		Vascular and connective tissue component of
		  most tumors
		Osteogenic sarcoma
		Astrocytoma
		Chondrosarcoma
		Epidermoid carcinoma of lung
		Liposarcoma
		Adenocarcinoma of breast, kidney, thyroid, colon,
		  liver, pancreas

Low	Mature hematopoietic cells Muscle cells Mature connective tissue Mature bone and cartilage Ganglion cells	Rhabdomyosarcoma Leiomyosarcoma Ganglioneuroma

be further divided into (1) acute or early and (2) delayed or late.

By convention, acute effects are those that produce signs and symptoms of radiation damage from the time of exposure to 30 to 60 days subsequent to exposure. In man, clinical evidence of acute effects occurs only after relatively high doses (above about 50 rad) delivered over a short period of time. Above this dose level, symptoms increase in severity with increasing dose. Although all major organs of the body probably are involved to varying degrees, symptoms during the acute phase generally reflect malfunction of rapidly proliferating tissues, the integrity of which is vital to homeostasis. These rapid renewal systems include the bone marrow, lymphoid organs, testes, and the epithelium of the gastrointestinal tract.

Late or delayed effects are those that manifest themselves many months or, more commonly, years after exposure. They tend to be manifest by an increased incidence of a specific lesion and are a function of dose. Radiation carcinogenesis is perhaps the best known of the delayed effects. Other life-threatening delayed effects involve the kidney (radiation nephritis), gastroin-

testinal tract (stricture, chronic ulcer), lung (radiation pneumonitis), bladder (ulcer and fistula formation), spinal cord (transverse myelitis), and the heart (constrictive pericarditis). These types of delayed effects are more often associated with repeated (fractionated) local exposures than from a single whole-body exposure.

The effects of radiation injury can also be classified as stochastic or nonstochastic. A stochastic (random) effect varies in frequency but not in severity with dose and fails to exhibit a threshold, a dose below which no effect is seen. Examples of stochastic effects are heritable effects on germ cells, teratogenic effects on the developing embryo, and some types of radiation-induced tumors. Nonstochastic effects vary in severity but not in frequency with dose and often exhibit a threshold. Many of the acute effects of radiation injury are stochastic in nature. Both stochastic and nonstochastic effects are discussed in more detail in subsequent sections of this chapter.

In this section, both genetic and somatic effects in humans are reviewed. Acute and delayed effects are considered as are the consequences of both local and whole-body exposures. By way of introduction, the human populations that have been exposed to significant amounts of ionizing radiation are summarized briefly because much of the subsequent information has been obtained from this experience.

Exposed populations

A significant number of persons have been accidentally or therapeutically exposed to biologically significant amounts of ionizing radiation. However, evaluation of many cases is not possible because of incomplete follow-up data or insufficient demographic data. Thus most of our current knowledge with respect to radiation injury in humans has been obtained from an evaluation of the populations summarized in Table 5-4. And even among these carefully studied groups, direct compari-

sons are often complicated by differences in age, variability in the conditions of exposure (extent, magnitude, time frame, external versus internal emitters, and so on), and the presence or absence of known preexisting disease. In reviewing the exposed human populations, specific mention will be made of some of these variables.

During the period 1935 to 1954, a significant number of persons were irradiated, primarily to the spine, for the relief of symptoms associated with ankylosing spondylitis. Subsequent evaluation of a group of British males treated in this fashion has revealed an increased frequency of malignant disease, especially leukemia, and persistent chromosome abnormalities. It is important to note that these people were afflicted with a

Table 5-4. Summary of irradiated human populations

Population and years of exposure	Primary type of radiation	Region primarily irradiated	Sample size	Comments
British adults irradiated for ankylosing spondylitis (1935-1954)	X rays	Spine	14,111	Increased frequency of malignant tumors
Children irradiated for suspected enlarged thymus and other benign lesions of head, neck, and scalp (1910-1959)	X rays	Mediastinum, scalp, tonsillar and nasopharyngeal regions	24,604*	Increased frequency of benign and malignant tumors, especially at thyroid
American radiologists (1905-1949)	X rays, radium	Partial to whole body	425 to 82,441*	Increased frequency of malignant tumors, decreased life span
Radium-dial painters and related workers; adults treated with radium (1905-1926; 1945-1955)	Gamma rays, alpha, and beta particles (^{226}Ra, ^{228}Ra, ^{224}Ra)	Skeleton	4532†	Increased frequency of malignant tumors, especially of bone
Thorium dioxide (1930-1951)	Alpha particles	Predominantly liver, spleen, bone marrow	16,074*	Increased frequency of hepatic and other neoplasms, cirrhosis, blood dyscrasias, and local granulomas at site of injection
Children irradiated in utero during diagnostic or therapeutic procedures involving the mother (1947-1954)	X rays	Whole body	14,294	Increased frequency of congenital abnormalities, mental retardation, leukemia, and solid tumors
Marshall Islanders (1954)	Gamma rays plus internally deposited radionuclides	Whole body but with disproportional irradiation of thyroid	7266*	Retardation of growth and development, benign and malignant thyroid tumors, chromosomal abnormalities, possible increased frequency of miscarriages and stillbirths
Japanese atomic bomb survivors (1945)	Gamma rays plus neutrons	Whole body	120,000*	Increased incidence of developmental abnormalities, benign and malignant tumors, and degenerative changes

*Includes comparable group of nonexposed ("control") individuals.
†Includes only American workers.

preexisting disease of significant magnitude. Although symptoms relate primarily to the spine, ankylosing spondylitis is currently believed to be a systemic disease with features common to the collagen disorders, and it is possible that the increased risk of colon cancer in these persons relates to a known relationship between this disease and ulcerative colitis, which, in turn, has been shown to predispose to colon cancer. However, no known association exists between other malignancies and spondylitis. In addition, these persons' exposures were restricted to one region of the body, and animal experiments have demonstrated that a standard dose administered to part of the body produces less pronounced acute and delayed effects than it would if administered to the whole body.

Similarly, infants treated with x rays for so-called status thymolymphaticus were exposed in a regional manner. These treatments were given to shrink a supposedly enlarged thymus gland, a procedure erroneously believed might alleviate respiratory distress or protect against the sudden infant death syndrome. An increased incidence of benign and malignant thyroid tumors has been documented in this population as well as a probable increase in lymphoma and leukemia and probably other types of tumors. In addition, thymic irradiation early in life may alter permanently the immunologic responsiveness of the recipient. An apparent increased incidence of asthma and a constellation of uncommon diseases with immunologic features has been noted among people irradiated for "status thymolymphaticus." Other groups of children were irradiated in comparable fashion for tinea capitis (ringworm of the scalp), cervical lymphadenitis, or unusually prominent pharyngeal tonsils.

An unknown number of early American radiologists were exposed to considerable radiation as a result of the poor shielding of their equipment. The magnitude of exposure in these persons is unknown. An increased prevalence of aplastic anemia, leukemia, lymphoma, multiple myeloma, and skin tumors has been documented in this population as well as a nonspecific decrease in life span.

Internally deposited radionuclides can also cause severe radiation injury. One of the first reports of this relationship concerned the early radium-dial painters. These workers, principally young women, applied luminescent radium-containing paint to watch and clock dials with fine camel's hair brushes, which they pointed with their tongue and lips. A significant portion of these radium compounds was ingested, absorbed from the gastrointestinal tract, and deposited in bone. In this location continuous radioactive decay led to bone necrosis, infection, and irradiation of adjacent structures. Of particular significance was the exposure of the respiratory epithelium in the nasal sinuses and air sacs from radium concentrated in the adjacent skull bones.

It is important to note that the paint used by the dial painters contained a relatively low concentration of radium. However, this element localizes very efficiently in teeth and bone, especially in those regions where new mineral is being formed. In addition, the radium incorporated in this fashion remains in the involved tissues for a long period of time. Thus the long-term consequences represent the cumulative effects of a relatively low dose and include malignant tumors of bone, the epithelial lining of the paranasal sinuses and the colon as well as a probable increased incidence of leukemia and blood dyscrasias.

Despite the above-mentioned experience, groups of patients, especially in Europe, were treated immediately after World War II with repeated injections of ^{224}Ra for ankylosing spondylitis, tuberculosis of bone, and degenerative joint disease. These persons exhibit an increased incidence of bone sarcomas and leukemias.

Because of its radiopacity, colloidal thorium dioxide (Thorotrast) was widely employed as a contrast medium from 1930 to 1945 by diagnostic radiologists. When administered intravenously, this radioactive substance localizes primarily in the liver, spleen, and bone marrow. Unfortunately, thorium dioxide is chemically inert, is poorly eliminated from the body, and has a long physical half-life and a biologic half-life in the liver of 200 to 400 years. It is phagocytosed by reticuloendothelial cells and remains there until the cell dies, whereupon it is often rephagocytosed by a neighboring cell. A variety of malignant tumors of the liver have been associated with thorium dioxide administration including hepatomas, cholangiocarcinomas, and hemangioendotheliomas; such tumors develop after an average latent period of approximately 20 years. Thorotrast is an alpha emitter and serves to illustrate the importance of the relationship between the way in which a radioactive substance is presented to the host and the probability of subsequent deleterious effects. Harmless externally because of a limited capacity to penetrate surface tissues, alpha particles are highly destructive when located within cells and may be responsible for the death of the host when they are deposited internally. In addition, evidence exists to suggest that Thorotrast and related colloids may also be carcinogenic chemically.

Radiation of the embryo or fetus in utero has long been recognized as injurious. After such exposure, small head circumference and mental retardation have been documented among the offspring of mothers irradiated therapeutically and of mothers exposed to the atomic bombs of Hiroshima and Nagasaki. More recently, in utero exposure has also been implicated in the subsequent development of leukemia and other tumors in the offspring of mothers receiving diagnostic x-ray exposures.

An unknown number of inhabitants of the Marshall Islands were accidentally exposed in 1954 to varying amounts of fallout released during the testing of a nuclear weapon on Bikini Atoll. A significant portion of the radiation absorbed by these islanders resulted from the deposition of a mixture of radioiodines. The maximum whole-body exposure from external radiation was estimated to be 175 rad and most of the 82 people located on the most proximal of the inhabited atolls (Rongelap) developed acute radiation sickness. Localized deposition of the various radioactive isotopes of iodine produced mean thyroid exposures of 1000 rad in young children, proportionately less in older children and adults. Subsequent follow-up examination has been extremely careful, and the population under evaluation now includes a control group and totals 7266 people. Problems thus far encountered by the exposed Marshall Islanders have involved primarily the thyroid gland, though disturbances of growth and development and increased numbers of chromosome abnormalities have also been noted. Up to now, irradiation of the thyroid gland has been manifest by an increased prevalence of benign thyroid nodules, frequently multiple and often associated with hypothyroidism, as well as an increased frequency of carcinoma. The growth retardation noted in these children probably relates to hypothyroidism.

The estimated civilian populations of Hiroshima and Nagasaki in August 1945 were 225,000 and 174,000, respectively. Of the total civilian population of both cities, approximately 106,200 died within the initial 12 weeks after exposure. Dosimetry is now available for almost all the survivors. The magnitude of possible exposure of an unshielded person, as a function of his or her distance from the hypocenter, is shown in Fig. 5-6. The hypocenter is the point on the ground immediately beneath the center of the explosion. The intercity discrepancies in Fig. 5-6 are primarily attributable to differences between the two bombs. The fissionable material in the Hiroshima bomb was uranium 235, and the resultant radiation spectrum contained somewhat more neutrons than the plutonium 238 bomb employed in Nagasaki. It is important to reemphasize the observation that fast neutrons are more effective than gamma rays in producing most of the delayed effects thus far studied.

Early deaths were caused by acute radiation sickness, flash burns, and mechanical injuries from falling buildings. Most victims and survivors sustained more than one type of injury. Table 5-5 shows the estimated distribution of the types of injury among the survivors.

Mechanical injuries were mostly of the "indirect" blast type; that is, they were produced by falling beams, flying glass, or other debris. Examples of trauma occurred at least as far as 4000 meters from the hypocenter.

Roughly 20% to 30% of the acute deaths were caused by "flash" or "profile" types of burns on the exposed areas of the skin that were in the direct path of the bomb's intense heat rays. Apart from other injuries, flash burns would have been fatal to all unshielded persons at distances up to 2000 meters from the hypocenter, and even beyond 4000 meters there were instances of burns severe enough to require treatment.

The direct effects of ionizing radiation were outlined by a local physician, Dr. Hachiya, for the Hiroshima newspaper on September 1, 1945.*

---

*From Hachiya, M.: Hiroshima diary—the journal of a Japanese physician, August 6–September 30, 1945, Chapel Hill, 1955, The University of North Carolina Press.

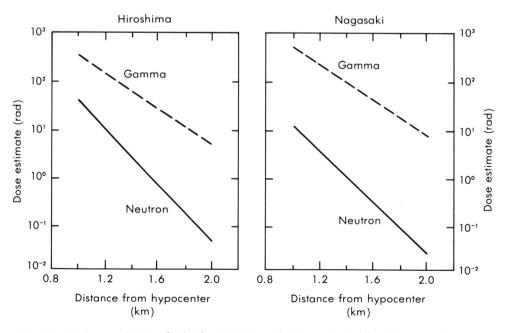

Fig. 5-6. Air dose estimates for both neutrons and gamma rays, Hiroshima and Nagasaki.

Table 5-5. Types of injury among atomic bomb survivors

Type of injury	Etiologic factor	Percent of survivors with injury*	Farthest distance injury reported (meters)
Mechanical trauma	Blast	70	4000
Burn	Heat	65	4000
Radiation sickness	Ionizing radiation	30	1500

Adapted from Key, C.R.: Hum. Pathol. **2:**475-484, 1971.
*Total exceeds 100% because of many persons with multiple injuries.

1. Those who were exposed within 500 meters out-of-doors were killed instantly or died within four or five days.
2. Some who were within 500 meters were protected by buildings and hence not burned. Within a period of two to 15 days many of these people developed a so-called "radiation sickness" and died. This sickness was manifested by anorexia, vomiting, hematemesis, and hemoptysis.
3. Those exposed in the 500 to 1000 meter zone have shown symptoms similar to those who were exposed within 500 meters but the onset of symptoms was later and insidious. The death rate in this group has been high.
4. I have studied the location of the in-patients and a great number of the out-patients and found most of them were exposed between 1000 and 3000 meters. Those in this group who were closest to the center became critically ill and some have died but the majority are in stable condition or well.
5. A great number of patients have complained of falling hair that began as late as two weeks following the explosion. Some of these patients have had an uneventful course while others have had a bad one.
6. The most serious clinical sign of radiation sickness is a decrease in white blood cells and pathologically great changes were found in the hematopoietic system, especially in the bone marrow. Those who received fatal injuries have died within the past month. Patients with low white blood counts who survived this period are now stable or convalescing. Within the past week the hospital has become very cheerful.

Dr. Hachiya's failure to mention decreased platelets, petechiae, and purpura was an oversight that he noted in a later entry in his diary. Most of those who developed severe signs and symptoms of acute radiation sickness were within 1500 meters of the hypocenter.

Other irradiated human populations include the following:

1. An unknown number of young women who received variable doses of radiation on one or both breasts for postpartum mastitis, unilateral hypertrophy, or fibrocystic disease; these individuals have developed excessive numbers of malignant breast tumors.
2. Women with pulmonary tuberculosis treated with pneumothorax to collapse the affected lung and then monitored with repeated chest fluoroscopies to ascertain the degree of collapse; these patients also developed increased numbers of malignant breast tumors.
3. Women with menometrorrhagia treated with radiation to cause an artificial menopause; these women showed an increased incidence of leukemia.
4. Persons with peptic ulcer treated with external irradiation for hyperactivity; these persons exhibited an increased frequency of malignancies of the portions of the gastrointestinal tract included in the treatment field (stomach, pancreas, large intestine).
5. Patients with certain malignant tumors, especially lymphoma and pediatric malignancies, cured with high-dose irradiation who then develop a second primary neoplasm, again located most commonly within the field of the initial treatment.

Genetic effects

Ionizing radiation was the first mutagenic agent discovered. In common with the spontaneous variety, radiation-induced mutations may affect either somatic cells, in which case the effects are limited to the irradiated individual, or germinal tissues, in which case the consequences may affect future generations. Mutations may also be classified as point mutations or chromosomal aberrations. Point mutations generally consist of small alterations in the sequence or composition of the DNA bases and are not evident by standard karyotyping. Most radiation-induced mutations of this type are recessive and therefore do not become expressed unless carried by both members of homologous chromosomes, a highly unlikely circumstance. For this reason, most of the available information about point mutations is derived from large numbers of carefully controlled breeding experiments on *Drosophila* and mice.

Chromosomal aberrations generally refer to changes that are evident by standard karyotyping with light microscopy. Although chromosomal and point mutations may occur simultaneously within the same cell, it is convenient to discuss them as separate entities.

Point mutations. Point mutations occur spontaneously but, at least in recognizable form, at a low natural rate. Of these spontaneous mutations, it is estimated that approximately 10% are attributable to the natural or background radiation that has always been a part of our environment; the remainder are believed to be caused by either mutagenic chemicals or the thermal movement of molecules. The frequency of radiation-induced point mutations is dose dependent.

Chromosomal aberrations. Chromosomal aberrations arise when radiation breaks a chromosome or a chromatid at one or more points along its length. Such an interruption may result in an alteration in the number of genes in the cell or in the linear sequence of the genes, or both. The broken ends of a chromosome may (1) rejoin with no resultant lesion, (2) heal without rejoining, (3) join with the broken ends of other chromosomes, or (4) fail to heal. It is estimated that 90% of individual chromosome breaks rejoin with no demonstrable lesion.

As might be expected, the frequency of nonviable chromosomal aberrations is greater than the frequency of nonviable gene (point) mutations. Chromosomes also exhibit increased stickiness just before or during metaphase when irradiated with doses of 100 rad or more. This poorly understood phenomenon often causes individual chromosomes to stick together and form loosely adherent clumps. At anaphase such clumps do not separate properly and such aberrant separation results in an unequal distribution of genes to the daughter cells.

Dose-response effects. In general, the number of detectable point mutations increases linearly with increasing dose and with no evidence of a threshold effect. Even very low doses, doses in the 1 rad range, may be associated with a small increase in the number of mutations. The relationship between dose and the rate of mutation of a specific somatic cell locus is shown in Fig. 5-7. The study group consisted of Hiroshima atomic bomb survivors and controls, and the locus evaluated is known to code for the expression of the polymorphic glycophorin A locus in erythroid precursor cells. The frequency of mutation (loss of gene expression) is directly proportional to the estimated dose absorbed by these persons in 1945. In the mouse, whole-body exposures in the 30 to 40 rad range are believed to produce about as many point mutations as are believed to occur from natural causes. This is known as the doubling dose.

In common with point mutations, single chromosome breaks, also known as single-hit aberrations, bear a linear relationship to dose. Two-hit chromosome breaks

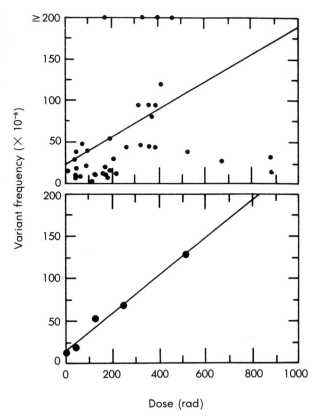

Fig. 5-7. Frequency of mutation of glycophorin A locus as a function of estimated dose among Hiroshima atomic-bomb survivors. (From Langlois, R.G., et al.: Science **236:**445-448, 1987.)

are the result of two single aberrations that occur in close proximity. As might be expected, two-hit breaks exhibit a threshold and then increase in frequency at a rate greater than the single power of the dose.

Geneticists are appropriately concerned about the hazards of the exposure of human beings to ionizing radiation, particularly with respect to the implications for future generations. Most radiation-induced mutations are transmitted as recessive traits; as such, they can be transmitted to large numbers of offspring, an occurrence that goes undetected until matings between carriers begin to occur. For this reason, deleterious recessive mutations, though not evident immediately, are more dangerous to a population than are harmful dominant mutations, particularly when the latter are damaging enough to prevent carriers from reproducing.

With respect to radiation exposure, geneticists are particularly concerned about the following categories of people:

1. *Radiology personnel.* The unfortunate experience of the pioneer American radiologists focused attention on some of the hazards in this regard and resulted in stringent safety precautions. Despite these precautions, however, lymphocytes from

the peripheral blood of radiologists and radiotherapy nurses occasionally demonstrate a significant increase in the frequency of chromosomal aberrations.

2. *Patients receiving radioactive isotopes.* Isotopes may be potentially hazardous depending on the distribution of the substance in the patient. For example, a person with thyrotoxicosis who is treated with an average therapeutic dose of iodine 131 will receive the following average tissue exposures: 4000 to 10,000 rad to the thyroid gland; 2 to 5 rad to the hematopoietic tissues; 1 rad to the testes or 2 rad to the ovary. The dose estimates for the testes and ovary are particularly significant to future generations.

3. *Workers in nuclear installations.* Studies on radiation workers in a nuclear installation have demonstrated that low levels of exposure over a prolonged period of time can significantly increase the number of chromosomal aberrations in peripheral blood lymphocytes.

4. *Patients exposed to x rays during diagnostic radiologic examinations.* At present, medical and dental exposures are the most significant source of iatrogenic radiation effects. Of particular importance are diagnostic procedures that involve repeated exposures or simultaneous fluoroscopic examinations. Many of these procedures involve exposures to the gonads that are 2 to 20 times the average natural background. The scope of the problem is evident from the following figures collected in the United States from a survey made in 1964: 600,000 patients received radiation therapy; 7.8 million were given fluoroscopic examinations; 46 million received dental x-ray examinations; 66 million were exposed during diagnostic medical radiographic examinations, this in a total population of approximately 181 million at that time. More recent data are not available.

Diagnostic radiology is an indispensable part of medical practice, but physicians must be aware of the genetic effects of radiation in order to balance the benefits of a specific procedure against the possible hazards.

Experience with Japanese atomic bomb survivors. Residual chromosomal aberrations have been documented in 61% of heavily exposed atomic bomb survivors. In addition, a variety of complex chromosomal aberrations (rings, dicentrics, acentric fragments, and translocations) were documented among 39% of the persons exposed in utero as compared with 1% of the controls. In contrast to the cytogenetic defects observed after intrauterine (postconception) exposure, no such effects have been associated thus far with preconception irradiation. Specific observations concerning this lack of a relationship are as follows:

1. No significant relationship could be documented between the frequency of congenital malformations and either maternal or paternal exposure.

2. Similarly, no consistent effect could be documented between maternal or paternal exposure and the frequency of stillbirths or neonatal deaths.

3. Up to now, no clear evidence exists for an increased death rate among children born to exposed parents.

4. Cytogenetic examination of the children of heavily exposed survivors has as yet failed to reveal any aberrations ascribable to radiation injury.

It is important, however, to introduce a note of caution in the interpretation of these four observations. Even with high doses to the reproductive tissues of the parents, the expected risk to an individual offspring is exceedingly small. Very large numbers of offspring must therefore be studied to detect any effect. In addition, both congenital abnormalities and stillbirths occur primarily on nongenetic bases, and therefore the effects of an alteration in the genetic component that influences these two phenomena would tend to be masked by a large number of "spontaneous" events. Finally, it is believed that mutations in immature germ-line cells result in cell death whereas similar lesions in more mature cells persist; thus only the latter may be available for conception. Needless to say, in the immediate postwar period, conditions in Japan were not conducive to procreation.

As noted above, the frequency of residual point mutations in irradiated germ cells is believed to be dependent on the time interval between exposure and mating. If mating occurs soon after exposure (within about 60 days in humans), fertilization will probably involve irradiated *mature* germ cells. The mutation rate for recessive genes in these cells is believed to be roughly twice that associated with irradiated immature germ cells possibly because many injured members die acutely.

On the basis of the above information, persons should be advised to avoid procreation during the initial few months after the exposure of unshielded gonads to radiation incurred either accidentally or for therapeutic purposes. After this initial period, fewer radiation-induced mutations are transmitted to the offspring by the female than by the male. This observation probably reflects either a more efficient repair mechanism or a difference in the relative radiosensitivity of oocytes and male germ cells.

Somatic effects

As noted before, the majority of radiation-induced chromosome breaks apparently rejoin immediately so that no lesion results. Permanent chromosomal alterations are generally of little significance to the host when they occur in an organ with a stable cell population such as adult liver cells. The lethal aspects of chromosomal aberrations become manifest at the time of cell division when one or more sets of genes are lost to a cell. This line of reasoning forms the basis of the law of Bergonié and Tribondeau, which states that dividing cells are more radiosensitive than nondividing cells. Thus hematopoietic cells and gastrointestinal epithelium are more radiosensitive than neurons or cardiac muscle are, and the embryo and fetus are more susceptible than the adult to radiation injury.

Somatic effects of radiation injury may be acute or delayed. Among the acute effects, early lethality is of prime concern. Among the important delayed effects are carcinogenesis, abnormalities of growth and development, alterations in life span, and a broad spectrum of injuries to individual organs.

Early lethality

Key to an understanding of early lethality is an appreciation of the concept of $LD_{50(30)}$. In toxicology the lethal dose 50, or LD_{50}, is the amount of an agent that causes a 50% mortality in the experimental group. The same approach has been applied to radiation injury, especially injury associated with whole-body exposure. However, death after whole-body exposure is often delayed for days or even weeks, depending on the magnitude of exposure. Therefore, with respect to radiation exposure, mortality is expressed in terms of a specific period of time, generally 30 days. The $LD_{50(30)}$ is defined as the dose associated with a 50% mortality within 30 days of exposure.

In humans the sequence of events after radiation injury is slower than that for experimental animals. For this reason, the frame of reference generally employed for man is the $LD_{50(60)}$ or the amount of radiation that would be expected to kill 50% of a population within 60 days of exposure.

A quantitative dose-response relationship for early lethality in humans is not known. Several investigators have derived hypothetical dose-response curves based upon experience with reactor accidents and the atomic explosions in Japan. From these observations, the $LD_{50(60)}$ for humans exposed to a single dose of highly penetrating electromagnetic radiation (x or gamma rays) delivered over a period of less than 24 hours is believed to be in the 225 to 270 rad range.

Within a given population, a variety of host and environmental factors are known to influence the response of the individual to whole-body irradiation. In general, males are more sensitive than females. Middle-aged persons appear to exhibit a greater degree of tolerance to radiation than the young and the old do. The presence of infection sharply increases the mortality from whole-body exposure. The microorganisms implicated in these infections appear to be of both exogenous and endogenous origin. The latter are the normal flora of the body, especially of the gastrointestinal tract, which gain entry through denuded mucosal surfaces. Dissemination of these opportunistic offenders is facilitated by the accompanying leukopenia. Finally, humans appear to vary considerably in their individual susceptibility to irradiation.

Of greater magnitude than the individual differences just outlined are the noticeable discrepancies among species. For example, the $LD_{50(30)}$ of sheep is about 150 rad, whereas that of one inbred strain of female mice is 689 rad. Even among the various inbred strains of mice there is a remarkable variation in radiosensitivity as expressed by the $LD_{50(30)}$. The basis for these interspecies and intraspecies differences is not known.

If an area of the body is shielded, the effects of a constant amount of radiation are decreased. Partial-body shielding can protect an individual from an otherwise lethal exposure to ionizing radiation. Shielding of the bone marrow, spleen, and gastrointestinal tract is especially efficacious.

The relationship between survival time and magnitude of whole-body exposure in terms of mode of death is illustrated in Fig. 5-8. The curve shows three distinct components. The first region covers the dose range of 400 to 1200 rad, over which survival time decreases exponentially with increasing dose. This range is generally referred to as the region of *hematopoietic death* because bone marrow damage is the most prominent

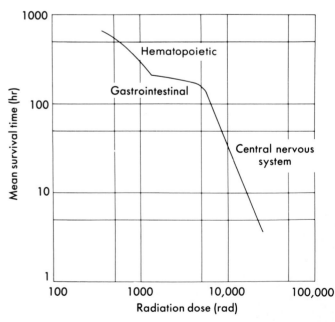

Fig. 5-8. Relationship between mean survival time, magnitude of whole-body exposure, and primary mode of death in humans. (After Langham, W.H., et al.: Aerospace Med. **36:**1, 1965.)

finding, both clinically and at autopsy. Designation of this component of the dose-response curve as the region of hematopoietic death should not, however, be interpreted as an indication that damage is confined to the bone marrow. Injury to hematopoietic cells is the most conspicuous finding, but destruction involving other organs also may contribute to the death of the patient. In particular, signs and symptoms attributable to necrosis of the mucosa of the gastrointestinal tract are often prominent in the 400 to 1200 rad dose range. Bacteremia, often resulting from ulceration of the gastrointestinal tract, contributes greatly to lethality in the hematopoietic range. The increasing contribution of gastrointestinal damage in the death of the patient is in part responsible for the exponential decrease in mean survival time over this portion of the dose-response curve.

Throughout the dose range of 1200 to 5000 rad there is a plateau in the mean survival curve (Fig. 5-8). This part of the dose-response curve is generally referred to as the region of *gastrointestinal death*. Again, this distinction is based on the most prominent clinical and morphologic findings. Morphologically, there is a progressive loss of gastrointestinal mucosa secondary to impaired proliferation of the stem cell or renewal population. Necrosis of mucosal cells leads to ulceration, bacteremia, hemorrhage, and loss of fluids and electrolytes. In this dose range the bone marrow is totally aplastic and numerous other tissues also show severe damage. However, damage to the gastrointestinal tract is the primary cause of death in the 1200 to 5000 rad dose range.

Above about 5000 rad, mean survival time again begins to decrease exponentially with increasing dose (Fig. 5-8), and death is characterized by a variety of central nervous system signs and symptoms. For this reason, the region of the survival curve associated with exposures in excess of 5000 rad is referred to as the region of *central nervous system death*. Incapacitation occurs relatively rapidly and is characterized by confusion, convulsions, apathy, and coma, followed by death.

Late somatic effects

Various somatic effects have been attributed to radiation injury; of these, the most important are carcinogenesis, abnormalities of growth and development, and changes in life span.

Carcinogenesis (see also Chapter 14). The carcinogenic effects of ionizing radiation have been recognized for almost a century. In fact, a significant number of the pioneer radiation workers developed epidermoid and basal cell carcinomas of the hands. These tumors generally arose in areas of radiation dermatitis caused by repeated exposures with massive accumulated doses, which often totaled several thousand rad. For example,

many of the early workers focused their equipment on the bones of their own hands and were also accustomed to positioning their patients with their unshielded hands while the equipment was in operation.

Despite the early recognition of this untoward effect of ionizing radiation, even today the mechanisms involved in radiation-induced neoplasia remain poorly understood in part because of our incomplete understanding of carcinogenesis in general.

Common to most theories of carcinogenesis are the concepts of monoclonality and stepwise progression. Studies of the genetics of neoplastic cells indicate that cancer cells may arise by the activation of oncogenes, or the inactivation of antioncogenes, through chromosomal rearrangements, point mutations, or related DNA alterations. As we have seen, changes of these types are readily inducible by radiation.

Despite the inadequacy of existing information, several generalizations with respect to radiation carcinogenesis appear warranted. First, all forms of ionizing radiation are carcinogenic. Second, multiple doses are more tumorigenic than is a single exposure of the same total magnitude. Third, tumors of almost any type may be induced by irradiation under appropriate conditions in susceptible subjects. Fourth, susceptibility to the carcinogenic action of radiation appears to be widely shared by many different species of animals including man. Fifth, indirect effects of radiation on the host are responsible for some types of neoplasms, indicating that radiation need not always be absorbed at the site of the subsequent tumor in order to be carcinogenic. Sixth, in most instances the incidence of radiation-induced neoplasms is correlated with the absorbed dose, dose rate, volume of tissue exposed, and the LET (linear energy transfer) of the radiation. However, the incidence of some neoplasms is greatly increased by relatively small amounts of radiation whereas others exhibit a pronounced dropoff in incidence at high dose levels, perhaps because of the sterilization of the target tissue.

Possible mechanisms of radiation carcinogenesis. Current available evidence from both human and animal studies indicates that (1) multiple factors may influence the genesis and evolution of most neoplasms and (2) the relative importance of these various genetic and environmental influences may vary as a function of the biologic experience of the host and the individual characteristics of specific tumors. An extension of this line of reasoning indicates that radiation may cause a tumor in one of several ways depending on the tumor type and that the dose-response relationship may be expected to vary from organ to organ and according to (1) the age and gender of the individual, (2) possible occupational or other exposure to cocarcinogens, (3) the genetic predisposition of the host, (4) diet, (5) socioeconomic factors, and in all probability (6) numerous other variables, the action of which is not yet understood. Depending upon the circumstances, radiation may act as an initiator, a promoter, or, most commonly, a complete carcinogen.

The character of the primary subcellular events induced by radiation that ultimately results in a tumor is not known. Two prime suspects are the activation of latent oncogenic viruses and permanent DNA aberrations. A considerable amount of experimental evidence exists to support both of these hypotheses, which are certainly not mutually exclusive. For example, viruses have been shown to induce tumors in experimental animals and probably unequivocally in man. Radiation is known to alter gene expression, and such alterations in virus-susceptible cells could facilitate the penetration of opportunistic latent viral genomes. However, it is important to note that in humans no direct relationships between the induction of cancer by radiation and the activation of latent oncogenic viruses has been demonstrated.

Radiation-induced somatic mutations have long been postulated to play an etiologic role in radiation carcinogenesis. Radiation is a potent mutagen, and many tumors are associated with chromosome abnormalities. Proponents of the somatic mutation theory suggest that these associations are causally related. Among the various chromosomal changes postulated to induce neoplasia are damage to specific genes, gene amplification, chromosomal imbalance, and disproportionate DNA replication. A current popular hypothesis implicates radiation-induced deletion of a regulating gene, a gene that normally represses the expression of oncogenes, in the genesis of radiation-related tumors.

An extension of the above line of reasoning is the single-hit hypothesis. The theoretical basis of this hypothesis is the concept that neoplastic transformation follows the passage of a single ionizing particle through a susceptible cell. This approach postulates a linear relationship between radiation dose and the incidence of cancer in a uniform population. However, because neoplasms appear to evolve stepwise through a succession of alterations, it appears unlikely that tumors arise from a single mutation. If this were the case, for example, age at exposure would not be expected to be a significant factor in radiation carcinogenesis. A mutation would be expected to result in a neoplasm irrespective of the age of the person involved. As shown in Fig. 5-9, which shows the relation among age, latent period, and risk of leukemia for atomic bomb survivors, such is not the case. The wavelike pattern in Fig. 5-9 reflects the relationship between latent period (the time between irradiation and the development of leukemia) and age at exposure. Experience with other tumors also shows age to be a factor. Nevertheless, assuming that tumors arise as the result of a series of alterations, some of which may involve mutations, it is eminently possible that a single radiation-induced mutation could act as a promoter in a suitably conditioned host.

A variety of indirect effects of radiation upon the induction of neoplasms has been well documented experimentally. For example, thymic lymphomas occur in susceptible strains of mice when nonirradiated thymus is transplanted into irradiated recipients. The mechanism involved has been only partially defined but is believed to involve either (1) activation of a tumorigenic virus that is released from a nonthymic site by the action of radiation, or (2) inactivation of a hypothetical repressor that normally restricts provirus transcription by radiation. In either circumstance, the released provirus is apparent widely disseminated throughout the host but has a predilection for dividing thymus cell. In this example, the thymus is regenerating from mechanical injuries sustained at the time of transplantation and ra-

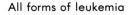

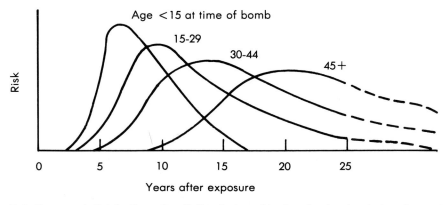

Fig. 5-9. Temporal distribution of radiation-induced leukemias in atomic-bomb survivors in relation to age at the time of irradiation. (From Ichimaru, M., and Ishimaru, T.: J. Radiat. Res. **16**(suppl.):89, 1975.)

diation is acting as a promoter or coleukemogenic agent. In similar fashion, the induction of pituitary tumors in irradiated mice is believed to relate in part to disturbances occurring elsewhere in the host, in this instance a hormonal disturbance caused by radiation-related injury to target organs such as the thyroid. The resultant hypothyroidism activates the pituitary by well-characterized feedback mechanisms, and hyperfunction ensues. Hyperfunction results in hyperplasia, and in some cases neoplasia eventually occurs. More recently, radiation-induced impairment of normal immunologic surveillance mechanisms has been implicated in select tumors.

To summarize, a variety of diverse effects must be contemplated in a consideration of the mechanisms involved in radiation carcinogenesis. Direct and indirect effects must be considered, the nature and relative importance of which probably vary with respect to the type of neoplasm in question as well as the conditions of irradiation. In a growing number of instances, however, carcinogenesis appears to be a multistep process and to involve interactions among the effects of radiation, viruses, chemicals, and a variety of poorly understood host factors.

Heredity. In man, a broad spectrum of inherited conditions have been associated with specific neoplasms, and in some of these tumor-prone disorders, radiation appears to potentiate the risk of tumorigenesis. For example, children with one form of retinoblastoma occasionally also develop osteogenic sarcoma at various sites including especially the extremities; however, patients irradiated for retinoblastoma not infrequently develop osteogenic sarcomas in the field of therapy. This finding indicates a genetic predisposition to osteogenic sarcoma in these children that is made manifest by the action of radiation. Similarly, several children with the hereditary multiple basal cell nevus syndrome have developed basal cell nevi concentrated in the field of previous irradiation for medulloblastoma. Cells from cancer-prone persons (such as persons with ataxia telangiectasia, Fanconi's anemia, dysplastic nevus syndrome) exhibit an enhanced sensitivity to irradiation during the G_2 phase of the cell cycle as manifest by an increased frequency of chromatic breaks and gaps. Certain types of fish have been shown to possess a gene responsible for the development of tumors, including neuroblastoma. Under normal circumstances, this gene appears to be repressed by a complementary series of regulating genes that are tissue specific. Irradiation of these fish causes the development of periocular neuroblastoma, as well as other neoplasms, presumably because of inactivation of the repressor gene. Finally, different strains of rodents develop distinctly different spectra of tumors after identical doses of radiation, and in at least one experimental situation, irradiation of parent mice causes a dose-dependent increase in neoplasms, as well as genetic abnormalities in their offspring. Thus the available evidence strongly indicates that heredity may play a major role in radiation carcinogenesis.

Differences among organs and cells. Under appropriate circumstances, most human tissues are believed to be susceptible to the carcinogenic effects of radiation. A well-recognized exception is the small lymphocyte. Thus chronic lymphocytic leukemia, a relatively common malignancy in western populations, is not increased in frequency after whole-body or local irradia-

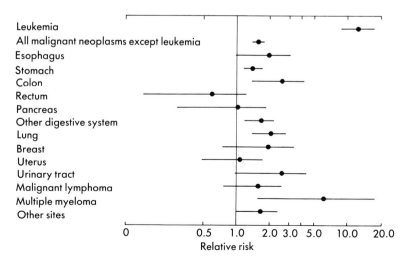

Fig. 5-10. Relative risk and 90% confidence intervals of mortality attributable to various types of neoplasms from 1950 to 1978 among atomic bomb survivors who received at least 200 rad in comparison with the population that received 0 rad. (Modified from Kato, H., and Schull, W.J.: Radiat. Res. **90:**395, 1982.)

tion. And even among susceptible organs, the dose of radiation required for tumorigenesis varies greatly. As a consequence, in an irradiated population, the relative risk (or the ratio between incidence in the irradiated group and that in the nonirradiated members of the population) differs greatly for various tumor types. Fig. 5-10 shows the relative risk for specific types of malignant tumors among Japanese atomic bomb survivors exposed to 200 or more rad. Notice that this figure is based upon mortality data, hence the absence of neoplasms such as carcinoma of the thyroid known to be radiation-induced but of low potential for death.

Dose-incidence relationships. Considerable effort has been given to an attempt to define in mathematical terms the relationships between dose of irradiation and tumor incidence especially at low dose levels. The latter are of particular importance in defining maximum permissible exposure levels for radiation workers. Unfortunately, the available data are insufficient to establish with confidence the shape of the dose-incidence curve at low doses. Hence efforts to estimate the possible risks of low-level irradiation involve extrapolation from observations made at higher dose levels. These extrapolations, based upon assumptions yet to be proved, yield three types of curves: linear nonthreshold, linear threshold, and linear-quadratic. These curves are represented schematically in Fig. 5-11.

The concept of threshold is of critical importance in a consideration of the carcinogenic effects of radiation. As depicted in Fig. 5-11, threshold implies a "safe" dose of radiation below which there is no increased incidence of the disease in question. At present the available evidence fails to support or refute the concept of a threshold in relation to the carcinogenic effects of radiation. For this reason, most authorities have recommended that the linear, nonthreshold dose-incidence model (Fig. 5-11) be employed to derive risk estimates for carcinogenesis among people exposed to low doses of radiation. This conservative approach assumes that any level of exposure is associated with some risk of harm. Corollaries to this axiom include the following: (1) no exposure to radiation is justifiable if it is avoidable or fails to provide a benefit commensurate with the presumed risk and (2) every exposure, even when amply justified, must be kept as low as possible.

In contrast with low dose effects, considerable data are available concerning the characteristics of the dose-incidence curve at intermediate and high exposure levels. In many instances the linear quadratic model (Fig. 5-11) appears to best describe stochastic effects at these dose levels.

Abnormalities of growth and development. Radiation is known to be especially injurious to rapidly dividing tissues. For this reason the developing embryo and the preadolescent child are particularly susceptible to radiation-induced disorders of growth and development. In general, the character of the defect reflects those tissues that are undergoing the most rapid growth and differentiation at the time of exposure. From this standpoint it is convenient to divide radiation-related disorders of growth and development into four phases: the preimplantation period, the period of major organogenesis, the fetal period, and the postnatal period.

Preimplantation period. Irradiation shortly after conception is associated with one of two extremes: it is likely to be either lethal or of no apparent significance

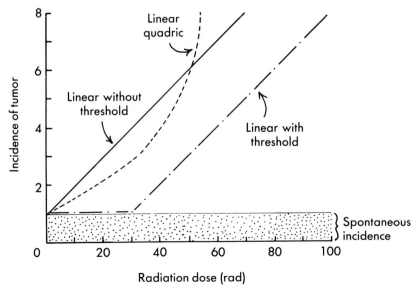

Fig. 5-11. Hypothetical dose-response curves for radiation carcinogenesis.

to the preimplantation embryo, which therefore survives without evidence of abnormality. When the organism consists of only a few cells, radiation-induced damage to only one cell is likely to be fatal to the embryo. Under such circumstances, the mother is generally unaware that she has even conceived.

Period of major organogenesis. This period, which begins at the time of implantation (day 8 or 9) and extends through the initial 6 weeks of gestation, is the time when the developing fetus is maximally radiosensitive. Exposure during this period of remarkable growth and differentiation is associated with one or more of a vast number of possible congenital malformations. Susceptibility to the induction of one of several specific types of developmental anomalies is sharply pinpointed in time, apparently as a function of the organ or organs that are undergoing major differentiation at the time of exposure. Thus the developing fetus is a mosaic of constantly changing, organ-specific radiosensitivities.

Fetal period. From the sixth week of gestation until the time of parturition, susceptibility to recognizable morphologic anomalies decreases. Most of the organ systems are structurally differentiated, and therefore exposure of the fetus would not be expected to result in gross congenital abnormalities. However, susceptibility to radiation-induced functional disabilities persists during this period. Such disturbances, which involve particularly the central nervous system and the gonads, are often difficult to recognize and identify, especially since development of these tissues continues until well after birth. Radiation during the fetal period apparently depletes the total number of functional nerve and reproductive cells. With respect to the central nervous system, such depletion may be manifest by a reduced IQ. Thus identification of the defect may be postponed until the child reaches school age. Even then the relationship of the deficit to previous radiation exposure may not be recognized by the parents or the teacher. And if the loss is slight, the reduced IQ may fall within the normal range and thus never be recognized as abnormal for the particular child.

Postnatal period. Radiation-induced abnormalities, especially of bone, are associated with the exposure of infants and children before the cessation of physical growth and development. With respect to bone, the magnitude of impairment appears to depend on the rate of growth at the time of exposure. Other tissues that continue to develop in the postnatal period, such as the eye, the central nervous system, and the teeth, are also susceptible to radiation-induced abnormalities in growth and development.

• • •

Additional radiation-induced defects that result from exposure of the developing fetus and the preadolescent child include (1) growth retardation, (2) neurologic effects, and (3) neoplasia. Much of our information about the consequences of in utero irradiation in humans is derived from two populations: (1) persons whose mothers in the late 1920s received pelvic radiotherapy during early pregnancy and (2) persons born of pregnant women who were located close to the site of the atomic bomb explosion in Hiroshima. The findings in these two groups of people are in accord with the results from a large number of animal experiments.

Exposure during the period of major organogenesis, the fetal period, or the postnatal period can result in a diffuse retardation of normal growth. When exposure occurs in utero, this retardation is manifested by subnormal head circumference, body height, and weight. The maximum effect appears to occur when the fetus is exposed between the third and twentieth weeks of gestation. Radiation-related retardation of growth induced during the postnatal period is almost always a consequence of local exposure and involves only the irradiated region, most often a limb.

With respect to neurologic defects, it has been estimated that 80% of malformed children with a history of irradiation in utero have a subnormal head circumference. As might be expected, mental retardation is also a sequela of fetal irradiation, with or without reduced head size. The period of increased risk of mental retardation is sharply circumscribed to exposures occurring during 8 to 15 weeks of gestational age. This is the period of rapid proliferation of neurons in the paraventricular region of the developing brain and the subsequent migration to their relatively distant final positions, a process largely completed by the sixteenth week after conception. A variety of other central nervous system defects can be produced by irradiation throughout the fetal period in experimental animals. The character of the malformation is determined by the stage of gestation at the time of exposure. Malformations after low doses of radiation have also been reported, but their significance is not known. In this connection it is important to note that the fetal nervous system is capable of significant repair of radiation-induced injury.

Moderate to high doses of radiation administered to the fetus are carcinogenic. With respect to low dose radiation, most investigators believe that in utero exposure during diagnostic radiographic procedures performed during pregnancy increases the risk of leukemia and other malignancies in human offspring. One study has implicated doses as low as 2 rad. However, other observers question this association at low doses, and the issue probably will not be resolved until more is known about the mechanisms involved in leukemia induction.

On the basis of some of the preceding observations, many institutions have adopted a policy that limits elective diagnostic medical radiographic examinations among women of childbearing age to the first 10 days after the start of the last menses. This approach is designed to prevent exposure of an unsuspected conceptus.

Finally, it should be emphasized that the discussion in this section has focused especially upon exposure from external sources. Fetal irradiation may also occur when radioactive isotopes are administered to the mother. Radioactive iodine, strontium, tritium, phosphorus, and plutonium are among the many isotopes that can cross the placenta to become incorporated into, and thereby injure, fetal tissues. For example, radioactive iodine administered late in pregnancy for maternal hyperthyroidism can be concentrated in the thyroid of the developing fetus and result in cretinism.

Life span. Sublethal whole-body irradiation of rodents causes shortened life span. This life shortening results from an increase in age-specific mortality and persists even when appropriate corrections are made for the early mortality associated with radiation sickness and the late deaths caused by radiation-induced neoplasms.

Up to now, however, experimental studies have not shown unequivocally that radiation truly accelerates the aging process. The possibility remains that radiation reduces life span by some other mechanism. Autopsies of irradiated animals reveal that death is generally caused by the same diseases that kill their nonexposed contemporaries. In particular, radiation hastens the development of a variety of degenerative and neoplastic diseases as well as autoimmune phenomena. Not all age-dependent alterations, however, are temporally advanced by irradiation, and even for those that are advanced, the magnitude of change is not necessarily uniform.

Comparable data pertinent to humans are fragmentary. One of the first suggestions of a similar life-shortening effect came from the observation that pioneer American radiologists experienced a higher age-specific death rate than other specialists did. The increase in mortality was not attributable to a specific lesion and was interpreted as a nonspecific shortening of life span from occupational exposure. Interestingly the excess mortality has progressively decreased in all but the oldest age groups, possibly because of improved shielding and other radiologic safety procedures.

ACUTE RADIATION SYNDROME
General effects

The clinical signs and symptoms produced by intensive exposure of the entire body to penetrating radiation are referred to as the acute radiation syndrome or radiation sickness. This syndrome is characterized by three successive phases.

1. *A transient prodromal phase, which develops within a few hours of exposure to as little as 75 to 100 rad.* In humans this phase is characterized by apathy, anorexia, nausea, and vomiting. As shown in Fig. 5-12, the incidence and duration of prodromal symptoms are dose dependent and therefore provide a rough indication of the degree of irradiation in persons accidentally exposed to a dose of unknown magnitude. The prodromal phase rarely exceeds 24 hours except in very severe cases.

2. *An ensuing asymptomatic latent period, which re-*

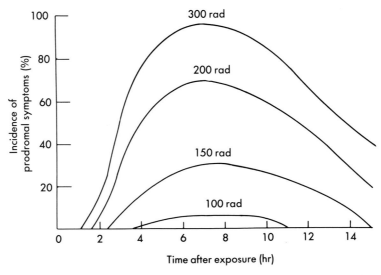

Fig. 5-12. Incidence and duration of prodromal symptoms as function of dose. (From Langham, W.H., et al.: Aerospace Med. **36:**1, 1965.)

flects the time required for the development of disturbances in specific organs. As will be seen subsequently, this period generally reflects the time required for the depletion of cells in mitotically active tissues through interference with normal renewal mechanisms. As such, the duration of the latent period is also dose dependent.

3. *The principal phase of the illness.* As noted previously, the acute radiation syndrome can be divided into three major categories on the basis of the organ system most conspicuously involved; these are the hematopoietic, gastrointestinal, and central nervous system syndromes. In varying degrees each syndrome is associated with death, and much of our understanding of the acute radiation syndrome has been gained from an evaluation of persons accidentally exposed during reactor accidents.

Some of the clinical and morphologic characteristics of the individual components of the acute radiation syndrome are summarized in Table 5-6. The most sensitive organ is the bone marrow, and symptoms relating to hematopoietic dysfunction are apparent after exposure to as little as 50 to 100 rad. Maximum expression of symptoms referable to the bone marrow is generally delayed until 2 to 3 weeks after exposure. At the other end of the spectrum is the central nervous system (CNS) syndrome, which follows very large doses (1000 rad or more) and where the clinical manifestations are often apparent within minutes of exposure. Intermediate between these extremes is the gastrointestinal syndrome.

Pathogenesis

The pathogenesis of the CNS component of the acute radiation syndrome is not known. Current evidence indicates that injury to small blood vessels may be the initiating event. Vacuolization of capillary endothelial cells, perivascular foci of hemorrhage, and perivascular collections of inflammatory cells have been described. Vascular permeability is known to be increased, and cerebral edema in uniformly present, among both persons exposed accidentally and animals exposed experimentally. It may well be that significant edema of other organs is associated with the high doses responsible for the CNS syndrome but that the rigid confines of the adult skull dictate that CNS symptoms precede those attributable to other organs. At extremely high dose levels, death may be caused by direct neuronal damage; the estimated intracerebral dose associated with this phenomenon is in excess of 100,000 rad for humans.

The cellular basis of the gastrointestinal and hematopoietic syndromes is directly related to the rate of cell turnover in these organs. The epithelial cells lining the digestive tract and the circulating leukocytes are short lived and therefore must be renewed at a rapid rate. In both instances renewal depends on a population of rapidly dividing stem cells that undergo a series of maturational steps to differentiate into the mature components that characterize these organs. Irradiation interferes with the proliferation of the stem cell population. Therefore replacements are not available after irradiation when normal biologic attrition causes the progressive loss of mature cells.

In the gastrointestinal tract, the stem cell population

Table 5-6. Important features of the acute radiation syndrome in man

Subcategory	Clinical threshold dose*	Latent period	Primary morphologic manifestations	Characteristic signs and symptoms	Mechanism of death	Time of death after exposure (mean)
Hematopoietic syndrome	100	2-3 weeks	Hypoplasia of bone marrow with leukopenia, thrombocytopenia and (occasionally) anemia	Petechiae, purpura, hemorrhage, infection	Infection	3 weeks
Gastrointestinal syndrome	500	3-5 days	Depletion of epithelium of small intestine with ulceration	Fever, diarrhea, fluid-electrolyte disturbances, infection	Dehydration, infection, electrolyte loss	10-14 days
Central nervous system syndrome	2000	15 minutes-3 hours	Edema, necrosis of neurons, vasculitis	Confusion, apathy, somnolence, tremor, ataxia, convulsions, coma	Increased central nervous system pressure	14-36 hours

*Air dose in roentgens.

is located in the crypts of Lieberkühn. Irradiation of these cells inhibits division or, if the dose is sufficiently large, kills them outright. The mature cells at the tips of the villi undergo spontaneous aging at the usual rate and are sloughed into the lumen of the intestine. Meanwhile, partially mature cells continue to migrate toward the tips of the villi to replace these senescent cells, thus depleting the crypts even further. In the absence of appropriate replacements, the villi become denuded and vital functions are compromised. In particular, loss of the normal mucosa permits fluid and electrolytes to escape from exposed tissue spaces and allows microorganisms, especially the normal intestinal flora, easy access to the bloodstream. Hemorrhage from exposed blood vessels may further complicate the clinical situation. If recovery is to occur, small foci of regenerating epithelium are generally evident by the end of the first week. This sequence of events is shown diagrammatically in Fig. 5-13.

The acute response of the stomach, colon, and rectum is similar to that of the small intestine. However, because cell turnover is highest in the small intestine, cell depletion occurs earlier there than elsewhere.

The pathogenesis of the events associated with the

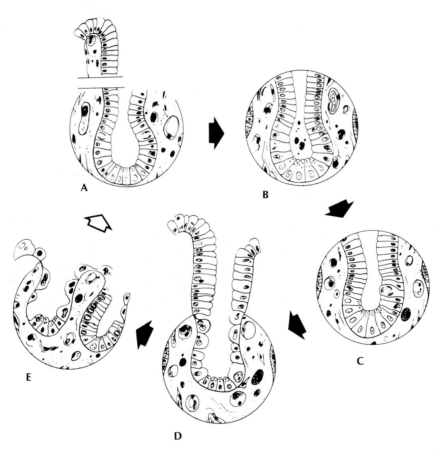

Fig. 5-13. Acute radiation injury to epithelium of small intestine. **A,** Normal state. Crypt area consists of basally situated Paneth cells, zone of proliferating cells, and narrow band of differentiating cells immediately beneath gland neck. Villus is lined by mature, epithelial cells, which undergo continuous migration to cell-extrusion zone at villus tip. **B,** Six hours after irradiation. Notice inhibition of mitosis and pronounced necrosis of immature cells in proliferative zone. **C,** Twelve to 24 hours after irradiation. Inhibition of mitosis ceases with large number of abortive cell divisions, many of which are abnormal and result in death of involved cells or abnormal daughter cells. **D,** One to 6 days after irradiation. In absence of effective cell division, epithelial cell population continues to diminish and many of residual cells are abnormally large and pleomorphic. Villi become progressively shortened, and residual abnormal cells spread out, possibly to preserve in part the integrity of the epithelial barrier. **E,** Six to 8 days after irradiation. If regeneration is to occur, small foci of regenerating epithelium are evident by end of first week. (After White, D.C.: Atlas of radiation histopathology, ERDA Report TID-26676.)

hematopoietic syndrome is very similar. With the exception of lymphocytes, the mature elements of the peripheral blood are remarkably resistant to the effects of radiation. However, they have a finite life span and cannot reproduce themselves. After whole-body exposure of sufficient magnitude, the majority of bone-marrow stem cells are damaged or dead and therefore are not available for division and maturation in order to replace those cells lost by natural attrition. The consequences of this situation, in order of appearance, are lymphopenia, thrombocytopenia, neutropenia, and anemia.

The severity of the acute radiation syndrome depends primarily on the number of surviving stem cells in mitotically active tissues. These cells constitute the only available source of the cells required for the restoration of tissue integrity.

Repair and regeneration

After whole-body exposure, recovery of damaged-cell populations occurs by two primary mechanisms: (1) repair of nonlethal injuries in individual cells and (2) proliferation of radioresistant or otherwise spared stem cells. The latter mechanism is of prime importance in the recovery of the bone marrow and the gastrointestinal tract after whole-body exposure. Stem cell proliferation begins almost immediately after irradiation, generally within 24 to 48 hours. In the bone marrow, recruitment of previously nondividing stem cells, which appear to serve as a reserve component for just such occasions, accelerates the process. Production of additional stem cells appears to have preference over the maturational phases. Some 2 to 3 weeks after exposure the absolute number of bone-marrow stem cells and other nucleated hematopoietic precursors exceeds preexposure levels. Over the subsequent several weeks this situation is reversed, and normal steady-state dynamics ensues.

RADIATION INJURY IN SPECIFIC TISSUES

In general, the effects of radiation in most tissues are quantitatively related to dose. The magnitude of the resultant loss of function reflects a balance among many factors but especially the number of cells irreparably damaged, the capacity of uninjured cells to undergo hypertrophy and thereby increase function, and the regenerative capability and reserve capacity of the irradiated tissue.

Highly differentiated and complex tissues have poorly developed regenerative capacities. Therefore radiation injury generally results in a dose-dependent loss of functional mass. As with other forms of necrosis, connective tissue proliferation often ensues and, when the involved organ is examined roentgenographically or at autopsy, may serve to mask the magnitude of the atro-

phy. Compensatory hypertrophy and hyperplasia are particularly apparent in the kidney where destruction of one kidney is accompanied by remarkable hypertrophy and hyperplasia of the nonirradiated, contralateral organ.

In some organs radiation injury is transiently associated with enhanced function. An increase in diffusion capacity after extensive exposure of the lung in humans has often been noted clinically. A transient increase in glomerular filtration rate has also been noted under similar circumstances. The basis of these unexpected observations is not clear, but radiation-related vasodilatation has been strongly implicated.

Finally, most organs are composed of a variety of interdependent cell types, each of which responds in a somewhat different fashion to the effects of radiation. Therefore, instead of referring to "radiation pneumonitis," for example, one would be more precise in speaking of radiation injury to the bronchial mucosa, to type I alveolar lining cells, or to capillary endothelial cells. Unfortunately, our knowledge of the response to radiation of the individual components of most organs is very limited. Therefore, despite the inherent oversimplications, much of the subsequent discussion is focused upon the response of an entire organ rather than the effects on individual components.

Skin

Radiation injury of the skin is the best known and most carefully studied of all radiation-induced responses in humans. During accidental or therapeutic exposures to most kinds of radiation, the skin generally receives the largest dose. The skin is also a good biologic dosimeter because of the great predictability of its response to various doses.

After sufficiently large exposures, there occurs a series of skin reactions, which often overlap. In chronological order, these are erythema, epilation, bleb formation, necrosis often accompanied by ulceration, and repair, which is generally associated with hyperpigmentation. The first sign of radiation damage to the skin is the development of an erythema, which resembles sunburn. Erythema occurs in 50% of persons who receive more than 600 rad to the skin. A dose of as little as 200 rad of soft radiation may produce temporary epilation. The scalp and face are especially sensitive. Regrowth of hair is usually complete in 3 to 6 months. Dry desquamation and wet desquamation (ulceration) occur after approximately 1000 and 2000 rad respectively. These effects are reliable end points for study as well as potential undesirable side effects for the radiotherapist to keep in mind.

Chronic radiodermatitis manifests itself in several ways: (1) an atrophic, thin, parchment-like tissue that exhibits hyperkeratosis with telangiectasia and increased pigmentation; (2) an unusual susceptibility to injury with poor healing capabilities and a propensity for ulcer formation; and (3) an increased incidence of malignant tumors.

Shortly after the discovery of x rays, radiation "burns" became an occupational as well as a therapeutic problem. In 1902 the first neoplasm attributed to radiation injury was reported. The tumor was an epidermoid carcinoma of the hand; the patient was an x-ray tube maker. Within the next decade more than 90 similar cases were reported among physicians and others exposed occupationally to ionizing radiation. The tumors generally involved the hands and arose in sites of antecedent radiodermatitis. The majority of the neoplasms were epidermoid carcinomas and were associated with a long latent period. With respect to neoplasia, latent period refers to the interval between irradiation and the appearance of the tumor. The peak incidence of radiation-induced skin tumors occurred approximately 8 years after the initial exposure.

With the advent of adequate protective measures, epidermoid carcinoma is no longer an occupational hazard among radiologists. More recently, however, there have been reports of radiodermatitis and radiation carcinogenesis among dentists and others who have used radiation equipment without strict adherence to protective guidelines.

The acute dose required to induce skin cancer is believed to be in excess of 1000 roentgens, which greatly exceeds the $LD_{50(60)}$ dose for humans. This discrepancy accounts for the fact that, up to now, the prevalence of skin cancer is not increased among the atomic bomb survivors, most of whom were exposed in whole-body fashion.

The mechanisms involved in radiation carcinogenesis of the skin are reasonably well known. A high incidence of neoplasia is associated with doses of radiation that result in ulcers with residual local vascular damage and scarring. Permanent damage to hair follicles also appears to be important. The subsequent neoplasms appear to arise from proliferating epithelial cells at the margin of ulcers or in association with irreparably damaged hair follicles. In approximately 30% of cases, multiple tumors are present.

Cardiovascular system

For a long time the heart was believed to be extremely radioresistant. Recently reexamination of this supposition has been prompted by a remarkable increase in cardiac complications among persons who have received large amounts of curative therapeutic radiation to the mediastinum for Hodgkin's disease and other neoplasms.

Radiation-induced heart disease has been reported in 5.8% of patients irradiated to the mediastinum for ma-

lignant lymphoma and 3.4% patients irradiated prophylactically after a simple or a radical mastectomy for carcinoma of the breast. The most common abnormality is fibrous pericarditis, often accompanied by effusion, which may organize, constrict the heart, and necessitate pericardectomy. Diffuse interstitial fibrosis of the myocardium is also not an infrequent finding. Although important, these abnormalities are rarely life threatening.

In contradistinction to the heart and major vessels, the smaller components of the vascular system have for some time been known to be extremely susceptible to both the acute and delayed effects of ionizing radiation. Erythema of skin is an early response to radiation injury and is believed to relate to vasodilatation and increased vascular permeability, probably secondary to endothelial injury. Endothelium is of intermediate radiosensitivity, and injury is manifest morphologically by swelling and necrosis. Such changes are particularly pronounced with respect to the nucleus. Endothelial injury is often accompanied by subintimal edema. Although the endothelium is the most radiosensitive component, no element of the vessel wall is immune to the effects of irradiation. Pronounced changes that involve each element of the vessel wall are shown in Fig. 5-14. The functional consequences of vascular injury probably relate to varying degrees of interstitial edema and, less commonly, perivascular hemorrhage and thrombosis.

Chronic vascular changes associated with radiation injury are most conspicuous in arterioles and capillaries. They consist in segmental sclerosis and thickening of the wall, narrowing of the lumen, and reduplication of the endothelial cells, which may also be increased in size. Some of these changes are shown in Fig. 5-15.

Animal experiments have demonstrated the arterial system to be more radiosensitive than the venous system and have also shown that arterioles and capillaries are more sensitive than arteries. Injury to arterioles and capillaries, with resultant relative ischemia, involves virtually every tissue and may be responsible for many of the delayed effects of radiation.

Some of the acute and chronic changes associated with radiation injury of blood vessels are summarized diagrammatically in Fig. 5-16.

Lung

Radiation injury to the lung is primarily associated with inhalation of radioactive substances or as a consequence of radiotherapy for carcinoma of the lung, esophagus, or breast or mediastinal tumors. The magnitude of injury appears to depend on several factors but especially the total dose, the dose rate, and the presence or absence of preexisting lung disease such as one of the pneumoconioses.

Little is known about the acute effects of radiation

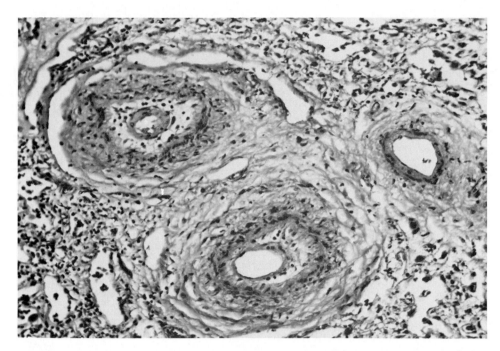

Fig. 5-14. Acute radiation injury involving pulmonary arterioles. A 2-year-old girl received 4000 rad of ionizing radiation for metastatic undifferentiated carcinoma 9 weeks before death. Arterioles show necrosis of endothelial cells, edema of subintimal region, edema and focal necrosis of media, and edema of adventitia. Acute and chronic inflammatory cells are present throughout vessel wall.

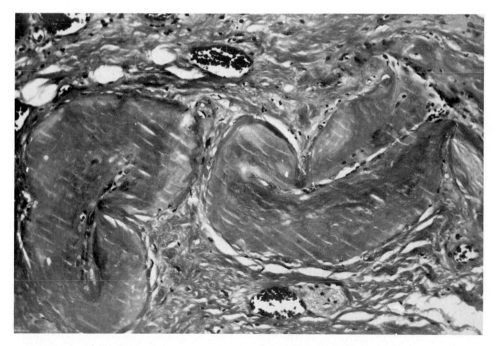

Fig. 5-15. Chronic radiation injury involving small artery of rectum of 66-year-old woman who received 4500 rad to uterus 22 years before death. Vessel shows thickening of wall with accumulation of hyaline-like substance and near complete occlusion of lumen.

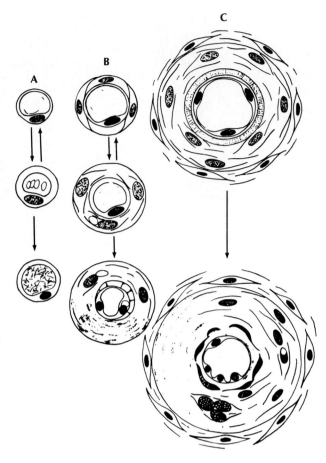

Fig. 5-16. Radiation injury involving capillary, arteriole, and small artery. **A,** Capillary. Acute response of capillary is dilatation accompanied by increased permeability. This is followed by narrowing of lumen from swelling of endothelial cells and sclerosis of vessel wall. Later a thrombus may form and occlude lumen completely. **B,** Arteriole. Changes in arteriole are similar to those noted in capillary. Initial vasodilatation is followed by endothelial swelling and edema of smooth muscle, both of which serve to narrow lumen. Subsequent degenerative changes include endothelial proliferation, subendothelial deposition of hyalin-like substance, and thickening of vessel wall with focal destruction of smooth muscle cells. **C,** Small artery. Because small arteries are fairly rigid structures, early changes are less pronounced. With passage of time, however, progressive damage to endothelium and media becomes evident. There is fragmentation and discontinuity of internal elastic lamella, degenerative changes in smooth muscle of media with large accumulations of hyalin-like substance, and fibrosis of the adventitia. (After White, D.C.: Atlas of radiation histopathology, ERDA Report TID-26676.)

injury to the human lung. Persons who die shortly after whole-body exposure generally exhibit significant alveolar damage, which may, at least in part, be related to systemic disturbances such as septicemia, fluid and electrolyte abnormalities, and shock. Experimentally, the primary acute local alterations in the lung consist of interstitial and intra-alveolar edema with hyaline membrane formation. The latter changes are associated with swelling of the endothelial cells of small blood vessels and are probably related to increased capillary permeability. Direct injury to type I alveolar lining cells is often manifested by necrosis. Organization and repair of the acute changes lead to interstitial fibrosis and vascular sclerosis. At autopsy, these lungs are pale, rubbery, and less crepitant than normal.

The morphologic abnormalities described above are summarized diagrammatically in Fig. 5-17. They are referred to as acute and chronic radiation pneumonitis, though they are associated with surprisingly little in the way of an inflammatory response. The functional correlates of these structural changes include a deterioration of most of the measures of pulmonary function, especially when reserve capacity is tested, as during exercise. Because the pathologic changes are distributed irregularly, the normal ventilation-perfusion relationships are altered, and impaired gas exchange re-

sults. A reduction in the compliance of the whole lung occurs as well. When severe, these functional abnormalities are associated with dyspnea, especially on exertion. As with any interstitial pulmonary inflammatory process, a nonproductive chronic cough is also a prominent feature of severe radiation pneumonitis.

External irradiation of the thorax is associated with a moderate increase in the incidence of carcinoma of the lung in humans, especially when combined with other carcinogenic influences such as smoking. Inhalation of radioactive particles of a size and configuration known to reach the gas-exchange zone distal to the terminal bronchioles results in a much higher incidence of pulmonary neoplasms than external irradiation does. In this connection, carcinoma of the lung has been recognized for some time to be an occupational disability among certain groups of miners. For example, in the period 1921 to 1926, 50% of the deaths among the miners in the Schneeberg region of Saxony were attributable to carcinoma of the lung. An increased mortality from lung cancer has also been reported among fluorspar miners in Newfoundland, iron ore miners in Britain, uranium miners of the Colorado Plateau of the United States, and tungsten, fluorspar, and lithium miners in Czechoslovakia. Only recently, however, has it been shown that the excessive number of deaths from

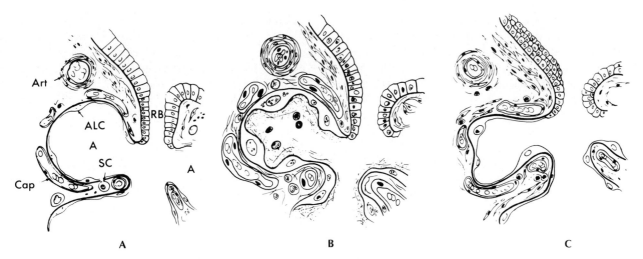

Fig. 5-17. Radiation injury to pulmonary parenchyma. **A,** Normal parenchyma. *A,* Alveolus; *ALC,* alveolar lining cell; *Art,* arteriole; *Cap,* capillary; *RB,* respiratory bronchiole; *SC,* septal cell. **B,** Acute radiation pneumonitis. Notice capillary dilatation and swelling of endothelial cells. This may result in interstitial edema and loss of proteinaceous fluid into alveoli with formation of hyaline membranes. Septal cells respond to pulmonary edema by migrating into alveoli. Notice also prominent enlargement and pleomorphism of alveolar lining cells and ciliated columnar epithelium that lines terminal bronchioles. **C,** Chronic radiation pneumonitis. Pronounced arteriolar sclerosis is associated with severe septal fibrosis. Bronchiolar epithelium is metaplastic. (After White, D.C.: Atlas of radiation histopathology, ERDA Report TID-26676.)

carcinoma of the lung is attributable to radiation. Underground mines, and especially uranium mines, contain variable amounts of the gaseous radionuclide radon. Radon 222 and its radioactive daughters attach to aerosol products in the environment. When inhaled, the aerosols are distributed throughout the tracheobronchial tree primarily on the basis of size. The smaller particles, particularly those between 0.1 and 1 μm in diameter, reach the bronchioles and alveoli where they remain trapped to deliver high-LET radiation to the surrounding lung parenchyma. Recently, radon in the home has caused citizen concern in some regions of the United States and Canada.

Determination of dose-incidence relationships among various groups of miners is complicated by uncertainties about the circumstances of irradiation. In addition to the usual demographic considerations, corrections need to be made for cigarette consumption and the relative proportions of individual radon daughters in the atmosphere. Therefore estimates of the cumulative dose received by a person over a prolonged period of time have until recently been fraught with uncertainty.

In miners who develop carcinoma of the lung, the average duration of exposure is 15 to 20 years. Small cell undifferentiated carcinoma is the most frequent type of tumor. Among the uranium miners, and perhaps other mining populations as well, cigarette smoking appears to be a potent cocarcinogen.

Cigarette smoke is known to contain several chemical carcinogens. Recently it has been suggested that one or more radionuclides may act as a synergistic agent in the cigarette-related carcinoma of the lung. Two radionuclides implicated in this regard are polonium 210 and lead 210. The former is an alpha emitter of the uranium series, which is present in trace amounts in most plants and foodstuffs. Lead 210 is also present in cigarette smoke in the form of insoluble particles of high specific activity that are derived from the combustion of trichromes in the tobacco leaf. The insoluble lead-210 particle, which is retained in the lung and has a physical half-life of 22 years, decays by beta emission to polonium 210.

Gastrointestinal tract

The sequence of radiation-induced alterations in the mucous membranes of the mouth and upper digestive tract is similar to that seen in the skin, but clinical evidence of injury appears much more quickly in the former site. Salivary gland exposure results in noticeable swelling of the gland, which may be associated with an elevation in serum amylase levels and dryness of the mouth (xerostomia). The response of the oral mucosa and salivary glands is of particular interest because radiotherapy appears to be the treatment of choice in many tumors of the head and neck, and these structures often must be included in the treatment field.

Some aspects of radiation damage to the alimentary tract have been discussed previously under the acute radiation syndrome. The onset of acute esophagitis, gastritis, enteritis, colitis, and proctitis occurs 1 to 3 weeks after exposure, depending primarily on how much of the gastrointestinal tract is irradiated and on the exposure level. The morphologic consequences of such exposure are the result of a loss of the regenerative capacity of stem cells, which are the precursors of the epithelial lining cells. The attendant symptoms resemble those associated with other ulcerative disorders.

The delayed sequelae of gastrointestinal exposure include strictures, chronic ulcers, and malignant tumors. Strictures are responsible for varying degrees of obstruction, whereas ulcers predispose to perforation and hemorrhage. Ulcers may involve any part of the alimentary tract, but the colon, rectum, and stomach are particularly susceptible. As shown in Fig. 5-18, radiation-induced injury to small blood vessels, and especially small arteries and arterioles, appears to be responsible for most of these late sequelae. The resultant

vascular insufficiency causes atrophy of the mucosa and reactive fibrosis. The atrophic mucosa is especially prone to ulcer formation. Corrective surgery is difficult because of vascular insufficiency and poor healing of anastomotic sites. Carcinogenesis has been implicated as a delayed effect of exposure of the gastrointestinal tract in humans. Primary sites include the colon, esophagus, stomach, and probably the pancreas.

Liver

The liver is of intermediate radioresistivity and well-defined morphologic alterations are associated with radiation doses employed clinically. Thus a significant number of patients who receive 4000 rad or more to the entire liver develop radiation hepatitis. Although still the subject of some controversy, the pathogenesis of this disorder appears to stem from occlusion of the small hepatic veins. The characteristic morphologic alterations include dilatation of the central veins, centrilobular congestion with focal hemorrhage, and variable degrees of necrosis and atrophy of parenchymal cells. Children are more susceptible than adults to radiation hepatitis. The nutritional status of the host also appears to influence the magnitude of the necrosis. Portal fibrosis may be a late sequela of radiation-induced necrosis.

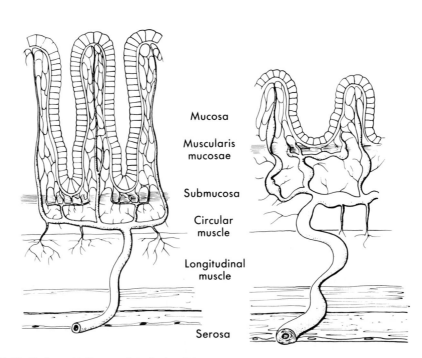

Fig. 5-18. Delayed effects of radiation injury to intestine. Majority of effects are related to abnormalities of vascular supply. Segmental sclerosis is most pronounced in small arteries and arterioles with secondary ectasia and loss of capillaries. Resultant relative tissue ischemia causes loss of the more differentiated cell populations, especially epithelial cells, and reactive fibrosis. Atrophic mucosa is particularly prone to ulceration. (After White, D.C.: Atlas of radiation histopathology, ERDA, Report TID-26676.)

The available evidence indicates that external irradiation of the liver is rarely associated with delayed sequelae. On the other hand, administration of thorium dioxide (Thorotrast) for diagnostic imaging purposes with subsequent localization and retention in the Kupffer cells has been associated with cirrhosis, hepatic cell carcinoma, cholangiocarcinoma, and hemangioendothelioma.

Bone marrow

The bone marrow is extremely sensitive to both the acute and the delayed effects of ionizing radiation. Acute necrosis of hematopoietic stem cells is primarily responsible for the panhypoplasia of the bone marrow and the cytopenias noted in the peripheral blood that are associated with whole-body exposure in the 200 to 1000 rad range. In terms of delayed effects, leukemia and related disorders are among the most frequently encountered malignancies after partial- or whole-body exposure. Degenerative changes, such as marrow fibrosis, are an infrequent complication of whole-body exposure but are not unusual after regional or local irradiation.

The leukemogenic action of radiation was initially recognized in 1911 in a report that dealt with five instances of leukemia among radiation workers. The authors of the report suggested that occupational exposure may have been a significant factor in the development of the disease. Since 1911, well over 500 cases of leukemia have been attributed to occupational, therapeutic, or accidental exposure. These cases involve most of the irradiated human populations. The type of leukemia depends primarily on the age at the time of exposure and the conditions of irradiation. In this connection, whole-body exposure is more leukemogenic than local irradiation, fractionated doses are more leukemogenic than single exposures, and irradiation primarily increases those types of leukemia that are most likely to occur in the age group at risk. Thus acute and chronic myelogenous leukemias are associated with irradiation in adult life, whereas acute lymphatic leukemia is more characteristic of the exposure of children. Up to now, no evidence exists to indicate that the incidence of chronic lymphocytic leukemia is influenced by irradiation.

In persons irradiated for ankylosing spondylitis and in the atomic bomb survivors, an increased incidence of leukemia first became evident 1 to 2 years after exposure, reached a peak after 3 to 7 years, and then declined to approximate background levels over the subsequent 15 to 35 years.

An increased rate of occurrence of malignant lymphoma has been reported among the pioneer American radiologists, persons irradiated for ankylosing spondylitis, and possibly the Hiroshima atomic bomb survivors.

Multiple myeloma is also increased in prevalence among the early American radiologists, persons irradiated for ankylosing spondylitis, atomic bomb survivors, radium-dial painters, workers in the nuclear industry, and patients given thorium dioxide. The magnitude of increase with respect to radiation-related lymphoma and multiple myeloma is less than that noted for leukemia.

Genitourinary system

The kidney is known to be moderately radiosensitive, but controversy exists with respect to the radiosensitivity of the various components and thus the pathogenesis of the acute and chronic effects. Injury to the convoluted tubules and small blood vessels has been most strongly implicated in this regard.

Acute radiation injury of the kidney is generally accompanied by tubular necrosis, vasodilatation, interstitial edema, and proteinuria. After a variable asymptomatic latent period, progressive vascular and tubular changes develop quite regularly in people and experimental animals exposed to large doses. In most cases, the sclerosis of the small blood vessels proceeds slowly, often accompanied by varying degrees of hypertension. The vascular lesions result in ischemia of nephrons with consequent hyalinization of glomeruli. Tubular injury is manifest by significant atrophy. Grossly the kidney of chronic radiation nephritis is small with a thin cortex and a finely irregular surface.

Clinically most instances of radiation nephritis terminate in renal failure with uremia, hypervolemia, dyspnea, headache, and vomiting. Rapid acceleration of the process with pronounced hypertension, evidence of increased intracranial pressure, and abnormalities of the optic fundus are suggestive of malignant hypertension. Recovery from radiation nephritis is possible only when the damage is unilateral and the involved kidney is removed.

Effects reminiscent of those described above have been documented experimentally with radioisotopes known to localize in the kidney; however, up to now, this has not been a significant problem in humans. Similarly, although rodents develop renal tumors as a consequence of whole-body or local exposure, radiation-induced tumors have not been reported in man, with the possible exception of a few cases associated with the administration of thorium dioxide.

In contrast with the kidney, where chronic effects are of paramount importance, the urinary bladder is highly susceptible to acute radiation injury. This is to be expected because the bladder mucosa undergoes constant replacement. The response of the urinary bladder to such injury is similar to that noted for skin except that the presence of urine, especially with a denuded mucosa, tends to exacerbate the situation. Initial hyperemia is often followed by suppression of normal cell division, loss of mucosal cells, and ulceration. Contracture, infection, and carcinogenesis are other important complications of chronic radiation injury of the bladder.

The germinal epithelium of the testes is extremely radiosensitive. Even after exposures at low dose levels, recovery is very slow and may never be complete. Acutely, radiation produces an immediate suppression of mitosis followed by necrosis of the germinal epithelial cells. Spermatogonia are more sensitive than spermatocytes and spermatids. Persistent effects include sclerosis of seminiferous tubules and hyalinization of blood vessels. In more severe cases there may be total tubular atrophy with hyalinization. Sertoli cells and interstitial cells are radioresistant.

The ovary is also very radiosensitive. Within several days after exposure to 300 rad, the human ovary shows a sharp increase in atretic follicles. However, a few primary primordial oocytes and their follicular epithelium are spared. Thus, about 6 months later, the cortex contains a few maturing follicles in an otherwise atrophic fibrous parenchyma.

Cartilage and bone

With respect to radiation-induced injury to cartilage and bone, it is important to distinguish between growing and mature tissues. Growing cartilage and bone are relatively radiosensitive, and exposure often results in growth abnormalities. Abnormal growth of the spine resulting in scoliosis is of particular importance because of the not infrequent exposure of this structure during the irradiation of abdominal tumors in children. The effect of externally applied radiation upon developing bone and cartilage is predictable: a reduction in the numbers of mitoses and disorderly maturation followed by the asymptomatic degeneration and necrosis of less mature elements. Proliferating chondroblasts are more sensitive than osteoblasts. Recovery is possible if there is a more radioresistant population of nondividing reserve cells unless there is also severe damage to the small blood vessels that supply the area. However, subtle abnormalities often persist in the form of a disoriented microstructure, which may be associated with a loss of normal tensile strength. In addition, even temporary interruption of normal growth results in a stunted bone.

In contradistinction to this, mature cartilage and bone are among the most radioresistant tissues of the body. Radionecrosis of mature bone and cartilage is unusual and when present appears to be related to injury to the arterioles and capillaries that supply these tissues. The resultant ischemia causes degeneration and necrosis of parenchymal cells and loss of tensile strength. Another consequence of such injury is an increased susceptibility to infection.

Bone-seeking radionuclides induce injury in a fashion similar to that described for external irradiation. Thus "radium jaw" among the early luminous-dial painters was first described in 1924 by Beum, a New York dentist. The changes in the maxilla and mandible of these patients consisted in arrested maturation of bone among young patients, localized regions of bone resorption, resorption of teeth, and foci of sclerosis, bone necrosis, and pathologic fractures. The abnormalities seen in the facial bones of these people were mirrored by comparable changes elsewhere in the skeleton. However, because of the frequent association of tooth decay and infection, the oral manifestations of osteoradionecrosis tended to become evident clinically while similar lesions elsewhere remained asymptomatic. In addition to these degenerative changes, a variety of malignant tumors have been documented among the radium-dial painters. The first reports, which concerned the development of osteogenic sarcoma, began to appear some 10 years after the initial exposure to this bone-seeking radionuclide.

Definition of a dose-incidence relationship for bone tumors induced by internal emitters such as radium is complicated by several factors. In the first place, the isotope is not distributed uniformly within the skeleton. Regions of intense localization result in "hot spots," which contain more radioactivity than the surrounding bone does, often by a factor of 10 or more. Second, changes occur with time in the distribution of the radioelement and its decay daughters. Such shifts result from the metabolic turnover of the bone constituents and the redistribution and excretion of the internal emitters. Last, the magnitude of exposure is influenced by the progressive diminution in the dose rate of the emitted radiation because of the physical decay of the isotope. Despite these problems in determining dose-response relationships, the incidence of bone tumors is believed to vary approximately as the square of the terminal concentration of radium in the skeleton. Such a relationship is consistent with comparable observations in experimental animals.

Tumors other than osteogenic sarcomas have been reported after radium exposure. They include not only soft-tissue tumors, such as fibrosarcomas, but also carcinomas of the epithelial cells that line the paranasal sinuses, the mastoid air cells, the gingival tissues, and the nasopharynx. These epithelial cells, because of their proximity to the bones of the skull, were also exposed to significant amounts of radiation. Recently, an apparent increase in the prevalence of blood dyscrasias, multiple myeloma, and malignant tumors of the central nervous system has also been noted in this group.

Lesions similar to those described have developed among patients treated with "radium water" and the inhabitants of regions of the world where the drinking water contains significant amounts of radium. Benign tumors, principally exostoses, have also been noted in children treated with radium.

Rare instances of osteosarcoma have been reported in association with therapeutic irradiation utilizing an external source. The doses have been extremely large, ranging from 3000 to more than 15,000 rad, with an average latent period of 9 years.

Thyroid

An increased incidence of thyroid tumors has been noted among Japanese atomic bomb survivors, the Marshallese who were accidently exposed to nuclear fallout, and children irradiated therapeutically for "status thymolymphaticus" or tinea capitis. Jewish persons, females, and children less than 10 years of age at the time of exposure appear to be particularly susceptible. An increased prevalence has also been noted among adult Japanese atomic bomb survivors, principally women, who were exposed to 50 rad or more. Papillary adenocarcinomas, adenomas, and hyperplastic nodules have been associated with exposure. The majority of the carcinomas noted among the Hiroshima and Nagasaki survivors were noted for the first time at autopsy and did not apparently cause symptoms before death. Some of the adenomas documented among the Marshall Islanders were associated with hypothyroidism.

The incidence of carcinoma of the thyroid appears to be increasing in the United States, perhaps as a result of prior irradiation of children for benign conditions of the head and neck. For this reason, persons with a history of exposure to this region should be carefully followed medically with particular attention to the thyroid. In addition, patients with suspected thyroid tumors should be questioned about prior irradiation of the head and neck region.

A relationship between iodine-131 administration for thyrotoxicosis and carcinoma of the thyroid has been postulated but not confirmed. If such a relationship exists, it must be rare. The reason for this may be the severe local destructive effect of the doses employed (5000 to 50,000 rad or more to the thyroid), which probably destroys entirely the epithelial component of the gland.

Breast

An increased incidence of carcinoma of the breast has been documented among several populations of women exposed to ionizing radiation: the Japanese atomic bomb survivors, tuberculous patients who received multiple chest fluoroscopies to monitor pneumothorax therapy, and persons in whom one or both breasts were irradiated for a variety of benign conditions including acute postpartum mastitis, unilateral hypertrophy, and fibroadenomatosis. Analysis of these data shows that the female breast is extremely sensitive to radiation carcinogenesis, with the risk of developing such tumors in-

creasing approximately linearly with increasing dose. Risk is also heavily dependent upon age at exposure, with women below 40 years particularly vulnerable. For this reason, mammographic screening of women below 40 is generally limited to persons with a history of breast cancer. Similarly, routine screening mammography for women ages 40 to 49 years is recommended only if they have a history of breast cancer or if a mother or a sister has breast cancer. In this context, a distinction must be made between screening and evaluation. Mammography is an important diagnostic tool in a woman with suspected breast cancer, irrespective of age.

Among irradiated persons an increased incidence of carcinoma of the breast begins within 10 years of exposure and persists for at least 30 years. The mean latent period is approximately 25 years. The vast majority of tumors are infiltrating ductal adenocarcinomas.

Central nervous system

As noted previously, the development of the brain may be severely disturbed by exposure to relatively small amounts of radiation during early embryonic development. Mature nervous tissue is relatively resistant to acute morphologic changes though functional abnormalities are often encountered, especially after wholebody exposure to doses in excess of 5000 rad (see under discussion of central nervous system syndrome). Late morphologic abnormalities of the brain are not uncommon, however, especially after local exposure. Focal necrosis, often associated with demyelination, is a frequent manifestation. The white matter is more susceptible than the gray matter to focal necrosis, perhaps because of its less abundant vasculature.

Irradiation of the spinal cord can also lead to acute necrosis. In such a situation, the cord usually has been unavoidably included in the treatment field of a thoracic or abdominal tumor. Vascular injury and thrombosis of small blood vessels are believed to be responsible for the necrosis of the spinal cord, which in its most severe form may result in permanent paraplegia and a syndrome known as transverse myelitis.

Eyes

Either single or multiple exposures of the optic lens can result in the formation of opacities, which may progress to clinically significant cataracts. Cataract formation depends on the magnitude of the dose and the character of the radiation; densely ionizing radiation is especially cataractogenic. A single acute exposure is more injurious and produces opacities sooner than the same dose administered in divided exposures.

Other tumors

Such a wide variety of neoplasms has been reported in exposed animals that radiation must be considered to be potentially carcinogenic for almost all tissues under the proper conditions of dose, shielding, host responsiveness, and exposure to the relevant cocarcinogens. Although most tissues may be potentially susceptible to radiation-induced carcinogenesis, individual organs vary greatly with respect to their relative susceptibility. Quantitation of relative susceptibility is not yet possible in humans because most of the irradiated populations have not been followed until the death of all members. In this connection, the risk of developing a malignant tumor is greatest when the exposed population enters the age span at which that particular form of neoplasm most commonly occurs. However, as shown in Fig. 5-10, among atomic bomb survivors, neoplasms of the hematopoietic system show the greatest increase in relative risk.

RADIOTHERAPY

Late in the nineteenth century, Wilhelm Konrad Roentgen's discovery of a "new kind of ray," coupled with the discovery of radium by Marie and Pierre Curie, launched a new era in medicine. Physicians quickly began to use x rays and radium diagnostically and therapeutically. X rays and radium became the treatment of choice for almost every type of illness imaginable. As a result, many tragic examples of radiation injury, of both patients and physicians, occurred and were subsequently documented. Unfortunately the untoward effects often were not manifest until many years later, and only recently have stringent controls been adopted to protect patients, physicians, and technical personnel.

On the positive side, the therapeutic value of radiation was quickly recognized, and the complete eradication of otherwise fatal tumors was reported. A new discipline of medicine was soon launched, and today radiotherapy, singly or with surgery and chemotherapy, represents the treatment of choice for several types of neoplasms. Before a more detailed consideration of radiation as a therapeutic modality is presented, it is important to review a few aspects of the radiobiology of tumors.

Tumor radiobiology

Fig. 5-19 shows a hypothetical dose-response curve for tumor cells grown in tissue culture and irradiated. The narrow shoulder indicates that these cells are relatively poorly equipped to repair sublethal damage. The steep slope of the linear portion of the curve indicates that the tumor cells are relatively radiosensitive. The exponential character of the curve indicates that most cells are killed by small amounts of radiation but that a large dose is required to kill the last viable malignant cell. Put another way, it requires the same dose to reduce the number of viable cells from 10^7 to 10^6 (a re-

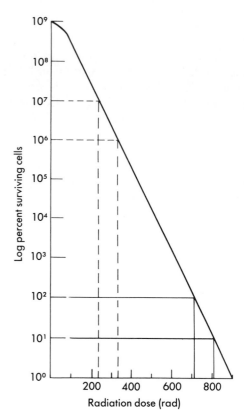

Fig. 5-19. Hypothetical survival curve for tumor cells.

duction of 9 million cells) as from 10^2 to 10^1 (a reduction of 90 cells). The critical task of the radiotherapist in attempting to eradicate a malignant tumor is either to kill all tumor cells or to reduce the number to such a level that host defense mechanisms can complete the task. The radiotherapist must accomplish this without undue injury to adjacent normal tissues and intervening vital structures. In balancing these competing objectives, the radiotherapist is greatly assisted by the difference between normal and abnormal cells with respect to repair of radiation-induced injury. This relationship is shown schematically in Fig. 5-20. The injury created among the normal and abnormal cells by each individual exposure dose, or fraction, is the same. However, the time interval (24 to 72 hours) between the completion of one radiation exposure and the start of the next provides a period for both the normal and abnormal cells to repair radiation-induced lesions. Since normal tissues generally possess a greater capability for repair than neoplastic cells do, a larger fraction of the former is present at the beginning of each subsequent treatment. For this reason, most radiation treatments are fractioned and protracted over a period of several weeks or months.

Fig. 5-21 depicts the effect of treatment, as a function

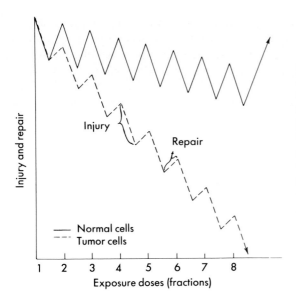

Fig. 5-20. Effect of fractionization on response of normal and neoplastic cells to radiation-induced injury. Although magnitude of injury is the same for most normal and neoplastic tissues, as illustrated by identical down segments of two curves, normal tissues generally have greater recovery ability, represented by up segments of curves. Therefore, with fractionization, normal tissue survives radiation injury more effectively than tumor does. (Modified from Kligerman, M.M.: Principles of radiation therapy. In Holland, J.F., and Frei, E., editors: Cancer medicine, Philadelphia, 1973, Lea & Febiger.)

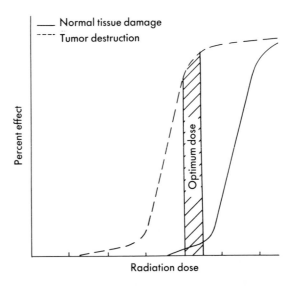

Fig. 5-21. Effect of treatment as function of dose with respect to normal and abnormal cells. Optimal dose for specific tumor-host system is amount of radiation that will cause greatest number of tumor cells to be destroyed in exchange for minimal amount of normal tissue damage. (After Kligerman, M.M.: Principles of radiation therapy. In Holland, J.F., and Frei, E., editors: Cancer medicine, Philadelphia, 1973, Lea & Febiger.)

of radiation dose, on normal and malignant cells. The optimal dose is the amount of radiation that will kill the greatest number of tumor cells while simultaneously injuring the smallest possible number of normal cells. Although a small amount of normal tissue destruction is acceptable, the dose must not be so large as to approach the linear portion of the "normal tissue damage" curve in Fig. 5-21.

Types of radiation generators

X and gamma rays cover a broad range of wavelengths. Within this range, the shorter the wavelength, the greater the energy and penetrating power of the rays. For this reason long wavelengths generated at 30 to 80 keV are used for routine diagnostic procedures in radiology. Although most of the radiation is absorbed by the skin, enough energy reaches the underlying structures to provide a satisfactory roentgenographic or fluoroscopic image. In radiation therapy, shorter wavelengths are generally employed to deliver a greater proportion of the energy to deeper structures. Hence, x-ray machines designed for diagnostic purposes are not used for radiotherapy. It also follows that a given dose of x rays from a diagnostic machine will produce greater skin damage and less injury to underlying tissues than the same dose delivered by a therapy machine.

On the basis of the foregoing discussion, it is evident that a variety of radiation energies must be available to treat patients with dissimilar tumors in optimal fashion. For example, energies in the lower ranges, 50 to 100 keV, are employed to treat superficial lesions such as the majority of skin tumors. On the other hand, energies in the orthovoltage range, 200 to 400 keV, are used to treat larger or more aggressive skin tumors such as carcinomas of the lower lip, whereas energies in the supervoltage range, 2 MeV or greater, are important in the treatment of most deep-seated tumors.

X rays are usually produced when electrons are accelerated to a variable degree and then are permitted to strike a tungsten target. Absorption of the energy by the target results in the production of electromagnetic radiation and heat. Depending on the energy imparted to the electrons, x rays in the superficial orthovoltage or supervoltage range are produced. The Van de Graaff generator and the linear accelerator are two machines used to accelerate electrons. The latter is the more common supervoltage machine in use today.

Currently there is considerable interest in the use of neutrons and other high-LET particles in radiotherapy because of their ability to kill anoxic tumor cells. So much ionization is produced when heavy particles pass through tissues that little recovery is possible regardless of the presence or absence of oxygen. Therefore the relative advantage enjoyed by tumor cells, which are generally less well oxygenated than the surrounding normal tissues, is largely abolished. Although neutrons were first employed to treat malignant tumors in the late 1930s, the initial experience was marred by significant injury to adjacent normal tissues. At that time, the concept of relative biologic effectiveness and the inhibition of normal tissue repair by heavy-particle irradiation had not yet been appreciated. Because of extensive injury to normal tissues and a variety of unfortunate complications, neutron therapy lost favor among radiotherapists until the past several years when interest again developed based upon a better understanding of the biologic effects of this particle.

Palliative and curative therapy

Radiation therapy may be employed to relieve symptoms caused by an inoperable tumor or to eradicate totally a malignant neoplasm. In many medical centers radiation represents the treatment of choice for stage I and stage II malignant lymphomas, certain epidermoid carcinomas of the laryngeal glottis, epidermoid carcinomas of the skin and lip, invasive epidermoid carcinomas of the pharynx, most carcinomas of the mouth, and select transitional cell carcinomas of the urinary bladder. Curative radiotherapy is also often employed with surgery in one of two ways: (1) prophylactically, when the surgeon believes that the tumor has been completely removed but cannot discount the possible presence of tumor cells in areas adjacent to the primary neoplasm such as the draining lymphatics or regional lymph nodes, and (2) therapeutically, when the surgeon is unable to totally resect the tumor because of adjacent vital structures.

Palliative radiotherapy is often employed to relieve symptoms or to abort impending complications. An example of the latter is the irradiation of a tumor metastasis in the neck of the femur or other weight-bearing bone that, if left untreated, might be expected to result in a pathologic fracture. Palliative radiotherapy is also used to relieve pain, which often occurs in association with bone tumor metastases, to relieve compression of a vital structure, such as the spinal cord, or to prevent ulceration by a subcutaneous or submucosal metastasis.

As with surgery, injury to normal tissues is an inevitable consequence of radiation therapy. A margin of normal tissue adjacent to a treatable tumor must be included in the treatment field in order to anticipate possible microscopic extension. Regional lymph nodes are often irradiated to eradicate possible metastases. Intervening tissues and structures are also injured by ionizations. The morphologic consequences of such injury in specific organs are discussed in the previous section.

Radiation therapy can also cause radiation sickness and depress the number of circulating platelets and leukocytes. Radiation sickness is associated with treatment of the thorax or abdomen, most frequently the latter. The symptoms of radiation sickness (fatigue, anorexia, vomiting) are short lived and are usually controlled by small reductions in the daily dose. Leukopenia and thrombocytopenia can occur when large portions of the bone marrow are included in the treatment field and may dictate temporary interruption of treatment.

A small but significant risk of inducing a new malignant tumor exists among irradiated patients. Other complications of radiotherapy include actinic conjunctivitis; cataract formation, especially in children; sterility; transverse myelitis; asymmetric growth retardation in children after exposure of long bones; radiation pneumonitis; radiation pericarditis; and constriction of a hollow viscus (especially the intestine) by fibrous connective tissue.

Radioisotopes

It was noted in the previous discussion that certain naturally occurring substances such as radium, thorium, and actinium give off radiant energy spontaneously. In addition, unstable isotopes of most known elements can be produced artificially. Since the radioactive isotope of an element is essentially identical chemically to the nonradioactive form, these substances have found widespread diagnostic and therapeutic application.

Diagnostic advantage is taken of the known propensity of organs to concentrate specific elements. For example, the thyroid gland concentrates iodine. By the administration of radioactive iodine, the physician can determine, with appropriate counting techniques, the capacity of this gland to concentrate iodine normally. More important, however, the organ can be scanned and the relative distribution of the isotope throughout the gland can be quantitated. Failure of the radioactive iodine to be distributed evenly throughout the gland indicates the possible displacement of normal thyroid by nonfunctioning tissue, for example, a cyst, an abscess, a nonfunctioning adenoma, or a carcinoma. Similar methods are used with other organs.

Radioisotopes are also used therapeutically. The administration of large doses of an isotope such as iodine 131, with a known propensity to concentrate in a specific organ, ensures the release of a significant amount of radioactivity within that organ. This approach may be employed to damage or destroy a malignant tumor or suppress a hyperfunctioning gland. In this connection, it is important to note that the selective concentration of most elements is not complete and therefore other tissues may be exposed, albeit to much smaller doses. This latter observation is of primary concern with the gonads and possible radiation-induced genetic effects.

Finally, it is important to remember that radiation may also be received by the fetus when a radioactive isotope is administered to the mother, who may or may not be aware that she is pregnant. Radioactive strontium, plutonium, phosphorus, tritium, iodine, and many other isotopes cross the placenta and can become incorporated into the fetus. Perhaps the most striking example is radioactive iodine, which, when administered to the mother late in pregnancy, is also concentrated in the fetal thyroid where the resultant radiation-induced injury can result in cretinism. Other examples have been documented experimentally in rodents and have been associated with malformations, neoplasms, and decreased life span in the fetus.

INJURY FROM NONIONIZING RADIATION

Thus far tissue injury caused by ionizing radiation has represented the primary focus of this chapter. In the past several years it has been recognized that tissues may also be injured by nonionizing forms of radiation. Table 5-7 lists some of the known deleterious effects of exposure to various types of nonionizing radiation. The industrial and medical applications of these forms of energy continue to increase dramatically. Therefore the potential for human injury from nonionizing radiation will also increase.

Numerous electronic devices represent potential sources of injury from nonionizing radiation. Currently, popular devices of this type include radar units, microwave ovens, and lasers. Despite the increasing use of these devices, surprisingly little attention has been paid to possible deleterious effects.

Microwaves represent a form of electromagnetic radiation in the frequency rate between ultrahigh frequency television and the infrared region of the spectrum. Potential sources of exposure to microwaves include microwave ovens and the high-output radar devices used in navigation and weather systems as well as burglar alarms. Animal experiments have shown that lens opacities and hematologic, endocrine, and possibly genetic effects can be caused by microwave radiations.

Microwave ovens appear to represent a particular health hazard for several reasons. In the first place, these ovens are becoming increasingly popular. Second, several surveys have documented detectable leakage around the door. And last, most owners and operators appear to be unaware of any radiation hazard.

The laser also represents a potential source of injury of nonionizing radiation. Because of the focusing characteristics of the lens of the eye, the retina is especially vulnerable to laser radiation. Even reflected beams represent a potential hazard. Pulsed lasers, which operate at very high power levels, can cause retina burns in 1 microsecond or less. The medical and industrial applications of lasers have increased dramatically in the past several years. Unfortunately, until recently, occu-

Table 5-7. Types of injury caused by types of nonionizing radiation

Type of radiation	Sources	Populations at particular risk	Effects
Ultraviolet	Sun; sun lamps; welder's arcs; industrial and medical applications	All mankind; sun worshipers; select occupational groups	Burns of skin and eye, malignant melanoma, benign skin tumors, senile keratoses
Visible light	Sun; artificial lights; lasers; communications, industrial, and medical applications	All mankind; occupational groups	Burns of retina, photosensitization
Infrared	Sun; industrial and military applications	All mankind; occupational groups	Cataracts
Microwaves; radio waves	Ovens; radar and other communications; industrial, military, and medical applications	Much of mankind; occupational groups	Thermal effects at high power levels; cataracts; possible behavioral effects and blood dyscrasias

From DHEW Publ. No. NIH 77-1277, 1977, U.S. Department of Health, Education and Welfare, p. 135.

pational safety measures lagged behind the technologic advancements.

Finally, it is often forgotten that ultraviolet (UV) radiation is a carcinogen especially when absorbed with exogenous photosynthesizers such as 8-methoxypsoralin (8-MOP), a chemical employed with UV radiation to treat certain skin diseases. The evidence in support of UV radiation as a carcinogen in man includes the following observations: (1) human fibroblasts can be transformed in vitro subsequent to exposure to UV irradiation; (2) persons with certain genetic diseases, such as xeroderma pigmentosum and albinism, exhibit strong sensitivity to the effects of UV irradiation that is matched by a sharp increase in the incidence of skin tumors that also tend to develop at an unusually early age; (3) persons who work outdoors have an increased frequency of skin tumors that preferentially develop on the exposed portions of the body; (4) in whites, the incidence of malignant melanoma is directly proportional to magnitude of sunlight exposure and again there is a strong predilection for these tumors to develop on the chronically exposed portion of the body. This body of human experience is buttressed by a large reservoir of data in rodents, where repeated UV irradiations also produce skin tumors as well as alterations in the proportion of several types of circulating lymphocytes.

RADIATION PROTECTION STANDARDS AND THE CONCEPT OF RELATIVE RISK

Recognition of some of the untoward effects of radiation occurred within months of Roentgen's discovery of x rays in 1895. Beginning soon thereafter various national and international committees developed radiation-protection standards. The efforts of these groups received significant impetus during the 1950s when large-scale testing of nuclear weapons led to widespread concern about the possible hazards of global contamination by radioactive fallout. More recently, the development of nuclear power as an energy source, in conjunction with our increasing knowledge of the risks associated with low-level exposure, has promoted a continuing assessment of radiation safety standards. Viewed in historical perspective, the evolution of these standards represents a movement toward progressively more cautious exposure limits both for the general public and for radiation workers.

As shown in Table 5-1, the average dose of radiation to the general public from medical and dental uses in medically advanced countries currently approaches that from natural background. Approaches for reducing the exposure to the patient include using radiography in preference to fluoroscopy whenever practical; proper installation and use of equipment; shielding tissues outside the area of interest, especially the gonads; using fast film to reduce the duration and intensity of exposure per radiograph; reducing the number of radiographs per procedure; limiting the size of the field to regions of prime interest; and the proper education of personnel working in the field.

Possible risks related to the nuclear power industry deserve special mention, especially in light of the American accident at Three Mile Island in 1979 and the Russian accident at Chernobyl in 1986. Both appear to have resulted from a combination of human error and technical problems. The release of radioactivity at Chernobyl was significant and resulted in at least 52 acute deaths. At the time of this writing, the size of the exposed population is not known but approximately 135,000 people were evacuated from the area, of whom 50 are believed to have received 50 or more rad; an additional 100, 300 or more rad; and 200, 100 or more rad. Roughly 24,000 persons received 40 or more rem. Thus it appears inevitable that a significant proportion of the survivors will develop malignant tumors.

The exposures at Three Mile Island were much smaller than Chernobyl, less than 100 mrem maximum dose; at these doses roughly two adverse health effects (fatal and nonfatal neoplasms and genetic effects) can be expected among the 2,000,000 people living within 50 miles of the facility.

CONCLUDING THOUGHTS

Radiation has always been and always will be a part of man's environment. The health-related effects of these environmental exposures are largely unknown. Except for malignant melanoma and other skin tumors induced by excessive ultraviolet exposures, it is generally assumed that, in most parts of the world, the deleterious consequences of exposure to background radiation are minimal.

Beginning with the discovery of the x ray by Roentgen, man has developed a series of technologies designed to utilize radiation for the diagnosis and treatment of patients. Because many of the deleterious side effects were not immediately recognized, both patients and their physicians suffered significantly and unnecessarily. In retrospect, it seems incredible that irradiation was the treatment of choice for such benign conditions as tinea capitis, plantar warts, gastric hyperacidity with peptic ulcer, postpartum mastitis, and so-called status thymolymphaticus. One can only hope that today we in medicine are more discriminate in our use of new technologies.

As with many diagnostic and therapeutic modalities, radiation has the potential both for great benefits (for example, the cure of a person with Hodgkin's disease) and for significant harm (mental retardation from in utero exposure). For every exposure, either for therapy or for diagnosis, the anticipated benefits must be carefully balanced against the inherent risks. Only when the former exceeds the latter should the responsible physician proceed, for the risks are inevitable while the benefits are often problematic.

REFERENCES
General

1. Behrens, C.F., King, E.R., and Carpender, J.W.J., editors: Atomic medicine, ed. 5, Baltimore, 1969, The Williams & Wilkins Co. (Selective review with timely references.)
2. Dalrymple, G.V., et al., editors: Medical radiation biology, Philadelphia, 1973, W.B. Saunders Co. (Excellent review, particularly with respect to molecular and cellular radiobiology.)
3. Ionizing radiation: sources and biological effects, United Nations Scientific Committee on the Effects of Atomic Radiation 1982 Report to the General Assembly, New York, 1982, United Nations.
4. Genetic and somatic effects of ionizing radiation, United Nations Scientific Committee on the Effects of Atomic Radiation 1986 Report to the General Assembly, New York, 1986, United Nations.
5. Upton, A.C.: Radiation injury: effects, principles and perspectives, Chicago, 1969, The University of Chicago Press. (Concise review of radiation pathology.)

Radiation spectrum; radioactive substances; radiation units

6. Hendee, W.R.: Medical radiation physics, ed. 2, Chicago, 1979, Year Book Medical Publishers.
7. Hendee, W.R.: Radiation therapy physics, Chicago, 1981, Year Book Medical Publishers.
8. Johns, H.E., and Cunningham, J.R.: Physics of radiology, ed. 4, Springfield, Ill., 1982, Charles C Thomas, Publisher.

Cellular and molecular radiobiology

9. Altman, K.I., Gerber, G.B., and Okada, S.: Radiation biochemistry, vol. 1, New York, 1970, Academic Press, Inc. (Broad discussion of biochemical effects.)
10. Bacq, Z.M., and Alexander, P.: Fundamentals of radiobiology, ed. 2, New York, 1971, Pergamon Press.
11. Cornforth, M.N., and Bedford, J.S.: X-ray–induced breakage and rejoining of human interphase chromosomes, Science **222**:1141, 1983.
12. Elkind, M.M., and Whitmore, G.F.: Radiobiology of cultured mammalian cells, New York, 1967, Gordon & Breach. (Classic reference on cellular radiobiology.)
13. Gantt, R., Parshad, R., Price, F.M., and Sanford, K.K.: Biochemical evidence for deficient DNA repair leading to enhanced G_2 chromatid radiosensitivity and susceptibility to cancer, Radiat. Res. **108**:117, 1986.
14. Puck, T.T.: Effect of radiation on mammalian cells. In Puck, T.T., editor: The mammalian cell as a microorganism, San Francisco, 1972, Holden-Day Inc., p. 102.
15. Puck, T.T., and Marcus, P.I.: Action of X-rays on mammalian cells, J. Exp. Med. **103**:653, 1956.
16. Sinclair, W.K.: Cyclic X-ray responses in mammalian cells in vitro, Radiat. Res. **33**:620, 1968.
17. Till, J.E., and McCulloch, E.A.: A direct measurement of the radiation sensitivity of normal mouse bone marrow cells, Radiat. Res. **14**:213, 1961.

General morphologic features of radiation injury

18. Bergonié, J., and Tribondeau, L.: Interprétation de quelques résultats de la radiothérapie et essai de fixation d'une technique rationnelle, Compt. Rend. Acad. Sci. **143**:983, 1906. (Radiosensitivity of tissues.)
19. Fajardo, L.F.: Pathology of radiation injury, New York, 1982, Masson Publishing. (Excellent review with emphasis on injury in man but with integration of appropriate experimental studies.)
20. Upton, A.C., and Lushbaugh, C.C.: The pathological anatomy of total-body irradiation. In Behrens, D.F., King, E.R., and Carpender, J.W.J., editors: Atomic medicine, ed. 5, Baltimore, 1969, The Williams & Wilkins Co., p. 154.

21. Warren, S.: Effects of radiation on normal tissues, Arch. Pathol. **34**:443, 562, 749, 917, 1070, 1942; **35**:121, 304, 1943. (A series of articles on the effects of radiation on normal tissues.)
22. Warren, S.: Histopathology of radiation lesions, Physiol. Rev. **24**:225, 1944.
23. White, D.C.: An atlas of radiation histopathology, Technical Information Center, Office of Public Affairs, U.S. Energy Research and Development Administration, Washington, D.C., 1975.

Radiation injury in humans

24. Advisory Committee on the Biological Effects of Ionizing Radiation: The effects on populations of exposure to low levels of ionizing radiation (BEIR Report), Washington, D.C., 1980, National Academy of Sciences–National Research Council.
25. Anderson, R.E.: The delayed consequences of exposure to ionizing radiation: pathology studies at the Atomic Bomb Casualty Commission, Hiroshima and Nagasaki, 1945-1970, Hum. Pathol. **2**:469, 1971.
26. Andrews, G.A.: Criticality accidents in Vinca, Yugoslavia, and Oak Ridge, Tennessee, JAMA **179**:191, 1962.
27. Berthrong, M., and Fajardo, L.F.: Radiation injury in surgical pathology. Part II. Alimentary tract, Am. J. Surg. Pathol. **5**:153, 1981.
28. Boice, J.D., and Fraumeni, J.F., editors: Radiation carcinogenesis: epidemiology and biological significance, Progress in cancer research and therapy, vol. 26, New York, 1984, Raven Press.
29. Borek, C., and Hall, E.J.: Effect of split doses of x-rays on neoplastic transformation of single cells, Nature **252**:499, 1974.
30. Brent, R.L.: Effects of radiation on the fetus, newborn and child. In Fry, R.J.M., et al., editors: Late effects of radiation, London, 1970, Taylor & Francis, p. 23.
31. Evans, R.D.: The effect of skeletally deposited alpha-ray emitters in man, Br. J. Radiol. **39**:881, 1966.
32. Fajardo, L.F.: Ionizing radiation and neoplasia. In Fenoglio-Preiser, C.M., Weinstein, R.S., and Kaufman, N., editors: The International Academy of Pathology, Baltimore, 1986, The Williams & Wilkins Co., p. 97.
33. Fajardo, L.F., and Berthrong, M.: Radiation injury in surgical pathology. Part I, Am. J. Surg. Pathol. **2**:159, 1978.
34. Hachiya, M.: Hiroshima diary—the journal of a Japanese physician, August 6–September 30, 1945, Chapel Hill, 1955, The University of North Carolina Press.
35. Hamilton, T.E., van Belle, G., and LoGerfo, J.P.: Thyroid neoplasia in Marshall Islanders exposed to nuclear fallout, JAMA **258**:629, 1987.
36. Harvey, E.B., Boice, J.D., Jr., Honeyman, M., and Flannery, J.T.: Prenatal x-ray exposure and childhood cancer in twins, N. Engl. J. Med. **312**:541, 1985.
37. Kato, H., et al.: Life span study report 9, Mortality from causes other than cancer among atomic bomb survivors, 1950-78, RERF TR S-81:1, 1982.
38. Kato, H., and Schull, W.J.: Studies of the mortality of A-bomb survivors. VII. Mortality, 1950-78. Part I, Cancer mortality, Radiat. Res. **90**:395, 1982.
39. Langham, W.H., Brooks, P.M., and Grahn, D.: Radiation biology and space environmental parameters in manned spacecraft design and operations, Aerospace Med. **36**:1, 1965.
40. Langlois, R.E., et al.: Evidence for increased somatic cell mutations at the glycophorin A locus in atomic bomb survivors, Science **236**:445, 1987.
41. Loewe, W.E., and Mendelsohn, E.: Revised dose estimates at Hiroshima and Nagasaki, Health Physics **41**:663, 1981.
42. Martland, H.S.: Occupational poisoning in manufacture of luminous watch dials, JAMA **92**:466, 1929.
43. Matanoski, G.M., Seltser, R., Sartwell, P.E., et al.: The current mortality rates of radiologists and other physician specialists: deaths from all causes and from cancer, Am. J. Epidemiol. **101**:188, 1975.
44. Matanoski, G.M., Seltser, R., Sartwell, P.E., et al.: The current mortality rates of radiologists and other physician specialists: specific causes of death, Am. J. Epidemiol. **101**:199, 1975.
45. Miller, R.W.: Delayed radiation effects in atomic-bomb survivors, Science **166**:569, 1969.
46. Neel, J.V., Kato, H., and Schull, W.J.: Mortality in the children of atomic bomb survivors and controls, Genetics **76**:311, 1974.

47. Okada, S., et al.: A review of thirty years study of Hiroshima and Nagasaki atomic bomb survivors, Radiat. Res. **16**(suppl.):1, 1975.
48. Otake, M., and Schull, W.J.: In utero exposure to A-bomb radiation and mental retardation: a reassessment, Br. J. Radiol. **57**:409, 1984.
49. Oughterson, A.W., and Warren, S.: Medical effects of the atomic bomb in Japan, New York, 1956, McGraw-Hill Book Co.
50. Polednak, A.P., Stehney, A.F., and Rowland, R.E.: Mortality among women first employed before 1930 in the U.S. radium dial–painting industry, J. Epidemiol. **107**:179, 1978.
51. Prentice, R.L., and Thompson, D.J.: Atomic bomb survivor data: utilization and analysis, Proceedings of a conference sponsored by SIAM Institute for Mathematics and Society, Philadelphia, 1984, Society for Industrial and Applied Mathematics.
52. Setlow, R.B., and Carrier, W.L.: The disappearance of thymine dimers from D.N.A.: an error-correcting mechanism, Proc. Natl. Acad. Sci. **51**:226, 1964.
53. Shore, R.E., Albert, R.E., Reed, M., Harley, N., and Pasternack, B.S.: Skin cancer incidence among children irradiated for ringworm of the scalp, Radiat. Res. **100**:192, 1984.
54. Shore, R.E., Woodard, E., Hildreth, N., Dvoretsky, P., Hempelmann, L., and Pasternack, B.: Thyroid tumors following thymus irradiation, J. Natl. Cancer Inst. **74**:1177, 1985.
55. Smith, P.G., and Doll, R.: Age and time-dependent changes in the rates of radiation-induced cancers in patients with ankylosing spondylitis following a single course of x-ray treatment. In Late biological effects of ionizing radiation, vol. 1, Vienna, 1978, International Atomic Energy Agency.
56. Spiers, F.W., Lucas, H.F., and Anast, G.A.: Leukaemia incidence in the U.S. dial workers, Health Physics **44**(suppl. 1):65, 1983.
57. United States Department of Health, Education and Welfare: Review of the use of ionizing radiation for treatment of benign diseases, Washington, D.C., 1977, U.S. Government Printing Office.
58. Upton, A.C.: Physical carcinogenesis: radiation history and sources. In Becker, F.F., editor: Cancer, a comprehensive treatise, vol. 1, New York, 1975, Plenum Press, p. 387.

Acute radiation syndrome

59. Bond, V.P., Cronkite, E.P., and Conard, R.A.: Acute whole body radiation injury: pathogenesis, pre- and postradiation protection. In Behrens, C.F., King, E.R., and Carpender, J.W.J., editors: Atomic medicine, ed. 5, Baltimore, 1969, The Williams & Wilkins Co., p. 221.
60. Bond, V.P., Fliedner, T.M., and Archambeau, J.O., editors: Mammalian radiation lethality: a disturbance in cellular kinetics, New York, 1965, Academic Press, Inc. (Cell turnover and acute radiation injury.)
61. Gerstner, H.B.: Acute clinical effects of penetrating nuclear radiation, JAMA **168**:381, 1958.
62. Hempelmann, L.H., Lisco, H., and Hoffman, J.G.: The acute radiation syndrome: a study of nine cases and a review of the problem, Ann. Intern. Med. **36**:279, 1952.

Radiation injury of select tissues

63. Anderson, R.E., Nishiyama, H., Ii, Y., et al.: Pathogenesis of radiation-related leukemia and lymphoma, Lancet **1**:1060, 1972.
64. Archambeau, J.O., Mathieu, G.R., Brenneis, H.J., et al.: The response of the skin of swine to increasing single exposures of X-rays (250 kVp), Radiat. Res. **37**:141, 1969.
65. Cuzick, J.: Radiation-induced myelomatosis, N. Engl. J. Med. **304**:204, 1981. (Multiple myeloma in irradiated populations.)
66. DeGroot, L., and Paloyan, E.: Thyroid carcinoma and radiation: a Chicago endemic, JAMA **225**:487, 1973.
67. Fajardo, L.F., and Stewart, J.R.: The pathogenesis of radiation-induced myocardial fibrosis, Lab. Invest. **29**:244, 1973.
68. Haley, T.J., and Snider, R.S.: Response of the nervous system to ionizing radiation, New York, 1962, Academic Press, Inc.
69. Hempelmann, L.H.: Risk of thyroid neoplasms after irradiations in childhood, Science **160**:159, 1968.
70. Ichimaru, M., and Ishimaru, T.: Leukemia and related disorders: a review of thirty years' study of Hiroshima and Nagasaki atomic bomb survivors. II. Biological effects, J. Radiat. Res. **16**(suppl.):89, 1975.
71. Knowlton, N.P., Jr., et al.: Beta ray burns of human skin, JAMA **141**:239, 1949.
72. Land, C.E., Boice, J.D., Jr., Shore, R.E., Norman, J.E., and Tokunaga, M.: Breast cancer risk from low-dose exposures to ionizing radiation: results of parallel analysis of three exposed populations of women, J. Natl. Cancer Inst. **65**:353, 1980.
73. Nishiyama, H., Anderson, R.E., Ishimaru, T., et al.: The incidence of malignant lymphoma and multiple myeloma in Hiroshima and Nagasaki atomic bomb survivors, Cancer **32**:1301, 1973.
74. Puck, T.T.: Cellular aspects of the mammalian radiation syndrome, Radiat. Res. **27**:272, 1966.
75. Saccomanno, G., Archer, V.E., Auerbach, O., et al.: Histologic types of lung cancer among uranium miners, Cancer **27**:515, 1971.
76. Shore, R.E., Hildreth, N., Woodard, E., Dvoretsky, P., Hempelmann, L., and Pasternack, B.: Breast cancer among women given X-ray therapy for acute postpartum mastitis, J. Natl. Cancer Inst. **77**:689, 1986.
77. Yamamoto, T., et al.: Lung cancer incidence among Japanese A-bomb survivors, 1950-80, J. Radiat. Res. **28**:156, 1987.

Injury from nonionizing radiation

78. Brill, A.B., and Johnston, R.E.: Exposure of man to radiation. In Fry, R.J.M., et al., editors: Late effects of radiation, Proceedings of a colloquium, University of Chicago, 1969, London, 1970, Taylor & Francis, Ltd.
79. Microwave hazards, Lancet **2**:694, 1975. (Editorial.)
80. Peyton, M.F., editor: Biological effects of microwave radiation, New York, 1961, Plenum Press.

6 Bacterial Diseases

JOHN M. KISSANE

Most bacteria are harmless; indeed, many are beneficial to humans. The essential preoccupation of medicine with disease tends to obscure the fact that microorganisms are ubiquitous and that interaction between humans and microorganisms is only a particular aspect in the complex interrelationship among all living things. Abnormal circumstances in which this interrelationship leads to disease in the human host must be examined for the circumstances related to both the host and the microorganism, whereby the more usual balance between host and parasite becomes disturbed. In this broad view, opportunism is merely an isolated component of the diverse patterns of parasitism.

INFECTION VERSUS DISEASE

Two terms, *pathogenicity* and *virulence*, are used to describe the relationship between a microorganism (for our purposes a bacterium) and disease in its host (for our purposes a human). Although the terms are often used synonymously, it is useful to distinguish their connotations.[12] *Pathogenicity* implies the ability of the organism to produce disease and is usually presented as an absolute. In point of fact, however, a cause-and-effect relationship between infection and disease is rarely inevitable. *Virulence* embodies the concept of degree and expresses the ability of an organism to produce disease in some circumstances but not in others, in some levels or routes of exposure but not in others, and in some species of host or even individuals within a species but not in others. The relationship between host and infecting microorganism is often symbiotic (*sym-*, 'together' + *bios*, 'life'), and disease results only when one or another component of the equilibrium is disturbed.

DISTINCTION BETWEEN INFECTION AND DISEASE

Several circumstances can be distinguished in which microbial infection remains inapparent or subclinical and is not accompanied by functional or clinical abnormalities recognizable as constituting a disease.

Incubation period

The interval between the lodgment of a pathogenic microorganism on or in its host and the appearance of signs or symptoms of disease is known as the incubation period. If appropriate cultures are made during the incubation period, often fortuitously the organisms may be detected. The individual who is incubating the microorganism may be infectious to others.

Three processes can be considered as occurring during the incubation period: (1) organisms are invading the body of the host from their site of lodgment through a portal of entry ultimately to reach tissue suitable for their proliferation or subject to damage by the organisms, (2) the infecting organisms are proliferating to a quantitative level that overwhelms factors in the resistance of the host, and (3) reactions are occurring in the host, most importantly immunologic, that require the passage of time. These host responses contribute to both the clinical aspects of the disease and the morphologic features of the lesions.

Carrier state

Relatively resistant individuals may harbor pathogenic organisms for an indefinitely prolonged period without manifesting symptoms or signs and without morphologic alterations. Such a prolonged period, in contrast to the relatively brief and less variable incubation period, is described as a carrier state.

Carrier states are of great importance in control of many diseases by public health measures. The carrier may, because of fluctuations in resistance, develop disease. Asymptomatic and mobile, this person may become a source of infection to others. An individual recovering from a disease may harbor organisms for varying periods as a "convalescent carrier." Often a convalescent carrier is demonstrably immune to the relevant microorganisms, but there may be morphologic factors in the failure of this person's defense mechanisms to eradicate the organisms (such as their lodgment in structures relatively inaccessible to immunologic or other defenses). A patient convalescing from typhoid fever, for example, may harbor typhoid bacilli in a chronically inflamed gallbladder.

DISTINCTION BETWEEN DISEASE AND LESION

Disease is a composite phenomenon—the collective deviations from normal of the patient, however manifested and however perceived. Lesions are morphologic abnormalities, which may be silent or clinical, to which signs and symptoms can be attributed.

Some infectious diseases are highly characteristic in the features by which they are recognized clinically. Meningitis, for example, is a relatively homogeneous clinical entity. Recognition of the disease "meningitis," however, does not have specific implications as to the etiologic agent. Many different microorganisms or even sterile irritants can produce meningitis if they gain access to the subarachnoid space. *Meningitis* therefore designates both the disease and the lesion. Many lesions are morphologically so nonspecific as to etiology that the morphologic designation of the lesion serves as the name of the disease—bronchopneumonia, acute appendicitis, acute cholecystitis.

Scarlet fever, on the other hand, not only is a quite specific clinical entity but also is almost always caused by specific erythrogenic strains of *Streptococcus pyogenes*. Even here, however, occasional cases of scarlet fever appear to be related to toxigenic strains of *Micrococcus pyogenes* var. *aureus* (staphylococcus).

FACTORS IMPORTANT IN PATHOGENESIS OF INFECTIOUS DISEASES (LESIONS)

Many factors enter into the equilibrium between host and bacterial parasite, which may be disturbed, resulting in disease. Among these are (1) access of the organism to the host, (2) portal of entry, (3) infectious dose, (4) host factors, and (5) factors intrinsic to the microorganism.

Access. In strictly "infectious" diseases the infecting organism must reach the body of the host before it can produce disease. Exceptions to this generality are the pure exotoxicoses (p. 292). Often the infecting organism is an invariable or at least frequent parasite on or in the human body. In other instances access of the organism to the potential host requires contact with contaminated objects (fomites) or transmission by vectors, often arthropods.

Portal of entry. The anatomic point at which a parasitic organism gains access to the body is referred to as the portal of entry. Rarely, highly virulent microorganisms may penetrate the intact skin. More frequently, organisms that normally subsist innocuously on the skin gain access to susceptible tissues through sites of injury either trivial and unrecognized or clinically significant and grossly obvious. Ingestion of infectious agents provides an alimentary portal of entry. Inhalation, usually of organisms colonizing microaerosols, provides a portal of entry to the respiratory tract. Instrumentation of the lower urinary tract may introduce organisms from the urethra into the bladder. The depth or extent of invasion by organisms beyond the portal of entry depends in turn on many factors: nature or size of the inoculum in which the organisms are introduced and propulsion of the inoculum as by peristalsis, the periodic flushing effect of the urinary voiding, or (more subtly) the mobility of the mucociliary blanket of the respiratory tract.

In some diseases the portal of entry defines the anatomic distribution of lesions. In others it is nonspecific, and organisms reach and produce lesions in susceptible tissues unrelated to the portal of entry. In still other diseases lesions may occur both at the portal of entry and systemically.

Infectious dose. The size of the infectious inoculum bears importantly, but variably, on the fluctuating equilibrium between host and parasite. Often host defenses can eradicate or at least counterpose considerable numbers of microorganisms before disease results. Alteration of the microbiologic population at a given site, often iatrogenically as by the administration of broad-spectrum antibiotics, may allow normally symbiotic species to proliferate to the extent that they become pathogenic.

Host factors. Almost innumerable factors in the host, many of them poorly understood, influence the pathogenicity of infecting organisms. These factors may be very specific and readily identifiable (such as species, previous experience with the microorganism, or immunologic competence) or quite nonspecific (such as age, general health, nutrition, or the presence of other diseases).

Organismic factors. The explication of mechanisms is particularly the province of pathology. Unfortunately the mechanisms whereby particular infections give rise to particular diseases (or lesions) is much less well understood than microbial metabolism, on the one hand, or the host's immune response on the other. No doubt the reason is that such mechanisms are exceedingly complex and represent the result of the interplay among many factors, some related to the infecting organism, others to the host.

Mechanical factors. Simple massive proliferation of microorganisms is rarely a factor in the production of lesions. Yet proliferation of *Bacillus anthracis* in bronchopulmonary lymph nodes has been assigned a mechanical role in the production of the pulmonary edema so characteristic of pulmonary anthrax. That lesion now seems, however, to result from the action of the exotoxin elaborated by *B. anthracis*.

Metabolic factors. Early in the twentieth century the discovery of the importance of trace nutrients, notably vitamins, raised the possibility that some features of infectious diseases might result from consumption of significant quantities of critical nutrients by the infecting agents. Although highly artificial animal models of such a mechanism have been devised, nutritional deficiency on this basis has been convincingly demonstrated only in cases of infestation by the fish tapeworm, *Diphyllobothrium latum*, and in abnormal circumstances of consumption by organisms of vitamin B_{12} in blind loops of the intestine. This is not to say, of course, that infectious diseases may not interfere with nutrition by other means.

Toxins. Bacterial toxins are products of bacterial metabolism that exert deleterious effects on cells of the host. It is at least didactically useful to recognize exotoxins, endotoxins, and other toxic bacterial products. *Exotoxins* are soluble products secreted by certain bacteria into the surrounding medium. Most are complex proteins secreted by gram-positive bacteria. Exotoxins mediate major specific features associated with certain bacterial diseases. Strongly antigenic, exotoxins or their nontoxic derivatives, toxoids, excite the production of humoral antibodies, antitoxins, which are strongly protective.

Endotoxins are either proteins or complex polymolecular aggregates of proteins, polysaccharides, and phospholipids. They are believed to be associated with the cell walls of many gram-negative bacteria. In contrast to the highly specific actions of exotoxins, the toxic effects of endotoxins are nonspecific, largely involving the host's cardiovascular system. Antibodies to endotoxins are generally not protective.

Other products of certain bacteria have been ascribed roles in pathogenicity. Many of these substances are chemically incompletely characterized and are identified chiefly by the procedures that isolate them or by their empirically observed effects on living cells on other assay systems. Among these are the staphylococcal and streptococcal leukocidins (enzymes that lyse certain human and other mammalian leukocytes) and hemolysins (which lyse erythrocytes). Pathogenic staphylococci elaborate a coagulase that, acting on a thermolabile factor in either human or rabbit plasma, converts fibrinogen to fibrin. A bound form of coagulase, clumping factor, is found on the surface of most coagulase-positive staphylococci. Coagulase and clumping factor are believed to contribute to the tendency of staphylococci to produce localized abscesses.

Many gram-positive organisms form hyaluronidases, enzymes that are capable of depolymerizing the hyaluronic acid polysaccharide that contributes to viscosity of extracellular tissue fluid. It is suggested that these agents facilitate the spread of infectious organisms such as streptococci through tissue spaces (Fig. 6-1).

Streptococci and staphylococci produce fibrinolytic agents known respectively as streptokinase and staphylokinase. The role of these agents in infections by the appropriate organisms is not known.

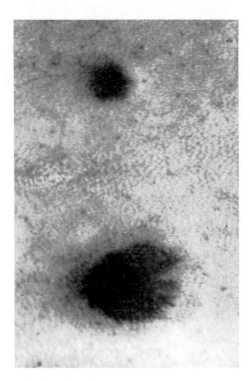

Fig. 6-1. Effect of hyaluronidase on spread of particulate carbon (india ink) of size comparable to staphylococci. Photograph taken 30 minutes after intradermal injections of 0.1 ml of carbon suspension into rabbit. Larger lesion represents increased spread of india ink because of added hyaluronidase.

Many bacteria produce proteolytic enzymes. Several gas-forming clostridia produce a potent collagenase, which liquefies collagen while leaving other components of connective tissue intact. Although collagenase might be considered as contributing to the tendency of certain clostridial infections to liquefy connective tissue, specific anticollagenase is not protective against experimental gas gangrene.

As implied in the foregoing summary, attribution of either the occurrence of a specific bacterial disease or the morphologic features of its lesions to specific biochemical activities of one or more bacterial products is largely conjectural. There has been little progress in this area since the assignment of several morphologic features of tuberculous infection to specific chemically defined fractions of tubercle bacilli.

Certain products of bacterial metabolism exert essentially mechanical effects on pathogenicity and virulence. Among these products are the polysaccharide capsules elaborated, for example, by pathogenic types of *Diplococcus pneumoniae*. Pathogenic and nonpathogenic strains of *Haemophilus influenzae* differ only in production by the former of a capsule that appears to interfere with phagocytosis by host leukocytes. Waxy components of the cell wall of *Mycobacterium tuberculosis* enable that organism to survive in an intracellular habitat after phagocytosis.

DISEASES AND LESIONS ASSOCIATED WITH INFECTIONS BY SPECIFIC BACTERIA

In the discussions that follow, results of infections by specific bacteria are described. Bacteriologic, serologic, epidemiologic, and clinical features are touched on only briefly and descriptively, since details of these aspects are more appropriate to works devoted to microbiology, immunology, public health, and clinical medicine. In contrast to the familiar presentation of these disorders in systems of classification based on microbiologic or clinical features, this presentation is, insofar as possible, along lines of similarity of pathogenic mechanism. Where possible, there is developed a system of classification that relates pathogenic mechanism and morphologic response of the host to the level of parasitism established by the infecting microorganisms (Table 6-1).

Exotoxicoses

There are several diseases in which bacterial toxins lead to profound systemic effects. In these diseases minimal parasitic interrelationships or even none at all exist between the causative microorganisms and the host. Most of the microorganisms responsible for diseases of this type are gram-positive cocci, usually spore bearing. Species, organ, and tissue specificities cannot really be described because there is such a minimal parasitic relationship. This is not to say, however, that the respective exotoxins do not have considerable species and organ specificities in their pharmacologic actions.

Botulism

Botulism results from the ingestion of the potent exotoxin produced by *Clostridium botulinum*—a soil anaerobe common throughout the world, particularly in the western United States. Contamination of foodstuffs, especially vegetables, by the organism is therefore relatively common. Spores of *C. botulinum* withstand dry heat as high as 180° C for as long as 15 minutes and 100° C for hours. If proper precautions are not taken in the preservation of food, conditions favorable to germination, proliferation, and toxin production by the organism may be established. Inadequate heating during

Table 6-1. General correlates of infectious processes with degree of parasitism

Degree of parasitism	Site of infection	Classification of disease	Tissue response	Organ/tissue specificity	Infectious processes
None	External	Exotoxicoses	Functional	None	Botulism Food poisoning Tetanus
Slight	Surface	Noninvasive infections	Surface exudation	Portal of entry	Diphtheria Gas gangrene Anthrax Pertussis Cholera Bacillary dysentery

Intermediate	Extracellular	Pyogenic infections	Necrosis and polymorphonuclear infiltration	Portal of entry and systemic	Infection by
					  Staphylococcus
					  Streptococcus
					  Pneumococcus
					  Neisseria
					  Enteric opportunists etc.
					Glanders
					Melioidosis

Intimate	Intracellular	Systemic infections (often species specific)	Proliferation (including granulomas)	Reticuloendothelial	Typhoid fever Brucellosis Tularemia Plague Tuberculosis
Obligatory	Intranuclear	Viral infections (viral tumors)	Neoplasia	Cell specific	Verrucae Papillomas Animal tumors Mitochondria?
	Ultrastructural	None (organelles, e.g., mitochondria?)			

processing, in fact, favors the growth of this organism by killing other bacteria that are less heat resistant and that cannot therefore overgrow and inhibit *C. botulinum.* Destruction of other organisms also prevents obvious warning features of spoilage such as bad odor and color. Most cases of botulism in the United States result from the ingestion of home-processed vegetables, especially nonacid ones such as beans or corn. In Europe most cases result from contamination of preserved meat such as ham and sausage (Latin *botulus,* 'sausage'). Five to 10 sporadic cases of botulism occur annually in the United States.

Botulism related to commercially processed food is rare. Its epidemiology may be difficult to elicit because of the wide distribution of processed foods. Rarely, systemic botulism follows infections of wounds by toxigenic *C. botulinum.*[23]

The rare occurrence of botulism in infants constitutes an exception to the generalization that botulism results from ingestion or rarely absorption of preformed toxin.[20,28] In infants, ingested spores of *C. botulinum* may germinate in the intestine and elaborate toxin, which gives rise to symptoms such as those of a hypotonic infant ("floppy baby"). Infant botulism exceptionally has been incriminated as a cause of the sudden infant death syndrome.[13]

Botulinus toxin is the most potent of all bacterial toxins. Because it resists destruction by proteolytic enzyme, it remains effective when ingested. Six types of botulinus toxin have been identified. Four are responsible for human disease. Type A, the most potent, carries a mortality of approximately 75%, and type B a mortality of approximately 20%. The promptness of onset of the symptoms depends on dose, usually beginning between 12 and 36 hours after ingestion, rarely as little as 3 to 4 hours. Nausea and vomiting, sometimes with a sense of abdominal distress but no real pain, are observed early. Diplopia and difficulty swallowing are usually the first features of the characteristic paralyses produced by the toxin. Paralysis of pharyngeal muscles leads to regurgitation of ingested food and liquids through the nose. This often causes aspiration pneumonia. The patient may be unable to hold the head erect because of involvement of the neck muscles. Death, if it occurs, usually results from respiratory failure. Specific antitoxin is the only therapeutic measure available and is of value only early. The toxin is bound to neural tissues once the disease becomes established and in those sites can no longer be neutralized by specific antitoxin.

Botulinus toxin acts something like curare, affecting principally the end plates of nerves and specifically the myoneural junctions of the motor apparatus. No morphologic changes occur that are specific for botulism. There may be petechiae and ecchymoses on serous surfaces and in the central nervous system as secondary effects of anoxia. The specific diagnosis depends on the demonstration of an antitoxin-neutralizable paralysis in rodents injected with the suspected food material or even with a sample of the patient's blood.

Staphylococcal exotoxicoses

Food poisoning that results from the ingestion of a potent exotoxin produced by certain strains of *Micrococcus pyogenes* (*Staphylococcus pyogenes*) is a common public health problem. Since the disease is not reportable, however, its frequency is unknown. In contrast to botulism, symptoms appear rapidly and are of short duration; recovery is usually prompt and complete. Excessive salivation is often the first sign of intoxication, followed shortly by nausea and vomiting, abdominal cramps, and diarrhea. Toxigenic strains of staphylococci produce toxin during their growth phase at temperatures above 40°F. Circumstances favorable for toxin production are most commonly encountered in cream-filled bakery goods or other foodstuffs with an approximately neutral reaction. Staphylococcal enterotoxin is extremely heat resistant and is also stable during prolonged refrigeration. Clinical and epidemiologic features of staphylococcal food poisoning are sufficiently characteristic to establish the diagnosis in most cases. Formal laboratory confirmation is difficult to achieve. Morphologic changes have not been described.

In 1978, Todd and Fishaut[33] reported a prostrating illness in seven children, five of whom were colonized by phage group I staphylococci.[14] What these workers styled the toxic-shock syndrome (TSS) included prostration, severe hypotension, a desquamative cutaneous eruption, and hepatorenal failure. Soon thereafter, highly characteristic epidemiologic features emerged.[18,24] Ninety-six percent of cases reported to the Centers for Disease Control from 1970 to 1982 were women and 92% were menstruating.[32] Many of these were using tampons. The rate of usually vaginal colonization in menstruating women with TSS by exotoxin-producing staphylococci of phage group I is several times the rate of colonization of asymptomatic women with this organism.[30] All males with TSS are colonized with exotoxin-producing staphylococci.[15] Proteins characterized as enterotoxin 2 and as exotoxin type C (probably identical) have been implicated though the mechanism of pathogenesis has not been elicited.[16] Some cases have been associated with colonization by exotoxin-producing streptococci.[17]

The mortality in TSS is currently about 3%. Pathologic features in fatal cases include desquamation of vaginal and cervical mucosae, acute renal tubular necrosis, portal infiltration in the liver, and pulmonary changes of diffuse alveolar injury.[25] Lesions of staphylococcal septicopyemia (multiple abscesses) are *not* characteristic.

Currently staphylococcal (as opposed to the more usual streptococcal form) of scarlet fever is regarded as a *forme fruste* of TSS in which only the desquamative cutaneous eruption is expressed.

Salmonellal food poisoning

Contamination of foods by any of the strains of *Salmonella* produces a self-limited nonspecific gastroenteritis often clinically and epidemiologically confused with staphylococcal food poisoning.

Tetanus

Tetanus (lockjaw) results from the absorption of the potent exotoxin produced by *Clostridium tetani*. This free-living saprophyte, widespread in nature, especially in cultivated soil, is commonly found in the feces of cattle and horses and less commonly of humans. It therefore tends to colonize manured areas of cultivation. Once introduced into an area, spores of *C. tetani* persist almost indefinitely. Tetanus is therefore particularly a hazard in intensively cultivated rural areas.

Tetanus results from the introduction of spores of *C. tetani* into tissue, where anaerobic conditions favorable to germination and toxin production may be present. Puncture wounds as from a nail or splinter are particularly dangerous. Tetanus was once a frequent complication of abortion and was also commonly seen in infants as *tetanus neonatorum*, which resulted from infection of the umbilical stump. Active immunization has contributed to a decline in the occurrence of tetanus, but 150 or so cases are reported annually in the United States.

Tetanus toxin is absorbed from the local site of production and is transmitted into the central nervous system along the axons of neurons. Tetanus toxin is a potent neurostimulatory agent. Clinical features of tetanus may appear several weeks or even months after the responsible injury, and in a considerable number of cases no injury can be demonstrated or recalled. Symptoms begin with headache, followed shortly by difficulty in swallowing and stiffness of the jaw. Muscle stiffness or spasm may initially be confined to the region of the local infection (*local tetanus*). Spasm of the muscles of the trunk may lead to opisthotonos. Contraction of facial muscles produces the characteristic *risus sardonicus*. Consciousness is undistributed, and perception of pain is undiminished. Death results from inanition or secondary complications such as bronchopneumonia. Specific morphologic changes have not been described. A reliable diagnostic procedure is the demonstration of muscle spasms in guinea pigs injected with wound scrapings suspended in a saline solution. The presence of tetanus bacilli established by culture is not diagnostic, since spores of *C. tetani* frequently contaminate wounds.

Infections of surfaces of the body

A small group of bacterial diseases results from infection of body surfaces by indigenous bacterial flora that may occasionally be introduced into deeper tissues and cause disease. The diseases discussed here result from infection of the surface itself. The systematically heterogeneous organisms responsible for this group of infections have little or no inherent capacity to invade deeper tissues and manifest a degree of parasitism with their human host only slightly more intimate than that manifested by organisms responsible for the exotoxicoses just described. Included in this group of diseases are diphtheria, gas gangrene, pertussis, bacillary dysentery, and Asiatic cholera.

Diphtheria

Diphtheria is amenable to virtually complete eradication by routine immunization with diphtheria toxoid. Even in medically advanced countries, however, diphtheria may occur when immunization procedures break down because of war, complacency, or cultism. An important epidemic occurred in Texas in 1970.[21,34]

The low-grade endemicity of diphtheria depends on the occurrence of toxigenic *Corynebacterium diphtheriae* in the nasopharynges of a small number (fewer than 1%) of asymptomatic human carriers. Transmission to nonimmune individuals usually occurs by the respiratory route.

In diphtheria, unlike food poisoning or tetanus, a parasitic relationship exists between the causative microorganism, *C. diphtheriae*, and its host. Diphtheria is a composite of a local inflammation and a systemic intoxication. Toxic produced locally by toxigenic strains of *C. diphtheriae* is responsible for an inflammatory reaction on body surfaces at the site of infection (usually the oral pharynx, from which the process often extends to the nose or larynx). Occasionally the tracheal, esophageal, or gastric mucosa is involved as well. Less commonly, but particularly in the tropics, cutaneous trauma or burns may be the site of diphtheria. The umbilical cord (in *diphtheria neonatorum*), the genital tract, and the conjunctivae are rare sites. Unlike streptococcal tonsilitis, diphtheria is often insidious in onset and may be preceded by 2 or 3 days of listlessness, malaise, and headache before local symptoms occur. Cervical adenopathy seems out of proportion to the pharyngeal lesion. Soon small gray or white patches of exudate appear on the pharyngeal mucosa, usually over the tonsils. These enlarge and coalesce and, with the accumulation of blood, become gray or black. This exudate constitutes the characteristic diphtheritic membrane, which consists of leukocytes and numerous bacteria enmeshed in a dense network of fibrin (Fig. 6-2). The epithelial surface becomes necrotic and densely adherent to the overlying membrane; this adherency explains

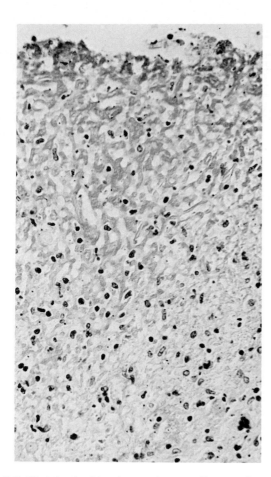

Fig. 6-2. Diphtheria. Membrane that overlies tonsil consists of feltwork of fibrin, necrotic debris, and sparse leukocytes. (From Kissane, J.M.: Pathology of infancy and childhood, ed. 2, St. Louis, 1975, The C.V. Mosby Co.)

why raw bleeding points are exposed when the membrane is forcibly removed. If particularly extensive, the local process may produce mechanical respiratory obstruction, stridor, and even asphyxiation.

The local inflammatory process and its mechanical consequences are less important in the evolution of diphtheria than is the profound toxemia that characterizes the infection. Diphtheria toxin, produced by *C. diphtheriae* in response to infection of that organism by a specific bacteriophage, is a potent inhibitor of cellular protein synthesis.[27] It is readily absorbed from the point of production into the bloodstream, and its effects are noted in many organs and systems throughout the body. The lymphoid tissues both in regional lymph nodes and systemically (as in the spleen) undergo hyperplasia with the development of prominent germinal centers that are often centrally necrotic.

Diphtheria toxin is particularly toxic to myocardium. In the early stages, interstitial edema, cloudy swelling of myocardial fibers, and the accumulation of fine cytoplasmic granules of lipid are seen microscopically. Later these changes become widespread and more severe. Myocardial fibers eventually undergo necrosis, and a focal interstitial myocarditis with exudation of mononuclear cells occurs. Cardiac involvement, either acutely in the form of cardiovascular collapse or as an arrhythmia or more chronically in the form of congestive heart failure, is the most common threat to life in diphtheria.

A nonspecific, nonsuppurative interstitial nephritis is frequent in diphtheria and is believed to be responsible for the proteinuria often observed. The renal lesion usually resolves completely in patients who recover. The liver is characteristically enlarged; hepatocytes exhibit cloudy swelling and less commonly focal necrosis.

Diphtherial toxin has a special affinity for peripheral nerves. Toxic effects are manifested in degeneration or even destruction of myelin sheaths. Axis cylinders undergo swelling and rarely necrosis. The paralytic effects of diphtheritic neuropathy are often sharply localized. Paralysis of the voluntary muscles of the palate may produce a peculiar nasal quality of the voice and a tendency to regurgitate fluids through the nose. Hypopharyngeal involvement may lead to aspiration pneumonia. Involvement of extraocular muscles may produce diplopia, and involvement of the ciliary body may result in defective visual accommodation. Clinically apparent weakness or paralysis of limbs is rare. Neuropathic manifestations of diphtheria are usually temporary and disappear within 2 or 3 months if the patient survives.

Gas gangrene

Three members of the genus *Clostridium*, *C. welchii* (*perfringens*), *C. novyi* (*oedematiens*), and *C. septicum*, may produce gas gangrene; at least three other members of this genus may contribute to such a process though incapable of producing it themselves. Infections associated with gas gangrene are often mixed and include various anaerobic organisms as well as toxicogenic clostridia. Gas-forming clostridia are strictly anaerobic, gram-positive, sporulating bacilli widely distributed in nature. Gas-forming clostridia may be introduced into wounds as spores that, devoid of toxin, are incapable of producing disease. Conditions that seem to favor germination of spores and subsequent toxin production include extensive necrosis (such as that produced by crushing injuries) or the presence of foreign particulate matter (especially that containing calcium salts or silicic acid).

A curious and interesting disease, known locally as *pig-bel*, occurs in the highlands of central New Guinea. In that locality pig-bel is the most common cause of acute abdominal emergencies. Anatomic lesions include enteritis with deep, often perforating, peculiarly serpiginous ulcers. Epidemiologic studies are ambiguous, but some emphasize the association of pig-bel with ritual feasts on putrid pork carcasses. Gas-forming clostridia have been cited as etiologically important.

The various toxins produced by gas-forming clostridia are locally toxic and perpetuate the local process while being available for absorption and systemic effects as well.[20] Appropriate surgical management, particularly débridement of all devitalized tissue from wounds subject to gas gangrene, and prompt initiation of antibiotic therapy have drastically reduced the incidence and morbidity of this bacterial disease. Hyperbaric oxygen has both advocates and skeptics.[27,29]

In peacetime, sporadic cases of gas gangrene are occasionally observed, particularly among agricultural workers. Features of gas gangrene usually appear within hours to days after the relevant injury. Tissues about the wound become swollen, edematous, and painful as a result of increased tension. Once established, the process often advances with great rapidity. The injured member becomes tense and crepitant because of the accumulation of gas bubbles within the tissues. A scanty serosanguineous fluid exudes from the wound. Rarely the fluid may be effervescent. Soon the wounded tissue becomes grayish black and extremely foul smelling. This local process, called clostridial cellulitis, may in itself occasionally threaten life. The syndrome, gas gangrene, however, includes the systemic toxic effects of several clostridial toxins and, once it develops, has a significant mortality.

The most conspicuous local effects involve muscle. The muscle fibers undergo coagulative necrosis and occasionally liquefy (Fig. 6-3). Large gram-positive bacilli are present in great numbers. In later cases a zone of intense leukocytic reaction and hyperemia confines the area of infection. In severe cases there is practically no leukocytic response about the region of frank necrosis but a wide zone of edema and congestion. Capillary and venous thrombi are common.

There are at least 12 immunologically distinct toxins produced by gas-forming clostridia. The most important of these are the potent lecithinase (alpha toxin) and another necrotizing toxin (sigma toxin). Potent hemolytic toxins may produce a precipitous drop in the number of circulating erythrocytes. Terminally, bacilli invade the bloodstream and are distributed widely throughout the body. Pulmonary edema and hyperemia are usually pronounced. If postmortem examination is delayed even a few hours, gas formation occurs in virtually any organ of the body.

Anthrax

The inclusion of anthrax among these diseases resulting from a minimal parasitic relationship between organism and host may seem inappropriate. In fact, anthrax organisms are found in great profusion in tissues of infected animals or humans. They excite almost no inflammatory response, however, and the hemorrhagic edema so characteristic of the lesions is now attributed to a very potent exotoxin.

A disease known since antiquity, anthrax was described in Homer's *Iliad*. It is of great historical interest for it was the first human disease of proved bacterial origin. Although numerous, large, rod-shaped organisms had been observed in the blood of animals dying of anthrax in 1850, it remained for Robert Koch to prove that these organisms were actually the cause of anthrax. This he did in 1876, at the same time formulating what we now accept as Koch's postulates. In 1881

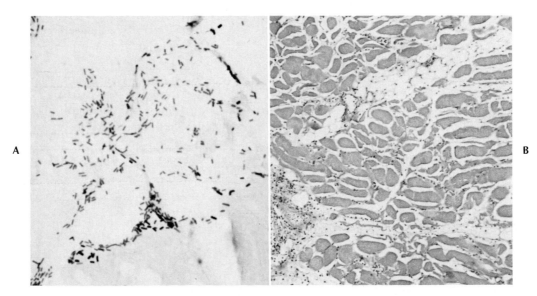

Fig. 6-3. Gas gangrene. **A,** Numerous *Clostridium welchii* and necrosis of muscle fiber. **B,** Large gas-filled spaces and separation of individual muscle fibers from their sarcolemmal sheaths.

Pasteur succeeded in attenuating the organism and produced an effective vaccine, the first successful practical application of active immunization in the control of disease.

Bacillus anthracis is a long (4.5 to 10 μm), square-ended, gram-positive rod that often grows in short chains. It is capable of forming very resistant spores, but spore forms do not occur in animals or humans with the disease. Many species of animals are susceptible to infection, but grazing animals are most commonly affected, especially sheep and cattle. The disease in animals almost invariably results in septicemia and death. In the so-called apoplectic form, death may occur within an hour or two after symptoms are first noticed. Animals, in contrast to humans, usually become infected by ingesting the spores. These pass unharmed through the stomach and invade the intestinal mucosa. The spore forms are so resistant that pastures once seeded with *B. anthracis* remain a source of infection indefinitely.

The disease is uncommon in the United States, with an average of four or five cases per year having been reported during the past 5 years.[39] However, it is interesting to note that during this period the number of cases of anthrax considerably exceeded that of smallpox. Among humans in the United States, most infections are occupational, appearing in textile workers and stevedores who handle wool, hides, or hair. Agricultural anthrax is very rare in the United States. Human gastrointestinal anthrax, unknown in the United States, occurs when unenlightened or impoverished people eat the carcasses of animals dead of anthrax. Farmers, butchers, and veterinarians are occasionally infected, and a small number of cases have been reported in which the disease followed the use of a shaving brush or hairbrush with contaminated bristles. Infection also occurs from the biting of flies (family Tabanidae).

Most commonly the disease occurs in the form of the malignant pustule (Fig. 6-4), as a result of entry of *B. anthracis* into an abrasion or scratch of the skin. In the majority of instances, the primary infection is of the head or neck.[36] The lesion first appears as a papule, soon surrounded by a zone of edema and hyperemia. Vesiculation occurs, and on rupture of the small blister an eschar forms. Soon there is central necrosis, and a small ragged black ulcer develops. This may be surrounded by minute vesicles or pustules. Sometimes the local lesion involves a large area. The lesion is not particularly painful, though characteristically there is intense itching. Regional lymph nodes are somewhat swollen and tender, but involvement is not comparable to that seen in tularemia or plague. In the majority of instances the disease remains localized, and in a week or two the small ulcer heals. The eschar may separate from the underlying tissue, leaving a suppurating slough. Especially if lymphadenopathy is a prominent feature, forces of localization may be overcome and septicemia may result. This is accompanied by profound systemic manifestations, and death is the usual consequence. Occasionally no ulcer forms at the site of initial infection, but rather an area of malignant edema. This may or may not be associated with acute hyperemia and other signs of acute inflammation. Generalization of the infection (septicemia) is more likely to occur here than in the case of the malignant pustule. Next in frequency is the pneumonic form (wool-sorter's disease), which occurs from inhalation of the spores. In this case the malignant pustule forms in a bronchus, and this soon leads to an extensive hemorrhagic consolidation of the involved lobe or lobes. There are striking systemic manifestations, progressive dyspnea, and cough productive of bloody sputum. Before antibiotic therapy was available, septicemia and death occurred in the majority of those affected. Rarely, in humans there is a third form—quite similar to that seen in cattle—the intestinal type. In this infection, also, septicemia and death usually result.

Morphologic changes are characterized principally by a bloody mucinous edema that affects many tissues and is found in most serous cavities. Meningitis may be a prominent feature. The damage wrought by *B. anthracis* in the septicemic form of anthrax is so overwhelming that there is relatively little cellular reaction, principally necrosis with massive bloody edema. In the acute septicemic forms death occurs in over 90% of the patients unless they are treated promptly with specific antiserum or sulfonamides.

Curiously, until recently anthrax—so extensively studied and the first bacterial disease for which an effective vaccine was produced—has resisted analyses to determine its lethal mechanism of action. Of the many toxins elaborated by *B. anthracis*, the "lethal factor" (LF) is an exotoxin, its concentration varying with the number of organisms present in the blood. This is an edema-producing toxin (EF), affecting capillary permeability, that is mainly responsible for the secondary shock, which in turn is the usual precipitating cause of death.

In persons with typical skin manifestations, the diagnosis is not difficult. Large numbers of the characteristic organisms can be seen in smears made from the pustule or from sputum in the pulmonic form. The organisms also should be cultured and their virulence ascertained by inoculation into guinea pigs or mice.

Pertussis (whooping cough)

Pertussis is traditionally attributed to superficial infection of the distal airway by *Bordetella pertussis* (formerly *Haemophilus pertussis*). *B. pertussis* is a short, gram-negative bacillus that produces both an endotoxin

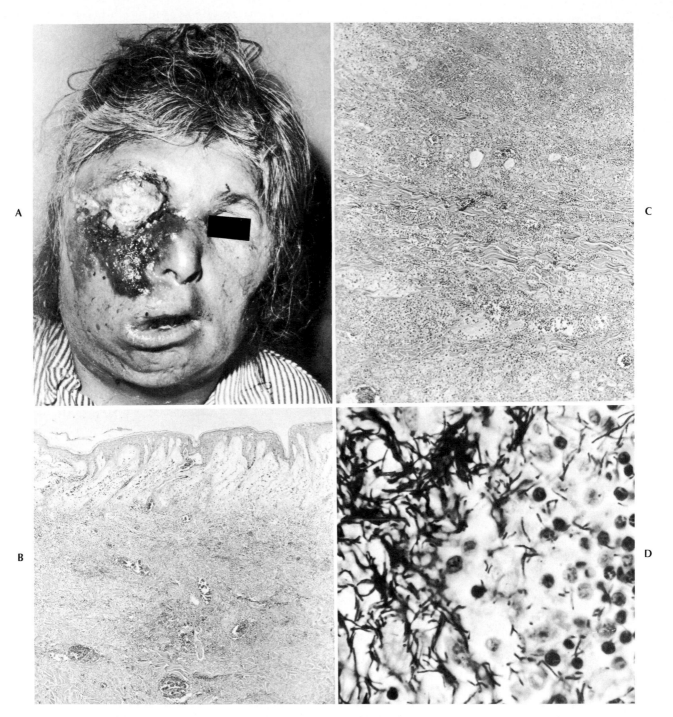

Fig. 6-4. Anthrax. **A,** Severe malignant pustule. **B** and **C,** Histopathologic appearance of skin. **D,** Bacilli. (**B** and **C,** Hematoxylin and eosin; **B,** 35×; AFIP 66-13163; **C,** 77×; AFIP 66-13164; **D,** Gram stain of tissue section; 800×; AFIP 66-13179; **A** to **D,** from Dutz, W.: Int. Pathol. **8:**38, 1967.)

and an exotoxin. A clinically indistinguishable disorder can be produced by numerous viruses. Some authorities have even challenged any etiologic role of *B. pertussis* in whooping cough. Formerly the most important acute infectious disease of childhood, pertussis has in the last few decades diminished in both frequency and severity. Only 2000 to 3000 cases are reported annually in the United States, with only seven deaths in 1985.

Morphologic changes, in the uncomplicated case, are mostly limited to the air passages and lungs (Fig. 6-5). Findings include laryngitis, tracheitis, bronchitis, and bronchiolitis; however, changes are most noticeable in the bronchi.[50] Bacterial stains reveal many of the specific organisms contained within the mucopurulent exudate that overlies the mucosa and is intertwined and tangled with the cilia of the columnar epithelium. Occasionally areas of superficial necrosis and erosion are evident. Hyperemia and excessive production of mucus occur. The smaller bronchi may contain dense plugs of mucus, and these will include a few inflammatory cells and many organisms. Peribronchitis and interstitial pneumonitis, especially around small bronchi, are characteristic findings but are not by any means pathognomonic, since they are seen also in other diseases (for instance, atypical pneumonia). Little exudate is to be found in alveoli unless there is secondary bronchopneu-

monia. Emphysema is almost always evident microscopically. Peribronchial lymph nodes are hyperemic and exhibit moderate hyperplasia.

Diseases caused by vibrios

Members of the genus *Vibrio* are responsible for Asiatic cholera and also for a form of food poisoning relatively prevalent in Japan. One of the great historical pestilences, Asiatic cholera has apparently been perennially endemic in the Indian subcontinent. Escaping from this homeland early in the nineteenth century, cholera has occurred in six pandemics elsewhere in the world—including the classic one in London, traced to the contamination of the Broad Street pump by John Snow.[42] Cholera occurred in eastern Europe until 1923. Epidemics also occurred in the United States during the nineteenth century, but there have been only three rigorously identified cases during the twentieth century, a fatal case in a longshoreman in New Orleans in 1941 and two laboratory infections in 1964.

In India, cholera has traditionally been caused by classic *Vibrio cholerae*. Infection by the El Tor biotype identified in Suez in 1906 was not considered "cholera" until 1961. In 1964 the disease produced by the El Tor organism essentially replaced that attributable to classic *V cholerae* in India, but not in Bangladesh. Since 1968

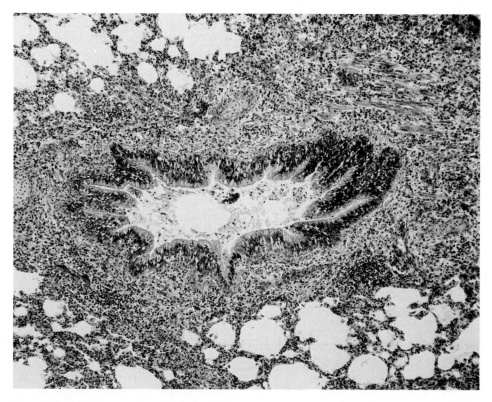

Fig. 6-5. Pertussis. Tenacious exudate clings to side of bronchus. Bronchitis, peribronchitis, and focal areas of emphysema are present. (From Kissane, J.M.: Pathology of infancy and childhood, ed. 2, St. Louis, 1975, The C.V. Mosby Co.)

the El Tor biotype has predominated there as well.[38]

The most recent sizable outbreak of cholera outside India occurred in Italy in 1972. The epidemiology of that contagion has not been firmly established, but contamination of shellfish imported from North Africa has been suggested.

The only significant natural reservoir of cholera appears to be humans, and the only clinically significant portal of entry is the alimentary tract by the fecal-oral route. *V. cholerae* are appreciably sensitive to normal gastric acidity. Oral infection can be produced by 10^8 ingested organisms, but that figure drops to 10^4 if gastric acidity is neutralized. Interestingly, a disproportionate number of patients afflicted in an outbreak in Israel had undergone surgical procedures (vagotomy, pyloroplasty, or gastrectomy), which tend to vitiate the protective effect of gastric acidity.[40]

The incubation period is usually 1 to 5 days, after which a profuse watery diarrhea occurs usually without tenesmus or abdominal distress. Fluid loss can exceed 10 liters per day. Prostration is therefore rapid and profound. The disease is ordinarily self-limited, with death or recovery occurring within a few days. An asymptomatic convalescent carrier state is uncommon but can occur.

Cholera can be reproduced in all essentials by cell-free extracts of cultures of *V. cholerae*. Manifestations of the disease are attributable to a very potent enterotoxin, choleragen, which has been highly purified as a protein with a molecular weight of about 90,000. Choleragen acts on the mucosal cells of isolated loops of rabbit intestine by reversing the normal direction of ion transport, thereby causing fluid to accumulate in the lumen. This action appears to be mediated by adenosine-3,5-cyclic monophosphate (cyclic AMP).[37] Either choleragen or cyclic AMP stimulates secretion of chloride by intestinal mucosal cells and inhibits absorption of sodium.[49] *V. cholerae* ordinarily does not invade beyond the intestinal mucosal surface, though infection of bile and the presence of organisms in the liver at least at autopsy have been reported.

Intestinal biopsy specimens from living patients with severe cholera have shown the mucosa of the intestine to be intact with only slight edema and hypercellularity of the lamina propria. Parenchymatous degeneration of solid viscera, traditionally described among findings at autopsy, appears to be a nonspecific feature of fluid and electrolyte loss.

Noncholera vibrios. The genus *Campylobacter* has recently been designated to include motile gram-negative curved organisms other than *V. cholerae*. There are two biotypes, *C. fetus* (var. *intestinalis*) and *C. fetus* (var. *jejuni*), both pathogenic for humans.

Initially recognized in the tropics, representatives of the genus *Campylobacter* are now known to be distributed throughout the world. Animal reservoirs are suspected, but the mode of transmission to humans has not been established. Human infections by *Campylobacter* are associated with three clinical syndromes: (1) *C. fetus* (usually var. *jejuni*) is responsible for about 6% of cases of infantile enteritis (enterocolitis) in the United States, and as much as 30% in the tropics. Most often self-limited, the disease may be severe and prostrating, even fatal. Morphologically *C. fetus* produces a nonspecific acute enterocolitis, occasionally hemorrhagic or necrotizing. (2) *C. fetus* (especially var. *intestinalis*) is responsible for occasional examples of localized infections in elderly adults debilitated by other diseases. Septicemia, meningoencephalitis, and infectious arthritis have been described. (3) *C. fetus* (especially var. *intestinalis*) causes some perinatal infections, presumably acquired by the infant from an asymptomatic carrier mother.

Diseases caused by Shigella

Members of the genus *Shigella* cause a readily communicable infectious colitis, bacillary dysentery, that has historically afflicted troops in the field, prisoners of war, victims of natural disasters, and those subject to unsanitary overcrowded conditions (as in orphanages or mental hospitals). The disease was distinguished from amebic dysentery in 1896 by Shiga, who recognized the first representative of the genus now known as *Shigella dysenteriae*.

The four species of *Shigella* (*S. dysenteriae*, *S. flexneri*, *S. boydii*, and *S. sonnei*) are nonmotile gram-negative bacilli distinguished from other Enterobacteriaceae by means of biochemical reactions and from each other by their biochemical and antigenic characteristics. All known species are pathogenic for humans.*[45]

The natural disease occurs only in primates, and shigellas are found only in the intestinal tracts of humans, subhuman primates, and rarely dogs.

Early in the twentieth century *S. dysenteriae* was the most common cause of bacillary dysentery. Since then, *S. sonnei* and *S. flexneri* have become more commonly recognized as causes of dysentery. *S. sonnei* now predominantes in medically more advanced countries, and *S. flexneri* in the less advanced. *S. boydii* is rarely isolated. *S. dysenteriae* had nearly disappeared from most parts of the world until the late 1960s, when epidemics caused by this agent appeared in Central America and subsequently spread to Mexico. Since 1968 bacillary dysentery from *S. dysenteriae* has occurred in tourists returning to the United States from Central America and Mexico and in their contacts.[53] The disease has remained a major public health problem in Central America. In the United States, bacillary dysentery develops most often in children younger than 10 years of

---

*Doubtful pathogens formerly designated *S. alkalescens* and *S. dispar* are now classified as *Escherichia coli*.

age, often from socioeconomically deprived segments of the population.

Transmission occurs by the fecal-oral route. Although shigellas compete poorly with other intestinal bacteria both in vitro and in vivo, as few as several hundred bacilli can produce disease in healthy volunteers. Factors responsible for pathogenicity are poorly understood.[35] *S. dysenteriae* produces a heat-labile neurotoxin and an enterotoxin (possibly the same product) that, like the enterotoxins of *E. coli* and *V. cholerae*, induce fluid accumulation in isolated segments of rabbit ileum.[43]

Lesions of the natural disease are confined to the terminal ileum and colon and consist of shallow ulcers, usually transversely arrayed, with serpiginous borders and coated by a delicate filmy membrane of fibrin, polymorphonuclear leukocytes, cell debris, and bacteria (Fig. 6-6). The ulcers probably result from entry of the bacilli into the lamina propria, where release of endotoxin causes death of host cells and an acute inflammatory response.[46] Further invasion is almost unknown. In some patients, almost always those with *S. dysenteriae*, encephalopathic manifestations that are usually transitory develop.

Extracellular infections

Most human bacterial infections are attributable to organisms to which the host response is acute inflammation characterized by the formation of pus. These organisms are therefore appropriately designated *pyogenic bacteria*. The most typical members of this group are gram-positive cocci, though gram-negative cocci of *Neisseria* species and *Haemophilus influenzae* also evoke typically purulent responses. Furthermore, many genera of gram-negative bacilli, particularly those whose normal habitat is the gastrointestinal tract, evoke a purulent response when they gain access to tissues of the host beyond their usual habitat. Morphologic features of lesions produced by pyogenic organisms include predominantly the polymorphonuclear leukocyte plus local necrosis and its consequences. These responses constitute acute inflammations, described elsewhere p. 87. The degree of parasitism manifested by agents that produce a purulent response is expressed by an almost entirely extracellular habitat, pathogenic aspects of the relationship being largely neutralized when organisms are phagocytosed and come to reside intracellularly. Although there is some variability in the response of different species to infections by members of this group of microorganisms, species specificity is not pronounced. Susceptibility of various organs and tissues within a given species to infection by organisms of this category is not highly specific and is usually related to the portal of entry or point of lodgment. Mechanisms by which these organisms produce lesions, though incompletely understood, seem to be related to the production of cell death—necrosis—both of migratory phagocytic cells of the host and of fixed cellular elements of the host's tissues. In general, the host's immunologic response to infections in this category is humoral. Endogenous humoral antibodies produced during these infections are often important in limiting the course of the disease. Humoral antibodies in the form of antisera have played important roles in therapy directed against certain of these diseases (for example, pneumococcal pneumonia and meningococcal meningitis), though in these roles they have largely been superseded by antibiotics.

Many, perhaps technically all, pyogenic infections represent expressions of virulence by organisms that are at least occasionally avirulent commensals in one or another compartment of the host's environment. This category of infections therefore introduces the concept of *opportunism* (that is, of diseases or lesions resulting when one set of circumstances leads to a given host's being parasitized by microorganisms of a given category).

Infections caused by staphylococci

Bacteria of the genus *Micrococcus (Staphylococcus)* are gram-positive, nonencapsulated, non–spore forming cocci that grow in grapelike clusters. Natural habitats of staphylococci include the human skin and nasopharynx. Smith[8] has estimated that 80% of people have a staph-

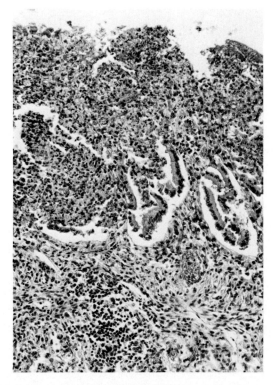

Fig. 6-6. Colon in bacillary dysentery. Acute inflammation of mucosal surface is in response to infection by essentially noninvasive organism *Shigella dysenteriae*.

ylococcal infection sometime during their lives and that a staphylococcal lesion develops in 5% in any one year. Staphylococci, especially the *aureus* variety, are the most common cause of purulent infections of the skin and subcutaneous tissues—lesions collectively designated *pyodermas*. These lesions bear such designations as *furuncle, carbuncle, impetigo, acne, paronychia, felon, phlegmon,* and *abscess*. The characteristic feature of dermal infection by staphylococci is necrosis of skin. Recent evidence indicates that this may result largely from ischemia, which in turn is a consequence of vasoconstrictive action of a toxin product of the staphylococcus. Other important toxins elaborated by this group of organisms, named according to their activities, include leukocidin, necrotoxin, hyaluronidase, and coagulase. Other features of staphylococci that contribute to virulence are (1) a surface constituent that enables the organism to resist phagocytosis and (2) the ability of certain strains of the organism to survive within leukocytes. Some strains of staphylococci elaborate an enterotoxic exotoxin, clinicopathologic aspects of which are described on p. 292.

Besides its primary, though in the broad sense opportunistic, role as a causative agent in pyodermas, *Staphylococcus*, especially the variant *aureus*, is a major cause of bacterial wound infections. *S. aureus* may complicate or contribute to chronicity of otherwise primary infections such as pneumonia, measles, pertussis, and scarlet fever.[66] The staphylococcus is frequently responsible for otitis media or paranasal sinusitis. From these loci related to the respiratory tract, the staphylococcus may secondarily cause meningitis or brain abscess. The organism may infect serous surfaces, producing purulent peritonitis, pericarditis (Fig. 6-7), or pleuritis (empyema). In infants and young children, primary staphylococcal pneumonia is a characteristic clinicopathologic entity with a relatively high mortality (see p. 929). Staphylococci may lodge in the kidney and cause hematogenous pyelonephritis. Staphylococci are the most common cause of purulent osteomyelitis.

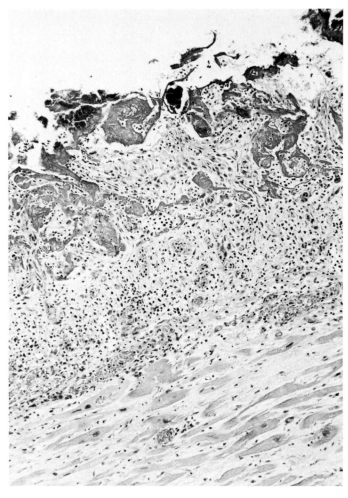

Fig. 6-7. Pyrogenic inflammation. Purulent pericarditis is produced by the staphylococcus *(Micrococcus pyogenes* var. *aureus).*

Impetigo contagiosa is an infectious and communicable disease largely restricted to children. Epidemic outbreaks occur in institutions such as nurseries or orphanages. Traditionally ascribed to infection by staphylococci, impetigo may also result from streptococcal infection of the skin.[27] Impetigo consists in the sequential development of pustules, vesicles, and crusted lesions (Fig. 6-8). Sometimes large confluent bullae occur. In newborn or debilitated infants, impetigo is occasionally fatal. The streptococcal form may be associated with glomerulonephritis (see Chapter 18).

Infections caused by streptococci

Streptococci are gram-positive organisms that grow in chains. Pathogenic varieties produce either alpha or beta hemolysis when cultured on blood agar. Alpha hemolysis results from incomplete lysis of blood cells in the culture medium and produces a green discoloration around the colony. Organisms that produce alpha hemolysis are customarily designated alpha-hemolytic streptococci (formerly *Streptococcus viridans*). This organism is a commensal in the mouth but gains clinical significance as the most common cause of subacute bacterial endocarditis (see p. 654).

Bacteria that produce beta hemolysis (complete hemolysis, with a clear, colorless halo about growing colonies) tend to be more invasive than alpha-hemolytic

streptococci. Nonhemolytic (delta) streptococci only exceptionally produce human disease.

In contrast to staphylococcal lesions, wherein thick purulent exudation is characteristic, streptococcal infections usually produce thin watery exudate, a reaction that has been attributed to the fact that streptococci elaborate streptokinase. This is by no means a rule, however. Pronounced diversity of reaction is an outstanding characteristic of streptococcal infection, and streptococci often produce pyogenic reactions. Examples of focal lesions include otitis media, appendicitis, impetigo, wound infections, tonsillitis, and pharyngitis. More generalized diseases are puerperal sepsis, brochopneumonia, meningitis, erysipelas, scarlet fever, and septicemia. In addition to these, streptococcal infection is undoubtedly concerned in (though not the immediate cause of) rheumatic fever and glomerulonephritis. It appears that immunologic reaction to the products of bacterial growth and the infectious process are direct causative mechanisms, though much remains to be explained (p. 811). The variation in reaction to streptococcal infection often pertains to the host, and age is an important factor, as has been emphasized by Powers and Boisvert.[64] In adults, streptococcal infections tend to be of a more spreading nature and produce less suppuration.

The high incidence of streptococcal infection is attributable not only to the pathogenicity of the streptococcus but also to its wide distribution in nature. *Streptococcus pyogenes* is found in the throat of 5% to 10% of the healthy adult population. Occurrence of this organism in the nose is a much more serious matter. Nasal carriers scatter large numbers of these organisms in the air and are also much more likely to infect their hands, clothing, and so on, than oral carriers are. Alpha-hemolytic streptococci are found almost invariably in the nasopharynx of healthy persons and are normal inhabitants of the small intestine.

Sore throat. Sore throat, when of infectious cause is more properly termed nasopharyngitis. Beta-hemolytic streptococci (*S. pyogenes*) are one of the most frequent causes and certainly the most important. As a rule the infection is superficial and characterized by a swollen, velvety, red pharyngeal mucosa, with swollen tonsils whose crypts exude purulent exudate. In addition to local pain, swelling, and tenderness, usually a generalized discomfort, headache, and malaise provide clinical evidence of toxemia. The process may extend further. Local extension may produce peritonsillar abscess (quinsy). With suppuration in or around the tonsil, there may be such swelling as to cause pronounced interference with eating and breathing. As a consequence of peritonsillar abscess, there may be wide dissemination of the infection through the soft tissues of the neck, resulting in cellulitis (Ludwig's angina). Before the ad-

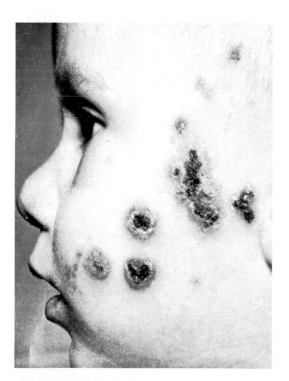

Fig. 6-8. Impetigo. Older lesions are dark and encrusted. (From Wehrle, P.F., and Top, F.H.: Communicable and infectious diseases, ed. 9, St. Louis, 1981, The C.V. Mosby Co.)

vent of chemotherapy and antibiotics, such a complication caused death in the majority of patients. Considerable regional extension may come about also as the result of suppuration with cervical lymph nodes, with spread along fascial planes to cause retropharyngeal or lateral pharyngeal abscess. Extension to tissues of other regions may occur as well, and both otitis media and sinusitis are frequent complications of streptococcal pharyngitis. Epidemic forms of streptococcal nasopharyngitis have occurred as a result of the ingestion of milk contaminated with S. *pyogenes*.

Septicemia is a complication especially feared. Finally, in considering complications of streptococcal nasopharyngitis and tonsillitis, one can hardly overemphasize the relationship these infections bear to rheumatic fever and glomerulonephritis.

Bronchopneumonia. Bronchopneumonia of streptococcal cause is almost always the result of streptococcal

pharyngitis or of infection superimposed on pertussis measles, influenza, or other viral pneumonitis. In the great influenza epidemic that occurred during World War I, most deaths were actually the result of streptococcal pneumonia. In these cases, tracheitis and bronchitis were striking features. The pneumonia was largely interstitial, tending to involve mostly the regions around bronchioles.

Erysipelas. Erysipelas, a specific form of cellulitis caused by beta-hemolytic streptococci, illustrates the diffusely spreading nature of many streptococcal infections. It usually begins without obvious portal of entry, though occasionally a primary injury can be demonstrated. The lesion is most often self-limited except in the very young or very old. The tissue involved is the subcutaneous, usually of the face but occasionally of the trunk or limbs. There is pronounced interstitial edema of subcutaneous tissues, and this exudate contains edema of subcutaneous tissues, and this exudate contains fibrin, some extravasated erythrocytes, and moderate numbers of inflammatory cells, mostly monocytes and lymphocytes (Fig. 6-9). Streptococci are present in great quantities in this fluid, especially in the zone of subepidermal tissue just ahead of the spreading lesion. Despite this, there is little evidence of necrosis. Suppuration does not occur except as a complication. The noticeable reddish discoloration that characterizes the

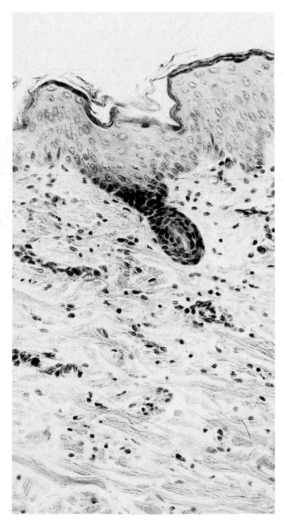

Fig. 6-9. Cellulitis in erysipelas. Cells of inflammation extending through loose, edematous, hyperemic, subcutaneous tissue.

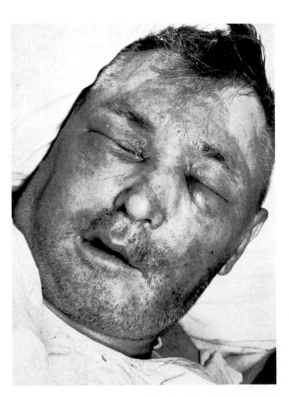

Fig. 6-10. Facial erysipelas. Notice sharp demarcation of discolored edematous area. (From Wehrle, P.F., and Top, F.H.: Communicable and infectious diseases, ed. 9, St. Louis, 1981, The C.V. Mosby Co.)

lesion, and from which the name erysipelas ('red skin') is derived, is an effect of great congestion. Direct injury to blood vessels is evident also in the hemorrhage that occurs through diapedesis. It is by this means that erythrocytes are contributed to the exudate and that blood pigment accumulates within macrophages. Usually within a week or 10 days there is spontaneous remission, and shortly thereafter complete healing occurs. Clinically, although the sharply circumscribed brawny edematous area discolored a fiery red (Fig. 6-10) is dramatic, the outstanding feature is profound toxemia.

Scarlet fever (scarlatina). The precise cause and pathogenesis of scarlet fever were not evident until the Dicks demonstrated in 1924 that an erythrogenic toxin obtained from broth filtrate of certain beta-hemolytic streptococci would, on injection into a susceptible individual, produce a typical erythematous reaction. As a result of widespread application of the Dick test, it became apparent that only a minority of adults were susceptible to scarlet fever and that the number who were "immune" was far greater than the number who had actually had the disease previously. Thus some of the difficulties in earlier experiments were explained. It appears that repeated experiences with *S. pyogenes* may confer immunity to scarlet fever even though the individual has not been exposed to the disease itself. Further evidence of the significance of erythrogenic toxin in the production of scarlet fever is furnished by the Schultz-Charlton phenomenon, and this is used also as a diagnostic test. When a patient with scarlet fever is given an intradermal injection of a small amount of specific antiserum (convalescent serum), blanching of the characteristic erythematous rash soon occurs in the immediate area of injection. Since the specific effect of such an injection is neutralization of the streptococcic toxin, it follows that the generalized skin reaction must be an effect of toxemia. The importance of individual variation in the host is illustrated by the fact that streptococcal pharyngitis may develop from the same strain of organism in several or all members of a family, yet scarlet fever may develop in only one of the group, the others manifesting only nasopharyngitis. It is apparent from this that scarlet fever may be contracted from a person who has only streptococcal pharyngitis.

In the early stages there is rather severe pharyngitis and tonsillitis. These, combined with fever, vomiting, and headache, make up the cardinal prodromal symptoms of scarlet fever. Because there is no specific strain of beta-hemolytic streptococci responsible for scarlet fever, bacteriologic studies do not provide a means for early diagnosis; in other words, a diagnosis of throat infection caused by *S. pyogenes* is not a diagnosis of scarlet fever. The diagnosis cannot be positively made until the second stage of the disease, which is reached 1 to 5

days after the onset. This is characterized by erythematous rash, and it is this skin reaction, more than any other feature, that defines scarlet fever as a distinct disease entity. The hyperemia and resultant red coloration of skin are manifestations of toxic injury (atony and dilatation) of vascular endothelium. This hyperemia blanches on pressure and disappears on death; thus little of the characteristic skin reaction is evident at autopsy. The skin is edematous, and particularly around hair follicles there are focal aggregations of lymphocytes and monocytes. In the middle layers of the epidermis an inflammatory exudate accumulates, and there is an accelerated keratinization at this level—pseudokeratosis. It is because of this that desquamation occurs sometime between the fifth and twenty-fifth days. The outer layers of skin separate from the intermediate zone, which has become keratinized. The tongue usually participates in this reaction too. During the first few days, it presents a "strawberry" appearance because of the erythematous papillae that project from a gray-coated background. When peeling occurs, the tongue becomes beefy red and glistening. Complications are divisible into three major categories:

1. The results of bacterial dissemination locally—otitis media, sinusitis, cervical adenitis, acute suppurative mastoiditis, and retropharyngeal abscess
2. The result of bacterial dissemination generally—metastatic foci of infection throughout the body, or frank septicemia
3. The manifestation of extraordinary reactions to toxins (this may be brought about by hypersensitivity)—interstitial nephritis or myocarditis, pericarditis, nonsuppurative arthritis, and glomerulonephritis

Puerperal sepsis. In the days before antiseptic surgery, puerperal sepsis was an important cause of death. In the maternity hospitals of that day, as many as one woman out of six died of septicemia. The very efforts that were exerted to determine the cause of this dread "childbed fever" served only to spread the disease, since the careful dissection and study of the dead women by their accoucheurs made gross contamination a certainty and increased the likelihood that the next patient would also be infected. Semmelweis, through his painstaking studies, and Oliver Wendell Holmes, by his brilliant writings, convinced the physicians and midwives of that day that childbed fever was the result of infection and that the etiologic agent was introduced by "unclean hands." Colebrook and Hare[55] reviewed 63 cases of puerperal sepsis of which approximately one third were shown to be the result of infection by *S. pyogenes* antigenically identical to that obtained from the patient's throat or nose. In slightly over half the cases, hemolytic streptococci of identical strain were isolated from the nose or throat of the physician in attendance or from other persons who had been in close contact with the patient.

Clinical signs of puerperal endometritis usually appear 3 or 4 days after labor but may be delayed for as long as 2 or 3 weeks. Symptoms are predominantly those of septicemia and include a septic type of fever, often with chills. Infection of the uterus as such does not ordinarily cause much discomfort, though this organ may be somewhat enlarged and tender to palpation. The vaginal discharge (lochia) may be either scanty or abundant but usually has a foul odor. Within the uterus, the inflammatory process is rather superficial and tends to be unimpressive. Thrombophlebitis is the really significant local change, since this is the means by which wide dissemination of the infection is accomplished. Uterine, pelvic, and ovarian veins may all be involved. Peritonitis is a frequent accompaniment of septic endometritis.

Endocarditis. Acute endocarditis, as a complication of septicemia, has been mentioned previously. Often this is caused by *S. pyogenes*, but it also commonly results from pneumococci, staphylococci, gonococci, and influenzal bacilli. Any organism that can cause septicemia may produce acute bacterial endocarditis. Subacute bacterial endocarditis (endocarditis lenta) is much more important, since the endocarditis in this instance represents the primary lesion and is a cause of bloodstream infection rather than a result. *Streptococcus viridans* is the organism responsible in approximately 95% of the cases and *Haemophilus influenzae* in approximately 3%. Infection of the heart valves results from bacteremia. Usually the cause of this bacteremia is not apparent. Often, however, it is a direct result of tooth extraction. Normal heart valves are practically never subject to the type of "chronic" infection (extending over months) that characterizes subacute bacterial endocarditis. Previous injury by rheumatic fever is by far the most common predisposing cause, though such congenital anomalies as bicuspid aortic valve, septal defects, and patent ductus arteriosus are also predisposing factors.

Infections caused by pneumococci

Diplococcus pneumoniae is responsible for most cases of lobar pneumonia (Fig. 6-11) and many cases of bronchopneumonia. Since the portal of entry for pneumococci is the respiratory tract, it is understandable that these organisms are often responsible for otitis media and paranasal sinusitis. Brain abscess may follow septic thrombosis of venous sinuses of the brain. The pneumococcus is an important cause of meningitis in both adults and children. In adults about half the cases occur without clinical evidence of a primary focus. In children, meningeal involvement is usually the result of an upper respiratory infection or otitis media.

Pneumococci have an antiphagocytic factor in their capsule, and they elaborate a hemolytic toxin, pneumolysin. However, neither of these, nor any other toxin that they produce, is known to be related to the virulence. Thus the pathogenesis of pneumococcal infection is not understood.

D. pneumoniae resembles alpha-hemolytic streptococci in many morphologic characteristics. However, its bile solubility and special antigenic properties serve to

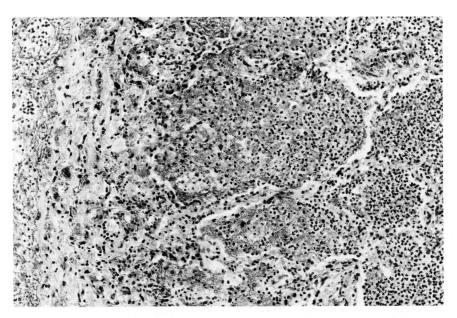

Fig. 6-11. Lobar pneumonia *(right)* and fibrinopurulent pleurisy *(left)*. Purulent inflammation is in response to infection by pneumococcus.

differentiate this oval or lance-shaped encapsulated gram-positive coccus. The organism usually occurs in diploform but may exist in short chains. Serologic studies have been concerned mostly with pneumococci isolated from patients with lobar pneumonia. Systematic studies have led to the establishment of specific types 1, 2, and 3, leaving a large residual group of unclassified types (group IV). Extension of these observations has separated from group IV 80 additional types. Approximately half of human infections result from types 1 through 8. There is an important practical aspect of this work, since these serologic differences—the result of specific capsular polysaccharides—determine antigenic behavior and are responsible for the fact that antibodies produced against one type are effective only for that type. Before chemotherapy and antibiotics proved effective, serum therapy was extensively used in the treatment of pneumococcal pneumonia, and it was essential that the type of organism be known so that type-specific antiserum could be given promptly.

Infections caused by meningococci

Neisseria meningitidis, a small, oval or bean-shaped, gram-negative coccus, usually occurs in pairs and occasionally in tetrads. It closely resembles the gonococcus morphologically. A capsule may be demonstrated but is not usually apparent. As in the case of pneumococcus, types based on antigenic differences are of practical importance, since immunity is largely type specific. Four serologic types have been described.

In addition to an antiphagocytic factor contained in the capsule, meningococci produce considerable endotoxin, and this is probably most important in the pathogenesis of meningococcal disease. The two major diseases resulting from meningococcal infection are meningitis and a fulminating form of septicemia.

Meningococcal meningitis. Meningococcal meningitis may be sporadic, endemic, or epidemic. It affects children and young adults most often. The source of infection is usually a healthy carrier or a person recently recovered from the disease. Ordinarily the population at large will include 2% to 5% of healthy individuals who harbor meningococci in the nasopharynx. When this figure approaches 20%, there is danger of an epidemic. During the height of an epidemic the carrier rate may reach 70%. Obviously the virulence of the prevailing strain of organisms will be of at least equal importance to the number of carriers. The disease is not highly contagious, and the infection rate rarely exceeds 1 in 1000, even during epidemics.

Meningococcal meningitis is conveniently considered under three stages. *Stage 1* consists in a local infection in the area of the portal of entry—the nasopharynx. This initial reaction is rarely given significance by the patient and may escape notice. *Stage 2* is characterized by septicemia (in approximately 25%, organisms are readily demonstrable in venous blood), and symptoms do not point toward any specific organ. There is fever, often associated with slight chills. The most striking feature is the rash, which has led to the term *spotted fever.* These "spots" begin as small areas of erythema. Soon, however, hemorrhage is evident as a result of thrombosis of arterioles and capillaries. Most of these are petechial in form (less than 2 mm), but there may be confluent areas as large as 1 cm in diameter. Fulminant forms often present massive purpuric hemorrhages, and the regions so involved may become gangrenous. At this time, should a spinal puncture be made, the fluid would appear essentially normal.

Stage 3 is the period of metastatic localization, principally to the cerebral meninges. Intense headache, vomiting, and prostration are followed by drowsiness or irritability and later by delirium or stupor, which may progress to coma. There is stiffness of the neck and, especially in children, a rigid posterior curvature of the back (opisthotonos).

Within the brain the first changes occur in the blood vessels of the leptomeninx (pia and arachnoid): hyperemia, slight serous exudation, and minute areas of hemorrhage. These progress, and soon cellular exudate becomes apparent. The pathologic picture varies depending on the duration and severity of the disease. In an advanced stage thick purulent exudate is present, most prominently over the base of brain, filling in around vessels and sulci and often obscuring cranial nerves. The vessels of the pia are engorged. The ventricles contain no great excess of fluid, but the fluid is turbid and filled with pus cells. Careful microscopic examination usually demonstrates the considerable efficiency of the pia as a mechanical barrier in preventing the spread of organisms into the brain substance. Degenerative changes are present in the superficial layers, however, as a result of the diffusion of toxins. The inflammatory exudate is composed principally of polymorphonuclear leukocytes enmeshed in numerous strands of fibrin (Fig. 6-12). Exudate is densest around blood vessels and may follow the vessels for some distance within the substance of the brain. These morphologic changes are similar to those occurring in most types of purulent meningitis. There is often focal encephalitis, evident as minute aggregations of leukocytes and, perhaps, tiny hemorrhages. In patients who die within the first few days, cerebrospinal fluid is increased in amount, but there is no evidence of hydrocephalus. In chronic forms internal hydrocephalus is often striking. Before specific therapy was developed, the mortality averaged 60% to 70%. Today the expected mortality is 5% to 10%.

Endocarditis and, occasionally, purulent monarthritis occur. The latter is to be differentiated from the tran-

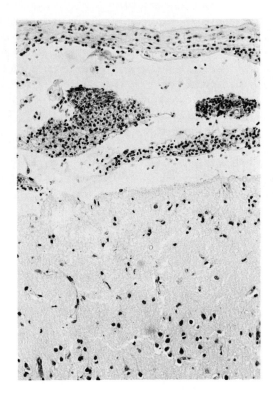

Fig. 6-12. Acute purulent meningitis caused by *Neisseria meningitidis.*

sient polyarthritis that frequently occurs, probably as an effect of hemorrhage within the joint. Pneumonia often complicates severe forms of the disease. Bacteria such as staphylococci and streptococci exert the major effect.

Rarely, there occurs a chronic meningococcemia that may persist as long as several months, often resolving spontaneously.

Fulminant meningococcemia. In fulminant meningococcemia the onset of symptoms is precipitous and the disease runs a violent and rapid course. Moritz and Zamcheck,[63] in their comprehensive study, found that meningococcemia was responsible for 110 of approximately 750 sudden and unexpected deaths in young soldiers. More than half the patients died within 6 hours after coming under medical observation. In all instances death occurred within 24 hours after onset of incapacitating symptoms, though approximately 70% of the patients had had prodromal signs in the form of a mild upper respiratory infection or subnormal feeling. Clinically the predominant manifestation was peripheral vascular collapse and shock; cyanosis was often a prominent feature, and cutaneous hemorrhages were observed in the majority (Fig. 6-13). This picture is essentially similar to that seen in infants and children. Clinical evidence of meningitis is not common because the rapid course of the disease usually leads to death before opportunity for noticeable involvement. Even though meningeal involvement does occur, symptoms

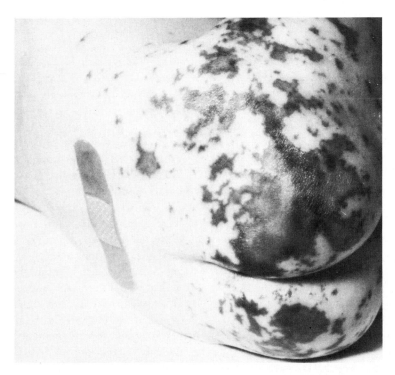

Fig. 6-13. Purpura in fulminating meningococcemia.

are frequently masked by the shocklike state of collapse. The term *Waterhouse-Friderichsen syndrome* is applied to this condition when, in addition to cutaneous hemorrhages, there is hemorrhage (usually massive and bilateral) into the adrenal glands. Some authorities have considered the state of collapse, which is so prominent in this condition, to be a manifestation of acute adrenocortical deficiency. However, complete cessation of adrenocortical function does not produce peripheral vascular collapse within so short a time. The action of bacterial toxins seems sufficient to explain the clinical picture in the majority of cases.

Infections caused by gonococci

Neisseria gonorrhoeae is the other important member of the group *Neisseria* and was the first to be described. Its detection by Neisser, in 1879, in inflammatory exudate from gonorrheal lesions settled the long controversy as to the true nature of this disease. The organism is very similar to the meningococcus. It is gram negative and most often occurs in diploform. There has been some question as to the character of toxins produced by this organism, but toxic action in experimental animals seems largely if not entirely a result of endotoxins, as is also the case with the meningococcus. Studies of serologic types have yielded very irregular results. Since the organism is fastidious in its growth requirements and dies quickly under unfavorable conditions, infection is almost always the result of direct personal contact. The gonococcus is quite restricted in its portal of entry. In human experiments, large quantities of virulent organisms have been injected subcutaneously without resultant disease.

The role of several surface components of gonococci in pathogenesis of gonorrheal infection has been productivity studied.[51,54] The outer envelope of gonococci, as of all gram-negative bacteria, consists of an inner cell membrane, a middle peptidoglycan cell wall, and an outer membrane. In pathogenic gonococci this triple envelope is traversed by elongated filamentous pili, polymers of protein subunits of molecular weight about 19,000. Pili mediate attachment of gonococci to susceptible cells.

The outer membrane contains a lipopolysaccharide and a variety of proteins. Among these is protein I immunologically heterogenous, some serotypes of which contribute to serum resistance and disseminated infection. Protein II is associated with colony opacity, which is correlated with virulence in a chick embryo model.

The only natural host of *N. gonorrhoeae* is humans, and the usual mode of transmission is sexual contact. Gonorrhea is the most common venereal disease. Approximately 1 million cases are reported in the United States annually, but because of underreporting and asymptomatic infections the annual occurrence of new cases may be nearer 3 million. The highest frequency is in men and women between 20 and 24 years of age, and the second highest is in the age group 15 to 19 years. Homosexuality and juvenile sexuality have recently become more important than prostitution in perpetuating gonorrhea in medically advanced societies.

The incubation period of genital gonorrhea is between 2 and 7 days depending, at least in part, on the number of infecting organisms. Gonorrhea is an acute purulent inflammation largely confined to mucus-secreting surfaces. Deep or systemic pyogenic infections are likewise pathologically nonspecific.

In males the earliest manifestation is an acute urethritis manifested by dysuria, frequency, and a purulent urethral discharge. Seminal vesiculitis and acute prostatis are now uncommon. In untreated cases an acute epididymitis, usually exquisitely painful, may occur. Late complications in males include periurethritis with urethral strictures, prostatic abscesses, and chronic epididymitis. Sterility may result.

In females the most common site of infection is the cervix. Urethritis and infection of accessory glands (Bartholin's and Skene's) may occur. At least half the infected women are asymptomatic. Gonococcal endometritis is virtually unknown, but infection of the mucosal surface of the uterine tubes is common. In many cases, fimbriae coalesce and purulent inflammation of the obstructed tube (pyosalpinx) results. In others, adherence of fimbriae to the ovary is followed by the development of an inflammatory mass (tubo-ovarian abscess). This constellation of clinicopathologic syndromes, of which gonorrhea is the major etiologic factor, is clinically designated *pelvic inflammatory disease* (PID).

Although usually confined to mucus-secreting surfaces, infection by gonococci may rarely spread as disseminated gonococcal infection (DGI) to joints,[41] the endocardium, or the meninges. The gonococcus is the most common agent identified in acute monarticular purulent arthritis. A variety of cutaneous and renal lesions, some of them probably immunologically mediated, have been described.

Gonococcal infection of the rectum occurs in women and homosexual men by penoanal intercourse with an infected partner and by secondary spread from the endocervix in women.[44,47,48] Stratified squamous anal epithelium is resistant to infection, but the columnar rectal mucosa is susceptible. Most cases of rectal gonorrhea are asymptomatic with minimal or nonspecific histologic features, but an acute mucopurulent or hemorrhagic proctitis may occur.

Gonococcal pharyngitis occurs in women and homosexual men who practice fellatio.[52] Most cases are asymptomatic, but histologically nonspecific pharyngitis, tonsillitis, and gingivitis have been described.

Gonococcal infection of the conjunctiva and an acute purulent conjunctivitis may occur in newborn infants during passage through the infected birth canal. Historically an important cause of blindness, gonococcal conjunctivitis has been largely prevented by such procedures as routine conjunctival instillation of silver nitrate solution at delivery.

Acute purulent gonococcal vulvovaginitis occurs in young girls in whom nonkeratinized epithelium of the reproductive tract is susceptible to invasion of gonococci. Although fomites such as contaminated underclothes or bed linens may occasionally be implicated, most cases result from sexual contact with adults.

Infections caused by Haemophilus

Haemophilus influenzae (Pfeiffer's bacillus), a minute gram-negative rod so short as to be almost coccal, often occurs in chains. It frequently exhibits pleomorphism, and pathogenic strains are almost always encapsulated. The species name, *influenzae*, was suggested by Pfeiffer in 1892 as a result of observations that led him to conclude, erroneously, that this was the causative organism of influenza. It is now established that influenza is caused by a virus and that the frequent association of *H. influenzae* with this disease is evidence of secondary infection. The genus name, *Haemophilus*, refers to the hemophilic nature of this group of organisms. Blood is a necessary part of their nutriment because it furnishes a coenzyme and also an iron-containing pigment from which the organism may synthesize cytochrome and related compounds.

H. influenzae normally inhabits the nasopharynx and tonsillar region of approximately 50% of individuals, and infections with this organism are usually secondary to some other disease. After a "cold" or other upper respiratory infection it commonly produces sinusitis or otitis media. *H. influenzae*, though a frequent cause of primary pneumonia in children, rarely causes pneumonia in adults except as a complication of influenza or primary atypical pneumonia. Pneumonia produced by the influenzal bacillus is characterized by bronchitis, bronchiolitis, and patchy bronchopneumonia. Purulent exudate may fill the bronchioles and lead to bronchiectasis. This picture contrasts sharply with that of interstitial pneumonia caused by *Streptococcus pyogenes*, which may also complicate influenza (see p. 363). In infants and young children, *H. influenzae* infection of the respiratory passages may cause pronounced edema, obstructive laryngitis or acute epiglottitis, and death within a few hours.

No exotoxin has been recovered from *H. influenzae*, and it appears that the serious effects of infection result from endotoxins. Most pathogenic strains have a capsule, and this is believed to offer protection against phagocytosis by leukocytes.

H. influenzae is responsible for approximately 3% of cases of subacute bacterial endocarditis. After bacteremia it may on occasion produce a variety of pyogenic infections (such as cholecystitis, pyelitis, arthritis, or osteomyelitis). Especially in children, this organism causes a particularly destructive meningitis.

One of the most common causes of acute infectious conjunctivitis is the so-called Koch-Weeks bacillus (*Haemophilus aegyptius*), an organism closely related to or identical with *H. influenzae*.

A more recently recognized variety of *Haemophilus* has been termed *Haemophilus vaginalis* because of its frequent occurrence in the vagina and its production of what was formerly considered nonspecific vaginitis.

Chancroid is an infection by *Haemophilus decreyi*. Now uncommon in medically advanced countries, it occurs in socioeconomically deprived societies in emerging cultures. The disease is almost always venereally transmitted.

Chancroid begins as a nonspecific papule in the genitourethral epithelium of either sex and progresses to ulceration and purulent inflammation on the penile corona of males or the genital vestibule of females. It then progresses to a purulent destructive lesion in the inguinal region. Ragged, often excavated, local genital ulcers occur (Fig. 6-14). Spontaneous resolution is accompanied by considerable fibroblastic distortion. During the evolution of the genital lesions, reactive hyperplasia of inguinal lymph nodes results in the production of buboes, which with purulent necrosis and the formation of abscesses become painful. Many inguinal swellings in chancroid are actually subcutaneous areas of inflammation (pseudobuboes) independent of regional lymph nodes.

Microscopically the genital lesions of chancroid present three zones: (1) a zone of ulceration and acute inflammation consisting of fibrin, pyknotic nuclear frag-

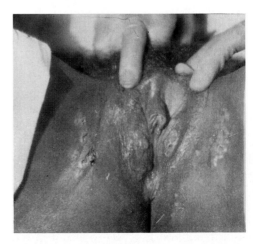

Fig. 6-14. Multiple chancroidal ulcers on vulva, perineum, and thighs.

ments, erythrocytes, and polymorphonuclear cells, (2) a deeper and peripherally spreading zone of actively inflamed granulation tissue, and (3) a zone of perivascular lymphocytic and plasmacytic infiltration. Tissue is rarely made available for microscopic examination but is occasionally examined when the clinical question of malignancy is raised.

Infections caused by Proteus

Highly pleomorphic gram-negative bacilli that are actively motile, *Proteus* organisms are widely dispersed in nature, especially in relation to decaying meat and manure. They are commonly found in the feces of humans but in small numbers as a rule.

As far as disease production is concerned, there are two main species: *P. vulgaris* and *P. morganii*. These organisms are principally saprophytes. However, *P. vulgaris* often produces cystitis. Frequently it can be recovered from the urine in pure culture. Because this organism produces ammonia from urea, infection is characterized by very alkaline urine. This may precipitate calcium, magnesium, and ammonium salts from the urine, resulting in alkaline-encrusted cystitis. Otitis media is occasionally produced by *P. vulgaris* and is characterized by rather widespread necrosis of both osseous and soft tissues. *Proteus* organisms can be recovered in approximately 10% of cases of appendicitis. These organisms often occur in abscesses, infected wounds, and burns as one component of a mixed infection, and their effects are obscured by the other, more predominant organisms.

P. morganii was originally isolated from the stools of infants with summer diarrhea and ever since that time (1906) has been considered one of the etiologic agents of summer diarrhea. Many careful studies would indicate that there is no single specific bacterial cause for this clinical entity.

Infections caused by Pseudomonas aeruginosa

Pseudomonas aeruginosa is a slender, gram-negative rod that varies considerably in length. It is a common cause of wound infection, and the nature of the infection is often recognized clinically by the greenish blue color imparted to the purulent exudate. It was formerly called *Bacillus pyocyaneus* because of this property. Particularly in the case of burns, infection with *P. aeruginosa* is often associated with delayed wound healing. Cruickshank and Lowbury[56] have shown that pyocyanine, the principal blue-gree pigment elaborated by *P. aeruginosa*, has a relatively high toxicity for human skin and human leukocytes in vitro. The level of concentration of this material, as measured in a series of infected human burns, was sufficient to account for such toxic effects. Infections of the nasal fossae, middle ear, and external ear are occasionally produced by this organism,

especially in children. These tissues may undergo extensive necrosis, leading to meningitis. Especially in infants and small children, a serious form of pneumonia may be produced.[59] Infection of the skin can lead to patchy areas of necrosis and ulceration sometimes referred to as *ecthyma gangrenosum* (Fig. 6-13). The organism is occasionally responsible for pyelonephritis and also infection of the eye and of joints.

As with *Proteus* infections, the frequency and importance of *P. aeruginosa* in mixed infections have been more fully appreciated since antibiotics have become widely used. Frequently the presence of *P. aeruginosa*, masked by other, antibiotic-sensitive organisms, is apparent only when these other organisms are destroyed. Particularly in debilitated persons (treated with antibiotics), *P. aeruginosa* is becoming a common cause of septicemia and death. In these cases there are many foci of necrosis, resembling the Shwartzman phenomenon, with exudation being minimal. Walls of small arteries and veins are necrotic and thrombosed, and large numbers of organisms are evident within the vessels. In one series of 23 cases reported by Forkner and associates,[60] abnormal neurologic manifestations occurred in more than half. In all, peripheral vascular collapse occurred as a terminal event.

As in the case of *Proteus* organisms, *P. aeruginosa* has been recovered frequently from the stools of those with summer diarrhea and is considered to be one of the etiologic agents of this disease.

Pseudomonas pseudomallei infection (that is, melioidosis) is discussed on p. 322.

Infections caused by Legionella

Legionella pneumophila is a fastidious gram-negative bacillus demonstrated with difficulty in diseased tissue. The organism causes Legionnaires' disease[69] (a sporadic pneumonic infection with an appreciable mortality) and Pontiac fever (a febrile, flulike illness with minimal mortality and nonpneumonic clinical features).[87]

Infections caused by Escherichia coli

Escherichia coli (Bacillus coli) is a gram-negative bacillus, varying in form from a short coccobacillus to a long slender rod, indistinguishable from the typhoid, dysentery, and paratyphoid group of organisms except by cultural or serologic characteristics. It is a normal inhabitant of feces, and the infections it produces are largely on the basis of opportunism (except in infants, in whom *E. coli*, particularly serogroups O 111 and O 55, may produce severe diarrhea—often of epidemic proportions and occasionally causing death, with minimal or no anatomic lesions).[57,67] This organism frequently is considered together with *Pseudomonas aeruginosa* and bacilli of the *Proteus* group, since it produces pyogenic infections of similar type. Resultant purulent exudate is ordinarily grayish green, in contrast to the blue-green color that characterizes infection by *P. aeruginosa.*

E. coli is of great importance as a cause of infections of the urinary tract, where it ranks first in frequency. It often acts alone and may be recovered in pure culture. Frequently, however, there is a mixed infection, and an important component is *Streptococcus faecalis* (group D hemolytic streptococcus). As in all ascending infections of the urinary tract, obstruction to the outflow of urine is an important predisposing factor. First, there is infection of the bladder, and cystitis may represent the total extent of bacterial involvement. Often, however, this is followed by ureteritis and pyelonephritis (p. 834).

Since *E. coli* normally inhabits the intestinal tract, fecal peritonitis invariably includes this organism as a part of the infectious mixture. Where there is mechanical injury, local injury from interference with blood supply (volvulus, obstructive appendicitis, diverticulitis, infarction of the bowel), or preliminary injury resulting from a primary hematogenous infection, *E. coli* avails itself of the opportunity provided and causes or contributes to infection.

In cholecystitis and cholangitis, *E. coli* is frequently demonstrable on culture. However, there is evidence that cholecystitis is usually of hematogenous origin and that streptococci most often initiate the disease. The failure to find streptococci more often may be because bile inhibits the growth of this organism, and culture of the bile fails to indicate the nature of infection within the wall of the gallbladder.

E. coli is an important cause of wound infection, especially in the region of the buttocks or thighs.

Infections caused by Klebsiella and Enterobacter aerogenes

Klebsiella pneumoniae (Friedländer's bacillus) is a short, gram-negative, encapsulated bacillus that often occurs in diploform, in which case it resembles the pneumococcus in appearance. As with the pneumococcus, the capsule contains an antigenic polysaccharide that is responsible for type specificity; nucleoprotein contained within the body of the organism (somatic antigen) confers species specificity. Three principal strains have been isolated and defined—A, B, and C. A large group (group X) remains unclassified. Type B of *K. pneumoniae* is similar immunologically to type 2 pneumococcus. Protective antibodies are type specific. The organism inhabits the nasopharynx of 5% to 25% of individuals.

Enterobacter aerogenes (an uncommon organism) is virtually identical to *K. pneumoniae.* Consequently, these organisms often are referred to as the *Klebsiella-Enterobacter* group. Traditionally *E. aerogenes* is con-

sidered to occur normally in the intestinal tract, whereas *K. pneumoniae* is found in the nasopharynx. Actually differentiation between the two often cannot be made on morphologic or antigenic grounds.

Pneumonia. Pneumonia caused by *K. pneumoniae* (Friedländer's pneumonia) probably accounts for 2% or 3% of all pneumonias, though estimates of frequency range from 0.4% to 18%. It most often affects those in the older age group, and its occurrence is favored by any condition of general debility, including chronic alcoholism. The early course of the disease, with its acute onset, resembles that of pneumococcal pneumonia, but prostration is usually more striking and is often associated with pronounced dyspnea and cyanosis. The sputum usually contains more blood than that in the case of pneumococcal pneumonia and appears mucinous. There may be frank hematemesis. Organisms are readily seen in the sputum and are there in great abundance. Characteristically the lung presents an area of massive consolidation that may exceed the limits of a single lobe. Grossly, the picture is similar to the one seen with pneumococcal lobar pneumonia except that cut surfaces of the lung appear slimy and the lung parenchyma is friable. Histologically the major point of difference between this and ordinary lobar pneumonia is necrosis of the alveolar walls (Fig. 6-15). It is this effect that makes the lung friable and greatly predisposes to such serious complications as lung abscess and organization. Fibrinous pleuritis is a characteristic feature of the disease, and empyema is another complication to be feared. Bacteremia is readily detectable in over half the cases and may lead to metastatic involvement of the meninges or joints. Septicemia with endocarditis has been observed. This may occur independent of pneumonia, and often the source of infection is obscure. The mortality of Friedländer's pneumonia was formerly very high, averaging 70% to 80%, and the majority of those who survived had major complications. Although antibiotics are effective in treatment, the mortality from Friedländer's pneumonia is still 20% to 25%.

Chronic pulmonic infections. Chronic pulmonic infections with Friedländer's bacillus often arise in patients with chronic bronchitis or bronchiectasis, tuberculosis, influenza, or pneumonia. Occasionally, acute pneumonia caused by this organism continues as a persistent chronic disease, leading to chronic abscesses, bronchiectasis, cavity formation, and extensive fibrosis. The condition often closely simulates pulmonary tuberculosis.

K. pneumoniae has been isolated from a wide variety of focal suppurative lesions (otitis media, salpingitis, subphrenic abscess, and cholecystitis). An epidemic of infectious diarrhea in infants, with high mortality, has been ascribed to this organism.

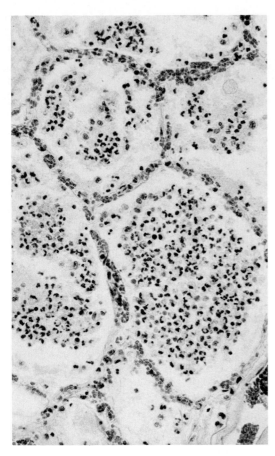

Fig. 6-15. Pneumonia caused by *Klebsiella pneumoniae* (Friedländer's bacillus).

Rhinoscleroma. Rhinoscleroma, a chronic and progressive granulomatous infection of the mucosa of the nose and pharynx, has been attributed to *Klebsiella rhinoscleromatis*, but more recent studies indicate that this organism may be identical to type C of *K. pneumoniae*.

Atrophic rhinitis. A persistent atrophic rhinitis, characterized by abundant encrusted purulent discharge and a foul odor, is apparently caused by *Klebsiella ozaenae*. This organism shares the somatic antigen of *K. pneumoniae* but has a different capsular antigen from A, B, or C.

Cat-scratch disease

A fastidious coccobacillus or cell wall–deficient bacillus has recently been incriminated in cat-scratch disease.[82]

Listeria and Erysipelothrix

Members of the genera *Listeria* and *Erysipelothrix* are small gram-positive rods that are nonsporulating, aerobic, facultative anaerobes of the family Corynebacteriaceae.

Infections caused by Listeria. *Listeria monocytogenes* is easily confused with diphtheroids and has often mistakenly been considered a contaminant. Although the importance of listeriosis as a disease of animals (especially cattle, sheep, goats, and rabbits) has been long recognized, the role of *L. monocytogenes* as a human pathogen has been appreciated only recently.[73,74] In humans there are four principal forms that the infection may take.[89] In order of decreasing importance these are as follows:

1. Listeria meningitis, an acute purulent meningitis that cannot be differentiated morphologically from several other purulent meningitides[64]
2. Granulomatosis infantiseptica, resulting from intrauterine infection complicating bacteremia or mild septicemia in the mother; usually causes death of the fetus or newborn infant; petechial hemorrhages of the skin often occur, progressing to purpura—a picture similar to the one seen with meningococcemia; most characteristic are the numerous and widely disseminated focal necroses that occur throughout organs and tissues
3. Listeria septicemia, which may resemble septicemia produced by numerous other organisms, including *Salmonella typhosa*, and requires isolation of the organism for specific diagnoses
4. Oculoglandular listeriosis

Infections caused by Erysipelothrix. In humans, *Erysipelothrix rhusiopathiae* causes erysipeloid, a skin infection that usually occurs on the hands and appears somewhat like erysipelas.[91] The infection is ordinarily localized, but occasionally lymphadenitis develops. In approximately 6% of cases, arthritis occurs in the joints adjacent to the area of primary infection. Rarely the infection becomes generalized, producing septicemia. *E. rhusiopathiae* principally affects animals. When human infection occurs, it is usually an occupational disease, developing in workers who pack meat (particularly swine), dress poultry (particularly turkeys), or process seafood (including crabs).

Infections caused by Mycoplasma

Mycoplasma is a genus of bacteria (PPLO organisms) that has only recently come to be recognized as pathogenic for humans, though for many years species have been known to produce disease in a variety of animals, some of which are of economic importance. These organisms are the smallest free-living cells yet recognized. They have no cell walls and are quite pleomorphic. Their range of size is considerable. Many are 0.2 to 0.5 μm, though the smallest infective unit is less than 0.2 μm, and colonies of organisms cluster together to form bodies larger than 0.5 μm.[92] Obviously, these organisms are beyond the resolution of light microscopy. They behave as intracellular parasites but grow on a variety artificial (including solid) media. Individual colonies are too small to be seen without magnification, though when grown on blood agar, the zone of hemolysis (produced by some species) is visible to the naked eye.

A causal relationship between *Mycoplasma pneumoniae* and primary atypical pneumonia has been proved. Although *Mycoplasma* organisms frequently have been recovered from affected tissues in several of the arthritides and certain ill-defined urogenital diseases, causal relationship has not been proved.

L (Lister Institute) forms of a variety of bacteria somewhat resemble *Mycoplasma* morphologically and in cultural characteristics. The role of L forms in human pathogenesis is controversial.

Intracellular infections

A limited number of bacterially mediated diseases constitute the next step of parasitic intimacy. In this group of bacterial infections a relatively close relationship between parasite and host is reflected by considerable species specificity, a relatively circumscribed habitat of microorganisms within their host (largely within cells of the reticuloendothelial system), and a tendency for these infections to be associated with proliferation of parasitized cells rather than necrosis of host cells. This group of bacterial infections constitutes the zoonoses—phenomenologically defined infectious diseases of defined animal species, including humans. Among these infections are the characteristic human zoonoses *Salmonella typhosa* typhoid fever and *Mycobacterium tuberculosis* (var. *hominis*) tuberculosis. Also included would be the inadvertent interposition of a human host along the chain of infectivity, for example, in the almost innumerable species-characteristic (if not species-specific) salmonelloses, brucellosis, tularemia, and plague.

Occurrence of many of these diseases in the human host requires the interposition of geographic, occupational, or other environmental exposures that make possible contact with infected fomites. Uncommon and exotic infections such as glanders and meliodosis may present features of either an acute septicopyemia or a disseminated reticuloendothelial granulomatous disease depending on a variety of factors, most important among which is probably the dose of infecting microorganisms.

The tendency of many diseases in this category to exist in nature as overt (epizootic) or latent (enzootic) zoonoses reflects considerable species specificity. It is perhaps worth reemphasis that this level of species specificity may recognize humans as in the case of typhoid fever or tuberculosis. In the category of infections under discussion, organ and tissue specificity is much less related to portal of entry than in the infections by pyogenic bacteria described previously. Infections in the category under discussion tend to produce systemic manifestations and are accompanied by lesions, particularly in components of the reticuloendothelial system, almost irrespective of or at least in concurrence with lesions at the portal of entry. Bacteria responsible for this group of diseases promptly tend to be phagocytosed by fixed phagocytic cells of the reticuloendothelial system and to stimulate responses by mononuclear cells, an inflammatory reaction characterized by infiltration and proliferation of fixed mononuclear cells and designated granulomatous. Many infectious lesions attributable to microorganisms in the category of this discussion therefore fall into the group of granulomatous inflammations.

The immunologic response of the host to infections of this class of microorganisms tends increasingly to be mediated by the cellular limb of the immune response and also to be less than completely protective. Often, however, immunologic aspects of these infections assume diagnostic importance, particularly inasmuch as formal isolation and identification of these organisms may be less easy than in the case of pyogenic infections.

Infections caused by salmonellas

The genus *Salmonella* contains species pathogenic for both animals and humans. Originally salmonellas were classified by the human diseases they caused, the species from which they were isolated, or the geographic location in which they were first isolated. Recent usage recognizes only three species: *S. choleraesuis*, *S. typhosa*, and *S. enteritidis*. The first two are serologically homogeneous. *S. enteritidis* is not, consisting of more than 1000 strains conventionally designated with nonitalicized characterizations, for example, *S. enteritidis* (serotype paratyphi A).

With respect to host preference, salmonellas fall into three groups: (1) *S. typhosa*, which is more or less strongly adapted to humans, (2) *S. choleraesuis*, of which the primary host is swine but which also occurs in other animals including humans, and (3) a very large number of salmonellas that produce disease in humans and other animals with equal facility.

Salmonellas cause three types of human disease: specific enteric fevers, septicemic diseases without specific organ-system localization, and gastroenteritis.

Enteric (typhoid and paratyphoid) fevers. In 1926 the death rate from typhoid fever in the United States was 20.54 per 100,000 population. In 1973 only 680 cases of typhoid fever were reported, with only 7 deaths. At present only a few hundred cases occur annually in the Unites States. Epidemics such as the one in Zermatt, Switzerland,[71] continue to occur, however, even in medically advanced countries.[78] As our vigilance relaxes, new and large epidemics may be expected as a reminder that *S. typhosa* is a highly pathogenic organism.

S. typhosa is a short, plump, gram-negative rod that is flagellated and actively motile. It is indistinguishable morphologically from other members of the enteric group. Its relative lack of resistance to common antiseptics, drying, sunlight, and heat is one reason why sanitary measures have been so effective in controlling the disease. Infection occurs directly or indirectly from an individual afflicted with or convalescing from the disease or from a healthy carrier. Contaminated food or water is the common medium of contagion. The "five F's" most concerned with spread of this disease are food, fingers, flies, fomites, and feces. Urine is often a more important source of infection than feces, since contamination of the hands is more likely to occur after urination, and the urine is more likely to be "deposited" in an unsuitable container or on the ground. Then, too, in those whose typhoid fever is complicated by pyeloureteritis, the number of organisms passed in the urine is greatly in excess of that commonly found in the feces.

S. typhosa is, for all practical purposes, restricted in portal of entry to the gastrointestinal tract. In human volunteers, 10^5 to 10^7 ingested bacilli are required to induce the disease. Typhoid bacilli have been injected subcutaneously without harm and, in fact, some vaccines have contained viable organisms. On penetrating the intestinal mucosa, the organisms quickly enter lymphatic vessels and mesenteric nodes, whence they reach the liver and then, by the thoracic duct, the bloodstream. All this occurs in the incubation period, usually 10 to 14 days. This is the first stage of the disease, in which generalization of the infection occurs before localizing lesions draw attention to the intestine.

In the second stage there are severe headaches; generalized aching, especially of the arms and legs; malaise; and fatigue. Shortly thereafter the picture changes to one of frank septicemia, with chills, fever, prostration, splenic enlargement, and the characteristic rose spots. The last usually occur during the second week of the disease and at first glance resemble petechial hemorrhages. The fact that they blanch on pressure reveals them to be an effect of severe hyperemia (capillary atony). Aggregations of macrophages and edema in these focal areas indicate that they represent sites of bacterial localization (embolization) and resultant local toxic injury. They disappear after a few days.

The third stage, after a week to 10 days, is dominated by effects of local bacterial injury, especially in the intestinal tract, mesenteric lymph nodes, spleen, and liver.

Last is the stage of lysis, in which the infectious process is gradually overcome. Symptoms slowly disappear and the temperature gradually returns to normal.

The four stages of the disease and their significance are illustrated in Fig. 6-16.

Although septicemia dominates the early stages of typhoid fever, significant local changes begin to occur during the third stage—7 to 10 days after clinical onset—first in the lymphoid tissue of the intestinal tract. Peyer's patches of the ileum and the solitary lymph follicles in the region of the cecum become hyperplastic and so swollen as to produce almost buttonlike protrusions (Fig. 6-17).[76] The mesenteric lymph nodes become hyperplastic too, as a result of infection through the lymphatics, and *S. typhosa* can usually be recovered in pure culture from these nodes. Along with this, the reticuloendothelial system as a whole is responding to septicemia, and there is hyperplasia of other lymph

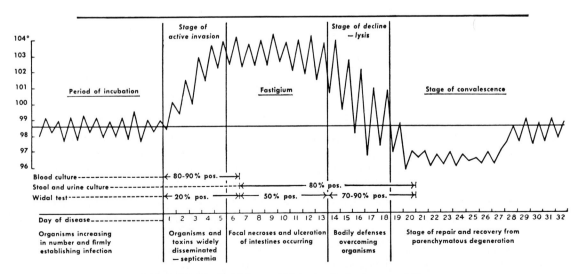

Fig. 6-16. Typhoid fever. Clinicopathologic correlation.

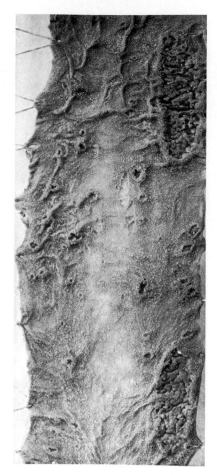

Fig. 6-17. Typhoid fever. Ulceration of ileum. Ulcerative lesions of ileum correspond in location to lymphoid follicles and Peyer's patches. Where they occur in Peyer's patches *(on right)*, their oval shape with long axis is parallel to that of intestine. (AFIP 2803.)

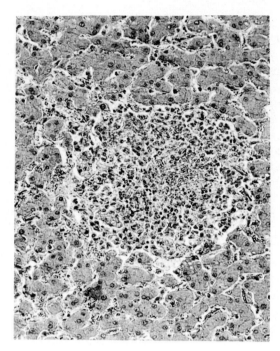

Fig. 6-18. Typhoid nodule in liver.

nodes, the spleen, reticular elements of the bone marrow, and the Kupffer cells of the liver. After 7 to 10 days, the picture in the intestine is complicated by necrosis and ulceration of areas that formerly exhibited lymphoid hyperplasia. Long oval ulcers in the ileum parallel the long axis of the bowel and correspond in shape and arrangement to Peyer's patches (Fig. 6-17). In the colon, ulcers are smaller and punctate, corresponding to the smaller lymphoid follicles there.

Microscopically an outstanding characteristic is the lack of polymorphonuclear leukocytes. The predominant cell of reaction is a large monocyte (macrophage) that somewhat resembles the blood monocyte. These are present in abundance in the base and margins of the ulcer. Lymphocytes and plasma cells are seen too. Lymph nodes exhibit foci of necrosis that may be as large as several millimeters in diameter. There is gross proliferation of the sinusoidal cells, and sinusoids are filled with macrophages similar to those observed in the

intestinal ulcers. Leukopenia is characteristic and an important clinical sign.

Among other organs, most changes occur in the spleen and liver. The spleen is greatly enlarged, frequently weighing 500 g or more. Its capsule is tense, and the parenchyma is soft. The organ is so soft and swollen that occasionally it ruptures during removal at autopsy. The striking cherry-red color is reflected microscopically by hyperemia. There is hyperplasia, especially of the red pulp. Areas of focal necrosis are seen, similar to those observed in mesenteric lymph nodes.

The liver also is enlarged and swollen, as evidenced by the tense capsule and rounded edges. It presents the picture of gross cloudy swelling. Parenchymatous degeneration is evident microscopically, and focal necrosis is a characteristic finding. This is a characteristic reaction of typhoid fever and occurs in lymph nodes, spleen, and bone marrow, as well as the liver (Fig. 6-18).

The heart and kidneys show cloudy swelling as a manifestation of toxemia. This change in the heart is reflected by a persistent bradycardia (an important diagnostic sign) that appears out of place alongside the patient's fever.

Skeletal muscles are particularly susceptible to these toxins and exhibit a pronounced degree of Zenker's (waxy) degeneration.

There are many other complications from this disease. Most feared is massive intestinal hemorrhage, which occurs in 5% to 10% of the patients. Next in importance is peritonitis resulting from perforation of the bowel. The most common site is the terminal ileum, and the most common time is during the second or third week. When perforation of the intestine occurs, the resultant fecal peritonitis is usually fatal. Rupture of a mesenteric lymph node will produce a specific *Salmonella typhosa* peritonitis, which is less severe and from which the patient often recovers. Intestinal obstruction as a sequel to ulceration rarely occurs because there is relatively little scar formation on healing. Since typhoid fever is a septicemic disease, focal metastatic infections can develop in a variety of places and may be responsible for osteomyelitis, meningitis, endocarditis, or nephritis. In approximately 5% to 10% of cases, thrombophlebitis of the femoral or saphenous veins occurs. This rarely develops before the fourth week and comes at a time when the patient appears well on the road to recovery. Infection of the gallbladder occurs almost invariably. This poses a special problem if the resultant cholecystitis becomes chronic, leading to a persistent carrier state. Focal paralysis sometimes occurs and seems to be an effect of toxemia. Relapses occur in 5% to 10% of the cases.

Death may result from one of the complications previously described but often simply from typhoid fever itself. The terminal phase is one of severe debility and wasting. The mortality, formerly 10% to 20%, has been greatly reduced by use of chloramphenicol.

Septicemia. *Salmonella* septicemias produce high remittent fevers ordinarily without gastrointestinal manifestations. Foci of suppuration may occur in almost any organ—kidneys, biliary tract, heart, meninges, bones, joints, or lungs. Predisposing factors include sickle cell disease, the hemolytic anemia of bartonellosis, and treatment of other conditions with broad-spectrum antibodies, which disturb the normal flora of the intestine.

Enteric fevers (paratyphoid fever) caused by salmonellas other than *S. typhosa* are milder than classic typhoid fever and usually have a shorter incubation period.

Gastroenteritis. Any of a very wide group of salmonellas can cause acute gastroenteritis. The source of infection is ingestion of organisms contained in contaminated food or drink, often meat or eggs. *Salmonella* gastroenteritis is one bacterial disease that is not decreasing in incidence in the United States. Annually 15,000 to 20,000 cases are reported. The incubation period is somewhat longer than in staphylococcal food poisoning, with which *Salmonella* gastroenteritis may be easily confused. Headache, chills, and abdominal pain are followed by nausea, vomiting, and diarrhea. The diagnosis depends on isolating the organism from stool or from the suspected food.

Brucellosis (undulant fever, Mediterranean fever, Malta fever)

The serious aspects of brucellosis, as it exists in the United States, have been generally appreciated only recently.[115] Despite its high incidence, brucellosis long escaped proper notice because of its protean nature and because of the many diseases that it commonly simulates—notably typhoid fever, tuberculosis, malaria, influenza or other viral disease, infectious mononucleosis, some hidden focus of pyogenic infection, appendicitis, and cholecystitis. Often it has paraded under the name "neurasthenia."

Three different members of the genus *Brucella* may cause the disease, and each has a different animal reservoir. The caprine (goat) strain, *B. melitensis*, is prevalent in the Maltese islands and the Mediterranean area, whence came the original name of Malta fever, or Mediterranean fever. It is the least common cause of brucellosis in the United States, occurring principally in the southwestern part. The bovine (cow) strain, *B. abortus*, is widespread among the dairy herds of the United States and produces in cattle what is commonly known as Bang's disease, or contagious abortion. *B. abortus* is responsible for the majority of human infections in the United States.[122] The porcine (pig) strain, *B. suis*, is also an important cause of human disease in the United States, especially in swine-raising areas. Two species relatively recently described, the canine (dog) strain, *B. canis*, and the ovine (sheep) strain, *B. ovis*, rarely cause human infections.

In each of these animals, symptoms commonly result from infection by *Brucella*. The predominant effect is abortion, but there may also be mastitis, lameness, and (especially in swine) vertebral abscesses. Sheep, horses, dogs, rats, guinea pigs, cats, and birds may be infected by and harbor *Brucella*.

These organisms are small, gram-negative coccobacilli that are difficult to cultivate on artificial media and are slow to grow. The natural host of each of the organisms is a common domestic animal, and humans contract brucellosis as a result of contact with these animals or their products. It has been demonstrated that the organisms may pass through the unbroken epidermis; thus the disease is a serious occupational hazard to meat packers, farmers who raise hogs and cows, and laboratory workers who handle the organisms. The respiratory route is a possibility too; the disease has been produced experimentally by inhalation of the organisms suspended in aerosol. Ingestion of infected milk, once an important means of contracting the disease, is now responsible for less than 10% of the cases in the United States.[116]

Brucella organisms elaborate no exotoxins but produce a potent endotoxin. An important factor in virulence is their ability to survive intracellularly—within polymorphonuclear leukocytes and monocytes.

Since there are no pathognomonic signs or symptoms of brucellosis, diagnosis rests primarily on bacteriologic or serologic studies. The simplest procedure is the skin test, in which 0.1 ml of protein nucleate fraction, Brucellergen, is injected intradermally. As with the tuberculin test, however, a positive reaction does not necessarily mean active disease, since this tests only the person's sensitivity to the infecting agent and may simply reflect an infection of long ago—one that may have been subclinical and thus unrecognized. Demonstration of a significantly high serum agglutination titer is probably the most helpful laboratory procedure, though many patients with brucellosis have no demonstrable serum agglutinins.

In the United States the majority of affected persons (81% in Spink's series[116]) acquire their infection directly through contact with diseased animals. After initial localization, usually in the skin, there is extension along lymphatics and involvement of regional lymph nodes. The organisms, phagocytosed first by granulocytes and, subsequently, by monocytes and macrophages, produce focal granulomatous reaction, often with minute areas of necrosis. Assuming that there is progressive infection, the organisms proliferate and spread from lymph nodes to the bloodstream, an event that can occur within hours or may require days depending on the virulence, dose of the organism, and resistance of the host. Once in the bloodstream, the organisms are widely disseminated, but with preferential localization to reticuloendothelial tissues such as bone marrow, spleen, and liver and to the kidneys. In these organs, as in the lymph nodes, multiple minute granulomas form (Fig. 6-19). These may provide a basis for diagnosing the disease, since they are sometimes apparent on histologic study of bone marrow aspirate or needle biopsy specimens of the liver or spleen. Since brucellosis is a septicemic disease, focal lesions may occur in almost any organ or tissue, producing meningitis, osteomyelitis, orchitis, vegetative endocarditis, or empyema. The spleen is often considerably enlarged, and splenomegaly is a characteristic physical finding. There may be hepatomegaly also, and lymph nodes (particularly those of the mesentery) are usually considerably enlarged, soft, and diffluent. Most epithelial tissues show parenchymatous degeneration.

Tularemia (rabbit fever)

Tularemia is a relatively recently recognized disease entity. McCoy and Chapin of the U.S. Public Health Service first identified the causative organism in 1911 and named it in species form *tularensis* after Tulare County, California. Shortly after this, Wherry recognized, and for the first time proved, infection in a human. The bulk of our knowledge and understanding of this disease we owe to the long and efficient work of Edward Francis. Tularemia is caused by *Francisella tularensis* (formerly *Pasteurella tularensis*), a small gramnegative bacillus that is pleomorphic, sometimes appearing in coccal form. It grows only on special culture

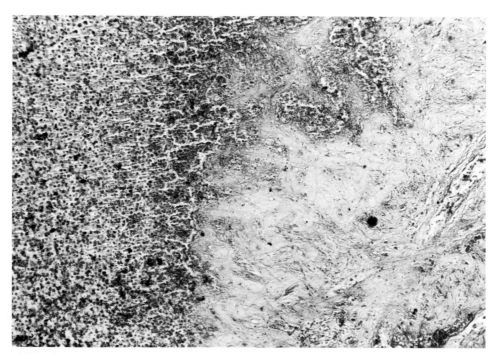

Fig. 6-19. Granulomatous inflammation produced by a bacillus, *Brucella abortus,* in bone.

media. Plague and tularemia have much in common. A variety of wild animals forms a natural reservoir for *F. tularensis*. Especially important in human infection are wild rabbits (cottontails), hares (jackrabbits), and ground squirrels. The disease is rapidly fatal in these animals. Francis has estimated that 1% of wild rabbits are infected. In Russia, outbreaks of the disease have occurred in those who obtain and prepare the skins of water rats for the fur industry. Infection will occur from direct contact with infected animals, and thus the disease is especially likely to occur among trappers, hunters, butchers, and laboratory workers. *F. tularensis* is capable of passing readily through the unbroken skin, and it is said to be the most dangerous of all infectious agents from the standpoint of the laboratory worker. The second most common method of infection is by the bite of insects, especially ticks (*Dermacentor andersoni, D. variabilis, D. occidentalis,* and *Haemaphysalis leporis palustris*), horseflies, or deerflies (*Chrysops discalis*). Ingestion of the poorly cooked meat of infected animals has also produced the disease. In at least one instance a small epidemic of tularemia occurred from drinking contaminated water. On the average, around 180 cases are reported in the United States each year.

According to Francis and Callender,[85] the mortality is nearly 4%, with slow convalescence in many cases. The occurrence of suppurative or granulomatous late lesions with attendant prostration and debility emphasized the seriousness of contracting this infection. The incubation period is ordinarily 3 to 5 days, after which there suddenly develop headache, chills, and high fever, along with generalized aching and the severe prostration characteristic of septicemia. Not until 36 to 48 hours later does the patient usually notice painful swollen lymph nodes, most often in an axilla. This may direct attention for the first time to the focus of primary infection, an area drained by the involved lymph nodes. Usually the lesion is on the finger or hand. It begins as a tender red papule. Soon there is central necrosis, and a "punched-out" ulcer develops. Over three fourths of the cases are associated with such a primary ulcerating lesion, which is slow to heal and persists, on the average, a month or so. Regional lymph nodes enlarge to a pronounced degree and resemble somewhat the buboes of plague. In about one fourth of the cases these enlarged lymph nodes suppurate and may spontaneously rupture and drain cheesy purulent material. This is the so-called ulceroglandular type of the disease, and approximately 75% of cases fall within this category.

Next in frequency, accounting for 10% or less of cases, is the oculoglandular type, essentially similar to the ulceroglandular type just described except that the focus of inoculation is the conjunctiva. Edema, severe hyperemia, itching, and pain are present. Multiple, small, discrete, yellowish nodules may be seen on the mucous membrane. These signs are accompanied by cervical lymphadenopathy. Corneal scarring and blindness are occasional sequelae.

Less common are the glandular and typhoidal forms, in which there is no evident site of initial infection. Pneumonic tularemia is rare.

Tularemia is a septicemic disease, and signs and symptoms often point to a variety of organs. Involvement of the lung, when it occurs, is usually quite evident clinically. Pulmonic lesions may be discrete and nodular, closely resembling those of tuberculosis, or they may occur in the form of confluent bronchopneumonia or lobar pneumonia.

Morphologic changes are essentially similar, regardless of which of the four clinical forms the disease has taken. Often there is a close resemblance to miliary tuberculosis, and minute (2 to 3 mm) hard "tubercles" may be found in the liver (Fig. 6-20), spleen, kidneys, lungs, and other organs. If the tularemic nodules are of larger size, central necrosis is quite evident, and the lesions may be mistaken for abscesses. Tissue changes depend largely on the stage of the disease. Early in its

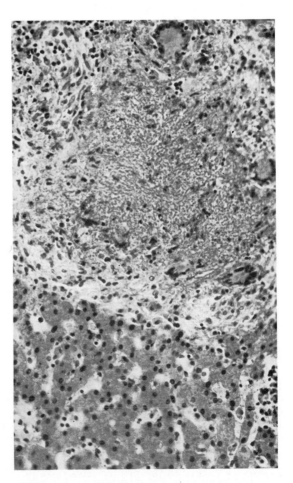

Fig. 6-20. Tularemia. Granulomatous reaction in liver closely simulates tuberculosis.

course the predominant change is focal necrosis. If there has been time for reaction to this, the granulomatous nature of the disease is readily evident. The predominant cell of reaction is the macrophage, and these cells often are arranged in a radial manner around a central area of caseous necrosis, the whole enclosed within a fibrous capsule. Occasional giant cells of the Langhans type are seen. Organisms cannot be demonstrated in histologic preparations of human tissues. In addition, there is generalized hyperplasia of the reticuloendothelial system. The spleen may be enlarged to 400 or 500 g and is often palpable on physical examination. Parenchymatous degeneration is found in many organs.

Sensitivity to bacterial proteins is a prominent feature of tularemia, and a small percentage of patients have spectacular cutaneous eruptions during the second or third week. The Foshay intradermal test is useful in establishing the diagnosis, as is the demonstration of specific agglutinins. A disadvantage of this latter test is that the disease must be a week or so old before antibodies can be demonstrated in the blood. Cross agglutination occurs between *F. tularensis* and organisms of the genus *Brucella*, and if either disease is suspected, agglutination titers should be determined against both; the specific titer will be much higher in one than the other. The organism may be cultured from the local external lesion, from the blood, or—in cases of tularemic pneumonia—from the sputum. In the absence of specific media, a guinea pig may be injected and will die of the disease within 5 to 7 days. Although the handling of infected patients is apparently without much hazard, anyone who attempts to culture the organisms is in serious danger of contracting the disease.

Infections caused by Yersinia

Plague (bubonic plague, black death, pest). This most dreaded of medieval diseases has ravaged Europe and Asia in numerous pandemics. One of the most serious of these began in China in 1374, killing 13 million people there and spreading to involve all of Europe. An estimated 25 million lives were lost to the disease within a 3-year period, approximately one fourth of the total population of Europe at that time. There have been recent pandemics, the most serious of which raged intermittently for 30 years, affecting principally India and costing 12 million lives there.

The causative organism is *Yersinia pestis*, a pleomorphic, gram-negative coccobacillus that presents bipolar bodies; it is often encapsulated. Depending on the animal reservoir, two forms of the disease are recognized. In murine plague, rats (most commonly the gray sewer rat) serve as the primary source of infection. As the rodent succumbs to the disease, it often enters some human dwelling to die. Infected fleas leave its

body, and an acceptable host is found in the common black house rat. In sylvatic plague, rodents of nondomestic habits are the source of infection. In the United States the ground squirrel is most dangerous, but infection has been reported in at least 72 different animal species.

The disease is endemic in India, China, East Africa, and South America.[75] In the United States, an endemic focus of wild rodent plague exists, and several outbreaks of human plague have been reported, all of them west of the 100th meridian.[83] According to Holmes,[5] in 1907 to 1908, within a 12-month period, 37 deaths from plague occurred in the San Franciso–Oakland area, and there have been cases in New Orleans, Beaumont and Galveston, Texas, and Pensacola, Florida. Infections also have been reported in New Mexico, southwestern Oregon, Idaho, Utah, and Nevada.[93]

The disease is transmitted to humans in two principal ways. More commonly, infection results from the bite of an infected flea (especially *Xenopsylla cheopsis* and *Pulex irritans*). The body louse and bedbug also may serve as vectors of infection. Less common is the pneumonic form of the disease, spread directly from person to person by droplets. Occasionally, especially in children who may handle dead rodents, there is direct infection of wounds or other lesions. The incubation period averages 2 to 4 days. Although there may be prodromal symptoms such as malaise and headache, more often the individual first responds with a sudden chill, fever, and other symptoms of severe toxemia or septicemia, including nausea and vomiting. As in the case of tularemia, it may be a day or two before onset of the obvious lymphadenitis. This occurs most commonly in the inguinal lymph nodes, less often in the axillary nodes, and only occasionally in the cervical nodes. The buboes (bubonic plague) are very painful and may attain great size, up to 4 or 5 cm in diameter. Within a day or two, organisms find their way into the bloodstream by entering blood vessels directly or in infected thoracic duct lymph, and the septicemic stage of the disease develops. Profound systemic manifestations progress, and the patient, at first very nervous and apprehensive, may sink into coma and die within a few days. There are three clinical forms of the disease. That just described represents the bubonic type, which is the most common. Death occurs in 60% to 90% of the patients. In the primary septicemic type there may or may not be buboes. This form of the disease is almost always quickly fatal, as is the highly infectious pneumonic type, in which death may occur within a few hours after first symptoms. A much milder form of the disease, pestis minor, is occasionally seen. In this type the organisms remain localized and septicemia does not occur.

Morphologic changes in those dying of plague represent the effects of overwhelming infection by bacteria that produce potent necrotizing toxins coupled with disseminated intravascular coagulation (DIC). The picture is much the same everywhere. Large areas of necrotic tissue are seen, and these tissues are teeming with organisms. In the fulminant forms of the disease, lesions include relatively little inflammatory exudate but much hemorrhage. When the infection is not so overwhelming, exudation of inflammatory cells may be prominent, even to the point of suppuration. For instance, in the pneumonic form of the disease, only severe hyperemia and sanguineous edema may be found in the lungs of persons dying quickly. If the process continues longer, lobular pneumonia develops and may progress to confluence, giving the picture of lobar pneumonia.

In involved lymph nodes (buboes), the gland is almost replaced by hemorrhagic necrotic tissue. This reaction spreads beyond the confines of the capsule, and in the surrounding tissues, necrosis, hemorrhage, and cellulitis also are evident (Fig. 6-21).

The disease may simulate tularemia, but its course is so fulminating that its true nature is usually soon evident. Smears may be made from contents of buboes and will usually reveal Y. *pestis* in great numbers. The organisms may be cultured or an animal (guinea pig or white rat) inoculated. Inoculation is accomplished when

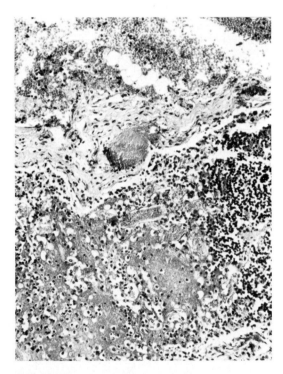

Fig. 6-21. Lymph node in plague. Hemorrhagic edematous cellulitis *(top)* extends from infected lymph node. Despite obvious acuteness of process, cellular reaction is almost exclusively mononuclear. Gray myxoid interstitial haze *(bottom)* is produced by profusion of microorganisms.

some of the infected material is rubbed into the shaved skin of the anterior abdominal wall. If the material contains Y. *pestis*, the animal will die within 3 to 5 days, presenting typical findings. Blood cultures are positive in approximately 50% of cases. Extreme caution must be taken in all such procedures and with the infected person to prevent direct infection of the person or an insect vector. Tetracycline and chloramphenicol are effective in early cases. Active immunization provides only relative temporary protection.

Other Yersinia infections. The genus *Yersinia* includes two human pathogens, Y. *entercolitica* and Y. *pseudotuberculosis*, other than the plague bacillus. Although the distribution of these organisms is worldwide, early reports were predominantly from Europe, particularly Scandinavia. The early reports of human cases emphasized contact with household pets or exotic species, but those reservoirs have recently been less emphasized though animal reservoirs are assumed.

Y. *enterocolitica* causes a usually self-limited, anatomically nonspecific enterocolitis, particularly in infants and young children. Y. *pseudotuberculosis* is more frequently incriminated in cases of mesenteric adenitis in older children and adolescents, in whom the disease may mimic acute appendicitis.[81]

Infections caused by Pasteurella

Members of the genus *Pasteurella* are frequent commensals of the oral cavity of animals (cats, dogs, and rodents). P. *multocida* causes occasional human infection in three circumstances: (1) victims of animal bites, (2) patients with chronic pulmonary disease, often with animal contacts but without a history of animal bites, and (3) patients with chronic gastrointestinal (especially hepatic) disease without a history of animal bites. Three categories of lesion are associated with infections by P. *multocida:* (1) an acute cellulitis or abscess at the site of a bite or scratch by a pet animal, (2) pulmonary suppuration complicating preexisting chronic pulmonary disease, or (3) peritonitis or sepsis in a patient with chronic hepatic disease, often with a history of animal contact.

Glanders

Glanders is another example of a disease that affects animals primarily; humans are rarely involved and then, it would seem, by accident. This is a disease of horses and mules principally, and in these animals it may assume either of two forms. *Glanders* is a relatively acute disease affecting principally the lungs and bringing death in the majority of cases, within 4 to 6 weeks. *Farcy* is a relatively chronic condition that involves primarily the skin, subcutaneous tissues, and their lymphatic vessels. The disease is caused by *Actinobacillus (Malleomyces) mallei*, a rather pleomorphic, usually slender, gram-negative rod. It does not produce an exotoxin. The disease is uncommon in humans and is almost always confined to those who work closely with horses and mules or to laboratory workers who cultivate the organism. Therefore its incidence has dropped sharply in recent years. *A. mallei* ranks with *Francisella tularensis* in the hazard it presents to laboratory workers. Although the organism can penetrate intact epithelium, the site of infection is usually an abrasion or other minor injury to the skin, after which there develops a small nodule that usually ulcerates. Regional lymph nodes become swollen and tender. Shortly thereafter, fever and frequently a mucopurulent nasal discharge occur. An important characteristic at this stage of the process is the exceptional prostration, disproportionate to other signs and symptoms. In many patients a generalized pustular rash develops involving skin and mucous membranes—not unlike that of smallpox. Focal areas of suppuration or nodular granulomas occur in many organs, the joints, and especially the subcutaneous tissues (farcy buds), where they ulcerate and discharge a thick, tenacious, bloody pus.

Morphologically the disease resembles pyemia, with abscesses to be found in many organs. Often, if it is chronic, a granulomatous reaction may predominate. This chronic form particularly may simulate other infectious diseases, and the condition may persist, with frequent remissions, for years. Formerly the disease in its acute form was almost always fatal; in its chronic form the mortality was 50% to 70%. The use of sulfonamides has reduced this figure somewhat.

Diagnosis rests on demonstration of complement-fixing antibodies, recovery of the organism from a subcutaneous lesion (preferably a recent one), or guinea pig inoculation (Straus reaction). Skin tests (mallein) become positive in 3 to 4 weeks and resemble a positive tuberculin test.

Melioidosis

Until a few years ago melioidosis was considered to be an uncommon, usually fatal, disease limited to Southeast Asia. Now it is recognized that the infection is much more common than the clinically apparent disease (7% to 10% of persons living in highly endemic areas have demonstrable antibodies) and that it occurs also in Australia, Africa, Malagasy, the Caribbean, and tropical America.[113] For a long time the causative agent was known as *Malleomyces pseudomallei* because it was believed to be of the same genus as the organism that causes glanders. Recently, however, its name has been changed to *Pseudomonas pseudomallei*. The organism is a small (0.5 × 1.5 to 2 μm), motile, pleomorphic, gram-negative rod with bipolar staining properties. It has no capsule, nor does it form spores. In the early 1900s, Whitmore collected and described some 38 cases

of the disease in Rangoon (Whitmore's disease). Thirty-one of these cases had occurred in drug addicts, and for a while the disease was called morphine addict's septicemia. Shortly after this time the disease virtually disappeared, except for rare sporadic cases. Interest was reawakened in connection with the experience of French troops in Indochina from 1948 to 1954, during which time approximately 100 cases of the disease were recognized. The experience of soldiers in Vietnam has stimulated further interest and extensive clinical and laboratory studies from which much new information has emerged.[106]

Melioidosis presents a broad clinical spectrum, varying from inapparent infection on the one extreme to fulminant septicemia on the other. Interrelationships among the various forms of the disease are shown diagrammatically in Fig. 6-22.

The precise mechanism by which infection occurs is not known. It has been hypothesized that the organism enters through a minute break in the skin or as a wound infection. The possibility of entry by inhalation and ingestion has also been considered. *P. pseudomallei* is widely dispersed in water and soil in endemic areas and also may be found in a variety of infected animals (reservoirs?), including domestic ones, where it often produces serious disease, sometimes occurring as epizootics.

Although the manifestations of melioidosis vary enormously, particular forms of the disease are recognized. The acute pulmonary form of infection is most common, and the picture is one of pronounced sepsis with high fever, profound fatigue, and often chest pain. Leukocytosis is variable in occurrence and degree, with the number of cells ranging from normal to around 20,000. X-ray findings include patchy infiltrations or even consolidation of a pulmonary lobe. With progression of the disease (without treatment), cavitation may develop within several days. The radiologic changes often simulate those of tuberculosis, and this is an important differential diagnostic consideration. The acute septicemic form of the disease usually begins as a pulmonary infection and may run a rapid course, terminating in death within several days. A form of chronic septicemia, which requires several months to run its course, is oc-

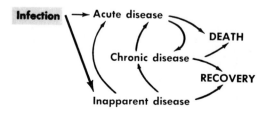

Fig. 6-22. Interrelationships among various forms of melioidosis.

casionally seen. The chronic condition is similar to glanders in that many abscesses occur, involving most tissues of the body. Still another form of the disease is characterized by localized suppurative infections, and almost any organ or tissue may be involved.

Pathologic changes cover as wide a range as clinical manifestations, their form depending in large measure on whether the disease is rapidly progressive, subacute, or chronic. In the acute progressive cases the characteristic lesion is a well-defined abscess that is usually small, firm, and yellow or yellowish. The exudate is composed primarily of neutrophils with lesser numbers of histiocytes and considerable fibrin. The abscesses are usually multiple and may affect virtually any organ, especially the lungs, lymph nodes (Fig. 6-23), liver, and spleen. In the less rapidly progressive disease the lesions are again focal but are granulomatous. Often the granulomas present central areas of caseous necrosis

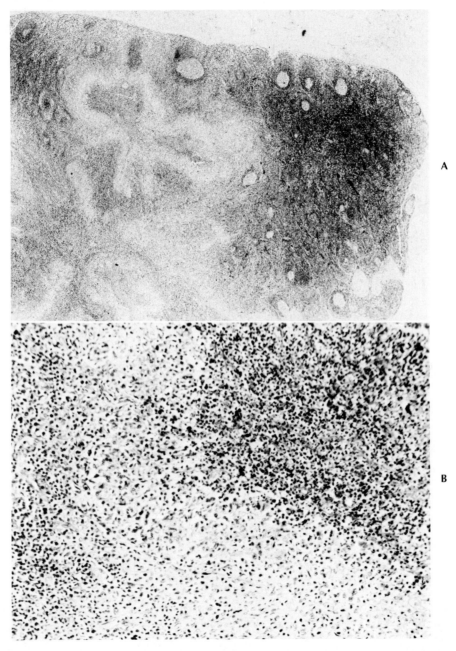

Fig. 6-23. Melioidosis. Lymph node from patient with progressive chronic melioidosis of 15 months' duration. **A,** Irregular "stellate" areas of necrosis. **B,** Small areas of necrosis with borders of epithelioid cells (lymphoid follicle to right). (Hematoxylin and eosin; **A,** 11×; AFIP 68-796; **B,** 67×; AFIP 68-3516.)

and contain Langhans' (or foreign body–type) giant cells. It may be impossible on histopathologic grounds alone to differentiate these lesions from those caused by tuberculosis. The larger granulomas frequently present extensive central necrosis, associated with purulent exudate, forming stellate abscesses—a response that closely stimulates the lesions produced by tularemia, cat-scratch disease, lymphogranuloma venereum, and sporotrichosis. Unfortunately, in the granulomatous lesions the causative organisms can rarely be demonstrated—in contrast to the acute suppurative lesions.

One of the treacherous aspects of the disease, which has earned it the name "Vietnamese time bomb," is that an isolated focus of the disease, often producing few if any signs or symptoms, may lie dormant for as long as several years and then, for no evident reason, suddenly become active to produce serious disease.

Positive diagnosis can be made only by demonstration of the organism, though serologic studies (especially hemagglutination) may be helpful. Chloramphenicol, in combination with other drugs, and tetracyclines are useful in treating the disease, but the more fulminant forms still carry a mortality of 90% and persistent chronic melioidosis may lead to death in 30% to 50% of the cases.

Clinical manifestations may appear after a latent period of many years.

Granuloma inguinale (donovanosis)

Uncommon in medically advanced countries, granuloma inguinale is caused by a minute negative coccobacillus now designated *Calymmatobacterium granu-lomatis*. This organism, which has been cultivated only on embryonated eggs or on media that contain egg yolk, is antigenically related to *Klebsiella* species, but its taxonomy remains unclear.[125-127]

Granuloma inguinale is very rare in the United States but is endemic in socioeconomically deprived tropical and subtropical populations, particularly in South America, the West Indies, India, Africa, and Southeast Asia.

Although the role of sexual transmission of granuloma inguinale has been debated, recent epidemiologic and clinical experience indicates that the disease may usually be venereally transmitted. The earliest lesion is an indurated papule that over several days to a few weeks ulcerates. Three types of lesions then may result: (1) virtually painless hyperplastic granulomatous lesions, (2) a chronically ulcerating form, often very painful (Fig. 6-24), or (3) a hypertrophic form that, by chronic obstruction of lymphatic vessels, may lead to genital elephantiasis. Extragenital lesions, such as a multifocal osteomyelitis, are very rare. Microscopically lesions of granuloma inguinale are nonspecific except for the demonstration of minute coccobacillary forms with bipolar hyperchromatic staining in large macrophages (Fig. 6-25).

Diseases caused by spirochetes

The order Spirochaetales includes three genera pathogenic for humans. The genus *Treponema* includes *T. pallidum*, *T. pertenue*, and *T. carateum*, which cause syphilis, yaws, and pinta, respectively. The genus *Borrelia* includes many species or strains that cause relapsing fever. The genus *Leptospira* comprises a large

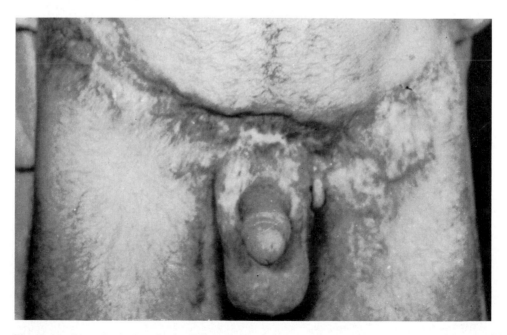

Fig. 6-24. Granuloma inguinale. Bilateral serpiginous ulcers with involvement of inguinal regions and scrotum.

number of immunologically heterogeneous organisms. A single species, *L. interrogans*, is systematically recognized, but the serology is complex, variously recognizing serotypes pathogenic for humans (among other mammals) and groups nonpathogenic for mammals.

Many representatives of this order are not readily cultured on artificial media. They are, moreover, not identifiable in routine stains of sectioned material but require special histologic techniques such as dark-field examination of fresh material or demonstration of organisms by immunofluorescence.

Mechanisms whereby spirochetes damage tissues of the host are not clearly established. Some, such as *Borrelia* or *Leptospira*, are believed to produce hemolysins, to which the destruction of erythrocytes in the appropriate diseases is attributed. No direct toxic mechanism has been incriminated in diseases produced by *Treponema*. Immunologic response by the host is a major mechanism of tissue injury in this group of diseases.

Syphilis. Syphilis, the archetypal spirochetal disease,

is of relatively recent occurrence in humans. Clinical features or lesions attributable to it were not clearly described in Western medicine until the late fifteenth and early sixteenth centuries. The Renaissance epidemiologist and poet Fracastoro left us the name of the disease as that of a shepherd, the protagonist in one of his narrative poems. This systematic designation abjures, or nearly so, ethnic attributions (*morbus gallicus*) as well as many that are more specific (the "great pox" as opposed to smallpox, then a less fearful disease) or euphemistic (*lues*, 'plague').

Many historically renowned medical scientists are associated with studies of syphilis: John Hunter, for his autoinoculation experiment, which he misinterpreted as establishing identity between syphilis and gonorrhea; the French physician Villemin, who recognized the unity of the many clinical expressions of syphilis and promulgated the clinical classification, variations of which are basic to discussions of the disease even today; Schaudinn and associates, who first identified the spirochete in syphilitic lesions; and Wasserman and co-workers, who established an immunologic diagnostic procedure based on nonspecific antibodies elaborated during treponemal infection.

T. pallidum, the causative agent of syphilis, is a tightly coiled, regularly spiraling organism 6 to 15 μm in length that moves with a distinctive rhythmicity as viewed in dark-field illumination. It is best demonstrated in sectioned material by silver impregnation (Fig. 6-26). Although *T. pallidium* may preserve viability and infectivity in artificial media for a few days and

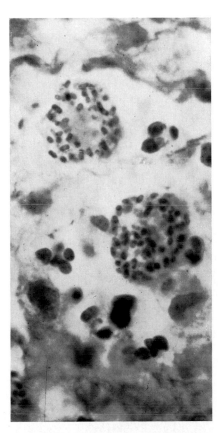

Fig. 6-25. Granuloma inguinale. Donovan bodies within macrophages stain with silver. Because of bipolar staining, "closed safety pin" appearance is observed in many. With this stain, cysts are not easily seen. (Dieterle's silver stain; 1900×; from Torpin, R., Greenblatt, R.B., and Pund, E.R.: Am. J. Surg. **44:**551, 1939.)

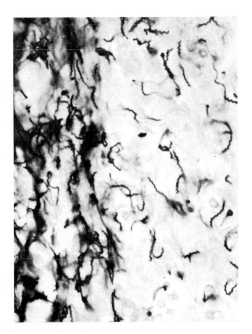

Fig. 6-26. Spirochetes *(Treponema pallidum)* in section from mucous patch of vulva.

there is some evidence of replication under these conditions, the organism is regarded as noncultivable by routine methods in artificial media. Experimental infection can be produced in primates and a few other species, but humans are the only natural reservoir. No endotoxin or exotoxin has been attributed to *T. pallidum*. The mechanisms of its pathogenicity are not known; however, the host's immunologic responses appear to be a major factor. Two broad groups of antigens are associated with treponemal infection: (1) a nonspecific group known as reagins and (2) a specific group known as antigen antibodies that immobilize treponemes (treponemal immobilization antibody) and that can be located by immunofluorescence studies. Although *T. pallidum* (the cause of syphilis), *T. pertenue* (the cause of yaws), and *T. carateum* (the cause of pinta) are given species designations, no morphologic or immunologic differences exist among these organisms, however geographically, epidemiologically, or clinically distinctive the respective diseases are.[139]

Except for congenital syphilis, an epidemiologic and clinically distinct problem, and for currently uncommon events such as transfusion of infected blood, syphilis is transmitted by intimate person-to-person contact, usually sexual. The organisms are believed to gain entry into the host through minute subclinical breaks in an epithelial surface, such as that of the glans penis, vulva, vagina, or cervix.

Fourteen to 21 days after infection a painless papule develops at the site of inoculation. This expands peripherally while it ulcerates centrally, producing a circular or ovoid indurated lesion with a clean central ulceration (unless secondarily infected), the chancre of primary syphilis. Hyperplasia of regional lymph nodes reflects lymphatic dissemination of spirochetes in the formation of usually inguinal buboes. One or more bouts of spirochetemia may disseminate organisms throughout the body and precede acquisition of host immunity. Lesions remote from the chancre and regional lymph nodes constitute the outward manifestations of secondary syphilis. It must be emphasized that some of these manifestations may appear before the primary chancre has healed. Within weeks, however, the chancre heals, usually without scarring.

Secondary syphilis produces lesions most conspicuously on mucocutaneous surfaces of the body, especially the skin and oropharynx. At this stage, too, systemic manifestations, generalized lymphadenopathy, and slight fever may occur. Grossly the lesions of secondary syphilis are highly variable and include maculopapular, usually nonpruritic, cutaneous patches characteristically involving the palms and soles. Epithelial proliferation may predominate on moist intertriginous locations, such as about the anus or on the perineum. The result is a lesion known as the condyloma latum (Fig. 6-27).

Microscopically both primary chancres and mucocutaneous secondary lesions manifest distinctly perivascular aggregates of mononuclear cells, particularly plasma cells. Hyperplastic lymph nodes in the secondary stage show considerable proliferation of sinus histiocytes and infiltration of mononuclear cells, especially plasma cells about afferent and efferent lymphatics.

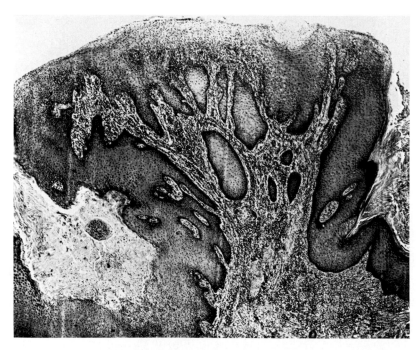

Fig. 6-27. Section from condyloma latum.

Treponemes can usually be demonstrated in primary or secondary lesions either by silver impregnation of sectioned material or, more important, by dark-field examination of wet-mounted specimens.

Although one or more mucocutaneous relapses may occur during "early syphilis," after 2 years beyond the primary infection such relapses no longer occur (if treatment has been adequate) and the patient enters the clinical stage referred to as late syphilis. Many of these patients remain asymptomatic (though pathologically recognizable lesions may develop) through the rest of their lives and are designated as having late latent syphilis. Clinically recognizable manifestations constitute tertiary syphilis, which in turn is classified as benign late syphilis, late cardiovascular syphilis, and late neurosyphilis; the incidence of these tertiary forms among untreated patients observed for many years is 15%, 10%, and 7%, respectively.

Benign late (gummatous) syphilis is characterized by the occurrence of solitary or (more commonly) multiple syphilitic granulomas, known as gummas, in bone or solid viscera, most commonly the liver, brain, or testis. Gummas are circumscribed, rubbery, opalescent, spherical lesions from a few millimeters to several centimeters in diameter. Microscopically the major part of a gumma consists of coagulative necrosis surrounded by a veil of epithelioid cells, lymphocytes, and plasma cells. Treponemes are occasionally demonstrable in gummas, unlike the lesions of late cardiovascular syphilis or late neurosyphilis, in which organisms are rarely identifiable.

Congenital syphilis. Congenital syphilis may develop in the fetus exposed in utero to an episode of maternal spirochetemia. Conventional teaching is that the fetus is subject to congenital syphilis only after about 16 weeks of gestation, when the Langhans layer of the placenta has disappeared. Treponemes have been identified in abortuses as early as 10 to 12 weeks of gestation, and so it appears that absence of lesions recognizable as congenital syphilis is a consequence of fetal immunologic nonreactivity rather than exclusion of organisms.

Fetuses with congenital syphilis may die in utero, be born prematurely, or be born alive but with features of congenital infection. Hepatosplenomegaly and lymphadenopathy are common, as are mucocutaneous lesions, often concentrated about the mouth (rhagades) or anus. Skeletal lesions (periostitis and osteochondritis) are common and account for such clinical features as saber shins and saddle nose. Disturbed dentition (Hutchinson's teeth and peg-shaped, screwdriver-shaped, or pumpkin seed–shaped incisors) is evident when eruption of deciduous teeth occurs.

In solid viscera, histologic maturation is retarded, and there is a distinctive, poorly collagenized, interstitial stromal expansion in such organs as the liver, heart, kidney, and pancreas. Treponemes are usually readily identified in fetal tissues and in the placenta. Without treatment, growth failure and marasmus lead to death after a few months to a few years. Long-term survivors may manifest the tartiary signs of acquired syphilis.

Nonvenereal treponematosis. Treponemes are the etiologic agents of a variety of infectious diseases be-

Table 6-2. Comparative features of treponematoses

	Pinta	Yaws	Nonvenereal syphilis	Venereal syphilis
Usual mode of transmission	Personal contact, arthropods (?)	Personal contact, arthropods (?)	Personal contact, fomites	Venereal
Congenital transmission	No	No	No	Yes
Primary	Yes, skin	Yes, skin	Rare	Skin or mucous membrane
Regional lymphadenopathy	Yes	Yes	Yes	Yes
Secondary lesions	Skin only	Skin, mucous membrane, rare	Skin, mucous membrane	Skin, mucous membrane
Latency	Probably	Yes	Yes	Yes
Tertiary lesions	Yes, but may resemble secondary lesions	Yes	Yes	Yes, visceral
Osseous lesions	No	Yes	Yes	Yes
Nasopharyngeal gummas	No	Yes	Yes	Yes
Aortitis and CNS disease	Undocumented	Undocumented	Undocumented	Yes
Visceral gummas	No	No	No	Yes
Juxta-articular nodules	Questionable	Yes	Yes	Yes
Ocular lesions	Undocumented	Undocumented	Undocumented	Yes

From Binford, C.H., and Connor, D.H., editors: Pathology of tropical and extraordinary diseases, Washington, D.C., 1976, Armed Forces Institute of Pathology. Reproduced with permission.

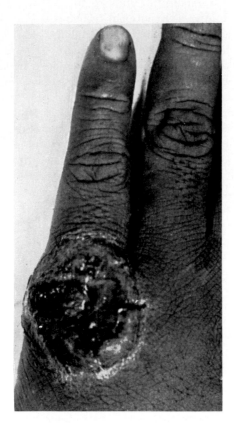

Fig. 6-28. Yaws. Primary lesion (mother yaw or chancre). (Courtesy Dr. Herbert S. Alden, Atlanta, Ga., and Dr. P.D. Gutiérrez.)

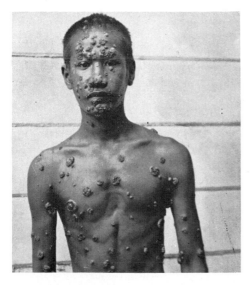

Fig. 6-29. Yaws. Secondary frambesiform lesions. (AFIP 39201.)

sides venereal (or congenital) syphilis. Although there are no morphologic or immunologic features that distinguish the agents of these diseases from *T. pallidum*, these agents are given specific designations on the basis of epidemiologic features. Thus the agent of yaws is designated *T. pertenue*, that of pinta *T. carateum*, and that of nonvenereal syphilis (bejel) *T. pallidum*. These are diseases of regional, especially tropical, significance with distinctive epidemiologic, geographic, and clinical features but no rigorous microbiologic, serologic, or morphologic distinctions from syphilis. (Salient features are compared with those of syphilis in Table 6-2.) Public health measures have greatly diminished the occurrence of yaws and pinta. The specialized literature should be consulted for clinicopathologic details.

Yaws. This disease of the arid tropics usually begins in childhood and progresses to chronic dermatologic or orthopedic manifestations in later life (Figs. 6-28 and 6-29).

Pinta. This chronic dermatologic disorder of the tropical Western Hemisphere features areas of cutaneous depigmentation.

Nonvenereal syphilis. This disease goes by a host of local vernacular designations, the most familiar of which is bejel in Arabia, Syria, and Iraq. Cutaneous and osseous lesions resemble those of syphilis.

Diseases caused by *Leptospira*. Leptospiras are helicoid organisms 6 to 20 μm in length with hooked ends. Some representatives are straight or have single hooks. Leptospiral infections are zoonoses widely distributed throughout the world. At least 180 mammalian species have been described as harboring leptospiras, the most important being rats, swine, dogs, and cattle. Currently a single species, *L. interrogans*, is recognized, of which there are many serologically distinctive variants.

Human leptospirosis results from contact of humans with infected animal products, usually urine with which the human subject comes into contact. In developed societies, therefore, most cases occur among dock workers, sewer workers, slaughterers, and so on. It is not clinically useful to distinguish epidemiologically characteristic leptospiroses by such designations as "Weil's disease," "swineherd's disease," and "swamp disease," since different biovars may be identified in identical epidemiologic situations.

Human leptospirosis is characterized by involvement of many organ systems in an acute febrile illness. Myalgia, focal meningoencephalitis, cutaneous purpura, and hepatic and renal failure may occur. Degenerative lesions in solid viscera (the liver, kidney, myocardium, and skeletal muscle) have been described. Organisms can be demonstrated in infected tissues, especially by silver impregnation techniques.

Diseases caused by *Borrelia*. Representatives of the genus *Borrelia* are coarsely and irregularly helical gram-negative organisms 10 to 20 μm in length. Some 18 species are distinguished, partially serologically but more importantly by the arthropod vectors (lice or ticks) responsible for their transmission from a primary rodent reservoir to humans. *Borrelia* causes relapsing fever, a clinically nonspecific recurring febrile illness distributed throughout the world but uncommon in the United States or Western Europe. In rare fatal cases foci of necrosis in the liver and kidneys have been described in which organisms can be demonstrated. Splenic microabscesses are typical.

Diseases caused by Spirillum minor and Streptobacillus moniliformis. *Spirillum minor* and *Streptobacillus moniliformis* are unrelated organisms that cause clinically similar diseases. Many cases follow bites of rats, other rodents, or species that eat rodents. *S. minor* is associated with sodoku, a disease chiefly in Japan. *S. moniliformis* causes rat-bite fever, a febrile illness that is accompanied by generalized lymphadenopathy and is distributed throughout the world. Cases lacking histories of rodent bites are designated Haverhill fever, after an outbreak in Haverhill, Massachusetts, attributed to drinking contaminated raw milk. Infections by both organisms are accompanied by rashes. Toxic changes and nonspecific inflammatory lesions in various solid viscera have been described in rare fatal cases.

Synergistic fusospirochetosis. In a variety of synergistic infections occurring in several organ systems, one component is a spirochete variously designated *Treponema* or *Borrelia vincentii*. These infections feature dirty indolent ulcerative processes, which are painful if they occur on mucocutaneous surfaces. Infections are usually found in circumstances of suboptimal local hygiene or other secondary predisposing factors. Examples are genital fusospirochetosis, oropharyngeal fusospirochetosis (trench mouth, Vincent's infection), orofacial gangrene (noma, cancrum oris), and fusospirochetal complications of chronic sinopulmonary infection.

REFERENCES
General

1. Ash, J.E., and Spitz, S.: Pathology of tropical diseases, Philadelphia, 1945, W.B. Saunders Co.
2. Binford, C.H., and Connor, P.H.: Pathology of tropical and extraordinary diseases, Washington, D.C., 1976, Armed Forces Institute of Pathology.
3. Braude, A.I., editor: Medical microbiology and infectious diseases, Philadelphia, 1981, W.B. Saunders Co.
4. Burnett, M.: The natural history of infectious disease, London, 1953, Cambridge University Press.
5. Holmes, W.H.: Bacillary and rickettsial infections, New York, 1940, The Macmillan Co.
6. Mackoweak, P.A.: Microbial synergism in human infections, N. Engl. J. Med. **298:**24, 1978.
7. Mandell, G.L., Douglas, G., Jr., and Bennett, J.E.: Principles and practice of infectious diseases, ed. 2, New York, 1985, John Wiley & Sons, Inc.
8. Smith, H.: Biochemical challenge of microbial pathogenicity, Bacteriol. Rev. **32:**164, 1968.
9. Symmers, W.S.: Opportunistic infections: the concept of opportunistic infections, Proc. R. Soc. Med. **58:**341, 1965.
10. van Heyningen, W.E., and Arseculeratne, S.N.: Exotoxins, Annu. Rev. Microbiol. **18:**195, 1964.
11. Wehrle, P.F., and Top, F.H., Sr., editors: Communicable and infectious diseases, ed. 9, St. Louis, 1981, The C.V. Mosby Co.
12. Wilson, G.S., and Miles, A.A.: Topley and Wilson's principles of bacteriology and immunology, ed. 6, Baltimore, 1975, The Williams & Wilkins Co.

Intoxications

13. Arnon, S.S., Midura, T.F., Damus, K., Wood, R.M., and Chin, J.: Intestinal infection and toxin production by *Clostridium botulinum* as one cause of sudden infant death syndrome, Lancet **1:**1273, 1978.
14. Altemeier, W.A., Lewis, S., Schlievert, P.M., and Bjornson, H.S.: Studies of the staphylococcal causation of toxic shock syndrome, Surg. Gynecol. Obstet. **153:**481, 1981.
15. Bartlett, P., Reingold, A.L., Graham, D.R., Dan, B.B., Seliger, D.S., Tank, G.W., and Wichterman, K.A.: Toxic shock syndrome associated with surgical wound infections, JAMA **247:**1448, 1982.
16. Bergdoll, M.S., Crass, B.A., Reiser, R.F., Robbins, R.N., Lee, A.C.-M., Chesney, P.J., Davis, J.P., Vergeront, J.M., and Ward, P.J.: An enterotoxin-like protein in *Staphylococcus aureus* strains from patients with toxic shock syndrome, Ann. Intern. Med. **96:**969, 1982.
17. Cone, L.A., Woodard, D.R., Schlievert, P.M., and Tomory, G.S.: Clinical and bacteriologic observations of a toxic shock–like syndrome due to *Streptococcus pyogenes*, N. Engl. J. Med. **317:**146-149, 1987.
18. Davis, J.P., Chesney, P.J., Wand, P.J., and LaVenture, M.: Toxic shock syndrome: epidemiologic features, recurrence, risk factors, and prevention, N. Engl. J. Med. **303:**1429, 1980.
19. Elder, J.M., and Miles, A.A.: The action of the lethal toxins of gas gangrene clostridia on capillary permeability, J. Pathol. Bacteriol. **74:**133, 1957.
20. Feldman, R.A., editor: A seminar on infant botulism, Rev. Infect. Dis. **1:**611, 1979.
21. Marcuse, E.K., and Grand, M.G.: Epidemiology of diphtheria in San Antonio, Texas, 1970, JAMA **224:**305, 1973.
22. McKenna, U.G., et al.: Toxic shock syndrome, a newly recognized entity, Mayo Clin. Proc. **55:**663, 1980.
23. Merson, M.H., and Dowell, V.R.: Epidemiologic, clinical and laboratory aspects of wound botulism, N. Engl. J. Med. **289:**1005, 1973.
24. Osterholm, M.T., Davis, J.P., Gibson, R.W., Mandel, L.A., Wintermeyer, L.A., Helms, C.M., Fortang, J.C., Rondeau, J., and Vergeront, J.M.: Tri-state toxic shock syndrome study. I. Epidemiologic findings, J. Infect. Dis. **145:**143, 1982.
25. Paris, A.L., Herwaldt, L.A., Blum, D., Schmid, G.P., Shands, K.N., and Broome, C.V.: Pathologic findings in twelve fatal cases of toxic shock syndrome, Ann. Intern. Med. **96:**852, 1982.
26. Parker, M.T., Tomlinson, A.J.H., and Williams, R.E.O.: Impetigo contagiosa: the association of certain types of *Staphylococcus aureus* and *Streptococcus pyogenes* in superficial skin infections, J. Hyg. Cambridge **53:**458, 1955.
27. Pappenheimer, A.M., Jr., and Gill, D.M.: Diphtheria, Science **182:**353, 1973.
28. Pickett, J., Berg, B., Chaplin, E., and Brunstetler-Shafer, M.A.: Syndrome of botulism in infancy: clinical and electrophysiologic study, N. Engl. J. Med. **295:**770, 1976.
29. Roding, B., Groenveld, P.H.A., and Boerema, I.: Ten years of experience in the treatment of gas gangrene with hyperbaric oxygen, Surg. Gynecol. Obstet. **134:**579, 1972.
30. Schlievert, P., Schoettle, D., and Watson, D.: Purification and physicochemical and biological characterization of a staphylococcal pyrogenic exotoxin, Infect. Immun. **23:**609, 1979.
31. Schlievert, P.M., Shands, K.N., Dan, B.B., Schmid, G.P., and Nishimura, R.D.: Identification and characterization of an exotoxin from *Staphylococcus aureus* associated with toxic-shock syndrome, J. Infect. Dis. **143:**509, 1981.

32. Shands, K.N., Schmid, G.P., Dan, B.B., Blum, D., Guidotti, R.J., Hargrett, N.T., Anderson, R.L., Hill, D.L., Broome, C.V., Band, J.D., and Fraser, D.W.: Toxic shock syndrome in menstruating women: its association with tampon use and *Staphylococcus aureus* and the clinical features of 52 cases, N. Engl. J. Med. **303**:1436, 1980.

33. Todd, J., and Fishaut, M.: Toxic-shock syndrome associated with phage-group-I staphylococci, Lancet **2**:1116, 1978.

34. Zalma, V.M., Older, J.J., and Brooks, G.F.: The Austin, Texas, diphtheria outbreak: clinical and epidemiological aspects, JAMA **211**:2125, 1970.

Noninvasive infections

35. DuPont, H.L., Hornick, R.B., Snyder, M.J., Libonati, J.P., Formal, S.B., and Ganganosa, E.J.: Immunity in shigellosis (in two parts), J. Infect Dis. **125**:5, 12, 1972.

36. Dutz, W., and Kohout, E.: Anthrax. In Sommers, S.C., editor: Pathology annual, vol. 6, New York, 1971, Appleton-Century-Crofts.

37. Field, M.: Intestinal secretion: effect of cyclic AMP and its role in cholera, N. Engl. J. Med. **284**:1137, 1971.

38. Finkelstein, R.A.: Cholera, CRC Crit. Rev. Microbiol. **2**:553, 1973.

39. Fox, M.D., Kaufmann, A.F., Zendel, S.A., et al.: Anthrax in Louisiana 1971: epizootiologic study, J. Am. Vet. Med. Assoc. **163**:446, 1974.

40. Gitelson, S.: Gastrectomy, achlorhydria, and cholera, Isr. J. Med. Sci. **7**:663, 1971.

41. Goette, D.K.: Gonococcal arthritis, Cutis **11**:337, 1973.

42. Hornick, R.B., Music, S.I., Wenzel, R., et al.: The Broad Street pump revisited: response of volunteers to ingested cholera vibrios, Bull. NY Acad. Med. **47**:1181, 1971.

43. Keusch, G.T., Grady, G.F., Mata, L.J., and McIver, J.: The pathogenesis of *Shigella* diarrhea. I. Enterotoxin production by *Shigella dysenteriae* 1, J. Clin. Invest. **51**:1212, 1972.

44. Klein, E.J., Fisher, L.S., Chow, A.W., and Guze, L.B.: Anorectal gonococcal infection, Ann. Intern. Med. **86**:340, 1977.

45. Levine, M.M., DuPont, H.L., Formal, S.B., Hornick, R.B., Takeuchi, A., Gangarosa, E.J., Snyder, M.J., and Libonati, J.P.: Pathogenicity of *Shigella dysenteriae* 1 (Shiga) dysentery, J. Infect. Dis. **127**:261, 1973.

46. Macumber, H.H.: Acute bacillary dysentery: clinico-pathologic study of 263 consecutive cases, Arch. Intern. Med. **69**:624, 1942.

47. McCormack, W.M., Stumacher, R.J., Johnson, K., and Donner, A.: Clinical spectrum of gonococcal infection in women, Lancet **1**:1182, 1977.

48. McMillan, A., McNeillage G., Gilmour, H.M., and Lee, F.D.: Histology of rectal gonorrhea in men, with a note on anorectal infection with *Neisseria meningitidis*, J. Clin. Pathol. **36**:511, 1983.

49. Pierce, N.F., Greenough, W.B., and Carpenter, C.C.J., Jr.: *Vibrio cholerae* enterotoxin and its mode of action, Bacteriol. Rev. **35**:1, 1971.

50. Smith, L.W.: Pathologic anatomy of pertussis with special reference to pneumonia caused by pertussis bacillus, Arch. Pathol. **4**:732, 1927.

51. Ward, M.E., Watt, P.J., and Robertson, J.N.: The human fallopian tube: a laboratory model for gonococcal infection, J. Infect. Dis. **129**:650, 1979.

52. Weisner, P.J., Tronca, E., Bonin, P., Pedersen, A.H.B., and Holmes, K.K.: Clinical spectrum of pharyngeal gonococcal infection, N. Engl. J. Med. **288**:181, 1973.

53. Weissman, J.B., Marton, K.I., Lewis, J.N., Friedman, C.T.H., and Gangarosa, E.J.: Impact in the United States of the Shiga dysentery pandemic of Central America and Mexico: a review of surveillance data through 1972, J. Infect. Dis. **129**:218, 1974.

Pyogenic infections

54. Britigan, B.E., Cohen, M.S., and Sparling, P.F.: Gonococcal infections: a model of molecular pathogenesis, N. Engl. J. Med. **312**:1683, 1985.

55. Colebrook, L., and Hare, R.: Anaerobic streptococci associated with puerperal fever, J. Obstet. Gynaecol. Br. Emp. **40**:609, 1933.

56. Cruickshank, C.N.D., and Lowbury, E.J.L.: The effect of pyocyanin on human skin cells and leucocytes, Br. J. Exp. Pathol. **34**:583, 1953.

57. DuPont, H.L., Formal, S.B., Hornick, R.B., Snyder, M.J., Libonati, J.P., Sheahan, D.G., Lebrec, E.H., and Kalas, J.P.: Pathogenesis of *E. coli* diarrhea, N. Engl. J. Med. **285**:1, 1971.

58. Felner, J.M., and Dowell, V.R.: "Bacteroides" bacteremia, Am. J. Med. **50**:787, 1971.

59. Fetzer, A.E., Werner, A.S., and Hagstrom, J.W.C.: Pathologic features of pseudomonal pneumonia, Am. Rev. Respir. Dis. **96**:1121, 1967.

60. Forkner, C.E., Jr., et al.: *Pseudomonas* septicemia: observations on twenty-three cases, Am. J. Med. **25**:877, 1958.

61. Gaisin, A., and Heaton, C.L.: Chancroid: alias the soft chancre, Int. J. Dermatol. **14**:188, 1975.

62. Gardner, H.L., and Dukes, C.D.: *Haemophilus vaginalis* vaginitis, Am. J. Obstet. Gynecol. **69**:962, 1955.

63. Moritz, A.R., and Zamcheck, N.: Sudden and unexpected deaths of young soldiers: diseases responsible for such deaths during World War II, Arch. Pathol. **42**:459, 1946.

64. Powers, G.F., and Boisvert, P.L.: Age as a factor in streptococcosis, J. Pediatr. **25**:481, 1944.

65. Rho, Y.M., and Josephson, J.E.: Epidemic enteropathogenic *Escherichia coli*, Newfoundland, 1963: autopsy study of 16 cases, Can. Med. Assoc. J. **96**:392, 1967.

66. Wollenman, O.J., Jr., and Finland, M.: Pathology of staphylococcal pneumonia complicating clinical influenza, Am. J. Pathol. **19**:23, 1943.

67. Zinserberg, A.: Dysentery and colienterocolitis: some aspects of pathogenesis and pathological anatomy, Virchows Arch. [Pathol. Anat.] **361**:19, 1973.

Bacillary infections

68. Annotations: listerial infection of the nervous system, Lancet **1**:362, 1968.

69. Balows, A., and Fraser, D.W., editors: International symposium on legionnaires' disease, Ann. Intern. Med. **90**:491, 1979.

70. Barber, M., Nellen, M., and Zoob, M.: Erysipeloid of Rosenbach: response to penicillin, Lancet **1**:125, 1946.

71. Bernard, R.P.: The Zermatt typhoid outbreak in 1963, J. Hyg. **63**:537, 1965.

72. Beyt, B.E., Sondag, J., Roosevelt, T.S., and Bruce, R.: Human pulmonary pasteurellosis, JAMA **242**:1647, 1979.

73. Buchner, L.H., and Schneierson, S.S.: Clinical and laboratory aspects of *Listeria monocytogenes* infections: with a report of ten cases, Am. J. Med. **45**:904, 1968.

74. Busch, L.A.: Human listeriosis in the United States, J. Infect. Dis. **123**:328, 1971.

75. Butler, T., Bell, W.R., Linn, N.N., Trep, N.D., and Arnold, K.: *Yersinia pestis* infection in Vietnam. I. Clinical and hematological aspects, J. Infect. Dis. **129**:578, 1974.

76. Chuttani, H.K., Jain, K., and Misra, R.C.: Small bowel in typhoid fever, Gut **12**:709, 1971.

77. Clasener, H.: Pathogenicity of the L-phase of bacteria, Annu. Rev. Microbiol. **26**:55, 1972.

78. Collins, R.N.: The 1964 epidemic of typhoid fever in Atlanta: clinical and epidemiologic observations, JAMA **197**:179, 1966.

79. Cox, C.D., and Arbogast, J.L.: Melioidosis, Am. J. Clin. Pathol. **15**:567, 1945.

80. Dannenberg, A.M., Jr., and Scott, E.M.: Melioidosis: pathogenesis and immunity to mice and hamsters. I. Studies with virulent strains of *Malleomyces pseudomallei*, J. Exp. Med. **107**:153, 1958.

81. Delorme, J., Laverdière, M., Martineau, B., and Lafleur, L.: Yersiniosis in children, Can. Med. Assoc. J. **110**:281, 1979.

82. English, C.K., Wear, D.J., Margileth, A.M., Lissner, C.R., and Walsh, G.P.: Cat-scratch disease, isolation and culture of the bacterial agent, JAMA **259**:1347, 1988.

83. Finegold, M.J.: Pathogenesis of plague: a review of plague deaths in the United States during the last decade, Am. J. Med. **45:**549, 1968.
84. Francis, D.P., Holmes, M.A., and Brandon, G.: *Pasteurella multocida* infections after domestic animal bites and scratches, JAMA **233:**42, 1975.
85. Francis, E., and Callender, G.R.: Tularemia: microscopic changes of lesions in man, Arch. Pathol. **3:**577, 1927.
86. Gerding, D.N., Khan, M.Y., Ewing, J.W., and Hall, W.H.: *Pasteurella multocida* peritonitis in hepatic cirrhosis with ascites, Gastroenterology **70:**413, 1976.
87. Glick, T.H., Gregg, M.B., Berman, B., Mallison, G., Rhodes, W.W., Jr., and Kassanoff, I.: Pontiac fever, an epidemic of unknown etiology in a health department. I. Clinical and epidemiologic aspects, Am. J. Epidemiol. **107:**149, 1978.
88. Goodpasture, E.W., and House, S.J.: Pathologic anatomy of tularemia in man, Am. J. Pathol. **4:**213, 1928.
89. Gray, M.L., and Killinger, A.H.: *Listeria monocytogenes* and listeric infections, Bacteriol. Rev. **30:**309, 1966.
90. Greenwald, G.A., Nash, G., and Foley, F.D.: Acute systemic melioidosis: autopsy findings in four patients, Am. J. Clin. Pathol. **52:**188, 1969.
91. Grieco, M.H., and Sheldon, C.: *Erysipelothrix rhusiopathiae*, Ann. NY Acad. Sci. **174:**523, 1970.
92. Hayflick, L., and Chanock, R.M.: *Mycoplasma* species of man, Bacteriol. Rev. **29:**185, 1965.
93. Hoekenga, M.T.: Plague in Americas, J. Trop. Med. **50:**190, 1947.
94. Hornick, R.B., Greisman, S.E., Woodward, T.E., DuPont, H.L., Dawkins, A.T., and Snyder, M.J.: Typhoid fever: pathogenesis and immunologic control, N. Engl. J. Med. **283:**686, 1970.
95. Howe, C., and Miller, W.R.: Human glanders: report of 6 cases, Ann. Intern. Med. **26:**93, 1947.
96. Howe, C., Sampath, A., and Spotnitz, M.: The pseudomallei group: a review, J. Infect. Dis. **124:**598, 1971.
97. Hunt, A.C., and Bothwell, P.W.: Histological findings in human brucellosis, J. Clin. Pathol. **20:**267, 1967.
98. Klauder, J.V.: Erysipeloid as an occupational disease, JAMA **111:**1345, 1938.
99. Kohn, L.A.: Experimental typhoid in man, N. Engl. J. Med. **278:**739, 1968.
100. Lavetter, A., Leedom, J.M., Mathies, A.W., Jr., Ivler, D., and Wehrle, P.F.: Meningitis due to *Listeria monocytogenes:* a review of 25 cases, N. Engl. J. Med. **285:**598, 1971.
101. Leino, R., and Kalliomaki, J.L.: Yersiniosis as an internal disease, Ann. Intern. Med. **81:**458, 1974.
102. Mair, I.W., Natvig, K., and Johannessen, T.A.: Otolaryngological manifestations of tularemia, Arch. Otolaryngol. **98:**156, 1973.
103. Medoff, G., Kunz, L.J., and Weinberg, A.N.: Listeriosis in humans: an evaluation, J. Infect. Dis. **123:**247, 1971.
104. Meyer, K.F.: The natural history of plague and psittacosis, Public Health Rep. **72:**705, 1957.
105. Mollaret, H.H.: Un domaine pathologique nouveau: l'infection à *Yersinia enterocolitica*, Ann. Biol. Clin. **30:**1, 1972.
106. Morrison, R.E., Lamb, A.S., Craig, D.B., and Johnson, W.M.: Meliodosis: a reminder, Am. J. Med. **84:**965, 1988.
107. Piggott, J.A.: Demonstriation for diagnosis: melioidosis, Int. Pathol. **9:**34, 1968.
108. Pollitzer, R.: Plague, WHO Monogr Ser. no. 22, 1954.
109. Prost, E., and Riemann, H.: Food-borne salmonellosis, Annu. Rev. Microbiol. **21:**495, 1967.
110. Pullen, R.L., and Stuart, B.M.: Tularemia: analysis of 225 cases, JAMA **129:**495, 1945.
111. Rubin, H.L., Alexander, A.D., and Yager, R.H.: Meliodosis—a military medical problem, Milit. Med. **128:**538, 1963.

112. Schultz, M.G.: A history of bartonellosis (Carrion's disease), Am. J. Trop. Med. Hyg. **17:**503, 1968.
113. Sheehy, T.W., Deller, J.J., Jr., and Weber, D.R.: Melioidosis, Ann. Intern. Med. **67:**897, 1967.
114. Smith, P.F.: The biology of mycoplasmas, New York, 1971, Academic Press, Inc.
115. Spink, W.W.: The nature of brucellosis, Minneapolis, 1956, University of Minnesota Press.
116. Stuart, B.M., and Pullen, R.L.: Tularemia pneumonia: review of American literature and report of 15 additional cases, Am. J. Med. Sci. **210:**223, 1945.
117. Stuart, B.M., and Pullen, R.L.: Typhoid: clinical analysis of 360 cases, Arch. Intern. Med. **78:**629, 1946.
118. Takeuchi, A.: Electron microscopic studies of experimental *Salmonella* infection. I. Penetration into the interstinal epithelium by *Salmonella typhimurium*, Am. J. Pathol. **50:**109, 1967.
119. Torin, D.E.: A typhoid fever outbreak on a university campus, Arch. Intern. Med. **129:**606, 1969.
120. Typhoid fever, Lancet **2:**416, 1972. (Editorial.)
121. Weber, J., Finlayson, N.B., and Mark, N.B.D.: Mesenteric lymphadenitis and terminal ileitis due to *Yersinia pseudotuberculosis*, N. Engl. J. Med. **283:**172, 1970.
122. White, P.C., Jr.: Brucellosis in a Virginia meat packing plant, Arch. Environ. Health **28:**263, 1974.
123. Zucker-Franklin, D., Davidson, M., and Thomas, L.: The interaction of mycoplasmas with mammalian cells. I. HeLa cells, neutrophils and eosinophils, J. Exp. Med. **124:**521, 1966.
124. Zucker-Franklin, D., Davidson, M., and Thomas, L.: The interaction of mycoplasmas with mammalian cells. II. Monocytes and lymphocytes, J. Exp. Med. **124:**533, 1966.

Donovanosis
125. Davis, C.M.: Granuloma inguinale: a clinical, histological, and ultrastructural study, JAMA **211:**632, 1970.
126. Kuberski, T.: Granuloma inguinale (donovanosis), Sex. Transm. Dis. **7:**29, 1980.
127. Stewart, D.B.: Ulcerative and hypertrophic lesions of the vulva, Proc. R. Soc. Med. **61:**363, 1968.

Spirochetal diseases
128. Arean, V.M.: The pathologic anatomy and pathogenesis of fatal human leptospirosis (Weil's disease), Am. J. Pathol. **40:**393, 1962.
129. Beeman, H., et al.: Syphilis: review of the recent literature, 1959-1960, Arch. Intern. Med. **107:**121, 1961.
130. Benirschke, K.: Syphilis—the placenta and the fetus, Am. J. Dis. Child. **128:**142, 1974.
131. Clark, E.G., and Danbolt, H.: The Oslo study of the natural course of untreated syphilis: an epidemiologic investigation based on a restudy of the Boeck-Brussgard material, Med. Clin. North Am. **48:**613, 1964.
132. Guthe, T.: The treponematoses as a world problem, Br. J. Vener. Dis. **36:**67, 1960.
133. Hager, W.D.: Transplacental transmission of spirochetes in congenital syphilis: a new perspective, Sex. Transm. Dis. **5:**122, 1978.
134. Harter, C.A., and Benirschke, K.: Fetal syphilis in the first trimester, Am. J. Obstet. Gynecol. **124:**705, 1976.
135. Hume, J.C.: Worldwide problems in the diagnosis of syphilis and other treponematoses, Med. Clin. North Am. **48:**721, 1964.
136. Jeerapaet, P., and Ackerman, A.B.: Histologic patterns in secondary syphilis, Arch. Dermatol. **107:**373, 1973.
137. Judge, D.M.: Louse-borne relapsing fever in man, Arch. Pathol. **97:**136, 1974.
138. Lees, R.E.M.: A selective approach to yaws control, Can. J. Public Health **64**(suppl. 2):52, 1973.
139. Willcox, R.R.: Changing patterns of treponemal disease, Br. J. Vener. Dis. **50:**169, 1974.

7 Leprosy

WAYNE M. MEYERS
CHAPMAN H. BINFORD

DEFINITION, HISTORY, AND PREVALENCE

Leprosy is a chronic infectious disease caused by *Mycobacterium leprae* and affecting chiefly the cooler parts of humans—skin, respiratory tract, anterior structures of the eyes, superficial segments of peripheral nerves, and testes.

Although leprosy dates to ancient times, Old Testament descriptions of lesions called leprosy (for example, *Leviticus* 13 and 14) do not fit the disease as we know it today. The Hebrew word *tsāra'ath,* translated 'leprosy,' probably referred to a variety of skin lesions of the nomadic Israelites. Leprosy was widely prevalent in Europe during the millennium between approximately the fall of the Roman Empire and the fifteenth century.

The World Health Organization (WHO) estimates that in 1985 there were 10 to 12 million leprosy patients in the world[49] (Fig. 7-1). Other estimates range up to 15 million patients. Registered cases in 1985 (5,368,000) increased by 89.6% over the total in 1976. The estimated total number of patients is based on whole population surveys that indicate that there are 1 to 2 undocumented patients for each one registered. The highest recorded prevalence rates are now in tropical Africa, South America, India, Southeast Asia, the Philippines, and some South Pacific islands. Although most patients live in warm climates, the spread of leprosy most likely depends more on the living conditions that prevail in many developing countries, rather than on the tropical climate. Although the predominant type of leprosy varies in different populations, there is no evi-

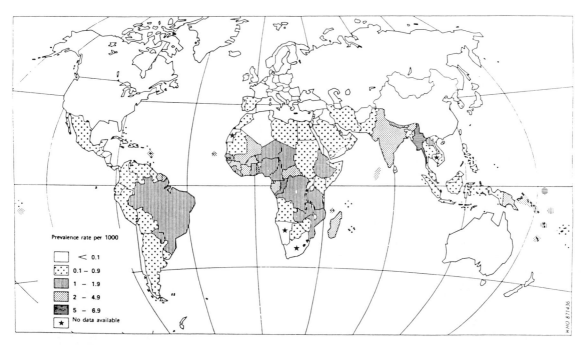

Fig. 7-1. Leprosy throughout the world. (Reproduced by permission from WHO Expert Committee on Leprosy: Sixth report, WHO Tech. Rep. Ser. no. 768, Geneva, 1988, World Health Organization. AFIP 88-7054.)

dence for racial or ethnic factors in overall susceptibility. The ratio of adult male to female patients is approximately 2:1, and in areas of high prevalence, onset of disease is most frequent in the second decade of life.

There are now approximately 6000 leprosy patients in the United States, with indigenous leprosy in California, Florida, Hawaii, Louisiana, and southeastern Texas. During the period 1976-1985, the Centers for Disease Control reported 2288 new leprosy patients in the United States.[7] The 361 new patients reported in 1985 represents a 150% increase over 1976. States reporting the highest number of patients were California with 155, Washington 37, Hawaii 31, New York 30 (with 29 in New York City), Texas 28, Illinois 24, and Louisiana 13. Although 88% (316) of all new cases reported in 1985 were imported, there is no known secondary case arising because of contacts with these patients. Thus immigrants with leprosy do not pose a public health problem in the United States.

LEPROSY BACILLUS[14]

Mycobacterium leprae resembles *M. tuberculosis* in morphology and staining but is less acid-fast. In tissues, *M. leprae* stains well by the Fite-Faraco[20] procedure but poorly by the Ziehl-Neelsen technique. In contrast to other mycobacteria, the acid-fastness of *M. leprae* is abolished by exposure to pyridine.[11] *M. leprae* in older lesions may be arranged in compact rounded masses (globi) or grouped in bundles, like cigarettes in a pack. Viable organisms stain solidly, but degenerating bacilli first stain irregularly, then become granular, and eventually lose acid-fastness completely. Non–acid fast carcasses of *M. leprae* stain by the Gomori methenamine-silver (GMS) method.

In 1873 Hansen[24] discovered the leprosy bacillus in skin lesions. Although the bacillus has been studied extensively, *M. leprae* has not been acceptably cultivated in vitro.

TRANSMISSION

Patients with untreated lepromatous leprosy may shed numerous bacilli from skin abrasions or ulcers and in nasal secretions. From unbroken skin a few bacilli may be shed via hair follicles, or even desquamating epidermal cells.[66] The traditional belief is that leprosy is spread by direct skin contact between infected and healthy persons without the aid of insect vectors or animal hosts. Indirect contact with recently contaminated objects may play a role. The prevailing view today, however, is that transmission of the bacillus is through the mucous membranes of the mouth or nose. *M. leprae* in nasal secretions are viable up to 9 days after drying in open petri dishes.[13]

Attack rates among healthy spouses of leprosy patients is approximately 6%. This prevalence in spouses is similar to the estimate that only 5% of people worldwide are susceptible to leprosy.

Placental transmission of leprosy has frequently been proposed, and recent observations on infants of patients and armadillos indicates the likelihood of intrauterine infection.[6,15,28] Milk of lepromatous patients contains *M. leprae;* thus infants could acquire the infection from this source.[53]

The incubation period of leprosy is usually 2 to 5 years but may be as long as 10 to 20 years.

Beginning shortly after Hansen discovered the leprosy bacillus, there have been numerous animal-transmission studies. In recent years, after investigators realized that in humans the leprosy bacillus grew best in cooler tissues, there have been important advances in developing animal models.[2,29,43] For example, Shepard[60] demonstrated multiplication of *M. leprae* in the footpads of mice, providing a useful method for determining the viability of *M. leprae.*

The nine-banded armadillo *(Dasypus novemcinctus)* is an excellent laboratory model for lepromatous leprosy.[33] A high percentage of inoculated armadillos develop a disseminated disease histopathologically resembling human leprosy, including invasion of nerves. The low body-core temperature of armadillos, 32° to 35° C, probably explains why viscera in the armadillo are more heavily infected than in human leprosy.

Mild infection with *M. leprae* has been obtained in several species of normal rodents,[3,4] and heavy lepromatous infections have been achieved in immunosuppressed[19,56] and immunodeficient[9] rodents.

LEPROSY AS A ZOONOSIS[64]

In 1975, indigenous leprosy was first reported in wild armadillos captured in Louisiana.[65] This disease cannot be distinguished histopathologically, bacteriologically, or immunologically from that in armadillos inoculated with *M. leprae* from patients. In a survey of 451 wild armadillos in Texas, Smith et al.[61] found that 4.66% had lepromatous leprosy. Because of their high susceptibility to leprosy, armadillos may have initially been infected through discarded dressings, secretions, or other materials from advanced lepromatous patients who lived at home in rural areas in the era before effective sulfone therapy was available. The disease probably then became focally endemic in armadillo populations by animal-to-animal passage. A few patients in Texas may have acquired leprosy by handling armadillos,[38] and armadillo contact is suspected to be an epidemiologic factor in patients in California.[62]

Three nonhuman primates from Africa, while being used in research unrelated to leprosy in laboratories in the United States, have spontaneously developed lepromatous leprosy, possibly from exposure before importation to untreated leprosy patients. Leininger and co-

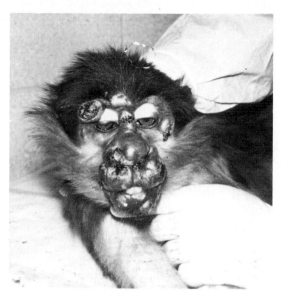

Fig. 7-2. Sooty mangabey monkey with naturally acquired lepromatous leprosy. (AFIP 80-9993-2.)

workers[37] at the University of Iowa reported a chimpanzee from Sierra Leone with advanced lepromatous leprosy. At the Delta Regional Primate Research Center in Covington, Louisiana, two mangabey monkeys from Nigeria with advanced, naturally acquired lepromatous leprosy have been studied[23,45] (Fig. 7-2). Transmission of the infection to other mangabey monkeys, rhesus, and African green monkeys has been successful, and primate models of leprosy are now under development.[1]

The large number of naturally infected armadillos in Louisiana and Texas establishes leprosy as an endemic zoonotic disease in those states, and the several wild nonhuman primates from Africa with naturally acquired leprosy indicates that they may be reservoirs of leprosy.

CLASSIFICATION

The Sixth International Congress of Leprosy in 1953 classified leprosy into two principal types: *lepromatous* and *tuberculoid*. Cases not falling into these types were classified into two other groups: *indeterminate* and *borderline*. With refinements, this classification is in use today.

The lepromatous and tuberculoid types represent opposite poles of host anergy and hyperergy, respectively.

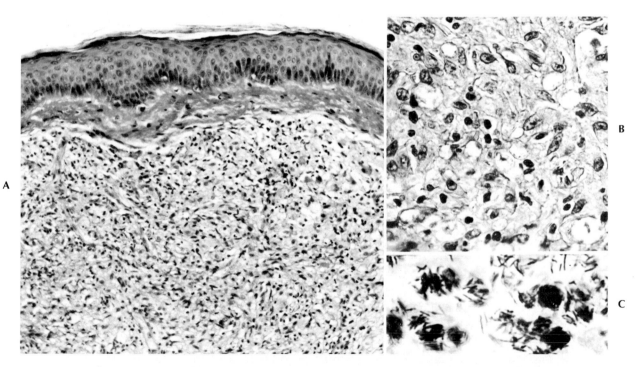

Fig. 7-3. Lepromatous leprosy. **A,** Section of skin in lesion of advanced lepromatous leprosy. Observe nearly total replacement of entire dermis by massive infiltrate but no encroachment on basal part of epidermis. **B,** Lepromatous infiltrate. Cells are histiocytes (lepra cells); many show no vacuolization, but in **C** observe cells filled with bacilli. **C,** Lepromatous infiltrate stained by Fite-Faraco acid-fast technique. (**A** and **B,** Hematoxylin and eosin; **A,** 145×; AFIP 65-1653; **B,** 400×; **C,** 1600×; AFIP 54-17674.)

In lepromatous leprosy, great numbers of bacilli inhabit histiocytes (Fig. 7-3, *C*), and in advanced cutaneous lesions, heavily bacillated histiocytes may replace nearly the entire dermis. In tuberculoid leprosy, a few bacilli or bacillary products elicit severe delayed type of hypersensitivity granulomas (Fig. 7-4, *D*).

Ridley and Jopling[57] divide the spectrum of leprosy into five groups based on the patient's ability to mount a cell-mediated immune response to *M. leprae*. There is good correlation between the clinical and histopathologic classifications if strict criteria are maintained.[44] The groups are tuberculoid (TT), borderline-tubercu-

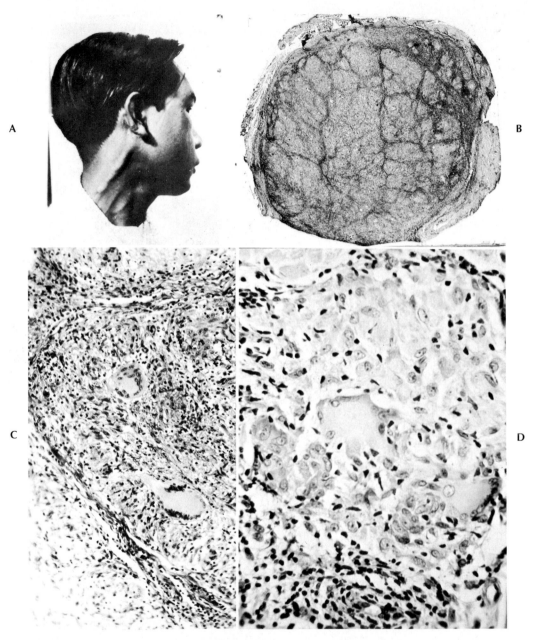

Fig. 7-4. Tuberculoid leprosy. **A,** Enlarged great auricular nerve in Hawaiian man. **B,** Cross section of enlarged nerve in tuberculoid leprosy. Almost entire nerve is replaced by epithelioid cell granulomatous infiltration. Few bacilli are seen. **C,** High magnification of section of nerve in tuberculoid leprosy showing epithelioid cells, Langhans' giant cells, and lymphocytes. **D,** Epithelioid cell granuloma with Langhans' giant cells in skin lesion of tuberculoid leprosy. Observe similarity to nodular granulomas seen in Boeck's sarcoid. (Hematoxylin and eosin; **B,** 9½×; AFIP 55-10845; **C,** approximately 100×; **D,** approximately 200×.)

loid (BT), borderline (BB), borderline-lepromatous (BL), and lepromatous (LL). The TT and LL groups are stable both clinically and histopathologically, but the borderline groups are unstable and may shift toward either pole during the course of the disease. *Indeterminate* leprosy (Fig. 7-5) is a nascent stage of the disease in which neither the clinical nor the histopathologic features clearly indicate the cellular immune status of the patient.

The first responsibility of the pathologist is to make or rule out a diagnosis of leprosy, but because each type of leprosy requires different treatment and management, precise classification is important. If unfamiliar with leprosy, the pathologist should consult those experienced in the recognition and management of leprosy.

Lepromin test. In 1919 Mitsuda introduced a skin test employing an homogenate of heat-treated lepromatous tissue.[26] This test is useful in classifying the disease in patients with known leprosy, but *it is not a diagnostic test* because many people who have never been exposed to leprosy react positively. Lepromin assesses host resistance to *M. leprae*, being nonreactive (negative) in patients with lepromatous leprosy and positive in those with tuberculoid leprosy. A positive lepromin test is biphasic, with an early erythematous indurated response at 24 to 48 hours (Fernandez reaction)[17] and a delayed nodular epithelioid cell granulomatous reaction after 3 to 4 weeks (Mitsuda reaction). Lepromin is available on an Investigational New Drug Application basis from the Laboratory Research Branch, Gillis W. Long Hansen's Disease Center, Carville, LA 70721.

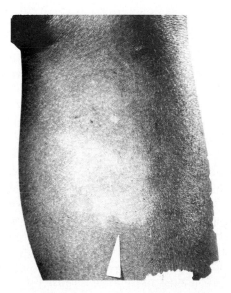

Fig. 7-5. Lesion of indeterminate leprosy on leg of Filipino patient. Lesion is flat and hypopigmented. (AFIP 74-9029-1.)

CLINICAL FEATURES

Lesions of *lepromatous* leprosy vary from slightly hypopigmented or erythematous macules to papules, nodules, plaques, or diffuse infiltrations (Fig. 7-6, *B* and *D*). Typically, the borders of lepromatous lesions are not sharply defined. Lesions tend to be numerous and symmetrically distributed and, with progression, become confluent and widespread. Early lesions of lepromatous leprosy are mildly hypesthetic and old lesions may be anesthetic, but sensory disturbances are not as distinct as in tuberculoid leprosy.

Lucio, or "spotted leprosy," first reported in 1852 by Lucio and Alvarado, is an interesting clinical and histopathologic variety of lepromatous leprosy.[36] This form, seen principally in patients of Mexican origin, is characterized by diffuse involvement of the skin without discrete lesions. A necrotizing cutaneous vasculitis may cause multiple small ulcers (Lucio phenomenon).

In *tuberculoid* leprosy (Fig. 7-9, *B*), the early macular lesions are sharply defined and, depending on natural skin color, hypopigmented or slightly erythematous, with distinct sensory impairment. Typically there is a single or only a few asymmetrically distributed lesions. During increased activity, the lesions may be plaquelike, or the borders may become elevated, papular, and erythematous, while the centers remain flat.

Borderline lesions begin as macules that may develop into plaques with elevated centers and streaming irregular sloping borders. Sensory changes are usually readily detectable. The central area may flatten, and the circinate or serpiginous borders become elevated. Tuberculoid features predominate in BT lesions, and lepromatous features in BL lesions. Damage to peripheral nerve trunks is often pronounced. The lepromin test (Mitsuda reaction) is positive in BT, weak in BB, and usually negative in BL. See Fig. 7-7.

Indeterminate lesions may first present as small erythematous or hypopigmented macules that may be mildly hypesthetic. The lepromin test (Mitsuda reaction) may be negative or positive.

REACTIONS

The clinical course of leprosy is often punctuated by acute episodes called *reactions* and fall into two groups: *reversal upgrading reactions* and *erythema nodosum leprosum* (ENL).

Reversal upgrading reactions. Reversal upgrading reactions are manifestations of increased cell-mediated immunity to *M. leprae*. Lesions become erythematous and edematous, and acute peripheral neuritis is common. By repeated reversal reactions, borderline patients often upgrade toward tuberculoid disease.

Erythema nodosum leprosum. Approximately 50% of lepromatous patients suffer outcroppings of tender cutaneous nodules called *erythema nodosum leprosum* (ENL). These episodes are usually accompanied by fe-

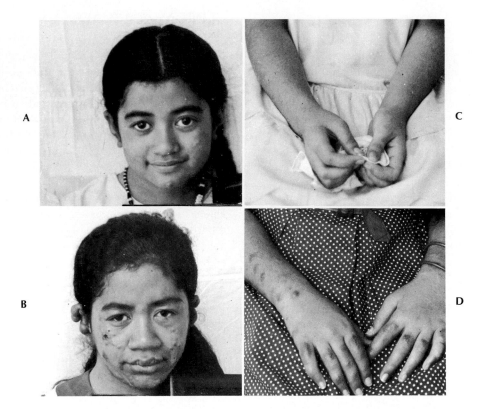

Fig. 7-6. Lepromatous leprosy. **A,** Hawaiian girl, 11 years of age, with early lepromatous leprosy. Hypopigmented, inconspicuous lesions can be seen on cheeks and chin. **B,** Same girl at 13 years of age. Observe nodular thickening of right ear, lesions of cheeks and chin, and conspicuous change in facial appearance. Diffuse infiltration of skin by lepra cells caused thickening of skin that distorted face. **C,** Forearms and hands when patient was 11 years of age. There are no obvious lesions. **D,** Hands when patient was 13 years of age. In 2-year period, nodular lesions have developed in skin of right forearm and fingers with diffuse thickening of entire skin of forearm.

ver and malaise and sometimes by synovitis and iridocyclitis. Multiple or recurrent attacks are not uncommon. Effective chemotherapy tends to precipitate ENL.

Amyloidosis. Before effective antileprosy treatment was available, secondary amyloidosis was a serious complication of lepromatous leprosy in some populations. Powell and Swan,[54] in a review of 50 consecutive autopsies of patients dying at the U.S. Public Health Service Hospital at Carville (1948-1954), found secondary amyloidosis in 23 patients. Renal insufficiency from amyloidosis was the cause of death in 38%. Although sulfone therapy was being used at Carville during this period, in many patients the disease was advanced and long-standing before effective treatment was started. By contrast, in 103 autopsies before 1942 at the Palo Seco leprosarium in the Canal Zone, Kean and Childress[31] found amyloidosis of the kidneys in only four cases; however there was a high incidence of glomerulonephritis. In Malaysia there was amyloidosis in 22% and glomerulonephritis in 13% of a series of autopsies of

leprosy patients between 1981 and 1985.[27] Amyloidosis is a late sequela of repeated ENL and may be related to the neutrophilic leukocytosis in these patients.[39]

HISTOPATHOLOGY

Biopsy specimens should be taken from the border of skin lesions. Hematoxylin-eosin and Fite-Faraco stained sections are usually sufficient for evaluation, but occasionally the Gomori methenamine-silver (GMS) stain will help detect carcasses of *M. leprae* in treated patients. A histopathologic diagnosis of leprosy must be made only on convincing evidence.

Lepromatous. Skin lesions in lepromatous leprosy develop by the proliferation of histiocytes that first form small infiltrations around blood vessels, nerves, and epidermal appendages. Because the histiocytes offer so little resistance to bacillary growth, large numbers of cells are required to accommodate this unimpeded multiplication. In advanced lesions, these infiltrations may replace almost the entire dermis (Fig. 7-3, *A* and *B*). The cellular infiltration of lepromatous leprosy,

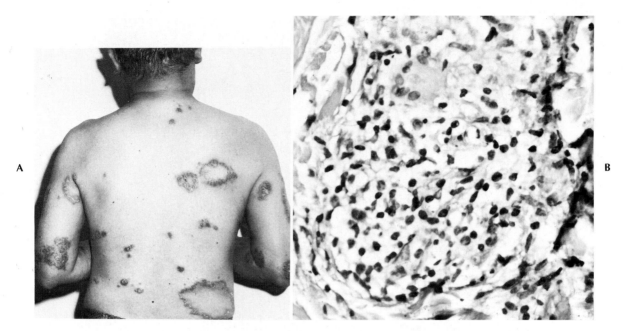

Fig. 7-7. A, Borderline leprosy. Lesions have hypopigmented and hypesthetic centers. Elevated borders are erythematous. Inner margins of ring lesions are sharp, whereas outer margins slope into normal skin. Exacerbation of these lesions appeared shortly after this Filipino man arrived in United States to attend school. **B,** Borderline leprosy with tuberculoid features. Nerves in this section showed mild round cell infiltrate and many macrophages with bacilli. (440×; AFIP 72-12458.)

though so prolific that nodules (lepromas) may form, characteristically does not encroach on the basal layer of the epidermis but is separated from it by a thin, sparsely cellular clear zone. Expanding lesions iron out rete ridges, flatten dermal papillae, and thin the epidermis, sometimes to ulceration. The histiocytic infiltrations are supported by a delicate stroma vascularized by a rich network of capillaries. Other inflammatory cells are not prominent in these lesions.

Aging vacuolated histiocytes contain many acid-fast bacilli (Fig. 7-3, *C*) and are commonly called "Virchow lepra cells," or simply "lepra cells." The bacilli are frequently arranged in clusters or compact globular masses (globi) that eventually replace nearly the entire intracellular space. When these histiocytes disintegrate, the freed bacilli may coalesce to form large, compact, rounded masses (giant globi), often found in foreign-body giant cells. In lepromatous leprosy there are usually large numbers of bacilli in nerves in the skin. Infected nerves may show only slight histopathologic changes other than increased numbers of bacilli-laden histiocytes and Schwann cells. Macrophages in walls of blood vessels and vascular endothelial cells are frequently heavily bacillated[47] (Fig. 7-8). The epithelial cells of hair follicles and arrector pili muscle cells may contain bacilli, but bacilli are rarely observed within the cells of sweat and sebaceous glands.

In effectively treated lepromatous leprosy, the intracellular bacilli lose acid-fastness but are well demonstrated by the GMS stain if the time in the silver solution is slightly prolonged. The persistence for long periods of these dead bacilli or their fragments contributes to the slow resolution of lepromatous lesions.

Tuberculoid. The intense cell-mediated immune response in tuberculoid leprosy is reflected in the granulomatous reaction (Fig. 7-9). Characteristic granulomas are made up of a central nest of epithelioid cells with a mantle of lymphocytes and may or may not contain Langhans' giant cells. Tuberculoid leprosy in the skin histopathologically resembles Boeck's sarcoid (Fig. 7-4, *D*), tuberculosis without caseation, and many other diseases in which the host reaction is that of delayed-type hypersensitivity granulomas. The infiltrate of tuberculoid leprosy extends into the papillary stroma up to and often invading the basal cells of the epidermis (Fig. 7-10, *A*). Thus, in contrast to lepromatous lesions, there is no clear zone between the infiltrate and the overlying epidermis.

In tuberculoid leprosy, dermal nerves are frequently damaged by the cellular reaction (Fig. 7-10, *B*). The infiltrate in small nerves may consist of epithelioid cells or lymphocytes. Nerve destruction is an early event, often leading to the absence of nerves in the histopathologic sections. Inability to demonstrate nerves in gran-

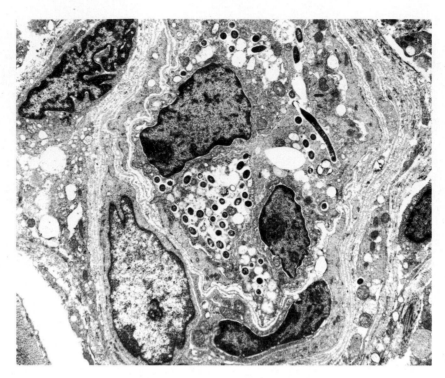

Fig. 7-8. Electron micrograph showing heavy bacillation of endothelial cells of a small blood vessel in dermis of a patient with untreated lepromatous leprosy. (14,000×; AFIP 87-5206.)

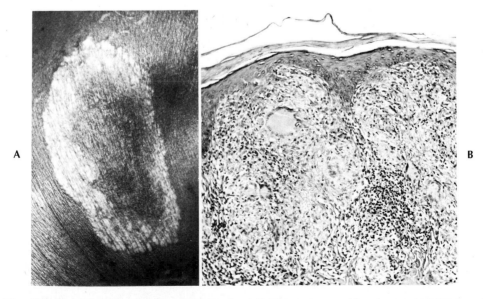

Fig. 7-9. A, Tuberculoid leprosy on back of Zaïrian woman. Margins are distinct and papular. Lesion is anesthetic. **B,** Tuberculoid leprosy. Compact infiltrate is composed of epithelioid cells, Langhans' giant cells, and lymphocytes. There is no clear zone as in lepromatous leprosy, but infiltrate extends to and erodes basal layer of epidermis. (84×; AFIP 72-12465.)

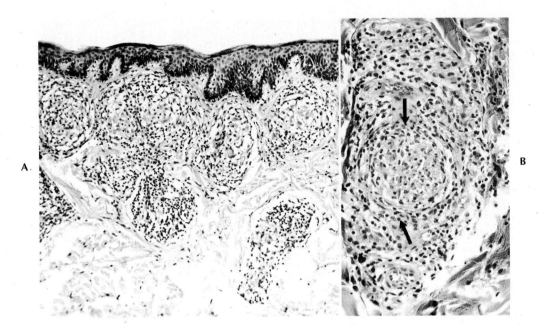

Fig. 7-10. Tuberculoid leprosy. **A,** Section of skin showing early tuberculoid leprosy. Observe small epithelioid cell granulomas, one with giant cell, and lymphocytes surrounding granulomas. Infiltrate extending into papillae. **B,** Small nerve in tuberculoid leprosy *(between arrows)* enveloped and almost completely infiltrated by epithelioid cells. Bacilli are scarce, but searching many sections stained by Fite-Faraco method usually reveals occasional bacillus. (Hematoxylin and eosin; **A,** 210×; AFIP 56-19556; **B,** approximately 200×; AFIP 65-8941.)

ulomatous skin lesions is suggestive of leprosy but is certainly not diagnostic. Bacilli are scarce but, if found, are usually within small nerves, or fragments of nerves in granulomas. If bacilli cannot be found in nerves, the papillary dermis and arrector pili muscle should be searched.

Indeterminate. The histopathologic features of indeterminate leprosy are nonspecific. Pathologists often make a diagnosis of mild, nonspecific dermatitis, or lymphocytic angiitis (Figs. 7-5 and 7-11, *A*). The nonspecific cellular reaction in lesions of indeterminate leprosy is attributed to the early phase of the disease and a lack of immunologic polarization. Usually there are mild round cell infiltrations around neurovascular channels or epidermal appendages. Small nerves, though usually intact, may show slight infiltration by round cells. Normal-appearing nerves may contain bacilli (Fig. 7-11, *B*). The demonstration of acid-fast bacilli in a nerve in a lesion of this form confirms a diagnosis of leprosy (Fig. 7-11, *C*).

Borderline. Borderline leprosy presents a broad spectrum of histopathologic variations. In the near-tuberculoid (BT) form, strong cell-mediated immunity is demonstrated by the large numbers of epithelioid cells and lymphocytes. Nerves are less severely dam-

aged than in polar tuberculoid (TT) leprosy, and acid-fast bacilli, though scarce, are usually easily found in nerves, in the subepidermal zone, or in an arrector pili muscle. Borderline-lepromatous (BL) lesions may contain a few epithelioid cells and irregularly distributed lymphocytes, but histiocytes usually prevail. The perineuria of nerves are infiltrated by the cellular exudates, but the nerves are usually readily identifiable. There are many acid-fast bacilli in nerves and histiocytes.

Some histopathologists do not recognize midborderline (BB) leprosy as an entity because of the high instability of this form, and examination of multiple sections often reveals features of either BT or BL disease. BB leprosy, however, may be perceived as intermediate between BT and BL. In BB there often are epithelioid cells and lymphocytes in the perineuria and in the surrounding dermis. Acid-fast bacilli are readily identified and most plentiful in nerves.

Reactions. In acute reversal upgrading reactions, there is edema within the granulomas, accompanied by increased numbers of lymphocytes and often Langhans' giant cells. In severe reversal reactions, there may be central necrosis in the granulomas, sometimes misleading the pathologist to consider other diagnoses.

Erythema nodosum leprosum is believed to be a lo-

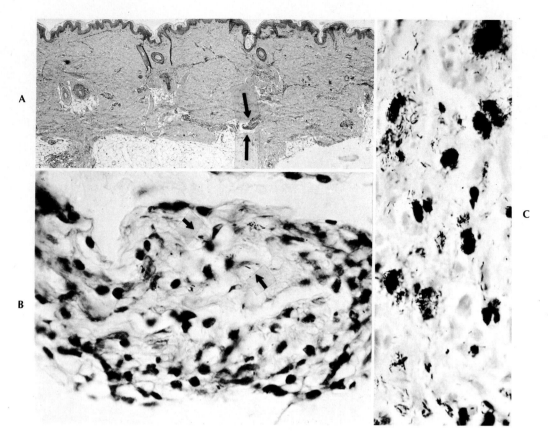

Fig. 7-11. Indeterminate leprosy, unrecognized. **A,** Skin of boy 6 years of age. Histopathologic diagnosis was chronic, mild dermatitis. At 14 years of age, condition was diagnosed as advanced lepromatous leprosy, at which time study of slides made 8 years before revealed several acid-fast bacilli in small dermal nerve *(arrows).* **B,** Nerve is that shown in **A** but stained for acid-fast bacilli. Observe increased number of nuclei within nerves. *Arrows,* Well-defined bacilli. **C,** Section of skin lesion of patient at 14 years of age when diagnosis of advanced lepromatous leprosy was made. (**A,** Hematoxylin and eosin, 16×; AFIP 63-2022; **B** and **C,** Fite-Faraco stain; **B,** 650×; AFIP 32-0211; **C,** 1100×; AFIP 59-255.)

calized reaction to immune complexes, usually involving the skin, but also may affect nerve, lymph node, synovium, and iris. Characteristically, there is an influx of neutrophils. Skin may be involved at any level, often with a severe panniculitis. In severe forms there is necrosis, with ulceration. Vasculitis within lesions is common but not an essential feature.

HISTOID VARIETY OF LEPROMATOUS LEPROSY

In 1963 Wade[63] described circumscribed nodules that clinically and histopathologically resembled dermatofibromas in patients with relapsed lepromatous leprosy. These nodules frequently are dome-shaped tumors elevated well above the surface of the surrounding skin (Fig. 7-12, *A*). Simulating fibromas, they are composed of whorls and fascicles of spindle cells (Fig. 7-12, *B*). The spindle cells resemble fibroblasts, but they are highly active proliferating histiocytes.[58] The active expansion of these histiocytic infiltrations pushes the collagen aside, often producing a pseudocapsule. Characteristically, the spindle cells contain many long, well-stained acid-fast bacilli arranged parallel to the long axis of the cell (Fig. 7-12, *C*). Occasionally there are local reactional sites with necrosis in the centers of the lepromas. Histoid lesions are more common in relapsing lepromatous leprosy than in primary infections but do not indicate drug-resistant disease as was originally postulated.[59]

NERVE INVOLVEMENT

Among pathogenic bacteria *M. leprae* seems unique in its predilection for peripheral nerves. All patients with leprosy have nerve involvement, even though in many only the small nerves in the skin are affected. Segments of large peripheral nerves lying near the skin

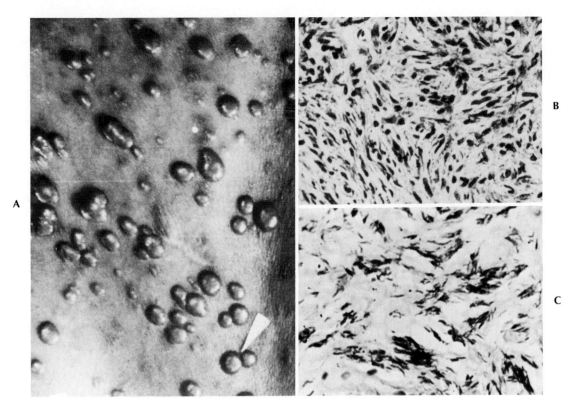

Fig. 7-12. A, Histoid lesions on back of 35-year-old Filipino patient with lepromatous leprosy who had received sulfone therapy regularly for 4 years and intermittently for following 5 years. *Arrow,* Lesion from which the biopsy specimen was taken. **B,** Hematoxylin and eosin–stained section of typical histoid lesion. Observe fascicular arrangement of spindle cells resembling dermatofibroma. **C,** Fite-Faraco– and acid-fast–stained section showing presence of large numbers of *Mycobacterium leprae* in spindle cells that compose lesion. Notice that bacilli usually are arranged parallel to long axis of spindle cells. (**A,** From Rodríguez, J.N.: Int. J. Leprosy **37:**1, 1969; **B,** 175×; **C,** 530×.)

surface are common sites of neuropathy, typically such segments of the ulnar, median, radial, common peroneal, posterior tibial, and great auricular nerves (see Fig. 7-4, *A* and *B*). In less advanced disease, nerve involvement may be appreciated only by microscopic examination; however, in more advanced leprosy, nerves are visibly or palpably enlarged.

Histopathologic changes in large nerves correspond to the skin lesions for each type of leprosy. In lepromatous leprosy histiocytes containing bacilli may replace a part of the nerve trunk and involve the perineural stroma. In the tuberculoid form, epithelioid cell granulomas may completely replace intraneural structures (Fig. 7-4, *C*). The result of nerve involvement in either form of leprosy may be total anesthesia of the skin of the anatomic region supplied by the nerve or nerves, together with paresis, or paralysis, of the relevant muscles. In tuberculoid leprosy caseous nerve abscesses of major nerves resemble the necrosis caused by *M. tuberculosis*. This is the one sit-

uation in which caseation is commonplace in leprosy.

A variety of factors secondary to direct invasion of the nerve by bacilli and inflammatory cells contribute to nerve damage: among these are entrapment in fibroosseus tissues, minor trauma, and stretching over articulations.[8,12]

In some persons there may be no evident skin lesions, the manifestations of disease being confined entirely to one or more peripheral nerve trunks. This is called *pure neural leprosy.*

Nerve damage causes most of the severe deformities in leprosy (such as mask face, lagophthalmos, claw hand, and drop foot) and may be largely responsible for the great fear and stigma of the disease. Because of anesthesia, patients may be unaware of cuts, puncture wounds, bruises, and burns of the skin, especially of the feet or hands. The combined effect of paralytic deformity and cutaneous anesthesia may lead to damage of soft tissues and bone and secondary infections that may gradually destroy the foot or hand.

TEMPERATURE SELECTIVITY AND GENERAL PATHOLOGY

M. leprae appears to grow best in tissues that are cool, and this is well demonstrated by the distribution and severity of the disease in different regions of the body. The cooler areas are ears, nose, mucous membranes of the upper respiratory tract (especially the turbinates and nasal septum), anterior segment of the eyes, testes, and the most superficial nerve trunks.[5] Although there are leprosy bacilli in peripheral blood monocytes of patients with advanced lepromatous leprosy, visceral lesions are not prominent. The reticuloendothelial cells of the liver and spleen phagocytose circulating bacilli producing microscopic aggregates of lepra cells. These organs may also contain small aggregates of inflammatory histiocytes that contain leprosy bacilli, but these visceral lesions are usually not progressive, even though the bacilli may be viable. Leprous orchitis is regularly seen in advanced lepromatous leprosy. The result of leprosy of the testes is hyalinization of the seminiferous tubules and replacement of the lumens of the tubules and interstitial tissues by lepromatous infiltrates. The testicular involvement is in sharp contrast to the virtual absence of lesions in the ovary.

In lepromatous leprosy, destructive cystic osteitis caused by *M. leprae* is occasionally observed in the bones of the hand and foot but not in the larger bones. In such lesions the trabeculas are atrophic with osteoid formation. The intratrabecular spaces contain macrophages and sometimes giant cells laden with acid-fast bacilli. Bone marrow aspirated from advanced lepromatous patients usually shows a few macrophages containing bacilli. There may be a proliferative periostitis.

In the lepromatous patient, *M. leprae* multiples profusely in the mucosa of the upper respiratory tract from the nares to the larynx. There are extensive infiltrations of *M. leprae*–laden histiocytes immediately beneath the epithelium of the mucosa. Even when there is no gross ulceration, there is a constant shedding of bacilli that contaminate the nasal discharge and sputum. Before effective chemotherapy, laryngeal obstruction was a well-known cause of death in leprosy. Leprosy does not affect the trachea below the larynx, or the lungs.

In untreated lepromatous patients, there are often sight-threatening complications of the eye. Commonly these are lagophthalmos, scleritis, corneal anesthesia, exposure keratopathy, and iritis.[18] These structures are cooler than the retina and optic nerve, which have not been reported to be infected by *M. leprae*.

There is no proof that leprosy affects the gastrointestinal tract, spinal cord, or the brain.

LYMPH NODE INVOLVEMENT

Lymph nodes draining skin and the hepatic portal areas in lepromatous patients show capsular thickening and replacement of the paracortical areas by bacilli-laden macrophages. In the erythema nodosum leprosum (ENL) reaction there is a suppurative lymphadenitis with many acid-fast bacilli. In tuberculoid leprosy, epithelioid cell granulomas may invade lymph nodes that drain the affected skin. The histopathologic reaction in these nodes resembles that in sarcoidosis.

IMMUNOLOGY

Modified lepromin tests using concentrated lepromin show that in lepromatous patients macrophages at the test site are incapable of clearing *M. leprae* whereas in tuberculoid patients the bacilli are rapidly digested.[10] Thus cell-mediated immunity to *M. leprae* is greatly suppressed in lepromatous leprosy, and this suppression is gradually less pronounced in forms of leprosy that are progressively nearer polar tuberculoid disease.[22] The immunosuppression is believed to be specific for *M. leprae*, though in far-advanced lepromatous leprosy skin-test reactions to antigens unrelated to *M. leprae* (such as that for dinitrochlorobenzene) are depressed.

There is a continuous decrease in the response of peripheral blood lymphocytes to *M. leprae* proceeding from tuberculoid to lepromatous patients. Lymphocyte subsets in lesions of tuberculoid leprosy reveal T-helper lymphocytes distributed within the granulomas, with T-suppressor lymphocytes predominating in the mantle of the granuloma. In lepromatous lesions, T-helper cells are greatly diminished throughout the cellular infiltrates.[46] Delayed-type hypersensitivity in the high-resistance forms of leprosy is believed to be conferred by T-helper cells, and cloned T-helper cells recognize several protein antigens of *M. leprae*.[51] Lepromin and the unique antigen of *M. leprae*, phenolic glycolipid-I, have been reported to induce suppressor T-cell activity in lymphocytes from lepromatous patients, but not those from tuberculoid patients[40]; however, this finding is controversial.[55] *M. leprae* thus contains both immunostimulating and immunosuppressive antigens, and possibly previous sensitization to homologous antigens or cross-reactive mycobacterial antigens determines the reactivity of T-cells to *M. leprae* antigens.[30] Interferon-gamma stimulates similar responses in macrophages from lepromatous patients and normal subjects, an indication that the immunologic defect in lepromatous leprosy may not be in the response of macrophages but in T-lymphocytes.[32] Interferon-gamma provokes features of delayed-type hypersensitivity in vivo in lesions of lepromatous leprosy, with apparent decreases in numbers of *M. leprae*.[48] Lepromatous patients show defects in interleukin-2 (IL-2), and IL-2 restores T-lymphocyte proliferation in response to specific antigens.[25]

Immunoglobulin production (IgG, IgA, and IgM) and antibody to mycobacterial antigens are greatly elevated in lepromatous patients but only slightly, if at all, in tuberculoid leprosy. These antibodies are not protective but do provide a basis for serologic detection of two *M. leprae*–specific antigens: phenolic glycolipid-I[21,35] and an epitope of the 36,000-dalton protein.[34] Nearly all untreated multibacillary leprosy patients have detectable antibody levels. Serologic testing, especially of contacts, may detect leprosy in a preclinical stage, and early treatment of these patients would prevent sequelae and help control the spread of leprosy.

There is genetic control of the type of leprosy that develops after infection, and this control resides in the HLA class II–linked genes. Ir genes regulating the immune response to *M. leprae* may code for restriction determinants that restrict and regulate the presentation of antigens of *M. leprae* to T-helper and T-suppressor cells. The majority of restriction determinants are believed to be in the polymorphic areas of HLA-DR molecules.[50,52]

Candidate antileprosy vaccines are now under development, and some are being tested under field conditions. These vaccines are composed of either heat-killed *M. leprae* alone or in combination with live BCG. Heat-killed *M. leprae* plus BCG is known to increase the cell-mediated immune response to *M. leprae* in lepromatous patients and has an immunotherapeutic effect.[42] A highly immunogenic cell wall protein–peptidoglycan complex of *M. leprae* offers promise for a purified vaccinogenic product for leprosy.[41] Because of the potentially long incubation periods of leprosy, the efficacy of candidate leprosy vaccines will probably not be known before the year 2000.

DIAGNOSIS

Many pathologists diagnose indeterminate leprosy histopathologically *only* if acid-fast bacilli are seen *within nerves*. Moderately advanced or advanced lepromatous skin lesions can be diagnosed histopathologically if the infiltrate contains macrophages laden with bacilli characteristically arranged in packets or globi and if persisting nerves contain bacilli. The diagnosis of borderline and tuberculoid leprosy must be based on typical histopathologic patterns and nerve involvement. In all types of leprosy the finding of acid-fast bacilli in nerves is pathognomonic.

Skin smears, obtained by splitting the skin and scraping the cut edges of the dermis, may be successfully stained by the techniques used for *M. tuberculosis* in sputum smears. Large numbers of acid-fast bacilli in such smears nearly always confirms a diagnosis of leprosy. Other mycobacterial infections, especially Buruli ulcer, may occasionally show large numbers of acid-fast bacilli in the skin. Smears from the nasal mucosa must be interpreted with caution because the small numbers of saprophytic acid-fast bacilli occasionally found in nasal smears of normal persons may be misleading. Special techniques such as the Fite-Faraco[20] stain must be

used for adequate staining of tissue sections. Histopathologic examination helps in the classification of the disease and thus in the establishment of appropriate therapeutic regimens and provides medicolegal documentation.

Fear of leprosy, irrespective of geographic location or race, is so deeply ingrained that a diagnosis of leprosy, even in its mildest form, may stigmatize a patient to such a degree that he or she can never again lead a normal life. A histopathologist uncertain of the diagnosis or inexperienced in the recognition and treatment of leprosy should obtain help from more experienced colleagues. The diagnoses "compatible with" or "consistent with" leprosy should *not be made* because of the stigmatizing potential of such a diagnosis for a person without leprosy.

DIFFERENTIAL DIAGNOSIS

Lesions of leprosy mimic many other diseases, both clinically and histopathologically. Lepromatous leprosy may be confused with xanthomatous lesions, and tuberculoid leprosy with the numerous diseases causing epithelioid cell granulomas. At the Armed Forces Institute of Pathology, when a diagnosis of leprosy is being established histopathologically, *intraneural cellular or bacterial involvement, or both, are of primary importance*. This is especially important when sarcoidosis and skin lesions caused by atypical mycobacteria[16] must be distinguished from leprosy.

LEPROSY CONTROL

After the administration of effective combined therapy with dapsone, clofazimine, or rifampin, *M. leprae* obtained from patients with lepromatous leprosy will no longer multiply in mouse footpads. These patients therefore are not considered infectious. Chemotherapy of patients is the only proved method of control of leprosy available today and where applied assiduously is effective. In most countries leprosy patients are no longer subject to compulsory segregation and are treated as outpatients. Physicians needing advice on the recognition, management, and treatment of leprosy should contact the Clinical Branch, Gillis W. Long Hansen's Disease Center, Carville, LA 70721, telephone (504) 642-4789, or (800) 642-2477.

REFERENCES

1. Baskin, G.B., Gormus, B.J., Martin, L.N., et al.: Experimental leprosy in a rhesus monkey: necropsy findings, Int. J. Lepr. **55**:109, 1987.
2. Binford, C.H.: Comprehensive program for the inoculation of human leprosy into laboratory animals, U.S. Public Health. Rep. **71**:955, 1956.
3. Binford, C.H.: Studies on a mycobacterium obtained from the golden hamster (*Cricetus auratus*) after inoculation with lepromatous tissue, Lab. Invest. **11**:942, 1962.
4. Binford, C.H.: The transmission of *M. leprae* to animals: attempts to find an experimental model, Int. J. Lepr. **36**:599, 1968.

5. Binford, C.H., Meyers, W.M., and Walsh, G.P.: Leprosy: state of the art, JAMA **247**:2283, 1982.
6. Brubaker, M.L., Meyers, W.M., and Bourland, J.: Leprosy in children one year of age and under, Int. J. Lepr. **53**:517, 1985.
7. Centers for Disease Control: Summary of notifiable diseases United States 1985, Morbidity Mortality Weekly Report **34**:6, 15, 1987.
8. Chandi, S.M., and Chacko, C.J.G.: An ultrastructural study of dermal nerves in early human leprosy, Int. J. Lepr. **55**:515, 1987.
9. Colston, M.J., and Hilson, G.R.F.: Growth of *Mycobacterium leprae* and *M. marinum* in congenitally athymic (nude) mice, Nature **262**:399, 1976.
10. Convit, J., Avila, J.L., Goihman, M., et al.: A test for the determination of competency in clearing bacilli in leprosy patients, Bull. WHO **46**:821, 1972.
11. Convit, J., and Pinardi, M.E.: A simple method for the differentiation of *Mycobacterium leprae* from other mycobacteria through routine staining techniques, Int. J. Lepr. **40**:130, 1972.
12. Dastur, D.K.: Pathology and pathogenesis of predilective sites of nerve damage in leprous neuritis: nerves in the arm and face, Neurosurg. Rev. **6**:139, 1983.
13. Desikan, K.V.: Viability of *Mycobacterium leprae* outside the human body, Lepr. Rev. **48**:231, 1977.
14. Draper, P.: The bacteriology of *Mycobacterium leprae*, Tubercle **64**:43, 1983.
15. Duncan, M.E., Melsom, R., Pearson, J.M.H., et al.: A clinical and immunological study of four babies of mothers with lepromatous leprosy, two of whom developed leprosy in infancy, Int. J. Lepr. **51**:7, 1983.
16. Feldman, R.A., and Hershfield, E.: Mycobacterial skin infection by an unidentified species: a report of 29 patients, Ann. Intern. Med. **80**:445, 1974.
17. Fernández, J.M.M.: The early reaction induced by lepromin, Int. J. Lepr. **8**:1, 1940.
18. ffytche, T.J., and McDougall, A.C.: Leprosy and the eye: a review, J. R. Soc. Med. **78**:397, 1985.
19. Fieldsteel, A.H., and Levy, L.: Dapsone chemotherapy of *Mycobacterium leprae* infection of the neonatally thymectomized Lewis rat, Am. J. Trop. Med. Hyg. **25**:854, 1976.
20. Fite, G.L., Cambre, P.J., and Turner, M.H.: Procedure for demonstrating lepra bacilli in paraffin sections, Arch. Pathol. **43**:624, 1947.
21. Fujiwara, T., Hunter, S.W., Cho, S.-N., et al.: Chemical synthesis and serology of disaccharides and trisaccharides of phenolic glycolipid antigens from the leprosy bacillus and preparation of a disaccharide protein conjugate for serodiagnosis of leprosy, Infect. Immun. **43**:245, 1984.
22. Gaylord, H., and Brennan, P.J.: Leprosy and the leprosy bacillus: recent developments in characterization of antigens and immunology of the disease, Annu. Rev. Microbiol. **41**:645, 1987.
23. Gormus, B.J., Wolf, R.H., Baskin, G.B., et al.: A second sooty mangabey monkey with naturally acquired leprosy: first reported possible monkey-to-monkey transmission, Int. J. Lepr. **56**:61, 1988.
24. Hansen, G.A.: Spedalskhedens årsager, Norsk Mag. Laegevidensk. **4**:76, 1874; reprinted in part in English translation as Causes of leprosy, Int. J. Lepr. **23**:307, 1955.
25. Haregewoin, A., Longley, J., Bjune, G., et al.: The role of interleukin-2 (IL-2) in the specific unresponsiveness of lepromatous leprosy to *Mycobacterium leprae*: studies in vitro and in vivo, Immunol. Lett. **11**:249, 1985.
26. Hayashi, F.: Mitsuda's skin reaction in leprosy, Int. J. Lepr. **1**:31, 1933.
27. Jayalakshmi, P., Looi, L.M., Lim, K.J., et al.: Autopsy findings in 35 cases of leprosy in malaysia, Int. J. Lepr. **55**:510, 1987.
28. Job, C.K., Sanchez, R.M., and Hastings, R.C.: Lepromatous placentitis and intrauterine fetal infection in lepromatous ninebanded armadillos *(Dasypus novemcinctus)*, Lab. Invest. **56**:44, 1987.
29. Johnstone, P.A.S.: The search for animal models of leprosy, Int. J. Lepr. **55**:535, 1987.
30. Kaplan, G., Gandhi, R.R., Weinstein, D.E., et al.: *Mycobacterium leprae* antigen-induced suppression of T-cell proliferation in vitro, J. Immunol. **138**:3028, 1987.
31. Kean, B.H., and Childress, M.E.: A summary of 103 autopsies on leprosy patients on the Isthmus of Panama, Int. J. Lepr. **10**:51, 1942.
32. Kaplan, G., Nathan, C.F., Gandhi, R., et al.: Effect of recombinant interferon-gamma on hydrogen peroxide–releasing capacity of monocyte-derived macrophages from patients with lepromatous leprosy, J. Immunol. **137**:983, 1986.
33. Kirchheimer, W.F., and Storrs, E.E.: Attempts to establish the armadillo *(Dasypus novemcinctus* Linn.) as a model for the study of leprosy. I. Report of lepromatoid leprosy in an experimentally infected armadillo, Int. J. Lepr. **39**:693, 1971.
34. Klatser, P.R., DeWit, M.Y.L., and Kolk, A.H.J.: An ELISA-inhibition test using monoclonal antibody for the serology of leprosy, Clin. Exp. Immunol. **62**:468, 1985.
35. Koster, F.T., Scollard, D.M., Umland, E.T., et al.: Cellular and humoral immune response to a phenolic glycolipid antigen (Phen GL-1) in patients with leprosy, J. Clin. Microbiol. **25**:551, 1987.
36. Latapí, F., and Chevez Zamora, A.: The "spotted" leprosy of Lucio (la lepra "manchada" de Lucio): an introduction to its clinical and histological study, Int. J. Lepr. **16**:421, 1948.
37. Leininger, J.R., Donham, K.J., and Meyers, W.M.: Leprosy in a chimpanzee: postmortem lesions, Int. J. Lepr. **48**:414, 1980.
38. Lumpkin, L.R., III, Cox, G.F., and Wolf, J.E., Jr.: Leprosy in five armadillo handlers, J. Am. Acad. Dermatol. **6**:899, 1983.
39. McAdam, K.P.W.J., Anders, R.F., Smith, S.R., et al.: Association of amyloidosis with erythema nodosum leprosum reactions and recurrent neutrophil leucocytosis in leprosy, Lancet **2**:572, 1975.
40. Mehra, V., Brennan, P.J., and Rada, E.: Lymphocyte suppression in leprosy induced by unique *M. leprae* glycolipid, Nature **308**:194, 1984.
41. Melancon-Kaplan, J., Hunter, S.W., and McNeil, M., et al.: Immunological significance of *Mycobacterium leprae* cell walls, Proc. Natl. Acad. Sci. USA **85**:1917, 1988.
42. Meyers, W.M., Binford, C.H., McDougall, A.C., et al.: Histologic responses in sixty multibacillary leprosy patients inoculated with autoclaved *Mycobacterium leprae* and live BCG, Int. J. Lepr. **56**:302, 1988.
43. Meyers, W.M., Binford, C.H., Walsh, G.P., et al.: Animal models in leprosy, Microbiology 1984, pp. 307-311, Washington, D.C., 1984, American Society for Microbiology.
44. Meyers, W.M., Heggie, C.D., Kay, T.L., et al.: The Ridley-Jopling five-group classification in 1,429 leprosy patients, Int. J. Lepr. **47**:683, 1979.
45. Meyers, W.M., Walsh, G.P., Brown, H.L., et al.: Leprosy in a mangabey monkey: naturally-acquired infection, Int. J. Lepr. **53**:1, 1985.
46. Modlin, R.L., Hofman, F.M., Taylor, C.R., et al.: T lymphocyte subsets in the skin lesions of patients with leprosy, J. Am. Acad. Dermatol. **8**:182, 1983.
47. Mukherjee, A., and Meyers, W.M.: Endothelial cell bacillation in lepromatous leprosy: a case report, Lepr. Rev. **58**:419, 1987.
48. Nathan, C.F., Kaplan, G., Levis, W.R., et al.: Local and systemic effects of intradermal recombinant interferon-gamma in patients with lepromatous leprosy, N. Engl. J. Med. **315**:6, 1986.
49. Nordeen, S.K., and López Bravo, L.: The world leprosy situation, World Health Stat. Q. **39**:122, 1986.
50. Ottenhof, T.H.M., and de Vries, R.R.P.: HLA class II immune response and suppression genes in leprosy, Int. J. Lepr. **55**:521, 1987.
51. Ottenhof, T.H.M., Klatser, P.R., Ivanyi, J., et al.: *Mycobacterium leprae*–specific protein antigens defined by cloned human helper T cells, Nature **319**:66, 1986.
52. Ottenhof, T.H.M., Neuteboom, S., Elferink, D.G., et al.: Molecular localization and polymorphism of HLA class II restriction determinants defined by *Mycobacterium leprae*–reactive helper T cell clones from leprosy patients, J. Exp. Med. **164**:1923, 1986.

53. Pedley, J.C.: The presence of *M. leprae* in human milk, Lepr. Rev. **38**:239, 1967.
54. Powell, C.S., and Swann, L.L.: Leprosy: pathologic changes observed in fifty consecutive necropsies, Am. J. Pathol. **37**:1131, 1955.
55. Prasad, H.K., Mishra, R.S., and Nath, I.: Phenolic glycolipid-I of *Mycobacterium leprae* induces general suppression of in vitro concanavalin A responses unrelated to leprosy type, J. Exp. Med. **165**:239, 1987.
56. Rees, R.J.W., Waters, M.F.R., Weddell, A.G.M., et al.: Experimental lepromatous leprosy, Nature **215**:599, 1967.
57. Ridley, D.S., and Jopling, W.H.: Classification of leprosy according to immunity: a five group system, Int. J. Lepr. **34**:255, 1966.
58. Ridley, M.J., and Ridley, D.S.: Histoid leprosy: an ultrastructural observation, Int. J. Lepr. **48**:135, 1980.
59. Rodriguez, J.N.: The histoid leproma: its characteristics and significance, Int. J. Lepr. **37**:1, 1969.
60. Shepard, C.C.: The experimental disease that follows the injection of human leprosy bacilli into footpads of mice, J. Exp. Med. **112**:445, 1960.
61. Smith, J.H., Folse, D.S., Long, E.G., et al.: Leprosy in wild armadillos *(Dasypus novemcinctus)* of the Texas Gulf Coast: epidemiology and mycobacteriology, J. Reticuloendothel. Soc. **34**:75, 1983..
62. Thomas, D.A., Mines, J.S., Thomas, D.C., et al.: Armadillo exposure among Mexican-born patients with lepromatous leprosy, J. Infect. Dis. **156**:990, 1987.
63. Wade, H.W.: The histoid variety of lepromatous leprosy, Int. J. Lepr. **31**:129, 1963.
64. Walsh, G.P., Meyers, W.M., Binford, C.H., et al.: Leprosy: a zoonosis, Lepr. Rev. **52**(suppl. 1):77, 1981.
65. Walsh, G.P., Meyers, W.M., and Binford, C.H.: Naturally acquired leprosy in the nine-banded armadillo: a decade of experience 1975-1985, J. Leukocyte Biol. **40**:645, 1986.
66. Weiner, M.A.: Leprosy: report of a case with a rare histopathological feature, A.M.A. Arch. Dermatol. **79**:709, 1959.

8 Rickettsial and Chlamydial Diseases

DAVID H. WALKER

Obligate intracellular bacteria, members of the genera *Rickettsia, Coxiella, Ehrlichia,* and *Chlamydia,* compose a unique group of infectious agents of human disease.[5,7,151,152,164] These microorganisms have never been cultivated outside of eukaryotic cells and thus occupy an interesting ecologic niche. Intracellular parasitism is necessary for their survival in nature. It should be recognized that bacterial interactions with human cells form a spectrum from free-living bacteria such as *Pseudomonas aeruginosa* to obligate intracellular rickettsiae and chlamydiae. Intermediate positions in the spectrum of bacteria-host cell interaction include facultative intracellular bacteria (for example, *Mycobacterium, Brucella, Listeria,* and *Salmonella*), which may grow within or outside of host cells, and extracellular organisms, such as *Bartonella,* which appear to grow best attached to the outside of the host cell. Other extracellular bacteria, such as *Escherichia coli,* have attachment mechanisms that anchor the bacteria in their ecologic niche with less chance of removal by the mechanical current of the local cleansing mechanism. Because rickettsiae and chlamydiae are in part defined by the negative characteristic of being unable to proliferate extracellularly, their members are constantly liable to being expelled by a scientist who discovers conditions permitting their cultivation in a cell-free environment. An example of this reclassification is *Rochalimaea quintana,* the etiologic agent of trench fever, which was considered a louse-born rickettsial disease until successful cell-free cultivation of the bacterium.[4]

Many of these obligate intracellular bacteria cause zoonoses. A *zoonosis* is a disease that is spread to humans from a reservoir in other animals. *Chlamydia psittaci* is spread to poultry workers from infected turkeys and other fowl and to those who own and sell infected pet birds. *Coxiella burnetii* is spread mainly via aerosol from infected ruminants, especially from the placentas of infected sheep, goats, and cattle. Rickettsiae are transmitted to humans from infected ticks, mites, chiggers, lice, and fleas.[1,5,7] As a group the zoonoses exist independent of humans, who are infected only accidentally and usually as a dead end from the point of view of the microorganism, which is rarely shed or transmitted from humans back into nature. *Chlamydia tracho-*matis is the only obligate intracellular bacterium that is usually transmitted directly from one person to another.

Rickettsia, Coxiella, and *Chlamydia* were all considered viruses before elucidation of their bacterial characteristics. At one time the term *virus* was used to mean "infectious agent." Subsequently, "virus" was often used to refer to an infectious agent that passed through a Berkefeld filter or required living host cells such as cell culture, embryonated eggs, or animals for its propagation. Except for intracellular proliferation, rickettsiae and chlamydiae share the properties of bacteria rather than viruses. They differ from viruses in that they contain DNA and RNA, ribosomes, and metabolic enzymes, have a gram-negative type of bacterial cell wall, replicate by binary fission, and are susceptible to antimicrobial agents. Because rickettsiae are cultivated with much more difficulty[2,46] and, in some instances, more danger than other bacteria, diagnosis of rickettsial infection is seldom documented by isolation of the agent.[2,42] More often a tentative diagnosis of rickettsiosis is made on clinical grounds, and later acute and covalescent sera are tested to demonstrate the appearance or rise in titer of specific antibodies.[30] In contrast, cultivation of *Chlamydia trachomatis* has become a routine procedure in many hospital laboratories. In the last decade rapid, clinically useful diagnostic tools have been developed that demonstrate specific rickettsial and chlamydial antigens in specimens from the patient.[50,65,137,148]

RICKETTSIAL DISEASES

Rickettsiae are small, obligate, intracellular coccobacilli measuring $0.3 \mu m \times 1$ to $2 \mu m$ that spend all or a portion of their life in an arthropod host and contain antigens of the spotted fever, typhus, or scrub typhus group. *Coxiella burnetii,* which has been isolated from 40 species of ticks, differs remarkably from the genus *Rickettsia. C. burnetii* appears to have a spore form[113] and intraphagolysosomal location,[104] and unrelated antigens and causes distinctly different pathologic lesions.[3] Organisms of *Rickettsia, Coxiella,* and *Ehrlichia* cause the infectious diseases of humans shown in Table 8-1.

Table 8-1. Rickettsial diseases of humans

Disease	Etiologic agent	Transmission	Pathologic lesion	Geographic distribution
SPOTTED FEVER GROUP				
Rocky Mountain spotted fever	*Rickettsia rickettsii*	Tick bite	Microvascular injury involving skin, brain, lungs, and other organs	North and South America
Rickettsialpox	*Rickettsia akari*	Mite bite	Microvascular injury with rash and eschar	U.S.A., U.S.S.R., Africa, Korea,
Boutonneuse fever	*Rickettsia conorii*	Tick bite	Microvascular injury with rash and eschar	Mediterranean basin, Africa, Indian subcontinent
North Asian tick typhus	*Rickettsia sibirica*	Tick bite	Microvascular injury with rash and eschar	Asiatic U.S.S.R., China, Mongolia,
Queensland tick typhus	*Rickettsia australis*	Tick bite	Microvascular injury with rash and eschar	Australia
TYPHUS GROUP				
Epidemic typhus	*Rickettsia prowazekii*	Louse feces	Microvascular injury involving skin, brain, and other organs	Potentially worldwide, recently in Africa, South America, Central America, Mexico, Asia
Brill-Zinsser disease	*Rickettsia prowazekii*	(See text)	Microvascular injury involving skin, brain, and other organs	Potentially worldwide, including U.S.A., U.S.S.R., Canada, and eastern Europe
Flying squirrel typhus	*Rickettsia prowazekii*	Ectoparasite of flying squirrel	Microvascular injury involving skin, brain, and other organs	U.S.A.
Murine typhus	*Rickettsia typhi*	Rat flea feces	Microvascular injury involving skin, brain, and other organs	Worldwide
SCRUB TYPHUS GROUP	*Rickettsia tsutsugamushi*	Chigger bite	Microvascular injury involving skin, brain, lungs, and other organs	Southern Asia, Japan, western Pacific, Indonesia, Australia, Korea, Asiatic U.S.S.R., India, Sri Lanka, China
Q FEVER	*Coxiella burnetii*	Inhalation of aerosol from infected animals	Pneumonia; granulomas of liver, spleen, and bone marrow; endocarditis	Worldwide
HUMAN EHRLICHIOSIS	*Ehrlichia* sp. closely related to *E. canis*	Tick bite	Not known	U.S.A., possibly worldwide
SENNETSU RICKETTSIOSIS	*E. sennetsu*	Not known	Not known	Japan, Malaysia

Spotted fever group infections
Rocky Mountain spotted fever

Rocky Mountain spotted fever (RMSF) is one of the severest infectious diseases, with a mortality in previously healthy persons of 20% before the advent of antimicrobial therapy. RMSF is the most important rickettsiosis in the United States from the aspects of morbidity and mortality.[10,25,26] However, contrary to its name, cases occur throughout the U.S.A. as well as in Central and South America with the majority of cases occurring in the Southeastern states. *R. rickettsii* are released from the salivary glands of a feeding *Dermacentor variabilis, D. andersoni, Rhipicephalus sanguineus,* or *Amblyomma cajennense* tick and are injected into the feeding blood pool in the host's skin. After an incubation period of 2 to 12 days the patient develops severe headache, fever, and frequently nausea, vomiting, or abdominal pain. A maculopapular rash appears on the wrists and ankles 2 to 5 days later, usually spreads to involve the trunk, palms, and soles, and may become petechial.[22,38] Nevertheless, delay or absence of rash and frequent lack of a history of tick bite make misdiagnosis and fatality a genuine problem. In severe cases the patient may manifest signs of encephalitis, noncardiogenic pulmonary edema, skin necrosis, coagulopathy with bleeding, acute renal failure, jaundice, and hypovolemic shock.[27,31] In fatal cases death usually ensues 8 to 15 days after onset of symptoms. There is a fulminant form of RMSF observed most often in glucose-6-phosphate dehydrogenase–deficient black males in which the patient may die before the fifth day of illness.[43] Early treatment with tetracycline or chloramphenicol cures most patients; however, late diagnosis and inappropriate treatment result in an overall mortality of 3% to 8%.[25-27]

Pathologic lesions. Rickettsiae spread via the bloodstream, enter endothelial cells, proliferate within the cytoplasm and nuclei of endothelial and vascular smooth muscle cells of the microcirculation of virtually all organs (Fig. 8-1), and directly injure the foci of infected cells.[49] The consequence is systemic vascular damage that is the pathologic basis for the rash, interstitial pneumonia, interstitial myocarditis, meningoencephalomyelitis, hepatic portal triaditis, and interstitial nephritis. Microscopically the vasculitis consists of swollen or necrotic endothelial cells; intramural and perivascular infiltration, predominantly by macrophages and T-lymphocytes with few polymorphonuclear (PMN) leukocytes; focal extravasation of erythrocytes; and occasionally, usually nonocclusive, eccentric thrombi in the foci of rickettsial infection (Fig. 8-2).[29,35,64] In the skin these foci are located principally in the dermis. In the brain the lesions assume a characteristic appearance, so-called typhus nodules, found most frequently in the brainstem (Fig. 8-3). These perivascular accumulations of mononuclear cells, which measure 100 to

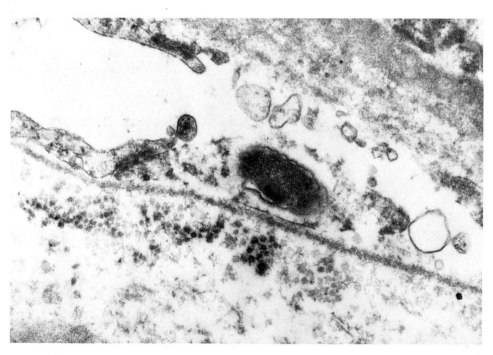

Fig. 8-1. Electron photomicrograph of *Rickettsia rickettsii* in cytoplasm of endothelial cell from patient with Rocky Mountain spotted fever. (From Walker, D.H.: Rickettsial diseases: an update. In Majno, G., and Cotran, R., editors: The inflammatory process and infectious diseases, Baltimore, 1981, The Williams & Wilkins Co.)

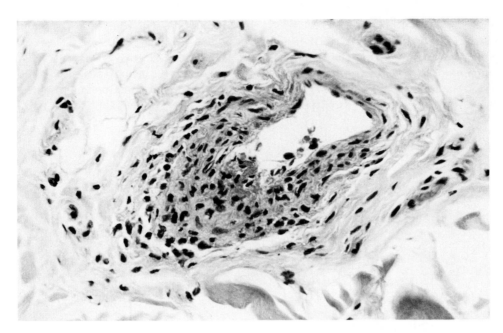

Fig. 8-2. Blood vessel from hemorrhagic skin lesion of patient with Rocky Mountain spotted fever shows characteristic rickettsial vasculitis with infiltration of blood vessel wall and perivascular tissue by mononuclear cells and with small, focal, nonocclusive thrombus. (From Green, W.R., Walker, D.H., and Cain, B.G.: Am. J. Med. **64:**523, 1978.)

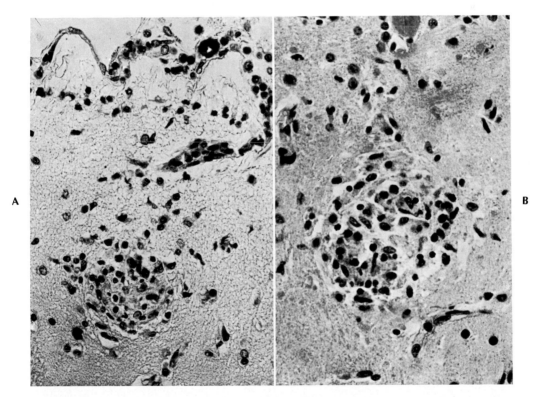

A   B

Fig. 8-3. A, Typhus nodules in gray matter of brain are generally considered to be adjacent to blood vessel, though vessel may not always be visible. **B,** Histologic components of these inflammatory foci are predominantly macrophages and lymphocytes. (AFIP 77543 and 78556; from Ash, J.E., and Spitz, S.: The rickettsial diseases. In Ash, J.E., and Spitz, S.: Pathology of tropical diseases, Philadelphia, 1945, W.B. Saunders Co.)

180 μm in diameter, indicate a probable rickettsial infection though they are not pathognomonic. Other neuropathologic lesions include microinfarcts of white matter and a mild mononuclear cell-rich leptomeningitis. Lungs are congested and heavy.[52] Microscopic pulmonary lesions include mononuclear interstitial pneumonia and interstitial and alveolar edema and hemorrhages (Fig. 8-4).

The heart is grossly normal except for epicardial petechiae, but it usually manifests a mild mononuclear interstitial myocarditis on microscopic examination (Fig. 8-5).[12,35,61] The hepatic portal triaditis and multifocal

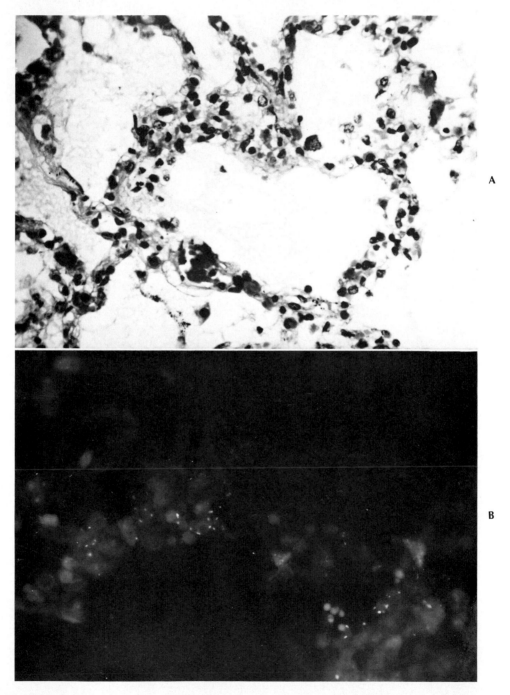

Fig. 8-4. A, Interstitial pneumonia of Rocky Mountain spotted fever with mononuclear infiltration of alveolar septa and proteinaceous edema fluid in alveolar spaces. **B,** Immunofluorescent *Rickettsia rickettsii* in thickened alveolar septum are cause of noncardiogenic pulmonary edema in Rocky Mountain spotted fever. (From Walker, D.H., and Mattern, W.D.: Am. Heart J. **100:**896, 1980.)

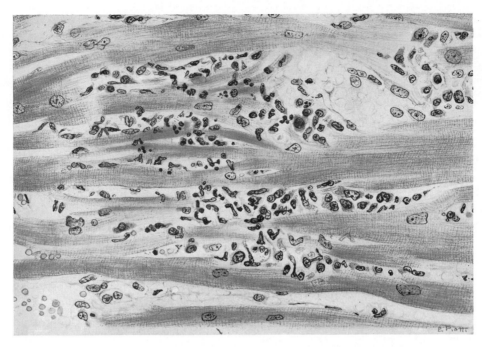

Fig. 8-5. Myocarditis in typhus fever. Infiltration of mononuclear cells and neutrophils between muscle fibers. (From Wolbach, S.B., Todd, J.L., and Palfrey, F.W.: The etiology and pathology of typhus, Cambridge, Mass., 1922, Harvard University Press.)

perivascular interstitial nephritis correspond to foci of infection of hepatic portal blood vessels and the renal microcirculation near the corticomedullary junction, respectively.[13,60] Erythrophagocytosis occurs in Kupffer cells and macrophages within sinuses of lymph nodes. In fulminant RMSF there are more thrombi and fewer intramural and perivascular leukocytes in foci of vascular injury.[57]

Clinicopathologic correlations. Disseminated vascular foci of rickettsial infection[51,65] and microvascular injury result in leakage of intravascular fluid into the interstitial space with consequent edema and hypovolemia.[6,23] Consumption of platelets and coagulation factors in thrombi at the sites of injury can cause thrombocytopenia and in very severe cases more severe coagulopathy. Focal lesions in the skin are the cause of the rash. Vasodilatation and petechiae are the basis of the cutaneous erythematous macules and central "spots" respectively. Increased vascular permeability of the infected pulmonary microcirculation may result in noncardiogenic pulmonary edema.[33,52] Myocardial injury is not a significant factor.[20,33,61] Central nervous system lesions are the cause of coma, seizures, multifocal, neurologic signs, and probably cardiorespiratory arrest. Jaundice correlates with hemolysis and portal triadal inflammation.[9] Acute renal failure results from hypovolemic prerenal azotemia or, in more severe cases, acute tubular necrosis.[60] Vasculitis in the gastrointestinal tract is the apparent pathologic basis for nausea, vomiting, and abdominal pain and tenderness.[44]

Pathogenesis. Immunopathology, coagulation, and inflammation have not been demonstrated experimentally as primary pathologic mechanisms in RMSF, though thrombosis and activation of the kallikrein-kinin pathways may exacerbate the disease and the acute-phase response presumably mediated by interleukin-1 is observed.[21,34,40,41,58,66] Moreover, *R. rickettsii* does not seem to produce a toxin.[32,55] On the other hand, direct injury of infected cells by rickettsiae has been documented.[50,54] The pathogenic mechanisms of the host cell injury have not been elucidated though cell membrane injury by phospholipase A and protease enzymes has been proposed.[53,63]

Other spotted fever group infections

Boutonneuse fever,[15,45,48,56,59,62] North Asian tick typhus,[16,19,36] Queensland tick typhus,[11] and rickettsialpox[14,18] are rickettsioses with similar clinical and pathologic features. In contrast to RMSF, these diseases are frequently associated with an eschar, a focus of skin necrosis at the original site of feeding by the arthropod vector.[39] Travelers return home from the Mediterranean basin and Africa with *R. conorii* infection.[24] In the indigenous areas, there is evidence for a high prevalence of undiagnosed infections.[37] Interestingly, several apparently nonpathogenic rickettsiae have been identified in a substantial proportion of ticks in the United States.[17] Their role in the ecology of *R. rickettsii* may include interference or competition for the niche in the tick host. Their role in human infections is currently unknown.

Typhus group infections
Typhus

Epidemic louse-borne typhus fever is one of the classic scourges of mankind. In times of war, famine, and other disasters, louse infestation, crowding, and malnutrition join forces with *R. prowazekii* to cause explosive epidemics of typhus. It has been postulated that more wars have been lost as a result of epidemic typhus than have been won by battlefield victories.[8] During and just after World War I, 15 million persons suffered from typhus and more than 3 million died. Infections by *R. prowazekii* occur in the United States as a zoonosis with a reservoir in flying squirrels and their fleas and lice.[67,70,73,81] A milder clinical type of typhus fever known as Brill-Zinsser disease occurs as recrudescence of an infection with *R. prowazekii* that has remained latent after acute typhus fever many years previously.[74,75,89] The reason for the recrudescence is not known.

Organisms of *R. prowazekii* proliferate in the intestinal epithelial cells of the human louse, are shed in its feces, and eventually kill the louse. After entry through human skin, the pathogenic events of typhus parallel those of RMSF and the other rickettsioses with spread via the bloodstream to skin, brain, and other organs. In contrast to RMSF, rickettsial infection involves only endothelial cells, and the rash begins on the trunk between days 4 and 8 of illness and spreads centrifugally to involve the arms and legs.[87] Pathologic lesions comprise disseminated mononuclear vasculitis of skin, typhus nodules of brain (Fig. 8-3), interstitial myocarditis, mild interstitial pneumonia, perivascular interstitial nephritis, and portal triaditis. Biopsy specimens of skin of patients with epidemic typhus in Poland during World War I were examined by Wolbach, thus providing a sequence of pathologic lesions. The earliest lesion was swelling of endothelial cells parasitized by rickettsiae. Subsequently, leukocytic infiltration of the vessel wall was observed. The pathophysiology of typhus fever is similar to that of RMSF.[88]

Typhus rickettsiae contain a lipopolysaccharide that is relatively nontoxic.[78,79] In vitro experiments have shown that cell membrane injury is associated with phospholipase activity.[84,85] The bursting of heavily infected cells is an overt cytolytic effect of *R. prowazekii* infection.[80] The so-called mouse toxin phenomenon is unlikely to be caused by a toxin. Intravenous injection of nonviable typhus rickettsiae does not cause a toxic death in mice.[68] Moreover, no toxin has been identified that produces this phenomenon. Some other mechanism, such as massive rickettsial penetration involving

phospholipase activity, may explain the mouse toxicity. Although immune mechanisms clearly act overall on behalf of the host in typhus group rickettsial infections,[83] evidence for immune-mediated lysis of infected cells and expression of rickettsial antigens on the surface of infected cells indicate that there may be an undetermined contribution of immunopathologic mechanisms to the disease state.[76,77,86]

Murine typhus

Another typhus group *Rickettsia* that causes human disease is *R. typhi* (*R. mooseri*).[71,72] Murine typhus is transmitted from rats to humans by the infected rat flea, which excretes rickettsiae in feces. Murine typhus is very rarely fatal, though it resembles the other rickettsial diseases clinically.[69,82] As with epidemic typhus, an eschar does not occur in murine typhus.

Scrub typhus group

Organisms of *R. tsutsugamushi* are transmitted to humans by the bite of a larval trombiculid mite.[91-93] As in the tick with *R. rickettsii*, transovarial infection of chiggers may account for the maintenance of *R. tsutsugamushi* in nature, though feral rodents do become infected and may amplify the distribution of rickettsiae. These rickettsiae have great diversity with many antigenically distinct strains that do not necessarily confer cross-protection. Scrub typhus occurs in southern and eastern Asia, Japan, Indonesia, northern Australia, and the islands of the western Pacific. The disease was of military importance during World War II and the Vietnam War with loss of manpower to the morbidity of the infection. The characteristic, but not uniformly present, eschar marks the site of feeding by the chigger. Regional lymph nodes draining the site of localized cutaneous necrosis and ulceration are swollen and inflamed. Diagnosis is facilitated by detection of the eschar. The pathologic lesions in blood vessels of skin, brain, lung, heart, and kidney resemble those of spotted fever and typhus except that there are even fewer capillary thrombi.[90,92,94,95]

Q fever

Q fever refers to the disease caused by *Coxiella burnetii*.[121] The letter Q is for *query*, designating the unknown etiology during the early days of recognition of the illness. Derrick[98] first described Q fever in 1937 as an occupational disease among slaughterhouse workers and dairy farmers in Australia. *C. burnetii* differs remarkably from organisms of genus *Rickettsia* in its capability to remain infectious under adverse extracellular conditions probably by the formation of spores. It differs also in its cellular location within phagolysosomes, where it functions most efficiently in the acid milieu.[96] In contrast, members of genus *Rickettsia* are usually found in cytosol, with spotted-fever group organisms occasionally in nucleoplasm.[47] Moreover, Q fever may have a chronic as well as an acute form, and pneumonia without vascular infection or rash contrasts with the disseminated vasculitis and microvascular injury of the rickettsioses. Chronic Q fever is a systemic granulomatous disease that may also include infective endocarditis.[101,123,126]

C. burnetii undergoes a transition when cultivated repeatedly in the absence of the immune system as in cell culture or embryonated eggs. This transition, called phase variation, is analogous to the conversion from smooth to rough of gram-negative enteric bacteria. Phase I, the smooth form found in nature, possesses the complete lipopolysaccharide and is virulent. The laboratory-generated rough form with truncated lipopolysaccharide is avirulent. Antibodies to phase I or phase II antigens carry different diagnostic and prognostic significance.[100] Early in acute Q fever the patient's plasma antibodies react only with phase II antigens. Patients with chronic Q fever endocarditis have a high titer of antibodies to phase I antigens.

Pathologic lesions. Because Q fever is rarely fatal, few tissues have been examined from the acute stage of the illness. Those cases have shown bronchopneumonia with a component of interstitial pneumonia also.[110,117,127] Alveolar, bronchiolar, and bronchial exudates contain many macrophages with variable quantities of lymphocytes, erythrocytes, and polymorphonuclear leukocytes. Alveolar septa are slightly to moderately thickened by mononuclear cell infiltration. The intracellular location of the *Coxiella* and the microscopic lesions resemble other unusual pneumonias such as psittacosis and Legionnaires' disease. Some patients develop granulomas of the liver or bone marrow.[115,116,119] The hepatic granulomas often have a characteristic doughnut appearance with a central clear zone surrounded by layers of fibrin and epithelioid macrophages (Fig. 8-6). Similar and other nonspecific granulomas have also been observed in bone marrow and spleen. Chronic Q fever may manifest chronic infective endocarditis, hepatic involvement, and thrombocytopenia.[119,126]

Pathogenesis. Humans acquire Q fever by inhalation of spores or aerosols of *C. burnetii*, usually from the highly infectious placentas of healthy-appearing sheep, goats, or cattle.[122] Ingestion of contaminated milk and tick bite are rarely implicated means of transmission. Illness follows a dose-dependent incubation period of 9 to 18 days with rickettsemia detectable 1 to 4 days prior to onset of symptoms.[125] Acute *C. burnetii* infection is usually self-limited and may be manifested as asymptomatic seroconversion, a nonspecific fever, atypical pneumonia, granulomatous hepatitis, or meningoencephalitis.[112] There are apparently geographic differences, since pneumonia is a frequent manifestation in North America and an unusual feature of Q fever in Australia. Chronic Q fever is generally considered synonymous

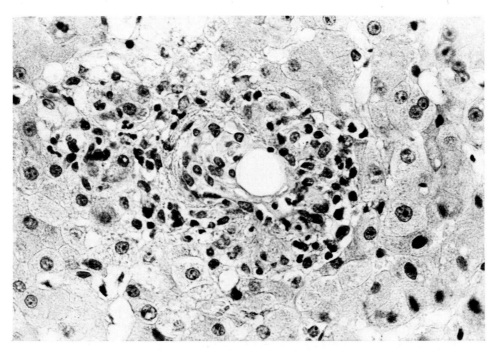

Fig. 8-6. Hepatic granuloma of Q fever with peripheral epithelioid macrophages and lymphocytes and characteristic central "doughnut" hole.

with *C. burnetii* endocarditis. Q fever endocarditis is diagnosed by demonstration of high titers of serum antibodies to the phase I variant of *C. burnetii*.[100] However, there are patients with such antibodies who do not have Q fever endocarditis. Patients with this chronic endocarditis may develop complications such as immune complex glomerulonephritis or systemic emboli.

The target cell of *C. burnetii* infection is the macrophage of the lung in pneumonia, of the liver, spleen, and bone marrow after hematogenous spread, and of the cardiac valves in endocarditis.[101,109,111,118] The organisms proliferate inside the phagolysosomes of these macrophages. Animal models have demonstrated that the disseminated infection of macrophages is controlled by formation of granulomas. Persistent infection of animals is reactivated by irradiation, steroids, immunosuppression, drugs, and pregnancy. Latently infected women may reactivate the infection with involvement of the placenta or abortus.[124] Immunocompromised patients may be at a higher risk of disease.[105] The mechanisms of cell and tissue injury are unclear. *C. burnetii* itself causes minimal injury to infected cells. Variants containing particular patterns of DNA homology with a plasmid of *C. burnetii*, Qph1, and particular lipopolysaccharide structure are associated with the most serious form of disease, endocarditis.[102,103,114,120] This evidence for virulence factors of the organisms must be viewed with the realization that overall the data favor host-mediated pathogenic mechanisms. The relatively nontoxic lipopolysaccharide might be hypothesized to stimulate the host-mediated acute-phase response including fever and increased hepatic synthesis of certain plasma proteins.[97,106,107] T-lymphocyte–mediated hypersensitivity to components of *C. burnetii* is responsible for granuloma formation and substantial tissue injury in studies of experimental animals.[108] Another pathogenic mechanism mediated by the host's immune system, immune complex disease, principally glomerulonephritis, occurs in some patients with chronic Q fever endocarditis.[99,128]

CHLAMYDIAL DISEASES

Chlamydias are 0.2 to 1 μm coccoid, obligate, intracellular bacteria that reside within a cytoplasmic vacuole.[151,152] They differ from rickettsiae in that they have two specialized morphologic and functional forms and are unable to synthesize ATP. The elementary body, with a diameter of 0.2 to 0.4 μm and a rigid cell wall, survives extracellularly without metabolic activity or replication. Moreover, this form is equipped for infectivity by its capability to induce its phagocytosis and to inhibit fusion of phagosome and lysosome. The reticulate particle has a diameter of 0.6 to 1 μm, and although unsuited for extracellular survival or infectivity, it is the metabolically active, replicative form of the organism. The chlamydial diseases of humans are shown in Table 8-2.

Psittacosis

Psittacosis occurs in humans as pneumonia, a toxic nonrespiratory illness with fever, myalgia, and headache, or a subclinical infection.[149] The mortality is low. The pathologic lesions are interstitial, predominantly mononuclear, pneumonia with gelatinous, sparsely cellular, mononuclear, alveolar exudates and focal hepatic and splenic necrosis.[159] Infection follows inhalation of infected dust or aerosols from infected birds.[134] The TWAR strain of *C. psittaci* has been implicated as the cause of febrile pneumonia, bronchitis, and pharyngitis in young adults without apparent exposure to infected birds. Penetration of host cells including macrophages by infective elementary bodies is followed by their reorganization into reticulate particles, which replicate by binary fission and eventually change again into elementary bodies. Release of elementary bodies from the host cell occurs by cytolysis, an apparent pathogenic mechanism.

Table 8-2. Chlamydial diseases of humans

Etiologic agent	Disease	Pathologic lesion	Transmission
Chlamydia psittaci	Psittacosis	Pneumonia, endocarditis	Aerosol from infected birds
Chlamydia trachomatis			
Serotypes A, B, Ba, and C	Trachoma	Chronic conjunctivitis	Contact
Serotypes L-1, L-2, L-3	Lymphogranuloma venereum	Inguinal lymph node abscesses and granulomas	Sexual contact
Serotypes D-K	Various sexually transmitted infections	Urethritis, epididymitis, prostatitis, cervicitis, endometritis, salpingitis, bartholinitis, perihepatitis, pharyngitis, proctitis	Sexual contact
	Neonatal infection	Conjunctivitis, pneumonia, otitis media	Contact with infection in birth canal

Large inocula of *C. psittaci* or *C. trachomatis* induce dose-dependent immediate cytotoxicity on cell cultures.[138,140] Cell injury requires chlamydial attachment and phagocytosis. Although heat-killed chlamydias are not toxic, large inocula of organisms with ability to replicate inhibited by an antibiotic or ultraviolet irradiation retain the capability to injure cell monolayers. The immediate cellular toxic effect is neutralized by immune sera. This pathogenic action resembles phospholipase A–mediated cell membrane injury by rickettsiae.

Trachoma

Trachoma, a major cause of blindness particularly in Africa, the Middle East, and southeastern Asia, is a chronic conjunctivitis caused by certain serotypes (A, B, Ba, and C) of *Chlamydia trachomatis*. Person-to-person spread occurs especially among children within families. Most cases of active trachoma heal spontaneously. Repeated infections seem to lead to conjunctival lymphoid follicle formation and subsequent scarring and distortion of the eyelid such that inturned lashes continually traumatize the cornea.[133] Corneal injury with secondary bacterial infections causes corneal opacification by scarring.

Experimental animal studies support the concept that immunopathologic responses in previously sensitized hosts are the pathologic basis of trachoma.[142,154,156] The hypersensitivity-associated antigens are soluble products secreted by *C. trachomatis* and *C. psittaci* rather than the major outer membrane or lipopolysaccharide. Repeated conjunctival inoculations cause chronic conjunctivitis with prominent lymphoid follicles with germinal centers, plasma cells, macrophages, and B- and T-lymphocytes.

Lymphogranuloma venereum

Serologically distinct, more invasive serogroups (L-1, L-2, and L-3) of *C. trachomatis* are the cause of lymphogranuloma venereum (LGV), a sexually transmitted disease. LGV occurs more often in males and is characterized by inguinal lymph node enlargement (buboes) and fever. The pathologic lesions in the inguinal lymph nodes are stellate abscesses surrounded by a granulomatous reaction of epithelioid macrophages.

LGV strains of *C. trachomatis* invade the subepithelial location and infect macrophages as well as epithelial cells. Colonic involvement is more severe distally with transmural chronic inflammation in the rectum, strictures in the rectosigmoid colon, and anorectal fistulas.[132] The chronic inflammation includes lymphocytes often in follicles, macrophages, plasma cells, and granulomas with giant cells. Fibrosis is a frequently observed feature. Experimental animals given a single inoculum of genital strains of chlamydias intrarectally develop self-limited lesions that resolve in 4 to 6

weeks.[147] Rechallenge after 4 weeks causes hemorrhagic ulcers, mucosal lymphoid follicles, and intense mucosal and submucosal follicular and granulomatous inflammation. Chlamydial inclusions diminish 4 to 6 weeks after inoculation.

Genital and neonatal infections

Another set of serogroups (D-K) of *C. trachomatis* are the etiologic agents of a variety of sexually transmitted infections of the male and female genitalia and of neonatal infections acquired during passage through the birth canal.[129,158] A large portion of cases of nongonococcal urethritis[153] and epididymitis[130] in males is caused by *C. trachomatis*, which also causes chronic prostatitis.[146] Females with this infection may be asymptomatic or manifest follicular cervicitis with mucopurulent exudate,[135] urethritis, chronic endometritis,[136] ascending acute salpingitis,[139,145] or inflammation of Bartholin's glands. Neonatal inclusion conjunctivitis occurs in 25% to 50% of infants of infected mothers, with onset 1 to 2 weeks after birth. This frequent infection is generally benign. Neonatal chlamydial pneumonia usually occurs at 1 to 4 months of age and is characterized by tachypnea, cough, hyperexpanded lungs with symmetric diffuse interstitial and alveolar infiltrates, and lack of fever.[131] Pneumonia is observed in 10% to 20% of infants of infected mothers. Chlamydias infect the mucosal epithelial cells of the genital and respiratory tracts in these diseases.[157,158] After intracellular proliferation, chlamydias are shed onto the mucosal surface and may be spread by direct contact such as sexual intercourse. Thus these obligate intracellular bacteria are able to spread to the appropriate ecologic niche in another host and to survive. These strains of *C. trachomatis* express their antigens on the surface of the infected cells from which they are released by a process resembling exocytosis.[155] The host cell repairs the surface membrane and does not die. Experimental animal models reproduce the lesions of acutely swollen, hyperemic fallopian tubes[150] that on repeated infection develop lymphoid follicles, scarring, luminal obstruction, and perihepatitis. Numerous cytotoxic T-lymphocytes are present in the mucosal and submucosal infiltrate. Immunopathologic mechanisms appear to be the major mechanism of tissue injury in chlamydial diseases with scarring as the final effect.[141,143,144] Fibrotic obstruction of the fallopian tubes may lead to infertility or ectopic pregnancy.

EHRLICHIAL DISEASES

Ehrlichiae are small, pleomorphic coccoid to ellipsoid bacteria (0.4 μm by 1.0 to 2.5 μm) that reside within cytoplasmic vacuoles of leukocytes where they multiply by binary fission.[164] Ehrlichial diseases affect dogs, horses, sheep, cattle, deer, and humans. The known vectors are ticks.

Sennetsu rickettsiosis has been diagnosed among patients in western Japan, and there is serologic evidence for a high prevalence in Malaysia.[164] Clinical manifestations including fever, malaise, anorexia, and lymphadenopathy resemble infectious mononucleosis. The reservoir and means of transmission are not known. The etiologic agent, *Ehrlichia sennetsu*, has been isolated from patients' blood.

Recently in the United States there has been recognized a new disease in which patients develop antibodies reactive with *E. canis*.[160-163] Diagnosed infections have ranged from asymptomatic to severe. Clinical features may include fever, chills, myalgia, headache, nausea, anorexia, relative bradycardia, leukopenia, lymphopenia, thrombocytopenia, anemia, elevated serum concentration of hepatic enzymes, hyperbilirubinemia, and acute renal failure. The disease is associated with tick bite. A severely ill patient was observed to have ehrlichial inclusions in peripheral white blood cells. Cytoplasmic membrane-bound vacuoles contained from few to 40 ehrlichiae measuring 0.2 to 0.8 μm. The lesions of human ehrlichiosis have not been described except for the observation of granulomas in hypocellular bone marrow of several cases. Canine ehrlichiosis, caused by this or a closely related organism, affects 11% to 58% of dogs in the United States and is transmitted by the tick *Rhipicephalus sanguineus*. The canine infection may progress to a subclinical carrier state and recrudescence. Terminally infected dogs manifest fever, lymphadenopathy, pneumonitis, edema, epistaxis, and pancytopenia. Necropsy of dogs reveals perivascular plasmacytic infiltration particularly in the lung, meninges, kidney, and spleen.

• • •

It is likely that the future holds a great expansion of knowledge about chlamydial and rickettsial diseases as techniques for their detection are refined and come into more general use. The final chapter on diseases caused by the obligate intracellular bacteria will not be written soon.

REFERENCES
General

1. Burgdorfer, W.: Tick-borne diseases in the United States: Rocky Mountain spotted fever and Colorado tick fever: a review, Acta Trop. **34**:103, 1977.
2. Elisberg, B.L., and Bozeman, F.M.: The rickettsiae. In Lennette, E.W., and Schmidt, N.J., editors: Diagnostic procedures for viral, rickettsial and chlamydial infections, Washington, D.C., 1979, American Health Association, p. 1061.
3. Moulton, F.R., editor: Rickettsial diseases of man, Washington, D.C., 1948, American Association for the Advancement of Science.
4. Vinson, J.W.: Etiology of trench fever in Mexico. In Industrial Counsel for Tropical Health: Industry and tropical health, Proc. Fifth Conf. of the Industrial Counsel for Tropical Health, Boston, 1964, Harvard School of Public Health.

5. Walker, D.H., editor: Biology of rickettsial diseases, Boca Raton, Fla., 1988, CRC Press.
6. Walker, D.H., and Mattern, W.D.: Rickettsial vasculitis, Am. Heart J. **100**:896, 1980.
7. Weiss, E.: The biology of rickettsiae, Annu. Rev. Microbiol. **36**:345, 1982.
8. Zinsser, H.: Rats, lice, and history, New York, 1935, Little, Brown & Co.

Rickettsial diseases
Spotted fever group infections

9. Adams, J.S., and Walker, D.H.: The liver in Rocky Mountain spotted fever, Am. J. Clin. Pathol. **75**:156, 1981.
10. Aikawa, J.: Rocky Mountain spotted fever, Springfield, Ill., 1966, Charles C Thomas, Publisher.
11. Andrew, R., Bonnin, J.M., and Williams, S.: Tick typhus in North Queensland, Med. J. Aust. **2**:255, 1946.
12. Bradford, W.D., Croker, B.P., and Tisher, C.C.: Kidney lesions in Rocky Mountain spotted fever: a light-, and immunofluorescence-, and electron-microscopic study, Am. J. Pathol. **97**:381, 1979.
13. Bradford, W.D., and Hackel, D.B.: Myocardial involvement in Rocky Mountain spotted fever, Arch. Pathol. Lab. Med. **102**:357, 1978.
14. Brettman, L.R., Lewin, S., Holzman, R.S., Goldman, W.D., Marr, J.S., Kechijian, P., and Schinella, R.: Rickettsialpox: report of an outbreak and a contemporary review, Medicine **60**:363, 1981.
15. Burgdorfer, W.: Boutonneuse fever (Marseilles fever, Kenya tick typhus, South African tick bite fever, Indian tick typhus). In Hubbert, W.T., McCulloch, W.F., and Schnurrenberger, P.R., editors: Diseases transmitted from animals to man, ed. 6, Springfield, Ill., 1975, Charles C Thomas, Publisher.
16. Burgdorfer, W.: North Asian tick typhus. In Hubbert, W.T., McCulloch, W.F., and Schnurrenberger, P.R., editors: Diseases transmitted from animals to man, ed. 6, Springfield, Ill., 1975, Charles C Thomas, Publisher.
17. Burgdorfer, W., Sexton, D.J., Gerloff, R.K., et al.: *Rhipicephalus sanguineus:* vector of a new spotted fever group rickettsia in the United States, Infect. Immun. **12**:205, 1975.
18. Dolgopol, V.B.: Histologic changes in rickettsialpox, Am. J. Pathol. **24**:119, 1948.
19. Fan, M.Y., Walker, D.H., Yu, S.R., and Liu, Q.H.: The epidemiology and ecology of rickettsial diseases in the People's Republic of China, Rev. Infect. Dis. **9**:823, 1987.
20. Feltes, T.F., Wilcox, W.D., Feldman, W.E., Lipskis, D.J., Carter, S.L., and Bugg, G.W.: M-mode echocardiographic abnormalities in Rocky Mountain spotted fever, South. Med. J. **77**:1130, 1984.
21. Hall, G.W., and Schwartz, R.P.: White blood cell count and differential in Rocky Mountain spotted fever, NC Med. J. **40**:212, 1979.
22. Harrell, G.T.: Rocky Mountain spotted fever, Medicine **28**:333, 1949.
23. Harrell, G.T., and Aikawa, J.K.: Pathogenesis of circulatory failure in Rocky Mountain spotted fever, Arch. Intern. Med. **83**:331, 1949.
24. Harris, R.L., Kaplan, S.L., Bradshaw, M.W., and Williams, T.W.: Boutonneuse fever in American travelers, J. Infect. Dis. **153**:126, 1986.
25. Hattwick, M.A.W., O'Brien, R.J., and Hanson, B.F.: Rocky Mountain spotted fever: epidemiology of an increasing problem, Ann. Intern. Med. **84**:732, 1976.
26. Hattwick, M.A.W., Retailliau, H., O'Brien, R.J., Slutzker, M., Fontaine, R.E., and Hanson, B.: Fatal Rocky Mountain spotted fever, JAMA **240**:1499, 1978.
27. Haynes, R.E., Sanders, D.Y., and Cramblett, H.G.: Rocky Mountain spotted fever in children, J. Pediatr. **76**:685, 1970.
28. Helmick, C.G., Bernard, K.W., and D'Angelo, L.J.: Rocky Mountain spotted fever: clinical, laboratory, and epidemiological features of 262 cases, J. Infect. Dis. **150**:480, 1984.
29. Herrero-Herrero, J.I., Walker, D.H., and Ruiz-Beltrán, R.: Immunohistochemical evaluation of the cellular immune re-

sponse to *Rickettsia conorii* in "taches noires," J. Infect. Dis. **155**:802, 1987.

30. Kaplan, J.E., and Schonberger, L.B.: The sensitivity of various serologic tests in the diagnosis of Rocky Mountain spotted fever, Am. J. Trop. Med. Hyg. **35**:840, 1986.

31. Kaplowitz, L.G., Fischer, J.J., and Sparling, P.F.: Rocky Mountain spotted fever: a clinical dilemma. In Remington, J.S., and Swartz, M.N., editors: Current clinical topics in infectious diseases, vol. 2, New York, 1981, McGraw-Hill Book Co.

32. Kaplowitz, L.G., Lange, J.V., Fisher, J.J., and Walker, D.H.: Correlation of rickettsial titers, circulating endotoxin and clinical features in Rocky Mountain spotted fever, Arch. Intern. Med. **143**:1149, 1983.

33. Lankford, H.V., and Glauser, F.L.: Cardiopulmonary dynamics in a severe case of Rocky Mountain spotted fever, Arch. Intern. Med. **140**:1357, 1980.

34. Li, H., Jerrells, T.R., Ault, M.L., Spitalny, G.L., and Walker, D.H.: Gamma interferon as a crucial host defense against *Rickettsia conorii in vivo*, Infect. Immun. **55**:1252, 1987.

35. Lillie, R.D.: The pathologic histology of Rocky Mountain spotted fever, Nat. Inst. Health Bull. **177**:1, 1941.

36. Lyskovtsev, M.M.: Tickborne rickettsiosis, Moscow, 1963, State Publishing House of Medical Literature, p. 43.

37. Mansueto, S., Vitale, G., Miceli, M.D., Tringali, G., Quartararo, P., Picone, D.M., and Occhino, C.: A sero-epidemiological survey of asymptomatic cases of boutonneuse fever in western Sicily, Trans. R. Soc. Trop. Med. Hyg. **78**:16, 1984.

38. Maxey, E.E.: Some observations on the so-called spotted fever of Idaho, Med. Sentinel **7**:433, 1899.

39. Montenegro, M.R., Mansueto, S., Hegarty, B.C., and Walker, D.H.: The histology of "taches noires" of boutonneuse fever and demonstration of *Rickettsia conorii* in them by immunofluorescence, Virchows Arch. [A] **400**:309, 1983.

40. Moe, J.B., Mosher, D.F., Kenyon, R.H., et al.: Functional and morphologic changes during experimental Rocky Mountain spotted fever in guinea pigs, Lab. Invest. **35**:235, 1976.

41. Mosher, D.F., Fine, D.P., Moe, J.B., et al.: Studies of the coagulation and complement systems during experimental Rocky Mountain spotted fever in rhesus monkeys, J. Infect. Dis. **135**:985, 1977.

42. Oster, C.N., Burke, D.S., Kenyon, R.H., Ascher, M.S., Harber, P., and Pederson, C.E., Jr.: Laboratory-acquired Rocky Mountain spotted fever, N. Engl. J. Med. **297**:859, 1977.

43. Parker, R.R.: Rocky Mountain spotted fever, JAMA **110**:1185, 1273, 1938.

44. Randall, M.R., and Walker, D.H.: Gastrointestinal and pancreatic lesions and rickettsial infection in Rocky Mountain spotted fever, Arch. Pathol. Lab. Med. **108**:963, 1984.

45. Raoult, D., Zuchelli, P., Weiller, P.J., Charrel, C., San Marco, J.L., Gallais, H., and Casanova, P.: Incidence, clinical observations, and risk factors of the severe form of Mediterranean spotted fever among hospitalized patients in Marseilles, 1983-1984, J. Infect. **12**:111, 1986.

46. Ricketts, H.T.: The study of "Rocky Mountain spotted fever" (tick fever?) by means of animal inoculations, JAMA **47**:33, 1906.

47. Silverman, D.J., and Wisseman, C.L., Jr.: In vitro studies of rickettsia-host cell interactions: ultrastructural changes induced by *Rickettsia rickettsii* infection of chicken embryo fibroblasts, Infect. Immun. **26**:714, 1979.

48. Vicente, V., Alberca, I., Ruiz, R., Herrero, I., González, R., and Portugal, J.: Coagulation abnormalities in patients with Mediterranean spotted fever, J. Infect. Dis. **153**:128, 1986.

49. Walker, D.H., and Bradford, W.D.: Rocky Mountain spotted fever in childhood, Perspect. Pediatr. Pathol. **6**:35, 1981.

50. Walker, D.H., and Cain, B.G.: The rickettsial plaque: evidence for direct cytopathic effect of *Rickettsia rickettsii*, Lab. Invest. **43**:388, 1980.

51. Walker, D.H., Cain, B.G., and Olmstead, P.M.: Laboratory diagnosis of Rocky Mountain spotted fever by immunofluorescent demonstration of *Rickettsia rickettsii* in cutaneous lesions, Am. J. Clin. Pathol. **69**:619, 1978.

52. Walker, D.H., Crawford, C.G., and Cain, B.G.: Rickettsial infection of the pulmonary microcirculation, the basis of interstitial pneumonitis of Rocky Mountain spotted fever, Hum. Pathol. **11**:263, 1980.

53. Walker, D.H., Firth, W.T., Ballard, J.F., and Hegarty, B.C.: Role of the phospholipase-associated penetration mechanism in cell injury by *Rickettsia rickettsii*, Infect. Immun. **40**:840, 1983.

54. Walker, D.H., Firth, W.T., and Edgell, C.-J.S.: Human endothelial cell culture plaques induced by *Rickettsia rickettsii*, Infect. Immun. **37**:301, 1982.

55. Walker, D.H., Firth, W.T., and Hegarty, B.C.: Injury restricted to cells infected with spotted fever group rickettsiae in parabiotic chambers, Acta Trop. **41**:307, 1984.

56. Walker, D.H., and Gear, J.H.S.: Correlation of the distribution of *Rickettsia conorii*, microscopic lesions, and clinical features in South African tick bite fever, Am. J. Trop. Med. Hyg. **34**:361, 1985.

57. Walker, D.H., Hawkins, H.L., and Hudson, R.P.: Fulminant Rocky Mountain spotted fever: its pathologic characteristics associated with glucose-6-phosphate dehydrogenase deficiency, Arch. Pathol. Lab. Med. **107**:121, 1983.

58. Walker, D.H., and Henderson, F.W.: Effect of immunosuppression on *Rickettsia rickettsii* infection in guinea pigs, Infect. Immun. **20**:221, 1978.

59. Walker, D.H., Herrero-Herrero, J.I., Ruiz-Beltrán, R., Bullón-Sopelana, A., and Ramos-Hidalgo, A.: The pathology of fatal Mediterranean spotted fever, Am. J. Clin. Pathol. **87**:669, 1987.

60. Walker, D.H., and Mattern, W.D.: Acute renal failure in Rocky Mountain spotted fever, Arch. Intern. Med. **139**:443, 1979.

61. Walker, D.H., Paletta, C.E., and Cain, B.G.: Pathogenesis of myocarditis in Rocky Mountain spotted fever, Arch. Pathol. Lab. Med. **104**:171, 1980.

62. Walker, D.H., Staiti, A., Mansueto, S., and Tringali, G.: Frequent occurrence of hepatic lesions in boutonneuse fever, Acta Trop. **43**:175, 1986.

63. Walker, D.H., Tidwell, R.R., Rector, T.M., and Geratz, J.D.: The effect of synthetic protease inhibitors of the amidine type on cell injury by *Rickettsia rickettsii*, Antimicrob. Agents Chemother. **25**:582, 1984.

64. Wolbach, S.B.: Studies on Rocky Mountain spotted fever, J. Med. Res. **41**:2, 1919.

65. Woodward, T.E., Pedersen, C.E., Jr., Oster, C.N., et al.: Prompt confirmation of Rocky Mountain spotted fever: identification of rickettsiae in skin tissues, J. Infect. Dis. **134**:297, 1976.

66. Yamada, T., Harber, P., Pettit, G.W., Wing, D.A., and Oster, C.N.: Activation of the kallikrein-kinin system in Rocky Mountain spotted fever, Ann. Intern. Med. **88**:764, 1978.

Typhus group infections

67. Agger, W.A., and Songsiridej, V.: Epidemic typhus acquired in Wisconsin, Wis. Med. J. **84**:27, 1985.

68. Allen, E.G., Bovarnick, M.R., and Snyder, J.C.: The effect of irradiation with ultraviolet light on various properties of typhus rickettsiae, J. Bacteriol. **67**:718, 1954.

69. Binford, C.H., and Ecker, H.D.: Endemic (murine) typhus: report of autopsy findings in three cases, Am. J. Clin. Pathol. **17**:797, 1947.

70. Bozeman, F.M., Masiello, S.A., Williams, M.S., et al.: Epidemic typhus rickettsiae isolated from flying squirrels, Nature **255**:545, 1975.

71. Dyer, R.E., Rumreich, A., and Badger, L.F.: Typhus fever: a virus of the typhus type derived from fleas collected from wild rats, Pub. Health Rep. **46**:334, 1931.

72. Maxcy, K.F.: An epidemiological study of endemic typhus (Brill's disease) in the southeastern United States: with special reference to its mode of transmission, Pub. Health Rep. **41**:2967, 1926.

73. McDade, J.E., Shephard, C.C., Redus, M.A., Newhouse, V.F., and Smith, J.D.: Evidence of *Rickettsia prowazekii* infections in the United States, Am. J. Trop. Med. Hyg. **29**:277, 1980.

74. Murray, E.S., et al.: Brill's disease, JAMA **142**:1059, 1950.

75. Murray, E.S., et al.: Brill's disease. IV. Study of 26 cases in Yugoslavia, Am. J. Pub. Health **41**:1359, 1951.

76. Rollwagen, F.M., Bakun, A.J., Dorsey, C.H., and Dasch, G.A.:

Mechanisms of immunity to infection with typhus rickettsiae: infected fibroblasts bear rickettsial antigens on their surfaces, Infect. Immun. **50**:911, 1985.

77. Rollwagen, F.M., Dasch, G.A., and Jerrells, T.R.: Mechanisms of immunity to rickettsial infection: characterization of a cytotoxic effector cell, J. Immunol. **136**:1418, 1986.

78. Schramek, S., Brezina, R., and Kazar, J.: Some biological properties of endotoxic lipopolysaccharide from the typhus group rickettsiae, Acta Virol. **21**:439, 1977.

79. Schramek, S., Brezina, R., and Tarasevich, I.V.: Isolation of lipopolysaccharide antigen from *Rickettsia* species, Acta Virol. **20**:270, 1976.

80. Silverman, D.J., Wisseman, C.L., and Waddell, A.: In vitro studies of rickettsia-host cell interactions: ultrastructural study of *Rickettsia prowazekii*-infected chicken embryo fibroblasts, Infect. Immun. **29**:778, 1980.

81. Sonenshine D.E., Bozeman, F.M., Williams, M.S., Masiello, S.A., Chadwick, D.P., Stocks, N.I., Lauer, D.M., and Elisberg, B.L.: Epizootiology of epidemic typhus (*Rickettsia prowazekii*) in flying squirrels, Am. J. Trop. Med. Hyg. **27**:339, 1978.

82. Stuart, B.M., and Pullen, R.L.: Endemic (murine) typhus fever: clinical observation of one hundred and eighty cases, Ann. Intern. Med. **23**:520, 1945.

83. Turco, J., and Winkler, H.H.: Cloned mouse interferon-γ inhibits the growth of *Rickettsia prowazekii* in cultured mouse fibroblasts, J. Exp. Med. **158**:2159, 1983.

84. Winkler, H.H.: Rickettsial phospholipase A activity. In Kazar, J., editor: Rickettsiae and rickettsial diseases, Bratislava, 1985, Publishing House of the Slovak Academy of Sciences.

85. Winkler, H.H., and Miller, E.T.: Phospholipase A activity in the hemolysis of sheep and human erythrocytes by *Rickettsia prowazekii*, Infect. Immun. **29**:316, 1980.

86. Wisseman, C.L., Jr., and Waddell, A.: Interferonlike factors from antigen- and mitogen-stimulated human leukocytes with anti-rickettsial and cytolytic actions on *Rickettsia prowazekii* infected human endothelial cells, fibroblasts, and macrophages, J. Exp. Med. **157**:1780, 1983.

87. Wolbach, S.B., Todd, J.L., and Palfrey, F.W.: The etiology and pathology of typhus, Cambridge, Mass., 1922, Harvard University Press.

88. Woodward, T.E., and Bland, E.F.: Clinical observations in typhus fever, with special reference to the cardiovascular system, JAMA **126**:287, 1944.

89. Zinsser, H.: Varieties of typhus virus and the epidemiology of the American form of European typhus fever (Brill's disease), Am. J. Hyg. **20**:513, 1934.

Scrub typhus group

90. Allen, A.C., and Spitz, S.: A comparative study of the pathology of scrub typhus (tsutsugamushi disease) and other rickettsial diseases, Am. J. Pathol. **21**:603, 1945.

91. Berman, S.J., and Kundin, W.D.: Scrub typhus in South Vietnam: a study of 87 cases, Ann. Intern. Med. **79**:26, 1973.

92. Blake, F.G., et al.: Studies on tsutsugamushi disease (scrub typhus, mite-borne typhus) in New Guinea and adjacent islands: epidemiology, clinical observations, and etiology in the Dobadura area, Am. J. Hyg. **41**:243, 1945.

93. Brown, G.W., Robinson, D.M., Huxsoll, D.L., et al.: Scrub typhus: a common cause of illness in indigenous populations, Trans. R. Soc. Trop. Med. Hyg. **70**:444, 1976.

94. Levine, D.H.: Pathologic study of thirty-one cases of scrub typhus fever with especial reference to the cardiovascular system, Am. Heart J. **31**:314, 1946.

95. Settle, E.G., Pinkerton, H., and Corbett, A.J.: A pathologic study of tsutsugamushi disease (scrub typhus) with notes on clinicopathologic correlation, J. Lab. Clin. Med. **30**:639, 1945.

Q fever

96. Baca, O.G., and Paretski, D.: Q fever and *Coxiella burnetii*: a model for host-parasite interactions, Microbiol. Rev. **47**:127, 1983.

97. Baca, O.G., and Paretsky, D.: Some physiological and biochemical effects of a *Coxiella burnetii* lipopolysaccharide preparation on guinea pigs, Infect. Immun. **9**:939, 1974.

98. Derrick, E.H.: "Q" fever, a new fever entity: clinical features, diagnosis and laboratory investigation, Med. J. Aust. **2**:281, 1937.

99. Coyle, P.V., Thompson, J., Adgey, A.A., Rutter, D.A., Fay, A., McNeill, T.A., and Connolly, J.H.: Changes in circulating immune complex concentrations and antibody titres during treatment of Q fever endocarditis, J. Clin. Pathol. **38**:743, 1985.

100. Dupuis, G., Péter, O., Peacock, M., Burgdorfer, W., and Haller, E.: Immunoglobulin responses in acute Q fever, J. Clin. Microbiol. **22**:484, 1985.

101. Ferguson, I.C., Craik, J.E., and Grist, N.R.: Clinical, virological, and pathological findings in a fatal case of Q fever endocarditis, J. Clin. Pathol. **15**:235, 1962.

102. Hackstadt, T., Peacock, M.G., Hitchcock, P.J., and Cole, R.L.: Lipopolysaccharide variation in *Coxiella burnetii*: intrastrain heterogeneity in structure and antigenicity, Infect. Immun. **48**:359, 1985.

103. Hackstadt, T.: Antigenic variation in the phase I lipopolysaccharide of *Coxiella burnetii* isolates, Infect. Immun. **52**:337, 1986.

104. Hackstadt, T., and Williams, J.C.: Biochemical stratagem for obligate parasitism of eukaryotic cells by *Coxiella burnetii*, Proc. Natl. Acad. Sci. USA **78**:3240, 1981.

105. Heard, S.R., Ronalds, C.J., and Heath, R.B.: *Coxiella burnetii* infection in immunocompromised patients, J. Infect. **11**:15, 1985.

106. Heggers, J.P., Billups, L.H., Hinrichs, D.J., and Mallavia, L.P.: Pathophysiologic features of Q fever–infected guinea pigs, Am. J. Vet. Res. **36**:1047, 1975.

107. Hickey, M.J., Gonzales, F.R., and Paretsky, D.: Ribosomal protein phosphorylation induced during Q fever or by lipopolysaccharide: in vitro translation is stimulated by infected liver ribosomes, Infect. Immun. **48**:690, 1985.

108. Kishimoto, R.A., Rozmiarek, H., and Larson, E.W.: Experimental Q fever infection in congenitally athymic nude mice, Infect. Immun. **22**:69, 1978.

109. Lillie, R.D.: Pathologic histology in guinea pigs following intraperitoneal inoculation with the virus of "Q" fever, Public Health Rep. **57**:296, 1942.

110. Lillie, R.D., Perrin, T.L., and Armstrong, C.: An institutional outbreak of pneumonitis. III. Histopathology in man and rhesus monkeys in the pneumonitis due to the virus of "Q" fever, Public Health Rep. **56**:149, 1941.

111. Marmion, B.P.: Subacute rickettsial endocarditis: an unusual complication of Q fever, J. Hyg. Epidemiol. Microbiol. Immunol. **6**:79, 1962.

112. Marrie, T.J.: Pneumonia and meningo-encephalitis due to *Coxiella burnetii*, J. Infect. **11**:59, 1985.

113. McCaul, T.F., and Williams, J.C.: Developmental cycle of *Coxiella burnetii* structure and morphogenesis of vegetative and sporogenic differentiations, J. Bacteriol. **147**:1063, 1981.

114. Moos, A., and Hackstadt, T.: Comparative virulence of intra- and interstrain lipopolysaccharide variants of *Coxiella burnetii* in the guinea pig model, Infect. Immun. **55**:1144, 1987.

115. Okun, D.B., Sun, N.C.J., and Tanaka, K.R.: Bone marrow granulomas in Q fever, Am. J. Clin. Pathol. **71**:117, 1979.

116. Pellegrin, M., Delsol, G., Auvergnat, J.C., Familiades, J., Faure, H., Guiu, M., and Voigt, J.J.: Granulomatous hepatitis in Q fever, Hum. Pathol. **11**:51, 1980.

117. Perrin, T.L.: Histopathologic observations in a fatal case of Q fever, Arch. Pathol. **47**:361, 1949.

118. Perrin, T.L.: The histopathology of experimental "Q" fever in mice, Public Health Rep. **57**:790, 1942.

119. Picchi, J., Nelson, A.R., Waller, E.E., Razavi, M., and Clizer, E.E.: Q fever associated with granulomatous hepatitis, Ann. Intern. Med. **53**:1065, 1960.

120. Samuel, J.E., Frazier, M.E., and Mallavia, L.P.: Correlation of plasmid type and disease caused by *Coxiella burnetii*, Infect. Immun. **49**:775, 1985.

121. Sawyer, L.A., Fishbein D.B., and McDade, J.E.: Q fever: current concepts, Rev. Infect. Dis. **9**:935, 1987.

122. Spelman, D.W.: Q fever: a study of 111 consecutive cases, Med. J. Aust. **1**:547, 1982.
123. Srigley, J.R., Vellend, H., Palmer, N., Phillips, M.J., Geddie, W.R., Van Nostrand, A.W., and Edwards, V.D.: Q-fever: the liver and bone marrow pathology, Am. J. Surg. Pathol. **9**:752, 1985.
124. Syrucek, L., Sobeslavsky, O., and Gutvirth, I.: Isolation of *Coxiella burnetii* from human placentas, J. Hyg. Epidemiol. Microbiol. Immunol. **2**:29, 1958.
125. Tigertt, W.D., and Benenson, A.S.: Studies on Q fever in man, Trans. Assoc. Am. Physicians **69**:98, 1956.
126. Turck, W.P.G., Howitt, G., Turnberg, L.A., et al.: Chronic Q fever, Q. J. Med. **45**:193, 1976.
127. Whittick, J.W.: Necropsy findings in a case of Q fever in Britain, Br. Med. J. **1**:979, 1950.
128. Yu, S.R., Yu, G.Q., Shi, J.Q., Zhang, X., and Su, Y.P.: Experimental Q fever glomerulonephritis in guinea pigs, Chin. J. Pathol. **15**:106, 1986.

Chlamydial diseases

129. Barry, W.C., Teare, E.L., Uttley, A.H., Wilson, S.A., McManus, T.J., Lim, K.S., Gamsu, H., and Price, J.F.: *Chlamydia trachomatis* as a cause of neonatal conjunctivitis, Arch. Dis. Child. **61**:797, 1986.
130. Berger, R.E., Alexander, E.R., Monda, G.D., Ansell, J., McCormick, G., and Holmes, K.K.: *Chlamydia trachomatis* as a cause of acute "idiopathic" epididymitis, N. Engl. J. Med. **298**:301, 1978.
131. Brasfield, D.M., Stagno, S., Whitley, R.J., Cloud, G., Cassell, G., and Tiller, R.E.: Infant pneumonitis associated with cytomegalovirus, *Chlamydia*, *Pneumocystis*, and *Ureaplasma*: follow-up, Pediatrics **79**:76, 1987.
132. De La Monte, S.M., and Hutchins, G.M.: Follicular proctocolitis and neuromatous hyperplasia with lymphogranuloma venereum, Hum. Pathol. **16**:1025, 1985.
133. Grayston, J.T., Wang, S.P., Yeh, L.J., and Kuo, C.C.: Importance of reinfection in the pathogenesis of trachoma, Rev. Infect. Dis. **7**:717, 1985.
134. Grayston, J.T., Kuo, C.C., Wang, S.P., and Altman, J.: A new *Chlamydia psittaci* strain, TWAR, isolated in acute respiratory tract infections, N. Engl. J. Med. **315**:161, 1986.
135. Hare, M.J., Toone, E., Taylor-Robinson, D., Evans, R.T., Furr, P.M., Cooper, P., and Oates, J.K.: Follicular cervicitis: colposcopic appearances and association with *Chlamydia trachomatis*, Br. J. Obstet. Gynaecol. **88**:174, 1981.
136. Jones, R.B., Mammel, J.B., Shepard, M.K., and Fisher, R.R.: Recovery of *Chlamydia trachomatis* from the endometrium of women at risk for chlamydial infection, Am. J. Obstet. Gynecol. **155**:35, 1986.
137. Kiviat, N.B., Wølner-Hanssen, P., Peterson, M., Wasserheit, J., Stamm, W.E., Eschenbach, D.A., Paavonen, J., Lingenfelter, J., Bell, T., Zabriskie, V., et al.: Localization of *Chlamydia trachomatis* infection by direct immunofluorescence and culture in pelvic inflammatory disease, Am. J. Obstet. Gynecol. **154**:865, 1986.
138. Kuo, C.-C.: Immediate cytotoxicity of *Chlamydia trachomatis* for mouse peritoneal macrophages, Infect. Immun. **20**:613, 1978.
139. Møller, B.R., Weström, L., Ahrons, S., Ripa, K.T., Svensson, L., von Mecklenburg, C., Henrikson, H., and Mårdh, P.A.: *Chlamydia trachomatis* infection of the fallopian tubes, Br. J. Vener. Dis. **55**:422, 1979.
140. Moulder, J.W., Hatch, T.P., Byrne, G.I., et al.: Immediate toxicity of high multiplicities of *Chlamydia psittaci* for mouse fibroblasts (L cells), Infect. Immun. **14**:277, 1976.
141. Patton, D.L.: Immunopathology and histopathology of experimental chlamydial salpingitis, Rev. Infect. Dis. **7**:746, 1985.
142. Patton, D.L., and Taylor, H.R.: The histopathology of experimental trachoma: ultrastructural changes in the conjunctival epithelium, J. Infect. Dis. **153**:870, 1986.
143. Patton, D.L., Kuo, C.C., and Wang, S.P.: Distal tubal obstruction induced by repeated *Chlamydia trachomatis* salpingeal infections in pig-tailed macaques, J. Infect. Dis. **155**:1292, 1987.
144. Patton, D.L., Kuo, C.C., Wang, S.P., Brenner, R.M., Sternfeld, M.D., Morse, S.A., and Barnes, R.C.: Chlamydial infection of subcutaneous fimbrial transplants in cynomolgus and rhesus monkeys, J. Infect. Dis. **155**:229, 1987.
145. Per-Anders, M., et al.: *Chlamydia trachomatis* infection in patients with acute salpingitis, N. Engl. J. Med. **296**:1377, 1977.
146. Poletti, F., Medici, M.C., Alinovi, A., Menozzi, M.G., Sacchini, P., Stagni, G., Toni, M., and Benoldi, D.: Isolation of *Chlamydia trachomatis* from the prostatic cells in patients affected by nonacute abacterial prostatitis, J. Urol. **134**:691, 1985.
147. Quinn, T.C., Taylor, H.R., and Schachter, J.: Experimental proctitis due to rectal infection with *Chlamydia trachomatis* in nonhuman primates, J. Infect. Dis. **154**:833, 1986.
148. Rapoza, P.A., Quinn, T.C., Kiessling, L.A., Green, W.R., and Taylor, H.R.: Assessment of neonatal conjunctivitis with a direct immunofluorescent monoclonal antibody stain for *Chlamydia*, JAMA **255**:3369, 1986.
149. Ridgway, G.L.: Chlamydial infections in man, Postgrad. Med. J. **62**:249, 1986.
150. Ripa, K.T., Møller, B.R., Mårdh, P.A., Freundt, E.A., and Melsen, F.: Experimental acute salpingitis in grivet monkeys provoked by *Chlamydia trachomatis*, Acta Pathol. Microbiol. Scand. **87B**:65, 1979.
151. Schaechter, J.: Chlamydial infections, N.Engl. J. Med. **298**:428, 490, 540, 1978.
152. Schaechter, J., and Caldwell, H.D.: Chlamydiae, Annu. Rev. Microbiol. **34**:285, 1980.
153. Swartz, S.L., Kraus, S.J., Herrmann, K.L., Stargel, M.D., Brown, W.J., and Allen, S.D.: Diagnosis and etiology of nongonococcal urethritis, J. Infect. Dis. **138**:445, 1978.
154. Taylor, H.R., Johnson, S.L., Schaechter, J., Caldwell, H.D., and Prendergast, R.A.: Pathogenesis of trachoma: the stimulus for inflammation, J. Immunol. **138**:3023, 1987.
155. Todd, W.J., and Caldwell, H.D.: The interaction of *Chlamydia trachomatis* with host cells: ultrastructural studies of the mechanism of release of a biovar II strain from HeLa 229 cells, J. Infect. Dis. **151**:1037, 1985.
156. Watkins, N.G., Hadlow, W.J., Moos, A.B., and Caldwell, H.D.: Ocular delayed hypersensitivity: a pathogenetic mechanism of chlamydial conjunctivitis in guinea pigs, Proc. Natl. Acad. Sci. USA **83**:7480, 1986.
157. Wilhelmus, K.R., Robinson, N.M., Tredici, L.L, and Jones, D.B.: Conjunctival cytology of adult chlamydial conjunctivitis, Arch. Ophthalmol. **104**:691, 1986.
158. Winkler, B., and Crum, C.P.: *Chlamydia trachomatis* infection of the female genital tract, Pathol. Annu. **22**:193, 1987.
159. Yow, E.M., Brennan, J.C., Preston, J., and Levy, S.: The pathology of psittacosis, Am. J. Med. **27**:739, 1959.

Ehrlichial diseases

160. Fishbein, D.B., Sawyer, L.A., Holland, C.J., Hayes, E.B., Okoroanyanwu, W., Williams, D., Sikes, K., Ristic, M., and McDade, J.E.: Unexplained febrile illnesses after exposure to ticks: infection with an *Ehrlichia*? JAMA **257**:3100, 1987.
161. Fishbein, D.B., et al.: Human ehrlichiosis in the United States. In Program and Abstracts of the Twenty-Seventh Interscience Conference on Antimicrobial Agents and Chemotherapy, sponsored by the American Society for Microbiology, Washington, D.C., 1987.
162. Maeda, K., Markowitz, N., Hawley, R.C., Ristic, M., Cox, D., and McDade, J.E.: Human infection with *Ehrlichia canis*, a leukocytic rickettsia, N. Engl. J. Med. **316**:853, 1987.
163. Rohrbach, B.W., et al.: Human ehrlichiosis, Oklahoma. In Program and Abstracts of the Twenty-Seventh Interscience Conference on Antimicrobial Agents and Chemotherapy, sponsored by the American Society for Microbiology, Washington, D.C., 1987.
164. Ristic, M., and Huxsoll, D.L.: Ehrlichiae. In Bergey's manual of systematic bacteriology, vol. 1, Kreig, N.R., and Holt, J.G., editors: Baltimore, 1984, Williams & Wilkins.

9 Viral Diseases

JOSÉ COSTA
ALAN S. RABSON

Illnesses now known to be caused by viruses have been recognized since antiquity. However, major advances in the study of viruses have been possible only in the twentieth century because of the development of tissue culture, electron microscopy, and immunologic techniques. In recent years molecular biology has given us a detailed understanding of the genetics and life cycles of some viruses.

To prove that a disease is caused by a specific viral agent, the postulates of Rivers (modified Koch's postulates) must be fulfilled. These are (1) isolation of a virus from diseased hosts, (2) cultivation of the agent in experimental host or host cells, (3) proof of filterability of the pathogen, (4) production of a similar disease in the original host species or an animal model, and (5) reisolation of the virus from the experimentally inoculated diseased host. In some instances these postulates have not been fulfilled because there is no known experimental host or no system in the laboratory to culture the virus. However, when sera from patients suffering from a particular clinical syndrome show a definite increase in antibodies reacting with a particular virus, an etiologic relationship of the virus to the syndrome is assumed. If, in addition, morphologic evidence of viral infection (such as inclusion bodies or visualization of capsids with the electron microscope) is found in the lesions that are characteristic of the disease, the etiologic relationship of the agent with a specific syndrome is reinforced. In situ hybridization is a powerful technique to identify the cells supporting viral replication in tissue sections (Fig. 9-1).

Viruses are organisms that can be characterized as having two distinct phases in their life cycle—an intracellular and an extracellular phase. The intracellular phase is the replicative phase during which the virus multiplies in the infected cell. There it borrows the metabolic machinery of the cell to direct the synthesis of proteins coded by the viral genome. The structural and nonstructural virion components are synthesized independently, and the structural proteins are assembled into whole virions during the final stages of reproduction. When virons leave the cell, they are particles of uniform size, shape, and chemical composition that in some cases can crystallize. This is the extracellular phase of the virus. The viral particles can initiate the infectious process of new cells, and hence they constitute the infectious form of the virus.

The morphology of the virions provides a good basis for their classification. Information about the morphology of viruses is gained through study of purified populations of particles with the electron microscope. The basic component of the virions is the capsid, which contains in its interior the genome of the virus. According to the structural characteristics of the capsid, viruses are divided into two major groups, viruses with helical symmetry and those with icosahedral symmetry. Some viruses also acquire an envelope as they bud through the cell membrane of the infected cells.

The genome of a virus can be either RNA or DNA, and the type of nucleic acid is one of the most important characteristics of any virus. Other characteristics of the genome, such as the size or the fact that in some RNA viruses the genome can be segmented, are also very important in the understanding of the life cycles and properties of the viruses (see discussion of influenza virus).

Most taxonomic systems for viruses rely on the morphology of the particles and the nucleic acid type of genome. Groups that reveal evolutionary and phylogenetic relationships among the members of the group are thus established.

Many of the disturbances that we recognize as symptoms and signs of viral diseases result from the direct effects of viruses on cells. There are three types of virus–host cell interaction: (1) cytocidal infection, (2) steady-state infection, and (3) transformation.

In *cytocidal infection* the virus kills the cells in which it reproduces. During viral replication different morphologic alterations of the cell can be shown to progress as the viral cycle proceeds. One of the best-known morphologic results of cytocidal infection is the formation of inclusion bodies. These inclusions are located either in the nucleus or in the cytoplasm and are seen in infections caused by the herpes simplex virus, cytomega-

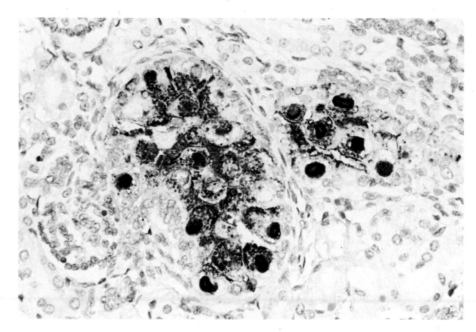

Fig. 9-1. In situ hybridization showing the presence of cytomegalovirus message in the cytoplasm of kidney tubular cells. (Biotinylated probe visualized with streptavidin-biotin complex coupled to horseradish-peroxidase; 320×.)

lovirus, rabies, vaccinia, adenovirus, measles, and papovaviruses (Fig. 9-2).

In *steady-state infection* the infected cells continuously produce virus without a drastic alteration of the cellular metabolism. In many cases of stady-state infection the progeny virions are released by budding through the cell membrane, and the cells can continue to divide and function.

The third type of virus cell interaction and perhaps one of the best studied is *transformation*. It is seen when oncogenic viruses (viruses capable of causing tumors when inoculated into laboratory animals) infect a cell. The main properties acquired by the transformed cell after infection are (1) that the cell becomes immortalized (can be passaged in vitro indefinitely) and (2) that the cells are capable of producing a tumor when injected into the animal of origin. Because many of the transforming viruses cause tumors when injected into animals, transformation of cultured cells provides an in vitro model for the study of carcinogenesis and has been extensively studied.

Study of RNA tumor viruses has led to the discovery of the genes responsible for their tumor-causing capacities. These genes, named oncogenes, turned out to be altered DNA sequences of the animal species in which the virus replicates.

Viral disease is not only the result of the cellular alterations caused by the virus but it is also in most instances the result of the interplay of host defense mechanisms with the infected cell. The effects of human

antibody on virus particles or virally infected cells are quite variable. Humoral immunity helps limit the infection when interaction of the antibody with the virus blocks the attachment of virus to susceptible cells, decreases the intracellular initiation of replication by interfering with uncoating of the genome, or damages the virus coat by activating complement. Lysis of infected cells by antibody and complement can result in clearance of cells supporting viral replication. Cell-mediated immunity is a very important determinant of host resistance to many virus infections. Different subsets of lymphocytes may be capable of killing virus-infected cells, may produce chemotactic factors that attract mononuclear phagocytes, or may produce interferon. The importance of the immune mechanism in viral disease is easily understood when one keeps in mind two observations: (1) most viral infections are asymptomatic, indicating that the host defense mechanisms are capable of limiting the infection with little consequence for the host, and (2) viral infections in naturally or iatrogenically immunosuppressed individuals are often devastating.

RNA VIRUSES
Orthomyxoviruses

Influenza is a disease characterized by abrupt onset, fever, sore throat, headache, muscle pains, and acute toxic state. Dry cough and nasal discharge are present but usually are overshadowed by systemic symptoms. In uncomplicated cases the illness lasts a few days, but

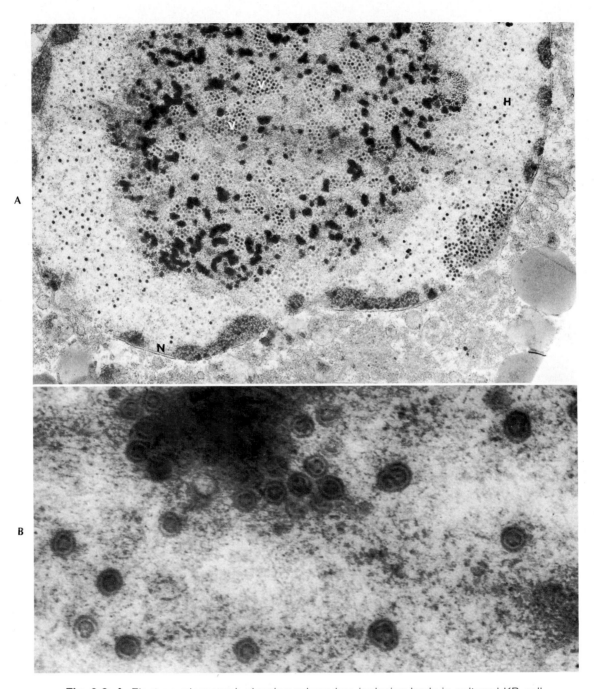

Fig. 9-2. A, Electron micrograph showing adenovirus inclusion body in cultured KB cell. Inclusion is composed of virions *(V)*, chromatin, and dense bodies of unknown nature. Between inclusion body and nuclear membrane *(N)* is halo *(H)*. **B,** Human cytomegalo-virions within nuclear inclusion in cultured human fibroblast line. Diameter is 100 nm; addition of lipid envelope from nuclear membrane gives complete virion diameter of 220 nm. (**A,** 10,000×; **B,** 50,000×.)

pulmonary complications such as influenza pneumonia and secondary bacterial infection of the lung may complicate and prolong the course. Epidemics of influenza have been recorded for the past 400 years. Between 1173 and 1875 there were at least 299 outbreaks of the disease at an average interval of 2.4 years. When epidemics are of worldwide scope they are referred to as pandemics. The greatest pandemic occurred in 1918 and caused 21 million deaths.[20] Influenza A virus was first isolated in ferrets by Smith and co-workers[116] in 1933. Influenza B virus was isolated by Francis[37] in 1936, and Taylor[124] isolated influenza C virus in 1970. The first vaccines for influenza were developed in the 1950s and have since been used in various parts of the world to protect selected segments of the population.

Influenza virus is a filamentous or spherical particle measuring from 80 to 100 nm in diameter when spherical. It exhibits projections or spikes at the surface of the envelope. The filamentous particles may measure up to 400 nm in length.[27] The surface spikes are glycoproteins with two biologic properties: a hemagglutinin and a neuraminidase.[111] The hemagglutinin is the molecular that mediates attachment of the virus to the susceptible host cell and also to erythrocytes. If the hemagglutinin spikes are removed by chymotrypsin, the infectivity is reduced to one thousandth of the original activity.[99] The neuraminidase spike may function to remove sialic acid from the mucins present at the surface of the cells lining the respiratory tract. It also is believed to play an important role in the release of mature virions from the infected cell.

Influenza virus has eight different segments of RNA in its genome. The genome shows high levels of recombination between genes located in different segments. The segmented nature of the influenza virus genome explains the antigenic variations observed among the isolates made in different epidemics. Minor changes in antigenicity are referred to as *antigenic drift*, and they occur frequently within a given influenza subtype. Major antigenic shifts usually herald pandemics and are likely to result from genetic recombination of viruses that have replicated in nonhuman reservoirs. Continual shifting of RNA segments between animal and human influenza viruses allows for the emergence of new antigenic types that infect the human population.[132] Thus new strains of influenza A, for example, can arise in nature by genetic reassortment in animal hosts. Once a new strain emerges it may be at a selective advantage, since there is a high level of immunity in the human population to the old strain but a lack of immunity to the new strain.

Infection in the human is usually acquired by transfer of virus-containing respiratory secretions from an infected to a susceptible person. Biopsy specimens from patients with acute influenza reveal desquamation of

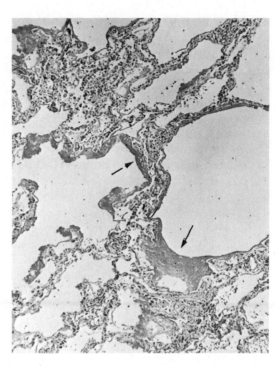

Fig. 9-3. Asian influenza. Pure viral lesion with interstitial pneumonia and hyaline membrane *(arrows)* lining air sacs.

the ciliated and columnar epithelium of the nasopharynx, nasal cavity, and bronchi. Individual cells show pyknosis of the nuclei and loss of cilia. If influenza pneumonia complicates the case, the lungs are dark red and firm with interstitial emphysema that may extend into the mediastinal tissue. Microscopically there is pronounced sloughing of the bronchial epithelial cells into the bronchial lumens. Intraalveolar hemorrhage and hyaline membrane formation can be seen in such cases (Fig. 9-3). The inflammatory infiltrate is sparse. If bacterial superinfection occurs, the picture is indistinguishable from that of ordinary bronchopneumonia or lobar pneumonia. Superinfection with hemolytic streptococci or *Haemophilus influenzae* results in a diffuse hemorrhagic consolidation. Myocarditis and pericarditis, as well as encephalitis, might be found at postmortem examination of fatal cases, but they are uncommon.

Paramyxoviruses

Paramyxoviruses are spherical enveloped particles with a diameter ranging from 100 to 800 nm containing a nucleocapsid with an RNA genome. In common with the influenza viruses (orthomyxoviruses) they have spikes in the envelope with hemagglutinin activity and in some cases also with neuraminidase activity. In contrast, however, to influenza viruses they are antigenically stable and genetic recombination does not occur. The paramyxoviruses that infect humans include the parainfluenza viruses 1, 2, 3, 4A, and 4B; the mumps virus; the measles virus; and the respiratory syncytial virus. Newcastle disease virus, which is a pathogen for chickens, may accidentally infect humans.

The *parainfluenza viruses* are important causes of respiratory disease in infants and young children. They are indeed the most common identifiable agents in the croup syndrome and are second only to respiratory syncytial virus as a cause of lower respiratory disease requiring hospitalization in infants.[83] The parainfluenza viruses are distributed worldwide, and the best evidence of infection is a fourfold rise of antibody titer in convalescent serum collected 3 to 4 weeks after infection. The clinical manifestations vary from no illness or a very minor cold episode to life-threatening croup and bronchiolitis. The most common symptom associated with parainfluenza is a "cold." The viruses are transmitted from person to person by transfer of respiratory tract secretions. The virus infects the cells of the upper respiratory tract mucosa, and multiplication of the viruses in those cells is probably the pathogenic substrate of the most common clinical manifestation. Parainfluenza virus antigens have been demonstrated by immunofluorescence in the ciliated columnar epithelial cells in the nasal secretions of ill children.[40] When the lung is involved, the pathologic changes are indistinguishable from those produced by other viral pneumonias.[138]

Mumps is an acute generalized benign and self-limited infection that occurs primarily in school-aged children and young adolescents. When it occurs in the postpubertal person, it is a more severe illness and more commonly leads to extrasalivary gland involvement. The complete mumps virion has an irregular spherical shape with a diameter ranging from 90 to 300 nm. The viral envelope exhibits glycoprotein spikes that possess hemagglutinin and neuraminidase activity. In addition, it also has a cell fusion activity. The genome of the virus consists of a continuous linear molecule of single-stranded RNA surrounded by symmetric repetitions of protein subunits.

Mumps is an endemic disease throughout the world. Humans are the only known natural host, but monkeys and other laboratory animals can be experimentally infected. The disease is naturally transmitted through direct contact, respiratory droplets, or fomites, which enter through the nose or mouth. Experimental infection in monkeys has been produced by direct instillation of the virus into Stensen's duct.[62]

The most common clinical manifestion of mumps is bilateral or unilateral parotiditis. It is proceeded by nonspecific prodromal symptoms. Involvement of the submaxillary, submandibular, and sublingual glands is uncommon but might occur. Meningitis and encephalitis are the most common extrasalivary gland manifestations of mumps in the preadolescent, whereas in the adult male epididymitis and orchitis are the most com-

monly encountered. Oophoritis, arthritis, and pancreatitis have also been reported. Many case reports can be found in the litrerature relating maternal mumps infection to a wide variety of congenital anomalies. However, there is no convincing evidence that mumps virus is a fetal pathogen. Manson and co-workers[76] in their classic study observed no significant difference in fetal complications between 501 cases of maternal mumps and a control group irrespective of the stage in which infection occurred. These results have also been confirmed in Siegel's studies.[114] St. Geme and others[108] have suggested that intrauterine mumps infection may be linked to endocardial fibroelastosis. Hutchins and Vie[58] suggest that endocardial fibroelastosis may be the result of interstitial myocarditis with persistent left ventricular dilatation, relative mitral valvular insufficiency, and increased endocardial tension leading to compensatory hypertrophy. This in turn causes the accumulation of the thick layer of collagen and elastic tissue beneath the endocardial lining resulting in the classic picture of endocardial fibroelastosis. This mechanism could be operating in myocarditis caused by a variety of viral agents.

The lesions of the salivary glands have been best characterized in experimentally infected monkeys. The affected glands are swollen, edematous, and show minute capsular hemorrhages. Microscopically there is pronounced interstitial edema with inflammatory infiltrate

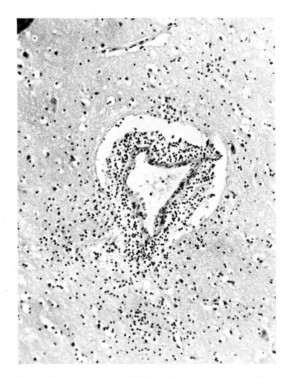

Fig. 9-4. Mumps encephalitis. Perivascular cuffing and spillage of phagocytic microglial cells into area of incipient demyelinization.

in the ducts and degenerative changes of the ductal epithelium. The glandular cells are spared but may be focally affected by the inflammatory reaction present in the interstitial tissue. Multinucleated cells are not seen in vivo.

In *orchitis* focal hemorrhages and necrosis are frequently seen. There are also microscopic areas of infarction and a conspicuous polymorphonuclear infiltrate. Healing is associated with focal testicular atrophy. *Encephalitis* is uncommon, and when it is of early onset in the disease it usually represents damage to the neurons caused by viral replication in the neuronal cells.[123] Late-onset encephalitis is usually a postinfectious demyelinating process or perivenular postinfectious encephalitis (Fig. 9-4).

Respiratory syncytial virus (RSV) was first isolated in 1956 by Morris and co-workers[85] who named it "chimpanzee coryza agent." Shortly thereafter, Chanock and co-workers[13] confirmed that the agent was able to cause respiratory illness in humans. Respiratory syncytial virus measures from 121 to 300 nm. It has an RNA genome, and like all members of the paramyxovirus family, the envelope exhibits spokes of glycoprotein.[8] RSV

is of worldwide distribution, and primary infection occurs in the very young.[100]

In the initial pulmonary infection there is a lymphocytic peribronchiolar infiltrate with some edema of the bronchial walls. Necrosis of the cells lining the bronchioles can be seen. Subsequently there is a proliferative response of the bronchial epithelium. The lumen of the small airways becomes narrowed because of sloughing of necrotic epithelium and an increase in mucin secretion. Obstruction of airflow occurs, resulting in hyperinflation and trapping of air. Complete bronchiolar obstruction may lead to atelectasis. In severe cases there is a prominent interstitial alveolar infiltrate accompanied by edema.[2,35] Other manifestations of RSV infection include otitis media, meningitis, myelitis, and myocarditis.

Measles (rubeola) is a highly communicable disease characterized by fever, cough, coryza, conjunctivitis, and an erythematous cutaneous eruption. The rash is composed of small, reddish, macular papules. It appears first on the face and spreads rapidly to the abdomen and limbs. Koplik spots are practically pathognomonic of the disease and consist of blue-gray specks

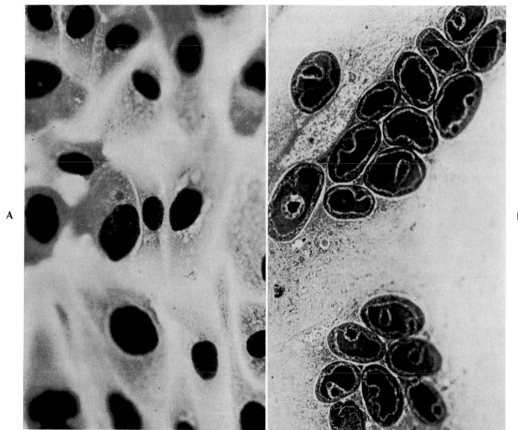

Fig. 9-5. Culture of human renal cells. **A,** Control. **B,** Cytopathogenic effect of measles giant cell pneumonia virus (strain 1) 12 days after inoculation, with giant cell formation and nuclear inclusions. (Hematoxylin and eosin; 500×; from Enders, J.F., et al.: N. Engl. J. Med. **261:**875, 1959.)

with a red base that appear in the mucosa. They are most often seen opposite the second molar, but in severe cases they can involve the entire mucous membrane of the mouth. These persist for several days and begin to disappear as the cutaneous rash appears. Involvement of the respiratory tract is common. Complications include involvement of the central nervous system. Measles virus is a pleomorphic agent but is usually spherical, ranging from 120 to 250 nm with hemagglutinin glycoprotein on the surface of the envelope but no neuraminidase.[30,59,90] The nuclear capsid contains an RNA genome with a molecular weight of 6.2×10^6 daltons. When grown in epithelial cells in tissue culture, measles virus produces two types of cytopathic effects. The first is the production of multinucleate giant cells with intranuclear and intracytoplasmic inclusions (Fig. 9-5). These cells are similar to giant cells seen in the lymphoid tissue of patients with the disease and are characteristic of the virus. The other type of cytopathic effect is the so-called spindle cell transformation; it is typically produced by the vaccine strains of the virus.

Humans are the only natural host for the wild type of measles virus, but monkeys may be experimentally infected. It is an endemic virus throughout the world, but the widespread use of measles vaccine has led to a sharp decrease in the incidence of the disease. The infection is spread by direct contact with droplets from the respiratory tract of infected individuals.

Measles virus first infects the upper respiratory tract of the patients. After multiplying locally there is a primary viremia with spread of the virus to the reticuloendothelial system and circulating lymphocytes, especially T lymphocytes. The selective infection of T lymphocytes may be responsible for the immune defects observed in patients with measles. When the virus replicates in the lymphoid tissue of the body, it gives rise to the Warthin-Finkeldey giant cells.[36,131] After replication of the virus in the lymphoid tissue, a secondary viremic phase occurs, and within a few days the Koplik spots appear followed by the development of the rash.

Pathologically the cutaneous lesions show vascular congestion, edema of the dermis, and perivascular lymphocytic infiltrate. The endothelial cells are swollen. Mitotic figures can be seen, and vascular thrombosis with extravasation of erythrocytes may occur. There is hyperkeratosis and vacuolization of the epidermal cells. The Koplik spots show a similar histologic picture but with more prominent necrosis of the epithelial mucosal cells and a more neutrophilic exudate.[68,69,109,118] Bronchopneumonia is the most common fatal complication of the disease. The histopathologic picture varies from almost pure interstitial pneumonitis to bacterial pneumonia. The diagnosis can be made if Warthin-Finkeldey cells are seen, though this is unusual. *Encephalitis* following measles may be acute or chronic[79] (see discussion of subacute sclerosing panencephalitis on the next page). The acute form is a result of viral infection of the central nervous system; mortality is estimated to be between 10% and 30%.

Measles giant cell pneumonia is a characteristic pulmonary lesion observed in hosts unable to mount an antibody response to the virus. The disease usually occurs as a massive pneumonia in children. Histologically the pulmonary parenchyma shows pronounced consoli-

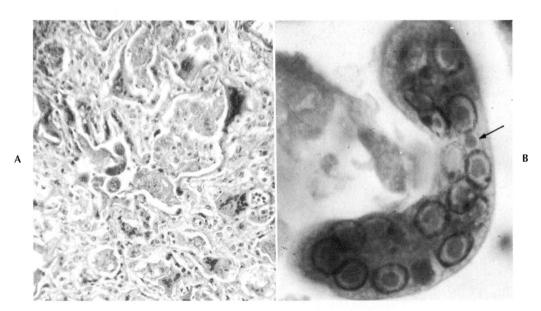

Fig. 9-6. Measles giant cell pneumonia. **A,** Low-power view showing syncytial giant cells lining alveoli and thickening of alveolar walls. **B,** High-power view of one giant cell seen in **A** showing many nuclear inclusions and one cytoplasmic inclusion *(arrow).*

dation with massive formation of syncytial giant cells showing the characteristic intranuclear eosinophilic inclusions surrounded by a halo, and intracytoplasmic inclusion bodies (Fig. 9-6). This picture was described under the term "giant cell pneumonia of infants" before the pathogenesis of the lesion was understood.

Subacute sclerosing panencephalitis (SSPE) is a progressive inflammatory brain disease of children and young adults first described by Dawson in 1934. Dawson suspected that it was a viral disease because of the inflammatory character of the lesions and the presence of intranuclear inclusion bodies in the cells about the lesion. These inclusion bodies are mainly found in neuroglial cells but also can be seen in neurons (Fig. 9-7). Cytoplasmic inclusions are less numerous but can be found. The virus recovered from specimens from cerebral biopsies and lymph node biopsies of patients with SSPE[49,56] is closely related to measles virus and probably represents a defective measles virus with a biochemical lesion that interferes with completion of the viral maturation process in the infected cell. The pathologic findings in SSPE are those of a subacute encephalitis involving both the white and gray matter of the cerebral hemispheres and the brainstem. There are perivascular lymphocytic infiltrates, and there is evidence of neuronal loss. In later stages diffuse proliferations of glial cells and degeneration of myelin occur. By electron microscopy the inclusions are seen to contain tubular paramyxovirus-like nucleocapsids. Measles virus antigen can be demonstrated in the nuclei and cytoplasm of infected neurons and glial cells.[44,125]

Coronaviridae

Coronaviruses cause disease in a variety of animals such as rats, mice, chickens, turkeys, cats, and pigs. In humans they were first isolated from patients with the common cold by inoculation of respiratory tract secretions into human embryonic tracheal organ cultures.[128] The viral particles have a diameter ranging from 60 to 200 nm. They are enveloped virions with widely spaced, petal-shaped projections 20 nm in length that give a crownlike appearance to the virion, hence the name coronavirus.[127] The genome is a single-stranded RNA molecule with a molecular weight of about 6×10^6 daltons. Coronavirus infections have been found throughout the world.

The human coronaviruses cause upper respiratory tract disease,[77] and several strains have been recovered from adults suffering from the common cold.

Rhabdoviridae

The rhabdoviruses are RNA viruses with a single-stranded RNA genome of 4 million daltons in molecular weight. The nuclear capsid is enclosed within a bullet-shaped capsid that measures approximately 175×75 nm. Rhabdoviruses infect vertebrates, insects, and plants. The most important rhabdovirus in humans is rabies virus. Other rhabdoviruses are vesicular stomatitis virus, the Mokola virus, the Lagos bat virus, the Obodhiang virus, and the Katonkan virus.

Rabies is one of the oldest known and most feared of human diseases.[6] It is primarily a disease of animals, and the epidemiology of human rabies closely parallels the epizoology of animal rabies. Where domestic animal rabies has not been controlled, dog or cat bites account for 90% of the reported human cases. In areas where the domestic animal rabies is well controlled, the majority of exposures are the consequence of wild animal bites such as bat, skunk, wolf, coyote, and raccoon bites. It is likely that rabies maintains itself as an endemic illness in each of these species. Rabies is transmitted to humans practically always as a result of a bite from a rabid domestic or wild animal. The disease has also rarely been transmitted through corneal transplants. Clinically the initial symptoms of the disease are nonspecific, such as malaise, fatigue, and headache, followed by a period of acute neurologic symptoms including hyperactivity, disorientation, hallucinations, seizures, and bizarre behavior, followed by coma and death. Combined immune serum and vaccine are the recommended postexposure prophylaxis of the disease in the United States. Specific chemotherapy for clinical rabies is not available, and treatment consists in intensive supportive care.

The rabies virus multiples at the site of the local bite and travels to the central nervous system through the peripheral nerves. Once in the central nervous system it replicates within the neurons.[87] Grossly the brain and spinal cord show edema and petechial hemorrhages. Involvement of the spinal cord is most conspicuous when the portal of entry is on the lower part of the body. Microscopically the predominant inflammatory lesion

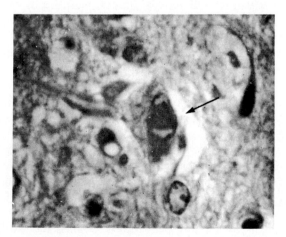

Fig. 9-7. Subacute sclerosing panencephalitis. *Arrow,* Neuron containing homogeneous eosinophilic nuclear inclusion with halo.

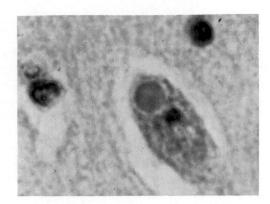

Fig. 9-8. Negri bodies of rabies.

consists in lymphocytic perivascular cuffing within the parenchyma of the nervous system. Little meningeal reaction is seen. Nodules of glial cells termed Babès nodes are often seen and consist of nonspecific glial aggregates. In about 75% of cases Negri bodies can be seen on hematoxylin and eosin–stained sections. These cytoplasmic inclusion bodies in the neurons are practically pathognomonic for rabies and are an important diagnostic finding (Fig. 9-8). They are most consistently present in the Purkinje cells of the cerebellum and in the large neurons of the hippocampus. They are found in intact neurons as round to oval eosinophilic bodies measuring 2 to 10 μm in diameter.[29,91] Ultrastructural studies have shown that the Negri body consists of a mass of nucleocapsids surrounded by viral particles budding from intracytoplasmic membranes.[122] Those bodies can be seen in axons, and it is in this way that the virus spreads from the central nervous system to many organs of the body. Because Negri bodies are usually seen in intact neurons, they are found away from the inflammatory, nonspecific lesions. Rabies viral antigens can be demonstrated in infected cells by means of fluorescent antibody techniques.[87] Antigens can be shown to be present in cells in the absence of Negri bodies, and hence this technique is much more sensitive than the search of sections of brain for the pathognomonic cytoplasmic inclusions.

Bunyaviridae

The *Bunyavirus* genus comprises over 80 antigenically related viruses of which the California encephalitis group is the most important.[102] The virions are enveloped spherical particles approximately 100 nm in diameter, and they contain a three-part segmented genome of single-stranded RNA segments. This allows for genetic recombination or reassortment to occur in doubly infected cels. The principal member of the California encephalitis virus group in the United States is the La Crosse (LAC) virus. It is transmitted to humans by *Aedes triseriatus*, a forest-dwelling mosquito of the north central and northeastern United States. Infection of humans may result in a mild febrile illness or sometimes a severe encephalitis or meningoencephalitis.[65] Most patients appear to recover completely, though personality changes and learning disorders have been reported as sequelae.

Togaviridae

Many viruses have been classified in the past based on their mode of transmission. The viruses transmitted from person to person or from animal to human by means of arthropods were classified as arthropod-borne animal viruses or arboviruses.[12] Information accumulated on the physical and biochemical properties of the viruses grouped under arboviruses indicates that several different virus families were included and that some members of those families were not transmitted by arthropod vectors. Viruses that are transmitted by arthropod vectors are now classified under one of the following families: Bunyaviridae, Togaviridae, Reoviridae, and Rhabdoviridae. Togaviridae are spherical, enveloped virions measuring 40 to 90 nm in diameter with a nuclear capsid that exhibits cubic symmetry.[34] There are two genera of Togaviridae that contain viruses transmitted to arthropod vectors, the alphaviruses and the flaviviruses.

Rubivirus

Rubella virus (German measles) is a spherical, enveloped virus measuring approximately 60 nm in diameter. It has an RNA genome, and it replicates in the cell cytoplasm maturing by budding from the cell membrane.[86] The virus is classified in the togavirus family as a separate genus, *Rubivirus*, based on the RNA genome, icosahedral capsule, and lipoprotein envelope. The virus is spread by droplets that are shed from respiratory secretions of infected persons. Infants born with congenital rubella shed large quantities of viruses from body secretions for many months.

Infection with rubella virus leads to very different diseases depending on the age at which the virus interacts with the host. Postnatally acquired rubella is generally an innocuous infection. Probably most cases are subclinical, and the patients who are symptomatic do not experience a prodromal phase. The major symptoms of infection by rubella virus in the adult are adenopathy, especially in the occipital and posterior cervical region, fever, malaise, leukopenia, and relative lymphocytosis. The picture is accompanied by a mild, generalized, macular eruption that is probably related to the antibody response. Rubella virus has been detected in leukocytes of patients during the viremic phase and has been recovered also from skin lesions at the time of the rash.[54] Contrasting with the benign, self-limited course of the postnatal infection, the fetus is at high risk for developing severe disease with long-standing sequelae if infected transplacentally.[16] In some cases infection will be incompatible with fetal life. Not all the consequences of fetal infection are evident at birth, and some lesions resulting from the viral infection become apparent years after birth. The effects of the virus on the fetus are in part dependent on the time of infection. The younger the fetus, the more severe the effects. During the first 2 months of fetal life, the fetus has a 40% to 60% chance of being affected with an outcome of either multiple congenital defects or spontaneous abortion. During the third month of the fetal life, rubella has been associated with 30% to 35% chance of developing a single defect such as deafness or congenital heart disease. Fetal infection during the fourth month carries a 10% risk of a single congenital defect.

The results of rubella infection are varied and multiple and involve the cardiovascular system, the ocular and auditory systems, the liver, the reticuloendothelial system, and (predominantly) the central nervous system.[28,32] To explain such varied lesions several mechanisms have been proposed. They include inhibition of cellular growth after infection, fetal vasculitis and placental angiopathy, and tissue necrosis. Human fibroblasts infected with rubella virus produce a growth inhibition factor, which could perhaps be related to retardation of fetal growth.

Alphaviruses

The *Alphavirus* genus includes 20 viruses. They are antigenically related and correspond to the group A arboviruses in Casals' serologic classification. There are enveloped spherical virions containing a single-stranded RNA genome of 4×10^6 daltons. Eastern, western, and Venezuelan equine encephalitis are the three significant diseases caused by these viruses in humans.[53] They are initiated by inoculation of the virus by a mosquito bite. In the laboratory alphaviruses can be transmitted by aerosol and have caused numerous infections in laboratory workers by this route. After inoculation the virus multiplies in the nonneuronal tissues causing a febrile illness. The infection may be eliminated by the host defense mechanisms after a subclinical infection or a benign febrile illness, or the virus may invade the central nervous system giving rise to an encephalitis. Alphaviruses replicate in the central nervous system causing cell destruction and a severe inflammatory response. The mortality for western equine encephalitis is approximately 10% and for eastern equine encephalitis 70%. Total recovery is uncommon, and patients are left with sequelae that include mental retardation, behavioral changes, and convulsive disorders. The mortality resulting from Venezuelan equine encephalitis is a general low, though a more severe form of the disease

has been recognized and is probably caused by the lymphocytolytic effect of the virus.

Gross examination of the brain in fatal cases of *eastern equine encephalitis* shows edema. Microscopically, there is a noticeable meningoencephalitis with a conspicuous, acute, neutrophilic infiltrate and an acute vasculitis with fibrinoid necrosis of the vessel wall. Neuronal necrosis and neuronophagia are very common. At later stages glial nodules and perivascular cuffing become prominent. The lesions involve all regions of the brain, but the rainstem and basal ganglia may be the most severely involved regions.

In *western equine encephalitis* the inflammatory response is less intense and composed of mononuclear cells. The greatest damage is seen in the basal ganglia and in the white matter of the cerebral hemispheres. Cystic degeneration of the white matter has been described in patients under 1 year of age.

Little is known about the pathology of *Venezuelan equine encephalitis* since the mortality is low. The encephalomyelitis is milder than the other types and morphologically consists mostly of the perivascular cuffing and microglial nodules. The inflammatory lesions may be most prominent in the putamen and cerebral white matter.

Establishing the diagnosis of alphavirus infection depends on clinical and epidemiologic information and obtaining the appropriate specimens for biologic and serologic tests. In fatal cases of encephalitis the virus may be isolated from the central nervous system tissues obtained at autopsy. As a rule, virus is not present in the cerebrospinal fluid.

Flaviviruses

Flaviviruses are immunologically distinguishable from alphaviruses. They are enveloped, spherical, and slightly smaller than alphaviruses, measuring 40 to 50 nm. All flaviviruses with the exception of dengue have complex primary cycles of transmission involving arthropod vectors, wild birds, and mammals. In many cases humans are an accidental end host because the levels of viremia produced are insufficient to infect vectors. Flaviviruses cause the following diseases in humans: dengue (breakbone fever), St. Louis encephalitis, Japanese B encephalitis, tick-borne encephalitis, and yellow fever. Dengue virus has a human-mosquito-human cycle.

Dengue virus infection causes a syndrome characterized by fever, rash, and muscle and joint pains. It also can cause a severe hemorrhagic disease (dengue hemorrhagic fever, which is now recognized as an epidemic disease in Southeast Asia). Biopsy studies of the rash seen in nonfatal dengue fever show a lymphocytic vasculitis in the dermis. In cases of fatal dengue hemorrhagic fever the gross findings are petechial hemorrhages in the skin and hemorrhagic effusions in the pleural, pericardial, and abdominal cavities. Hemorrhage and congestion are seen in many organs. Histologic studies show hemorrhage, perivascular edema, and focal necrosis but no vasculitic or endothelial lesions. It is believed that most of the morphologic abnormalities seen result from disseminated intravascular coagulation and shock.[133]

St. Louis encephalitis was recognized in 1933 when an epidemic occurred in southern Illinois and in the area of St. Louis, Missouri. The virus was recovered from brain tissue at autopsy from persons who died of the disease during the 1933 epidemic. The St. Louis encephalitis virus replicates at the site of inoculation and probably gains access to the central nervous system through viremia. In fatal cases of St. Louis encephalitis the brain may appear normal at gross examination. The histologic features are those of a meningoencephalitis, with leptomeningeal mononuclear cell infiltration and parenchymal lesions consisting of perivascular cuffing and reactive microglial nodules. The lesions are more intense in the substantia nigra and thalamic nuclei.[94]

Severe epidemics of encephalitis have occurred in Japan since 1871. The mortality in acute cases is between 30% and 40%, and epidemics are caused by the *Japanese encephalitis* virus transmitted by an arthropod. Cases have been reported in Japan, Korea, China, Southeast Asia, and India. Pathologically the meningoencephalitis involves especially the subcortical zone of the white matter. In patients surviving for a long time the lesions may become heavily calcified. Neuronophagia is commonly seen in the ventral horns of the spinal cord.

Tick-borne encephalitis virus is responsible for epidemics of *Russian spring-summer encephalitis*. The disease occurs in the U.S.S.R., central Europe, and Finland. The virus is maintained between ticks and various warm-blooded mammals. Most clinical cases occur in people exposed to infections in forests or in the laboratory. The clinical disease ranges from meningeal irritation to frank meningoencephalitis with paralysis. In fatal cases there is congestion of the brain; microscopically lesions are found in the gray matter of the precentral cortex, basal ganglia, brainstem, cerebellum, and spinal cord. In the spinal cord the lesions are more severe in the cervical and lower lumbar segments.

Yellow fever is an acute illness manifested by abrupt onset of chills and fever, conjunctival injection, leukopenia, a brief period of remission, and then reappearance of fever with jaundice, punctate hemorrhages of the soft palate, epistaxis, and gingival and gastrointestinal bleeding (black vomit). Approximately 50% of the patients develop relative bradycardia in relation to the degree of fever. The yellow fever virus is viscerotropic,

causing the most damage in the liver, kidney, heart, and gastrointestinal tract. The gross features in fatal cases are not specific. The heart when involved is flabby and pale with scattered pericardial and petechial hemorrhages. Microscopically there is degeneration of myocardial fibers and accumulation of fat. The kidneys may show edema; microscopically the features are those seen in cases of acute tubular necrosis. Hemoglobin casts may be seen. The most characteristic pathologic changes are seen in the liver.[11,115] The appearance of the lesions is typical between the seventh and ninth day of the illness. The liver is grossly normal in size, pale, and yellow because of fatty metamorphosis. Microscopically there is extensive midzonal necrosis, which in severe cases may extend to become panlobular (Fig. 9-9). Intracellular condensations of cytoplasm that appear as round to oval, well-demarcated, eosinophilic inclusions are termed *Councilman bodies*. These are also found in the cytoplasm of Kupffer cells. These inclusions are not composed of virus particles and are nonspecific for the disease. They are periodic acid–Schiff (PAS) positive. A hallmark of the hepatitis caused by yellow fever virus is the absence of an inflammatory component. Also distinctive of the lesion is the fact that despite massive necrosis, the reticulin framework of the hepatic lobule is preserved. Fatty metamorphosis of the microvacuolar type is invariably seen.

Arenaviridae

Arenaviruses are round, oval, or pleomorphic with a range in size between 100 and 130 nm. They are enveloped particles, and the envelope contains club-shaped projections at its surface. Electron-dense granules are found in variable numbers in the interior of the virions. These granules are 20 to 25 nm in diameter and represent host ribosomes. The sandlike granules gave the name to this group of viruses (*arēna*, Latin for 'sand').[87] The genome of arenaviruses consists of four pieces of single-stranded RNA and several small pieces of RNA, some of which may be of host origin. Rodents are the natural host of arenaviruses, and humans are accidentally infected when they come into contact with infected urine. Person-to-person spread is unusual except for Lassa virus. The relevant members of the Arenaviridae family are lymphocytic choriomeningitis virus, Lassa virus, Junín virus, and Machupo virus.

Lymphocytic choriomeningitis (LCM) virus infection is probably widespread throughout the world, though it has been rigorously documented only in North America and Europe.[71] The mode of spread of LCM virus in most sporadic human cases is unknown, but studies suggest direct contact with rodents or spread by infected aerosols. The clinical disease produced by LCM is a meningitis, a meningoencephalitis, or a self-limited

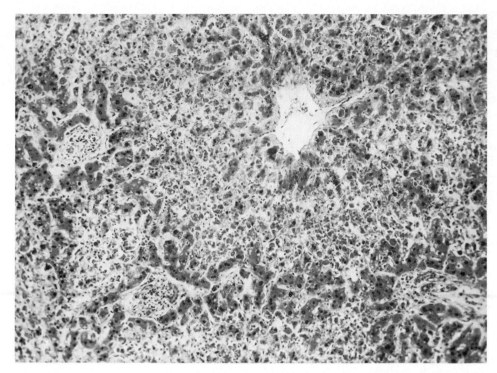

Fig. 9-9. Yellow fever. Liver lesion characterized by midzonal necrosis as shown here. However, damage may involve other portions of lobule or even entire lobule. Early degeneration and necrosis of hepatic cells are attended by relatively little inflammatory reaction. (AFIP 68426; from Ash, J.E., and Spitz, S.: Pathology of tropical diseases, Philadelphia, 1945, W.B. Saunders Co.)

febrile illness, Arthritis, parotiditis, orchitis, and myopericarditis have also been reported. Fatal cases in humans are extremely rare. In monkeys infected by inhalation, virus can be recovered from the lungs and hilar lymph nodes 2 days after infection. Lymphocytic meningitis is often the most conspicuous lesion, but hemorrhagic necrosis may also be seen in liver, kidney, heart, adrenal gland, and other organs. The spleen and the lymph nodes show hyperplasia.

Lassa fever is a disease that ranges in severity from mild and perhaps even subclinical infection to an inexorably progressive, multisystem illness with a mortality of over 45%. The early symptoms of Lassa fever are nonspecific. The diagnosis may be made serologically or by isolation of the virus from serum, throat washings, pleural or ascitic fluid, or urine. Attempts to isolate the virus should be made only in a maximum containment laboratory.

Junín and Machupo viruses are the etiologic agents of the Argentine and Bolivian hemorrhagic fevers. These fevers have similar clinical features, which result from involvement of the hematopoietic, cardiovascular, and central nervous systems. Mortality averages 10% to 20%. The illness begins with fever, malaise, pro-

nounced myalgia, retro-orbital headache, and cutaneous hyperesthesia. As the illness progresses, there is hypertension, diaphoresis, and neurologic manifestations ranging from irritability to seizures. The diagnosis is established by isolation of the virus or by demonstration of significant rises in neutralizing antibody in the serum of the patient. Virus can be recovered from blood, throat, and less commonly urine.

The pathology of hemorrhagic fevers caused by arenaviruses (Lassa, Argentine, and Bolivian hemorrhagic fevers) varies.[14, 129, 135, 139] Interstitial pneumonitis sometimes with hyaline membrane disease is prominent. Morphologic evidence of encephalitis is unusual and inconspicuous when present even though the clinical picture may include encephalopathy and other central nervous system symptoms. The reticuloendothelial system appears activated, and phagocytic activity in Kupffer cells is a common finding. In all three diseases there are focal areas of central and pericentral hepatic necrosis. Eosinophilic or acidophilic bodies similar to Councilman bodies are present in the hepatocytes and Kupffer cells. The fatty metamorphosis observed in almost all cases of yellow fever is not present in Lassa fever.

Picornaviridae

The picornaviruses are characterized by nonenveloped virions with icosahedral capsids 20 to 30 nm in diameter. They contain a single-stranded RNA genome with a molecular weight of 2.6×10^6 daltons. Two genera of picornaviruses that commonly infect humans are the enteroviruses, which have at least 67 recognized immunologic types, and the rhinoviruses, with more than 100 types infecting the human. Enteroviruses have been subdivided on the basis of antigenic relationships and differences in host range into polioviruses, coxsackieviruses groups A and B, and echoviruses.

Coxsackieviruses were first isolated in suckling mice from the feces of two children suffering from a poliomyelitis-like syndrome in the town of Coxsackie, New York.[137] When additional agents of the same group were isolated, it was recognized that some, called group A, produced generalized myositis and flaccid paralysis in the mice used for isolation. Others, classified as group B, produced a focal myositis but also affected the myocardium, brown fat, pancreas, and central nervous system. Damage to the central nervous system results in spastic paralysis. Coxsackieviruses, like most members of the enterovirus group, are transmitted predominantly by the fecal-oral route rather than by respiratory secretions. They have been associated with the following diseases of children: aseptic meningitis, encephalitis, herpangina, pleurodynia, hand-foot-mouth syndrome, pericarditis, lymphonodular pharyngitis, epidemic conjunctivitis, and myocarditis.

The *echoviruses* (enteric cytopathogenic human orphan viruses) were isolated from fecal specimens of healthy children.[137] They produce cytopathic effects in primate cell cultures, but at isolation they were nonpathogenic for suckling mice or primates. They are immunologically distinct from polioviruses and have been associated with a variety of diseases including nonspecific febrile illnesses with or without respiratory symptoms, aseptic meningitis, paralysis and encephalitis, exanthema, generalized disease of newborn, and neonatal diarrhea. They also have been associated with chronic meningoencephalitis in agammaglobulinemic patients.

Three immunotypes of **polioviruses** can be distinguished on the basis of neutralization tests. Most paralytic disease in the prevaccine era was caused by type 1. Humans are the only natural host and reservoir of polioviruses, though in the laboratory polioviruses infect other primates. Early after infection in humans the virus replicates in the gut and adjacent lymphoid tissues, spreading to the regional lymph nodes. From there, there is a minor viremia that disseminates the virus to all susceptible reticuloendothelial tissues. At this point, in many patients, there is an antibody response that limits the infection, which remains subclinical. In some, however, extensive viral replication in the reticuloendothelial system gives rise to a second major viremia, which corresponds with the clinical minor illness or abortive poliomyelitis. These viremias may result in meningitis. It is probably through viremia—though spread through the nervous system has not been ruled out—that the viruses reach the central nervous system and replicate in the neurons of the gray matter, destroying them.

Before the late 1800s poliomyelitis was predominantly sporadic. Early in the nineteenth century epidemics were recognized in Scandinavia and western Europe, and in the first half of the twentieth century epidemics of the disease occurred in developed countries. In the early 1950s around 20,000 cases of paralytic disease were being reported annually in the United States. The introduction of inactivated vaccines in 1955 and attenuated oral vaccines in 1962 brought a dramatic reduction in incidence of paralytic poliomyelitis in the developed countries of the world. In the postvaccine era an increasing proportion of cases of paralytic poliomyelitis in the United States are associated with the use of oral poliovaccines. This vaccine-associated disease is seen not only in the recipients of the vaccine but occasionally in their contacts. The estimated risk of vaccine-associated disease is one recipient case and two contact cases per 10 million doses of trivalent oral polioviruses distributed.[93]

The manifestations of infection by polioviruses are extremely variable. The varieties of illness are inapparent infection; abortive, nonparalytic, spinal paralytic, or bulbar poliomyelitis; and encephalitis. Several risk factors are known to influence the likelihood that an individual will develop paralysis once infected with poliovirus. Boys are more commonly paralyzed than girls, and exercise, trauma, tonsillectomy, and pregnancy all increase the risk of paralytic forms of the disease. Tonsillectomized persons have a risk of acquiring bulbar poliomyelitis that is approximately eight times that in those with intact tonsils. The risk is true not only for those with onset of infection shortly before or after tonsillectomy but also when tonsillectomy is remote.

The gross pathologic condition in both acute and chronic cases of poiliomyelitis infection may be inconspicuous. The most severe lesions are usually found in the anterior two thirds of the gray matter of the spinal cord.[19] They vary from level to level and might be asymmetric in the same section of spinal cord. The ventral horns and the base of the dorsal horns are infiltrated by lymphocytes and hypertrophied microglial cells. Polymorphonuclear leukocytes are often numerous in the neuronophagic nodules that are seen in the early stages of the disease (Fig. 9-10). The leptomeninges show a varying degree of infiltration with inflammatory cells. The earliest lesion in neurons is loss of Nissl substance in the cytoplasm. There is subsequent

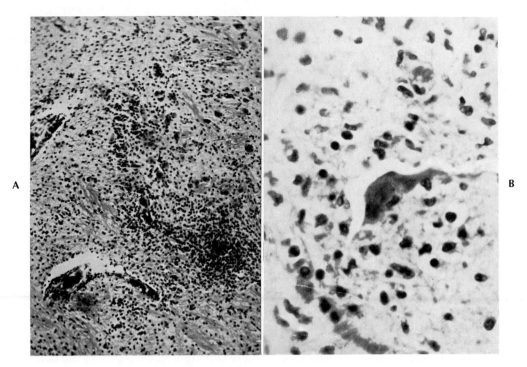

Fig. 9-10. Poliomyelitis. **A,** Focal and diffuse inflammatory cell infiltration in anterior horn of spinal cord. **B,** Degenerating neuron in anterior horn, surrounded by inflammatory cells, some of which are neutrophils. (**A,** From Anderson, W.A.D., and Scotti, T.M.: Synopsis of pathology, ed. 7, St. Louis, 1968, The C.V. Mosby Co.)

progression to eosinophilic necrosis with presence of type B intranuclear inclusions. Death of the neuron is followed by neuronophagia. The perivascular infiltration with lymphocytes and plasma cells in the leptomeninges and parenchyma may persist for weeks or even months. In cases that come to autopsy long after onset of paralysis the most obvious change is loss of neurons in the ventral horns. The axons of the neurons that have been destroyed undergo wallerian degeneration, and the affected muscle shows the typical features of denervation atrophy. Lesions outside the nervous system are less striking. In patients dying in the acute stage of the disease there is generalized lymph node enlargement with disseminated petechial hemorrhages.

Rhinoviruses

Rhinoviruses share many of the properties of the picornavirus group.[48] Human rhinoviruses will infect only humans and higher primates, and epidemiologic studies have shown that rhinoviruses are the major cause of the common cold. They have also been implicated in acute paranasal sinus infection. Currently over 90 types of rhinoviruses have been identified. The identification of new types of rhinoviruses may continue, since it is possible that antigenic drift occurs in this virus. Rhinovirus colds are one of the most common infections in humans, with a rate of 1.2 infections per person per year

in children under 1 year of age and 0.7 infections per year in young adults. The major site for rhinovirus transmission is the home, and the infection is often introduced by a child of school age. Efficient transmission of the rhinoviruses probably depends on close contact.

Human retroviruses

Retroviruses are RNA viruses that contain a reverse transcriptase, an enzyme that uses the viral RNA as a template for making DNA. This DNA copy integrates into the chromosomes of the host cell and serves then as the basis of viral replication. Retroviruses propagate by transmission from host to host, but some members of this group will integrate in the chromosomes of their host and will be transmitted through the germ line. These viruses named "endogenous retroviruses" give rise to infectious particles only under special circumstances and are of little clinical importance.

Human retroviruses have been isolated from human malignancies and from AIDS patients. The first group is termed "human T-cell leukemia virus" (HTLV) and the second "human immunodeficiency virus" (HIV).

The HTLV group has two members: HTLV I, isolated from cells of cutaneous T-cell lymphoma, is linked to adult T-cell leukemia, mycosis fungoides, and Sézary's syndrome. HTLV II was isolated from a patient with "hairy-cell leukemia." Both viruses have similar genetic structure. HTLV I is endemic to southwestern Japan and to the Caribbean basin and is transmitted by placental route, sexual contact, blood transfusion, and among drug addicts shared needles. The latency between infection and emergence of a lymphoproliferative disorder is several years, and viral infection is one of the steps necessary to cause the proliferation leading to leukemia or lymphoma. HTLV-associated malignancies show a broad range of morphologic expressions. In Japan as well as in the western countries[49,61] the most specific feature is the presence of greatly pleomorphic lymphoid cells in the peripheral blood. The pathologic condition of the leukemia and the lymphoma seen in association with HTLV is characteristic of peripheral T-cell lymphomas in general and does not allow distinction from "HTLV-negative" cases, but HTLV-negative lymphomas most often lack the leukemic pattern of infiltration.

The second group of human retroviruses is the human immunodeficiency virus (HIV) family first isolated in 1983. HIV infects and replicates in helper-inducer lymphocytes and in macrophages. This specific cell tropism is attributable to the presence on the surface of these cells of a specific receptor the T4 molecule. Once in the cell the integrated viral genome can replicate or remain latent. Cell death is probably caused by massive replication. The replication of HIV in T4-positive helper lymphocytes is responsible for the depletion of these cells and the subsequent functional depletion of the immune system.

The clinical spectrum of HIV infection is now recognized to comprise (1) acute viral infection sometimes associated with immune complex disease, (2) persistent generalized lymphadenopathy, (3) chronic active viral infection with constitutional symptoms or AIDS-related complex (ARC), (4) immunodeficiency leading to opportunistic infection or tumors (AIDS), (5) chronic encephalopathy caused by HIV, and (6) chronic active viral infection with immune-complex disease (such as thrombocytopenic purpura). New manifestations of HIV infection will probably be recognized in the future.

Infection with HIV constitutes a worldwide problem. Whereas in the European and American continents HIV is transmitted mostly among homosexual men and intravenous drug abusers, in Africa HIV is mainly acquired as an heterosexually transmitted disease.

Neurologic complications, especially the AIDS-dementia complex is an important cause of morbidity in patients in advanced stages of infection. The pathologic abnormalities in patients with AIDS-dementia complex are variable. Multinucleated cells in the brain are found in a subgroup of patients with severe disease. These cells are derived from macrophages and support viral replication. These are thus markers of productive infection. All histopathologic abnormalities are most promi-

nent in the subcortical structures, and besides multinucleated cells they include diffuse pallor of the white matter and vacuolar myelopathy.[103]

At autopsy the gross pathology of AIDS can be split into three general categories as follows: (1) the morphologic manifestations of profound lymphoid depletion, (2) infections caused by opportunistic pathogens, and (3) unusual neoplasms such as Kaposi's sarcoma and high-grade lymphoma.[105] The histopathologic lesions of the lymphoid system are nonspecific and vary from pronounced follicular hyperplasia to severe depletion of lymphoid cells. In some cases the lymph-node appearance is reminiscent of toxoplasma lymphadenitis, angioimmunoblastic lymphadenopathy, and Castleman's disease.

Other RNA viruses

Marburg and *Ebola viruses* are pleomorphic RNA viruses that are distinct from all other viruses and from each other serologically. Their natural reservoir remains undetermined. The initial Marburg virus outbreak in 1967 resulted in 31 infections in Marburg and Frankfurt, Germany, and in Yugoslavia. All patients had contact with infected monkey kidneys. The source of the virus was African green monkey cells imported from Uganda for use in the preparation of vaccines. Additional cases of Marburg virus disease were reported from Johannesburg, South Africa, in 1975. The epidemiology and epizootiology of Ebola virus are unclear. The only reported outbreaks of the disease occurred in Sudan and Zaïre in 1976. Both Marburg and Ebola viruses produce hemorrhagic fevers.[64,75] Death usually results from hemorrhagic complications, renal failure, or shock. Epidemics have been controlled by strict isolation procedures.

Orbiviruses belong to the family of Reoviridae. The genus *Orbivirus* was created to classify a group of about 25 arthropod-borne viruses with distinctive physical, chemical, and serologic properties. Three viruses in this genus are known to cause disease in humans. They are the *Colorado tick fever virus*, the *Kemerovo virus*, and the *Orungo virus*. The Colorado tick and Kemerovo viruses are transmitted by ticks, whereas the Orungo virus is mosquito borne. Colorado tick fever is a self-limited disease characterized by fever, chills, lethargy, and prostration.[119] The duration of the acute illness is 7 to 10 days, and the fever is characteristically biphasic in about 15% of the cases. Encephalitis, meningoencephalitis, and meningitis are possible complications in children. Kemerovo and Orungo viruses produce myalgias, headache, and febrile illnesses.

Electron microscopy and immune electron microscopy of stool filtrates from patients suffering from viral gastroenteritis have identified two classes of agents, the Norwalk group of viruses and the rotavirus group. The *rotavirus group* is very likely a major etiologic agent of infantile gastroenteritis in many parts of the world. It has been associated with about 50% of acute diarrheal illnesses in hospitalized pediatric patients.[67,68] Rotaviruses are non–lipid containing RNA viruses with a double-stranded RNA genome composed of 11 segments. The human rotavirus induces a diarrheal illness in various newborn animals. In the few cases that have been pathologically studied the changes observed include infiltration of the lamina propria of the small intestine with mononuclear cells and shortening of the mucosal villi.[110] Ultrastructurally, mitochondrial swelling, irregularities in the microvilli, and dilatation of the endoplasmic reticulum have also been observed.

The term **Norwalk-like agents** refers to a group of viruses detected in stools from patients with acute gastroenteritis. These agents are named in most instances for the location of the outbreak of illness from which they have been identified. The Norwalk-like agents have not been cultivated in vitro but are identified by electron microscopy and immune electron microscopy. They appear as nonenveloped particles 25 to 27 nm in diameter with cubic symmetry. Gastrointestinal illness has been transmitted to normal volunteers after oral administration of Norwalk and Hawaii agents. Infection with the Norwalk and Hawaii agents results in jejunal lesions characterized by blunting of the villi and inflammatory cell infiltrate in the lamina propria.[26]

Human hepatitis delta virus (HDV) is a replication-defective agent that infects humans only in the presence of a co-infecting hepatitis B virus (a DNA virus). When HDV superinfects a chronic HBV carrier, the resultant is often severe chronic hepatitis and cirrhosis, whereas when there is HDV and HBV acute co-infection, the resultant is fulminant hepatitis. The HDV consists of a 36 nm particle with an envelope containing HBV surface antigen, a nucleocapsid with HD antigen, and a 1.75 kilobase RNA genome.

Hepatitis A virus

The visualization by Feinstone and co-workers[33] in 1973 of a viral particle by immune electron microscopy in the acute phase of experimentally and naturally infected individuals indicated that infectious hepatitis had at least two etiologic agents: the hepatitis A virus, a spherical particle 27 to 29 nm in diameter with icosahedral symmetry, and the hepatitis B virus (see p. 387).

Hepatitis A virus purified from stool has been found to be infectious in the chimpanzee and has been used as an immunogen for production of monospecific antibodies in rabbits.[10] Using this antibody, researchers can detect hepatitis A antigen in hepatocytes of experimentally infected chimpanzees. The staining is finely granular, which is localized in cytoplasm and not in the nucleus. Examination of other tissues including small and large bowel mucosa reveals no evidence of antigen synthesis.

The hepatitis A virus is usually transmitted by close person-to-person contact, probably almost always by the fecal-oral route. Patients are probably most infectious in the late incubation period or about the time symptoms begin. No cases of chronic hepatitis A virus shedding have been documented. The histopathology of acute viral hepatitis is discussed in Chapter 25.

DNA VIRUSES
Adenoviruses

Adenoviruses were first isolated in 1953 by Rowe and co-workers[107] frum human adenoids removed at surgery. At present 41 serotypes have been described. Many serotypes are not linked to a specific disease. Human adenoviruses have a capsid with icosahedral symmetry. Rodlike structures with knobs at the ends protrude from the capsid. The genome of the virus is a double-stranded DNA linear molecule with a weight of 23×10^6 daltons. When infecting cells in vitro, adenoviruses are capable of lytic infection, latent infection, and transformation. Because of the ability to transform cells and to produce tumors in rodents, they have been considered possible human tumor viruses, but up to now there has been no evidence that links adenoviruses to human tumors. Adenoviruses are associated with the following diseases: coryza and pharyngitis in infants; upper respiratory disease, pharyngoconjunctival fever, and hemorrhagic cystitis in children; acute respiratory disease and pneumonia in young adults; and epidemic keratoconjunctivitis and pneumonia in immunocompromised and normal adults. Adenoviruses that are difficult to culture have been associated with 7% to 17% of cases of diarrhea in children.

The histopathology of *adenovirus pneumonia* was described by Goodpasture and co-workers[46] in a paper reporting five cases of pneumonia in infants up to 2½ years of age. Goodpasture postulated the viral cause of the disease based on the presence of intranuclear inclusion bodies. Adenovirus pneumonia is characterized by a necrotizing bronchitis and bronchiolitis. There is intense necrosis and desquamation of the respiratory epithelium into the bronchial lumens.[121,136] These foci of bronchiolitis are surrounded by areas of consolidation, hemorrhage, and atelectasis. At low power the appearance may be confused with bacterial bronchopneumonia. In the areas of consolidation and among the necrotizing bronchiolar epithelial lesions, cells with intranuclear inclusion bodies may be found. In the early stages cytopathic effects are manifested by granular, slightly enlarged nuclei containing eosinophilic bodies intermixed with clumped basophilic chromatin (Fig. 9-11). The eosinophilic bodies coalesce, forming larger masses to end as a central, granular, ill-defined

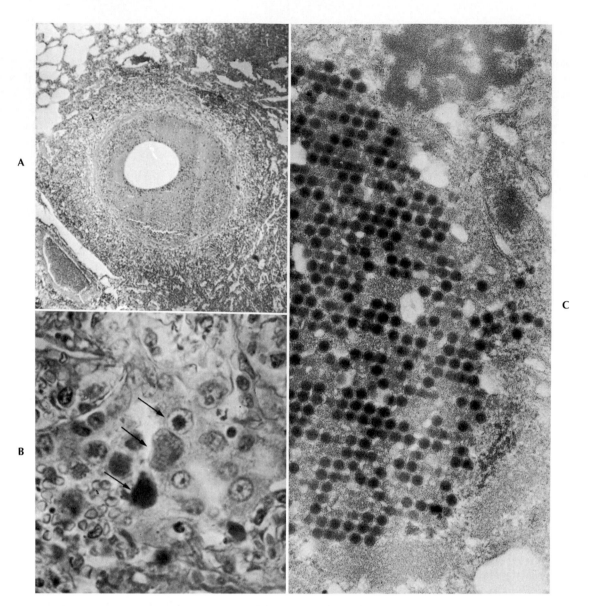

Fig. 9-11. Adenovirus pneumonia. **A,** Necrotizing bronchiolitis with inspissated secretion. **B,** *Arrows from above downward,* Nuclear inclusion of rosette type, hypertrophied nucleus, and smudge cell, with fusion of nucleus and cytoplasm. **C,** Electron micrograph of smudge cell, showing spillage of adenovirions and other nuclear components in cytoplasm. (**A,** AFIP 971609; **C,** 36,000×.)

mass surrounded by a halo. The second type of inclusion, which is more common and probably corresponds to a late-stage infected cell, is designated the "smudge cell." The nucleus is rounded or ovoid, large, and completely occupied by a granular amphophilic to deeply basophilic mass. There is no halo, and the nuclear membrane and nucleus are indistinct. Electron microscopy of the lung demonstrates viral particles in the bronchiolar and alveolar lining cells.

Herpesviruses

The family of herpesviruses consists of a large group of enveloped DNA viruses measuring approximately 120 nm in diameter. Inside the capsid there is a nucleoprotein core that contains a linear, double-stranded DNA molecule with a molecular weight of 100 million daltons. Herpesviruses multiply in the nucleus of the host cell and mature by budding from the cell membranes. The members of the herpesvirus family of relevance to human disease are herpes simplex virus, cytomegalovirus, varicella-zoster virus, Epstein-Barr virus, and herpes simiae virus (B virus). The first four viruses have humans as their natural host, herpes simiae virus infects humans only as a laboratory accident. One pathogenetic property of importance that is shared by all human herpesviruses is the ability to produce latent infections. After a primary infection, infectious virus can no longer be recovered from the host tissues, but the virus resides in an inactive form in cells from which it can be reactivated at a later time. The exact nature of the latent state and the factors triggering reactivation are not clear.

Herpes simplex virus can be divided into two types on the basis of antigenicity, pathogenicity, and genetic properties. Herpes simplex type II is the major cause of urogenital infections, whereas type I is more often isolated from nongenital infections. Herpes simplex viruses have a worldwide distribution, and direct contact with infected secretions is the principal mode of spread. Herpes simplex causes diseases of the skin and mucosa such as acute gingivostomatitis, recurrent stomatitis, oral ulcers (cold sores), herpetic keratoconjunctivitis, herpetic esophagitis, and genital herpes. It also causes systemic disease as in disseminated herpetic infection of infants, acute necrotizing encephalitis of the adult, and infections in the immunodeficient host.

The two types of cytopathology seen in herpes simplex infections are rounding and degeneration of the cells with inclusion body formation and cell fusion with formation of syncytia. The intranuclear inclusion is the characteristic cellular lesion, and it consists of a single, eosinophilic, well-demarcated inclusion body surrounded by a halo and marginated chromatin. By electron microscopy the inclusion body consists of paracrystalline arrays of viral capsids and electron-dense glycoprotein.

Herpetic infection of skin and mucosa is manifested by the appearance of red papules that quickly become vesiculated. Histologically there is degeneration of the cells in the stratum malpighii and the stratified squamous epithelium. In early stages one observes ballooning of the epidermal cells and clearing of the nuclear chromatin. There is acantholysis and formation of a unilocular vesicle. The typical inclusion bodies (Cowdry type A) can be seen in epidermal cells. The upper dermis or submucosal portions of the affected regions show an inflammatory infiltrate around capillaries. The histologic lesion of herpes simplex in the skin and mucosa is practically indistinguishable from that caused by herpes zoster. Immunohistochemistry using fluorescent antibodies or immunoperoxidase can, however, make the distinction between these viruses and even allows typing of the herpesvirus.[96]

Disseminated herpetic infection of the newborn affects neonates in the first 4 weeks of life as well as an older group of infants in whom it causes hepatoadrenal necrosis.[89] Autopsies of infants dying from disseminated herpetic disease show multiple miliary foci of necrosis surrounded by hemorrhagic borders in the liver, adrenal gland, and brain (Fig. 9-12). Microscopically these foci consist of a zone of central coagulative necrosis surrounded by an area of hyperemia with a sparse mono-

nuclear inflammatory reaction. Inclusion bodies characteristic of the herpetic infection are found in nuclei of the parenchymal cells surrounding the necrotic zone. The pathologic combination may be complicated by the presence of gram-negative septicemia.[72,126] Morphologic manifestations of disseminated intravascular coagulation (DIC) may be also prominent. The virus can be easily demonstrated in the lesions by electron microscopic examination.[103]

Herpes simplex virus has been shown to be a cause of *acute necrotizing encephalitis of the adult*.[51] Patients with this syndrome may display a picture of encephalitis or a clinical picture of an expanding lesion, often of the temporal lobe. In fatal cases the brain shows asymmetric necrosis particularly prominent in the temporal lobes but also involving the hippocampus and the posterior occipital cortex. Hemorrhage may be prominent. In the early stages of the disease the histopathologic picture is that of acute necrosis associated with a diffuse meningoencephalitis. Inclusion bodies within the nuclei of neurons and glial cells can be seen but on occasion are difficult to find (Fig. 9-13).

Reactivation and dissemination of herpetic lesions are not uncommon in immunocompromised hosts. Esophageal and upper respiratory tract lesions are commonly found at autopsy in patients who have undergone intense chemotherapy. Dissemination occasionally occurs, and a picture similar to the disseminated disease in newborns can be seen. Dissemination with a fatal outcome also occurs in some severely burned patients.

Cytomegaloviruses are a group of species-specific agents capable of causing asymptomatic infections to severe or fatal illnesses in mammalian species. In vivo and in vitro infection with human cytomegalovirus is characterized by a specific cytopathic effect consisting of distinctly enlarged cells (cytomegaly), 25 to 40 µm in diameter, containing an intranuclear reniform or ovoid inclusion body that measures 8 to 10 µm (Fig. 9-14). The inclusion body is often surrounded by a clear halo and is Feulgen positive. Punctate amphophilic. PAS-positive, cytoplasmic inclusions can also be found in the cytomegalic cells. Ultrastructural studies of both in vivo and in vitro infected cells show herpesvirus capsids forming the inclusion body in the nucleus. The cytoplasmic inclusions are formed by aggregates of dense osmiophilic material surrounding enveloped virions.

Cytomegalovirus (CMV) is a ubiquitous infection and, depending on the socioeconomic condition of the population, the prevalence of antibodies in the adult ranges from 40% to 100%. CMV is usually transmitted by close contact. It may be venerally transmitted and is one of the agents that can be transmitted by blood transfusions.

Infection of the fetus in utero or of the newborn produces a disease that may vary from asymptomatic to a serious and often fatal syndrome. The clinical manifes-

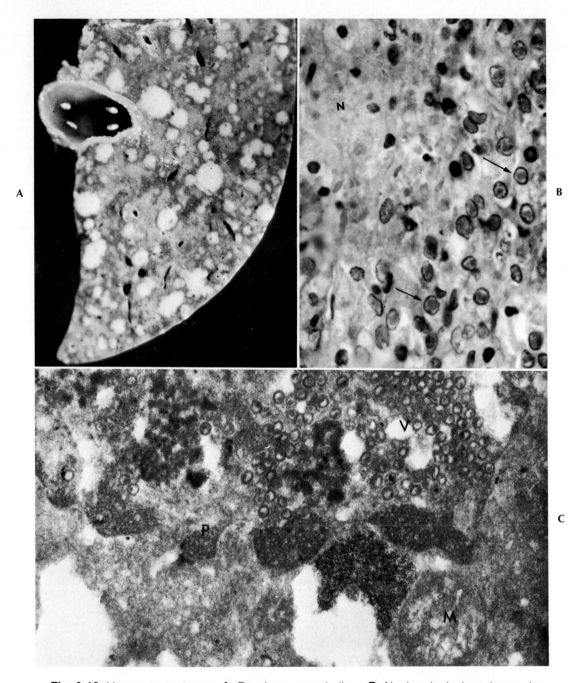

Fig. 9-12. Herpes neonatorum. **A,** Focal necroses in liver. **B,** Nuclear inclusions *(arrows)* at edge of necrotic lesion. **C,** Electron micrograph of inclusion-bearing cell. *M,* Mitochondrion; *P,* peripheral nuclear chromatin; *V,* herpes virions, probably type 2, in nuclear inclusion. Some contain nucleoids, but enveloped forms are not seen. (**A,** 4×; AFIP 997583; **B,** 800×; **C,** 30,000×.)

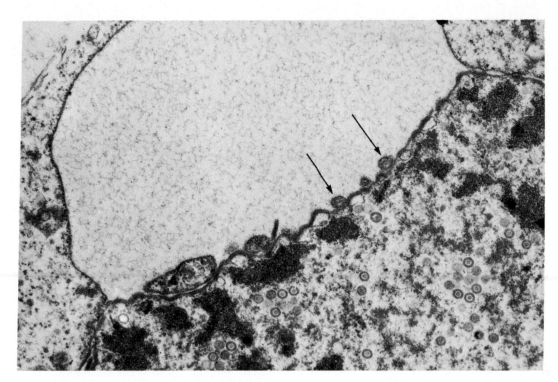

Fig. 9-13. Fatal herpes simplex encephalitis in 18-year-old person. Electron micrograph of formalin-fixed brain tissue showing intranuclear herpes virions, separation of outer and inner nuclear membranes, and acquisition of envelope from latter *(arrows)*. (32,000×; courtesy Drs. Vincent G. Palermo and J.R. Taylor, St. Louis, Mo.)

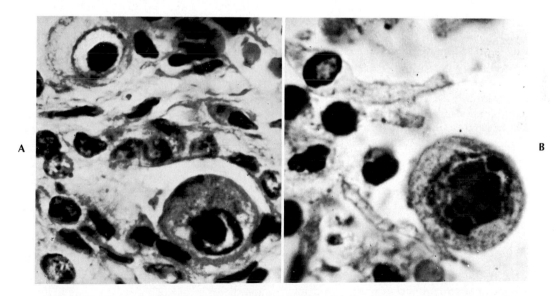

Fig. 9-14. Cytomegalovirus infection of kidney. **A,** Section showing two huge nuclear inclusions in tubular epithelium. **B,** Diagnostic cell in hematoxylin and eosin–stained urinary sediment *(lower right)*. Compare with normal-appearing tubular epithelial cell *(upper left)*.

tations of congenital cytomegalovirus infection appear to be a reflection of the duration of the infection in utero.[50,82] Cytomegalic inclusion disease of the newborn is manifested by jaundice, petechiae, chorioretinitis, microcephaly, thrombocytopenia, diarrhea, and central nervous system disease. The pathologic changes in newborn infants with cytomegalic inclusion disease are usually severe in the liver, kidneys, lungs, and brain. In the liver one observes persistence of hematopoietic tissue and periportal necrosis of hepatocytes with a dense mononuclear inflammatory cell infiltrate. In some cases the histologic picture is that of giant cell hepatitis. Inclusion bodies are difficult to find. The classic lesion in the cerebral nervous system is destruction with subsequent calcification of the cerebral tissue beneath the ependyma of the ventricles. In most cases gross and microscopic evidence of interference with the normal brain development is manifested by abnormal patterns of development of cerebral convolutions. Other organs such as adrenal glands, pancreas, thyroid, pituitary, bone marrow, and myocardium may be found to have cells with the characteristic inclusion bodies.

Cytomegalovirus in the adult is most often seen associated with *gastrointestinal tract disease*[24] or as an opportunistic agent in the immunosuppressed patient. Recent studies indicate that cytomegalovirus may be a common latent infection of the human gastrointestinal tract. Overt infection with viral replication is most often associated with ulcerative diseases such as Crohn's disease and ulcerative colitis. In those cases viral inclusions can be found in cells at the ulcer bed and in the endothelial cells underlying the ulcerated area. Occasionally the inclusion bodies are found in cells lining the mucosa surrounding the ulcer.

CMV pneumonitis is seen in the debilitated adult and in patients who are immunosuppressed.[76] It may be evident on chest radiographs as a reticular nodular density; the diagnosis is established through lung biopsy. The histopathologic picture is that of an interstitial pneumonitis in which the alveolar lining cells show the features of cytomegalovirus infection. It is often associated with a combined infection of the lungs with other organisms such as *Candida, Aspergillus, Nocardia, Mycobacterium tuberculosis*, and quite often *Pneumocystis carinii*. In patients dying with neoplasms, CMV was isolated in 8.8% of 502 unselected autopsy cases at the Mayo Clinic.[116] CMV inclusion bodies in this series with or without associated inflammation were found in descending order of frequency in the lung, kidney, liver, pancreas, adrenal, esophagus, prostate, testes, thyroid gland, parathyroid, stomach, small intestine, and heart.

Varicella-zoster virus (VZ virus) is the etiologic agent of two clinically distinct entities in the human. Chick-enpox (varicella) is an acute infectious disease of childhood characterized by crops of vesicles on the face and tongue. Herpes zoster (shingles) is typified by a painful vesicular eruption restricted to one or more segmental dermatomes in adults. It is often seen in debilitated patients or in immunosuppressed patients. Initial infection with VZ virus at a young age results in the acute disease and dissemination of the agent. It is believed that during the viremic phase the virus infects the neurons of the dorsal root ganglia and is capable of remaining there in a latent state.[7] Zoster (shingles) is the manifestation of the reactivation of the latent infection in the ganglion cells in a partially immune host.

The cutaneous lesion of *varicella* is characterized by crops of vesicles, which may become confluent in severe cases. Microscopically the vesicles of varicella are indistinguishable from the lesions caused by herpes simplex. In fatal cases the predominant lesion is pneumonia.[63,95] It usually occurs within 1 to 5 days after the appearance of rash, with chest pain, cyanosis, and hemoptysis. Radiologically it is characterized by nodular densities throughout the lung fields. Clinical resolution might occur in 2 to 3 weeks, but if the case is fatal, autopsy will demonstrate heavy edematous lungs with dark color and pale areas throughout the parenchyma resembling foci of consolidation. The bronchi are usually filled with hemorrhagic mucus. Microscopically there is hemorrhagic intra-alveolar exudate with hyaline membrane formation and desquamation of alveolar epithelial cells. The desquamated cells may contain inclusion bodies (Fig. 9-15). Nodular calcification has been described as a late sequela to lung necrosis. Varicella is particularly severe in neonates who have acquired infection in utero. Babies dying from the disease usually show disseminated visceral lesions that grossly resemble miliary tuberculosis or disseminated herpes simplex.

The pathology of the *zoster* cutaneous lesion is similar to that of varicella and herpes simplex.[80] The virus may be identified specifically as zoster by means of immunofluorescence or immunohistochemical techniques. In the acute stage the dorsal root ganglion affected by the virus is swollen and hemorrhagic. Microscopically there is an intense inflammation composed of round cells, and the neurons show chromatolysis, with eosinophilia of the cytoplasm. Neuronophagia may also be observed. Inclusion bodies may be seen in the neurons, but as a rule they are hard to demonstrate. Disseminated forms of zoster may be seen in severely immunocompromised patients.[22]

The *Epstein-Barr virus* (EBV) was discovered by Epstein, Achong, and Barr in the course of ultrastructural examination of cell lines derived from patients with Burkitt's lymphoma. Epstein-Barr virus has the characteristic morphology of the herpes group of viruses.

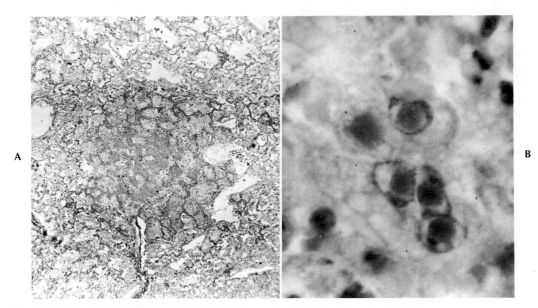

Fig. 9-15. Varicella pneumonia. **A,** Focal hemorrhagic lesion in lung. **B,** Four cells from lesion shown in **A,** each containing inclusion body that partially fills nucleus. Giant cells, though present in cutaneous lesions, are seen only very rarely in varicella pneumonia. (**A,** 30×.)

The host range is limited, and in nature EBV infects only humans. In vitro cultivation of the virus can be carried out only in human B lymphocytes. After infection some of the lymphocytes are "immortalized" (that is, they acquire the ability to grow continuously and indefinitely in culture). Cells infected with Epstein-Barr virus express a variety of antigens that can be detected by sera of different specificity. These antigens are a nuclear antigen (EBNA), early viral antigens (EA), viral capsid antigens (VCA), and antigens present on the membrane of infected and immortalized cells (MA). Antibodies to Epstein-Barr virus have been found in all population groups studied. In the United States and Great Britain EBV seroconversion occurs before 5 years of age in about 50% of the population. A second wave of seroconversion occurs midway through the second decade of life. Lower socioeconomic groups have a higher EBV antibody prevalence than more affluent matched controls do. The immune response to Epstein-Barr virus infected or immortalized lymphocytes is complex and involves both humoral and cell-mediated immune mechanisms.

EBV induces a broad spectrum of illness. Classic *infectious mononucleosis* is an acute disease characterized by sore throat, fever, lymphadenopathy, transient heterophil antibodies, and leukocytosis, which consists in part of atypical lymphocytes. The age of the patient has a profound influence on the clinical expression of EBV expression. However, EBV infection in the young is often asymptomatic.

The atypical lymphocytes seen in peripheral blood of patients with EBV mononucleosis are slightly larger than normal lymphocytes with a pale blue vacuolated cytoplasm and scalloped border (Dutch skirt appearance). The oval nucleus contains a coarse chromatin network. The atypical lymphocytes are heterogeneous in morphologic appearance as opposed to those malignant diseases such as leukemia or lymphosarcoma. It is now known that the atypical cells that circulate in patients with infectious mononucleosis represent activated T-cells that are mounting a cell-mediated immune response against infected B lymphocytes.[101] Lymph node biopsy samples in patients with mononucleosis and a clinically typical course usually show pronounced follicular hyperplasia with atypical lymphocytes in the sinuses. Foci of necrosis may be observed. Atypical cells may be prominent and together with architectural effacement may mislead pathologists into a diagnosis of malignancy.[15] Cells indistinguishable from Reed-Sternberg cells have been noted.

One of the complications of mononucleosis can be a ruptured spleen resulting from minor trauma.[116] In such a case gross examination reveals a capsular tear with a subcapsular hematoma. Histologic examination shows the red pulp and the capsule to be infiltrated by atypical lymphocytes. The autopsy findings of a patient who died of mononucleosis have been described by Custer and Smith.[20] Liver biopsy specimens in patients with mononucleosis almost always show abnormality. Microscopically Kupffer cell activation is prominent as is infiltration of the portal triads with mononuclear cells.[92] Occasionally small foci of necrosis with eosinophilic bodies can be observed. Bone marrow granulomas have been reported in patients with infectious mononucleosis.[57]

Epstein-Barr virus reactivation can be detected serologically in immunosuppressed allograft recipients. Lack of control of cellular proliferation induced by Epstein-Barr virus may result in lymphoproliferative-disorders. This has been best documented in patients with the X-linked recessive lymphoproliferative syndrome.[104]

Papovaviruses

The name *papova* is an acronym derived from papilloma, polyoma, and simian vacuolating virus. This family of viruses can be divided in two genera, *Polyomarivirus* and *Papillomavirus*. Viruses of the polyoma genus have been studied the most because they have been known to cause tumors in experimental animals. Polyomaviruses can also transform cells in vitro, rendering oncogenic. The polyomavirus of mouse and the SV40 virus of monkeys have been intensely studied by molecular biologists. The genomes of SV40 and polyoma (3 × 10⁶ daltons) have been completely sequenced. The relevant human members of the family are JC and BK virus in the polyoma genus and human papillomavirus or human wart virus. All members replicate in the nuclei of mammalian cells and form nonenveloped nucleocapsids, 30 to 50 nm in diameter, containing the DNA genome.

Progressive multifocal leukoencephalopathy (PML) is a rare neurologic disease primarily affecting adults between 50 and 70 years of age. The neurologic manifestations of the disease indicate diffuse asymmetric involvement of the cerebral hemispheres. The duration from onset of symptoms to death is usually less than 6 months. PML is most often seen in immunocompromised hosts, especially in patients with leukemia, lymphoma, Hodgkin's disease, diffuse carcinomatosis, sarcoidosis, or tuberculosis. It has also been reported in patients with congenital immunodeficiencies. The incidence of PML is low; of 3000 consecutive autopsy cases studied by Del Duca and Morningstar,[23] PML was diagnosed in only two instances. The pathologic diagnosis of PML is usually established at postmortem examination, but it can be made on brain biopsy. At autopsy the lesions appear most often in the cerebrum, beneath the cortical ribbon, and look like small necrotic areas.[5] They tend to coalesce to form larger foci of demyelination. When several months old, the lesions appear as retracted foci grossly resembling a cerebral infarct. The distribution in the central nervous system is variable, with the cerebrum being the most frequently affected site.

Histopathologically the hallmark of the disease is the presence of oligodendrocytes with enlarged nuclei containing basophilic intranuclear inclusion bodies. Reactive hypertrophic astrocytes with giant hyperchromatic nuclei that often contain a cytoplasmic invagination are also typical, especially of the late stage of the lesion. No cytologic abnormalities are seen in neurons, ependymal cells, endothelial cells, or macrophages. Ultrastructural examination reveals the presence of viral capsids in the nuclei of the oligodendrocytes.[140] They are seldom seen in the giant astrocytes. A polyomavirus, named *JC virus*, has been consistently isolated in PML cases from brain tissue at biopsy or at autopsy.[98] Viral antigens can be shown to be present in the abnormal oligodendrocytes by immunohistochemical techniques. The disease has not been transmitted to experimental animals, but monkeys have a pathologic lesion identical to PML that has been shown to be caused by the SV40 virus, the polyomavirus of the monkey. Inoculation of JC virus into newborn hamsters causes a variety of tumors, often in the nervous system.[130]

BK virus, the other human polyomavirus, was first isolated by Gardner and co-workers[41] from the urine of a renal allograft recipient on immunosuppressive therapy. It has also been isolated from the urine of patients with Wiskott-Aldrich syndrome and from a biopsy specimen of a cerebral lymphoma in a child with Wiskott-Aldrich syndrome. Recent studies indicate that BK virus may be latent in the kidney and may be reactivated during the immunosuppressed state. BK virus, like JC virus, is capable of inducing tumors in the newborn hamster and transforming cells in vitro. No specific clinical syndrome has been unequivocally linked to BK infection. In patients with kidney transplants, urinary cytology may show cells with intranuclear inclusions very similar to those seen in the oligodendrocytes infected with JC virus. Similar inclusions have been observed in the urothelium of the renal pelvis and have been shown by electron microscopy to contain papovavirus capsids. Both BK and JC viruses are found throughout the world, and judged by the levels of antibody in sera, the prevalence of infection is high.

Papillomaviruses are distinguished from the polyoma group by the size of their capsid (55 nm in diameter) and the molecular weight of their genome—5 × 10⁶ daltons, compared to 3 × 10⁶ daltons in the polyoma genus. In addition, the genetic organization of papilloma virus differs in that in polyoma viruses separate DNA strands code for vegetative functions and structural proteins whereas in papilloma viruses there is only one coding strand.

Papillomaviruses are classified according to host range and relatedness of nucleic acid, and serology plays little role in the taxonomy of this group of viruses.

Over 30 types of human papillomavirus have been characterized, and they are classed into 15 groups, from A to O, the members of which cross-hybridize among themselves but show no significant homology to other groups when tested under stringent conditions.

Papillomaviruses are highly species specific and tissue specific. They are capable of inducing epithelial and mesenchymal proliferative lesions in a variety of animals. In the human the papillomaviruses are epitheliotropic and the benign virus-induced proliferative lesions have the potential for malignant conversion. Carcinomas can develop in long-lasting lesions when additional factors such as ultraviolet rays (for epidermodysplasia verruciformis) or x rays (for laryngeal papillomas) act on cells infected by human papillomavirus.

The role of papillomaviruses in cancer of the uterine cervix has received much attention in the recent years. The human papillomavirus types 16 and 18 are closely associated with human genital cancer, and expression of integrated viral genome or genomes is most likely necessary for the maintenance of the malignant state.[112] These two HPV types have also been associated with bowenoid papulosis.

The human diseases that are linked with productive infection of epithelial cells are warts (HPV types 1, 2, 3, 4, 7, 28, 29, 41), genital condylomas (HPV types 6, 16, 31, 18), bowenoid papulosis (HPV types 16, 18), laryngeal papillomas (HPV type 11), focal oral epithelial hyperplasia of Heck (HPV type 13), epidermodysplasia verruciformis (HPV types 5, 8, 9, 12, 19, 25), and dysplasia of the uterine cervix (HPV types 6, 11, 16, 18).

The viral genome is found in an episomal form in nontumoral or preneoplastic lesions whereas the genome is integrated in the host chromosome in cell lines derived of epidermoid carcinoma of the cervix.

Cutaneous warts (verruca vulgaris) are found anywhere on the skin. They are circumscribed nodular growths having a hyperkeratotic surface. Histologically, there is thickening of the epidermis caused by proliferation of epidermal cells. In some of the cells the nuclei are deeply basophilic, are surrounded by a clear halo, and can be shown by electron microscopy and immunocytochemistry to contain HPV particles or antigens.[3] Warts also often contain cells with vacuolated clear cytoplasm called "koilocytes" (Fig. 9-16). Skin warts may regress spontaneously, and at least two thirds of the cases do so. There is a high incidence of warts in immunosuppressed patients or patients with congenital immune deficiencies. Malignant transformation does not occur except in some patients with epidermodysplasia verruciformis.

Condylomata acuminata are verruciform anogenital lesions that are venerally transmitted.[84] They occur in young adults and are not associated with skin warts. Some of the condylomas may become very large (giant condyloma of Buschke-Löwenstein). Verrucous carcinoma may also be seen in large condylomatous lesions.

Papillomaviruses have also been implicated in *cervical dysplasia*, and they are often the cause of well-known cytologic alterations such as koilocytosis. The koilocytic cells have been shown by electron microscopy to contain papilloma particles in their nuclei.[78]

Multiple *laryngeal papillomas* occurring during infancy and childhood have also been linked epidemiologically and by means of immunocytochemistry to papilloma viruses.[17] The lesions appear grossly as thin,

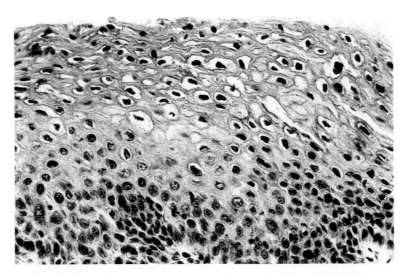

Fig. 9-16. Flat condylomatous lesion in a 20-year-old woman showing prominent koilocytic change in the superior layers of the epithelium. (Hematoxylin and eosin; 350×.)

whitish nodules, either sessile or pedunculated. Histologically they are composed of a fibrovascular core covered by thick, stratified, squamous epithelium. The lesions may exhibit malignant potential if irradiated.

Poxviridae

The poxviruses of mammals are a complex group of agents that produce vesicular skin lesions. They are the largest animal viruses, containing a double-stranded DNA genome of 200 million daltons. They are brick shaped, measuring 380 × 260 nm, and are very resistant to chemical and physical inactivation. They multiply in the cytoplasm of cells, and the virions mature in cytoplasmic foci or "viral factories." Some of the important pox-viruses are the etiologic agents for vaccinia, variola, ectromelia, monkeypox, and molluscum contagiosum.

As a result of the successful campaign sponsored by the World Health Organization (WHO), *smallpox* (variola) has been eradicated worldwide.[25,134] Variola infection is limited to humans, and study of the virus has been somewhat limited because of the laboratory hazards. There are at least two strains of variola virus; the most virulent causes variola major with a mortality of 20% to 50%. Variola minor, or alastrim, has a mortality of less than 1%. The two strains can be differentiated by their temperature-sensitive growth characteristics on chorioallantoic membrane. Variola virus is transmitted by close contact and is spread through the air, gaining entrance to the respiratory tract where it multiplies in the epithelium and regional lymph nodes. This first replicative period is followed by viremia with dissemination of the virus to the reticuloendothelial system. There follows a second replicative phase, in which a second viremia spreads to the skin, lymphatics, and internal organs. This secondary viremia marks the beginning of clinical symptoms. Clinically smallpox is characterized by fever followed a few days later by a centrifugal papular rash that appears first on the face and the skull and spreads to the back, chest, arms, and legs. The macules become papules, vesicles, and finally pustules (Fig. 9-17). The pustules dry up, forming scabs during the second week of the rash. The clinical disease produced by smallpox has a spectrum of severity that ranges from the very mild to the very severe and often fatal form. WHO describes four clinical types of smallpox: ordinary, modified, flat, and hemorrhagic. The third and fourth are the most severe.

The cutaneous lesions in the papular stage have a diameter of 2 to 4 mm and are partially buried in the skin. Microscopically the cutaneous lesions first show vascular congestion with mononuclear cell infiltrate in the dermis. The epidermal cells show ballooning degeneration with formation of an intraepidermal vesicle.[81] There is involvement of the adnexal elements.

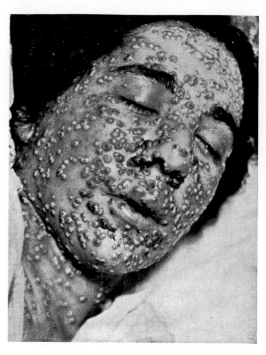

Fig. 9-17. Smallpox in unvaccinated woman. (Courtesy Dr. Samuel Sweitzer; from Sutton, R.I., Jr.: Diseases of the skin, ed. 11, St. Louis, 1956, The C.V. Mosby Co.)

Cells with cytoplasmic inclusion bodies (Guarnieri bodies) can be found in early vesicles and disappear with healing. These inclusion bodies are variable in size, granular, eosinophilic, round to oval, and surrounded by a halo. Electron microscopic examination of the epidermal lesions demonstrates the presence of "viral factories" in the cytoplasm of the infected cells.[19] In fatal cases pneumonia of the interstitial type is often seen. The viral lesions are often obscured by superimposed bacterial infection.

The present *vaccinia virus* is probably derived from the cowpox virus by the process of person-to-person vaccination. Jenner was the first to observe in 1798 that pustular material from the lesions of cowpox protected humans from infection with smallpox. Jenner's observations form the basis for vaccination. Vaccination results in a modified swelling at the site of vaccination and regional lymphadenopathy. Primary vaccination sites develop a vesicle within 3 to 5 days that will become pustular and reach maximum size after approximately 9 days. The lesion will form a scab and leave a small circular scar approximately 1 cm in diameter. Complications that result from vaccination are postvaccination encephalitis, vaccinia gangrenosa seen in patients with T-cell immune deficiencies, eczema vaccinatum seen in patients with atopic dermatitis, generalized vaccinia, and erythematous urticarial lesions.

Molluscum contagiosum is a benign skin disease of worldwide distribution characterized by the occurrence

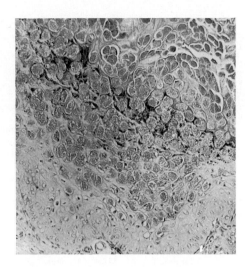

Fig. 9-18. Molluscum contagiosum.

of raised, umbilicated, waxy, cutaneous nodules. The lesions may be multiple or solitary. Histologically moluscum contagiosum is a proliferative lesion of the epidermal cells, which form a lobulated mass. The infected cells contain large intracytoplasmic eosinophilic inclusion bodies (Fig. 9-18).[52,73]

Two additional poxviruses that cause disease in humans are the paravaccinia virus of cattle, which produces milker's nodules, and orf virus of sheep, which causes contagious pustular dermatitis.

Hepatitis B virus

Hepatitis B virus infection is widespread throughout the world. Infection often occurs at very young ages. It is one of the most common persistent viral infections of humans. The hepatitis B virion is a complex structure measuring approximately 42 nm in diameter, possessing in its surface the hepatitis B surface antigen (HBsAg), an envelope, and an electron-dense 28 nm internal core or nucleocapsid containing a small DNA genome. Hepatitis B virus is a most unusual virus, and one of its unique properties is the configuration of the small circular DNA within the core of the virion (Dane particle). The circular DNA molecule is double stranded for about two thirds of its length and single stranded for the remainder. The DNA polymerase enzyme present in the core is probably responsible for closing the single-stranded gap upon infection and making a double-stranded circular DNA molecule of approximately 3200 nucleotide pairs. Present in the blood of infected patients are small spherical particles, 16 to 25 nm in diameter, that bear surface antigenic activity. Two additional antigenic activities are found associated with hepatitis B. One is the hepatitis B core antigen found associated with the dense nucleoprotein core of the viral particles (Dane particles).[21] Structures with the

morphology of the viral cores can be seen by electron microscopy in nuclei of hepatocytes infected with hepatitis B virus.[4,42] Another is the activity of the e antigen, which exists in serum as a large protein of approximately 300,000 daltons. Immunofluorescence straining of tissue sections for viral antigens indicates that hepatocytes may be the only cell type infected with hepatitis B virus during the persistent infection. During the acute phase of disease the majority of the hepatocytes appear to be infected.[47]

Blood and blood products are the best-documented vehicles for transmission of hepatitis B virus. In addition to serum, saliva and semen have been also shown to contain infectious virus in experimental transmission studies. Before screening of blood donors for hepatitis B antigen was introduced, from 1% to 10% of transfused patients acquired hepatitis. The pathology of hepatitis B is discussed in Chapter 25.

UNNAMED VIRUS-LIKE AGENTS PRODUCING DISEASE OF THE CENTRAL NERVOUS SYSTEM

The *spongiform encephalopathies* (kuru, Creutzfeldt-Jakob disease, scrapie, and transmissible mink encephalopathy) are caused by transmissible agents of very small size and of great resistance to inactivation with chemical and physical agents. These transmissible agents lack a demonstrable nucleic acid.[43] They have been termed by Gajdusek[38] "unconventional viruses," but it is still uncertain whether they should be considered viruses or members of a new group of microorganisms, perhaps similar to the viroids of plants.

Epidemiologically *kuru* has been confined to a primitive population in eastern New Guinea. The studies by Gajdusek suggested that kuru was transmitted by inoculation of infected tissue through skin cuts during participation of children and women in ritual cannibalism.[38] *Creutzfeldt-Jakob* disease is found throughout the world with a prevalence of approximately one case per million population. About 10% of the cases have an apparent inherited transmission, but the pattern is equivocal. Creutzfeldt-Jakob disease has been transmitted from human to human by corneal transplant and by contaminated sterotactic brain electrodes. No cases have been diagnosed among virologists working with the disease or pathologists studying Creutzfeldt-Jakob cases. The unusual resistance of the agents to inactivation by physical and chemical agents necessitates special precautions in dealing with patients and pathologic specimens.[39]

Both kuru and Creutzfeldt-Jakob disease are spongiform encephalopathies[45,70] showing diffuse loss of neurons, pronounced gliosis with proliferation of astrocytes, and vacuolization of the neuronal and glial processes. The lesions in kuru are most frequent in the cerebellar, cortex, pons, thalamus, and basal nuclei. Electron microscopic study of the neurons demonstrates fragments of curled membranous material within the vacuoles of the cytoplasm. No viral organisms can be visualized.

REFERENCES

1. Adams, J.H.: Virus diseases of the nervous system. In Blackwood, W., and Corseless, J.A.N., editors: Greenfield's neuropathology, Chicago, 1976, Year Book Medical Publishers.
2. Aherne, W., Bird, T., Court, S.D.M., Gardner, P.S., and McQuillin, J.: Pathological changes in virus infections of the lower respiratory tract in children J. Clin. Pathol. **23**:7, 1970.
3. Almeida, J.D., Howartson, A.F., and Williams, M.G.: Electron microscope study of human wart: sites of virus production and nature of the inclusion bodies, J. Invest. Dermatol. **38**:337, 1962.
4. Almeida, J.D., Waterson, A.P., and Trowell, J.M.: The findings of virus-like particles in two Autralian antigen positive human livers, Microbiology **2**:145, 1970.
5. Astrom, K.E., Mancall, E.L., and Richardson, E.P., Jr.: Progressive multifocal leukoencephalopathy, Brain **81**:93, 1958.
6. Baer, G.M., editor: The natural history of rabies, vols. I and II. New York, 1975, Academic Press.
7. Bastian, F.O., Rabson, A.S., Yee, C.L., and Tralka, T.S.: Herpes virus varicellae: isolated from human dorsal root ganglia, Arch. Pathol. **97**:331, 1974.
8. Berthiaume, L., Joncas, J., and Pavilanis, V.: Comparative structure, morphogenesis, and biological characteristics of the respiratory syncytial (RS) virus and the pneumonia virus of mice (PVM), Arch. Virol. **45**:39, 1974.
9. Bodian, D.: Histopathologic basis of the clinical findings poliomyelitis, Am. J. Med. **6**:563, 1949.
10. Bradley, D.W.: Hepatitis A virus infection: pathogenesis and serodiagnosis of acute diseases, J. Virol. Meth. **2**:31, 1960.
11. Camain, R., and Lambert, D.: Histopathologie des foies amarils prélevés post mortem et par ponction-biopsie hépatique, Bull. WHO **36**:129, 1967.
12. Casals, J., and Clarke, H.: Arboviruses group A. In Horsfall, F.L., and Tamm, I., editors: Viral and rickettsial infections of man, ed. 4, Philadelphia, 1965, J.B. Lippincott Co.
13. Chanock, R.M., Roydsman, B., and Meyers, R.: Recovery from infants with respiratory illness of a virus related to chimpanzee coryza agent (CCA). I. Isolation: properties and characterization, Am. J. Hygiene **66**:281, 1957.
14. Child, P.L., MacKenzie, R.B., Valverde, L.R., and Johnson, K.M.: Bolivian hemorrhagic fever, Arch. Pathol. **83**:434, 1967.
15. Childs, C.C., Parham, D.M., and Berard, C.W.: Infectious mononucleosis: the spectrum of morphologic changes simulating lymphoma in lymph nodes and tonsils, Am. J. Surg. Pathol. **11**:122-132, 1987.
16. Cooper, L.Z.: Congenital rubella in the United States. In Krugman, S., and Gershon, A., editors: Infections of the fetus and the newborn infant, New York, 1975, Alan R. Liss.
17. Costa, J., Howley, P.M., and Howard, R.B.: Presence of human papilloma viral antigens in juvenile multiple laryngeal papilloma, Am. J. Clin. Pathol. **75**:194, 1981.
18. Crosby, A.W.: Epidemic and peace, 1918, part IV, Westport, Conn., 1976, Greenwood Press.
19. Cruickshank, J.G., Bedson, H.S., and Watson: D.H.: Electron microscopy and the rapid diagnosis of smallpox, Lancet **2**:527, 1966.
20. Custer, R.P., and Smith, E.B.: Pathology of infectious mononucleosis, Blood **3**:830, 1948.
21. Dane, D.S., Cameron, C.H., and Briggs, M.: Virus-like particles in serum of patients with Australian antigen associated hepatitis, Lancet **1**:695, 1970.
22. Dayan, A.D., and Wilson, I.B.: Disseminated herpes zoster in the reticuloses, Am. J. Roentgenol. **92**:116, 1964.
23. Del Duca, V., and Morningstar, W.A.: Multiple myeloma associated with progressive multifocal leukoencephalopathy, JAMA **199**:671, 1967.
24. Dent, D.M., Duys, P.J., Bird, A.R.: Cytomegalic virus infection of bowel in adults, S. Afr. Med. J. **49**:669, 1975.
25. Dickson, C.W.: Smallpox, London, 1962, Churchill.
26. Dolin, R., Levy, A.G., Wyatt, R.G., et al.: Viral gastroenteritis induced by the Hawaii agent: jejunal histopathology and serologic response, Am. J. Med. **59**:761, 1975.
27. Dowdle, W.R., Noble, G.R., and Kendal, A.P.: Orthomyxovirus—influenza comparative diagnosis unifying concept. In Kurstak, E., and Kurstak, C.H., editors: Comparative diagnosis of viral diseases, New York, 1977, Academic Press, Inc.
28. Driscoll, S.G.: Histopathology of gestational rubella, Am. J. Dis. Child. **118**:49, 1969.
29. Dupont, J.R., and Earle, K.M.: Human rabies encephalitis: a study of 49 fatal cases with a review of the literature, Neurology (Minneap.) **15**:1023, 1965.
30. Enders, J.F.: Measles virus historical review isolation and behavior in various systems, Am. J. Dis. Child. **103**:282, 1962.
31. Enders, J.F., McCarthy, K., Mitus, A., and Cheatham, W.J.: Isolation of measles virus at autopsy in cases of giant cell pneumonia without rash N. Engl. J. Med. **261**:875, 1959.
32. Esterley, J.R., and Oppenheimer, E.H.: Intrauterine rubella infection. In Rosenberg, H.S., and Bolande, R.P., editors: Perspective in pediatric pathology, vol. I. Chicago, 1973. Year Book Medical Publishers.
33. Feinstone, S.M., Kapikian, A.Z., and Purcell, R.H.: Hepatitis A: detection by immune electron microscopy of a virus-like antigen associated with acute illness, Science **182**:1026, 1973.
34. Fenner, F.: The classification and nomenclature of viruses. Summary of results of meetings of the International Committee on Taxonomy of Viruses in Madrid, Sept. 1975, Virology **71**:371, 1976.
35. Ferris, J.A.J., Aherne, W.A., Locke, W.S., McQuillan, J., and Gardner, P.S.: Sudden and unexpected death in infants: histology and virology, Br. Med. J. **2**:439, 1973.
36. Finkeldey, W.: Über Riesenzellbefunde in den Gaumenmandeln, zugleich ein Beitrag zur Histopathologie der Mandelveränderungen im Maserninkubationsstadium, Virchows Arch. **281**:323, 1931.
37. Francis, T., Jr.: A new type of virus from epidemic influenza, Science **92**:405, 1914.
38. Gajdusek, D.C.: Unconventional viruses and the origin and disappearance of kuru, Science **197**:943, 1977.
39. Gajdusek, D.C., Gibbs, C.J., Jr., Asher, D.M., Brown, P., Diwan, A., Hoffman, P., Nemo, G., Rohwer, R., and White, L.: Precautions in medical care of, and in handling materials from patients with transmissible virus dementia (Creutzfeldt-Jakob disease), N. Engl. J. Med. **297**:1253, 1977.
40. Gardner, P.S., McQuillin, J., McGuckin, R., and Ditchburn, R.K.: Observations on clinical and immunofluorescent diagnosis of parainfluenza virus infections, Br. Med. J. **2**:1, 1971.
41. Gardner, S.D., Field, A.M., Coleman, D.V., and Hulme, B.: New human papovavirus (BK) isolated from urine after renal transplantation, Lancet **1**:1253, 1971.
42. Gerber, M.A., Hadziyannis, S., Vissoulis, C., Schaffner, F., Paronetto, F., and Popper, H.: Electron microscopy and immune electron microscopy of cytoplasmic hepatitis B antigen in hepatocytes, Am. J. Pathol. **75**:489, 1974.
43. Gibbs, C.J., and Gajdusek, D.C.: Studies on the viruses of acute spongiform encephalopathies using primates, the only available indicator, First Inter-American Conference on Conservation and Utilization of American Non-human Primates in Biomedical Research, Pan American Health Organization Scientific Publication **317**:831, 1976.
44. Gonatas, N.K.: Subacute sclerosing leucoencephalitis: electron microscopic and cytochemical observations on a cerebral biopsy, J. Neuropathol. Exp. Neurol. **25**:177, 1966.
45. Gonatas, N.K., Terry, F.D., and Vice, M.: Electron microscopic study in two cases of Jakob-Creutzfeldt disease, J. Neuropathol. Exp. Neurol. **25**:575, 1965.

46. Goodpasture, E.W., Auerbach, S.H., Swanson, H.S., and Cotter, E.F.: Virus pneumonia of infants secondary to epidemic infections, Am. J. Dis. Child. **57**:997, 1939.

47. Gudat, F., Bianchi, L., Sonnabend, W., Thiel, G., Aenishänslin, W., and Stadler, G.A.: Pattern of core and surface expression in liver tissue reflects state of specific immune response in hepatitis B, Lab. Invest. **32**:1, 1975.

48. Hamre, D.: Rhinoviruses. In Melnick, J.L., editor: Monographs in virology, 1, Basel, 1968, S. Karger AG.

49. Hanaoka, M.: Progress in adult T-cell leukemia research, Acta Pathol. Jpn. **32**(suppl. 1):171-185, 1982.

50. Hanshaw, J.B.: Congenital cytomegalovirus infection, N. Engl. J. Med. **288**:1406, 1973.

51. Harland, W.A., Adams J.H., and McSweeney, D.: Herpes simplex virus in acute necrotizing encephalitis, Lancet **2**:581, 1967.

52. Hasegawa, T., Fujiwara, E., Ametani, T., et al.: Further electron microscopic observation of molluscum contagiosum virus, Arch. Klin. Exp. Dermatol. **235**:319, 1969.

53. Haymaker, W.: Mosquito borne encephalitides. In Van Bogaert, L., et al., editors: Encephalitides, Amsterdam, 1961, Elsevier.

54. Heggie, A.D.: Pathogenesis of rubella exanthem: isolation of rubella virus from skin, N. Engl. J. Med. **285**:664, 1971.

55. Horta-Barbosa, L.H., Fucillo, D.A., and Sever, J.L.: Subacute sclerosing panencephalitis: isolation of measles virus from a brain biopsy, Nature **221**:974, 1969.

56. Horta-Barbosa, L., Hamilton, R., Wittig, B., Fucillo, D.A., and Sever, J.L.: Subacute sclerosing panencephalitis: isolation of suppressed measles virus from lymph node biopsies, Science **173**:840, 1971.

57. Hovder, F., and Sundberg, R.D.: Granulomatous lesions in the bone marrow in infectious mononucleosis, Blood **5**:209, 1950.

58. Hutchins, G.M., and Vie, S.A.: The progression of interstitial myocarditis to idiopathic endocardial fibroelastosis, Am. J. Pathol. **66**:483, 1972.

59. Imagaba, D.T.: Relationships among measles, canine distemper and rinderpest virus, Prog. Med. Virol. **10**:116, 1968.

60. Jacobson, I.M., Dienstag, J.L., Werner, B.G., Brettler, D.B., Levine, P.H., and Mushahwar, I.K.: Epidemiology and clinical impact of hepatitis D virus (delta) infection, Hepatology **5**:188, 1985.

61. Jaffe, E.S., Blattner, W.A., Blayney, D.W., Bunn, P.A., Jr., Cossman, J., Robert-Guroff, M., and Gallo, R.C.: The pathologic spectrum of HTLV-associated leukemia/lymphoma in the United States, Am. J. Surg. Pathol. **8**(4):264, 1984.

62. Johnson, C.B., and Goodpasture, E.W.: An investigation of the etiology of mumps, J. Exp. Med. **59**:1, 1934.

63. Johnson, H.N.: Visceral lesions associated with varicella, Arch. Pathol. **30**:292, 1944.

64. Johnson, K.M., Lange, J.V, Webb, P.A., and Murphy, F.A.: Isolation and partial characterization of a new virus causing acute hemorrhagic fever in Zaire, Lancet **1**:599, 1977.

65. Johnson, K.P., Lepov, M.L., and Johnson, R.T.: California encephalitis. I. Clinical and epidemiological studies, Neurology **8**:250, 1968.

66. Kapikian, A.Z., Kim, H.W., Wyatt, R.G., Cline, W.L., and Arrobio, J.O.: Human reovirus-like agent as the major pathogen associated with winter gastroenteritis and hospitalized infants and young children, N. Engl. J. Med. **294**:965, 1976.

67. Kapikian, A.Z., Wyatt, R.G., Dolin, R., Thornhill, T.S., Kelica, A.R., and Chanock, R.M.: Visualization by immune electron microscopy of a 27 nm. particle associated with acute infectious nonbacterial gastroenteritis, J. Virol. **10**:1075, 1972.

68. Kimura, A., Tosaka, K., and Nakao, T.: An immunofluorescence and electron microscopic study of measles skin eruptions, Tohoku J. Exp. Med. **117**:245, 1975.

69. Kimura, A., Tosaka, K., and Nakao, T.: Measles rash. I. Light and electron microscopic study of skin eruptions, Arch. Virol. **47**:95, 1975.

70. Klatzo, I., Gajdusek, D.C., and Zigas, V.: Pathology of kuru, Lab. Invest. **8**:799, 1959.

71. Lehmann-Grube, F.: Lymphocytic choriomeningitis virus, New York, 1971, Springer-Verlag.

72. Lin, J.H., Duffy, J.L., and Palladino, V.S.: Disseminated neonatal herpes simplex infection, NY State J. Med. **75**:608, 1975.

73. Lutzner, M.A.: Molluscum contagiosum, verruca and zoster viruses, Arch. Dermatol. **87**:436, 1963.

74. McIntosh, K., McQuillin, J., Reed, S.E., and Gardner, P.S.: Diagnosis of human coronavirus infection by immune fluorescence: method and application to respiratory disease in hospitalized children, J. Med. Virol. **2**:341, 1978.

75. McSorley, J., Shapiro, L., Brownstein, M.H., and Hsu, K.C.: Herpes simplex and varicella zoster: comparative histopathology of 77 cases, Int. J. Dermatol. **13**:69, 1974.

76. Manson, M.M., and Logan, W.P.D.: Rubella and other virus infections in pregnancy: reports on public health and medical subjects, No. 101, London, 1960, Ministry of Health.

77. Martini, G.A.: Marburg virus disease: the clinical syndrome. In Martini, G.A., and Siegert, R., editors: Marburg virus disease, Berlin, 1971, Springer-Verlag.

78. Meisels, A., Morin, C., and Casas-Cordero, M.: Lesions of the uterine cervix associated with papillomavirus and their clinical consequences. In Koss, L.G., and Coleman, D.C., editors: Advances in clinical cytology, vol. 2, New York, 1981, Butterworth & Co.

79. Meulen, V. ter, Müller, D., Käckell, M.Y., Katz, M., and Meyermann, R.: Isolation of infectious measles virus in measles encephalitis, Lancet **2**:1172, 1972.

80. Meyers, J.D., Spencer, H.C., Watts, J.C., Gregg, M.B., Stewart, J.A., Troupin, R.H. and Thomas, E.D.: Cytomegalovirus pneumonia after human marrow transplantation, Ann. Intern. Med. **82**:181, 1975.

81. Michaelson, H.E., and Ikeda, K.: Microscopic changes in variola, Arch. Belg. Dermatol. Syphiligr. **15**:138, 1927.

82. Moniff, G.R.G., Egan, E.A., II, Held, B., and Eitzman, D.V.: The correlation of maternal cytomegalovirus infection during varying stages in gestation with neonatal involvement, J. Pediatr. **80**:17, 1972.

83. Monto, A.S.: The Tecumseh study of respiratory illness. V. Patterns of infection with the parainfluenza viruses, Am. J. Epidemiol. **97**:338, 1973.

84. Morin, C., Brown, L., Casas-Cordero, M., Shah, K.V., Roy, M., Fortier, M., and Meisels, A.: Confirmation of the papilloma virus etiology of condylomatous cervix lesions by the peroxidase antiperoxidase technique, J. Natl. Canc. Inst. **66**:831, 1981.

85. Morris, J.A., Blunt, R.E., and Savage, R.E.: Recovery of cytopathogenic agent from chimpanzees with coryza, Proc. Soc. Exp. Biol. Med. **92**:544, 1956.

86. Murphy, F.A., Halomen, P.E., and Harrison, A.K.: Electron microscopy of the devolopment of rubella virus in BHK-21 cells, J. Virol. **2**:1223, 1968.

87. Murphy, F.A., and Whitfield, S.G.: Morphology and morphogenesis of arenaviruses, Bull. WHO **52**:408, 1975.

88. Murphy, F.A., Harrison, A.K., Winn, W.C., and Bauer, S.P.: Comparative pathogenesis of rabies and rabies-like viruses, Lab. Invest. **29**:1, 1973.

89. Nahmias, J.A.: Disseminated herpes simplex infection, N. Engl. J. Med. **282**:684, 1970.

90. Nakai, M., and Imagaba, D.T.: Electron microscopy of measles virus replication, J. Virol. **3**:187, 1969.

91. Negri, A.: Beitrag zum Studium der Aetiologie der Tollwuth, Z. Hyg. Infektionskrankh. **43**:507, 1903.

92. Nelson, R.S., and Darragh, J.H.: Infectious mononucleosis hepatitis: a clinicopathological study, Am. J. Med. **21**:26, 1956.

93. Neurotropic diseases surveillance, Poliomyelitis Summary 1974-1976, Atlanta, 1977, Center for Disease Control.

94. Nieberg, K.C., and Blumberg, J.M.: Viral encephalitides. In Minckler, J., editor: Pathology of the nervous system, vol. 3, New York, 1972, McGraw-Hill Book Co.

95. Nisenbaum, C., Wallis, K., and Henzey, E.: Varicella pneumonia in children, Helv. Paed. Acta **24**:212, 1969.

96. Olding-Stenkvist, E., and Grandien, M.: Early diagnosis of virus caused vesicular rashes by immunofluorescence on skin biopsy. I. Varicella zoster and herpes simplex virus, Scand. J. Infect. Dis. **8**:27, 1976.

97. Olding-Stenkvist, E., and Kreuger, A.: Clinical features of acute gastroenteritis associated with rotavirus, enteric adenoviruses and bacteria, Arch. Dis. Child. **61:**732, 1986.

98. Padgett, B.L., Walker, D.L., ZuRhein, G.M., and Eckroade, R.J.: Cultivation of papova-like virus from human brain with progressive multifocal leukoencephalopathy, Lancet **1:**1257, 1971.

99. Palese, P., and Compans, R.W.: Characterization of temperature sensitive influenza virus mutants defective in neuroaminidase, Virology **61:**397, 1974.

100. Parrott R.H., Kim, H.W., Arrobio, J.O., Hodes, D.S., Murphy, B.R., Brandt, C.D., Camargo, E.R., and Chanock, R.M.: Epidemiology of respiratory syncytial virus infection in Washington, D.C. II. Infection and disease with respect to age, immunological status, race and sex, Am. J. Epidemiol. **98:**289, 1973.

101. Pattengale, P.K., Smith, R.W., and Perlin, E.: Atypical lymphocytes in acute infectious mononucleosis identification by multiple T and B lymphocyte markers, N. Engl. J. Med. **291:**1145, 1974.

102. Porterfield, J.S., et al.: Bunyaviruses and Bunyaviridae, Intervirology **2:**270, 1974.

103. Price, R.W., Brew, B., Sidtis, J., Rosenblum, M., Scheck, A.C., and Cleary, P.: The brain in AIDS: central nervous system HIV-I infection and AIDS dementia complex, Science **239:**586, 1988.

104. Purtillo, D.T., Yang, J.P., Allegra, S., DeFlorio, D., Hutt, L.M., Soltani, M., and Vawter, G.: Hematopathology and pathogenesis of the X-linked recessive lymphoproliferative syndrome, Am. J. Med. **62:**219, 1977.

105. Reichert, C.M., O'Leary, T.J., Levens, D.L., Simrell, C.R., and Macher, A.M.: Autopsy pathology in acquired immune deficiency syndrome, Am. J. Pathol. **112:**357, 1983.

106. Rose, A.G., and Becker, W.B.: Disseminated herpes simplex infection: retrospective study by light microscopy and electron microscopy of paraffin embedded tissues, J. Clin. Pathol. **25:**79, 1972.

107. Rowe, W.P., et al.: Isolation of a cytopathogenic agent from human adenoids undergoing spontaneous degeneration in tissue culture, Proc. Soc. Exp. Biol. Med. **84:**570, 1958.

108. St. Geme, J.W., Peralta, H., Farias, E., Davis, C.W.C., and Noren, G.R.: Experimental gestational mumps virus infection and endocardial fibroelastosis, Pediatrics **48:**821, 1971.

109. Salvador, A.H., Harrison, E.G., and Kyle, R.A.: Lymphadenopathy due to infectious mononucleosis: its confusion with malignant lymphoma, Cancer **27:**1029, 1971.

110. Schellmann, J., and Samson, J.G.: Prodromal stages of measles diagnosed at autopsy, J. Pediatr. **67:**39, 1965.

111. Schreiber, D.S., Blacklow, N.R., and Trier, G.S.: Mucosa lesion of the proximal small intestine in acute infectious non-bacterial gastroenteritis, N. Engl. J. Med. **228:**1318, 1973.

112. Schneider-Gadicke, A., and Schwarz, E.: Transcription of human papillomavirus type-18 DNA in human cervical carcinoma cell lines, Hämatol. Bluttransfus. **31:**380, 1987.

113. Schulze, I.T.: The structure of influenza virus. I. The polypeptides of the virion, Virology **42:**890, 1970.

114. Siegel, M.S.: Congenital malformations following chicken pox, measles, mumps and hepatitis: results of a cohort study, JAMA **226:**1521, 1973.

115. Smetana, H.F.: The histopathology of experimental yellow fever, Virchows Arch. [Pathol. Anat.] **335:**411, 1962.

116. Smith, E.B., and Custer, R.P.: Rupture of spleen in infectious mononucleosis: clinical pathological report of seven cases, Blood **1:**317, 1946.

117. Smith, T.F., Holley, K.E., Keys, T.F., and Macasaet, F.F., Cytomegalovirus studies of autopsy tissue. I. Virus isolation, Am. J. Clin. Pathol. **63:**854, 1975.

118. Smith, W., Andrewes, C.H., and Laidlaw, P.P.: A virus obtained from influenza patients, Lancet **2:**66, 1933.

119. Solinga, D.W.R., Bang, L.J., and Ackerman, A.B.: Role of measles virus in skin lesions and Koplick spots, N. Engl. J. Med. **283:**1139, 1970.

120. Spurance, S.L., and Bailey, A.: Colorado tick fever: a review of 115 laboratory confirmed cases, Arch. Intern. Med. **131:**228, 1973.

121. Strano, A.J., and Henson, D.E.: Fatal adenovirus pneumonia: a study of 17 cases, Lab. Invest. **31:**346, 1975. (Abstract.)

122. Sung, J.H., Hayano, M., Mastri, A.R., and Okagaki, T.: A case of human rabies and ultrastructure of the Negri body, J. Neuropathol. Exp. Neurol. **35:**541, 1976.

123. Taylor, F.B., and Torenson, W.E.: Primary mumps meningeal encephalitis, Arch. Intern. Med. **112:**216, 1963.

124. Taylor, R.M.: A further note on 1233 (influenza C) virus, Arch. Gesamte Virusforschung **4:**85, 1951.

125. Telle, Z., Nagol, J., and Harter, D.H.: Subacute sclerosing leukoencephalitis: ultrastructure of intranuclear and intracytoplasmic inclusions, Science **154:**899, 1966.

126. Tucker, E.S., and Scofield, G.E.: Hepatoadrenal necrosis: fatal systemic herpes simplex virus infection: review of the literature and report of two cases, Arch. Pathol. **71:**538, 1961.

127. Tyrrell, D.A.J., and Bynoe, M.L.: Cultivation of a novel type of common-cold virus in organ cultures, Br. Med. J. **5448:**1467, 1965.

128. Tyrrell, D.A.J., Almeida, J.D., Berry, D.M., Cunningham, C.H., Hamre, D., Hofstad, M.S., Mallucci, L., and McIntosh, K.: Coronaviruses, Nature **220:**650, 1968.

129. Walker, D.H., Wulff, H., Lange, J.V., and Murphy, F.A.: Comparative pathology of Lassa virus infection in monkeys, guinea pigs, and *Mastomys natalensis*, Bull. WHO **52:**523, 1975.

130. Walker, D.L., Padgett, B.L., ZuRhein, G.M., and Albert, A.E.: Human papovavirus (JC): induction of brain tumors in hamsters, Science **187:**674, 1973.

131. Warthin, A.S.: Occurrence of numerous large giant cells in tonsils and pharyngeal mucosa in prodromal stage of measles: report of four cases, Arch. Pathol. **11:**864, 1931.

132. Webster, R.G., Campbell, C.H., and Granoff, A.: In vivo production of new influenza A viruses. I. Genetic recombination between avian and mammalian influenza viruses, Virology **44:**317, 1971.

133. WHO Memorandum: Pathogenic mechanism in dengue hemorrhagic fever: report of an international collaborative study, Bull. WHO **48:**117, 1973.

134. WHO Technical Report, Series no. 493, WHO Expert Committee on Smallpox Irradication, second report, Geneva, 1972, World Health Organization.

135. Wind, W.C., Jr., and Walker, D.H.: Pathology of human Lassa fever, Bull. WHO **52:**535, 1975.

136. Wright, H.D., Jr., Beckwith, J.B., and Guinn, J.L.: A fatal case of inclusion body pneumonia in an infant infected with adenovirus type III, Gen. Pediatr. **64:**528, 1964.

137. Young, N., Coxsackievirus and echovirus. In Mandell, G.L., Douglas, G., and Bennett, J.E., editors: Principles and practice of infectious diseases, New York, 1979, John Wiley & Sons.

138. Zingerling, A.: Pecularities of lesions in viral and mycoplasma infections of the respiratory tract, Virchows Arch. [Pathol. Anat.] **356:**259, 1972.

139. Zimmerman, L.E., and Binford, C.H.: Pathology of epidemic hemorrhagic fever, AFIP Syllabus, Oct. 1953, Armed Forces Institute of Pathology.

140. ZuRhein, G.M., and Aron, J.M.: Particles resembling papovaviruses in human cerebral demyelinating disease, Science **148:**1477, 1965.

10 Mycotic, Actinomycotic, and Algal Infections

FRANCIS W. CHANDLER
JOHN C. WATTS

Fungi are eukaryotic, unicellular, or filamentous organisms that are ubiquitous in nature. Most are saprophytes that live in organic debris or in soil enriched with organic matter. Of over 100,000 fungal species, only about 150 are pathogenic for humans. Their ability to cause disease depends on the virulence and dose of the agent, the route of infection, and the immunologic status of the host. Fungal diseases can be grouped arbitrarily into three broad categories based on the predominant location of infection within the body: superficial, cutaneous and subcutaneous, and systemic. The histopathologic features of the more common mycoses (fungal diseases) in each of these categories are summarized in Table 10-1.

The *superficial mycoses* are those in which the fungus is usually confined to the keratinized layer of the skin and its appendages. Because fungal growth is superficial, there is little or no inflammatory response. These infections are the more common of the mycoses, cause minor discomfort, and are primarily of cosmetic importance. They are rarely encountered by the histopathologist. The *cutaneous* and *subcutaneous mycoses* are a polymorphic group of diseases caused by a wide variety of fungi. These fungi enter the skin and subcutaneous tissues as a result of traumatic implantation or contamination of open wounds. Although infections usually remain localized, they occasionally spread through the lymphatics to involve other sites. The *systemic mycoses* usually have a pulmonary inception, from where they may disseminate to other organs. The gastrointestinal tract is occasionally a primary focus of infection, and primary cutaneous forms of the systemic mycoses rarely occur as a result of direct inoculation of an agent after injury. In some patients, systemic infections are asymptomatic. In other patients, they produce severe disease, which can be fatal if not promptly diagnosed and treated.

Traditionally, actinomycosis and nocardiosis have fallen within the province of medical mycology and are therefore included in this chapter, even though their etiologic agents are filamentous bacteria in the order Actinomycetales and not true fungi. Diseases caused by the *Prototheca* spp. are also included, though these agents are considered by most taxonomists to be achloric mutants of green algae. For further information on the taxonomy of the fungi and classification of mycotic and actinomycotic diseases, several references are recommended.[4,8,11,13]

Except for tinea versicolor, the dermatophytoses, and candidiasis in the newborn, there is no clear-cut evidence that the mycoses are communicable. Most mycoses are contracted by exposure to environmental sources. A few, such as actinomycosis and candidiasis, are endogenous. The agents of these endogenous infections occur as commensals on the skin and mucous membranes and in the gastrointestinal tract.

Although some of the systemic mycoses, such as coccidioidomycosis and histoplasmosis, are caused by fungi that are familiar pathogens, many others are caused by "opportunistic" fungi. These opportunists are saprophytes that are usually innocuous and assume the role of pathogens only under conditions that render a host abnormally susceptible to infection.[2,9,16] They rarely infect the noncompromised, healthy person. During the past two decades, there has been an alarming increase in the incidence of opportunistic infections, particularly candidiasis, aspergillosis, cryptococcosis, zygomycosis, and nocardiosis. Contributing to this increased incidence is the widespread use of modern medical treatments that predispose patients to infection, such as cancer chemotherapeutic agents, irradiation, immunosuppressive agents, hyperalimentation, and the prolonged and frequent use of broad-spectrum antibiotics. Persons with malignancies (especially leukemia and lymphoma), burns, organ transplants, metabolic diseases, malnutrition, the acquired immunodeficiency syndrome, or inborn immunologic deficiencies, and those who have undergone abdominal or cardiac surgery or who have received repeated intravenous injections are at special risk for mycotic infections. Some of the basic alterations

Table 10-1. Histologic features of the more common mycoses

Disease	Biologic agent(s)	Typical morphology in tissue	Usual host reaction
SUPERFICIAL MYCOSES			
Black piedra	*Piedraia hortae*	Pigmented, closely septate hyphae, 4-6 μmD, organized as nodules surrounding hair shaft; asci containing ascospores may also be present	None; involves the hair exclusively
Tinea nigra	*Phaeoannellomyces werneckii, Stenella araguata*	Pigmented, branched, septate hyphae, 1-3 μmD; elongated budding cells, 1-5 μmD	Mild to moderate hyperkeratosis; little or no dermatitis
Tinea versicolor	*Malassezia furfur*	Short, curved, and bent, hyaline hyphae, 2-4 μmD; clusters of oval or round, thick-walled cells (phialoconidia), 3-8 μmD	Like tinea nigra
White piedra	*Trichosporon beigelii*	Hyaline hyphae, 2-4 μmD; arthroconidia and blastoconidia organized as nodules surrounding hair shaft; invades and destroys hair	Like black piedra
Dermatophytosis	Pathogenic members of the genera *Epidermophyton, Microsporum,* and *Trichophyton*	Hyaline, septate hyphae that break up into chains of arthroconidia	Hyperkeratosis, acanthosis, and mild mononuclear infiltrate in dermis; rarely, suppurative or granulomatous
CUTANEOUS AND SUBCUTANEOUS MYCOSES			
Chromoblastomycosis	*Cladosporium carrionii, Fonsecaea compacta, F. pedrosoi, Phialophora verrucosa, Rhinocladiella aquaspersa*	Large, 6-12 μmD, spherical to polyhedral, thick-walled, dark brown muriform cells (sclerotic bodies) with septations along one or two planes; pigmented hyphae sometimes present	Mixed suppurative and granulomatous
Lobomycosis	*Loboa loboi*	Spherical, budding yeastlike cells, 5-12 μmD, that form chains of cells connected by tubelike isthmuses; secondary budding may be present	Granulomatous
Mycetoma (actinomycotic)	*Actinomadura madurae, A. pelletieri, Streptomyces somaliensis, Nocardia* spp., and others	Granules, 0.1 to several mmD, composed of delicate filaments (about 1 μmD) that are often branched and beaded	Like actinomycosis
Mycetoma (eumycotic)	*Pseudallescheria boydii, Madurella grisea, M. mycetomatis, Curvularia geniculata, Exophiala jeanselmei, Leptosphaeria senegalensis,* and others	Granules, 0.2 to several mm D, composed of broad (2-6 μm), hyaline (white to yellow granules) or dematiaceous (black granules) septate hyphae that often branch and form chlamydoconidia	Like actinomycosis
Prototheca	*Prototheca wickerhamii, P. zopfii*	Spherical, oval, or polyhedral sporangia, 2-25 μmD, that, when mature, contain 2 to 20 sporangiospores	Varies from little or no reaction to granulomatous

D, Diameter.

Table 10-1. Histologic features of the more common mycoses—cont'd

Disease	Biologic agent(s)	Typical morphology in tissue	Usual host reaction
CUTANEOUS AND SUBCUTANEOUS MYCOSES—cont'd			
Rhinosporidiosis	*Rhinosporidium seeberi*	Large sporangia, 100-350 μmD, with thin walls (3-5 μm) that enclose numerous sporangiospores, 6-8 μmD	Nonspecific chronic inflammatory or granulomatous
Sporotrichosis	*Sporothrix schenckii*	Pleomorphic, spherical to oval and, at times, cigar-shaped yeastlike cells, 2-10 μmD, that produce single and, rarely, multiple buds	Mixed suppurative and granulomatous; Splendore-Hoeppli material surrounds fungus in some cases (asteroid body)
Subcutaneous phaeohyphomycosis	*Exophiala jeanselmei, Phialophora parasitica, P. richardsiae, Wangiella dermatitidis,* and others	Pigmented (brown) hyphae, 2-6 μmD, branched or unbranched, and often constricted at their frequent and prominent septations; yeast forms and chlamydoconidia sometimes present	Subcutaneous cystic or solid granulomas; overlying epidermis rarely affected
Subcutaneous zygomycosis (entomophthoromycosis)	*Basidiobolus ranarum, Conidiobolus coronatus*	Short, poorly stained hyphal fragments, 6-25 μmD, with nonparallel sides, infrequent septa, and random branches	Eosinophilic abscesses and granulation tissue; hyphal fragments bordered by prominent Splendore-Hoeppli material
SYSTEMIC MYCOSES			
Actinomycosis	*Actinomyces israelii, A. naeslundii, A. viscosus, A. odontolyticus, A. bovis, Arachnia propionica, Rothia dentocariosa*	Organized aggregates (granules) composed of delicate, branched filaments about 1 μmD; entire granules 30-3000 μmD	Suppurative with multiple abscesses, extensive fibrosis, and formation of sinus tracts; Splendore-Hoeppli material usually borders granules
Adiaspiromycosis	*Chrysosporium (Emmonsia) parvum* var. *crescens*	Large adiaconidia, 200-400 μmD, with thick (20-70 μm) walls	Granulomatous, fibrotic, and noncaseating
Aspergillosis	*Aspergillus fumigatus* group, *A. flavus* group, *A. niger* group, and other aspergilli	Septate, dichotomously branched hyphae of uniform width (3-6 μm); conidial heads may be formed in cavitary lesions	Nodular infarcts; rarely granulomatous or suppurative; tendency for angioinvasion
Blastomycosis	*Blastomyces dermatitidis*	Spherical, multinucleated yeastlike cells, 8-15 μmD, with thick walls and single, broad-based buds	Mixed suppurative and granulomatous
Candidiasis	*Candida albicans, C. tropicalis, C. parapsilosis, C. krusei, C. pseudotropicalis, C. guilliermondii, C. stellatoidea*	Oval, budding yeastlike cells, 2-6 μmD, and pseudohyphae; septate hyphae may also be present	Suppurative, less commonly granulomatous or infarctive; minimal inflammation in preterminal infections
Coccidioidomycosis	*Coccidioides immitis*	Spherical, thick-walled, endosporulating spherules, 30-200 μmD; mature spherules contain small, 2-5 μD, uninucleate endospores; arthroconidia and hyphae may be formed in cavitary lesions	Mixed suppurative and granulomatous

Continued.

Table 10-1. Histologic features of the more common mycoses—cont'd

Disease	Biologic agent(s)	Typical morphology in tissue	Usual host reaction
SYSTEMIC MYCOSES—cont'd			
Cryptococcosis	*Cryptococcus neoformans*	Pleomorphic yeastlike cells, 2-20 μmD, with gelatinous, carminophilic capsules and single or multiple narrow-based buds; some strains poorly encapsulated and may not be carminophilic	Varies from minimal reaction ("cystic" or "mucoid" lesion) to granulomatous
Fusariosis	*Fusarium moniliforme, F. oxysporum, F. solani*	Septate hyphae that are uniform in width (3-8 μm) and branch at right angles	Like aspergillosis
Geotrichosis	*Geotrichum candidum*	Septate, infrequently branched hyphae, 3-6 μm wide; spherical yeastlike cells; and rectangular or oval arthroconidia, 4-10 μm wide, with rounded or squared ends	Varies from minimal reaction to acute suppurative inflammation and necrosis
Histoplasmosis capsulati	*Histoplasma capsulatum* var. *capsulatum*	Spherical to oval budding yeastlike cells, 2-4 μmD; often clustered because of growth within mononuclear phagocytes (reticuloendothelial mycosis)	Granulomatous, caseating or noncaseating; parasitization of histiocytes may cause bland necrosis
Histoplasmosis duboisii	*Histoplasma capsulatum* var. *duboisii*	Spherical to oval, uninucleate, thick-walled yeastlike cells, 8-15 μmD, that bud by a narrow base, creating typical "hourglass" or "figure-eight" forms	Granulomatous; many fungi in cytoplasm of huge multinucleated giant cells
Nocardiosis	*Nocardia asteroides, N. brasiliensis, N. otitidis-caviarum*	Long, delicate (about 1 μmD), branched filaments that are gram-positive, weakly acid-fast, and often beaded	Suppurative
Paracoccidioidomycosis	*Paracoccidioides brasiliensis*	Large spherical yeastlike cells, 5-60 μmD, with multiple buds attached by narrow necks ("steering wheel" forms)	Mixed suppurative and granulomatous; like blastomycosis

believed to be responsible for this increased susceptibility are leukopenia, suppression of humoral and cellular immunity, suppression of the acute inflammatory response, neutrophil or mononuclear phagocyte dysfunction, disruption of mucosal and cutaneous barriers, and reduction of the bacterial flora of the body that normally inhibit fungal overgrowth. Other factors contributing to the increased incidence of certain mycoses include migration of susceptible persons into highly endemic areas, aging of the population, and greater awareness of fungal infections in compromised hosts. In the future, "new" opportunists will surely be recognized as agents of disease in the abnormal host.

There are four basic approaches to the diagnosis of mycotic diseases: (1) clinical, (2) mycologic, (3) immunologic, and (4) pathologic.[1,5-8,11-14] Diseases caused by fungi may be difficult to distinguish, both clinically and pathologically, from those caused by other microbial agents. Because serologic tests have certain limitations and have not been developed for some fungal diseases, a definitive diagnosis of a mycotic disease often rests on direct microscopic demonstration of a fungus in tissues and exudates, or on the isolation and identification of it in culture. Histopathology should not be a substitute for microbiologic culture, but rather the two should complement each other whenever possible. When cultural studies are not possible, as when only fixed tissues are available, a histopathologist can nevertheless provide a presumptive or specific diagnosis of a mycotic

Table 10-1. Histologic features of the more common mycoses—cont'd

Disease	Biologic agent(s)	Typical morphology in tissue	Usual host reaction
SYSTEMIC MYCOSES—cont'd			
Penicilliosis marneffei	*Penicillium marneffei*	Spherical to oval yeastlike cells, 2.5-5 μmD, with a single transverse septum; short hyphal forms and elongated, curved "sausage" forms with one or more septa may be formed in necrotic and cavitary lesions	Like histoplasmosis capsulati
Pseudallescheriasis	*Pseudallescheria boydii*	Septate, randomly branched hyphae, 2-5 μm wide; conidia of scedosporium type may be formed in cavitary lesions	Like aspergillosis
Systemic phaeohyphomycosis	*Xylohypha bantiana, Bipolaris hawaiiensis,* and others	Pigmented (brown) hyphae, 2-6 μm wide, that may be branched or unbranched and are often constricted at their frequent and prominent septations	Mixed suppurative and granulomatous; large abscesses surrounded by giant cells
Torulopsosis	*Torulopsis glabrata*	Spherical to oval yeastlike cells, 2-5 μmD	Varies from minimal reaction to suppurative and granulomatous
Trichosporonosis	*Trichosporon beigelii, T. cutaneum*	Blastoconidia, 3-8 μmD, septate hyphae, and arthroconidia	Like candidiasis
Zygomycosis (mucormycosis)	*Absidia corymbifera, Apophysomyces elegans, Cunninghamella bertholletiae, Mucor ramosissimus, Rhizomucor pusillus, Rhizopus oryzae, R. rhizopodiformis, Saksenaea vasiformis,* and others	Broad, thin-walled, infrequently septate hyphae, 6-25 μm wide, with nonparallel sides and random branches	Suppurative necrosis, less commonly granulomatous; tendency for angioinvasion and infarction

disease if the agent can be detected in a tissue section and accurately identified. The agents of some mycoses, such as lobomycosis and rhinosporidiosis, have not yet been isolated in culture on synthetic media, and the only means of establishing a diagnosis is by direct microscopic examination of tissue or exudate. Although certain inflammatory patterns indicate the possible presence of a fungus, the diagnosis of a mycotic infection can never be based on the tissue reaction alone.[1,3-5,15]

Histopathologic evaluation provides indisputable evidence of tissue invasion and therefore can confirm the pathogenic significance of a cultural isolate that belongs to the normal body flora or that is usually encountered as an environmental contaminant in culture. Histopathology can also confirm the presence of coexisting infections by other fungi, bacteria, viruses, and protozoa, thus guiding the clinician in selecting the most appropriate therapy and management for the patient. No other diagnostic approach can assess whether the host response signifies tissue invasion or a purely allergic reaction, such as invasive versus allergic pulmonary aspergillosis.

Even though most fungi can be isolated from clinical materials, the cultivation and characterization of an isolate may take weeks, and the clinician usually cannot wait to begin therapy. Because the management of one mycosis may be entirely different from that of another, the pathologist must often play a key role in recognizing the mycoses and identifying their etiologic agents. In attempting to identify fungi using conventional histologic methods, it is helpful to remember that these microbes appear in tissue either as hyphae, yeastlike cells, endosporulating spherules, or a combination of these forms. Based on the morphologic distinctiveness of their etiologic agents in tissue, the mycoses can be grouped as follows[4,5]:

1. *Those caused by fungi that can be identified because they have a distinctive morphology in tissue.* If typical forms are observed, a specific diagnosis can be made (for example, adiaspiromycosis, blastomycosis, coccidioidomycosis, cryptococcosis, histoplasmosis capsulati, histoplasmosis duboisii, lobomycosis, paracoccidioidomycosis, protothecosis, rhinosporidiosis, sporotrichosis).

2. *Those caused by any one of several species of a genus that are so similar morphologically that they can be identified only to the genus level.* Nevertheless, the diseases they cause can be diagnosed generically (for example, aspergillosis, candidiasis, nocardiosis).

3. *Those caused by any of a number of fungi belonging to various genera that appear similar if not identical to one another in tissue.* Although the agent cannot be specifically identified, the mycosis can still be named (for example, actinomycosis, chromoblastomycosis, dermatophytosis, phaeohyphomycosis, zygomycosis).

4. *Mycetomas, which are special cases that constitute a group by themselves.* Because most agents of mycetoma form their own distinctive type of granule, the experienced microscopist can often identify the etiologic agent by observing the size, shape, architecture (morphology of mycelial elements and their arrangement), and color of a granule. One can determine if the granule is composed of an actinomycete (filamentous bacterium) or a eumycete (true fungus), and whether it is hyaline (white grain) or dematiaceous (black grain).

Although some fungi can be detected in hematoxylin and eosin—stained tissue sections, special histologic stains are usually necessary to demonstrate their morphology in detail. A list of these stains and their diagnostic applications are given in Table 10-2.

Direct fluorescent antibody (DFA) staining of tissue sections is a valuable adjunctive procedure that can be used to confirm a presumptive histopathologic diagnosis.[4,5,10,12] Formalin-fixed, paraffin-embedded tissues are adequate for DFA studies of fungi because the polysaccharide antigens in fungal cell walls are not destroyed by formalin fixation. Because of the added dimension of serologic specificity, DFA can greatly increase the accuracy of conventional histologic evaluation, especially when only atypical forms of a fungus are present. A broad battery of sensitive and specific fluorescent antibody (FA) reagents is available for detecting and identifying many of the common pathogenic

Table 10-2. Useful stains for demonstrating fungi and actinomycetes in tissue sections

Stains	Diagnostic applications
Hematoxylin and eosin (H&E)	Demonstrates tissue response and some fungi, including those that are naturally pigmented; stains nuclei of some yeastlike cells
Special stains for fungi 　Gomori methenamine-silver (GMS) 　Periodic acid–Schiff (PAS) 　Gridley fungus (GF) 　GMS with H&E counterstain (GMS/H&E)	Excellent for detecting fungi and studying their morphology in detail; GMS is best for screening, and it also stains the actinomycetes; GMS/H&E demonstrates fungi and tissue components simultaneously
Mucin stains 　Mayer's mucicarmine 　Southgate's mucicarmine 　Alcian blue	Demonstrate mucoid capsule of *Cryptococcus neoformans,* thus differentiating this fungus from others of similar morphology
Modified Gram stains 　Brown and Brenn (B&B) 　Brown-Hopps (Humberstone)	Demonstrate gram-positive filaments of the actinomycetes and nonfilamentous bacteria of botryomycosis; some fungi, especially the *Candida* spp., are gram-positive
Modified acid-fast stains 　Fite-Faraco 　Kinyoun's 　Ziehl-Neelsen	Demonstrate filaments of the *Nocardia* spp., most of which are weakly acid-fast; fungal cell walls and the agents of actinomycosis are not acid-fast
Giemsa stains 　May-Grunwald 　Wolbach's	Demonstrate kinetoplast of leishmanial forms and intracystic sporozoites of *Pneumocystis carinii;* both are protozoans that may be mistaken for fungi
Melanin stains 　Fontana-Masson	Confirms and accentuates the presence of melanin or melanin-like substances in the lightly pigmented agents of phaeohyphomycosis; stains the cell wall of *Cryptococcus neoformans,* which contains silver-reducing substances, possibly melanin precursors

fungi, actinomycetes, and protothecae in tissue sections.[10,12] Only a few specialized diagnostic centers can presently perform these tests. In the future, however, specific FA reagents should become readily available to most hospital and public health laboratories.

Because mycologic terminology is highly specialized and essential for a discussion of fungi, actinomycetes, and algae in tissue sections, the following terms that pertain to these agents are defined:

arthroconidium Conidium formed by mycelial disarticulation

bud (blastoconidium) Conidium produced by lateral outgrowth from a parent cell; buds may be single or multiple

chlamydoconidium Thick-walled, rounded, resistant conidium formed by direct differentiation of the mycelium

conidium Asexual spore formed on but easily detached from a conidiophore

conidiophore Specialized hypha that produces and bears conidia

dematiaceous Term applied to naturally pigmented, usually brown or black, fungi

dimorphic Term applied to fungi that grow as hyphae in vitro at 25° C and as budding yeastlike cells or spherules in infected tissues or in vitro at 37° C on special media

endospore Asexual spore formed within a closed structure such as a spherule

germ tube Tubelike process, produced by a germinating conidium, that eventually develops into a hypha

granule Compact mass of organized mycelium that may be embedded in a cementlike substance; formed in actinomycosis and in actinomycotic and eumycotic mycetomas; also formed by nonfilamentous bacteria in botryomycosis

hypha Filament that forms the thallus, or body, of most fungi

mycelium Mass of intertwined and branched hyphae

pseudohypha Short hyphalike filament produced by the successive buds of a yeast that elongate and fail to separate

septate Having cross walls

spherule Closed, thick-walled, spherical structure within which asexual endospores are produced by progressive cytoplasmic cleavage

Splendore-Hoeppli material Eosinophilic, refractile substance that surrounds some fungi and represents a localized antigen-antibody reaction in the hypersensitized host

yeast Round to oval unicellular fungus that reproduces by budding

SUPERFICIAL MYCOSES

The superficial mycoses are a group of fungal diseases that are usually confined to the outermost layers of the skin or its appendages.[18,19] Two of these diseases, black piedra and white piedra, involve the hair exclusively, and histopathology is not ordinarily used for their diagnosis. The agents of tinea nigra and tinea versicolor grow in the stratum corneum and rarely invade the deeper skin layers. The histopathologist seldom encounters these infections unless the lesions are atypical and the clinician suspects another disease (tinea nigra has been mistaken for junctional nevus or malignant melanoma). The histologic features of these mycoses are summarized in Table 10-1. For more detailed information, several texts are recommended.[8,13,18,19]

Dermatophytosis

The most important superficial mycosis is dermatophytosis, a clinical entity caused by any of 31 recognized species of pathogenic and taxonomically related fungi (dermatophytes) of the genera *Epidermophyton*, *Microsporum*, and *Trichophyton*.[20] This mycosis involves the skin, hair, and nails to a greater degree than the other superficial mycoses do. Diseases produced by the dermatophytes occur worldwide and are known as tineas, or ringworm. The more common tineas include (1) tinea capitis (that is, tinea of the head: scalp, eyebrows, and eyelashes) (Fig. 10-1, *A*); (2) tinea corporis (of the body); (3) tinea cruris (of the groin) (Fig. 10-2); (4) tinea pedis (of the foot); and (5) tinea unguium (of the nails) (onychomycosis). Tineas of the hairy skin often present as circular or ring-shaped patches of alopecia with erythema and scaling, or as more diffusely distributed papules, pustules, vesicles, and kerions. Ringworm of the glabrous skin also commonly appears as erythematous and scaling patches, but more severe forms of tinea corporis may resemble other dermatologic disorders. Tinea unguium presents as thickening, discoloration, and deformity of the nails (Fig. 10-3).

Histopathologic features of dermatophytosis are summarized in Table 10-1. Tissue forms of the dermatophytes are similar to one another. They usually stain with hematoxylin and eosin but are best demonstrated with special stains for fungi. Hyphae and arthroconidia invade the stratum corneum, hair follicles, and hair shafts (Fig. 10-1, *B*). The pattern of hair invasion is either ectothrix, endothrix, endoectothrix, or favic, depending on the etiologic agent.[18-20] Occasionally, rupture of a hair follicle and release of fungal elements into the dermis elicits acute suppurative inflammation that eventually becomes granulomatous.[17] The term "Majocchi's granuloma" refers to nodular, granulomatous lesions in the dermis that contain individual dermatophyte hyphae. Aggregates of hyphae embedded in and surrounded by abundant Splendore-Hoeppli material in the dermis and subcutaneous tissue have been misinterpreted by some investigators as grains or granules and therefore the infection as a mycetoma (Fig. 10-4, *A*). These aggregates consist of clustered dermatophyte hyphae, each ensheathed by Splendore-Hoeppli material, and are actually pseudogranules (Fig. 10-4, *B*). Their microscopic appearance is strikingly similar from case to case, irrespective of the dermatophytic agent.[4,5,21]

Agents of the superficial mycoses are routinely demonstrated by direct microscopic examination of skin scrapings or hair in 10% potassium hydroxide. Cultural

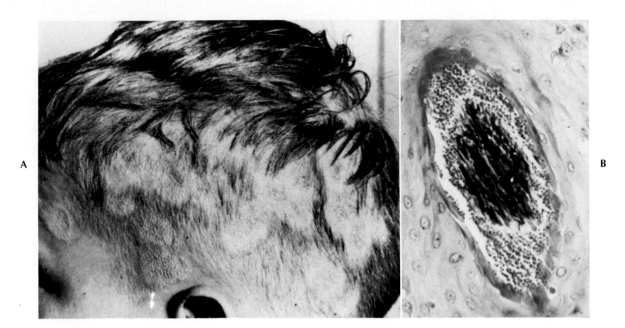

Fig. 10-1. A, Tinea capitis caused by *Microsporum canis.* **B,** Arthroconidia of *M. canis* surrounding a partially degenerated hair. (Hematoxylin and eosin; 600×; **A,** courtesy Dr. William Kaplan, Centers for Disease Control, Atlanta.)

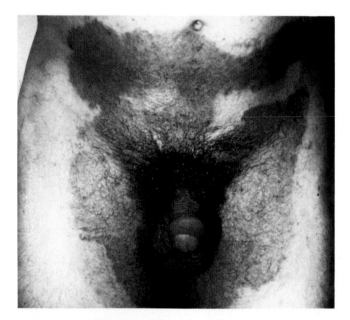

Fig. 10-2. Tinea cruris and tinea corporis caused by *Trichophyton rubrum.* (Courtesy Dr. Libero Ajello, Centers for Disease Control, Atlanta.)

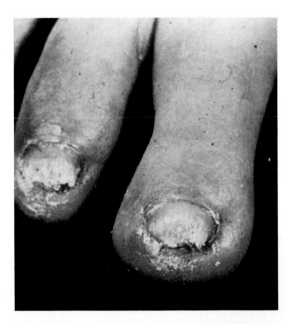

Fig. 10-3. Tinea unguium caused by *Trichophyton rubrum* in an adult male. Notice thickening and discoloration of the nails.

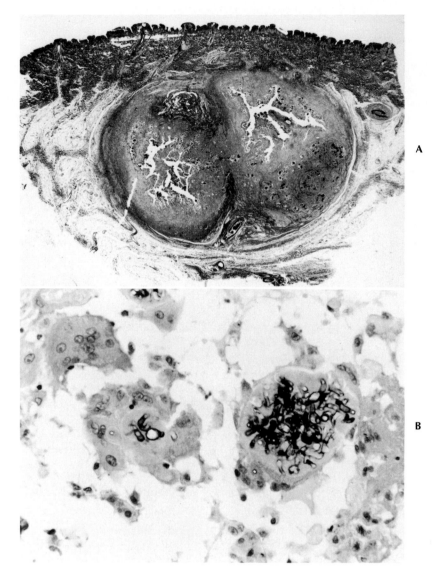

Fig. 10-4. Deep dermatophytic granuloma caused by *Microsporum canis.* **A,** Dermis and subcutaneous tissue contain multiple hyphal aggregates (pseudogranules) that stimulate an intense granulomatous reaction. **B,** Aggregates of dermatophytic hyphae (pseudo-granules) ensheathed by Splendore-Hoeppli material. (**A,** Periodic acid–Schiff; 5×; **B,** Gomori methenamine-silver/hematoxylin and eosin; 350×.)

studies are required for their definitive identification.[11,13,20]

CUTANEOUS AND SUBCUTANEOUS MYCOSES

Certain fungi that commonly infect internal organs may also involve the skin and mucous membranes. The cutaneous and subcutaneous manifestations of these mycoses are discussed separately under the respective disease headings. Included here are those diseases that involve the skin and subcutaneous tissue predominantly or exclusively.

Chromoblastomycosis

Chromoblastomycosis is an indolent cutaneous infection caused by any of several related dematiaceous (pigmented) fungi. The most common etiologic agents are *Fonsecaea pedrosoi, F. compacta, Phialophora verrucosa, Rhinocladiella aquaspersa,* and *Cladosporium carrionii.*[23,25] The disease is cosmopolitan, but most cases are encountered in tropical or subtropical regions. A locally spreading verrucous plaque or solid nodule develops in the skin at the site of traumatic implantation of the fungus, usually on an extremity.[24] Satellite lesions may develop as a consequence of regional lym-

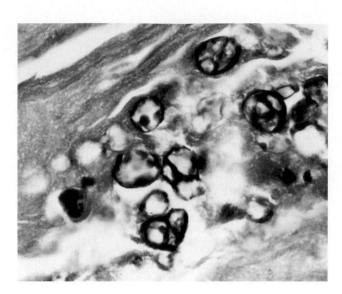

Fig. 10-5. Cutaneous chromoblastomycosis. Pigmented sclerotic bodies in keratin layer. Notice septation in one or two planes. (Hematoxylin and eosin; 760×.)

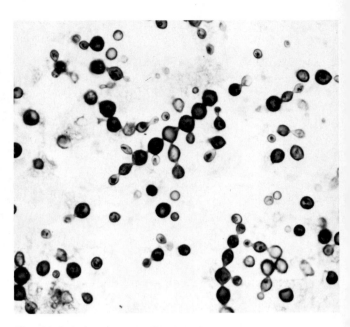

Fig. 10-6. Lobomycosis. Chains of budding cells with secondary budding. Nonbudding and single-budding cells are also present. (Gridley stain; 480×.)

phatic spread or autoinoculation, but internal dissemination is rare.[23,25]

Although the agents of chromoblastomycosis can be distinguished from one another in culture, their tissue forms are identical. Round, thick-walled, dark brown muriform cells ("sclerotic bodies"), 5 to 12 μm in diameter, are grouped within the dermis where they elicit a granulomatous and suppurative inflammatory reaction.[24] These cells reproduce by septation in one or two planes (Fig. 10-5). Nonseptate cells and, rarely, septate hyphae are also observed in the lesions. Associated epidermal changes include hyperplasia and hyperkeratosis, and transepidermal elimination of the pigmented sclerotic bodies may be observed.[22]

Lobomycosis

Lobomycosis is a cutaneous mycosis that occurs in South America, especially in Brazil and Surinam, and in parts of Central America. Natural infection occurs only in humans and dolphins[26] and produces locally enlarging cutaneous nodules that become verrucous.[27] These lesions are best treated by surgical excision. *Loboa loboi*, the etiologic agent, cannot be grown in culture.

The yeastlike cells of *L. loboi* are abundant in the dermis of the cutaneous nodules. These thick-walled cells, 6 to 12 μm in diameter, are remarkably uniform in size and shape. They reproduce by progressive budding in chains, three to eight cells in length, each of which resembles a "string of pearls" (Fig. 10-6). Adjacent cells are connected to one another by tubelike

isthmuses, and secondary budding may be observed. Nonbudding and single-budding cells are also present. The surrounding dermis contains a dispersed epithelioid and giant cell granulomatous inflammatory reaction.

Mycetoma (Madura foot, maduromycosis)

Mycetomas are tumorous lesions of the subcutaneous tissues and bone caused by a wide variety of geophilic actinomycetes and fungi that form granules (compact mycelial aggregates) within tissue (Fig. 10-7). Patients are infected when these exogenous organisms are introduced into some part of the body, usually the lower extremities or the trunk, as the result of trauma. Most cases of mycetoma occur in tropical regions such as Asia, Africa, and Central and South America; the disease is rarely encountered in the United States.[29,33] There are two distinct types of mycetomas: actinomycotic and eumycotic. Their principal agents are listed in Table 10-1.[4]

Accurate histologic differentiation between the granules formed by actinomycetes and fungi is crucial in determining the form of treatment and the prognosis of mycetoma. Actinomycotic mycetomas usually respond to antibiotics or sulfonamides, but eumycotic mycetomas do not. Treatment of the latter is limited primarily to surgical excision and débridement.[31,32]

Special stains for bacteria and fungi (Table 10-2) may be needed to determine whether a granule is actinomycotic or eumycotic. Granules of actinomycotic mycetomas contain delicate, gram-positive, branched fila-

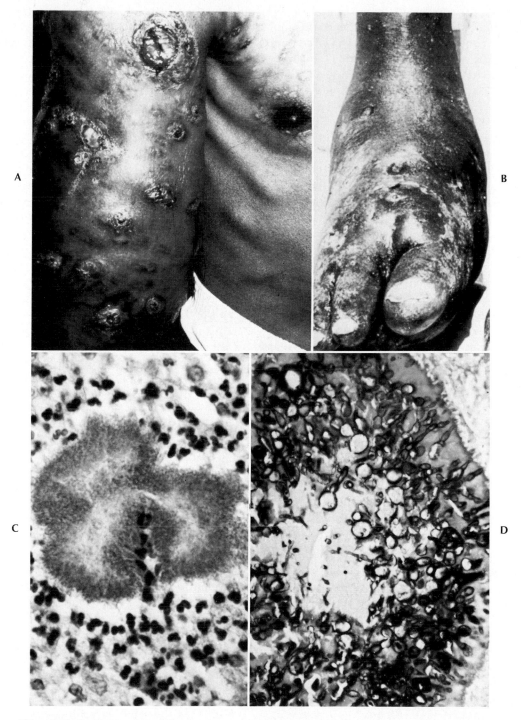

Fig. 10-7. A, Mycetoma of upper arm caused by *Nocardia brasiliensis.* Notice tumefaction and multiple openings of draining sinuses. **B,** Mycetoma (Madura foot). **C,** Granule of *N. brasiliensis* in biopsy of lesion shown in **A. D,** Granule of *Madurella mycetomatis* bordered by Splendore-Hoeppli material. Radially oriented hyphae and vesicular chlamydoconidia form the granule. (**C,** Hematoxylin and eosin; 600×; **D,** periodic acid–Schiff; 300×.)

ments, about 1 μm in width, whereas those of eumycotic mycetomas contain broad, septate, fungal hyphae, 2 to 6 μm or more in width[28,34] (Fig. 10-7, C and D). Chlamydoconidia are sometimes found near the periphery of eumycotic granules. Granules may be pigmented (black grain) or hyaline (white grain) and may contain an amorphous cementlike substance, depending on the etiologic agent. Because many granules have a characteristic architecture, presumptive etiologic identification can often be made histologically. However, cultural studies are needed for definitive identification. Immunofluorescence conjugates are available for detecting *Pseudallescheria boydii*, the most common agent of eumycotic mycetoma in the United States.

The inflammatory reaction in mycetoma is similar regardless of the causative agent.[28,30,34] Lesions contain multiple sinus tracts that usually discharge serosanguinous fluid and, at times, grossly visible granules of various colors, sizes, and degrees of hardness depending on the agent involved. Histologically, the dermis and subcutaneous tissue contain localized abscesses, each of which contains one or more granules in its center. Eosinophilic, clublike Splendore-Hoeppli material may border the granules (Fig. 10-7, C and D). Between abscesses, there is extensive formation of granulation tissue, resulting in tumefaction and deformity that is often so severe as to be mistaken clinically for a neoplasm (Fig. 10-7, A and B). Mycetomas are insidious, localized infections, but they do not respect tissue planes. Infections often involve contiguous bone, resulting in destructive osteomyelitis. Lymphatic or hematogenous dissemination from the primary subcutaneous lesion rarely occurs.

Phaeohyphomycosis (subcutaneous and systemic)

Phaeohyphomycosis comprises those subcutaneous and systemic diseases caused by opportunistic naturally pigmented fungi that develop in tissue as dark-walled (brown), septate hyphae.[24,35,41] The inclusive name "phaeohyphomycosis" replaces the misleading and inappropriate term "phaeosporotrichosis" formerly applied to such infections. A wide variety of polymorphous fungi that are saprophytes of soil and wood can cause phaeohyphomycosis, for example, *Exophiala (Phialophora) jeanselmei, Phialophora* spp., *Xylohypha (Cladosporium) bantiana*, and *Bipolaris (Drechslera)* spp. Infections are encountered in healthy persons, but those who are immunosuppressed or chronically debilitated are at increased risk.

Phaeohyphomycosis has two clinical forms: subcutaneous and systemic. The subcutaneous form (phaeomycotic cyst) usually occurs as a single, firm to fluctuant, painless abscess, up to 7 cm in diameter, in the deep dermis or subcutaneous tissue.[36,42,44] Lesions occur on exposed parts of the body after penetrating injury by a wood splinter or other foreign object, which acts as a vehicle of infection. Infection remains localized, and lymphangitis is uncommon. Microscopically, the overlying skin is unaffected. The subcutis contains a large, cystic granuloma composed of compact multinucleated giant cells and histiocytes enclosed by granulation tissue or a well-defined, fibrotic capsule. The centrally located abscess or cyst contains cellular debris, fibrin, polymorphonuclear leukocytes, and, at times, plant fibers or other foreign material.[39] Short, closely septate hyphae, 2 to 6 μm in width, and chains of budding yeastlike cells are present in the wall of the abscess and amidst the centrally located exudate. These moniliform fungi appear light brown when stained with hematoxylin and eosin, and they are well demonstrated with special stains for fungi. However, special stains mask their natural brown color. *Phialophora* and *Exophiala* spp. are most often found in cystic lesions, whereas other genera, such as *Wangiella* and *Bipolaris*, are associated with solid granulomas, which may contain small, stellate abscesses.[38]

In the systemic form (cerebral phaeohyphomycosis), infection generally occurs by the respiratory tract, and the most commonly encountered agent is *Xylohypha (Cladosporium) bantiana*.[37,40,43] This fungus is extremely neurotropic, and most infections are confined to the brain and meninges; the lung and other organs are rarely involved. Cerebral lesions appear as encapsulated abscesses or generalized inflammatory infiltrates (Fig. 10-8, A). Symptoms include headache, nausea, vomiting, fever, and nuchal rigidity. The inflammatory reaction is similar to that seen in subcutaneous lesions.

The agents of phaeohyphomycosis are morphologically and tinctorially similar in tissue sections, where they cannot be differentiated from each other. However, a disease diagnosis can be based on the natural brown color of morphologically typical fungi (Fig. 10-8, B). Culture is needed for specific identification of the etiologic agents.

Protothecosis

Protothecosis is an infection caused by achlorophyllous algae of the genus *Prototheca*. Although they do not contain chloroplasts, these saprophytic algae are believed to be related to green algae of the genus *Chlorella*.[51] Three species of protothecae are recognized, of which two, *P. wickerhamii* and *P. zopfii*, are known to cause disease. Almost all authenticated cases of human protothecosis have been caused by *P. wickerhamii*.[46] Human infections are cosmopolitan in distribution, but most have occurred in the United States.[46] The source of infection is often not apparent but can be related to penetrating injury in some cases.

Two clinically distinct forms of protothecosis are rec-

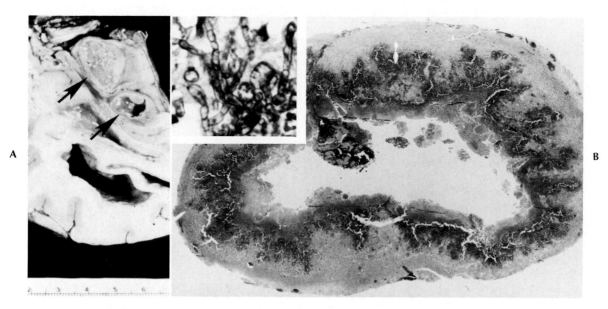

Fig. 10-8. Systemic (cerebral) phaeohyphomycosis. **A,** Two sharply circumscribed, encapsulated abscesses *(arrows)* caused by *Xylohypha bantiana* in brain of adult. **B,** Abscess caused by *X. bantiana* enucleated from left frontal lobe. The suppurative and necrotic center was lost during processing. (AFIP 62-5502; courtesy Dr. C.H. Binford, Armed Forces Institute of Pathology, Washington, D.C.) *Inset,* Dermatiaceous hyphae in wall of abscess are branched and constricted at their prominent septations. (**B,** Hematoxylin and eosin; 10×; *inset, 900×*.)

ognized: cutaneous infection and olecranon bursitis. Cutaneous protothecosis, which occurs preferentially in debilitated or compromised patients, presents as spreading papulonodular or verrucous lesions, usually involving the distal extremities or head.[52] Infection may extend into the subcutaneous tissue and rarely spreads to regional lymph nodes.[48,52] Olecranon bursitis, which occurs in otherwise healthy hosts, presents as a subcutaneous nodule adjacent to the elbow.[50,52] Bursectomy is the treatment of choice. Chemotherapy alone has not effectively eradicated localized infection in most cases. The single reported case of disseminated human protothecosis occurred in a patient with transient depression of specific cell-mediated immunity to *Prototheca*. He recovered after therapy with transfer factor and amphotericin B.[47]

The protothecae are found in tissue sections in the form of endosporulating sporangia. Their asexual reproductive cycle in tissue is similar to that of the endosporulating fungi. Small, uninucleate, immature sporangia undergo nuclear division followed or accompanied by progressive cytoplasmic cleavage to produce mature sporangia that contain sporangiospores. Characteristically, the sporangiospores are polygonal or wedge shaped, fill the parent cell, and may be radially arranged around a central sporangiospore, producing the distinctive "morula" form (Fig. 10-9, *A*). The sporangia of the two pathogenic protothecae differ in size but are

otherwise similar in morphology. Sporangia of the small form, *P. wickerhamii*, measure 2 to 12 μm in diameter, whereas those of *P. zopfii* measure 10 to 25 μm in diameter. Morula forms are uncommon in infections caused by *P. zopfii*. Endosporulating cells of *P. zopfii* are oval, and their larger nuclei are more conspicuous than those of *P. wickerhamii* (Fig. 10-9, *B*).

The cell walls of both the sporangia and the sporangiospores are stained with the special stains for fungi. With hematoxylin and eosin, these cells are hyaline, but their contents may be eosinophilic or basophilic. The two species are more reliably distinguished from one another in tissue sections by direct immunofluorescence and in culture by their patterns of carbohydrate assimilation.

Cutaneous lesions often show hyperkeratosis, parakeratosis, and acanthosis, and they may be ulcerated. Algal cells are abundant in the dermis and may also be found in the epidermis and keratin layer as a result of transepidermal elimination. An inflammatory reaction, when present, may be granulomatous or may consist of a mixture of acute and chronic inflammatory cells. Infection of the olecranon bursa produces necrotizing granulomatous inflammation. The bursal lining consists of a stellate zone of necrotic debris, neutrophils, and fibrin that is surrounded by palisaded epithelioid histiocytes and multinucleated giant cells. The adjacent soft tissue contains granulation tissue, acute and chronic in-

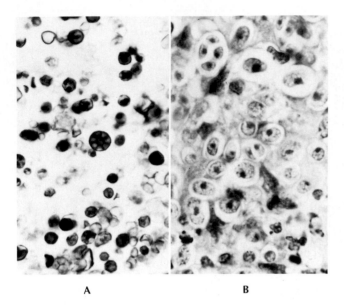

Fig. 10-9. Prototothecosis. **A,** Distinctive endosporulating sporangium ("morula form") of *Prototheca wickerhamii (center).* **B,** Oval cells of *P. zopfii.* Nuclei are visible in most cells. One endosporulating cell is present *(top left).* (**A,** Gridley stain; 760×; **B,** hematoxylin and eosin; 760×.)

flammatory cells, and small granulomas. *Prototheca* cells are difficult to find in these lesions, which can be misinterpreted as rheumatoid nodules if special stains are not used to detect the algae. Endosporulating fungi such as *Coccidioides immitis* and *Rhinosporidium seeberi* are distinguished from the protothecae in tissue sections on the basis of their size and distinctive morphology (see Table 10-1).

Green algae of the genus *Chlorella* cause cutaneous and systemic infections in animals, but human green algal infection has been recognized only recently.[49] In tissue sections, the cells of *Chlorella,* 6 to 14 μm in diameter, appear similar to those of *P. zopfii.* However, infections caused by the two algae can be differentiated by other criteria.[45] The protothecae can be distinguished from each other and from *Chlorella* in tissue sections by direct immunofluorescence.

Rhinosporidiosis

Rhinosporidiosis is a mucosal and cutaneous mycosis caused by *Rhinosporidium seeberi.* The disease is endemic in India, Sri Lanka, and parts of Africa, but sporadic cases occur in the western hemisphere, including the United States.[55] Infection produces bulky, friable mucosal polyps in the nasal cavity and nasopharynx and on the palate. The conjunctiva, larynx, genitalia, rectum, and skin are involved less commonly.[57]

Since *R. seeberi* cannot be isolated on synthetic me-

dia, diagnosis of the disease depends on recognition of its distinctive morphology in tissue sections. The sporangia of *R. seeberi* are located predominantly in the stroma of the mucosal polyps. Spherical, uninucleate trophic forms (immature sporangia), 10 to 100 μm in diameter, develop into mature sporangia, 100 to 350 μm in diameter, by a process of progressive enlargement and endosporulation[56] (Fig. 10-10). Sporangiospores are uninucleate, and the larger, mature sporangiospores contain globular eosinophilic inclusions. Maturation and zonation of sporangiospores within the sporangium is frequently observed.[53]

Cylindrical cell papillomas of the paranasal sinuses and nasal cavity that contain numerous intraepithelial mucous cysts can be mistaken for rhinosporidial polyps.[54]

Sporotrichosis

Sporotrichosis is a subacute or chronic disease caused by the dimorphic fungus *Sporothrix schenckii.* The disease occurs worldwide, but most reported cases have originated from the United States, South Africa, Mexico, and South America. Infection usually results from the traumatic implantation of the fungus, growing in soil or on plant materials, into the skin and subcutaneous tissue. In rare instances, a primary cutaneous infection may disseminate to the bones, joints, lungs, and other organs.[63,65] Even more rarely, inhalation of the fungus results in primary pulmonary infection, which may disseminate.[58,60,67] Sporotrichosis is not conta-

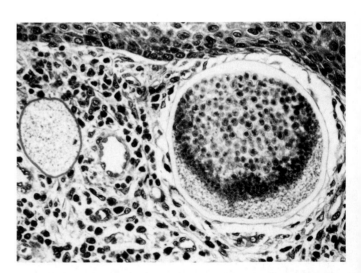

Fig. 10-10. Rhinosporidiosis. A trophic form and a mature sporangium of *Rhinosporidium seeberi* in the stroma of a nasal polyp. Notice zonation of immature and mature sporangiospores within sporangium. Mature sporangiospores contain small, globular inclusions. (Hematoxylin and eosin; 300×.)

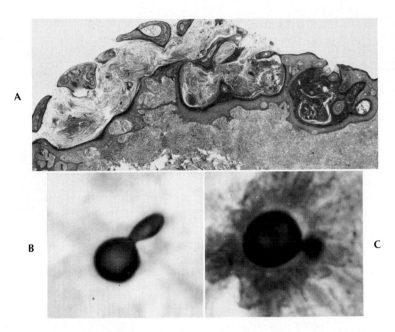

Fig. 10-11. Cutaneous sporotrichosis. **A,** Hyperplasia of epidermis and mixed suppurative and granulomatous inflammation in dermis. **B,** Single yeastlike cell of *Sporothrix schenckii* with elongated bud in dermal granuloma. **C,** Asteroid body composed of fungal cell surrounded by irregular spicules of Splendore-Hoeppli material. (**A,** Hematoxylin and eosin; 10×; **B,** Gomori methenamine-silver; 1500×; **C,** Gomori methenamine-silver/hematoxylin and eosin; 1500×.)

gious, but infection can result from contamination of skin wounds with exudates from humans or animals with sporotrichosis. There is no evidence that underlying disease or immunosuppression predispose a person to infection.

The most common form of sporotrichosis is lymphocutaneous.[59,66] Clinically, this form is manifested as a chain of subcutaneous nodules along the course of lymphatics draining a primary skin lesion that may be nodular and ulcerated. Lymphocutaneous lesions develop within 7 to 90 days or longer after penetrating injury to an exposed part of the body, such as the hand, arm, neck, or foot. Eventually, the subcutaneous nodules soften, ulcerate, and discharge pus. Solitary, ulcerated, and verrucous lesions of the skin without lymphatic involvement also occur. They are sometimes mistaken for a neoplasm and excised surgically. The treatment of choice for sporotrichosis is potassium iodide, especially for lymphocutaneous infection. Amphotericin B and other antifungals may also be useful in systemic infection.[63,65] If untreated, the infection may persist for years.

S. schenckii usually elicits a mixed suppurative and granulomatous inflammatory reaction accompanied by microabscess formation and fibrosis[59,62,64] (Fig. 10-11, A). This type of inflammation is typical of all forms of the disease, but it is not specific. In tissue sections, *S. schenckii* appears as spherical, oval, or elongated (cigar-shaped) yeastlike cells, 2 to 6 μm or more in diameter. The fungal cells often bear buds with narrow-based attachments to the parent cells (Fig. 10-11, *B*). Multiple budding is seen rarely. Although considered by some to be the classic tissue form of the fungus, cigar-shaped organisms are not commonly found. When present, they are most often observed in disseminated lesions. Hyphae are rarely formed in tissue.

The presence of asteroid bodies (fungal cells surrounded by Splendore-Hoeppli material) within microabscesses is helpful in making a presumptive histologic diagnosis of sporotrichosis[59,62] (Fig. 10-11, *C*). However, the asteroid body is not pathognomonic for this disease. Splendore-Hoeppli material may surround parasite ova, actinomycotic granules, eumycotic granules, foreign objects such as silk sutures, and other species of fungi, especially *Coccidioides immitis*, the *Aspergillus* spp., the *Candida* spp., and the agents of entomophthoromycosis.[61] In many cases of sporotrichosis, asteroid bodies cannot be detected. Generally, few *S. schenckii* cells are found in cutaneous lesions, and special stains for fungi, complemented by immunofluorescence staining, are needed to identify the fungus in fixed tissues. When immunofluorescence tests are not available, microbiologic culture or mouse inoculation is essential for an accurate diagnosis.

SYSTEMIC MYCOSES
Actinomycosis

Actinomycosis is a chronic suppurative disease caused by anaerobic, filamentous bacteria in the order Actinomycetales.[71,72] The disease occurs worldwide, and males are affected three times as frequently as females. The principal agent of actinomycosis in humans is *Actinomyces israelii*. This species and others listed in Table 10-1 have never been isolated from environmental sources. Rather, they occur as commensals in the mouth, and "sulfur" granules are commonly found in the tonsillar crypts of healthy persons. The actinomycetes are ordinarily of low pathogenicity. Underlying disease and interruption of mucocutaneous barriers predispose a person to actinomycosis by providing a medium in which these endogenous organisms can invade, proliferate, and disseminate. Unlike nocardiosis, actinomycosis does not occur preferentially in patients with defective immunity.[68,72]

Based on the anatomic site of the lesions, four clinical forms of actinomycosis are recognized: cervicofacial, thoracic, abdominal, and pelvic.[68,72] Most commonly involved is the cervicofacial area, where the disease is often a sequel to dental caries, periodontal disease, or injury to the oral mucosa, such as a tooth extraction. The localized lesion enlarges, abscesses form, and draining sinus tracts emerge (Fig. 10-12). If untreated, the infection may extend into the mandible, paranasal sinuses, orbit, cranial bones, and thorax, where it may then disseminate to the central nervous system, skin, and other bones. Thoracic infection may follow aspiration of infectious materials. Abdominal actinomycosis (Fig. 10-13) is frequently mistaken clinically for advanced malignancy. It may result from direct extension

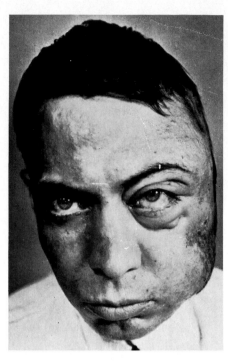

Fig. 10-12. Cervicofacial actinomycosis. Notice swelling and openings of draining sinuses. (Courtesy Dr. Antonio González-Ochoa, Mexico City.)

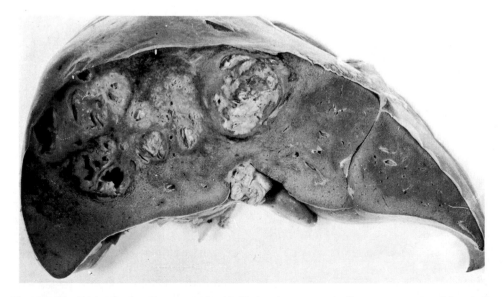

Fig. 10-13. Abdominal actinomycosis. Multiple abscesses in liver were caused by *Actinomyces israelii*. Primary infection in cecum or appendix resulted in retrocecal abscess that extended to skin surface in right inguinal region. (Courtesy Dr. Roger D. Baker, Silver Spring, Md.)

of a thoracic infection but is more commonly seen as a consequence of a ruptured appendix or bowel perforation by swallowed foreign bodies, such as toothpicks or needles.[69] Pelvic actinomycosis is a well-recognized complication of intrauterine contraceptive devices.[70,76] Primary skin infections may develop after human bites.

The inflammatory reaction in actinomycosis is suppurative, with the formation of abscesses that contain one or more granules (organized aggregates of filaments), 30 to 3000 μm in diameter, that are bordered by eosinophilic, clublike, Splendore-Hoeppli material[71,73] (Fig. 10-14, A). Bacterial stains reveal that the granules are composed of delicate, branched, gram-positive filaments, about 1 μm in diameter, haphazardly arranged in an amorphous matrix of uncertain composition (Fig. 10-14, B). The filaments may be fragmented and, unlike those of the *Nocardia* spp., are not acid-fast.[73-75] Gomori methenamine-silver staining is also useful for demonstrating the filaments, which are not stained by the hematoxylin and eosin, periodic acid–Schiff, and Gridley stains. Specific identification requires culture or immunofluorescence staining because, in tissue sections, the agents of actinomycosis cannot be distinguished from each other. Both gram-positive and gram-negative bacilli and cocci may be found in close association with actinomycete filaments within a granule, but it is generally believed that these bacteria are secondary pathogens.

Penicillin is the drug of choice for treating actinomycosis.[68,72] It is speculated that fewer cases are seen today because of the widespread use of antibacterial antibiotics for treating minor, unrelated infections.

Adiaspiromycosis

Adiaspiromycosis is an uncommon pulmonary mycosis caused by *Chrysosporium parvum* var. *crescens (Emmonsia crescens)*. Human infection is usually asymptomatic, self-limited, and confined to the lungs.[77,78] The inhaled conidia of *C. parvum* var. *crescens*, 2 to 4 μm in diameter, progressively enlarge within the lungs to a diameter of 200 to 400 μm at maturity, with chitinous walls 20 to 30 μm or more in width[78,79] (Fig. 10-15). No other fungus of medical importance has a wall this thick. Each mature adiaconidium is enclosed within a fibrotic granuloma that compresses the surrounding lung tissue. Since *C. parvum* var. *crescens* does not replicate within the human host, the degree of impairment of pulmonary function is related to the number of conidia inhaled and the frequency of exposure.[79]

Aspergillosis

The broad spectrum of disease caused by fungi of the genus *Aspergillus* includes allergic bronchopulmonary disease; colonization of pulmonary cavities; indolent superficial infection of the skin and mucosal surfaces; chronic, progressive pulmonary infection in mildly compromised hosts; and fulminant, invasive pulmonary infection with systemic dissemination in severely immunosuppressed patients. Aspergillosis is the second most common opportunistic mycosis among patients with malignant disease, accounting for up to 30% of fungal infections found at autopsy in these patients.[82] *A. fumigatus* is the species most frequently isolated from patients with invasive or disseminated infec-

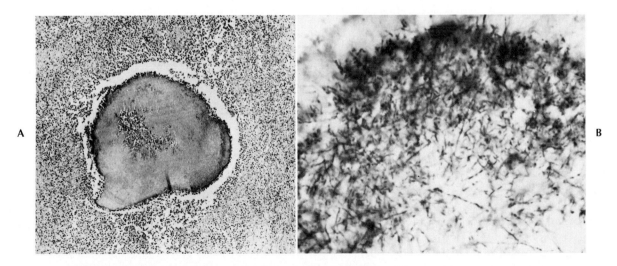

Fig. 10-14. Actinomycosis. **A,** Granule of *Actinomyces israelii* in hepatic abscess. **B,** Gram-positive, branched filaments and coccoid elements, 1 μm or less in diameter, in replicate section of granule in **A.** (**A,** Hematoxylin and eosin; 40×; **B,** Brown and Brenn; 480×.)

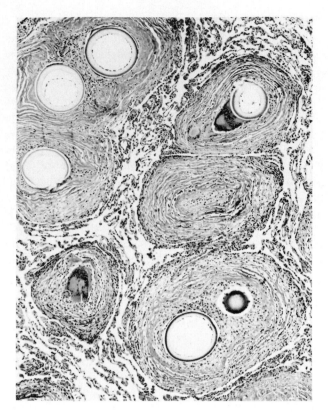

Fig. 10-15. Adiaspiromycosis. Fibrotic pulmonary granulomas contain large, thick-walled adiaconidia of *Chrysosporium parvum* var. *crescens*. Outer portion of each adiaconidium wall is eosinophilic; inner portion is hyaline. (Hematoxylin and eosin; 50×.)

tions,[92] but *A. flavus*, *A. niger*, and other *Aspergillus* spp. can also cause disease.[93] Since the conidia of the aspergilli are ubiquitous in the environment, isolation of an *Aspergillus* sp. in microbiologic culture must be interpreted cautiously.[90] Proof of its etiologic role in infection is best confirmed by demonstration of characteristic hyphae in tissue sections. A detailed account of the mycology of the aspergilli is provided by Raper and Fennell.[89]

Typical hyphae of the *Aspergillus* spp. have a characteristic appearance in tissue sections (Fig. 10-16, *A*). The hyphae are uniform, narrow (3 to 6 μm in width), tubular, and regularly septate. Branching is regular, progressive, and dichotomous. Hyphal branches tend to arise at acute angles from parent hyphae. Viable hyphae may be deeply basophilic, whereas degenerated or necrotic hyphae are often hyaline or eosinophilic. Hyphal morphology is demonstrated better with the special stains for fungi than with hematoxylin and eosin.

Under certain circumstances, the hyphae of the aspergilli may have an unusual or bizarre appearance in tissue sections. Degenerated hyphae encountered in pulmonary fungus balls and in indolent, granulomatous lesions assume bizarre shapes with globose varicosities

and inconspicuous septa (Fig. 10-16, *B*). Such hyphae may be mistaken for those of the zygomycetes.[90] Conidial (fruiting) heads may be produced in lesions exposed to air, for example, in pulmonary fungus balls and in superficial infections involving the skin and bronchial mucosa (Fig. 10-16, *C*). Calcium oxalate crystals may accumulate within the mycelium of fungus balls in the lungs or paranasal sinuses.[86] Hyphal fragments in chronic granulomatous lesions are often coated with eosinophilic Splendore-Hoeppli material.

The clinical course and pathologic manifestations of aspergillosis are determined, for the most part, by the integrity of host defense mechanisms. In the hypersensitized host, the aspergilli can stimulate a variety of allergic pulmonary reactions, which includes the syndrome of allergic bronchopulmonary aspergillosis, chronic eosinophilic pneumonia, mucoid impaction of proximal bronchi, bronchocentric granulomatosis with asthma, and microgranulomatous hypersensitivity pneumonitis.[85,91] There is considerable clinical and pathologic overlap among these allergic reactions, which seldom occur in pure form. Pathologic findings include mucus hypersecretion, eosinophil infiltration with Charcot-Leyden crystals, bronchiolitis, and destructive granulomatous lesions of the airways.[85] Hyphae, which are difficult to find in these lesions, are fragmented and degenerated, and they do not invade adjacent pulmonary parenchyma or blood vessels.

The colonizing form of aspergillosis is typified by the pulmonary aspergilloma, or fungus ball. This is a compact mass of hyphae that forms within a preexisting, usually tuberculous, pulmonary cavity. The clinical diagnosis of aspergilloma is suggested by radiographic demonstration of an intracavitary mass, hemoptysis, and a positive serum precipitin reaction to aspergillus antigens.[84] The mycelial ball measures up to 5 cm in diameter and is composed of tangled, often bizarre hyphae, which may produce conidial heads. Erosion of the cavity wall by the mobile fungus ball results in recurrent or life-threatening hemoptysis, which may necessitate surgical resection of the cavity or involved pulmonary lobe. Because the aspergilli in these lesions are noninvasive colonizers that are confined within the cavity by host defenses, antifungal chemotherapy is not required. Fungus balls are occasionally produced by other fungi, notably *Coccidioides immitis* and *Pseudallescheria boydii*.

A recently described form of pulmonary aspergillosis, termed chronic necrotizing pulmonary aspergillosis[81] or semi-invasive pulmonary aspergillosis,[83] shares some features of both the colonizing and invasive forms of aspergillosis. It is a locally progressive and destructive infection that occurs in mildly compromised patients who have underlying noncavitary structural lung disease. Chest radiographs disclose parenchymal infiltrates and thick-walled cavities, about 40% of which contain

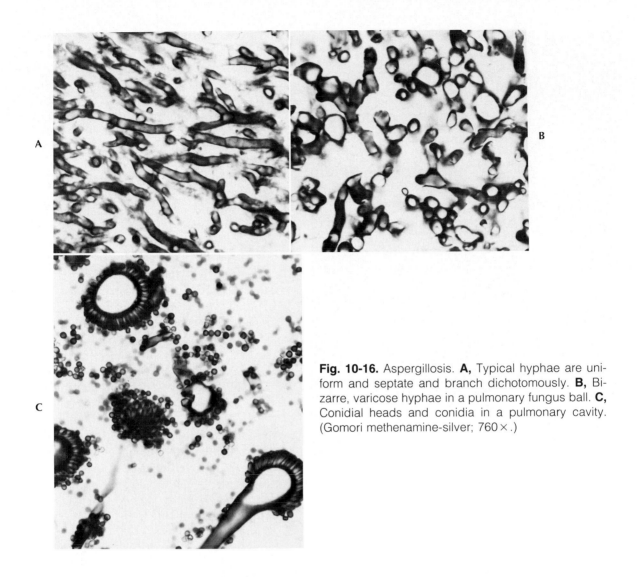

Fig. 10-16. Aspergillosis. **A,** Typical hyphae are uniform and septate and branch dichotomously. **B,** Bizarre, varicose hyphae in a pulmonary fungus ball. **C,** Conidial heads and conidia in a pulmonary cavity. (Gomori methenamine-silver; 760×.)

intracavitary fungus balls. The pathologic features of chronic necrotizing pulmonary aspergillosis have not yet been described in detail. Major findings include large cavities that contain fungus balls or amorphous mycelial aggregates, and limited invasion and destruction of adjacent noncavitary lung tissue.

Invasive pulmonary aspergillosis is a fulminant opportunistic infection that occurs almost exclusively in patients whose defense mechanisms are severely compromised by hematologic malignancy, corticosteroids, cytotoxic chemotherapy, and granulocytopenia.[87,93] Clinical findings are nonspecific, and sputum cultures are positive in only about one third of cases. Hyphae proliferate within the bronchial tree, invade through the walls of distal airways, and extend into adjacent arteries and veins. Vascular invasion and thrombotic occlusion result in characteristic nodular infarcts, several millimeters to 3 cm or more in diameter, that may replace much of a lobe (Fig. 10-17). Each of these nodules is composed of a central zone of ischemic necrosis, an intermediate zone of fibrinous exudate, and a periph-

eral zone of parenchymal hemorrhage.[88] Hyphae radiate throughout these nodules from a central, occluded blood vessel. Hyphal invasion and occlusion of larger, proximal arteries and veins results in large, wedge-shaped hemorrhagic infarcts. Suppurative bronchopneumonia may occur in nongranulocytopenic patients.[88]

Disseminated infection develops in about 25% of patients with invasive pulmonary aspergillosis. The gastrointestinal tract, central nervous system, heart, kidneys, and liver are frequently involved, but lesions may be found in any organ.[87,93] The systemic lesions are infarctive, less often suppurative or granulomatous. Endocarditis of native or prosthetic cardiac valves results in bulky, friable vegetations and is usually accompanied by myocardial lesions.[80]

The aspergilli cause a variety of indolent, superficial infections in mildly compromised hosts. Localized granulomatous infections can occur in the lungs, subcutaneous tissue, paranasal sinuses and orbit of diabetics or patients treated with corticosteroids. Cutaneous lesions

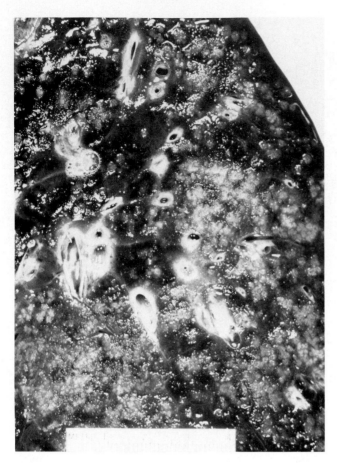

Fig. 10-17. Invasive pulmonary aspergillosis. Confluent, granular nodules occupy much of the sectioned surface. From a pancytopenic patient with disseminated aspergillosis that involved the lungs and brain and complicated chemotherapy for acute granulocytic leukemia.

may result from disseminated infection or can occur primarily in burned patients. The aspergilli also cause superficial infections of the external ear canal and nails.

Other pathogenic fungi that form branched, septate hyphae can be mistaken for the aspergilli in tissue sections. These fungi include *Pseudallescheria boydii*, the *Fusarium* spp., and, on occasion, the *Candida* spp. and the zygomycetes. Recognition of subtle differences in the morphology of these fungi may enable one to differentiate them from the aspergilli. However, unless typical conidial heads are observed, a histopathologic diagnosis of aspergillosis must be considered presumptive unless confirmed by direct immunofluorescence or microbiologic isolation of an *Aspergillus* sp. from the lesion.

Blastomycosis

Blastomycosis is a chronic granulomatous and suppurative infection caused by the dimorphic fungus *Blastomyces dermatitidis*.[95,99,101] This mycosis was long believed to be restricted to North America, but autochthonous cases are now known to occur in the Middle East and in several African countries. Although clinical and epidemiologic evidence indicates that persons contract blastomycosis from sources in nature such as soil, the natural habitat of *B. dermatitidis* has not yet been discovered. Most infections result from inhalation of the conidia of the saprophytic fungus, and thus the disease usually has a pulmonary inception.

Blastomycosis has two clinical forms: systemic and cutaneous.[94,98,103] Infection is often confined to the lungs in the systemic form or may spread by the bloodstream to other organs, especially the skin, bones, joints, male genital tract,[96] urinary bladder, brain, and spinal cord.[100,102,103] Pulmonary lesions are occasionally inapparent. Cutaneous blastomycosis presents as indolent, ulcerated or verrucous, granulomatous lesions that generally occur on exposed surfaces (Fig. 10-18, *A* and *B*). Both forms of the disease are best treated with amphotericin B; 2-hydroxystilbamidine has also been effective.[97]

In tissue, *B. dermatitidis* appears as spherical, single-budding, yeastlike cells, 8 to 15 μm in diameter, with thick, "doubly contoured" walls[100] (Fig. 10-18, *C*). Several basophilic nuclei may be visible when optimally fixed tissues are stained with hematoxylin and eosin. The broad-based budding of this fungus is diagnostic and aids in differentiating it from other yeast forms of similar size, such as *Histoplasma capsulatum* var. *duboisii* and *Cryptococcus neoformans*. These agents can also be distinguished from each other by direct immunofluorescence. Occasionally, small but morphologically typical forms of *B. dermatitidis*, 2 to 4 μm in diameter, are found in tissue sections, but they are always present as part of a continuous series of sizes ranging from the unusually small to the larger forms characteristic of the fungus. This mixture of small and typical forms should not be mistaken for coexisting mycoses. Hyphae are rarely formed in tissue.

Blastomyces dermatitidis usually elicits a mixed suppurative and granulomatous inflammatory reaction.[100,102] Early lesions are predominantly suppurative, whereas older ones tend to be granulomatous, with abscess formation and caseation. Although diffuse fibrosis is common in chronic infections, solitary fibrocaseous nodules, as seen in histoplasmosis capsulati, are extremely rare in blastomycosis. Florid pseudoepitheliomatous hyperplasia of skin lesions can mimic squamous cell carcinoma (Fig. 10-18, *B*).

Botryomycosis (bacterial pseudomycosis)

Botryomycosis is a chronic, localized infection of the skin and subcutaneous tissues or viscera caused by nonfilamentous bacteria that form granules.[104] Disseminated infection is rare.[105] In hematoxylin and eosin–

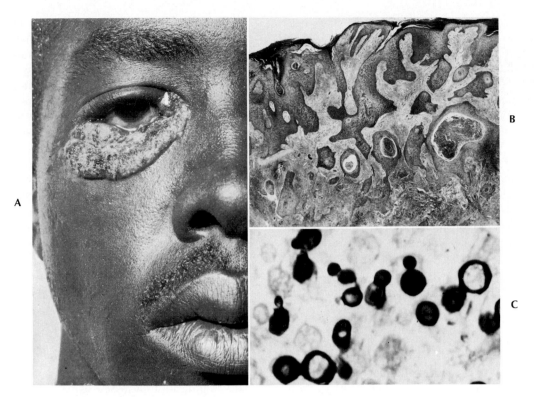

Fig. 10-18. Cutaneous blastomycosis. **A,** Elevated ulcer. **B,** Pseudoepitheliomatous hyperplasia of epidermis and mixed suppurative and granulomatous inflammation in dermis. **C,** Single and budding *Blastomyces dermatitidis* cells in dermal abscess. Notice characteristic broad-based budding of yeastlike cells. (**A,** Courtesy Dr. Roger D. Baker, Silver Spring, Md.; **B,** hematoxylin and eosin; 10×; **C,** Gomori methenamine-silver; 600×.)

stained tissue sections, the granules may be mistaken for those of actinomycosis and actinomycotic mycetoma. Bacteria most commonly implicated include *Pseudomonas aeruginosa, Staphylococcus aureus, Escherichia coli,* and species of *Streptococcus* and *Proteus.* Botryomycotic granules and those of actinomycosis and mycetoma (see discussion of mycetomas) can be differentiated from each other if appropriate bacterial and fungal stains are used. Differentiation is important because each of these diseases is managed differently.

Candidiasis

Candidiasis is a superficial, mucocutaneous, or systemic mycosis most often caused by the endogenous species *Candida albicans. C. tropicalis* is the next most frequently isolated pathogen in this genus, and occasional human infections are caused by other saprophytic species, including *C. guilliermondii, C. krusei, C. parapsilosis,* and *C. pseudotropicalis.*[111,115,117,118] Although *Torulopsis glabrata* was tentatively merged with the genus *Candida* as *C. glabrata,* it is now considered taxonomically distinct and is discussed separately.

C. albicans is found among the normal flora of the oral cavity, upper respiratory tract, digestive tract, and vagina. The other *Candida* spp. are saprophytes or commensals that can be isolated from both human and environmental sources. Infection caused by the *Candida* spp. is almost always preceded by compromise of host defense mechanisms. Factors that predispose to infection by these fungi include disruption of cutaneous barriers caused by trauma, burns, surgery, or indwelling vascular catheters; genitourinary or gastrointestinal mucosal ulceration; prolonged broad-spectrum antibiotic therapy that alters the normal balance of endogenous microflora; and impairment of cellular or humoral immunity as a result of underlying disease or its therapy, such as diabetes mellitus, acute leukemia, granulocytopenia, corticosteroid therapy, and cytotoxic chemotherapy.[107,115,117,120] Candidiasis is the most frequent opportunistic mycosis in the United States, accounting for more than 75% of fungal infections in patients with neoplastic diseases.[115]

Superficial candidal infections involve the skin and the mucosal surfaces of the oral cavity and vagina. Intertriginous cutaneous infections occur in obese, diabetic, and alcoholic persons. Maceration of the skin attributable to prolonged, repeated immersion in water may predispose to cutaneous candidiasis, paronychia, and onychomycosis. Vulvovaginal candidiasis occurs in patients with diabetes mellitus and during pregnancy. Infection of the oral cavity (thrush) is encountered in newborns, in patients treated with broad-spectrum antibiotics, and as a complication of diabetes mellitus, the acquired immunodeficiency syndrome, or other debilitating diseases. Thrush manifests as soft, friable, white patches on the tongue and oral mucosae that are composed of yeastlike cells, pseudohyphae, and hyphae enmeshed in an inflammatory pseudomembrane. Invasion of submucosal tissue does not ordinarily occur.

Chronic mucocutaneous candidiasis, a protracted superficial infection of the skin, nails, oral cavity, oropharynx, and vagina, usually afflicts patients who have underlying defects in cell-mediated immunity.[106] Five clinically distinct forms are recognized, one of which is associated with endocrine abnormalities, most commonly hypoparathyroidism and adrenal failure.[109] Mucocutaneous infection begins early in life and is particularly resistant to topical or parenteral antifungal chemotherapy. About 25% of patients with chronic mucocutaneous candidiasis have no demonstrable abnormality of cell-mediated immunity. Defective neutrophil chemotaxis can be demonstrated in some cases. The mucosal lesions of chronic mucocutaneous candidiasis resemble those of thrush. Disfiguring cutaneous lesions, termed "Candida granulomas," are warty, hyperkeratotic papules and plaques within which the fungal elements remain confined to the superficial epidermis.

Systemic candidiasis is an opportunistic mycosis that usually involves the gastrointestinal tract, kidneys, heart, and central nervous system but can involve almost any organ.[117,120] Within the gastrointestinal tract the distal esophagus and stomach are involved most frequently.[110] The Candida spp. often colonize preexisting

ulcers without giving rise to disseminated infection.[114] However, once invasion into underlying viable tissue occurs, the risk of vascular invasion and hematogenous dissemination increases, particularly in patients who are immunosuppressed. Invasive gastrointestinal lesions consist of punctate mucosal erosions or diffuse mucosal ulcers covered by friable inflammatory pseudomembranes that contain yeastlike cells and mycelial elements (Fig. 10-19, A). The fungal elements invade into the submucosa and submucosal blood vessels.

Primary infection of the urinary tract by the Candida spp. results in cystitis and ascending pyelonephritis that is often complicated by papillary necrosis. Sloughed necrotic papillae containing fungal elements form "fungus balls" that can cause ureteropelvic obstruction with secondary hydronephrosis. Infection of the kidneys during the course of hematogenous dissemination results in bilateral miliary lesions, either abscesses or necrotic nodules, that contain abundant yeastlike cells and mycelial elements.

Cerebral candidiasis is the most frequent mycosis of the central nervous system, accounting for about one half of such infections encountered at autopsy.[121] It is a late complication of disseminated candidiasis in patients with cardiac and renal involvement. Cerebral lesions consist of multifocal microabscesses sometimes accompanied by noncaseating granulomas and localized meningitis.[122] Diffuse leptomeningitis does not occur.

The pathologic features of pulmonary candidiasis are largely determined by the route of infection.[108,113,116,124] Aspiration of Candida spp. from the oral cavity or upper respiratory tract, termed "endobronchial pulmonary candidiasis," results in asymmetrically distributed, nodular areas of bronchopneumonia involving predominantly the lower lobes. This form of pulmonary infection is not commonly associated with disseminated candidiasis. Hematogenous pulmonary candidiasis is

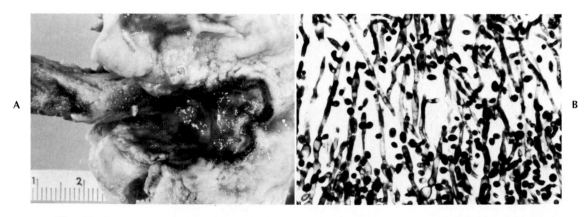

Fig. 10-19. Candidiasis. **A,** Ulcer at esophagogastric junction caused by Candida albicans. The 5-year-old patient was pancytopenic as a result of treatment for acute lymphocytic leukemia. At autopsy the lungs, liver, and spleen contained friable, yellow, necrotic nodules. **B,** Yeastlike cells, pseudohyphae, and hyphae of C. albicans. (**B,** Gomori methenamine-silver; 480×.)

characterized by round, hemorrhagic, grayish-tan necrotic nodules, 2 to 4 mm in diameter, distributed randomly but symmetrically throughout both lungs.[108] Endobronchial and respiratory mucosal involvement is uncommon in this form of pulmonary infection, whereas extrapulmonary involvement is frequently found in the esophagus, stomach, liver, spleen, and kidneys. A third form, embolic pulmonary candidiasis, occurs in children who have indwelling venous catheters.[113] Occlusion of small and medium-sized pulmonary arteries by mycotic emboli results in hemorrhagic pulmonary infarcts.

The *Candida* spp. are the most frequent etiologic agents of cardiac fungal infection.[125] Microabscesses or necrotic nodules involving the myocardium are a sequela of disseminated candidiasis and may coexist with endocardial vegetations.[119] The latter are typically bulky and friable and may give rise to arterial emboli. Preexisting valvular deformity is not a necessary prerequisite for candidal endocarditis, which can develop in immunosuppressed patients, drug addicts, and patients with indwelling central venous catheters whose valves are otherwise normal. Candidal infection of prosthetic cardiac valves develops on neoendocardium that grows onto the sewing cloth and struts of the prostheses, and systemic arterial emboli are a frequent complication.[123]

The lesions of invasive candidiasis contain yeastlike cells and mycelial elements (Fig. 10-19, *B*). The oval yeastlike cells, 2 to 6 μm in diameter, reproduce by budding. The mycelial elements consist of both pseudohyphae and true hyphae. Pseudohyphae are formed by progressive budding of yeastlike cells that elongate and remain attached to one another in chains. There are segmental constrictions in these chains where adjacent cells remain apposed (Fig. 10-20, *A*). The branched, septate, tubular hyphae are narrower than the pseudohyphae and do not have conspicuous constrictions at sites of septation (Fig. 10-20, *B*). An inflammatory response is minimal within superficial mucosal ulcers and in mucocutaneous lesions where the *Candida* spp. are colonizers or do not deeply invade viable tissue. The inflammatory response to invasive candidiasis in the nongranulocytopenic host is typically suppurative, but it may be both granulomatous and suppurative in chronic, indolent infections. Disseminated candidiasis in the granulocytopenic host produces nodular infarcts, a result of invasion and occlusion of small blood vessels.[108] Occlusion of large blood vessels and parenchymal infarction, which typify the lesions of aspergillosis and zygomycosis, are found infrequently in disseminated candidiasis.

On occasion, the *Candida* spp. can be mistaken for other fungal pathogens in tissue sections, notably the *Trichosporon* spp. and weakly pigmented agents of phaeohyphomycosis. If microbiologic culture is not available, the *Candida* spp. can be identified generically in tissue sections by immunofluorescence or immunohistochemistry.[112] The individual species are not morphologically distinguishable from each other in tissue sections.

Coccidioidomycosis

Coccidioidomycosis is a pulmonary infection caused by the dimorphic pathogen *Coccidioides immitis*. The disease is endemic in semiarid regions of the southwestern United States, northern and central Mexico, and in parts of Central and South America, where the mycelial form of *C. immitis* resides in desert soil.[132] Infection is acquired by inhalation of airborne arthroconidia.

The epidemiology and clinical aspects of coccidioidomycosis have been extensively reviewed elsewhere.[126,127,133,141] About 60% of patients who have pri-

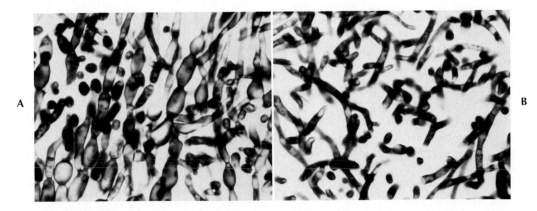

Fig. 10-20. Candidiasis. **A,** Yeastlike cells and pseudohyphae of *Candida albicans*. Notice constrictions between adjacent cells that form the pseudohyphae. **B,** Septate hyphae of *C. albicans* are uniform and narrow and lack prominent constrictions. (Gomori methenamine-silver, 760×.)

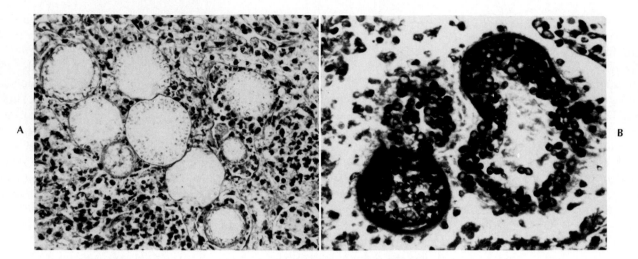

Fig. 10-21. Coccidioidomycosis. **A,** Endosporulating spherules in primary pulmonary coccidioidomycosis. **B,** Endospores released after rupture of spherules. (**A,** Hematoxylin and eosin; 300×; **B,** Gomori methenamine-silver/hematoxylin and eosin; 480×.)

mary pulmonary coccidioidomycosis are asymptomatic; the other 40% develop a mild influenza-like illness that resolves spontaneously in most. Symptoms or radiographic abnormalities persist beyond 6 to 8 weeks in a few patients, who may require treatment with amphotericin B. Chronic progressive coccidioidal pneumonia, an indolent but destructive fibrocavitary disease, occurs in about 1% of patients, and miliary pulmonary infection develops in about 4% of patients. Both forms require systemic antifungal chemotherapy. Benign residual pulmonary nodules, or coccidioidomas, are a late manifestation of pulmonary infection by *C. immitis* that do not ordinarily require antifungal chemotherapy. Disseminated coccidioidomycosis develops in less than 1% of patients with symptomatic primary pulmonary infection. Risk factors for the development of disseminated infection include pregnancy, extremes of age, race (blacks, Filipinos, and American Indians), and immunosuppression.[130,133] Frequent sites of dissemination include the skin and subcutaneous tissue, bones, joints, lymph nodes, spleen, kidneys, and meninges,[128,135] and fatality is high. Primary extrapulmonary (cutaneous) coccidioidomycosis is exceedingly rare; most patients with skin lesions have disseminated infection from an inapparent pulmonary focus.

Primary pulmonary coccidioidomycosis is an acute suppurative and granulomatous pneumonitis. Diagnostic tissue forms of *C. immitis*, usually abundant in active lesions, consist of thin-walled, mature spherules, 30 to 200 μm in diameter (Fig. 10-21, *A*). Rupture of the spherules releases packets of endospores into the surrounding tissue[134] (Fig. 10-21, *B*), where they enlarge progressively to become immature spherules and, after

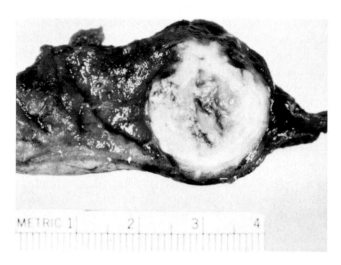

Fig. 10-22. Residual pulmonary coccidioidal nodule. The subpleural fibrocaseous nodule is sharply circumscribed.

endosporulation, mature spherules. The ultrastructure and developmental sequence of *C. immitis* in tissue have been reported by Donnelly and Yunis.[131]

The residual pulmonary coccidioidal nodule, or coccidioidoma, is a peripheral, sharply circumscribed and centrally necrotic granuloma that measures up to 3.5 cm in diameter[129] (Fig. 10-22). About 25% of these nodules are centrally cavitated. Diagnostic endosporulating spherules are found in only about half the nodules, and a specific histopathologic diagnosis may require confirmation by direct immunofluorescence[136] or culture. Mycelium and arthroconidia are occasionally produced in cavitary lesions that communicate with the

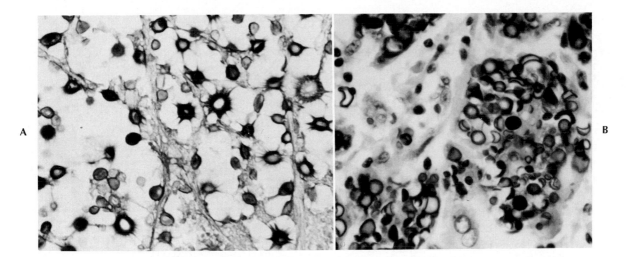

Fig. 10-23. A, Cerebromeningeal cryptococcosis. Numerous single and budding cryptococci have mucicarmine-positive capsules that have a spinous appearance because of shrinkage during processing of tissue. **B,** Granulomatous pneumonia caused by a poorly encapsulated strain of *Cryptococcus neoformans*. The pleomorphic yeast forms do not have conspicuous capsules. (**A,** Mayer's mucicarmine; 600×; **B,** Gomori methenamine-silver; 480×.)

bronchial tree.[138] The lesions of disseminated coccidioidomycosis are granulomatous or suppurative and granulomatous.[135,140]

Characteristic endosporulating spherules of *C. immitis* can be reliably distinguished from the sporangia of *Rhinosporidium seeberi* and the adiaconidia of *Chrysosporium parvum* var. *crescens* in tissue sections on the basis of size, wall thickness, and morphology of endospores (see Table 10-1). The "parent bodies" and "endobodies" found in myospherulosis, a pseudomycosis of the upper respiratory tract and middle ear,[137] are similar in both size and morphology to the spherules and endospores of *C. immitis* but are distinguished by their inherent brown color. The structures of myospherulosis are derived from altered erythrocytes.[139]

Cryptococcosis

Cryptococcosis begins as a pulmonary disease that is usually acquired by inhalation of the soil-inhabiting yeast *Cryptococcus neoformans*.[149,150] This saprophytic fungus is ubiquitous in nature and cosmopolitan in distribution. It is most abundant in habitats that are heavily contaminated by pigeon excreta. Cryptococcosis is not contagious. Although the disease occurs in apparently healthy persons, those with defective immunity and severe underlying diseases, such as hematologic malignancies, are particularly at risk.[145,149]

Clinically, two forms predominate: pulmonary cryptococcosis[147,151] and, by hematogenous dissemination from a pulmonary focus, cerebromeningeal cryptococcosis.[149,150] Dissemination from a primary pulmonary

infection less often results in cutaneous, mucocutaneous, osseous, and visceral forms. In disseminated cryptococcosis, primary lung infection is frequently undetected, and the incubation period is unknown. A primary pulmonary–lymph node complex develops in approximately 1% of the cases of first-infection cryptococcosis.[142] Rarely, cutaneous infection results from direct inoculation of the skin.[143,152]

For reasons that are poorly understood, *C. neoformans* is extremely neurotropic.[150] The clinical course of cerebromeningeal cryptococcosis varies from a few days to 20 years or more. However, it is usually fulminant and, if untreated, is almost invariably fatal. A diagnosis can be made by demonstration of *C. neoformans* cells in cerebrospinal fluid (CSF) or tissue, by isolation of the fungus in culture, or by demonstration of cryptococcal polysaccharide antigen in the CSF by the latex agglutination test. About 25% of patients with cerebromeningeal infection undergo exploratory surgery before the disease is detected. These patients are usually afebrile and have an expanding intracranial lesion that mimics a brain tumor. Amphotericin B is the drug of choice for the treatment of cryptococcosis, and 5-fluorocytosine is effective in some cases.

In tissue sections, *C. neoformans* is a spherical, oval, or elliptical yeastlike fungus that ranges from 5 to 20 μm in diameter.[154] The cell walls of cryptococci are lightly basophilic when stained with hematoxylin and eosin, but they are demonstrated better with the special stains for fungi. Typically, a clear zone of varying width surrounds each fungal cell, representing the space occupied by a mucoid capsule before fixation and processing of the tissue. When stained by mucicarmine, the clear zone contains carminophilic material that often has a spinous appearance because of irregular shrinkage of the mucopolysaccharide capsule during fixation (Fig. 10-23, *A*). Budding cells are numerous in lesions that contain abundant, rapidly proliferating cryptococci. Cryptococci usually have single buds that are attached to parent cells by narrow bases, and multiple buds are occasionally seen. Pseudohyphae and, rarely, true hyphae may be formed in tissue.

Because *C. neoformans* is unusually pleomorphic, and its encapsulated forms are not always conspicuous, cryptococcosis should be considered in the differential histologic diagnosis of virtually any yeast infection.[146] When the capsules of typical cryptococci are carminophilic, a histopathologic diagnosis of cryptococcosis can be made with confidence. Capsule-deficient cryptococci or those with attenuated capsules produced by the so-called "dry variants" can be specifically identified by fluorescent antibody staining of tissue sections. In most instances, however, at least some cryptococci will have capsules that are detectable with stains for mucin.[144,148] Because cryptococcal cell walls contain silver-reducing substances that react positively with melanin stains, a modified Fontana-Masson procedure can be used to identify capsule-deficient cryptococci in histologic sections.[153] Positive staining does not depend on the presence of capsular mucopolysaccharide.

The spectrum of the inflammatory response to *C. neoformans* is broad and varies from little or no inflammation to a purely granulomatous reaction. At times, particularly in terminal or disseminated infections, cryptococci multiply profusely with no apparent host response (Fig. 10-23, *A*). Yeastlike cells displace normal parenchyma and form "cystic" lesions filled with myriad, compact cryptococci whose wide mucoid capsules impart a glistening appearance and slimy consistency to lesions on gross examination. Generally, poorly encapsulated cryptococci elicit granulomatous inflammation in which numerous yeastlike cells without conspicuous capsules are seen within huge multinucleated giant cells and histiocytes[144,148] (Fig. 10-23, *B*).

Pulmonary infection by *C. neoformans* may occasionally result in solitary or multiple fibrocaseous granulomas (cryptococcomas) that, in hematoxylin and eosin–stained sections, are indistinguishable from those caused by infection with *Histoplasma capsulatum* var. *capsulatum* and *Coccidioides immitis*[149,151] (Fig. 10-24). In these cryptococcomas, the yeastlike cells are usually atypical, fragmented, and stain poorly with the special stains for fungi (Fig. 10-24, *inset*). Their capsules may not be carminophilic, and it is often difficult to culture cryptococci from these lesions. Immunofluorescence staining is a valuable diagnostic tool in these cases.

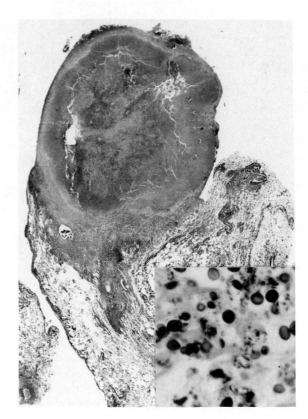

Fig. 10-24. Solitary fibrocaseous nodule (cryptococcoma) in lung of adult woman. *Inset,* Fragmented and unevenly stained cryptococci within central caseous material of nodule. (Hematoxylin and eosin; 10×; *inset,* Gomori methenamine-silver; 480×.)

Fusariosis

The *Fusarium* spp. are responsible for a variety of ocular, cutaneous, and invasive opportunistic fungal infections. These fungi have recently emerged as opportunists among patients with cutaneous burns[157] and patients whose systemic defense mechanisms are compromised by hematologic malignancy or its therapy.[155,156,158] The three major pathogens in this genus are *F. moniliforme, F. oxysporum,* and *F. solani.*[157]

Disseminated fusariosis is usually preceded or accompanied by cutaneous infection in the form of burn wound colonization or painful, erythematous, and necrotic nodules. Local invasion of cutaneous or subcutaneous blood vessels then leads to hematogenous spread to the lungs, liver, kidneys, brain, and other organs.[155] Systemic lesions are abscesses, granulomas, or nodular infarcts.

The hyphae of the *Fusarium* spp. are similar to those of the *Aspergillus* spp., from which they cannot be reliably distinguished in tissue sections. The septate hyphae, 3 to 8 μm in width, do not display the progressive pattern of branching that typifies the hyphae of the *Aspergillus* spp. Instead, hyphal branches are haphaz-

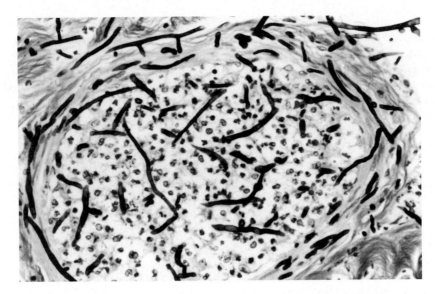

Fig. 10-25. Invasive fusariosis involving a cutaneous burn wound. Septate hyphae of *Fusarium oxysporum* invade a dermal blood vessel. Most hyphal branches arise at right angles to parent hyphae. (Gomori methenamine-silver; 300×.)

ardly distributed along the mycelium and often arise perpendicular to parent hyphae (Fig. 10-25). Intercalated or terminal chlamydoconidia and hyphal varicosities can be seen in some cases, but definitive diagnosis requires isolation and identification of the fungus on synthetic media.

Geotrichosis

Geotrichosis, a rare opportunistic mycosis, is caused by *Geotrichum candidum*, a ubiquitous environmental saprophyte and transient commensal of the human oropharynx, tracheobronchial tree, and gastrointestinal tract. The spectrum of disease caused by this fungus includes transient fungemia[164]; transient or persistent colonization of the respiratory tract, especially the bronchi and preexisting pulmonary cavities[160,161]; and, rarely, cutaneous, oropharyngeal, gastrointestinal, and invasive systemic infections.[159,162,163] Patients who are profoundly immunosuppressed or who have serious underlying disease are predisposed to infection.

In histologic sections, the host response to *G. candidum* is similar to that seen in invasive candidiasis. *G. candidum* appears as hyaline, septate, infrequently branched hyphae, 3 to 6 μm wide, with irregular contours; thick-walled spherical cells up to 12 μm in diameter; and dissociated rectangular or oval arthroconidia, 4 to 10 μm wide, with rounded or squared ends (Fig. 10-26). Fungal elements are poorly stained with hematoxylin and eosin but are readily demonstrated with any of the special stains for fungi.

A definitive diagnosis of geotrichosis is made by obtainment of multiple positive cultures of the fungus

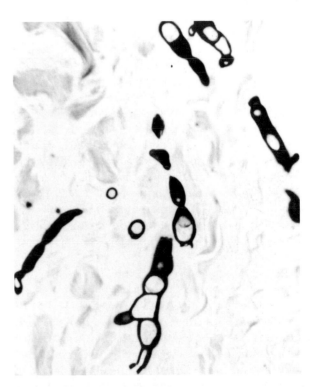

Fig. 10-26. Cutaneous geotrichosis. Hyphae of *Geotrichum candidum* have prominent septations and irregular contours and branch at acute angles. (Gomori methenamine-silver; 850×.)

from blood, respiratory secretions, or tissue, combined with demonstration of typical fungal elements in corresponding specimens using conventional stains and direct immunofluorescence. Severe bronchopulmonary geotrichosis has been successfully treated with oral potassium iodide and aerosolized nystatin, combined with the elimination of predisposing conditions. Bronchopulmonary and disseminated infections may also respond to treatment with amphotericin B and 5-fluorocytosine.

Histoplasmosis capsulati

This systemic mycosis is a respiratory disease contracted by inhalation of airborne infectious conidia of the dimorphic fungus, *Histoplasma capsulatum* var. *capsulatum*.[167,170,176] Conidia and hyphae of this fungus are found in soil, where avian and chiropteran habitats such as blackbird roosts, chicken coops, caves, and attics, favor their growth and multiplication. The disease occurs worldwide, but it is not contagious. In the United States, highly endemic areas include the broad region of the Ohio and Mississippi river valleys. Other countries with high endemicity include Guatemala, Mexico, Peru, and Venezuela. Disease caused by *H. capsulatum* var. *duboisii* is discussed separately (see "Histoplasmosis duboisii") because it is a distinct clinical and pathologic entity. It is confined to the African continent, where both varieties of *H. capsulatum* exist. The two varieties can be distinguished only by the difference in size of their tissue forms.

Epidemiologists estimate that approximately 90% of human infections by *H. capsulatum* var. *capsulatum* are asymptomatic. Confirmation of either current or past infection is based on a positive reaction to the skin test antigen histoplasmin. In time, many asymptomatic persons develop multiple lung calcifications. Symptomatic infections in the remaining 10% fall into three clinical categories: (1) acute pulmonary,[178] (2) disseminated,[173,175] and (3) chronic pulmonary (cavitary).[169,177] About half of all patients with disseminated histoplasmosis capsulati have no apparent immunologic defects.[173,174,179]

In patients who have the acute pulmonary disease, influenza-like symptoms develop after an incubation period of about 15 days. With supportive therapy, these infections either resolve or progress to solitary fibrocaseous nodules (histoplasmomas), and treatment with amphotericin B is only occasionally required. Hematogenous dissemination occurs in a small percentage of patients who have acute pulmonary infections. The yeastlike fungus disseminates by way of the mononuclear phagocyte system and infects various organs, particularly the lungs, lymph nodes, spleen, liver, bone marrow, gastrointestinal tract, and adrenals. It also tends to invade mucosal ulcers.[175] Hepatomegaly and spleno-

megaly are common in this most severe and life-threatening form of the disease. Early diagnosis and antifungal therapy are imperative. The chronic cavitary form of histoplasmosis capsulati is seen primarily in adults, and it may become clinically apparent only after a long dormancy. Radiographs usually reveal unilateral cavities in the upper lung lobes that resemble those seen in tuberculosis. Sclerosing mediastinitis may complicate chronic infection.[168]

In tissue, the yeastlike cells are spherical to oval, 2 to 4 μm in diameter, and reproduce by single budding.[165,166] In active lesions, fungal cells are readily detected with hematoxylin and eosin. Their basophilic cytoplasm is retracted from the rigid but thin and poorly stained cell wall, creating a clear space or "halo" that gives the false impression of an unstained capsule (Fig. 10-27, *A*). Cell walls stain deeply with the special stains for fungi, and the "halo" is not evident (Fig. 10-27, *B*). Pseudohyphae are occasionally seen, and hyphae have been rarely observed near the surface of valvular vegetations in patients with endocarditis.[172]

In the disseminated form of the disease, numerous yeastlike cells replicate within mononuclear phagocytes in the nonimmune or compromised host,[171,173,179] whereas the fungus elicits an epithelioid and giant cell granulomatous reaction in the immune host.[166,176] Necrotic lesions may calcify, and epithelioid cell granulomas resemble those seen in sarcoidosis and tuberculosis.[165,166,176] Because of their intracellular confinement, fungal cells occur in prominent clusters.

Asymptomatic disease may not be detected until old fibrocaseous nodules are found incidentally at autopsy[165] or are suspected of being neoplasms on the basis of chest radiographs and are resected. Microscopically, these nodules (histoplasmomas) consist of a large central zone of caseous necrosis surrounded by a thick wall of dense collagenous connective tissue that may contain epithelioid and multinucleated giant cells (Fig. 10-27, *C*). In the caseous portion, small numbers of distorted and unevenly stained yeastlike cells are usually demonstrated with the Gomori methenamine-silver stain (Fig. 10-27, *D*). The Gridley, periodic acid–Schiff, and hematoxylin and eosin stains do not reliably demonstrate the yeast cells in these lesions, and attempts to culture the fungus are usually unsuccessful. The organisms can be specifically identified by immunofluorescence staining.

Poorly encapsulated cryptococci and small tissue forms of *Blastomyces dermatitidis* can resemble yeast forms of *Histoplasma capsulatum* var. *capsulatum*. However, cryptococci are usually carminophilic, and *B. dermatitidis* cells are multinucleated, have thick walls, and bud by a broad base. When these differentiating features are equivocal, immunofluorescence staining is

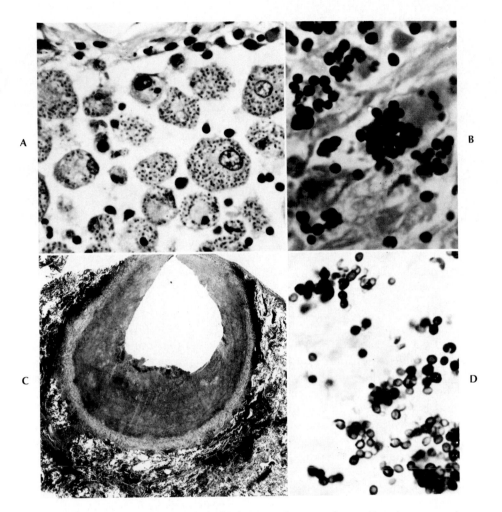

Fig. 10-27. Histoplasmosis capsulati. **A,** Acute pulmonary form. Alveolar macrophages are filled with small yeast forms, 2 to 4 μm in diameter, whose dark cytoplasm is retracted, creating a clear space or "halo." **B,** Disseminated form in adrenal gland. Notice clustering of fungal cells. There is no "halo" effect when special fungal stains are used. **C,** Subpleural solitary nodule (histoplasmoma) in lung of adult man. **D,** Replicate section of nodule in **C** demonstrates distorted, poorly stained *Histoplasma* cells in central caseous material. (**A,** Hematoxylin and eosin; 480×; **B,** Gomori methenamine-silver; 600×; **C,** Hematoxylin and eosin, 10×; **D,** Gomori methenamine-silver; 600×.)

invaluable. In hematoxylin and eosin–stained sections, intracellular forms of the *Leishmania* spp. and *Trypanosoma* spp. can mimic *Histoplasma* spp. The distinguishing barshaped kinetoplast of these two protozoans can sometimes be seen under oil immersion but is best demonstrated by Giemsa and Wilder's reticulum stains. Cells of *Toxoplasma gondii*, which can also be confused with *Histoplasma*, are smaller, stain entirely with hematoxylin and eosin, and are usually not found within phagocytes. The *Leishmania* spp., *Trypanosoma* spp., and *Toxoplasma gondii* are not reliably stained with the special stains for fungi.

Histoplasmosis duboisii (African histoplasmosis)

Histoplasmosis duboisii is a pulmonary disease with a pronounced tropism for bones and skin.[180-185] It is caused by the large-celled form or *duboisii* variety of *Histoplasma capsulatum*. When grown in vitro, mycelial and yeast forms of this fungus are indistinguishable from those of the classical, small-celled form or *capsulatum* variety of this species. The two can be distinguished from each other only when the size of the yeastlike cells that develop in tissue is observed. Diseases caused by the two varieties of *Histoplasma cap-*

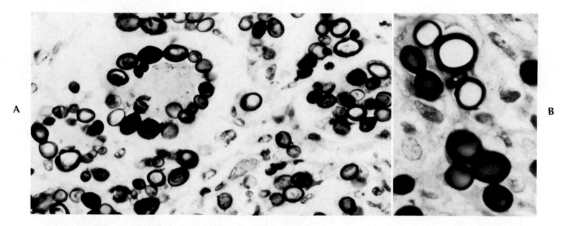

Fig. 10-28. Cutaneous histoplasmosis duboisii. **A,** Single and budding yeast forms within histiocytes and large multinucleated giant cells in dermis. **B,** Details of classical hourglass or double-cell yeast forms, 8 to 15 μm in diameter, with narrow based buds and thick cell walls. (Gomori methenamine-silver/hematoxylin and eosin; **A,** 480×; **B,** 900×.)

sulatum are clinically and pathologically distinct.

Other than one autochthonous case from Japan, natural infection caused by *H. capsulatum* var. *duboisii* has been reported only in humans and nonhuman primates from Africa. The disease is rarely seen in the United States in persons who previously lived or traveled in Africa.[184] Clinically, patients usually present with one or more of the following: lymphadenopathy; mucocutaneous lesions that may be abscessed and ulcerated; and insidious osteolytic lesions, particularly of the ribs, long bones, and cranium. Disseminated disease may also involve the lungs, liver, spleen, and intestine. Amphotericin B and excision of isolated skin lesions are treatments of choice for disseminated and localized infection, respectively.

Lesions typically contain a dispersed granulomatous inflammatory reaction in which large numbers of yeastlike cells are seen within the cytoplasm of histiocytes and huge multinucleated giant cells[180,185] (Fig. 10-28, *A*). The spherical to oval fungal cells are uninucleate and 8 to 15 μm in diameter, have thick walls, and bud by a relatively narrow base. Classical "hourglass" and "double-cell" forms are created when budding daughter cells enlarge until they equal the size of the parent cells, to which they remain connected by a narrow base (Fig. 10-28, *B*). Tissue forms of *H. capsulatum* var. *duboisii* and *Blastomyces dermatitidis* are of similar size and shape and thus may be mistaken for each other. However, the latter buds by a broader base and is multinucleated. Histoplasmosis capsulati also occurs in Africa, but its causative agent is much smaller (2 to 4 μm) in tissue than the large-celled *duboisii* variety.

Malasseziasis (systemic)

Malassezia furfur is usually encountered as the etiologic agent of tinea versicolor, a common superficial mycosis that occurs worldwide and is primarily of cosmetic importance. In rare instances, however, this lipophilic and lipid-dependent fungus can cause fungemia and systemic infection that is usually a specific complication of prolonged intralipid infusion through central venous catheters.[186-188] Most systemic infections have occurred in infants less than 14 weeks old and in older patients with severe, chronic gastrointestinal disease.[187] Although patients may be asymptomatic, they usually present with fever and signs and symptoms of sepsis and thrombocytopenia. The lungs are most frequently involved, apparently because of increased lipid deposition in the walls of pulmonary blood vessels.[188]

In deep infections, elements of *M. furfur* appear as spherical or oval, thick-walled, budding yeastlike cells, 3 to 8 μm in diameter, that are considered to be phialoconidia (Fig. 10-29). Often, a small, unipolar, phialidic collarette can be seen at the point where a conidium (bud) was extruded from a parent cell; short, curved hyphae are rarely produced in deep infections. Fungal elements are either basophilic or amphophilic in hematoxylin and eosin–stained tissue sections but are best demonstrated with the special stains for fungi.

Prompt removal of colonized vascular catheters may be the only treatment necessary for *M. furfur* fungemia. Severe systemic infections have been treated successfully with miconazole and amphotericin B after catheter removal.[187]

Nocardiosis

Between 500 and 1000 new cases of nocardiosis, a subacute or chronic bacterial infection, are diagnosed annually in the United States.[189,192] In about 85% of these cases, infection is caused by *Nocardia asteroides*. The remaining 15% are caused by *N. brasiliensis* and *N. otitidiscaviarum (caviae)*.[191,192] Infections by these filamentous bacteria of the order Actinomycetales occur worldwide and are usually seen in persons with underlying immunologic deficiency. Well-recognized conditions that predispose patients to nocardial infection include lymphoma, Hodgkin's disease, chronic granulomatous disease of childhood, and pulmonary alveolar proteinosis.[193,195,199] Unlike actinomycosis, nocardiosis is an exogenous disease, and infections are usually contracted by inhalation of nocardiae that live as saprophytes in nature. The disease is not contagious.

The clinical manifestations of nocardiosis are extremely variable.[192-194] All three *Nocardia* species may cause mycetoma, which is discussed elsewhere in this chapter. More commonly, the disease is systemic with a pulmonary inception. Lung lesions may occur as large cavitating abscesses or as diffuse fibrinopurulent pneumonia similar to that caused by certain nonfilamentous bacteria. Fibrosis is usually minimal. There may be hematogenous dissemination to other body sites from a primary focus in the lungs. About 20% of patients with pulmonary nocardiosis have central nervous system involvement, usually in the form of cerebral abscesses.[191,192,198] Meningitis, a rare complication, results from rupture of an intracerebral abscess or direct extension of nocardial osteomyelitis. Nocardiosis may also present as solitary or multiple subcutaneous lesions that are attributable either to traumatic implantation or to systemic infection.[190,196] These localized lesions, with chains of nodules leading from a primary skin ulcer, can mimic those of cutaneous sporotrichosis.[192] This entity is known as the sporotrichoid form of nocardiosis. Sulfonamides are useful for treating all forms of the disease. Because of a strong tendency for relapse, prolonged therapy may be required.[192,197]

In systemic infections, the *Nocardia* spp. almost never form granules. Rather, these organisms occur as individual, gram-positive, beaded filaments, about 1 μm in width, that branch at approximately right angles (Fig. 10-30). The delicate filaments are not stained by hematoxylin and eosin, periodic acid–Schiff, or Gridley stains. However, they are readily demonstrated with the Gomori methenamine-silver and tissue Gram stains. All three *Nocardia* spp. are often partially acid-fast in tissue sections when stained with modified acid-fast procedures using a weak decolorizing agent. They lose their acid-fastness when cultured on artificial media. Usually, the agents of actinomycosis are not acid-fast.

Paracoccidioidomycosis (South American blastomycosis)

Paracoccidioidomycosis is a progressive pulmonary infection caused by the single dimorphic species *Paracoccidioides brasiliensis*. The disease is highly endemic in South America, particularly in Brazil, Colombia, and Venezuela. Autochthonous cases have also been re-

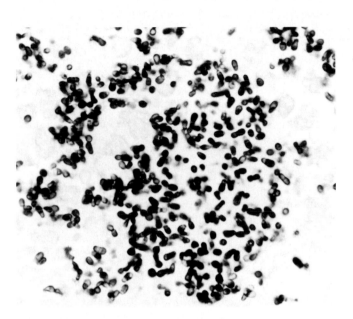

Fig. 10-29. Systemic malasseziasis in an infant. A pulmonary thromboembolus contains numerous yeastlike cells of *Malassezia furfur*, 3 to 8 μm in diameter, with single buds (phialoconidia). (Gomori methenamine-silver; 560×.)

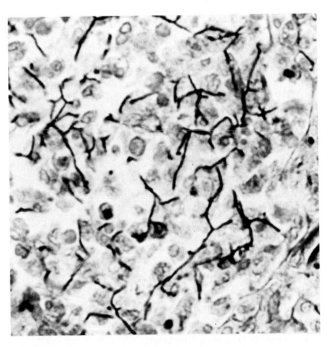

Fig. 10-30. Pulmonary nocardiosis. Delicate filaments that branch at approximately right angles are embedded in fibrinopurulent, alveolar exudate. (Gomori methenamine-silver/hematoxylin and eosin; 600×.)

ported from Central America and Mexico, but cases discovered in the United States have all been acquired within endemic areas of Latin America.[205]

Paracoccidioidomycosis is predominantly a disease of rural adult males.[206] The primary focus of infection occurs in the lungs, but pulmonary involvement may be overshadowed clinically by manifestations of limited or widespread lymphatic and hematogenous dissemination.[200] Paracoccidioidomycosis of childhood is an acute, progressive pulmonary infection that rapidly disseminates to lymph nodes, liver, and spleen.[201] In adults, the infection pursues a more chronic course with variable periods of clinical latency.[200,202,203]

Acute progressive pulmonary paracoccidioidomycosis is an acute suppurative pneumonitis that contains scattered multinucleated giant cells and yeast forms of *P. brasiliensis.* The chronic progressive form is characterized by granulomatous inflammation with extensive interstitial and conglomerate fibrosis, necrosis, and arterial intimal fibrosis leading to cor pulmonale.[207,208] At autopsy, disseminated lesions are found in extrathoracic sites in the majority of patients, chiefly involving the oropharyngeal mucosa, larynx, trachea, skin, lymph nodes, liver, spleen, adrenal glands, intestines, and kidneys.[207,208] These disseminated lesions are granulomatous, or suppurative and granulomatous. Cutaneous and mucosal lesions also exhibit pseudoepitheliomatous hyperplasia similar to that typically found in the lesions of blastomycosis and sporotrichosis.

In tissue sections, *P. brasiliensis* occurs predominantly as pleomorphic yeastlike cells, 5 to 60 μm in diameter, that reproduce by budding. Small yeast forms and hyphae are occasionally found.[204] Thick-walled, effete "mosaic" cells with fractured walls are often numerous in chronic pulmonary lesions. A definitive histopathologic diagnosis of paracoccidioidomycosis requires identification of characteristic multiple-budding cells that resemble a ship's steering wheel (Fig. 10-31). The blastoconidia produced by these cells have an oval, tubular, or teardrop configuration and are attached to parent cells by narrow necks.

Penicilliosis marneffei

Penicilliosis marneffei is a rare progressive and disseminated mycosis caused by *Penicillium marneffei,* a ubiquitous saprophyte of soil and decomposing organic matter.[213] Of the more than 150 recognized species of *Penicillium,* only *P. marneffei* is known to be dimorphic and to cause invasive infection. This mycosis is endemic in Southeast and Far East Asia, and most human infections probably have a pulmonary inception after inhalation of airborne infectious conidia of *P. marneffei* produced in the environment.[209-212] Persons who are debilitated or immunocompromised appear to be at increased risk of infection.[214]

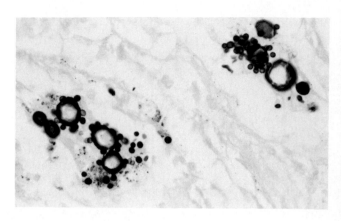

Fig. 10-31. Paracoccidioidomycosis. Several thick-walled cells have produced multiple blastoconidia. (Gomori methenamine-silver; 480×.)

Patients with disseminated penicilliosis marneffei often present with chronic productive cough, mucoid sputum, chest pain, generalized lymphadenopathy, hepatosplenomegaly, draining skin ulcers, subcutaneous abscesses, osteolytic lesions, anemia, leukocytosis, and a history of weight loss and prolonged intermittent fever.[209] The course of the disease can range from 2 months to 3 years or more. Organs most frequently involved include the lungs, liver, intestine, lymph nodes, tonsils, skin, bone marrow, kidneys, and spleen.[209,211]

The host response in penicilliosis marneffei is similar to that seen in histoplasmosis capsulati, where numerous small yeastlike cells proliferate within and distend histiocytes (Fig. 10-32). Slowly evolving pulmonary abscesses and granulomas can lead to fibrosis and cavitation, but calcification has not been reported. In histologic sections, the cells of *P. marneffei* are spherical to oval, 2.5 to 5μm in diameter, and resemble those of *Histoplasma capsulatum* var. *capsulatum* (Fig. 10-32). However, unlike histoplasma and other invasive yeastlike fungi, *P. marneffei* does not bud. Reproduction is by fission (schizogony) with the formation of a single transverse septum that stains more intensely with the special stains for fungi and is wider than the external wall (Fig. 10-32, *inset*). Short hyphal forms and elongated, curved sausage-like forms with rounded ends and one or more septa are also occasionally produced, especially in necrotic and cavitary lesions.

A definitive diagnosis of penicilliosis marneffei can be made by demonstration of typical yeastlike cells in clinical specimens and by microbiologic culture on standard mycologic media. The mycosis must be aggressively treated with amphotericin B, 5-fluorocytosine, or ketoconazole. Because relapse is common, antifungals should be given for several months.

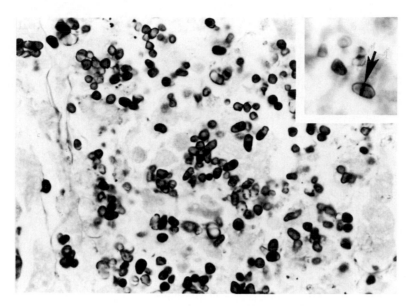

Fig. 10-32. Disseminated penicilliosis marneffei. Hepatic abscess contains individual and clustered yeastlike cells of *Penicillium marneffei*, 2.5 to 5 μm in diameter. *Inset, P. marneffei* cell with single, wide, transverse septum *(arrow)* and rounded ends. (Gomori methenamine-silver/hematoxylin and eosin; 850×; *inset,* 1200×.)

Pseudallescheriasis

Pseudallescheria boydii is the most frequent etiologic agent of eumycotic mycetoma in the United States and is an occasional agent of otomycosis, keratitis, endophthalmitis, meningitis, brain abscess, and osteomyelitis.[219] This fungus can be isolated from clinical specimens in either of two forms: the asexual (anamorphic) form, designated *Scedosporium* (formerly *Monosporium) apiospermum,* and the sexual (teleomorphic) form, designated *Pseudallescheria* (formerly *Allescheria* and *Petriellidium) boydii.* By convention, the disease is named for the sexual form.

P. boydii can colonize preexisting pulmonary cavities and form intracavitary fungus balls that resemble those produced by the *Aspergillus* spp.[215] The intracavitary mycelium consists of amorphous hyphal aggregates or of compact, concentrically laminated and intertwined hyphae. Invasive pulmonary and disseminated pseudallescheriasis are rare opportunistic infections that occur preferentially in patients treated for acute leukemia who are granulocytopenic.[216-218] Invasive lesions are infarctive as a consequence of mycelial invasion of blood vessels, but abscesses have also been reported.[217] Disseminated pseudallescheriasis frequently involves the brain, thyroid gland, heart, and kidneys.

In tissue sections, the hyphae of *P. boydii* resemble those of the *Aspergillus* spp. The septate hyphae, 2 to 5 μm wide, branch in a dichotomous but haphazard pattern and may produce vesicles, truncated terminal conidia, and terminal or intercalated chlamydoconidia (Fig. 10-33). Hyphal vascular invasion is conspicuous in the invasive and disseminated lesions. Because the morphologic features of pulmonary and disseminated pseudallescheriasis and the morphologic features of the hyphae in tissue sections closely resemble those of aspergillosis, the diagnosis is best confirmed by culture or immunofluorescence.

Torulopsosis

Torulopsosis is a rare opportunistic mycosis caused by the small (2 to 5 μm), budding, spherical to oval, yeastlike fungus *Torulopsis glabrata*—a dominant member of the body's natural flora.[220,221] Fungemia, the most common form of *T. glabrata* infection, has been associated with prolonged intravenous alimentation, severe abdominal trauma, and appendiceal abscesses.[222-225] Often, the source of fungemia is unexplained. Tissue invasion by *T. glabrata* is uncommon. When it occurs, the endocardium, kidneys, lungs, and central nervous system, are sites most frequently involved with suppurative or, rarely, granulomatous inflammation.[222,223] The morphologic features of *T. glabrata* are similar to those of *Histoplasma capsulatum* var. *capsulatum*, especially when cells of the former are clustered within histiocytes (Fig. 10-34). However, unlike histoplasma, the yeastlike cells of *T. glabrata* are amphophilic when stained

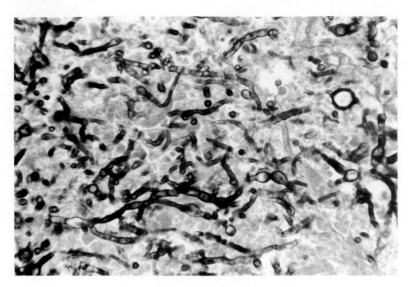

Fig. 10-33. Disseminated pseudallescheriasis. Slender hyphae of *Pseudallescheria boydii* are segmentally vesicular. A thick-walled, terminal chlamydoconidium is visible at upper right. (Gomori methenamine-silver; 480×.)

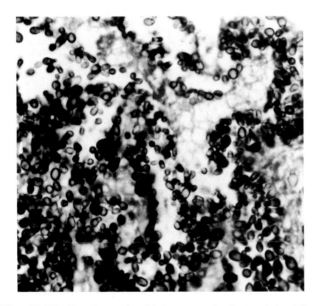

Fig. 10-34. Torulopsosis. Numerous single and budding yeastlike cells of *Torulopsis glabrata,* 2 to 5 μm in diameter, are embedded in an arterial thrombus. (Gomori methenamine-silver; 850×.)

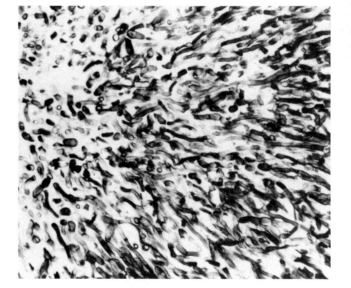

Fig. 10-35. Disseminated trichosporonosis. Hyphae and oval or rectangular arthroconidia of *Trichosporon beigelii* in a splenic nodular infarct. Blastoconidia are not clearly visible in this field. (Gomori methenamine-silver; 480×.)

with hematoxylin and eosin, and no "halo" or pseudocapsular effect is evident. Culture or immunofluorescence is needed for definitive identification.

Trichosporonosis

The *Trichosporon* spp., like the agents of fusariosis, have recently emerged as significant systemic pathogens in compromised patients. These yeastlike fungi are soil saprophytes that also form a minor component of

normal skin flora. Only two species are known to cause disseminated opportunistic infection. *T. beigelii (T. cutaneum),* the more frequent pathogen, is better known as the agent of white piedra, a nodule-forming trichomycosis. The other species, *T. capitatum,* has only rarely been implicated as an agent of disseminated infection.[231]

Disseminated trichosporonosis occurs principally in patients who are neutropenic as a result of treatment

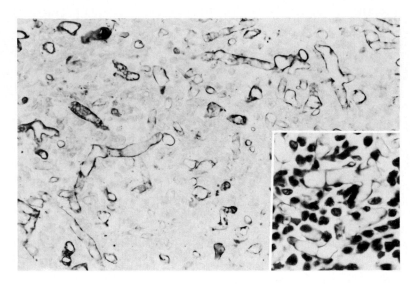

Fig. 10-36. Zygomycosis (mucormycosis). Broad, irregular hyphae of *Saksenaea vasiformis*. Notice haphazard branching at right angles and absence of septa. Round and oval forms are hyphae sectioned transversely. *Inset,* Septa are occasionally present in some hyphae. (Gomori methenamine-silver; 300×; *inset,* periodic acid–Schiff; 480×.)

for acute leukemia, lymphoma, or solid tumors,[228,230] but it has also been reported in immunosuppressed transplant recipients. Purpuric cutaneous nodules are a frequent clinical manifestation, and the lungs, kidneys, myocardium, liver, spleen, and bone marrow are also frequently involved. Systemic lesions consist of abscesses,[229] granulomas,[226] or nodular infarcts,[227] the last a consequence of mycotic vascular invasion and occlusion.

In tissue sections, the *Trichosporon* spp. can be recognized as pleomorphic blastoconidia, 3 to 8 μm in diameter, septate hyphae, and arthroconidia that are produced by fragmentation of hyphal segments (Fig. 10-35). These fungi may be difficult to distinguish from some other opportunistic pathogens, such as the *Candida* spp., if arthroconidia are inconspicuous. A presumptive histopathologic diagnosis of trichosporonosis is therefore best confirmed by culture or immunofluorescence.

Zygomycosis

Zygomycosis is a generic term used to designate a variety of infectious diseases caused by members of the class Zygomycetes (formerly Phycomycetes). Pathogenic fungi belonging to this class are grouped in the orders Mucorales and Entomophthorales, and the diseases caused by these fungi are often referred to respectively as mucormycosis and entomophthoromycosis.

Mucormycosis

Mucormycosis is a sporadic but cosmopolitan opportunistic infection that occurs in patients with serious underlying diseases, such as diabetic acidosis and acute leukemia, and in patients treated with corticosteroids or cytotoxic drugs.[239,242] Well-authenticated agents of human mucormycosis include species within the genera *Rhizopus, Absidia, Mucor, Rhizomucor, Apophysomyces, Cunninghamella,* and *Saksenaea.* These saprophytic fungi are widely distributed in nature, and infection is acquired by exposure to their sporangiospores. Although relatively uncommon, mucormycosis is the third most frequent opportunistic mycosis in patients with neoplastic diseases.

The hyphae of the mucoraceous zygomycetes have a characteristic appearance in tissue sections (Fig. 10-36). Typical hyphae are broad (6 to 25 μm wide), thin-walled, and pleomorphic, with irregular, nonparallel contours. Branches arise haphazardly, often at right angles to the parent hyphae. Septa can be found in some of the hyphae (Fig. 10-36, *inset*), though most of the hyphae appear nonseptate (cenocytic). Because the hyphae have little structural stability, they are often folded, twisted, wrinkled, or collapsed. The thin hyphal walls stain as well with hematoxylin as with the special stains for fungi. Thick-walled, ovoid chlamydoconidia are rarely formed in tissues,[235] but sporangia are almost never produced.

Invasive opportunistic infections caused by the mucoraceous zygomycetes are characterized by tissue infarction and, in the nongranulocytopenic host, acute suppurative inflammation. Infarcts are caused by thrombosis complicating hyphal invasion of arteries and veins. Angioinvasion may also lead to hematogenous dissemination. Microscopically the lesions are characterized by coagulative necrosis and neutrophilic infiltra-

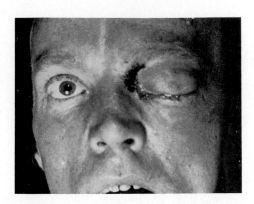

Fig. 10-37. Cellulitis of left orbit in a diabetic patient with rhinocerebral form of mucormycosis. (Courtesy Dr. Roger D. Baker, Silver Spring, Md.)

tion. Rarely a granulomatous reaction is observed in localized, indolent, or partially treated infections.

Several clinical forms of mucormycosis are recognized.[239,245] Rhinocerebral mucormycosis begins as a fulminant infection of the nasal cavity, paranasal sinuses, and soft tissues of the orbit (Fig. 10-37). The infection, often unilateral, may extend directly from these sites to involve the meninges and brain, and it may be complicated by thrombosis of the cavernous sinus and internal carotid artery. Patients with diabetic acidosis or leukemia are predisposed to rhinocerebral infection, which is most often caused by *Rhizopus oryzae*. Once established, this infection is difficult to treat and is rapidly fatal.

Invasive pulmonary mucormycosis and disseminated mucormycosis occur preferentially in patients with acute leukemia or lymphoma.[242] Pulmonary mucormycosis is a progressive infection characterized by pulmonary vascular invasion, parenchymal infarction, and hematogenous dissemination. A more limited endobronchial form, which occurs in diabetics, causes bronchial obstruction and may eventuate in serious hemorrhage after hyphal invasion into adjacent blood vessels.[234] Gastrointestinal mucormycosis usually begins as a secondary infection of preexisting ulcers in malnourished persons, but it may also be a manifestation of disseminated infection.[240] The stomach is involved most frequently, followed by the colon and small intestine.[243] The mucosal lesions are blackened, necrotic ulcers, and local vascular invasion may lead to ischemia of adjacent segments of the stomach or intestine.

Cutaneous mucormycosis can be a manifestation of disseminated mucormycosis or can occur as a primary infection of burned patients[233] or patients whose surgical wounds are dressed with contaminated elastic bandages.[236,241] Many of the bandage-associated nosocomial infections have been caused by *Rhizopus rhizopodiformis*. Cutaneous lesions are necrotic nodules that ulcer-

ate and become covered with blackened exudate.[233] Disseminated mucormycosis can involve almost any organ, most frequently the lungs, central nervous system, spleen, kidneys, heart, and gastrointestinal tract.[242] Septic thrombosis of the coronary arteries produces mycotic myocardial infarction.[246]

Successful treatment of mucormycosis depends on early recognition of the infection and control of the underlying disease coupled with radical débridement or excision of devitalized tissue and systemic antifungal chemotherapy with amphotericin B. Greater awareness of this opportunistic infection and rapid clinical intervention have resulted in improved prognosis.[244]

Entomophthoromycosis (subcutaneous and rhinofacial zygomycosis)

Entomophthoromycosis is a sporadic subcutaneous infection that is largely restricted to tropical areas of Africa, Asia, and South America.[232,247] Neither of the two clinically distinct forms of this mycosis occurs preferentially in patients with underlying disease or defective immunity.

Subcutaneous zygomycosis, caused by *Basidiobolus ranarum*, manifests clinically as a firm, painless, disciform nodule on the trunk or extremities.[233,238] If untreated, the nodule may enlarge and spread locally, but systemic dissemination is extremely uncommon. The infection is probably initiated by penetrating trauma. Rhinofacial zygomycosis, caused by *Conidiobolus coronatus*, is a locally progressive infection of the nasal cavity, paranasal sinuses, and soft tissues of the face.[232]

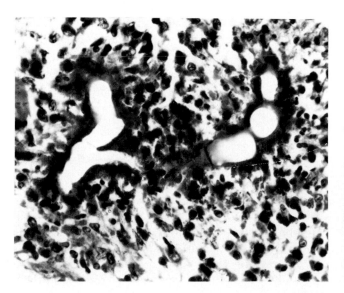

Fig. 10-38. Subcutaneous zygomycosis (entomophthoromycosis). Hyphal fragments of *Basidiobolus ranarum*, coated with Splendore-Hoeppli material, are surrounded by granulation tissue rich in eosinophils. (Hematoxylin and eosin; 480×.)

Extension of the infection to the mediastinum has been reported.[237]

The microscopic features of both forms of entomophthoromycosis are similar, but they differ altogether from those of mucormycosis.[237,247] Relatively few, broad, thin-walled, and infrequently septate hyphal fragments are found in the lesions. Each hyphal fragment is enveloped by eosinophilic Splendore-Hoeppli material (Fig. 10-38). The inflammatory reaction immediately surrounding each hyphal fragment is eosinophilic and granulomatous, and the adjacent stroma consists of granulation tissue with acute and chronic inflammatory cells. Unlike the agents of mucormycosis, those of entomophthoromycosis do not aggressively invade blood vessels, which accounts for the rarity of infarction and dissemination in this form of zygomycosis.

REFERENCES
General

1. Baker, R.D., senior editor: The pathologic anatomy of mycoses: human infection with fungi, actinomycetes and algae, New York, 1971, Springer-Verlag.
2. Baker, R.D., and Chick, E.W.: Proceedings of International Symposium on Opportunistic Fungus Infections, Lab Invest. **11:**1017, 1962.
3. Binford, C.H., and Connor, D.H., editors: Pathology of tropical and extraordinary diseases, Washington, D.C., 1976, Armed Forces Institute of Pathology, pp. 551-609.
4. Chandler, F.W., Kaplan, W., and Ajello, L.: Color atlas and text of the histopathology of mycotic diseases, Chicago, 1980, Year Book Medical Publishers.
5. Chandler, F.W., and Watts, J.C.: Pathologic diagnosis of fungal infections, Chicago, 1987, American Society of Clinical Pathologists Press.
6. Chandler, F.W., and Watts, J.C.: Fungal infections. In Dail, D.H., and Hammar, S.P., editors: Pulmonary pathology, New York, 1988, Springer-Verlag.
7. Conant, N.F., et al.: Manual of clinical mycology, ed. 3, Philadelphia, 1971, W.B. Saunders Co.
8. Emmons, C.W., et al.: Medical mycology, ed. 3, Philadelphia, 1977, Lea & Febiger.
9. Grieco, M.H., editor: Infections in the abnormal host, New York, 1980, Yorke Medical Books, pp. 325-359.
10. Kaplan, W., and Kraft, D.E.: Demonstration of pathogenic fungi in formalin-fixed tissues by immunofluorescence, Am. J. Clin. Pathol. **52:**420, 1969.
11. McGinnis, M.R.: Laboratory handbook of medical mycology, New York, 1980, Academic Press.
12. Palmer, D.F., et al.: Serodiagnosis of mycotic diseases, Springfield, Ill., 1977, Charles C Thomas, Publisher.
13. Rippon, J.W.: Medical mycology: the pathogenic fungi and the pathogenic actinomycetes, ed. 3, Philadelphia, 1988, W.B. Saunders Co.
14. Roberts, S.O.B., Hay, R.J., and Mackenzie, D.W.R.: A clinician's guide to fungal disease, New York, 1984, Marcel Dekker.
15. Schwarz, J.: The diagnosis of deep mycoses by morphologic methods, Hum. Pathol. **13:**519, 1982.
16. Warnock, D.W., and Richardson, M.D., editors: Fungal infection in the compromised patient, New York, 1982, John Wiley & Sons.

Superficial mycoses

17. Alteras, I., Feuerman, E.J., David, M., and Shvili, D.: Unusual aspects of granulomatous dermatophytosis, Mycopathologia **86:**93, 1984.
18. Graham, J.H.: Superficial fungus infections. In Graham, J.H.,

Johnson, W.C., and Helwig, E.G., editors: Dermal pathology, Hagerstown, Md., 1972, Harper & Row.
19. Graham, J.H., and Barroso-Tobila, C.: Dermal pathology of superficial fungus infections. In Baker, R.D., editor: The pathologic anatomy of mycoses: human infection with fungi, actinomycetes and algae, New York, 1971, Springer-Verlag.
20. Rebell, G., and Taplin, D.: Dermatophytes: their recognition and identification, ed. 2, Coral Gables, Fla., 1970, University of Miami Press.
21. West, B.C., and Kwon-Chung, K.J.: Mycetoma caused by *Microsporum audouinii:* first reported case, Am. J. Clin. Pathol. **73:**447, 1980.

Cutaneous and subcutaneous mycoses
Chromoblastomycosis

22. Batres, E., Wolf, J.E., Jr., Rudolph, A.H., and Knox, J.M.: Transepithelial elimination of cutaneous chromomycosis, Arch. Dermatol. **114:**1231, 1978.
23. Carrion, A.L.: Chromoblastomycosis and related infections, Int. J. Dermatol. **14:**27, 1975.
24. McGinnis, M.R.: Chromoblastomycosis and phaeohyphomycosis: new concepts, diagnosis, and mycology, J. Am. Acad. Dermatol. **8:**1, 1983.
25. Vollum, D.I.: Chromomycosis: a review, Br. J. Dermatol. **96:**454, 1977.

Lobomycosis

26. Caldwell, D.K., Caldwell, M.C., Woodard, J.C., et al.: Lobomycosis as a disease of the Atlantic bottle-nosed dolphin, Am. J. Trop. Med. Hyg. **24:**105, 1975.
27. Wiersema, J.P.: Lobo's disease (keloidal blastomycosis). In Baker, R.D., editor: The pathologic anatomy of mycoses: human infection with fungi, actinomycetes and algae, New York, 1971, Springer-Verlag.

Mycetoma

28. Cameron, H.M., Gatei, D., and Bremner, A.D.: The deep mycoses in Kenya: a histopathological study. 1. Mycetoma, East Afr. Med. J. **50:**382, 1973.
29. Green, W.O., and Adams, T.E.: Mycetoma in the United States: a review and report of seven additional cases, Am. J. Clin. Pathol. **42:**75, 1964.
30. Magana, M.: Mycetoma, Int. J. Dermatol. **23:**221, 1984.
31. Mahgoub, E.S.: Medical management of mycetoma, Bull. WHO **54:**303, 1976.
32. Mahgoub, E.S., and Murray, I.G.: Mycetoma, London, 1973, William Heinemann Medical Books.
33. Tight, R.R., and Bartlett, M.S.: Actinomycetoma in the United States, Rev. Infect. Dis. **3:**1139, 1981.
34. Winslow, D.J., and Steen, F.G.: Considerations in the histologic diagnosis of mycetoma, Am. J. Clin. Pathol. **42:**164, 1964.

Phaeohyphomycosis (subcutaneous and systemic)

35. Ajello, L.: Phaeohyphomycosis: definition and etiology. In Mycoses, Scientific Publication no. 304:126, Washington, D.C., 1975, Pan American Health Organization.
36. Bambirra, E.A., Miranda, D., Nogueira, A.M., and Barbosa, C.S.: Phaeohyphomycotic cyst: a clinicopathologic study of the first four cases described from Brazil, Am. J. Trop. Med. Hyg. **32:**794, 1983.
37. Crichlow, D.K., Enrile, F.T., and Memon, M.Y.: Cerebellar abscess due to *Cladosporium trichoides (bantianum):* case report, Am. J. Clin. Pathol. **60:**416, 1973.
38. Estes, S.A., Merz, W.G., and Maxwell, L.G.: Primary cutaneous phaeohyphomycosis caused by *Drechslera spicifera,* Arch. Dermatol. **113:**813, 1977.
39. Iwatsu, T., and Miyaji, M.: Phaeomycotic cyst: a case with a lesion containing a wooden splinter, Arch. Dermatol. **120:**1209, 1984.
40. Masini, T., Riviera, L., Cappricci, E., and Arienta, C.: Cerebral phaeohyphomycosis, Clin. Neuropathol. **4:**246, 1985.
41. McGinnis, M.R.: Human pathogenic species of *Exophiala, Phialophora* and *Wangiella.* In The black and white yeasts, Sci-

entific Publication no. 356:37, Washington, D.C., 1978, Pan American Health Organization.

42. Moskowitz, L.B., Cleary, T.J., McGinnis, M.R., and Thomson, C.B.: *Phialophora richardsiae* in a lesion appearing as a giant cell tumor of the tendon sheath, Arch. Pathol. Lab. Med. **107**:374, 1983.

43. Riley, O., Jr., and Mann, S.H.: Brain abscess caused by *Cladosporium trichoides:* review of three cases and report of fourth case, Am. J. Clin. Pathol. **33**:525, 1960.

44. Ziefer, A., and Connor, D.H.: Phaeomycotic cyst: a clinicopathologic study of twenty-five patients, Am. J. Trop. Med. Hyg. **29**:901, 1980.

Prototothecosis

45. Chandler, F.W., Kaplan, W., and Callaway, C.S.: Differentiation between *Prototheca* and morphologically similar green algae in tissue, Arch. Pathol. Lab. Med. **102**:353, 1978.

46. Connor, D.H., Gibson, D.W., and Ziefer, A.: Diagnostic features of three unusual infections: micronemiasis, phaeomycotic cyst, and prototothecosis. In Majno, G., Cotran, R.S., and Kaufman, N., editors: Current topics in inflammation and infection, IAP Monogr. no. 23, Baltimore, 1982, Williams & Wilkins.

47. Cox, G.E., Wilson, J.D., and Brown, P.: Prototothecosis: a case of disseminated algal infection, Lancet **2**:379, 1974.

48. Davies, R.R., and Wilkinson, J.L.: Human prototothecosis: supplementary studies, Ann. Trop. Med. Parasitol. **61**:112, 1967.

49. Jones, J.W., McFadden, H.W., Chandler, F.W., Kaplan, W., and Conner, D.M.: Green algal infection in a human, Am. J. Clin. Pathol. **80**:102, 1983.

50. Nosanchuk, J.S., and Greenberg, R.D.: Prototothecosis of the olecranon bursa caused by achloric algae, Am. J. Clin. Pathol. **59**:567, 1973.

51. Sudman, M.S.: Prototothecosis: a critical review, Am. J. Clin. Pathol. **61**:10, 1974.

52. Tindall, J.P., and Fetter, B.F.: Infections caused by achloric algae (prototothecosis), Arch. Dermatol. **104**:490, 1971.

Rhinosporidiosis

53. Bader, G., and Grueber, H.L.E.: Histochemical studies of *Rhinosporidium seeberi*, Virchows Arch. [Pathol. Anat.] **350**:76, 1970.

54. Hyams, V.J.: Papillomas of the nasal cavity and paranasal sinuses, Ann. Otol. Rhinol. Laryngol. **80**:192, 1971.

55. Jimenez, J.F., Young, D.E., and Hough, A.J., Jr.: Rhinosporidiosis: a report of two cases from Arkansas, Am. J. Clin. Pathol. **82**:611, 1984.

56. Kannan-Kutty, M., and Teh, E.C.: *Rhinosporidium seeberi:* an electron microscopic study of its life cycle, Pathology **6**:63, 1974.

57. Karunaratne, W.A.E.: Rhinosporidiosis in man, London, 1964, Athlone Press.

Sporotrichosis

58. Berson, S.D., and Brandt, F.A.: Primary pulmonary sporotrichosis with unusual fungal morphology, Thorax **32**:505, 1977.

59. Bullpitt, P., and Weedon, D.: Sporotrichosis: a review of 39 cases, Pathology **10**:249, 1978.

60. England, D.M., and Hochholzer, L.: Primary pulmonary sporotrichosis: report of eight cases with clinicopathologic review, Am. J. Surg. Pathol. **9**:193, 1985.

61. Liber, A.F., and Choi, H.S.: Splendore-Hoeppli phenomenon about silk sutures in tissue, Arch. Pathol. **95**:217, 1973.

62. Lurie, H.I.: Histopathology of sporotrichosis, Arch. Pathol. **75**:92, 1963.

63. Lynch, P.J., Voorhees, J.J., and Harrell, E.R.: Systemic sporotrichosis, Ann. Intern. Med. **73**:23, 1970.

64. Marrocco, G.R., Tihen, W.S., Goodnough, C.P., et al.: Granulomatous synovitis and osteitis caused by *Sporothrix schenckii*, Am. J. Clin. Pathol. **64**:345, 1975.

65. Smith, P.W., Loomis, G.W., Luckasen, J.L., and Osterholm, R.K.: Disseminated cutaneous sporotrichosis: three illustrative cases, Arch. Dermatol. **117**:143, 1981.

66. Sperling, L.C., and Read, S.I.: Localized cutaneous sporotrichosis, Int. J. Dermatol. **22**:525, 1983.

67. Watts, J.C., and Chandler, F.W.: Primary pulmonary sporotrichosis, Arch. Pathol. Lab. Med. **111**:215, 1987.

Systemic mycoses
Actinomycosis

68. Bennhoff, D.F.: Actinomycosis: diagnostic and therapeutic considerations and a review of 32 cases, Laryngoscope **94**:1198, 1984.

69. Berardi, R.S.: Abdominal actinomycosis, Surg. Gynecol. Obstet. **149**:257, 1979.

70. Bhagavan, B.S., and Gupta, P.K.: Genital actinomycosis and intrauterine contraceptive devices, Hum. Pathol. **9**:567, 1978.

71. Brown, J.R.: Human actinomycosis: a study of 181 subjects, Hum. Pathol. **4**:319, 1973.

72. Causey, W.A.: Actinomycosis. In Handbook of clinical neurology, vol. 35, p. 383: Infections of the nervous system, Part 3, Amsterdam, 1978, North Holland Publishing Co.

73. Hotchi, M., and Schwarz, J.: Characterization of actinomycotic granules by architecture and staining methods, Arch. Pathol. **93**:392, 1972.

74. Oddó, D., and González, S.: Actinomycosis and nocardiosis: a morphologic study of 17 cases, Pathol. Res. Pract. **181**:320, 1986.

75. Robboy, S.J. and Vickery, A.L.: Tinctorial and morphologic properties distinguishing actinomycosis and nocardiosis, N. Engl. J. Med. **282**:593, 1970.

76. Schiffer, M.A., et al.: Actinomycosis infections associated with intrauterine contraceptive devices, Obstet. Gynecol. **45**:67, 1975.

Adiaspiromycosis

77. Kodousek, R., Vortel, V., Fingerland, A., et al.: Pulmonary adiaspiromycosis in man caused by *Emmonsia crescens:* report of a unique case, Am. J. Clin. Pathol. **56**:394, 1971.

78. Schwarz, J.: Adiaspiromycosis, Pathol. Annu. **13**(1):41, 1978.

79. Watts, J.C., Callaway, C.S., Chandler, F.W., et al.: Human pulmonary adiaspiromycosis, Arch. Pathol. **99**:11, 1975.

Aspergillosis

80. Atkinson, J.B., Connor, D.H., Robinowitz, M., McAllister, H.A., and Virmani, R.: Cardiac fungal infections: review of autopsy findings in 60 patients, Hum. Pathol. **15**:935, 1984.

81. Binder, R.E., Faling, L.J., Pugatch, R.D., Mahasen, C., and Snider, G.L.: Chronic necrotizing pulmonary aspergillosis: a discrete clinical entity, Medicine (Baltimore) **61**:109, 1982.

82. Cho, S.Y., and Choi, H.Y.: Opportunistic fungal infection among cancer patients, Am. J. Clin. Pathol. **72**:617, 1979.

83. Gefter, W.B., Weingrad, T.R., Epstein, D.M., Ochs, R.H., and Miller, W.T.: "Semi-invasive" pulmonary aspergillosis: a new look at the spectrum of aspergillus infections of the lung, Radiology **140**:313, 1981.

84. Glimp, R.A., and Bayer, A.S.: Pulmonary aspergilloma: diagnostic and therapeutic considerations, Arch. Intern. Med. **143**:303, 1983.

85. Katzenstein, A.L., Liebow, A.A., and Friedman, P.J.: Bronchocentric granulomatosis, mucoid impaction, and hypersensitivity reactions to fungi, Am. Rev. Respir. Dis. **111**:497, 1975.

86. Kurrein, F., Green, G.H., and Rowles, S.L.: Localized deposition of calcium oxalate around a pulmonary *Aspergillus niger* fungus ball, Am. J. Clin. Pathol. **64**:556, 1975.

87. Meyer, R.D., Young, L.S., Armstrong, D., et al.: Aspergillosis complicating neoplastic disease, Am. J. Med. **54**:6, 1973.

88. Orr, D.P., Myerowitz, R.L., and Dubois, P.J.: Patho-radiologic correlation of invasive pulmonary aspergillosis in the compromised host, Cancer **41**:2028, 1978.

89. Raper, K.B., and Fennell, D.I.: The genus aspergillus, Baltimore, 1965, Williams & Wilkins.

90. Schwarz, J.: Aspergillosis, Pathol. Annu. **8**:81, 1973.

91. Warnock, M.L., Fennessy, J., and Rippon, J.: Chronic eosinophilic pneumonia, a manifestation of allergic aspergillosis, Am. J. Clin. Pathol. **62**:73, 1974.

92. Young, R.C., Jennings, A., and Bennett, J.E.: Species identification of invasive aspergillosis in man, Am. J. Clin. Pathol. **58**:554, 1972.
93. Young, R.C., Bennett, J.E., Vogel, C.L., et al.: Aspergillosis: the spectrum of disease in 98 patients, Medicine (Baltimore) **49**:147, 1970.

Blastomycosis
94. Cush, R., Light, R.W., and George, R.B.: Clinical and roentgenographic manifestations of acute and chronic blastomycosis, Chest **69**:345, 1976.
95. Drake, R.G., Jr.: North American blastomycosis: a review, J. Ky. Med. Assoc. **83**:77, 1985.
96. Inoshita, T., Youngberg, G.A., Boelen, L.J., and Langston, J.: Blastomycosis presenting with prostatic involvement: report of 2 cases and review of the literature, J. Urol. **130**:160, 1983.
97. Lockwood, W.R., Allison, F., Jr., Batson, B.E., et al.: The treatment of North American blastomycosis: ten years' experience, Am. Rev. Respir. Dis. **100**:314, 1969.
98. Recht, L.D., Davies, S.F., Eckman, M.R., and Sarosi, G.A.: Blastomycosis in immunosuppressed patients, Am. Rev. Respir. Dis. **125**:359, 1982.
99. Sarosi, G.A., and Davies, S.F.: Blastomycosis, Am. Rev. Respir. Dis. **120**:911, 1979.
100. Schwarz, J., and Salfelder, K.: Blastomycosis: a review of 152 cases, Curr. Top. Pathol. **65**:165, 1977.
101. Tenenbaum, M.J., Greenspan, J., and Kerkering, T.M.: Blastomycosis, CRC Crit. Rev. Microbiol. **9**(3):139, 1982.
102. Vanek, J., Schwarz, J., and Haken, S.: North American blastomycosis, Am. J. Clin. Pathol. **54**:384, 1970.
103. Witorach, P., and Utz, J.P.: North American blastomycosis: a study of 40 patients, Medicine (Baltimore) **47**:169, 1968.

Botryomycosis
104. Winslow, D.J.: Botryomycosis, Am. J. Pathol. **35**:153, 1959.
105. Winslow, D.J., and Chamblin, S.A.: Disseminated visceral botryomycosis: report of a fatal case probably caused by *Pseudomonas aeruginosa*, Am. J. Clin. Pathol. **33**:43, 1960.

Candidiasis
106. Aronson, I.K., and Soltani, K.: Chronic mucocutaneous candidosis: a review, Mycopathologia **60**:17, 1976.
107. Bodey, G.P., and Fainstein, V.: Systemic candidiasis, New York, 1985, Raven Press.
108. Dubois, P.J., Myerowitz, R.L., and Allen, C.M.: Pathoradiologic correlation of pulmonary candidiasis in immunosuppressed patients, Cancer **40**:1026, 1977.
109. Dwyer, J.M.: Chronic mucocutaneous candidiasis, Annu. Rev. Med. **32**:491, 1981.
110. Eras, P., Goldstein, M.J., and Sherlock, P.: *Candida* infection of the gastrointestinal tract, Medicine (Baltimore) **51**:367, 1972.
111. Hughes, W.T.: Systemic candidiasis: a study of 109 fatal cases, Pediatr. Infect. Dis. **1**:11, 1982.
112. Humphrey, D.M., and Weiner, M.H.: Candidal antigen detection in pulmonary candidiasis, Am. J. Med. **74**:630, 1983.
113. Kassner, E.G., Kauffman, S.L., Yoon, J.J., Semiglia, M., Kozinn, P.J., and Goldberg, P.L.: Pulmonary candidiasis in infants: clinical, radiologic, and pathologic features, AJR **137**:707, 1981.
114. Katzenstein, A.L.A., and Maksem, J.: Candidal infection of gastric ulcers: histology, incidence, and clinical significance, Am. J. Clin. Pathol. **71**:137, 1979.
115. Maksymiuk, A.W., Thongprasert, S., Hopfer, R., Luna, M., Fainstein, V., and Bodey, G.P.: Systemic candidiasis in cancer patients, Am. J. Med. **77**(4D):20, 1984.
116. Masur, H., Rosen, P.P., and Armstrong, D.: Pulmonary disease caused by *Candida* species, Am. J. Med. **63**:914, 1977.
117. Myerowitz, R.L., Pazin, G.J., and Allen, C.M.: Disseminated candidiasis: changes in incidence, underlying diseases, and pathology, Am. J. Clin. Pathol. **68**:29, 1977.
118. Odds, F.C.: *Candida* and candidosis, Baltimore, 1977, University Park Press.
119. Parker, J.C., Jr.: The potentially lethal problem of cardiac candidosis, Am. J. Clin. Pathol. **73**:356, 1980.

120. Parker, J.C., Jr., McCloskey, J.J., and Knauer, K.A.: Pathologic features of human candidiasis: a common deep mycosis of the brain, heart, and kidney in the altered host, Am. J. Clin. Pathol. **65**:991, 1976.
121. Parker, J.C., Jr., McCloskey, J.J., and Lee, R.S.: The emergence of candidosis: the dominant postmortem cerebral mycosis, Am. J. Clin. Pathol. **70**:31, 1978.
122. Parker, J.C., Jr., McCloskey, J.J., and Lee, R.S.: Human cerebral candidosis: a postmortem evaluation of 19 patients, Hum. Pathol. **12**:23, 1981.
123. Robboy, S.J., and Kaiser, J.: Pathogenesis of fungal infection on heart valve prostheses, Hum. Pathol. **6**:711, 1975.
124. Rose, H.D., and Sheth, N.K.: Pulmonary candidiasis: a clinical and pathological correlation, Arch. Intern. Med. **138**:964, 1978.
125. Walsh, T.J., Hutchins, G.M., Bulkley, B.H., and Mendelsohn, G.: Fungal infections of the heart: analysis of 51 autopsy cases, Am. J. Cardiol. **45**:357, 1980.

Coccidioidomycosis
126. Bayer, A.S.: Fungal pneumonias; pulmonary coccidioidal syndromes (part 1): primary and progressive primary coccidioidal pneumonias—diagnostic, therapeutic, and prognostic considerations, Chest **79**:575, 1981.
127. Bayer, A.S.: Fungal pneumonias: pulmonary coccidioidal syndromes (part 2): miliary, nodular, and cavitary pulmonary coccidioidomycosis: chemotherapeutic and surgical considerations, Chest **79**:686, 1981.
128. Bouza, E., Dreyer, J.S., Hewitt, W.L., and Meyer, R.D.: Coccidioidal meningitis: an analysis of thirty-one cases and review of the literature, Medicine (Baltimore) **60**:139, 1981.
129. Deppisch, L.M., and Donowho, E.M.: Pulmonary coccidioidomycosis, Am. J. Clin. Pathol. **58**:489, 1972.
130. Deresinski, S.C., and Stevens, D.A.: Coccidioidomycosis in compromised hosts, Medicine (Baltimore) **54**:377, 1974.
131. Donnelly, W.H., and Yunis, E.J.: The ultrastructure of *Coccidioides immitis*, Arch. Pathol. **98**:227, 1974.
132. Drutz, D.J., and Catanzaro, A.: Coccidioidomycosis, part I, Am. Rev. Respir. Dis. **117**:559, 1978.
133. Drutz, D.J., and Catanzaro, A.: Coccidioidomycosis, part II, Am. Rev. Respir. Dis. **117**:727, 1978.
134. Drutz, D.J., and Huppert, M.: Coccidioidomycosis: factors affecting the host-parasite interaction, J. Infect. Dis. **147**:372, 1983.
135. Huntington, R.W., et al.: Pathologic and clinical observations on 142 cases of fatal coccidioidomycosis with necropsy. In Ajello, L., editor: Coccidioidomycosis, Tucson, 1967, University of Arizona Press.
136. Kaplan, W.: Application of the fluorescent antibody technique to the diagnosis and study of coccidioidomycosis. In Ajello, L., editor: Coccidioidomycosis, Tucson, 1967, University of Arizona Press.
137. Kyriakos, M.: Myospherulosis of the paranasal sinuses, nose, and middle ear: a possible iatrogenic disease, Am. J. Clin. Pathol. **67**:118, 1977.
138. Meyer, P.R., Hui, A.N., and Biddle, M.: *Coccidioides immitis* meningitis with arthroconidia in the cerebrospinal fluid: report of the first case and review of the arthroconidia literature, Hum. Pathol. **13**:1136, 1982.
139. Rosai, J.: The nature of myospherulosis of the upper respiratory tract, Am. J. Clin. Pathol. **69**:475, 1978.
140. Sobel, R.A., Ellis, W.G., Nielsen, S.L., and Davis, R.L.: Central nervous system coccidioidomycosis: a clinicopathologic study of treatment with and without amphotericin B, Hum. Pathol. **15**:980, 1984.
141. Stevens, D.A., editor: Coccidioidomycosis: a text, New York, 1980, Plenum Medical Book Co.

Cryptococcosis
142. Baker, R.D.: The primary pulmonary lymph node complex of cryptococcosis, Am. J. Clin. Pathol. **65**:83, 1976.
143. Chu, A.C., Hay R.J., and MacDonald, D.M.: Cutaneous cryptococcosis, Br. J. Dermatol. **103**:95 1980.

144. Farmer, S.G., and Komorowski, R.A.: Histologic response to capsule-deficient *Cryptococcus neoformans*, Arch. Pathol. **96**:383, 1973.

145. Gal, A.A., Koss, M.N., Hawkins, J., Evans, S., and Einstein, H.: The pathology of pulmonary cryptococcal infections in the acquired immunodeficiency syndrome, Arch. Pathol. Lab. Med. **110**:502, 1986.

146. Gutierrez, F., Fu, Y.S., and Lurie, H.I.: Cryptococcus histologically resembling histoplasmosis: a light and electron microscopical study, Arch. Pathol. **99**:347, 1975.

147. Hammerman, K.J., Powell, K.E., Christianson, C.S., et al.: Pulmonary cryptococcosis: clinical forms and treatment: a Center for Disease Control cooperative mycoses study, Am. Rev. Respir. Dis. **108**:1116, 1973.

148. Harding, S.A., Scheld, W.M., Feldman, P.S., and Sande, M.A.: Pulmonary infection with capsule-deficient *Cryptococcus neoformans*, Virchows Arch. [Pathol. Anat.] **382**:113, 1979.

149. Lewis, J.L., and Rabinovich, S.: The wide spectrum of cryptococcal infections, Am. J. Med. **53**:315, 1972.

150. Littman, M.L., and Walter, J.E.: Cryptococcosis: current status, Am. J. Med. **45**:922, 1968.

151. McDonnell, J.M., and Hutchins, G.M.: Pulmonary cryptococcosis, Hum. Pathol. **16**:121, 1985.

152. Noble, R.C., and Fajardo, L.F.: Primary cutaneous cryptococcosis: review and morphologic study, Am. J. Clin. Pathol. **57**:13, 1972.

153. Ro, J.Y., Lee, S.S., and Ayala, A.G.: Advantage of Fontana-Masson stain in capsule-deficient cryptococcal infection, Arch. Pathol. Lab. Med. **111**:53, 1987.

154. Stoetzner, H., and Kemmer, C.: The morphology of *Cryptococcus neoformans* in human cryptococcosis: a light-, phase-contrast and electron-microscopic study, Mycopathol. Mycol. Appl. **45**:327, 1971.

Fusariosis

155. Anaissie, E., Kantarjian, H., Jones, P., Barlogie, B., Luna, M., Lopez-Berestein, G., and Bodey, G.P.: *Fusarium*: a newly recognized fungal pathogen in immunosuppressed patients, Cancer **57**:2141, 1986.

156. Blazar, B.R., Hurd, D.D., Snover, D.C., Alexander, J.W., and McGlave, P.B.: Invasive *Fusarium* infections in bone marrow transplant patients, Am. J. Med. **77**:645, 1984.

157. Wheeler, M.S., McGinnis, M.R., Schell, W.A., and Walker, D.H.: *Fusarium* infection in burned patients, Am. J. Clin. Pathol. **75**:304, 1981.

158. Young, N.A., Kevon-Chung, K.J., Kubota, T.T., Jennings, A.E., and Fisher, R.I.: Disseminated infection by *Fusarium moniliforme* during treatment for malignant lymphoma, J. Clin. Microbiol. **7**:589, 1978.

Geotrichosis

159. Chang, W.W.L., and Buerger, L.: Disseminated geotrichosis, Arch. Intern. Med. **113**:356, 1964.

160. Fishbach, R.S., White, M.L., and Finegold, S.M.: Bronchopulmonary geotrichosis, Am. Rev. Respir. Dis. **108**:1388, 1973.

161. Ghamande, A.R., Landis, F.B., and Snider, G.L.: Bronchial geotrichosis with fungemia complicating bronchial carcinoma, Chest **59**:98, 1971.

162. Jagirdar, J., Geller, S.A., and Bottone, E.J.: *Geotrichum candidum* as a tissue invasive human pathogen, Hum. Pathol. **12**:668, 1981.

163. Kassamali, H., Anaissie, E., Ro, J., Rolston, K., Kantarjian, H., Fainstein, V., and Bodey, G.P.: Disseminated *Geotrichum candidum* infection, J. Clin. Microbiol. **25**:1782, 1987.

164. Sheehy, T.W., Honeycutt, B.K., and Spency, J.T.: *Geotrichum* septicemia, JAMA **235**:1035, 1976.

Histoplasmosis capsulati

165. Baker, R.D.: Histoplasmosis in routine autopsies, Am. J. Clin. Pathol. **41**:457, 1964.

166. Binford, C.H.: Histoplasmosis: tissue reactions and morphologic variations of the fungus, Am. J. Clin. Pathol. **25**:25, 1955.

167. Domer, J.E., and Moser, S.A.: Histoplasmosis: a review, Rev. Med. Vet. Mycol. **15**:159, 1980.

168. Eggleston, J.C.: Sclerosing mediastinitis, Progr. Surg. Pathol. **2**:1, 1980.

169. Goodwin, R.A., Jr., Owens, F.T., Snell, J.D., et al.: Chronic pulmonary histoplasmosis, Medicine (Baltimore) **55**:413, 1976.

170. Goodwin, R.A., Jr., and Des Prez, R.M.: Histoplasmosis: state of the art, Am. Rev. Respir. Dis. **117**:929, 1978.

171. Hemochowicz, S., et al.: Histoplasmosis diagnosed on peripheral blood smear from a patient with AIDS, JAMA **253**:3148, 1985.

172. Hutton, J.P., Durham, J.B., Miller, D.P., and Everett, E.D.: Hyphal forms of *Histoplasma capsulatum*: a common manifestation of intravascular infections, Arch. Pathol. Lab. Med. **109**:330, 1985.

173. Kauffman, C.A., Israel, K.S., Smith, J.W., White, A.C., Schwarz, J., and Brooks, G.F.: Histoplasmosis in immunosuppressed patients, Am. J. Med. **64**:923, 1978.

174. Mandell, W., Goldberg, D.M., and Neu, H.C.: Histoplasmosis in patients with the acquired immune deficiency syndrome, Am. J. Med. **81**:974, 1986.

175. Miller, R.L., Gould, A.R., Skolnick, J.L., and Epstein, W.M.: Localized oral histoplasmosis, Oral Surg. **53**:367, 1982.

176. Schwarz, J.: Histoplasmosis, New York, 1981, Praeger Publishers.

177. Straus, S.E., and Jacobson, E.S.: The spectrum of histoplasmosis in a general hospital: a review of 55 cases diagnosed at Barnes Hospital between 1966 and 1977, Am. J. Med. Sci. **279**:147, 1980.

178. Vanek, J., and Schwarz, J.: The gamut of histoplasmosis, Am. J. Med. **50**:89, 1971.

179. Wheat, L.J., Slama, T.G., and Zeckel, M.L.: Histoplasmosis in the acquired immune deficiency syndrome, Am. J. Med. **78**:203, 1985.

Histoplasmosis duboisii

180. Clark, B.M., and Greenwood, B.M.: Pulmonary lesions in African histoplasmosis, J. Trop. Med. Hyg. **71**:4, 1968.

181. Cockshott, W.P., and Lucas, A.O.: Histoplasmosis duboisii, Q. J. Med. **33**:223, 1964.

182. Lanceley, J.L., Lunn, H.F., and Wilson, A.M.M.: Histoplasmosis in an African child, J. Pediatr. **59**:756, 1961.

183. Lunn, H.F.: A case of histoplasmosis of bone in East Africa, J. Trop. Med. Hyg. **63**:175, 1960.

184. Shore, R.N., Waltersdorff, R.L., Edelstein, M.V., and Teske, J.H.: African histoplasmosis in the United States, JAMA **245**:734, 1981.

185. Williams, A.O., Lawson, E.A., and Lucas, A.O.: African histoplasmosis due to *Histoplasma duboisii*, Arch. Pathol. **92**:306, 1971.

Malasseziasis (systemic)

186. Dankner, W.M., Spector, S.A., Fierer, J., and Davis, C.E.: Malassezia fungemia in neonates and adults: complication of hyperalimentation, Rev. Infect. Dis. **9**:743, 1987.

187. Marcon, M.J., and Powell, D.A.: Epidemiology, diagnosis, and management of *Malassezia furfur* systemic infection, Diagn. Microbiol. Infect. Dis. **7**:161, 1987.

188. Redline, R.W., Redline, S.S., Boxerbaum, B., and Dahms, B.B.: Systemic *Malassezia furfur* infections in patients receiving intralipid therapy, Hum. Pathol. **16**:815, 1985.

Nocardiosis

189. Beaman, B.L., Burnside, J., Edwards, B., et al.: Nocardial infections in the United States, 1972-1974, J. Infect. Dis. **134**:286, 1976.

190. Boudoulas, O., and Camisa, C.: *Nocardia asteroides* infection with dissemination to skin and joints, Arch. Dermatol. **121**:898, 1985.

191. Bradsher, R.W., Monson, T.P., and Steele, R.W.: Brain abscess due to *Nocardia caviae*: report of a fatal outcome associated with abnormal phagocyte function, Am. J. Clin. Pathol. **78**:124, 1982.

192. Causey, W.A., and Lee, R.: Nocardiosis. In Vinken, P.J., and Bruyn, G.W., editors: Handbook of clinical neurology, Amsterdam, 1978, North Holland Publishing Co., pp. 517-530.

193. Curry, W.A.: Human nocardiosis: a clinical review with selected case reports, Arch. Intern. Med. **140:**818, 1980.
194. Frazier, A.R., Rosenow, E.C., III, and Roberts, G.D.: Nocardiosis: a review of 25 cases occurring during 24 months, Mayo Clin. Proc. **50:**657, 1975.
195. Jonsson, S., Wallace, R.J., Jr., Hull, S.I., and Musher, D.M.: Recurrent *Nocardia* pneumonia in an adult with chronic granulomatous disease, Am. Rev. Respir. Dis. **133:**932, 1986.
196. Kalb, R.E., Kaplan, M.H., and Grossman, M.E.: Cutaneous nocardiosis: case reports and review, J. Am. Acad. Dermatol. **13:**125, 1986.
197. Palmer, D.L., Harvey, R.L., and Wheeler, J.K.: Diagnostic and therapeutic considerations in *Nocardia asteroides* infection, Medicine (Baltimore) **53:**391, 1974.
198. Pizzolato, P., Ziskind, J., Derman, H., and Buff, E.E.: Nocardiosis of the brain: report of three cases, Am. J. Clin. Pathol. **36:**151, 1961.
199. Young, L.S., Armstrong, D., Blevins, A., et al.: *Nocardia asteroides* infection complicating neoplastic disease, Am. J. Med. **50:**356, 1971.

Paracoccidioidomycosis

200. Giraldo, R., Restrepo, A., Gutiérrez, F., et al.: Pathogenesis of paracoccidioidomycosis: a model based on a study of 46 patients, Mycopathologia **58:**63, 1976.
201. Londero, A.T., and Melo, I.S.: Paracoccidioidomycosis in childhood: a critical review, Mycopathologia **82:**49, 1983.
202. Londero, A.T., Ramos, C.D., and Lopes, J.O.S.: Progressive pulmonary paracoccidioidomycosis: a study of 34 cases observed in Rio Grande do Sul (Brazil), Mycopathologia **63:**53, 1978.
203. Londero, A.T., and Severo, L.C.: The gamut of progressive pulmonary paracoccidioidomycosis, Mycopathologia **75:**65, 1981.
204. Londero, A.T., Severo, L.C., and Ramos, C.D.: Small forms and hyphae of *Paracoccidioides brasiliensis* in human tissue, Mycopathologia **72:**17, 1980.
205. Murray, H.W., Littman, M.L., and Roberts, R.B.: Disseminated paracoccidioidomycosis (South American blastomycosis) in the United States, Am. J. Med. **56:**209, 1974.
206. Restrepo, A., Robledo, M., Gutiérrez, F., et al.: Paracoccidioidomycosis (South American blastomycosis): a study of 39 cases observed in Medellín, Colombia, Am. J. Trop. Med. Hyg. **19:**68, 1970.
207. Salfelder, K., Doehnert, G., and Doehnert, H.R.: Paracoccidioidomycosis: anatomic study with complete autopsies, Virchows Arch. [Pathol. Anat.] **348:**51, 1969.
208. Tuder, R.M., el Ibrahim, R., Godoy, C.E., and De Brito, T.: Pathology of the human pulmonary paracoccidioidomycosis, Mycopathologia **92:**179, 1985.

Penicilliosis marneffei

209. Deng, Z., and Connor, D.H.: Progressive disseminated penicilliosis caused by *Penicillium marneffei*: report of eight cases and differentiation of the causative organism from *Histoplasma capsulatum*, Am. J. Clin. Pathol. **84:**323, 1985.
210. DiSalvo, A.F., Fickling, A.M., and Ajello, L.: Infection caused by *Penicillium marneffei*: description of first natural infection in man, Am. J. Clin. Pathol. **60:**259, 1973.
211. Jayanetra, P., et al.: Penicilliosis marneffei in Thailand: report of five human cases, Am. J. Trop. Med. Hyg. **33:**637, 1984.
212. Pautler, K.B., Padhye, A.A., and Ajello, L.: Imported penicilliosis marneffei in the United States: report of a second human infection, Sabouraudia **22:**433, 1984.
213. Pitt, J.I.: The genus *Penicillium* and its teleomorphic states *Eupenicillium* and *Talaromyces*, New York, 1979, Academic Press, Inc.
214. So, S., Chau, P.Y., Jones, B.M., Wu, P.C., Pun, K.K., Lam, W.K., and Lawton, J.W.: A case of invasive penicilliosis in Hong Kong with immunologic evaluation, Am. Rev. Respir. Dis. **131:**662, 1985.

Pseudallescheriasis

215. Bakerspigel, A., Wood, T., and Burke, S.: Pulmonary allescheriasis: report of a case from Ontario, Canada, Am. J. Clin. Pathol. **68:**299, 1977.
216. DeMent, S.H., Smith, R.R., Karp, J.E., and Merz, W.G.: Pulmonary, cardiac, and thyroid involvement in disseminated *Pseudallescheria boydii*, Arch. Pathol. Lab. Med. **108:**859, 1984.
217. Enggano, I.L., Hughes, W.T., Kalwinsky, D.K., Pearson, T.A., Parham, D.M., and Stoss, S.A.: *Pseudallescheria boydii* in a patient with acute lymphoblastic leukemia, Arch. Pathol. Lab. Med. **108:**619, 1984.
218. Smith, A.G., Crain, S.M., Dejongh, C., Thomas, G.M., and Vigorito, R.D.: Systemic pseudallescheriasis in a patient with acute myelocytic leukemia, Mycopathologia **90:**85, 1985.
219. Travis, L.B., Roberts, G.D., and Wilson, W.R.: Clinical significance of *Pseudallescheria boydii*: a review of 10 years' experience, Mayo Clin. Proc. **60:**531, 1985.

Torulopsosis

220. Aisner, J., Schimpff, S.C., Sutherland, J.C., et al.: *Torulopsis glabrata* infections in patients with cancer: increasing incidence and relationship to colonization, Am. J. Med. **61:**23, 1976.
221. Grimley, P.M., Wright, L.D., and Jennings, A.E.: *Torulopsis glabrata* infection in man, Am. J. Clin. Pathol. **43:**216, 1965.
222. Heffner, D.K., and Franklin, W.A.: Endocarditis caused by *Torulopsis glabrata*, Am. J. Clin. Pathol. **70:**420, 1978.
223. Hickey, W.F., Sommerville, L.H., and Schoen, F.J.: Disseminated *Candida glabrata*: report of a uniquely severe infection and a literature review, Am. J. Clin. Pathol. **80:**724, 1983.
224. Rodríguez, R., et al.: *Torulopsis glabrata* fungemia during prolonged intravenous alimentation, N. Engl. J. Med. **284:**540, 1971.
225. Valdivieso, M., Luna, M., Bodey, G.P., et al.: Fungemia due to *Torulopsis glabrata* in the compromised host, Cancer **38:**1750, 1976.

Trichosporonosis

226. Evans, H.L., Kletzel, M., Lawson, R.D., Frankel, L.S., and Hopfer, R.L.: Systemic mycosis due to *Trichosporon cutaneum*: a report of two additional cases, Cancer **45:**367, 1980.
227. Gold, J.W.M., Poston, W., Mertelsmann, R., Lange, M., Kiehn, T., Edwards, F., Bernard, E., Christiansen, K., and Armstrong, D.: Systemic infection with *Trichosporon cutaneum* in a patient with acute leukemia, Cancer **48:**2163, 1981.
228. Hoy, J., Hsu, K.C., Rolston, K., Hopfer, R.L., Luna, M., and Bodey, G.P.: *Trichosporon beigelii* infection: a review, Rev. Infect. Dis. **8:**959, 1986.
229. Leblond, V., Saint-Jean, O., Datry, A., Lecso, G., Frances, C., Bellefiqh, S., Gentilini, M., and Binet, J.L.: Systemic infections with *Trichosporon beigelii (cutaneum)*: report of three new cases, Cancer **58:**2399, 1986.
230. Walsh, T.J., Newman, K.R., Moody, M., Wharton, R.C., and Wade, J.C.: Trichosporonosis in patients with neoplastic disease, Medicine (Baltimore) **65:**268, 1986.
231. Winston, D.J., Balsley, G.E., Rhodes, J., et al.: Disseminated *Trichosporon capitatum* infection in an immunosuppressed host, Arch. Intern. Med. **137:**1192, 1977.

Zygomycosis

232. Baker, R.D.: The phycomycoses, Ann. NY Acad. Sci. **174:**592, 1970.
233. Baker, R.D., Seabury, J.H., and Schneidau, J.D.: Subcutaneous and cutaneous mucormycosis and subcutaneous phycomycosis, Lab. Invest. **11:**1091, 1962.
234. Bigby, T.D., Serota, M.L., Tierney, L.M., Jr., and Matthay, M.A.: Clinical spectrum of pulmonary mucormycosis, Chest **89:**435, 1986.
235. Chandler, F.W., et al.: Zygomycosis: report of four cases with formation of chlamydoconidia in tissue, Am. J. Clin. Pathol. **84:**99, 1985.

236. Gartenberg, G., Bottone, E.J., Keusch, G.T., and Weitzman, I.: Hospital acquired mucormycosis *(Rhizopus rhizopodiformis)* of skin and subcutaneous tissue: epidemiology, mycology, and treatment, N. Engl. J. Med. **299:**1115, 1978.

237. Gilbert, E.F., Khoury, G.H., and Pore, R.S.: Histopathological identification of *Entomophthora* phycomycosis: deep mycotic infection in an infant, Arch. Pathol. **90:**583, 1970.

238. Joe, L.K., and Eng, N.I.T.: Subcutaneous phycomycosis: a new disease found in Indonesia, Ann. NY Acad. Sci. **89:**4, 1960.

239. Lehrer, R.I., moderator: Mucormycosis, Ann. Intern. Med. **93**(part 1): 93, 1980.

240. Lyon, D.T., Schubert, T.T., Mantia, A.G., and Kaplan, M.H.: Phycomycosis of the gastrointestinal tract, Am. J. Gastroenterol. **72:**379, 1979.

241. Marchevsky, A.M., et al.: The changing spectrum of disease, etiology, and diagnosis of mucormycosis, Hum. Pathol. **11:**457, 1980.

242. Meyer, R.D., Rosen, P., and Armstrong, D.: Phycomycosis complicating leukemia and lymphoma, Ann. Intern. Med. **77:**871, 1972.

243. Neame, P., and Rayner, D.: Mucormycosis: a report on twenty-two cases, Arch. Pathol. **70:**261, 1960.

244. Parfrey, N.A.: Improved diagnosis and prognosis of mucormycosis: a clinicopathologic study of 33 cases, Medicine (Baltimore) **65:**113, 1986.

245. Straatsma, B.R., Zimmerman, L.E., and Gass, J.D.M.: Phycomycosis: a clinicopathologic study of fifty-one cases, Lab. Invest. **11:**963, 1962.

246. Virmani, R., Connor, D.H., and McAllister, H.A.: Cardiac mucormycosis: a report of five patients and review of 14 previously reported cases, Am. J. Clin. Pathol. **78:**42, 1982.

247. Williams, A.O.: Pathology of phycomycosis due to *Entomophthora* and *Basidiobolus* species, Arch. Pathol. **87:**13, 1969.

11 Protozoal and Helminthic Diseases

MANUEL A. MARCIAL
RAÚL A. MARCIAL-ROJAS

PROTOZOAL DISEASES
Diseases caused by amebas
Amebiasis

Amebiasis is caused by *Entamoeba histolytica*, a protozoan whose life cycle involves several changes in structure. From the medical standpoint the most important of these are the cystic and the trophozoite or motile forms. The infection is acquired by the ingestion of food or water containing the cysts of *E. histolytica*. Homosexual practices[42] and colonic irrigation with contaminated water[9,44] have been identified as other modes of infection of amebiasis.

The cysts are spherical and have a refractile wall that protects them against the hazards of the environment. In humans the cyst wall is resistant to destruction by the acid content of the stomach; however, it is destroyed by the alkaline intestinal medium. When the alkaline content of the small intestine digests the wall of a cyst, a quadrinucleated parasite is liberated, which, after cytoplasmic division, gives rise to four amebulas. These develop into adult trophozoites. The adult trophozoite or motile form moves downstream and colonizes the large intestine, particularly the cecum. Once in the colon, *E. histolytica* can behave either as a commensal or as a highly invasive pathogen. Although the determinants of which host-parasite interaction will be established have not been completely elucidated, the specific protozoal strain and its virulence seem to be the major factors. The pathogenicity and the spectrum of virulence of amebic strains have been determined in vitro using liver cell monolayers and in vivo using experimental animals such as the hamster.[24,25,37] In addition, by studying the electrophoretic patterns of four enzymes isolated from amebic trophozoites, characteristic isoenzyme patterns have been identified as markers of pathogenicity.[14,41] The degree of virulence, as determined by bioassays, has been correlated with both cytotoxic and proteinase activity present in the amebic trophozoite of that particular strain.[17,18,25,41] Furthermore, a positive correlation between the degree of virulence and the rate of erythrophagocytosis has been observed.[26] Host defense mechanisms against protozoal invasion include both humoral and cellular immune responses.[46] The induced circulating antibodies, mostly of the IgG class, have protective effects, since they have in vitro amebicidal properties, and passive immunity in animal models partially protects the host against invasion.[43] Cell-mediated immune mechanisms include antigen-specific cytotoxic T-cell activity and the activation of monocyte-derived macrophages by lymphokines, such as interferon-gamma.[33,39]

The pathogenic effect of *E. histolytica* is believed to be the result of a lectin-mediated, cytoskeleton-dependent adhesion of trophozoites to epithelial cells followed by the release of cytotoxins and the eventual phagocytosis of lysed cells by the ameba.[12,36,43] However, no specialized attachment organelle has been unequivocally identified by ultrastructural methods.[8] Cytotoxic-enterotoxic substances isolated from lysates of axenic cultures of *E. histolytica* have included proteolytic enzymes such as cathepsin and collagenase and neurohumoral substances such as serotonin.[6,15,16,19,25] Their cytopathic effects have been determined in monolayer cultures of mammalian cells, and their enterotoxic properties have been assayed in ligated intestinal loops and in Ussing chambers by demonstration of toxin-induced fluid secretion.

Incidence and prevalence rates of amebiasis are difficult to estimate, since the majority of infected persons are asymptomatic. Furthermore, false-positive and false-negative results are not uncommon when unskilled laboratory technologists perform stool examination for intestinal protozoa.[13] In the United States, although the prevalence in the general population is probably less than 5%, prevalence rates in populations of homosexual men have ranged from 21% to 36%.[21,27,32,35] *E. histolytica* is usually found in association with other intestinal pathogens, and its presence as part of the gay bowel syndrome correlates with oroanal sexual practices.[21,32] Fortunately for these persons, it seems that the strains of amebas colonizing their large intestines are of low virulence. A large number of these patients are asymptomatic, and the presence of symptoms does not correlate with amebic infection.[3,21,27,32,35]

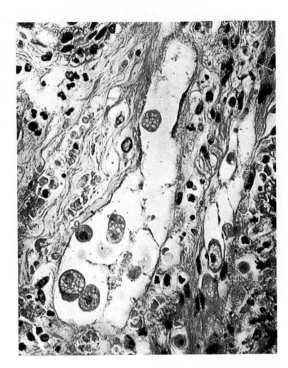

Fig. 11-1. Amebic colitis. Amebas are within lymphatic vessel and in tissues of submucosa; there is scant infiltration with neutrophils and lymphocytes. (360×.)

The isoenzyme patterns of the amebas isolated from homosexual men have been of the zymodeme type regarded as nonpathogenic.[14,20,23] Moreover, erythrophagocytosis is seldom detected in the trophozoite-containing stools of these patients.[21] Thus, although amebiasis is an endemic infection among homosexual men, these persons are not at a high risk of developing invasive complications such as amebic liver abscess.

In invasive intestinal amebiasis the inflammatory reaction is usually minimal[30,31] (Fig. 11-1). This paucity of inflammation has been partially attributed to the production of leukocyte locomotion–inhibitory factors by the protozoon.[7] However, recent data from experimental models (see next column) indicates that the paucity of polymorphonuclear cells may be the result of ameba-mediated lysis of neutrophils.[40,47] Occasionally, when there is secondary infection, there is a severe inflammatory response.

The muscle coats of the intestine form a barrier to the penetrating trophozoites, which then extend along the surface of the muscle coat, producing an undermined, flask-shaped ulcer with a narrow neck. In the early stages the colonic ulcers have a narrow neck and thus appear as small nodules with a minute surface opening averaging 5 mm in diameter (Fig. 11-2). As the ulcers enlarge, they always retain their undermined base, but the ulcerated area of the mucosa becomes larger and covered by grayish white exudate. Only

rarely do amebic ulcerations coalesce. There is always undenuded mucosa between the ulcers. This ulcerative process may be very severe and diffuse (Fig. 11-3). It is usually more prominent in the cecum and ascending colon, followed by the sigmoid and rectum in order of frequency. Only occasionally will one of these ulcers penetrate through the muscularis and produce perforation. Symptoms include abdominal pain and diarrhea, which may contain blood and mucus.[1,10,29]

In 40% of the cases of amebic colitis the trophozoites enter the circulation and are filtered in the liver, where they produce solitary or multiple abscesses (Fig. 11-4). The right lobe is involved in 50% to 68% of such cases, and the abscesses are multiple in 40% of cases. They are usually between 8 and 12 cm in diameter and are frequently located close to the dome of the right lobe of the liver or near its inferior surface, in proximity to the hepatic flexure of the colon. The outline of the abscesses is irregular. Abscesses compress the liver parenchyma around them, and a pseudocapsule of pale fibrous tissue is formed. The contents of the abscesses have been likened to anchovy sauce. The amebas are rarely demonstrable in the necrotic material. When demonstrable, they are found in the area near the capsule.

Hepatic amebiasis can be produced experimentally in hamsters by injection of pathogenic amebas intraportally.[4] Animal models of amebic liver abscess have permitted the elucidation of the sequence of morphologic changes taking place during abscess formation.[45,47,48] The initial host response to the invasive trophozoite consists in a polymorphonuclear reaction surrounding the sinusoid localized amebas. Many of these polymorphonuclear leukocytes undergo lysis with release of ly-

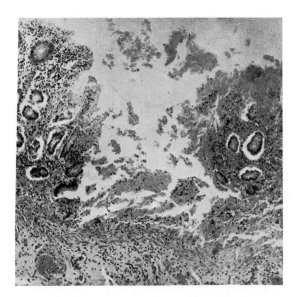

Fig. 11-2. Amebic colitis. This is very early ulcer with initial undermining shown at right. (800×.)

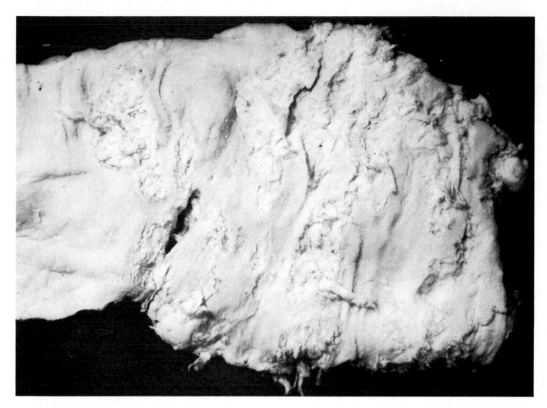

Fig. 11-3. Amebic colitis. Despite extensive ulcerations, mucosa in between remains unaffected. (Courtesy Dr. Gustavo A. Ramírez de Arellano, San Juan, Puerto Rico.)

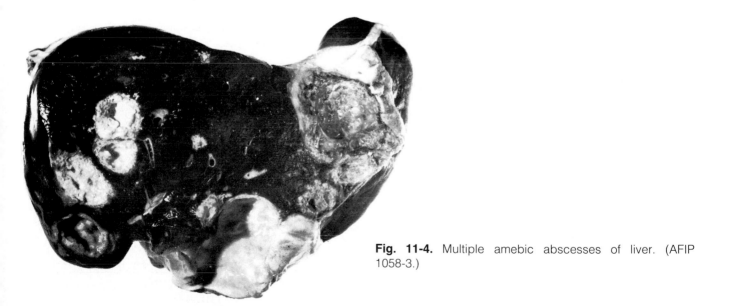

Fig. 11-4. Multiple amebic abscesses of liver. (AFIP 1058-3.)

sosomal enzymes, a process that apparently results in the necrosis of adjacent hepatocytes. Subsequently there is a decrease in neutrophils and an increase in mononuclear cells, lymphocytes, and macrophages, with the formation of a rim of granulomatous inflammation around these necrotic foci. The trophozoites are always located at the edge of this necrotic zone. The coalescence of multiple foci results in extensive areas of necrosis circumscribed by a layer of atrophied compressed hepatocytes and a zone of fibrosis. Studies using hepatocyte cell cultures support the concept that neutrophils, instead of being protective, enhance tissue damage.[40] Thus the ameba-mediated lysis of neutrophils with the subsequent release of lysosomal products may play a major role in the pathogenesis of invasive amebiasis.[40,47]

The hepatic abscesses may rupture into the right pleural cavity, into the right lung, or into the pericardial sac.[2,11,34] The abscesses usually appear 1 to 2 months after the onset of acute amebic colitis but may appear earlier or much later.

Hematogenous pulmonary abscesses may develop as a result of amebic emboli transported in the bloodstream. These emboli originate in the branches of the hepatic vein or in the colonic blood vessels. Direct extension of hepatic abscesses through the diaphragm into the right lobe of the lung is the most frequent mechanism in the production of pulmonary abscesses. Amebic

abscesses of the brain are usually solitary and located in either cerebral hemisphere; the cerebellum is rarely involved. The amebas also reach the meninges and the cerebral substance, where they produce encephalomalacia. In the central nervous system they elicit very little inflammatory response. Cerebral abscesses may reach a diameter of 10 cm. Patients with cerebral abscesses usually die 1 or 2 weeks after the clinical onset of the complication, and at autopsy concomitant amebic abscesses of the liver or lung are encountered.

E. histolytica may produce ulcers of the skin that discharge an anchovy sauce–like material. Cutaneous ulcers are usually secondarily infected and for this reason reveal severe polymorphonuclear infiltration. Amebas are present in the tissue at the base of the ulcer and in the exudate. The amebic skin ulcers develop more commonly in the subcutaneous tissue adjacent to a surgical incision for the drainage of an amebic abscess or in an appendectomy scar in the case of amebiasis of the cecum and appendix. In children, especially girls, they may develop in the perianal or perivulvar region from self-contamination (Fig. 11-5).

In rare instances a proliferative type of granulation tissue resulting from the amebic infection may produce an ulcerated area in the colon, with pronounced thickening of the wall. Such an area may be confused with carcinoma of the colon on roentgenographic study. The most commonly involved areas are the cecum, hepatic and splenic flexures, and sigmoid colon. The granulation tissue forming an amebic granuloma (ameboma) undergoes fibrosis, and the mass thus becomes firm.

It is important to remember that the presence of *E. histolytica* in the stools is not necessarily accompanied by clinical amebiasis.

Distinction of *Entamoeba histolytica* from *Entamoeba coli* and other amebas that are commensal inhabitants of the colon is important. The trophozoites of *E. histolytica* frequently phagocytose red blood cells and contain one to four nuclei in the encysted form, whereas the trophozoites of *E. coli* do not phagocytose erythrocytes and contain up to eight nuclei in the encysted form. *E. coli* does not penetrate the intestinal wall.

Sigmoidoscopic examination is useful to evaluate the mucosa and to obtain fresh specimens in which hematophagous trophozoites can be identified.[28] It is also helpful in the differential diagnosis of other conditions, such as inflammatory bowel disease.

Because stool examination is difficult and can lead to both underdiagnosis and overdiagnosis, serodiagnosis has become very useful and important.[13]

Serologic diagnosis depends on the detection of antibodies that arise only as a result of invasive amebiasis. Methods available include indirect immunofluorescence, indirect hemagglutination, enzyme-linked immunosorbent assay, counterelectrophoresis, and the gel

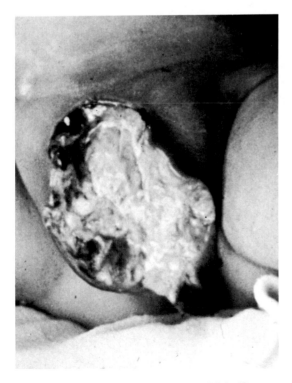

Fig. 11-5. Amebiasis of skin of vulva in child. (Courtesy Dr. Francisco Biaggi, Mexico City.)

diffusion precipitin test.[22] The indirect hemagglutination (IHA) test is the most widely used, and it is the standard method performed at the Centers for Disease Control (CDC). Results are positive in 85% of patients with amebic colitis and in 95% of patients with amebic liver abscess.[49] Test results remain positive for a long time. The gel diffusion precipitin (GDP) test has an accuracy comparable to that of the IHA method,[28] and since its positivity correlates better with active disease, the IHA test should be used for epidemiologic studies and the GDP method as a test for symptomatic infection.[45] A recently described highly specific and sensitive solid-phase radioimmunoassay for *E. histolytica* antigens in human serum promises to be of great value in the diagnosis and monitoring of patients with colonic or hepatic amebiasis.[33]

Amebic meningoencephalitis

Amebic meningoencephalitis, caused by free-living amebas, has been recognized as a clinicopathologic entity only since the report of Fowler and Carter in 1965.[51,52,59] Butt[50] proposed the name "primary amebic meningoencephalitis," which has been adopted by most subsequent investigators. The disease has been recognized in many parts of the world.

The disease is caused by free-living amebas of the genera *Naegleria* and *Acanthamoeba*. The clinicopathologic findings differ depending on the etiologic agent.

The ameboflagellate *Naegleria fowleri* is the organism most commonly cultured from cerebrospinal fluid of patients with amebic meningoencephalitis. The route of entry is through the nasal mucosa via the cribriform plate, from which organisms can be cultured. Those affected are usually young, healthy persons with a history of practicing aquatic sports in fresh water 3 to 7 days before the onset of symptoms. This disease resembles a fulminant bacterial meningitis with symptoms of headache, stiffness of the neck, fever, nausea, and vomiting.

The pathologic changes include a purulent exudate involving the base of the brain, the cerebellum, the frontal lobes, and the olfactory bulbs. Microscopically numerous trophozoites are seen in the fibrinopurulent exudate around the perivascular (Virchow-Robin) spaces. There is hemorrhagic necrosis, most prominent in the olfactory bulbs and in the cortical gray matter and occasionally also involving the spinal cord.[58] Histologic diagnosis of *Naegleria* can be confirmed by culture and by either indirect immunofluorescence or immunoperoxidase studies of brain sections.[65]

Amebic meningoencephalitis caused by the members of the genus *Acanthamoeba* is usually a disease of chronically ill or immunosuppressed patients.[56,57] The organisms can be identified both histologically and by immunologic techniques and have recently been cultured.[67,69]

The incubation period is longer and the route of entry is unknown for *Acanthamoeba* infections. There is no recent history of swimming in freshwater, and the clinical course is prolonged. The neuropathologic lesions reveal areas of hemorrhage with necrotizing granulomas containing amebas.[60,61,62,64] Thus *Acanthamoeba* brain infections have been termed "granulomatous amebic encephalitis."[60] In patients with AIDS, however, the lesions can resemble those seen with *Naegleria* infections.[53,68]

Acanthamoeba has also been shown to cause pulmonary disease, uveitis, and keratitis, the last associated with the use of contact lenses.[54,55,63,66]

Balantidiasis

Balantidium coli, a parasite of cosmopolitan distribution, is found mostly in pigs but also may be found in monkeys and rats. The organism has two stages, trophozoite and cyst. The trophozoite is the largest of the protozoa parasitizing humans, with reported lengths up to 200 μm. Their size, ciliary covering, and characteristic macronuclei and micronuclei (Fig. 11-6) make their recognition an easy task. The spherical cyst, which is about 50 μm in diameter, is the resting and transfer stage. Humans are infected by ingestion of the cyst forms in contaminated food or water. The human infection prevails in hot humid climates in persons who are on a high caloric diet and have multiple intestinal parasitoses.

The symptoms in balantidiasis vary from fulminating, sometimes fatal, dysentery to an essentially asymptomatic carrier state. The most severe cases in our experience were seen in hospitalized mental patients. These patients may also have fever, abdominal pain, nausea, and vomiting. Because of the presence of blood and mucus in the stools, balantidial infections must be differentiated from ulcerative colitis and amebic dysentery. Intestinal ulcers may develop. Hemorrhage, perforation, and peritonitis[72] may complicate the picture.

B. coli usually inhabits the cecal level of the large intestine but can also occur at lower levels. The ulcerative lesions are encountered predominantly in the cecum, ascending colon, sigmoid colon, and rectum.[70,71] The ulcers resemble amebic ulcers morphologically, but because *B. coli* is a much larger, sturdier organism than *E. histolytica*, it produces a bigger opening in the intestinal mucosa as it enters the wall. The invasion seems to be facilitated by the production of proteolytic enzymes such as hyaluronidase. The parasites are readily identified in the mucosa and submucosa of the affected areas (Fig. 11-7). A zone of coagulation necrosis is evident at the base and margins of the ulcers. The adjacent submucosa is edematous and infiltrated with chronic inflammatory cells. Neutrophilic infiltration is usually scanty or absent. Despite the fact

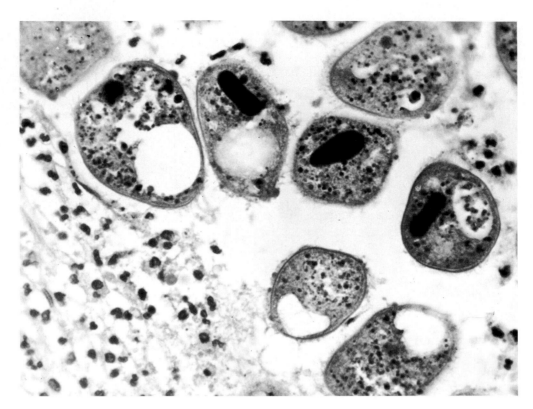

Fig. 11-6. Numerous balantidia in appendix. Notice large characteristic macronuclei in some. (Hematoxylin and eosin; 430×.)

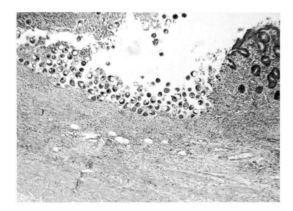

Fig. 11-7. Balantidiasis of appendix. Ulcer shows undermining borders. Wall of appendix discloses acute suppurative process. (Hematoxylin and eosin; 35×.)

that *B. coli* enters the venules, the occurrence of hepatic abscess has not been reported. In very unusual cases the organism has caused extraintestinal infections in the urinary tract and vagina.[73]

Diseases caused by flagellate protozoa

Some flagellates live in the human digestive tract,[87] others are found in the genital tract, and still others have become parasites in the blood and tissues.

Diseases caused by flagellates of the digestive tract and genital organs

Giardiasis. Giardiasis is caused by the ingestion of viable cysts of *Giardia lamblia* present in contaminated food or water.[76,79,93] Reports have identified ororectal sexual practice in homosexuals as a mode of transmission for both giardiasis[5] and amebiasis.[42,98]

G. lamblia has both trophozoite and cystic stages. Trophozoites inhabit the duodenum and jejunum, from which myriad organisms may be sampled either by duodenal aspiration or by small bowel biopsy. The stage commonly recovered in the feces is the cyst; trophozoites are seen only in frankly diarrheic stool. Since the passage of cysts in the feces is intermittent, multiple stool examinations should be performed.[104] A trichrome stain of a stool smear has been shown to improve the sensitivity of the examination.[105] The most efficient method of diagnosis is microscopic examination of a duodenal aspirate, endoscopic brush cytology, or small intestinal biopsy.[90,102] An immunofluorescence test and an enzyme-linked immunosorbent assay have been developed to detect antibodies to *G. lamblia*.[99,100,106,107]

The changes in the mucosa of the small intestine can range from normal to total villous atrophy[81,88] with an increased mononuclear cellular infiltrate of the lamina propria. In our experience mucosal alterations are minimal; at the most a mild enteritis occurs with focal mild villus shortening, crypt hyperplasia, and focal epithelial damage.

The organisms are usually seen only in the lumen, either attached to the surface or within the unstirred mucus layer.[81,94] The predilection of this protozoan for inhabiting the upper small intestine is partially explained by the fact that bile salts promote the growth of Giardia.[80]

The most commonly reported symptoms are epigastric or right upper quadrant pain and persistent steatorrhea.[74] However, the infection is usually asymptomatic.[96] Manifestation of symptoms or increase in their severity has been correlated with host factors such as achlorhydria and low secretory IgA levels.[108]

This correlation between giardiasis and low IgA levels indicated that humoral immunity played an important role in the intestinal clearance of Giardia. Experimental studies have shown the development of a specific secretory IgA immune response against surface antigens of Giardia lamblia.[78,83,89] However, it is unclear whether cell-mediated immune mechanisms have any role in the luminal clearance of this protozoon.[75,82,85]

The pathogenic mechanism by which Giardia causes malabsorption has not been elucidated. Theories include mechanical barrier to absorption, toxin production, competition for nutrients, damage to the microvilli, and bacterial overgrowth and bile salt deconjugation.[77,86,92,97,100,103]

Trichomoniasis. Of the several species of Trichomonas inhabiting humans, only T. vaginalis may become pathogenic to this host. This flagellate is found only in the trophozoite stage, and it multiplies by longitudinal binary fission. T. vaginalis is a common inhabitant of the vagina in females and the genital tract in males. Transmission of the infection is accomplished principally through sexual intercourse.

In men the infection is usually asymptomatic but may occasionally produce a urethritis. In women T. vaginalis is an important contributor to a distinct type of vaginitis characterized by leukorrhea, pruritus and burning of the vagina and vulva, and chafing of the vulva. The disease is much more severe during certain hormonal states, such as pregnancy, the late luteal phase, and menstruation. A definite diagnosis can be made by the identification of the trophozoite in a cervicovaginal smear or by its growth in culture media.[95,101] A fairly sensitive and specific enzyme immunoassay has recently been developed for the detection of Trichomonas vaginalis antigen in cervicovaginal swabs.[109] The organism can also be recovered from the urethra.

Chronic infection with Trichomonas, particularly when the parasite settles in the endocervical canal, may produce certain atypical cellular changes that can be disturbing to the cytologist because they can be distinguished from true malignant change only with difficulty. Trichomonas vaginalis has recently been reported as an unusual etiologic agent for neonatal pneumonia.[84,91]

Diseases caused by flagellates of blood and tissues

African trypanosomiasis. African trypanosomiasis, or sleeping sickness, is a disease caused by Trypanosoma brucei gambiense or T. brucei rhodesiense. It is transmitted by the bite of various species of Glossina, the tsetse fly. The trypanosomes give rise to two distinct clinical entities, Gambian trypanosomiasis and Rhodesian trypanosomiasis. African trypanosomiasis is limited to a wide belt of territory in the African continent between the latitudes of 10° north and 25° south. Cases seen in the United States have occurred in persons returning from trips to endemic areas.[119] The Gambian variety is much more widely distributed than the Rhodesian, which is limited to areas in East Africa. Neither type is present at elevations over 7000 feet above sea level. Humans are the main reservoir of both forms.

A firm, tender, reddened nodule may develop in a matter of a few days at the site of the bite. Trypanosomes may be identified in Giemsa-stained smears of fluid aspirated from the nodule. The ulcerated nodule, or "trypanosomal chancre," is accompanied by a regional lymphadenitis that lasts 1 or 2 weeks. The rapidity of the development of the chancre is related to the number of trypanosomes transmitted. The chancre precedes parasitemia. The hemoflagellates apparently reach the bloodstream via the lymphatics. This is followed within 1 to 5 weeks by the onset of fever, sweating, general malaise, and a generalized lymphadenitis often involving primarily the posterior cervical glands. Frequently there are transient skin eruptions characterized by erythema or edema. These symptoms and signs may progress to the phase of central nervous system involvement, or they may ablate and then recur.

Numerous trypanosomes are found in the blood soon after the infection, especially after symptoms have developed. Other hematologic findings may include anemia granulocytopenia, and thrombocytopenia.[116,119,122] There is an increase in sedimentation rate and a hypergammaglobulinemia especially of the IgM class. Patients have high levels of circulating immune complexes,[120] which are believed to lead to immune complex–mediated vasculitis.

Lymph node enlargement, particularly of the posterior cervical lymph nodes (Winterbottom's sign), is a common clinical feature. The lymph nodes contain numerous parasites, and there is a generalized hyperplasia of lymphoid and reticular elements. Fibrosis of the lymph nodes develops later, with reduction in their size.

Trypanosomes evade the immunologic response of the host by presenting to the immune system progressively different surface glycoprotein constituents.[111,112,121] By the time the host mounts an immune response, the trypanosome has new surface antigens to which the formed antibodies are not specific. This phenomenon of antigenic variation is accomplished by the trypanosome through a mechanism of gene conversion and DNA rearrangement.[110,115] Trypanosomes also are known to cause immunosuppression by limiting specific antibody response, especially of the IgG type.[118] The host is left with nonspecific IgM production to combat the infection. This partially explains the rise in IgM levels in this chronic infection.

Although there is considerable overlap between the clinical manifestations of *T. brucei gambiense* and *T. brucei rhodesiense* infections, the latter usually follows a much more acute course. Untreated persons with *T. brucei rhodesiense* infection frequently die within 6 to 9 months after onset of the disease. The systemic stage is often characterized by serous effusions and evidence of pancarditis. The parasites in the Rhodesian variety, after entering the lymph nodes, produce toxic substances that cause hyperplasia of the endothelial lining of the blood sinuses and perivascular infiltration of leukocytes. Only rarely does the victim survive long enough for the trypanosomes to invade the central nervous system and produce lesions characteristic of the third stage of *T. brucei gambiense* infection. The neurologic symptoms and signs, when present, are similar to those of gambian trypanosomiasis. The latter is characteristically a chronic disease.

In the third stage the patient becomes indifferent, apathetic, and drowsy. Focal neurologic signs are uncommon, though athetosis, chorea, and sphincter disturbances may become apparent. The syndrome resulting from invasion of the central nervous system is commonly referred to as "sleeping sickness," but this designation suggests only one of the more advanced neurologic symptoms.

In the majority of cases there are no major macroscopic alterations in the brain substance other than edema and occasionally petechiae. Microscopically the picture is that of a diffuse meningoencephalitis. There is mononuclear infiltration of the superficial leptomeninges, sulci, and Virchow-Robin spaces. The cellular infiltrate, composed of lymphocytes and plasma cells in various proportions, may also infiltrate the white matter and to a lesser extent the gray matter.

The morular cell described by Mott[114] is a plasma cell whose cytoplasm contains numerous Russell bodies, which coalesce and partially or totally hide the nucleus of the cell. Although these cells are not pathognomonic of trypanosomiasis, their presence in large numbers is fairly characteristic of the disease.[113]

The simplest diagnostic test is the demonstration of the trypanosomes in the circulating blood during febrile episodes. Lymph node imprints may be useful for the identification of the parasite. Examination of the cerebrospinal fluid reveals trypanosomes as the disease progresses and may serve as an index of the course of the disease.

The great elevation of IgM in both the serum and cerebrospinal fluid can be used as a screening diagnostic test. Inoculation of blood into mice and blood culture are also reliable diagnostic methods. Serodiagnosis is available by indirect immunofluorescence, complement fixation, and enzyme-linked immunosorbent assay (ELISA).[117]

American trypanosomiasis (Chagas' disease). Existing as an acute or chronic disease, American trypanosomiasis, or Chagas' disease, is caused by *Trypanosoma cruzi*, a pleomorphic trypanosome. It occurs in the blood as a trypomastigote and in reticuloendothelial and other tissue cells typically as a leishmanial form, the amastigote. The amastigote form lacks flagella but retains the kinetoplast, which permits its differentiation from other intracellular organisms such as *Toxoplasma* and *Histoplasma*.

The disease occurs in North and South America, mostly in the area from Mexico to Argentina. It has never been reported outside the Western Hemisphere, though the vectors and the animal reservoirs are common to many parts of the world. The vectors are large biting insects of the genus *Triatoma*. These insects are found in areas where there are unhygienic conditions associated with poverty. They bite only at night. During the day they hide in cracks in the walls of primitive country dwellings.

The organism is sucked up by the triatomid bug as a free flagellate or as an intracellular leishmanial form within a macrophage. In the midgut of the insect the organism becomes flagellated, and binary multiplication occurs. It migrates to the hindgut, where it is transformed into the metacyclic trypanosome form infective for the vertebrate host. Since the *Triatoma* defecates at the time of biting, the infection is usually acquired by rubbing the feces containing the metacyclic trypanosome stage of the parasite into the tiny skin puncture or into other abrasions of the skin in the area. Infections through the intact mucous membranes occur most frequently in the lips or in the conjunctivae, when the eyes are rubbed with fingers soiled with the insect's feces.

T. cruzi enters macrophages by parasite-specified phagocytosis.[129,130,138] Phagocytosis is partially dependent on macrophage cell surface receptors.[123,135] The protozoon does not remain within the phagocytic vacuole but escapes into the cytoplasm where it multiplies.[131] By leaving the parasitophorous vacuole, the organism escapes the action of microbicidal lysosomal enzymes. The circulating forms are susceptible to the trypanosomal activity of the lysosomal enzymes and major basic protein of eosinophils.[132]

Specific diagnosis of American trypanosomiasis may be accomplished by the finding of the typical trypanosome stage of *T. cruzi* in the blood during febrile episodes. Aspiration of spleen, liver, lymph nodes, or bone marrow will frequently reveal the leishmanial form of the organism in fixed macrophages. In reticuloendothelial cells *T. cruzi* cannot be easily distinguished from species of *Leishmania*, but only *T. cruzi* invades myocardial and neuroglial cells as a leishmanial type of organism. Xenodiagnosis can be performed, but it takes approximately 2 weeks to obtain the results. Serologic methods include complement fixation, indirect immunofluorescence, hemagglutination, enzyme-linked immunosorbent assay, and thin-layer immunoassay.[126,137,133]

Acute Chagas' disease. The acute form is the more common of the two types of Chagas' disease. It occurs predominantly in small children and is characterized by fever, slight generalized lymph node enlargement, moderate hepatosplenomegaly, facial edema, tachycardia, and the presence of *T. cruzi* in peripheral blood. In 50% of cases the primary site is the outer canthus of one eye, with unilateral palpebral edema and satellite preauricular lymph node enlargement (Romaña's sign) (Fig. 11-8, *A*). In 25% of cases the portal of entry is represented by a nodular or ulcerative skin lesion (chagoma), accompanied by enlargement of regional lymph nodes.[124]

Histologically the primary lesion is characterized by numerous histiocytes, chronic inflammatory cells, and areas of fat necrosis throughout which numerous leishmanial forms are encountered (Fig. 11-8, *B*). Multiplication of the organisms that have been engulfed by nearby macrophages is soon followed by the invasion of other structures such as smooth and striated muscle (including cardiac muscle), glial and nervous cells, and fat cells. Parasites are found in almost all organs, and their presence is accompanied by mononuclear cell infiltration, congestion, and edema and occasionally by granulomatous areas. Reticuloendothelial activity and increase in the number of fixed macrophage cells cause splenomegaly, hepatomegaly, adenopathy, and hyperplasia of bone marrow. The process is then a reticulopathy similar to kala-azar and histoplasmosis.

Death during the acute phase is caused by acute myocarditis with congestive cardiac failure, meningoencephalitis, or complications such as bronchopneumonia. A recent study showed that *T. cruzi* readily enters the central nervous system during the acute infection. Cerebrospinal fluid findings include pleocytosis and high protein levels.[128]

The heart is enlarged and flabby with pronounced dilatation of the left ventricle. The myocardium is pink and shows yellowish gray streaks. Microscopically the myocardium is diffusely involved but reveals only spotty cell destruction. The myocardial fibers are separated by intense edema, proliferation of histiocytes, and infiltration with chronic inflammatory cells and few polymorphonuclear cells. Within the muscle fibers are leishmanial forms either arranged in rows or in cystlike dilatations (Fig. 11-9). Cardiac fibers show degenerative

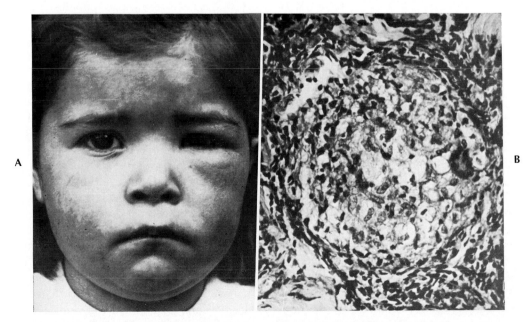

Fig. 11-8. Chagas' disease in child. **A,** Romaña's sign. Ophthalmoganglionary chagoma on left side, 16 days after insect bite. **B,** Initial lesion (chagoma) in arm. Focal histiocytic proliferation with formation of giant cells and peripheral infiltration with lymphocytes. (Courtesy Professor Mazza and the Misión de Estudios de Patología Regional del Norte, Argentina, Pub. 46.)

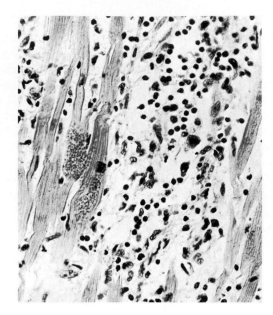

Fig. 11-9. Acute Chagas' disease. There is interstitial myocarditis, with loss of muscle fibers and dense infiltration with round cells and eosinophils. Colonies of *Trypanosoma* in two myocardial fibers appear at left of center. (360×.)

changes, the most important of which is hyaline necrosis of isolated fibers. Inflammatory changes in the myocardium also may involve the bundle of His and its ramifications.[95,136]

Chronic Chagas' disease. The dominant factor in the chronic stages of Chagas' disease is almost always some degree of myocardial fibrosis. Many patients report a previous acute attack. However, in a number of cases there is no history of a previous attack. The chronic cardiac form of Chagas' disease is a leading cause of cardiac failure and sudden death in endemic areas.

The heart is enlarged, with generalized hypertrophy and dilatation. Mural endocardial thromboses are usually present, most frequently in the right auricle and at the apex of the left ventricle. Apical thrombosis, with focal endomyocardial fibrosis at its base, represents the most important single gross finding suggestive of Chagas' myocarditis. In the absence of thrombosis the myocardium at the apex frequently appears distended and thinned, sometimes even to the point of aneurysmal formation.[124] Embolic phenomena, both pulmonary and systemic, are present in about 75% of autopsied cases.[124] The main sources of emboli are intracardiac thrombi, which are also found at autopsy in approximately 75% of cases.

Microscopically the myocardium shows chronic, nonspecific, mononuclear inflammation. Hypertrophy of cardiac fibers, small focal areas of necrosis and granular degeneration of cardiac fibers, focal and diffuse fibrosis, vascular dilatation and congestion, and interstitial and interfibrillary edema are other common microscopic features. Parasites (leishmanial forms in pseudocysts) are identified with difficulty in a very limited percentage of cases. Thus the pathogenesis of myocardial fiber damage in chronic Chagas' disease is still unclear. Autoimmunity and intravascular platelet aggregation have both been proposed as having a pathogenetic role.[127,139,141] Animal models will hopefully help in the elucidation of pathogenetic mechanisms.[127,140,142]

Digestive form of Chagas' disease. Megaesophagus and megacolon are manifestations of chronic Chagas' disease. Fibrosis and degeneration of autonomic ganglia in the heart have been demonstrated in persons with megaesophagus, as well as considerable diminution in the number of ganglionic cells in the Auerbach plexus of the esophagus and intestine.

Congenital Chagas' disease. The transplacental transmission of *T. cruzi* infection has been well documented in both humans and experimental animals, though its epidemiologic importance and frequency are not fully understood. Congenital Chagas' disease can lead to premature birth and fetal death. A chronic placentitis, similar in some respects to the syphilitic placenta, with bulky and ischemic villi, has been described. Leishmanial forms are found within the cytoplasm of macrophages in variable numbers. Interstitial pneumonitis with a prominent mononuclear histiocytic infiltrate can develop in infants.[134]

Leishmaniasis. Leishmaniasis is a group of diseases caused by one or another of several species of protozoa belonging to the genus *Leishmania*.[151] All of these protozoa are transmitted to humans by the bite of a small sand fly of the genera *Phlebotomus* in the Old World and *Lutzomya* in the New World. Each of the species of *Leishmania* is transmitted only by a specific sand fly species.

The protozoon exists in humans as an obligate intracellular parasite.[158] The process of entry of the amastigote into a host macrophage begins with attachment of the parasite to the host cell membrane, an interaction that is believed to depend on surface protein determinants.[167] The protozoon then enters the macrophages by phagocytosis and multiplies in them by binary fission.[148] The amastigote has developed mechanisms for survival within the phagolysosome. These are believed to be inactivation of the microbicidal lysosomal enzymes and the capacity for parasite-specified phagocytosis. Induced or facilitated phagocytosis is a mechanism of entry that leishmanias share with *Toxoplasma gondii* and *Trypanosoma cruzi*. They are able to parasitize nonactivated macrophages without triggering a respiratory burst. The activated phagocytes can produce toxic oxygen metabolites that are leishmanicidal.[156,162]

The diseases caused by the leishmanias are subdivided into two types—visceral and cutaneous—based on the clinical picture. The organisms recovered from patients with these three diseases show differences in culture characteristics, in experimental animal inoculation, and especially in sensitivity or immunologic reactions.

Visceral leishmaniasis (kala-azar). Visceral leishmaniasis, or kala-azar, is a disease heralded by loss of weight, weakness, enlargement of the abdomen because of prominent splenomegaly and hepatomegaly, fever, cough, and pain over the spleen. The onset is insidious, and the course is chronic.[147]

Visceral leishmaniasis is caused by the species *Leishmania donovani*, *L. infantum*, and *L. chagasi*. The latter two have been identified as the causative agents of Mediterranean and New World kala-azar, respectively.[165]

Some authors regard *L. infantum* and *L. chagasi* as subspecies of *L. donovani*.[153] We hope that the use of newly developed molecular, biochemical, and immunologic methods (such as isoenzyme electrophoresis, monoclonal antibodies, and DNA probe analysis) will clarify the taxonomic classification in the very near future.[150]

The sand fly ingests leishmanias with the blood of an infected person bitten. The promastigotes multiply rapidly in the midgut and then migrate to the pharynx and buccal cavity of the vector. When the fly attempts to obtain blood from a healthy individual, many of the flagellated promastigotes (leptomonads) are introduced into the outer dermis.

The incubation period varies from 2 weeks to 18 months. The onset may be sudden, with acute manifestations, but is usually insidious, and many patients have pronounced splenomegaly and hepatomegaly on examination.[166]

Kala-azar is endemic in many areas of India and in parts of China. It is also encountered in the countries bordering the Mediterranean and in parts of West Africa. It is sparsely distributed in South and Central America. In Mediterranean countries and China it is primarily a disease of infants and young children. In India and South America young adults are most frequently infected. In the Sudan a particularly fulminating type is observed commonly in young adults.

The injected flagellates rapidly change to the oval amastigote form in the host, and after colonizing in the dermis, they gain access to the bloodstream or lymphatics and are transported to the viscera. The leishmanias parasitize reticuloendothelial cells in all parts of the body. The disease is manifested primarily in organs with reticuloendothelial tissue such as the spleen, liver, bone marrow, and lymph nodes.[166] The outstanding characteristics of the parasitized reticuloendothelial cells are the distension of the cell membrane and the great multiplication of amastigotes (Leishman-Donovan bodies) within the cytoplasm.

The spleen is the most severely affected organ and may be involved to the point of losing all architectural detail, both grossly and microscopically (Fig. 11-10). The spleen may weigh several kilograms, and infarcts are not uncommon. In the liver there is pronounced Kupffer cell hyperplasia, and an inflammatory cell infiltrate may be found in the portal areas and in the sinusoids. The bone marrow is replaced by parasitized macrophages. The hematologic findings of anemia, leukopenia, and thrombocytopenia are believed to be the result of decreased production in the marrow and increased sequestration because of hypersplenism. Destruction by immunologic factors has also been proposed.

Severe secondary infections, especially cancrum oris or noma, develop terminally in patients with agranulocytosis. The presence of IgG hypergammaglobulinemia and hypoalbuminemia leads to an inverted albumin/globulin ratio. Most of this IgG is nonspecific and thus not protective. Proteinuria and microhematuria associated with mesangial proliferation and immunoglobulin deposition have been reported.[164] Evidence of circulating immune complexes in kala-azar has recently been presented.[152] Skin macular and nodular lesions resembling those of leprosy may be a sequela to kala-azar. This is known as post–kala-azar dermal leishmaniasis.

The definite diagnosis of kala-azar is made by identification of the parasite in tissue sections or smears.[144] *Leishmania* is distinguished from other intracellular organisms, like *Histoplasma* and *Toxoplasma* by its two basophilic dots, its nucleus, and its kinetoplast. Bone marrow aspiration yields a diagnosis in 90% of the cases, whereas liver biopsy shows positive results in 70% of them. Splenic puncture is a very high yield procedure with positive results in 95% of the cases. Although most physicians would prefer the bone marrow aspirate, for safety reasons, in expert hands splenic aspiration is a low-risk procedure that allows quantitation of parasite load.[149] Culture of aspirated samples and the use of immunofluorescence and immunoperoxidase techniques increase the yield of diagnosis.[154]

Serodiagnosis of kala-azar is possible by several methods, including the indirect hemogglutination antibody (IHA) test, the indirect fluorescent antibody (IFA) test, ELISA, complement fixation (CF), and direct agglutination (DA) test.[145,146,155,157] Both IFA and DA are available in the United States through the Centers for Disease Control. The DA test is the most sensitive of all. A dilution titer of 1:64 or more is considered positive.

Cutaneous and mucocutaneous leishmaniasis. Cutaneous leishmaniasis is encountered in both the New and Old World. The *Leishmania* organisms responsible for these related diseases cannot be differentiated mor-

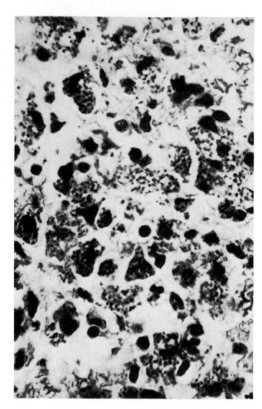

Fig. 11-10. Kala-azar. In this spleen of an Indian patient, reticuloendothelial cells of pulp and sinuses have become distended with *Leishmania*. (776×.)

phologically or serologically. The differentiation among varieties of cutaneous leishmaniasis is based on clinical, epidemiologic, geographic, and immunologic grounds.

The primary lesion in all variants is usually an ulcer, which develops most frequently at the site of the bite of an infected sand fly *(Phlebotomus* or *Lutzomya)*. It starts as a macule within 2 to 6 months after the bite and then becomes a papule, and finally the lesion breaks down in the center leaving an ulcer with sharply defined and elevated borders (Fig. 11-11). Biopsy of the lesion reveals a granulomatous reaction with lymphocytes, plasma cells, epithelioid histiocytes, and Langhans' giant cells.[160] Organisms may be identified within tissue biopsy macrophages or isolated from biopsy or aspirate cultures.[143,161,163]

There are no systemic manifestations, and the symptoms in cutaneous leishmaniasis result from the primary skin lesion and from the metastatic lesions, if any. Characteristically there is only one ulcer for each infected sand fly bite, developing at or near the point of inoculation on the exposed skin. Two varieties of cutaneous leishmaniasis have been distinguished in the Old World, an urban or "dry" type and a rural or "wet" type. They are both known as "oriental sore." The wet type is caused by *L. tropica major* and the dry type by

L. tropica minor. Lymphatic spread may rarely occur in the wet type, with the formation of metastatic nodules along the lymphatic vessel, and leishmanias can be found in the regional lymph nodes.

Cutaneous leishmaniasis in South and Central America is similar in many respects to the Old World disease, but metastatic spread is more frequent and the disease is mutilating, since frequently there is involvement of the nasal and mucosal surfaces of the mouth and upper respiratory tract. When this occurs, the disease is referred to as mucocutaneous leishmaniasis.

There are four clinical, epidemiologic, and geographic types in the New World. In Mexico, mainly in the Yucatán Peninsula, and in the jungles of Guatemala and Honduras, one encounters the *chiclero ulcer*. It is a self-limiting disease with no metastatic spread. The ulcer is most frequently found in the pinna of the ear but sometimes in the skin of the cheek, forehead, and less commonly other exposed areas of the body. It is ascribed to a separate species of leishmania, *L. tropica mexicana.*

The Andean or Peruvian lesion, known as *uta*, is similar to the chiclero ulcer, and metastases are uncommon. It is caused by *L. braziliensis.*

Pian bois, or forest yaws, may cause a single ulcerative lesion but often metastasizes along lymphatic chan-

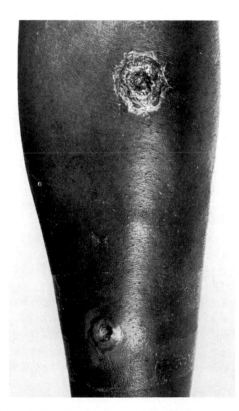

Fig. 11-11. Oriental sore. These two well-developed sores of lower leg have excavated centers and swollen borders. (AFIP 1440-1.)

nels, producing multiple cutaneous ulcers or nodules. Nasopharyngeal spread does not occur. It is also caused by *L. braziliensis.*

Another type of cutaneous leishmaniasis is found in Central America and the upper half of South America. It is known as *espundia* and is also caused by *L. braziliensis.* It is characterized by a high incidence of metastatic lesions, with migration of the organisms to secondary foci, mainly in mucocutaneous areas, particularly the nasal septum. Because of this mucosal tropism, the disease is referred to as the classical type of American mucocutaneous leishmaniasis. Extensive destruction of soft and underlying hard tissues of the nose and pharynx occurs, producing severe mutilation of the face. The organism's tropism for the nose cartilage is believed to result from the parasite's growth pattern, which is dependent on low skin temperature, and from the lack of a cellular immune response in the host tissue.

A diffuse, chronic variant of cutaneous leishmaniasis with numerous nodular, fleshy swellings resembling lepromatous leprosy is known as *leishmaniasis tegmentaria diffusa.* It occurs mostly in Venezuela but is found in both the Old and New World. Destructive mucocutaneous lesions do not occur. The lesions consist of organisms proliferating within macrophages. There is no granulomatous response because of the host's depressed cell-mediated immunity.

Results of the leishmanin test are negative, hence the names *anergic* or *disseminated cutaneous leishmaniasis* occasionally used for this entity. The patient's anergy is specific to the leishmanin skin test, since a delayed hypersensitivity reaction is elicited by other common skin test antigens. A lymphocyte proliferative response, though present for several mitogens, is not elicited by leishmanial antigens. This selective anergy could be modulated by an adherent suppressor cells mechanism.[159]

Diseases caused by sporozoans
Isoporiasis (coccidiosis)

Coccidia are parasites of the intestinal tract of many vertebrate species. They are usually transmitted by the ingestion of the sporulated oocyst in contaminated water or food. The life cycle of these sporozoans in humans has not been completely elucidated, but they have the distinguishing feature of undergoing both schizogony and gametogony in the small bowel epithelium.[169]

Isospora belli has been the most commonly identified *Isospora* species in the small bowel of patients with mucous diarrhea, fever, weight loss, abdominal pain, peripheral eosinophilia, and malabsorption.[172,178] Small intestinal biopsy reveals a moderate to severe enteritis with villous shortening, crypt hyperplasia, and infiltra-

tion of the lamina propria with eosinophils, neutrophils, lymphocytes, and plasma cells.[169,187,193] Stages of both asexual (schizonts) and sexual (gametocytes) cycles are identifiable within the absorptive cells. Although the organisms are usually restricted to the epithelial cells of the small intestine, a case of disseminated extraintestinal isosporiasis in an AIDS patient has recently been reported.[186]

The sporozoan formerly called *I. hominis* has been reclassified under the genus *Sarcocystis* because sexual and asexual reproduction takes place in different hosts.

Cryptosporidiosis

Cryptosporidium, the agent of cryptosporidiosis, formerly a rare zoonotic disease in immunosuppressed hosts,[182,184,192] has recently been recognized as a cause of diarrhea in both immunocompetent and immunodeficient patients.[171,194]

Although the clinical course in immunocompromised hosts, such as AIDS patients, is one of chronic protracted diarrhea, cryptosporidiosis presents as an acute, self-limited diarrheal disease in immunocompetent persons.[171,175-177]

This 2 to 4 μm protozoon, which belongs to the order Coccidia, may involve the gastrointestinal, pancreatobiliary, or respiratory epithelium.[168,183,188] The small intestinal lesion is very similar to that just described for isosporiasis. However, unlike *Isospora,* which multiplies deep within the absorptive cell, *Cryptosporidium* seems restricted to the apical portion of the enterocyte. The brush-border localization led many investigators to consider *Cryptosporidium* a luminal parasite. We have recently confirmed its intracellular localization.[180,190]

The development and use of techniques that permit the identification of *Cryptosporidium* oocysts in stool specimen[170,173,179,191] have shown that cryptosporidiosis may account for up to 20% of the diarrheal disease among the population at large.[174,181,185] A recently developed enzyme immunoassay for the detection of antibodies to *Cryptosporidium* promises to be a useful adjunct in epidemiologic studies.[189]

Malaria

Malaria is a disease of worldwide distribution and is probably the most widespread of all diseases. It is caused by a protozoan parasite belonging to the genus *Plasmodium.* Humans are infected by four common species, the distribution of which is not uniform. *P. vivax* causes tertian malaria; *P. malariae,* quartan malaria; *P. ovale,* ovale malaria; and *P. falciparum,* the most severe form of the disease, known as pernicious, subtertian, malignant, or estivoautumnal malaria. The natural reservoir of the disease is humans. The vector is the female *Anopheles* mosquito. Recently the possibility of congenitally acquired malaria has been reported.[220] Plasmodia are found in great numbers in the intervillous spaces of the placenta of infected mothers. The disparity between the approximate 30% incidence of placental malaria in endemic areas[223] and the rarity of congenital malaria reports is believed to be related to an immunologically dependent placental barrier mechanism. The disease has been associated epidemiologically with many hematologic conditions. Inherited erythrocyte abnormalities, such as sickle hemoglobinopathy and glucose-6-phosphate dehydrogenase deficiency, are extremely common in malarial areas. Genetic selection for these conditions is believed to be the result of the abnormal red blood cells' resistance to infection, leading to a survival advantage for the heterozygous gene defect carrier. Studies have shown that sickle hemoglobin restricts both parasite invasion and growth.[217] The prevalence of Burkitt's lymphoma in malarious areas has led to the proposal that malaria may enhance the oncogenic potential of the Epstein-Barr virus.[210]

The life cycle of the malarial organism is divided into the asexual or endogenous cycle in the human (schizogony) and the sexual or exogenous cycle in the mosquito (sporogony). The asexual cycle begins with the introduction of the sporozoites by the bite of the infected mosquito. A preerythrocytic phase, which occurs within hepatic cells in the liver, antedates bloodstream invasion by the parasite. At the end of approximately 1 week for *P. falciparum*, the schizonts rupture the liver cells and free merozoites into the bloodstream. This damage to the liver parenchyma does not give rise to any significant functional alteration.

The erythrocytic cycle, the most important pathogenetically, begins with the merozoite invasion of red blood cells. Whereas *P. vivax and P. ovale* invade only reticulocytes, *P. falciparum* merozoites can invade any erythrocyte.

The merozoites attach to the red blood cell membrane by specific receptors, such as the Duffy blood group determinant for *P. vivax* and glycophorin A and B for *P. falciparum*.[202,214,215] Subsequently, a "junction" is formed between the cell membranes of the host and parasite, and the protozoon enters the cell by a cytoskeleton-mediated process.[195] The merozoites become trophozoites, which in turn undergo either shizogony or gametogony within the erythrocyte. During its development the sporozoon digests hemoglobin, which becomes the malarial pigment hemozoin, an iron porphyrin–proteinoid complex, which is birefringent under polarized light.[209] When the erythrocyte ruptures, the merozoites liberated will parasitize other red blood cells and the hemozoin pigment will be phagocytized by reticuloendothelial cells.

The pathogenesis of the anemia in acute malaria is far from settled.[218] Most investigators agree that rupture of parasitized cells and destruction of nonparasitized cells by activated reticuloendothelial cells of the spleen, liver, and bone marrow contribute to the anemia. The controversy concerns whether immunologic factors, such as complement-mediated hemolysis, have a role in the cause of anemia.[204,225]

The debris of the ruptured cells, together with the merozoites and their metabolic by-products, is set free in the bloodstream and acts as a pyrogen. When the pyrogen accumulates, it produces the characteristic chills and fever of a malarial attack.

Some of the trophozoites within red blood cells become differentiated into round or crescentic sexual forms called microgametocytes and macrogametocytes. These gametocytes are taken up by the *Anopheles* mosquito and undergo maturation in 7 to 12 days. The male microgamete then fertilizes the female macrogamete, producing a fertilized cell or zygote. The zygote penetrates the wall of the stomach and forms an oocyst. Large numbers of spores (sporozoites) develop within this cyst. The oocyst ruptures, and the sporozoites then reach the body cavity of the mosquito. From the body cavity the sporozoites invade other parts of the mosquito's body. Those reaching the salivary glands pass down the proboscis when the insect bites, thus infecting a human.

The clinical picture in the benign types of malaria is characterized by periodic paroxysms of shaking chills, followed by high fever and pronounced diaphoresis as the patient's body temperature falls. The paroxysms last from 4 to 10 hours and recur every third day in vivax and ovale infections and every fourth day in quartan malaria.

Our knowledge of the lesions of benign malaria is derived mainly from cases of death in the course of natural and blood transfusion–related malarial infection. The main pathologic alterations are those of reticuloendothelial response to the malarial parasite and its pigment and a secondary anemia. The spleen is enlarged and is a slate gray as a result of deposition of malarial pigment. The latter is most abundant in the reticuloendothelial cells and in the macrophages of the red pulp. Parasites occasionally are demonstrable within some of the macrophages and reticuloendothelial cells. The liver is also enlarged and congested. The Kupffer cells show prominent phagocytic activity and contain abundant pigment and occasional parasites. The bone marrow discloses erythroid hyperplasia, mostly normoblastic. It also shows increased myeloid activity, but despite this, there is no leukocytosis in the peripheral blood.

Malignant pernicious malaria. Much more frequently than in the other types, falciparum malaria is accompanied by pernicious manifestations. The paroxysms in falciparum malaria are less regular than in other types.

Severe parasitemia and multiple infection of red blood cells, though not diagnostic, are common in falciparum infections. The plasmodium evades the host's immune system by a combination of mechanisms that include antigenic variation, antigenic complexity, and intracellular development.[200,212]

The parasitized erythrocytes are less deformable and tend to adhere to endothelial walls by surface "knobs."[207,211,216] These knobs on parasitized erythrocytes seem to bind specifically to an endothelial receptor, possibly involving thrombospondin (thrombin-sensitive protein).[221] This phenomenon, known as the "visceral tide," leads to prominent accumulation of parasitized red blood cells within the visceral and cerebral capillaries.[203,211,216]

The progressive decrease in circulating erythrocytes, the severe engorgement of small visceral capillaries with red blood cells, and the decrease in circulating blood volume are responsible for the severe anoxia of important organs in pernicious malaria. Although the red blood cells give the impression of being clumped, actual thrombosis is rare. Occasionally infarcts occur as the result of thrombosis of blood vessels. The accumulation of parasitized red cells is more common in the small vessels of the spleen, liver, bone marrow, brain, and lungs than in the kidneys, small intestine, pancreas, heart, and testes.

In the brain, perivascular "ring" hemorrhages and necrosis of surrounding parenchyma are seen (Fig. 11-12). These lesions, predominantly of the white matter, are believed to be the result of vascular damage by sludged, parasitized red blood cells.[211,216] The damage leads to a reactive gliosis with the formation of malarial granulomas, known as Dürck's glial nodes. The role of monokines and of oxygen metabolites released by activated monocyte macrophages in the pathogenesis of cerebral malaria is presently under investigation.[199] Alterations in host-mediated responses have been documented in patients with cerebral malaria and high parasitemia.[198] Mechanisms proposed for the induction of the immunosuppression in malaria have included clonal deletion of antigen-specific cells, responses to polyclonal activation, antigenic competition, and non-specific activation of suppressor cells.[226]

Abundant pigment and parasites are observed within reticuloendothelial cells and macrophages (Fig. 11-13). Pigmentation of the liver is not as noticeable as that in the spleen. The hepatic cells show cloudy swelling and fatty change. Kupffer cells are large and actively phagocytic. They contain parasites, erythrocytes, and malarial pigment (Fig. 11-13).

A disseminated intravascular coagulopathy may occasionally develop in patients with malaria.[206] This has been associated with the adult respiratory distress syndrome seen in some fatal cases of malaria.[219] An immune complex glomerulonephritis formed by *P. falciparum* antigen and corresponding antibodies has been documented by electron microscopy and immunofluorescence.[197]

Blackwater fever. Blackwater fever, or hemoglobinuric fever, is a very dangerous complication of malignant malaria. It occurs among persons previously infected with falciparum malaria or in persons living in areas where this disease abounds. Within a few days of

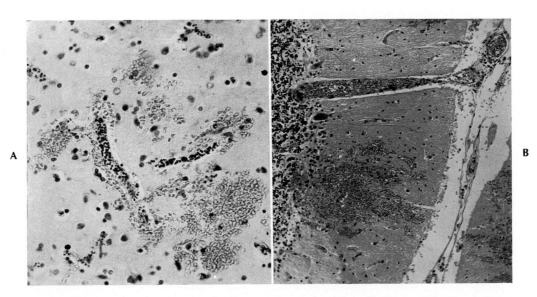

Fig. 11-12. Cerebral malaria. **A,** Multiple hemorrhages into brain. Capillaries are engorged with pigmented and parasitized erythrocytes. **B,** Hemorrhages may be as numerous in cerebellar cortex as in cerebrum. Smaller blood vessels are laden with parasitized erythrocytes. (80×.)

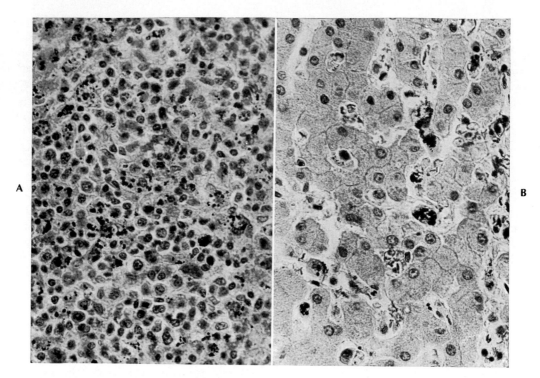

Fig. 11-13. Acute falciparum malaria. **A,** Spleen shows pronounced reticuloendothelial hyperplasia and loss of outline of sinuses. Finely divided malarial pigment appears within red blood cells and phagocytes. **B,** Liver shows cloudy swelling and some disarrangement of hepatic cords. Kupffer cells are swollen with malarial pigment and cellular debris. (360×.)

onset there are severe chills, with rigor, high fever, jaundice, vomiting, rapidly progressive anemia, and the passage of dark red or black urine.

The condition is more common in patients who have been subject to excessive fatigue, privation, exposure, exhaustion, shock, or injury; intercurrent infection; childbirth; or alcoholic excess; or who have received inadequate treatment with quinine.

The cause of the hemolytic crises that characterize the disease is unknown. There is rapid and massive destruction of red blood cells with the production of hemoglobinemia, hemoglobinuria, intense jaundice, anuria, and finally death in the majority of cases. The most probable explanation for blackwater fever is an autoimmune reaction. Grossly and microscopically the kidneys are similar to those of "hemoglobinuric or tubular nephrosis" or acute tubular necrosis as seen in other conditions such as the crush syndrome.

Diagnosis

The diagnosis of malaria depends on the demonstration of malarial parasites on a Giemsa-stained thick or thin blood smear. Erythrocytes containing multiple ring forms and the presence of banana-shaped gametocytes are diagnostic of *P. falciparum*. Because of fluctuations in degree of parasitemia, multiple periodic blood-smear examinations should be performed. A diagnosis can be corroborated by serologic tests. The methods currently available include the indirect hemagglutination antibody (IHA), the ELISA, the indirect fluorescent antibody test (IFA), radioimmunoassay (RIA), and the complement fixation (CF) test.[196,208,222] The IFA test, because of its specificity and sensitivity, is the preferred method for serodiagnosis and the one presently used by the Centers for Disease Control.[224] An enzyme-linked DNA probe has recently been developed for the diagnosis of falciparum malaria.[213] Serodiagnosis is also very useful for epidemiologic studies and for the investigation and identification of donors responsible for transfusion-related malaria cases.[201,205]

Toxoplasmosis

Toxoplasmosis is caused by the obligate intracellular protozoan *Toxoplasma gondii*. The parasite was originally identified in the small North African rodent *Ctenodactylus gundi*, hence its name. "*Toxo-*" refers to the curved or arcuate shape of the organism, not to a toxin. It is widely distributed among domestic animals and humans throughout the world.

Toxoplasma is a tissue coccidium. Both coccidian stages, schizogonic and gametogonic, are found in the epithelium of the small intestine of cats. The *Toxo-*

plasma oocyst, similar in morphology to that of *Isospora belli*, is excreted in cat feces. The oocysts, millions of which may be shed in a single stool of an infected cat, survive for months in moist environments, water, or soil.

In human tissues proliferating tachyzoites (trophozoites) and cysts may be identified (Fig. 11-14). The presence of tachyzoites is diagnostic of acute infection. Cysts containing hundreds and sometimes thousands of bradyzoites make their appearance in brain, skeletal muscles, and other tissues with the development of immunity. Rupture of these cysts has been proposed as a pathogenetic mechanism for the development of inflammatory lesions.[233]

Toxoplasma tachyzoites enter the cells by both phagocytosis and active invasion.[230,244] The latter mode of entry depends on specialized organelles, called rhoptries, and on "penetration-enhancing factor." During this infectious process an oxidative respiratory burst is not stimulated; thus no oxygen metabolites are formed to kill the protozoan. *T. gondii* also alters the membrane of the parasitophorous vacuole so that lysosomal fusion does not take place.[238]

Oocysts and cysts are the principal infective forms. Infection occurs when a person eats undercooked or raw meat of animals with chronic toxoplasmosis or in-

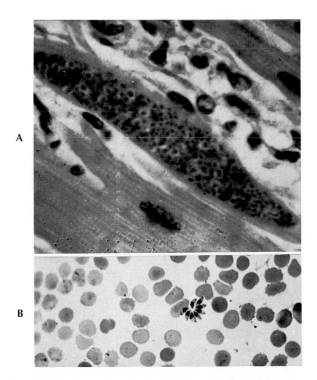

Fig. 11-14. Toxoplasmosis. **A,** *Toxoplasma* cyst in human heart muscle. **B,** Toxoplasma tachyzoites in smear from omentum of guinea pig. (From Pinkerton, H., and Henderson, R.G.: JAMA **116:**807, copyright 1941, American Medical Association.)

gests oocysts from the feces of cats. Recently an outbreak of acute toxoplasmosis associated with ingestion of contaminated water was reported.[228] Most of these primary infections are asymptomatic and result in a chronic carrier stage, again mostly symptomless.

Transplacental transmission occurs rarely but accounts for the majority of patients. Infection of the fetus is seen in 30% to 40% of cases of acquired toxoplasmosis during pregnancy.[234] The yearly incidence of gestational infection in the United States is said to be two to six cases per 1000 pregnancies.[239]

Relatively few cases of human disease have been reported in immunocompetent hosts, but results of the skin test for *Toxoplasma* and the Sabin-Feldman dye test[246] have been positive in 10% to 50% of the adults tested, indicating that although disease is rare infection is common. Actually the prevalence can be less than 10% in dry areas such as Arizona and close to 100% in moist, lowland tropical areas such as Costa Rica and Guatemala. Prevalence increases with age. The majority of immunocompetent individuals infected with *Toxoplasma* have minimal or no symptoms. However, in immunocompromised patients disseminated disease can occur and it is often fatal.[236,240,245,247] Central nervous system toxoplasmosis is the major form of involvement in these patients.[242,249,253] Patients with the acquired immunodeficiency syndrome (AIDS) frequently develop neurologic manifestations resulting from toxoplasmic encephalitis or brain abscess, or both.[237,253] The risk of toxoplasmic encephalitis in seropositive AIDS patients has been estimated to be as high as 12% in New York City and 25% in San Francisco.[237,253]

The clinicopathologic presentation in toxoplasmosis varies according to the age and the immune status of the patient. Three distinct presentations are described: congenital toxoplasmosis in neonates, *Toxoplasma* lymphadenitis in immunocompetent adults, *Toxoplasma* encephalitis in immunocompromised host.

Congenital toxoplasmosis. Congenital or neonatal toxoplasmosis should be strongly suspected when the characteristic ocular lesions and the presence of cerebral calcifications in roentgenographic examinations are associated with hydrocephalus and pleocytosis of the cerebrospinal fluid. The pathologic lesions are those of hydrocephalus caused by necrotic foci in the brain, usually located in the periventricular areas. These lesions are microglial nodules surrounded by areas of vasculitis and necrosis. Calcium deposits in these focal lesions and bilateral chorioretinitis are evident. Focal areas of necrosis may be seen in viscera, leading to myocarditis, pneumonitis, and rarely hepatitis.

Toxoplasma lymphadenitis. The clinical picture of adult toxoplasmosis is undoubtedly uncommon. It consists in lymphadenitis (usually posterior cervical), fever, and malaise. A biopsy of the firm, rubbery nodes is commonly done to rule out lymphoproliferative diseases, and it is the pathologist who first suggests the diagnosis of toxoplasmosis.[243] The architecture of the lymph node is preserved. There is pronounced follicular hyperplasia, sinus histocytosis, and clusters of epithelioid histiocytes inside and surrounding the follicles. Organisms are rarely seen.

Pathologic diagnosis can be confirmed by the Sabin-Feldman dye test or by more recent serologic methods such as indirect immunofluorescence, indirect hemagglutination, complement fixation, and enzyme-linked immunosorbent assay.[232,250,251] Some of these serologic tests have been suggested as screening methods for toxoplasmosis in pregnancy.[229] Acute infection is diagnosed on the basis of a fourfold rise in antibody titer or detection of IgM antibodies by the indirect immunofluorescence method. A Paul-Bunell test for heterophil antibodies is usually done to rule out infectious mononucleosis.

Toxoplasma encephalitis. Well-circumscribed areas of hemorrhage and necrosis are frequently identified by CT scan and on gross inspection. Microscopic examination usually reveals necrosis, vascular thrombosis, and the presence of tachyzoites. Immunoperoxidase and immunofluorescence methods have recently been developed for the diagnosis of toxoplasmosis in tissue sections.[231,248]

Other, less common manifestations of toxoplasmosis are interstitial pneumonitis, myocarditis, and hepatitis.[252] Chorioretinitis and uveitis sometimes occur.[235,241]

Pneumocystosis

Pneumocystosis (*Pneumocystis* pneumonia) is an endemic or epidemic disease caused by the organism *Pneumocystis carinii*. Although some investigators claim that *P. carinii* should be classified as fungus,[264] most authors consider it a protozoon. The organism's life-cycle forms and their interaction with host cells have been studied ultrastructurally in human tissues, animal models, and tissue culture systems.[266,279,284]

The protozoon has trophozoite and cyst stages, and both are identified in the pulmonary lesions. The organisms do not invade but remain extracellular, attached to the pulmonary alveolar epithelial cells, Type I pneumocytes.[272,282,283] Occasionally they may be phagocytosed by alveolar cells.

The epidemic disease occurs chiefly in premature infants and debilitated children who are malnourished at a time when the immunologic mechanisms are incompletely developed. These patients have an interstitial plasma cell pneumonia, which was once believed to be characteristic of pneumocystosis. Since then, there have been many reports of endemic cases of pneumocystosis in immunosuppressed patients in which a plasma cell infiltrate is not prominent.

Any disease process or form of therapy that sharply reduces the immunologic defenses predisposes the patient to pulmonary pneumocystosis. The disease is usually encountered in patients with congenital immunodeficiency states and in patients receiving corticosteroids or cytotoxic agents.[268] The incidence is high in transplant patients and in persons receiving chemotherapy for malignancy. *Pneumocystis carinii* pneumonia is the most frequent fatal opportunistic infection seen in AIDS patients, occurring at least once in more than 60% of these patients.[257,259,260,262,275,277] Concomitant infection with other opportunistic organisms such as *Aspergillus, Cryptococcus, Candida,* and cytomegalovirus (CMV) has been observed.[254,255,265]

The transmission of pneumocystosis is believed to be airborne,[254,269] but a case of transplacental transmission has been reported.[280] Experimental evidence indicates that the disease may occur by activation of a latent infection.

The disease's symptoms include fever, cough, shortness of breath, and less commonly chills and chest pain.[270] The onset of symptoms in immunosuppressed patients may be abrupt and fulminant. However, in AIDS patients, *Pneumocystis carinii* pneumonia seems to present as a more subtle slowly progressive illness.[270] The disease in marasmic children has an insidious onset characterized by progressive dyspnea, weight loss, and failure to thrive.[273]

Despite the severity of the respiratory symptoms, physical findings are minimal. Dullness to percussion is practically never elicited. A few moist rales occasionally may be heard. Laboratory findings include leukocytosis, hypoxemia, and increase in the alveolar-arterial PO_2 gradient as a result of alveolocapillary diffusion abnormalities and ventilation-perfusion mismatches.

Roentgenographic examination early in the disease discloses ground glass–like infiltration of the pulmonary parenchyma, which is more conspicuous toward the hilar region and spreads peripherally in a butterfly pattern. Subsequently, the infiltrate assumes a nodular pattern, with intervening areas of radiolucency attributable to compensatory emphysema.

Pathologic changes are predominantly limited to the lungs, which are firm, rubbery, and noncrepitant. The cut surface is whitish or brownish and discloses several firm nodules with a granular mucinous appearance. These nodules may be separated from each other by spongy areas of emphysematous pulmonary parenchyma, but often they are confluent. On microscopy the respiratory bronchioles and alveoli are distended by a honeycombed foamy material that stains brightly eosinophilic (Fig. 11-15). On special stains the organisms are identified lining the alveolar walls. The cyst wall is best outlined with the methenamine-silver method,

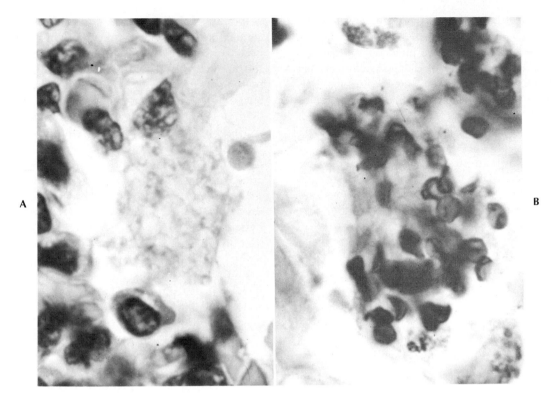

Fig. 11-15. A, Pneumocystosis. Foamy mass of organisms appears in alveolus of lung. **B,** Pneumocystosis. (**A,** Hematoxylin and eosin; **B,** Gomori methenamine-silver.)

whereas the free trophozoites and cystic contents are best seen on Giemsa stains. There is a minimal inflammatory reaction composed mainly of monocytes, occasional plasma cells, and histiocytes. Plasma cells are numerous only in cases of the "epidemic type" of disease. The disease seldom spreads to extrapulmonary sites.[258,263,267]

Diagnosis of pneumocystosis is established by examining tissue obtained by transbronchial, percutaneous, or open lung wedge biopsy, or by identification of the organisms in tracheobronchial secretions obtained by bronchial washings or bronchioalveolar lavage.[256,278,281] The latter method has replaced open-lung biopsy as the diagnostic method of choice.[261,271,276]

Babesiosis (piroplasmosis)

Babesiosis, formerly called piroplasmosis, is a serious hemolytic disease that affects cattle. Since the first case of human babesiosis was described by Skrabalo[299] in 1957, many other clinical and subclinical cases have been identified.[289,298]

The most common *Babesia* species to infect humans are *B. bovis* in Europe and *B. microti* in North America. The vector for this zoonosis and for Lyme disease (see pp. 357 and 2075 in ref. 152 there) is the tick *Ixodes dammini;* thus both diseases can sometimes affect the same patient.[286,293] Babesiosis can also be transmitted by transfusion of infected erythrocytes.[292,300,303]

Babesia merozoites invade erythrocytes with an entry process that requires the presence of complement factor[291,302] in a manner similar to the blood group determinant requirements of some plasmodia.[202,214,215] The protozoon multiplies inside the red blood cell by budding rather than by schizogony.[288] The absence of schizonts and gametocytes and the lack of hemozoin pigment in *Babesia*-parasitized erythrocytes are the fundamental points in its differential diagnosis with malarial infections.[290,301] No exoerythrocytic cycle has been documented in babesiosis.

The initial cases reported occurred in splenectomized individuals. The clinical course was hemoglobinuria, hemoglobinemia, jaundice, anemia, and renal failure frequently with a fatal outcome. Postmortem findings included bile staining of viscera and serosal membranes, acute tubular necrosis, and a generalized reticuloendothelial response most prominent in the Kupffer cells.[288]

Recent cases[297] in nonsplenectomized patients followed a milder course with viral syndrome–like symptoms. That the absence of the spleen leads to a more severe illness[294-296,304] has been confirmed in experimental animals. Older age also predisposes to clinical infection. In addition, the competence of the host's cell-mediated immune system is believed to play a major role in the control of parasitemia and the development of immunity.[285,295]

The diagnosis of babesiosis is confirmed by identification of the ring and tetrad forms in Giemsa-stained thick or thin blood smears. As in malaria, multiple examinations increase the yield of diagnosis. Smears are also helpful in quantitation of parasitemia to follow response to drug therapy. In cases of high suspicion in which parasites are not seen in smears, the patient's blood can be injected into a hamster for confirmation. This bioassay has also been used in the evaluation of drug therapy to distinguish complete eradication from lowering of parasitemia to undetectable levels by blood-smear examination.[300] Serodiagnosis for babesiosis, based on an indirect fluorescent antibody test, is now available.[287]

HELMINTHIC DISEASES
Diseases caused by trematodes (flukes)
Distomiases

Hepatic distomiasis. Hepatic distomiasis is caused mainly by the trematodes of *Fasciola hepatica* (sheep liver fluke), *Clonorchis sinensis* (Chinese liver fluke), *Opisthorchis felineus* (cat liver fluke), and *Opisthorchis viverrini.*

Fascioliasis. The trematode *Fasciola hepatica* is found most commonly in sheep- and cattle-raising countries, where it produces the disease known as liver rot. The operculated ova are passed in the feces. They mature in fresh water, after which they hatch a miracidium, which invades a freshwater snail. Cercariae are produced, which, instead of swimming freely as do those of the schistosomes, form cysts (metacercariae) that attach themselves to aquatic vegetation. Most infections are acquired by eating watercress. On ingestion metacercariae are liberated in the upper small intestine of humans or more frequently of sheep and cattle, and the parasites penetrate directly through the gut to the peritoneal cavity and into the hepatic parenchyma until they reach their usual habitat in the large biliary ducts. The disease is usually manifested by a pronounced leukocytosis and eosinophilia; eosinophils may reach a value of 70%.[324] Hepatomegaly, splenomegaly, and lymphadenopathy are frequently encountered. In some cases the symptoms and signs are those of chronic cholecystitis or cholangitis. Intermittent jaundice may develop occasionally because of obstruction by the adult parasite. We have seen three cases in which the adult parasite or ova were incidental findings when tissue was studied after cholecystectomy (Fig. 11-16).

The adult parasites produce epithelial hyperplasia of the biliary epithelium,[316] with periductal infiltration by eosinophils, lymphocytes, and plasma cells and eventual extensive fibrosis.[305] However, it is extremely rare for cirrhosis to develop as the result of this parasitic infection. Aberrant migration of *Fasciola* larvae can occasionally lead to ectopic fascioliasis, with abscess for-

mation involving almost any organ.[306,326] These complications are not seen in other liver fluke diseases because their excysted larvae reach the biliary tree via the ampulla of Vater. Experimentally, the host's immunologic response to *Fasciola* is similar to that described for *Schistosoma* and *Trichinella* with eosinophil degranulation and release of toxic substances.[311]

The diagnosis is established when the ova are found in the feces or in the duodenal contents. Serodiagnostic tests have been developed and include complement fixation, hemagglutination, and the enzyme-linked immunosorbent assay.[313,319,321] Although not very specific, they can be useful as supportive evidence when a radiologic diagnosis of *F. hepatica* is suggested either by nuclear scans, by computerized tomography, or by endoscopic retrograde cholangiopancreatography (ERCP).[309,312,330] Thus the widespread use of sensitive immunodiagnostic methods such as ELISA will depend on the isolation of a genus-specific antigen that would increase diagnostic specificity.[318]

Clonorchiasis. The liver fluke *Clonorchis sinensis* is parasitic in cats, dogs, and humans. Two intermediate hosts are required, a freshwater mollusk and one of several species of freshwater fish. The eggs passed in the feces do not hatch in freshwater but within the first host, a freshwater snail. The miracidium is transformed into a cercaria within the snail. The cercaria then leaves the snail and swims until it finally penetrates beneath the scales of the second host, a freshwater fish. Here it develops into a metacercaria. Humans are infected by

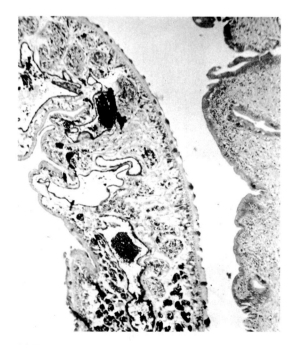

Fig. 11-16. *Fasciola hepatica* encountered accidentally in common bile duct in course of exploration for chronic cholecystitis. (Hematoxylin and eosin; 35×.)

eating raw fish. The liberated metacercariae adhere to the duodenal mucosa and migrate into the common duct and the intrahepatic ducts, where they develop into adult worms. When the parasites are numerous, they may block biliary flow.[317] Roentgenographic examination of the biliary tract sometimes leads to the diagnosis.[333]

Severe adenomatous hyperplasia of biliary duct epithelium is far more common in this disease than in fascioliasis[328] (Fig. 11-17). These changes are believed to be the result of both mechanical injury, caused by the suckers of the parasite, and chemical stimulation by parasitic metabolic products.[329] Periductal inflammation with eosinophils and round cells also is seen. Severe portal fibrosis ensues, followed by cirrhosis with portal hypertension.

The clinical course is characterized by relative absence of symptoms. The symptoms and signs of cirrhosis are evident as late complications. Diagnosis is based on recovery of the ova in the feces or duodenal contents.

Carcinoma of the liver is often found in association with clonorchiasis.[323,327] Their association is most probably the result of the high incidence of both parasitism and hepatitis B infection in the same communities. On the other hand, clonorchiasis may play an etiologic role in cholangiocarcinoma as implied by both epidemiologic and animal studies.[328]

Opisthorchiasis. The cat liver fluke, *Opisthorchis felineus,* occurs endemically in Liberia, parts of the Orient, and Eastern Europe. *O. viverrini* is endemic in northeast Thailand, where 25% to 75% of the population is infected.[331]

As in clonorchiasis, the disease is acquired when raw fish are eaten. The adult parasite invades not only the bile ducts but also the pancreatic duct. The pathologic changes and symptoms are similar to those of clonorchiasis.[336]

Experimental data indicate that the host's immunologic response may be important in the development of portal fibrosis in a manner similar to schistosomiasis.[308] The same investigators have implied that the combined effect of nitrosamine compounds in the diet and of liver fluke infection may play an etiologic role in the pathogenesis of cholangiocarcinoma.[307,314,315,320,332] The diagnosis is based on finding the ova in the feces or duodenal contents.[334,335]

Intestinal distomiasis. An infection limited to the Far East, intestinal distomiasis is caused by the trematode *Fasciolopsis buski.* The adult fluke lives in the duodenum and upper jejunum and occasionally may be found in the colon. The ova are deposited in the stools. If the latter come into contact with freshwater, miracidia are liberated from the ova. These miracidia swim freely until they invade a freshwater snail and mature

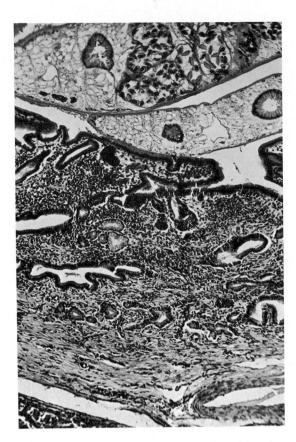

Fig. 11-17. *Clonorchis sinensis* within dilated intrahepatic bile duct. Wall of duct shows adenomatous proliferation and pronounced round cell infiltration. There is fibrosis of portal space. (80×.)

into infective cercariae. The cercariae, like those of *Fasciola hepatica,* leave the snail and become encysted on water plants. Humans acquire the disease by ingestion of aquatic vegetation. The metacercariae are liberated from the cyst wall by the gastric juice and then mature. The adult subsequently becomes attached to the mucosa of the duodenum.

The main pathologic changes are ulceration in the intestinal mucosa and hemorrhages at the areas of attachment. Abscesses may develop occasionally. Both local tissue and peripheral eosinophilia may occur. The symptoms usually are limited to the gastrointestinal tract and include abdominal pain and diarrhea.

Pulmonary distomiasis (paragonimiasis). Paragonimiasis, or endemic hemoptysis is caused by trematodes of the genus *Paragonimus,*[322] mainly *P. westermani.*[325] The disease occurs in the Far East, parts of Africa, the South Pacific, and the northern countries of South America. The operculated ova of the parasite pass to the outside with the sputum of the infected individual or in the feces if the sputum has been swallowed. As in all trematodes pathogenic to humans, the ova need a freshwater snail in which to mature to infective forms. The metacercariae liberated by action of gastric juice penetrate the wall of the duodenum and traverse the peritoneal cavity, diaphragm, pleural cavity, and pleura until they reach the lungs, where they mature. The parasite produces cystic spaces or cavities in the lungs, more numerous in the periphery. The adult worms are surrounded by a dense zone of eosinophilic, polymorphonuclear, and chronic inflammatory cell infiltration. A dense fibrous capsule envelops the area. The cavities produced by the presence of the worms contain brownish fluid that is rather viscid and resembles anchovy sauce. The fluid is composed of the inflammatory exudate, erythrocytes, eosinophils, and numerous ova.

Chronic cough productive of brownish sputum, thoracic discomfort, and recurring hemoptysis are the dominant clinical features of this disease. Other organs such as the brain, liver, intestine, and muscles may be affected. Secondary pulmonary infections, with consequent development of pneumonitis, pulmonary abscesses, and destruction of bronchi, occur rather frequently. In the later stages of the disease there are diffuse areas of focal fibrosis, which may adversely affect pulmonary function and produce chronic cor pulmonale. Pulmonary osteoarthropathy may be present in long-standing cases. The metacercariae that do not reach the lungs but remain in other organs produce small granulomas. These granulomas contain large numbers of eosinophils. Definite diagnosis of this condition rests on finding the characteristic ova in the sputum or the feces.[310] Immunologic tests have been developed for diagnosis.[318]

Schistosomiasis (bilharziasis)

Several different species of blood flukes, or schistosomes, are pathogenic to humans and are distributed in different regions of the globe. The urinary form of schistosomiasis, caused by *Schistosoma haematobium*, occurs mostly in Africa. In the Far East the responsible agent is *S. japonicum*. *S. mansoni* is seen in Africa, in parts of the Antilles, and in the northern part of South America. Blood flukes are known as schistosomes because of the "split body" on the ventral side of the male, in which the female is held during insemination and egg laying.

The ova of the different schistosomes are passed in the feces or urine of the infected mammal, usually a human. If they gain access to freshwater, free-swimming miracidia are hatched, and they penetrate certain species of freshwater snails. Numerous cercariae are liberated from the mollusk and enter the intact skin or mucosa of a person bathing in or wading through an infected pond, stream, or irrigation canal. Infection is far more frequent during the middle of the day when sunlight is very strong, for these cercariae are phototropic.

The fork-tailed cercariae lose their tails while entering the skin and thus become known as schistosomula.

The latter enter through the lymphatics of the dermis and pass through the regional lumph nodes, apparently reaching the circulation through the thoracic duct. They pass through the pulmonary circuit, from the right to the left side of the heart, and finally enter the systemic circulation. The schistosomula, insofar as is known, can mature only in the intrahepatic portal veins, where each schistosomulum develops into an adult male or female worm. Apparently only those able to pass from the arterial to the venous side survive. This takes place for the most part in the abdominal organs drained by the portal system. The adult worms travel against the mesenteric circulation, where they copulate and where the females deposit their ova. Oviposition takes place in the urinary plexuses in the case of schistosomiasis haematobia and in the mesenteric and the hemorrhoidal plexuses in schistosomiasis japonica and mansoni. The ova are laid in narrow venules in the submucosa of the intestine or the urinary bladder, depending on the species. The ova are retained in these organs, swept back into the liver, or passed with the urine or feces.

Schistosomiasis has been referred to as an immunologic disease.[382] The pathogenesis of both acute and chronic schistosomiasis appears to involve immunologic mechanisms, either humoral or cell mediated. The major component of the host immune response against the schistosomula is the eosinophil.[381] Eosinophils have been shown to adhere to the surface of the schistosomulum in the presence of antibody or complement. This is followed by degranulation and the release of granule contents, which include lysosomal hydrolytic enzymes, peroxidase, and major basic protein. Major basic protein is an arginine-rich cationic protein that seems to be the main effector of schistosomal damage.[344] The role of other effectors of eosinophil-mediated damage, such as the generation of the toxic oxygen metabolites superoxide and hydrogen peroxide, is uncertain.[360,374] Although neutrophils[358] and macrophages[341] have been shown in vitro to be cytotoxic to schistosomula, their role as effector cells in schistosome immunity is unclear.

The schistosomula attempt to evade the host's immune system by several mechanisms.[342,383] They lose some of their surface antigens and mask others with a coat of host molecules[380] that include blood group and major histocompatibility antigens.[343,377] The schistosomula also develop an outer tegument or cytoplasmic syncytium composed of two lipid bilayers, which is resistant to immune damage.[377]

The definitive diagnosis of schistosomiasis can be made only when schistosome eggs are found in urine or feces or in a proctoscopic mucosal biopsy specimen. Serodiagnostic methods are available and include indirect immunofluorescence, circumoval precipitin test,[356] radioimmunoassay, and enzyme-linked immunosorbent assay.[355,362] These tests are valuable in epidemiologic studies or in diagnosis of ectopic or central nervous system schistosomiasis where results of routine tests would be negative. Sonography has also been suggested as an adjunct in the diagnosis of schistosomal hepatic fibrosis and other schistosomal syndromes.[357]

Schistosomiasis mansoni

Acute schistosomiasis mansoni. The entrance of cercariae into the skin has been associated with immediate cutaneous manifestations. The pruritic papular rash or swimmer's itch is believed to be a hypersensitivity reaction, since it is uncommon among previously unexposed persons. When present it is highly suggestive of reinfection.

Four to 8 weeks after infection a syndrome known as Katayama fever may develop, which includes fever, chills, sweating, headache, and cough. Hepatomegaly accompanied by pronounced eosinophilic infiltration of the portal areas has been encountered in the few cases in which liver biopsies have been performed. The spleen and lymph nodes are enlarged as a result of reticuloendothelial hyperplasia. The classic bilharzial pseudotubercles (Fig. 11-18) with centrally located ova are evident in biopsy specimens obtained 80 days after infection. The liver parenchyma is well preserved, and no biliary duct proliferation or portal fibrosis is evident.

This syndrome, which coincides with the beginning of oviposition, is more commonly seen in heavy infections. Although recovery is the rule, some fatal cases have occurred, especially with *S. japonicum* infections. This serum sickness–like syndrome is believed to be the result of immune complex formation that follows the antigenic challenge of oviposition.[363]

Chronic schistosomiasis mansoni

INTESTINAL SCHISTOSOMIASIS. The distal parts of the colon are more frequently and severely affected in intestinal schistosomiasis. In most cases no gross changes are seen. To be grossly discernible, the infection has to be very severe, producing abundant fibrosis or localized polypoid inflammatory lesions.

The lesions are composed of granulation tissue within which are innumerable ova of *S. mansoni* containing living embryos. Numerous chronic inflammatory cells, including moderate numbers of eosinophils, are encountered. These inflammatory polyps may reach 8 cm and may produce bleeding from their ulcerated surfaces. Occasionally a narrow segment of colon may be involved, with ulceration and dense fibrosis of the wall and a reduction in size of the intestinal lumen. The roentgenographic findings resemble those in granulomatous colitis or carcinoma. In the material available at the University of Puerto Rico School of Medicine, no etiologic relationship could be established between schistosomiasis mansoni and the development of adenocarcinoma of the colon.[365] The small intestine is rarely affected grossly.

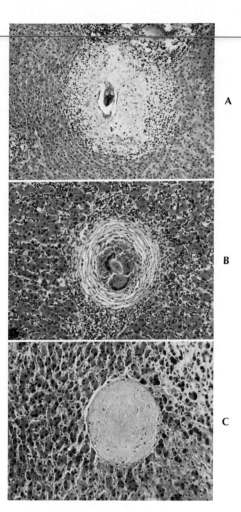

Fig. 11-18. Sequence of changes in pseudotubercles developing about eggs in Manson's schistosomiasis. **A,** Pseudotubercle at height of development is composed mainly of histiocytes (epithelioid cells). **B,** Peripheral capsule of concentric fibroblasts slowly replaces area previously occupied by epithelioid cells as foreign body giant cells digest egg shell. **C,** Ultimate results is fibrous nodule. (**A** and **B,** 80×; **C,** 100×; **A** from Koppisch, E.: Puerto Rico J. Public Health **13:**1, 1937.)

HEPATOSPLENIC SCHISTOSOMIASIS. Hepatosplenic schistosomiasis is seen in a small subset of patients chronically infected with *S. mansoni* and *S. japonicum.* The ova lodged in the small intrahepatic portal radicles contain a living embryo that can survive for a period of 2 to 3 weeks.[384] During this period it continues to secrete soluble antigens that induce a granulomatous type of reaction. The granulomatous response in *S. mansoni* is an immunologic reaction of the cell-mediated type with delayed sensitivity.[384] The host's response interferes with the egg metabolic and immunologic activities.[346,347]

The most frequently encountered vascular lesion is that in which the intrahepatic portal radicle is totally replaced by a granuloma that occludes the lumen (Fig. 11-19). Occasionally an acute endophlebitis of the intrahepatic radicles is encountered, which is probably most important in the final causation of the intrahepatic vascular block.[361] Inflammation and destruction of the coats of the vessels lead to thrombosis. The thrombi become recanalized, and the newly formed blood vessels communicate through the wall of the vein with adjacent vessels outside, forming telangiectasias in the portal areas.

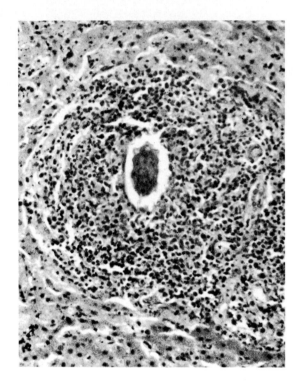

Fig. 11-19. Schistosomiasis mansoni. Granuloma with centrally located living ovum replaces radicle of portal vein. Portal branch of hepatic artery and common duct are visible to right of ovum. (Hematoxylin and eosin; 100×.)

Because of the prominent vascular and fibrotic changes in the portal areas, the latter are moderately broadened and lengthened and stand out in cross section, justifying the gross descriptive term of "pipestem" fibrosis (Fig. 11-20). Although a positive correlation between worm burden, fecal egg counts, and fibrosis has been documented, it is apparent that the reparative fibrosis that follows the destruction caused by the intravascular and perivascular portal granulomas is not sufficient to explain the extensive fibrosis seen in the classic pipestem pattern. Thus it seems that the egg granulomas can induce collagen formation through a mechanism other than necrosis followed by reparative fibrosis.[337,345] In vitro studies have shown that egg granulomas can secrete soluble products that alter collagen metabolism.[340,354,372]

The liver is enlarged, and the surface is smooth or only slightly nodular but not hobnailed. Occasionally the surface is bosselated, forming so-called mountains separated by moderately deep valleys, which correspond to the areas of retraction in the fibrosed portal spaces. These pathologic changes in the liver lead to portal hypertension.

Findings in the adjacent liver parenchyma and the majority of the liver function tests in uncomplicated schistosomiasis mansoni are negative, contrary to the findings in classic liver cirrhosis.[375] The liver block in schistosomiasis mansoni is at the intrahepatic or presinusoidal level, whereas in Laennec's cirrhosis the blockage is at the suprahepatic circulation. We have not noted a parallelism between hepatic schistosomal involvement and liver cell carcinoma. Other workers have reached similar conclusions for both S. *mansoni*[367] and S. *japonicum.*[370]

Massive congestive splenomegaly develops, with subsequent fibrosis of the pulp and formation of Gamna-Gandy bodies. Esophageal varices complicate

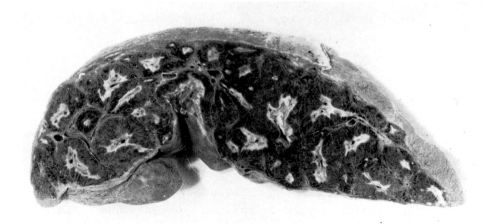

Fig. 11-20. Hepatic fibrosis of "pipestem" type in advanced schistosomiasis mansoni.

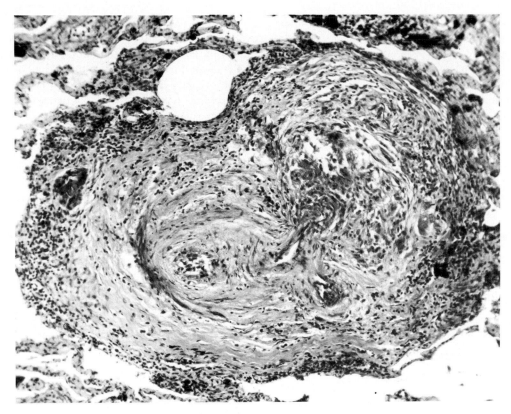

Fig. 11-21. Schistosomiasis mansoni. Newly formed blood vessels in para-arterial granuloma in lung communicate with original, partially destroyed pulmonary arteriole. (Hematoxylin and eosin; 100×.)

the picture of portal hypertension. Death in patients with hepatosplenic involvement usually is attributable to rupture of these varices. Hepatic coma is unusual in the uncomplicated case.[350,351] The same can be said for liver cell necrosis and regeneration.

CARDIOPULMONARY SCHISTOSOMIASIS. Although ova may frequently be found in the lungs of patients with schistosomiasis, the finding of pulmonary obstructive arteriolitis leading to cor pulmonale is less common. This condition is rare, probably because considerable egg emboli must reach the lungs before the development of pulmonary arterial schistosomal disease. For sufficient numbers of ova to reach the lungs, portal hypertension with collateral venous channels must be present to allow direct passage of eggs to the right side of the heart and from there to the pulmonary arterial tree. For this reason cardiopulmonary bilharziasis almost always develops in patients with hepatosplenic schistosomiasis.

The wall of the artery is destroyed by an inflammatory process characterized by a granulomatous reaction, with chronic inflammatory cells and occasional eosinophils. This reaction surrounds the ova and extends toward the lumen of the vessel as well as through its wall. Finally it obliterates the lumen of the artery and, in the process of extending through its wall, pushes the frag-

mented elastic lamina ahead of it, producing a pseudoaneurysm. The results is a dumbbell type of granuloma formed by the intra-arterial and the para-arterial components, joined by a granulomatous isthmus in the destroyed arterial wall. Proliferation of endothelial cells with neoformation of blood vessels occurs in both the intra-arterial and the para-arterial granulomas. These blood vessels form communications among themselves and also with branches of the pulmonary veins destroyed by the para-arterial granulomas (Fig. 11-21). The newly formed blood vessels have been named "intra-arterial angiomatoids."[364] The newly formed blood vessels in the para-arterial granulomas, which form an anastomosis with the pulmonary veins and cause areas of dilatation because of their arteriovenous nature, are the classic angiomatoids considered characteristic of pulmonary schistosomal endarteritis. The occlusion of the arterioles by granulomatous tissue, the pseudoaneurysms, and the arteriovenous communications play a vital role in the causation of hypertension in the lesser circulation and finally right-sided cardiac failure (cor pulmonale).[376]

A schistosomal glomerulopathy mediated by immune complex deposition has been described. The majority of cases have histopathologic findings consistent with a diffuse membranoproliferative glomerulonephritis in which immune complexes are detected by both immunofluorescence and electron microscopy.[338]

ECTOPIC GRANULOMATOUS SCHISTOSOMIASIS. Isolated granulomas have been found in practically every organ,[359,386] including the heart. These granulomas do not give rise to clinical manifestations. The term "granulomatous schistosomiasis" is better reserved for those usually solitary lesions composed of numerous eggs, pseudotubercles, granulation tissue, and varying amounts of fibrous tissue that are always located in an ectopic site. These solitary lesions are usually large enough to produce replacement of normal tissues or protrusion into lumens or cavities, which accounts for their symptoms. The lesions considered ectopic are those encountered outside the portocaval venous circulation, including the extension of the latter into the pulmonary arterioles.

Symptomatic ectopic granulomas in our experience have been most commonly localized to the spinal cord, producing a transverse myelitis.[366]

Schistosomiasis japonica. In the human host the habitat of *S. japonicum* is essentially the lower mesenteric venous system, although it often may be found in the veins of the small and large intestines. Occasionally it may limit itself to the veins of the small intestine. In general, schistosomiasis japonica is characterized by similar but more serious symptoms than those of schistosomiasis mansoni, probably because of the larger number of eggs produced by the parasite.[369,385]

The small intestine is far more frequently affected than in the mansoni type, and fibrotic stenotic lesions of the bowel are more common. Intestinal polyp formation is likewise more frequent and severe, as in involvement of the liver and lungs. The clinical signs and symptoms are thus usually more pronounced than those of schistosomiasis mansoni. As association between schistosomiasis and colonic carcinoma has been reported from the People's Republic of China.[368,387] Since the investigators fail to show convincing evidence of dysplastic changes in the epithelium away from the carcinomas, we agree with others[371,388] that the proposed association is inadequately documented.

Schistosomiasis haematobia. *S. haematobium* is widely distributed throughout Africa. It is also encountered in the Middle East. The vesical and the pelvic venous plexuses constitute the final habitat of *S. haematobium*. Occasionally the parasites may be retained in the hemorrhoidal plexus of veins or in the terminal tributaries of the inferior mesenteric vein, producing lesions in the rectosigmoid as in other schistosomal infections.

The adult female parasite leaves the vesical and pelvic plexuses of veins and migrates into the venules, usually of the submucosa of the urinary bladder, where it lays its eggs. These eggs produce the classic bilharzial granulomas. The latter may coalesce and form larger "bilharzial nodules." These appear as polypoid or pla-

teaulike elevations covered by granular or ulcerated mucosa. The adjacent mucosa becomes hyperplastic and undergoes glandular metaplasia, giving rise to the classic picture of cystitis glandularis. In other areas the mucosa may undergo squamous metaplasia, giving rise to a white patch known as "leukoplakic patch."[352]

The sharp reduction of blood supply caused by the granulomatous process and subsequent fibrosis may produce prominent ulcerations. The atrophy of the surface epithelium overlying plaques of calcified ova accounts for the formation of the "sandy patch." This process is followed by severe cicatrization, which may lead to obstruction. Obstruction is very prominent at the bladder neck and around the urethral orifices. Hydronephrosis[373] and hydroureter[378,379] may result. Calcifications may eventually occur.

In many of these patients carcinoma of the urinary bladder may develop.[348] The general consensus is that cancer of the bladder is related to urinary bilharziasis, but the exact relationship still remains obscure.[349] The disease also may affect the prostate, seminal vesicles, spermatic cord, epididymis, testes, penis, penile urethra, and female urethra.

Diseases caused by cestodes (tapeworms)
Taeniasis saginata

Taenia saginata (beef tapeworm), a flatworm averaging 4 to 12 m (12 to 36 feet) in length, grows in the human intestinal tract; humans are the only definitive host. It attaches itself to the mucosa of the small intestine, usually in the jejunum, by four suckers. The worm contains from 1000 to 2000 proglottids. Ova develop in the distal half of the worm. The proglottids containing developing ova are cast off. Cattle ingest the liberated eggs or gravid proglottids occasionally released in the fecal stream. Within cattle the embryos hatch in the intestinal tract and finally migrate to skeletal muscle, where they develop to the next larval stage (cysticerus). Humans become infected by eating uncooked or poorly cooked meat harboring these larvae, which develop into adult worms in the intestine. Usually there is only one adult worm, but occasionally numerous adult worms are present. The symptoms are either allergic or nervous in nature, but in 72% of cases symptoms also are referable to the digestive system.[393]

Taeniasis solium

T. solium (pork tapeworm) ranges in length from 2 to 7 m (7 to 23 feet) and lives in the human small intestine. In contrast to *T. saginata*, it attaches itself to the mucosa of the small intestine by its head or scolex, which contains hooklets. In cases of taeniasis solium, generally only one worm is found, as the name implies, but occasionally there may be two or three. The ova or proglottids passed by humans in the feces are ingested by the intermediate host, the pig. The liberated em-

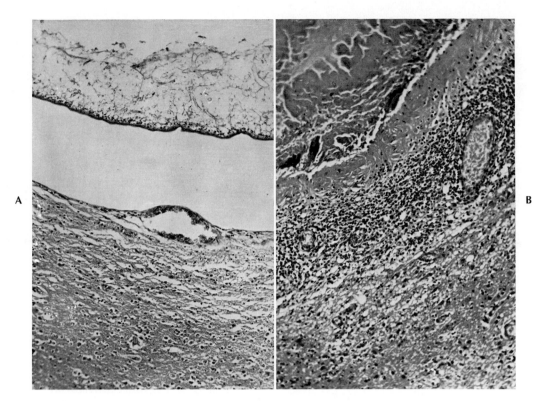

Fig. 11-22. Cerebral cysticercosis. **A,** Part of wall of larval cyst is included above. As long as cyst is alive, cerebral substance, below, shows only compression atrophy. **B,** When cyst dies, it is converted into formless debris that evokes granulomatous inflammatory reaction in surrounding cerebral tissues. (80×.)

bryos or oncospheres penetrate the venules in the intestinal wall of the pig, enter the blood, and are carried to various organs and tissues. The embryo develops into the next larval stage, a cysticerus (formerly called *Cysticercus cellulosae*). A cysticercus consists of a small ovoid vesicle about 5 mm long and 10 mm wide, having an invagination on one side containing a small white spot that represents the scolex and its hooklets. Humans acquire the intestinal infection by the ingestion of viable cysticerci in undercooked pork. The cysticercus matures into the adult *T. solium* in the human intestine.

Cysticercosis. When a person ingests food or water contaminated with the feces of another person harboring the eggs of *T. solium*, the cysticerci develop in the tissues. Individuals infected with *T. solium* may infect themselves when their fingers convey ova to the mouth. It is possible, although not probable, that in a few cases autoinfection may take place when ova or ripe proglottids are regurgitated into the stomach or duodenum. The larvae are liberated in the stomach or duodenum and penetrate through the wall, gaining access to the circulation. They travel in the bloodstream and subsequently develop into encysted larvae of cysticerci in tissue.[389] In order of frequency, the tissues affected are the subcutaneous tissue, brain, muscles, heart, liver, lungs, and peritoneum. When the cysticerci are

alive (Fig. 11-22, *A*), very slight inflammatory reaction, lymphocytic in type, is elicited. As soon as the larvae die, the cysticercus is surrounded by a dense infiltration composed of polymorphonuclear leukocytes, chronic inflammatory cells, epithelioid cells, and occasional foreign-body giant cells (Fig. 11-22, *B*). Outside this zone is a zone of fibrosis and chronic inflammatory cell infiltration. Calcification is the result. In the subcutaneous tissue the larvae are palpable and firm. Roentgenograms of the soft tissues will disclose foci of calcification representing the end stage of the cysticerci. The average period of time for calcification to take place is 5 years.

Cysticerci do most damage to the brain and meninges. The larvae may project from the ependymal lining into the ventricles or may be located within the cerebral substance (Fig. 11-23). The symptoms produced by the cerebral cysticerci depend on the number of larvae present and their anatomic location.[409] They may manifest themselves as space-occupying lesions, giving rise to symptoms of a cerebral neoplasm, or they may cause obstruction to the cerebrospinal fluid, with subsequent hydrocephalus.[391,404,415] There is glial proliferation around the larvae, and there also may be fibrosis of the leptomeninges. Occasionally cysticerci tend to grow as grapelike clusters, and such grouping is then termed cysticercus racemosus. Epileptic seizures frequently are

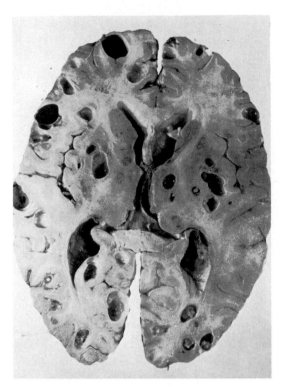

Fig. 11-23. Cerebral cysticercosis. Larval cysts may still be seen within some cavities, whereas they have dropped out of others. (From Ash, J.E., and Spitz, S.: Pathology of tropical diseases, Philadelphia, 1945, W.B. Saunders Co.; AFIP.)

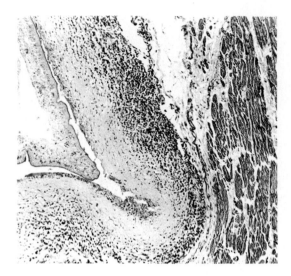

Fig. 11-24. Cysticercosis of myocardium. (Hematoxylin and eosin; 100×.)

associated with cerebral cysticercosis.[405] Occasionally cysticerci develop beneath the retina, and the subsequent inflammation leads to iridocyclitis and secondary glaucoma.[406] When the heart is involved (Fig. 11-24), the cysticerci occur within the myocardium and valves. There may be cardiac arrhythmias.

Radiologic tests, including computerized tomography scan[392,395,411] and arteriography, can be used for the diagnosis of cysticercosis. Serodiagnostic tests are useful in confirming the diagnosis. Methods available include indirect hemagglutination, complement fixation, indirect immunofluorescence and enzyme-linked immunosorbent assay.[396,407,413]

Diphyllobothriasis

Diphyllobothriasis is found principally among fish-eating people in the Scandinavian countries, in Russia, and in parts of Asia. In the United States it is found in northern Michigan, Wisconsin, and Minnesota. The infection is extremely rare in tropical areas. The causative agent, *Diphyllobothrium latum* (fish tapeworm), measures between 3 and 10 m (10 and 33 feet) in length and is composed of 3000 or more proglottids. Humans and other mammals, especially dogs, acquire the infection by eating undercooked fish or fish products. The

worm lives in the small intestine; the presence of multiple worms is not uncommon.

Infected persons may be symptomless or may be asthenic and suffer from gastrointestinal disorders, especially abdominal pain. Occasionally a megaloblastic anemia (bothriocephalus anemia) is seen, especially when the worm is implanted high in the small intestine. The exact mechanism for the production of anemia has not been fully elucidated. One explanation for the anemia is that the worm produces an enzyme that interferes with the association between vitamin B_{12} and the intrinsic factor.[417] The uncomplexed vitamin B_{12} is not absorbed in the ileum and is available for the tapeworm's utilization.[418] Megaloblastic hyperactivity of the bone marrow and even central nervous system degeneration may be encountered in some patients.

Differential diagnosis should be made primarily between tapeworm anemia and genuine pernicious anemia. Free hydrochloric acid in the gastric juice, remission after the worm cure without additional therapy, and a Schilling test value that becomes normal after the expulsion of the parasite constitute evidence of tapeworm anemia.[416]

Echinococcosis (echinococcal disease, hydatid disease)

Echinococcosis, or hydatidosis, is one of the most important zoonoses. The species *Echinococcus granulosus* is the cause of cystic hydatid disease, the hydatid disease most commonly seen throughout the world. Areas of high incidence include East Africa, Spain, Greece, the Middle East, Iran, western Australia, Chile, Argentina, and Uruguay. *E. multilocularis* causes alveolar hydatid disease that is seen mostly in Alaska, Canada, the Soviet Union, and central Europe. A third species, *E.*

vogeli, has recently been identified as the cause of polycystic hydatid disease in Colombia, a disease with features similar to those of alveolar hydatid disease.[394]

The definitive hosts for the adult cestode are carnivores, commonly the domestic dog for *E. granulosus* and the fox for *E. multilocularis.* The adult tapeworms, which may number several thousands in the heavily infected dog intestine, shed both eggs and gravid proglottids, which can be found in the host's stool. Human and the natural intermediate hosts become infected when they swallow these immediately infective eggs. In the duodenum the larvae or oncospheres are freed and, using their hooklets, find their way through the intestinal mucosa into the lumen of blood vessels. They are then carried by the blood until they lodge in capillaries at almost any site. In 60% of cases, the larvae are retained in the sinusoids of the liver. The remainder pass through the hepatic circulation, and 20% are retained in the lung; the others gain access to the systemic circulation.

The embryos of *E. granulosus* that survive develop into hydatid cysts containing numerous scolices provided with hooklets. These scolices represent the future head of the adult tapeworm. The cysts have an outer laminated, elastic layer and an inner germinal layer. They enlarge gradually for several months until they attain a diameter of 10 to 20 cm. Abundant clear fluid is contained within the cysts. The germinal layer develops numerous papillae, which become pedunculated vesicles (brood capsules) containing scolices (Fig. 11-25). Cysts of echinococcosis occur more frequently in the liver or in the lung. Approximately 70% of primary

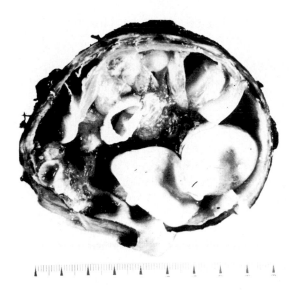

Fig. 11-26. Large echinococcal cyst of liver. (Courtesy Dr. Diego Ribas-Mujal; from Marcial-Rojas, R.A.: Parasitic diseases of the liver. In Schiff, L., editor: Diseases of the liver, Philadelphia, 1969, J.B. Lippincott Co.)

echinococcal cysts are found in the liver (Fig. 11-26), and four out of every five of these are in the right lobe.

It has been estimated that approximately 25% of people infected with *Echinococcus* go through life without any symptoms referable to the tapeworm. Symptoms may take a long time to develop, for the disease progresses slowly. The cysts may become secondarily infected, suppurate, and produce the clinical picture of hepatic abscess. Some of the cysts may collapse and undergo fibrosis and, not infrequently, calcification. The hydatid fluid, when liberated into the circulation, gives rise to pronounced eosinophilia. There may be allergic manifestations such as urticaria and angioneurotic edema. Diffuse implantation in the peritoneal or pleural cavities may develop after rupture of subpleural and subperitoneal cysts.[402]

In *E. multilocularis,* the daughter cysts, which arise from the germinal membrane by budding, develop on the outside of the original (mother) cyst. This results in invasion of surrounding parenchyma by the new scolices, which are not contained by the laminated cuticular membrane. The pattern of growth resembles that of malignant neoplastic lesions. The disease is fatal in most untreated patients and in a significant percentage of those treated with surgery.[398-419]

The diagnosis of hepatic hydatid disease is suggested by the presence of an abdominal mass detected by palpation and confirmed by sonography,[397,408] liver scans, or computerized tomography scans.[390,410,403] The diagnosis must then be comfirmed serologically. Of the multiple methods available,[414] which include complement fixation, enzyme-linked immunosorbent as-

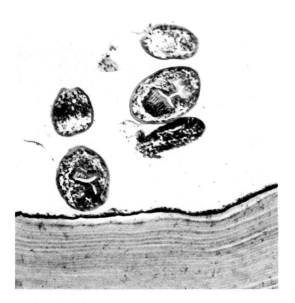

Fig. 11-25. Wall of echinococcal cyst disclosing numerous scolices, with hooklets evident in some. (Hematoxylin and eosin; 100×.)

say,[399,401,412] and indirect hemagglutination, the last is the test of choice.[400]

Diseases caused by nematodes
Diseases caused by nematodes of the digestive tract

Ascariasis. *Ascaris lumbricoides* is a nematode of worldwide distribution, most prevalent in tropical and subtropical countries. The incidence and severity of the infection are closely related to hygienic levels. The incidence in some areas of Europe and the Orient is reported to be as high as 90% to 94%. Endemic regions exist in the United States, especially in the Southeast, where 30% to 40% of the rural population has been found to be infected.

The adult worms range from 15 to 30 cm in length and from 3 to 5 mm in diameter. The eggs are deposited in the soil, where they undergo a period of incubation. The infection is acquired by ingestion of the fully embryonated ova. The larvae are hatched in the small intestine and penetrate the wall, reaching the lungs by way of venules or lymphatics. They pass into the alveoli from the alveolar capillaries and migrate up the main bronchial tree and down the esophagus with the swallowed saliva. In the small intestine they grow into adult males or females. In severe infections, during the period of lung migration, the larvae produce areas of hemorrhage and inflammatory reaction characterized by the presence of neutrophils and eosinophils. A clinical picture resembling bronchial asthma and diffuse peribronchitis, with occasional hemoptysis, is sometimes encountered.[433,525]

Ascariasis is usually a benign and self-limited disease because of the short life span of the adult worm (6 to 12 months). The most frequent complications of ascariasis are caused by the adult parasite. Large masses of worms may produce intestinal obstruction[421,433] (Fig. 11-27) and rarely may lead to perforation[497] and peritonitis.[512] Although ascariasis has been shown to have an adverse effect on nutritional status,[432,434] there is little evidence that it can cause intestinal malabsorption.[436]

Ascaris worms have a tendency to wander into natural passages and may migrate into the biliary system, pancreatic duct, or lumen of the appendix.[478] They may obstruct the extrahepatic biliary tree and produce jaundice, ascending cholangitis, or acute cholecystitis.[476] Single or multiple abscesses of the liver are sometimes produced. Occasionally the adult worms migrate into the upper respiratory passages.

Diagnosis is based on fecal examination. Serologic tests have been developed but are rarely used for diagnostic purposes. Endoscopic and radiologic techniques have been helpful in establishing the accurate diagnosis of biliary ascariasis.[475,578,539]

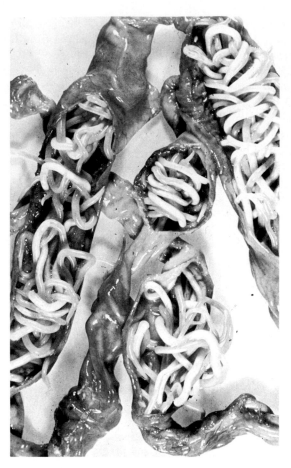

Fig. 11-27. Intestinal obstruction caused by masses of *Ascaris* adult worms in young child. (Courtesy Dr. Rafael Ramírez-Weiser, San Juan, Puerto Rico.)

In addition to *A. lumbricoides*, the closely related pig roundworm, *Ascaris suis*, can sometimes infect humans. In humans, *A. suis* develops to the larval tissue–migratory stages and rarely reaches the adult intestinal stage.[506] The true incidence of *A. suis* infection in humans is unknown. In a recent report from a nonendemic rural area, four of five children with ascariasis were infected with *A. suis*.[484] Thus in such communities the *A. suis* may be of epidemiologic importance.

Anisakiasis. Anisakiasis is a gastrointestinal parasitic infection caused by larvae of the nematode family Anisakidae. The adult form of this nematode inhabits the intestine of sea mammals and the larval stages are found in a variety of fish, such as haddock, mackerel, cod, herring, Alaskan pollack, squid, and salmon.[420,514] Humans are accidentally infected when they eat raw, lightly salted or pickled fish harboring the infective larvae. The infection is not uncommon in the Netherlands, where slightly salted herring ("green herring") is consumed, and in Japan, where *sushi* (vinegared fish and rice), *sashimi* (raw-fish slices), and *sunomono* (pickled fish) are favorite dishes.

The disease manifestations will depend on the type and site of involvement. In the luminal form, the most commonly seen in the United States, the noninvasive larvae are either removed manually by the patient or expelled by coughing or vomiting.[477,483] Although invasive gastric anisakiasis presents as an acute abdominal pain shortly after ingestion of the larvae containing fish, in the invasive intestinal form the symptoms appear more than 1 week after infection.[445] In the latter form patients are not infrequently operated upon with a diagnosis of acute appendicitis, diverticulitis, or regional enteritis.[508,575]

Trichuriasis (trichocephaliasis). One of the most common intestinal parasites of humans in tropical areas is *Trichuris trichiura*, formerly *Trichocephalus trichiurus*, also known as the whipworm.

Trichuriasis is contracted through the ingestion of food or water containing the ova. The larvae are released from the embryonated ova into the small intestine and become attached to the mucosa. Subsequently, they migrate downward to their usual habitat in the ileocecal region (Fig. 11-28). The anterior tip of the whipworm rarely penetrates below the muscularis mucosae, thus eliciting practically no reaction on the part of the tissues. In case of massive infection with *T. trichiura*, prominent hyperemia and edema of the mucosa with occasional ulcerations may be produced, but in the majority of cases the infection does not produce symptoms. Although in severe cases blood-streaked stools

are observed, there is controversy as to whether this amount of intestinal blood loss is enough to cause anemia.[460,464,481,486] In the most severe cases rectal prolapse may occur. Colonic obstruction, because of a tangle of worms, and perforation have been reported.[450] Rapid, severe dehydration and concomitant electrolyte imbalance may cause death. Peripheral eosinophilia is practically never seen in pure *Trichuris* infection. Diagnosis is made when the characteristic ova are found on stool examination.

Ancylostomiasis (uncinariasis, hookworm disease). Hookworm disease is one of the most prevalent diseases in the world. It is not limited to tropical and subtropical areas but may be encountered in temperate climates. The disease is caused by *Ancylostoma duodenale*, the Old World hookworm, or by *Necator americanus*, the New World hookworm.

From the ova deposited in the ground, rhabditiform larvae are hatched. These develop into the infective filariform larvae in about 5 to 8 days. The latter penetrate the skin, much like the filariform larvae of *Strongyloides*. The passage of the filariform larvae through the skin produces a sometimes severe irritation or dermatitis known as ground itch.[491] This generally occurs in the feet, between and beneath the toes, since most peole who acquire the infection live in impoverished and unsanitary areas and usually walk barefoot. The filariform larvae gain access to the lymphatics or the venules and finally reach the pulmonary circulation. From

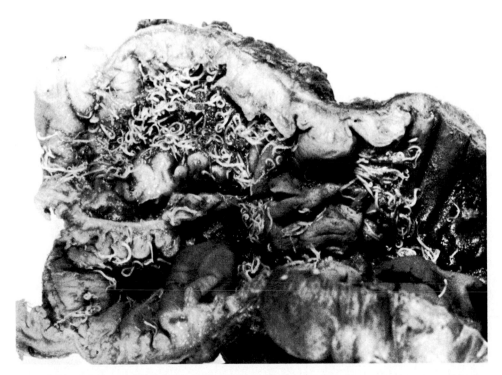

Fig. 11-28. Massive infestation with *Trichuris,* which produced severe hemorrhagic diarrhea and death in very young child.

the interalveolar capillaries, they pass into the alveolar sacs, up the tracheobronchial tree, and eventually into the gastrointestinal tract. In the passage through the lungs, petechial hemorrhages and areas of transient bronchopneumonia are produced. On reaching the small intestine, especially the duodenum and first portion of the jejunum, the adult parasites attach themselves to the mucosa by means of a well-developed buccal capsule (Fig. 11-29). In so doing, they damage small areas of the mucosa, producing punctate hemorrhages, and at the same time they draw blood from the mucosa. In heavy infections there is considerable blood loss as a result of both direct continuity between the oropharynx of the parasite and mucosal blood vessels and free bleeding from multiple points of attachment of the parasites, since they migrate from one area to another. The resulting classic picture of hookworm disease is characterized by severe, hypochromic microcytic anemia with deficiency of iron. The anemia usually is complicated by other nutritional deficiencies that are prevalent in economically poor, underdeveloped areas.[530]

Small intestinal mucosal changes of villous atrophy and crypt hyperplasia have been described in cases of hookworm disease. However, these morphologic features and the malabsorptive state that is commonly present are probably unrelated to the infection.[436] When the severe sideropenic anemia occurs in young children, it retards growth as well as sexual and mental development. The presence of characteristic ova in the stools establishes the diagnosis. Serologic tests are available but play little role in clinical diagnosis.[504]

Enterobiasis (oxyuriasis). Enterobiasis is a very common parasitic disease of cosmopolitan distribution. The causative nematode is *E. vermicularis*, formerly known as *Oxyuris vermicularis*, or commonly as the pinworm or threadworm. The disease is acquired by ingestion of the fully embryonated ova deposited by the female worm about the anus and transferred to other hosts by fecal contamination or to the same host to produce reinfection. The ova are very resistant to destruction, and the infection occasionally affects all persons in the same household. The life span of the worm is short (1½ to 2 months), and the chief problem is reinfection. The larvae are hatched from the fully embryonated ova in the region of the duodenum and then pass downward while they molt twice and mature, until they reach the ileocecal area. The adult worms attach themselves to the superficial portion of the mucosa of the terminal ileum, cecum, and appendix by their anterior end.

The pathologic changes produced by the adult worms in this area are minimal, and their role in the pathogenesis of appendicular symptoms in some cases is by no means settled. It is our impression that, even when adult worms are present in acute appendicitis, they are not a significant cause of inflammation but merely represent a fortuitous association (Fig. 11-30).

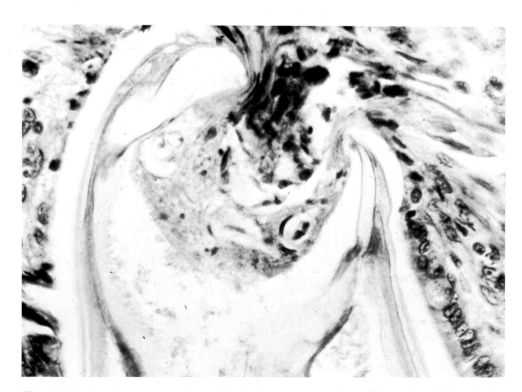

Fig. 11-29. *Ancylostoma caninum* attached to mucosa of small intestine of dog by its well-developed buccal capsule. (Hematoxylin and eosin; 430×.)

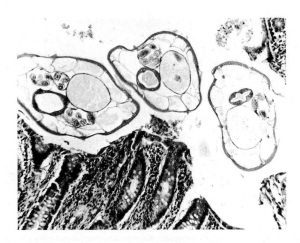

Fig. 11-30. *Enterobius vermicularis* in appendix. (Hematoxylin and eosin; 100×.)

The most important symptoms of this disease is intense pruritus ani caused by the migration of the adult female worm to the perianal region, where she lays her eggs. The adult male worm is unimportant in the pathogenesis, since it dies after copulation.

Rarely, *E. vermicularis* can be seen in extraintestinal sites.[438] In females the nematode migrates up the uterus and fallopian tubes to produce a foreign-body type of granulomatous inflammation most commonly seen in the surface of the ovaries, omentum, and peritoneum.[429,493,492] This parasite apparently cannot survive outside its natural habitat, and the granulomatous reaction described occurs after death of the worms.[529]

Other less common ectopic sites include the urinary bladder, lung, and liver.[427,444,482] An association has been reported between enterobiasis and lower urinary tract infections, with the nematode acting as a carrier of enteric bacteria when it migrates from the perianal region to the urinary bladder.[520] Diagnosis is made by identification of the ova by a cellophane-tape test.

Trichiniasis (trichinosis, trichinelliasis). A cosmopolitan disease, trichiniasis is most common in the temperate areas of the United States and Europe and is caused by *Trichinella spiralis*. The infection, though not as common as it was in the past, is still encountered in approximately 5% of the autopsies performed in the United States.[544] An average of 150 new cases are reported annually[526] to the Centers for Disease Control.

Humans usually become infected by eating raw or undercooked pork. Other sources of infection are walrus and bear meat.[442,532]

The larvae of the parasite become encysted in the muscles of the infected animal and are ingested by humans. During ingestion these larvae are liberated by proteolytic enzymes and pass on to the small intestine. The larvae attach themselves to the mucosa and attain sexual maturity within 2 days. Electron microscopic studies have identified the intracellular nature of both the enteric larvae and the adult worm.[541] The parasite inhabits the cytoplasm of either absorptive or goblet cells.

During its development the parasite expresses different surface antigenic constituents to which the host humoral and cellular immune system responds.[488,498] The multiple responses directed against the infectious larvae, the developing larvae, and the adult worm act synergistically to protect the host.[430]

The adult male worm dies soon after copulation, and the female adult dies after larviposition is completed.

Between 1000 and 1500 larvae may be produced by the female. Most of these larvae enter the lymphatics or the venules of the lamina propria. After traversing the pulmonary circulation, they enter the systemic circulation and are carried to all organs and tissues of the body.

The symptoms during the period of invasion of the intestinal wall are the result of gastrointestinal irritation by the adult worm, which produces nausea, vomiting, diarrhea or constipation, and abdominal cramps. During the stage of hematogenous dissemination or migration, the symptoms are rather variable and are more frequently characterized by muscle aches, fever, chemosis of the conjunctivae, and occasionally prostration. Severe peripheral eosinophilia is frequently seen. The eosinophilic cell count may reach a value of 70% or more of the total white blood cell count.

The larvae become encysted only in striated voluntary muscles, though they also reach the heart, lungs, brain, and meninges. Once they penetrate individual muscle fibers, they grow in size and then coil in corkscrew fashion and proceed to encyst.

The muscles most frequently affected are the diaphragmatic, gastrocnemius, intercostal, deltoid, gluteal, and pectoral. The parasitized muscle fiber becomes strongly basophilic. This process, once mislabeled "basophilic degeneration," is the result of increased muscle fiber endoplasmic reticulum and ribosomal RNA content.[446] The parasitized muscle fiber, called a "nurse cell," lives for extended periods. An inflammatory reaction in which lymphocytes and eosinophils predominate develops around the nurse cell–parasite unit. As in other helminthic infections, eosinophil leukocytes play a major role in the host immune response.[466] Elevated IgE levels are partially responsible for this level of eosinophilia.[448] Eosinophils adhere to the migrating parasite by an antibody-mediated process. Being unable to phagocytose the parasite, the eosinophil degranulates, releasing hydrolytic enzymes, cationic proteins such as major basic protein, and hydrogen peroxide, which destroy the larvae.[426,437,472,473,533]

The infected muscle fiber is destroyed by the inflam-

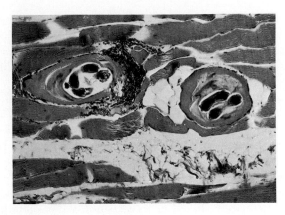

Fig. 11-31. Two *Trichinella* larvae encysted in voluntary muscle of rat infected experimentally. (180×.)

matory process, and adjacent muscle fibers undergo hyaline degeneration. A fibrous wall or capsule develops around the larvae, producing small cysts averaging 1 mm or less in diameter (Fig. 11-31). The wall of these cysts subsequently may calcify after 6 months to 2 years. The trichinas themselves also may undergo calcification.

Growth of larvae and encystation do not occur in cardiac muscles. In the cardiac muscle, acute inflammatory changes may be seen in the early stage of the infection, leading to a patchy or diffuse interstitial myocarditis. The larvae in the myocardium undergo necrosis and usually cannot be identified. Foci of necrosis in the muscle fibers of the myocardium and the nonspecific myocarditis are most noticeable in the area close to the epicardium.

The central nervous system usually reacts to invasion by the larvae with a diffuse leptomeningeal round cell type of infiltration.[499] Minute foci of gliosis around capillaries occasionally are seen. Renal involvement by an immune-mediated glomerulonephritis has been recently described.[521] Immune complex deposition in vessels has been suggested as a cause of vasculitis.[451]

The mortality in this disease is extremely low. Death may ensue in very severe, overwhelming infections as a result of involvement of the respiratory muscles, with secondary pulmonary complications. Involvement of the myocardium is the most common cause of death; massive involvement may lead to cardiac failure.[469,528] A recent case report recognized trichiniasis as a possible fatal infection in the immunosuppressed host.[468]

The best method for diagnosis is muscle biopsy obtained from the tendinous insertions of the deltoid or gastrocnemius muscles. Serologic tests are available and usually show positive results after the third week of disease. Methods include the bentonite flocculation test, immunofluorescence, enzyme-linked immunosorbent assay, counterimmunoelectrophoresis, and gel diffusion.[447]

Capillariasis

Capillariasis hepatica. This disease is caused by the nematode *Capillaria (Hepaticola) hepatica.* This helminth is common in the liver of rats and, less frequently, in mice, hares, dogs, muskrats, beavers, and some species of monkeys. Human infections are rare; only about 30 authenticated cases have been reported in the world's literature.[424]

The eggs are discharged in fecal matter or are released from the decaying carcasses of affected animals. The ova are nonembryonated and must attain maturity and infectivity when they reach the soil. They require certain conditions of humidity. Humans acquire the disease by ingesting food or dirt contaminated with embryonated ova. The ova hatch in the cecum; the free larvae penetrate venules of the portal system and ultimately reach the liver, where they mature. About 4 weeks after infection the adult worms disintegrate and release large numbers of ova in the liver substance.

Spurious infections are occasionally present in humans and are acquired by eating the undercooked or raw liver of a habitual host. In these instances the eggs are nonembryonated and are passed in the stools without undue harm to the individual.

The majority of cases occur in children or institutionalized mental patients. As would be expected from the life cycle of this organism, instances of the human disorder appear in persons who have dirt-eating habits or live in substandard sanitary conditions.

The clinical picture of an enlarged liver and a high-grade eosinophilia in a young patient must be differentiated from that of toxocariasis or visceral larva migrans.[454] The diagnosis of this disease can be established only by liver biposy, since ova are present only in the liver substance and are not detectable in intestinal content.[423]

The liver is enlarged with a smooth surface, and beneath the capsule are numerous grayish or yellowish white nodules measuring 0.1 to 0.2 cm. Many of these coalesce and form lesions 2 to 3 cm in diameter. The granulomas are composed of epithelioid cells and multinucleated giant cells surrounding parasites or ova. Occasionally necrosis is apparent with or without cuticular fragments of the disintegrated worms or ova. Peripheral portions of the granulomas exhibit a heavy infiltration of plasma cells, eosinophils, and macrophages. The adjacent liver plates undergo degeneration and contain a similar inflammatory cell infiltration. Ultimately there may be extensive scarring in which ova may be preserved. Many eggs are engulfed by multinucleated giant cells. An experimental model has been developed in mice for a *C. hepatica* egg granuloma. The model indicates that granuloma formation may have an immunologic basis in which both cell- and humoral-mediated immune responses participate.[510,511,523,524]

The ova of *C. hepatica* are barrel shaped, as are those of *Trichuris trichiura*, but possess a double shell containing visible radiations between the two layers.

Most cases reported in the literature have been fatal, since infections tend to be severe. In all probability, however, there are many unreported infections of lesser severity that remain clinically inapparent with mild and nonspecific manifestations.

Capillariasis philippinesis. Capillaria philippinesis has been held responsible for a severe form of protein-losing enteropathy associated with a malabsorption syndrome.[439,505,534] The disease may lead to death in 20% of cases, especially when severe bacterial infections supervene because of the hypogammaglobulinemic state.[500] The disease may acquire epidemic proportions.[449,534,537]

It has been shown that the worm reproduces by internal autoinfection,[453] as the presence of larviparous female parasites in the lumen of the intestine has suggested.[449] The life cycle of *C. philippinensis* is still unknown. It is suggested by clinical evidence and animal experimentation that the disease is acquired by eating small uncooked fish.[441,537]

The parasites may penetrate the surface intestinal mucosa and that of the crypts but are not seen beyond the muscularis mucosae.[423] The parasite induces only a very mild inflammatory response, composed mostly of plasma cells and lymphocytes with some eosinophils. The exact mechanism by which the parasite produces the severe protein-losing enteropathy remains to be elucidated.[536] Roentgenographic examination reveals a classical malabsorption pattern in the small intestine.[500]

Diagnosis is based on the identification of the parasite in stool examination or mucosal biopsy of the small intestine.

Larva migrans

Cutaneous larva migrans. The localized or cutaneous form of larva migrans, also known as creeping eruption, results from infection with the canine or feline strains of *Ancylostoma braziliense* and less commonly with *A. caninum*. The disease is usually contracted at beaches or sandy playgrounds where cats or dogs have deposited their feces. The infective larvae penetrate the skin and migrate at a rate of about 2.5 cm daily, producing serpiginous tunnels between the stratum germinativum and the stratum spinosum. The elevated tunnels frequently become vesicular, and the involved tissue is infiltrated by chronic inflammatory cells and numerous eosinophils. Because of severe pruritis and scratching, secondary infection frequently occurs.

Visceral larva migrans. Visceral larva migrans is a syndrome seen primarily in children under 4 years of age. It is characterized by pronounced and prolonged eosinophilia (in virtually 100% of cases), hepatomegaly (87%), pulmonary symptoms (50%), fever, and other systemic manifestations. This condition was frequently referred to in the literature as tropical infiltrative eosinophilia, Löffler's syndrome, and even benign eosinophilic leukemia until the specific larva of *Toxocara canis* were identified by Beaver and associates.[428]

In addition to high serum immunoglobulin levels, anti-A and anti-B titers are detected because the *Toxocara* larvae contain surface antigens that stimulate isohemagglutinins.[461,517]

This clinical syndrome can be produced by (1) human helminthic infections having an extraintestinal cycle but with localization in the intestine, (2) such infections but with localization outside the intestine, and (3) animal helminth infections that occasionally affect humans. Examples of the first group are ascariasis, strongyloidiasis, and hookworm disease. Examples of the second are schistosomiasis and fascioliasis. The third group, diseases caused by larvae of nematodes normally parasitic in lower animals, is the most interesting one and the one to which the term *visceral larva migrans* is specifically applied. Secondary stage *T. canis* and *T. catis* larvae have been recognized as etiologic agents of visceral larva migrans.[428] The third-stage larva of *Ancylostoma caninum* is probably also an etiologic agent. *Capillaria hepatica* may also cause visceral larva migrans.

Only a few postmortem examinations of patients with visceral larva migrans have been performed.[422] The liver usually is enlarged with small gray-white nodules, 2 to 4 mm in diameter, scattered throughout the parenchyma (Fig. 11-32). Microscopically the nodules are composed of numerous eosinophils, Langhans' giant cells, and larvae. In patients with severe hyperergy, eosinophilic abscesses and adjacent hepatic necrosis are prominent. Other viscera may be affected. Massive fatal myocarditis has resulted from the presence of larvae within the myocardium.[422] Larvae also may localize in the eye, usually in the posterior chamber. They give rise to a granuloma that can cause detachment of the retina. The granuloma may simulate retinoblastoma clinically.[538] The granulomatous response, as in schistosomiasis, seems to be a cell-mediated process.[471]

The diagnosis of visceral larva migrans is difficullt. We have been able to confirm the diagnosis by liver biopsy in several cases. In one case the larvae were seen in biopsy samples from a cervical lymph node. Of the serologic tests available, enzyme-linked immunosorbent assay is suffcently sensitive and specific to be clinically useful in the diagnosis of toxocariasis.[443,462,463,531]

Strongyloidiasis (strongyloidosis). *Strongyloides stercoralis* is a parasite with a complicated life cycle. Strongyloidiasis occurs not only in tropical and subtropical areas but also in more northerly latitudes. It is not as common as ascariasis, trichuriasis, and ancylostomiasis.

The free-living, nonparasitic, rhabditiform larvae de-

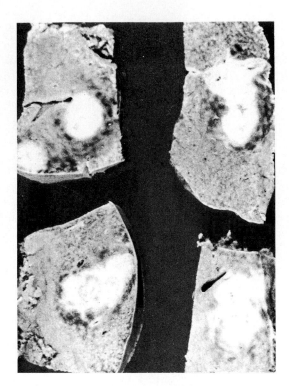

Fig. 11-32. Multiple, confluent, grayish white granulomas in liver of patient with visceral larva migrans. (Courtesy Dr. Manuel de Jesús; from Marcial-Rojas, R.A.: Parasitic diseases of the liver. In Schiff, L., editor: Diseases of the liver, Philadelphia, 1969, J.B. Lippincott Co.)

velop from ova in the intestine of humans and are passed in the stools to the soil, where they mature into adult males and females. After copulation of the adult worms, more ova are laid, and rhabditiform larvae hatch from them. This is known as the direct cycle. Under favorable conditions in the soil, the indirect cycle begins by the transformation of the rhabditiform larvae into infective filariform larvae. The infective filariform larvae penetrate the skin or oral mucosa of humans, gain access to venules, and finally reach the alveolar capillaries. In the lungs they mature into adult worms and pass into the alveoli, finally making their way through the tracheobronchial tree into the gastrointestinal tract.

The major anatomic changes are produced in the mucosa of the duodenum and jejunum by the female worms. The mucosa of the intestine becomes hyperemic and edematous. In severe infections, ulcerations are produced. The female worm deposits her eggs in the mucosa, where more rhabditiform larvae develop. Gastrointestinal symptoms include epigastric pain or tenderness, anorexia, nausea and vomiting, diarrhea, and malabsorption.[494,519]

Occasionally the noninfective rhabditiform larvae metamorphose into infective filariform larvae within the intestinal lumen and penetrate either the mucosa of the colon (endogenous autoinfection) or the perianal skin (exogenous autoinfection). The cycle of autoinfection can lead to clinical illness manifested many years after the patient has left an endemic area.[490,494,501,507]

The lungs are affected by the migratory phase of the maturing larvae through the alveoli. Areas of edema, congestion, and consolidation, not unlike those in the migratory phase of ascariasis, may develop.[458,489] Signs of bronchospasm or pneumonia and episodes of hemoptysis are sometimes seen.

The inflammatory reaction at the site of entrance of the larvae into the skin is similar to that in the intestinal mucosa. It is characterized by a mixed leukocytic infiltration containing numerous eosinophils. The larvae may be seen migrating in the dermis as a type of cutaneous larva migrans.

In immunosuppressed patients the process of endogenous autoinfection can lead to disseminated disease known as hyperinfection.[435,513,540] In hyperinfection there are several inflammatory changes in the intestinal mucosa (mostly of the distal parts of the sigmoid and rectum), and numerous larvae are seen within the mucosa and submucosa (Figs. 11-33 and 11-34). A massive inflammatory reaction develops, characterized by a predominantly eosinophilic infiltrate. These filariform larvae migrate through the systemic circulation and may produce an inflammatory reaction in other organs similar to that occurring in visceral larva migrans. The predominant feature is pulmonary involvement, which leads to respiratory failure and a 90% mortality.[431]

It is apparent that the alterations in the immune mechanism of the host brought about by diseases, such as lymphoma, AIDS, leprosy, uremia, and severe malnutrition, or by drugs, such as steroids or cytotoxic agents, disturb the immunologic balance between the host and the parasite.[456] This alteration in the immune mechanism of the host, especially of the cell-mediated responses, allows for increased pathogenicity and virulence of the parasite.

Diagnosis of the disease rests on the identification of the rhabditiform or the infective filariform larvae in the stools, duodenal aspirates, or small-bowel biopsy specimens. Occasionally the diagnosis is made by demonstration of the larvae in the sputum.[474] Serologic methods of diagnosis include indirect hemagglutination, complement fixation, immunofluorescence, and enzyme-linked immunosorbent assay[457,465,502] The last two appear to be the most sensitive and specific diagnostic methods.[455,459]

Angiostrongyliasis. Eosinophilic meningoencephalitis is acquired by eating land snails and slugs, which are the intermediate hosts of *Angiostrongylus cantonensis*, a lungworm of rats.[509] The first-stage larvae develop from eggs deposited in the lungs of rats by the adult worm living in the pulmonary arteries.[543] The larvae

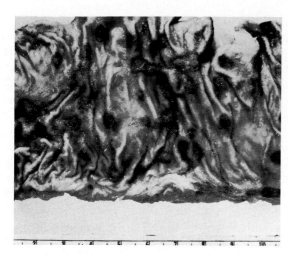

Fig. 11-33. Lesions of intestinal mucosa associated with *Strongyloides* infection. (From Anderson, W.A.D., and Scotti, T.M.: Synopsis of pathology, ed. 10, St. Louis, 1980, The C.V. Mosby Co.)

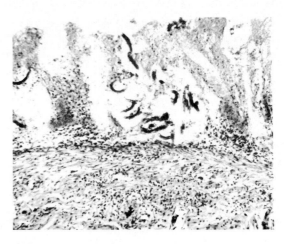

Fig. 11-34. Numerous strongyloidal larvae in mucosa and submucosa of intestine. Hemorrhage and inflammatory cells are evident. (Hematoxylin and eosin; 100×.)

migrate up the trachea and are eventually passed in the feces. The intermediate molluskan hosts acquire the infection by ingesting the feces of infected rats. The third-stage infective larvae develop in mollusks in about 3 weeks.

When humans become infected, the third-stage larvae and the young adult worms usually die, most frequently in the brain (Fig. 11-35), spinal cord, and meninges.[480,503] Larvae sometimes migrate to the eye.[470]

The tissue reaction is characterized by severe eosinophilic infiltration, which is also frequently manifested in the peripheral blood and cerebrospinal fluid. The symptoms are those of a meningoencephalitis[440] indistinguishable from that caused by cysticercosis, trichiniasis, paragonimiasis, and schistosomiasis. Gastrointestinal symptoms are also seen.[542] Serodiagnostic methods include a complement fixation test and an indirect fluorescent antibody test[535]; the latter is the more sensitive.

A. costaricensis has been described in Costa Rica[495] other Central and South American countries,[487] and the United States.[527] It lives as a parasite in the mesenteric arteries of wild rats. The life cycle is similar to that of *A. cantonensis*, though *A. costaricensis* larvae develop in the wall of the intestine. The species affects humans at the level of the wall of the intestine. It is seen usually in young children, who have acute abdominal symptoms, fever, and eosinophilia.[485] Laparotomy reveals an inflammatory granulomatous mass in the appendix, cecum, or terminal ileum.[425] The disease does not affect the central nervous system. Fecal examination is useless because neither eggs nor larvae appear in stools.[452] A precipitin test is available for serodiagnosis of chronic infection and for epidemiologic studies.[516]

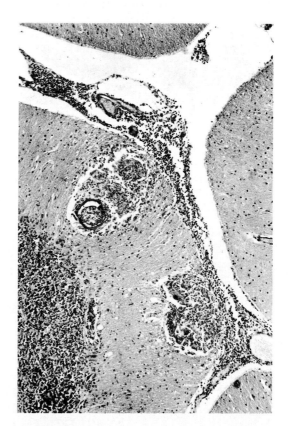

Fig. 11-35. Eosinophilic meningoencephalitis. Remnants of *Angiostrongylus cantonensis* may be seen in cerebellar fissure and cortex. Diffuse infiltration with eosinophils is evident in meninges. (Hematoxylin and eosin; 63×; from Rosen, L., et al.: JAMA **179:**620, copyright 1962, American Medical Association.)

Diseases caused by filarial nematodes (filariasis)

Bancroftian filariasis. Bancroftian filariasis is commonly referred to as filariasis. It is caused by *Wuchereria (Filaria) bancrofti.* The mature female worm measures up to 10 cm in length and 3 mm in width, whereas the male is only about one third this size.

The microfilariae are taken up with the blood of humans by mosquitoes of the genus *Culex* and occasionally of the genera *Aedes* and *Anopheles.* The microfilariae penetrate the stomach wall of the mosquito and reach the thoracic muscles. They undergo multiple changes in the mosquito until they mature and are transmissible to humans. The larve move down to the proboscis of the mosquito, migrate out of the labium, and are implanted on the human skin. They enter the dermal lymphatics and pass to the regional lymph nodes. Maturity occurs either within the lymph nodes or, more frequently, within the larger lymphatic trunks near the regional lymph nodes (Fig. 11-36). The adult worms copulate, and each female worm produces numerous microfilariae. The microfilariae are liberated into the lymphatics and eventually enter the bloodstream, producing a microfilaremia. In the bloodstream they are again available to complete their cycle if they are taken up by the mosquito.

There is a definite microfilarial periodicity, occurring toward midnight, in most endemic foci. This may be an adaptation to the feeding habits of the vector, which is a night-biting mosquito. A diurnal strain occurs in the South Pacific.

The most frequently involved lymphatic vessels are those of the lower limbs, retroperitoneal tissues, spermatic cord, epididymis, and mammary gland.[546,566] The presence of worms in these areas, especially in the region of the spermatic cord, does not necessarily imply that the clinical symptoms fever, lymphadenitis, headache, and epididymitis will eventually develop.

In approximately 20% of necropsies on men in Puerto Rico, histopathologic evidence of filariasis is found in the spermatic cord even though there is no clinical history of the disease.[552] We have seen patients who have massive microfilaremia without the slightest symptoms of the disease.

The pathologic changes in the lymphatics and lymph nodes are attributable to the presence of the adult worm.[549] While the worm is alive, there is minimal reaction on the part of the lymphatics, and the most frequent changes are those of polypoid endolymphangitis and distension of lymphatics. Death of the adult filarial worm is followed by a severe inflammatory reaction that is characterized by fibrinoid necrosis and pronounced eosinophilic infiltration (Fig. 11-37). The inflammatory reaction develops in nodular fashion around fragmented and necrotic worms. Epithelioid cells and foreign body giant cells appear subsequently. These filarial granulomas eventually undergo fibrosis, leaving a concentrically lamellated, hyalinized structure that frequently calcifies (Fig. 11-38). Numerous lymphocytes and plasma cells also are seen in the lesion, mostly in the periphery.

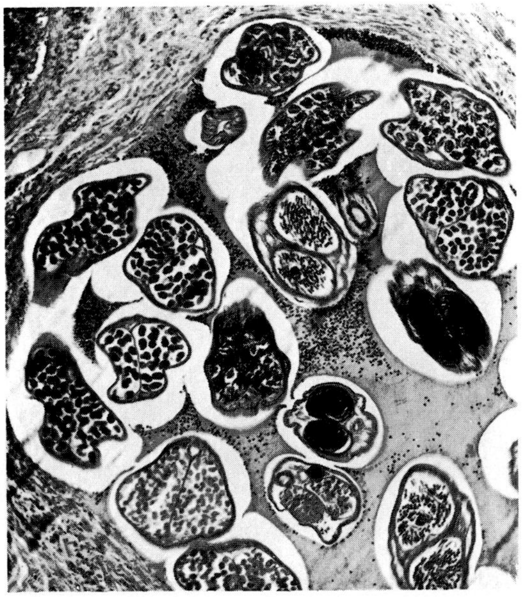

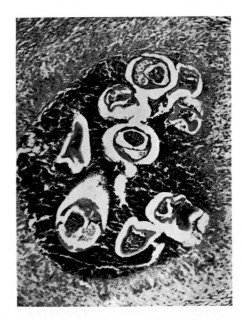

Fig. 11-36. Bancroftian filariasis. Living worms coiled in dilated afferent lymphatic vessel of greatly fibrosed inguinal node provoke only scant inflammatory reaction in wall of lymph vessel. (80×.)

Fig. 11-37. Filarial funiculitis. Eosinophilic pseudoabscess and granulomatous reaction about dead filarial worm, with obliteration of lymphatic vessel. (80×.)

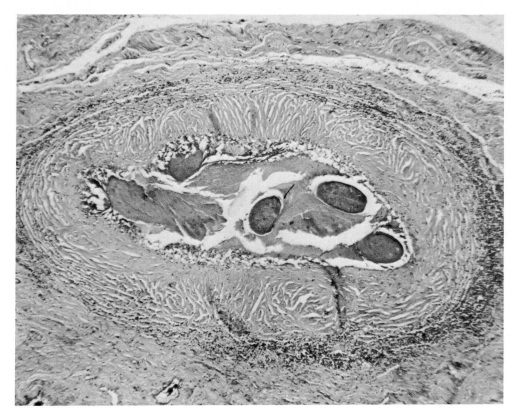

Fig. 11-38. Well-defined filarial granuloma in spermatic cord. Peripheral zone of dense fibrous tissue surrounds fragments of dead parasite. (Hematoxylin and eosin; 35×; courtesy Dr. Lorenzo Galindo, San Juan, Puerto Rico.)

It is evident from the pathologic processes described that lymphatics will be obstructed and that the severity of this obstruction will depend on the number of worms present. When numerous lymphatics are obliterated by fibrosis, lymphedema results. The classical chronic edema of subcutaneous tissues and the consequent proliferation of fibrous connective tissue and thickening of the epidermis are characteristic of elephantiasis. The full-blown picture of elephantiasis usually develops after repeated episodes of lymphadenitis and ascending lymphangitis. In all probability, secondary streptococcal or other type of bacterial infection plays an important role in the pathogenesis of ascending lymphangitis and elephantiasis. In tropical areas the frequency of hydrocele of the tunica vaginalis testis is at least partially related to the incidence of filariasis.

The microfilariae only rarely produce visible damage. Occasionally small granulomas, measuring 1 to 2 cm in diameter, are discovered in lymph nodes or spleen, and they may contain microfilariae. The granulomas are composed of prolifrating reticuloendothelial cells, fibroblasts, and eosinophils.

Malayan filariasis is caused by *Brugia malayi*, a species closely related to *W. bancrofti*. The clinical and pathologic findings are similar to those described for bancroftian filariasis.

An immunosuppressive state, with altered cell- and humoral-mediated immune response, has been reported in patients infected with filariasis.[558,573] Since lymphatic obstruction is believed to be the result of allergic tissue reactions to the nematode, such immune unresponsiveness would be beneficial to the host and would explain the lack of correlation between infestation and clinical symptoms.

Tropical (filarial) eosinophilia is a syndrome characterized by cough, wheezing, hypereosinophilia, and pulmonary infiltrates.[568] It is believed to be a form of occult filariasis that results from hypersensitivity to circulating microfilaria.[571,572]

The diagnosis of filariasis is made by identification of the microfilaria on Giemsa-stained blood smears. Serodiagnostic methods available are enzyme-linked immunosorbent and indirect hemaglutination tests.[557,562,564]

Onchocerciasis (onchocercosis). The filarial worm that causes onchocerciasis is known as *Onchocerca volvulus*. The disease is seen in west and central Africa and in circumscribed areas of Mexico, Guatemala, Venezuela, and Colombia and in parts of Yemen.[548]

Onchocerciasis is transmitted by small flies of the genus *Simulium* (gnat or black fly). These tiny flies ingest the microfilariae when they bite an infected person. After undergoing several transformations in the body of the fly, the microfilariae finally reach the thoracic muscles and develop into infective larvae. The larvae migrate into the proboscis and are introduced into the skin of a person who is bitten by the fly. The organisms travel freely along the dermis but appear only rarely in the blood or internal organs. They have been identified in the lungs, liver, spleen, and kidneys.[547,567]

The larvae mature in the dermis and produce solitary or multiple cutaneous nodules called onchocercomas, which are characteristic of this disease. In the African variant of the disease the nodules are limited to the skin over the pelvic bones and lower limbs, whereas in the Central American variant the nodules are usually located in the scalp (Fig. 11-39, *A*) and the skin of the face and neck. There is, however, considerable overlapping between these two variants of the disease. The nodules (Fig. 11-39, *B*) represent an inflammatory reaction to the adult worms. Adult worms in small clefts are present in the onchocercomas, usually in a proportion of two or more males to each female. The worms may be alive or dead. The inflammatory reaction is greater around dead worms. Histiocytic proliferation and foreign-body giant cell reaction are seen around many of the dead parasites. There is an accompanying pronounced leukocytic infiltration, mostly polymorphonuclear in type, but also chronic, with occasional eosinophils. Dense fibrosis ensues, so that the nodule is replaced by dense collagenous fibroconnective tissue. The nodules may even erode adjacent bone. Variable numbers of microfilariae are present in the nearby areas. Migration of the microfilariae from the onchocercotic nodules to the adjacent dermis produces irritation of the skin. Small hemorrhages and an inflammatory reaction are seen microscopically. Eosinophils, through the release of eosinophil-granule major basic protein, are believed to play a role in the host defense against microfilariae.[556,565] Edema and thickening of the skin and subcutaneous tissue develop after several months. Itching is occasionally present and in some cases may be severe. When the onchodermatosis is conspicuous in the facial region, leonine facies may develop (Fig. 11-40).

The most serious complication of the migratory phase of the microfilariae in onchocerciasis is the ocular involvement so frequently encountered in Central America. In 5% to 20% of cases in Guatemala and Mexico the microfilariae invade the eyeball.[551] A prominent horizontal punctate keratitis produced by the reaction of the corneal tissue to microfilariae is the most common finding. The keratitis does not appreciably reduce the visual acuity of these patients. When microfilariae reach the vitreous humor and penetrate the ciliary body, however, visual impairment develops. Photophobia, lacrimation, and finally blindness result. Secondary

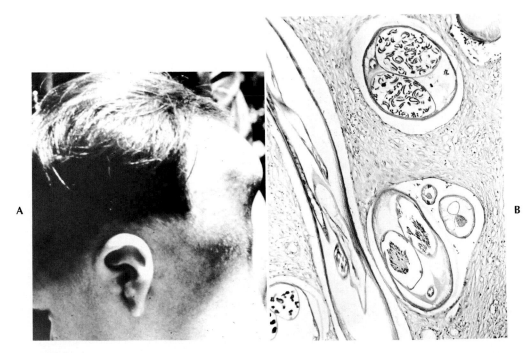

Fig. 11-39. Onchocercoma. **A,** Classic appearance in scalp of Guatemalan child. **B,** Microscopic section disclosing numerous *Onchocerca volvulus*. Interstitial tissue is fibrotic. (Hematoxylin and eosin; 100×; courtesy Dr. E. Pérez-Guisasola, Guatemala City, Guatemala.)

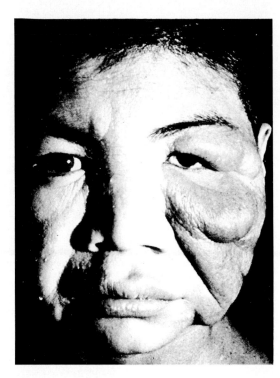

Fig. 11-40. Leonine facies in Guatemalan woman with onchocerciasis. (Courtesy Dr. E. Pérez-Guisasola, Guatemala City, Guatemala.)

changes of a degenerative type develop in the crystalline lens; anterior synechiae are formed after exudation of fibrin and leukocytes into the anterior chamber. The posterior chamber and optic nerve also are occasionally affected. The outcome of all these processes is total blindness, with glaucoma and phthisis bulbi. For this reason the disease entity is commonly referred to as "river blindness."

Lymphadenitis and rarely elephantiasis may develop in African patients. Obstructive lymphadenitis is believed to be the result of inflammation and fibrosis caused by immune complex deposition.[554]

Diagnosis is made by identification of the microfilariae in skin snips, in urine, or by slitlamp examination.[555] A skin test[561] and the serologic methods of complement fixation and enzyme immunoassay[545] are also available for diagnosis and epidemiologic studies.

Loaiasis (loiasis). Loaiasis is a form of filariasis limited to tropical West Africa. The causative organism, *Loa loa*, also known as the eye worm, travels through the subcutaneous tissue and occasionally in internal organs. The worms travel at the rate of about 1 cm per minute and produce serpiginous burrows that occasionally are evident externally. They sometimes migrate to the anterior chamber of the eye and appear beneath the ocular conjunctiva. The dead worms, as in other filarial diseases, cause a severe inflammatory response and eventually become calcified.

In contrast to bancroftian filariasis, the microfilariae in loaiasis appear in the peripheral bloodstream mostly during the daytime. The intermediate host and vector, the female *Chrysops* fly, bites during the day.

The so-called fugitive or Calabar swellings are subcutaneous nodules that develop suddenly in any part of the body in the course of this disease. They are painless, last for a few days, and disappear slowly. Occasionally they persist and become cystic. Calabar swellings are believed to represent an allergic manifestation to the parasite or its products.[569]

A pronounced peripheral eosinophilia is frequently present during the course of the disease, the usual range being 30% to 40%.[576] The extensive fibrosis and obstruction of lymphatics commonly seen in bancroftian filariasis do not occur in loaiasis. Nodular areas of fibrosis are found in the spleen, together with eosinophilic infiltration. These are probably the result of rapid destruction of microfilariae.[575]

Dirofilariasis. Dirofilariasis is a zoonosis caused mainly by *Dirofilaria immitis*, the dog heartworm, and *D. tenuis*, a parasite from raccoons.[559,577] The disease is transmitted to humans by mosquitoes, which inoculate the microfilariae into the skin.

D. immitis infection in man presents as a solitary lung nodule or radiographic "coin lesion".[550,563] Histologically the usually well-circumscribed lesion reveals a central zone of coagulation necrosis surrounded by granulomatous inflammation and fibrosis.[550] Identification of the parasite, with its characteristic cuticle, is diagnostic.

Dirofilaria tenuis infection leads to subcutaneous or conjunctival lesions.[559,560] Microscopically the parasite is seen within a necrotic granulomatous nodule.

Dracunculiasis (dracunculosis, dracontiasis, guinea worm infection, Medina worm infection). Dracunculiasis affects an estimated 10 to 48 million persons in the Near East, western India, and some parts of northwestern Africa. The parasite is *Dracunculus medinensis*, or the guinea worm. It is commonly referred to as a filaria, but it lacks a microfilarial stage and the adult worms are distinctly different from the true filariae.

The larvae are taken up by a freshwater crustacean of the genus *Cyclops*. They mature within the crustacean into elongated larvae infective for humans. These larvae are liberated by the gastric digestive juices when a person drinks water contaminated with infected *Cyclops*. The larvae migrate through the wall of the stomach or small intestine into the connective tissue of the abdominal wall. The male worm is small and probably dies after copulation. The female worm, which averages 1 m in length, wanders out to the subcutaneous tissue, especially that of the feet and legs. A small papule appears, which later becomes a vesicle with a small ulceration in the center through which the embryos are liberated. The latter usually are present in milky fluid contained in a segment of the worm's uterus that is extruded and breaks away from the body of the parasite.[574] On rare occasions the worms may be found in joints and serosal cavities.[553]

The signs and symptoms of dracunculiasis are limited to the period of liberation of embryos. Pruritus and moderate edema may be accompanied by low-grade fever and urticarial rash, caused by an anaphylatic reaction to the products of the worm. If the worm dies or if the embryos are liberated into the tissues, a severe inflammatory reaction with abscess formation ensues.

REFERENCES
Protozoal diseases
Amebiasis

1. Adams, E.B., and MacLeod, I.N.: Invasive amebiasis. 1. Amebic dysentery and its complications, Medicine 56:315-323, 1977.
2. Adams, E.B., and MacLeod, I.N.: Invasive ambiasis. II. Amebic liver abscess and its complications, Medicine 56:325-334, 1977.
3. Allason-Jones, E., Mindel, A., Sargeaunt, P., and Williams, P.: *Entamoeba histolytica* as a commensal intestinal parasite in homosexual men, N. Engl. J. Med. 315:353-356, 1986.
4. Chadee, K., and Meerovitch, E.: The pathogenesis of experimentally induced amebic liver abscess in the gerbil *(Meriones unguiculatus),* Am. J. Pathol. 117:71, 1984.
5. Chadee, K., and Meerovitch, E.: The pathology of experimentally induced cecal amebiasis in gerbils *(Meriones unguiculatus):* Liver changes and amebic liver abscess formation, Am. J. Pathol. 119:485-494, 1985.
6. Gadasi, H., and Kessler, E.: Correlation of virulence and collagenolytic activity on *Entamoeba histolytica,* Infect. Immunol. 39:528, 1983.
7. Giménez-Scherer, J.A., Pacheco-Cano, M.G., Cruz de Lavín, E., Hernández-Jáuregui, P., Merchant, M.T., and Kretschmer, R.R.: Ultrastructural changes associated with the inhibition of monocyte chemotaxis caused by products of axenically grown *Entamoeba histolytica,* Lab. Invest. 57:45-51, 1987.
8. González-Robles A., and Martínez-Palomo, A.: Scanning electron microscopy of attached trophozoites of pathogenic *Entamoeba histolytica,* J. Protozool. 30:692-700, 1983.
9. Istre, G.F., Kreiss, K., Hopkins, R.S., Healy, G.R., Benziger, M., Canfield, T.M., Dickinson, P., Engelbert, T.R., Compton, R.C., Mathews, H.M., and Simmons, R.A.: An outbreak of amebiasis spread by colonic irrigation at a chiropractic clinic, N. Engl. J. Med. 307:339-342, 1982.
10. Knight, R., and Wright, S.G.: Progress report: intestinal protozoa, Gut 19:940-953, 1978.
11. Knight, R.: Hepatic ambiasis, Semin. Liver Dis. 4:277-292, 1984.
12. Kobiler, D., and Mirelman, D.: Adhesion of *Entamoeba histolytica* to monolayers of human cells, J. Infect. Dis. 144:539-546, 1981.
13. Krogstad, D.J., Spencer, H.C., Jr., Healy, G.R., Gleason, N.N., Sexton, D.J., and Herron, C.A.: Amebiasis: epidemiologic studies in the United States, 1971-74, Ann. Intern. Med. 88:89-97, 1978.
14. Krogstad, D.J.: Isoenzyme patterns and pathogenicity in amebic infection, N. Engl. J. Med. 315:390-391, 1986. (Editorial.)
15. Lushbaugh, W.B., Kairalla, A.B., Cantey, J.R., Hofbauer, A.F., and Pittman, F.E.: Isolation of a cytotoxin-enterotoxin from *Entamoeba histolytica,* J. Infect. Dis. 139:9-17, 1979.
16. Lushbaugh, W.B., Hofbauer, A.F., and Pittman, F.E.: Proteinase activities of *Entamoeba histolytica* cytotoxin, Gastroenterology 87:17-27, 1984.
17. Lushbaugh, W.B., Hofbauer, A.F., Kairalla, A.A., Cantey, J.R., and Pittman, F.E.: Relationship of cytotoxins of axenically cultivated *Entamoeba histolytica* to virulence, Gastroenterology 86:1488-1495, 1984.
18. McGowan, K., Deneke, C.F., Thorne, G.M., and Gorbach, S.L.: *Entamoeba histolytica* cytotoxin: purification, characterization, strain virulence and protease activity, J. Infect. Dis. 146:616-625, 1982.
19. McGowan, K., Kane, A., Asarkof, N., Wicks, J., Guerina, V., Kellum, J., Baron, S., Gintzler, A.R., and Donowitz, M.: *Entamoeba histolytica* causes intestinal secretion: role of serotonin, Science 221:762-764, 1983.
20. McMillan, A., Gilmour, H.M., McNeillage, G., and Scott, G.R.: Amoebiasis in homosexual men, Gut 25:356-360, 1984.
21. Markell, E.K., Havens, R.F., Kuritsubo, R.A., and Wingerd, J.: Intestinal protozoa in homosexual men of the San Francisco Bay area: prevalence and correlates of infection, Am. J. Trop. Med. Hyg. 33:239-245, 1984.
22. Mathews, H.M., Walls, K.W., and Huong, A.Y.: Microvolume kinetic-dependent enzyme-linked immunosorbent assay for amoeba antibodies, J. Clin. Microbiol. 19:221-224, 1984.
23. Mathews, H.M., Moss, D.M., Healy, G.R., and Mildvan, D.: Isoenzyme analysis of *Entamoeba histolytica* isolated from homosexual men, J. Infect. Dis. 153:793-795, 1986.
24. Mattern, C.F.T., and Keister, D.B.: Experimental amebiasis. II. Hepatic amebiasis in the newborn hamster, Am. J. Trop. Med. Hyg. 26:401, 1977.
25. Muñoz, M.L., Rojkind, M., Calderón, J., Tanimoto, M., Arias-Negrete, S., and Martínez-Palomo, A.: *Entamoeba histolytica:* collagenolytic activity and virulence, J. Protozool. 31:468, 1984.
26. Orozco, E., Guarneros, G., Martínez-Palomo, A., and Sánchez, T.: *Entamoeba histolytica:* phagocytosis as a virulence factor, J. Exp. Med. 158:1511-1521, 1983.
27. Ortega, H.B., Borchardt, K.A., Hamilton, R., Ortega, P., and Mahood, J.: Enteric pathogenic protozoa in homosexual men from San Francisco, Sex. Transm. Dis. 11:59-63, 1984.
28. Patterson, M., Healy, G.R., and Shabot, J.M.: Serologic testing for amoebiasis, Gastroenterology 78:136-141, 1980.
29. Patterson, M., and Schoppe, L.E.: The presentation of amoebiasis, Med. Clin. North Am. 66:689-705, 1982.
30. Pérez-Tamayo, R.: Pathology of amebiasis. In Martínez Palomo, A., editor: Amebiasis, Amsterdam, 1986, Elsevier Biomedical.
31. Pérez-Tamayo, R., and Brandt, H.: Amebiasis. In Marcial-Rojas, R.A., editor: Pathology of protozoal and helminthic diseases, Baltimore, 1971, The Williams & Wilkins Co.
32. Phillips, S.C., Mildvan, D., William, D.C., Gelb, A.M., and White, M.C.: Sexual transmission of enteric protozoa and helminths in a venereal-disease-clinic population, N. Engl. J. Med. 305:603-606, 1981.
33. Pillai, S., and Mohimen, A.: Solid-phase sandwich radioimmunoassay for *Entamoeba histolytica* proteins and the detection of circulating antigens in amoebiasis, Gastroenterology 83:1210-1216, 1982.
34. Plorde, J.J., and Matlock, M.L.: Amebic liver abscess, Med. Grand Rounds 2:45-56, 1983.
35. Quinn, T.C., et al.: Prospective study of infectious agents isolated from the intestines of symptomatic and asymptomatic male homosexuals: the polymicrobial origin of intestinal infections in homosexual men, N. Engl. J. Med. 309:576-582, 1983.
36. Ravdin, J.I., and Guerrant, R.L.: Role of adherence in cytopathogenic mechanisms of *Entamoeba histolytica:* study with mammalian tissue culture cells and human erythrocytes, J. Clin. Invest. 68:1305-1313, 1981.
37. Rodríguez, M.A., and Orozco, E.: Isolation and characterization of phagocytosis and virulence-deficient mutants of *Entamoeba histolytica,* J. Infect. Dis. 154:27-32, 1986.
38. Salata, R.A., Martínez-Palomo, A., Murray, H.W., Conales, L., Trevino, N., Segovia, E., Murphy, C.F., and Ravdin, J.I.: Patients treated for amebic liver abscess develop cell mediated immune responses effective in vitro against *Entamoeba histolytica,* J. Immunol. 136:2633-2639, 1986.
39. Salata, R.A., Murray, H.W., Rubin, B.Y., and Ravdin, J.I.: The role of gamma interferon in the generation of human macrophages cytotoxic for *Entamoeba histolytica* trophozoites, Am. J. Trop. Med. Hyg. 37:72-78, 1987.
40. Salata, R.A., and Ravdin, J.I.: The interaction of human neutrophils and *Entamoeba histolytica* increases cytopathogenicity for liver cell monolayers, J. Infect. Dis. 154:19-26, 1986.

41. Sargeaunt, P.G., Jackson, T.F., and Simjee, A.: Biochemical homogenicity of *Entamoeba histolytica* isolates, especially those from liver abscess, Lancet **1**:1386-1388, 1982.
42. Schmerin, M.J., Gelston, A., and Jones, T.C.: Amebiasis: an increasing problem among homosexuals in New York City, JAMA **238**:1386-1387, 1977.
43. Sepúlveda, B.: Amebiasis: host-pathogen biology, Rev. Infect. Dis. **4**:836-842, 1982.
44. Simmons, R., et al.: Amebiasis associated with colonic irrigation: Colorado, MMWR **30**:101-102, 1981.
45. Stamm, W.P.: The value of amebic serology in an area of low endemicity, Trans. R. Soc. Trop. Med. Hyg. **70**:49-53, 1976.
46. Trisse, D.: Immunology of *Entamoeba histolytica* in human and animal hosts, Rev. Infect. Dis. **4**:1154-1184, 1982.
47. Tsutsumi, V., and Martínez Palomo, A.: Inflammatory reaction in experimental hepatic amebiasis: an ultrastructural study, Am. J. Pathol. **130**:112-119, 1988.
48. Tsutsumi, V., Mena-López, R., Anaya-Velázquez, F., and Martínez-Palomo, A.: Cellular basis of experimental amebic liver abscess formation, Am. J. Pathol. **117**:81, 1984.
49. Walls, K.W., and Smith, J.W.: Serology of parasitic infections, Lab. Med. **10**:329-336, 1979.

Amebic meningoencephalitis

50. Butt, C.G.: Primary amebic meningocephalitis, N. Engl. J. Med. **274**:1473-1476, 1966.
51. Duma, R.J., Helwig, W.B., and Martínez, A.J.: Meningoencephalitis and brain abscess due to free-living amoeba, Ann. Intern. Med. **88**:468-473, 1978.
52. Fowler, M., and Carter, R.F.: Acute pyogenic meningitis probably due to *Acanthamoeba*, Br. Med. J. **2**:740-742, 1965.
53. González, M.M., Gould, E., Dickinson, G., Martínez, A.J., Visvesvara, G.S., Cleary, T.J., and Hensley, G.T.: Acquired immunodeficiency syndro e associated with *Acanthamoeba* infection and other opportunistic organisms, Arch. Pathol. Lab. Med. **110**:749-751, 1986.
54. Jones, D.B., Visvesvara, G.A., and Robinson, N.M.: *Acanthamoeba* uveitis associated with fatal meningoencephalitis, Trans. Ophthalmol. Soc. UK **5**:221-224, 1975.
55. Margo, C.E.: *Acanthamoeba* keratitis, Arch. Pathol. Lab. Med. **111**:759-760, 1987.
56. Martínez, A.J.: Acanthamoebiasis and immunosuppression: case report, J. Neuropathol. Exp. Neurol. **41**:548-557, 1982.
57. Martínez, A.J.: Is *Acanthamoeba* encephalitis an opportunistic infection? Neurology **30**:567-574, 1980.
58. Martínez, A.J., et al.: Primary amebic meningoencephalitis, Pathol. Annu. **12**:225-250, 1977.
59. Martínez, A.J.: Free-living amoebae: pathogenic aspects, a review, Protozoological Abstracts **7**:293-306, 1983.
60. Martínez, A.J., García, C.A., Halks-Miller, M., and Arce-Vela, R.: Granulomatous amebic encephalitis presenting as a cerebral mass lesion, Acta Neuropathol. **51**:85-91, 1980.
61. Martínez, A.J., Sotelo-Avila, C., Alcalá, H., and Willaert, E.: Granulomatous encephalitis, intracranial arteritis, and myotic aneurysm due to a free-living ameba, Acta Neuropathol. **49**:7-12, 1980.
62. Martínez, A.J., Sotelo-Avila, C., García-Tamayo, J., Moron, J.T., Willaert, E., and Stamm, W.P.: Meningoencephalitis due to *Acanthamoeba* Sp.: pathogenesis and clinico-pathological study, Acta Neuropathol. **37**:183-191, 1977.
63. *Acanthamoeba* keratitis associated with contact lenses: United States, MMWR **35**:405-408, 1986.
64. Ofori-Kwakye, S.K., Sidebottom, D.G., Herbert, J., Fischer, E.G., and Visvesvara, G.S.: Granulomatous brain tumor caused by *Acanthamoeba*, J. Neurosurg. **64**:505-509, 1986.
65. Seidel, J.S., Harmatz, P.H., Visvesvara, G.S., Cohen, A., Edwards, J., and Turner, J.: Successful treatment of primary amebic meningoencephalitis, N. Engl. J. Med. **306**:346-348, 1982.
66. Theodore, F.H., Jakobiec, F.A., Juechter, K.B., Ma, P., Troutman, R.C., Pang, P.M., and Iwamoto, T.: The diagnostic value of a ring infiltrate in acanthamoebic keratitis, Ophthalmology **92**:1471-1479, 1985.
67. Visvesvara, G.S., Mirra, S.S., Brandt, F.H., Moss, D.M., Mathews, H.M., and Martínez, A.J.: Isolation of two strains of *Acanthamoeba castellanii* from human tissue and their pathogenicity and isoenzyme profiles, J. Clin. Microbiol. **18**:1405-1412, 1983.
68. Wiley, C.A., Safrin, R.E., Davic, C.E., Lampert, P.W., Braude, A.I., Martínez, A.J., and Visvesvara, G.S.: *Acanthamoeba* meningoencephalitis in a patient with AIDS, J. Infect. Dis. **155**:130-144, 1987.
69. Willaert, E., Stevens, A.R., and Healy, G.R.: Retrospective identification of *Acanthamoeba culbertsoni* in a case of amoebic meningoencephalitis, J. Clin. Pathol. **31**:717-720, 1978.

Balantidiasis

70. Areán, V.M., and Echevarría, R.: Balantidiasis. In Marcial-Rojas, R.A., editor: Pathology of protozoal and helminthic diseases, Baltimore, 1971, The Williams & Wilkins Co.
71. Areán, V.M., and Koppisch, E.: Balantidiasis: a review and report of cases, Am. J. Pathol. **32**:1089-1115, 1956.
72. Lahiri, V.L., Elhence, B.R., and Agarwal, B.M.: *Balantidium* peritonitis diagnosed on cytologic material, Acta Cytol. **21**:123-124, 1977.
73. Neafie, R.C.: Balantidiasis. In Binford, C.H., and Connor, D.H., editors: Pathology of tropical and extraordinary diseases, Washington, D.C., 1976, Armed Forces Institute of Pathology.

Flagellates of digestive tract and genital organs

74. Anand, B.S.: *Giardia lamblia:* clinical and immunological aspects, Trop. Gastroenterol. **1**:180-184, 1980.
75. Aggarwal, A., and Nash, T.E.: Lack of cellular cytotoxicity by human mononuclear cells to *Giardia*, J. Immunol. **136**:3486-3488, 1986.
76. Brandborg, L.L., et al.: Giardiasis and traveler's diarrhea, Gastroenterology **78**:1602-1614, 1980.
77. Brasitus, T.A.: Parasites and malabsorption, Am. J. Med. **67**:1058-1065, 1979.
78. Brogan, M.D.: Mucosal immunity and infection, pp. 859-862. In Targan, S.R., moderator: Immunologic mechanisms in intestinal diseases, Ann. Intern. Med. **106**:853-870, 1987.
79. Dykes, A.C., Juranek, D.D., Lorenz, R.A., Sinclair, S., Jakubowski, W., and Davies, R.: Municipal waterborne giardiasis: an epidemiologic investigation: beavers implicated as a possible reservoir, Ann. Intern. Med. **92**:165-170, 1980.
80. Farthing, M.J.G., Keusch, G.I., and Carey, M.C.: Components of bile effect growth of *Giardia lamblia*, J. Clin. Invest. **76**:1727-1732, 1985.
81. Hartong, W.A., Courley, W.K., and Arvanitakis, C.: Giardiasis: clinical spectrum and functional-structural abnormalities of the small intestinal mucosa, Gastroenterology **77**:61-69, 1979.
82. Heyworth, M.F., Owen, R.L., and Jones, A.L.: Comparison of leukocytes obtained from the intestinal lumen of *Giardia*-infected immunocompetent mice and nude mice, Gastroenterology **89**:1360-1365, 1985.
83. Heyworth, M.: Antibody response to *Giardia muris* trophozoites in mouse intestine, Infect. Immun. **52**:568-571, 1986.
84. Hiemstra, I., Van Bel, F., and Berger, H.M.: Can *Trichomonas vaginalis* cause pneumonia in newborn babies? Br. Med. J. **289**:355-356, 1984.
85. Kanwar, S.S., Ganguly, N.K., Walia, B.N., and Mahajan, R.C.: Direct and antibody dependent cell mediated cytotoxicity against *Giardia lamblia* by splenic and intestinal lymphoid cells in mice, Gut **27**:73-77, 1986.
86. Khosla, S.N., Sharma, S.V., and Srivastava, S.C.: Malabsorption in giardiasis, Am. J. Gastroenterol. **69**:694-700, 1978.
87. Knight, R., and Wright, S.G.: Progress report: intestinal protozoa, Gut **19**:940-953, 1978.
88. Levinson, J.D., and Nastro, L.J.: Giardiasis with total villous atrophy, Gastroenterology **74**:271-275, 1978.
89. Loftness, T.J., Erlandsen, S.L., Wilson, I.D., and Meyer, E.A.: Occurrence of specific secretory immunoglobulin A in bile after inoculation of *Giardia lamblia* trophozoites into rat duodenum, Gastroenterology **87**:1022-1029, 1984.
90. Marshall, J.B., Kelley, D.H., and Vogele, K.A.: Giardiasis: diagnosis by endoscopic brush cytology of the duodenum, Am. J. Gastroenterol. **79**:517-519, 1984.

91. McLaren, L.C., Davis, L.E., Healy, G.R., and James, C.G.: Isolation of *Trichomonas vaginalis* from the respiratory tract of infants with respiratory disease, Pediatrics **71**:888-890, 1983.
92. Meyer, E.A., and Radulescu, S.: *Giardia* and giardiasis, Adv. Parasitol. **17**:1-47, 1979.
93. Osterholm, M.T., et al.: An outbreak of foodborne giardiasis, N. Engl. J. Med. **304**:24-28, 1981.
94. Owen, R.L., Nemanic, P.C., and Stevens, D.P.: Ultrastructural observations on giardiasis in a murine model, Gastroenterology **76**:757-769, 1979.
95. Philip, A., Caster-Scott, P., and Rogers, C.: An agar culture technique to quantitate *Trichomonas vaginalis* from women, J. Infect. Dis. **155**:304-308, 1987.
96. Pickering, L.K., et al.: Asymptomatic *Giardia* in day care centers, J. Pediatr. **104**:522-526, 1984.
97. Rogers, A.I.: *Giardia* and steatorrhea, Gastroenterology **76**:224, 1979.
98. Schmerin, M.J., Jones, T.C., and Klein, H.: Giardiasis: association with homosexuality, Ann. Intern. Med. **88**:801-803, 1978.
99. Smith, P.D., Gillin, F.D., Brown, W.R., and Nash, T.E.: IgA antibody to *Giardia lamblia* directed by enzyme-linked immunosorbent assay, Gastroenterology **80**:1476-1480, 1981.
100. Smith, P.D., Gillin, F.D., Spira, W.M., and Nash, T.E.: Chronic giardiasis: studies on drug sensitivity, toxin production, and host immune response, Gastroenterology **83**:797-803, 1982.
101. Spence, M.R., Hollander, D.H., Smith, J., McCaig, L., Sewell, D., and Brockman, M.: The clinical and laboratory diagnosis of *Trichomonas vaginalis* infection, Sex. Transm. Dis. **7**:168-171, 1980.
102. Sun, T.: The diagnosis of giardiasis, Am. J. Surg. Pathol. **4**:265-271, 1980.
103. Tandon, B.N., Tandon, R.K., Satpathy, B.K., et al.: Mechanism of malabsorption in giardiasis: a study of bacterial flora and bile salt deconjugation in upper jejunum, Gut **18**:176-181, 1977.
104. Thomson, R.B., Haas, R.A., and Thompson, T.H.: Intestinal parasites: the necessity of examining multiple stool specimens, Mayo Clin. Proc. **59**:641-642, 1984.
105. Thornton, S.A., West, A.H., DuPont, H.L., and Pickering, L.K.: Comparison methods for identification of *Giardia lamblia*, Am. J. Clin. Pathol. **80**:858-860, 1983.
106. Visvesvara, G.S., Smith, P.D., Healy, G.R., and Brown, W.R.: An immunofluorescence test to detect antibodies to *Giardia lamblia*, Ann. Intern. Med. **93**:802-804, 1980.
107. Wittner, M., Maayan, S., Farrer, W., and Tanowitz, H.B.: Diagnosis of giardiasis by two methods, Arch. Pathol. Lab. Med. **107**:524-527, 1983.
108. Wolfe, M.S.: Symptomatology, diagnosis and treatment. In Erlandsen, S.L., and Meyer, E.A., editors: *Giardia* and giardiasis: biology, pathogenesis, and epidemiology, New York, 1984, Plenum Press Inc.
109. Yule, A., Gellan, M.C., Oriel, J.D., and Ackers, J.P.: Detection of *Trichomonas vaginalis* antigen in woman by enzyme immunoassay, J. Clin. Pathol. **40**:566-568, 1987.

Flagellates of blood and tissues
African trypanosomiasis

110. Bernards, A.: Transposable genes for surface glycoproteins in trypanosomes, TIBS, pp. 253-255, July 1982.
111. Borst, P., and Cross, G.A.M.: Molecular basis for trypanosome antigenic variation, Cell **29**:291-303, 1982.
112. Cross, G.A.M.: Antigenic variation in trypanosomes, Proc. R. Soc. Lond. (Biol.) **202**:55-72, 1978.
113. Hutt, M.S.R., and Wilks, N.E.: African trypanosomiasis. In Marcial-Rojas, R.A., editor: Pathology of protozoal and helminthic diseases, Baltimore, 1971, The Williams & Wilkins Co.
114. Mott, F.W.: Histological observations of sleeping sickness and other trypanosome infections, Reports of the Sleeping Sickness Commission, no. 7, 1906.
115. Pays, E., Van Assel, S., Laurent, M., Darville, M., Vervoort, T., Van Meirvenne, N., and Steinert, M.: Gene conversion as a mechanism for antigenic variation in trypanosomes, Cell **34**:371-381, 1983.
116. Robins-Browne, R.M., Schneider, J., and Metz, J.: Thrombocytopenia in trypanosomiasis, Am. J. Trop. Med. Hyg. **24**:225-231, 1975.
117. Ruitenberg, E.J., and Buys, J.: Application of the enzyme-linked immunosorbent assay (ELISA) for the serodiagnosis of human African trypanosomiasis (sleeping sickness), Am. J. Trop. Med. Hyg. **26**:31-36, 1977.
118. Sacks, D.L., Gross Kinsky, C.M., and Askonas, B.A.: Immune dysfunction caused by African trypanosomes: effect on parasite-specific responses and analysis of active fractions. In Van den Bossche, H., editor: The host invader interplay, Amsterdam, 1980, Elsevier/North Holland.
119. Spencer, H.C., Gibson, J.J., Jr., Brodsky, R.E., et al.: Imported African trypanosomiasis in the United States, Ann. Intern. Med. **82**:633-638, 1975.
120. Van Marck, E.A.E., Beckers, A., Deelder, A.M., Jacob, W., Wery, M., and Gigase, P.L.: Renal disease in chronic experimental *Trypanosoma gambiense* infections, Am. J. Trop. Med. Hyg. **30**:780-789, 1981.
121. Vickerman, K., et al.: Antigenic variation in trypanosomes, In Van den Bossche, H., editor: The host invader interplay, Amsterdam, 1980, Elsevier/North Holland.
122. Wery, M., Mulumba, P.M., Lambert, P.H., and Kazyumba, L.: Hematologic manifestations, diagnosis and immunopathology of African trypanosomiasis, Semin. Hematol. **19**:83-92, 1982.

American trypanosomiasis (Chagas' disease)

123. Alcántara, A., and Brener, Z.: *Trypanosoma cruzi:* role of macrophage membrane components in the phagocytosis of bloodstream forms, Exp. Parasitol. **50**:1-6, 1980.
124. Andrade, Z.A., and Andrade, S.G.: American trypanosomiasis. In Marcial-Rojas, R.A., editor: Pathology of protozoal and helminthic diseases, Baltimore, 1971, The William & Wilkins Co.
125. Andrade, Z.A., Andrade, S.G., Oliveira, G.B., and Alonso, D.R.: Histopathology of the conducting tissue of the heart in Chagas' myocarditis, Am. Heart J. **95**:316-324, 1978.
126. Brener, Z.: Immunity to *Trypanosoma cruzi*, Adv. Parasitol. **18**:247-292, 1980.
127. Cossio, P.M., Laguens, R.P., Kreutzer, E., et al.: Chagasic cardiopathy: immunopathologic and morphologic studies in myocardial biopsies, Am. J. Pathol. **86**:533-544, 1977.
128. Hoff, R., Teixeira, R.S., Carvalho, J.S., and Mott, K.E.: *Trypanosoma cruzi* in the cerebrospinal fluid during the acute stage of Chagas' disease, N. Engl. J. Med. **298**:604-606, 1978.
129. Hudson, L.: Immunobiology of *Trypanosoma cruzi* infection in Chagas' disease, Trans. R. Soc. Trop. Med. Hyg. **75**:493-498, 1981.
130. Jones, T.C.: Interactions between murine macrophages and obligate intracellular protozoa, Am. J. Pathol. **102**:127-132, 1981.
131. Jones, T.C., and Masur, H.: Survival of *Toxoplasma gondii* and other microbes in cytoplasmic vacuoles. In Van den Bossche, H., editor: The host invader interplay, Amsterdam, 1980, Elsevier/North Holland.
132. Kierszenbaum, F., Ackerman, S.J., and Gleich, G.J.: Destruction of bloodstream forms of *Trypanosoma cruzi* by eosinophil granule major basic proteins, Am. J. Trop. Med. Hyg. **30**:775-779, 1981.
133. Kirchhoff, L.V., Gam, A.A., Gusmao, R.A., Goldsmith, R.S., Rezende, J.M., and Rassi, A.: Increased specificity of serodiagnosis of Chagas' disease by detection of antibody to the 72- and 90-kilodalton glycoproteins of *Trypanosoma cruzi*, J. Infect. Dis. **155**:561-564, 1987.
134. Lisboa Bittencourt, A., Rodrigues de Freitas, L.A., Galvão de Araujo, M.O., and Jácomo, K.: Pneumonitis in congenital Chagas' disease, Am. J. Trop. Med. Hyg. **30**:38-42, 1981.
135. McCabe, R.E., Remington, J.S., and Araujo, F.G.: Mechanisms of invasion and replication of the intracellular stage in *Trypanosoma cruzi*, Infect. Immun. **46**:372-376, 1984.
136. Mott, K.E., and Hagstrom, J.W.C.: The pathologic lesions of the cardiac autonomic nervous system in chronic Chagas' myocarditis, Circulation **31**:273, 1965.
137. Nilsson, L.A., and Voller, A.: A comparison of thin layer immunoassay (TIA) and enzyme linked immunosorbent assay (ELISA) for the detection of antibodies to *Trypanosoma cruzi*, Trans. R. Soc. Trop. Med. Hyg. **76**:95-97, 1982.

138. Nogueira, N., and Cohn, Z.: *Trypanosoma cruzi* mechanism of entry and intracellular fate in mammalian cells, J. Exp. Med. **143:**1402-1420, 1976.

139. Rossi, M.A., Gonçalves, S., and Ribiro-dos-Santos, R.: Experimental *Trypanosoma cruzi* cardiomyopathy in BALB/c mice: the potential role of intravascular platelet aggregation in its genesis, Am. J. Pathol. **114:**209-216, 1984.

140. Teixeira, A.R.L.: Chagas' disease in inbred III/J rabbits, Am. J. Pathol. **124:**363-365, 1986.

141. Teixeira, A.R.L.: Chagas' disease: trends in immunologic research and prospects for immunoprophylaxis, Bull. WHO **57:**697, 1979.

142. Teixeira, A.R.L., Figueiredo, F., Rezende Filho, J., and Macêdo, V.: Chagas' disease: a clinical parasitologic, immunologic and pathologic study in rabbits, Am. J. Trop. Med. Hyg. **32:**258-272, 1983.

Leishmaniasis

143. Andrade, Z.A., Reed, S.G., Roters, S.B., and Sadigursky, M.: Immunopathology of experimental cutaneous leishmaniasis, Am. J. Pathol. **114:**137-148, 1984.

144. Anthony, R.L., Grogl, M., Sacci, J.B., and Ballou, R.W.: Rapid detection of *Leishmania* amastigotes in fluid aspirates and biopsies of human tissues, Am. J. Trop. Med. Hyg. **37:**271-276, 1987.

145. Badaró, R., Reed, S.G., and Carvalho, E.M.: Immunofluorescent antibody test in American visceral leishmaniasis: sensitivity and specificity of different morphological forms of two *Leishmania* species, Am. J. Trop. Med. Hyg. **32:**480, 1983.

146. Badaró, R., Reed, S.G., Barral, A., Orge, G., and Jones, T.C.: Evaluation of the microenzyme linked–immunosorbent assay (ELISA) for antibodies in American visceral leishmaniasis, Am. J. Trop. Med. Hyg. **35:**72, 1986.

147. Badaró, R., Jones, T.C., Lorenço, R., Cerf, B.J., Sampaio, D., Carvalho, E.M., Rocha, H., Teixeira, R., and Johnson, W.D., Jr.: A prospective study of visceral leishmaniasis in an endemic area of Brazil, J. Infect. Dis. **154:**639-649, 1986.

148. Chang, K.P., and Dwyer, D.M.: *Leishmania donovani:* hamster macrophages interactions in vitro: cell entry, intracellular survival and multiplication of amastigotes, J. Exp. Med. **147:**515-530, 1978.

149. Chulay, J.D., and Bryceson, A.D.M.: Quantitation of amastigotes of *Leishmania donovani* in smears of splenic aspirates from patients with visceral leishmaniasis, Am. J. Trop. Med. Hyg. **32:**475-479, 1983.

150. Grimaldi, G., David J.R., and McMahon-Pratt, D.: Identification and distribution of New World *Leishmania* species characterized by serodeme analysis using monoclonal antibodies, Am. J. Trop. Med. Hyg. **36:**270-287, 1987.

151. Haghighi, P., and Rezai, H.R.: Leishmaniasis: a review of selected topics, Pathol. Annu. **12:**63-89, 1977.

152. Kharazmi, A., Rezai, H.R., Fani, M., and Behforouz, N.C.: Evidence for the presence of circulating immune complexes in serum and C3b, and C3d on red cells of kala-azar patients, Trans. Trop. Med. Hyg. **76:**793-796, 1982.

153. Lainson, R.: The American leishmaniasis: some observations on their ecology and epidemiology, Trans. R. Soc. Trop. Med. Hyg. **77:**569, 1983.

154. Lightner, L.K., Chulay, J.D., and Bryceson, A.D.: Comparison of microscopy and culture in the detection of *Leishmania donovani* from splenic aspirates, Am. J. Trop. Med Hyg. **32:**296, 1983.

155. Luzzio, A.J., et al.: Quantitative estimation of leishmanial antibody titers by enzyme linked immunosorbent assay, J. Infect. Dis. **140:**370, 1979.

156. Murray, H.W.: Susceptibility of *Leishmania* to oxygen intermediates and killing by normal macrophages, J. Exp. Med. **153:**1302-1315, 1981.

157. Pappas, M.G., Hajkowski, R., Diggs, C.L., and Hockmeyer, W.T.: Disposable nitrocellulose filtration plates simplify the Dot-ELISA for serodiagnosis of visceral leishmaniasis, Trans. R. Soc. Trop. Med. Hyg. **79:**136, 1985. (Letter.)

158. Pearson, R.D., Wheeler, D.A., Harrison, L.H., and Kay, H.D.: The immunobiology of leishmaniasis, Rev. Infect. Dis. **5:**907, 1983.

159. Peterson, E.A., et al.: Specific inhibition of lymphocyte-proliferation responses by adherent suppressor cells in diffuse cutaneous leishmaniasis, N. Engl. J. Med. **306:**387-391, 1982.

160. Ridley, D.S., and Ridley, M.J.: The evolution of the lesion in cutaneous leishmaniasis, J. Pathol. **141:**83-96, 1983.

161. Ridley, M.J., and Wells, C.W.: Macrophage-parasite interaction in the lesions of cutaneous leishmaniasis, Am. J. Pathol. **123:**79-85, 1986.

162. Sacks, D.L., Lal, S.L., Shrivastava, S.N., Blackwell, J., and Neva, F.A.: An analysis of T-cell responsiveness in Indian kala-azar, J. Immunol. **138:**908-913, 1987.

163. Weigle, K.A., de Dávalos, M., Heredia, P., Molineros, R., Saravia, N.G., and D'Alessandro, A.: Diagnosis of cutaneous and mucocutaneous leishmaniasis in Colombia: a comparison of seven methods, Am. J. Trop. Med. Hyg. **36:**489-496, 1987.

164. Weisinger, J.R., Pinto, A., Velázquez, G.A., Bronstein, I., Dessene, J.J., Duque, J.F., Montenegro, J., Tapanes, F., and de Rousse, A.R.: Clinical and histological kidney involvement in human kala-azar, Am. J. Trop. Med. Hyg. **27:**357-359, 1978.

165. Werner, J.K., and Barreto, P.: Leishmaniasis in Colombia: a review, Am. J. Trop. Med. Hyg. **30:**751-761, 1981.

166. Winslow, D.J.: Kala-azar (visceral leishmaniasis). In Marcial-Rojas, R.A., editor: Pathology of protozoal and helminthic diseases, Baltimore, 1971, The Williams & Wilkins Co.

167. Wyler, D.J., and Suzuki, K.: In vitro parasite-monocyte interactions in human leishmaniasis: effect of enzyme treatment on attachment, Infect. Immunol. **42:**356, 1983.

Isosporiasis and cryptosporidiosis

168. Angus, K.W.: Cryptosporidiosis in man, domestic animals and birds: a review, J. R. Soc. Med. **76:**62-70, 1983.

169. Brandborg, L.L., Goldberg, S.B., and Breidenbach, W.C.: Human coccidiosis: a possible cause of malabsorption, N. Engl. J. Med. **283:**1306-1313, 1970.

170. Current, W.L., and Haynes, T.B.: Complete development of *Cryptosporidium* in cell culture, Science **224:**603-605, 1984.

171. Current, W.L., Reese, N.C., Ernst, J.V., Bailey, W.S., Heyman, M.B., and Weinstein, W.M.: Human cryptosporidiosis in immunocompetent and immunodeficient persons, N. Engl. J. Med. **308:**1252-1257, 1983.

172. Forthal, D.N., and Guest, S.S.: *Isospora belli* enteritis in three homosexual men, Am. J. Trop. Med. Hyg. **33:**1060-1064, 1984.

173. García, L.S., Bruckner, D.A., Brewer, T.C., and Shimizu, R.Y.: Techniques for the recovery and identification of *Cryptosporidium* oocysts from stool specimens, J. Clin. Microbiol. **18:**185-190, 1983.

174. Holten-Andersen, W., Gerstoft, J., Henriksen, S.A., et al.: Prevalence of *Cryptosporidium* among patients with acute enteric infection, J. Infect. **9:**277-282, 1984.

175. Jokipii, L., and Jokipii, A.M.M.: Timing of symptoms and oocyst excretion in human cryptosporidiosis, N. Engl. J. Med. **315:**1643-1647, 1986.

176. Jokipii, L., Pohjola, S., and Jokipii, A.M.: Cryptosporidiosis associated with traveling and giardiasis, Gastroenterology **89:**838-842, 1985.

177. Jokipii, L., Pohjola, S., and Jokipii, A.M.: *Cryptosporidium:* a frequent finding in patients with gastrointestinal symptoms, Lancet **2:**358-361, 1983.

178. Liebman, W.M., Thaler, M.M., DeLorimier, A., Brandborg, L.L., and Goodman, J.: Intractable diarrhea of infancy due to intestinal coccidiosis, Gastroenterology **78:**579-584, 1980.

179. Ma, P., and Soave, R.: Three step stool examination for cryptosporidiosis in 10 homosexual men with protracted watery diarrhea, J. Infect. Dis. **147:**824-828, 1983.

180. Marcial, M.A., and Madara J.L.: *Cryptosporidium:* cellular localization, structural analysis of absorptive cell-parasite membrane-membrane interactions in guinea pigs, and suggestion of protozoan transport by M cells, Gastroenterology **90:**583-594, 1986.

181. Mathan, M.M., Venkatesan, S., George, R., Mathew, M., and Mathan, V.I.: *Cryptosporidium* and diarrhea in southern Indian children, Lancet **2:**1172-1175, 1985.

182. Meisel, J.L., Perera, D.R., Meligro, C., et al.: Overwhelming watery diarrhea associated with a cryptosporidium in an immunosuppressed patient, Gastroenterology **70:**1156-1160, 1976.

183. Navin, T.R., and Juranek, D.D.: Cryptosporidiosis: clinical, epidemiologic, and parasitologic review, Rev. Infect. Dis. **6:**313-327, 1984.

184. Nime, F.A., Burek, J.D., Page, D.L., et al.: Acute enterocolitis in a human being infected with the protozoan *Cryptosporidium*, Gastroenterology **70:**592-598, 1976.

185. Pape, J.W., Levine, E., Beaulieu, M.E., Marshall, F., Verdier, R., and Johnson, W.D., Jr.: Cryptosporidiosis in Haitian children, Am. J. Trop. Med. Hyg. **36:**333-342, 1987.

186. Restrepo, C., Macher, A.M., and Radamy, E.H.: Disseminated extraintestinal isosporiasis in a patient with acquired immune deficiency syndrome. Am. J. Clin. Pathol. **87:**536-542, 1987.

187. Trier, J.S., Moxey, P.C., Schimmel, E.M., et al.: Chronic intestinal coccidiosis in man: intestinal morphology and response to treatment, Gastroenterology **66:**923-935, 1974.

188. Tzipori, S.: Cryptosporidiosis in animals and humans, Microbiol. Rev. **47:**84-96, 1983.

189. Ungar, B.L.P., Soave, R., Fayer, R., and Nash, T.E.: Enzyme immunoassay detection of immunoglobulin M and G antibodies to *Cryptosporidium* in immunocompetent and immunocompromised patients, J. Infect. Dis. **153:**570-578, 1986.

190. Vetterling, J.M., Takeuchi, A., and Madden, P.A.: Ultrastructure of *Cryptosporidium wrairi* from the guinea pig, J. Protozool. **18:**248-260, 1971.

191. Waldman, E., Tzipori, S., and Forsyth, J.R.L: Separation of *Cryptosporidium* species oocysts from feces by using a percoll discontinuous density gradient. J. Clin. Microbiol. **23:**199-200, 1986.

192. Weinstein, L., Edelsten, S.M., Madara, J.L., Falchuk, K.R., McManus, B.M., and Trier, J.S.: Intestinal cryptosporidiosis complicated by disseminated cytomegalovirus infection, Gastroenterology **81:**584-591, 1981.

193. Whiteside, M.E., Barkin, J.S., May, R.G., Weiss, S.D., Fischl, M.A., and MacLeod, C.L.: Enteric coccidiosis among patients with the acquired immunodeficiency syndrome, Am. J. Trop. Med. Hyg. **33:**1065-1072, 1984.

194. Wolfson, J.S., Richter, J.M., Waldron, M.A., et al.: Cryptosporidiosis in immunocompetent patients, N. Engl. J. Med. **312:**1278-1282, 1985.

Malaria

195. Aikawa, M., Miller, L.H., Rabbege, J.R., and Epstein, N.: Freeze fracture study on the erythrocyte membrane during malarial parasite invasion, J. Cell Biol. **91:**55, 1981.

196. Avidor, B., Golenser, J., Schutte, C.H., Cox, G.A., Isaacson, M., and Sulitzeanu, D.: A radioimmunoassay for the diagnosis of malaria, Am. J. Trop. Med. Hyg. **37:**225-229, 1987.

197. Broompucknavig, V., and Sitprija, V.: Renal disease in acute *Plasmodium falciparum* infection in man, Kidney Int. **16:**44-52, 1979.

198. Brasseur, P.H., Agrapart, M., Ballet, J.J., Druilhe, P., Warrell, M.J., and Tharavanij, S.: Impaired cell-mediated immmunity in *Plasmodium falciparum*-infected patients with high parasitemia and cerebral malaria, Clin. Immunol. Immunopathol. **27:**38, 1983.

199. Clark, J.A., et al.: Possible roles of tumor necrosis factor in the pathology of malaria, Am. J. Pathol. **129:**192-199, 1987.

200. Cohen, S.: *Plasmodium:* mechanisms of survival. In Van den Bossche, H., editor: The host invader interplay, Amsterdam, 1980, Elsevier/North Holland.

201. Deroff, P., Reguer, M., Simitzis, A.M., Boudon, A., and Saleun, J.P.: Screening blood donors for *Plasmodium falciparum* malariae, Vox Sang. **45:**392, 1983.

202. Facer, C.A.: Erythrocyte sialoglycoproteins and *Plasmodium falciparum*, Trans. R. Soc. Trop. Med. Hyg. **77:**724, 1983.

203. Franz, D.R., Lee, M., Seng, L.T., Young, G.D., Baze, W.B., and Lewis, G.E., Jr.: Peripheral vascular pathophysiology of *Plasmodium berghei* infection: a comparative study in the cheek pouch and brain of the golden hamster, Am. J. Trop. Med. Hyg. **36:**474-480, 1987.

204. Greenwood, B.M., Stratton, D., Williamson, W.A., and Mohammed, I.: A study of the role of immunological factors in the pathogenesis of the anaemia of acute malaria, Trans. R. Soc. Trop. Med. Hyg. **72:**378-385, 1978.

205. Guerrero, I.C., et al.: Transfusion malaria in the United States, 1972-1981, Ann. Intern. Med. **99:**221, 1984.

206. Hall, A.P.: The treatment of severe falciparum malaria, Trans. R. Soc. Trop. Med. Hyg. **71:**367-379, 1977.

207. Igarashi, I., Oo, M.M., Stanley, H., Reese, R., and Aikawa, M.: Knob antigen deposition in cerebral malaria, Am. J. Trop. Med. Hyg. **37:**511-515, 1987.

208. Kagan, I.G.: Evaluation of indirect hemagglutination test as an epidemiologic technique for malaria, Am. J. Trop. Med. Hyg. **21:**683-698, 1972.

209. Lawrence, C., and Olson, J.A.: Birefringent hemozoin identifies malaria, Am. J. Clin. Pathol. **86:**360-363, 1986.

210. MacKowiak, P.A.: Microbial synergism in human infections. Part I. N. Engl. J. Med. **298:**21-25, 1978.

211. MacPherson, G.G., Warrell, M.J., White, N.J., Looareesuwan, S., and Warrell, D.A.: Human cerebral malaria: a quantitative ultrastructural analysis of parasitized erythrocyte sequestration, Am. J. Pathol. **119:**385-401, 1985.

212. McBride, J.S., Walliker, D., and Morgan, G.: Antigenic diversity in the human malaria parasite *Plasmodium falciparum*, Science **217:**254-257, 1982.

213. McLaughlin, G.L., Ruth, J.L., Jablonski, E., Steketee, R., and Campbell, G.H.: Use of enzyme-linked synthetic DNA in diagnosis of falciparum malaria, Lancet **1:**714-716, 1987.

214. Miller, L.H., Haynes, J.D., McAuliffe, F.M., et al.: Evidence for differences in erythrocyte surface receptors for the malarial parasites, *Plasmodium falciparum* and *Plasmodium knowlesi*, J. Exp. Med. 146:277-280, 1977.

215. Miller, L.H., McGinniss, M.H., Holland, P.V., and Sigmon, P.: The Duffy blood group phenotype in American blacks infected with *Plasmodium vivax* in Vietnam, Am. J. Trop. Med. Hyg. **27:**1069-1072, 1978.

216. Oo, M.M., Aikawa, M., Than, T., Aye, T.M., Myint, P.T., Igarashi, I., and Schoene, W.C.: Human cerebral malaria: a pathological study, J. Neuropathol. Exp. Neurol. **46:**223-231, 1987.

217. Pasvol, G.: The interaction between sickle hemoglobin and the malarial parasite *Plasmodium falciparum*, Trans. R. Soc. Trop. Med. Hyg. **74:**701-705, 1980.

218. Perrin, L.H., Mackey, L.J., and Miescher, P.A.: The hematology of malaria in man, Semin. Hematol. **19:**70-82, 1982.

219. Punyagupta, S., et al.: Acute pulmonary insufficiency in falciparum malaria: summary of 12 cases with evidence of disseminated intravascular coagulation, Am. J. Trop. Med. Hyg. **23:**551-559, 1974.

220. Quinn, T.C., Jacobs, R.F., Mertz, G.J., Hook, E.W., III, and Locksley, R.M.: Congenital malaria: a report of four cases and a review, J. Pediatr. **101:**229-232, 1982.

221. Sherwood, J.A., Roberts, D.D., Marsh, K., Harvey, E.B., Spitalnik, S.L., Miller, L.H., and Howard, R.J.: Thrombospondin binding by parasitized erythrocyte isolates in falciparum malaria, Am. J. Trop. Med. Hyg. **36:**228-233, 1987.

222. Spencer, H.C., Collins, W.E., Warren, M., Jeffery, G.M., Mason, J., Huong, A.Y., Stanfill, P.S., and Skinner, J.C.: The enzyme-linked immunosorbent assay (ELISA) for malaria. III. Antibody response in documented *Plasmodium falciparum* infections, Am. J. Trop. Med. Hyg. **30:**747-750, 1981.

223. Walter, P.R., Garin, Y., and Blot, P.: Placental pathologic changes in malaria: a histologic and ultrastructural study, Am. J. Pathol. **109:**330-342, 1982.

224. Wilson, M., Fife, E.H., Jr., Mathews, H.M., et al.: Comparison of complement fixation, indirect immunofluorescence and indirect hemagglutination test for malaria, Am. J. Trop. Med. Hyg. **24:**755-759, 1975.

225. Woodruff, A.W., Ansdell, V.E., and Pettiff, L.E.: Cause of anemia in malaria, Lancet **1:**1055-1057, 1979.

226. Wyler, D.J.: Malaria resurgence, resistance and research, N. Engl. J. Med. **308:**875, 1983.

Toxoplasmosis

227. Anders, K.H., Guerra, W.F., Tomiyasu, U., Verity, M.A., and Vinters, H.V.: The neuropathology of AIDS, Am. J. Pathol. **124:**537-558, 1986.
228. Benenson, M.W., Takafuji, E.T., Lemon, S.M., Greenup, R.L., and Sulzer, A.J.: Oocyst-transmitted toxoplasmosis associated with ingestion of contaminated water, N. Engl. J. Med. **307:**666-669, 1982.
229. Broadbent, E.J., Ross, R., and Hurley, R.: Screening for toxoplasmosis in pregnancy, J. Clin. Pathol. **34:**659-664, 1981.
230. Chiappino, M.L., Nichols, B.A., and O'Connor, G.R.: Scanning electron microscopy of *Toxoplasma gondii:* parasite torsion and host-cell responses during invasion, J. Protozool. **31:**288-292, 1984.
231. Conley, F.K., Jenkins, K.A., and Remington, J.S.: *Toxoplasma gondii* infection of the central nervous system, Hum. Pathol. **12:**690-698, 1981.
232. Cursons, R.T.M.: DIG-ELISA for the serologic diagnosis of toxoplasmosis, Am. J. Clin. Pathol. **77:**459-461, 1982.
233. Frenkel, J.K., and Escajadillo, A.: Cyst rupture as a pathogenic mechanism of toxoplasmic encephalitis, Am. J. Trop. Med. Hyg. **36:**517-522, 1987.
234. Frenkel, J.K., Nelson, B.M., and Arias-Stella, J.: Immunosuppression and toxoplasmic encephalitis: clinical and experimental aspects, Hum. Pathol. **6:**97-111, 1975.
235. Gump, D.W., and Holden, R.A.: Acquired chorioretinitis due to toxoplasmosis, Ann. Intern. Med. **90:**58-60, 1979.
236. Hakes, T.B., and Armstrong, D.: Toxoplasmosis: problems in diagnosis and treatment, Cancer **52:**1535-1540, 1983.
237. Hofflin, J.M., Conley, F.K., and Remington, J.S.: Murine model of intracerebral toxoplasmosis, J. Infect. Dis. **155:**550-557, 1987.
238. Jones, T.C.: Interactions between murine macrophages and obligate intracellular protozoa, Am. J. Pathol. **102:**127-132, 1981.
239. Krick, J.A., and Remington, J.S.: Toxoplasmosis in the adult: an overview, N. Engl. J. Med. **208:**550-553, 1978.
240. Luft, B.J., Naot, Y., Araujo, F.G., Stinson, E.B., and Remington, J.S.: Primary and reactivated *Toxoplasma* infection in patients with cardiac transplants, Ann. Intern. Med. **99:**27-31, 1983.
241. Masur, H., Jones, T.C., Lempert, J.A., and Cherubini, T.D.: Outbreak of toxoplasmosis in a family and documentation of acquired retinochoroiditis, Am. J. Med. **64:**396-402, 1978.
242. McLeod, R., Berry, P.F., Marshall, W.H., Jr., Hunt, S.A., Ryning, F.W., and Remington, J.S.: Toxoplasmosis presenting as brain abscess: diagnosis by computerized tomography and cytology of aspirated purulent material, Am. J. Med. **67:**711-714, 1979.
243. Miettinen, M.: Histological differential diagnosis between lymph node toxoplasmosis and other benign lymph node hyperplasia, Histopathology **5:**205-216, 1981.
244. Nichols, B.A., and O'Connor, G.R.: Penetration of mouse peritoneal macrophages and protozoon *Toxoplasma gondii:* new evidence for active invasion and phagocytosis, Lab. Invest. **44:**324-335, 1981.
245. Ruskin, J., and Remington, J.S.: Toxoplasmosis in the compromised host, Ann. Intern. Med. **84:**193-199, 1976.
246. Sabin, A.B., and Feldman, H.A.: Dyes as microchemical indicators of a new immunity phenomenon affecting a protozoon parasite *(Toxoplasma),* Science **108:**660-663, 1948.
247. Shepp, D.H., Hackman, R.C., Conley, F.K., Anderson, J.B., and Meyers, J.D.: *Toxoplasma gondii* reactivation identified by detection of parasitemia in tissue culture, Ann. Intern. Med. **103:**218-221, 1985.
248. Sun, T., Greenspan, J., Tenenbaum, M., Farmer, P., Jones, T., Kaplan, M., and Peacock, J.: Diagnosis of cerebral toxoplasmosis using fluorescein-labeled antitoxoplasma monoclonal antibodies, Am. J. Surg. Pathol. **10:**312-316, 1986.
249. Tang, T.T., Harb, J.M., Dunne, W.M., Jr., Wells, R.G., Meyer, G.A., Chusid, M.J., Casper, J.T., and Camitta, B.M.: Cerebral toxoplasmosis in an immunocompromised host: a precise and rapid diagnosis by electron microscopy, Am. J. Clin. Pathol. **85:**104-110, 1986.
250. Van Knapsen, F., and Panggabean, S.O.: Detection of *Toxoplasma* antigen in tissues by means of enzyme-linked immunosorbent assay (ELISA), Am. J. Clin. Pathol. **77:**755-757, 1982.
251. Walls, K., Bullock, S., and English, D.: Use of the enzyme-linked immunosorbent assay (ELISA) and microadaptation for the serodiagnosis of toxoplasmosis, J. Clin. Microbiol. **5:**273-277, 1977.
252. Weitberg, A.B., Alper, J.C., Diamond, I., and Fligiel, Z.: Acute granulomatous hepatitis in the course of acquired toxoplasmosis, N. Engl. J. Med. **300:**1093-1096, 1979.
253. Wong, B., Gold, J.W., Brown, A.E., Lange, M., Fried, R., Grieco, M., Mildvan, D., Giron, J., Tapper, M.L., Lerner, C.W., et al.: Central-nervous-system toxoplasmosis in homosexual men and parenteral drug abusers, Ann. Intern. Med. **100:**36-42, 1984.

Pneumocystosis

254. Areán, V.M.: Pulmonary pneumocystosis. In Marcial-Rojas, R.A., editor: Pathology of protozoal and helminthic diseases, Baltimore, 1971, The Williams & Wilkins Co.
255. Ariztia, A., et al.: Interstitial plasma cell pneumonia and *Pneumocystis carinii,* J. Pediatr. **51:**639-645, 1957.
256. Broaddus, C., Dake, M.D., Stulbarg, M.S., Blumenfeld, W., Hadley, W.K., Golden, J.A., and Hopewell, P.C.: Bronchoalveolar lavage and transbronchial biopsy for the diagnosis of pulmonary infections in the acquired immunodeficiency syndrome, Ann. Intern. Med. **102:**747-752, 1985.
257. Centers for Disease Control Update: Acquired immunodeficiency syndrome—United States, MMWR **35:**542, 1986.
258. Coulman, C.U., Greene, I., and Archibald, R.W.R.: Cutaneous pneumocystosis, Ann. Intern. Med. **106:**396-398, 1987.
259. De Vita, V.T., Jr., Broder, S., Fauci, A.S., Kovacs, J.A., and Chabner, B.A.: Developmental therapeutics and the acquired immunodeficiency syndrome, Ann. Intern. Med. **106:**568-581, 1987.
260. Follansbee, S.E., Busch, D.F., Wofsy, C.B., Coleman, D.L., Gullet, J., Aurigemma, G.P., Ross, T., Hadley, W.K., and Drew, W.L.: An outbreak of *Pneumocystis carinii* pneumonia in homosexual men, Ann. Intern. Med. **96:**705-713, 1982.
261. Gal, A.A., Klatt, E.C., Koss, M.N., Strigle, S.M., and Boylen, C.T.: The effectiveness of bronchoscopy in the diagnosis of *Pneumocystis carinii* and cytomegalovirus pulmonary infections in acquired immunodeficiency syndrome, Arch. Pathol. Lab. Med. **111:**238-241, 1987.
262. Gottlieb, M.S., Schroff, R., Schanker, H.M., Weisman, J.D., Fan, P.T., Wolf, R.A., and Saxon, A.: *Pneumocystis carinii* pneumonia and mucosal candidiasis in previously healthy homosexual men, N. Engl. J. Med. **305:**1425-1431, 1981.
263. Grimes, M.M., LaPook, J.D., Bar, M.H., Wasserman, H.S., and Dwork, A.: Disseminated *Pneumocystis carinii* infection in a patient with acquired immunodeficiency syndrome, Hum. Pathol. **18:**307-308, 1987.
264. Haque, A., et al.: *Pneumocystis carinii:* taxonomy as viewed by electron microscopy, Am. J. Clin. Pathol. **87:**504-510, 1987.
265. Hamperl, H.: *Pneumocystis* infection and cytomegaly of lungs in newborn and adult, Am. J. Pathol. **32:**1-13, 1956.
266. Henshaw, N.G., Carson, J.L., and Collier, A.M.: Ultrastructural observations of *Pneumocystis carinii* attachment to rat lung, J. Infect. Dis. **151:**181-186, 1985.
267. Heyman, M.R., and Rasmussen, P.: *Pneumocystis carinii* involvement of the bone marrow in acquired immunodeficiency syndrome, Am. J. Clin. Pathol. **87:**780-783, 1987.
268. Hofflin, J.M., Potasman, I., Baldwin, J.C., Oyer, P.E., Stinson, E.B., and Remington, J.S.: Infectious complications in heart transplant recipients receiving cyclosporine and corticosteroids, Ann. Intern. Med. **106:**209-216, 1987.
269. Hughes, W.T.: Natural mode of acquisition for de novo infection with *Pneumocystis carinii,* J. Infect. Dis. **145:**842, 1982.
270. Kovacs, J.A., Hiemenz, J.W., Macher, A.M., Stover, D., Murray, H.W., Shelhamer, J., Lane, H.C., Urmacher, C., Honig, C., Longo, D.L., et al.: *Pneumocystis carinii* pneumonia: a comparison between patients with the acquired immunodeficiency syndrome and patients with other immunodeficiencies, Ann. Intern. Med. **100:**663-671, 1984.
271. Linder, J., Vaughan, W.P., Armitage, J.O., Ghafouri, M.A., Hurkman, D., Mroczek, E.C., Miller, N.G., and Rennard, S.I.: Cytopathology of opportunistic infection in bronchoalveolar lavage, Am. J. Clin. Pathol. **88:**421-428, 1987.
272. Long, E.G., Smith, J.S., and Meier, J.L.: Attachment of *Pneumocystis carinii* to rat pneumocytes, Lab. Invest. **54:**609-615, 1986.

273. Lunseth, J.H.: Interstitial plasma cell pneumonia, J. Pediatr. 46:137-155, 1955.

274. Masur, H.: New concepts in the therapy of infections in the acquired immunodeficiency syndrome, pp. 802-804. In Fauci, AS., editor: The acquired immunodeficiency syndrome: an update, Ann. Intern. Med. 102:800-813, 1985.

275. Masur, H., Michelis, M.A., Greene, J.B., Onorato, I., Stouwe, R.A., Holzman, R.S., Wormser, G., Brettman, L., Lange, M., Murray, H.W., and Cunningham-Rundles, S.: An outbreak of community-acquired *Pneumocystis carinii* pneumonia, N. Engl. J. Med. 305:1431-1438, 1981.

276. Martin, W.J., II, Smith, T.F., Sanderson, D.R., Brutinel, W.M., Cockerill, F.R., II, and Douglas, W.W.: Role of bronchoalveolar lavage in the assessment of opportunistic pulmonary infections: utility and complications, Mayo Clin. Proc. 62:549-557, 1987.

277. Mildvan, D., Mathur, U., Enlow, R.W., Romain, P.L., Winchester, R.J., Colp, C., Singman, H., Adelsberg, B.R., and Spigland, I.: Opportunistic infections and immune deficiency in homosexual men, Ann. Intern. Med. 96:700-704, 1982.

278. Mones, J.M., Saldana, M.J., and Oldham, S.A.: Diagnosis of *Pneumocystis carinii* pneumonia: roentgenographic-pathologic correlates based on fiberoptic bronchoscopy specimens from patients with the acquired immunodeficiency syndrome, Chest 89:522-526, 1986.

279. Murphy, M.J., Jr., Pifer, L.L., and Hughes, W.T.: *Pneumocystis carinii* in vitro: a study by scanning electron microscopy, Am. J. Pathol. 86:387-394, 1977.

280. Pavlica, F.: The first observation of congenital pneumocystic pneumonia in a fully developed stillborn child, Ann. Paediatr. 198:177-184, 1962.

281. Schwartz, D.A., Munger, R.G., and Katy, S.M.: Plastic embedding evaluation of *Pneumocystis carinii* pneumonia in AIDS, Am. J. Surg. Pathol. 11:304-309, 1987.

282. Walzer, P.D.: Attachment of microbes to host cells: relevance of *Pneumocystis carinii*, Lab. Invest. 54:589-592, 1986. (Editorial.)

283. Yoneda, K., and Walzer, P.D.: Attachment of *Pneumocystis carinii* to type I alveolar cells studied by freeze-fracture electron microscopy, Infect. Immun. 40:812-815, 1983.

284. Yoshida, Y., Matsumoto, Y., Yamada, M., Okabayashi, K., Yoshikawa, H., and Nakazawa, M.: *Pneumocystis carinii*: electron microscopic investigation of the interaction of trophozoite and alveolar lining cell, Zentralbl. Bakteriol. Mikrobiol. Hyg. [A] 256:390-399, 1984.

Babesiosis (piroplasmosis)

285. Benach, J.L., Habicht, G.S., and Hamburger, M.I.: Immunoresponsiveness in acute babesiosis in humans, J. Infect. Dis. 146:369-380, 1982.

286. Benach, J.L., Coleman, J.L., and Habicht, G.S.: Serological evidence for simultaneous occurrences of Lyme disease and babesiosis, J. Infect. Dis. 152:473-477, 1985.

287. Chisholm, E.S., Ruebush, T.K., II, Sulzer, A.J., and Healy, G.R.: *Babesia microti* infection in man: evaluation of an indirect immunofluorescent antibody test, Am. J. Trop. Med. Hyg. 27:14, 1978.

288. Dammin, G.J.: Babesiosis. In Weinstein, L., and Fields, B.N., editors: Seminars in Infectious Disease, vol. 1, pp. 168-199, New York, 1978, Stratton Intercontinental Medical Book Corp.

289. Dammin, G.J., Spielman, A., Benach, J.L., and Piesman, J.: The rising incidence of clinical *Babesia microti* infection, Hum. Pathol. 12:398-400, 1981.

290. Healy, G.R., and Ruebush, T.K.: Morphology of *Babesia microti* in human blood smears, Am. J. Clin. Pathol. 73:107-109, 1980.

291. Jack, R.M., and Ward, P.A.: *Babesia rhodaini* interactions with complement: relationship to parasitic entry into red cells, J. Immunol. 124:1566-1573, 1980.

292. Jacoby, G.A., Hunt, J.V., Kosinski, K.S., Demirjian, Z.N., Huggins, C., Etkind, P., Marcus, L.C., and Spielman, A.: Treatment of transfusion-transmitted babesiosis by exchange transfusion, N. Engl. J. Med. 303:1098-1100, 1980.

293. Marcus, L.C., Steere, A.C., Duray, P.H., Anderson, A.E., and Mahoney, E.B.: Fatal pancarditis in a patient with coexistent Lyme disease and babesiosis, Ann. Intern. Med. 103:374-376, 1985.

294. Rosner, F., Zarrabi, M.H., Benach, J.L., and Habicht, G.S.: Babesiosis in splenectomized adults: review of 22 reported cases, Am. J. Med. 76:696-701, 1984.

295. Rowin, K.S., Tanowitz, H.B., Rubinstein, A., Kunkel, M., and Wittner, M.: Babesiosis in asplenic hosts, Trans. R. Soc. Trop. Med. Hyg. 78:442-444, 1984.

296. Ruebush, T.K., II, Colling, W.F., and Warren, M.: Experimental *Babesia microti* infections in *Macaca mulatta*: recurrent parasitemia before and after splenectomy, Am. J. Trop. Med. Hyg. 30:304-307, 1981.

297. Ruebush, T.K., II, et al.: Human babesiosis on Nantucket Island: clinical features, Ann. Intern. Med. 86:6-14, 1977.

298. Ruebush, T.K., II, Juranek, D.D., Chisholm, E.S., et al.: Human babesiosis on Nantucket Island: evidence for self-limited and sub-clinical infections, N. Engl. J. Med. 297:825-829, 1977.

299. Skrabalo, Z.: Babesiosis (piroplasmosis). In Marcial Rojas, R.A., editor: Pathology of protozoal and helminthic diseases, Baltimore, 1971, The Williams & Wilkins Co.

300. Smith, R.P., Evans, A.T., Popovsky, M., Mills, L., and Spielman, A.: Transfusion-acquired babesiosis and failure of antibiotic treatment, JAMA 256:2726-2727, 1986.

301. Sun, T., Tenenbaum, M.J., Greenspan, J., Teichberg, S., Wang, R.T., Degnan, T., and Kaplan, M.H.: Morphologic and clinical observations in human infection with *Babesia microti*, J. Infect. Dis. 148:239, 1983.

302. Ward, P.A., and Jack, R.M.: The entry process of *Babesia* merozoites into red cells, Am. J. Pathol. 102:109-113, 1981.

303. Wittner, M., Rowin, K.S., Tanowitz, H.B., Hobbs, J.F., Saltzman, S., Wenz, B., Hirsch, R., Chisholm, E., and Healy, G.R.: Successful chemotherapy of transfusion babesiosis, Ann. Intern. Med. 96:601-604, 1982.

304. Zwart, D., and Brocklesby, D.W.: Babesiosis: non-specific resistance, immunological factors and pathogenesis, Adv. Parasitol. 17:50-113, 1979.

Helminthic diseases
Distomiases

305. Acosta-Ferreira, W., Vercelli-Retta, J., and Falconi, L.M.: *Fasciola hepatica* human infection: histopathological study of sixteen cases, Virchows Arch. [Pathol. Anat.] 383:319, 1979.

306. Acuna-Soto, R., and Braun, Roth, G.: Bleeding ulcer in the common bile duct to *Fasciola hepatica*, Am. J. Gastroenterol. 82:560-562, 1987.

307. Bhamarapravati, N., and Thammavit, W.: Animal studies on liver fluke infection, dimethyl nitrosamine and bile duct carcinoma, Lancet 1:206-207, 1978.

308. Bhamarapravati, N., and Thammavit, W., and Vajrasthira, S.: Liver changes in hamsters infected with liver fluke of man, *Opisthorchis viverrini*, Am. J. Trop. Med. Hyg. 27:787-794, 1978.

309. Bynum, T.E., and Hauser, S.C.: Abnormalities on ERCP in a case of human fascioliasis, Gastrointest. Endosc. 30:80-82, 1984.

310. Chung, C.H.: In Marcial-Rojas, R.A., editor: Pathology of protozoal and helminthic diseases, Baltimore, 1971, The Williams & Wilkins Co.

311. Davies, C., and Goose, J.: Killing of newly encysted juveniles of *Fasciola hepatica* in sensitized rats, Parasite Immunol. 3:81-86, 1981.

312. de Miguel, F., Carrasco, J., García, N., Bustamante, V., and Beltrán, J.: CT findings in human fascioliasis, Gastrointest. Radiol. 9:157-159, 1984.

313. Espino, A.M., Duménigo, B.E., Fernández, R., and Finlay, C.M.: Immunodiagnosis of human fascioliasis by enzyme-linked immunosorbent assay using excretory-secretory products, Am. J. Trop. Med. Hyg. 37:605-608, 1987.

314. Flavell, D.J.: Liver fluke infection as an aetiological factor in bile-duct carcinoma in man, Trans. R. Soc. Trop. Med. Hyg. 75:814, 1981.

315. Fravell, D.J., and Lucas, S.B.: Potentiation by the human liver fluke, *Opisthorchis viverrini*, of the carcinogenic action of *N*-nitrosodimethylamine upon the biliary epithelium of the hamster, Br. J. Cancer 46:985, 1982.

316. Foster, J.R.: A study of the initiation of biliary hyperplasia in rats infected with *Fasciola hepatica*, Parasitology **83**:253, 1981.

317. Gibson, J.B., and Sun, T.: Clonorchiasis. In Marcial-Rojas, R.A., editor: Pathology of protozoal and helminthic diseases, Baltimore, 1971, The Williams & Wilkins Co.

318. Hillyer, G.V.: Fascioliasis, paragonimiasis, clonorchiasis and opistorchiasis. In Walls, K.W., and Schantz, P.M., eds.: Immunodiagnosis of parasitic diseases, New York, 1986, Academic Press Inc.

319. Hillyer, G.V.: Fasciliasis in Puerto Rico: a review, Bol. Asoc. Med. P.R. **73**:94, 1981.

320. Kurathong, S., Lerdverasirikul, P., Wongpaitoon, V., Pramoolsinsap, C., Kanjanapitak, A., Varavithya, W., Phuapradit, P., Bunyaratvej, S., Upatham, E.S., and Brockelman, W.Y.: *Opisthorchis viverrini* infection and cholangiocarcinoma, Gastroenterology **89**:151, 1985.

321. Levine, D.M., Hillyer, G.V., and Flores, S.I.: Comparison of counter electrophoresis, the enzyme-linked immunosorbent assay and Kato fecal examination for the diagnosis of fascioliasis in infected mice and rabbits, Am. J. Trop. Med. Hyg. **29**:602-608, 1980.

322. Mariano, E.G., Borja, S.R., and Vruno, M.J.: A human infection with *Paragonimus kellicoti* (lung fluke) in the United States, Am. J. Clin. Pathol. **86**:685-687, 1986.

323. Nakashima, T., Sakamoto, K., and Okuda, K.: Hepatocellular carcinoma and clonorchiasis, Cancer **39**:1306-1311, 1977.

324. Náquira-Vildoso, F., and Marcial-Rojas, R.A.: Fascioliasis. In Marcial-Rojas, R.A., editor: Pathology of protozoal and helminthic diseases, Baltimore, 1971, The Williams & Wilkins Co.

325. Pachucki, C.T., et al.: American paragonimiasis treated with praziquantel, N. Engl. J. Med. **311**:582-583, 1984.

326. Park, C.I., Kim, H., Ro, J.Y., and Gutiérrez, Y.: Human ectopic fascioliasis in the cecum, Am. J. Surg. Pathol. **8**:73-77, 1984.

327. Purtillo, D.T.: Clonorchiasis and hepatic neoplasms, Trop. Geogr. Med. **28**:21-27, 1976.

328. Schwartz, D.A.: Cholangiocarcinoma associated with liver fluke infection: a preventable source of morbidity in Asian immigrants, Am. J. Gastroenterol. **81**:76-79, 1986.

329. Sun, T.: Pathology and immunology of *Clonorchis sinesis* infection of the liver, Ann. Clin. Lab. Sci. **14**:208-215, 1984.

330. Takeyama, N., Okumura, N., Sakai, Y., Kamma, O., Shima, Y., Endo, K., and Hayakawa, T.: Computed tomography findings of hepatic lesions in human fascioliasis: report of two cases, Am. J. Gastroenterol. **81**:1078-1081, 1986.

331. Tansurat, P.: Opisthorchiasis. In Marcial-Rojas, R.A., editor: Pathology of protozoal and helminthic diseases, Baltimore, 1971, The Williams & Wilkins Co.

332. Thammavit, W., et al.: Effects of dimethylnitrosamine on induction of cholangiocarcinoma in *Opisthorchis viverrini*-infected Syrian golden hamsters, Cancer Res. **38**:4634-4639, 1978.

333. Uflacker, R., Wholey, M.H., Amaral, N.M., and Lima, S.: Parasitic and mycotic causes of biliary obstruction, Gastrointest. Radiol. **7**:173-179, 1982.

334. Upatham, E.S., Viyanant, V., Kurathong, S., Brockelman, W.Y., Menaruchi, A., Saowakontha, S., Intarakhao, C., Vajrasthira, S., and Warren, K.S.: Morbidity in relation to intensity of infection in *Opisthorchis viverrini*: study of a community in Khon Kaen, Thailand, Am. J. Trop. Med. Hyg. **31**:1156, 1982.

335. Viyanant, V., Brockelman, W.Y., Lee, P., Ardsungnoen, S., and Upatham, E.S.: A comparison of a modified quick-Kato technique and the Stoll dilution method for field examination for *Opisthorchis viverrini* eggs, J. Helminthol. **57**:191-195, 1983.

336. Wong, R.K.H., Peura, D.A., Mutter, M.L., Heit, H.A., Birns, M.T., and Johnson, L.F.: Hemobilia and liver flukes in a patient from Thailand, Gastroenterology **88**:1958-1963, 1985.

Schistosomiasis (bilharziasis)

337. Andrade, Z.A., and Grimaud, J.A.: Evolution of schistosomal hepatic lesions in mice after curative chemotherapy, Am. J. Pathol. **124**:59-65, 1986.

338. Andrade, Z.A., and Rocha, H.: Schistosomal glomerulopathy, Kidney Int. **16**:23-29, 1979.

339. Attah, E.B., and Nkposong, E.O.: Schistosomiasis and carcinoma of the bladder: a critical appraisal of causal relationship, Trop. Geogr. Med. **28**:268-272, 1976.

340. Biempica, L., Dunn, M.A., Kamel, I.A., Kamel, R., Hait,

P.K., Fleischner, C., Biempica, S.L., Wu, C.H., and Rojkind, M.: Liver collagen–type characterization in human schistosomiasis: a histological, ultrastructural, and immunocytochemical correlation, Am. J. Trop. Med. Hyg. **32**:316, 1983.

341. Bout, D.T., Joseph, M., David, J.R., and Capron, A.R.: In vitro killing of S. *mansoni* schistosomula by lymphokine-activated mouse macrophages, J. Immunol. **127**:1-5, 1981.

342. Butterworth, A.E., Taylor, D.W., Veith, M.C., Vadas, M.A., Dessein, A., Sturrock, R.F., and Wells, E.: Studies on the mechanisms of immunity in human schistosomiasis, Immunol. Rev. **61**:1-39, 1982.

343. Capron, A., et al.: Schistosome mechanisms of evasion. In Van den Bossche, H., editor: The host invader interplay, Amsterdam, 1980, Elsevier/North Holland.

344. Caulfield, J.P., Lenzi, H.L., Elsas, P., and Dessein, A.J.: Ultrastructure of the attack of eosinophils stimulated by blood mononuclear cell products on schistosomula of *Schistosoma mansoni*, Am. J. Pathol. **120**:380-390, 1985.

345. Cheever, A.W., Duvall, R.H., Hallack, T.A., Jr., Minker, R.G., Malley, J.D., and Malley, K.G.: Variation of hepatic fibrosis and granuloma size among mouse strains infected with *Schistosoma mansoni*, Am. J. Trop. Med. Hyg. **37**:85-97, 1987.

345a. Chen, M.C., Chuang, C.Y., Chang, P.Y., and Hu, J.C.: [These are proper surnames for reference 368, which see.]

346. de Brito, P.A., Kazura, J.W., and Mahmoud, A.A.: Host granulomatous response in schistosomiasis mansoni: antibody and cell-mediated damage of parasite eggs in vitro, J. Clin. Invest. **74**:1715, 1984.

347. Doenhoff, M.J.: The schistosome egg granuloma: immunopathology in the cause of host protection or parasite survival? Trans. R. Soc. Trop. Med. Hyg. **80**:503-514, 1986.

348. El-Bolkainy, M.N., Mokhtar, N.M., Ghoneim, M.A., and Hussein, M.H.: The impact of schistosomiasis on the pathology of bladder carcinoma, Cancer **48**:2643-2648, 1981.

349. Elsebai, I.: Parasites in the etiology of cancer, CA **27**:100-106, 1977.

350. García-Palmieri, M.R., and Marcial-Rojas, R.A.: Portal hypertension due to schistosomiasis mansoni, Am. J. Med. **27**:811-816, 1959.

351. García-Palmieri, M.R., and Marcial-Rojas, R.A.: The protean manifestations of schistosomiasis mansoni: a clinicopathological correlation, Ann. Intern. Med. **57**:763-775, 1962.

352. Gazayerli, M., Khalil, H.A., and Gazayerli, I.M.: Schistosomiasis hematobium (urogenic bilharziasis). In Marcial-Rojas, R.A., editor: Pathology of protozoal and helminthic diseases, Baltimore, 1971, The Williams & Wilkins Co.

353. Gentile, J.M.: Possible basic mechanisms of carcinogenesis in schistosomiasis and other trematode infections, Bull. WHO/ Schisto/ **83**:74, 1983.

354. Grimaud, J.A., Boros, D.L., Takiya, C., Mathew, R.C., and Emonard, H.: Collagen isotypes, laminin and fibronectin in granulomas of the liver and intestines of *Schistosoma mansoni*-infected mice, Am. J. Trop. Med. Hyg. **37**:335-344, 1987.

355. Hillyer, G.V., Ramzy, R.M., El Alamy, M.A., and Cline, B.L.: Immunodiagnosis of infection with *Schistosoma haematobium* and S. *mansoni* in man, Am. J. Trop. Med. Hyg. **29**:1254-1257, 1980.

356. Hillyer, G.V., Ramzy, R.M., El Alamy, M.A., and Cline, B.L.: The circumoval precipitin test for the serodiagnosis of human schistosomiasis mansoni and haematobia, Am. J. Trop. Med. Hyg. **30**:121-126, 1981.

357. Homeida, M., Abdel-Gadir, A.F., Cheever, A.W., Bennett, J.L., Arbab, B.M., Ibrahim, S.Z., Abdel-Salam, I.M., Dafalla, A.A., and Nash, T.E.: Diagnosis of pathologically confirmed Symmers' periportal fibrosis by ultrasonography: a prospective blind study, Am. J. Trop. Med. Hyg. **38**:86-91, 1988.

358. Incani, R.N., and McLaren, D.J.: Neutrophil-mediated cytotoxicity to schistosomula of *Schistosoma mansoni* in vitro: studies on the kinetics of complement and/or antibody-dependent adherence and killing, Parasite Immunol. **3**:107-126, 1981.

359. Jakobiec, F.A., Gress, L., and Zimmerman, L.E.: Granulomatous dacryoadenitis caused by *Schistosoma hematobium*, Arch. Ophthalmol. **95**:278-280, 1977.

360. Jong, E.C., Mahmoud, A.A.F., and Klebahoff, S.J.: Peroxidase-mediated toxicity to schistomula of *Schistosoma mansoni*, J. Immunol. **126**:468-471, 1981.

361. Lichtenberg, F.: Lesions of intrahepatic portal radicles in Manson's schistosomiasis, Am. J. Pathol. **31**:757-771, 1955.

362. Long, E.G., McLaren, M., Goddard, M.J., Bartholomew, R.K., Peters, P., and Goodgame, R.: Comparison of ELISA radioimmunoassay and stool examination for *Schistosoma mansoni* infection, Trans. R. Soc. Trop. Med. Hyg. **75**:365-371, 1981.

363. Mahmoud, A.A.F.: Schistosomiasis: In Warren, K.S., and Mahmoud, A.A.F., editors: Tropical and geographical medicine, New York, 1984, McGraw Hill Book Co.

364. Marchand, E.J., et al.: The pulmonary obstruction syndrome in *Schistosoma mansoni* pulmonary endarteritis, Arch. Intern. Med. **100**:965-980, 1957.

365. Marcial-Rojas, R.A.: Schistosomiasis mansoni. In Marcial-Rojas, R.A., editor: Pathology of protozoal and helminthic diseases, Baltimore, 1971, The Williams & Wilkins Co.

366. Marcial-Rojas, R.A., and Fiol, R.E.: Neurologic complications of schistosomiasis: review of the literature and report of two cases of transverse myelitis due to *S. mansoni*, Medicine **59**:215-230, 1963.

367. Martínez-Maldonado, M., Girod, C.E., Ramírez de Arellano, G., et al.: Liver cell carcinoma (hepatoma) in Puerto Rico: a survey of 26 cases, Am. J. Dig. Dis. **10**:522, 1965.

368. Ming-Chai, C., Chi-Yuan, C., Pei-Yu, C., and Jen-Chun, H. [see reference 345a for proper surnames]: Evolution of colorectal cancer in schistosomiasis: transitional mucosal changes adjacent to large intestinal carcinoma in colectomy specimens, Cancer **46**:1661-1675, 1980.

369. Miyake, M.: Schistosomiasis japonicum: In Marcial-Rojas, R.A., editor: Pathology of protozoal and helminthic diseases, Baltimore, 1971, The Williams & Wilkins Co.

370. Nakashima, T., Okuda, K., Kojiro, M., et al.: Primary liver cancer coincident with schistosomiasis japonica: a study of 24 necropsies, Cancer **36**:1483-1489, 1975.

371. Nash, T.E., Cheever, A.W., Ottesen, E.A., and Cook, J.A.: Schistosome infections in humans: prospectives and recent findings, Ann. Intern. Med. **97**:740-754, 1982.

372. Olds, G.R., Finegan, C., and Kresina, T.F.: Dynamics of hepatic glycosaminoglycan accumulation in murine *Schistosoma japonicum* infection, Gastroenterology **91**:1335-1342, 1986.

373. Oyedrian, A.B.O.O.: Renal disease due to schistosomiasis of the lower urinary tract, Kidney Int. **16**:15-22, 1979.

374. Pincus, S.H., Butterworth, A.E., David, J.R., Robbins, M., and Vadas, M.A.: Antibody-dependent eosinophil-mediated damage to schistosomula of *Schistosoma mansoni*: lack of requirement for oxidative metabolism, J. Immunol. **126**:1794-1799, 1981.

375. Rodríguez, H.F., García-Palmieri, M.R., Rivera, J.V., and Rodríguez-Molina, R.: A comparative study of portal and bilharzial cirrhosis, Gastroenterology **29**:235-246, 1955.

376. Sadisgursky, M., and Andrade, Z.A.: Pulmonary changes in schistosomal cor pulmonale, Am. J. Trop. Med. Hyg. **31**:779-783, 1982.

377. Sher, A., and Moser, G.: Schistosomiasis: immunologic properties of developing schistosomula, Am. J. Pathol. **102**:121-126, 1981.

378. Smith, J.H., Kelada, A.S., Khalil, A., et al.: Surgical pathology of schistosomal obstructive uropathy: a clinicopathologic correlation, Am. J. Trop. Med. Hyg. **26**:96-108, 1977.

379. Smith, J.H., and Christie, J.D.: The pathobiology of *Schistosoma hematobium* infection in humans, Hum. Pathol. **17**:333-345, 1986.

380. von Lichtenberg, F., Sher, A., and McIntyre, S.: A lung model of schistosome immunity in mice, Am. J. Pathol. **87**:105-124, 1977.

381. von Lichtenberg, F., Sher, A., Gibbons, N., et al.: Eosinophil-enriched inflammatory response to schistosomula in the skin of mice immune to *Schistosoma mansoni*, Am. J. Pathol. **84**:479-500, 1976.

382. Warren, K.S.: Hepatosplenic schistosomiasis mansoni: an immunologic disease, Bull. NY Acad. Med. **51**:545-550, 1975.

383. Warren, K.S.: Schistosomiasis: host-pathogen biology, Rev. Infect. Dis. **4**:771, 1982.

384. Warren, K.S.: The kinetics of hepatosplenic schistosomiasis, Semin. Liver Dis. **4**:293, 1984.

385. Warren, K.S., Su, D.L., Xu, Z.Y., Yuan, H.C., Peters, P.A., Cook, J.A., Mott, K.E., and Houser, H.B.: Morbidity in schistosomiasis japonica in relation to intensity of infection: a study of two rural brigades in Anhui Province, China, N. Engl. J. Med. **309**:1533, 1983.

386. Wright, E.D., Chiphangwi, J., and Hutt, M.S.R.: Schistosomiasis of the female tract: a histopathological study of 176 cases from Malawi, Trans. R. Soc. Trop. Med. Hyg. **76**:822-849, 1982.

387. Xu, Z., and Su, D.L.: *Schistosoma japonicum* and colorectal cancer: an epidemiological study in the People's Republic of China, Int. J. Cancer, **34**:315-318, 1984.

388. Zuckerman, M.J., Goldfarb, J.P., Cho, K.C., and Molnar, J.J.: An unusual pedunculated polyp of the colon: association with schistosomiasis, J. Clin. Gastroenterol. **5**:169-172, 1983.

Diseases caused by cestodes (tapeworms)

389. Abraham, J.L., Spore, W.W., and Benirschke, K.: Cysticercosis of the fallopian tube: histology and microanalysis, Hum. Pathol. **13**:665-670, 1982.

390. Beggs, I.: The radiology of hydatid disease, AJR **145**:639-648, 1985.

391. Berman, J.D., Beaver, P.C., Cheever, A.W., and Quindlen, E.A.: Cysticercus of 60-millimeter volume in human brain, Am. J. Trop. Med. Hyg. **30**:616-619, 1981.

392. Carbajal, J.R., Palacios, E., Azar-Kia, B., et al.: Radiology of cysticercosis of the central nervous system including computed tomography, Radiology **125**:127-131, 1977.

393. Castillo, M.: Intestinal taeniasis. In Marcial-Rojas, R.A., editor: Pathology of protozoal and helminthic diseases, Baltimore, 1971, The Williams & Wilkins Co.

394. D'Alessandro, A., et al.: *Echinococcus vogeli* in man, with a review of polycystic hydatid disease in Colombia and neighboring countries, Am. J. Trop. Med. Hyg. **28**:303, 1979.

395. de Ghetaldi, L.D., Norman, R.M., and Douville, A.W., Jr.: Cerebral cysticercosis treated biphasically with dexamethasone and praziquantel, Ann. Intern. Med. **99**:179-181, 1983.

396. Diwan, A.R., Coker-Vann, M., Brown, P., Subianto, D.B., Yolken, R., Desowitz, R., Escobar, A., Gibbs, C.J., Jr., and Gajdusek, D.C.: Enzyme-linked immunosorbent assay (ELISA) for the detection of antibody to cysticerci of *Taenia solium*, Am. J. Trop. Med. Hyg. **31**:249-369, 1982.

397. Hadidi, A.: Sonography of hepatic echnicoccal cysts, Gastrointest. Radiol. **7**:349-354, 1982.

398. Honma, K., Sasano, N., Andoh, N., and Iwai, K.: Hepatic alveolar echinococcosis invading pancreas, vertebrae and spinal cord, Hum. Pathol. **13**:944, 1982.

399. Iacona, A., Pini, C., and Vicari, G.: Enzyme-linked immunosorbent assay (ELISA) in the serodiagnosis of hydatid disease, Am. J. Trop. Med. Hyg. **29**:95-102, 1980.

400. Kune, G.A., Jones, T., and Sali, A.: Hydatid disease in Australia: prevention, clinical presentation and treatment, Med. J. Aust. **2**:385, 1983.

401. Lanier, A.P., Trujillo, D.E., Schantz, P.M., Wilson, J.F., Gottstein, B., and McMahon, B.J.: Comparison of serologic tests for the diagnosis and follow-up of alveolar hydatid disease, Am. J. Trop. Med. Hyg. **37**:609-615, 1987.

402. Lewall, D.B., and McCorkell, S.J.: Rupture of echinococcal cysts: diagnosis, classification and clinical implications, AJR **146**:391-394, 1986.

403. Maier, W.: Computed tomographic diagnosis of *Echinococcus alveolaris*, Hepato-gastroenterology **30**:83, 1983.

404. Márquez-Monter, H.: Cysticercosis. In Marcial-Rojas, R.A., editor: Pathology of protozoal and helminthic diseases, Baltimore, 1971, The Williams & Wilkins Co.

405. McCormick, G.F., Zee, C.S., and Heiden, J.: Cysticercosis cerebri: review of 127 cases, Arch. Neurol. **39**:534-539, 1982.

406. Messner, K.H., and Kammerer, W.S.: Intraocular cysticercosis, Arch. Ophthalmol. **97**:1103-1105, 1979.

407. Mohammad, I.N., Heiner, D.C., Miller, B.L., Goldberg, M.A., and Kagan, I.G.: Enzyme-linked immunosorbent assay for the diagnosis of cerebral cysticercosis, J. Clin. Microbiol. **20**:775-779, 1984.

408. Nakhla, N.B., Rais, K.J., Hasafa, T.M., Mosa, M.K., and Salem, H.H.: Ultrasound and the monitoring of the medical treatment of hepatic hydatid disease, J. Trop. Med. Hyg. 84:121-124, 1981.
409. Nash, T.E., and Neva, F.A.: Recent advances in the diagnosis and treatment of cerebral cysticercosis, N. Engl. J. Med. 311:1492, 1984.
410. Pandolfo, I., Blandino, G., Scribano, E., Longo, M., Certo, A., and Chirico, G.: CT findings in hepatic involvement by *Echinococcus granulosus*, J. Comput. Assist. Tomogr. 8:839, 1984.
411. Rangel, R., Torres, B., Del Bruto, O., and Sotelo, J.: Cysticercotic encephalitis: a severe form in young females, Am. J. Trop. Med. Hyg. 36:387-392, 1987.
412. Rausch, R.L., Wilson, J.F., Schantz, P.M., and McMahon, B.J.: Spontaneous death of *Echinococcus multilocularis*: cases diagnosed serologically (By EM₂ ELISA) and clinical significance, Am. J. Trop. Med. Hyg. 36:576-585, 1987.
413. Téllez-Girón, E., Ramos, M.C., Dufour, L., Alvarez, P., and Montante, M.: Detection of *Cysticercus cellulosae* antigens in cerebrospinal fluid by Dot enzyme-linked immunosorbent assay (Dot-ELISA), Am. J. Trop. Med. Hyg. 37:169-173, 1987.
414. Varela-Díaz, V.M., Coltorti, E.A., Prezioso, U., et al.: Evaluation of three immunodiagnostic tests for human hydatid disease, Am. J. Trop. Med. Hyg. 24:312-319, 1975.
415. Vijayan, G.P., Venkataraman, S., Suri, M.L., Seth, H.N., and Hoon, R.S.: Neurological and related manifestations of cysticercosis, Trop. Geogr. Med. 29:271-278, 1977.
416. Vik, R.: Diphyllobothriasis. In Marcial-Rojas, R.A., editor: Pathology or protozoal and helminthic diseases, Baltimore, 1971, The Williams & Wilkins Co.
417. von Bonsdorff, B.: *Diphyllobothrium latum* as a cause of pernicious anemia, Exp. Parasitol. 5:207-230, 1956.
418. von Bonsdorff, B.: Diphyllobothriasis in man, London, 1977, Academic Press, Inc.
419. Wilson, J.F., Rausch, R.L.: Alveolar hydatid disease: a review of clinical features of 33 indigenous cases of *Echinococcus multilocularis* infection in Alaskan Eskimos, Am. J. Trop. Med. Hyg. 29:1340, 1980.

Diseases caused by nematodes of the digestive tract

420. Areán, V.M.: Anisakiasis. In Marcial-Rojas, R.A., editor: Pathology of protozoal and helminthic diseases, Baltimore, 1971, The Williams & Wilkins Co.
421. Areán, V.M., and Crandall, C.A.: Ascariasis. In Marcial-Rojas, R.A., editor: Pathology of protozoal and helminthic diseases, Baltimore, 1971, The Williams & Wilkins Co.
422. Areán, V.M., and Crandall, C.A.: Toxocariasis. In Marcial-Rojas, R.A., editor: Pathology of protozoal and helminthic diseases, Baltimore, 1971, The Williams & Wilkins Co.
423. Areán, V.M.: Capillariasis. In Marcial-Rojas, R.A., editor: Pathology of protozoal and helminthic diseases, Baltimore, 1971, The Williams & Wilkins Co.
424. Attah, E.B., Nagarajan, S., Obineche, E.N., and Gera, S.C.: Hepatic capillariasis, Am. J. Clin. Pathol. 79:127, 1983.
425. Baird, J.K., Neafie, R.C., Lanoie, L., and Connor, D.H.: Abdominal angiostrongylosis in an African man: case study, Am. J. Trop. Med. Hyg. 37:353-356, 1987.
426. Bass, D.A., and Szejda, P.: Mechanisms of killing of newborn larvae of *Trichinella spiralis* by neutrophils and eosinophils: killing by generators of hydrogen peroxide in vitro, J. Clin. Invest. 64:1558-1564, 1979.
427. Beaver, P.C., Kriz, J.J., and Lau, T.J.: Pulmonary nodule caused by *Enterobius vermicularis*, Am. J. Trop. Med. Hyg. 22:711-713, 1973.
428. Beaver, P.C., et al.: Chronic eosinophilia due to visceral larva migrans: report of three cases, Pediatrics 9:7-19, 1952.
429. Beckman, E.N., and Holland, J.B.: Ovarian enterobiasis: a proposed pathogenesis, Am. J. Trop. Med. Hyg. 30:74-76, 1981.
430. Bell, R.G., McGregor, D.D., and Despommier, D.D.: *Trichinella spiralis*: mediation of the intestinal component of protective immunity in the rat by multiple phase-specific antiparasitic responses, Exp. Parasitol. 47:140-157, 1979.
431. Berger, R., Kraman, S., and Paciotti, M.: Pulmonary strongyloidiasis complicating therapy with corticosteroids, Am. J. Trop. Med. Hyg. 29:31-34, 1980.
432. Blumenthal, D.S.: Intestinal nematodes in the United States, N. Engl. J. Med. 297:1437-1439, 1977.
433. Blumenthal, D.S., and Schultz, M.G.: Incidence of intestinal obstruction in children infected with *Ascaris lumbricoides*, Am. J. Trop. Med. Hyg. 24:801-805, 1975.
434. Blumenthal, D.S., and Schultz, M.G.: Effects on *Ascaris* infection on nutritional status in children, Am. J. Trop. Med. Hyg. 25:682-690, 1976.
435. Boram, L.H., Keller, K.F., Justus, D.E., and Collins, J.P.: Strongyloidiasis in immunosuppressed patients, Am. J. Clin. Pathol. 76:778-781, 1981.
436. Brasitus, T.A.: Parasites and malabsorption, Am. J. Med. 67:1058-1065, 1979.
437. Butterworth, A.E., and David, J.R.: Eosinophil function, N. Engl. J. Med. 304:154-156, 1981.
438. Chandrasoma, P.T., and Mendis, K.N.: *Enterobius vermicularis* in ectopic sites, Am. J. Trop. Med. Hyg. 26:644-649, 1977.
439. Chitwood, M.B., Velásquez, C., and Salazar, N.G.: *Capillaria philippinensis*, sp. n. (Nematoda: Trichinellida) from the intestine of man in the Philippines, J. Parasitol. 54:368-371, 1972.
440. Cross, J.H.: Clinical manifestations and laboratory diagnosis of eosinophilic meningitis syndrome associated with angiostrongyliasis, Southeast Asian J. Trop. Med. Public Health 9:161-170, 1978.
441. Cross, J.H., Banzon, T., Clarke, M.D., et al.: Studies on the experimental transmission of *Capillaria philippinensis* in monkeys, Trans. R. Soc. Trop. Med. 66:819-827, 1972.
442. Currier, R.W., Herron, C.A., Hendricks, S.L., and Zimmermann, W.J.: A trichinosis outbreak in Iowa, JAMA 249:3196-3199, 1983.
443. Cypress, R.H., Karol, M.H., Zidian, J.L., et al.: Larva-specific antibodies in patients with visceral larva migrans, J. Infect. Dis. 135:633-636, 1977.
444. Daly, J.J., and Baker, G.F.: Pinworm granuloma of the liver, Am. J. Trop. Med. Hyg. 33:62, 1984.
445. Deardorff, T.L., Fukumura, T., and Raybowne, R.B.: Invasive anisakiasis: a case report from Hawaii, Gastroenterology 90:1047-1050, 1986.
446. Despommier, D.: Adaptive changes in muscle fibers infected with *Trichinella spiralis*, Am. J. Pathol. 78:477-496, 1975.
447. Despommier, D., Müller, M., Jenks, B., et al.: Immunodiagnosis of human trichinosis using counterimmunoelectrophoresis and agar gel diffusion techniques, Am. J. Trop. Med. Hyg. 23:41-44, 1974.
448. Dessein, A.J., Parker, W.L., James, S.L., and David, J.R.: IgE antibody and resistance to infection. I. Selective suppression of the IgE antibody response in rats diminishes the resistance and the eosinophil response to *Trichinella spiralis* infection, J. Exp. Med. 153:423-436, 1981.
449. Detels, R., Gutman, L., Jaramillo, J., et al.: An epidemic of intestinal capillariasis in man: a study in a barrio in northern Luzon, Am. J. Trop. Med. Hyg. 18:676, 1969.
450. Fishman, J.A., and Perrone, T.L.: Colonic obstruction and perforation due to *Trichuris trichiura*, Am. J. Med. 77:154-156, 1984.
451. Frayha, R.A.: Trichinosis-related polyarteritis nodosa, Am. J. Med. 71:307-312, 1981.
452. Frenkel, J.K.: *Angiostrongylus costaricensis* infections. In Binford, C.H., and Connor, D.H., editors: Pathology of tropical and extraordinary diseases, Washington, D.C., 1976, Armed Forces Institute of Pathology.
453. Fresh, J.W., Cross, J.H., Reyes, V., et al.: Necropsy findings in intestinal capillariasis, Am. J. Trop. Med. Hyg. 21:169-173, 1972.
454. Galvão, V.A.: Estudios sobre *Capillaria hepatica*: uma avaliação do seu papel patogénico para o homem, Mem. Inst. Oswaldo Cruz 76:415, 1981.
455. Gam, A.A., Neva, F.A., and Krotoski, W.A.: Comparative sensitivity and specificity of ELISA and IHA for serodiagnosis of strongyloidiasis with larval antigens, Am. J. Trop. Med. Hyg. 37:157-161, 1987.

456. Genta, R.M.: Immunobiology of strongyloidiasis, Trop. Geogr. Med. **30:**223, 1984.
457. Genta, R.M., Ottesen, E.A., Poindexter, R., Gann, A.A., Neva, F.A., Tanowitz, H.B., and Wittner, M.: Specific allergic sensitization to *Strongyloides* antigens in human strongyloidiasis, Lab. Invest. **48:**633-638, 1983.
458. Genta, R.M., and Ward, P.A.: The histopathology of experimental strongyloidiasis, Am. J. Pathol. **99:**207-220, 1980.
459. Genta, R.M., and Weil, G.J.: Antibodies to *Strongyloides stercoralis* larval surface antigens in chronic strongyloidiasis, Lab. Invest. **47:**87-90, 1982.
460. Gilman, R.H., Chong, Y.H., Davis, C., Greenberg, B., Virik, H.K., and Dixon, H.B.: The adverse consequences of heavy *Trichuris* infection, Trans. R. Soc. Trop. Med. Hyg. **77:**432-438, 1983.
461. Glickman, L.T.: Toxocariasis. In Warren, K.S., and Mahmoud, A.A.F., editors: Tropical and geographical medicine, New York, 1984, McGraw Hill Book Co.
462. Glickman, L.T., and Schantz, P.M.: Epidemiology and pathogenesis of zoonotic toxocariasis, Epidemiol. Rev. **3:**20, 1981.
463. Glickman, L.T., Schantz, P., Dombroske, R., and Cypess, R.: Evaluation of serodiagnostic tests for visceral larva migrans, Am. J. Trop. Med. Hyg. **27:**492-498, 1978.
464. Greenberg, E.R., and Cline, B.L.: Is trichuriasis associated with iron deficiency anemia? Am. J. Trop. Med. Hyg. **28:**770-772, 1979.
465. Grove, D.I., and Blair, J.: Diagnosis of human strongyloidiasis by immunofluorescence, using *Strongyloides ratti* and *S. stercoralis* larvae, Am. J. Trop. Med. Hyg. **30:**344-349, 1981.
466. Grove, D.I., Mahmoud, A.A.F., and Warren, K.S.: Eosinophils and resistance to *Trichinella spiralis*, J. Exp. Med. **145:**755-759, 1977.
467. Hsiu, J.G., Gamsey, A.J., Ives, C.E., D'Amato, N.A., and Hiller, A.N.: Gastric anisakiasis: report of a case with clinical, endoscopic and histological findings, Am. J. Gastroenterol. **81:**1185-1187, 1986.
468. Jacobson, E.S., and Jacobson, H.G.: Trichinosis in an immunosuppressed human host, Am. J. Clin. Pathol. **68:**791-794, 1977.
469. Kaimal, K.P., and Beyt, B.E., Jr.: Cardiac dysfunction in trichinosis, N. Engl. J. Med. **307:**374-375, 1982.
470. Kanchanaranya, C., Prechanond, A., and Punyagupta, S.: Removal of living worm in retinal *Angiostrongylus cantonesis*, J. Ophthalmol. **74:**456-458, 1972.
471. Kayes, S.G., and Oaks, J.A.: Development of the granulomatous response in murine toxocariasis, Am. J. Pathol. **93:**277-294, 1978.
472. Kazura, J.W.: Host defense mechanisms against nematode parasites: destruction of *Trichinella spiralis* newborn larvae by parasite stage specific human antibody and granulocytes, J. Infect. Dis. **143:**712-718, 1981.
473. Kazura, J.W., and Aikawa, M.: Host defense mechanism against *Trichinella spiralis* infection in the mouse: eosinophil-mediated destruction of larvae in vitro, J. Immunol. **124:**355-361, 1980.
474. Kenney, M., and Webber, C.A.: Diagnosis of strongyloidiasis in Papanicolaou-stained sputum smears, Acta Cytol. **18:**270-273, 1974.
475. Khuroo, M.S., Zargar, S.A., Mahajan, R., Bhat, R.L., and Javid, G.: Sonographic appearances in biliary ascariasis, Gastroenterology **93:**267-272, 1987.
476. Khuroo, M.S., and Zargar, S.A.: Biliary ascariasis: a common cause of biliary and pancreatic disease in an endemic area, Gastroenterology **88:**418, 1985.
477. Kliks, M.M.: Anisakiasis in the western United States: four new case reports from California, Am. J. Trop. Med. Hyg. **32:**526-532, 1983.
478. Krige, J.E.J., Lewis, G., and Bornman, P.C.: Recurrent pancreatitis caused by a calcified ascaris in the duct of Wirsung, Am. J. Gastroenterol. **82:**256-257, 1987.
479. Kusuhara, T., Watanabe, K., and Fukuda, M.: Radiographic study of acute gastric anisakiasis, Gastrointest. Radiol. **9:**305-309, 1984.
480. Laqueur, G.L.: Eosinophilic meningitis (*Angiostrongylus cantonensis*). In Marcial-Rojas, R.A., editor: Pathology of protozoal and helminthic diseases, Baltimore, 1971, The Williams & Wilkins Co.
481. Layrisse, M., Aparcedo, L., Martínez-Torres, C., et al.: Blood loss due to infection with *Trichuris trichiura*, Am. J. Trop. Med. Hyg. **16:**613-619, 1967.
482. Little, M.D., Cuello, C.J., and D'Alessandro, A.: Granuloma of the liver due to *Enterobius vermicularis*, Am. J. Trop. Med. Hyg. **22:**567-569, 1973.
483. Little, M.D., and Mast, H.: Anisakid larva from the throat of a woman in New York, Am. J. Trop. Med. Hyg. **22:**609-612, 1973.
484. Lord, W.D., and Bullock, W.L.: Swine ascaris in humans, N. Engl. J. Med. **306:**1113, 1982.
485. Loria-Cortés, R., and Lobo-Sanahuja, J.F.: Clinical abdominal angiostrongylosis: a study of 116 children with intestinal eosinophilic granuloma caused by *Angiostrongylus costaricensis*, Am. J. Trop. Med. Hyg. **29:**538-544, 1980.
486. Lotero, H., Tripathy, K., and Bolaños, O.: Gastrointestinal blood loss in *Trichuris* infection, Am. J. Trop. Med. Hyg. **23:**1203-1204, 1974.
487. Malek, E.A.: Presence of *Angiostrongylus costaricensis* Morera and Céspedes 1971 in Colombia, Am. J. Trop. Med. Hyg. **30:**81-83, 1981.
488. Manson-Smith, D.F., Bruce, R.G., and Parrott, D.M.V.: Villous atrophy and expulsion of intestinal *Trichinella spiralis* are mediated by T cells, Cell. Immunol. **47:**285-292, 1979.
489. Marcial-Rojas, R.A.: Strongyloidiasis. In Marcial-Rojas, R.A., editor: Pathology of protozoal and helminthic diseases, Baltimore, 1971, The Williams & Wilkins Co.
490. Marsden, P.D.: Strongyloidiasis: a replicating human helminthic infection, Trop. Gastroenterol. **3:**9-14, 1982.
491. Maxwell, C., Hussain, R., Nutman, T.B., Poindexter, R.W., Little, M.D., Schad, G.A., and Ottesen, E.A.: The clinical and immunologic responses of normal human volunteers to low dose hookworm (*Necatur americanus*) infection, Am. J. Trop. Med. Hyg. **37:**126-134, 1987.
492. McMahon, J.N., Connolly, C.E., Long, S.V., and Meehan, F.P.: *Enterobius* granulomas of the uterus, ovary and pelvic peritoneum: two case reports, Br. J. Obstet. Gynaecol. **91:**289-290, 1984.
493. Mendoza, E., Jordà, M., Rafel, E., Simón, A., and Andrada, E.: Invasion of human embryo by *Enterobius vermicularis*, Arch. Pathol. Lab. Med. **111:**761-762, 1987.
494. Milder, J.E., Walzer, P.D., Kilgore, G., Rutherford, I., and Klein, M.: Clinical features of *Strongyloides stercoralis* infection in an endemic area of the United States, Gastroenterology **80:**1481-1488, 1981.
495. Morera, P.: Life history and redescription of *Angiostrongylus costaricensis* Morera and Céspedes, Am. J. Trop. Med. Hyg. **22:**613-621, 1973.
496. Morera, P., Pérez, F., Mora, F., et al.: Visceral larva migrans–like syndrome caused by *Angiostrongylus costaricensis*, Am. J. Trop. Med. Hyg. **31:**67-70, 1982.
497. Morgan, O., James, O., and Sahoy, R.: Intestinal perforation in ascariasis: case report, Trans. R. Soc. Trop. Med. Hyg. **73:**183-184, 1979.
498. Most, H.: Trichinosis—preventable yet still with us, N. Engl. J. Med. **298:**1178-1180, 1978.
499. Most, H., and Abeles, M.M.: Trichiniasis involving nervous system: clinical and neuropathologic review with report of 2 cases, Arch. Neurol. **37:**589-616, 1937.
500. Neafie, R.C., Connor, D.H., and Cross, J.H.: Capillariasis. In Binford, C.H., and Connor, D.H., editors: Pathology of tropical and extraordinary diseases, Washington, D.C., 1976, Armed Forces Institute of Pathology.
501. Neva, F.A.: Biology and immunology of human strongyloidiasis, J. Infect. Dis. **153:**397-406, 1986.
502. Neva, F.A., Gam, A.A., and Burke, J.: Comparison of larval antigens in an enzyme-linked immunosorbent assay for strongyloidiasis in humans, J. Infect. Dis. **144:**427, 1981.

503. Nye, S.W., Tangchai, P., Sundarakiti, S., et al.: Lesions of the brain in eosinophilic meningitis, Arch. Pathol. 89:9-19, 1970.

504. Ogilvie, B.M., Bartlett, A., Godfrey, R.C., Turton, J.A., Worms, M.J., and Yeates, R.A.: Antibody responses in self-infections with Necator americanus, Trans. R. Soc. Trop. Med. Hyg. 72:66-71, 1978.

505. Paulino, G.B., Jr., and Wittenberg, J.: Intestinal capillariasis: a new cause of a malabsorption pattern, Am. J. Roengenol. Radium Ther. Nucl. Med. 117:340-345, 1973.

506. Pawloski, F.S.: Ascariasis: host-pathogen biology, Rev. Infect. Dis. 4:806, 1982.

507. Pelletier, L.L., and Gabre-Kidan, T.: Chronic strongyloidiasis in Vietnam veterans, Am. J. Med. 78:139-140, 1985.

508. Pinkus, G.S., Coolidge, C., and Little, M.D.: Intestinal anisakiasis: first case report from North America, Am. J. Med. 59:114-120, 1975.

509. Punyagupta, S., Juttijudata, P., and Bunnag, T.: Eosinophilic meningitis in Thailand: clinical studies of 484 cases probably caused by Angiostrongylus cantonensis, Am. J. Trop. Med. Hyg. 24:921, 1975.

510. Raybourne, R., and Solomon, C.B.: Capillaria hepatica: granuloma formation to eggs. III. Anti-immunoglobulin augmentation and reagin activity in mice, Exp. Parasitol. 38:87-95, 1975.

511. Raybourne, R.B., Solomon, G.B., and Soulsby, E.J.L.: Capillaria hepatica: granuloma formation to eggs, II. Peripheral immunological responses. Exp. Parasitol. 36:244-252, 1974.

512. Reddy, C.R.R., Venkateswar Rao, D., Sarma, E.N., et al.: Granulomatous peritonitis due to Ascaris lumbricoides and its ova, J. Trop. Med. Hyg. 78:146, 1975.

513. Rivera, E., Maldonado, N., Vélez-García, E., et al.: Hyperinfection syndrome with Strongyloides stercoralis, Ann. Intern. Med. 72:199, 1970.

514. Rosset, J.S., McClatchey, K.D., Higashi, G.I., and Knisely, A.S.: Anisakis larval type I in fresh salmon, Am. J. Clin. Pathol. 78:54-57, 1982.

515. Rushovich, A.M., Randall, E.L., Caprini, J.A., and Westenfelder, G.O.: Omental anisakiasis: a rare mimic of acute appendicitis, Am. J. Clin. Pathol. 80:517-520, 1983.

516. Sauerbrey, M.: A precipitin test for the diagnosis of human abdominal angiostrongyliasis, Am. J. Trop. Med. Hyg. 26:1156-1158, 1977.

517. Schantz, P.M., and Glickman, L.T.: Toxocaral visceral larva migrans, N. Engl. J. Med. 298:436-439, 1978.

518. Schulman, A., Loxton, A.J., Heydenrych, J.J., and Abdurahman, K.E.: Sonographic diagnosis of biliary ascariasis, AJR 139:485, 1982.

519. Scowden, E.B., Schaffner, W., and Stone, W.J.: Overwhelming strongyloidiasis: an unappreciated opportunistic infection, Medicine 57:527-544, 1978.

520. Simon, R.D.: Pinworm infestation and urinary tract infection in young girls, Am. J. Dis. Child. 128:21-22, 1974.

521. Sitprija, V., Keoplung, M., Boonpucknavig, V., and Boonpucknavig, S.: Renal involvement in human trichinosis, Arch. Intern. Med. 140:544-546, 1980.

522. Smith, J.W., and Wooten, R.: Anisakis and anisakiasis, Adv. Parasitol. 16:93-163, 1978.

523. Solomon, C.B., and Crigonis, C.J., Jr.: Capillaria hepatica: relation of structure and composition of egg shell to antigen release, Exp. Parasitol. 40:298-307, 1976.

524. Solomon, G.B., and Soulsby, E.J.L.: Granuloma formation to Capillaria hepatica eggs. I. Descriptive definition, Exp. Parasitol. 33:458-467, 1973.

525. Spillman, R.K.: Pulmonary ascariasis in tropical communities, Am. J. Trop. Med. Hyg. 24:791-800, 1975.

526. Trichinosis surveillance annual summary 1979, Atlanta, 1980. Centers for Disease Control, U.S. Department of Health and Human Services.

527. Ubelaker, J.E., and Hall, N.M.: First report of Angiostrongylus costaricensis Morera and Céspedes 1971 in the United States, J. Parasitol. 65:307, 1979.

528. Ursell, P.C., Habib, A., Babchick, O., Rottolo, R., Despommier, D., and Fenoglio, J.J.: Myocarditis caused by Trichinella spiralis, Arch. Pathol. Lab. Med. 108:4-5, 1984. (Letter.)

529. Vafai, M., and Mohtt, P.: Granuloma of the anal canal due to Enterobium vermicularis, Dis. Colon Rectum 26:349-350, 1983.

530. Variyam, E.P., and Banwell, J.G.: Nutrition implications of hookworm infection, Rev. Infect. Dis. 4:830-835, 1982.

531. van Knapen, F., van Leusden, J., Polderman, A.M., and Franchimont, J.H.: Visceral larva migrans: examination by means of enzyme-linked immunosorbent assay of human sera for antibodies to excretory-secretory antigens of the second-stage larvae of Toxocara canis, Z. Parasitenkd. 69:113, 1983.

532. Viallet, J., MacLean, J.D., Goresky, C.A., Staudt, M., Routhier, G., and Law, C.: Arctic trichinosis presenting as prolonged diarrhea, Gastroenterology 91:938-946, 1986.

533. Wasson, D.L., and Gleida, C.J.: Damage to Trichinella spiralis newborn larvae by eosinophil major basic protein, Am. J. Trop. Med. Hyg. 28:860-863, 1979.

534. Watten, R.H., Beckner, W.M., Cross, J.H., et al.: Clinical studies of capillariasis philippinensis, Trans. R. Soc. Trop. Med. Hyg. 66:828-834, 1972.

535. Welch, J.S., Dobson, C., and Campbell, G.R.: Immunodiagnosis and seroepidemiology of Angiostrongylus cantonensis zoonoses in man, Trans. R. Soc. Trop. Med. Hyg. 74:614-623, 1980.

536. Whalen, G.E., Rosenberg, E.B., and Stickland, G.T.: Circulating immunoglobulins, intestinal protein loss, and malabsorption in intestinal capillariasis, Ann. Intern. Med. 70:1072, 1969.

537. Whalen, G.E., Rosenberg, E.B., Strickland, G.T., et al.: Intestinal capillariasis: a new disease in man, Lancet 1:13, 1969.

538. Wilder, H.C.: Nematode endophthalmitis, Trans. Am. Acad. Ophthalmol. 55:99-109, 1950.

539. Winters, C., Chobanian, S.J., Benjamin, S.B., Ferguson, R.K., and Cattau, E.L., Jr.: Endoscopic documentation of Ascaris-induced pancreatitis, Gastrointest. Endosc. 30:83, 1984.

540. Wong, B.: Parasitic diseases in immuno-compromised hosts, Am. J. Med. 76:479, 1984.

541. Wright, K.A.: Trichinella spiralis: an intracellular parasite in the intestinal phase, J. Parasitol. 65:441-445, 1979.

542. Yii, C.Y.: Clinical observations of eosinophilic meningitis and meningoencephalitis caused by Angiostrongylus cantonensis on Taiwan, Am. J. Trop. Med. Hyg. 25:233-249, 1976.

543. Yii, C.Y., and Cross, J.H.: Human angiostrongyliasis in Taiwan, Southeast Asian J. Trop. Med. Public Health 1:154-155, 1970.

544. Zimmerman, W.J., Steele, J.H., and Kagan, I.G.: Trichinosis in the U.S. population, 1966-1970: prevalence and epidemiologic factors, Health Serv. Rep. 88:606-623, 1973.

Diseases caused by filarial nematodes (filariasis)

545. Bartlett, A., Bidwell, D., and Voller, A.: Preliminary studies on the application of enzyme-immunoassay in the detection of antibodies in onchocerciasis, Trop. Med. Parasitol. 26:370-374, 1975.

546. Chen, Y.H., and Qun, X.: Filarial granuloma of the female breast: a histopathological study of 131 cases, Am. J. Trop. Med. Hyg. 30:1206-1210, 1981.

547. Connor, D.H.: Onchocerciasis, N. Engl. J. Med. 298:379-381, 1978.

548. Connor, D.H., Gibson, D.W., Neafie, R.C., Merighi, B., and Buck, A.A.: Sowda—onchocerciasis in north Yemen: a clinicopathologic study of 18 patients, Am. J. Trop. Med. Hyg. 32:123-137, 1983.

549. Connor, D.H., Palmieri, J.R., and Gibson, D.W.: Pathogenesis of lymphatic filariasis in man, Z. Parasitenkd. 72:13-18, 1986.

550. Darrow, J.C., and Lack, E.F.: Solitary lung nodule due to Dirofilaria immates (dog "heartworm"), J. Surg. Oncol. 16:219-224, 1981.

551. de Buen, S.: Onchocerciasis. In Marcial-Rojas, R.A., editor: Pathology of protozoal and helminthic diseases, Baltimore, 1971, The Williams & Wilkins Co.

552. Galindo, L.: Bancroftian filariasis. In Marcial-Rojas, R.A., editor: Pathology of protozoal and helminthic diseases, Baltimore, 1971, The Williams & Wilkins Co.

553. Gentilini, M., Carme, B., Smith, M., Brucker, G., and Nosny, Y.: A case of eosinophilic pleurisy due to *Dracunculus medinensis* infection, Trans. R. Soc. Trop. Med. Hyg. **72:**540-541, 1978.

554. Gibson, D.W., and Connor, D.H.: Onchocercal lymphadenitis: clinicopathologic study of 34 patients, Trans. R. Soc. Trop. Med. Hyg. **72:**137-153, 1978.

555. Gibson, D.W., Heggie, C., and Connor, D.H.: Clinical and pathological aspects of onchocerciasis, Pathol. Annu. **15:**195-240, 1980.

556. Greene, B.M., Taylor, H.R., and Aikawa, M.: Cellular killing of microfilariae of *Onchocerca volvolus:* eosinophil and neutrophil mediated immune serum dependent destruction, J. Immunol. **127:**1611-1618, 1981.

557. Grove, D.I., and Davis, R.S.: Serological diagnosis of bancroftian and malaysian filariasis, Am. J. Trop. Med. Hyg. **27:**508-513, 1978.

558. Grove, D.I., and Forbes, I.J.: Immunosuppression in bancroftian filariasis, Trans. R. Soc. Trop. Med. Hyg. **73:**23-26, 1979.

559. Gutiérrez, Y.: Diagnostic features of zoonotic filariae in tissue sections, Hum. Pathol. **15:**514-525, 1984.

560. Gutiérrez, Y., and Paul, G.M.: Breast nodule produced by *Dirofilaria tenuis*, Am. J. Surg. Pathol. **8:**463-465, 1984.

561. Hashiguchi, Y., Kawabata, M., Zea, G., Recinos, M.M., and Flores, O.: The use of an *Onchocerca volvulus* microfilarial antigen skin test in epidemiological survey of onchocerciasis in Guatemala, Trans. R. Soc. Trop. Med. Hyg. **73:**543-548, 1979.

562. Reference moved to 578.

563. Kahn, F.W., Wester, S.M., and Agger, W.A.: Pulmonary dirofilariasis and transitional cell carcinoma, Arch. Intern. Med. **143:**1259-1260, 1983.

564. Kaliraj, P., Ghirmikar, S.N., and Harinath, B.C.: Immunodiagnosis of bancroftian filariasis: Comparative efficiency of the indirect hemagglutination test, indirect fluorescent antibody test and enzyme-linked immunosorbent assay done with *Wuchereria bancrofti* microfilarial antigens, Am. J. Trop. Med. Hyg. **30:**982-987, 1981.

565. Kephart, G.M., Gleich, G.J., Connor, D.H., Gibson, D.W., and Ackerman, S.J.: Deposition of eosinophil granule major basic protein onto microfilariae of *Onchocerva volvolus* in the skin of patients treated with diethylcarbamazine, Lab. Invest. **50:**51-61, 1984.

566. Lang, A.P., Luchsinger, I.S., and Rawling, E.G.: Filariasis of the breast, Arch. Pathol. Lab. Med. **111:**757-759, 1987.

567. Meyers, W.M., Neafie, R.C., and Connor, D.H.: Onchocerciasis invasion of deep organs by *Onchocerca volvolus*, autopsy findings, Am. J. Trop. Med. Hyg. **26:**650-657, 1977.

568. Neva, F.A., and Ottensen, E.A.: Tropical (filarial) eosinophilia, N. Engl. J. Med. **298:**1129-1131, 1978.

569. Nutman, T.B.: *Loa loa* infection in temporary residents of endemic regions: recognition of hyperresponsive syndrome with characteristic clinical manifestations, J. Infect. Dis. **154:**10-18, 1986.

570. Ottesen, E.A.: Immunopathology of lymphatic filariasis in man, Springer Semin. Immunopathol. **2:**373-385, 1980.

571. Ottesen, E.A.: Immunological aspects of lymphatic filariasis and onchocerciasis in man, Trans. R. Soc. Trop. Med. Hyg. **78**(suppl.):9-18, 1984.

572. Ottesen, E.A., Neva, F.A., Paranjape, R.S., Tripathy, S.P., Thiruvengadam, K.V., and Beaven, M.A.: Specific allergic sensitization to filarial antigens in tropical eosinophilia syndrome, Lancet **1:**1158-1161, 1979.

573. Piessens, W.F., Partono, F., Hoffman, S.L., Ratiwayanto, S., Piessens, P.W., Palmieri, J.R., Koiman, I., Dennis, D.T., and Carney, W.P.: Antigen-specific suppressor T lymphocytes in human lymphatic filariasis, N. Engl. J. Med. **307:**144-148, 1982.

574. Price, D.L., and Child, P.L.: Dracontiasis (dracunculiasis, dracunculosis, Medina worm, Guinea worm). In Marcial-Rojas, R.A., editor: Pathology of protozoal and helminthic diseases, Baltimore, 1971, The Williams & Wilkins Co.

575. Price, D.L., and Hopps, H.C.: Loiasis (the eyeworm, loa worm). In Marcial-Rojas, R.A., editor: Pathology of protozoal and helminthic diseases, Baltimore, 1971, The Williams & Wilkins Co.

576. Sacks H.N., Williams, D.N., and Eifrig, D.E.: Loiasis: report of a case and review of the literature, Arch. Intern. Med. **136:**914-915, 1976.

577. Thompson, J.H., and Harrison, E.G.: Dirofilariasis. In Marcial-Rojas, R.A., editor: Pathology of protozoal and helminthic diseases, Baltimore, 1971, The William & Wilkins Co.

578. Zheng, H.J., Tao, Z.H., Reddy, M.V., Harinath, B.C., and Piessens, W.F.: Parasite antigens in sera and urine of patients with Bancroftian and Brugian filariasis detected by sandwich ELISA with monoclonal antibodies, Am. J. Trop. Med. Hyg. **36:**554-560, 1987.

12 Immunopathology (Hypersensitivity Diseases)

STEWART SELL

Immunity means protection or security from diseases or poisons. Immunopathology is the study of diseases caused by immune mechanisms. The word *immunopathology* illustrates the paradox of immune reactions. On one hand, immune reactions provide efficient protection against infectious organisms; on the other hand, they may destroy the host's own tissues and cause disease.

Specific immune protection is mediated by products generated as a result of an immune response, which involves proliferation and differentiation of cells in the lymphoid system. This specific protection depends on previous exposure of the individual to the particular noxious agent or organism (antigen). As a result of this primary exposure to antigen, there develop serum proteins (antibodies) or altered cells (specifically sensitized cells) that have the capacity to recognize, react with, and neutralize the noxious agent or infecting organism.

The term *allergy* has different meanings depending on how it is used. Von Pirquet originally coined the term in 1906 to mean altered reactivity to a given agent because of a previous exposure to it, without judging whether the altered effect was good or bad. In Britain allergy designates any nonprotective immune reaction; in the United States the term usually refers to atopic reactions. *Hypersensitivity* implies destructive effects of any immune reaction.

Many examples of altered reactivity because of a previous exposure are not reactions of allergy or immunity. Some of these phenomena include the Shwartzman reaction (alteration in the state of blood coagulation), adaptive enzyme synthesis (substrate selection of enzyme production), anaphylactoid reactions (pseudoallergic reactions attributable to nonallergic liberation of pharmacologically active agents that may also be liberated by allergic reactions), untoward reactions to drugs attributable to physiologic hyperreactivity (idiosyncrasy), and other types of adaptations to environmental parameters (heat adaptation, cold adaptation, altitude adaptation, emotional adaptation, and so on).

BASIC IMMUNOLOGY
Antigenicity

In all types of immunologic or allergic reactions an individual's immune system acquires specific information (learns) from contact with an antigen (Ag). The acquisition and expression of this immunologic knowledge consists in afferent, central, and efferent phases. The afferent phase is the delivery of antigen to specifically reactive cells usually but not always in lymph nodes. The central phase is proliferation and differentiation of cells in the lymphoid system leading to the production of antibody or cells that recognize and react with the antigen. The efferent phase is the delivery of the immune products to tissues that contain the antigen and is initiated by the reaction of antibody or sensitized cells with the antigen in situ. The result of this reaction is protective if the antigen is an infecting agent or noxious material; it may be destructive if the antigen is associated with normal tissue.

Essential to an immune response is the capacity of the individual's immune system to recognize an antigen. Most natural antigens are other organisms (bacteria, viruses, fungi). Experimental or therapeutic procedures provide contact with other potential antigens, such as exogenous macromolecules (drugs), serum proteins, blood cells, or tissues (grafts) from individuals of the same or other species. An antigen that can induce an immune response is termed an *immunogen*. The capacity of an individual to respond to a given immunogen depends on several factors, such as dose, route, form, degree of foreignness, and number of previous exposures to the immunogen. The products of the immune response are humoral (immunoglobulin) antibody and cellular (specifically sensitized cells).

Haptens

Some antigens are unable to induce an immune response but are able to react with products of an immune response generated as a result of immunization with the nonimmunogenic molecule complexed to a complete antigen (carrier).

487

Hapten   → No response
Carrier   → Anticarrier
Carrier + Hapten → Anticarrier + Antihapten

Such an antigen (hapten) is called an incomplete antigen. Some drugs and chemicals responsible for allergic reactions, such as penicillin metabolites, nickel, or the poison ivy allergen, act as haptens by conjugating to host proteins, which act as carriers.

Immunoglobulins and antibodies

Circulating antibodies belong to one or more of several groups of structurally related proteins known collectively as immunoglobulins. The structural features of an immunoglobulin molecule are presented in Fig. 12-1. Immunoglobulins may be divided into several major classes (Table 12-1). The manifestations of the reaction of antibody with antigen in vivo depends on the class of immunoglobulin to which the antibody belongs, as well as the location of the tissue in which the reaction takes place.

Epitopes, paratopes, and idiotopes

The antigenic structure (determinant) that is recognized by an antibody combining site is termed an *epitope*. The antibody binding site is called a *paratope*. The paratope is formed by folding of the variable regions of the light and heavy chains of an Ig molecule so that the hypervariable segments form a site that will fit over the epitope and provide charge, hydrogen, and hydrophilic fields that hold the epitope. Most antigens contain many epitopes. The composit reactivity of the epitopes of an antigen is called an *epitype*.

Idiotypes

Antibodies that recognize determinants in another antibody molecule may be produced. These anti-antibodies that are specific for a given antibody species are

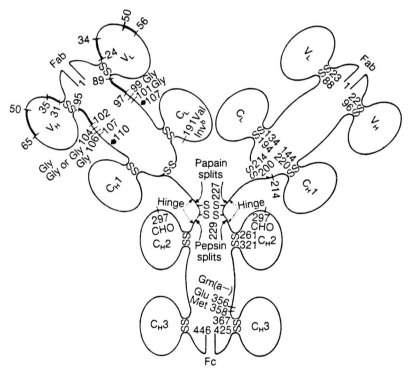

Fig. 12-1. Schema of four-chain structure of human IgG molecule. Numbers *on right side* are actual residues of myeloma protein EU; numbers of Fab fragments *on left side* aligned for maximum homology; light chains numbered as by Kabat (J. Immunol. **125**:961, 1980). Hypervariable regions, complementarity-determining regions (CDR) that form paratope when IgG molecule is folded, are indicated by the *heavy lines* in the V_H and V_L domains. V_L and V_H, Light- and heavy-chain variable regions: C_H1, C_H2, and C_H3, domains of constant region of heavy chain; C_L, constant region of light chain. Hinge region in which two heavy chains are linked by disulfide bonds is indicated approximately. Attachment of carbohydrate is at residue 297. Arrows at residues 107 and 110 denote transition from variable to constant regions. Sites of action of papain before the hinge region and pepsin after the hinge region show why papain produces Fab monomers and pepsin produces F(ab)2 dimers. Locations of several inheritable allotypic differences, *Gm, Inv,* are given.

Table 12-1. Some properties of immunoglobulins

Ig class	Structure	Serum concentration (mg/ml)	Size (mol. wt.)	Antigen-binding sites	Complement fixation	Antibody activity	Immune effector function
IgG		12	140,000	2	+	Major class, precipitating	Toxic complex, neutralization, cytotoxic
IgA		2.5	160,000 to 320,000 (dimer)	4	−	Secretory	Toxic complex (rare)
IgM		1	900,000* (pentamer)	10	+ +	First formed, highly lytic, B cell surface	Cytotoxic
IgE	Mast cell	0.0005	180,000	2	−	Binds to mast cells	Anaphylactic
IgD	B cell	0.03	200,000*	2	−	B cell surface	?

−, None; +, some; + +, more.
*μ and α chains contain an N-derived polypeptide associated with B-cell membrane insertion.

called *anti-idiotypes*. Three major classes of anti-idiotypic antibodies are possible (Fig. 12-2). The most important of these is an anti-idiotope that reacts specifically with the paratope of the first antibody. The antigen binding site of this anti-idiotope may be structurally identical to the antigen (epitope) with which the first antibody reacts.

Antigen   →   Antibody 1   →   Antibody 2a
(Epitope)   (Anti-idiotype)

This is called molecular mimicry and has important implications for some autoimmune diseases (see discussion of idiotype networks, internal images and hormone receptors, p. 508).

Immunoglobulin genes and their expression

The variable and constant regions of immunoglobulin molecules are coded by a string of exons separated by noncoding introns. The genes for the heavy chains for human Ig are on chromosome no. 8; κ chains on chromosome no. 2, and λ chains on chromosome no. 22. In addition to variable (V), and constant (C) genes, heavy-chain genes have a diversity (D) and joining (J) region; light-chain genes, a J region but no D region. Immunoglobulin gene rearrangements occur during B-cell differentiation. Juxtaposition of the exons by looping out or removal of introns is required for transcription of immunoglobulin genes by B-cells.

Antibody-antigen reactions

Primary antibody-antigen reaction. The combination of antigen with antibody to form an antigen-antibody

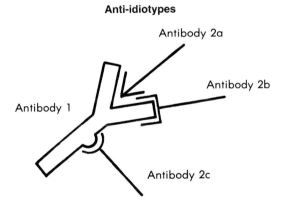

Anti-idiotypes

Fig. 12-2. Anti-idiotypic antibodies to an antibody may react with the paratope (anti-idiotype 2a), with part of the paratope and part of the adjacent nonparatope variable region (anti-idiotype 2b) or with nonparatopic variable region (anti-idiotype 2c). The paratope of anti-idiotype 2a may mimic the antigen to which the original antibody reacts and has been termed the internal image of the antigen. Anti-idiotype 2a will block the binding of the antigen to the antibody completely. Anti-idiotype 2b will block partially and anti-idiotype 2c may not block at all unless the tertiary structure is changed by binding of anti-idiotype 2c. (From Sell, S.: Basic immunology, New York, copyright 1987, Elsevier Science Publishing Co., Inc.)

complex is termed the *primary reaction of antibody.* The primary reaction may be considered an equilibrium between free antigen and free antibody on the one hand and bound antigen and antibody (that is, antigen-antibody complex) on the other.

Primary reaction	Secondary reactions	In vivo reaction
	Precipitation →	Tissue damage
	Agglutination	
	Lysis	
	Complement fixation	
	Immobilization	
	Neutralization etc.	

Ag + Ab ⇌ AgAb complex (Affinity / Avidity)

Secondary antibody-antigen reactions. On formation of antibody-antigen complexes in vitro, several different phenomena may be observed, depending on the conditions under which the primary reaction takes place. These phenomena are termed *secondary reactions.* Secondary reactions depend on the nature of the antigen, the nature of the antibody, and other factors such as the presence of complement. A partial list of secondary reactions includes precipitation of the antigen-antibody complex, agglutination of antigen-containing cells or organisms; complement fixation; immobilization of motile organisms; and neutralization of organisms or biologically active molecules.

In vivo antibody-antigen reaction. If antibody-antigen reactions occur in a living animal, tissue damage may occur. This effect of antibody-antigen reactions in vivo is considered later in the chapter as antibody-mediated immunopathologic mechanisms.

LYMPHOCYTES
B- and T-cells

Functionally the properties of the two major lymphocyte populations are fairly well defined: B-cells are the precursors of plasma cells, and T-cells assist in antibody production and in mediating the various phenomena associated with cell-mediated immunity (delayed hypersensitivity). The regulation of the immune response is a complex phenomenon involving participation of both B- and T-cells. Several different functions have been attributed to different subpopulations of T-cells (see p. 492).

Distinguishing a normal T- and B-lymphocytes morphologically is impossible. Various techniques that have been found empirically to correlate with functional indices of T- and B-cell activity have been developed. Table 12-2 presents a list of classically defined T- and B-cell markers as well as a summary of other features.

B-cells have an easily recognized product (cell surface immunoglobulin), making their recognition relatively straightforward. T-cells do not have surface immuno-

Table 12-2. Some properties of T- and B-lymphocytes

	T-cells	B-cells
Site of origin	Thymus	Fetal liver, gastrointestinal tract
Tissue location	Diffuse cortex	Primary follicles, germinal centers
Surface markers		
T antigens	+	−
E rosettes	+	−
EAC rosettes (C receptor)	−	+
Surface Ig	−	+
HLA-A, -B, -C	+	+
HLA-D (Ia)	−	+
FC receptor	−	+
Frequency		
Blood	70%	20%
Lymph node	85%	15%
Spleen	65%	35%
Bone marrow	Rare	Many
Thymus	90%	2%-3%
Mitogen responses		
Soluble conA	+	−
Insoluble conA	+	+
PHA	+	+
Functions	T_H (helper)	Precursor of plasma cell
	T_S (suppressor)	
	T_K (killer)	
	T_D (delayed hypersensitivity)	

+, Present; −, absent.

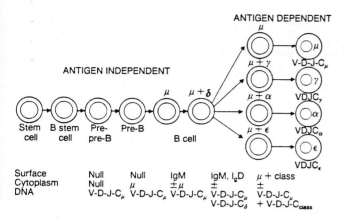

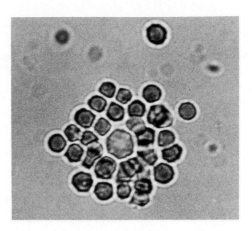

Fig. 12-3. Model of B-cell differentiation. There are two major phases of B-cell development: antigen independent and antigen dependent. B-cell maturation from a multipotent hematopoietic stem cell to mature B-cells expressing cell surface IgM and IgD is believed to be antigen independent. By rearranging a given V-D-J combination one may determine the antigen-recognizing specificity of the B-cell at these steps before antigen enters the system. The first identifiable cell in the B-cell lineage is the pre-pre-B cell, in which rearrangement of immunoglobulin heavy chain genes with a juxtaposition of V_H-D-J-Cμ has occurred but rearrangement of the light chain genes has not. The pre-pre-B cell does not express either cytoplasmic or cell surface immunoglobulin. The next cell, the pre-B cell, expresses cytoplasmic μ-chains but not cell surface immunoglobulin and still has not rearranged or expressed light chain genes. Immature B-cells have rearranged heavy and light chain genes and express both. They exist in two classes, those that express cell surface IgM only and those that express cell surface IgM and IgD. Upon antigenic stimulation and given appropriate signals from helper T-cells, B-cells proliferate to expand the clone and differentiate into plasma cells that express the same V-D-J combination as before but may now use a different constant region gene, which results in the same antigen recognition specificity but a different isotype (IgG, IgA, or IgE) or subclass of the secreted antibody molecule. Plasma cells have little surface immunoglobulin but rapidly synthesize and secrete antibody of only one immunoglobulin class. (From Sell, S.: Basic immunology, New York, copyright 1987, Elsevier Science Publishing Co., Inc.

Fig. 12-4. Lymphoid rosette. Central lymphocyte is surrounded by adherent erythrocytes. (Courtesy Antonino Cantanzaro, University of California School of Medicine, San Diego, La Jolla, Calif.)

the availability of hybridoma monoclonal antibodies has enhanced our ability to define and recognize human T-cells and T-cell subsets. Groupings of similar epitopes identified on lymphocytes by different monoclonal antibodies have been given the name *cluster designation* (Table 12-3). By using antibody preparations containing a single antibody species directed against T-cell membrane antigens, we are now able to identify thymus-derived cells as to degree of maturation as well as proposed function.

Monoclonal antibodies to monocyte antigens are also available. These new reagents together with conventional techniques provide the capacity to distinguish different subpopulations of macrophage lineage (Table 12-4).

The identification of monoclonality and polyclonality is of great use in dissecting both benign and malignant B-lymphocytic lesions. B-lymphocytes bear immunoglobulin receptors in their cell membranes. Although these may be of various heavy or light chain types, any given B-cell makes only one light-chain type. In humans, kappa and lambda light chains are about equally distributed among lymphocytes. A reactive process to a foreign material, since it arises from the stimulation of several clones by foreign material, contains some B-cells bearing kappa and some bearing lambda light chains (that is, polyclonal). Malignant B-lymphocytic proliferations, on the other hand, usually contain only the progeny of one malignant clone and thus show only one light-chain type (that is, monoclonal). Antibodies labeled specifically to kappa and lambda chains on unfixed preparations can be used to determine if a lesion is polyclonal (benign) or monoclonal (malignant). The demonstration of monoclonal rearrangement of Ig genes in lymphoid tissue may be used to identify pre-pre-B-cell tumors when monoclonal Ig expression is not

globulin though they insert an immunoglobulin-like fragment into their cell surface as an antigen receptor. Cell surface immunoglobulin is identified by use of anti-immunoglobulin reagents. Identification of cytoplasmic or membrane-bound immunoglobulin suffices to classify a cell as a B-cell. Primitive B-cell precursors are more difficult to identify (Fig. 12-3). B-cells also possess receptors for the Fc fragment of IgG and for complement, as indicated in Table 12-2.

Human T-cells are recognized by their ability to form rosettes with sheep erythrocytes (Fig. 12-4). Recently

Table 12-3. Some important T-lymphocyte subsets identified by monoclonal antibodies

Cluster designation*	Subpopulation	Monoclonal antibodies
CD1	Cortical thymocytes	T_6, Leu6
CD2	Pan T-cell	T_{11}, Leu5
CD3	Mature T-cells, medullary thymocytes	T_3, Leu4
CD4	Most thymocytes 50%-60% of peripheral T-cells (helper)	T_4, Leu3
CD5	Mature T-cells, medullary thymocytes	T_1, Leu1
CD8	Most thymocytes, 25%-35% of peripheral T-cells (suppressor)	T_8, Leu2
T_i	T-cell receptor	—
CD25	IL-2 receptor	anti-TAC

*Cluster designation refers to the set of monoclonal antibodies that identify a given population of lymphocytes.

Table 12-4. Macrophage subpopulations

Macrophage subpopulation	Organ	Presumed function
Stem cell	Bone marrow	Precursor
Monocyte	Blood	Circulating macrophage
Fixed histiocyte	Reticuloendothelial cells	Phagocytic cells in tissue
Dendritic histiocytes	Lymphoid organs	Process antigen for B-cells
Interdigitating reticulum cells	Lymphoid organs	Process antigen for T-cells
Langerhans' cells	Skin, epithelium	Process antigen for T-cells

Table 12-5. Effector lymphocyte populations

Population	Phenotype	Functional activity
T_D	CD4 T cell	Specific; release lymphokines, mediate delayed hypersensitivity reactions, and activate macrophages
T_{CTL}	CD8 T cell	Specific; react with and lyse target cells
NK	Null (large granular lymphocytes)	Nonspecific; react with and lyse target cells
K	Fc or IgG receptors (large granular lymphocytes)	Antibody-dependent cell-mediated cytotoxicity

found, but Ig gene rearrangements are identifiable. In normal or hyperplastic B-cell proliferation the Ig gene rearrangements will be mixed and not clearly detectable by cDNA probes, whereas in monoclonal proliferation clearly identifiable DNA band will be demonstrated by Southern blotting. Exceptions to the monoclonality rule for lymphomas are seen in the polyclonal B-cell proliferative diseases that occur in immunosuppressed individuals (AIDS, cyclosporine).

Effector lymphocytes. The second major effector aim of the immune response is mediated by sensitized lymphocytes.

Lymphocytes that indicate immune reactions belong to several different subpopulations (Table 12-5). The major populations involved in cell-mediated reactions in vivo are T_D and T_{CTL} (cytotoxic) lymphocytes. Both of these T-lymphocyte populations are able to recognize antigen through the T-cell receptor and are increased by specific immunization. The T-cell receptor consists of two chains (α and β), which have variable and constant regions similar to antibody molecules as well as intramembranous and cytoplasmic domains (Fig. 12-5). The complete T-cell receptor consists of the α and β chains but also of a set of other proteins (δ, γ, ϵ, and ξ chains, the T3 complex).

Natural killer (NK) cells are present in nonimmu-

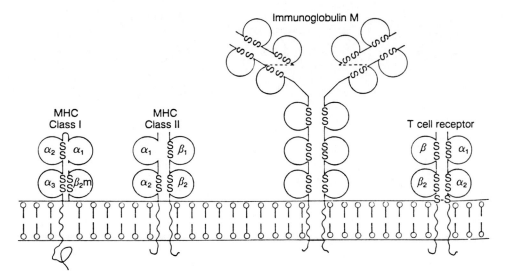

Fig. 12-5. Similarities in structure of lymphoid cell surface receptors: MHC (major histocompatability complex) class I, MHC class II, IgM, and T-cell receptor. Receptors contain extracellular, transmembrane, and cytoplasmic domains.

nized individuals and are able to react with and lyse certain target cell lines in vitro. NK activity is increased by infections and in vitro by treatment with IL-2, a product of activated T helper cells (see next page). So-called LAK (lymphokine-activated killer cells) have shown some promise in effecting rejection of transplanted tumors in animals, but clinical trials in humans have not yielded significant results.

Antibody-dependent cell-mediated cytotoxic cells (ADCC) have receptors for IgG or Fc of antibody. By this mechanism they are directed to target cells with which the antibody reacts. This mechanism may play a role in some immune-mediated human diseases, such as autoimmune thyroiditis.

Major histocompatibility complex (MHC) and the immunoglobulin gene superfamily

The human MHC includes class I, class II, and class III markers. Class I genes code for markers found on all nucleated cells and are recognized by sensitized cells that effect tissue graft rejection. Class II markers are found primarily on B-cells and macrophages and are recognized during induction of immune responses (see next page). Class III genes code for certain components of the complement system. The class I MHC markers are also designated HLA-A, HLA-B, and HLA-C (HLA = human lymphocyte antigen). Class II MHC markers are also called HLA-D.

The structures of the class I and class II markers are compared to the T-cell receptor and IgM in Fig. 12-5. The class I MHC consists of an α and β chain. Both markers have two variable regions and two constant regions as well as intramembranous and cytoplasmic domains.

MHC and tissue transplantation

Historically, the major importance of the human MHC is in matching donor and recipients for tissue transplantation. At present there are at least 23A, 50B, 8C, and 14D specificities. Since the D region contains four allelic subregions, this alone may contribute up to 10 different specificities in a heterozygous individual. In addition, some tissue alloantigens are controlled by other genetic regions (so-called minor histocompatibility antigens) and are not included in present testing methods. It is estimated that this contributes to 15% of rejected renal grafts. Thus it is not surprising that at present tissue typing does not always correlate precisely with graft survival. HLA (MHC) markers are inherited within members in a family. The HLA-A, B, C, and D genes carried on one chromosome are termed a haplotype. In a monogenous family each parent will contribute two haplotypes (diplotype) to the children. The chances are one in four that the children within a family will have identical MHC diplotypes.

	Mother		Father	
	Haplotype 1	×	Haplotype 3	
	Haplotype 2		Haplotype 4	

		Children		
1	**2**	**3**	**4**
Haplotype 1	*Haplotype 1*	*Haplotype 2*	*Haplotype 2*
Haplotype 3	Haplotype 4	Haplotype 3	Haplotype 4

Thus, in a family with more than four children, at least two children will have identical HLA matches.

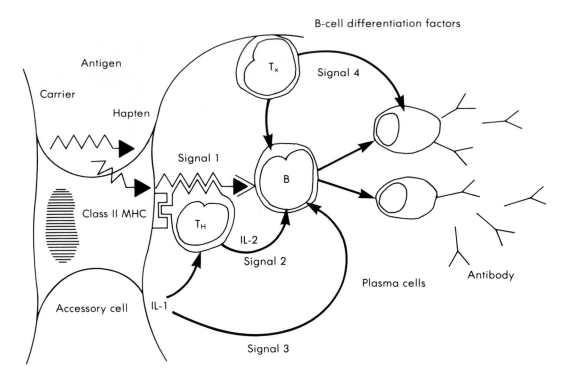

Fig. 12-6. Macrophage–T-B cell cooperation in induction of antibody formation to haptens. Macrophages process the antigen nonspecifically and provide activation signals to T- and B-cells. T-cells recognize the immunogenic carrier molecule in association with class II MHC markers, whereas B-cells recognize the hapten. The reaction of the B-cell to the hapten occurring in the presence of reaction of the T-cell with the carrier along with the macrophage provides the required set of signals for B-cell stimulation. It is postulated that at least three signals are required to stimulate B-cells: one signal supplied by the antigen (hapten), one by the macrophage, and one by the T-cell. *IL,* Interleukin. Further signals are required to induce differentiation of B-cells. During induction of these responses, antibodies to the carrier antigen will also be produced (that is, B-cells to the carrier as well as to the hapten are stimulated), as well as memory B-cells. (From Sell, S.: Basic immunology, New York, copyright 1987, Elsevier Science Publishing Co., Inc.)

Cellular interactions during induction of antibody formation

A model of the cellular interactions during induction of antibody formation by B-cells is given in Fig. 12-6. Depicted is an antigen molecule composed of a carrier and a hapten. Dendritic macrophages process the antigen and present the antigen in the form of smaller peptides in association with class II MHC markers. This associated marker and antigen is termed an *aggretope.* T helper cells are activated by the T-cell reaction of the receptor that reacts with class II MHC and antigen and by a product of the macrophage (interleukin-1, IL-1). At least four signals are believed to be required for B-cell proliferation and differentiation into antibody-secreting plasma cells. Signal 1 is provided by reaction of the B-cell receptor with antigen, signal 2 by interleukin-2 produced by the activated T helper cell, and signal 3 by IL-1. Signal 4 is provided by differentiation factors produced by activated T-cells. Up to eight such

factors have been described in different B-cell activation systems in vitro, but the role of these in vivo has not yet been clearly established.

The ability to fuse B-cells from immunized mice with plasma cell tumor lines to produce hybridomas that secrete large amounts of a single "monoclonal" antibody has revolutionized the techniques used to provide specific antibodies for diagnostic, therapeutic, and experimental use. Until a few years ago reagent antibodies had to be produced by immunization of animals. The antisera produced included a mixture of molecules with different biologic properties and antigen-binding specificities. Hybridoma cell lines produce a homogeneous reactant with antigen-binding specificities that can be clearly defined. The B-cells (spleen cells) from the immunized mouse provide the mechanism for production of the antibody (an activated gene). The plasma cell tumor cells provide the mechanism for continued proliferation and immunoglobulin production. Clones are isolated from population of hybridoma cells by cellular dilution and are grown in vitro. The culture fluids contain large amounts of specific monoclonal antibody that can be harvested and used for a variety of purposes.

Control of the immune response

The extent of proliferation of lymphocytes after antigenic stimulation in vivo must be controlled. If the stimulated cells continued to proliferate, the individual would eventually become overwhelmed by lymphocytes. This may actually occur in some immunosuppressed individuals who develop polyclonal B-cell tumors. Some postulated mechanisms for control of the immune response include the following: (1) Continued presence of antigen is required to drive reactive cells; degradation of antigen results in withdrawal of stimulation. (2) Specific circulating antibody provides a feedback signal to block further proliferation of cells. (3) A population of specific T-cells (T-suppressors) is produced that acts to inhibit both T- and B-cell proliferation. (4) Antibody to the specific antibody (anti-idiotype) is produced, and it acts on similar "idiotypic" antigenic immunoglobulin structures on certain T- and B-cells. (5) Reactive T- and B-cell populations may have an inherent refractory period after stimulation. The availability of so many hypotheses is indicative of our poor understanding of this important phenomenon. Loss of control of proliferation of lymphocytes is one of the postulated mechanisms for development of lymphocytic leukemia or lymphoma and production of autoallergic or autoimmune diseases.

Lymphoid tissue and immune response

The introduction of an immunogen into a responsive individual leads to changes in the individual's tissues. These changes characteristically occur in lymphoid organs, which contain large numbers of lymphocytes, macrophages, and plasma cells. Lymphoid organs include lymph nodes, spleen, thymus, and the gastrointestinal tract in which lymphoid tissue is concentrated such as tonsils, Peyer's patches, appendix and isolated submucosal lymphoid aggregates, and bone marrow.

A feature of active immune responses is the enlargement of small lymphocytes into immature blast cells. Blast cells are found in lymphoid organs that drain sites of antigen injection and in active inflammatory lesions, particularly those of delayed hypersensitivity reactions. Blast cells may also be induced in cultures of small lymphocytes by certain mitogenic agents in vitro. Blast cells are a manifestation of the proliferative phase of the immune response.

Functions of lymphoid organs

The *bone marrow* contains the progenitor cells for the other lymphoid organs. Progenitor cells produced in the bone marrow circulate to the thymus or gastrointestinal tract where they develop into more mature lymphoid cells. Populations of bone marrow cells that may have recirculated back to the bone marrow can respond to antigens. The *thymus* produces small lymphocytes *(thymus-derived lymphocytes*, or *T-cells)*, necessary for cellular hypersensitivity and cooperative effects in the induction of circulating antibody. The *gastrointestinal lymphoid tissue*, or fetal liver, is believed to be required for the maturation of plasma cell precursors necessary for antibody production (B-cells); these plasma cell precursors may be produced by the bone marrow or the gastrointestinal tract in the adult. The lymph nodes and spleen contain sites where cells from the thymus (T-cells) and cells from the bone marrow or gastrointestinal tract (B-cells) are organized into a functional unit for the production of circulating antibody or specifically sensitized cells.

Structure of lymphoid tissue

The size and microscopic appearance of lymphoid organs depend on antigenic stimulation. The structure and the lymph node is an example. Lymph nodes are bean-shaped organs with two layers. The outside layer (cortex) is denser in cells than the inside (medulla). Lymphatic vessels enter through the cortex, drain through the medulla, and exit through a single lymphatic vessel at an indentation in the node known as the *hilum*. In the medulla, cords of lymphocytes alternate with lymphatic sinusoids that connect the afferent and efferent lymphatics. Lymphoid cells in the lymph node cortex are organized into ball-like clusters called *follicles*. If the follicle has a less dense center with a rim of lightly packed cells, it is called a *secondary follicle;* if it is composed of tightly packed cells without a dense center, it is a *primary follicle.*

The induction of an immunoglobulin antibody response is associated with the development of germinal centers (secondary follicles) in the responding lymphoid organs. Lymphoid follicles form around dendritic macrophages that contain antigen. Dendritic macrophages are elongated, spindle-shaped cells with cytoplasmic extensions that are closely associated with lymphocytes of the cortex, or white pulp. Cell proliferation leads to development of a spherical mass of cells that pushes the nonreacting cells to the edge of the proliferation (marginal zone). The proliferating B-cells in the germinal center are characterized by cell types seen in various B-cell lymphomas (Fig. 12-7) (see Chapter 28). With 5 to 7 days after immunization, plasma cells appear below the germinal center and migrate into the medullary cords where they produce and secrete antibody, which is then released into the medullary sinusoids. Plasma cells may be observed in large numbers in the adjacent medullary cords or splenic red pulp for at least 10

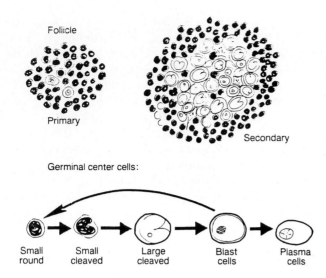

Fig. 12-7. Germinal center cells. The cells seen in a germinal center range in size and shape from small round cells to large irregular "cleaved" cells on the basis of nuclear morphology. Primary follicles consist primarily of small round cells. Germinal centers contain a mixture of cells: small round, intermediate round, large round, small cleaved, medium cleaved, and large cleaved. Cleaved cells may represent "activated" B-cells, with large round cells being "blast" cells that divide to form two daughter B-cells that are small and round. These morphologic cell types have been used to classify tumors arising from B-cells (B-cell lymphomas). Small round B-cell tumors have a good prognosis; large cleaved B-cell tumors have a poor prognosis; large cleaved B-cell tumors have a poor prognosis; cell types in between have an intermediate prognosis. (From Sell, S.: Basic immunology, New York, copyright 1987, Elsevier Science Publishing Co., Inc.)

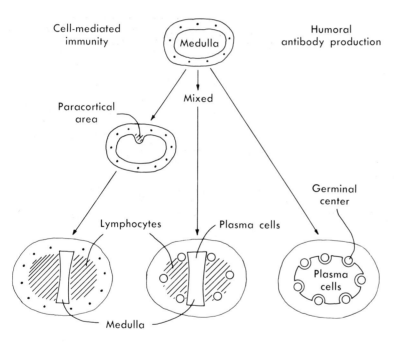

Fig. 12-8. Response of lymphoid tissue to antigenic stimulation. Induction of antibody production is associated with prominent germinal center development in lymph nodes and plasma cell production in medullary cords; delayed hypersensitivity is associated with hyperplasia of paracortical zones. (Modified from Turk, J.L., and Oort, J.: Germinal centers activity in relation to delayed hypersensitivity. In Cottier, H., et al., editors: Germinal centers in immune responses, New York, 1967, Springer-Verlag.)

weeks after immunization. In addition to plasma cells, germinal centers produce memory B-cells. On reexposure to antigen these enable the "immunized" individual to produce larger amounts of antibody more quickly.

Morphologic changes that occur in a lymph node during the development of specifically sensitized T-cells (delayed hypersensitivity) differ from those that occur during the production of circulating antibody (Fig. 12-8). During the development of delayed hypersensitivity, changes occur not in the follicles or germinal centers but in the other areas of the cortex, which contain tightly packed lymphocytes (the paracortical area). Here, a few days after contact with an antigen, large

pyroninophilic "immature" blast cells and mitotic figures may be recognized. A temporary increase in the number of small lymphocytes occurs in this area 2 to 5 days after immunization. Probably these are the specifically sensitized cells that are rapidly released into the draining lymph and disseminated throughout the body.

The role of antigenic stimulation in determining the structure of lymph nodes is illustrated by the effect of immunization in germ-free animals that have little antigenic contact. In germ-free animals, lymph nodes contain few primary follicles, essentially no secondary follicles, and sparse paracortical areas (Fig. 12-9). Serum immunoglobulin levels may be only one tenth to one hundredth those of conventional animals. The

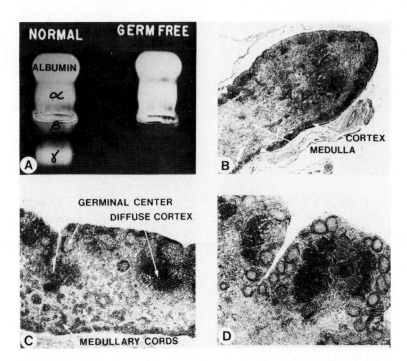

Fig. 12-9. Serum globulin and lymph nodes of germ-free and normal animals. Serum γ-globulin levels of germ-free animals remain very low, and lymph nodes remain undeveloped because of lack of antigenic stimulation. Normal animals have well-developed germinal centers and diffuse cortex. These zones become enlarged and more permanent after antigenic stimulation in germ-free animals. **A,** Agar gel electrophoresis of normal and germ-free guinea pig sera. From the top the major protein bands are albumin, α-, β-, and γ-globulin. **B,** Lymph node from germ-free guinea pig. There is a narrow rim of cortical tissue with no germinal centers and poorly developed medullary cords. **C,** Normal lymph node (guinea pig). **D,** Lymph node from recently immunized guinea pig.

medullary sinusoids are relatively depleted of mononuclear cells. If antigen is introduced, a sharp increase in cortical follicles and paracortical tissue occurs, and the serum immunoglobulin levels may increase to almost normal levels.

Autoimmunity and tolerance

If the immune system serves to recognize, react with, and reject organisms or tissues foreign to the host, it would be expected that an individual would not make an immune response to his own tissues. In fact, the possibility that an individual might make an autoimmune reaction was considered such a terrible and irrational event that Paul Ehrlich in 1902 used the term "horror autotoxicus" for such a possibility. However, it is now clear that many autoimmune reactions do occur. (Diseases caused by autoimmune reactions are discussed in more detail later in this chapter.) Specific mechanisms normally prevent an individual from making an immune response to his own tissue antigens and may also prevent a reaction to foreign antigens. The operation of these mechanisms results in immune tolerance. A break in natural tolerance to self-antigens produces an autoimmune reaction.

Immune tolerance

Immune tolerance is a state of unresponsiveness to a substance that is normally capable of inducing an immune response. It is specific for a given antigen; the immune response to other unrelated antigens remains intact. *Natural tolerance* develops during fetal life so that an individual will not make an immune response to his own tissue antigens but retains the ability to react to tissue antigens from other individuals. *Acquired tolerance* may be induced to foreign antigens if these are contacted when the immune system is compromised, as early in life or after secondary suppressive events such as irradiation or administration of large doses of immunosuppressive drugs.

The mechanisms responsible for immune tolerance are incompletely understood. Some postulate mechanisms are as follows:

1. *Clonal elimination.* The cells responsible for recognizing and responding to the specific antigen are eliminated from the tolerant animal.
2. *Suppressor cells.* Tolerant animals contain a population of specific suppressor cells, which inhibit the reactive cells present from proliferation or differentiation on reactions with antigen.

3. *Blocking antibody.* Specific circulating antibody or antigen-antibody complexes block the response of potentially responding cells.
4. *Anti-idiotype network control.* Circulating antibodies develop that react with the specific antibody to the antigen because of antigenic determinants on the specific antibody (idiotypes). These idiotypes also are found on the cells responding to the original antigen. Reaction of anti-idiotypes with the cell surface receptors may inhibit the response of these cells.
5. *Antigen processing.* The antigen is not made available to the potentially responding cells because of catabolism in the tolerant animal that bypasses reactive cells.

No single theory explains all the natural and experimental phenomena that are included under tolerance or immune unresponsiveness. Different mechanisms may be operative in different situations. Tolerance is most likely an active process involving either the production of tolerant cells or some controlling mechanism that inhibits potentially responding cells.

Tolerance should be clearly differentiated from desensitization. *Desensitization* is a temporary state of immune unresponsiveness induced in an already immunized animal by large doses of antigen administered in a relatively innocuous manner. Desensitization results from consumption of reactive antibodies or cells, thus exhausting the specific immune reactants. Since the antigen is degradable, continued production of antibody or sensitized cells will result in overcoming the desensitized state. Desensitization to IgE reactivity is one of the desired results of immunotherapy for atopic reactions (see p. 520).

Immune paralysis

An effect similar to tolerance may be induced by injection of moderate amounts of nondegradable antigen (Felton's immunologic paralysis). In such cases, antibody-producing cells may be identified if they are removed from the animal, but secreted antibody is rapidly bound to the circulating antigen. Usually antigens bound to antibody (complexes) are taken up by macrophages (phagocytosis) and both antigen and antibody are degraded. With an undegradable antigen, only the antibody is destroyed and the antigen is released so that it may again combine with antibody. Thus any antibody formed is removed rapidly by antigen, and so circulating antibody is not detectable.

Autoimmunity

The opposite side of the coin of tolerance is autoimmunity. Autoimmune disease is caused by an immune response to one's own tissues or tissue products. Autoimmunity is a loss of tolerance to one's own tissue antigens. At least eight mechanisms that may explain how self-tolerance may be broken have been identified. They are as follows:

Sequestered antigens released from tissue
Alteration of self-antigens
Increased T helper activity
Decreased T suppressor activity
Polyclonal activation of B-cells
Generation of self-reactive B-cell clones
Fluctuation of idiotype network
Increased expression of class II MHC on tissues

Some specific diseases caused by autoimmunity are attributable to different immune effector mechanisms and are presented subsequently.

Immune effector mechanisms

The essence of an immune response is that, as a result of the production of specific antibody or of specifically sensitized cells, the immune individual reacts differently on subsequent exposure to the antigen. This altered reactivity is expressed by the activation of immune effector mechanisms either individually or in combination. Immune effector mechanisms may be divided into six categories: (1) neutralization or inactivation, (2) cytotoxic or cytolytic, (3) atopic or anaphylactic, (4) immune complex, (5) cellular (delayed), and (6) granulomatous. The first four types of immunopathologic mechanisms result from circulating antibody combining with a given antigen in vivo. Cellular or delayed reactions are not mediated by humoral antibodies but by specifically sensitized T-lymphocytes. Granulomatous reactions may be initiated by reaction of either sensitized effector cells or antibody with poorly degradable antigens and are distinguished from the usual cellular or delayed reactions by morphologic differences in the tissue reaction.

Each immune effector mechanism has a defensive function beneficial for the host (Table 12-6). Antibody-mediated effector mechanisms generally operate against bacteria or bacterial products; cellular effector mechanisms operate against viruses or fungi. The contributions of these mechanisms may vary from one individual to another. Neutralization or inactivation of biologically active toxins by antibody is highly desirable. This is precisely what is accomplished by active immunization

Table 12-6. Principle immune defense reactions to infective agents

Type of infection	Immune defense mechanism
Bacterial	Antibody
Viral	Delayed and antibody
Mycobacterial	Granulomatous (delayed)
Protozoal	Delayed and antibody
Worms	Anaphylactic and granulomatous
Fungal	Delayed (granulomatous)

with diphtheria toxoid. Cytotoxic or lytic reactions may have direct effect on infecting organisms leading to the death of the offender. The effect of histamine release (the anaphylactic mechanism) at the usual dose level can result in slight vasodilatation and increased capillary permeability, both effects interpreted in classic pathology as aiding defense. Spasmodic contractions and massive diarrhea produced as a result of gastrointestinal anaphylaxis may serve to eliminate intestinal parasites.

The inflammatory effect of Ag-Ab precipitate in the Arthus mechanism produces stickiness among leukocytes, platelets, and vascular endothelium and results in increased vascular permeability. These effects promote defense by localization, diapedesis of leukocytes, and increased phagocytosis. The delayed types of sensitivity (for example, to tuberculin) at the dose level that occurs in the infection result in local mobilization of phagocytic cells. Granulomatous hypersensitivity may function to isolate or localize insoluble toxic materials or microorganisms. A beneficial effect of granulomatous reactivity occurs in tuberculoid leprosy.

At the abnormal dose level used in the laboratory or in medical practice, or with the use of nonphysiologic routes of entry (such as intravenous), one may observe disorders that rarely occur naturally, such as anaphylaxis, tuberculin shock, serum sickness, transfusion reaction, and graft rejection. With frequent administration, ingestion, and contact with drugs and other chemicals, other unnatural or iatrogenic diseases occur. There are, however, a large number of naturally occurring immune-mediated diseases: hemolytic anemias, leukopenias, purpura, erythroblastosis fetalis, neonatal thrombocytopenic purpura, atopy, hay fever, polyarteritis nodosa, glomerulonephritis, contact dermatitis, sarcoidosis, and so on. In these naturally occurring diseases, infectious agents do not appear to be primarily involved, and it may properly be said that they occur because the immune apparatus is being used for the wrong purpose.

Immune deficiency diseases

Since immune mechanisms protect the human body against infection, malfunctions of the immune system may be manifested by infections. Thus the occurrence of repeated infections in an individual may reflect a deficiency in defense mechanisms. Such deficiencies especially must be considered if the infecting organism is one that is not usually responsible for human diseases. Immune deficiency diseases may be classified as primary or secondary. *Primary immune deficiencies* result from genetic or developmental abnormalities in the acquisition of immune maturity. *Secondary deficiencies* result from diseases or drugs that interfere with the expression of a mature immune system.

Multiple levels of defensive reactions must be considered in the evaluation of resistance to infection. Infections may occur with increased frequency in elderly individuals, in debilitated patients, or when natural nonimmune barriers are affected. The depression of pulmonary clearing mechanisms because of the loss of the ciliary activity of bronchial lining cells found associated with exposure to cigarette smoke is an example. In addition there is a genetic disorder resulting in a microtubule defect that affects the mobility of cilia, the immotile cilia syndrome. Affected patients also have immobile sperm and chronic respiratory infections, frequent *Haemophilus influenzae* infection and abundant mucus secretions. Because of the complexity of immune deficiencies and the diverse clinical presentation of deficiency states, a careful systematic diagnostic workup must be carried out in order to select appropriate therapy.

Primary immune deficiencies

Primary immune deficiencies may be understood as defects in the development of the immune system. The development of the immune system is depicted in Fig. 12-10. A common ancestral cell for all white cells, including immunologically competent cells, arises from a bone marrow precursor. For potentially immunologically competent cells to mature and obtain the capacity to recognize antigen they must come into contact with or be affected by products of endodermal tissue. The embryonal gut-associated (endodermal) lymphoid tissue, termed the *central* lymphoid tissue, consists of the thymus, tonsils, appendix, Peyer's patches, liver, and, in fowl, the bursa of Fabricius. The peripheral lymphoid tissue includes the spleen and lymph nodes.

Primary immune deficiency may be classified into the following four general groups depending on the stage in development at which the defect occurs:
1. Combined (T- and B-cell) deficiencies
2. B-cell deficiencies
3. T-cell deficiencies
4. Deficiency in inflammatory cells (agranulocytosis)

Secondary deficiencies occur after full development of the immune system. Some of these are secondary to immunosuppressive therapy or infections (such as AIDS). Others occur without known cause and are termed "common variable immune deficiencies."

A brief listing of some of the major immune deficiencies is given in Table 12-7.

The type of infection observed is determined by the kind of immune abnormality present. Deficiencies in T-cell immunity usually result in fatal viral, fungal, or mycobacterial infections. Defects in B-cell immunity (humoral antibody) are associated with fatal bacterial infections. Defects in production of inflammatory cells, particularly polymorphonuclear leukocytes (agranulocytosis) are also associated with bacterial infections.

Defects in purine metabolism are responsible for a small number of immune deficiencies. Such deficien-

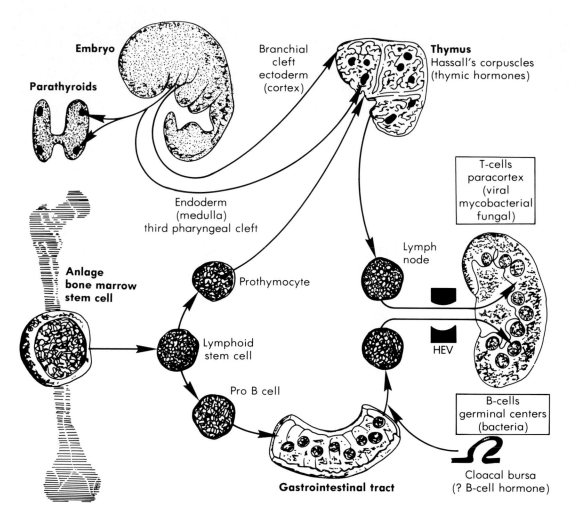

Fig. 12-10. Development of the immune system. A common bone marrow hematopoietic stem cell gives rise to all elements in the blood and in the lymphoid system. In the stromal microenvironment of the lymphoid organs, specific differentiation of T- and B-cells occurs. The epithelial cells of the thymus provide "thymic hormones" believed to drive maturation of thymocytes to T-cells. In mammals B-cells may mature in bone marrow, in fetal liver, or in the gastrointestinal-associated lymphoid tissues (GALT).

Table 12-7. Features of immune deficiency diseases

| Designation | Usual phenotypic expression | | | | | Presumed nature of basic defect | Inheritance |
	Serum Ig	Serum antibodies	Circulating B-cells	Circulating T-cells	Cell-mediated immunity		
SEVERE COMBINED IMMUNE DEFICIENCY DISEASES (SCIDS)							
Reticular dysgenesis	None	None	None	None	None	No anlage	?
Swiss type of agammaglobulinemia	Decreased or absent	Absent	Decreased or absent	Decreased or absent	Absent	No lymphoid stem cell	Autosomal recessive
Thymic alymphoplasia	Decreased or absent	Absent	Decreased or absent	Decreased or absent	Absent	No lymphoid stem cell	X-linked
Wiskott-Aldrich syndrome*	Increased IgA, IgE, decreased IgM	Decreased	Normal	Progressive decrease	Progressive decrease	Cell membrane defect affecting all hematopoietic stem cell derivatives	X-linked
Ataxia telangiectasia†	Often decreased IgA, IgE, and IgG; increased IgM (monomers)	Variably decreased	Normal	Decreased	Decreased	Unknown: defective T-cell maturation	Autosomal recessive
SCID with adenosine deaminase deficiency	Decreased	Decreased	Decreased	Decreased	Decreased	Toxic metabolites due to enzyme deficiency	Autosomal recessive
Bare lymphocyte syndrome	Decreased	Decreased	Decreased	Decreased	Decreased	Lack of MHC‡ determinant on T- and B-cells	Autosomal recessive
PREDOMINANTLY T-CELL DEFECTS							
DiGeorge syndrome	Normal	Decreased	Normal	Decreased	Decreased	Failure of development of epithelial component of thymus	—
CID with predominant T-cell defect	Normal	Decreased	Normal	Decreased	Decreased	Failure of T-cell development (? absence of prothymocyte)	Unknown
Purine nucleoside phosphorylase (PNP) deficiency	Normal	Normal	Normal	Decreased	Decreased	T-cell defects due to toxic metabolites	Autosomal recessive
PREDOMINANTLY ANTIBODY DEFECTS							
Bruton's X-linked agammaglobulinemia*	All isotypes decreased	Decreased	Usually absent	Normal	Normal	Intrinsic defect, pre-B- to B-cell differentiation	X-Linked
Autosomal recessive agammaglobulinemia	All isotypes decreased	Decreased	Decreased	Normal	Normal	Intrinsic defect in pre-B- to B-cell differentiation	Autosomal recessive
Ig deficiency with increased IgM (and IgD)	IgM and IgD increased, IgG and IgA decreased	IgM increased, IgG + IgA decreased	Normal IgM- and IgD-, no IgG- or IgA-bearing cells	Normal	Normal	Intrinsic isotype switch defect: failure of IgM+ and IgD+ B-cell maturation to IgG+, IgA+, IgE+ B cells	X-linked or autosomal recessive or autosomal dominant or unknown

*Characteristic associated features: thrombocytopenia, eczema.
†Characteristic associated features: cerebellar ataxia, telangiectasia, ovarian dysgenesis, chromosomal instability, decreased α-fetoprotein.
‡*MHC*, Major histocompatibility complex.   *Continued.*

Table 12-7. Features of immune deficiency diseases—cont'd

Designation	Usual phenotypic expression					Presumed nature of basic defect	Inheritance
	Serum Ig	Serum antibodies	Circulating B-cells	Circulating T-cells	Cell-mediated immunity		
IgA deficiency	IgA decreased	IgA decreased	Immature sIgA B cells	Usually normal	Usually normal	Defective IgA (±IgG subclass) B-cell maturation	Unknown: some autosomal recessive
Selective deficiency of other Ig isotypes	Decrease in IgM, IgE, or IgD	Decrease of deficient isotype	Normal	Normal	Normal	Differentiation defect of IgM B-cell to isotype-specific plasma cell	Unknown
Immune deficiency with thymoma	All isotypes decreased	Decreased	Absent or very low	Variable	Variably decreased	Unknown defect in pre-B-cell maturation	None
Transcobalamin 2 deficiency	All isotypes decreased	Decreased	Normal	Normal	Normal	Defect in B_{12} transport resulting in defective cell proliferation; B-cell to plasma cell differentiation	Autosomal recessive

COMMON VARIABLE IMMUNODEFICIENCY

Designation	Serum Ig	Serum antibodies	Circulating B-cells	Circulating T-cells	Cell-mediated immunity	Presumed nature of basic defect	Inheritance
Common variable immunodeficiency with predominant B-cell defect	Decreased	Decreased	Decreased or near-normal numbers but abnormal proportions of subtypes	Variable	Variable	Intrinsic defect in cell differentiation of immature to mature B-cells	Unknown: autosomal recessive, autosomal dominant
Common variable immunodeficiency with predominant immunoregulatory T-cell disorder:							
1. Deficiency of T helper cells	Decreased	Decreased	Normal	Variable	Variable	Immunoregulatory T-cell disorder: defect in thymocyte to T helper cell differentiation	Unknown
2. Presence of activated T suppressor cells	Decreased	Decreased	Normal	Variable	Variable	Immunoregulatory T-cell disorder: cause unknown	Unknown
Common variable immunodeficiency with autoantibodies to B- or T-cells	Decreased	Decreased	Decreased	Decreased	Variable	Variable; differentiation defect unknown	Unknown

cies may result in a loss of T-cell (purine nucleoside phosphorylase, PNP, deficiency) or T- and B-cell (adenosine deaminase, ADA, deficiency) function because of accumulation of toxic metabolites (inosine and guanosine with PNP deficiency; AMP and deoxy-AMP with ADA deficiency). Other purine metabolizing enzyme deficiencies are hypoxanthine-guanine phosphoribosyl transferase (Lesch-Nyhan syndrome) and ecto-5'-nucleotidase, which may be associated with a B-cell deficiency.

Secondary immune deficiencies

Secondary immune deficiencies are associated with debilitating diseases, such as cancer, or with treatment with immunosuppressive drugs.

The most common immune deficiencies are those that are secondary to immune suppressive therapy, as in graft recipients or cancer patients. Less common are immune deficiencies secondary to infections, such as AIDS or infection with Epstein-Barr virus. Many chemotherapeutic agents for cancer are antimetabolites that also depress the immune system. Frequently cancer patients die from infections that are treatment related. Particularly important are steroids, which are used for therapy of a variety of diseases. High doses of steroids are particularly dangerous because they are directly toxic to lymphocytes and suppress phagocytosis.

Deficiencies in inflammatory mechanisms

Defects may also occur in the accessory inflammatory systems activated by immune effector mechanisms. Defects in complement are listed in Table 12-8. These are very rare but may be associated with particular infections, as with *Neisseria*. Also rare, but more severe, are disorders in phagocytosis (Table 12-9).

Phagocytic disorders frequently lead to the accumulation of large collections of foamy macrophages in tissues. These may occur with fibrosis and scarring so that the lesion resembles a granuloma.

Two diseases of particular interest from the standpoint of immune deficiency are chronic mucocutaneous candidiasis and lepromatous leprosy. In these diseases there is a selective defect in the T-cell response to the specific antigen of the infecting organisms; humoral antibody responses are intact and active. This may be considered a form of "split tolerance," that is, a specific

Table 12-8. Complement deficiencies

Component	Increased susceptibility to infection	Associated with SLE	Comments
C1 esterase inhibitor	No	No	Hereditary angioedema
C1q	Yes	No	Associated with hypogammaglobulinemia,
C1r	Yes	Yes	AR
C1s	No	Yes	
C2	Yes and no	Yes	Usually normal, AR antibody infections
C3	Yes	Yes	Very rare, AR, infections
C3b inhibitor	Yes	No	Depletion of C3 and C5-9
C4	Yes	Yes	Infections
C5	Yes	Yes	Phagocytic dysfunction, infections
C6	Yes	No	AR, infections, especially *Neisseria*
C7	Yes	Yes	AR, infections, especially *Neisseria*
C8	Yes	Yes	AR, infections

SLE, Systemic lupus erythematosus; *AR*, autosomal recessive.

Table 12-9. Phagocytic disorders

Stage of phagocytosis	Defect
1. Opsonization	Antibody, complement deficiency
2. Recognition, patching	LFA1, MAC1 deficiency (surface-adherence glycoproteins)*
3. Ingestion	Job's syndrome (glutathione reductase deficiency, etc.)
4. Superoxide formation	Chronic granulomatous disease of children
5. Formation of phagolysosome	Chediak-Higashi (microtubule defect)
6. Digestion	Myeloperoxidase deficiency

*LFA1 and MAC1 are cell surface adhesion molecules detected by monoclonal antibodies.

Table 12-10. Characteristics of immune effector mechanisms

Mechanism	Immune reactant	Accessory component	Skin reaction	Protective function	Examples of protection	Pathologic mechanism	Disease states
Inactivation or activation	IgG antibody			Inactivate toxins	Tetanus, diphtheria	Inactivation of biologically active molecules or cell surface receptors	Insulin-resistant diabetes, myasthenia gravis, hyperthyroidism (LATS, LATSP)
Cytotoxic or cytolytic reactions	IgM > IgG antibody	Complement, macrophages		Kill bacteria	Bacterial infections	Cell lysis or phagocytosis (opsonization)	Hemolytic anemias, vascular purpura, transfusion reactions, erythroblastosis fetalis
Toxic complex reactions	IgG	Complement polymorphonuclear leukocytes	Arthus peaks at 6 hours, fades by 24	Mobilize neutrophils to sites of infection	Bacterial and fungal infections	Polymorphonuclear leukocyte infiltrate, release or lysosomal enzymes	Glomerulonephritis, vasculitis, arthritis, rheumatoid diseases
Anaphylaxis	IgE antibody	Mast cells, mediators, end-organ cell	Cutaneous anaphylaxis, peak at 15 to 30 min, fades in 2 to 3 hours; hives	Open vessels, delivery of blood components to inflammation sites	Parasitic infections	Bronchoconstriction, edema, shock	Anaphylactic shock, hives, asthma, hay fever, insect bites
Delayed hypersensitivity	T$_{CTL}$ and T$_D$ cells	Lymphokines, macrophages	Delayed reaction (tuberculin), peaks at 24 to 48 hours	Kill organisms, virus-infected cells	Virus, fungal, microbacterial infections, ? cancer	Mononuclear cell infiltrate, target cell killing	Viral skin rashes, graft rejection, autoallergic disease, demyelination
Granulomatous lesions	T$_D$ cells	Macrophages (epithelioid and giant cells)	Granuloma (weeks)	Isolate infectious agents	Leprosy, tuberculosis	Replacement of tissue by granulomas	Sarcoidosis, berylliosis, tuberculosis

T$_{CTL}$, Killer cells; T$_D$, delayed hypersensitivity cells.
LATS, Long-acting thyroid stimulator; *LATSP,* long-acting thyroid stimulator protector.

loss of one arm of the immune response to an antigen, with other components of the immune response remaining intact. In these diseases there is a poor response to therapy and gradual progression to more severe lesions unless a cellular immune response takes place. These diseases illustrate the importance of cell-mediated immunity in protective immune responses.

Immunopathologic (allergic) diseases

Tissue alterations that result from the various immune mechanisms may be considered variations of the inflammatory reaction. Allergic (immunopathologic) mechanisms are identical to the protective immune effector mechanisms listed previously. A summary of the features of each type of reaction is presented in Table 12-10.

Antibody-mediated disease

The first four types of allergic reactions result from circulating or humoral antibody combining in vivo with antigen. They share the following properties: (1) The hypersensitive state results from the formation of antibody after exposure to antigen. (2) The first exposure to antigen is followed by a definite induction or latent period (1 to 2 weeks). (3) The allergic reaction occurs only after exposure to the specific antigen or to closely related chemical substances that cross-react. (4) The reaction depends not only on the characteristics of the antigen but also on characteristics of the antibody or species of animal (for example, features of anaphylaxis depend on distribution of smooth muscle). (5) The degree of hypersensitivity tends to diminish with time; reexposure to antigen results in the reappearance of hypersensitivity more rapidly and more intensely than primary exposure does (secondary or anamnestic response). (6) The hypersensitive state can be passively transferred with serum or antibody. (7) Administration of antigen with proper precautions can result in temporary desensitization, that is, loss of the ability to react because of saturation of antibody available at the given time.

Cell-mediated disease

Classic delayed hypersensitivity is characterized by the reaction of specifically sensitized cells (lymphocytes) with antigen. As a result of such reactions there may be a release of several mediators that increase the intensity of the tissue response by the recruitment of other mononuclear cells. In contrast to reactions characterized in the preceding discussion, delayed hypersensitivity reactions cannot be initiated or transferred by circulating immunoglobulin antibody.

Granulomatous hypersensitivity is characterized by the formation of organized collections of altered mononuclear cells (granulomas). Antigen recognition in granulomatous hypersensitivity may be by T-cells or by antibody. Granulomatous lesions develop when activated macrophages are unable to clear poorly degradable antigens. In tissues the macrophages assume a resemblance to epithelial cells and are termed *epithelioid cells.*

Neutralization or inactivation of biologically active molecules

Neutralization reactions (Fig. 12-11) occur when antibody reacts with the antigen that performs a vital function. Inactivation may occur by reaction of antibody to soluble molecules, such as hormones or enzymes, or by reaction of antibody with cell surface receptors. Reactions with soluble molecules produce changes in the tertiary structure of the biologically active molecule so that it no longer performs its biologic function or is cleared from the circulation by the reticuloendothelial

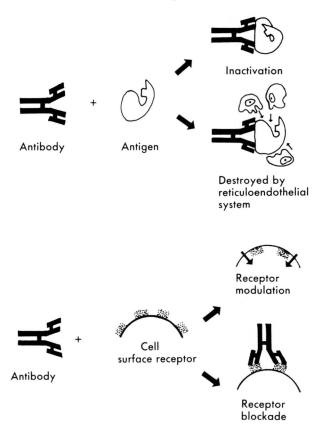

Fig. 12-11. Inactivation and activation of biologically active molecules. (1) Reaction of antibody with antigen results in alteration of tertiary structure of antigen. If antigen is a biologically active molecule such as a hormone or enzyme, this may result in inactivation of active molecule or activation of inactive form. (2) Indirect inactivation occurs as antibody-coated antigen is removed from circulation by reticuloendothelial system. (3) Antibodies may react with cell surface receptors resulting in blockage or (4) modulation of cell surface receptor. Antibodies reacting with some cell surface receptors may also activate cell.

Table 12-11. Some diseases associated with neutralization reactions

Disease	Target antigen
Diabetes	Insulin
	Insulin receptors
	Islet cells
Clotting deficiencies	Clotting factors
Pernicious anemia	Parietal cells
	Intrinsic factor
Myasthenia gravis	Acetylcholine receptor
Hyperthyroidism	Thyroid-stimulating hormone receptor (LATS, LATSP)
Hypothyroidism	Thyroid hormone
Chronic asthma	β-adrenergic receptor

LATS, Long-acting thyroid stimulator; *LATSP,* long-acting thyroid stimulator protector.

Table 12-12. Immunologic and nonimmunologic factors in diabetes mellitus

Type	Factors
IMMUNE	
Type Ia juvenile onset	Early anti–islet cell antibody
Type Ib juvenile onset	Both early and late anti–islet cell antibody, associated with polyendocrinopathy
Insulin resistant	Anti-insulin antibodies in response to therapy
Insulin receptor	Anti-antireceptors
NONIMMUNE	
Type II maturity onset	Lack of receptor response
Secondary	Pancreatic disease (type III); hormonal; drug induced

system as an immune complex. Reaction of antibody with cell surface receptors blocks or induces loss of receptor from the cell surface by modulation. Some of the diseases in which neutralization reactions are significant are listed in Table 12-11.

In some of these diseases the patient lacks or has lost the ability to produce a given hormone or factor and is treated by replacement of the missing hormone or factor. Thus the individual is being injected and immunized by *exogenous* molecules. These are recognized as foreign by the immune system, and antibodies are produced that have the capacity to neutralize the hormone or factor used for therapy. In other diseases, antibodies are produced to self-antigen (autoimmune reaction).

Reactions of antibodies with cellular receptors for biologically active molecules have produced both a loss of the ability of the affected cells to respond to stimulatory molecules in some diseases, and the activation of cells by the antibody reaction in other diseases. Antibody to insulin receptors or to acetylcholine receptors blocks the response of the affected cells. On the other hand, antibodies to the thyroid-stimulating hormone receptors (long-acting thyroid stimulator, LATS, and long-acting thyroid stimulator protector, LATSP) may *stimulate* the thyroid cells and produce hyperthyroidism presumably by mimicking the action of thyroid-stimulating hormone. These are called thyroid-stimulating autoantibodies (TSaab).

Insulin resistance

An example of the variety of antibodies against biologically active materials is antibody-mediated insulin

resistance in diabetic patients (Table 12-12). Patients receiving heterologous insulin preparations usually produce antibodies with reactivity to the insulin molecule itself. The functional significance of most of these antibodies is dubious. Large numbers of people have antibodies to insulin without evidence of insulin resistance. Nevertheless, there are people with documented antibodies to insulin in which at least part of the antibody activity is directed to the functional sites on the hormone molecule. Such people develop profound insulin resistance, requiring massive doses of the hormone to activate hypoglycemic activity. It is anticipated that these reactions may be reduced by the use of recombinant-DNA techniques to produce a human insulin for therapy. In another form of diabetes, autoantibodies are directed to the receptor sites for insulin. These antibodies may competitively bind the end-organ receptor for insulin and prevent effective insulin-receptor binding. In this circumstance massive amounts of insulin are necessary to produce an acceptable blood glucose level.

Thyroid disease

Antibodies found associated with thyroid disease are listed in Table 12-13. Many individuals have antibodies to thyroid antigens without demonstrable clinical signs or symptoms. Autoantibodies to thyroid-stimulating hormone may cause hypothyroidism, whereas antibodies to thyroid-stimulating hormone (TSH) receptor may cause hyperthyroidism. Transplacental transfer of antibodies to the TSH receptor during pregnancy may cause transient neonatal hyperthyroidism. Anti-immune thyroiditis (inflammation of the thyroid) may be produced in animals by immunization with thyroid antigens and is associated with a variety of antibodies to thyroid antigens. However the lesions of autoimmune

Table 12-13. Autoantibodies to thyroid antigens

Antigen	Effect of antibody
Thyroxine and triiodothyronine	Blocks thyroid hormone action—hypothyroidism
TSH (thyroid-stimulating hormone)	Blocks effect of TSH—hypothyroidism
TSH receptor	Stimulates receptor—hyperthyroidism (LATS), inhibits TSH binding—hypothyroidism, or both
Not defined (TSH related)	Stimulates growth of thyroid cells
Cell surface antigen	Cytotoxic with lymphocytes (ADCC); associated with thyroiditis
Microsomal antigen	Cytotoxic with lymphocytes, thyroiditis
Thyroglobulin	Not clearly understood, associated with thyroiditis
Colloid antigen	Not known, associated with thyroiditis

TSH, Thyroid-stimulating hormone; *LATS,* long-acting thyroid stimulator; *ADCC,* antibody-dependent cell-mediated cytotoxicity.

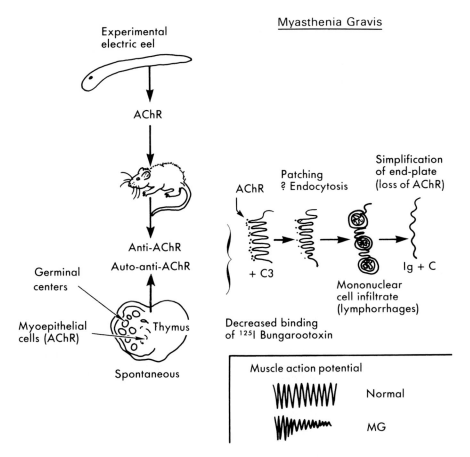

Fig. 12-12. Comparison of experimental allergic and naturally occurring myasthenia gravis. Antibody to acetylcholine receptors (AChR) may be induced in experimental animals by immunization with AChR from electric eel or autologous AChR. Autoantibodies to AChR occur spontaneously in humans with myasthenia gravis. Both experimental animals and affected humans demonstrate progressive muscle weakness, decrease in AChR, associated immunoglobulin and complement deposition, and mononuclear infiltrate at neuromuscular junction. On restimulation, muscle action potential reveals rapid decline. Thymus of affected humans may contain germinal centers not normally found in thymus. Since thymus contains myoepithelial cells with AChR, it is possible that autoantibody production to AChR occurs in thymus. (Modified from Sell, S.: Immunology, immunopathology and immunity, ed. 3, New York, 1980, Harper & Row, Publishers, Inc.)

thyroiditis are most likely attributable to specifically sensitized lymphocytes (T_D or T_{CTL}).

Myasthenia gravis

A comparison of the naturally occurring disease myasthenia gravis with experimental autoallergic myasthenia and the postulated role of antibodies to acetylcholine receptors (AChR) are illustrated in Fig. 12-12. In this disease, antibodies to AChR result in a loss of receptors at the motor end plate either because of modulation (endocytosis) or because of an associated lymphocyte inflammation. The lymphocyte infiltrate may be T_{CTL} or ADCC mediated. The loss of receptors is demonstrable by a decreased binding of radiolabeled bungaro toxin, which also binds to AChR.

Drugs

Neutralizing antibodies to drugs may be used to treat overdoses. For instance, $F(ab)_2$ fragments of the digitoxin antibody have been used to reduce digitoxin levels rapidly in cases of digitoxin overdose. Other antibodies that inhibit drugs include antibodies to steroids, chloramphenicol, morphine, oxytoxin, and vasopressin.

Idiotype networks, internal images, and hormone receptors

As previously discussed, idiotypes are antigenic determinants that are specific for the V_H domains of an antibody and are specific for a given antibody. Immunization of an animal with an antibody (Ab_1) can result in the production of an antiantibody (Ab_2), and in an individual producing a given antibody autoanti-idiotypic antibodies can be detected, usually transiently and in low amounts. Such anti-idiotypic antibodies may react with the portion of the folded V_H region that is the antigen binding site, with adjacent determinants that are not in the antigen binding site, or with portions of both.

IDIOTYPES

Nonantigen binding site

Antigen binding site

For the present discussion the anti-idiotype that reacts with the antigen binding site will be emphasized, that is, Ab_{2a}. If Ab_{2a} does react with the antigen binding site of Ab_1, it may essentially duplicate the structure of the antigenic determinant to which Ab_1 reacts. Thus animals immunized with Ab_{2a} will be stimulated to produce Ab_1. This implies that Ab_{2a} (anti-idiotype) contains antigenic determinants (epitopes) conformationally similar to those on the original antigen used to stimulate Ab_1 (idiotype of Ab_{2a} mimics antigen). It has been shown experimentally that antibodies to viral antigens can be induced by immunization with anti-idiotypic antibody (Ab_{2a}) that was made in response to immunization with antiviral antibody (Ab_1). In this instance Ab_2 acts like the original viral antigen and competes with viral antigen in binding to Ab_1. These observations fulfill Jerne's hypothesis of internal images in idiotype networks: Ab_{2a} contains the internal image of the viral antigen.

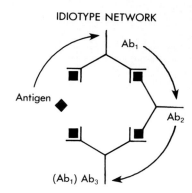

IDIOTYPE NETWORK

Hormones and neurotransmitter receptors share several conceptual analogies with antibodies. Both receptors and antibodies have a recognition domain (for hormone or antigen respectively) and a functional domain that interacts with a unit able to transmit a biologic signal to an effector system. Both receptors and antibodies have the capacity to distinguish fine specificity among ligands (hormones or antigens) with very similar structures. The binding properties of antibodies and receptors for their respective ligands are very similar.

There is convincing evidence that anti-idiotypic antibodies to antihormone or antineurotransmitter antibodies that have antigen binding sites mimicking ligand structure (Ab_{2a}) can actually function biologically as the hormone or neurotransmitter. Other anti-idiotypic antibodies may react to sites on the receptor that are not involved in ligand binding (Ab_{2c}) similar to the anti-idiotypes that react with the nonantigen portion of the V_H domain of antibody. These antibodies may block receptors by conformation changes or steric hindrance. Thus anti-idiotypes to antiligand antibodies may either stimulate or block receptors.

LIGANDS, RECEPTORS, AND IDIOTYPES

Some examples of molecular mimicry between biologically active ligands and anti-idiotypic antibodies to antiligands follow:

1. Anti-idiotypic antibody to antibodies against insulin receptors interact with the membrane-bound insulin receptor and mimic insulin action in vitro.
2. Anti–beta-adrenergic ligand anti-idiotype antibodies bind to the beta-adrenergic receptor and stimulate adenyl cyclase.
3. Antibodies to an agonist of the acetylcholine receptor mimic the binding characteristics of acetylcholine receptor; that is, the antagonist antibody binding site binds the same ligands as the receptor. Immunization of rabbits with this antibody produces an anti-idiotypic antibody that recognizes acetylcholine receptor, presumably by mimicking the structure of the agonist. This antibody blocks reaction of acetylcholine and a myasthenia gravis–like condition is produced in animals making the anti-idiotypic antibody.
4. Rabbits immunized with rat anti–human thyroid-stimulating hormone (TSH) antibodies produce antibodies that inhibit the binding of TSH to the TSH receptor.

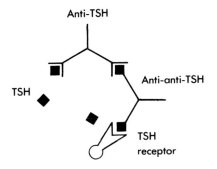

The introduction of hormones and neurotransmitters into the idiotype network opens the door for analyzing a variety of activating and inactivating antibodies, as well as providing a rationale for therapy, since anti-idiotypes can inhibit the production of the antibody to which they are directed (idiotype network).

Cytotoxic or cytolytic reactions

In cytotoxic or cytolytic reactions, circulating antibody reacts with either an antigenic component of a cell or an antigen that has become intimately associated with a cell (Fig. 12-13). As a result of this reaction, the complement system is usually activated, with the subsequent death or lysis of the target cell. The ultimate clinical effect depends on the type of cell involved and the severity of the allergic reaction. Cytotoxic or cytolytic reactions caused by humoral antibodies usually affect cells in suspension in the blood (erythrocytes, leukocytes, or platelets) or in the lining of the blood vessels (vascular endothelium). Therefore diseases attributable to this mechanism are often called "immunohematologic diseases."

The nature of the clinical disease depends on the type of cell being destroyed and the amount of antibody produced. Destruction of erythrocytes leads to loss of red cells (anemia) and accumulation of released cell contents (hemoglobinemia and hemoglobinuria) and their breakdown products (jaundice and hemosiderosis). The destruction of leukocytes causes increased susceptibility to infection. Platelet loss leads to purpura (purple hemorrhagic lesions caused by the accumulation of red blood cells in the tissues) and other hemorrhagic manifestations. Similar lesion may be produced by antibodies to vascular endothelium.

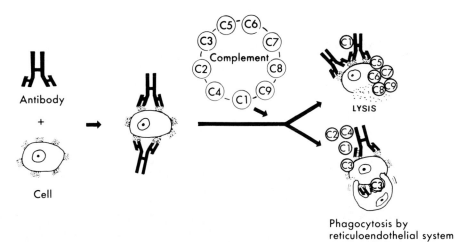

Fig. 12-13. Cytotoxic or cytolytic reactions. Circulating humoral antibody reacts with cell membrane antigens. Through action of complement system, cell membrane integrity is compromised and cell is lysed or altered cell is subject to phagocytosis. These reactions most often affect cells in intimate contact with circulating plasma, such as erythrocytes, leukocytes, platelets, or vascular endothelium.

Table 12-14. Sequence and mechanism of immune hemolysis

Reaction	Biochemical event
$E + A \rightleftharpoons EA$	Erythrocyte reacts with antierythrocyte antibody
$EA + C1 \rightarrow EAC1q^*$	C1 attaches to antibody at a site on C1q and Fc portion of Ig antibody
$C1r \rightarrow \overline{C1r}$	Bound C1q* converts C1r to active form by cleavage of C1r
$C1s \rightarrow \overline{C1s}$	$\overline{C1r}$ activates C1s by cleavage of C1s
$\left.\begin{array}{l} C4 \rightarrow \overline{C4a} + C4b^* \\ C2 \rightarrow C2a + C2b \end{array}\right\}$	$\overline{C1s}$ cleaves C4 into $\overline{C4a}$ and C4b* and C2 into $\overline{C2a}$ and C2b*; $\overline{C4a}$ has anaphylatoxin activity
$C4b^* + C2a^* \rightarrow \overline{C4b2a}$	C4b* and C2a* combine to form C3 convertase
$C3 \rightarrow \overline{C3a} + C3b^*$	$\overline{C4b2b}$ cleaves C3 into $\overline{C3a}$ and C3b; C3a causes degranulation of mast cells (anaphylatoxin)
$C3b^* + C4b2b \rightarrow \overline{C4b2b3b}$	C3b* binds to activated bimolecular complex of C4b2b to form a trimolecular complex that is a specific enzyme for C5, C5 convertase, C3b*; macrophages have receptors for C3b, so that C3b acts as opsonin; C3b on cell surfaces is cleaved by C3b inactivated into C3c and C3d; C3c is released into the fluid phase, whereas C3d remains bound to the cell where it may be detected by antibody to C3d
$C5 \rightarrow \overline{C5a} + c5b^*$	C5 is cleaved into C5a and C5b* by C5 convertase; $\overline{C5a}$ has anaphylactic and chemotactic activity for polymorphonuclear neutrophils
$C5b^* + C6789 \rightarrow \overline{C5b.9}$	C5b* reacts with other complement components to produce a macromolecular complex that has the ability to alter cell membrane permeability; $\overline{C8}$ is most likely the active component with $\overline{C9}$ increasing efficiency of $\overline{C8}$ and producing maximal cell lysis

Modified from the lectures of Hans Müller-Eberhard, Scripps Clinic and Research Foundation, La Jolla, Calif. In Sell, S.: Immunology, immunopathology and immunity, ed. 3, New York, 1980, Harper & Row, Publishers, Inc.
E, Erythrocyte; *A,* antibody to erythrocyte; $\overline{C1}$, $\overline{C4}$, *etc.,* line above the C number indicates the active form of the component; *C4a, C4b, etc.,* small letters indicate cleavage products of the parent complement molecule; *C4b*, C3b*,* asterisk indicates the cleavage product that contains an active binding site for other complement components.

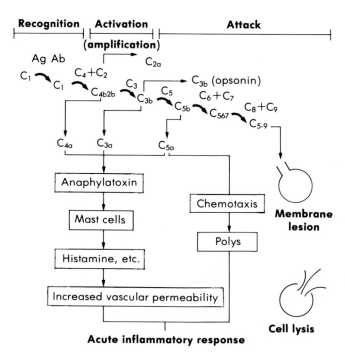

Fig. 12-14. Classical pathway of complement activation. After reaction of antibody with antigen, cascade of complement components is activated. C_1 functions as recognition unit for altered Fc of two IgG molecules or one IgM molecule that have reacted with antigen. C_2 and C_4 function as activation unit leading to cleavage of C_3. C_3 fragments have several biologic activities: C_{3a} is anaphylatoxin, and C_{3b} is recognized by receptors on macrophages (opsonin). C_{3b} also joins with fragments of C_4 and C_2 to form C_3 convertase, which cleaves C_5. C_5 then reacts with C_6 through C_9 to form membrane attack unit that produces lesion in cell membranes through which intracellular components may escape (lysis). *Polys,* Polymorphonuclear neutrophils.

Complement

Complement is made up of at least 11 proteins found is normal serum that interact to produce fragments of complexes with different biologic activities. The first stage of complement activation involves reaction with a receptor site on the Fc portion of an antibody molecule after formation of an antibody-antigen complex. The activation of the entire complement sequence causes alteration of a target cell membrane that permits excess fluid to enter the cell and leads to lysis of the cell. Although the role of complement in inducing cell lysis has been studied for many years, it is now recognized that the activated fragments and complexes of the complement components provide mechanisms for activation or attraction of inflammatory cells (see discussion of toxic complex reactions on next page). C1 is a macromolecular complex consisting of three components: C1q, C1r, and C1s and serves as a *recognition unit;* C2, C3, C4, and C5 serve as an enzymatic *activation unit* resulting in a macromolecular assembly of C5, C6, C7, C8, and C9, which serve as an *attack unit (for alteration of the cell membrane).* C1 has the ability to bind to the activated Fc receptor of antibody by a reversible ionic reaction through the C1q component. The sequence of events involved in the classical pathway of complement activation is shown in Table 12-14 and illustrated in Fig. 12-14.

An alternative pathway for complement activation bypassing the requirement for antibody-antigen complex activation may occur by the C3 shunt mechanism. C3 is cleaved by a system of serum proteins known as properdin. Properdin may be activated by endotoxin or other microbial products as well as by IgA. Therefore the properdin system is a non–antibody activated alternative mechanism of defense.

Antibody-induced hemolytic diseases

A brief summary of hemolytic diseases caused by antibodies is given in Fig. 12-15. This summary emphasizes the source of the antigen and the origin of the antibody response. For example, in autoimmune hemolytic animals both the antigen and the antibody are endogenous.

Drug-induced hemolytic reactions

Hemolytic reactions to drugs may be caused by at least five mechanisms (Table 12-15): (1) Drugs may attach to cell membranes and function as haptens. The red blood cell–hapten complex induces an immune response, and the antibody to the drug reacts with the drug on the cell surface causing lysis of the cell by activation of complement. (2) Immune complexes of antibody and drugs found in the circulation may adhere to cell membranes, cause lysis by complement, and then pass to another cell. In such cases the red blood cell is

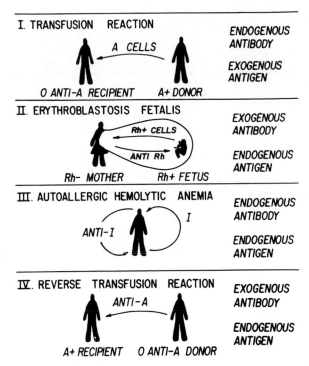

Fig. 12-15. Hemolytic reactions. Shown are four types of hemolytic reactions caused by antibody-mediated complement activation and the source of the antibody and antigen: *I,* Transfusion reactions. Erythrocytes from a donor (A+) that are antigenic for a recipient whose serum contains antibody to the donor's erythrocyte antigen (0 anti-A) will be lysed immediately upon transfusion, resulting in release of hemoglobulin and a clinical syndrome known as a "transfusion reaction." Exogenous antigen and endogenous antibody. *II,* Erythroblastosis fetalis. Rh+ erythrocytes cross the placenta and stimulate the production of antibody to Rh if the mother is not Rh+. These antibodies will cross back through the placenta to attack fetal erythrocytes. Endogenous antigen and exogenous antibody. *III,* Autoallergic hemolytic anemia. An individual becomes sensitized to the antigens of his own erythrocytes (autoantibody). Endogenous antigen and endogenous antibody. *IV,* Reverse transfusion reaction. Antibodies are transfused from a donor to a recipient those red blood cells contain the antigen. This passively transferred antibody caused lysis of recipient red blood cells. Endogenous antigen and exogenous antibody.

an "innocent bystander," since it does not contain the antigen responsible for the hemolytic reaction. (3) Drugs may induce changes in developing cells so that the mature cell expresses a "new" antigen that is autoimmunogenic. The antibody produced reacts with the patient's own cells in the absence of bound drug. (4) Normal erythrocytes may be destroyed by complement components formed by reaction of antibody with another cell if the complement components are not inactivated rapidly or are produced in such large amounts that inactivation of all active components cannot be ac-

Table 12-15. Types of hemolytic drug reactions

Type	Mechanism	Antibody producing direct antiglobulin test positivity	Examples of causative drugs
Hapten	Antibody reactions with drug on cell membrane	Anti-IgG	Penicillin
Immune complex	Antibody-drug complex binds to cells	Anticomplement (C3d)	Quinidine, stibophen
Neoantigen	Antibody reacts to new antigen (frequently Rh)	Anti-IgG	α-Methyldopa
Complement transfer	Complement binds to normal cells after antibody activation	Anticomplement (C3d)	Penicillin
Nonspecific	IgG attaches to altered membrane	Anti-IgG and anticomplement (C3d), or both	Cephalosporins

complished quickly. (5) Some drugs appear to alter the cell membrane nonspecifically so that plasma proteins attach to the membrane. If immunoglobulin attaches and forms aggregates, complement activation may occur.

Antiglobulin (Coombs') test

The Coombs' antiglobulin test detects immunoglobulin or complement on the surface of affected cells by agglutination of coated cells by antibodies. There are two tests. In the *direct* Coombs' test, cells taken from the patient are placed with antibody to IgG or complement in vitro. If the cells in the patient's circulation have been coated with IgG or complement, they will agglutinate in vitro when the antibody is added. In the *indirect* Coombs' test the patient's serum is added to test cells believed to contain the antigen. These cells are then washed to remove serum proteins, and an antiserum to IgG is added. If the patient's serum contains free antibody that binds to, but does not agglutinate, erythrocytes, the addition of anti-IgG will cause agglutination of serum-treated cells. If agglutination occurs, the test demonstrates the presence of antibody in the patient's serum. The results of the direct Coombs' test in the drug-induced hemolytic anemias are listed in Table 12-15. Antibodies to complement are also frequently used to detect the inactivated fragment of C3b on red blood cells (C3d).

Toxic complex reactions

A toxic immune complex reaction is initiated when antibody reacts directly with antigens of basement membranes, when soluble antigen reacts in the tissue spaces with precipitating antibody forming microprecipitates in and around small vessels, or when antigen in excess reacts in the bloodstream with potentially precipitating antibody, forming soluble circulating complexes, which are deposited in the walls of blood vessels. These antigen-antibody complexes fix complement with activation of C3a, C4a, and C5a (anaphylatoxic and chemotactic factors). C3a and C5a are the major anaphylatoxins. C5a is the major chemotactic factor and

C3b attached to cells enhances phagocytosis. This results in accumulation of polymorphonuclear leukocytes, which release cathepsins, granulocytic substances, and other permeability factors (Fig. 12-16). These agents cause destruction of the elastic lamina of arteries, alterations in basement membrane (such as glomerulonephritis, p. 812), or dissolution of the basement membranes of vessels (Arthus reaction). Activation of complement chemotactic factors by the alternative pathway may also cause tissue destruction.

Arthus reaction

The Arthus reaction is a dermal inflammatory reaction occurring upon injection of an antigen into the skin of an individual with circulating antibody. The reaction consists in edema, erythema, and hemorrhage, which develop over a few hours, reaching a maximum in 2 to 5 hours or even later if the reaction is severe. Gross necrosis occurs in a reaction of high intensity (Fig. 12-17, A). Histologically there are polymorphonuclear leukocyte and platelet thromboses, edema, hemorrhage, vascular fibrinoid necrosis, and massive diapedesis of neutrophils (Fig. 12-17, B). The same lesions may be produced in any vascular organ including the stomach, kidney, brain, and joints. The mechanism of this type of reaction involves formation of antigen-antibody precipitates in the vessel wall leading to accumulation of polymorphonuclear leukocytes and damage to vascular endothelium, followed by blockage of flow in small vessels and ischemic necrosis of the surrounding tissue.

The Arthus reaction differs from the anaphylactic reaction in its time course, gross and histologic features, and physiologic basis. Typical lesions may be produced by preformed antigen-antibody complexes and are usually distributed in vessels throughout the body. This type of lesion resembles polyarteritis nodosa and glomerulonephritis in humans.

Serum sickness

The syndrome of serum sickness, first recognized in 1905, includes arthritis, vasculitis (Fig. 12-18), and glomerulonephritis (Fig. 12-19), appearing 10 days to 2

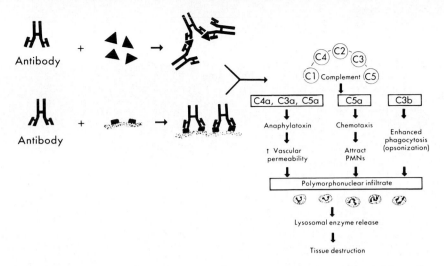

Fig. 12-16. Antibody (usually circulating soluble IgG) reactions with soluble antigens to produce soluble circulating immune complexes or with basement membranes (such as renal glomerular basement membrane). This antibody-antigen complex causes activation of complement with formation of complement fragments. Fragments C3a, C4a, and C5a cause constriction of vascular endothelium (increase vascular permeability). C5a is chemotactic for polymorphonuclear leukocytes and causes degranulation of polymorphonuclear neutrophils. Released lysosomal polymorphonuclear enzymes digest tissues, producing "fibrinoid" necrosis. C3b stimulates phagocytosis.

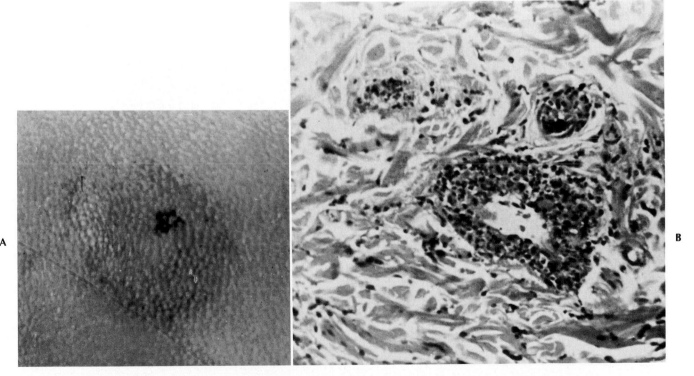

Fig. 12-17. Arthus skin reaction. **A,** Gross appearance of Arthus reaction 6 hours after intradermal injection of antigen into sensitized guinea pig. Dark color in center is caused by escape of red blood cells in places where blood vessels have been severely damaged and may be much larger in more severe reactions. **B,** Microscopic appearance. There is infiltrate of polymorphonuclear leukocytes into wall or small arterioles and fibroid necrosis. Vascular damage permits leakage of blood cells and fluid into dermis, producing edema and erythema. If reaction is severe, thrombosis of affected vessels occurs and may lead to central necrotic area in skin reaction.

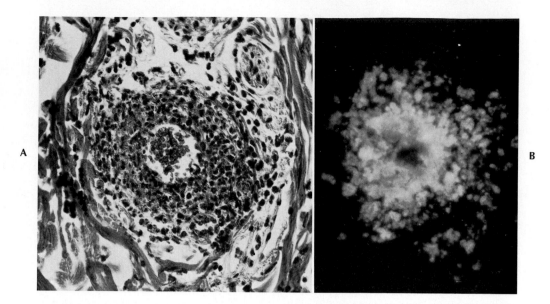

Fig. 12-18. Typical vascular (coronary artery) lesion occurring during course of serum sickness in rabbit after single large intravenous injection of bovine serum albumin (BSA). Photomicrographs of different sections from same block of tissue stained by hematoxylin and eosin, **A,** and fluorescent, anti-BSA, rabbit serum, **B,** with latter demonstrating specific localization of BSA. (Approximately 450×; courtesy Dr. Frank J. Dixon, La Jolla, Calif.)

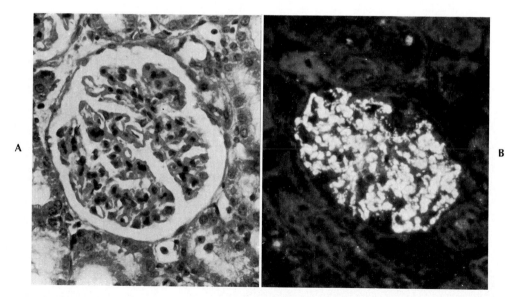

Fig. 12-19. Membranous glomerulonephritis that developed in rabbit after daily small intravenous injections of bovine serum albumin (BSA). Photomicrographs of different sections from same block of tissue stained by hematoxylin and eosin, **A,** and fluorescent, anti-BSA, rabbit serum, **B,** with latter demonstrating specific localization of BSA. (Approximately 450×; courtesy Dr. Frank J. Dixon, La Jolla, Calif.)

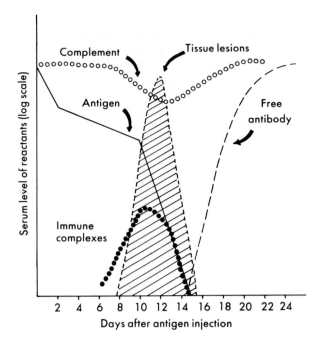

Fig. 12-20. Serum levels of antigen, complement, immune complexes, and antibody during course of experimental acute serum sickness of rabbits. After intravascular injection of antigen, there are three phases of elimination of antigen from serum: rapid fall because of equilibration between intravascular and extravascular fluids, a more gradual fall as a result of nonimmune catabolism, and finally rapid immune elimination as antibody is formed. Heart, kidney, or joint lesions are observed shortly after appearance of immune complexes in circulation and are associated with fall in serum complement.

weeks after passive immunization with horse serum (horse tetanus antitoxin). The disease results from the production of circulating, precipitating antibody to horse serum by the treated individual. The disease may be replicated by injection of large amounts of soluble antigen into rabbits. Lesions appear at the time of immune elimination of labeled antigen when soluble complexes are in the serum (Fig. 12-20). By a continuous infusion of antigen, three different immune responses occur in rabbits: (1) Some animals do not respond (immunologic paralysis, a type of tolerance), do not make antibody, and do not develop serum sickness. (2) Some animals make large amounts of antibody and form complexes in antibody excess, which are rapidly cleared from the bloodstream and do not induce lesions. (3) Most animals produce a moderate amount of antibody, form soluble antigen-antibody complexes in antigen excess, and develop lesions of serum sickness. Complexes formed in vitro and injected into animals can also produce lesions but only if the complexes are formed in antigen excess.

Antibody excess or complexes in equivalence are

cleared by the reticuloendothelial system (RES). The RES recognizes aggregated Ig through Fc receptors. Soluble immune complexes in antigen excess do not have aggregated Ig and are not cleared by the RES. In contrast, since Arthus skin reactions occur locally when antigen is injected into the skin, the RES does not play a clearing role and complexes of different composition may induce lesions.

Immune complex disease in humans

Organs of the body that contain capillary basement membrane exposed to the circulating blood (not completely covered by endothelium) are particularly prone to deposition of soluble immune complexes or binding of antibodies to basement membrane. Such organs include the renal glomerulus, lung, choroid plexus of the brain, and uveal tract of the eye, as well as joint synovial membrane.

Glomerulonephritis. The renal glomerular basement membrane is a frequent site for immune complex deposition because of its role as a molecular sieve. Various forms of glomerulonephritis depend on the type of immune complex deposition that occurs. In membranous glomerulonephritis, immune complexes are initially deposited within the basement membrane, resulting in a granular pattern when viewed by immunofluorescence. In the glomerulonephritis occurring after infection with certain serotypes of beta-hemolytic streptococci, subepithelial deposits of complexes that give a "lumpy-bumpy" pattern are seen. Several different patterns are found in systemic lupus erythematosus. One of these, lupus glomerulitis, is characterized by subendothelial deposits. The location of the deposit of immune complexes within the glomerulus appears to depend on the physical and chemical properties of the complexes. Acute inflammation of the glomerulus is caused by complement activation and elaboration of chemotactic fragments that attract and activate polymorphonuclear neutrophils. Glomerular damage is produced by lysosomal enzymes released from these cells. Subacute and chronic inflammation results from a more prolonged deposition of complexes (see next page).

Anti–glomerular basement membrane glomerulonephritis. Experimental allergic glomerulonephritis is induced by immunization of animals with glomerular basement membrane, resulting in the production of antibody to glomerular basement membrane. This antibody then localizes on the endothelial side of the basement membrane and may be observed by immunofluorescence as a diffuse, thin layer along the endothelial side of the basement membrane (in contrast to the subepithelial location and form of the soluble immune complex deposition just described). This linear pattern is seen in about 5% of patients with glomerulonephritis. The reaction to this antibody with the basement membrane results in the binding of complement, polymorphonuclear leukocyte infiltration, and basement membrane destruction.

Alternative-pathway glomerulonephritis. Nonimmune activation of the C3 shunt of the complement system may be the pathogenic mechanism for some cases of glomerulonephritis. Immunofluorescent examination of the glomeruli in these cases may fail to reveal immunoglobulin or antigen, but properdin and complement components above C3 may be detected. It is possible that toxic complexes initiate complement deposition but are undetectable when the examination takes place. Since this type of glomerulonephritis is associated with low serum concentrations of complement, it has been termed *hypocomplementemic glomerulonephritis.*

IgA nephritis. Deposition of IgA antibody–immune complexes in the mesangium of the glomerulus is found with a form of glomerulonephritis often associated with Henoch-Schönlein purpura or cirrhosis of the liver. The pathogenic mechanism is not well understood. Experimental models indicate that large IgA-immune complexes tend to deposit in the mesangium and produce nephritis. The role of complement in this form of nephritis appears to be through the alternative pathway.

Relationship of immunopathologic mechanisms to clinical findings. Glomerulonephritis is classified as acute, subacute, or chronic according to clinical and pathologic features. Each of the immunopathologic mechanisms—antibody to glomerular basement membrane, deposition of toxic complexes, or alternative pathway deposition of complement—can produce acute, subacute, or chronic glomerulonephritis. The type of lesion depends on the degree of injury produced in a given period of time. Extensive damage from the accumulation of a large number of polymorphonuclear leukocytes in a short period of time results in the pathologic features of focal necrosis and infiltration with leukocytes. Clinical features are caused by extensive destruction of the basement membrane, which permits passage of serum proteins of different sizes (proteinuria) or red blood cells (hematuria). Subacute glomerulonephritis is associated with proliferation of glomerular cells and smaller lesions in the basement membrane, permitting the passage of only smaller serum proteins (albuminuria) and the clinical picture of nephrosis (hypoproteinemia). Chronic glomerulonephritis may result from continued scarring of glomeruli or from pronounced thickening of the glomerular basement membrane caused by the gradual deposition of small amounts of immune complexes over a long period of time (membranous glomerulonephritis). This leads to failure of glomerular filtration, retention of nitrogen (azotemia), and gradual renal failure. The immunopathologic mechanism cannot be identified by routine pathologic examination but requires careful clinical doc-umentation and immunofluorescence or electron microscopic studies. A summary of some forms of immune-mediated glomerulonephritis in man is given in Table 12-16.

Collagen diseases. An important group of human diseases variously referred to as "collagen diseases," "connective tissue diseases," or "rheumatoid diseases" has been largely attributed to variations of immune complex mechanisms. These diseases include polyarteritis nodosa, systemic lupus erythematosus, scleroderma, dermatomyositis, rheumatoid arthritis and its variants, and Sjögren's syndrome (Fig. 12-21).

Other immune complex diseases. Other diseases caused by antibody to basement membrane or deposition of immune complexes include the following: *Goodpasture's disease* is glomerulonephritis associated with pulmonary hemorrhage caused by an antibody that reacts with both pulmonary and renal basement membrane. *Cellular interstitial pneumonia* is a inflammatory disease of the alveolar walls associated with deposition of immunoglobulin and complement in the lung and circulating soluble immune complexes. *Arthritis* is frequently seen transiently during infections. It is believed to be caused by deposition of immune complexes.

Immune complexes have been observed in the choroid plexus in experimental animals injected with immune complexes and in patients with systemic lupus erythematosus. Their role in producing neurologic symptoms remains undefined.

Inflammation of the uveal tract may also be caused by immune complex deposition. In humans acute uveitis is associated with circulating immune complexes and immune complexes in the aqueous humor of the anterior chamber of the eye. Other forms of uveitis are caused by cellular reactions. The role of immune complex in skin disease is discussed below.

Atopic and anaphylactic reactions

Anaphylaxis was used by Porter and Richet in 1902 to indicate adverse reactions to horse serum used for passive immunization (anaphylaxis is the opposite of prophylaxis). The term atopy (strange reaction) was coined by Coca in 1930 for a variety of adverse reactions in humans. In 1906 von Pirquet applied allergy to designate altered reactivity as a result of prior exposure to an elicitating agent (that is, antigen or allergen). These are now used interchangably for acute allergic reactions.

These reactions are caused by pharmacologically active substances released by the reaction of allergen (antigen) with cells passively sensitized by antibody (Fig. 12-22). The cell type responsible is the mast cell (tissue) or basophil (peripheral blood). The cell-bound antibody is of the IgE class. After reaction with antigen, at least

Table 12-16. Some forms of human glomerulonephritis

Type	Mechanism	Pathologic findings		Immunofluorescence	Clinical features	Prognosis
Postinfectious glomerulone-phritis (human counterpart of acute serum sickness)	Immune complex	LM:	diffuse cellular prolifer-ation, neutrophils	Coarse granular or lumpy bumpy pattern in base-ment membranes (IgG, C3)	Acute nephritis	Good
		EM:	subepithelial deposits ("humps")			
Membranous neophropathy (human counterpart of chronic serum sickness)	Immune complex	LM:	diffuse basement membrane thickening	Fine granular along basement mem-branes (IgG, C3)	Nephrotic syndrome	Slowly progressive (renal failure)
		EM:	subepithelial deposits, several, small			
Minimal change disease	Immunologic (exact mechanism unknown)	LM:	normal glomeruli	Negative or non-specific	Nephrotic syndrome	Good
		EM:	effacement of epithelial cell foot processes			
IgA nephropa-thy (Berger's disease)	Immune complex (IgA)	LM:	increase in mesangial matrix and cells	Positive in the mes-angium (IgA, IgG, C3)	Hematuria	Usually good
		EM:	electron-dense depos-its in the mesargium			
Goodpasture's disease	Anti–basement membrane (kid-ney,lung)	LM:	crescentic glomerulo-nephritis	Linear positively along basement membranes (IgG, C3)	Acute renal failure Hemoptysis (lung hemorrhage)	Rapidly progressive (renal failure)
		EM:	no evidence of depos-its			
Membrano-proliferative GN (type I)	Immune complex	LM:	mesangial proliferation, basement membrane alteration	Granular irregular pattern in base-ment membranes (IgG, C3)	Variable (nephrotic syndrome, ne-phritis)	Progressive (renal failure)
		EM:	split basement mem-branes, subendothelial deposits			
Dense deposit disease (membrano-proliferative GN, type II)	Alternative pathway of complement	LM:	mesangial proliferation, basement membrane alteration	Focal C3 (IgG, and early-acting com-plement compo-nents absent)	Variable (nephrotic syndrome, ne-phritis, hypocom-plementemia)	Progressive (renal failure)
		EM:	very dense material of unknown nature de-posited in basement membranes			

NOTE: These are basic characteristic features; variations occur in pathologic and clinical findings:
   nephrotic syndrome: proteinuria >3.5 g/24 hr
   nephritis: hematuria, red blood cell casts, hypertension
LM, Light microscopy; *EM,* electron microscopy.

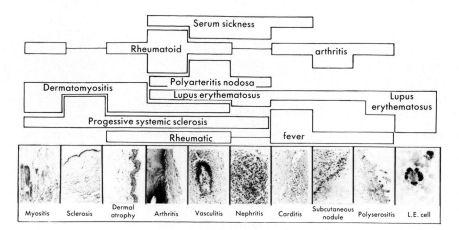

Fig. 12-21. Pathologic features of collagen (rheumatoid) diseases. Lesions associated with collagen diseases are shown at bottom of figure. Relative frequency of these lesions within each disease complex is indicated by thickness of overlying bars. Serum sickness is included to illustrate commonality of lesions of known cause (immune complex–mediated vasculitis, glomerulonephritis, arthritis, and carditis) with lesions of the various naturally occurring collagen diseases. This may indicate a role for immune complexes in most collagen disease, but other mechanisms, such as cellular reactions in rheumatoid arthritis, may also be active.

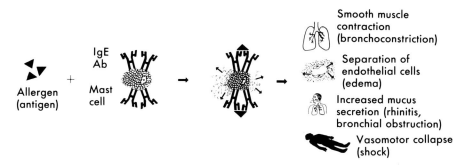

Fig. 12-22. Atopic (immediate-type) reactions. Reaction of allergen (antigen) with IgE antibody fixed to mast cells results in release of pharmacologically active agents. These agents are responsible for an acute reaction consisting in constriction of smooth muscle or endothelial cells. Primary manifestations of this are bronchoconstriction and systemic shock caused by increased vascular permeability. Delayed manifestations of this reaction are caused by other mediators, which induce a cellular inflammatory reaction (see Table 12-17).

nine pharmacologically active agents may be released or activated (Table 12-17). The exact role of each of the anaphylactic mediators is unclear, though histamine and arachidonic acid metabolites appear to be the most important in humans. The effects of these agents include contraction of smooth muscle, increased vascular permeability, an early increase in vascular resistance (vasoconstriction) followed by collapse (shock), increased gastric secretion, and increased nasal and lacrimal secretions. The lesions observed may be acute because of the sudden release of pharmacologically ac-

tive agents, or chronic because of the delayed effects of cellular inflammatory infiltrates, primarily polymorphonuclear neutrophils and eosinophils, as in nasal polyps and chronic asthma. Such chronic inflammatory reactions are often associated with repeated contact with small amounts of allergen. Sensitivity may be determined by injection of the antigen into the skin of an affected person. This results in a central swollen raised area (wheal) surrounded by a red rim (flare) caused by the local release of anaphylactic mediators in the skin (cutaneous anaphylaxis) (Fig. 12-23).

Table 12-17. Mast cell mediators

Mediator	Structure/chemistry	Source	Effects
Histamine	β-Imidazolylethylamine	Mast cells, basophils	Vasodilatation, increase in vascular permeability (venules), mucus production
Serotonin	5-Hydroxytryptamine	Mast cells (rodent), platelets, platelets, cells of enterochromaffin system	Vasodilatation, increase in vascular permeability (venules)
Neutrophil chemotactic factor	MW > 750,000	Mast cells	Chemotaxis of neutrophils
Eosinophil chemotactic factor A	Tetrapeptide	Mast cells	Chemotaxis of eosinophils
Vasoactive intestinal peptide	28-amino-acid peptide	Mast cells, neutrophils, cutaneous nerves	Vasodilatation, potentiate edema produced by bradykinin and C5a des-arg
Thromboxane A_2		Arachidonic acid (cyclooxygenase pathway)	Vasoconstriction, bronchoconstriction, platelet aggregation
Prostaglandin E_2 (or D_2)		Arachidonic acid (cyclooxygenase pathway)	Vasodilatation, potentiate permeability effects of histamine and bradykinin, increase permeability when acting with leukotactic agent, potentiate leukotriene effect, hyperalgesia
Leukotriene B_4		Arachidonic acid (lipoxygenase pathway)	Chemotaxis of neutrophils, increase vascular permeability in the presence of prostaglandin E_2
Leukotriene D_4		Arachidonic acid (lipoxygenase pathway)	Increase in vascular permeability
Platelet-activating factor	Acetylated glycerol ether phosphocholine	Basophils, neutrophils, monocytes, macrophages	Release of mediators from platelets, neutrophil aggregation, neutrophil secretion, superoxide production by neutrophils, increase vascular permeability

Reaginic antibody (IgE). The antibody responsible for atopic or anaphylactic sensitivity is called reagin. The term "reagin" was originally applied to the Wassermann reagin, a serum reactant found in patients with syphilis. However, in current terminology reagin is used to designate antibody that has a special ability to bind to mast cells in skin or other tissues, the so-called homocytotropic antibody. This type of activity may be found in any of the major immunoglobulin groups (IgA, IgG, IgM), but in most cases reaginic antibody is found in a separate immunoglobulin class, IgE. In humans atopic or anaphylactic reactions are almost always caused by IgE antibody.

Skin tests are commonly used to detect reaginic antibody activity. Suspected allergens are injected into the skin, and the local reaction is observed within 30 minutes. Skin testing must be done under careful supervision because systemic anaphylactic shock may be induced. Antianaphylactic drugs (epinephrine) must be kept on hand for rapid use if necessary. The local transfer of skin-fixing antibody may be used to demonstrate reaginic activity in serum (passive cutaneous anaphylaxis, Prausnitz-Küstner test).

In vitro tests include the Schultz-Dale test, which uses organs containing smooth muscle (guinea pig intestine or rat uterus) in an organ bath. When the organ is taken from a sensitized animal or incubated with serum from a sensitized individual, contraction will occur when the specific antigen is added. Contraction may also be induced by the addition of mediators (histamine). The release of histamine from mast cells in vitro may be induced by contact of sensitized mast cells with antigen. Histamine release may be quantitated spectrophotometrically or by observation of mast cell degranulation. Mast cells may be passively sensitized by incubation with reagin-containing serum. The reactivity of sensitized mast cells to antigen may be inhibited by the addition of blocking serum containing IgG antibody to the same antigen as the IgE antibody. The passive leukocyte-sensitizing (PLS) activity of a given serum is determined by incubation of a reaginic serum with blood leukocytes from nonallergic donors. The cells are

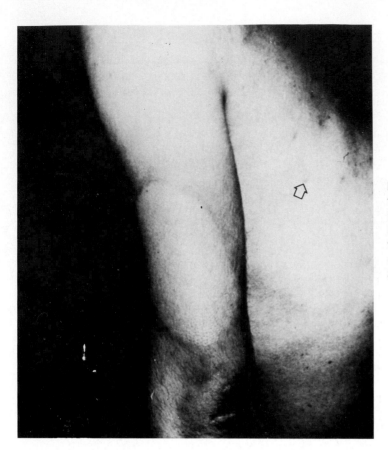

Fig. 12-23. Wheal-and-flare reaction. Massive wheal reaction to bee sting. Central, raised, pale, spongy area (wheal) is surrounded by thin, red flat rim (flare). Wheal is caused by edema, flare by microvascular congestion. Small more typical reactions are present on other areas of skin *(arrow)*. (Courtesy Macy Levine, University of Pittsburgh Medical School, Pittsburgh, Pa.)

then washed and treated with antigen. The extent of histamine release is used as an index of the serum reagin content. The PLS activity of ragweed-sensitive individuals is highest in the early fall (during the pollen season) and lowest in summer just before the pollen season.

The radioallergosorbent test (RAST) depends on the binding of radiolabeled antibody specific for IgE by an antigen-IgE antibody complex. The suspected antigen is first attached to insoluble particles and then added to samples of serum. In sera containing antibodies to the antigen, antibody immunoglobulin binds to the insoluble antigen. Antibody of classes other than IgE may also bind, and so excess insoluble antigen is used. The particles are washed and treated with a radiolabeled antibody to IgE. The labeled anti-IgE will bind to the IgE antibody, which is bound to the insoluble antigen. An estimation of the amount of IgE antibody to the antigen may then be made by determination of the amount of labeled anti-IgE bound.

The release of mediators from mast cell granules may occur by one of two mechanisms, nonlytic or lytic. Nonlytic release occurs by fusion of membranes of basophil granules with each other and with the cell membrane, resulting in externalization of granule contents (degranulation) (Fig. 12-24). The mast cell is not destroyed, and the granules reform. Lytic release is caused by antibody-antigen fixation of complement on the mast cell surface, leading to complement-mediated lysis of the cell. IgE-mediated nonlytic release is responsible for almost all anaphylactic reactions. Lytic release provides a mechanism whereby IgG or IgM antibody may produce anaphylactic symptoms. The mechanism of nonlytic release after reaction of allergen with reaginic antibody fixed to the mast cell is illustrated in Fig. 12-25.

Mast cells also contain and release arachidonic acid upon degranulation. Arachidonic acid is metabolized by cells other than mast cells to form prostaglandins and a group of biologically active metabolites called leukotrienes (Fig. 12-26). Some leukotrienes and prostaglandins are responsible for delayed inflammatory effects.

Anaphylactic reactions

The acute phase of allergic reactions is primarily manifested in five organ systems as the result of the action of histamine on cells with histamine receptors (Table 12-18). The acute phase is characterized by immediate smooth-muscle constriction or dilatation. Smooth muscle of pulmonary bronchi, gastrointestinal tract, and genitourinary tract and endothelial cells as well are stimulated to contract though activation of H1 receptors: the

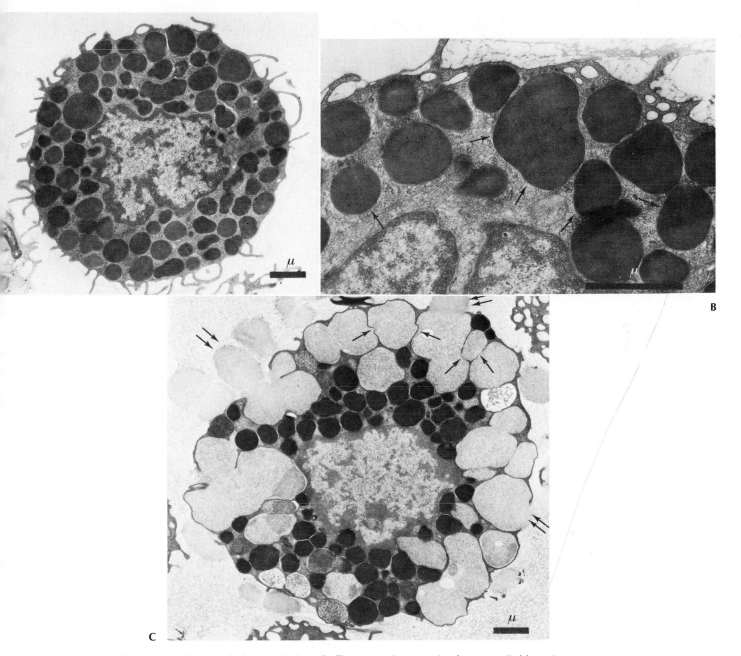

Fig. 12-24. Mast cell degranulation. **A,** Electron micrograph of mast cell. Many homogeneous, electron-dense granules are seen in cytoplasm. **B,** Higher magnification of mast cell granules surrounded by perigranular membranes *(arrows).* **C,** Degranulation of sensitized mast cell 60 seconds after exposure to antigens *(double arrows).* Granule membranes oppose *(single arrows)* and fuse with each other and with cell membrane *(double arrows).* (**A,** 9000×; **B,** 26,000×; **C,** 8000×; from Anderson, P., Slorach, S.A., and Uvnäs, B.: Acta Physiol. Scand. **88:**359, 1973. Courtesy Börje Uvnäs, Karolinska Institutet, Stockholm, Sweden.)

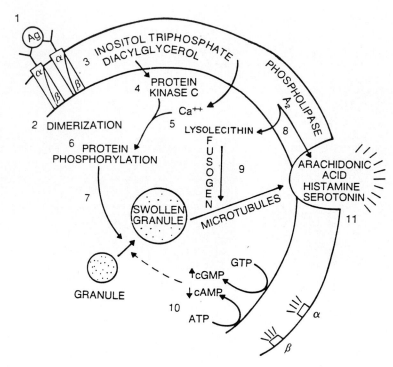

Fig. 12-25. Postulated steps in mast cell degranulation. *1,* Binding of antigen (allergen), cross-linking two IgE molecules on mast cell surface. *2,* Dimerization of IgE receptors: α, 50,000 daltons, attached to IgE; β, 30,000 daltons. *3,* Activation of phospholipase C; action of phospholipase C on membrane phosphatidylinositol-4,5-biphosphate to form inositol triphosphate and diacylglycerol. *4,* Activation of protein kinase C. *5,* Mobilization of intracellular Ca^{++}. *6,* Phosphorylation of protein. *7,* Enlargement of granules by protein kinases. *8,* Activation of phospholipase A_2 with formation of lysolecithin and arachidonic acid. *9,* Lysolecithin acts as "fusogen," causing granule to fuse with membrane and release contents. *10,* Activation of granules dependent on levels of cAMP and cGMP, which in turn are regulated by α and β adrenergic receptors. *11,* Release of histamine and membrane phospholipids (arachidonic acid).

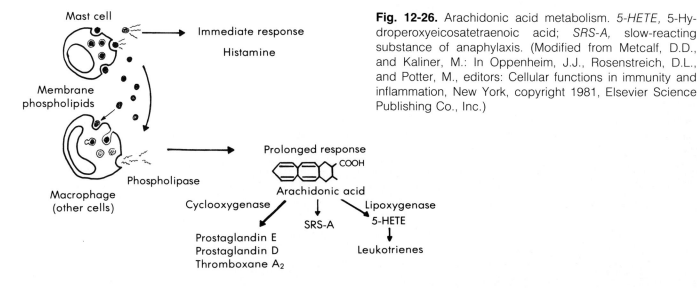

Fig. 12-26. Arachidonic acid metabolism. *5-HETE,* 5-Hydroperoxyeicosatetraenoic acid; *SRS-A,* slow-reacting substance of anaphylaxis. (Modified from Metcalf, D.D., and Kaliner, M.: In Oppenheim, J.J., Rosenstreich, D.L., and Potter, M., editors: Cellular functions in immunity and inflammation, New York, copyright 1981, Elsevier Science Publishing Co., Inc.)

Table 12-18. Anaphylactic symptoms: five organ systems

Histamine receptor	Reactive tissue	Constriction	Dilatation	Symptoms
H1	Lung	X		Asthma
	Gastrointestinal tract	X		Vomiting and diarrhea
	Genitourinary system	X		Involuntary urination
	Vascular endothelium	X		Edema
H2	Vascular smooth muscle		X	Shock

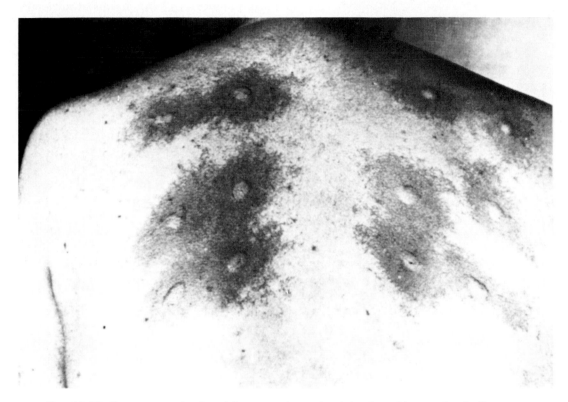

Fig. 12-27. Cutaneous wheal-and-flare reactions after injection of horse dandruff extract into skin sites on back of nonreactive person who has previously been injected with dilutions of sera from person sensitive to horse dandruff (Prausnitz-Küstner test). Central raised edematous area (wheal) is surrounded by flat erythematous zone (flare). (Courtesy Dr. Dennis R. Stanworth, University of Birmingham, Eng.)

smooth muscle of arterioles is stimulated to dilate by activation of H2 receptors. The effect of activation is cutaneous anaphylaxis (wheal and flare), systemic anaphylaxis (shock), acute bronchial asthma, and so on.

Cutaneous reactions. Cutaneous anaphylaxis (urticaria, wheal and flare, hives) is elicited in a sensitive individual by skin test (scratch or intradermal injection of antigen). Grossly visible manifestations include erythema, formation of a wheal with pseudopods, and a spreading flare that reaches a maximum in 15 to 20 minutes and fades in a few hours (Fig. 12-27). Histolog-

ically there is dermal edema with essentially no cellular infiltration. The mechanism is the same as in systemic anaphylaxis, but the reaction is localized because of antibody fixation in the skin. The release of histamine or histamine-like substances into the skin produces local changes in vascular permeability. Cutaneous anaphylaxis should be differentiated from the Arthus reaction in terms of time, appearance, and morphology of the reaction.

Systemic reactions. Anaphylactic shock may occur in an atopic individual after either systemic or local expo-

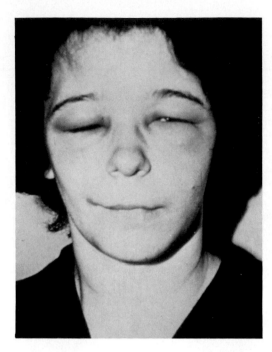

Fig. 12-28. Angioedema. Massive swelling of face occurs with rapid onset and resolves quickly. Swelling shown here was gone 24 hours later. (Courtesy Macy Levine, Pittsburgh, Pa.)

sure to allergen. Systemic vascular dilatation is prominent, with increased permeability of small vessels, leukopenia, fall in temperature, hypotension, incoagulability of blood, bradycardia, and decreased serum complement levels. Circulatory shock with dizziness and faintness may be the only manifestation, but collapse, unconsciousness, and death can occur. Death may result from hypotension or from obstruction and edema of the upper respiratory tract. Acute systemic anaphylaxis in humans is usually iatrogenic, that is, produced by injection of drugs (penicillin), but may occur naturally, as after an insect (bee, wasp, fire ant) sting.

Angioedema. Angioedema is a hereditary condition in which edema and swelling are more extensive than in localized hives. The lesion may involve the eyelids, lips, tongue, or area of the trunk (Fig. 12-28). Involvement of the gastrointestinal tract may produce acute abdominal distress. The symptoms almost always disappear in a few days without surgical intervention. A potentially life-threatening complication is severe pharyngeal involvement that may lead to asphyxia. The pathologic lesion is a firm, nonpitting edema of the dermis and subcutaneous tissue that differs from the wheal-and-flare reaction, which has no erythema. Antihistamines have no effect on angioedema, and the lesions cause a burning or stinging sensation rather than itching. Urticaria may accompany angioedema but is clearly a separate lesion.

Angioedema is inherited as an autosomal dominant trait in which C1 esterase inhibitor is either deficient or inactive. C1 esterase is the active form of the first component of complement. During attacks the C4 and C2 levels in the serum are decreased, indicating that activation of the complement system is important in this phenomenon. The injection of C1 esterase into the skin of normal individuals produces a wheal-and-flare reaction, but the injection of C1 esterase into the skin of patients with angioedema produces a firm, nonpitting induration with no flare (localized angioedema). Therefore production of the lesions of angioedema must involve factors other than lack of C1 esterase inhibitor. C1 esterase inhibitor is also an inhibitor of the kinin system. Thus interactions of different inflammatory systems may be responsible for the clinical picture observed.

Atopic reactions

Other human atopic (allergic) reactions include asthma, rhinitis, conjunctivitis, and eczema. These are termed "atopic" when IgE mediated and "anaphylactoid" when not IgE mediated. The mechanisms are essentially the same as those involved in cutaneous and systemic anaphylaxis. The clinical features of atopic allergy are itching and the production of wheals, sneezing, and respiratory distress. The pathologic features include edema, smooth muscle contraction, and leukopenia. The pharmacologic characteristics are histamine release and partial protection by antihistamines. The type of reaction seen clinically depends on four factors:

1. *Route of contact with antigen.* If contact occurs with the skin, hives (wheal and flare) predominate. If contact is with respiratory mucous membranes, asthma and rhinitis occur. If contact occurs with the eyes, conjunctivitis will predominate, or if with the ears, serous otitis. If contact occurs in the gastrointestinal tract, food allergy with cramps, nausea, vomiting, and diarrhea results.

2. *Dose of antigen.* In systemic anaphylaxis, large doses of antigen are introduced. In other atopic allergies the doses are relatively small and are repeated.

3. *Shock organ.* Individual differences in reactivity depend on individual idiosyncrasy, pharmacologic abnormality of the target tissue (increased histamine content), or increased susceptibility of a given organ because of nonspecific inflammation or adrenergic balance. Many affected individuals have an atopic reaction that involves primarily one organ system (such as the lungs in asthma) while sparing other organs.

4. *Familial susceptibility.* Members of atopic families have an increased incidence of atopic reactions. It

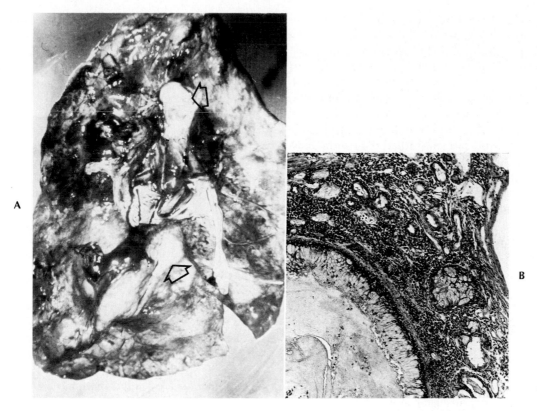

Fig. 12-29. Lung in asthma. **A,** Whole lung. Major bronchi are completely occluded with mucus *(arrows)*. **B,** Microscopic view. Bronchus illustrates characteristic features of asthma: mucus occluding lumen, hyperplastic mucous glands and goblet cells lining bronchus, thickened basement membrane, and infiltration of bronchial wall with inflammatory cells. (**A,** Courtesy William M. Thurlbeck, University of British Columbia, Vancouver.)

is possible, though not yet established, that genetic control of the immune responses may extend to the IgE immunoglobulin class; certain individuals inherit genes that select an IgE antibody response to a given antigen rather than a response with another immunoglobulin class.

Asthma. Patients with asthma have repeated attacks of respiratory distress because of obstruction of the airway that results from constriction of the smooth muscle in the small bronchi and increased secretion of mucus (Fig. 12-29). There are at least two forms of asthma: one clearly mediated by the anaphylactic mechanism ("allergic" or "extrinsic" asthma) and a nonallergic "intrinsic" form in which the mechanism is not well understood but is probably the result of an imbalance in smooth muscle tone. Specific external antigens cannot be identified and immune mechanisms are not believed to be involved.

Hay fever (seasonal allergic rhinitis). Seasonal upper respiratory reactions to pollen are commonly referred to as hay fever. The eliciting antigens represent a variety of airborne plant pollens that cause a reaction in the nasal passages and eyes of affected individuals. Symptoms include sneezing, nasal congestion, watery discharge from the eyes, conjunctival itching, and cough with mild bronchoconstriction. Usually there is edema of the submucosal tissue with an infiltration of eosinophils, which is entirely reversible. The degree of reaction and severity of symptoms are directly related to the amount of exposure of the allergen responsible.

Nasal polyps. Nasal polyps may form in the nasal air passages, causing chronic airway obstruction and rendering nasal breathing difficult or impossible. The relationship between nasal polyps and allergic rhinitis (inflammation of the nasal mucous membranes because of atopic reactivity) is uncertain though some observers believe that sinusitis and polyps may be caused by bacterial allergy. Surgical removal is the most consistently effective therapy.

Food allergy. Ingestion of allergens may lead to gastrointestinal reactions known collectively as food allergy. The relationship of the gastrointestinal reaction to atopic sensitivity is not clear, since many individuals with positive skin reactions to an allergen do not react to ingestion of the allergen whereas individuals with repeated episodes of vomiting or diarrhea after eating a given food do not produce a skin reaction to the food. Allergy to cow's milk protein is the most frequently suspected gastrointestinal reaction to food. In addition, unsuspected additives to cattle food, such as penicillin, may be present in milk and elicit allergic reactions. Food allergy may lead to hypoproteinemia attributable to loss of protein in the gastrointestinal tract and persistent diarrhea. Other manifestations of food allergy are extensive skin eruptions (urticaria or eczema) and systemic shock.

Aspirin intolerance. Aspirin, one of the world's most widely used drugs, is responsible for a variety of atopic and anaphylactic reactions, including asthma, rhinitis, nasal polyps, and even anaphylactic shock. Aspirin is a chemically active molecule that acetylates serum proteins, including human serum albumin; therefore it is possible that chronic aspirin intolerance may be caused by alteration in the antigenicity of albumin or by aspirin acting as a hapten. However, an idiosyncratic effect of aspirin in disruption of the physiologic control of smooth muscle and mucus secretion is more likely to be responsible for aspirin intolerance. Aspirin intolerance may develop in children or appear in adults with no history of atopy.

Insect allergy. Atopic anaphylactic reactions to contact with insects may be divided into three groups: (1) inhalant or contact reactions to insect body parts or products, (2) skin reactions (wheal and flare) to bites by insects, and (3) systemic reactions to insect stings. Asthmatic or hay fever–like reactions may result from airborne exposure of sensitive individuals to large numbers of insects or their body parts. This occurs outdoors with insects that periodically appear in large numbers, such as cicadas or grasshoppers, and more chronically indoors with beetles, flies, spiders, and so on. Biting insects may produce delayed hypersensitivity or acute wheal-and-flare skin reactions. In a given individual a delayed reaction may convert with age to an anaphylactic one. The common reaction to a mosquito or flea bite is a localized cutaneous anaphylactic reaction; there is a very limited, direct toxic effect of the saliva introduced by the insect bite. Systemic reactions occur frequently from stinging insects, such as bees and wasps; more people die each year as a result of insect stings than from snake bites. Deaths from stinging insects usually occur within 1 hour of the sting. Therefore immediate therapy is required. This may be provided by injection of epinephrine.

Atopic allergens. Atopic reactions may occur to very unusual antigens. Systemic anaphylactic reactions have been unleashed by ingestion of beans, rice, shrimp, fish, milk, cereal mixes, potatoes, Brazil nuts, and tangerines. Men have complained about being allergic to

their wives, but usually they are reacting to some component of makeup, hair spray, or other cosmetic agent. There are documented cases of wives who developed systemic anaphylactic symptoms shortly after intercourse; appropriate tests demonstrated that they are anaphylactically sensitive to their husband's seminal fluid. Many individuals who work with laboratory animals develop anaphylactic reactions to the dander from these animals. The incidence of such sensitivity increases with the amount of contact with the animals. During the days of cavalry, as many as 20% of cavalrymen had to be discharged or assigned to different tasks because of allergic reactions to horse dander. Documentation of allergic reactions of horses to humans has not been found.

Atopic eczema. This is a chronic skin eruption of varied cause that usually occurs in young individuals who develop atopic reactions (hay fever) at a later age. The pathologic changes in the skin are consistent with those of a severe contact dermatitis. Erythema, papules, and vesicles are accompanied by intense pruritus. There often follows a more acute wheal-and-flare reaction. There is perivascular accumulation of mononuclear cells, followed by infiltration into the epidermis with epidermal spongiosis. As the affected child becomes older, thickening of the skin of the affected areas occurs (lichenification). Identification of an antigen that elicits the eczema is very difficult, but in some cases there is evidence that the antigens are those that also elicit atopic 'reactions (pollen, house dust, animal dander). Atopic eczema is morphologically more like a reaction of cellular or delayed hypersensitivity but is discussed here because of its association with atopic conditions. It is believed to occur in individuals with a predisposition to atopic reactivity. An allergic etiology of all eczema must be questioned, since typical eczema may occur in children with severe combined immunologic deficiency and typical atopic eczema may occur in individuals with no personal or family history of atopy.

Anaphylactoid reactions. Any event causing histamine release may cause atopic symptoms that may be confused with a true allergic reaction. Anaphylactoid shock can be produced in normal (nonimmune) animals by injection of a variety of agents capable of releasing histamine, without the mediation of an antigen-antibody reaction. The clinical, physiologic, and pathologic picture that results is virtually indistinguishable from true anaphylaxis but is not produced by an immune reaction. Physical agents (heat, cold), trauma (dermatographic), emotional disturbances, or exercise may evoke pharmacologic mechanisms that mimic allergic reactions. Dermatographia is caused by the release of anaphylactic mediators from mast cells of susceptible individuals by a degree of physical trauma that does not induce a reaction in normal individuals. Such a reaction may confuse the results of skin testing, since a wheal may result simply from insertion of a needle. Cholinergic urticaria is believed to be produced by an abnormal response to acetylcholine released from efferent nerves after exposure to emotional stress, physical activity, or trauma. Cholinesterase levels of the skin may be reduced in cholinergic urticaria leading to prolonged persistence of acetylcholine, which may act to release histamine from tissue mast cells.

The clinical findings in an atopic reaction are often complicated by associated nonimmune factors. Thus asthma is frequently complicated by infection or bronchiectasis, which may overshadow the allergic condition. The severity and duration of asthmatic attacks may be greatly influenced by psychologic conditions, and typical attacks may occur during periods of emotional stress with no known contact with an allergen. These anaphylactoid reactions may be mediated by nonimmunologic mediator release, an imbalance of the sympathetic nervous system, or hyperreactivity of end-organ smooth muscle.

Control of atopic and anaphylactic reactions

The severity of an anaphylactic reaction depends not only on the amount of allergen and reaginic antibody present but also on the reactivity of mast cells, the responsiveness of the end organ (such as smooth muscle), and the influences of the autonomic nervous system (Fig. 12-30). Imbalances among these homeostatic control mechanisms may explain how exposure to various nonimmunologic stimuli, such as heat, cold, physical exercise, light, or psychologic stress, may in some individuals excite reactions that mimic allergic reactions (anaphylactoid reactions). Atopic individuals are more sensitive to histamine than are nonatopic individuals. The lymphocytes of atopic individuals have a decreased ability to respond to certain stimuli by increasing cyclic-AMP levels. Thus atopic individuals may not be able to balance the effects of alpha-receptor stimulation or allergen contact (decreased cyclic AMP).

The pharmacologic treatment of atopic reactions may be effective at the level of the mast cell, end organ, or autonomic nervous system. Agents that stimulate beta receptors or sympathetic nerves or agents that block alpha receptors or the parasympathetic system should alleviate the effects of atopic reactions.

Cellular or delayed hypersensitivity

Delayed hypersensitivity reactions are mediated by specifically modified lymphocytes capable of responding specifically to allergen at a local site (Fig. 12-31). It is manifested by the infiltration of cells, beginning as a perivascular accumulation of lymphocytes and monocytes. The main pathologic feature is the direct destruction of tissue elements (target cells) that contain the antigen. The time course is measured in days or even weeks, in contrast to the cutaneous anaphylactic reaction, which peaks in a few minutes, and to the Arthus type of lesion, which occurs in 4 to 6 hours. The term *tuberculin type of hypersensitivity* is applied because for many years the study of delayed hypersensitivity was the study of the response to tubercle bacilli. It is now known that delayed hypersensitivity also contributes to graft rejection and autoimmune diseases and can be induced by purified protein antigens. It differs from the allergic reactions mentioned previously in that (1) humoral antibody is not involved and reactivity cannot be transferred by serum but only by cells, (2) the development of the lesion is prolonged, and (3) the gross and microscopic appearance of the lesions are different from those mediated by circulating antibody.

Delayed skin reaction

After injection of antigen into the skin of a sensitive individual, there is little or no reaction for 4 to 6 hours. Induration and swelling usually reach a maximum at 24 to 48 hours (Fig. 12-32). Histologically there is accumulation of mononuclear cells around small veins. Later mononuclear cells may be seen throughout the area of the reaction with massive infiltration in the dermis (Fig. 12-33). Polymorphonuclear cells usually constitute less than one third of the cells at any time, and very few are present at 24 hours or later unless the reaction is severe enough to cause necrosis. The skin reaction is firmer than that in the Arthus reaction. Deposition of fibrin may be seen between collagen fibers in the dermis. Delayed reactions may occur in tissues other than skin. A schema of a delayed hypersensitivity skin reaction is given in Fig. 12-34.

Lymphocyte mediators

The immunologic activity of lymphocytes (T-cells) as effector cells in delayed hypersensitivity reactions is amplified and extended by a variety of mediators (lymphokines). These mediators may either be extracted from sensitized cells or released from sensitized cells after reaction with specific antigen; some mediators may also be released from unsensitized lymphocytes activated by mitogens. Some of the lymphokines believed to have activities in inflammation are listed in Table 12-19. Extractable factors include transfer factor, a low-molecular-weight material extractable from sensitized lymphocytes that can confer specific reactivity to a previously unsensitized person; lymphocyte permeability factor, which increases vascular permeability when injected into skin; and interferon, a factor that inhibits viral growth. Antigen-stimulated factors released from sensitized cells include migration inhibitory factor (MIF), which suppresses the movement of macrophages

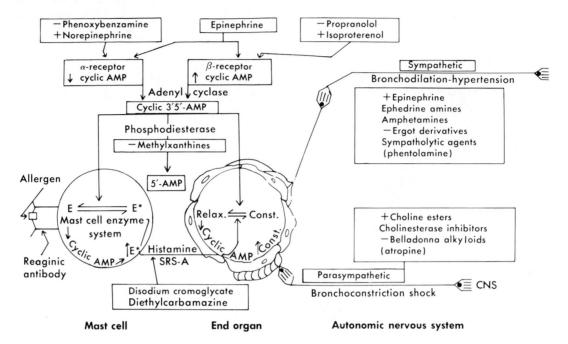

Fig. 12-30. Pharmacologic control of atopic-anaphylactic reactions. Effects of atopic or anaphylactic reactions are mediated by biologically active mediators released by mast cells and affecting end-organ smooth muscle. Amount of mediators released and reactivity of end organ to mediators are controlled by cellular messenger systems. Mast cell sensitivity depends on amount of reaginic antibody sensitizing the cell and on intracellular level of cyclic AMP. Cyclic AMP levels are controlled by adrenergic receptors. Stimulation of α-receptors causes decrease of cyclic AMP and increased reactivity; stimulation of β-receptors activates adenyl cyclase and produces increased cyclic AMP and decreased reactivity. Similar mechanism is operative for end-organ smooth muscle. Degree of mast cell and end-organ excitability may be modified by pharmacologic agents that operate through adrenergic or autonomic systems. Cyclic AMP is broken down to 5′-AMP by phosphodiesterase, so that inhibition of phosphodiesterase activity by methyxanthines increases cyclic AMP and decreases sensitivity of mast cell and end organs. Epinephrine stimulates both α- and β-receptors but generally has pronounced ability to reverse acute allergic reactions at the usual therapeutic dose. Disodium cromoglycate and diethylcarbamazine inhibit histamine release from mast cells. Excitation of end organs is controlled by a balance of autonomic nervous system. Parasympathetic effects are smilar to anaphylactic effects (bronchial constriction, endothelial contraction, increased peristalsis, dilatation of bladder sphincter, and so on), whereas sympathetic effects are the opposite. Certain situations may result in temporary imbalance of these systems and increase severity of reaction, as in patients with chronic asthma. (From Sell, S.: Immunology, immunopathology, and immunity, ed. 3, New York, 1980, Harper & Row, Publishers, Inc.)

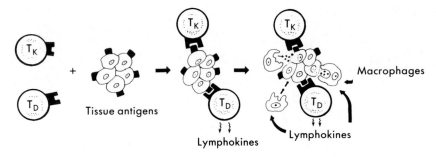

Fig. 12-31. Delayed hypersensitivity (cellular) reactions are mediated by specifically sensitized lymphocytes capable of recognizing antigen. Most likely mechanism is through activation of T_D (delayed hypersensitivity) cells. T_D cells, upon reacting with antigen, release variety of inflammatory mediators (lymphokines), which mainly attract and activate macrophages. Tissue destruction occurs when macrophages phagocytose and digest cells or other tissue components. In some cases antigen is on target cell surface; in others cells are destroyed because macrophages have been activated by lymphokines released from T_D cells reacting with ambient antigen ("innocent bystander effect"). Another T cell, T_{CTL} or T cytotoxic cell, which has been demonstrated to kill target cells in vitro without macrophages, may also cause tissue damage, but role of T_{CTL} cells in vivo is unclear.

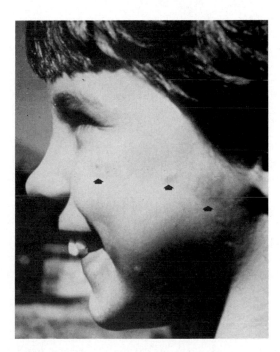

Fig. 12-32. Delayed dermal reactions to mosquito bites. Arrows indicate three reactions at different stages of development or resolution. Just in front of ear is firm, erythematous raised lesion that represents reaction to bite occurring approximately 24 hours previously. Just in front of this is resolving reaction of about 5 to 7 days' duration. Under eye is reaction of 3 to 4 days' duration.

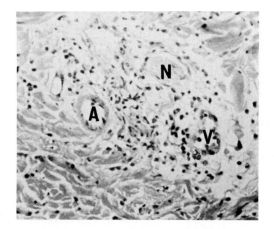

Fig. 12-33. Delayed skin reaction in sensitized guinea pig (microscopic view). There is accumulation of mononuclear cells in and around small venules; later these extend into adjacent dermal tissue. Arterioles (primary site of involvement in Arthus reactions) are not involved. *A*, Arterioles; *N*, nerve; *V*, venule.

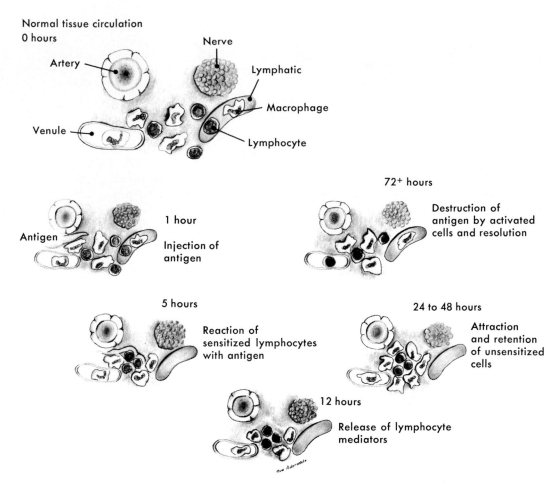

Fig. 12-34. Evolution of delayed hypersensitivity skin reaction. Lymphocytes normally pass through skin from venules to lymphatics, but sensitized lymphocytes in presence of specific antigen become immobilized and activated at site of antigen. These activated lymphocytes release mediators that attract, hold, and activate macrophages. After 24 to 48 hours macrophages destroy antigen and lesion resolves as reacting cells either disintegrate or return to circulation. (From Sell, S.: Immunology, immunopathology and immunity, ed. 2, New York, 1975, Harper & Row, Publishers, Inc.)

in vitro; skin reactive factor, which produces an inflammatory reaction when injected into skin; cytotoxic factor, which kills certain target cells; macrophage chemotactic factor; lymphocyte blastogenic factor; macrophage aggregation factor, which causes clumping of macrophages and lymphocytes; macrophage activation factor, which causes macrophages to adhere to plastic surfaces more avidly; and proliferation inhibitory factor, which inhibits growth of certain target cells.

Lymphokines are identified by their activity. The role that these mediators might play in delayed hypersensitivity reactions remains uncertain, but it is likely that they have significant function. On contact with antigen, sensitized lymphocytes might release factors that attract, hold, and activate macrophages. The number of reacting cells may be increased by transfer factor, cytophilic antibody, or blastogenic factor. Cytotoxic or proliferation inhibitory factors may act on target cells.

Each of these may contribute to the protective or destructive effects of delayed hypersensitivity reactions by amassing effector cells or products that serve to kill invading organisms or tissue target cells.

Cutaneous basophil hypersensitivity. A group of lymphocyte-mediated tissue reactions that contain a large number of cells with basophilic granules has been termed *cutaneous basophil hypersensitivity* (CBH). Basophils are infrequent in pure delayed hypersensitivity but may make up 50% of the cells in CBH reactions. Basophils may also be observed in graft rejections, viral reactions, and contact allergic reactions. The ultrastructural appearance of the granules of basophils in CBH seems to be different from that of mast cells responsible for anaphylactic reactions. The basophils in CBH do not degranulate. Their role in the tissue reaction is not known, but they may serve as a phagocytic cell to supplement the macrophage.

Table 12-19. Lymphokines

Factor	Molecular weight (daltons)	Produced by	Effect
Migration-inhibitory factor	15,000-70,000	Activated T_D cells	Inhibit migration of microphages
Macrophage-activating factor	35,000-55,000	Activated T_D cells	Increase lysosomes in macrophages; increases phagocytic activity
Macrophage chemotactic factor	12,500	1. Activated T_D cells 2. Lysates of PMNs 3. Ag-Ab complexes (complement)	Attracts macrophages; gradient chemotaxis
Lymphotoxin	Multiple (10,000-200,000)	Activated T_{CTL} or NK cells	Causes lysis of target cells
Lymphocyte-stimulating factor	85,000	Activated T_D cells	Stimulates proliferation of lymphocytes
Proliferation-inhibitory factor	70,000	Activated T_D cells	Inhibits proliferation of lymphocytes
Aggregation factor		Activated T_D cells	Causes lymphocytes and macrophages to adhere together
Interferon	20,000-25,000	Activated T_D cells	Inhibits growth of viruses; activates NK cells
Lymphocyte-permeability factor	12,000	Lymph node cells	Increases vascular permeability
Transfer factor	10,000	Activated T_D cells	Induces antigen-specific delayed hypersensitivity after passive transfer
Skin reactive factor	10,000	Activated T_D cells	Induces inflammation upon injection into skin
Cytophilic antibody	160,000	Plasma cells	Binds to macrophages; stimulates phagocytosis of specific antigen
Leukocyte-inhibitory factor	68,000	Activated T-cells	Inhibits neutrophil mobility
Osteoclast-activating factor	17,000	T- and B-cells	Stimulates osteoclasts to absorb bone

NK, Natural killer; *PMN*, polymorphonuclear neutrophil; T_D, delayed hypersensitivity; T_{CTL}, cytotoxic.

Contact dermatitis. Contact dermatitis (contact eczema, dermatitis venenata) is best represented by the reaction to poison ivy. It also occurs as an allergic response to a wide variety of simple chemicals in ointments, clothing, cosmetics, dyes, adhesive tape, and so on. The allergens are all highly reactive chemical compounds capable of combining with proteins, but they also have lipid solubility, which permits them to penetrate the epidermis. These allergens combine with some constituent of the epidermis to form complete antigens (allergen acting as hapten).

The characteristic skin reaction is elicited in sensitized individuals by exposure of the skin to allergen (natural exposure, patch tests). It is a sharply delineated, superficial skin inflammation with an onset as early as 24 hours after exposure and a maximum at 48 to 72 hours. Its appearance is characterized by redness, induration, and vesiculation. Histologically the dermis shows characteristic perivenous accumulation of lymphocytes and histiocytes and some edema. The epidermis is invaded by these cells and reveals intraepidermal edema (spongiosis), progressing to vesiculation and death of epidermal cells (Fig. 12-35). Hematogenous lymphocytes are the carriers of sensitivity, and epidermal cell death is comparable to the destruction of parenchyma (that is, of the cell bearing the antigen) in graft rejection and the cell-mediated autoallergies.

Graft rejection. The solid tissue from one individual of a species transplanted to a genetically different individual of the same species will evoke a characteristic *allograft* (homograft) rejection. If transplantation occurs from one part of the body of an individual to another part of the same individual *(autograft)* or between two genetically identical individuals *(syngraft)* such as monozygotic twins, this reaction will not take place. If transplantation is made between individuals of different species *(xenograft)*, rejection is generally similar to that of an allograft but surprisingly is sometimes less intense.

The reaction is perhaps best illustrated by the rejection of two skin grafts from the same donor to the same recipient with the second graft placed about 1 month after the first graft. Revascularization begins during the second or third day after the first grafting procedure

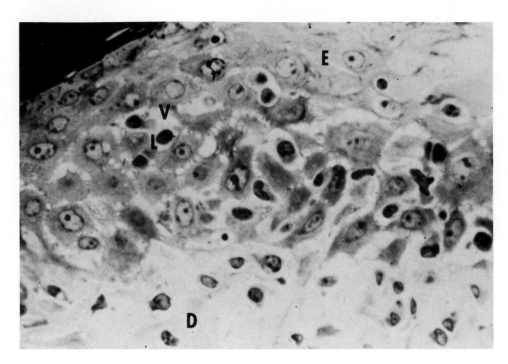

Fig. 12-35. Minimal lesion in contact dermatitis. Mononuclear cells pass from veins in dermis through basement membrane into epidermis where they separate and detach the epidermal cells, producing small spaces (vesicles) that coalesce to form larger vesicles seen grossly. Notice separation of epidermal cells as indicated by prominent intracellular bridges. Resolution occurs by regeneration of epidermal cells from basal layer and sloughing of upper epidermis. *D*, Dermis; *E*, epidermis; *L*, lymphocyte; *V*, microscopic vesicle. (Courtesy Martin Flax, Tufts University, Boston, Mass.)

and is complete by the sixth or seventh day. A similar response is observed in autografts, syngrafts, allografts, or xenografts, in that each of these grafts will become vascularized. However, after about a week, the first signs of rejection appear in the deep layers of an allograft or a xenograft. A perivascular (perivenular) accumulation of mononuclear cells occurs similar to that seen in the early stages of a tuberculin skin reaction. The infiltration steadily intensifies, and the graft becomes grossly edematous. The lymphocytic infiltrate extends into the epidermis resulting in an appearance similar to that of contact dermatitis. After 9 to 10 days, thrombosis of the dermal vessels occurs with necrosis and sloughing of the graft. This entire process usually requires 11 to 14 days and is called a *first-set rejection.* (A syngraft or autograft does not undergo this process but remains viable with little or no inflammatory reaction.) When a second graft from the same genetically unrelated donor who provided the first graft is transplanted, a more rapid and more vigorous rejection occurs *(second-set rejection).* During the first 3 days after the second transplant the second graft is handled in essentially the same way as the first graft. However, vascularization is abruptly halted at 4 to 5 days with the sudden onset of ischemic necrosis. Because the graft

never becomes vascularized and the blood supply is cut off by the second-set rejection, there is little chance for cellular infiltration to occur. The primary target for the second-set rejection appears to be the capillaries taking part in revascularization. Similar events occur after grafting other solid organs such as the kidney or heart.

Although graft rejections are more closely linked to delayed or cellular hypersensitivity than to humoral reactions, there is some evidence that circulating antibody plays a role in graft rejection. An acute necrotic rejection of skin allografts occurs when specific antiserum to the graft is injected directly into the site of the skin graft. The failure of any circulation to be established results in complete ischemic necrosis, the "white graft" reaction.

The role that different immune mechanisms play in graft rejection can be seen in the morphologic changes observed in rejected renal allografts. The morphology of first-set rejections in untreated recipients is entirely consistent with cellular mechanisms. The main feature is the accumulation of mononuclear cell infiltrate. Within a few hours small lymphocytes collect around small venules. Later many more mononuclear cells appear in the stroma. After a few days these mononuclear cells are much more varied in structure with many

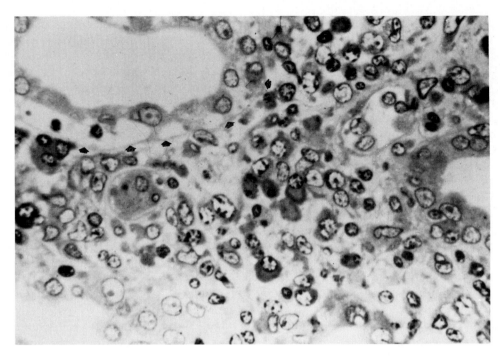

Fig. 12-36. Renal graft rejection. Mononuclear cells have invaded renal stroma and have passed through basement membrane of renal tubule *(arrows)* causing separation, detachment, and death of tubular lining cells. Stroma contains lymphocytes, macrophages, and plasma cells. (Courtesy Martin Flax, Tufts University, Boston, Mass.)

small and large lymphocytes, immature blast cells, and typical mature plasma cells. Invasion of the renal tubular cells occurs with isolation, separation, and death of these cells and is morphologically very similar, if not identical, to that described for tissue-culture monolayers (Fig. 12-36). The interstitial tissue of the rejecting kidney accumulates large quantities of fluid (edema). Finally the afferent arterioles and small arteries become swollen and occluded by fibrin–white cell thrombi. Occasionally these vessels show fibrinoid necrosis and contain immunoglobulins and complement consistent with deposition of antibody-antigen complexes. Therefore the first-set renal allograft rejection by a untreated recipient appears to occur primarily by cellular mechanisms though there is evidence that humoral antibody may play a role.

A second renal allotransplant from the same donor who provided the first graft may be rejected much more rapidly (within 1 to 3 days). There is little mononuclear cell infiltrate, presumably because adequate circulation for the accumulation of blood mononuclear cells is never established. There is destruction of peritubular capillaries and fibrinoid necrosis of the walls of the small arteries and arterioles. By 24 hours there is widespread tubular necrosis, and the kidney never assumes any functional activity. Perfusion of a renal homotransplant with plasma from an animal hyperimmunized against the donor of the kidney produces a similar

reaction. Therefore the hyperacute second-set rejection of renal allografts is mediated by preformed circulating antibodies. This type of hyperacute rejection of a renal allograft has been observed in humans when grafting was attempted across ABO blood group types. A renal allograft from an A or a B donor to an O recipient resulted in a complete failure of circulation in the graft with distension and thrombosis of afferent arterioles and glomerular capillaries with sludged red cells, presumably because of the action of cytotoxic anti–blood group antibodies on blood group antigens in the vasculature of the grafted kidney.

Immunosuppressive therapy is now widely used to postpone allograft rejection, and the use of immunosuppressive agents has resulted in a prolonged survival of human renal allografts. Such therapy appears to be effective in suppressing the early development of rejection but does not prevent later rejection. Many patients have now survived for several years with renal allografts. However, rejection may still occur. Morphologically the major finding in such late rejected kidneys is a pronounced intimal proliferation and scarring of the walls of medium-sized arteries. The appearance is much like that of a healed or late-stage polyarteritis nodosa. These late rejections are most likely caused by a slowly accumulating antibody-mediated immune-complex reaction.

An important factor in the survival of a renal transplant is the original disease that caused renal failure. In some recipients whose renal failure was caused by glomerulonephritis, glomerulonephritis also develops in the transplanted kidney. This may result from the continued presence of circulating antibody in the recipient's blood that reacts with glomerular antigens. It supports the concept that some stages of poststreptococcal glomerulonephritis are caused by antibodies that react directly with glomerular antigens and not streptococcal antigen deposited on the membranes.

Graft facilitation (tumor enhancement). Humoral antibody to grafted tissue may suppress or block the rejection of a graft by the cellular mechanism (blocking antibody). This paradoxical effect was first noted when transplanted tumor tissue that should have been rejected actually survived longer if the recipient had humoral antibody to the tumor before transplantation (tumor enhancement). Nontumor tissue grafts also survive longer if the recipient has humoral antibody to the graft, either by active or passive immunization (graft facilitation). The enhancement-facilitation effect may interfere with a potential delayed hypersensitivity–mediated rejection reaction (1) by blocking delivery of antigen to the potentially responding cells (afferent effect), (2) by preventing responding cells from recognizing the antigen (central effect), or (3) by protecting the target graft or tumor cells from reaction with a sensitized cells that might be produced (efferent effect). Interference with effector cells is supported by the fact that humoral antibodies may block immune attack of sensitized killer cells in vitro. The exact mechanism of facilitation or enhancement many vary from one situation to another so that no single explanation covers all facilitation-enhancement phenomena.

Graft-versus-host reactions. Graft-versus-host reactions result when immunologically competent cells from allogenic or xenogenic donors are transferred to a recipient whose own immune response is impaired. The transferred lymphoid cells colonize and react to the histocompatibility antigens in the recipient. Graft-versus-host reactions become important clinically when grafts of lymphoid tissue, such as bone marrow, which contains immunologically reactive cells, are made. In some situations when the lymphoid tissue of the recipient is not completely destroyed, regeneration of this tissue in the presence of the proliferating donor tissue produces a state of mutual tolerance in which the recipient maintains both its own and the donor lymphoid components.

The reaction of grafted immunoreactive cells produces a wasting syndrome (runting) or a secondary disease in the recipient. This consists of two components: (1) infiltration of tissues, especially the skin, intestine, spleen, and liver with proliferating lymphocytes, resulting in hepatosplenomegaly, diarrhea, and scaly contact dermatitis–like skin lesions, and (2) loss of immune

reactivity to other antigen (immune deficiency). Hyperplasia of spleen and other lymphoid tissue is followed by atrophy, presumably because the grafted cells have attacked and destroyed the host's lymphoid tissue. Proliferating host cells make the major contribution to the lymphoid hyperplasia, and it is the recipient's lymphopoietic tissue that bears the brunt of the attack. The success of bone marrow grafting depends on preventing a graft-versus-host reaction.

Bone marrow transplantation. Bone marrow grafts are used to treat patients with aplastic anemia (failure of blood cell production), with immune deficiencies, and with leukemia after radiation treatment. With careful matching and follow-up monitoring, good results are obtained in about half the cases of aplastic anemia or immune deficiency if an HLA-identical sibling donor is used.

Unless an identical twin is available, some degree of graft-versus-host reactivity seems inevitable. Efforts in improving bone marrow transplantation have centered on reducing the severity of the graft-versus-host reaction while providing sufficient bone marrow stem cells to reconstitute the recipient. Techniques used have included HLA matching, particularly using HLA-matched siblings; the use of mixtures of cells from several related donors with the hope that the most compatible donor cells will survive; the administration of immunosuppressive agents such as cyclophosphamide or antilymphocyte serum; the fractionation of cells in an attempt to eliminate the immunologically reactive cells that would produce the graft-versus-host reaction; the use of preserved autologous bone marrow obtained during a remission and treatment of the cells to be transferred with monoclonal antibody to remove T-cell subpopulations. None of these procedures can be considered satisfactory as yet, though long-term remissions have been obtained in some patients. In most remissions, a transient graft-versus-host reaction occurs and the treated individual demonstrates both host and donor cells after the reaction (chimerism).

Autoimmune diseases

The criterion for inclusion of a disease process in the autoimmune category is the demonstration of an endogenous immune response to an endogenous antigen. Acquired hemolytic anemia, idiopathic thrombocytopenic purpura, experimental allergic glomerulonephritis, rheumatoid arthritis, and systemic lupus erythematosus are examples of diseases caused by autoantibodies. Many other autoallergic diseases are believed to be the result of a delayed type of reaction. Experimentally, lesions are produced by immunization of an animal with constituents of its own tissues. When the hypersensitive state appears, reactions occur where antigen is situated in its tissues and result in lesions. Thus far, le-

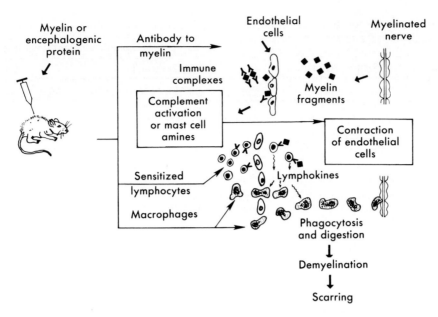

Fig. 12-37. Possible pathogenic events in experimental allergic encephalomyelitis. Immunization of experimental animals with myelin or encephalogenic protein results in production of humoral antibody and specifically sensitized cells, which together lead to demyelination by macrophages. Antibody reacting with myelin released into circulation through endothelial venules in white matter (that is, myelinated area of brain and spinal cord) activates either anaphylatoxin (complement) or mast cell (IgE) degranulation. Contraction of endothelial cells opens up gaps in small venule walls. Sensitized small lymphocytes move into white matter, react with myelin antigen, and release lymphocyte mediators. Macrophages, attracted and activated by these mediators, phagocytose and digest antibody-coated myelin or myelin affected by reaction with sensitized lymphocytes. If zones of demyelination are large, fibrosis will occur and permanent loss of function will result. (From Sell, S.: Immunology, immunopathology, and immunity, ed. 3, New York, 1980, Harper & Row, Publishers, Inc.)

sions have been produced by immunization of animals with lens, uvea, central nervous system (CNS) myelin, peripheral nervous system myelin, acetylcholine receptors, thyroid, adrenal, testes, glomerular basement membrane, and salivary gland. The lesions are irregularly distributed in regions of high antigen concentration, as in the white matter of the CNS in experimental allergic encephalomyelitis (Fig. 12-37). Local inflammatory reactions occur around small veins and consist of lymphocytes, histiocytes, and giant cells. Necrosis, hemorrhage, and polymorphonuclear infiltration occur in severe acute reactions, and these reactions may be initiated by humoral antibody (toxic complex reaction). Parenchymal destruction is coexistent with inflammation (that is, demyelination, destruction of uveal pigment, thyroid colloid, and so on). Within the involved tissue, the degree of destruction is determined to a great extent by blood-tissue barriers. Antibody and sensitized cells may act synergistically or antagonistically in the autoimmune process.

The experimental autoimmune diseases provide good models for the human disease of unknown cause (Table 12-20). The acute monocyclic diseases may result from allergic reactions to viruses or bacterial product–tissue combinations.

Autoantibodies. A variety of autoantibodies have been described in different human diseases. The pathogenic significance of most autoantibodies is unknown. A pathogenic importance has been convincingly demonstrated for some of these in vivo, but until more evidence is obtained, it is more likely that most such antibodies are the result of tissue alteration or breakdown rather than the cause of the lesion. It has been postulated that such antibodies actually function to clean up or clear the body fluids of abnormal or damaged tissue components, since it is known that the presence of circulating antibody results in a rapid clearance of antigen from the bloodstream.

Autoimmune mechanisms. The reasons why autoimmune reactions develop are many. When an immunotolerant animal becomes responsive to an antigen to which it was previously tolerant, tolerance is said to have been broken. Autoimmunization is braking of natural tolerance to self-antigens (see discussion of toler-

Table 12-20. Relation of experimental autoimmune diseases to human diseases

		Histologically similar human disease	
Experimental disease	**Tissue involved**	**Acute monocyclic**	**Chronic relapsing**
Allergic encephalomyelitis	Myelin (central nervous system)	Postinfectious encephalomyelitis	Multiple sclerosis
Allergic neuritis	Myelin (peripheral nervous system)	Guillain-Barré polyneuritis	
Phacoanaphylactic endophthalmitis	Lens		Phacoanaphylactic endophthalmitis
Allergic uveitis	Uvea	Postinfectious iridocyclitis	Sympathetic ophthalmia
Allergic orchitis	Germinal epithelium	Mumps orchitis	Nonendocrine chronic infertility
Allergic thyroiditis	Thyroglobulin	Mumps thyroiditis	Subacute and chronic thyroiditis
Allergic sialadenitis	Glandular epithelium	Mumps parotitis	Sjögren's syndrome
Allergic adrenalitis	Cortical cells		Cytotoxic contraction of adrenal
Allergic gastritis	Gastric mucosa		Atrophic gastritis
Experimental allergic nephritis	Glomerular membrane	Acute glomerulonephritis	Chronic glomerulonephritis

Modified from Waksman, B.H.: Int. Arch. Allergy Appl. Immunol. **14**(suppl.):1, 1959.

Table 12-21. Some HLA disease associations

HLA specificity	**Disease**
B27	Reiter's syndrome, ankylosing spondylarthritis, psoriatic rheumatism
DR3 (A1, B8)	Myasthenia gravis, Graves' disease, Addison's disease, Sjögren's syndrome, systemic lupus erythematosus, chronic active hepatitis, juvenile diabetes dermatitis herpetiformis, sprue
DR2	Multiple sclerosis, systemic lupus
DR4	erythematosus, rheumatoid arthritis, juvenile diabetes, and pemphigus
DR5, DR8, DR6	Juvenile arthritis

ance, p. 497). The etiology of many autoimmune diseases is still obscure, even if the pathophysiology of the diseases is becoming clear. As is true for the induction of tolerance, breaking tolerance need not proceed by only one mechanism in a given disease. Only when these mechanisms are sorted out on a disease-by-disease, patient-by-patient basis can progress toward understanding and preventing some of these diseases occur.

MHC and autoimmune diseases

The association of some diseases believed to have an autoimmune cause with certain HLA types strongly indicates that the human MHC may control the type and extent of the immune response to certain antigens (Ta-

ble 12-21). For example, an inflammatory disease of spinal articulations, termed "ankylosing spondylitis," develops in persons who are HLA-B27 positive after infection with certain gram-negative bacteria, such as *Shigella, Salmonella,* and *Yersinia.* Although ankylosing spondylitis also develops in HLA-B27–negative individuals, the incidence is much lower. Thus there may be an immune response gene region in the human MHC that corresponds to the mouse IR region. This immune response (IR) region may determine that susceptibility to a variety of autoimmune diseases.

Granulomatous hypersensitivity

Granulomatous hypersensitivity produce space-occupying masses of inflammatory cells in reactions to antigens or foreign bodies that cannot be easily degraded by macrophages (Fig. 12-38). Granulomatous hypersensitivity reactions are identified by the appearance of reticuloendothelial cells, including phagocytes, histiocytes, epithelioid cells, and giant cells. The characteristic epithelioid cell has a prominent eosinophilic amorphous cytoplasm and a large, oval, pale-staining nucleus with a sharp, thin, nuclear membrane and large nucleoli. These cells have been called "epithelioid cells" because of their morphologic resemblance to epithelial cells. The epithelioid cells are arranged into tubercles or granulomas, the most characteristic feature of granulomatous hypersensitivity reactions. Granulomatous reactions are responses to poorly degradable substances and may arise in response to foreign bodies or be ascribed to a hypersensitivity reaction to insoluble antigens. If soluble protein antigen from a tuberculin extract is injected into the skin of a sensitive individual, a

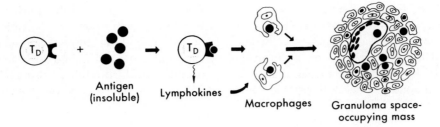

Fig. 12-38. Granulomatous hypersensitivity reactions. Reaction of sensitized cells with poorly degradable antigens results in focal collection of macrophages, lymphocytes, epithelioid cells, and giant cells arranged in oval laminated structure called a granuloma. Granulomas are space-occupying lesions that result in loss of tissue function.

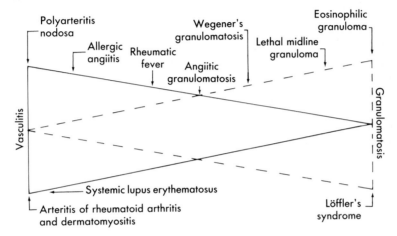

Fig. 12-39. Spectrum of diseases with mixed features of granulomatous lesions and vasculitis. Lesions of Löffler's syndrome and eosinophilic granuloma are essentially pure granulomas with little or no vasculitis. Lesions of polyarteritis nodosa and other rheumatoid diseases are primarily vascular, though some granulomatous lesions (subcutaneous nodules) are associated with these diseases. Other diseases demonstrate different mixtures of vasculitis and granulomatous lesions. (Modified from Alarcón-Segovia, D., and Brown, A.L., Jr.: Mayo Clin. Proc. **39**:205, 1964.)

typical delayed skin reaction is elicited. However, if a poorly soluble, waxy preparation is used, a granulomatous lesion is produced.

Granulomatous reactions may follow sensitized T-cell or antibody reactions with antigen in tissues. Epithelioid cells are believed to be "activated" macrophages or to represent macrophages that have already performed phagocytosis and partial digestion of antigen. The onset of granulomatous hypersensitivity reactions is much more delayed than that of true delayed hypersensitivity, requiring weeks or even months to develop. Granulomas frequently form around foreign bodies such as suture material. These may or may not be immune mediated. Granulomatous reactions may also occur to antibody-antigen complexes if the antigen is not readily catabolized.

The diseases in which granulomatous reactions are involved include tuberculosis, histoplasmosis, sarcoidosis, leprosy, many parasitic infections, zirconium granulomas, berylliosis, and granulomatoses associated with vasculitis (Fig. 12-39). The morphologic features of these diseases are discussed in other chapters of this book.

Tuberculosis is a classic example of the role of granulomatous reactivity in producing tissue damage. Infection with tubercle bacilli leads to different types of immune reactivity, including antibody formation, classic delayed hypersensitivity, increased macrophage activity (activated macrophages), and granulomatous reactivity. Granulomatous reactivity is necessary for isolation of infectious organisms. Persons who have recovered from tuberculosis usually have evidence of old granulomas in tissue that were infected. In some persons the infection may become disseminated before the immune response is able to localize it, or a previously localized infection may become disseminated if there is a decrease in granulomatous reactivity. That fatal tuberculosis is associated with multiple granulomatous lesions does not mean that granulomatous reactivity is not protective. Immune reactivity is not always successful in limiting an infection, particularly if the infection is well established before full immune reactivity develops or if other factors such as age, immune suppression, or poor condition contribute to a lowered resistance.

Allergic granulomatosis, or Churg-Strauss syndrome, includes necrotizing vasculitis, extravascular granulomas, and tissue infiltration with eosinophils occurring in association with bronchial asthma. Such a combination of allergic lesions may indicate the involvement of different immune effector mechanisms—such as toxic complex, anaphylactic, and granulomatous mechanisms—in a single individual.

The *protective function* of granulomatous reactivity is best exemplified by leprosy. It is clear that a favorable response to therapy occurs in patients with granulomatous lesions (tuberculoid leprosy), whereas the prognosis and response to therapy are not good in patients without granulomatous reactivity (lepromatous leprosy). The granulomatous form is associated with low tissue content of the organism and a high resistance, whereas the opposite is true for the lepromatous form. Lepromatous leprosy is associated with high titers of serum antibodies and immune complex–mediated lesions. Granulomatous reactivity most likely plays a similar role in tuberculosis and other infections, particularly chronic mucocutaneous candidiasis.

Drug allergy

True allergic reactions to drugs fall into one of the preceding categories. Many drug allergies involve in vivo combination of drugs with body constituents to produce complete antigens. This is apparently almost always true in contact allergies and probably is also the case with atopic disease attributable to aspirin and other chemicals. Drugs reactions may produce asthma and vasomotor rhinitis, urticaria and angioneurotic edema, serum sickness, drug rashes, agranulocytosis, aplastic anemia and thrombocytopenia, contact dermatitis, fixed eruptions, exfoliative dermatitis, photosensitization, erythema nodosum, and drug-induced hemolytic anemia.

Penicillin reaction are excellent examples of the complexities of drug allergies. Penicillin metabolites act as haptens (incomplete antigen) that combine with serum or tissue proteins to form complete antigens. Such combinations may be found in three different chemical forms because of the ability of benzylpenicillin (penicillin G) to attach to proteins by different bonds. The administration of the simple compound benzylpenicillin to experimental animals and to humans may lead to the production of antibodies with at least three different specificities. This opens the possibility of a given individual's producing reaginic type (atopic type) of antibody to one determinant and delayed sensitivity or precipitating antibodies (Arthus type) to another, or even different types of hypersensitivity to the same determinant, thus causing a complex clinical picture because of a combination of different types of allergic reactions.

Immune-mediated skin diseases

A variety of skin lesions illustrate the wide range of manifestations of immune mechanisms. A classification of some skin disease on the basis of immune mechanism is given in Table 12-22. Of particular interest are those mediated by humoral antibodies and associated with deposition of immunoglobulin in the skin. Intraepithelial separation (bullae) in pemphigus is associated with intraepithelial Ig; basement membrane lesions in phemphigoid and herpes gestationis is associated with basement membrane deposition of Ig. Deposition of IgA in dermal microfibers is seen with dermatitis herpetiformis and deposition of immunoglobulin and complement in vascular walls in cutaneous vasculitis.

CONCLUSIONS

Immune mechanisms that serve as defensive reactions to invasion of the body by foreign organisms or to the effects of toxic agents may actually cause disease in certain circumstances. When immune mechanisms are used in a destructive way, the reactions are termed "allergic" or "hypersensitivity" reactions. In most cases of human disease in which immune reactions are believed to play a role, it is difficult to rule out other possible inflammatory mechanisms. The characteristics found in experimental immune responses can rarely if ever be exactly duplicated for human diseases. These include (1) a well-defined immunizing event (infection, immunization, or vaccination), (2) a latent period (usually 6 to 14 days), (3) a secondary response (a more rapid and intense reaction on second exposure to the antigen), (4) passive transfer of the disease state with cells or serum from an affected individual, (5) specific depression of the disease by large amounts of antigen (desensitization), and (6) identification and isolation of the antigen.

Presumptive findings consistent with but not proving an allergic mechanism in disease states include (1) a morphologic picture consistent with known allergic reactions, (2) the demonstration of antibody or a positive delayed skin reaction, (3) a depression of complement during some stage of the disease, (4) a beneficial effect

Table 12-22. Immune mechanism in some skin diseases

Disease	Lesion	Association	Immune mechanism
CYTOTOXIC LESIONS			
Dermatitis herpetiformis	Subepidermal bullae	Gluten enteropathy (sprue)	IgA and complement deposition in dermal microfibers and basement membrane (autoantibody or immune complex)
Herpes gestationis	Subepidermal bullae	Pregnancy	Properdin, C3 and IgG in basement membrane (autoantibody, or immune complex)
Pemphigus	Intraepithelial bullae	Autoallergic diseases	Autoantibody to epithelial cell surfaces
Pemphigoid	Subepidermal bullae	Neoplasm, autoallergy	Autoantibody to basement membrane
Psoriasis	Corneum parakaratosis, acanthosis	Psoriatic arthritis	?Autoantibody to keratin
Cutaneous lupus	Basement membrane degeneration, subcutaneous vasculitis	Systemic and discoid lupus	Autoantibody to basement membrane, immune complex deposition or membrane attack complex
Vitiligo	Melanocytes, depigmentation	Autoallergic diseases	Antibody to melanocytes
Alopecia areata	Loss of hair	Endocrinopathy	Antibody to capillary of endothelium hair bulb
VASCULAR LESIONS (IMMUNE COMPLEX)			
Erythema nodosum	Subcutaneous vasculitis	Infection	Immune complex
Erythema marginatum	Subcutaneous vasculitis	Rheumatic fever	Immune complex (?anaphylactic)
Erythema multiforme	Subcutaneous vasculitis	Drug reaction	Immune complex
Cutaneous vasculitis	Subcutaneous vasculitis	Infection, systemic lupus erythematosus	Immune complex
ANAPHYLACTIC REACTIONS			
Cutaneous anaphylaxis	Wheal and flare	Mosquito bite, allergic reaction	IgE-mediated mast cell degranulation—histamine
Giant urticaria	Wheal	?Allergy	IgE
Angioedema	Nonpitting edema	—	C1 inhibitor deficiency
DELAYED HYPERSENSITIVITY LESIONS			
Contact dermatitis	Vesiculation, induration, spongiosis	Poison ivy, poison oak	Delayed hypersensitivity
Viral exanthema	Vesiculation, induration, spongiosis	Measles, smallpox, etc	Delayed hypersensitivity
Tuberculin test	Perivascular mononuclear cell infiltrate, induration	Tuberculosis	Delayed hypersensitivity
Syphilis (chancre)	Perivascular and diffuse mononuclear cell infiltrate	Syphilis	Delayed hypersensitivity
GRANULOMATOUS LESIONS			
Zirconium granulomas	Axillary granuloma	Stick deodorants	Granulomatous hypersensitivity
Tuberculoid leprosy	Cutaneous granulomas	Leprosy	Granulomatous hypersensitivity
Sarcoidosis	Granulomas	Sarcoid	Granulomatous hypersensitivity

of agents that are known to inhibit some portion of the allergic reaction (steroids, radiation, nitrogen mustard, aminopterin, and so on), (5) identification of a reason-able experimental model in animals that mimics the human disease, (6) an association with other possible allergic diseases, and (7) an increased familial susceptibility to the same disease or other allergic diseases. An immune cause for many other diseases not included in this chapter, such as inflammatory bowel disease, is suspected but not yet proved. With further understanding of both normal and abnormal immune reactions, many other diseases of unknown cause may well be shown to be caused by immune mechanisms.

REFERENCES
General

Barrett, J.T.: Textbook of immunology, ed. 4, St. Louis, 1983, The C.V. Mosby Co.

Bellanti, J.A.: Immunology, Philadelphia, 1971, W.B. Saunders Co.

Boyd, W.C.: Fundamentals of immunology, ed. 4, New York, 1966, Interscience Publishers.

Eisen, H.N.: Immunology, ed. 2, Hagerstown, Md., 1980, Harper & Row, Publishers, Inc.

Golub, E.S.: The cellular basis of the immune response, ed. 2, Sunderland, Mass., 1981, Sinauer Associates, Inc.

Hood, L.E., Weissman, I.L., and Wood, W.B.: Immunology, ed. 2, Menlo Park, Calif., 1984, The Benjamin/Cummings Publishing Co.

Kimball, J.W.: Introduction to immunology, ed. 2, New York, 1986, MacMillan Publishing Co.

Lachmann, P.J., and Peters, D.K., editors: Clinical aspects of immunology, ed. 4, Oxford, Eng., 1982, Blackwell Scientific Publications.

McConnel, I., Monroe, A., and Waldmann, H.: The immune system, ed. 2, Oxford, Eng., 1975, Blackwell Scientific Publications.

Miescher, P.A., and Müller-Eberhard, H.J.: Textbook of immunopathology, ed. 2, New York, 1976, Grune & Stratton, Inc.

Roitt, I.M.: Essential immunology, ed. 5, Oxford, Eng., 1984, Blackwell Scientific Publications.

Sampter, M., editor: Immunological diseases, ed. 3, Boston, 1988, Little, Brown & Co.

Sell, S.: Immunology, immunopathology, and immunity, ed. 4, New York, 1987, Elsevier Science Publishing Co., Inc.

Stites, D.P., et al.: Basic and clinical immunology, ed. 5, Los Angeles, 1984, Lange Medical Publishers.

Basic immunology
Antigenicity

Benjamin, D.C., et al.: The antigenic structure of proteins: a reappraisal, Annu. Rev. Immunol. 2:67, 1984.

Heidelberger, M.: Lectures in immunochemistry, New York, 1956, Academic Press, Inc.

Kabat, E.A.: The nature of an antigenic determinant, J. Immunol. 97:1, 1966.

Kabat, E.A.: Structural concepts in immunology and immunochemistry, New York, 1986, Holt, Rinehart & Winston.

Landsteiner, K.: The specificity of serological reactions, New York, 1962, Dover Publications.

Sela, M.: Immunological studies with synthetic polypeptides, Adv. Immunol. 5:30, 1969.

Immunoglobulins and antibodies

Amzel, L.M., and Poljak, R.J.: Three dimensional structure of immunoglobulins, Am. Rev. Biochem. 48:961, 1979.

Bernier, B.M.: Structure of human immunoglobulins: myeloma proteins as analogues of antibody, Prog. Allergy 14:1, 1970.

Binz, H., Lindeman, J., and Wigzell, H.: Cell-bound receptors for alloantigens on normal lymphocytes. II. Antialloantibody serum contains specific factors reacting with relevant immunocompetent T lymphocytes, J. Exp. Med. 140:731, 1974.

Cosenza, H., and Kohler, H.: Specific suppression of the antibody response by antibodies to receptors, Proc. Natl. Acad. Sci. USA 69:2710, 1972.

Davis, J., et al.: Structural correlates of idiotypes, Annu. Rev. Immunol. 4:147, 1986.

Edelman, G.M., Cunningham, B.A., Gall, W.E., et al.: The covalent structure of an entire γG-immunoglobulin molecule, Biochemistry 63:78, 1969.

Gell, P.G.H., and Kelus, A.S.: Anti-antibodies, Adv. Immunol. 6:461, 1967.

Kabat, E.A.: Origins of antibody complementarity and specificity-hypervariable regions and the multigene hypothesis, J. Immunol. 125:961, 1980.

Kelus, A.S., and Gell, P.G.H.: Immunoglobulin allotypes of experimental animals, Prog. Allergy 11:141, 1967.

Kindt, T.S., and Capra, J.D.: The antibody enigma, New York, 1984, Plenum Press.

Liu, C.-P., et al.: Structure of the genes that rearrange in development, Science 209:1348, 1980.

Natvig, J.B., and Kunkel, H.G.: Human immunoglobulins: classes, subclasses, genetic variants and idiotypes, Adv. Immunol. 16:1, 1973.

Nisonoff, A., Hopper, J.E., and Spring, S.R.: The antibody molecule, New York, 1975, Academic Press, Inc.

Novotný, J., Bruccoleri, R., Newell, J., Murphy, D., Haber, E., and Karplus, M.: Molecular anatomy of the antibody binding site, J. Biol. Chem. 258:14433, 1983.

Ohno, S., Nori, N., and Matsunaga, T.: Antigen binding specificities of antibodies are primarily determined by seven residues of VH, Proc. Natl. Acad. Sci. USA 82:2945, 1985.

Winkelnake, J.L.: Immunoglobulin structure and effector functions, Immunochemistry 15:695, 1978.

Immunoglobulin genes

Calame, K.L.: Mechanisms that regulate immunoglobulin gene expression, Annu. Rev. Immunol. 3:159, 1985.

Cushley, W., and Williamson, A.R.: Expression of immunoglobulin genes, Essays Biochem. 18:1, 1982.

Honjo, T.: Immunoglobulin genes, Annu. Rev. Immunol. 1:499, 1983.

Hood, L., Campbell, J.H., and Elgin, S.C.R.: The organization, expression, and evolution of antibody genes and other multigene families, Annu. Rev. Genet. 9:305, 1975.

Möller, G., editor: Control of immunoglobulin gene expression, Immunol. Rev. 89, 1986.

Seidman, J.G., Leder, A., Nau, M., Norman, B., and Leder, P.: Antibody diversity: the structure of cloned immunoglobulin genes suggests a mechanism for generating new sequences, Science 202:11, 1978.

Wall, R., and Kuehl, M.: Biosynthesis and regulation of immunoglobulins, Annu. Rev. Immunol. 1:393, 1983.

Yancopoulos, G.D., and Alt, F.W.: Regulation of the assembly and expression of variable-region genes, Annu. Rev. Immunol. 4:339, 1986.

Antibody-antigen reactions

Benjamin, D.C., et al.: The antigenic structure of proteins: a reappraisal, Annu. Rev. Immunol. 2:67, 1984.

Coons, A.H.: Histochemistry with labeled antibody, Int. Rev. Cytol. 5:1, 1956.

Cotton, R.G.H.: Monoclonal antibodies in the study of structure-functional relationships of proteins, Med. Res. Rev. 5:77, 1985.

Crowle, A.J.: Immunodiffusion, New York, 1961, Academic Press, Inc.

Farr, R.S.: A quantitative immunochemical measure of the primary interaction between I*BSA and antibody, J. Infect. Dis. 103:239, 1958.

Gill, T.J., III: Methods for detecting antibody, Immunochemistry 7:997, 1970.

Heidelberger, M.: Lectures in immunochemistry, New York, 1956, Academic Press, Inc.

Kabat, E.A., and Mayer, M.M.: Experimental immunochemistry, ed. 2, Springfield, Ill., 1961, Charles C Thomas, Publisher.

Karush, F.: Immunological specificity and molecular structure, Adv. Immunol. **2**:1, 1962.

Kitagawa, M., Yagi, Y., and Pressman, D.: The heterogeneity of combining sites of antibodies as determined by specific immunoabsorbents, J. Immunol. **95**:446, 991, 1965.

Lymphocytes
B-cells

Cooper, M.D., and Lawton, A.R.: The development of the immune system, Sci. Am. **231**:58, 1974.

Cebra, J.J., Komisar, J.L., and Schweitzer, P.A.: CH isotype "switching" during normal B cell development, Annu. Rev. Immunol. **2**:493, 1984.

Dutton, R.W.: Separate signals for the initiation of proliferation and differentiation in the B cell response to antigen, Transplant. Rev. **23**:66, 1975.

Howard, M., and Paul, W.E.: Regulation of B cell growth and differentiation by soluble factors, Annu. Rev. Immunol. **1**:307, 1983.

Möller, G., editor: B cell lineages, Immunol. Rev., vol. 93, 1986.

Parkhouse, R.M.E., and Cooper, M.D.: A model for the differentiation of B lymphocytes with implications for the biological role of IgD, Immunol. Rev. **37**:105, 1977.

Whitlock, C., Denis, K., Robertson, D., and Witte, O.: In vitro analysis of murine B-cell development, Annu. Rev. Immunol. **3**:213, 1985.

T-cells

Barth, R.K., Kim, B.S., Lan, N.C., Hunkapiller, T., Sobieck, N., Winoto, A., Gershenfeld, H., Okada, C., Hansburg, D., Weissman, I.L., et al.: The murine T-cell receptor uses a limited repertoire of expressed Vβ gene segments, Nature **316**:517, 1985.

Cantrell, P.A., and Smith, K.A.: The interleukin-2 T cell system: a new cell growth model, Science **224**:1312, 1984.

Fitch, F.T.: Cell clones and T cell receptors, Microbiol. Rev. **50**:50, 1986.

Haskins, K., Kappler, J., and Marrack, P.: The major histocompatibility complex–restricted antigen receptor on T-cells, Annu. Rev. Immunol. **2**:51, 1984.

Haynes, B.F.: Phenotypic characterization and ontogeny of components of the human thymic microenvironment, Clin. Res. **32**:500, 1984.

Van Ewjk, W.: Immunohistology of lymphoid and non-lymphoid cells in the thymus in relation to T cell differentiation, Am. J. Anat. **170**:311, 1964.

Weiss, A., Imboden, J., Hardy, K., Manger, B., Terhorst, C., and Stobo, J.: The role of T3/antigen receptor complex in T-cell activation, Annu. Rev. Immunol. **4**:593, 1986.

Effector lymphocytes

Adams, D.O., and Hamilton, T.A.: The cell biology of macrophage activation, Annu. Rev. Immunol. **2**:283, 1984.

David, J.R.: Delayed hypersensitivity in vitro: its mediation by cell free substances formed by lymphoid cell–antigen interaction, Proc. Natl. Acad. Sci. USA **56**:72, 1966.

George, M., and Vaughn, J.H.: In vitro cell migration as a model for delayed hypersensitivity, Proc. Soc. Exp. Biol. Med. **111**:514, 1962.

Henney, C.S.: On the mechanism of T-cell mediated cytolysis, Transplant. Rev. **17**:37, 1973.

Herbermann, R.N., Reynolds, C.W., and Ortaldo, J.: Mechanisms of cytotoxicity by natural killer cells, Annu. Rev. Immunol. **4**:651, 1986.

Mackaness, G.B.: Resistence to intercellular infection, J. Infect. Dis. **123**:429, 1971.

Perlmann, P., and Holm, G.: Cytotoxic effects of lymphoid cells in vitro, Adv. Immunol. **11**:117, 1969.

Major histocompatibility complex

Bodmer, J., and Bodmer, W.: Histocompatibility 1984, Immunol. Today **5**:251, 1984.

Hildemann, W.H., Clark, E.A., and Raison, R.L.: Comprehensive immunogenetics, New York, 1981, Elsevier Scientific Publishing Co.

Hood, L., Kronenberg, M., and Hunkapiller, T.: T cell antigen receptors and the immunoglobulin supergene family, Cell **40**:225, 1985.

Klein, J., Figueroa, F., and Nagy, G.: Genetics of the major histocompatibility complex: the final act, Annu. Rev. Immunol. **1**:119, 1983.

Lew, A.M., Lillehoj, E.P., Cowan, E.P., Maloy, W.L., van Schravendijk, M.R., and Coligan, J.E.: Class I genes and molecules: an update, Immunology **57**:3, 1986.

McDevitt, H.O.: The HLA system and its relation to disease, Hosp. Pract. **20**:57, 1985.

Steinmetz, M., and Hood, L.: Genetics of the major histocompatibility complex, Science **222**:727, 1983.

Cellular interactions during the immune response

Altman, A., and Katz, D.H.: The biology of monoclonal lymphokines secreted by T cells and hybridomas, Adv. Immunol. **33**:73, 1982.

Burnet, F.M.: The clonal selection theory of acquired immunity, London, 1959, Cambridge University Press.

Claman, H.N., and Mosier, D.E.: Cell-cell interactions in antibody production, Prog. Allergy **16**:40, 1972.

Durun, S.K., Schmidt, J.A., and Oppenheim, J.J.: Interleukin 1: an immunological perspective, Annu. Rev. Immunol. **3**:263, 1985.

Ehrlich, P.: On immunity, with special reference to cell life, Proc. R. Soc. Lond. (Biol.) **66**:424, 1900.

Hildemann, W.H., Clark, E.A., and Raison, R.L.: Comprehensive immunogenetics, New York, 1981, Elsevier Scientific Publishing Co.

Jerne, N.K.: The natural selection theory of antibody formation, Proc. Natl. Acad. Sci. USA **41**:849, 1955.

Mitchison, N.A.: The carrier effect in the secondary response to hapten-protein conjugates. II. Cellular cooperation, Eur. J. Immunol. **1**:18, 1971.

Mosier, D.E., and Coppleson, L.W.: A three-cell interaction required for the induction of the primary response in vitro, Proc. Natl. Acad. Aci. USA **61**:542, 1968.

Nossal, G.J.V., and Ada, G.L.: Antigens, lymphoid cells and the immune response, New York, 1971, Academic Press, Inc.

Sell, S.: Development of restrictions in the expression of immunoglobulin specificities by lymphoid cells, Transplant. Rev. **5**:19, 1970.

Singer, A., and Hodes, R.J.: Mechanisms of T-cell B-cell restrictions, Annu. Rev. Immunol. **1**:211, 1983.

Szilard, L.: The molecular basis of antibody formation, Proc. Natl. Acad. Sci. USA **46**:293, 1960.

Control of the immune response

Asherson, G.L., Colizzi, V., and Zembala, M.: An overview of T-suppressor cell circuits, Annu. Rev. Immunol. **4**:37, 1986.

Green, D.R., Flood, P.M., and Gershon, R.: Immunoregulatory T-cell pathways, Annu. Rev. Immunol. **1**:439, 1983.

Jerne, N.K.: The immune system: a network of V domains, Harvey Lect. **70**:93, 1975.

Möller, G., editor: Idiotype networks, Immunol. Rev., vol. 79, 1984.

Lymphoid tissue and immune response

Benditt, B.P., and Lagunoff, D.: The mast cell: its structure and function, Prog. Allergy **8**:195, 1964.

Cohen, Z.A.: The structure and functions of monocytes and macrophages, Adv. Immunol. **9**:163, 1968.

Goldschneider, I., and McGregor, D.D.: Anatomical distribution of T and B lymphocytes in the rat, J. Exp. Med. **138**:1443, 1973.

Gowans, J.L., and McGregor, D.D.: The immunological activities of lymphocytes, Prog. Allergy **9**:1, 1965.

Gutman, G.A., and Weissman, I.L.: Lymphoid tissue architecture: experimental analysis of the origin and distribution of T-cells and B-cells, Immunology **23**:465, 1972.

Lukes, R.J., and Collins, R.D.: New observations in follicular lymphoma, Gann. Monogr. Cancer Res. **15**:209, 1973.

Miller, J.R.A.P., and Osoba, D.: Current concepts of the immunological function of the thymus, Physiol. Rev. **47**:437, 1967.

Nossal, G.J.V., Ada, G.L., and Austin, C.M.P.: Antigens in immunity. IV. Cellular localization of ^{125}I-labeled flagella in lymph nodes, Aust. J. Exp. Biol. Med. Sci. **42**:311, 1964.

Sell, S., and Asofsky, R.: Lymphocytes and immunoglobulins, Prog. Allergy **12:**86, 1968.

Turk, J.L., and Oort, J.: Germinal center activity in relation to delayed hypersensitivity. In Cottier, H., et al., editors: Germinal centers in immune responses, New York, 1967, Springer-Verlag.

Waksman, B.H.: The homing pattern of thymus-derived lymphocytes in calf and neonatal mouse Peyer's patches, J. Immunol. **111:**878, 1973.

Yoffey, J.M., and Courtice, F.D.: Lymphatics, lymph and the lymphomyeloid complex, New York, 1970, Academic Press, Inc.

Autoimmunity and tolerance

Argyris, B.F.: Adoptive tolerance: transfer of the tolerant state, J. Immunol. **90:**29, 1963.

Burnet, F.M.: The clonal selection theory of acquired immunity, London, 1959, Cambridge University Press.

Burnet, F.M.: The integrity of the body: a discussion of modern immunological ideas, Cambridge, Mass., 1962, Harvard University Press.

Dorf, M.E., and Benacerraf, B.: Suppressor cells and immunoregulation, Annu. Rev. Immunol. **2:**126, 1984.

Dresser, D.W., and Mitchison, N.A.: The mechanism of immunological paralysis, Adv. Immunol. **8:**129, 1968.

Felton, L.D.: The significance of antigen in animal tissue, J. Immunol. **61:**107, 1949.

Gershon, R.K., Cohen, P., Hencin, R., et al.: Suppressor T cells, J. Immunol. **108:**586, 1972.

Grabar, D.: Antibodies and the physiologic role of immunoglobulin, Immunol. Today **4:**337, 1983.

Hasek, M., Langerova, A., and Hraba, T.: Transplantation immunity and tolerance, Adv. Immunol. **1:**1, 1961.

Katz, D.H., and Benacerraf, B.: Immunological tolerance: mechanisms and potential therapeutic applications, New York, 1974, Academic Press, Inc.

Kripke, M.L.: Immunological unresponsiveness induced by ultraviolet irradiation, Immunol. Rev. **80:**87, 1984.

Mitchison, N.A.: Induction of immunological paralysis with two zones of dosage, Proc. R. Soc. Lond. (Biol.) **161:**275, 1966.

Möller, G., editor: Auto-immunity, Immunol. Rev., vol. 94, 1986.

Owen, R.D.: Immunogenetic consequence of vascular anastomoses between bovine twins, Science **102:**400, 1945.

Parks, D.E., and Weigle, W.O.: Current perspectives on the cellular mechanisms of immunologic tolerance, Clin. Exp. Immunol. **39:**257, 1980.

Smith, H.R., and Steinberg, A.D.: Autoimmunity: a perspective, Annu. Rev. Immunol. **1:**175, 1983.

Immune effector mechanisms

Gell, P.G.H., and Coombs, R.R.A.: Clinical aspects of immunology, Oxford, 1963, Blackwell.

Roitt, I.M.: Essential immunology, Oxford, 1971, Blackwell.

Sell, S.: Immunology, immunopathology and immunity, Hagerstown, Md., 1972, Harper & Row.

Immune deficiency diseases

Afzelius, B.A.: The immobile-cilia syndrome: a microtubule associated object, CRC Crit. Rev. Biochem. **19:**63, 1985.

Barton, R.W., and Goldschneider, I.: Neocleotide-metabolizing enzymes and lymphocyte differentiation, Mol. Cell. Biochem. **28:**135, 1979.

Cooper, M.D., and Lawton, A.R., III: The development of the immune system, Sci. Am. **231:**58, 1974.

Cooper, M.D., Peterson, R.D.A., South, M.A., and Good, R.A.: The functions of the thymus system and the bursa system in the chicken, J. Exp. Med. **123:**75, 1966.

Davis, S.D., Schallar, S., and Wedgewood, R.J.: Job's syndrome: recurrent "cold" staphylococcal abscesses, Lancet **1:**10134, 1966.

DeGraff, P.A., et al.: The primary response in patients with selective IgA deficiency, Clin. Exp. Immunol. **54:**778, 1983.

Fundenberg, H.H., Good, K.A., Goodman, H.C., Hitzig, W., Kunkel, H.G., Roitt, I.M., Rosen, F.S., Rowe, D.S., Seligmann, M., and Soothill, J.R.: Primary immunodeficiencies: report of a World Health Organization committee, Pediatrics **47:**927, 1971.

Good, R.A., and Gabrielsen, A.E., editors: The thymus. In Immunobiology, New York, 1964, Harper & Row.

Good, R.A., Quie, P.G., Windhorst, D.B., Page, A.R., Rodey, G.E., White, J., Wolfson, J.J., and Holmes, B.H.: Fatal (chronic granulomatous disease of children: a hereditary defect of leukocyte function, Semin. Hematol. **5:**215, 1968.

Kellems, R.E., Yeung, C.Y., and Ingolia, D.E.: Adenosine deaminase deficiency and severe combined immune deficiencies, Trends Genet. **1:**278, 1985.

Kohl, S., Springer, T.A., Schmalstieg, F.C., Loo, L.S., and Anderson, D.C.: Defective natural killer cytotoxicity and polymorphonuclear leukocyte antibody-dependent cellular cytotoxicity in patients with LFA-1/OKM-1 deficiency, J. Immunol. **133:**2972, 1984.

Komura, K., and Boyse, E.A.: Induction of T lymphocytes from precursor cells in vitro by a product of the thymus, J. Exp. Med. **138:**479, 1973.

Landing, B.H., and Shirkey, H.S.: A syndrome of recurrent infection and infiltration of viscera by pigmented lipid histiocytes, Pediatrics **20:**431, 1957.

Lederman, H.M., and Winkelstein, J.A.: X-linked agammaglobulinemia: an analysis of 96 patients, Medicine **64:**145, 1985.

Lurie, H.I., and Duma, R.S.: Opportunistic infections of the lungs, Hum. Pathol. **1:**233, 1970.

Miller, J.F.A.P., and Osoba, D.: Current concepts of the immunological function of the thymus, Physiol. Rev. **47:**437, 1967.

Parrott, D.M., DeSousa, M.A.B., and East, J.: Thymus-dependent areas in lymphoid organs of neonatally thymectomized mice, J. Exp. Med. **123:**191, 1966.

Peterson, R.D.A., Cooper, M.D., and Good, R.A.: The pathogenesis of immunological deficiency diseases, Am. J. Med. **38:**579, 1965.

Roberts, R., and Gallin, J.I.: The phagocyte cell and its disorders, Ann. Allergy **50:**330, 1983.

Rosen, F.S., et al.: Primary immunodeficiency diseases: WHO meeting report, Clin. Immunol. Immunopathol. **28:**450, 1983.

Ross, S.C., and Densen, P.: Complement deficiency states and infections: epidemiology, pathogenesis and consequences of neisserial and other infections in an immune deficiency, Medicine **63:**243, 1984.

Sell, S.: Immunological deficiency diseases, Arch. Pathol. **86:**95, 1968.

Touraine, J.L., Betuel, H., Souillet, G., and Jenne, M.: Combined immunodeficiency disease associated with absence of cell surface HLA-A and B antigens, J. Pediatr. **93:**47, 1978.

Waksman, B.H., Arnason, B.G., and Jankovic, B.D.: Role of the thymus in immune reactions in rats. III. Changes in the lymphoid organs of thymectomized rats, J. Exp. Med. **116:**187, 1962.

Waldmann, T.A., Broder, S., Goldman, C.K., Frost, K., Korsmeyer, S.J., and Medici, M.A.: Disorders of B cells and helper T cells in pathogenesis of the immunoglobulin deficiency of patients with ataxia telangiectasia, J. Clin. Invest. **71:**282-295, 1983.

Warner, N.L., and Szenberg, A.: The immunological function of the bursa of Fabricius in the chicken, Annu. Rev. Microbiol. **18:**253, 1964.

Wong, B.: Parasitic diseases in immunocompromised hosts, Am. J. Med. **76:**479, 1984.

Immunopathologic (allergic) diseases
Neutralization or inactivation of biologically active molecules

Courand, P.O., Lu, B.Z., Schmutz, A., et al.: Immunologic studies of β-adrenergic receptors, J. Cell. Biochem. **21:**187, 1983.

Fraser, C.M., and Venter, J.C.: Autoantibodies to beta-adrenergic receptors and asthma, J. Allerg. Clin. Immunol. **74:**227, 1984.

Goldberg, L.S., et al.: Human autoimmunity, with pernicious anemia as a model, Ann. Intern. Med. **81:**372, 1974.

Grob, D., editor: Myasthenia gravis, Ann. NY Acad. Sci. **274:**1, 1976.

Harrison, L.C., and Kahn, L.C.: Autoantibodies to the insulin receptor: clinical significance and experimental applications, Clin. Immunol. **4:**107, 1985.

Kelly, R.B., and Hail, Z.W.: Immunology of the neuromuscular function. In Brokes, J., editor: Neuroimmunology, New York, 1982, Plenum Press Inc.

Kriss, J.P.: Graves' ophthalmopathy: etiology and treatment, Hosp. Pract. **10:**124, 1975.

Lennon, V.A., Lindstrom, J., and Seybold, M.E.: Experimental autoimmune myasthenia: a model of myasthenia gravis in rats and guinea pigs, J. Exp. Med. **141**:1365, 1975.

Margolius, A., Jackson, D.P., and Ratnoff, O.D.: Circulating anticoagulants: a study of 40 cases and a review of the literature, Medicine **40**:197, 1961.

McKenzie, J.M., and Zakarija, M.: LATS in Graves' disease, Rec. Prog. Horm. Res. **33**:29, 1977.

Nash, H.A., Chang, C.C., and Tsong, Y.Y.: Formulation of a potential antipregnancy vaccine based on the β-subunit of human chorionic gonadotropin in humans, J. Reprod. Immunol. **7**:151, 1985.

Patrick, J., and Lindstrom, J.: Autoimmune response to acetylcholine receptor, Science **180**:821, 1973.

Pope, C.C.: The immunology of insulin, Adv. Immunol. **5**:209, 1966.

Rotman, M.B., and Celada, F.: Antibody mediated activation of a defective β-D-galactosidase extracted from an *Escherichia coli* mutant, Proc. Natl. Acad. Sci. USA **60**:660, 1968.

Smolarz, A., Roesch, E., Lanz, E., et al.: Digoxin specific antibody (Fab) fragments in 34 cases of severe digitalis intoxication, Clin. Toxicol. **23**:327, 1985.

Solomon, D.H., and Beall, G.N.: Thyroid-stimulating activity in the serum of immunized rabbits. II. Nature of the thyroid-stimulating material, J. Clin. Endocrinol. Metab. **28**:1496, 1968.

Strickroot, F.L., Schaeffer, R.L., and Bergo, H.L.: Myasthenia gravis occurring in an infant born of a myasthenic mother, JAMA **120**:1207, 1942.

Strosberg, A.D.: Anti-idiotype and anti-hormone receptor antibodies, Springer Semin. Immunopathol. **6**:67, 1983.

Talwar, G.P.: Immunology of gonadotropin-releasing hormone, J. Steroid Biochem. **23**:795, 1985.

Taylor, K.B., Roitt, I.M., Doniach, D., Couchman, K.G., and Shapland, C.: Autoimmune phenomena in pernicious anemia: gastric antibodies, Br. Med. J. **5316**:1347, 1962.

Volpe, R.: Autoimmune thyroid disease, Hosp. Pract. **19**:141, 1984.

Volpe, R.: The role of autoimmunity in hypoendocrine and hyperendocrine function, Ann. Intern. Med. **87**:86, 1977.

Cytotoxic or cytolytic reactions

Abramson, N., Eisenberg, P.D., and Aster, R.H.: Post-transfusion purpura: immunologic aspects and therapy, N. Engl. J. Med. **291**:1163, 1974.

Ackroyd, J.F.: Sedormid purpura: an immunologic study of a form of drug hypersensitivity, Prog. Allergy **3**:531, 1952.

Aster, R.H.: Immune thrombocytopenias, Hosp. Pract. **18**:187, 1983.

Baldini, M.: Idiopathic thrombocytopenic purpura, N. Engl. J. Med. **274**:1245, 1966.

Bowman, J.M.: Fetomaternal ABO incompatibility and erythroblastosis fetalis, Vox Sang. **50**:104, 1986.

Dacie, J.V., and Wolledge, S.M.: Autoimmune hemolytic anemia, Prog. Hematol. **6**:1, 1969.

Freda, V.J., Gorman, J.G., and Pollack, W.: Suppression of the primary Rh immune response with passive Rh IgG immunoglobulin, N. Engl. J. Med. **277**:1022, 1967.

Gorman, J.G., Freda, V.J., and Pollack, W.: Prevention of rhesus isoimmunization, Clin. Immunol. Allergy **4**:473, 1984.

Humphrey, J.H., and Dourmashkin, R.R.: The lesions in cell membranes caused by complement, Adv. Immunol. **11**:75, 1969.

Karpatkin, S.: Autoimmune thrombocytopenic purpura, Blood **56**:329, 1980.

Kerr, R.O., Cardamone, J., Dalmasso, A.P., et al.: Two mechanisms of erythrocyte destruction in penicillin-induced hemolytic anemia, N. Engl. J. Med. **287**:1322, 1972.

Levine, P.: The discovery of Rh hemolytic disease, Vox Sang. **47**:187, 1984.

Müller-Eberhard, H.J.: Chemistry and reaction mechanisms of complement, Adv. Immunol. **8**:1, 1968.

Pirofsky, B.: Clinical aspects of autoimmune hemolytic anemia, Semin. Hematol. **13**:251, 1976.

Poschmann, A., and Fisher, K.: Autoimmune hemolytic anemia: recent advances in pathogenesis, diagnosis and treatment, Eur. J. Pediatr. **143**:253, 1985.

Race, R.R., and Sanger, R.: Blood groups in man, Philadelphia, 1962, F.A. Davis Co.

Waksman, B.H.: Cell lysis and related phenomena in hypersensitivity reactions, including immunohematologic diseases, Prog. Allergy **5**:340, 1958.

Watkins, W.M.: Blood group substances, Science **152**:172, 1966.

Zmijewski, C.M.: Immunohematology, New York, 1968, Appleton-Century-Crofts.

Immune complex diseases

Adler, S., Baker, P., Pritzl, P., and Couser, W.G.: Effects of alterations in glomerular charge on deposition of cationic and anionic antibodies to fixed glomerular antigens in the rat, J. Lab. Clin. Med. **106**:1, 1985.

Andres, G., et al.: Biology of disease: formation of immune deposits and disease, Lab. Invest. **55**:510, 1986.

Arthus, M.: Injections répétées de sérum de cheval chez le lapin, C.R. Soc. Biol. (Paris) **55**:817, 1903.

Benoit, F.L., Rulon, D.B., Theil, G.B., et al.: Goodpasture's syndrome: a clinicopathologic entity, Am. J. Med. **37**:424, 1964.

Couser, W.G., and Salant, D.J.: In situ immune complex formation and glomerular injury, Kidney Int. **17**:1, 1980.

Crawfore, J.P., Movat, H., Ranaddive, N.S., and Hay, J.B.: Pathways to inflammation induced by immune complexes: development of the Arthus reaction, Fed. Proc. **41**:2583, 1982.

Dixon, F.J., et al.: Pathogenesis of serum sickness, Arch. Pathol. **65**:18, 1958.

Gauthier, V.J., Striker, G.E., and Mannik, M.: Glomerular localization of preformed immune complexes prepared with anionic antibodies or cationic antigens, Lab. Invest. **50**:636, 1984.

Griswold, W.R., Brans, M., and McNeal, R.: The rapidly changing nature of acute immune complex disease, J. Lab. Clin. Med. **96**:57, 1980.

Hargraves, M.M., Richmond, H., and Morton, R.: Presentation of 2 bone marrow elements: the "tart" cell and the "LE" cell, Mayo Clin. Proc. **23**:25, 1948.

McCombs, R.P.: Systemic "allergic" vasculitis: clinical and pathological relationships, JAMA **194**:1059, 1965.

Ploth, D.W., Fitz, A., Schnetzler, D., Seidenfeld, J., and Wilson, C.B.: Thyroglobulin–anti-thyroglobulin immune complex glomerulonephritis complicating radioiodine therapy, Clin. Immunol. Immunopathol. **9**:327, 1978.

Rich, A.R., and Gregory, J.E.: The experimental demonstration that polyarteritis nodosa is a manifestation of hypersensitivity, Bull. Johns Hopkins Hosp. **72**:63, 1943.

Rose, G.A., and Spencer, H.: Polyarteritis nodosa, Q. J. Med. **26**:43, 1957.

Stevenson, J.A., Leona, L.A., Cohen, A.H., and Border, W.A.: Henoch-Schoenlein purpura, Arch. Pathol. Lab. Med. **106**:192, 1982.

Theofilopoulos, A.N.: Evaluation and clinical significance of circulating immune complexes, Clin. Immunol. **4**:63, 1980.

Vaughn, J.J.: Rheumatologic disorders due to immune complexes, Postgrad. Med. **54**:129, 1973.

von Pirquet, C.F., and Schick, B.: Serum sickness, 1905, Baltimore, 1951, The Williams & Wilkins Co. (Translated by B. Schick.)

Wilson, C.B., and Dixon, F.J.: Immunopathology and glomerulonephritis, Annu. Rev. Med. **25**:83, 1974.

Zabriskie, J.B.: The role of streptococci in human glomerulonephritis, J. Exp. Med. **134**:180, 1971.

Zvailfer, N.J.: Rheumatoid arthritis: a dissertation of its pathogenesis and future directions for research, Aust. NZ J. Med. **8**(suppl.):44, 1978.

Atopic and anaphylactic reactions

Aas, K.: Heterogeneity of bronchial asthma, Allergy **36**:3, 1981.

Austen, K.F., and Lichtenstein, K.M., editors: Asthma: physiology, immunopharmacology and treatment, New York, 1973, Academic Press, Inc.

Bach, M.K.: Mediators of anaphylaxis and inflammation, Annu Rev. Microbiol. **36**:371, 1982.

Barr, S.E.: Allergy to Hymenoptera stings: review of the world literature: 1953-1970, Ann. Allergy **29**:49, 1971.

Block, K.S.: The anaphylactic antibodies of mammals including man, Prog. Allergy **10**:84, 1967.

Chakrin, L., and Bailey, D.: Leukotrienes, Orlando, Fla., 1984, Academic Press, Inc.

Coca, A.F., and Grove, E.F.: Studies on hypersensitiveness. XIII. A study of the atopic reagins, J. Immunol. 10:445, 1925.

Davis, P., Bailey, P.J., Goldenberg, M.M., et al.: The role of arachidonic acid oxygenation products in pain and inflammation, Annu. Rev. Immunol. 2:335, 1983.

Epstein, J.H.: Photoallergy: a review, Arch. Dermatol. 106:741, 1972.

Fein, B.T.: Aspirin shock associated with asthma and nasal polyps, Ann. Allergy 29:589, 1971.

Frazier, C.A.: Biting insect survey: a statistical report, Ann. Allergy 32:200, 1974.

Golbert, T.M., Patterson, R., and Pruzansky, J.J.: Systemic allergic reactions to ingested antigens, J. Allergy 44:96, 1969.

Grolnick, M.: An investigative and clinical evaluation of dermatographism, Ann. Allergy 28:395, 1970.

Halpern, B.N., Ky, T., and Robert, B.: Clinical and immunological study of an exceptional case of reaginic type sensitization to human seminal fluid, Immunology 12:247, 1967.

Hinson, R.F.W., Moon, A.J., and Plummer, N.S.: Bronchopulmonary aspergillosis, Thorax 7:317, 1952.

Ishizaka, K., Ishizaka, T., and Hornbrook, M.H.: Physico-chemical properties of human reaginic antibody. IV. Presence of a unique immunoglobulin as a carrier of reaginic activity, J. Immunol. 97:75, 1966.

James, L.P., and Austen, K.F.: Fatal systemic anaphylaxis in man, N. Engl. J. Med. 270:597, 1964.

Kay, A.B., Austen, K.F., and Lichtenstein, L.M., editors: Asthma: physiology, immunopharmacology and treatment, New York, 1984, Academic Press, Inc.

Kay, J.W.: Atopic dermatitis: an immunologic disease complex and its therapy, Ann. Allergy 38:345, 1977.

Killby, V.A., and Silverman, P.H.: Hypersensitive reactions in man to specific mosquito bites, Am. J. Trop. Med. Hyg. 16:374, 1967.

Lewis, R.A., and Austen, K.F.: Mediation of local homeostasis and inflammation by leukotrienes and other mast cell–dependent compounds, Nature 293:103, 1981.

Morley, J., editor: Beta-adrenergic receptors in asthma, New York, 1984, Academic Press, Inc.

Moller, G., editor: Immunoglobulin E, Immunol. Rev. 41:1, 1978.

Paterson, J.W., and Lulich, K.M.: Pharmacology of asthma: a review of certain aspects, Prog. Respir. Dis. 14:112, 1980.

Prausnitz, C., and Küstner, H.: Studies on sensitivity, Zentralbl. Bakteriol. (Orig. A) 86:160, 1921. (English translation in Gell, P.G.H., and Coombs, R.R.A.: Clinical aspects of immunology, Philadelphia, 1963, F.A. Davis Co.)

Rowe, A.H., and Rowe, A., Jr.: Food allergy, Springfield, Ill., 1972, Charles C Thomas, Publisher.

Sheffer, A.L., Austen, K.F., and Gigli, I.: Urticaria and angioedema, Postgrad. Med. 54:81, 1973.

Stebbings, J.H., Jr.: Immediate hypersensitivity: a defense against arthropods, Perspect. Biol. Med. 17:233, 1974.

Steinberg, P., Ishizaka, K., and Norman, P.S.: Possible role of IgE-mediated reaction in immunity, J. Allergy Clin. Immunol. 54:359, 1974.

Szentivanyi, A.: The beta adrenergic theory of the atopic abnormality in bronchial asthma, J. Allergy 42:203, 1968.

Wasserman, S.I., and Center, D.M.: The relevance of neutrophil chemotactic factors to allergic disease, J. Allergy Clin. Immunol. 64:231, 1979.

Cellular or delayed hypersensitivity

Ahmed, A.R., and Blose, D.A.: Delayed-type hypersensitivity skin testing: a review, Arch. Dermatol. 119:934, 1983.

Arnason, B.G., and Waksman, B.H.: Tuberculin sensitivity: immunologic considerations, Adv. Tuberc. Res. 13:1, 1964.

Beer, A.E., and Billingham, R.E.: Immunobiology of mammalian reproduction, Adv. Immunol. 14:1, 1971.

Biberfeld, P., Holm, G., and Perlmann, P.: Morphologic observations on lymphocyte peripolesis and cytotoxic action in vitro, Exp. Cell Res. 52:672, 1968.

Billingham, R.E., and Beer, A.E.: Reproductive immunology: past, present and future, Prospect. Biol. Med. 27:259, 1984.

Bloom, R.R., and Jiménez, L.: Migration inhibitory factor and the cellular basis of delayed hypersensitivity reactions, Am. J. Pathol. 60:453, 1970.

Cerottini, J.-C., and Brunner, K.T.: Cell-mediated cytotoxicity, allograft rejection and tumor immunity, Adv. Immunol. 18:67, 1974.

Cohen, S.: Symposium on cell mediated immunity in human disease, Hum. Pathol. 17:111, 1986.

Cohen, S.: The role of cell mediated immunity in the induction of inflammatory responses, Am. J. Pathol. 88:502, 1977.

Deeg, H.J., and Storb, R.: Graft versus host disease: pathophysiological and clinical aspects, Annu. Rev. Med. 35:11, 1984.

Doniach, D.: Autoimmune aspects of liver disease, Br. Med. Bull. 28:145, 1972.

Dvorak, H.F., et al.: Morphology of delayed type hypersensitivity reactions in man. I. Quantitative description of the inflammatory response, Lab. Invest. 31:111, 1974.

Flax, M.H.: Experimental allergic thyroiditis in the guinea pig. II. Morphologic studies on the development of the disease, Lab. Invest. 12:199, 1963.

Flax, M.H., Jankovic, D.B., and Sell, S.: Experimental allergic thyroiditis in the guinea pig. I. Relationship of delayed hypersensitivity and circulating antibody to the development of thyroiditis, Lab. Invest. 12:119, 1963.

Gale, R.P., and Opelz, G.: Second International Symposium on Immunobiology of Bone Marrow Transplantation, Transplant. Proc., vol. 10, no. 1, 1978.

Galli, S.J., and Dvorak, A.: What do mast cells have to do with delayed hypersensitivity? Lab. Investig. 50:365, 1984.

Hellström, K.E., and Hellström, I.: Lymphocyte-mediated cytotoxicity and blocking serum activity to tumor antigens, Adv. Immunol. 18:209, 1974.

Henkart, P.A.: Mechanism of lymphocyte mediated cytotoxicity, Annu. Rev. Microbiol. 3:31, 1985.

Henney, C.S.: On the mechanism of T-cell mediated cytolysis, Transplant. Rev. 17:37, 1973.

Jones, T.D., and Mote, J.R.: The phases of foreign sensitization in human beings, N. Engl. J. Med. 210:120, 1934.

Kaliss, N.: Immunological enhancement of tumor homografts in mice: a review, Cancer Res. 18:992, 1958.

Kaplan, M.H.: Autoimmunity to heart and its relation to human disease, Prog. Allergy 13:408, 1969.

Lampert, P.W.: Autoimmune and virus-induced demyelinating diseases, Am. J. Pathol. 91:176, 1978.

Lawrence, H.S., and Valentine, F.T.: Transfer factor and other mediators of cellular immunity, Am. J. Pathol. 60:437, 1970.

Leonard, J.E., Taetle, R., To, D., and Rhyneu, K.: Preclinical studies on the use of selective antibody-ricin conjugates in bone marrow transplantation, Blood 65:1149, 1985.

Levy, G.A., and Chisari, F.V.: The immunopathogenesis of hepatitis B virus induced liver disease, Springer Semin. Immunopathol. 3:439, 1981.

Nakamura, R.M., and Weigle, W.O: Transfer of experimental thyroiditis by serum from thyroidectomized donors, J. Exp. Med. 130:263, 1969.

Paterson, P.Y.: The demyelinating diseases: clinical and experimental correlates. In Sampter, M., editor: Immunological diseases, ed. 2, Boston, 1971, Little, Brown & Co.

Perlmann, P., and Holm, G.: Cytotoxic effects of lymphoid cells in vitro, Adv. Immunol. 11:117, 1970.

Rappaport, F.T., Converse, J.M., and Billingham, R.E.: Recent advances in clinical and experimental transplantation, JAMA 237:2835, 1977.

Rose, N.R., and Mackey, I.: The autoimmune diseases, Orlando, Fla., 1985, Academic Press, Inc.

Storb, R.: Bone marrow transplantation for the treatment of hematologic malignancy and of aplastic anemia, Transplant. Proc. 13:221, 1981.

Stroop, W.G., and Baringer, J.R.: Persistant, slow and latent viral infections, Prog. Med. Virol. 28:1, 1982.

Szulman, A.E.: The A, B and H blood-group antigens in the human placenta, N. Engl. J. Med. **286:**1028, 1972.

Voisin, G.A.: Immunological facilitation, a broadening concept of the enhancement phenomenon, Prog. Allergy **15:**328, 1971.

Waksman, B.H.: Experimental allergic encephalomyelitis and the "autoallergic" diseases, Int. Arch. Allergy Appl. Immunol. **14**(suppl.):1, 1959.

Waksman, B.H.: Autoimmunization and the lesions of autoimmunity, Medicine **41:**93, 1962.

Waksman, B.H., and Namba, Y.: On soluble mediators of immunologic regulation, Cell. Immunol. **21:**161, 1976.

Zwaan, F.E., Hermans, J., Barrett, A.J., and Speck, B.: Bone marrow transplantation for acute lymphoblastic leukemia: a survey of the European Group for Bone Marrow Transplantation, Br. J. Hematol. **58:**33, 1984.

Granulomatous hypersensitivity

Adams, D.O.: The granulomatous inflammatory response, Am. J. Pathol. **84:**164, 1976.

Albert, D.A., Weisman, M.H., and Kaplan, R.: The rheumatic manifestations of leprosy (Hansen disease), Medicine **59:**442, 1980.

Boros, D.L.: Basic and clinical aspects of granulomatous disease, New York, 1981, Elsevier Scientific Publishing Co.

Chaparas, S.D.: The immunology of mycobacterial infections, CRC Crit. Rev. Microbiol. **9:**139, 1982.

Chumbley, L.C., Harrison, E.C., Jr., and Deremee, R.A.: Allergic granulomatosis and angitis (Churg-Strauss syndrome): report of analysis of 300 cases, Mayo Clin. Proc. **52:**477, 1977.

Churg, J.: Allergic granulomatosis and granulomatous vascular syndromes, Ann. Allergy **21:**619, 1963.

Daniele, R.P., Dauber, J.H., and Rossman, M.D.: Immunologic abnormalities in sarcoidosis, Ann. Intern. Med. **92:**406, 1980.

Dannenberg, A.M.: Cellular hypersensitivity and cellular immunity in the pathogenesis of tuberculosis specificity, systemic and local nature, and associated macrophage enzymes, Bacteriol. Rev. **32:**85, 1968.

Deodhar, S.D., Barna, B., and Van Ordstrand, H.S.: A study of the immunologic aspects of chronic berylliosis, Chest **73:**309, 1973.

Epstein, W.L.: Granulomatous hypersensitivity, Prog. Allergy **11:**36, 1967.

Kaplan, G., Weinstein, D.E., Steinman, R.M., Levis, W.R., Elvers, U., Patarroyo, M.E., and Cohn, Z.A.: An analysis of in vitro T cell responsiveness in lepromatous leprosy, J. Exp. Med. **162:**917, 1985.

Larson, G.: Hypersensitivity lung disease, Annu. Rev. Immunol. **3:**59, 1985.

Mackaness, G.B., and Blanden, R.V.: Cellular immunity, Prog. Allergy **11:**89, 1967.

McCombs, R.P.: Diseases due to immunologic reactions in the lungs, N. Engl. J. Med. **286:**1186, 1972.

Postlethwait, A.E., Jackson, B.K., Beachey, E.H., and Kang, A.H.: Formation of multinucleated giant cells from human monocyte precursors: mediation by a soluble protein from antigen- and mitogen-stimulated lymphocytes, J. Exp. Med. **155:**168, 1982.

Skinsnes, O.K.: Immunopathology of leprosy: the century in review—pathology, pathogenesis and the development of classification, Int. J. Lepr. **41:**329, 1973.

Tepper, L.B., Hardy, H.L., and Chamberlin, R.I.: Toxicity of beryllium compounds, Amsterdam, 1961, Elsevier Publishing Co.

Turk, J.L., and Bryceson, A.D.M.: Immunological phenomena in leprosy and related disease, Adv. Immunol. **13:**209, 1971.

Warren, K.S.: Modulation of immunopathology and disease in schistosomiasis, Am. J. Trop. Med. Hyg. **26:**113, 1977.

Immune skin diseases

Beutner, E.H., Jordon, R.E., and Chorzelski, T.P.: The immunopathology of pemphigus and bullous pemphigoid, J. Invest. Dermatol. **51:**63, 1968.

Chorzelski, T.P., Von Weiss, J.F., Lever, W.F.: Clinical significance of autoantibodies in pemphigus, Arch. Dermatol. **93:**570, 1966.

Clark, W.H., Reed, R.J., and Mihm, M.C.: Lupus erythematosus: histopathology of cutaneous lesions, Hum. Pathol. **4:**157, 1975.

Cochran, R.E.I., Thompson, J., and MacSween, R.N.M.: An autantibody profile in alopecia totalis and diffuse alopecia, Br. J. Dermatol. **95:**61, 1976.

Cormane, R.H.: Diagnostic procedures in immunodermatology, J. Invest. Dermatol. **67:**129, 1976.

Hertz, K.C., Gazze, L.A., Kirkpatrick, C.H., and Katz, S.I.: Autoimmune vitiligo: detection of antibodies to melanin-producing cells, N. Engl. J. Med. **297:**634, 1977.

Holubar, K., Konrad, K., Stingl, G.: Detection by immuno-electron microscopy of immunoglobulin G deposits in skin of patients with herpes gestationis, Br. J. Dermatol. **96:**569, 1977.

Jordon, R.E., Heine, K.G., Tappeiner, G., Bushkell, L.L., and Provost, T.T.: The immunopathology of herpes gestationis: immunofluorescence studies and characterization of "HG factor," J. Clin. Invest. **57:**1426, 1976.

Katz, S.I., and Strober, W.: The pathogenesis of dermatitis herpetiformis, J. Invest. Dermatol. **70:**63, 1978.

Krogh, H.K., and Tonder, O.: Immunoglobulins and anti-immunoglobulin factors in psoriatic lesions, Clin. Exp. Immunol. **10:**623, 1972.

Lever, W.F.: Histopathology of the skin, ed. 3, Philadelphia, 1961, J.B. Lippincott Co.

Murphy, G.F., Guillen, F.J., and Flynn, T.C.: Cytotoxic T lymphocyte and phenotypically abnormal epithelial dendritic cells in fixed cutaneous eruptions, Hum. Pathol. **16:**1264, 1985.

Person, J.R., and Rogers, R.S.: Bullous and cicatricial pemphigoid: clinical, histopathologic and immunologic correlations, Mayo Clin. Proc. **53:**54, 1977.

Provost, T.T., and Tomasi, T.B., Jr.: Evidence for the activation of complement via the alternate pathway in skin diseases. II. Dermatitis herpetiformis, Clin. Immunol. Immunopathol. **3:**178, 1974.

Schultz, J.R.: Pemphigus acantholysis: a unique immunologic injury, J. Invest. Dermatol. **74:**359, 1980.

Tan, E.M., and Kunkel, H.G.: An immunofluorescent study of the skin lesions in systemic lupus erythematosus, Arthritis Rheum. **9:**37, 1966.

Yaoita, H., Briggaman, R.A., Lawley, T.J., et al.: Epidermolysis bullosa acquisita: ultrastructural and immunological studies, J. Invest. Dermatol. **76:**288, 1981.

13 Malnutrition and Deficiency Diseases

HERSCHEL SIDRANSKY

The role of nutrition in the pathogenesis of disease has been of great concern to scientists and physicians for many years. The importance of nutrition to well-being has been understood by civilized societies for centuries. Indeed, the state of nutrition in a society has usually correlated well with its socioeconomic development and advancement. Thus humans have been greatly concerned with the availability of adequate and balanced nutrition. Diseases that are consequences of inadequate diets have long plagued humankind. Unfortunately, they remain with us today and most probably will be with us for years to come.

Historically nutrition gained eminence as a medical science with the discoveries that the absence of essential nutrients, such as single vitamins, induced a variety of important and specific nutritional deficiency diseases. These monumental findings led to a clearer understanding of how essential nutrients play vital roles in the normal functioning of cells, tissues, and organs of animals and humans.

In recent years, as knowledge has rapidly expanded in many areas of biologic and medical science, it has become apparent that the nutritional intake and utilization by any host, animal or human, are important not only in the prevention of deficiency states but also in the host's adaptation and responses to environmental stresses and strains. This chapter is a brief review of the way malnutrition and deficiency diseases develop, the manifestations of certain deficiency states, nutritional imbalances, and the way nutritional alterations may influence the host's responses to certain environmental manifestations.

As an introduction to malnutrition and deficiency diseases, it is essential to mention briefly the dietary components involved in normal and adequate nutrition. The human body requires some 50 to 60 organic and inorganic compounds in quantities ranging from micrograms to grams.[5,47,67] These are included in six basic groups: proteins, carbohydrates, fats, vitamins, minerals, and water. Proteins are made up of amino acids, eight of which must be supplied by dietary intake because they cannot be synthesized by the body in the amounts needed. These are isoleucine, leucine, lysine, methionine, phenylalanine, threonine, tryptophan, and valine. In addition, an exogenous supply of histidine is needed for early growth and development and therefore may be considered essential. Carbohydrates in themselves are not essential, but they provide needed dietary calories. Fats or their constituent fatty acids also provide calories. However, three fatty acids, linolenic, arachidonic, and especially linoleic, are currently considered essential. Vitamins, certain minerals, and water are indispensable dietary components. The consequences of the absence or imbalance (altered relationships) of these components, leading to malnutrition or deficiency states, are considered later in the chapter.

In an attempt to characterize the various types of malnutrition or deficiency diseases as they affect individuals, one may consider them as (1) single deficiency states, (2) multiple deficiency states, (3) imbalances, and (4) excesses. The term *single deficiency states* implies that the disease results from the absence of a single essential or indispensable compound. Much of the information regarding such deficiency states has been derived from animal experimentation in which the variables were carefully monitored. Single vitamin deficiencies are the best examples. *Multiple deficiency states* develop when more than one necessary component is lacking in the diet. In humans, multiple deficiencies occur frequently because a diet deficient in one component is usually deficient in others. Thus the pathologic changes may reflect each deficiency to some degree. *Nutritional imbalances* occur when the proportion of one dietary component to another or others is such that pathologic changes occur. Nutritional imbalances can occur under a variety of conditions. One example is the disease kwashiorkor, in which there is a protein deficiency in the presence of adequate or even high caloric intake. In contrast, marasmus occurs when there is a deficiency of total food intake (protein and all other components). Experimentally, amino acid imbalances have been demonstrated to induce a variety of pathologic changes.[40] The concept of nutritional imbalances is relatively new but has been gaining recognition. It stresses that the quantity of intake of each dietary component in relation to other components is of great importance and must be carefully evaluated. *Nu-*

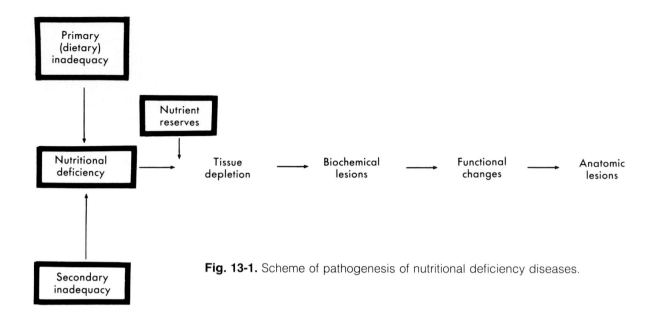

Fig. 13-1. Scheme of pathogenesis of nutritional deficiency diseases.

tritional excesses, single or multiple, are becoming increasingly important, especially in affluent societies. Obesity caused by excessive intake, particularly of calories, is a common condition. Hypervitaminosis occurs when specific vitamins are given in excessive amounts and can have serious pathologic manifestations.

PATHOGENESIS OF DEFICIENCY DISEASES

A nutritional deficiency disease develops when the amounts of essential nutrients provided to the cells are inadequate for their normal metabolic functions. The deficiency may be primary or secondary in origin. A primary nutritional inadequacy is induced by a poor diet—one that lacks essential nutrients in either kind or amount or that provides an imbalance of nutrients. A secondary nutritional inadequacy comes about from factors that interfere with the ingestion, absorption, or utilization of nutrients, as well as from metabolic or functional conditions that increase the requirement for nutrients or cause unusual destruction or abnormal excretion of nutrients.

Fig. 13-1 presents a diagrammatic scheme of the pathogenesis of nutritional deficiency diseases. After a nutritional inadequacy (primary or secondary) begins, there is a time lapse before the onset of a nutritional deficiency disease. The time interval may depend on the degree of nutritional inadequacy and the level of nutrient reserves. An important safety factor is the nutrient reserves on which the tissues may draw during temporary lapses in the supply of nutrients. These reserves may be large or small, depending on the specific nutrient and the overall state of the reserve tissues. Tissue depletion follows the exhaustion of nutrient reserves and may occur rapidly or slowly, depending on the degree of nutritional inadequacy, the amount of nu-

trient reserves, and the requirement of the body for essential nutrients.

Biochemical lesions develop as a consequence of tissue depletion. Such lesions can best be illustrated by deficiencies of vitamins that are involved with enzyme systems dealing with the disease of energy and other metabolic reactions. Biochemical alterations develop and may result in the accumulation of certain metabolites and in the altered metabolism of others. Functional changes in tissues and organs may then occur. Anatomic lesions develop and often are specific for or related to the missing nutritional component or components. Although this sequence has been presented in a stepwise manner, no one step in the chain of events from nutritional inadequacy to anatomic lesions need necessarily be complete before the next begins.

PRIMARY AND SECONDARY NUTRITIONAL INADEQUACY

Primary nutritional inadequacy is caused by a diet that lacks essential nutrients in either kind or amount or that provides an imbalance of nutrients. Such inadequacy has always existed at one time or another in some parts of the world. It has been especially prevalent during and after wars, after crop failures, and in relation to poverty, ignorance, faddism, and cultural taboos. Throughout the world today, protein-calorie malnutrition is the most prominent example of this form of nutritional inadequacy. This is reviewed in a subsequent section.

Although malnutrition and nutritional deficiency diseases are usually considered to arise solely from an inadequate diet, under certain circumstances these may occur in the presence of dietary adequacy. Secondary nutritional inadequacy is caused by a variety of factors other than a poor diet. This type of nutritional inadequacy is of special importance in affluent societies as in the United States. Factors that may be involved are as follows:

1. Interference with ingestion: gastrointestinal disorders (acute gastroenteritis, gallbladder disease, peptic ulcers, diarrheal diseases, obstructive lesions of the bowel), neuropsychiatric disorders (neurasthenia, psychoneurosis, migraine), anorexia (alcoholism, congestive heart failure, cancer therapy, infectious diseases), food allergy, loss of teeth, pregnancy

2. Increased nutritive requirement: abnormal activity, abnormal environmental factors, fever, hyperthyroidism, pregnancy and lactation

3. Interference with absorption: gastrointestinal diseases (associated with hypermotility or reduction of absorbing surfaces), achlorhydria, biliary diseases

4. Interference with utilization: hepatic dysfunction, hypothyroidism, malignancy

5. Increased excretion: polyuria, lactation, excessive perspiration

6. Increased destruction: achlorhydria

All of the preceding can be influenced by a variety of therapeutic agents that may indirectly induce secondary nutritional inadequacies.

STARVATION

Starvation occurs in individuals of all ages. Much information about this condition was gained from postmortem studies in prison camps during World War II.[49] In general, the overall pathologic changes are minimal; atrophy is the main feature. The changes caused by inanition include great loss of weight, serous atrophy of fat throughout the body, reduced amounts of lymphoid tissue, and pronounced atrophy of testes or ovaries, cardiac and skeletal muscle, thymus, and liver. Hemosiderosis of the spleen and lipid depletion of adrenal glands are common findings.

PROTEIN-CALORIE MALNUTRITION[12,16,69]

The most prevalent form of primary nutritional deficiency disease is protein-calorie malnutrition. According to the World Health Organization (WHO), protein-calorie malnutrition is rampant throughout the world. The two diseases associated with this malnutrition, marasmus and kwashiorkor, affect preschool-age children in the developing countries of the world. Marasmus is a form of childhood starvation caused by inadequate total food intake. Its manifestations are those of starvation in which pathologic changes are minimal.[12,48,53] Kwashiorkor, the most important and widespread nutritional deficiency disease in the world today (affecting more than 100 million children) according to WHO, has long been attributed to protein deficiency.

In the 1950s it was established that kwashiorkor is caused by a combination of protein deficiency and relatively high carbohydrate intake.[17,26] Such a nutritionally deficient and imbalanced diet leads rapidly to pathologic changes in several organs.[103] Many children throughout the world die from this disease. In addition, it has been speculated that children who survive may later develop an enhanced susceptibility to hepatic injury caused by viruses, toxins, or chemical carcinogens, and as adults may have an increased incidence of cirrhosis and primary liver cancer.

In recent years some authors have reported that protein-calorie malnutrition is being recognized with increasing frequency in hospitalized patients as well as in the geriatric population.[14,15,93] Also, in nursing home populations there has been reported to be cases in protein-calorie malnutrition.[72] These considerations relating to the occurrence of protein-calorie malnutrition are derived from evaluations based upon biochemical and anthropometric measurements. Whether these parameters correlate with morphologic findings characteristic or diagnostic of protein-calorie malnutrition still needs to be established.

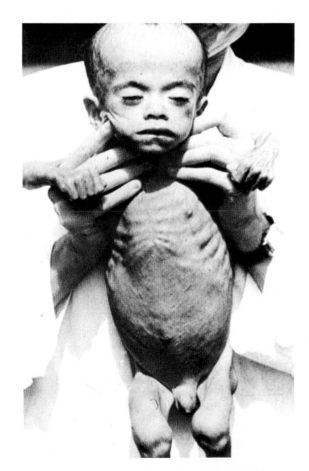

Fig. 13-2. Marasmus. Extreme wasting in child from Netherlands during World War II. (From Latham, M.C., et al.: Scope manual on nutrition, Kalamazoo, Mich., 1972, The Upjohn Co.)

Marasmus

Marasmus (Fig. 13-2) is a form of starvation that occurs during childhood. It results from an overall deficit in food intake, including all dietary components (protein, carbohydrate, lipid, vitamins, salts). Therefore it has often been referred to as "balanced starvation."

Marasmus occurs most commonly during the first year of life and is found in most developing countries. A common cause is early cessation of breast feeding with lack of food intake. The clinical features and findings in marasmus are growth failure (low weight and height, prominent ribs, monkeylike face, protuberant abdomen, thin limbs), muscle wasting and loss of subcutaneous fat, anemia, and diarrhea (common but not a constant feature). Edema is absent, mental changes are uncommon, and appetite is good. Serum protein levels are reduced. Other than the small size or atrophy of organs, no specific gross or microscopic (pathologic) changes are present. The liver is not fatty.

Kwashiorkor[17,26,69,103]

Kwashiorkor (Fig. 13-3) has been recognized for centuries and has been referred to by many names throughout the world. In 1936 Dr. Cicely Williams of the Gold Coast of Africa first described kwashiorkor in detail in the medical literature. Since that time kwashiorkor has gained notoriety as the most widespread and important dietary deficiency disease in the world.

Although kwashiorkor was at first considered to result from protein deficiency alone, the cause is now recognized to be a nutritional imbalance, consisting in protein deficiency and adequate or high carbohydrate intake. The disease occurs mainly in children 6 months to 3 years of age. It usually follows weaning when the infant is fed the poor and limited foods of the area (corn, cassava, or other grains and vegetables), which are relatively high in carbohydrate but contain inadequate amounts of proteins that are often of poor quality.

The clinical features and findings in kwashiorkor are growth failure; wasting of muscles of arms and legs but preservation of subcutaneous fat; edema; mental changes, such as apathy, irritability, and lack of interest in surroundings; changes in hair color, texture, and strength; depigmentation of skin; hepatomegaly; diarrhea; and anemia. The main pathologic findings consist in an enlarged, fatty liver with periportal distribution of lipid and atrophy of the pancreas, salivary glands, small intestine glands, and skeletal muscles.

Consequences of kwashiorkor

Although many children die from kwashiorkor, others survive as a consequence of mild involvement or treatment with a well-balanced diet containing adequate and good-quality proteins. Thus in the developing countries there are many adults who have had this nutritional deficiency disease during childhood. In the past, epidemiologists suggested that the fatty liver of kwashiorkor would progress directly to nutritionally induced cirrhosis in adult life. Such adults were believed to have a higher than normal predilection for primary hepatocellular carcinoma. More current views indicate that the liver damage from kwashiorkor may make these individuals more susceptible in later life to injury by hepatotoxic agents (such as viruses or aflatoxin), which then progresses to cirrhosis and in some cases to primary liver cancer.

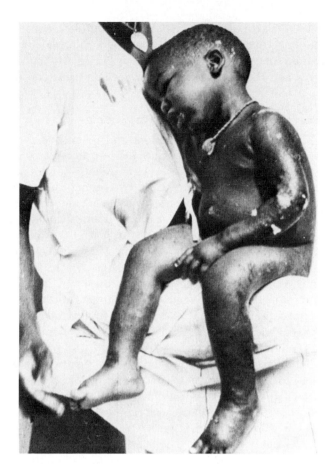

Fig. 13-3. Kwashiorkor. African child showing edema and dermatosis. (From Latham, M.C., et al.: Scope manual on nutrition, Kalamazoo, Mich., 1972, The Upjohn Co.)

Much interest has developed in the possibility that stunted mental development may occur as a consequence of kwashiorkor during childhood. In several studies children who had kwashiorkor during early childhood scored lower on IQ tests than did their siblings who did not have kwashiorkor.[13,57]

Although the conclusions from the preceding two examples are still speculative, they deal with important and significant problems that may be consequences of malnutrition during childhood. Absolute proof that these associations are valid is difficult to document. Therefore many investigators have attempted to use experimental kwashiorkor-like models[25,34,73,89,95] in animals to probe the pathogenesis of the induced lesions and the possible consequences of these alterations in later life. Such studies have provided valuable information concerning nutritional deficiencies and imbalances and their effects both on specific organs and on the whole organism.

Experimental kwashiorkor-like models

A number of investigators have developed experimental models of kwashiorkor to attempt to understand the pathogenesis of the lesions in children with this disease. This has been approached by feeding diets deficient in amino acids or protein to experimental animals. The experimental model that probably most closely resembles the pathologic changes reported in infants dying from kwashiorkor[103] is one in which animals are force-fed by stomach-tube purified diets devoid of single essential amino acids.[89] Lesions develop within 3 to 10 days in these force-feeding experiments and resemble those described in children with kwashiorkor. The morphologic changes consist in a periportal fatty liver, excess hepatic glycogen, and atrophy of the pancreas, submaxillary gland, stomach, spleen, and thymus. Some of the major conclusions based on these experimental studies are the following:

1. Both total intake and caloric intake of a deficient diet must be adequate to induce pathologic changes. Rats fed a deficient diet ad libitum eat little and develop a marasmus-like rather than a kwashiorkor-like condition. This explains the need for force-feeding the deficient or imbalanced diet to maintain an adequate intake and induce the pathologic changes.
2. Overall, the pathologic changes are similar regardless of which single essential amino acid is eliminated from the diet. This indicates that the results reflect protein deficiency rather than deficiency of a single essential amino acid. Use of poor-quality plant proteins as the sole source of protein with adequate amounts of all other components in force-feeding experiments substantiates this.
3. The pathologic changes are not mediated through adrenal or pituitary hormonal stimulation.
4. Loss of skeletal muscle protein occurs early and is important. Hepatic protein synthesis is maintained at a high level. Pronounced alterations in hepatic lipid and glycogen metabolism occur.
5. Treatment with a complete, balanced, purified diet rapidly reverses the condition.

VITAMINS

For practical purposes vitamins may be defined as organic catalysts of exogenous origin that are effective in relatively minute amounts and that are essential for the maintenance of the normal structure and function of cells. Vitamins themselves are not utilized to furnish energy but are essential components of the chemical machinery by which the true food substances are metabolized. With certain exceptions they are not synthesized in the body and must be supplied in the diet or from other external sources. Some compounds are vitamins in the above-defined sense for practically all mammals, whereas others are vitamins only for those that are unable to manufacture them. For example, humans, other primates, and guinea pigs are the only mammals that require vitamin C as a dietary component. In these mammals the synthesis of vitamin C from D-glucose proceeds normally except for the final step, the conversion of gluconate to ascorbate. The enzyme necessary for the final step is missing.

Mechanism of action

The biologic action of many vitamins is intimately related to intracellular enzyme systems. Certain vitamins represent components of essential enzyme systems that cannot be synthesized in the body. Moreover, many hormones act through the medium of the intracellular enzyme systems,[33,38] either by regulating their synthesis and breakdown or by stimulating or inhibiting them. An essential difference between hormones and vitamins is that the former are endogenous (synthesized in certain organs for the maintenance of others), whereas the latter are entirely of exogenous origin. The failure of certain enzyme systems also depends on the inheritance of defective genes.[10]

Thus living cells, with normal genic composition and with the aid of hormones and vitamins, may be said to construct and maintain the cytologic machinery that carries out the complex metabolic reactions necessary for their normal life, function, and reproduction. In their efforts to learn the details of these vital processes, investigators have been concerned with morphologic and biochemical events that occur normally and abnormally. With the availability of advanced tools and methods, such as electron microscopy, subcellular fractionation, and biochemical analysis, the intricate picture of the cell as a molecular factory has been developed.

Sources, requirements, and modern uses

Most vitamins are primarily of plant origin and normally enter the body as constituents of ingested plant or animal food. They may be added to the diet or injected parenterally in concentrated or pure form for both prophylactic and therapeutic purposes. The minimum daily requirements of many vitamins for the maintenance of health in normal individuals have been more or less accurately established,[5,47,67] and range from a fraction of a milligram to about 150 mg. The therapeutic dosage necessary to correct certain pathologic states may be many times the prophylactic dose. Although some moderate excess over the minimum requirements is desirable for normal people, there is definite evidence that large doses of vitamins A and D are harmful.

Paths of investigation in humans and animals

Early knowledge of vitamin deficiency was obtained largely by clinical observation of disease entities and empiric discovery that certain foods had preventive or curative value. Based on extensive studies of dietary deficiencies in experimental animals, the complexity of the problem has become evident. The isolation of vitamins in chemically pure form has led to the determination of the structural formulas and in many instances to chemical synthesis. The final step, determination of the mode of action, is under way in many laboratories. Recent developments relating to vitamins A and D have been most revealing.[27-29,36]

The pathologic lesions resulting from vitamin deficiencies are of two types: primary changes caused by metabolic disturbance in the tissues or organs physiologically served by the vitamin involved and secondary effects (notably inanition, organ atrophy, and arrest of growth) on the body as a whole.

Morphologic studies of the primary types of lesions have played an important role in attempts to understand the physiologic action of vitamins. Some vitamins often control the function of specific types of tissue, it has been possible to study not only the retrogressive changes resulting from deficiency but also the mechanisms of repair that occur when the deficiencies are corrected. Studies of this type have made unique contributions to our knowledge of normal cell physiology as well as that of abnormal cell responses. Correlations between morphologic and biochemical alterations are beginning to emerge.

As previously mentioned, vitamins function by entering into complex cytologic mechanisms that also involve enzymes, hormones, and genes. Important vital processes such as detoxication, electron transport, and immune body formation are implemented by these mechanisms. Thus the symptoms of secondary deficiency may appear as a result of disturbances of cellular metabolism from many different causes—from dietary lack to congenital or acquired defects in the intracellular machinery.

Antivitamins

Chemical compounds that are closely related to vitamins will in some cases compete with and replace active vitamins in enzyme systems and thus produce the effects of vitamin deficiences. Analogs acting in this way have been discovered for ascorbic acid, nicotinic acid, riboflavin, thiamine, pyridoxine, pantothenic acid, vitamin K, and folic acid. Folic acid analogs have been extensively studied because they are beneficial in certain cases of acute leukemia. Different in their mode of action are certain enzymes that destroy vitamins. The best-known example of the latter is thiaminase, which is present in certain types of raw fish and which has been responsible for a rapidly fatal disease in foxes known as Chastek paralysis.

Nomenclature

Chemical names have to some extent replaced letters for the nomenclature of vitamins, but the alphabetic designation is still widely used. All of the well-recognized vitamins are included under the following headings: vitamin A, vitamin B complex (composed of many specific factors), vitamin C (ascorbic acid), vitamin D, vitamin E (alpha-tocopherol and its congeners), and the K vitamins.

Vitamins A, D, E, and K are fat soluble, whereas vitamin C and the members of the B complex are water soluble. Pancreatic disease, hepatobiliary disorders, and prolonged diarrhea are particularly likely to interfere with the absorption of the fat-soluble vitamins. Because vitamins A and D are stored in the liver in large amounts, evidence of deficiencies appears only after malabsorption has existed for many months.

Vitamin A[9,59,85,98,114]
Chemistry and physiology

Vitamin A is a fat-soluble, colorless, primary alcohol that is derived from certain yellow plant pigments known as carotenes. It is available in the diet in two forms, as the vitamin itself or as the provitamin precursors, the carotenes. The carotene molecules are composed of a long chain of carbon and hydrogen atoms, with a ring at each end. In the intestinal mucosa and liver these carotene molecules are split in the center to form, with the addition of two molecules of water, two molecules of vitamin A. Fish-liver oils are important sources of vitamin A itself, whereas the carotenes, primarily of vegetable origin, make up most of the usual dietary intake.

In the small intestine vitamin A esters are hydrolyzed and packaged into micelles with the assistance of bile salts. Carotene is converted into vitamin A and, along with the preformed vitamin A, is esterified preferentially with palmitic acid. Retinyl palmitate is carried in chylomicrons through the lymphatic system to the blood and is stored in the liver. After hydrolysis in the liver, it enters the blood where it is bound to retinol-binding protein and is transported to the tissues where it is needed. Retinoid-binding proteins have also been found to exist in the intracellular compartment in many tissues.

The known physiologic activities of vitamin A are as follows:

1. Maintenance of the structure and function of certain of the specialized types of epithelium
2. Formation, by combination with a protein, of expendable photosensitive pigments in the rods and cones of the retina, which transform radiant energy into nerve impulses
3. Maintenance of normal skeletal growth
4. Regulation of cell membrane structure and function

Experimental lesions in animals

The most characteristic effects of experimental vitamin A deficiency are seen in epithelial structures. Many types of epithelium, including that of the salivary glands, respiratory tract, genitourinary tract, pancreatic ducts, skin, conjunctivae, and enamel organs of the teeth, are affected. The epithelial cells involved undergo atrophy, reparative proliferation of the basal layer, and then, regardless of their original structure and function, replacement by stratified keratinizing epithelium. Correction of the deficiency results in autolysis of the keratinized cells and restoration of the original type of epithelium by differentiation of the persisting basal layer.

Vitamin A deficiency in experimental animals causes cessation of endochondral growth, but periosteal bone formation continues normally, so that the long bones become shorter and thicker. Wolbach and Bessey[113] have shown that paralysis and nerve degeneration result not from a direct effect of the deficiency on nerve tissue but from continued growth of the central nervous system after skeletal growth has been arrested. This disproportionate growth rate causes overcrowding of the cranial cavity and spinal cord, with resulting herniation of the brain tissue and nerve roots into the venous sinuses and intervertebral foramina. In this way mechanical damage and degeneration of nerve tissue are brought about.

Recent experimental studies have implicated vitamin A deficiency in enhanced susceptibility to cancer induction by chemical carcinogens. Also, high levels of vitamin A have been found to inhibit the induction of certain cancers in experimental animals. Many studies dealing with vitamin A and its role in chemoprevention of cancer are in progress.[96,97]

Lesions in humans

Vitamin A deficiency leads to retarded growth in children and emaciation in persons of all ages. Atrophy of the skeletal muscles and lymphatic tissue and moderate anemia, probably as a result of bone marrow atrophy, occur.

Xerophthalmia, a dry scaly lesion of the scleral con-

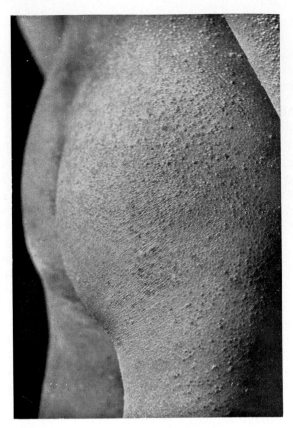

Fig. 13-4. Cutaneous lesions often seen in vitamin A deficiency showing general xeroderma and follicular hyperkeratosis in Chinese patient with xerophthalmia. (Courtesy Dr. Chester N. Frazier; from Sutton, R.L., and Sutton, R.L., Jr.: Diseases of the skin, ed. 10, St. Louis, 1939, The C.V. Mosby Co.)

junctiva, is the most obvious lesion and often establishes the diagnosis during life. Corneal ulceration may occur, with consequent bacterial infection (keratomalacia). Melanotic pigmentation of the cornea is often seen. Triangular grayish areas in the scleral conjunctiva (*Bitot spots*) represent accumulations of keratinized epithelium. This lesion may be seen in cases of prolonged mild deficiency.

Night blindness, or loss of visual acuity in dim light, is common in vitamin A deficiency. A pigment known as visual purple, or rhodopsin, must be present in the retina for normal vision in partial darkness. This pigment is formed by the combination of vitamin A aldehyde with a protein. The dissociation of this union by light results in an appropriate nerve impulse. Cyclic resynthesis of rhodopsin occurs in the dark, but some of the vitamin A is converted to an inactive compound in the process, and for this reason a continuous source of vitamin A is essential. It has been shown that rhodopsin is the specific stimulator of the retinal rods, which control vision in a weak light, whereas combination of vitamin A aldehyde with a different protein gives rise to iodopsin, which stimulates the cones. The cones react to light of high intensity and are necessary for color vision.

A common type of skin lesion is *follicular hyperkeratosis*. Multiple firm papules, 1 to 5 mm in diameter, which may be almost confluent, develop as a result of the formation of keratin plugs in the sebaceous glands, giving the characteristic "toad-skin" appearance (Fig. 13-4). Dryness and scaliness of the skin and furunculosis also are commonly present. These skin lesions have been described only in adults, and their specificity for vitamin A deficiency has been debated, since they have been found in scurvy and occasionally in general undernutrition. Histologially degeneration of the sweat glands and hyperkeratinization of the ducts and hair follicles are seen (Fig. 13-5).

Squamous metaplasia is most often seen in the trachea and bronchi and in the pelves of the kidneys, but the uterus, pancreatic ducts, and certain other epithelial structures also may be affected. Death often results from bronchopneumonia. Obstruction of pancreatic ducts by keratotic plugs may lead to cystic dilatation of the ducts and acini. All of these metaplastic epithelial lesions are far more common in children than in adults. The consequences of long-standing squamous metaplasia with possible progression to anaplasia under certain circumstances have been considered in the pathogenesis of some neoplasms.

Renal calculi are common in vitamin A–deficient animals. In humans, however, there is no evidence that this deficiency is a common cause of nephrolithiasis. The effect of vitamin A deficiency on human teeth is not yet entirely clear. In the continuously growing incisor teeth of rats and guinea pigs, important abnormalities occur as a result of atrophy and squamous metaplasia of the enamel organ. Similar changes in the tooth germs of an infant have been described.

Clinicopathologic correlation

The disease occurs at all ages but has a higher morbidity and mortality in infants. The papular cutaneous lesions, which are seen chiefly in adults, are most numerous on the thighs and forearms but also may involve the shoulders, chest, back, and buttocks. Acnelike lesions may appear on the face, but an etiologic relationship between vitamin A deficiency and acne vulgaris has not been demonstrated.

Bacterial infections, notably conjunctivitis, furunculosis, bronchopneumonia, and pyelonephritis, are common in vitamin A deficiency. There is, however, no proof that such infections are the result of a specific loss of resistance. The development of infection is always explainable on the basis of mechanical effects consequent to the epithelial changes.

The finding of keratinized epithelial cells in the urine, vaginal secretions, and corneal and nasal scrapings is helpful in establishing a diagnosis. Chemical tests for vitamin A concentration in the serum have been applied, but these tests do not have diagnostic value. The most valuable test for vitamin A deficiency is determination of the speed of adaptation to vision in a feeble light. The diagnostic significance of night blindness is increased if there are other reasons for suspecting vitamin A deficiency.

In both naturally occurring and experimentally produced cirrhosis of the liver there is decreased conversion of carotene to vitamin A with decreased storage of vitamin A. The level of vitamin A in the blood falls sharply, and in humans night blindness is often, though not invariably present. Other types of liver damage may cause similar changes.

Effect of excessive doses[37,92]

The administration of large amounts of pure vitamin A to experimental animals accelerates the maturation and degeneration of epiphyseal cartilage and the remodeling processes. Because of the excessive loss of cortical bone by increased osteoclastic activity (an exaggeration of the normal sequences), multiple fractures occur. Cutaneous lesions that resemble those seen in deficiency of the B group of vitamins also occur. A clinical picture in children characterized by irritability, anorexia, pruritus, hepatosplenomegaly, bulging fontanels, and painful swelling over the long bones has been ascribed to hypervitaminosis A.

In infants an intake of only 12 times the recommended daily allowance has apparently caused such

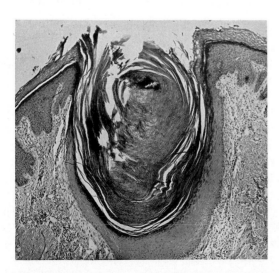

Fig. 13-5. Hyperkeratosis of hair follicle often associated with vitamin A deficiency but found in other nutritional disorders. (Courtesy Dr. Chester N. Frazier; from Sutton, R.L., Jr.: Diseases of the skin, ed. 11, St. Louis, 1956, The C.V. Mosby Co.)

toxic manifestations.[4,71] In adults toxic symptoms appear only after prolonged ingestion of 20 to 30 times the recommended daily allowance.[67,99] Such huge doses, nearly always self-administered, occasionally result in hospital admission for hyperexcitability, bone pain, and headache. Increased cerebrospinal fluid pressure, together with the history, indicates the correct diagnosis. Symptoms usually disappear shortly after the excessive intake is discontinued.

Vitamin D

Since the pathologic lesions of vitamin D deficiency are manifested almost entirely in the bones, this vitamin is discussed in Chapter 38. Note here that vitamin D is one of the factors involved in the absorption and transportation of calcium and in its normal deposition and maintenance in bone. Deficiency causes rickets in infants and one type of osteomalacia in adults.

Recently, major advances in regard to the biochemistry of vitamin D have been made by DeLuca.[27,28] He demonstrated the existence of biologically active metabolites of vitamin D and that vitamin D must be metabolically altered before it can function. In an attempt to elucidate the mechanism of action of vitamin D, DeLuca studied physiologic control mechanisms that regulate conversion of vitamin D to its various metabolites and characterized the cellular receptors in the vitamin D target tissues. Transport of vitamin D metabolites from the cytosol to the nucleus in these tissues has been demonstrated. Strong similarities between these metabolites and the steroid hormones have been observed. These findings stress the importance of basic biochemical research, which has now been directed toward clinical applications in attempts to correct metabolic bone diseases of major importance, such as renal osteodystrophy,[91] hypoparathyroidism,[50] glucocorticoid-induced osteoporosis, and vitamin D–resistant rickets.[94]

Hypervitaminosis D

The recommended daily allowance of vitamin D is 400 international units for most age groups. Huge overdosages (1000 to 3000 units/kg body weight/day) lead to hypercalcemia, hypercalciuria, and metastatic calcification.[67] There is some evidence of predisposition to renal calculus formation. Calcium is mobilized from the bones, with resulting osteoporosis. Symptoms include nausea, vomiting, and diarrhea. There is circumstantial evidence that as little as 2000 units per day (only five times the recommended daily allowance) may cause hypercalcemia in infants.[2,3]

Vitamin E (tocopherols)

Alpha-tocopherol is biologically the most active of the naturally occurring tocopherols and is prepared com-

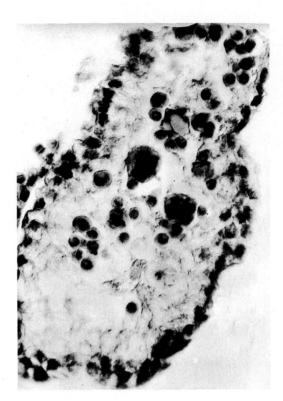

Fig. 13-6. Seminiferous tubule from rat fed diet deficient in vitamin E. Cells have atrophied and desquamated. Crescentic chromatin masses and huge multinucleated cells are typical of advanced vitamin E deficiency. (From Eddy, W.H., and Dalldorf, G.: The avitaminoses, ed. 3, Baltimore, copyrighted 1944 by The Williams & Wilkins Co.)

mercially. It is generally accepted that vitamin E acts in metabolism as an antioxidant.[107] Striking effects of vitamin E deficiency are seen in experimental animals of several species. These effects include cessation of growth, complete sterility in both male and female animals, and weakness of the muscles. In male animals degeneration of the seminiferous tubular epithelium occurs, resulting in aspermatogenesis (Fig. 13-6). In female animals the fertilized ova become implanted, but the young embryos become necrotic and are resorbed. The formation of the fetal placenta is retarded, and the maternal-fetal circulation is not properly established. In several species of animals, including guinea pigs and rabbits, degenerative changes occur in skeletal muscle as a result of vitamin E deficiency. Although the pathologic lesions are similar to those seen in the muscular dystrophies of humans, vitamin E has not been found to be of therapeutic value in these diseases.

In vitamin E–deficient animals, particularly if 20% cod-liver oil is present in the diet, an acid-fast lipid material known as *ceroid* is found in fat tissue and also in and about many other types of cells. Apparently this material represents oxidized fat of the unsaturated type, and one function of vitamin E is believed to be its ability to prevent the oxidation of such fats. The greatly increased oxygen consumption by striated muscle in vitro as a result of experimental vitamin E deficiency indicates that this vitamin may have general antioxidant properties.

Infants with cystic fibrosis sometimes show lesions in striated muscle similar to those seen in experimental animals deficient in vitamin E, as well as excessive creatinuria and the presence of ceroid in the intestinal wall. Certain types of megaloblastic anemia in severely undernourished infants have been reported to respond to vitamin E therapy.[8,55,60] The administration of vitamin E to patients with symptoms of porphyria decreases the urinary excretion of aminolevulinic acid, porphobilinogen, coproporphyrins, and uroporphyrins to normal levels.[66] Such observations have indicated that, in humans, vitamin E may have important functions other than the prevention of oxidation of unsaturated fatty acids.[45]

Vitamin K[70,87]

Vitamin K was named from the Danish word *Koagulations-Vitamin*. It occurs in several closely related forms, its activity apparently being dependent on the component 2-methyl-1,4-naphthoquinone. Although vitamin K is fat soluble, certain active compounds that are water soluble can be prepared. This vitamin was discovered by Dam in 1934 as a result of careful study of a hemorrhagic disease that he observed in chickens. It was later isolated by Doisy and associates. Physiologically it is necesary for the formation of prothrombin (factor II) and three other coagulation factors, VII, IX, and X; in its absence the mechanism of blood coagulation breaks down. In bacterial and plant cells vitamin K is important in electron-transport mechanisms.

Clinically vitamin K is of great importance in preventing hemorrhagic disease of the newborn. In adults simple deficiency is rare because of the abundance of this vitamin in leafy vegetables and other common foods and because of its formation by intestinal bacteria, which are absent for several days in newborn infants. Vitamin K deficiency can occur when there are great alterations in the intestinal flora or defects in fat absorption. Secondary deficiency occurs frequently in obstructive jaundice, since vitamin K is not absorbed satisfactorily in the absence of bile from the intestine. In the presence of severe liver damage, administration of vitamin K usually is ineffective in preventing hemorrhage. However, it is effective in correcting hemorrhagic lesions resulting from bishydroxycoumarin (Dicumarol) and other anticoagulants that inhibit prothrombin. Although much is known about vitamin K deficiency, the potential contribution of this disorder to the morbidity and mortality of hospitalized patients is often overlooked.[1]

Vitamins of B group

The term "vitamin B" was originally applied to the substance capable of curing experimental beriberi, which Funk isolated from rice polishings in 1911. This substance was not chemically pure, and it is now known that thiamine is its most important active component. Concentrates derived from yeast, wheat germ, rice polishings, and other sources contain several factors that collectively are known as the vitamin B complex. This complex comprises a group of essential compounds that are chemically unrelated but occur together in certain foods such as liver, milk, and leafy green vegetables. Most compounds in this group are involved in the metabolism of proteins, carbohydrates, and fats. Vitamin B_{12} and folic acid play important roles in blood formation.

Much of our knowledge of the specific effects of deficiency of single members of the B group is derived from studies carried out in experimental animals. To demonstrate the effect of deficiency of a single component, all other componens must be supplied in adequate amounts, and the animal must live long enough to become depleted of the component that one desires to study. The effects of riboflavin deficiency, for example, are not seen in animals deprived of the entire B complex. In humans, although deficiency in several of these factors commonly exists simultaneously, several disease entities are associated more or less specifically with the lack of individual factors. No specific disease is recognized as being attributable to lack of the entire B complex, and it is therefore desirable to discuss each factor in the group separately. Thiamine deficiency causes beriberi and is believed to be a factor in Wernicke's disease (see next page). Deficiency of niacin (nicotinic acid) is an important factor, though probably not the sole factor, in pellagra. The clinical picture of riboflavin deficiency includes cheilosis, a condition characterized by fissures at the angles of the mouth. Folic acid and vitamin B_{12} are important in hematologic disorders. Pyridoxine, pantothenic acid, biotin, choline, and inositol are also believed to be essential nutrients for humans. Certain effects produced in experimental animals by deprivation of other specific factors will be considered, even though they have not been duplicated in humans.

Thiamine

Chemistry and physiology. Thiamine is found in the thermolabile portion of the B complex, whereas the other members of the B complex that will be considered are thermostable. Thiamine hydrochloride, which was synthesized in 1937, is composed of a pyrimidine base united to a nitrogen-carbon-sulfur ring containing a pentavalent nitrogen. This compound is phosphorylated to form thiamine pyrophosphate, which acts intracellularly as the coenzyme for carboxylase. The latter enzyme decarboxylates pyruvic acid and participates in the synthesis of fat from carbohydrate. Thus in thiamine deficiency carbohydrate metabolism is interrupted at the pyruvic acid stage, and pyruvic acid accumulates in the tissues and the blood. The lesions of thiamine deficiency are not, however, produced by the simple injection of pyruvic acid, and it is probable that the failure of complete combustion of carbohydrate is the important factor, with the accumulation of pyruvic acid being incidental.

Thiamine is not stored in the body in large amounts. The depletion period before the onset of symptoms is variable, however, depending on the metabolic rate and unknown factors. Recently there have been reports that antithiamine factors in food may play a role in the development of beriberi.

Lesions resulting from deficiency. Human diseases in which thiamine deficiency plays an important role are beriberi, Wernicke's encephalopathy, and Korsakoff's psychosis.

In fatal cases of *beriberi* the findings are somewhat variable. On gross examination the most common lesions are emaciation, muscle atrophy, dilatation (with or without hypertrophy) of the right side of the heart, generalized edema, serous effusions, and chronic passive congestion of the viscera. Death may be caused by high-output cardiac failure, by acute pulmonary edema, or by pneumonia or other complicating infections. The edema is caused in part by cardiac failure, but hypoproteinemia is probably a contributory factor in many cases. This cardiovascular picture is particularly characteristic of the so-called wet type of beriberi, which is usually acute. Microscopically loss of striation and fatty degeneration of the myocardial fibers are noted. There is diffuse edema, often with slight lymphocytic infiltration of the intestinal tissue of many organs. Skeletal muscles show hyaline and fatty degenerative changes.

Degenerative changes in nerves are more characteristic of the dry or chronic form of the disease, which is seen chiefly in adults. Myelin degeneration and, in severe cases, fragmentation of the axis cylinders are seen in the affected nerves, which may be those of the extremities, the vagi, or the cranial nerves. In thiamine-deficient pigeons, axis cylinder degeneration begins distally and progresses until the neurons are involved. If thiamine is given before neuron death, regeneration of axis cylinders occurs at the usual normal rate. In dogs similar degenerative changes have been described in the central nervous system.

Wernicke's disease, which is associated with chronic alcoholism, is characterized by ganglion cell degeneration and focal demyelinating lesions and hemorrhage in the nuclei surrounding the ventricles and aqueduct, particularly in the nuclei of the extrinsic muscles of the eye. There is also some reparative proliferation of neuroglial cells. The picture is often complicated by symptoms of beriberi, scurvy, riboflavin deficiency, and pellagra. An apparently identical lesion may be produced in thiamine-deficient pigeons. In view of the experimental evidence, thiamine deficiency is now believed to be the most important etiologic factor in Wernicke's disease and in the pathologically similar Wernicke-Korsakoff syndrome.[31] Adding thiamine to the diet causes prompt clearing of the neurologic symptoms. *Korsakoff's psychosis,* the result of brain damage after recovery from coma in Wernicke's syndrome, improves more slowly, and underlying psychotic elements often remain.

Clinicopathologic correlation. The mechanism by which thiamine deficiency produces its characteristic lesions is not clear. The degenerative changes in the peripheral nerves and central nervous system are perhaps the result of interrupted carbohydrate metabolism as described previously. This seems logical in view of the fact that the metabolism of nervous tissue is believed to be totally dependent on carbohydrate oxidation. The cardiac manifestations may be related to the experimental observation that the oxygen uptake in vitro of the auricles of thiamine-deficient rats is significantly lower than that of the control animals.

A diet consisting largely of carbohydrate is an important contributing factor in the development of thiamine deficiency, since thiamine requirements are proportional to carbohydrate combustion. Symptoms of peripheral neuritis and mental confusion are explained on the basis of nervous tissue degeneration or anoxia, and cardiorespiratory symptoms such as tachycardia, edema, cyanosis, and pulmonary congestion are at least partially explained by the cardiac lesions. In the infantile form of beriberi, vomiting, cyanosis, and tachycardia may be followed by death (probably from pulmonary edema) in 24 to 36 hours. The mortality of beriberi varies from 5% to 50%, depending on the severity of symptoms and on the promptness and adequacy of treatment.

Niacin

Chemistry and physiology. Niacin, or nicotinic acid, is prepared by oxidation of the alkaloid nicotine. It is β-pyridine carboxylic acid and is active only in the amide form. Niacin is an essential molecular constituent of diphosphopyridine nucleotide and triphosphopyridine nucleotide, which act as cofactors for several dehydrogenases. Studies have shown that niacin may be synthesized from dietary tryptophan. Pyridoxine aids in this process.

Etiology of pellagra. Although divergent views still exist concerning the etiology of pellagra, there is general agreement that the major factor is deficiency of certain members of the B group of vitamins, particularly niacin. Some investigators believe that niacin deficiency should be regarded as the cause of pellagra, despite the fact that most affected individuals show evidence of multiple dietary deficiencies. The pathologic changes of uncomplicated niacin deficiency have not been described in either humans or experimental animals. Lesions that heal on administration of niacin are assumed to have been caused largely by lack of that compound. Pellagra is apparently a nutritional disease of the "conditioned" type; conditioning factors include exposure to sunlight, alcoholism, organic diseases, and infectious diseases. About 50% of persons with pellagra show achlorhydria. Macrocytic anemia, which is not uncommon, is probably the result of concomitant folic acid deficiency. Qualitative deficiency in the amino acid composition of the protein supply is probaby a conditioning factor in pellagra. The relationship of a cornmeal diet to pellagra is probably explainable on the basis of the fact that cornmeal is deficient in tryptophan, which is a precursor of nicotinic acid. There is also some evidence that cornmeal may contain an antagonist of nicotinic acid. Diphosphopyridine nucleotide and triphosphopyridine nucleotide, which have an abnormally low value in the blood and urine of persons with pellagra, rise to normal levels or higher when niacin is administered.

Pellagra occurs frequently in parts of Central America, Yugoslavia, Rumania, and Egypt. In the southern United States, where it was formerly common, it has largely disappeared.[79]

Lesions resulting from deficiency. The pathologic lesions of pellagra involve the skin, mucous membranes, gastrointestinal tract, and nervous system. Emaciation usually is present.

The *cutaneous lesions*, which may be absent in some cases, are seen particularly in areas exposed to sunlight but may occur in any region exposed to irritation. They show a striking tendency to symmetric distribution, and the affected areas are sharply demarcated from the normal. In the early stages the lesions resemble sunburn, but later the skin becomes roughened, keratotic, scaly, and pigmented (Fig. 13-7). Microscopically congestion of the papillary blood vessels and edema of the papillae are seen. There is moderate lymphocytic infiltration in the corium. The most striking feature is the noticeable thickening of the keratinized layer of the epidermis.

The *tongue*, buccal membranes, gums, and palate become swollen and red, with eventual ulceration. Infection with Vincent's organisms often causes a gray membrane to form. Microscopically the lesions resemble those of the skin.

In the *colon* thickening of the wall with edema and lymphocytic infiltration is seen. Membraneous enteritis, with or without ulceration, is often present. Atro-

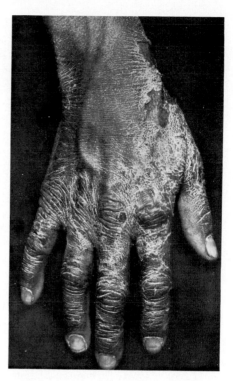

Fig. 13-7. Pellagra. Dermatitis and pigmentation of back of hand. (Courtesy Dr. Grover W. Wende; from Sutton, R.L., Jr.: Diseases of the skin, ed. 11, St. Louis, 1956, The C.V. Mosby Co.)

phy and cystic dilatation of the crypts of Lieberkühn are said to be characteristic (Fig. 13-8).

Lesions in the nervous system appear late in the course of the disease. Demyelinization of the posterior and lateral columns of the spinal cord and focal demyelinization and ganglion cell degeneration in the cerebrum have been described. Neurologic and even psychotic manifestations are common and clear up rapidly if niacin is administered early. They may be the only manifestations of the deficiency.

The possible occurrence of simultaneous lesions of beriberi or ariboflavinosis has already been mentioned. Nonspecific lesions seen on postmortem examination may include generalized emaciation, visceral atrophy, fatty infiltration and focal necrosis of the liver, and terminal bronchopneumonia.

The key to the production of certain of the lesions in pellagra is undoubtedly the role of niacin in cellular oxidation processes, but this physiologic principle has not been translated into terms that clearly explain the specific lesions found. The occasional appearance of pellagrous dermatitis in the carcinoid syndrome (see p. 1185) is of interest. It has been explained on the theory that the formation of serotonin from tryptophan makes less of this amino acid available for niacin synthesis.

The mucous membrane lesions and the gastrointes-

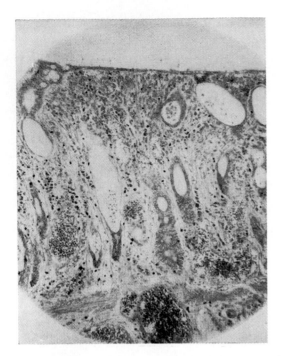

Fig. 13-8. Lesion in colon from patient with pellagra. Photograph of specimen is from collection of Dr. James Denton illustrating cystic glands characteristically found in pellagra, sprue, and possibly other related deficiency diseases. Lesion was formerly known as colitis cystica superficialis and is associated with malnutrition. (From Eddy, W.H., and Dalldorf, G.: The avitaminoses, ed. 3, Baltimore, copyrighted 1944 by The Williams & Wilkins Co.)

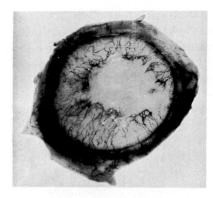

Fig. 13-9. Vascularization of cornea caused by riboflavin deficiency. Photograph of rat eye injected with india ink to demonstrate plexus of newly formed blood vessels. (From Eckardt, R.E., and Johnson, L.V.: Arch. Ophthalmol. **21:**315, 1939.)

tinal and mental symptoms usually respond promptly to niacin administration. Certain residual signs and symptoms are of the type associated with thiamine, pyridoxine, or riboflavin deficiency, and these often respond to the appropriate treatment.

Riboflavin

Riboflavin (empiric formula $C_{17}H_{20}N_4O_6$) was isolated in 1933 and synthesized in 1935. Historically it was the first vitamin to be identified as a constituent of an enzyme system. It forms the prosthetic group of several flavoprotein enzymes, including the "yellow respiratory enzyme" (Warburg), now known as cytochrome oxidase, which, together with the cytochromes, forms an enzyme system of outstanding importance in cellular respiration.

Experimental lesions. The lesions of riboflavin deficiency in young rats are produced only after a period of several weeks during which all other dietary factors are present in adequate amounts. Depletion will occur if rats are allowed to eat their feces, since the intestinal bacteria synthesize considerable amounts of riboflavin. Failure to gain weight, progressive loss of hair, and swelling and redness of the ears and paws are the out-

standing external manifestations. In the late stages extreme weakness and coma develop, with only one or two respirations per minute. From this moribund state, rats recover a considerable amount of vitality and strength almost instantaneously when small doses of crystalline riboflavin are injected. This dramatic result is apparently attributable to the sudden resumption of intracellular respiration.

Lesions in humans. Vascularization of the cornea by capillary sprouts from the limbic plexus (Fig. 13-9) was first noted in riboflavin-deficient rats and later was recognized as an important and early sign of deficiency of the vitamin in humans. In the later stages conjunctivitis develops. The ingrowth of capillaries into the normally avascular cornea probably is an attempt to compensate for the breakdown of oxidation processes in the corneal cells. The ocular lesions in humans and experimental animals progress to the formation of keratitis and ulceration of the cornea.

Ariboflavinosis in humans is characterized also by cheilosis (fissure formation and crusts at the angles of the mouth) and by redness and irritation of the tongue and lips. Of less common occurrence are circumoral pallor and seborrheic dermatitis of the nasolabial folds and ears (Fig. 13-10). Rarely the dermatitis has a more generalized distribution. Riboflavin deficiency may occur in a pure form or in patients with pellagra or various multiple deficiencies.

Pyridoxine (B₆)[86]

Pyridoxine, a pyridine derivative with the empiric formula $C_8H_{11}NO_3$, was differentiated from other heat-stable members of the B complex by György and associates in 1933. These investigators showed that a characteristic dermatitis in rats is caused specifically by the absence of this vitamin. The paws, snout, and ears be-

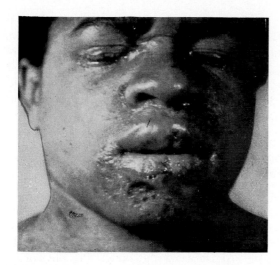

Fig. 13-10. Ariboflavinosis. Cheilosis, nasolabial lesion, and blepharospasm. (From Sydenstriker, V.P., et al.: JAMA **114:**2437, 1940.)

come hyperemic and swollen, with eventual desquamation and ulceration. Although the dermatitis has been described as "acrodynia-like," there is no evidence that human acrodynia is caused by pyridoxine deficiency.

Pyridoxine refers to three naturally occurring ring substances: pyridoxine, pyridoxal, and pyridoxamine. All three are converted to the active coenzyme form, pyridoxal 5'-phosphate, whose major function is related to protein or amino acid metabolism. Some metabolic processes in which pyridoxine is involved include transamination, amino acid decarboxylation, transmethylation of methionine, metabolism of tryptophan, and formation of melanin.

In several experimental animals, including pigs, prolonged pyridoxine deficiency causes severe microcytic anemia, which is improved but not entirely alleviated by the administration of pyridoxine. Other lesions found in experimentally induced deficiency in animals are demyelination of peripheral nerves, dorsal root ganglia, and dorsal columns of the spinal cord and fatty infiltration and hemosiderosis of the liver.

The importance of pyridoxine in human nutrition is not clear. Certain residual symptoms in persons with pellagra occasionally respond to pyridoxine administration, apparently because it is a coenzyme for the conversion of tryptophan to niacin. Hyperirritability and convulsions in infants, without other discoverable cause, have been associated rather definitely with pyridoxine deficiency in a commercial formula.

Experimental pyridoxine deficiency has been produced in humans by administration of the antivitamin deoxypyridoxine. The lesions noted include seborrheic dermatitis of the nasolabial folds, cheilosis, and glossitis, as well as a mild normochromic hypoplastic anemia.

Thus several of the lesions appear to overlap with those ascribed to riboflavin and niacin deficiency.

The treatment of tuberculosis with isoniazid sometimes results in a conditioned pyridoxine deficiency, with cheilosis and peripheral neuritis. These lesions are resolved by the administration of pyridoxine. Also, pyridoxine deficiency has been reported in patients receiving antihypertensive drugs, patients with Parkinson's disease being treated with L-dopa, and women taking oral contraceptives.[80]

Several B₆-dependency syndromes have been described.[35] They respond only to pyridoxine in very large doses, 200 to 600 mg of pyridoxine HCl per day in contrast to the normal requirement of 1.5 to 2 mg per day. These syndromes are as follows:

1. Convulsions in infants who have become dependent because their mothers were given large doses of the vitamin for hyperemesis gravidarum
2. Hypersideritis anemia with deposition of hemosiderin in the marrow and liver
3. Xanthurenic aciduria
4. Cystothionuria
5. Homocysteinura

The last four conditions usually are related to an inherited enzymatic defect and are examples of "genetically conditioned" deficiencies.

Pantothenic acid

Pantothenic acid is a component of coenzyme A. It prevents or cures a type of dermatitis peculiar to chickens. In rats deficiency of this compound causes a dermatitis, intestinal ulceration, and hemorrhagic necrosis in the adrenal cortex. There is evidence that pantothenic acid may be of importance in preventing the graying of hair that occurs in certain laboratory animals with nutritional deficiencies.

Pantothenic acid is present in most animal tissues and in yeast, and evidence indicates that it may be a growth-promoting substance of almost universal importance. The pantothenate level of the blood is below normal in pellagra, beriberi, and ariboflavinosis. Experimental pantothenic acid deficiency in humans causes malaise, headache, insomnia, and nausea but no significant interference with adrenal function. Despite the physiologic importance of this vitamin, evidence for the spontaneous occurrence of lesions resulting from deficiency remains inconclusive.

Biotin[86]

Biotin (vitamin H or coenzyme R) is a compound essential for the respiration of certain lower organisms and probably of all cells. It combines with avidin, a substance present in uncooked egg white, to form a compound that is not absorbed in the intestines. Our present knowledge of biotin deficiency has been gained largely through observations of animals or humans who have ingested large amounts of raw egg white. In human volunteers fed a diet in which egg white furnished 30% of the total caloric intake, a fine "branny" cutaneous desquamation developed in 3 to 4 weeks. Later, anemia, dryness of the skin, lassitude, mental depression, muscle pains, and other symptoms appeared.[110]

Choline[88]

Choline can be synthesized from dietary methionine. It is an important factor in fat metabolism, and many experimental studies have been concerned with the mechanisms by which it acts.[58,88] It is an essential component of lecithin, a phospholipid that is a constituent of all cells. Lecithin is probably formed in the liver as a preliminary step in the oxidation of fatty acids. Choline deficiency in experimental animals (dogs, rats, and rabbits), particularly when combined with a high intake of fats with saturated fatty acids, reduces the oxidation of fats in the liver and leads to the accumulation of fat in the liver cord cells (central lobular distribution) and eventually to cirrhosis. Recent experimental studies have suggested that a choline-deficient diet may act as a promoter in liver carcinogensis induced by chemical carcinogens.[88] In young rats, hemorrhagic cortical necrosis of the kidneys, hemorrhages in other organs, and involution of the thymus are found in addition to fatty livers. Cystine-rich diets intensify the liver and kidney lesions, whereas methionine, like choline, reverses the process. Lipocaic, which is obtained by extraction from pancreatic tissue, has a similar effect in removing fat accumulation from the liver (lipotropic action). It is a crude extract, containing choline and inositol, as well as some other lipotropic factor that has not been identified. Choline deficiency has not been shown to occur in humans, and whether choline is an essential dietary factor for humans is not known.

Folic acid and vitamin B₁₂[42,86]

Folic acid apparently is identical to the *Lactobacillus casei* factor, a compound essential for the growth of *L. casei*. It is composed of several related substances, containing glutamic acid and pteroyl groups, joined together by *para*-aminobenzoic acid and known collectively as pteroylglutamates. The physiologically active form is a reduction product, tetrahydrofolic acid, formed during absorption.

Folic acid deficiency in monkeys causes a nutritional anemia, with reversal of the lymphocyte-neutrophil ratio. In humans, folic acid is useful in the treatment of sprue and megaloblastic nutritional anemia. It brings about hematologic remission in pernicious anemia but, unlike vitamin B₁₂, does not prevent or improve the degenerative lesions in the spinal cord.

Vitamin B₁₂ is the extrinsic factor in pernicious ane-

mia. Its absorption is dependent on the intrinsic factor in gastric mucosa. Like folic acid, vitamin B₁₂ consists of a family of compounds. Since a cyano group or cobalt, or both, is present in the molecules, a generic name is the cyanocobalamins. The relation of vitamin B₁₂, liver extract, and folic acid to blood regeneration in various types of anemia is an intricate one (see p. 1375).

Vitamin C (ascorbic acid)
Chemistry and physiology

Ascorbic acid exists in natural sources chiefly in the form of L-ascorbic acid, a six-carbon compound closely related to glucose. In this form, it readily loses two hydrogen atoms to become dehydroascorbic acid, which is reversibly oxidizable in the body. The physiologic action of vitamin C therefore probably depends on its ability to carry out oxidation-reduction reactions, but its role in cellular physiology is incompletely known. There is good evidence that it is essential for the metabolism of phenylalanine and tyrosine and that it maintains certain important sulfhydryl enzymes in the active state.

Ascorbic acid concentration is particularly high in the adrenal glands, but its role in adrenal hormone production is not known. In severe scurvy, it remains in the adrenal glands after it has been depleted in other organs. It is clear that ascorbic acid is necessary for the production and maintenance of several intercellular substances, notably collagen, osseomucin, chondromucin, dentin, and probably the cement substances that hold vascular endothelial cells together in certain animals, including humans and guinea pigs.

Wound repair in scorbutic guinea pigs was studied by Wolbach.[112] The wound fills in normally with blood clot. The clot is then organized by fibroblasts but without blood vessels. No collagen is formed as long as the scorbutic diet is maintained. With the correction of the deficiency, collagen formation begins within 24 hours and proceeds rapidly. The newly formed intercellular material is homogeneous for a time, but argyrophilic fibers and true collagen fibers soon appear. Fibrin is not changed to collagen but is liquefied and removed, and the collagen is laid down independently.

It is apparent that the "homogeneous substance" described in healing wounds by Wolbach is the mucopolysaccharide ground substance of connective tissue from which reticulin and collagen fibrils normally are formed.[32] In scurvy this formation of fibrils does not occur. There is evidence that ascorbic acid is essential for the formation of hydroxyproline, the most characteristic and essential component of collagen. Radioisotopic studies have shown that the incorporation of labeled sulfur into the chondroitin sulfate of the ground substance is sharply reduced in scurvy, indicating that a basic defect in ground substance formation may exist. Ascorbic acid is vital for collagen formation, serving in the preservation and maturation of fibroblasts and the incorporation of hydroxyproline and hydroxylysine.

In recent years ascorbic acid has been linked to many areas of human health. It is now known that the beneficial effects of ascorbic acid go far beyond its role in the prevention of scurvy. New developments in research have focused on the vitamin's involvement in neuromodulation, neuropeptide synthesis, immune response, overall nutrition, as well as collagen synthesis.[18] Ascorbic acid appears to have a role as a cofactor in dopamine β-hydroxylase and peptidylglycine α-amidating monooxygenase enzyme systems, important in the synthesis of neurotransmitters and hormones respectively. Considerable attention has been given to the antioxidant function of ascorbic acid in neutralizing extracellular reactive oxidants produced during phagocytic activity and in protecting cell membranes from free-radical damage.

Lesions resulting from deficiency

Essentially similar lesions are found in humans and in guinea pigs. The oustanding features are hemorrhages and lesions in the skeleton, including the teeth.

Cutaneous hemorrhage, ranging from petechial to massive extravasation, is almost constantly found at autopsy in adults with vitamin C deficiency. The larger hemorrhages correspond to areas of trauma. Hemorrhage into muscles or along fascial planes is seen particularly at points of mechanical stress. Bleeding occurs from capillaries, presumably because of rupture of the loosened endothelial cells. In infants with vitamin C deficiency, massive subperiosteal hemorrhage is almost always present, especially in the legs. Massive areas of hemorrhage may become infected and suppurate. Ulceration of the gums, loosening of the teeth, and massive hemorrhage from the gums are commonly seen in adults but rarely in infants.

The skeletal lesions, which likewise are the result primarily of the failure to produce intercellular substances, are seen most conspicuously at the ends of growing tubular bones. The changes are described on p. 1982.

Anemia of various types is common in scurvy, particularly in infancy. Although hemorrhage may be a factor, it is rarely the sole cause. Interference with the formation of folic acid compounds has been postulated, and severe megaloblastic anemia in scurvy may respond only to folic acid.

Death most often results from secondary infection, with fatal hemorrhage being a rare cause. Sudden death may follow physical exertion, perhaps from addisonian crisis resulting from stress. Fulminating tuberculosis is particularly common. The failure of the normal localization and repair of tubercles by collagenous scar tissue is a logical explanation for this.

Clinicopathologic correlation

The mortality from scurvy is high in untreated cases but low in recognized cases given adequate therapy.

In infants, pain from subperiosteal hemorrhage is the chief symptom. In general, the symptoms in adults are merely general weakness and depression.

Roentgenographic examination of the bones is an important diagnostic feature in infantile scurvy. Capillary fragility, brought out by means of the tourniquet test or other tests, is of some diagnostic value. Chemical determination of the level of ascorbic acid in the serum and leukocyte layer of centrifuged blood and in the urine is also helpful, but in doubtful cases the response to antiscorbutic treatment often gives the best evidence of deficiency. Experienced clinicians believe that mild cases of anorexia and mental depression that are promptly relieved by vitamin C therapy often are caused by deficiency of that vitamin. In patients with extensive wounds or burns the ascorbic acid level in the blood falls rapidly (perhaps because of mobilization in granulation tissue), and replacement of therapy is often indicated.

Vitamins and congenital abnormalities[34,37,44,83,102]

Although definite relationships of dietary deficiencies to congenital abnormalities in humans have not been established, a wide variety of congenital lesions have been produced and studied in lower mammals, notably in rats. The basic principle established by this experimental work is that nutritional factors, particularly vitamins, are more important for fetal differentiation and development than for maternal health. Defects resulting from maternal deficiency in vitamin A, riboflavin, folic acid, vitamin B_{12}, pantothenic acid, and vitamin E and from general undernutrition have been well documented. In general, the similarities between the lesions caused by various dietary deficiencies are more striking than the differences. The lesions involve the eyes and the skeletal, central nervous, cardiovascular, and genitourinary systems. Also included are anophthalmia, cleft palate, exencephaly, hydrocephalus, spina bifida, and ectopia of the abdominal viscera. In the case of vitamin A, defects are caused not only by maternal deficiency but also by excessive maternal intake. Excess intake frequently causes cranial deformities with extrusion of the brain and, sporadically, ocular defects, harelip, and cleft palate. Further study of these phenomena should throw light on the complex and varied (and probably interrelated) mechanisms involved in the production of congenital abnormalities.

SPECIFIC AMINO ACID DEFICIENCIES

In rats and dogs 10 of the amino acids are indispensable for normal growth: tryptophan, lysine, histidine, arginine, phenylalanine, isoleucine, leucine, threonine, methionine, and valine. With the exception of arginine and histidine, these amino acids are essential to produce a positive nitrogen balance in humans. A few specific lesions have been described in animals as a result of deficiency of these elements. However, as mentioned previously in the discussion of experimental kwashiorkor-like models, the pathologic changes with diets deficient in a single essential amino acid are generally similar in rats to those observed with the intake of low-quantity or poor-quality proteins. Thus it may not be worthwhile to review some of the specific single essential amino acid deficiencies as described in the literature.[34,95]

A few specific essential amino acids, particularly tryptophan and the branched-chain amino acids (valine, isoleucine, and leucine) appear to have specific effects other than being mere building blocks for protein synthesis. Tryptophan, in addition to serving as a precursor to serotonin, nicotinic acid, and other metabolites, has been found to have an important regulatory role in hepatic protein synthesis in animals.[90] The branched-chain amino acids, particularly leucine, have been described as having an important role in skeletal muscle protein synthesis.[76]

SPECIFIC FATTY ACID DEFICIENCIES

Linoleic acid deficiency in rats causes scaling of the skin, alopecia, and injury to renal and testicular tubular epithelium. Some infants fed a formula containing less than 0.1% of calories as linoleic acid failed to grow and showed scaly skin changes.[64] At present there is little evidence for the occurrence of essential fatty acid deficiency in humans under natural conditions. In addition to linoleic acid, linolenic and arachidonic acids are believed necessary for humans.

ESSENTIAL ELEMENTS*

In addition to carbon, hydrogen, oxygen, and nitrogen, 16 elements are considered essential for life: calcium, magnesium, potassium, sodium, sulfur, phosphorus, chlorine, iron, copper, cobalt, manganese, zinc, iodine, selenium, molybdenum, and probably fluorine. Many other elements, however, are present in tissues, and studies of their possible importance are far from complete. In addition to the more obvious functions of calcium, magnesium, phosphorus, sodium, and chlorine—in acting as structural components and in maintaining the electrolyte balance—trace amounts of

*References 7, 11, 21, 56, 74, 75, 82, 104, 117.

several metallic elements, such as zinc, copper, manganese, selenium, molybdenum, and magnesium, are of vital importance, since they form essential components of certain enzyme systems. The function of iron as a component of hemoglobin and of intracellular oxidizing enzymes is too well known to require discussion here.

Calcium is important for the contraction of heart muscles and for blood coagulation. Its importance in rickets and osteomalacia and its relation to the parathyroid glands are discussed on p. 1570. Calcium and phosphorus metabolism are discussed in connection with rickets on pp. 1945 and 1983.

Sulfur is extremely important physiologically. However, it would be difficult to produce inorganic sulfur deficiency because, although this element occurs in methionine and cystine, inorganic sulfur cannot be used in the formation of these compounds. Sulfur is most important in the sulfhydryl (—SH) form, in which state it is an active component of many enzymes, vitamins, and hormones. Oxidation of this group to the inactive (S—S) form is believed to be the mechanism of action of many enzyme inhibitors.

Copper is important in hemopoiesis and is an essential constituent of several important enzymes. Experimental deficiency in rats, for example, leads to a microcytic hypochromic anemia, and the rats often die before the anemia becomes severe. Deficiency of this element also causes graying of the hair, which is not prevented by large amounts of pantothenic acid or *para*-aminobenzoic acid (the other anti–gray hair factors). Certain cases of hyperchromic anemia in children are believed to respond to copper supplementation. The relation of copper metabolism to Wilson's disease is discussed on p. 1269. Copper is also essential for the normal development of bone, the central nervous system, and connective tissue.

Cobalt deficiency in sheep and cattle is the cause of a severe anemia with hemosiderosis of the spleen. Deficiency of this element causes enzootic marasmus in Australian aborigines. Cobalt is a component of vitamin B_{12}.

Manganese deficiency has been largely neglected from the histologic viewpoint. In experimental animals disturbance of growth occurs in the offspring of deficient mothers, with frequent death and osseous defects in surviving animals. Lesions in the humans are unknown.

Zinc is an important component of carbonic anhydrase, uricase, insulin, and phosphatase. Dietary deficiency in rats causes corneal vascularization, alopecia, keratinization of the skin and esophagus, and death in a few weeks. Studies in the Middle East have strongly indicated a relationship of zinc deficiency to dwarfism and hypogonadism, as well as to iron-deficiency anemia and hepatosplenomegaly.[74] These abnormalities are corrected in response to zinc feeding.

Iodine deficiency[43] is related to lesions of the thyroid gland and is discussed in Chapter 31.

Fluorine inactivates phosphatase and several other enzyme systems. Experimental fluorine deficiency in rats has been reported to cause dental caries. For discussion of the effects of fluorine on teeth and bones, see pp. 1098 and 1945.

Selenium apparently substitutes for vitamin E as an antioxidant. *Manganese, chromium, molybdenum,* and *cadmium* have been shown to be active in enzyme systems of plants and lower animals.

MALNUTRITION AND BRAIN FUNCTION

In an earlier section the possibility that stunted mental development occurs secondarily to kwashiorkor was mentioned. Indeed, several studies have shown that many types of malnutrition retard the development of the human brain and adversely affect the patterns of learning and behavior in early life.[24,54,65,77,84] Whether the deficiency is in total calories, total protein, specific amino acids, micronutrients, or combinations of these factors, the result too often is a brain that is far below average size for the age of the child. When the underprivileged are better nourished (and viral and other infections of the central nervous system better controlled), the accepted level of human performance will be raised, and the problems of the social scientist will be considerably simplified.

NUTRITION AND CANCER

Much attention has been given to the possible association between nutrition and cancer (see also Chapter 14). Of the many environmental factors considered to be influential in the induction of cancer, diet and nutrition have gained much notoriety. This association has been derived mainly from diverse epidemiologic data but also from limited experimental studies with animals.*

In relating dietary factors and cancer one must consider the following:
1. Food additives or contaminants, as well as the nutrients themselves, may act as carcinogens, cocarcinogens, promoters, or combinations of these.
2. Nutritional deficiencies or imbalances may lead to biochemical abnormalities that in turn promote neoplastic processes.
3. Excessive intake of certain nutrients may produce metabolic abnormalities that promote neoplasms.

A few of the suspected food contaminants are mycotoxins (specifically aflatoxin) and nitrosamines, which are

*References 19, 23, 30, 68, 78, 100, 101, 111, 115, 116.

being investigated as important suspected carcinogens in humans. Studies have revealed that the charred parts of broiled meat and fish contain a series of new heterocyclic amines in the pyrolyzate of amino acids and proteins, which are mutagenic, and that two amines from tryptophan pyrolyzates—3-amino-1,4-dimethyl-5*H*-pyrido(4,3-*b*)indole and 3-amino-1-methyl-5*H*-pyrido(4,3-*b*)indole—are carcinogenic in animals.[62] Also, the amounts and type of fiber in the diet have been considered to be influential in the induction of bowel cancer in experimental animals.[68,105,111] Deficiencies of iron, iodine, riboflavin, vitamin A, pyridoxine, and choline have been considered to play a role in the induction of certain types of neoplasms. Based on epidemiologic data and also on animal studies, high dietary fat intake has been reported to increase breast cancer incidence in females.[20,116] In general, it is believed that the dietary effects occur mainly in relation to promotion, the second stage of the process of carcinogenesis.

Several experimental studies have revealed that diet or dietary components may act to *prevent* the induction of certain cancers.[109] Certain dietary components have been demonstrated to induce enzyme systems that detoxify chemical carcinogens. Also, some food additives, which are antioxidants, have been demonstrated to act in an inhibitory manner in chemical carcinogenesis. Studies with vitamin A treatment in animals have also indicated an inhibitory effect, particularly in relation to changes in cell differentiation, on the induction of certain types of cancers. Several experimental studies revealed that selenium supplementation protects against certain neoplasms induced by carcinogens.[68]

Overall, the present knowledge of the association between nutrition and cancer is limited. Further information is needed before their association may be used rationally in the prevention and treatment of cancer in humans.

This chapter has been limited to selected topics dealing with how altered nutrition may induce and influence disease states. It has not covered many important areas dealing with nutrition and its interrelationships, such as those with obesity,[106] heart and vessel diseases,[6,52] infection and the immune system,[22,39,61,108] aging,[46,51,118] and drugs.[41,63,80,81]

REFERENCES

1. Alperin, J.B.: Coagulopathy caused by vitamin K deficiency in critically ill, hospitalized patients, JAMA **258:**1916, 1987.
2. American Academy of Pediatrics, Committee on Nutrition: The prophylactic requirement and the toxicity of vitamin D, Pediatrics **31:**512, 1963.
3. American Academy of Pediatrics, Committee on Nutrition: The relation between infantile hypercalcemia and vitamin D—public health implications in North America, Pediatrics **40:**1050, 1967.
4. American Academy of Pediatrics, Committee on Nutrition: The use and abuse of vitamin A, Pediatrics **48:**455, 1971.

5. American Academy of Pediatrics, Committee on Nutrition: Commentary on breast-feeding and infant formulas, including proposed standards for formulas, Pediatrics **57**:278, 1976.

6. American Heart Association Committee Report: Diet and coronary heart disease, Circulation **58**:762A, 1978.

7. Avioli, L.V.: Major minerals: A. Calcium and phosphorus. In Goodhart, R.S., and Shils, M.E., editors: Modern nutrition in health and disease, ed. 6, Philadelphia, 1980, Lea & Febiger.

8. Baker, S.J., Pereira, S.M., and Begum, A.: Failure of vitamin E therapy in the treatment of anemia of protein calorie malnutrition, Blood **32**:717, 1968.

9. Bauernfeind, C., editor: Vitamin A deficiency and its control, Orlando, Fla., 1986, Academic Press, Inc.

10. Beadle, G.W.: Genes and the chemistry of the organism, Am. Sci.**34**:31, 1946.

11. Bentler, E.: Iron. In Goodhard, R.S., and Shils, M.E., editors: Modern nutrition in health and disease, ed. 6, Philadelphia, 1980, Lea & Febiger.

12. Bhattacharyya, A.K.: Protein-energy malnutrition (kwashiorkor-marasmus syndrome): terminology, classification and evolution, World Rev. Nutr. Diet. **47**:80, 1986.

13. Birch, H.G., et al.: Relation of kwashiorkor in early childhood and intelligence at school age, Pediatr. Res. **5**:579, 1971.

14. Bistrian, B.R., Blackburn, G.L., Hallowell E., and Heddle, R.: Protein status of general surgical patients, JAMA **230**:858, 1974.

15. Bistrian, B.R., Blackburn, G.L., Vitale, J., Cochran, D., and Naylor, J.: Prevalence of malnutrition in general medical patients, JAMA **235**:1567, 1976.

16. Blix, G., editor: Mild-moderate forms of protein-calorie malnutrition, I, Symposia of the Swedish Nutrition Foundation, Uppsala, 1963, Almqvist & Wiksells.

17. Brock, J.F., and Autret, M.: Kwashiorkor in Africa, WHO Monogr. Ser. **8**:36, 1952.

18. Burns, J.J., Rivers, J.M., and Macklin, L.J., editors: Third conference on vitamin C, Ann. NY Acad. Sci. **498**:1, 1987.

19. Calories and energy expenditure in carcinogenesis, Am. J. Clin. Nutr. **45**(suppl.):149, 1987.

20. Carroll, K.K.: Dietary fat and cancer. In Horisberger, M., and Bracco, U., editors: Lipids in modern nutrition, New York, 1987, Raven Press.

21. Cavalieri, R.C.: Trace elements: A. Iodine. In Goodhart, R.S., and Shils, M.E., editors: Modern nutrition in health and disease, ed. 6, Philadelphia, 1980, Lea & Febiger.

22. Chandra, P.K.: Interactions of nutrition, infection and immune response: immunocompetence in nutritional deficiency, methodological considerations and intervention strategies, Acta Paediatr. Scand. **68**:137, 1979.

23. Conference on Nutrition and Cancer Therapy, Cancer Res. **37**(7, part 2):2322, 1977.

24. Cravioto, J., and De Licardie, E.R.: Nutrition and behavior and learning, World Rev. Nutr. Diet. **16**:80, 1973.

25. David, H.: Die Leber bei Nahrungsmangel und Mangelernährung, Berlin, 1961, Akademie-Verlag.

26. Davies, J.N.P.: Nutrition and nutritional diseases, Annu. Rev. Med. **3**:99, 1952.

27. De Luca, H.F.: The metabolism and function of vitamin D, Adv. Exp. Med. Biol. **196**:361, 1986.

28. De Luca, H.F.: Vitamin D metabolism and function, Monogr. Endocrinol. **13**:1, 1979.

29. De Luca, L.M., and Shapiro, S.S., editors: Modulation of cellular interactions by vitamin A and derivatives (retinoids), Ann. NY Acad. Sci. **359**:1, 1981.

30. Diet, nutrition, and cancer, Washington, D.C., 1982, National Academy Press.

31. Dreyfus, P.M.: In Beeson, P.B., McDermott, W., and Wyngaarden, J.B., editors: Cecil-Loeb textbook of medicine, ed. 15, Philadelphia, 1979, W.B. Saunders Co.

32. Edwards, L.C., and Dunphy, J.E.: Wound healing, II. Injury and abnormal repair, N. Engl. J. Med. **259**:275, 1958.

33. Einstein, A.B., and Singh, S.P.: Hormonal control of nutrient metabolism. In Goodhart, R.S., and Shils, M.E., editors: Modern nutrition in health and disease, ed. 6, Philadelphia, 1980, Lea & Febiger.

34. Follis, R.H., Jr.: Deficiency disease, Springfield, Ill., 1958, Charles C Thomas, Publisher.

35. Frimpter, G.W., Andleman, R.J., and George, W.F.: Vitamin B₆-dependency syndromes: new horizons in nutrition, Am. J. Clin. Nutr. **22**:794, 1969.

36. Ganguly, J., et al.: Systemic mode of action of vitamin-A. In Vitamins and hormones, New York, 1980, Academic Press, Inc.

37. Geelen, J.A.G.: Hypervitaminosis A induced teratogenesis, CRC Crit. Rev. Toxicol. **6**:351, 1971.

38. Goodhart, R.S., and Shils, M.E., editors: Modern nutrition in health and disease, ed. 6, Philadelphia, 1980, Lea & Febiger.

39. Gross, R.L., et al.: Role of nutrition in immunologic function, Physiol. Rev. **40**:188, 1980.

40. Harper, A.E., Benevenga, N.J., and Wohlhueter, R.M.: Effects of ingestion of disproportionate amounts of amino acids, Physiol. Rev. **50**:428, 1970.

41. Hathcock, J.N., and Coon, J., editors: Nutrition and drug interrelations, New York, 1978, Academic Press, Inc.

42. Herbert, V., Coleman, N., and Jacob, E.: Folic acid and vitamin B₁₂. In Goodhart, R.S., and Shils, M.E., editors: Modern nutrition in health and disease, ed. 6, Philadelphia, 1980, Lea & Febiger.

43. Hetzel, B.S., Dunn, J.T., and Stanbury, J.B., editors: Prevention and control of iodine deficiency disorders, Amsterdam, 1987, Elsevier Science Publishers.

44. Hillman, R.W., and Goodhart, R.S.: Nutrition in pregnancy. In Goodhart, P.S., and Shils, M.E., editors: Modern nutrition in health and diseases, ed. 5, Philadelphia, 1973, Lea & Febiger.

45. Horwitt, M.K.: Vitamin E. In Goodhart, R.S., and Shils, M.E., editors: Modern nutrition in health and disease, ed. 6, Philadelphia, Lea & Febiger.

46. Hutchinson, M.L., and Munro, H., editors: Nutrition and aging, New York, 1986, Academic Press, Inc.

47. Irwin, M.I.: Nutritional requirements of man: a conspectus of research, New York, 1980, The Nutrition Foundation, Inc.

48. Jeliffe, D.D., and Welbourn, H.F.: Clinical signs of mild-moderate protein-calorie malnutrition of early childhood. In Blix, G., editor: Mild-moderate forms of protein-calorie malnutrition, Uppsala, 1963, Almqvist & Wiksell.

49. Keys, A., et al.: The biology of human starvation, vols. 1 and 2, Minneapolis, 1950, The University of Minnesota Press.

50. Koch, S.W., et al.: Treatment of hypoparathyroidism and pseudo-hypoparathyroidism with metabolites of vitamin D: evidence for impaired conversion of 25-hydroxyvitamin D to 1,25-dihydroxy-vitamin D, N. Engl. J. Med. **293**:840, 1975.

51. Kritchevsky, D.: Diet, lipid metabolism, and aging, Fed. Proc. **38**:2001, 1978.

52. Kritchevsky, D.: Nutrition and cardiovascular disease. In Sidransky, H., editor: Nutritional pathology, New York, 1985, Marcel Dekker, Inc.

53. Latham, M.C.: Human nutrition in tropical Africa, Rome, 1965, Food and Agriculture Organization of the United Nations.

54. Latham, M.C.: Protein-calorie malnutrition in children and its relations to psychological development and behavior, Physiol. Rev. **54**:541, 1974.

55. Leonard, P.J., and Losowsky, M.S.: Effect of alpha-tocopherol administration on red cell survival in vitamin E–deficient human subjects, Am. J. Clin. Nutr. **24**:388, 1971.

56. Li, T.K., and Vallee, B.L.: The biochemical and nutritional roles of other trace elements. In Goodhard, R.S., and Shils, M.E., editors: Modern nutrition in health and disease, ed. 6, Philadelphia, 1980, Lea & Febiger.

57. Lloyd-Still, J.D.: Clinical studies on the effects of malnutrition during infancy and subsequent physical and intellectual development. In Lloyd-Still, J.D., editor: Malnutrition and intellectual development, Littleton, Mass., 1976, Publishing Sciences Group, Inc.

58. Lombardi, B.: Effects of choline deficiency on rat hepatocytes, Fed. Proc. **30**:139, 1971.

59. Lui, N.S.T., and Roels, O.A.: The vitamins: A. Vitamin A and carotene. In Goodhart, R.S., and Shils, M.E., editors: Modern nutrition in health and disease, ed. 6, Philadelphia, 1980, Lea & Febiger.

60. Majaj, A.S., et al.: Vitamin E responsive megaloblastic anemia in infants with protein-calorie malnutrition, Am. J. Clin. Nutr. **12:**374, 1963.
61. Mata, L.: The malnutrition-infection complex and its environment factors, Proc. Nutr. Soc. **38:**29, 1979.
62. Matsukura, N., et al.: Carcinogenicity in mice of mutagenic compounds from a tryptophan pyrolyzate, Science **213:**346, 1981.
63. McDanell, R.E.M., and McLean, A.E.M.: Role of nutritional status in drug metabolism and toxicity. In Sidransky, H., editor: Nutritional pathology, New York, 1985, Marcel Dekker, Inc.
64. McLaren, D.S.: The vitamins. In Bondy, P.K., editor: Duncan's disease of metabolism: endocrinology and nutrition, ed. 6, Philadelphia, 1969, W.B. Saunders Co.
65. Morgan, B.L.G., and Winick, M.: Pathological effects of malnutrition on the central nervous system. In Sidransky, H., editor: Nutritional pathology, New York, 1985, Marcel Dekker, Inc.
66. Nair, P.P., et al.: Vitamin E and porphyrin metabolism in man, Arch. Intern. Med. **128:**411, 1971.
67. National Academy of Science–National Research Council, Food and Nutrition Board: Recommended dietary allowances, rev. ed. 9, Washington, D.C., 1980, U.S. Government Printing Office.
68. Newell, G.R., and Ellison, N.M., editors: Nutrition and cancer: etiology and treatment, Prog. Cancer Res. Ther. **17:**1, 1981.
69. Olson, R.E.: Protein-calorie malnutrition, New York, 1975, Academic Press, Inc.
70. Olson, R.E.: Vitamin K. In Goodhard, R.S., and Shils, M.E., editors: Modern nutrition in health and disease, ed. 6, Philadelphia, 1980, Lea & Febiger.
71. Persson, B., Tunnell, R., and Ekengren, K.: Chronic vitamin A intoxication during the first half year of life: description of 5 cases, Acta Paediatr. Scand. **54:**49, 1965.
72. Pinchcofsky-Devin, G.D., and Kaminski, M.V., Jr.: Incidence of protein calorie malnutrition in the nursing home population, J. Am. Coll. Nutr. **6:**109, 1987.
73. Platt, B.S., Heard, C.R.C., and Stewart, R.J.C.: Experimental protein-calorie deficiency. In Munro, H.N., and Allison, J.B., editors: Mammalian protein metabolism, vol. 2, New York, 1964, Academic Press, Inc.
74. Prasad, A.S., editor: Trace elements in human health and disease: zinc and copper, New York, 1976, Academic Press, Inc.
75. Prasad, A.S., editor: Trace elements in human health and disease: essential and toxic elements, vol. 2, New York, 1976, Academic Press, Inc.
76. Rannels, D.E., McKee, E.E., and Morgan, H.E.: Regulation of protein synthesis and degradation in heart and skeletal muscle. In Litwack, G., editor: Biochemical actions of hormones, vol. 4, New York, 1977, Academic Press, Inc.
77. Read, M.S.: Behavioral correlation of malnutrition. In Brazier, M.A.B., editor: Growth and development of the brain, New York, 1975, Raven Press.
78. Reddy, B.S.: Nutrition and its relationship to cancer, Adv. Cancer Res. **32:**238, 1980.
79. Rivlin, R.S.: Disorder of vitamin metabolism: deficiencies, metabolic abnormalities, and excesses. In Wyngaarden, J.B., and Smith, L.H., Jr., editors: Cecil-Loeb textbook of medicine, ed. 17, Philadephia, 1985, W.B. Saunders Co.
80. Roe, D.A.: Drug-induced nutritional deficiencies, Westport, Conn., 1978, The AVI Publishing Co., Inc.
81. Roe, D.A.: Pathological changes associated with drug-induced malnutrition. In Sidransky, H., editor: Nutritional pathology, New York, 1985, Marcel Dekker, Inc.
82. Sanstead, H.H.: Trace metals in human nutrition, Curr. Concepts Nutr. **13:**37, 1984.
83. Schardein, J.L.: Chemically induced birth defects, New York, 1985, Marcel Dekker, Inc.
84. Scrimshaw, N.S., and Gordon, J.E., editors: Malnutrition, learning and behavior, Cambridge, Mass., 1968, MIT Press.
85. Sebrell, W.H., Jr., and Harris, R.S., editors: The vitamins, ed. 2, vol. 1, New York, 1967, Academic Press, Inc.
86. Sebrell, W.H., Jr., and Harris, R.S., editors: The vitamins, ed. 2, vol. 2, New York, 1968, Academic Press, Inc.

87. Sebrell, W.H., Jr., and Harris, R.S., editors: The vitamins, ed. 2, vol. 3, New York, 1971, Academic Press, Inc.
88. Shinozuka, H., and Katyal, S.L.: Pathology of choline deficiency. In Sidransky, H., editor: Nutritional pathology, New York, 1985, Marcel Dekker, Inc.
89. Sidransky, H.: Chemical and cellular pathology of experimental acute amino acid deficiency, Methods Achiev. Exp. Pathol. **6:**1, 1972.
90. Sidransky, H.: Tryptophan: unique action by an essential amino acid. In Sidransky, H., editor: Nutritional pathology, New York, 1985, Marcel Dekker, Inc.
91. Silverberg, D.S., et al.: Effect of 1,25-dihydroxycholecalciferol in real osteodystrophy, Can. Med. Assoc. J. **112:**190, 1975.
92. Smith, F.R., and Goodman, D.S.: Vitamin A transport in human vitamin A toxicity, N. Engl. J. Med. **294:**805, 1976.
93. Smith, J.L., Wickiser, A.A., Korth, L.L., Grandjean, A.C., and Schaefer, A.E.: Nutritional status of an institutionalized aged population, J. Am. Coll. Nutr. **3:**13, 1984.
94. Sockalosky, J.J., et al.: Vitamin D–resistant rickets: end-organ unresponsiveness to $1,25-(OH)_2D_3$, J. Pediatr. **96:**701, 1980.
95. Sos, J.: Die Pathologie der Eiweissernährung, Budapest, 1964, Verlag der Ungarischen Akademie der Wissenschaften.
96. Sporn, M.B.: Retinoids and cancer prevention, Carcinog. Compr. Surv. **5:**99, 1980.
97. Sporn, M.B., and Newton, D.L.: Chemoprevention of cancer with retinoids, Fed. Proc. **38:**2528, 1979.
98. Sporn, M.B., Roberts, A.B., and Goodman, D.S., editors: The retinoids, New York, 1984, Academic Press, Inc.
99. Stimson, W.H.: Vitamin A intoxication in adults: report of a case with a summary of the literature, N. Engl. J. Med. **265:**369, 1961.
100. Symposium on nutrition and cancer, Fed. Proc. **35:**1307, 1976.
101. Symposium on nutrition in the causation of cancer, Cancer Res. **35**(II, part 2):3231, 1975.
102. Teratology Society position paper: Recommendation for vitamin A during pregnancy, Teratology **35:**269, 1987.
103. Trowell, H.C., Davies, J.N.P., and Dean, R.F.A.: Kwashiorkor, New York, 1982, Academic Press.
104. Underwood, E.J.: Trace elements in human and animal nutrition, ed. 4, New York, 1977, Academic Press, Inc.
105. Vahouny, G.V.: Dietary fibers. In Sidransky, H., editor: Nutritional pathology, New York, 1985, Marcel Dekker, Inc.
106. Van Itallie, T.B.: Obesity: adverse effects on health and longevity, Am. J. Clin. Nutr. **32**(12 suppl.):2723, 1979.
107. Wasserman, R.H., and Taylor, A.N.: Metabolic roles of fat-soluble vitamins D, E, and K, Annu. Rev. Biochem. **41:**179, 1972.
108. Watson, R.S., editor: Nutrition, disease resistance, and immune function, New York, 1984, Marcel Dekker, Inc.
109. Wattenberg, L.W.: Inhibitors of chemical carcinogenesis, Adv. Cancer Res. **26:**197, 1978.
110. Williams, R.H.: Clinical biotin deficiency, N. Engl. J. Med. **228:**247, 1943.
111. Winick, M., editor: Nutrition and cancer, Curr. Concepts Nutr., vol. 6, New York, 1977, John Wiley & Sons, Inc.
112. Wolbach, S.B.: Controlled formation of collagen and reticulum: study of source of intercellular substance in recovery from experimental scorbutus, Am. J. Pathol. **9**(suppl.):689, 1933.
113. Wolbach, S.B., and Bessey, O.A.: Tissue changes in vitamin deficiencies, Physiol. Rev. **22:**233, 1942.
114. Wolf, G.: Multiple functions of vitamin A, Physiol. Rev. **64:**873, 1984.
115. Workshop conference on nutrition in cancer causation and prevention, Cancer Res. **43:**2385, 1983.
116. Workshop on fat and cancer, Cancer Res. **41**(9):3677, 1981.
117. World Health Organization: Trace elements in human nutrition: report of a WHO expert committee, Geneva, 1973, WHO Tech. Rep. Ser. no. 532.
118. Young, V.R.: Diet as a modulator of aging and longevity, Fed. Proc. **38:**1994, 1979.

14 Neoplasia

MICHAEL W. LIEBERMAN
RUSSELL M. LEBOVITZ

All ignorance toboggans into know
and trudges up to ignorance again
e. e. cummings

The last decade has seen dramatic advances in our understanding of neoplasia but also an accelerating list of unanswered questions. Spectacular developments in cell and molecular biology have changed many basic concepts in neoplasia as well as experimental approaches and diagnostic strategies. Who could have foreseen that we could account for many aspects of neoplastic change by the action of a small collection of altered cellular genes (oncogenes) (see glossary for definitions, p. 610) or that their analysis would hold promise as a powerful diagnostic adjunct to microscopy? Or that the early observation of a chromosomal rearrangement in chronic myelogenous leukemia (the Philadelphia chromosome) would be the harbinger of a series of chromosomal rearrangements at oncogene loci in many leukemias and lymphomas? Or that one could identify and clone a gene that when inactivated gives rise to a familial tumor (retinoblastoma)? Yet the impact of these advances must be understood against a backdrop of observations in tumor biology, for it is the behavior of tumors, as they are observed microscopically, biochemically, and clinically, that embodies neoplasia and defines many challenging questions.

The commitment to understanding the process of neoplastic change and its implications for diagnosis and treatment underlie the organization of this chapter. Time-honored subjects such as the definition of neoplasia (still not easily defined), nomenclature, tumor behavior, and grading and staging are covered; most of the emphasis, however, is placed on understanding in cell and molecular terms the phenomena that constitute neoplasia. The section on etiology and pathogenesis (p. 586) deals extensively with viruses, oncogenes, growth factors, and chemical carcinogens. It covers both their molecular actions and, when possible, as much as we know about how these explain the development and behavior of neoplastic cells. A section on new diagnostic approaches aims to put in perspective the application of developments in cell and molecular biology to diagnosis. Family studies and geographic analyses continue to provide valuable clues for analysis of neoplasia and to document emerging public health problems; a section on these studies is included. An unfortunate didactic consequence of the emphasis on mechanism and the interrelatedness of many apparently disparate phenomena is that on occasion we have had to introduce concepts or terms before they are covered in detail.

We hope that this chapter will stimulate pathologists and pathologists-in-training to study the cell and molecular biology of neoplasia in detail. Opportunities to analyze fundamental mechanisms of neoplastic change and to sharpen diagnostic and predictive indicators exist to a degree unimagined only a few years ago. It is a time of opportunity in the pathology of neoplasia unrivaled since the revolution set in motion by Virchow.

DEFINITION OF NEOPLASIA

No completely satisfactory definition of neoplasia exists. The difficulty arises from the fact that neoplastic growth shares many features with other disturbances in cell growth (see next section) and even normal growth and therefore is hard to distinguish from these semantically. Advances in our understanding of the regulation of cell growth and differentiation have emphasized the similarities among different types of growth and have not as yet identified properties that unequivocally distinguish neoplastic growth, thus exacerbating the problem of definition. The definition of Willis, however, remains one of the most widely cited and useful: "A neoplasm is an abnormal mass of tissue, the growth of which exceeds and is uncoordinated with that of the normal tissues and persists in the same excessive manner after cessation of the stimuli which evoked the change."[162] What makes neoplasia much more than an interesting process is that the persistence and growth of a neoplastic mass often has catastrophic consequences for the host; in the United States in 1988 there

Work from our laboratories cited in this chapter was supported by NIH grants CA-39392 and CA-40263.

were almost one million new cases of cancer (exclusive of nonmelanotic skin cancer) and almost 500,000 deaths from cancer.[23] In practice, the clinical behavior of these disturbances in cell growth and their microscopic appearance define neoplastic change operationally. For the experimentalist, the situation is more complicated: If cells, suspected of being neoplastic, are transplanted to a syngeneic host, for example, and they persist at the transplantation site, is the investigator observing a neoplastic mass, a homograft, or some combination of the two? The study of neoplasia, like much of biology, remains a descriptive enterprise in which description (however sophisticated or molecular) replaces definition.

VARIATIONS IN CELL GROWTH

Textbooks of pathology usually define a series of alterations in cell growth (such as hyperplastic, dysplastic, hypertrophic) and offer examples of each. We retain this organization but introduce experimental findings to help illuminate these phenomena and suggest mechanistic relationships that cross these (often arbitrary) boundaries.

Tissue regeneration and repair. In response to injury many tissues are capable of restoration of approximately normal structures. Thus, if the epidermis is denuded by abrasion, it is replaced by new epidermis, which grows in from the margins of the lesion. Or, if part of the liver is lost through injury or partial hepatectomy (in rodents), it regenerates to its preinjury mass. Likewise, broken bones and damaged connective tissue undergo similar regeneration. What characterizes these and similar phenomena is the restoration of structures that approximate those present before injury and the cessation of growth after restoration. All these processes result from cell division and thus share features with hyperplastic responses to injury (see below). In the adult mammal, some organs and tissues are incapable of any appreciable regeneration under normal circumstances and respond to injury or degeneration by replacement with scar tissue or hypertrophy or both (see p. 586). Examples include the central nervous system, striated muscles, and cartilage.

Hyperplasia. An increase in the number of cells in a tissue or organ is termed "hyperplasia." It follows that only cells and tissues capable of cell division undergo hyperplasia and that some additional stimulus or increased responsiveness to an existing stimulus must be present. The epidermis, for example, in response to abrasion or pressure shows increased mitotic activity and an increase in cell number. Experimentally this process may be induced by the application of acetic acid or tumor-promoting chemicals (such as tetradecanoyl-phorbol acetate, benzoyl peroxide, mezerein; see section on etiology and pathogenesis).[7] Although the in-

duction of hyperplasia by these agents is often associated with changes that might be expected to accompany proliferation of epidermal cells (such as increased ornithine decarboxylase activity and altered transcription of epidermis-specific keratins,[47,91] etc.), the molecular basis for these changes is unknown.

In the prostate, hyperplasia of both glandular (epithelial) and stromal (fibromuscular) elements occurs with advancing age (Fig. 14-1). Prostatic hyperplasia is associated with increased conversion of androgens to dihydrotestosterone[61,123] and administration of androgens or high levels of dihydrotestosterone to castrated dogs results in prostatic hyperplasia.[92] However, the degree to which conversion of androgens to dihydrotestosterone is causal in men remains to be established. As in epidermal hyperplasia, the molecular basis of prostatic hyperplasia remains unknown. This hyperplastic response is important clinically because it may result in urethral obstruction and urinary retention; it also illustrates that both stromal and glandular elements in an organ may undergo hyperplasia. Finally it raises the possibility that stromal elements that often appear monotonously similar from organ to organ by light microscopy may have very discrete, specialized physiologic processes.

Hyperplastic responses in endocrine organs are often

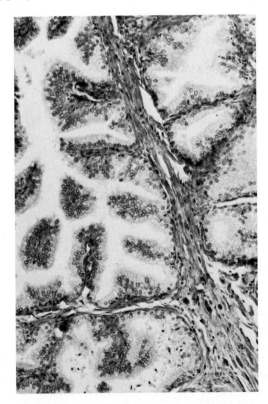

Fig. 14-1. Hyperplasia of prostate. In this example the process mainly involves epithelium, which because of increased number of cells is arranged in fronds with vascular stalk. (200×.)

dramatic. Thyroid-stimulating immunoglobulin (that is, antibodies to the thyroid-stimulating hormone receptor) or, rarely, increased levels of circulating TSH result in thyroid hyperplasia and thyrotoxicosis. Hyperplasia of the adrenal cortex results from increased levels of circulating adrenocorticotropic hormone (ACTH) and leads to clinical hypercorticoidism.

Compensatory hyperplasia may occur in response to lost parenchymal mass. This phenomenon is seen after unilateral nephrectomy: the contralateral kidney responds by an increase in cellularity and an increase in cell size (hypertrophy, see below).

Hyperplasia can place an organ at increased risk for neoplasia, especially if a chronic condition continues to stimulate cell division. An increase in the total number of cells and the percentage in the cell cycle increases the possibility of chromosomal change, of alterations in oncogene structure and function, and of mutation and other changes induced by chemical carcinogens (see section on etiology and pathogenesis). It has been suggested, for example, that the hyperplastic response of epidermis to tumor promoters increases the pool of cells at risk for papilloma formation and that these in turn provide increased numbers of cells for malignant tumor (that is, carcinoma) formation.[7,165] Agents that damage liver cells (such as alcohol, hepatitis viruses, chemical toxins) cause a loss of hepatic mass followed by regeneration and local hyperplasia (hyperplastic nodules).[36] These stimuli, which are often chronic, result in an increase in actively dividing cell populations, which are at risk for subsequent neoplastic change.

Hypertrophy. Organs or tissues that respond to stimuli by an increase in cellular mass without an increase in cell number are said to undergo hypertrophy. Often these are tissues in which regenerative capacity is limited. Thus in response to increased work load resulting from cardiac valvular deformity, individual myocardial fibers thicken and the heart hypertrophies. Exercise routines and anabolic steroids result in similar changes in skeletal muscle. Mixed hypertrophic-hyperplastic responses may occur as in the kidney after unilateral nephrectomy and in the response of the thyroid to thyroid-stimulating immunoglobulin. These examples illustrate that similar or identical signals can stimulate hyperplasia and hypertrophy, but the mechanism that determines the relative balance between increases in cell size and cell number is unknown.

Interrelatedness of different cellular growth patterns. The degree to which different patterns of cell growth may share related features can be illustrated by considering responses to a growth factor termed "transforming growth factor β" (TGF-β) (see also p. 591 and Table 14-4). This polypeptide originally discovered in supernatants from cultures of tumor cells is now known to stimulate proliferation of both fibroblasts and trans-

formed derivatives in cell culture and to inhibit the proliferation of many types of cultured epithelial cells. TGF-β plays a key role in the repair of connective tissue in vivo after wounding by promoting fibroblastic growth, capillary formation, and collagen synthesis.[110,128] After wounding, platelets, macrophages, and lymphocytes are attracted to the wound. All of these are known to secrete TGF-β,[110,128] which stimulates the restoration of dermal structure. Two other known growth factors (epidermal growth factor and platelet-derived growth factor) are considered not to be involved in this process,[23] but these and other growth factors and hormones (such as insulin-like growth factor, fibroblast growth factor) may play other roles in wound healing and in the other examples cited later.[2,31]

It is instructive to consider related pathologic conditions that occur in different contexts. A hyperplastic response of skin to injury termed "keloid formation" results in extensive local overproduction of connective tissue with thick collagenous bands. Local oversecretion of TGF-β or heightened sensitivity to it may be in part responsible. A similar pattern of connective tissue proliferation, termed "desmoplasia," is observed in association with the growth of several different tumors; common examples include the desmoplastic response seen in pancreatic cancer and in breast cancer (scirrhous carcinoma; Fig. 14-2). Many neoplastic cells secrete TGF-β, and it is reasonable to suppose that this desmoplastic response results at least in part from TGF-β release. TGF-β may also play an important role in the growth of tumors derived from fibroblasts (that is, fibrosarcomas) through a mechanism known as autocrine stimulation (see p. 591). However, as mentioned above, many epithelial cells are inhibited in cell culture by TGF-β, whereas their neoplastic counterparts are often resistant to the inhibitory effects of TGF-β. There is one example of escape from this regulatory control by loss of surface receptors for TGF-β: loss of TGF-β sensitivity correlates with a loss of receptors in a childhood tumor of retinal cells, retinoblastoma.[67] How other epithelial tumors escape regulation by TGF-β is not known, but it may involve the shutting off of a system that converts an inactive form of this growth factor to an active one. The role or potential role of TGF-β in many phenomena illustrates how closely related seemingly different patterns of cell growth can be. Many apparently disparate phenomena may have a common molecular basis, and undoubtedly in the next few years other regulatory pathways will become better understood.

Atrophy. A diminution in the size of an organ is termed "atrophy." This change may occur as a result of a reduction in cell size or cell number or both. Thus, for example, through disuse, age, or loss of innervation, skeletal muscle fibers may lose much of their bulk. In

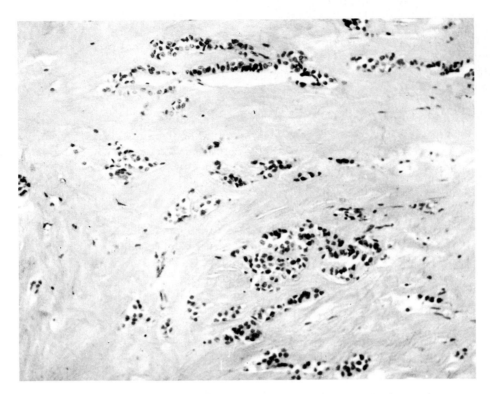

Fig. 14-2. Carcinoma of breast with extensive desmoplasia. (125×.)

each of these cases a loss of positive trophic stimuli leads to a reduction in myofiber size. Atrophy within the glandular elements of breast and endometrial tissue after menopause represents a reduction in cell number subsequent to loss of hormonal stimuli. Atrophy may also result from stimuli that actively cause regression. Programmed cell death as part of development may be viewed in this light.[107] Recently the gene for müllerian inhibiting substance has been cloned.[24] The protein, secreted by the developing testis, causes involution of the müllerian duct—the embryonic origin of the uterus, fallopian tubes, and upper third of the vagina. The protein shows a partial amino acid identity with TGF-β, which, though stimulatory for fibroblastic cells, is inhibitory for many epithelial cells. Cachexia, or "wasting" (actually atrophy), which accompanies many chronic diseases including cancer, is brought about in part by a protein known as "tumor necrosis factor," or "cachectin."[103] Thus atrophy, like hyperplasia and hypertrophy, can be an active response to external stimuli as well as a response to loss of trophic factors.

Metaplasia. A change in cell type (usually resulting from an identifiable stimulus) is referred to as metaplasia. It is seen most frequently in epithelial cells but may occur in other cell types as well. Bone (osteoid) formation, for example, may occur in connective tissue or muscle during tissue repair after trauma. Chronic irritation, including smoking, results in squamous metaplasia of the bronchial epithelium in which the normal

pseudostratified columnar lining is replaced by squamous epithelium. Avitaminosis A results in the replacement of many epithelial structures with keratinized squamous epithelium. Metaplastic change usually involves the loss or destruction of the normal cell population and its replacement during "tissue repair" with another. There are two potential sources of replacement cells: "reserve cells," which undergo metaplastic change, and surviving cells with proliferative capacity, which respond to the stimulus. The relative contribution of each is unknown. The change may be permanent, or tissues may revert if the stimulus is removed. Metaplasia is not usually thought of as a preneoplastic lesion, since the replacement cells are morphologically normal; however, in some instances it precedes neoplasia. For example, cigarette smoke–induced squamous metaplasia precedes bronchogenic carcinoma including squamous cell carcinoma. It is likely that metaplasias produced by different agents are not equivalent.

Metaplasia represents another example of cellular plasticity. In cell culture it is possible to stimulate the conversion of one cell type into another. Several lines of mouse fibroblasts convert spontaneously to adipocytes, myocytes, and chondrocytes.[137] Agents that demethylate DNA (such as 5-azacytidine), and thus alter the regulation of gene expression greatly increase the percentage of converted cells.[137] Part of the process has been studied in detail and appears to be under the control of a single gene, the expression of which is sufficient to convert mouse fibroblasts to myoblasts.[28] Although this phenomenon has been viewed as a model for differentiation, it is also reasonable to view it as a model for a metaplasia within a mesenchymal lineage especially if metaplasia in vivo results from reserve cells that differentiate. At present in vitro systems do not model all the complexities of in vivo change, but they provide a perspective for how the process might be studied.

Dysplasia. Tissues may contain atypical cells and display a disorganized growth pattern; this phenomenon is known as "dysplasia." In dysplasia, cells are often *pleomorphic* (varying in size and shape) with *hyperchromatic* (darkly staining) nuclei and show an increase in the ratio of nucleus to cytoplasm. The number of mitoses may be increased. Dysplastic tissues are disorganized and lack or partially lack the polarity and progression of their normal counterparts. Thus, in dysplastic squamous epithelium, mitoses are not confined to the basal cell layer, and progressive keratinization and nuclear dissolution are partially lost. Although, in theory, any disorganized, altered cells might be thought of as dysplastic, the term is usually confined to epithelial lesions. Dysplasia is reversible. It is also a precancerous change, and distinguishing severe dysplasia from early malignant neoplasia or *carcinoma in situ* can be difficult (Fig. 14-3). Although this distinction may be very important clinically, biologically one may view normal growth, dysplastic growth, and neoplastic growth as a continuum.

Recent work in cell culture illustrates the lack of discrete boundaries on this continuum and how fluid the conversions can be.[108,120] If one introduces a fusion gene consisting of an easily regulated gene control region and an oncogene into cultured fibroblasts or epithelial cells, it is possible to show that morphologic and growth characteristics vary directly with oncogene expression[108,120] (Fig. 14-4). Furthermore, the changes in morphology and growth are reversible if oncogene RNA synthesis is reduced. The clinical relevance of these observations may be that discontinuities of regulation (such as the point at which oncogene expression becomes constitutive at an elevated level) rather than morphologic discontinuities define permanent changes in cellular behavior (phenotype) (see p. 586).

Anaplasia. The term "anaplasia" is used to describe malignant tumors (see glossary) that lack histologically identifiable features (such as gland formation in epithe-

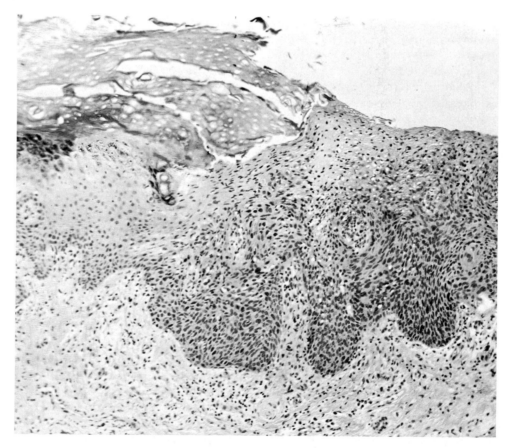

Fig. 14-3. Carcinoma arising in arsenical keratosis showing hyperkeratosis, dysplasia (atypical hyperplasia), and early carcinoma. (125×.)

lial cells or stainable fat in adipocytes) and are therefore said to be poorly differentiated (Fig. 14-5). However, the term also connotes extreme pleomorphism and rapid growth.

Inappropriate placement of normal tissues. Rarely minor developmental anomalies may be confused with neoplasms. These foci probably have their origin in various developmental rests, which are the vestiges of cell migration and differentiation during embryogenesis.

They are generally without significance, except that tumors may rarely arise from them (such as retrosternal thyroid tissue). *Hamartomas* occur in many organs and are composed of foci or nodules of tissues normally found there. In the lung, for example, it is not unusual to find discrete foci composed of mature cartilage and bronchial epithelium (Fig. 14-6). The distinction between hamartomas and nonmalignant tumors (see nomenclature and taxonomy section) is not always clear.

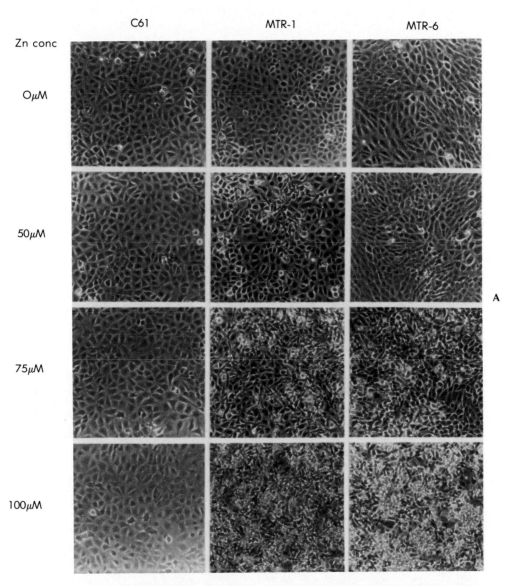

Fig. 14-4. Effect of variation of oncogene expression in morphology. **A,** Rat liver epithelial cells (C61) were transfected with a zinc-regulatable mutant *ras* gene consisting of the mouse metallothionein promoter (Zn-responsive) placed in front of the human bladder oncogene *ras*T24. Two of the derived cell lines (MTR-1 and MTR-6) show a progressive loss of organization with increasing ZnSO₄ concentrations, whereas control C61 cells are unchanged in the presence of ZnSO₄.   *Continued.*

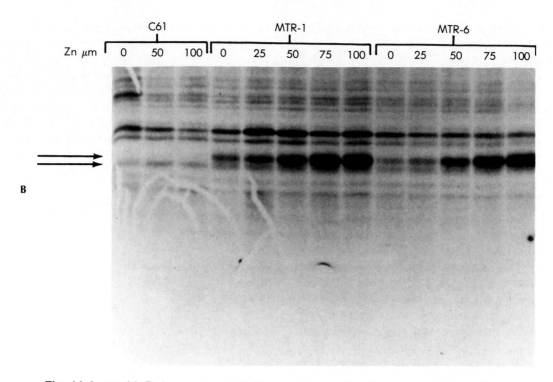

Fig. 14-4, cont'd. B, Immunoprecipitation experiment showing increased rate of synthesis of mutant *ras* protein *(upper arrow)* in response to $ZnSO_4$ in MTR-1 and MTR-6 cells. (From Seyama, T., et al.: Mol. Carcinogenesis **1:**89, 1988.)

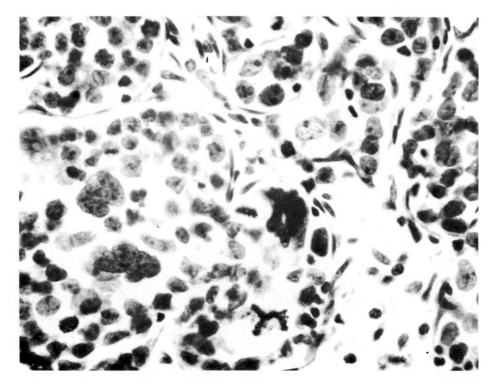

Fig. 14-5. Extremely anaplastic cancer showing abnormal mitoses, multinucleated tumor giant cells, and extensive pleomorphism. (800×.)

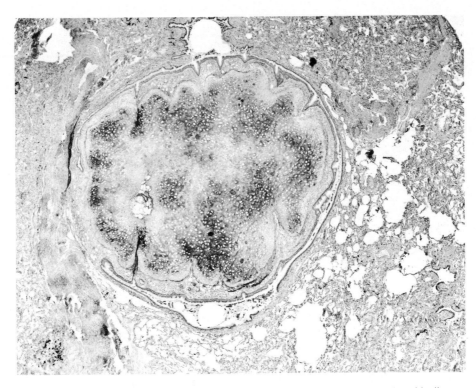

Fig. 14-6. Hamartoma of lung. Although overgrowth contains bronchial epithelium and mucous glands, its chief component is cartilage. (22×.)

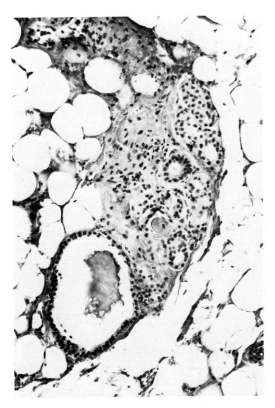

Fig. 14-7. Ectopic thyroid tissue in mediastinal fat. (150×.)

For example, a focus of normal-appearing vascular tissue (thus a hamartoma) is referred to as an angioma (the designation for a benign tumor); and a collection of pigmented cells in the skin (a pigmented nevus) may be thought of as a benign neoplasm (the usual case) or a hamartoma. A *choristoma* is similar to a hamartoma except that the tissues of which it is composed are not normally present in the part of the body in which it is found: for example, benign chondromas of the skin may occur on the foot. The term *ectopic* is sometimes applied to normal-appearing tissue in an abnormal location. Thus, when a focus of apparently normal thyroid tissue is found in mediastinal fat, it is referred to as ectopic thyroid tissue (Fig. 14-7); similarly adrenal gland tissue may be found in the urinary bladder.

NOMENCLATURE AND TAXONOMY

Tumor classification and the nomenclature that derives from it provide a convenient shorthand for communication among pathologists, clinicians, and researchers. Current usage is a hybrid of terms based on biologic behavior, function, histogenesis, embryogenesis, site of origin, and eponyms (Table 14-1).

Assessing the biologic behavior of tumors provides the single most important piece of information about them. *Benign tumors* are, in general, slow-growing, innocuous tumors (Table 14-2) that are usually of little consequence to the host unless they secrete excessive

Table 14-1. Nomenclature of tumors*

Cell or tissue of origin	Benign	Malignant
TUMORS OF EPITHELIAL ORIGIN		
Squamous cells	Squamous cell papilloma	Squamous cell carcinoma
Basal cells		Basal cell carcinoma
Glandular or ductal epithelium	Adenoma	Adenocarcinoma
	Papillary adenoma	Papillary adenocarcinoma
	Cystadenoma	Cystadenocarcinoma
Transitional cells	Transitional cell papilloma	Transitional cell carcinoma
Bile duct	Bile duct adenoma	Bile duct carcinoma (cholangiocarcinoma)
Islets of Langerhans	Islet cell adenoma	Islet cell carcinoma
Liver cells	Liver cell adenoma	Hepatocellular carcinoma
Neuroectoderm	Nevus	Malignant melanoma
Placental epithelium	Hydatidiform mole	Choriocarcinoma
Renal epithelium	Renal tubular adenoma	Renal cell carcinoma (hypernephroma)
Respiratory tract		Bronchogenic carcinoma
Skin adnexal glands:		
Sweat glands	Syringoadenoma, sweat gland adenoma	Syringocarcinoma, sweat gland carcinoma
Sebaceous glands	Sebaceous gland adenoma	Sebaceous gland carcinoma
Germ cells (testis and ovary)		Seminoma (dysgermanoma)
		Embryonal carcinoma, yolk sac tumor
TUMORS OF MESENCHYMAL ORIGIN		
Hematopoietic/lymphoid tissues		Leukemias
		Lymphomas
		Hodgkin's disease
		Multiple myeloma
Neural and retinal tissue		
Nerve sheath	Neurilemoma, neurofibroma	Malignant peripheral nerve sheath tumor
Nerve cells	Ganglioneuroma	Neuroblastoma
Retinal cells (cones)		Retinoblastoma
Connective tissue		
Fibrous tissue	Fibroma	Fibrosarcoma
Fat	Lipoma	Liposarcoma
Bone	Osteoma	Osteogenic sarcoma
Cartilage	Chondroma	Chondrosarcoma
Muscle		
Smooth muscle	Leiomyoma	Leiomyosarcoma
Striated muscle	Rhabdomyoma	Rhabdomyosarcoma
Endothelial and related tissues		
Blood vessels	Hemangioma	Angiosarcoma
		Kaposi's sarcoma
Lymph vessels	Lymphangioma	Lymphangiosarcoma
Synovia		Synoviosarcoma (synovioma)
Mesothelium	Benign mesothelioma	Malignant mesothelioma
Meninges	Meningioma	
Uncertain origin		Ewing's tumor
OTHER ORIGINS		
Renal anlage		Wilms' tumor
Trophoblast	Hydatidiform mole	Choriocarcinoma
Totipotential cells	Benign teratoma	Malignant teratoma

*No classification of tumors can be complete. Rather this list is intended to introduce a nomenclature scheme. As indicated in the text, the extant nomenclature is very mixed. More extensive classifications (with synonyms) may be found in the fascicles of the *Atlas of Tumor Pathology,* published by the Armed Forces Institute of Pathology, Washington, D.C., and in the *International Histologic Classification of Tumors,* published by the World Health Organization, Geneva.

Table 14-2. Some characteristics of typical benign and malignant tumors

	Benign	Malignant
Growth rate	Slow	Rapid
Mitoses	Few	Many
Nuclear chromatin	Normal	Increased
Differentiation	Good	Poor
Local growth	Expansive	Invasive
Encapsulation	Present	Absent
Destruction of tissue	Little	Much
Vessel invasion	None	Frequent
Metastases	None	Frequent
Effect on host	Often insignificant	Significant

amounts of bioactive molecules or are strategically placed (Fig. 14-8). For example, benign tumors of the β cells of the islets of Langerhans ("β-cell tumors") can result in life-threatening hypoglycemia (Fig. 14-9), and ependymal tumors blocking the aqueduct of Sylvius can result in hydrocephalus. *Malignant tumors* have more rapid growth rates, *invade* and destroy adjacent tissue (Fig. 14-10), and seed and grow at distant sites (*metastasize*) (Fig. 14-11). A *neoplasm* (new growth) may be benign or malignant, whereas malignant tumors are referred to as *cancers.*

Epithelial tumors, which constitute a majority of both benign and malignant lesions (see section on demographic and familial aspects of cancer), may be derived from any of the three germ layers (see Table 14-1). Malignant tumors of epithelial or organ parenchymal derivation are referred to as *carcinomas.* If the cells are of glandular or ductular origin, they are referred to as *adenocarcinomas* (see Fig. 14-10). If they are of squamous cell origin, they are referred to as *squamous cell,* or *epidermoid, carcinomas* (Fig. 14-12). The nomenclature for benign epithelial lesions is more varied (see Table 14-1), but the suffix *-oma* is often used. Thus a benign tumor of glandular epithelium is usually referred to as an adenoma (Fig. 14-13), whereas a benign tumor of squamous or transitional cell epithelium with a papillary conformation is referred to as a papilloma. The nomenclature of tumors derived from specific types of epitheliums is more direct, such as renal cell carcinoma, sweat gland carcinoma. Two important exceptions are "melanoma" and "hepatoma," which are malignant tumors of melanocytes and hepatocytes respectively and should be designated as malignant melanoma and hepatocellular carcinoma. Tumors that are clearly carcinomas but lack defining characteristics are referred to as undifferentiated or anaplastic carcinomas.

Malignant tumors of mesenchymal origin are referred

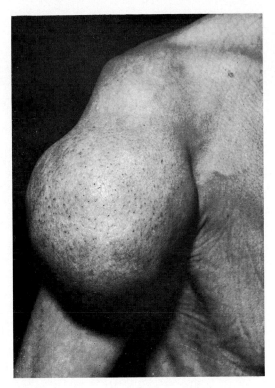

Fig. 14-8. Subcutaneous lipoma that had gradually increased in size over period of 6 to 8 years in 70-year-old man. Notice stretching of skin as evidenced by widely separated pores.

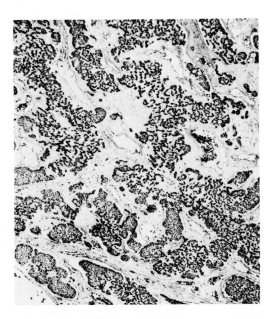

Fig. 14-9. Islet cell tumor. Solid clusters and ribbonlike growth are reminiscent of normal islet of Langerhans. (30×.)

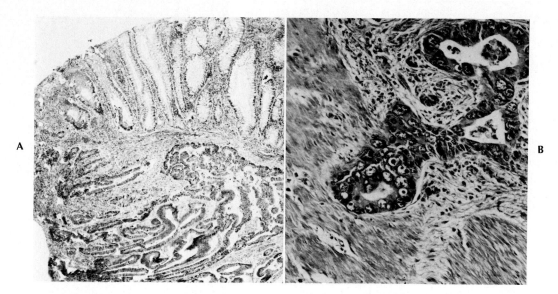

Fig. 14-10. A, Invasion of submucosa and muscularis by well-differentiated adenocarcinoma of colon. Notice glandular pattern typical of an adenocarcinoma. Some normal mucosa remains. **B,** Colonic adenocarcinoma invading muscularis. Same case as **A.** (**A,** 125×; **B,** 300×.)

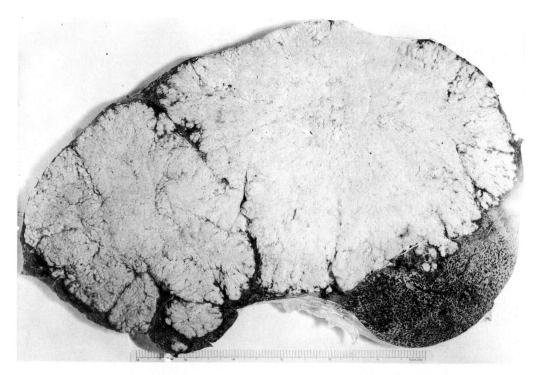

Fig. 14-11. Section of liver showing almost complete replacement of parenchyma by metastatic carcinoma. Primary tumor was in colon.

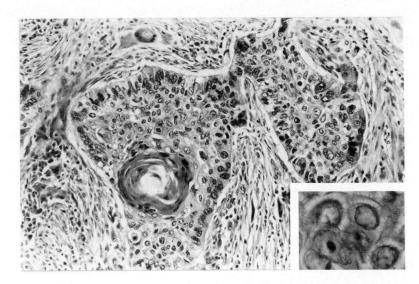

Fig. 14-12. Well-differentiated squamous cell carcinoma showing irregular margins, keratin pearls, and intercellular bridges (550×). *Inset,* 1250×. (Courtesy Dr. Ibrahim Ramzy, Houston, Texas.)

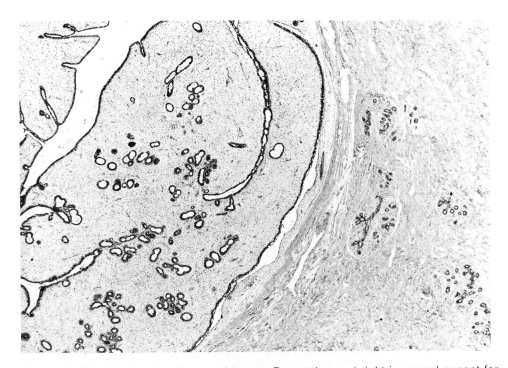

Fig. 14-13. Portion of adenofibroma of breast. Breast tissue at right is normal except for compression by tumor. (26×.)

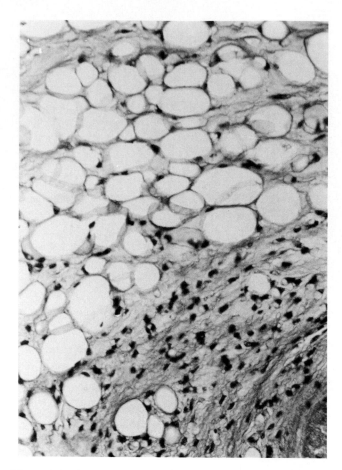

Fig. 14-14. Liposarcoma showing well-differentiated lipid-containing cells and more primitive cells. (550×; courtesy Dr. Ibrahim Ramzey, Houston, Texas.)

to as *sarcomas,* whereas their benign counterparts simply bear the suffix *-oma.* A malignant tumor of fat cells, for example, is termed a "liposarcoma," whereas a benign tumor is known as a "lipoma" (Fig. 14-14). As with carcinoma the so-called rules sometimes break down, and a malignant tumor of mesothelium—the cells lining the pleural and peritoneal surfaces—is often referred to as a mesothelioma, though it should be referred to as a malignant mesothelioma to distinguish it from a benign counterpart (benign fibrous mesothelioma). Notice that malignant tumors of the hematopoietic system have no benign counterparts. The latter group is named idiosyncratically: thus all leukemias are malignant, and the term "lymphoma" (more properly "malignant lymphoma") always refers to a malignant process (however, see "adenolymphoma" of the salivary gland, p. 579).

Tumors derived from all three germ layers are designated "teratomas" and are classified as "mature" or "immature" (Figs. 14-15 and 14-16).

This basic scheme has several modifications. A tumor of pancreatic β cells referred to previously as a "β cell tumor" can also be called an "insulinoma," reflecting its function, and an "islet cell adenoma" in reference to its anatomic origin (see Fig. 14-9). Another example of omission of the cell of origin in favor of an anatomic designation is the term "bronchogenic carcinoma," which may refer to several different histologic types. Often, however, designations are prefaced and convey more complete information, as in "papillary adenocarcinoma," which defines the growth pattern of the tumor, or "mucinous cystadenoma," which provides explicit information about differentiation. The suffix *-blastoma* is used to designate tumors of embryonic or-

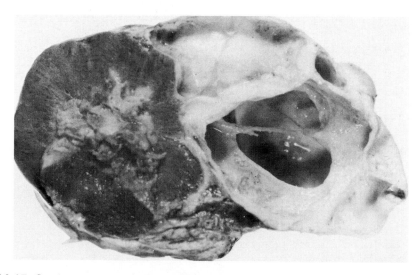

Fig. 14-15. Cystic teratoma of ovary. This benign neoplasm shows both solid and cystic foci. Microscopically various types of tissue composed tumor.

igin. The terms medulloblastoma (brain), hepatoblastoma (liver), nephroblastoma (kidney), retinoblastoma (retina), and neuroblastoma (adrenal) are in common use. Time-honored eponyms remain. Some, like Hodgkin's disease, a malignant neoplasm possibly derived from dendritic reticulum cells, and Ewing's sarcoma, a malignant neoplasm of uncertain origin, have no systematic equivalent. Others like Wilms' tumor have equivalents that are rarely used (nephroblastoma). Other eponyms, largely holdovers from another era, are sometimes used: a variant of renal cell carcinoma ("hypernephroma") is occasionally referred to as a Grawitz tumor, and a benign tumor of the salivary gland with both epithelial and lymphoid elements (papillary cystadenoma lymphomatosum or adenolymphoma) is often designated a Warthin tumor.

CHARACTERISTICS OF NEOPLASTIC CELLS

Proliferation and differentiation are normally tightly controlled so that in the adult some cells do not replicate (such as neurons, chondrocytes), others replicate only very slowly and probably only at a rate sufficient to replace lost cells (such as hepatocytes, renal tubular cells), whereas others replicate more or less continuously in response to continuous cell loss (such as intestinal epithelial cells, hematopoietic cells). The proliferation and maturation of these cells is always controlled and results only in a net replacement of cells. In contrast, neoplastic cells escape this regulation and accumulate to form a mass. This escape from feedback control is one of the important attributes of neoplastic change. While such cells are at the extremes, differences in regulation and growth pattern between normal cells and neoplastic cells are obvious; at the boundaries differences can be very subtle. Traditional distinctions between benign and malignant patterns of cell growth are presented in Table 14-2.

Growth rate and differentiation. In general, benign tumors tend to be slow growing and well differentiated, often resembling their tissue of origin to a remarkable degree. Thus a lipoma on microscopic examination may be composed of mature adipocytes, which are hardly distinguishable from normal fat cells. The only clue that the tissue is neoplastic may be that the mass has increased slowly in size over many years (see Fig. 14-8). In contrast, malignant tumors grow much more rapidly and may bear only slight resemblance to the parent tissue; hence a liposarcoma may grow rapidly, and the only clue to its origin may be the identification of occasional cells that stain positively for fat.

The accumulation of tumor mass is dependent on several factors, including transit time through the cell

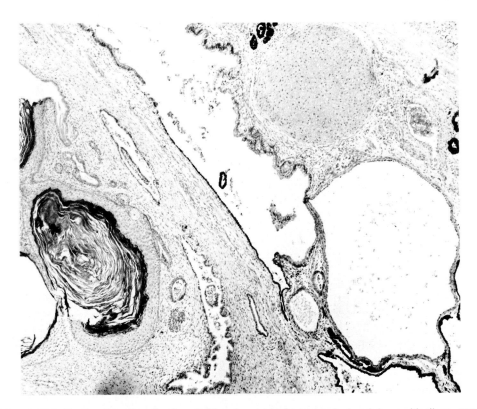

Fig. 14-16. Teratoma of testis. In addition to several types of glandular epithelium centrally, nodule of cartilage is present in upper right and masses of keratinizing squamous epithelium at left. (50×.)

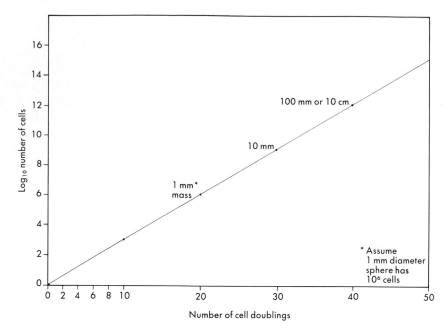

Fig. 14-17. Theoretical growth curve relating number of tumor doublings to number of tumor cells present and size of tumor.

cycle, the fraction of cells that remain in the cycle to proliferate in contrast to those that differentiate, and "spontaneous," intermittent growth arrest. Cell cycle time is probably only a minor factor in tumor growth. It has been known for many years that normal cells may traverse the cell cycle faster than some tumor cells.[12] A more important factor is retention of cells in the cell cycle. Normally in the small intestine, for example, the division of every crypt cell is followed by a partition in which one daughter cell remains in the proliferating compartment and the other differentiates and migrates toward the luminal surface. In neoplasia this partition is altered, and so too many cells remain in the proliferating compartment. It is worth noting here that, within tumors, cells often differentiate normally into mature postmitotic cells; a good example is the maturation seen in squamous and basal cell carcinomas of the skin (see Fig. 14-12). Occasionally neuroblastomas have been reported to differentiate into ganglioneuromas. One of the current goals of experimental cancer therapy is to devise ways to induce malignant cells to differentiate and exit from the cell cycle. Although there is little experimental work on intermittent variable growth rates in tumors, clinical observations indicate that this phenomenon may not be infrequent. It is known, for example, that after removal of a primary malignant melanoma recurrence can appear many years later. The erratic course of many breast cancers may be another example of intermittent growth. Factors extrinsic to these tumors (such as changes in levels of hormones and growth factors) and intrinsic factors (such as

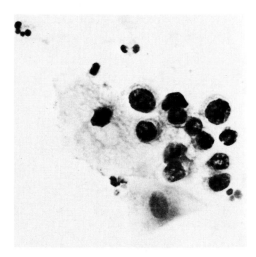

Fig. 14-18. Exfoliated cancer cells in Papanicolaou smear from uterine cervix. (500×.)

changes in receptor levels or level of oncogene expression) are probably involved. Thus linear correlations between cell doubling times and tumor mass represent an idealized model of tumor growth (Fig. 14-17). They do not encompass intermittent variations in growth rate, "progression" (the acquisition of more aggressive characteristics; see section on progression), or necrosis.

Cytologic features. As tumor cells acquire increased autonomy and aggressiveness, they may develop many characteristics of primitive blast cells and often acquire

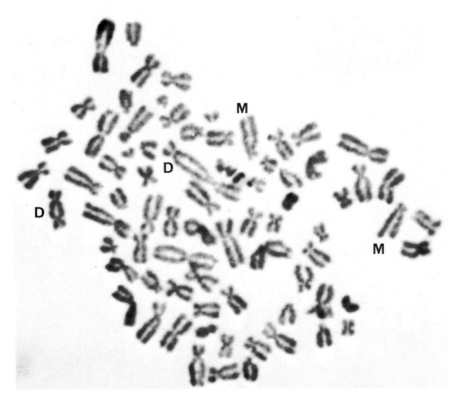

Fig. 14-19. Chromosome preparation of tumor cell from patient with breast cancer. Cell is hyperdiploid showing 74 chromosomes, including two markers, *M,* and two dicentrics, *D.*

bizarre, atypical features. Neoplastic cells that vary greatly in size and shape are said to be *pleomorphic* (see Fig. 14-5). Malignant cells may show increased *nuclear hyperchromicity* (basophilia) and size—reflective of increased DNA content and alterations in chromatin structure (Fig. 14-18). At some stage, many malignant tumors show abnormalities of karyotype and dramatic changes in ploidy (Fig. 14-19; see also p. 591 and Table 14-5).[55] Abnormal mitoses may be seen (Fig. 14-20). Nuclear and cell contours may vary sharply from the parental cell type, and the cytoplasm often becomes scant and somewhat hyperchromatic—reflective of increased ribosomal RNA and synthetic activity. Giant cells may develop. All these changes must be judged with reference to the cells of origin, since there is considerable variation among neoplasms; pleomorphism is not an absolute criterion of malignancy.

Angiogenesis and stromal support. For tumors, whether benign or malignant, to expand beyond a small mass, vascularization and often the development of stromal support are necessary. Tumor cells secrete growth factors like TGF-β (see p. 591 and Table 14-4), which stimulate capillary ingrowth and fibroblastic growth.[2,31,48,110,116,128] These nonneoplastic tissue elements are present in most tumors though they are often more prominent in carcinomas. When the fibroblastic response is intense, the process is said to be desmoplastic (see Fig. 14-2). The development of vascular and stromal support represents regulation of the growth of normal cells by neoplastic cells, a phenomenon that may be more prevalent than suspected and one that might offer a novel approach to therapy.

Local growth. When benign tumors expand, they compress surrounding tissue (see Fig. 14-13) and are often "*encapsulated*" (that is, surrounded by a rim of fibrous tissue). Local growth of malignant tumors is characterized by *invasion* of the surrounding tissue, often with extensive tissue destruction. Malignant tumors are unencapsulated, though when malignant foci arise in benign tumors capsular invasion may be seen. This invasiveness is well illustrated by thyroid carcinoma. *Invasion* and *metastasis* (spread to distant sites) are important characteristics that unambiguously distinguish malignant from benign tumors (Figs. 14-10, 14-11, 14-21, and 14-22). In carcinomas local invasion involves penetration of the basement membrane, followed by infiltration of deeper tissues. Carcinomas sometimes acquire all the morphologic characteristics of malignant tumors without showing invasion of the basement membrane. This lesion is referred to as *carcinoma in*

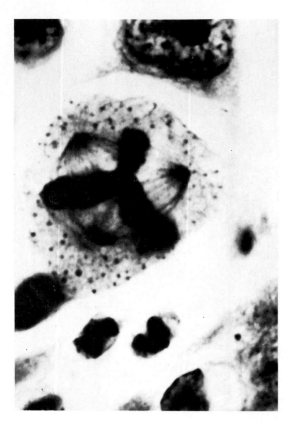

Fig. 14-20. Abnormal tripolar mitosis occurring in malignant melanoma. (Phosphotungstic acid–hematoxylin; 2350×.)

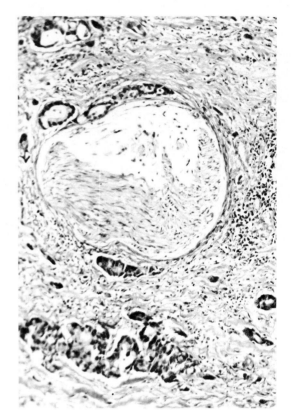

Fig. 14-21. Adenocarcinoma of lung with perineural invasion. Part of nerve shows degeneration. (125×.)

situ and is often seen in the uterine cervix (Fig. 14-23).

Local invasion. Local invasion is a complicated balance between tissue destruction and the synthesis of vascular and stromal support. The ability to synthesize and secrete extracellular proteases is clearly a prerequisite for invasion.[38,79,88] Tumor cells are known to secrete proteases including transin (stromolysin) and collagenases, which can attack components of basement membranes and extracellular matrix (laminin, fibronectin, and collagen).[44,79,85,86] Other proteases like fibrinolysin also participate in invasion. These clearly aid in destruction of extracellular matrix and probably destroy normal cells as well. As mentioned previously, TGF-β, which is secreted by many tumor cells (including epithelial tumors), stimulates fibroblastic growth but inhibits epithelial growth. One may imagine that factors like TGF-β and müllerian inhibiting substance might play a role in the local spread of tumors by inhibiting the growth of normal cells and stimulating the growth of stromal support. Presumably, epithelial tumors that secrete TGF-β are not inhibited by it. Though loss of TGF-β receptors has been implicated in one example of escape from TGF-β inhibition,[67] in most cases the mechanism of escape remains unknown. Frequently inflammation accompanies invasion. Since inflammatory

cells secrete proteases as well as growth factors, it is likely that the contribution of inflammatory cells to both invasion and metastasis is substantial.

Yet invasiveness also involves recognition of extracellular matrices and perhaps other cell types by tumor cells; tissue destruction may provide access to new areas, but recognition of substratum and binding are necessary for most tumors to establish growth. Tumor cells are known to attach more readily to laminin[63] than nontumor cells do, and this property (presumably related to increased numbers of laminin receptors or increased affinity of existing receptors) is probably in part responsible for increased tumor migration.[63,158] Similarly, fibronectin receptors may play a role in the migration of malignant cells.[59] TGF-β is also known to stimulate fibronectin synthesis and cell-adhesion-protein receptors (integrins), which may be involved in cell migration and the ability to grow in semisolid medium (a prominent in vitro property of tumor cells).[60] It is also known that the cytoskeleton of tumor cells differs greatly from that of their nontransformed counterparts and that communication between cytoskeleton and extracellular matrix occurs at points of cell adherence.[60] Thus local invasion requires a balance between the degradation of the local environment and preservation (or

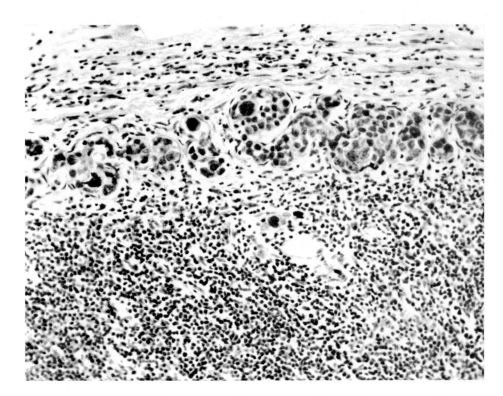

Fig. 14-22. Metastatic carcinoma in peripheral sinus of inguinal lymph node. Tumor lies just beneath capsule and is beginning to invade pulp. (250×.)

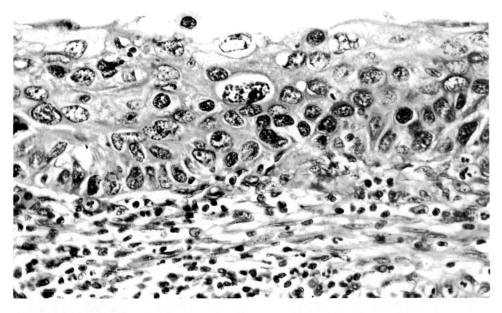

Fig. 14-23. Carcinoma in situ of cervix. Notice extreme atypicality of cells near surface and that one cell has desquamated. From such desquamated cells, cytologic diagnosis of cancer can be made. (500×.)

resynthesis) of a crucial molecular substratum. This balance appears to be achieved by a transmembrane feedback system involving the cytoskeleton, which itself is responsible for cell motility.

The degree to which all the aforementioned factors affect the behavior of individual tumors is extremely variable. Thus, for example, the need for some stromal support for tumor cells is more apparent in papillary carcinoma of the thyroid than in a giant cell carcinoma, which grows with little apparent organization and with significant tissue destruction. Invasion can be very extensive; as a pure biologic phenomenon it is best appreciated in basal cell carcinomas of the skin and malignant tumors of the central nervous system that do not metastasize and that spread without vascular or lymphatic entry.

Regional extension of tumors beyond their organ of origin. Tumors may infiltrate so extensively that they breach the surface of an organ. This phenomenon is frequently seen in colon and ovarian carcinomas as well as in bronchogenic carcinomas. The result is a seeding of the serosal surface of the peritoneal cavity and its organs or the pleural surfaces with tumor cells, some of which grow to form nodules. Local seeding requires a hospitable site. In carcinomas of the gastrointestinal tract, for example, it is extremely rare to find colonial spread distal to a primary tumor within the lumen even though the sloughing of viable tumor cells must be frequent. The movement of gastrointestinal contents, their

destructive character, and the resistance of epithelium to intrusion prevent such spreading.

Metastasis. The spread of malignant tumors to distant sites (metastasis) occurs through the lymphatics or the venous system and requires the acquisition of additional properties that are at least partially independent of one another. These include the ability to gain access to the vessel, to survive in the vasculature, and to exit and grow in a foreign organ. Usually carcinomas metastasize through lymphatic channels, whereas sarcomas metastasize through venous and capillary channels. Careful sampling of routine surgical pathologic material often reveals lymphatic invasion by carcinomas, including common tumors such as those in the colon and breast. In some organs (such as the prostate and pancreas) the perineural space including the lymphatics are frequently involved. Fig. 14-21 shows this process in an adenocarcinoma of the lung. The consequence of lymphatic invasion is often metastasis to regional lymph nodes and then to more distant sites. In contrast, sarcomas rarely metastasize to regional lymph nodes. Many important exceptions to these generalizations have been observed: renal cell carcinomas and hepatocellular carcinomas, for example, are often found invading renal and hepatic veins respectively and epithelioid sarcoma and synovial sarcoma frequently metastasize to lymph nodes. Careful inspection of routine surgical pathologic material may show vascular spread of carcinomas (Fig. 14-24). The microvasculature of tumors is

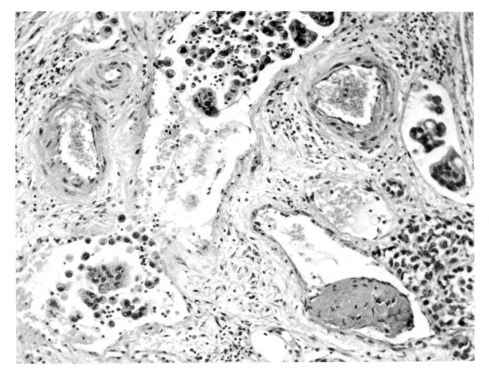

Fig. 14-24. Extensive blood vessel invasion by carcinoma of pancreas. Notice thrombus in one small vein. (250×.)

often more accessible to parenchymal cells than that of normal tissues is, and, in the case of some lymphomas, tumor cells may be shed directly into it.[155] As a result, many of our preconceived notions about invasion and metastasis based on normal tissues may not be directly applicable to tumor biology. Particular types of tumors often show strong predilection for metastatic sites. Breast and bronchogenic carcinomas metastasize disproportionately frequently to the central nervous system and adrenal glands, whereas metastasis of carcinomas to the spleen is not common.

The acquisition of metastatic potential and the distribution of metastases have been the subject of many studies. Regardless of whether the initial entry is by the lymphatic or venous system, many tumors gain access to larger veins and then to the microvasculature of the venous system in different organs. This interaction between distant microvasculature and clusters of tumor cells appears to be one critical factor in metastasis formation.[155] The inflammation resulting from damage caused by the lodging of foreign cells in the microvasculature leads to the release of proteases and growth factors which help access to foreign tissues. A common assay for metastatic potential involves analysis of colonization. Tumor cells (carcinomas or sarcomas) are injected into the tail vein of a nude or syngeneic mouse and the ability of cells to colonize tissues is scored several weeks or months later.[37] Although the assay only partially mimics the metastatic process, the assay represents a reasonable way to assess the metastatic potential of cells. Some aspects of organ specificity have been analyzed with this assay. If a mouse "melanoma" cell line is injected into the tail vein, colonies are observed in many organs. If a colony is recovered from a given organ (such as lung or brain) and the cells are reinjected, the proportion of lung or brain colonies is much higher in the second set of mice.[37,38] Although the biochemical basis of this specificity is not yet known, some progress has been made in understanding the mechanism of colonization. Recognition and specific binding of basement membrane and fibronectin (in the extracellular matrix) appear to be critical to invasion and colony establishment in the lung, since these phenomena can be blocked by either antibodies to cellular laminin receptors or peptides, which compete with laminin and fibronectin for receptor binding.[59,63,158] There is some evidence that an "active" form of the *ras* oncogene (see pp. 587 and 589) predisposes to metastasis,[49,98] but it has been difficult to control these studies for other factors like growth rate and local invasiveness. A report describing the identification of a gene associated with metastases has yet to be confirmed.[14]

Progression. The acquisition of increasingly aggressive characteristics by premalignant or malignant tumors is termed "progression." The changes manifest themselves most frequently by changes in morphology (from better differentiated to more poorly differentiated) or growth rate (from slower to faster). At accessible sites like the uterine cervix or skin, successive cytologic examination (see Glossary), biopsy or even careful clinical evaluation (especially in malignant melanoma) may reveal the increasingly aggressive nature of a neoplasm.[26] In lesions of the uterine cervix, cytologic and histologic evaluation over time may show increasing cellular atypia and tissue disorganization (increasing dysplasia), eventually carcinoma in situ and then invasive carcinoma, followed by metastatic spread. These changes often take many years to develop, and up to a point (moderate to severe dysplasia) they may regress spontaneously. (There is also preliminary evidence that retinoids can reverse cervical dysplasia in some women.) This general pattern of progressive change can also be documented in less accessible tissues (colon and prostate) and in carcinogen-induced skin and liver tumors in animals.[36]

Progression results from selection of characteristics that enhance survival and may be viewed as analogous to natural selection in population biology. Thus cell lineages within tumors that retain the largest fraction of cells in the cell-cycle compartment or secrete increased amounts of extracellular proteases, for example, with time come to predominate and to endow the tumor with new characteristics (in this example, a faster growth rate and invasiveness). The changes that are selected are, of course, properties of some tumor cells within the population and probably reflect cells in which the expression of only a few regulatory genes could have profound consequences for cellular behavior (see section on variation in cell growth and Fig. 14-4). Progression occurs on a continuum, and observed discontinuities represent the need of pathologists to identify "stages" in order to communicate the behavior of tumors. When large discontinuities occur rapidly, they may result from rapid selection of cells that show sudden large increases in the expression of regulatory genes (for example, as a result of amplification or insertion of the gene behind a strong promoter).

The question whether benign tumors progress to malignant tumors often arises. Experimental evidence indicates that malignant tumors may arise from benign tumors but that malignant tumors sometimes appear to develop in the absence of an identifiable benign lesion (that is, de novo): For example, when mouse skin is treated with carcinogens, squamous cell carcinomas develop both in benign papillomas (which themselves may regress fully) and in areas of skin that lack papillomas. In some human cancers (such as small cell carcinoma of the lung) benign precursors cannot be identified. Many benign lesions (such as lipomas, leiomyomas of the uterus, and dermal nevi) are only rarely precursors for malignant lesions, whereas others like tubular and villous adenomas of the colon often give rise to adenocarcinomas. Thus some benign tumors are clearly precursors for malignant tumors. Whether they are obligatory precursors cannot be determined with certainty, since it is always possible to argue that the original benign lesion was very small or was destroyed by its malignant progeny.

ETIOLOGY AND PATHOGENESIS

Throughout the twentieth century, many experimental and epidemiologic observations have indicated that neoplastic disease may result from somatic mutations occurring after physical or chemical damage to nuclear DNA. These observations have included (1) the correlation of specific chromosomal changes with certain types of cancer,[55] (2) the transfer of the neoplastic phenotype between organisms via oncogenic viruses,[156] and (3) the recognition that most chemical and physical carcinogens are also potent mutagens.[87] Until recently, however, the basis for these observations remained obscure, since investigators could measure only gross changes in total nuclear DNA and analysis of specific mutations affecting individual genes was technologically impossible.

Oncogenes. The past decade has witnessed a revolution in our ability to isolate, purify, and analyze the fine structure of individual genes. Subsequently, several ingenious approaches have been devised to identify the nuclear targets for carcinogens and oncogenic viruses. This work, in turn, has led to the important discovery of a class of growth-related genes that are referred to collectively as "oncogenes."[138] Concomitant with our heightened awareness of oncogenes and their role in normal growth control, important insights have been gained into mechanisms leading to the disruption of growth control by carcinogens and viruses. Two strategies in particular, the detailed genetic analysis of oncogenic viruses and the use of purified tumor-cell DNA fragments to transfer the neoplastic phenotype between cells, have been especially successful. In the following section we summarize some of the highlights of oncogene research; many recent reviews provide more detailed information.[16,149]

Identification of viral oncogenes. The first oncogenic virus to be described, the Rous sarcoma virus, was identified in 1911 as a filterable agent capable of transferring sarcomas among different chickens.[112] Peyton Rous, an experimental pathologist at the Rockefeller Institute, won the 1968 Nobel Prize for these efforts, which led to speculation that many human tumors might result from infection with oncogenic viruses. By preparing soluble extracts from each of the spontaneously occurring chicken sarcomas he encountered, Rous demonstrated that a cell-free filtrate from one of these sarcoma extracts could induce similar sarcomas when injected into healthy chickens. Subsequent analy-

ses revealed Rous sarcoma virus as an RNA-containing retrovirus capable of stably integrating its genome into that of its host. Many different oncogenic retroviruses were subsequently discovered in a variety of species, and each of these viruses was observed to induce a characteristic type of tumor (that is, sarcomas, myeloblastosis, osteosarcomas, etc.[16]). These observations indicated that oncogenic retroviruses may be able to carry a "transforming" gene capable of inducing the neoplastic phenotype in stably infected host cells. However, identification of the transforming components of these viruses, as well as their mechanism or mechanisms of action, awaited further advances in genetics and molecular biology.

Fittingly, the first viral transforming gene to be isolated and characterized was the *src* gene of Rous sarcoma virus, in 1976.[130] Approximately 40 different retroviral oncogenes have been identified at present, and a partial list appears in Table 14-3.

Identification of cellular oncogenes as homologs of viral oncogenes. Although most of the viral oncogenes exhibit little structural homology with one another, each of the retrovirus-derived oncogenes (v-*onc*) is closely related to a homologous cellular gene present within the nuclear DNA of most eukaryotic organisms (c-*onc*). These cellular homologs are referred to as cellular or proto-oncogenes, and the striking similarities with retroviral oncogenes indicate that the latter may have been derived by viral transduction of cellular oncogenes.[139] Preliminary studies indicate that cellular oncogenes may play a regulatory role within pathways related to cell growth and differentiation. However, when they are altered by point mutations, truncations, gene rearrangements, or other genetic insults, expression of these genes may result in loss of growth control and, ultimately, neoplastic transformation. As such, cellular oncogenes probably represent the predominant nuclear targets for the action of carcinogens.[132] It is worth noting that most of the original oncogenes were identified as viral homologs of cellular genes in RNA (retro)viruses. We now know that many oncogenic DNA viruses also carry oncogenes that have similar functions but do not have obvious cellular homologs (see Table 14-7).

Somatic mutations in cellular oncogenes can cause neoplastic growth. The role of mutated cellular oncogenes in human neoplasia has been dramatically underscored by an elegant series of experiments in which purified nuclear DNA from various human tumor-cell lines (such as T24 bladder carcinoma cells) is used to transform a second, morphologically normal cell line to the neoplastic phenotype.[104] In most experiments of this type, stable introduction of tumor-cell DNA into normal, growth-regulated recipient cells leads to dramatic changes in the growth pattern of the recipient

Table 14-3. Human proto-oncogenes and their approximate chromosomal locations

Oncogene	Origin	Chromosomal location
fgr	Gardner-Rasheed feline sarcoma	1p36
src 2	Rous chicken sarcoma	1p36
L-myc	Human lung carcinoma	1p32
N-ras	Human neuroblastoma	1p11-13
ski	SKV avian virus tdB77	1q22-24
arg	Abelson-related gene	1q24-25
N-myc	Human neuroblastoma	2p23-24
raf 1	3611 murine sarcoma	3p25
fms	McDonough feline sarcoma	5q34
pim	Mouse T-cell lymphoma	6p21-22
K-ras 1	Kirsten murine sarcoma	6p11-12
ras	Avian sarcoma	6q16-22
myb	Avian myeloblastosis	6q22-24
erb B	Avian erythroblastosis	7p11-12
met	Human osteosarcoma	7q22
mos	Moloney murine sarcoma	8q11 or 8q22
myc	MC29 avian myelocytomatosis	8q24
abl	Abelson murine leukemia	9p34
H-ras 1	Harvey murine sarcoma	11p15
int 2	Mouse mammary tumor	11q13
bcl-1	Human B-cell tumors	11q13
ets 1	Avian E26 leukemia	11q23
K-ras 2	Kirsten murine sarcoma	12p12
fes	Snyder-Theilen feline sarcoma	15q25-26
erb A	Avian erythroblastosis	17q11-12
neu	Rat neuroglioblastoma	17q11-12
erb B2	Avian erythroblastosis	17q21
yes 1	Avian Yamaguchi (Y73) tumor	18q21
bcl-2	Human B-cell tumor	18q21
src 1	Rous chicken sarcoma	20q13
ets	Avian E26 leukemia	21q22
sis	Simian sarcoma	22q13
fos	Finkel-Biskis-Jinkins murine osteosarcoma	—
jun	Avian sarcoma (ASV-17)	—

Modified from Heim, S., and Mitelman, F.: Cancer cytogenetics, New York, 1987, Alan R. Liss, Inc.

Chromosomal locations are designed as A(p or q)B, where *A* represents the chromosome number, *p* or *q* represents the long, *p*, or short, *q*, arm respectively, and *B* represents the chromosomal band.

cells, whereas introduction of DNA from normal cells has no detectable effect. The observed alterations in growth pattern include (1) the ability to grow at high cell densities, (2) the ability of "transformed" cells to grow directly on top of one another (that is, focus formation), and (3) the ability to grow in semisolid media (that is, anchorage-independent growth). The low frequency of neoplastic transformation that is observed in these experiments indicates that a single copy of a mu-

tant gene may be responsible for the initiation and maintenance of the neoplastic phenotype in T24 cells. Interestingly, the tumor-inducing gene present in T24 cells has been shown to be a mutated form of the previously characterized cellular oncogene known as c-Ha-*ras*. In this case, however, a single base change in codon 12 converts c-Ha-*ras* from a regulatory gene controlling growth and development to a "transforming" oncogene promoting uncontrolled growth.[104,135]

Subsequent studies have demonstrated that cellular oncogenes may be activated by many different molecular mechanisms including point mutations, gene rearrangements, and gene amplification.[16,139,149] Some cellular oncogenes, such as *ras*, can be activated by mutations within coding regions that enhance the specific activity of the oncogene products. Other oncogenes, in contrast, tend to be activated primarily by mutations within regulatory regions of the gene, leading to either increased or aberrant expression. Furthermore, except for the *ras* oncogenes, most cellular oncogenes require multiple mutations in order to become activated.[139] For example, expression of the cellular oncogene c-*fos* is induced to very high levels by a variety of growth factors and hormones, and in many cases this appears to stimulate cell growth and replication. However, the induction of c-*fos* by these factors is transient, and c-*fos* levels return to base-line values within 2 hours, even if the hormone remains present throughout the induction period. The transient nature of c-*fos* induction is tightly controlled by sequences at both the 5′ and 3′ ends of the gene.[142] If both of these regulatory sequences are inactivated concomitantly by somatic mutation, c-*fos* is expressed constitutively, and neoplastic transformation may result.[89]

Neoplastic transformation of some cells requires the activation of more than one oncogene. Although experiments utilizing oncogenic retroviruses or transfection with mutated *ras* genes indicate that expression of a single activated oncogene may be sufficient to cause neoplastic transformation, additional observations indicate that this may not always be true. For example, expression of the mutated *ras* gene derived from T24 cells (*ras*T24) is sufficient to transform cultures of immortalized cell lines but insufficient for transformation of primary (that is, freshly isolated) cultures. However, when primary cultures are transformed simultaneously with activated *ras* and *myc* oncogenes, neoplastic transformation is readily observed.[74] These results are consistent with the idea that, in some cells, growth regulation must be overridden at two or more control points in order to cause neoplastic transformation. It is interesting to note in this respect that the avian erythroblastosis viruses contain two different viral oncogenes, *erb*-a and *erb*-b, which are derived from separate regions of the host genome.[150]

Functions and intracellular locations of oncogene products. As a group, the cellular oncogenes appear to encode polypeptides that are involved in the initiation and intracellular transduction of signals related to cell growth and differentiation.[75,76,97] Most of the cellular oncogenes identified at present fall into one of the following categories: (1) those encoding known or suspected trophic (growth) factors (such as c-*sis*, transforming growth factors α and β), (2) those encoding membrane-bound receptors for extracellular growth factors (such as c-*fms* and c-*erb*-b), (3) those encoding polypeptides associated with the inner surface of the plasma membrane and transducing signals between membrane and cytoplasmic proteins (such as c-*src*, c-*ras*, c-*abl*), (4) those encoding soluble cytoplasmic receptors for hormones such as steroids and thyroid hormones (such as c-*erb*-a), (5) those encoding nuclear polypeptides that bind specifically to regulatory DNA regions and presumably modulate transcription and replication (such as c-*fos*, c-*myc*, c-*myb*, c-*jun*).

In addition to the growth-promoting effects of oncogenes, expression of activated oncogenes, in some cell types, results in cessation of cell division and the acquisition of differentiated phenotypes. For example, PC12 pheochromocytoma cells stop dividing and assume the shape of differentiated nerve cells in response to expression of an activated *ras* (*ras*T24) gene.[11,101] Nerve growth factor has an identical effect on PC12 cells. Similarly, expression of c-*fos* in myeloid precursor cells is associated with a decreased growth rate as well as the induction of markers characteristic of monocytic differentiation.[96] It is difficult to understand how a single gene (such as *ras*T24) could have growth-stimulating effects in one cell type and growth-inhibitory effects in another. However, the overall data indicate that cellular oncogenes may form an intracellular communications network that is triggered by extracellular trophic factors. Some of these factors may have either growth-promoting or growth-inhibiting effects, depending on the target cell. The particular response of a cell to the binding of these trophic factors depends on the developmental lineage of that cell rather than any inherent stimulatory or inhibitory properties of a particular oncogene.[75]

Two important corollaries of this model for oncogene action have significant implications for the diagnosis and treatment of neoplastic diseases. The first corollary predicts that since various cell types respond differently to the expression of any one oncogene each cell type may be susceptible to neoplastic transformation by only a limited subset of cellular oncogenes. The strikingly consistent correlations of N-*myc* with neuroblastoma,[118] c-*abl* with chronic myelogenous leukemia,[121] and c-*myc* with B-cell lymphomas[30,136] support this idea. The second corollary predicts that for a given cell type, two different activated oncogenes may induce neoplastic transformation by entirely different mechanisms. As a result, the optimal therapy for an individual tumor should be determined only after the mechanism of neoplastic transformation, that is, the activated oncogene, has been identified. Past therapies have taken advantage of increased rates of cell division in tumor cells because this represents a final common pathway for the activities of growth-promoting oncogenes. However, future therapies directed toward the action of a particular oncogene may prove, in some cases, to be more effective.

Analysis of oncogenes in the diagnosis of neoplasia. Later we present a section that focuses on new diagnostic approaches to neoplasia; however, because these approaches are so intimately related to tumor biology, aspects of this subject are presented here. Since alterations in the structure of cellular oncogenes can be detected routinely by molecular probes, hope has been expressed that such analyses may be clinically useful in assessment of the diagnosis, prognosis, and optimal therapy for a variety of different tumors. The value of this approach has been demonstrated clearly for neuroblastomas, in which expression of the N-*myc* oncogene correlates well with both the clinical stage at the time of diagnosis and the prognosis of each case.[22,118,143] Activation of N-*myc* in these tumors occurs almost exclusively by amplification of the N-*myc* gene, and the degree of amplification can be detected easily by use of small amounts of tumor tissue. Either fresh tissue or stored paraffin blocks can be used as a source of neuroblastoma DNA.[143]

Molecular diagnostic approaches have also been shown to be useful in certain cases of chronic myelogenous leukemia (CML). Most cases of CML carry a specific translocation between chromosomes 9 and 22 that is present only in tumor cells and disappears during clinical remissions (see p. 591). The (9;22) translocation results in the formation of an atypically small chromosome 22, referred to as the "Philadelphia chromosome," which frequently aids in the diagnosis of CML.[102] Unfortunately, only 75% to 85% of CML cases exhibit the Philadelphia chromosome, and this results occasionally in a difficult diagnostic dilemma. Recent investigations have shown that the (9;22) translocation alters the structure of the c-*abl* oncogene, leading to inappropriate expression of this gene.[50] Molecular analysis of c-*abl* gene structure by Southern blots has identified rearrangements characteristic of CML in many cases that lack a recognizable Philadelphia chromosome.[94]

Although some tumors, such as CML, neuroblastoma, and Burkitt's lymphoma, appear to be associated consistently with the activation of a specific oncogene, other tumors, such as lung, colon, and breast carcinomas, may result from activation at one of several different oncogene loci.[9,19,35,39,111,124] For these tumors, it would be useful to determine whether different oncogenes induce tumors with different natural histories or responses to chemotherapy. In addition, if successful oncogene-based, mechanistically oriented therapies are to be developed and applied, it will be essential to identify the specific activated oncogene for each individual case.

In one study of breast carcinomas, amplification of the *neu* oncogene was observed in approximately 30% of the primary tumors. Interestingly, when the tumors in this study were separated into groups based on the presence or absence of lymph node metastases, 40% of node-positive tumors exhibited amplification of the *neu* locus, whereas amplification was observed in only 10% of node-negative tumors.[124] Among several potential prognostic factors including size of the primary tumor, age at diagnosis, and estrogen-progesterone receptor status, the overall survival and time to relapse correlated most significantly with either the presence of nodal metastases or amplification of the *neu* oncogene. Furthermore, the shortest time to relapse and the shortest overall survival were observed in patients whose tumors contained the highest levels of amplified *neu*. The correlation of poorer prognosis with higher levels of oncogene amplification is also seen with N-*myc* amplification in human neuroblastomas.[118]

In a second study, amplification of the c-*myc* oncogene was observed in approximately 30% of primary breast carcinomas. However, amplification of c-*myc* does not appear to correlate with the presence of nodal metastases. Since transformation of cultured cell lines frequently requires the simultaneous action of two or more activated cellular oncogenes, it would be useful to learn whether significant overlap exists between subpopulations of breast tumors containing amplified *neu* and *myc* oncogenes.

In addition to the aforementioned studies, other investigators have focused their efforts on the association of activated *ras* with a variety of epithelial and mesenchymal tumors. The *ras* gene is of particular interest in these studies, since it can become activated by a single point mutation occurring at any of several possible sites. Analysis of primary human colon carcinomas indicates that activating ras mutations are present in greater than 30% of these tumors.[19,39] Surprisingly, most of these mutations occur in the K-*ras* gene; activating mutations in other members of the *ras* gene family, which includes K-*ras*, H-*ras*, N-*ras*, and R-*ras*, occur infrequently in colonic tumors. Furthermore, mutant K-*ras* genes were also observed within apparently benign adenomas located adjacent to the colonic carcinomas, and these results indicate that activated *ras* genes may be present in premalignant lesions as well. Similar studies have reported activated *ras* genes in both benign papillomas and malignant carcinomas of the skin.[9]

The list of human tumors whose development is associated with one or more activated oncogenes is growing at an increasing rate, and the examples presented in this section are intended to be instructive rather than comprehensive. Other notable examples include the association of activated K-*ras* genes with adenocarcinomas of the lung[111] and the association of activated K- and N-*ras* genes with myelodysplastic syndrome and preleukemia.[57,80]

Antioncogenes and neoplasia. Although abundant evidence supporting an etiologic role for activated cellular oncogenes in neoplastic disease has accrued, recent studies of retinoblastoma cells indicate that a second mechanism, ostensibly independent of cellular oncogenes, may also be important. Retinoblastoma cells have frequently been observed to harbor simultaneous deletions within both copies of chromosome 13, whereas nonneoplastic cells from the same individual contain at least one unaltered copy of this chromosomal region. On the basis of these and other related observations, Knudson[71] has proposed the existence of one or more antioncogenes that prevent uncontrolled cell growth, possibly by regulating the activity of cellular oncogenes. Since the first presumptive antioncogene has only recently been isolated and characterized,[42] the mechanism of action of these genes and their synergy with cellular oncogenes await further experimentation.

Future prospects for the diagnosis and treatment of neoplasia. The identification of viral oncogenes as the transforming component of oncogenic viruses and the subsequent discovery of homologous cellular oncogenes have radically altered our understanding of neoplastic diseases. At present, the considerable abilities of molecular biologists to produce data on the structure and function of oncogene products has greatly outstripped that of pathologists to assimilate these data into a clinically and diagnostically useful approach toward human neoplastic diseases. Although traditional approaches based on histology will continue to provide invaluable diagnostic information and insights, future therapies will undoubtedly address the structure and function of specific molecules, most of which cannot be detected histologically. Despite limited formal training of most pathologists in the area of molecular biology, techniques such as immunohistochemistry and in situ hybridization have become standard diagnostic procedures in an increasing number of laboratories. In addition, Southern blots are now used routinely in a few pathology departments for the diagnosis of certain lymphomas,[27] and additional applications are developing rapidly.

Growth factors. Growth factors are polypeptides or

Table 14-4. Some representative growth factors

Growth factor	Primary translation product	Mature factor size	Cell source	Target cell	Receptor
EGF	1168 or 1217 aa*	6 kDa (53 aa)	Submaxillary gland, Brunner's gland, possibly parietal cells	Wide variety of epithelial and mesenchymal cells	c-*erb* B gene; 170 kDa tyrosine kinase
TGF-α	160 aa	5.6 kDa (50 aa)	Transformed cells, placenta, embryos	Same as EGF	Same as EGF
PDGF	241 aa (B chain); A chain unknown; B chain encoded in c-*sis* proto-oncogene	32 kDa (16 kDa B chain; 14-18-kDa A chain); +CHO	Blood platelets, endothelial cells, placenta	Mesenchymal cells, smooth muscle, placental trophoblast	185 kDa tyrosine kinase
TGF-β	391 aa	25 kDa (2 × 112 aa)	Blood platelets, kidney, placenta, cultured cells	Fibroblastic cells, keratinocytes, mammary epithelial cells, carcinoma, and melanoma lines	565-615 kDa complex (2 × 280-290 kDa)
IGF-I	130 aa	7 kDa (70 aa)	Adult liver and other sites, smooth muscle cells	Epithelial, mesenchymal	450 kDa complex (2 α chains of 130 kDa; 2 β chains of 85 kDa)
IGF-II	180 aa	7 kDa (67 aa)	Fetal liver placenta	Epithelial, mesenchymal	Single polypeptide chain of 260 kDa
IL-2	153 aa (mouse); 169 aa (human)	15 kDa (133 aa); some CHO	T-helper cells	Cytotoxic T-lymphocytes	55 kDa (33 kDa protein + 22 kDa CHO)
FGF	Unknown	14-18 kDa (basic FGF is 146 aa)	Brain, pituitary, chondrosarcoma	Endothelial cells, fibroblasts	Unknown
β-NGF	307 aa	26 kDa (2 × 118 aa)	Submaxillary gland	Sympathetic and sensory neurons	130 kDa (possibly kinase)
CSF-1	252 aa	70 kDa (2 × 35 kDa); 60% CHO	Mouse L-cells	Macrophage progenitors	c-*fms* proto-oncogene; 170 kDa tyrosine kinase
CSF-2 (granulocyte-macrophage CSF)	144 aa	15-28 kDa (127 aa) (1-50% CHO)	Endotoxin-induced lung; placenta	Macrophage and granulocyte progenitors	Unknown
Multi-CSF (IL-3)	144 aa	28 kDa (134 aa) (50% CHO)	T-lymphocytes	Eosinophil, mast cell, granulocyte, macrophage progenitors; T-lymphocytes	Unknown

Modified from Goustin, A.S., Leof, E.B., Shipley, G.D., and Moses, H.L.: Cancer Res. **46:**1015, 1986.

*aa, Amino acid residues; CHO, carbohydrates, kDa, kilodaltons.

small proteins that are released by cells into the local environment and exert powerful regulatory effects on nearby cells ("paracrine effects") or on the secreting cells themselves ("autocrine effects")[48] (Table 14-4). They differ from polypeptide hormones in that they act locally and usually do not circulate (growth factors such as platelet-derived growth factor, PDGF, which is found in serum, are released during clotting). Growth factors are recognized by specific receptors on the plasma membrane of the target cell and exert their effects by triggering receptors to "transduce" signals to cytoplasmic pathways (such as protein kinase-mediated effects) and then to the nucleus.[48,113] Thus the biologic effects of growth factors may result from increased levels of the growth factor, increased numbers of receptors, altered receptors (that is, they behave as if they were "occupied"), or altered pathways.

In cell culture, transformed cells have reduced or absent growth factor requirements, and this loss of dependence is probably an important aspect of autonomous growth of tumors in vivo. It is believed that tumor cells respond in both an autocrine and paracrine manner. Their relative independence from exogenously supplied factors represents phenomena such as increased rates of synthesis of growth factors or their receptors or the development of altered receptors. This view is supported by the previously mentioned relationship between oncogenes and growth factors and their receptors and hormones; thus the *erb* B oncogene encodes the cytoplasmic and transmembrane portion of the TGF-α/EGF receptor, the *sis* oncogene is similar to the B-chain of the PDGF, *erb* A encodes part of the thyroid hormone receptor, and the c-*fms* proto-oncogene encodes the receptor for colony-stimulating factor-1 (CSF-1). Cells are usually responsive to several different growth factors that may (TGF-α and EGF) or may not (TGF-β and FGF) share the same receptors. Because of this overlap, it is often difficult even in vitro to unravel regulatory interactions.

One result of stimulation of growth factor pathways is cell proliferation. This phenomenon is well illustrated by the effects of IL-2 on T-lymphocyte proliferation or the effects of EGF on the growth of cultured cells. However, growth factors also produce changes in differentiation and maturation, as evidenced by NGF-stimulated neurite (axon) outgrowth from PC12 cells and the stimulation of precocious eye-opening and tooth eruption by EGF. They sometimes have opposite effects in different cells: we have mentioned the stimulation of fibroblast lineages by TGF-β and the inhibition of many epithelial lines, and lymphotoxin not only inhibits the growth of many transformed cells but also stimulates B-lymphocyte proliferation.[66] Thus as part of the acquisition of the neoplastic phenotype the escape from growth-factor regulation may involve escape from inhibition as well as loss of dependence on positive stimulating factors.

The foregoing discussion has focused on how growth factors might be involved in the growth of tumor cells themselves. We have mentioned that for tumors to grow they often require stromal and vascular support, and they frequently destroy or invade surrounding tissue. Part of these processes may be achieved by paracrine signaling to surrounding cells. Thus TGF-α, TGF-β, FGF, EGF, PDGF and endothelial cell growth factor (ECGF) stimulate angiogenesis or fibroblast growth, or both,[2,64,110,128,116] and TGF-β, lymphotoxin, EGF, IL-2, and TNF-α can be cytostatic or cytotoxic.[48,66] As a result, growth factors may be powerful modulators of tumor biology by virtue of their paracrine effects on heterologous cells.

Chromosomal changes in cancer. Chromosomes have been suspected as the cellular elements responsible for neoplastic transformation since the early part of the twentieth century. Boveri and von Hansemann were the first to postulate that the high frequency of abnormal mitotic figures observed in stained tumor sections were directly related to the acquisition of the neoplastic phenotype.[20,152] Further advances were severely constrained until reproducible preparations of mammalian chromosomes were achieved in the late 1950s. Soon afterwards, in 1960, a specific chromosomal abnormality associated with a particular cancer was reported by Nowell and Hungerford.[102] This abnormality consisted of an unusually small G-group chromosome (later identified as 22), which has become known as the Philadelphia chromosome. Since that time higher-resolution chromosome-banding methods have been developed to allow identification of relatively small and subtle structural abnormalities, and a rapidly growing field of cancer cytogenetics has emerged.

Chromosome structure and the origins of chromosomal abnormalities. The normal human karyotype contains 46 chromosomes, 22 pairs of autosomes and one pair of sex chromosomes (XX for females; XY for males) (Fig. 14-25). Genetic information is normally transmitted from parent to offspring as whole chromosomes; one member of each homologous chromosome pair is inherited from each parent.

The analysis of chromosomes from a single tissue or individual usually requires the preparation of intact chromosomes from a suspension of growing cells. Chromosome preparations are produced by controlled osmotic lysis of mitotic cells followed by specific staining techniques that produce, for each pair of homologous chromosomes, a unique and characteristic pattern of horizontal bands. An example of a banded preparation of normal human chromosomes is shown in Fig. 14-25. In many cases, the only indication of chromosomal abnormality is an alteration in the banding pattern for one

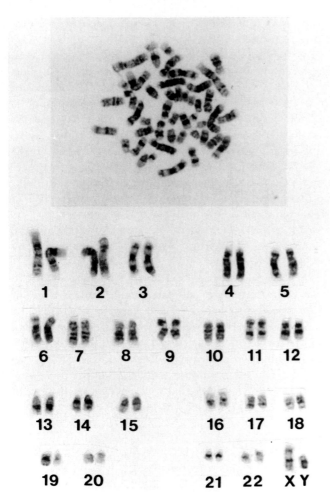

Fig. 14-25. Normal human karyotype. Chromosomes are banded using a combination of trypsin and Giemsa stain.

The rapid growth in cancer cytogenetics has resulted primarily from fortuitously coincidental advances in the molecular biology of neoplasia and the high-resolution analysis of chromosomal structure.[163] As discussed in a previous section, recent advances in molecular biology have led to the discovery and characterization of cellular oncogenes and their products. Simultaneous advances in cytogenetic analysis have permitted the chromosomal mapping of each cellular oncogene. In addition, these concomitant advances have expedited the detailed analysis of DNA from chromosomal breakpoint regions.[144] Results indicate that chromosomal rearrangements can activate cellular oncogenes by juxtaposition of inactive oncogenes within transcriptionally active chromosomal regions.[30,50,136,144] As such, chromosomal rearrangements represent alternative mechanisms of somatic mutation, analogous to point mutations and deletions, but that are detectable at the karyotypic level. Since a single chromosomal band contains approximately 100 to 300 genes, only rearrangements involving very large fragments can be detected. A list of chromosomal abnormalities associated with specific human malignancies is presented in Table 14-5. For a more detailed and comprehensive treatment of this subject, see reference 55.

Although the resolution of somatic mutations at the chromosomal level is considerably less than that available using molecular probes, chromosomal analysis offers the distinct advantage of a wider scope and greater sensitivity. Whereas a single Southern blot can allow identification of genomic alterations within the vicinity of a single gene, one high-resolution karyotype can allow identification of rearrangements (albeit large ones) arising anywhere within the genome. The most successful approaches therefore utilize karyotypic analysis to scan the entire genome for rearrangements and Southern blots to focus on the fine structure of karyotypically suspicious regions. As described previously, transformation by cellular oncogenes occurs when a particular cellular oncogene is activated by somatic mutation in a cell type that is susceptible to the action of that oncogene. The mechanisms that can lead to activation are determined primarily by the genetic structure of each oncogene. As a result, some cellular oncogenes are more likely than others to become activated by chromosomal rearrangements, and diseases associated with these particular oncogenes are more frequently associated with chromosomal translocation. In addition, most diseases associated with chromosomal rearrangements should also be associated with more localized gene rearrangements, since both mechanisms can generate similar changes in gene structure. Two examples illustrate this point clearly. Chronic myelogenous leukemia (CML) apparently results from inappropriate expression of the c-*abl* oncogene in immature hematopoietic

or more chromosomes. Somatic changes in chromosomal structure, as seen with many tumors, usually occurs in only one member of an homologous chromosome pair. The precise mechanisms by which chromosome segments are broken and rejoined are not completely understood at present. However, it is clear that the frequency of these events can be increased by agents that damage DNA, such as radiation, chemical carcinogens, and viruses.[114]

One of the most provocative observations related to the origin of cancer cells has been the consistent association of specific chromosomal abnormalities with certain types of cancer. Subsequent to the discovery of the Philadelphia chromosome in CML, investigators have uncovered many other examples of this phenomenon. In many cases, the specific chromosomal abnormality affects only the neoplastic cells, disappears with clinical remission, and reappears immediately before relapse.[55,114]

Table 14-5. Chromosomal aberrations in selected human cancers

Type of tumor	Chromosomal aberration	Frequency
Chronic myelogenous leukemia	t(9;22)(q34;q11)	75%-85%
Acute nonlymphocytic leukemia		
Subtype M1	t(9;22)(q34;q11)	9%
	del(5q)	10%
	−5	9%
	−7	17%
	+8	13%
Subtype M2	t(8;21)(q22;q22)	38%
	−7	11%
	+8	11%
Subtype M3	t(15;17)(q22;q11-12)	92%
Subtype M4	inv,del,t(16)(q13-22)	26%
	−7	11%
	+8	15%
Subtype M5	del,t(11)(q13-14)	30%
	+8	26%
Subtype M6	−7	26%
	+8	14%
	del(5q)	14%
Burkitt's lymphoma	t(8;14)(q24;q32)	75%-85%
	t(8;22)(q24;q11)	10%-20%
	t(2;8)(p12;q24)	5%
Retinoblastoma	Structural changes of 1	50%
	i(6p)	30%
	del(13)(q14)	20%
Small cell lung carcinoma	del(3)(p14p2)	>90%
Wilms' tumor	Structural changes of 1	50%
	del(11)(p13)	30%

Modified from Heim, S., and Mitelman, F.: Cancer cytogenetics, New York, 1987, Alan R. Liss.
The terminology used to described abnormal karyotypes is defined in ICSN: an international system for human cytogenetic nomenclature, Birth defects, Orig. Art. Ser. vol. 21, no. 1, New York, 1985, National Foundation–March of Dimes. Briefly, chromosomal abnormalities are designated by the form MOD(A;B)(c;d) where MOD represents a particular type of structural modification (such as *t,* translocation; *i,* isochromosome; *del,* deletion; *inv,* inversion; −/+, absence of extra presence of an entire chromosome); *A* and *B* represent the chromosome or chromosomes involved; and *c* and *d* represent specific chromosomal breakpoints.

cells.[121] In greater than 75% of patients with CML, c-*abl* is activated by a chromosomal translocation between chromosomes 9 and 22, in which the c-*abl* oncogene from chromosome 9 is fused to the control region of a gene known as *bcr* on chromosome 22.[50] One result of this translocation is a distinctively small remnant of chromosome 22 that is known as the Philadelphia chromosome.[102] In contrast, 15% to 25% of CML cases do not exhibit this translocation and are referred to as Philadelphia chromosome–negative CML. Recent experimental evidence, however, indicates that most cases of Philadelphia chromosome–negative CML contain a *bcr*/c-*abl* gene fusion, which is similar or identical to that observed in Philadelphia chromosome–positive CML.[94] These results demonstrate that the development of CML depends primarily on the formation of a *bcr*/c-*abl* fusion gene and that this occurs most frequently (75% to 80%) as a result of a specific translocation between chromosomes 9 and 22.

The second example concerns chromosomal alterations associated with the hereditary and sporadic forms of retinoblastoma. Approximately 5% of patients with hereditary retinoblastoma have a heterozygous deletion of band 13q14 within the long arm of chromosome 13.[55] This deletion, inherited at the time of conception, is present in every cell and is therefore referred to as a constitutional deletion. Subsequent studies have shown that the other 95% of patients with hereditary retinoblastoma also have a heterozygous deletion of genetic material from band 13q14, but this deletion is too small to be visible karyotypically. As discussed in a previous section, retinoblastoma results when the remaining copy of genetic material from band 13q14 is deleted or inactivated by a somatic mutation that may or may not be visible karyotypically. Thus, although karyotypically visible deletions are present only in a minor subpopulation of retinoblastoma patients, intensive study of these deletions has led to the isolation and characteri-

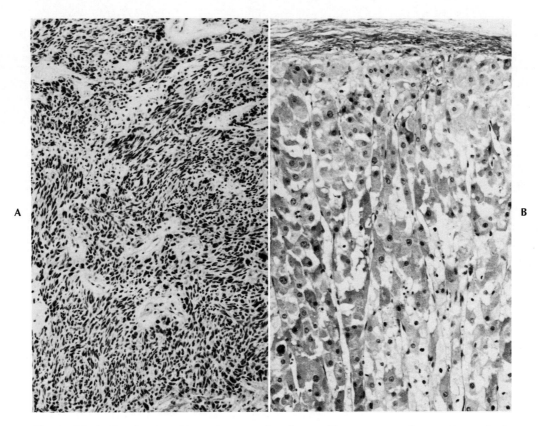

Fig. 14-26. A, Carcinoma of bronchus, small-cell type. Since tumor cells are often spindle shaped, cancer is sometimes called "oat cell." This tumor secreted excessive ACTH resulting in adrenocortical hyperplasia, **B,** and Cushing's syndrome. (**A,** 125×; **B,** 300×.)

zation of a gene responsible for the majority of retinoblastomas.[42]

In conclusion, both karyotypically detectable and nondetectable gene rearrangements may result in alterations in the expression of oncogenes and antioncogenes. Some cell types, such as lymphoid cells, contain specific DNA recombinases and may therefore be particularly susceptible to chromosomal rearrangements.[115]

Chemical and physical carcinogens. A majority of all cancer in humans results from exposure to chemical and physical carcinogens.[32,33; also 22,146] In the United States about 30% of all cancer deaths in both men and women have a single cause—exposure to tobacco products[32,33]! In addition to the well-known link between lung cancer and tobacco use (Fig. 14-26), individuals who smoke or chew tobacco are at increased risk for the development of cancers of the oral cavity, larynx, esophagus (in heavy drinkers), pancreas, and urinary system.[53] One interesting finding to emerge from epidemiologic studies is that other chemical carcinogens often act synergistically with tobacco: thus not only is asbestos a carcinogen for mesothelium and bronchial epithelium, but also in

combination with smoking it results in astronomical incidence rates for bronchogenic carcinoma in exposed workers. Radon-gas exposure (uranium miners) also results in bronchogenic carcinoma and acts synergistically with tobacco smoke to increase risk in an exponential fashion. Petrochemical smog does not increase the risk of lung cancer in the Los Angeles basin in nonsmokers, but results in a small (about twofold) increased risk in smokers. The most common cause of (nonfatal) cancers in the United States is exposure to solar radiation (primarily ultraviolet B, 290 to 330 nm), which results in hundreds of thousands of squamous and basal cell carcinomas on exposed areas of skin each year. It is also a major contributor to the incidence of malignant melanoma, which is now increasing in incidence faster than any other cancer in the United States (Fig. 14-27). Although there is much discussion about industrial exposure to chemicals as a cause of cancer in the United States and there have been several well-described "epidemics," only a small percentage of human cancer is traceable to such exposure. Most of the increased risk of cancer from exposure to chemicals and radiation is a result of life style and personal choice, not industrial or

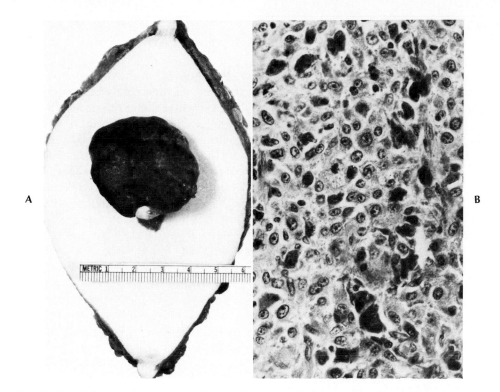

Fig. 14-27. Malignant melanoma of skin of back. **A,** Dark color is attributable to formation of large amounts of melanin by tumor cells. **B,** Photomicrograph of same tumor as **A.** Dark tumor cells contain much melanin pigment. (400×.)

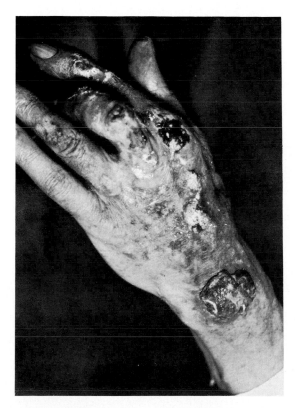

Fig. 14-28. X-ray dermatitis and multiple carcinomas of 5 years' duration in 83-year-old male physician after 15 years of repeated small exposure to x irradiation.

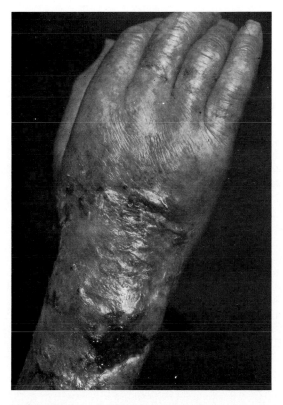

Fig. 14-29. Multiple epidermoid carcinomas and keratoses that developed as a result of repeated exposure to oil and tar over 30 years in 68-year-old man. Carcinoma had previously been excised from same area.

environmental exposure.[33] It is often easier, however, to identify occupational causes of cancer because of the clustering of cases and intense or protracted exposure (Figs. 14-28 and 14-29).

Most chemical carcinogens may be divided into two large classes, each with a different set of actions: those that, like radiation, produce covalent modification of cellular constituents and those that do not. Because DNA is believed to be the crucial cellular target for the former group, these carcinogens are sometimes referred to as genotoxic carcinogens whereas the latter group is referred to as nongenotoxic carcinogens. The list of agents that are known animal carcinogens runs into the hundreds,[161] and a subset of these and related compounds are known to be human carcinogens (Table 14-6).

Chemical carcinogens that form covalent bonds with cellular constituents (genotypic carcinogens) either do so directly ("direct-acting carcinogens") or are metabolized from "precarcinogens" to direct-acting intermediates ("ultimate carcinogens").[117,165] Bio-organic transformation usually occurs in mammalian cells, but sometimes is the result of action by intestinal flora (such as cycasin, Fig. 14-6). The result is the generation of electrophilic intermediates or free radicals, which attack most cellular constituents. Although DNA may not be the only cellular target for this class of chemical carcinogens and radiation, there is little doubt that it is a significant one.

Chemical carcinogens are ubiquitous (Fig. 14-30). Many are natural products, including, for example, cycasin (present in the cycad fern), safrole (found in the sassafras tree and present in extracts that were once used in flavoring root beer), aflatoxin B_1 (a mold product contaminating grains stored under moist conditions), and mitomycin C (a mold product used as an anticancer drug) (Fig. 14-30). Carcinogens like benzo[a]pyrene, 7,12-dimethylbenz[a]anthracene, and other polycyclic hydrocarbons are found among the combustion products of wood and fossil fuels. Nitrogen mustard is a direct-acting alkylating agent, synthesized as an anticancer agent, whereas bis(chloromethyl) ether is an industrial alkylating agent.

Metabolism of precarcinogens to ultimate carcinogens is an unfortunate by-product of cellular attempts to detoxify organic xenobiotics and render them water soluble. Usually only a small percentage of total metabolites is carcinogenic; the rest are inactive and excreted.

Table 14-6. Chemicals and mixtures carcinogenic or probably carcinogenic in humans

Agent	Site
LIFE-STYLE/PERSONAL-CHOICE EXPOSURE	
Tobacco	Lung, pancreas, oral cavity and pharynx, larynx, urinary tract
Tobacco quids and betel nut	Oral mucosa
Ethanol with smoking	Esophagus
INDUSTRIAL EXPOSURE	
Arsenic compounds	Skin, lungs
p-Biphenylamine and o-nitrobiphenyl	Urinary bladder
Asbestos	Pleura, peritoneum, lung
Asbestos with cigarette smoking	Synergistic increase in lung
Benzidine (4,4′-diaminobiphenyl)	Urinary bladder
Bis(chloromethyl) ether	Lung
Bis(2-chloroethyl) sulfide	Respiratory tract
Chromium compounds	Lung
2(or β)-Naphthylamine	Urinary bladder
Nickel compounds	Lungs, nasal sinuses
Soots, tars, oils	Skin, lung
Vinyl chloride	Liver mesenchyme
Radon gas (radiation)	Lung
Radon gas with cigarette smoking	Synergistic increase in lung
DRUGS AND THERAPEUTIC EXPOSURE	
N,N-Bis(2-chloroethyl)-2-naphthylamine (Chlornaphazine)	Urinary bladder
Cancer chemotherapy regimens	Leukemias, lymphomas, solid tumors
Diethylstilbestrol	Vagina
Estrogen	Breast, uterus
Phenacetin	Renal pelvis
Psoralen with ultraviolet radiation	Skin

Many dietary compounds affect carcinogen metabolism and often can decrease the already small percentage of carcinogenic metabolites of precarcinogens; these agents are sometimes referred to as "anticarcinogens."[126,127,154] Many have paradoxical effects in different species or organs or with different precarcinogens. Nevertheless agents like these along with those, like retinoic acid, that modify differentiation and gene expression are under active investigation as protective agents against cancer.[15,90,106,126,127,154]

Genotoxic carcinogens, as well as ultraviolet and ionizing radiation, damage cellular DNA in a variety of ways, including formation of covalent adducts with the DNA bases and the phosphodiester backbone, single- and double strand breaks, loss of purines and pyrimidines, and formation of photohydrates. Human cells are able to repair or partially repair DNA damage.[40] The significance of DNA repair is illustrated by persons with the rare autosomal recessive disorder *xeroderma pigmentosum* who lack to varying degrees of the ability either to excise damaged regions or to bypass them during DNA replication: Severely affected individuals develop numerous carcinomas on skin exposed to sunlight as early as their teens or even younger.

The cellular consequences of unrepaired DNA damage are mutations, including point mutations (base substitution, insertions, or deletions), rearrangements, deletions, insertions, or amplifications. Although the importance of mutation in the mechanism of action of carcinogens has long been postulated, until recently genomic targets were unknown. It is now clear that an important mode of action of chemical carcinogens is alteration of the structure or regulation of oncogenes. Several studies have demonstrated that in experimental chemical carcinogenesis in rodents, a majority of breast, liver, and skin cancers show point mutations in codon 12 or 61 of the c-H-*ras* oncogene.[10] It also seems likely that carcinogens may be involved in some of the rearrangements and amplifications now known to be associated with other forms of oncogene activation in humans (see p. 589 and Table 14-5), but few detailed model studies in animal systems are available. It cannot be stressed too strongly, however, that many changes in addition to oncogene modification occur as a result of administration of carcinogens. These include damage and modification of many genes besides the *known* oncogenes, the induction of metabolizing enzymes and repair systems, effects on DNA replication, and effects on noninitiated surrounding parenchymal cells. Many or all of these may be crucial in the generation and progression of neoplastic change.

Some agents known to be involved in carcinogenesis in either human or animal systems do not appear to form covalent bonds with cellular constituents: these include a variety of agents classified as nongenotoxic carcinogens and tumor promoters[166] (Fig. 14-31). The latter are agents that are not carcinogenic by themselves but greatly enhance the rapidity of onset or the yield of tumors (both benign and malignant) after carcinogen administration. The most potent of these are the phorbol esters (such as tetradeconylphorbol acetate, TPA) and structurally unrelated compounds with a similar mode of action, such as teleocidins and aplysiatoxin.[165,166] At the biochemical level this class of promoters seems to act by the protein kinase C pathway[165] and triggers the synthesis or activation of several transcription-regulating nuclear binding factors (AP-1 and AP-3), which regulate many cellular genes.[25] The molecular mechanism of action of other tumor promoters is not known in detail, but all tumor promoters stimulate cell division to some degree.

Carcinogens that do not appear to bind covalently to cellular DNA include estrogens, saccharin, inert plastic films, and asbestos. The molecular action of these agents is unclear, but many along with tumor promoters have common effects on cells. In the appropriate

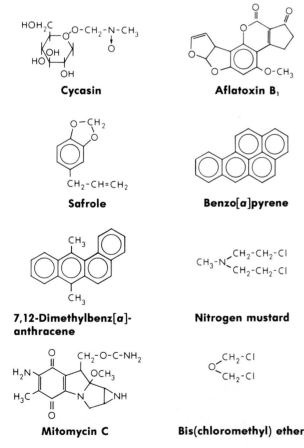

Cycasin

Aflatoxin B₁

Safrole

Benzo[a]pyrene

7,12-Dimethylbenz[a]-anthracene

Nitrogen mustard

Mitomycin C

Bis(chloromethyl) ether

Fig. 14-30. Examples of chemical carcinogens. All these chemicals are genotoxic (for covalent bonds with DNA). Cycasin, aflatoxin B₁, safrole, benzo[a]pyrene, and 7,12-dimethylbenz[a]anthracene require metabolic activation, whereas the others are direct acting.

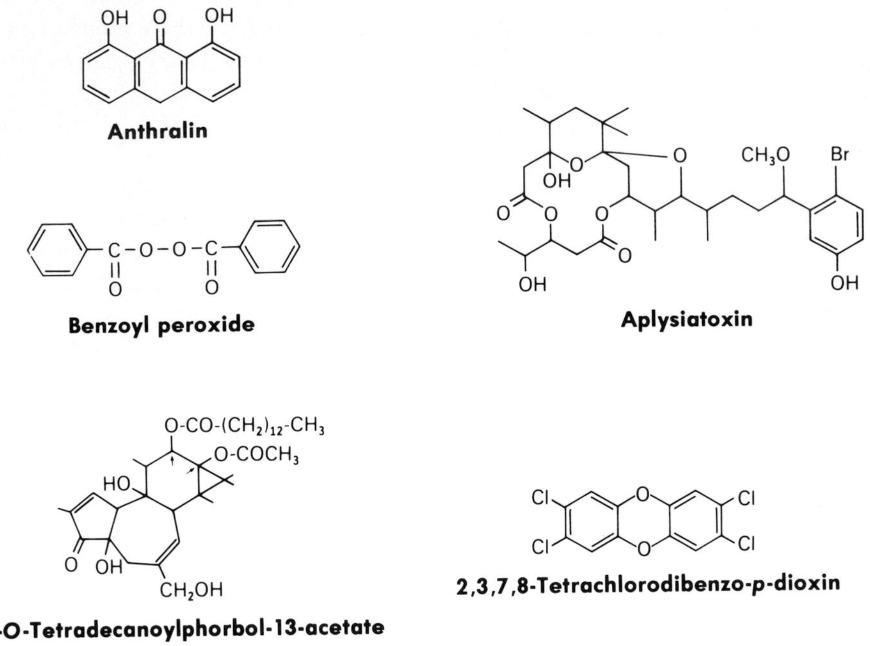

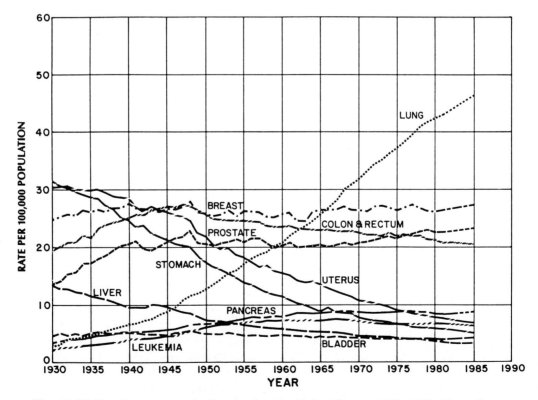

Anthralin

Benzoyl peroxide

Aplysiatoxin

12-O-Tetradecanoylphorbol-13-acetate

2,3,7,8-Tetrachlorodibenzo-p-dioxin

Fig. 14-31. Chemical structures of skin tumor–promoting agents. (From Yuspa, S.H.: J. Amer. Acad. Dermatol. **15**:1031, 1986.)

Fig. 14-32. Trends in cancer death rates by site, United States, 1930-1985. (From Cancer facts and figures—1988, New York, 1988, American Cancer Society.)

cell type, most of these agents stimulate cell division and the accumulation of a mass of proliferating cells, such as phorbol esters (mouse epidermal cells), estrogens (mouse breast parenchymal cells), saccharin (rat urothelium), plastic films (rat fibroblasts), and asbestos (mesothelial cells). The commonality may be that the probability of significant mutation or mutations (either spontaneous or induced) occurring in a large mass of proliferating cells is greater than in a few dividing cells; thus one action of these agents is to increase the number of cells at risk for neoplastic change. Some agents like the estrogens and TPA probably also alter the spectrum of expressed genes during proliferation. There may be a degree of overlap in the mode of action of these agents and some viruses associated with neoplasia. As suggested elsewhere, *part* of the action of hepatitis B virus in liver cells and HTLV-I in lymphoid tissue may relate to the enlarged pool of proliferating cells that they stimulate. However, stimulation of proliferation alone is unlikely to account for the entire action of these chemicals or viruses. It may be that some of these agents also have other effects; asbestos, for example, may stimulate free-radical formation in macrophages and thus result in DNA damage.

Several metals and metallic compounds including arsenic, beryllium, chromium state IV, and nickel are known to be carcinogenic in humans[46] (Table 14-6). Others have been shown to be cocarcinogenic or inhibitors of carcinogenesis in animals. Many effects of metals on biologic systems have been observed, including mutagenesis in short-term tests like the Ames' test and reduced fidelity of DNA synthesis; however, no comprehensive theory of metal carcinogenesis exists. In fact, it is likely that a variety of mechanisms, both genotoxic and nongenotoxic, are responsible for the carcinogenicity of these chemicals.

Estimating risk from exposure to chemical carcinogens for the entire United States population is difficult because it involves extrapolating from high-dose animal experiments across species barriers or from relatively small numbers of humans exposed to high levels of carcinogens (often in the workplace).[1,5] Yet it is clear that, except for smoking-related cancers and malignant melanoma, the incidence rates for cancer have not climbed despite a large increase in the manufacture of chemicals since World War II (Fig. 14-32). (Another exception may be the incidence of prostatic cancer, which has risen rapidly especially among blacks in the last 15 to 18 years.) Although there are undeniable examples of industrially generated cancers (Table 14-6), the total number of known cases does not begin to approach the number of smoking-associated cancers in the United States in a year.[23,32,117] The reason for this observation is not that many industrial agents are not potent—many are extremely effective experimental carcinogens—but

rather that thousands of workers exposed to varying levels of carcinogen often for only a few years do not develop as many cancers as millions of Americans smoking as many as two or more packs of cigarettes a day from an early age.

Many aspects of habit, diet, and environment alter the risk of developing cancer. Recently attempts have been made to assess this risk on the basis of both the potency of individual carcinogens and human exposure to them.[1] One may estimate daily exposure to agents like chloroform in municipal tap water (an unavoidable by-product of chlorination as protection against pathogenic bacteria), aflatoxin (in peanut butter), or formaldehyde (in mobile-home air) and the level of agent that produces tumors in 50% of exposed rodents. The possible implications are sobering: the amount of ethanol from a single glass of wine is many times more hazardous than the average American's daily exposure to polychlorinated biphenyls (PCBs) and the daily exposure to formaldehyde in mobile-home air is much more hazardous than exposure to the residue of ethylene dibromide on grain products consumed in an average day. An approach of this type should allow eventual elimination of unnecessary exposure to carcinogens and a better understanding of the trade-offs when exposures are unavoidable.

We have already mentioned the importance of *progression* in the development of neoplastic phenotypes (see p. 585). Two experimental systems, the development of skin cancer in mice and liver cancer in rats after the administration of tumor promoters and carcinogens, form the basis of much of our understanding of this process.[36,166] It is clear that often cancer develops as part of a selective process after the generation of papillomas (skin) or early nodules (liver) and that only a minority of these lesions progress to more aggressive lesions and finally to cancer. Experiments in which rats are exposed to carcinogen for a relatively brief period (2 to 3 weeks) indicate that, in liver at least, although the continued presence of carcinogen is not necessary, the development of frank hepatocellular carcinoma takes many months; also only a few carcinomas develop despite the presence of thousands of putative preneoplastic lesions.[36,65] There has been much speculation on how many steps are required to generate a malignant tumor and what the role of carcinogens is. However, it is also known that after carcinogen administration carcinomas in mouse skin or rat liver[119] can develop without identifiable preneoplastic lesions. These observations and present knowledge of oncogene function render these questions, as formulated, largely moot. Rather it is more appropriate to ask what properties must be acquired by individual cell types to make them identifiable as neoplastic or malignant and, in molecular terms, how these properties are acquired. What is required to generate a central nervous system ependymal tumor, a locally invasive squamous cell carcinoma of the skin, and a potentially metastatic hepatocellular carcinoma may be very different. Further, the degree to which a given oncogene, growth factor, or other gene is involved varies with cell type. For example, transplantation of cultured rat liver epithelial cells transfected with an activated H-*ras* construction results in metastatic adenocarcinoma, whereas cells transfected with a similar *myc* construction do not give rise to tumors[120] (also Lebovitz and Lieberman, unpublished data). Yet mice carrying the appropriate *myc* transgene develop adenocarcinoma of the breast.[77,148] Like so many questions in biology, questions about the number of "steps" or number of "hits" involved in the production of cancer must be examined carefully in an appropriate context and on a case-by-case basis.

Viral carcinogenesis. In the past decade, both DNA and RNA viruses have been implicated in human cancers[58,78,109] (Table 14-7). Although it has been known for over 75 years from work by Ellermann and Bang and by Rous that avian leukemias and sarcomas can be transmitted by filterable agents, only the careful epidemiology and molecular biology of many workers established an unequivocal role for viruses in the etiology of human cancer.[13,58,81] Unlike the original work on avian tumors and the investigation of the oncogenic action of active transforming retroviruses that grew out of it, analysis of human cancer has indicated that often only a small percentage of infected individuals develop cancer. The seminal observation from which explanatory hypotheses have flowed is the finding in the 1930s by Rous and his collaborators that a synergy existed between the Shope papilloma virus (CRPV) and chemical carcinogens in the development of cutaneous tumors. What has also become apparent with the advent of mo-

Table 14-7. Oncogenic viruses

Viruses	Animal tumors	Human tumors	Growth factor etc.
Adenoviruses	Fibrosarcomas (hamsters)	None identified	E1A protein E1B protein
Hepadenoviruses			
Hepatitis B virus		Hepatocellular carcinoma	None identified
Woodchuck hepatitis virus	Hepatocellular carcinoma (woodchuck)		None identified
Herpesviruses			
Epstein-Barr virus		Burkitt's lymphoma, nasopharyngeal carcinoma	?EBNA antigen ?LYDMA antigen
Frog herpes virus	Renal adenocarcinoma (frog)		
Papillomaviruses			
Bovine papilloma virus	Dermal and esophageal papillomas and squamous cell carcinomas		
Human papilloma virus		Cutaneous and genital carcinomas	E5 protein E6 protein
Polyomaviruses	Mouse adenocarcinomas, fibrosarcomas	None identified	Large T, small t antigens
Simian virus 40 (SV40)	Fibrosarcomas (hamster), lymphomas, osteosarcomas	None identified	Large T, middle t, small t antigens
Poxviruses	Shope fibroma (rabbit)	None identified	Vaccinia growth factor (EGF-like)
Retroviruses (RNA)			
Acute leukemia and sarcoma viruses	Leukemias, sarcomas	None identified	Common oncogenes (*ras, sarc, myc,* etc.)
Chronic leukemia viruses	Leukemias	None identified	None
Transregulating viruses			Transregulator of tat
Bovine leukemia virus	B-cell leukemias		
HTLV-1 HTLV-2		Some T-cell leukemias, T-cell variant of hairy cell leukemia	

EBNA, Epstein-Barr nuclear antigen; *HTLV,* human T-lymphocyte virus; *LYDMA,* lymphocyte determined membrane antigen.

lecular biology is that viruses play a variety of different roles in the carcinogenic process—roles that differ substantially from tumor to tumor.

Strong epidemiologic evidence links hepatitis B virus (HBV) with hepatocellular carcinoma.[13,81] Although relatively rare in the United States, worldwide it is one of the most common tumors, and its distribution is closely associated with the prevalence of HBV carriers. Only a small percentage of those infected with HBV become carriers (hepatitis B surface antigen positive), but their relative risk of developing hepatocellular carcinoma compared to noncarriers is about 200. Because of the long lag between infection and identifiable tumors (about 35 years) and the presence of chronic hepatitis and often cirrhosis, it is likely that events in addition to the presence of the HBV genome are necessary for tumor formation. Of interest in this regard is that no oncogene or growth factor–like functions have yet been identified for this small DNA virus. It seems plausible that chronic infection and the elaboration of surface antigen result in chronic destruction of the immunogenic hepatocytes with continual cell proliferation for replacement. These replicating cells are probably at risk for other events (such as mutation) that lead to neoplastic progression. One identifiable risk factor is the presence of aflatoxin, a powerful carcinogen in many species, in areas with a high incidence of hepatocellular carcinoma. Because an effective vaccine is available, hepatocellular carcinoma like lung cancer and skin cancer may be in large part preventable.

The relation between Epstein-Barr virus (EBV) and Burkitt's lymphoma (a B-cell lymphoma) is similar in broad detail to the HBV story. Although EBV infects more than 90% of all people worldwide by adulthood, Burkitt's lymphoma occurs most frequently in equatorial East Africa, a region in which malaria is endemic. Since African Burkitt's lymphoma appears to be a monoclonal proliferation of EBV-positive cells, it has been hypothesized that somehow malarial infection simulates the immune-cell proliferation from which these clones emerge or perhaps limits T-cell inhibition of B-cell growth. Whether or not two antigens encoded by HBV (EBNA and LYDMA) function as regulatory molecules remains to be seen (Table 14-7). As mentioned earlier, the characteristic chromosomal translocation and *myc* activation may represent a late or final step in the process.[68,69]

EBV-DNA is almost invariably found in biopsy specimens of nasopharyngeal carcinoma, and the incidence is especially high in Chinese.[56] This observation provides an interesting counterpoint to many demographic studies of cancer (see p. 607) in that these individuals regardless of locale seem to be at increased risk for this cancer. There is also an association between nasopharyngeal carcinoma and exposure to carcinogens or sub-stances suspected of harboring carcinogens (nitrosamines, fumes, smoke), and like the Shope papilloma-carcinogen model in rabbits, EBV and identifiable carcinogens may be synergistic in human nasopharyngeal carcinoma.

The human papillomaviruses (HPV) represent a family of over 50 related DNA viruses of intermediate size (8000 base pairs).[10] Papillomaviruses have been known to be oncogenic since the work of Shope in the 1930s.[10] Although there is a strong association between HPV-5 and HPV-6 and carcinomas that arise in the rare skin disease epidermoplasia verruciformis, the epidemiologic relationship of importance is between certain HPVs (especially HPV-16 and HPV-18) and genital cancers.[58,84] As with other human cancers, only a small portion of women with cervical infections develop neoplasia. The virus may be sexually transmitted, since in different geographical areas with differing incidences the ratio of incidence between cervical carcinoma and penile carcinoma remains similar. In the Scottish Highlands, cattle exposed to bovine papillomavirus (BPV4 or possibly other BPVs) show a high incidence of carcinomas of the esophagus and foregut only if they graze on bracken fern (known to contain several strongly carcinogenic pyrrolizidine alkaloids). Although this dependence on *known* chemical carcinogens is not obligatory (such as Shope papillomavirus, CRPV), it may provide a partial paradigm for explaining why not all infected women and men develop genital cancer. It is known, for example, that cervical carcinoma is higher in women who smoke than in those who do not. Since a large majority of women who develop cervical cancer have lesions that are HPV-positive, it may be that carcinogens in vaginal fluids from cigarette smoke act synergistically with HPV.[58] Normally HPV replicates episomally, but in several studies it has been found integrated into the tumor cell genome and transcribed, leading to relaxed expression of two presumed oncogenes—E6 and E7 proteins.

Two (RNA) retroviruses, HTLV-I and HTLV-II, are associated with two different human leukemias—adult T-cell leukemia and the T-cell variant of hairy cell leukemia respectively. They and a related bovine virus are unusual in that their 3' ends code for a transregulating factor, hence the designation "transregulating retroviruses." These genes appear to enhance transcription from the viral promoter and possibly cellular genes. What is at first examination surprising is that of all the known oncogenic retroviruses, only this small subclass is associated with human cancer. This observation may in part be explained by the suggestion that most of the acute transforming retroviruses (that is, those that carry known oncogenes and produce tumors rapidly) are inadvertent laboratory artifacts.

At present, only a very small percentage of human

leukemias are associated with a virus. HTLV-I may be transmitted through sexual contact (blood) and to infants during breast feeding. In areas where HTLV-I is endemic (as in Japan), less than 1% of seropositive individuals develop leukemia and the latent period may be many years. Although site of integration varies from individual to individual, there may be preferred sites that predispose to malignancy, but exactly how integration, transregulation, and host factors interact to lead to leukemia is unknown at present. Nontransregulating, chronic leukemia retroviruses appear to transform at least in part, by a mechanism known as promoter insertion, that is, by inserting a viral transcription start in front of cellular genes with oncogenic properties such as oncogenes and growth factors. What role this mechanism plays in HTLV-I or HTLV-II oncogenesis remains unknown.

It is also worth noting that some associations between viruses and human neoplasms are not casual. Rather the transformation process allows these cells to serve as hosts for viral growth. A well-known example is the recovery of herpes simplex virus from some cervical cancers.

GRADING AND STAGING

An estimate of the degree or grade of malignancy of a cancer is often useful for prognosis and for determination of the type of treatment. In this section we present the standard approach to *grading* and *staging* malignant tumors. In the next we suggest expansion of grading to encompass nonmorphologic criteria (such as information about tumor genotype and oncogene phenotype).

Cancers in some locations may be *graded* roughly by their appearance because often those that show an exophytic or fungating type of growth are less malignant than those that are diffusely infiltrating. More frequently, tumors are graded microscopically, with two factors being considered: (1) the degree of anaplasia or undifferentiation of the tumor and (2) an estimate of the rate of growth. Customarily tumors are graded numerically into three or four grades, with the low numbers implying a lesser degree of malignancy. Evidence of differentiation is based on the resemblance of the tumor to the normal tissue prototype. For example, a well-differentiated tumor arising from squamous epithelium would be expected to form considerable amounts of keratin and intercellular bridges. The estimate of rapidity of growth is based on the number of mitoses per unit of tissue (as per high-power microscopic field) and changes in nuclear chromatin patterns. Table 14-8 shows as an example the histologic grading of squamous cell carcinoma of the oral mucosa.

Grading may also depend primarily on the overall growth pattern and degree of invasion. With carcinoma

Table 14-8. Grading of squamous cell carcinoma of oral mucosa

Grouping	Grade		
	I	II	III
Evidence of differentiation			
Intercellular bridges	+	±	—
Keratinization	+	+	±
Epithelial pearls	+	±	—
Evidence of rapid, abnormal proliferation			
Mitoses per high-power field	<2	2-4	>4
Atypical mitoses	—	±	+
Nuclear and cellular pleomorphism	±	+	+
Multinucleated and tumor giant cells	—	—	+

+, Present; ±, may or may not be present; —, absent

of the thyroid gland, for example, the important distinctions are whether there is capsular invasion (grade 0-I) and whether the tumor is papillary or anaplastic. The usefulness of any grading system depends on the degree to which it provides prognostic information. With prostatic cancer, for example, three grading systems have been proposed, but the degree to which any is superior remains in question.[105]

Sometimes tumors that were once low grade become increasingly malignant with the passage of time so that a cancer that was once growing very slowly becomes high grade and invades and metastasizes widely and rapidly. For example, well-differentiated follicular carcinoma of the thyroid may transform itself into a giant cell carcinoma, which is one of the most highly malignant of all tumors; chronic myelogenous leukemia may progress into myeloblastic leukemia ("blast crisis"), which is much more malignant. Rarely, tumors become more differentiated and of a lower grade; an example is neuroblastoma that can differentiate into a benign ganglioneuroma.

Grading of tumors is common; however, it has limited clinical usefulness because of several difficulties. Although, in general, tumors are uniform throughout in histologic appearance, some vary considerably from portion to portion; hence sampling may be a problem. The prognosis achieved by gross or histologic grading obviously does not take into account such factors as the duration of the tumor, the presence or absence of metastasis, and the age of the patient, all of which are of great clinical importance in determining prognosis. Consequently, grading is most useful when combined with staging.

The *stage* of a cancer is an evaluation of its extent, based usually on gross and clinical findings, not the grade of the tumor. Consideration is given to the size and extent of the primary tumor (T), the presence and extent of lymph node (N) metastases, and the presence of distal metastases (M). By combining these three evaluations a staging system (TNM) has been developed as a useful method of describing the extent of spread of an individual tumor at a given time. Different staging schemes have been developed for different organs; thus the Gleeson and the Dohm staging systems are used for prostate cancer, the Dukes system for colon cancer, the FIGO system for gynecologic cancer, etc. Staging of cancer is treated for specific neoplasms in individual chapters on organ pathology. In treatment planning and the design of clinical trials accurate and complete staging is critical; a recent text on the management of lung cancer illustrates this point.[17] In the next section we suggest additions to current grading systems based on molecular subtyping.

NEW DIAGNOSTIC APPROACHES TO NEOPLASIA

In light of current understanding of the etiology of neoplasia, diagnostic strategies are changing. Molecular biology and molecular genetics, once considered the arcane purview of the experimentalist, have proved powerful adjuncts to standard diagnostic microscopy. Refinement of cytogenetic techniques has led to examination of solid tumors as well as leukemias. Immunohistochemistry and flow cytometry are in routine use in most major medical centers, and the increasing reliance on the interpretation of fine-needle aspirates has blurred the distinction between surgical pathology and cytopathology. In the following paragraphs we offer some examples of the application of these techniques to diagnostic pathology.

Diagnostic molecular biology. Pediatric rhabdomyosarcomas may be classified as embryonal or alveolar rhabdomyosarcomas. These tumors appear to arise by different mechanisms, since embryonal rhabdomyosarcomas show a loss of heterozygosity on the short arm of chromosome 11 (as determined by Southern blotting), whereas alveolar rhabdomyosarcomas maintain this heterozygosity.[116a] In addition to indicating that the origin of these two entities is different, this approach may provide a means for distinguishing embryonal rhabdomyosarcomas from other primitive small cell tumors of childhood.

Most follicular lymphomas show a rearrangement that juxtaposes the proto-oncogene *bcl-2* locus with the heavy-chain immunoglobulin locus; this feature is shared by a fraction of diffuse large cell lymphomas with no history of follicular lymphoma but not by small cell lymphomas, plasmacytomas, or Hodgkin's disease (including those that are rich in Reed-Sternberg cells and show immunoglobulin rearrangements).[157] Thus molecular genotyping may be useful in defining the origins of subclasses of diffuse large cell lymphomas. Although *bcl-2* rearrangement alone does not correlate with clinical behavior, additional genetic events, possibly including activation of c-*myc*, appear to relate to tumor aggressiveness.[29,164]

An analysis of breast cancers from women revealed a significant fraction with acquired hemizygosity on the short arm of chromosome 11, including many that have lost a c-H-*ras*-1 allele.[3,141] Further these losses tend to be associated with higher histopathologic grade, loss of hormonal receptors, and metastases. It would be of great interest to know the prognostic importance of deletions of part of 11p in cases of low histopathologic grade that are receptor positive. A smaller study involving premenopausal women revealed loss of heterozygosity on chromosome 13 in tumors from three of eight women with ductal breast carcinomas and maintenance of heterozygosity in four other tumors of varying histologic type.[82] Two additional studies show a correlation between alterations (usually amplifications) of oncogene structure (c-*myc* or *neu*) in breast cancer and poor prognosis[124,148] (see p. 586 and Table 14-3).

Although similar examples might be cited for other common tumors including colon, lung, and kidney cancer (such as references 19, 21, 39, 125, 167) or rarer childhood tumors (such as references 72 and 116a), the implication from the above examples is clear: Studies involving molecular biology are providing a new way of classifying tumors; this information relates to the underlying biology and has the potential to be clinically relevant. Standard histopathologic grading techniques may, in many cases, be inadequate to convey information to clinicians and may need to be augmented by a molecular grading scheme or replaced with a comprehensive grading or "pathologic staging" scheme that includes molecular biological and cytogenetic data, as well as findings from standard light microscopy, immunohistochemistry, and flow cytometry (see below). This contention is bolstered by numerous reports of changes in oncogene structure or function in human tumors or cells derived from them (as in references 3, 10, 19, 21, 29, 39, 72, 82, 100, 124, 125, 141, 157, 164, 167).

Cytogenetics. Although cytogenetics has been a valuable adjunct in the diagnosis of leukemias for many years, it is only recently that technical advances have made cytogenetic analysis of solid tumors possible on a selected basis. This approach has proved valuable in the diagnosis of Ewing's sarcoma in which a translocation [t(11;22)] has been found.[159] This translocation is absent in many other tumors of bone and soft tissue but present in peripheral neuroectodermal tumors. These data indicate a possible common mechanism and the possibility of treating Ewing's sarcoma with regimens designed for peripheral neuroectoderm tumors.

Immunohistochemistry. The use of immunohisto-chemistry (and immunocytochemistry) is expanding rapidly.[160] It is now hard to imagine classifying leuke-mias and lymphomas without either immunohistochem-istry or immunophenotyping by flow cytometry. Im-munohistochemistry has also found widespread use in general diagnostic pathology. Currently, for example, immunostaining for cytokeratins to help determine if an undifferentiated lesion is epithelial and staining for S100 proteins in the differential diagnosis of malignant melanoma are in widespread use. Staining for chromo-grainin is in use to determine if tumors have neurose-cretory granules (carcinoids, pheochromocytomas, etc.). An antigen termed "HMB45" is being evaluated as a possible way to distinguish nevi from malignant mela-noma.[39] Antibodies to oncogene products are becoming available: recently increased staining with anti-*neu* pro-tein (which appears similar to the epidermal growth fac-tor receptor) has been shown to correlate with gene amplification in human breast tumors,[147] and studies with anti-*bcl*-2 protein have also been useful.[99] To the extent that immunohistochemistry proves useful in pre-dicting the natural history of individual lesions, inclu-sion of such data in a grading or "pathologic staging" system may at times be appropriate.

Flow cytometry. Flow cytometry adds a degree of precision to immunodiagnostic techniques. It allows not only a more quantitative assessment of the presence of individual antigens, but also the opportunity to deter-mine if individual cells carry a second or even a third marker. It also allows analysis of the relative levels of expression of an antigen within a cell population and the possibility of correlating expression with other cell properties such as cell size or DNA content. The other major use of flow cytometry is the analysis of cell-cycle parameters in tumor specimens and even nuclei prepared from fixed tissues. Correlations be-tween the fraction of mitotically active cells and clini-cal behavior can be performed more rapidly and less tediously by flow cytometry than by conventional light-microscopic techniques and have proved clini-cally useful.[54,131,140]

In situ hybridization. In situ hybridization (the use of probes for detection of specific RNAs or DNAs in tissue sections) has received prominent attention re-cently. However, in general, investigators have found nucleic acid hybridization on filters (Southern or north-ern blotting) or immunohistochemistry to be more sat-isfactory. One important exception is the detection of viruses, including oncogenic viruses or potentially on-cogenic viruses like human papillomavirus.[51,153]

Tumor markers. Tumor markers are frequently used in cancer diagnosis or in following the course of therapy (Table 14-9).[134,145,151] In general parlance the term re-fers to circulating molecules in serum or occasionally plasma. Markers associated with the cell surface (such as the immunophenotypic markers of leukemias) or with tumors themselves are not usually referred to as "tumor markers." Tumor markers may be of two types: those elaborated by the tumors themselves and those produced by the host in response to the tumor. The former are the most useful group of markers. Many of these represent fetal gene products that are normally unexpressed or marginally expressed in adult tissues. In general, no markers are absolutely specific: most are made at low levels in the disease-free state, in nonneo-plastic disease, and in a variety of different tumors. For example, circulating α-fetoprotein, normally abundant in fetal liver, is frequently seen in hepatocellular carci-noma; however, serum levels are also high in some yolk sac–derived tumors (testis) and other gastrointestinal tumors. It is present at low levels in sera from normal persons and can rise in cirrhosis, hepatocellular necro-sis, hepatitis, and metastatic liver disease and in new-borns with spina bifida. In addition to α-fetoprotein, carcinoembryonic antigen (CEA; colon, lung breast), human chorionic gonadotropin (HCG; trophoblastic and germ cell tumors), calcitonin (medullary carcinoma of

Table 14-9. Some useful tumor markers

Marker	Common designation	Cancers
Alpha-fetoprotein	AFP	Liver, testis
CA-125 glycoprotein	CA-125	Ovary
Calcitonin		Medullary carcinoma of thyroid
Carcinoembryonic antigen	CEA	Colon, lung, breast
Gamma-glutamyl transferase	GGT	Liver, gastrointestinal tumors, lung cancer
Human chorionic gonadotropin	HCG	Trophoblastic tumors, germ cell tumors (testis)
Immunoglobulins (spike)		Multiple myeloma
Neuron-specific enolase	NSE	Small-cell carcinoma (lung), neuroblastoma, other tumors
Prostate-specific antigen	PSA	Adenocarcinoma of prostate
Prostatic acid phosphatase		Adenocarcinoma of prostate

Modified from Virji, M., Mercer, D.W., and Herberman, R.B.: CA **38**:104, 1988; Tseleni-Balafoura, S., and Kittas, C.: Arch. Pathol. Lab. Med. **112**:115, 1988; Taniguchi, N., Iizuka, S., Zhe, Z.N., House, S., Yokosawa, N., Ono, M., Kinoshita, K., Makita, A., and Sekiya, C.: Cancer Res. **45**:5835-5839, 1985.

the thyroid), prostatic acid phosphatase (prostate), and immunoglobulins (multiple myeloma) are in routine use. Other newer tumor markers including prostate-specific antigen (PSA; prostate), CA-125 (ovary), and neuron-specific enolase (small-cell carcinoma of the lung, neuroblastoma) are also useful, though the specificity of the last marker has been called into question (summarized in reference 145).

INTERRELATIONSHIP OF TUMOR AND HOST

Benign tumors affect the host primarily because of their size or location; a small but important minority may have life-threatening effects through products they secrete. A large benign tumor may be only a nuisance or a cosmetic problem. Because benign tumors, especially the larger ones, often undergo retrogressive changes, such as infarction and hemorrhage, they may show a sudden increase in size, giving the false impression of rapid cellular growth. Even a small benign tumor, however, may at times be of importance to the host because of location. For example, a tumor in the region of the ampulla of Vater may be less than 1 cm in diameter and still cause severe biliary obstruction, and an ependymal tumor near the sylvian aqueduct may result in hydrocephalus. Some benign endocrine tumors, even when small, may produce excessive amounts of hormone and result in life-threatening symptoms. The production of insulin by some islet cell adenomas with its resulting hypoglycemia and the secretion of parathyroid hormone by parathyroid adenoma with its resulting hypercalcemia are two examples.

Malignant neoplasms produce major effects on the host as they increase in mass and destroy normal tissues both locally and at distant sites. These effects are in general the result of several features in addition to loss of function after tissue destruction: the release of toxic metabolites or bioactive molecules after tissue destruction or tumor necrosis; the release of hormones, growth factors, and regulatory molecules by the tumor; psychosocial responses to cancer (anxiety, depression, listlessness); destruction of normal tissues during treatment (hematopoietic and lymphoid tissues and oral and gastrointestinal mucosa are particularly sensitive to chemotherapy and radiotherapy). Sometimes the molecular basis of symptoms is easily understood, as with endocrine tumors, the products of which are well characterized. In other cases such as the action of tumor- or host-synthesized growth factors we are nearing an understanding of effects in selected instances; the analysis of TGF-β and its effects is an example. However, it will probably be many years before all these factors are known and characterized and their host effects are fully appreciated (see the following paragraph and Table 14-4).

More complicated are conditions like anemia and cachexia, the generalized wasting seen in cancer patients mentioned earlier. Anemia may result from replacement of large portions of the marrow by tumor (metastasis), destruction of hematopoietic cells by therapy, or marrow shutdown resulting from synthesis of negative regulatory factors by tumors and so on. Similarly cachexia probably results in part from the action of powerful inhibitors of cell growth (cachectin/tumor necrosis factor, and other as yet undiscovered factors; it is worth noting again that TGF-β and müllerian inhibiting substance have selective inhibitory actions) and in part from lack of appetite, anemia, and infection as a result of the more general systemic effects of cancer, psychosocial factors, and treatment. Another consequence of advanced disease is infection, and cancer patients frequently die of bronchopneumonia, often caused by opportunistic bacteria or fungi.

There are innumerable other but inconstant systemic effects produced by tumors ("paraneoplastic epiphenomena"). Since the mechanisms of their development are poorly understood, only a few are mentioned as examples: dermatomyositis may develop in patients with various types of cancer; unexplained peripheral neuritis and degenerative brain changes may occur in cancer patients; and acanthosis nigricans (a hyperpigmented, keratotic skin lesion) indicates the likelihood of carcinoma, usually of the stomach. Many tumor effects are biochemical. For example, there may be a disturbed salt metabolism in some patients who have small-cell carcinoma of the lung; there may be a diminution or elevation of various serum enzymes, such as the acid phosphatase that often is elevated in patients with prostatic cancer. Many changes in the blood, especially in serum proteins, have been reported in cancer patients, such as a deficiency in specific proteins or the presence of abnormal proteins. Since increased coagulability of the blood may complicate cancers, particularly those of the pancreas and stomach, the development of sudden unexplained thrombotic episodes indicates the possibility of cancer of the upper abdomen.

The following are some additional examples of inconsistent effects produced by tumors:

Hematologic
    Anemia, erythrocytosis, thrombocytopenia, thrombocytosis, leukemoid reaction, abnormal serum proteins
Dermatologic
    Pruritus, urticaria, erythema, hyperpigmentation, dermatomyositis
Neurologic
    Neuropathy, myelopathy, encephalopathy
Skeletal
    Osteoporosis, osteomalacia
Systemic
    Fever, night sweats

One of the interesting challenges of clinical investigation is the analysis of these effects in molecular terms. There is also a large number of endocrine syndromes that result from ectopic hormone production by tumors. Thus tumors may secrete ACTH, vasoactive peptides, somatomedins, gastrin, parathyroid hormone–like polypeptides, serotonin, calcitonin, vasopressin (ADH), renin, glucocorticoids, sex hormones, glucagon, and insulin.

COURSE AND TREATMENT

Benign tumors not only grow slowly but also at times reach a point where they seem to become dormant or even to regress. This is true, for example, with leiomyomas of the uterus, which often cease growing after menopause. Occasionally even malignant tumors enter a stage of dormancy, and in rare but well-documented instances they may regress spontaneously. Spontaneous regression is defined as the complete or partial disappearance of cancer that cannot be attributed to treatment. The explanations for the phenomenon are inconclusive. Cancers of many different sites and types have shown such regression, the more common being renal cell carcinoma, neuroblastoma, choriocarcinoma, and malignant melanoma; however, complete spontaneous disappearance of a malignant tumor is extremely rare.

The more typical and usual course of untreated cancer is continuous local and metastatic extension with progressive systemic effects, all of which combine to weaken the host in diverse ways until cachexia and death from sepsis or bronchopneumonia, or both, ensue. About half of the deaths in cancer patients result from infections, the most common being bronchopneumonia, septicemia, and peritonitis. The majority of infections are caused by gram-negative bacilli or fungi. Other causes of death in these patients include organ failure, tumor infarction and hemorrhage, and carcinomatosis (widespread dissemination of the tumor).

With treatment, many tumors, though not cured, may persist for years before ultimately causing death. Some patients live many years with cancer even without treatment. Daland studied 100 cases of untreated cancer of the breast and found that 22% of the patients were alive at the end of 5 years and 5% at the end of 10 years; the last surviving patients died 13 years after their first symptoms.

Although an extensive description[93] of cancer therapy is beyond the scope of this chapter, we present a broad outline of general principles. First, no therapy of any sort should be initiated without a definitive diagnosis including histopathologic or appropriate cytopathologic examination accompanied or followed by appropriate grading and staging procedures. For some tumors, surgery remains the only effective treatment, and the extent to which surgical management of recurrences is possible will reflect survival. Thus for adenocarcinoma of the colon or malignant melanoma surgical treatment is essential, since there are no standard effective chemotherapies or radiotherapies for these diseases. However, in other cases such as Hodgkin's disease, Wilms' tumor, choriocarcinoma, and acute lymphocytic leukemia various combinations of chemotherapy, radiotherapy, and surgery often achieve cures. Most tumors show some response to chemotherapy or radiation therapy, and treatment sometimes results in cures and usually gives symptomatic relief (palliation). For example, the severe pain of carcinoma of the prostate metastatic to bone may be controlled for a time by the lowering of androgen levels (orchiectomy). Cancer of the breast in premenopausal women may respond favorably to antiestrogens (tamoxifen), removal of estrogen (oophorectomy, adrenalectomy, hypophysectomy), or testosterone administration.

Anticancer drugs now in use, in addition to hormones and other steroid compounds, include alkylating agents (cisplatin), antimetabolites (5-fluorouracil), and miscellaneous drugs, such as urethan and actinomycin D. In some instances chemotherapeutic drugs produce a favorable and even a prolonged response. Since such agents interfere with the synthesis of nucleic acids and proteins, not only tumor cells but also normal cells are often destroyed, and one of the elusive goals of drug development is identification of agents that have more selective anticancer effects. Standard practice is to rotate anticancer drugs as patients become refractory. Often, however, patients show cross-resistance of chemically unrelated drugs; this phenomenon, known as "multidrug resistance," results from more efficient drug efflux and metabolism.[95]

Radiation therapy is often very effective because treatment can be delivered to precise areas without systemic effects. Thus, for example, in some series the survival rates for prostatic cancer after radiation therapy are comparable to surgery. Radiosensitivity refers to the responsiveness of a tumor to ionizing radiation, which like alkylating agents brings about cell death by damaging cellular targets (DNA, the mitotic apparatus, cell membranes). In general, poorly differentiated tumors respond to radiation well and better-differentiated tumors respond poorly. There are, however, major exceptions to this. It is important to remember that radiosensitivity and radiocurability are not synonymous. In fact, some of the most radiosensitive tumors are seldom cured by this treatment. This apparent paradox results from the fact that poorly differentiated tumors are often fast growing and have a high proportion of cells in sensitive phases of the cell cycle (the S, M, and G_2) whereas slow-growing well-differentiated tumors may consist largely of G_0 and G_1 cells.

Recently agents referred to under the generic rubric

of biologic response modifiers have been used in cancer therapy and chemoprevention. These include the tumor-specific antibodies, interferons, the interleukins, and autologous cells activated in vitro by these and similar factors. There is great enthusiasm among oncologists for the use of these biologic response modifiers, but judged against standard therapies, gains have been modest. Clinical trials are also underway to determine the effectiveness of vitamin A and retinoids in chemoprevention.[15,90,106,126,127,154] These agents presumably act by promoting differentiation.

DEMOGRAPHIC AND FAMILIAL ASPECTS OF CANCER

Demographic and geographic factors. In this section we examine demographic and geographic aspects of cancer and, where possible, relate them to etiology. In the introduction we mentioned that in 1988 about 500,000 people died of cancer in the United States. For all ages cancer was the second leading cause of death behind heart disease. Lung cancer is now estimated to be the leading cause of cancer death in men, whereas in women lung and breast cancer are tied for first place (Table 14-10 and Fig. 14-32). In men lung cancer as a cause of death is followed by colon and rectal cancer, prostate cancer, and leukemias and lymphomas, in that order. Death rates, however, tell only part of the story: for example, the incidence of clinically significant prostate cancer and lung cancer in men is equal, but prostatic cancer is more easily controlled albeit with considerable morbidity. In women after lung and breast cancer, colon and rectal cancer and leukemias and lymphomas are the leading causes of death.

Over the past 50 years there have been dramatic changes in death rates from some cancers. Lung cancer death rates have increased more than tenfold in men and almost tenfold in women and probably reflect primarily increases in smoking during this period (Fig. 14-32). Recently in men the rate of increase has slowed, and this change may reflect a decline in smoking which began in the 1970s. Other important trends include a long-term decline in death rates for gastric cancer in both men and women, a change in the death rates for cancer of the uterus, and a dramatic rise in deaths from malignant melanoma in men and women. The decline in gastric cancer is believed to relate to some change in life-style, perhaps diet, but no generally accepted explanation has emerged. Reduced death rates from uterine cancer probably reflect better diagnosis and treatment as well as changes in life-style. Increases in the incidences of malignant melanoma and other skin cancers reflect population shifts to the sun belt and a more outdoor life-style among Americans. The disease is rare among blacks.

It is also instructive to look at death rates from cancer in different countries (Table 14-11). Even when differences in reporting and diagnosis and treatment are allowed for, differences in death rates can be dramatic. The death rate in Japan from stomach cancer is about eight times that in the United States, whereas death rates from breast and prostatic cancer are one fourth to one fifth the United States rate. Worldwide, liver cancer (hepatocellular carcinoma) is one of the commonest causes of death from cancer, yet in the U.S. only a small fraction of cancer deaths (about 1% to 2%) are the result of hepatocellular carcinoma.[23,81] In some parts of Africa cancer of the penis is very common, whereas it is rare in the United States.[105]

Over the decades, investigators have learned much about the etiology of cancer from these observations. For example, an analysis of Americans of Japanese descent indicated that their death rates from gastric and colonic cancer reflected those of the United States population not Japan's, thus ruling out a genetic component and suggesting an important role for life-style and environment. The distribution of liver cancer worldwide reflects the distribution of hepatitis B virus and, to some extent, aflatoxin contamination of foodstuffs and has implicated these agents as causes of hepatocellular carcinoma in humans.[8,81] Cancer of the penis is rare in circumsized men; its prevalence in some areas may reflect poor personal hygiene (and exposure to carcinogens and irritants) and endemic papillomavirus infections.

Occasionally there are strong regional trends within a country. In China, Linhsien in Honan Province has an extremely high incidence of cancer of the esophagus, which appears to be related to nitrosamines consumed in local pickled vegetables. In Uganda, Burkitt's lymphoma is confined to the humid lowlands and is believed to be related to mosquito-borne malarial infections (superimposed upon EBV infection). The role of infection is unknown, but one may speculate that it stimulates cell proliferation in the immune system under circumstances that are favorable for translocations (see section on etiology and pathogenesis).

Familial and genetic factors. Analysis of inherited and familial patterns of cancer incidence have provided important clues to etiology and contributed to prevention. A large number of tumors of childhood and infancy have a familial form; these include retinoblastoma, Wilms' tumor, and hepatoblastoma and are frequently associated with chromosomal abnormalities.[71,72] In retinoblastoma, tumors have been associated with deletions on chromosome 13 (some of which are detectable only by genetic probes).[71] It appears that most familial cases can be explained by the inheritance of a mutation in one copy of a gene and a somatic mutation in the second. It has been suggested that this gene functions to prevent the development of neoplasia

Table 14-10. Estimated cancer deaths by sex for all sites—United States, 1987

Site	Total	Male	Female
All sites	483,000	259,000	224,000
Buccal cavity and pharynx (oral)	9,400	6,350	3,050
Lip	175	150	25
Tongue	2,100	1,400	700
Mouth	2,825	1,800	1,025
Pharynx			
Digestive organs	119,900	62,400	57,500
Esophagus	8,800	6,400	2,400
Stomach	14,200	8,300	5,900
Small intestine	800	400	400
Large intestine	52,000	25,000	27,000
Rectum	8,000	4,100	3,900
Liver and biliary passage	10,600	5,300	5,300
Pancreas	24,300	12,300	12,000
Other and unspecified digestive	1,200	600	600
Respiratory system	141,250	96,000	45,250
Larynx	3,800	3,100	700
Lung	136,000	92,000	44,000
Other and unspecified respiratory	1,450	900	550
Bone	1,400	800	600
Connective tissue	2,800	1,300	1,500
Skin	7,800*	4,800	3,000
Breast	41,300	300	41,000
Genital organs	50,150	27,650	22,500
Cervix, uterus	6,800	—	6,800
Corpus, endometrium	2,900	—	2,900
Ovary	11,700	—	11,700
Other and unspecified genital, female	1,100	—	1,100
Prostate	27,000	27,000	—
Testis	400	400	—
Other and unspecified genital, male	250	250	—
Urinary organs	20,000	12,900	7,100
Bladder	10,600	7,200	3,400
Kidney and other urinary	9,400	5,700	3,700
Eye	300	150	150
Brain and central nervous system	10,200	5,500	4,700
Endocrine glands	1,800	750	1,050
Thyroid	1,100	400	700
Other endocrine	700	350	350
Leukemias	17,800	9,800	8,000
Lymphocytic leukemia	6,800	3,900	2,900
Granulocytic leukemia	10,500	5,600	4,900
Monocytic leukemia	500	300	200
Other blood and lymph tissues	24,900	12,800	12,100
Hodgkin's disease	1,500	900	600
Multiple myeloma	8,000	4,100	3,900
Other lymphomas	15,400	7,800	7,600
All other and unspecified sites	34,000	17,500	16,500

From Cancer facts and figures—1988, New York, 1988, American Cancer Society.
*Melanoma 5,800; other skin 2,000.

Table 14-11. Age-adjusted cancer death rates per 100,000 people—selected countries, 1980-1981

Country	Colon and rectum		Stomach		Breast	Prostate	Leukemia	
	Males	Females	Males	Females	Females	Males	Males	Females
United States	25.1	18.2	8.2	3.9	26.6	22.7	8.7	5.2
Brazil	2.4	2.5	9.0	4.2	5.3	3.7	2.5	2.0
Greece	7.3	6.6	15.5	8.9	17.4	10.9	8.1	4.9
Japan	16.4	11.6	63.1	30.3	6.4	4.1	4.9	3.2
Singapore	21.8	20.6	32.3	17.2	17.3	5.0	3.3	3.9

From Cancer facts and figures—1988, New York, 1988, American Cancer Society.

(that is, as an "antioncogene," or suppressor gene) and its inactivation by mutation results in tumors. Recently the gene has been cloned and is now being studied.[41,43]

Another class of inherited disorders associated with an increased incidence of tumors includes syndromes associated with increased rates of mutation or chromosomal instability, or both. Xeroderma pigmentosum, ataxia telangiectasia, Fanconi's anemia, and Bloom's syndrome are members of this group. Xeroderma pigmentosum is associated with more than a 1000-fold increased risk of skin cancer on exposed skin surfaces.[73] Although the causes of the genetic instability are unknown in the latter three syndromes, all show increased incidences of neoplasia. Patients with ataxia telangiectasia have an increase in leukemias and lymphomas as well as other cancers.[52,133] There is a large increase in leukemia rates in patients with Fanconi's anemia and in heterozygotic relatives and carriers.[4] Patients with Bloom's syndrome are particularly susceptible to the development of leukemia and to a lesser extent other cancers.[45] Because rearrangements are common in leukemias, cancer development may be related to the high rates of sister-chromatic exchange seen in this syndrome.

A variety of uncommon syndromes is also associated with an increased incidence of human cancer.[70] Two multiple endocrine adenomatosis syndromes predispose to pituitary, parathyroid, and islet cell adenomas (type 1) and to pheochromocytoma, medullary carcinoma of the thyroid and parathyroid hyperplasia/adenoma (type 2). Because the type and occurrence of tumors is so varied in the first of these syndromes, it has been proposed that a mechanism similar to that described for retinoblastoma may be responsible, except that the gene is expressed in many tissues.[70] Type 2 is inherited in a dominant fashion, and one of the genes involved has been localized to chromosome 10.[122] Neurofibromatosis (von Recklinghausen's disease) is a dominant condition that predisposes to neurofibroma (and sarcoma), pheochromocytoma, meningioma, and glioma. Different pedigrees appear to have different tumor dis-

tributions, a finding that may implicate different genes or different allelic variants. Basal cell nevus syndrome is dominantly inherited and results in a high frequency of basal cell carcinomas as well as osseous, neurologic, and endocrine stigmas. The relation between a dominant mode of inheritance and the appearance of basal cell carcinomas during the second decade on skin exposed to solar radiation is not understood.[70]

Breast cancer, colon cancer, and renal cancer are known to be familial (though not necessarily inherited) to varying degrees. Female relatives of breast cancer patients have a two- to threefold increased risk of developing breast cancer.[83] There are also pedigrees in which cancer of both the female and male breast are inherited, thus demonstrating that genetic events are involved in at least some cases.[170] Studies of changes in oncogene expression and loss of heterozygosity (see section on etiology and pathogenesis) should be helpful in unraveling the relation among hereditary factors, somatic cell mutation, and other factors (such as hormonal status, ethanol consumption, and fat consumption) in the etiology of breast cancer. Although colon cancer is not strongly familial, in patients with multiple polyposis (a dominantly inherited disorder) the incidence of colon cancer approaches 100%. This observation is significant because most colonic carcinomas are thought to arise in polyps and prophylactic colectomy is warranted in patients with polyposis. Further, the gene predisposing to familial polyposis is on the long arm of chromosome 5 and about 20% of colonic carcinomas show loss of heterozygosity in this region.[18,125] This finding provides a valuable link between inherited predisposition to colon cancer and nonfamilial cancer; it is easy to imagine, for example, that dietary mutagens (carcinogens) might act at this locus as well as others such as K-ras.[19,39] Finally, occasional families in which renal cell carcinoma is inherited show translocations on chromosome 3; in 11 cases of nonhereditary renal cell carcinoma, tumor tissue showed loss of alleles from this chromosome,[167] once again providing a valuable link between inherited and acquired neoplasia.

ACKNOWLEDGMENT

We thank Paul H. Duray, Anwar Farhood, Peter M. Howley, Alfred G. Knudson, W. Thomas London, Harold L. Moses, Ibrahim Ramzy, J.J. Steinberg, Thomas S. Winokur, and Stuart H. Yuspa for their valuable suggestions.

Glossary

allele The designation of a gene copy to indicate that it differs in sequence from other copies of the same gene.

adenocarcinoma Malignant tumor of glandular epithelium.

adenoma Benign tumor of glandular epithelium.

anaplasia State of being undifferentiated or primitive, lacking identifiable features.

aplasia Lack of development of an organ or tissue.

atrophy Diminution in size of cells, organ, or tissue after full development has been attained.

benign Pertaining to a neoplasm that grows slowly, remains localized, and usually does little harm; rarely used synonym, benignant.

cachexia Severe wasting of body tissues because of a chronic disease such as cancer.

cancer Malignant neoplasm.

carcinogen An agent that produces tumors or cancer, often used as a synonym for chemical carcinogen.

carcinoma Malignant tumor of epithelium.

carcinoma in situ Malignant epithelial tumor showing no invasion.

carcinosarcoma A cancer containing a mixture of carcinomatous and sarcomatous elements.

cystadenoma Benign tumor of glandular epithelium forming cysts.

cytology Literally, study of cells; in current usage, study of exfoliated cells for purpose of diagnosing cancer.

desmoplasia Excessive fibrous tissue formation in tumor stroma.

differentiated Possessing cellular maturity and organization similar to normal.

dysplasia Abnormal, atypical cellular proliferation; not tumor.

epidermoid carcinoma Cancer of squamous epithelium; synonym, squamous cell carcinoma.

grade Estimate of the degree of malignancy of a tumor.

hamartoma Malformation of tissues indigenous to area resembling and having some features of tumor.

hyperplasia Increase in number of cells per unit of tissue.

hypertrophy Increase in size of cells, organ, or tissue.

invasion Local extension of tumor into surrounding tissue, a hallmark of cancer.

lymphoma A cancer (malignant neoplasm) arising in lymphoid tissue; unless specified, synonymous with malignant lymphoma.

malignant Pertaining to a neoplasm with ability to invade, metastasize, and cause death; synonym rarely used, malign.

medullary 'Marrowlike'; gross description term for soft and presumably highly cellular tumor.

metaplasia Change of a type of adult cell to one not normally present in that tissue.

metastasis Growth of a tumor at a distant (discontinuous) site, a hallmark of cancer.

mixed tumor Literally, tumor with mixed elements; in common usage, term often applied to specific type of tumor arising mostly in salivary glands.

neoplasm New growth, tumor.

oncogene A gene capable of transforming cells in culture or inducing tumors in animals and often first identified in an oncogenic virus.

oncogenic That which produces tumors, such as oncogenic virus.

oncology Study of tumors.

papilloma Benign epithelial tumor in which neoplastic cells cover fingerlike processes of stroma; also any benign epithelial tumor growing outward from surface.

pearls Collections of keratins formed in well-differentiated epidermoid carcinomas.

pleomorphism Variability in morphology, especially in size and shape.

polyp Tumor or tumorlike mass projecting from mucosal surface.

promoter Region of a gene that controls its transcription (RNA synthesis); see also *tumor promoter*.

proto-oncogene A genomic sequence capable of being converted to an oncogene by mutation, deletion, or rearrangement.

sarcoma Nonepithelial malignant tumor; includes most cancers of mesodermal tissues, such as connective tissue, muscle, and lymphoid tissue.

scirrhous (pronounced skir′us or sir′us) Gross descriptive term for tumor that is firm because of extensive desmoplasia.

squamous cell carcinoma Cancer of squamous epithelium; synonymous with epidermoid carcinoma.

stage Estimate of extent of spread of cancer.

teratology Study of abnormal embryonic development and congenital malformations.

teratoma True neoplasm arising from totipotential cells and composed therefore of numerous types of tissues.

transcription The process by which RNA is copied from DNA.

tumor In older usage, any swelling; current usage, synonym for neoplasm.

tumor promoter An agent that enhances the rate of appearance or yield of tumors.

REFERENCES

1. Abelson, P.H.: Cancer phobia, Science **237**:473, 1987.
2. Abraham, J.A., Mergia, A., Whang, J.L., and Tumolo, A., Friedman, J., Hjerrild, K.A., Gospodarowicz, D., and Fiddes, J.C.: Nucleotide sequence of a bovine clone encoding the angiogenic protein, basic fibroblast growth factor, Science **233**:545, 1986.
3. Ali, I.U., Lidereau, R., Theillet, C., and Callahan, R.: Reduction to homozygosity of genes on chromosome 11 in human breast neoplasia, Science **238**:185, 1987.
4. Alter, B.P., and Potter, N.U.: Long-term outcome in Fanconi's anaemia: description of 26 cases and review of the literature. In German, J., editor: Chromosome mutation and neoplasia, New York, 1983, Alan R. Liss, Inc.
5. Ames, B.N., Magaw, R., and Gold, L.S.: Ranking possible carcinogenic hazards, Science **236**:271, 1987.
6. Anzano, M.A., Roberts, A.B., De Larco, J.E., Wakefield, L.M., Assoian, R.K., Roche, N.S., Smith, J.M., Lazarus, J.E., and Sporn, M.B.: Increased secretion of type β transforming growth factor accompanies viral transformation of cells, Mol. Cell. Biol. **5**:242, 1985.
7. Argyris, T.S.: Regeneration and the mechanism of epidermal tumor promotion, CRC Crit. Rev. Toxicol. **14**:211, 1985.
8. Autrup, H., Seremet, T., Wakhisi, J., and Wasunna, A.: Aflatoxin exposure measured by urinary excretion of aflatoxin B_1-guanine adduct and hepatitis B virus infection in areas with different liver cancer incidence in Kenya, Cancer Res. **47**:3430, 1987.
9. Balmain, A., and Pragnell, I.: Mouse skin carcinomas induced in vivo by chemical carcinogens have a transforming Harvey-ras oncogene, Nature **303**:72, 1983.
10. Barbacid, M.: ras genes, Annu. Rev. Biochem. **56**:779, 1987.
11. Bar-Sagi, D., and Feramisco, J.R.: Microinjection of the ras oncogene protein into PC12 cells induces morphological differentiation, Cell **42**:841, 1985.
12. Baserga, R.: The relationship of the cell cycle to tumor growth and control of cell division: a review, Cancer Res. **25**:581, 1965.
13. Beasely, R.P., Lin, C.C., Hwang, L., and Chien, C.: Hepatocellular carcinoma and hepatitis B virus: a prospective study of 22,707 men in Taiwan, Lancet **2**:1129, 1981.
14. Bernstein, S.C., and Weinberg, R.A.: Expression of the metastatic phenotype in cells transfected with human metastatic tumor DNA, Proc. Natl. Acad. Sci. USA **82**:1726, 1985.
15. Bertram, J.S., Kolonel, L.N., and Meyskens, F.L.: Rationale and strategies for chemoprevention of cancer in humans, Cancer Res. **47**:3012, 1987.
16. Bishop, J.M.: Cellular oncogenes and retroviruses, Annu. Rev. Biochem. **52**:301, 1983.
17. Bitran, J.D., Golomb, H.M., Little, A.G., and Weichselbaum, R.R.: Lung cancer: a comprehensive treatise, New York, 1988, Grune & Stratton, Inc.
18. Bodmer, W.F., Bailey, C.J., Bodmer, J., Bussey, H.J.R., Ellis, A., Gorman, P., Lucibello, F.C., Murday, V.A., Rider, S.H., Scambler, P., Sheer, D., Solomon, E., and Spurr, N.K.: Localization of the gene for familial adenomatous polyposis on chromosome 5, Nature **328**:614, 1987.
19. Bos, J.L., Fearon, E.R., Hamilton, S.R., Verlaan-de Vries, M., van Boom, J.H., van der Eb, A.J., and Vogelstein, B.: Prevalence of ras gene mutations in human colorectal cancers, Nature **327**:293, 1987.
20. Boveri, T.: Zur Frage der Entstehung maligner Tumoren, Jena, 1914, Gustav Fischer.
21. Brauch, H., Johnson, B., Hovis, J., Yano, T., Gazdar, A., Pettengill, O.S., Graziano, S., Sorensen, G.D., Poiesz, B.J., Minna, J., Linehan, M., and Zbar, B.: Molecular analysis of the short arm of the chromosome 5 in small-cell and non–small-cell carcinoma of the lung, N. Engl. J. Med. **317**:1109, 1987.
22. Brodeur G., Seeger, R., Schwab, M., Varmus, H.E., and Bishop, J.M.: Amplification of N-myc in untreated human neuroblastomas correlates with advanced disease stage, Science **224**:1121, 1984.
23. Cancer facts and figures—1988, New York, 1988, American Cancer Society, pp. 32.
24. Cate, R.L., Mattaliano, R.J., Hession, C., Tizzard, R., Farber, N.M., Cheung, A., Ninfa, E.G., Frey, A.Z., Gash, D.J., Chow, E.P., Fisher, R.A., Bertonis, J.M., Torres, G., Wallner, B.P., Ramachandran, K.L., Ragin, R.C., Manganaro, T.F., MacLaughlin, D.R., and Donahoe, P.K.: Isolation of the bovine and human genes for müllerian inhibiting substance and expression of the human gene in animal cells, Cell **45**:685, 1986.
25. Chiu, R., Imagawa, M., Imbra, R.J., Bockoven, J.R., and Karin, M.: Multiple cis- and trans-acting elements mediate the transcriptional response to phorbol esters, Nature **329**:648, 1987.
26. Clark, W.H., Jr., Elder, D.E., Guerry, D., Epstein, M.N., Greene, M.H., and Van Horn, M.: A study of tumor progression: the precursor lesions of superficial spreading and nodular melanoma, Hum. Pathol. **15**:1147, 1984.
27. Cossman, J., Uppenkamp, M., Sundeen, J., Coupland, R., and Raffeld, M.: Molecular genetics and the diagnosis of lymphoma, Arch. Pathol. Lab. Med. **112**:117, 1988.
28. Davies, R.L., Weintraub, H., and Lassar, A.B.: Expression of a single transfected cDNA converts fibroblasts to myoblasts, Cell **51**:987, 1987.
29. De Jong, D., Voetdijk, B.M.H., Beverstock, G.C., van Ommen, G.J.B., Willemze, R., and Kluin, P.M.: Activation of the c-myc oncogene in a precursor-B-cell blast crisis of follicular lymphoma, presenting as composite lymphoma, N. Engl. J. Med. **318**:1373, 1988.
30. Della-Favera, R., Bregni, M., Erikson, J., Patterson, D., Gallo, R.C., and Croce, C.M.: Human c-myc onc gene is located on the region of chromosome 8 that is translocated in Burkitt lymphoma cells, Proc. Nat. Acad. Sci. USA **79**:7824, 1982.
31. Deuel, T.F., and Senior, R.M.: Growth factors in fibrotic disease, N. Engl. J. Med. **317**:236, 1987.
32. Doll, R., and Peto, R.: The causes of cancer, Oxford, 1981, Oxford University Press.
33. Doll, R., and Peto, R.: The causes of cancer: quantitative estimates of avoidable risks of cancer in the United States today, J. Natl. Cancer Inst. **66**:1191, 1981.
34. Duray, P.H., Palazzo, J., Gown, A.M., and Ohuchi, N.: Melanoma cell heterogeneity: a study of two monoclonal antibodies compared to S-100 protein in paraffin sections, Cancer **61**(12):2460, 1988.
35. Escot, C., Theillet, C., Lidereau, R., Spyratos, F., Champeme, M.-H., Gest, J., and Callahan, R.: Genetic alteration of the c-myc protooncogene (MYC) in human primary breast carcinomas, Proc. Natl. Acad. Sci. USA **83**:4834, 1986.
36. Farber, E., and Cameron, R.: The sequential analysis of cancer development, Adv. Cancer Res. **31**:125, 1980.
37. Fidler, I.J.: Selection of successive tumour lines for metastasis, Nature **242**:148, 1973.
38. Fidler, I.J., Gerstein, D.M., and Hart, I.R.: The biology of cancer invasion and metastasis, Adv. Cancer Res. **28**:149, 1978.
39. Forrester, K., Almoguera, C., Han, K., Grizzle, W.E., and Perucho, M.: Detection of high incidence of K-ras oncogenes during human colon tumorigenesis, Nature **327**:298, 1987.
40. Friedberg, E.C.: DNA repair, New York, 1984, W.H. Freeman & Co.
41. Friend, S.H., Bernards, R., Rogelj, S., Weinberg, R.A., Rapaport, J.M., Albert, D.M., and Dryja, T.P.: A human DNA segment with properties of the gene that predisposes to retinoblastoma and osteosarcoma, Nature **323**:643, 1986.
42. Friend, S.H., Dryja, T.P., and Weinberg, R.A.: Oncogenes and tumor-suppressing genes, N. Engl. J. Med. **318**:618, 1988.
43. Friend, S.H., Horowitz, J.M., Gerber, M.R., et al.: Deletions of a DNA sequence in both retinoblastoma and mesenchymal tumors: organization of the sequence and its encoded protein, Proc. Natl. Acad. Sci. USA **84**:9059, 1987.
44. Garbisa, S., Pozzatti, R., Muschel, R.J., Saffotti, U., Ballin, M., Khoury, G., and Liotta, L.A.: Secretion of type IV collagenolytic protease and metastatic phenotype: induction by transfection with c-Ha-ras but not c-Ha-ras plus AD2-E1a, Cancer Res. **47**:1523, 1987.
45. German, J.: Bloom's syndrome. II. The prototype of human genetic disorders predisposing to chromosome instability and can-

cer. In German, J., editor: Chromosomes and cancer, New York, 1974, John Wiley & Sons.

46. Gilman, J.P.W., and Swierenga, S.H.H.: Inorganic carcinogenesis. In Searle, C.E., editor: Chemical carcinogens, American Chemical Society Monogr. 182, Washington, D.C., 1984, pp. 577.

47. Gilmour, S.K., Verma, A.K., Madara, T., and O'Brien, T.G.: Regulation of ornithine decarboxylase gene expression in mouse epidermis and epidermal tumors during two-stage tumorigenesis, Cancer Res. 47:1221, 1987.

48. Goustin, A.S., Leof, E.B., Shipley, G.D., and Moses, H.L.: Growth factors and cancer, Cancer Res. 46:1015, 1986.

49. Grieg, R.G., Koestler, T.P., Trainer, D.L., Corwin, S.P., Miles, L., Kline, T., Sweet, R., Yokoyama, S., and Poste, G.: Tumorigenic and metastatic properties of "normal" and ras-transfected NIH/3T3 cells, Proc. Natl. Acad. Sci. USA 82:3698, 1985.

50. Groffen, J., Stephenson, J.R., Heisterkamp, N., De Kline, A., Bartram, C.R., and Grosveld, G.: Philadelphia chromosome breakpoints are clustered within a limited region, bcr, on chromosome 22, Cell 36:93, 1984.

51. Grussendorf-Conen, E.-I., Deutz, F.J., and de Villiers, E.M.: Detection of human papillomavirus-6 in primary carcinoma of the urethra in men, Cancer 60:1832, 1987.

52. Harnden, D.G.: Ataxia telangiectasia syndrome: cytogenetic and cancer aspects. In German, J., editor: Chromosomes and cancer, New York, 1974, John Wiley & Son.

53. Health Consequences of Smoking, Public Health Service Publication no. 1696, 1967, pp. 227.

54. Hedley, D.W., Rugg, C.A., and Gelber, R.D.: Association of DNA index and S-phase fraction with prognosis of nodes positive early breast cancer, Cancer Res. 47:4729, 1987.

55. Heim, S., and Mitelman, F.: Cancer cytogenetics, New York, 1987, Alan R. Liss, pp. 309.

56. Henle, W., and Henle, G.: Epstein-Barr virus and human malignancies, Adv. in Viral Oncology 5:201, 1985.

57. Hirai, H., Kobayashi, Y., Mano, H., Hagiwara, K., Maru, Y., Omine, M., Mizoguchi, H., Nishida, J., and Takatsu, F.: A point mutation at codon 13 of the N-ras oncogene in myelodysplastic syndrome, Nature 327:430, 1987.

58. Howley, P.M.: Principles of carcinogenesis (viral). In Devita, V.P., Jr., Hellman, S., and Rosenberg, S.A., editors: Cancer: principle and practice of oncology, ed. 3, Philadelphia, 1989, J.B. Lippincott Co.

59. Humphries, M.J., Olden, K., and Yamada, K.M.: A synthetic peptide from fibronectin inhibits experimental metastasis of murine melanoma cells, Science 233:467, 1986.

60. Ignotz, R.A., and Massagué, J.: Cell adhesion protein receptors as targets for transforming growth factor-β action, Cell 51:189, 1987.

61. Isaacs, J.T., Brendler, C.B., and Walsh, P.C.: Changes in the metabolism of dihydrotestosterone in the hyperplastic human prostate, J. Clin. Endocrinol. Metab. 56:139, 1983.

62. ISCN: An international system for human cytogenetic nomenclature, Birth defects: Original Art. Ser., vol. 21, no. 1, New York, National Foundation–March of Dimes.

63. Iwamoto, Y., Robey, F.A., Graf, J., Sasaki, M., Kleinman, H.K., Yamada, Y., and Martin, G.R.: YIGSR, a synthetic laminin pentapeptide, inhibits experimental metastasis formation, Science 238:1132, 1987.

64. Jaye, M., Howk, R., Burgess, W., Ricca, G.A., Chiu, M.C., Ravera, M.W., O'Brien, S.J., Modi, W.S., Maciag, T., and Drohan, W.N.: Human endothelial cell growth factor: cloning, nucleotide sequence, and chromosome localization, Science 233:541, 1986.

65. Kaufmann, W.K., Mackenzie, S.A., and Kaufman, D.G.: Quantitative relationship between hepatocytic neoplasms and islands of cellular alteration during hepatocarcinogenesis in the male F344 rat, Am. J. Pathol. 119:171, 1985.

66. Kehrl, J.H., Alvarez-Mon, M., Delsing, G.A., and Fauci, A.S.: Lymphotoxin is an important T cell–derived growth factor for human B cells, Science 238:1144, 1987.

67. Kimchi, A., Wang, X.F., Weinberg, R.A., Cheifetz, S., and Massagué, J.: Absence of TGF-β receptors and growth inhibitory responses in retinoblastoma cells, Science 240:196, 1988.

68. Klein, G.: Lymphoma development in mice and human: diversity of initiation is followed by convergent cytogenetic evolution, Proc. Natl. Acad. Sci. USA 76:2442, 1979.

69. Klein, G., and Klein, E.: Evolution of tumors and the impact of molecular oncology, Nature 315:190, 1985.

70. Knudson, A.G.: Genetics and etiology of human cancer, Adv. Hum. Genet. 8:1, 1977.

71. Knudson, A.G., Jr.: Genetics of human cancer, Annu. Rev. Genet. 20:231, 1986.

72. Koufos, A., Hansen, M.F., Copeland, N.G., Jenkins, N.A., Lampkin, B.C., and Cavenee, W.K.: Loss of heterozygosity in three embryonal tumours suggests a common pathogenetic mechanism, Nature 316:330, 1985.

73. Kraemer, K.H., Lee, M.M., and Scotto, J.: Xeroderma pigmentosum: cutaneous, ocular, and neurologic abnormalities in 830 published cases, Arch. Dermatol. 123:241, 1987.

74. Land, H., Parada, L.F., and Weinberg, R.A.: Tumorigenic conversion of primary embryo fibroblasts requires at least two cooperating oncogenes, Nature 304:596, 1983.

75. Lebovitz, R.M.: Oncogenes as mediators of cell growth and differentiation, Lab. Invest. 55:249, 1986.

76. Lebovitz, R.M., and Lieberman, M.W.: Modulation of gene expression by oncogenes, Prog. Nucleic Acid Res. Mol. Biol. 35:73, 1988.

77. Leder, A., Pattengale, P.K., Kuo, A., Stewart, T.A., and Leder, P.: Consequences of widespread deregulation of the c-myc gene in transgenic mice: multiple neoplasms and normal development, Cell 45:485, 1986.

78. Levine, A.J.: Oncogenes of DNA tumor viruses, Cancer Res. 48:493, 1988.

79. Liotta, L.A.: Tumor invasion and metastasis: role of the extracellular matrix, Rhoads Memorial Award Lecture, Cancer Res. 46:1, 1986.

80. Liu, E., Hjelle, B., Morgan, R., Hecht, F., and Bishop, J.M.: Mutations of the Kirsten-ras proto-oncogene in human preleukemia, Nature 330:186, 1987.

81. London, W.T.: Primary hepatocellular carcinoma: etiology, pathogenesis, and prevention, Hum. Pathol. 12:1085-1097, 1981.

82. Lundberg, C., Skoog, L., Cavenee, W.K., and Nordenskjöld, M.: Loss of heterozygosity in human ductal breast tumors indicates a recessive mutation on chromosome 13, Proc. Natl. Acad. Sci. USA 84:2372, 1987.

83. MacMahon, B., Cole, P., and Brown, J.: Etiology of human breast cancer: a review, J. Natl. Cancer Inst. 50:21, 1973.

84. Macnab, J.C.M., Walkinshaw, S.A., Cordiner, J.W., and Clements, J.B.: Human papillomavirus in clinically and histologically normal tissue of patients with genital cancer, N. Engl. J. Med. 315:1052, 1986.

85. Matrisian, L.M., Leroy, P., Ruhlmann, C., Gesnel, M.-C., and Breathnach, R.: Isolation of the oncogene and epidermal growth factor–induced transin gene: complex control in rat fibroblasts, Mol. Cell. Biol. 6:1679, 1986.

86. Matrisian, L.M., Bowden, G.T., Krieg, P., Furstenberger, G., Briand, J.-P., Leroy, P., and Breathnach, R.: The mRNA coding for the secreted protease transin is expressed more abundantly in malignant than in benign tumors, Proc. Natl. Acad. Sci. USA 83:9413, 1986.

87. McCann, J., and Ames, B.N.: The salmonella/microsome mutagenicity test: predictive value for animal carcinogenicity. In Hiatt, H.H., Watson, J.D., and Winsten, J.A., editors: Origins of human cancer, Cold Spring Harbor, N.Y., 1977, Cold Spring Harbor Laboratory.

88. McCarthy, J.B., Basara, M.L., Palm, S.L., Sas, D.F., and Furcht, L.T.: The role of cell adhesion proteins—laminin and fibronectin—in the movement of malignant and metastatic cells, Cancer Metastasis Rev. 4:125, 1985.

89. Meijlink, F., Curran, T., Miller, A.D., and Verma, I.: Removal of a 67-base-pair sequence in the noncoding region of protoon-

cogene *fos* converts it to a transforming gene, Proc. Nat. Acad. Sci. **82**:4987, 1985.

90. Menkes, M.S., Comstock, G.W., Vuilleumier, J.P., Helsing, K.J., Rider, A.A., and Brookmeyer, R.: Serum beta-carotene, vitamins A and E, selenium, and the risk of lung cancer, N. Engl. J. Med. **315**:1250, 1986.

91. Molloy, C.J., and Laskin, J.D.: Specific alterations in keratin biosynthesis in mouse epidermis *in vivo* and in explant culture following a single exposure to the tumor promoter 12-O-tetradecanoylphorbol-13-acetate, Cancer Res. **47**:4674, 1987.

92. Moore, R.J., Gazak, J.M., Quebbeman, J.F., and Wilson, J.D.: Concentration of dihydrotestosterone and 3α-androstanediol in naturally occurring and androgen-induced prostatic hyperplasia in the dog, J. Clin. Invest. **64**:1003, 1979.

93. Moossa, A.R., Robson, M.C., and Schimpff, S.C.: Comprehensive textbook of oncology, Baltimore, 1986, The Williams & Wilkins Co.

94. Morris, C.M., Reeve, A.E., Fitzgerald, P.H., Hollings, P.E., Beard, M.E.J., and Heaton, D.C.: Genomic diversity correlates with clinical variation in Ph₁-negative chronic myeloid leukaemia, Nature **320**:281, 1986.

95. Moscov, J.A., and Cowan, K.H.: Multidrug resistance, J. Natl. Cancer Inst. **80**:14, 1988.

96. Müller, R., Curran, T., Müller, D., and Guilbert, L.: Induction of c-*fos* during myelomonocytic differentiation and macrophage proliferation, Nature **314**:546, 1985.

97. Müller, R.: Proto-oncogenes and differentiation, Trends Biochem. Sci. **11**:129, 1986.

98. Muschel, R.J., Williams, J.E., Lowy, D.R., and Liotta, L.A.: Harvey *ras* induction of metastatic potential depends upon oncogene activation and the type of recipient cell, Am. J. Pathol. **121**:1, 1985.

99. Ngan, B.-Y., Chen-Levy, Z., Weiss, L.M., Warnke, R.A., and Cleary, M.L.: Expression in non-Hodgkin's lymphoma of the *bcl*-2 protein associated with the t(14;18) chromosomal translocation, N. Engl. J. Med. **318**:1638, 1988.

100. Nishimura, S., and Sekiya, T.: Human cancer and cellular oncogenes, Biochem. J. **243**:313, 1987.

101. Noda, M., Ko, M., Ogura, A., Liu, D.-G., Amano, T., Takano, T., and Ikawa, Y.: Sarcoma viruses carrying *ras* oncogenes induce differentiation-associated properties in a neuronal cell line, Nature **318**:73, 1985.

102. Nowell, P.C., and Hungerford, D.A.: A minute chromosome in human chronic granulocytic leukemia, Science **132**:1497, 1960.

103. Old, L.J.: Tumor necrosis factor (TNF), Science **230**:630, 1985.

104. Parada, L.F., Tabin, C.J., Shih, C., and Weinberg, R.A.: Human EJ bladder carcinoma oncogene is homologue of Harvey sarcoma virus *ras* gene, Nature **297**:474, 1982.

105. Petersen, R.O.: Urologic pathology, Philadelphia, 1986, J.B. Lippincott Co.

106. Peto, R., Doll, R., Buckley, J.D., and Sporn, M.B.: Can dietary beta-carotene materially reduce human cancer rates? Nature **290**:201, 1981.

107. Potten, C.S., editor: Prospectives on mammalian cell death, Oxford, 1987, Oxford University Press.

108. Reynolds, V.L., Lebovitz, R.M., Warren, S.L., Hawley, T.S., Godwin, A.K., and Lieberman, M.W.: Regulation of a metallothionein-*ras*T24 fusion gene by zinc results in graded alterations in cell morphology and growth, Oncogene **3**:323, 1987.

109. Rigby, P.W.J., and Wilkie, N.M.: Viruses and cancer, Cambridge, 1985, Cambridge University Press.

110. Roberts, A.B., Sporn, M.B., Assoian, R.K., Smith, J.M., Roche, N.S., Wakefield, L.M., Heine, U.I., Liotta, L.A., Falanga, V., Kehrl, J.H., and Fauci, A.S.: Transforming growth factor type β: rapid induction of fibrosis and angiogenesis *in vivo* and stimulation of collagen formation *in vitro*, Proc. Natl. Acad. Sci. USA **83**:4167, 1986.

111. Rodenhuis, S., van de Wetering, M.L., Mooi, W.J., Evers, S.G., van Zandwijk, N., and Bos, J.L.: Mutational activation of the K-*ras* oncogene, N. Engl. J. Med. **317**:929, 1987.

112. Rous, P.: A sarcoma of the fowl transmissible by an agent separable from the tumor cells, J. Exp. Med. **13**:397, 1911.

113. Rozengurt, E.: Early signals in the mitogenic response, Science **234**:161, 1986.

114. Sandberg, A.A.: The chromosome in human cancer and leukemia, New York, 1980, Elsevier/North Holland, Inc.

115. Schatz, D.G., and Baltimore, D.: Stable expression of immunoglobulin gene V(D)J recombinase activity by gene transfer into 3T3 fibroblasts, Cell **53**:107, 1988.

116. Schreiber, A.B., Winkler, M.E., and Derynck, R.: Transforming growth factor-α: a more potent angiogenic mediator than epidermal growth factor, Science **232**:1250, 1986.

116a. Scrable, H., Witte, D., Shimada, H., Wang-Wuu, S., Soukup, S., Koufos, A., Houghton, P., Lampkin, B., and Cavanee, W.: Molecular genetic differential pathology of small tumors. (Submitted.)

117. Searle, C.E.: Chemical carcinogens, American Chemical Society Monogr. 182, Washington, D.C., 1984.

118. Seeger, R.C., Brodeur, G.M., Sather, H., Dalton, A., Siegel, S.E., Wong, K.Y., and Hammond, D.: Association of multiple copies of the N-*myc* oncogene with rapid progression of neuroblastomas, N. Engl. J. Med. **313**:1111, 1985.

119. Sell, S., Hunt, J.M., Knoll, B.J., and Dunsford, H.A.: Cellular events during hepatocarcinogenesis in rats and the question of premalignancy, Adv. Cancer Res. **48**:37, 1987.

120. Seyama, T., Godwin, A.K., DiPietro, M., Winokur, T.S., Lebovitz, R.M., and Lieberman, M.W.: In vitro and in vivo regulation of liver epithelial cells carrying a metallothionein-*ras*T24 fusion gene, Molecular Carcinogenesis **1**:89, 1988.

121. Shtivelman, E., Lifshitz, B., Gale, R.P., and Canaani, E.: Fused transcript of *abl* and *bcr* genes in chronic myelogenous leukemia, Nature **315**:550, 1985.

122. Simpson, N.E., Kidd, K.K., Goodfellow, P.J., McDermid, H., Myers, S., Kidd, J.R., Jackson, C.E., Duncan, A.M.V., Farrer, L.A., Brasch, K., Castiglione, C., Genel, M., Gertner, J., Greenberg, C.R., Gusella, J.F., Holden, J.J.A., and White, B.N.: Assignment of multiple endocrine neoplasia type 2A to chromosome 10 by linkage, Nature **328**:528, 1987.

123. Sitteri, P.K., Wilson, J.D., and Mayfield, J.A.: Dihydrotestosterone in prostatic hypertrophy, J. Clin. Invest. **49**:1737, 1970.

124. Slamon, D.J., Clark, G.M., Wong, W.G., Levin, W.J., Ullrich, A., and McGuire, W.L.: Human breast cancer: correlation of relapse and survival with amplification of the HER-2/*neu* oncogene, Science **235**:177, 1987.

125. Solomon, E., Voss, R., Hall, V., Bodmer, W.F., Jass, J.R., Jeffreys, A.J., Lucibello, F.C., Patel, I., and Rider, S.H.: Chromosome 5 allele loss in human colorectal carcinomas, Nature **328**:616, 1987.

126. Sparnins, V.L., Barany, G., and Wattenberg, L.W.: Effects of organosulfur compounds from garlic and onions on benzo[a]pyrene-induced neoplasia and glutathione S-transferase activity in the mouse, Carcinogenesis **9**:131, 1988.

127. Sparnins, V.L., Venegas, P.L., and Wattenberg, L.W.: Glutathione S-transferase activity: enhancement by compounds inhibiting chemical carcinogenesis and by dietary constituents, J. Natl. Cancer Inst. **68**:493, 1982.

128. Sporn, M.B., Roberts, A.B., Wakefield, L.M., and Assoian, R.K.: Transforming growth factor-β: biological function and chemical structure, Science **233**:532, 1986.

129. (Reference withdrawn.)

130. Stehelin, D., Guntaka, R.V., Varmus, H.E., and Bishop, J.M.: Purification of DNA complementary to nucleotide sequences required for neoplastic transformation of fibroblasts by avian sarcoma viruses, J. Mol. Biol. **101**:349, 1976.

131. Stephenson, R.A., James, B.C., Gay, H., Fair, W.R., Whitmore, W.F., and Melamed, M.R.: Flow cytometry of prostate cancer: relationship of DNA content to survival, Cancer Res. **47**:2504, 1987.

132. Sukumar, S., Notario, V., Martin-Zanca, D., and Barbacid, M.: Induction of mammary carcinomas in rats by nitroso-methylurea involves malignant activation of H-*ras*-1 locus by single point mutations, Nature **306**:658, 1983.

133. Swift, M., Reitnauer, P.J., Morrell, D., and Chase, C.L.: Breast and other cancers in families with ataxia-telangiectasia, N. Engl. J. Med. **316**:1289, 1987.

134. Taniguchi, N., Iizuka, S., Zhe, Z.N., House, S., Yokosawa, N., Ono, M., Kinoshita, K., Makita, A., and Sekiya, C.: Measurement of human serum immunoreactive γ-glutamyl transpeptidase in patients with malignant tumors using enzyme-linked immunosorbent assay, Cancer Res. **45**:5835, 1985.

135. Taparowsky, E., Suard, Y., Fasano, O., Shimuzu, K., Goldfarb, M., and Wigler, M.: Activation of the T24 bladder carcinoma transforming gene is linked to a single amino acid change, Nature **300**:762, 1982.

136. Taub, R., Kirsch, I., Morton, C., Lenoir, G., Swan, D., Tronick, S., Aaronson, S., and Leder, P.: Translocation of the c-*myc* gene into the immunoglobulin heavy chain locus in human burkitt lymphoma and murine plasmacytoma cells, Proc. Nat. Acad. Sci. USA **79**:7837, 1982.

137. Taylor, S.M., and Jones, P.A.: Multiple new phenotypes induced in 10T1/2 and 3T3 cells treated with 5-azacytidine, Cell **17**:771, 1979.

138. Temin, H.M.: The protovirus hypothesis: speculations on the significance of RNA-directed DNA synthesis for normal development and for carcinogenesis, J. Nat. Cancer Inst. **46**:3, 1971.

139. Temin, H.M.: Evolution of cancer genes as a mutation-driven process, Cancer Res. **48**:1697, 1988.

140. Têtu, B., Katz, R.L., Kalter, S.P., von Eschenbach, A.C., and Barlogie, B.: Acridine-orange flow cytometry of urinary bladder washings for the detection of transitional cell carcinoma of the bladder, Cancer **60**:1815, 1987.

141. Theillet, C., Lidereau, R., Escot, C., Hutzell, P., Brunet, M., Gest, J., Schlom, J., and Callahan, R.: Loss of a c-H-ras-1 allele and aggressive human primary breast carcinomas, Cancer Res. **46**:4776, 1986.

142. Treisman, R.: Transient accumulation of c-*fos* RNA following serum stimulation requires a conserved 5' element and c-*fos* 3' sequences, Cell **42**:889, 1985.

143. Tsuda, H., Shimosato, Y., Upton, M.P., Yokota, J., Terada, M., Ohira, M., Sugimura, T., and Hirohashi, S.: Retrospective study on amplification of N-*myc* and c-*myc* genes in pediatric solid tumors and its association with prognosis and tumor differentiation, Lab. Invest., vol. 59, no. 3, 1988.

144. Tsujimoto, Y., Finger, L.R., Yunis, J.J., Nowell, P.C., and Croce, C.M.: Cloning of the chromosomal breakpoint of neoplastic B-cells with the t(14;18) chromosomal translocation, Science **226**:1097, 1984.

145. Tseleni-Balafouta, S., and Kittas, C.: Neuron-specific enolase reactivity in hyperplasias and neoplasms of the thyroid, Arch. Pathol. Lab. Med. **112**:115, 1988.

146. Upton, A.C., Albert, R.E., Burns, F.J., and Shore, R.E.: Radiation carcinogenesis, New York, 1986, Elsevier Science Publishing Co.

147. Van de Vijer, M.J., Mooi, W.J., Wiseman, P., Peterse, J.L., and Nusse, R.: Immunohistochemical detection of the *neu* protein in tissue sections of human breast tumors with amplified *neu* DNA, Oncogene **2**:175, 1988.

148. Varley, J.M., Swallow, J.E., Brammer, W.J., Whittaker, J.L., and Walker, R.A.: Alterations to either c-*erb*B-2 (*neu*) or c-*myc* proto-oncogenes in breast carcinomas correlate with poor short-term prognosis, Oncogene **1**:423, 1987.

149. Varmus, H.E.: The molecular genetics of cellular oncogenes, Annu. Rev. Genet. **18**:553, 1984.

150. Vennström, B., and Bishop, J.M.: Isolation and characterization of chicken DNA homologous to the two putative oncogenes of avian erythroblastosis virus, Cell **28**:135, 1982.

151. Virji, M., Mercer, D.W., and Herberman, R.B.: Tumor markers in cancer diagnosis and prognosis, CA **38**:104, 1988.

152. von Hansemann, D.: Ueber asymmetrische Zelltheilung in Epithelkrebsen und deren biologische Bedeutung, Virchows Arch. A [Pathol. Anat.] **119**:299, 1890.

153. Wagner, D., Ikenberg, H., Böhm, N., and Gissman, L.: Identification of human papillomavirus in cervical smears by DNA *in situ* hybridization, Obstet. Gynecol. **64**:767, 1984.

154. Wattenberg, L.W.: Inhibition of neoplasia by minor dietary constituents, Cancer Res. **43**:2448s, 1983.

155. Weiss, L., Orr, F.W., and Honn, K.V.: Interactions of cancer cells with the microvasculature during metastasis, FASEB J. **2**:12, 1988.

156. Weiss, R., Teich, N., Varmus, H., and Coffin, J.: Molecular biology of tumor viruses, ed. 2, Cold Spring Harbor, N.Y., 1984, Cold Spring Harbor Laboratory.

157. Weiss, L.M., Warnke, R.A., Sklar, J., and Cleary, M.L.: Molecular analysis of the t(14;18) chromosomal translocation in malignant lymphomas, N. Engl. J. Med. **317**:1185, 1987.

158. Wewer, U.M., Taraboletti, G., Sobel, M.E., Albrechtsen, R., and Liotta, L.A.: Role of laminin receptor in tumor cell migration, Cancer Res. **47**:5691, 1987.

159. Whang-Peng, J., Triche, T.J., Knutsen, T., Miser, J., Kao-Shan, S., Tsai, S., and Israel, M.A.: Cytogenetic characterization of selected small round cell tumors of childhood, Cancer Genet. Cytogenet. **21**:185, 1986.

160. Wick, M.R., and Siegal, G.P., editors: Monoclonal antibodies in diagnostic immunohistochemistry, New York, 1988, Marcel Dekker, Inc.

161. Wilbourn, J., Haroun, L., Heseltine, E., Kaldor, J., Partensky, C., and Vainio, H.: Response of experimental animals to human carcinogens: an analysis based upon the IARC Monographs programme, Carcinogenesis **7**:1853, 1986.

162. Wills, R.A.: The spread of tumors in the human body, London, 1952, Butterworth & Co.

163. Yunis, J.J.: High resolution of human chromosomes, Science **191**:1268, 1976.

164. Yunis, J.J., Frizzera, G., Oken, M.M., McKenna, J., Theologides, A., and Arnesen, M.: Multiple recurrent genomic defects in follicular lymphoma: a possible model for cancer, N. Engl. J. Med. **316**:79, 1987.

165. Yuspa, S.H.: Cutaneous chemical carcinogenesis, J. Am. Acad. Dermatol. **15**:1031, 1986.

166. Yuspa, S.H., and Poirier, M.C.: Chemical carcinogenesis: from animal models to molecular models in one decade, Adv. Cancer Res. **50**:25, 1988.

167. Zbar, B., Brauch, H., Talmadge, C., and Linehan, M.: Loss of alleles of loci on the short arm of chromosome 3 in renal cell carcinoma, Nature **327**:721, 1987.

15 Heart

DONALD B. HACKEL
KEITH A. REIMER

Heart disease is a major cause of illness and disability in the United States, and although the age-adjusted death rate for heart disease has progressively declined during the past 20 years, heart disease remains today the leading cause of death in the United States. In 1984, there were about 2,047,000 deaths from all causes in the United States.[1] Among these, 986,000 were attributed to diseases of the heart and blood vessels, including stroke. The four major categories of heart disease are coronary (ischemic) heart disease, hypertensive heart disease, rheumatic heart disease, and congenital heart disease. In 1984, about 540,000 deaths (55% of cardiovascular deaths and 26% of all deaths) were attributed to coronary heart disease.[1] Thus considerable attention will be devoted to this subject. Congenital heart disease is discussed in Chapter 16.

Before the various heart diseases are discussed, it is fitting to review briefly some pertinent aspects of cardiac failure, since frequent reference is made to this condition.

CARDIAC FAILURE

Cardiac failure is a clinical state in which the heart is unable to maintain an adequate circulation for bodily needs.[2,3] The basic factors that cause or contribute to heart failure may be summarized as follows:

1. The heart muscle may be weakened by disease processes that cause sufficient loss of muscle tissue or impairment of contractility so that the heart is unable to function as an efficient pump. Among the lesions producing myocardial weakness are myocardial infarction, myocardial fibrosis, coronary insufficiency, myocarditis, and metabolic disorders.
2. There may be a mechanical overload of the heart that in time may lead to myocardial failure. Such an increased demand on the myocardium results from (a) an increased resistance to ejection of blood, as in valvular stenosis or systemic hypertension (pressure overload), or (b) an excessive demand for increased cardiac output, as in valvular

insufficiency, arteriovenous shunts, and increased tissue needs such as thyrotoxicosis (volume overload).
3. Impaired filling of the heart chambers, as may result from cardiac tamponade or constrictive pericarditis, may be responsible for a decreased cardiac output.

In some instances heart failure results from a combination of these basic factors.

Cardiac failure is either acute or chronic. Acute failure is caused by conditions such as coronary occlusion, obstruction to cardiac outflow as in massive pulmonary embolism, or cardiac tamponade resulting from sudden hemopericardium incident to rupture of the heart. In acute heart failure there is a sudden reduction or cessation of cardiac output. Dyspnea, orthopnea, and pulmonary edema may be present, and in some instances the symptoms of shock develop. Chronic heart failure is most commonly seen in association with coronary atherosclerosis, hypertensive cardiopathy, and valvular deformities. However, it may occur as a result of any disease that *weakens the heart* directly or *causes an increased demand* on the myocardium.

Whenever the cardiovascular system makes sufficient adjustments to maintain adequate output, a state of compensation is reached. The principal compensatory phenomena are tachycardia, cardiac dilatation, and cardiac hypertrophy. When these adjustments are inadequate, a state of cardiac decompensation is said to exist.

Heart failure may involve one side of the heart more than the other. In *left-sided heart failure* the major manifestations are those associated with passive congestion and edema of the lungs. In more severe cases, pulmonary hypertension results, leading to failure of the right side of the heart. Although failure of the right side of the heart is usually combined with that of the left, there are instances of isolated right-sided failure. The manifestations of *right-sided heart failure* include subcutaneous edema (particularly in the dependent parts of the body), hydrothorax, ascites, passive congestion of the liver and spleen, generalized venous congestion, cyanosis, and, usually, increased blood volume.

The clinical syndrome with the foregoing features is termed *congestive heart failure*. The cardiac output in typical congestive heart failure usually is reduced though in some patients at rest it may be normal. Cardiac failure associated with certain diseases (such as hyperthyroidism, severe anemias, and arteriovenous shunts, including arteriovenous fistulas and the shunts in the bones of osteitis deformans) may be accompanied by an elevated cardiac output; thus it is given the designation *high-output heart failure*.

The terms *backward failure* and *forward failure* have been applied to the manifestations of congestive heart failure. In *backward failure* there is an increase in diastolic pressure within the failing ventricle or ventricles, followed by a rise in atrial pressure that is transmitted backward, producing an elevated pressure in the veins. In *forward failure* the manifestations result from failure of the heart to pump a sufficient output, causing a diminished flow of blood to the tissues, particularly to the kidneys. The clinical manifestations of either forward or backward failure may predominate in an individual patient. However, it should be apparent that, given a continuous closed circulatory system, these two mechanisms do not function independently of each other.

The pathogenesis of edema in cardiac failure is an intriguing problem that has held the interest of investigators for a long time but is still not completely solved. For many years the edema has been explained as a *consequence of increased* venous pressure, leading to a rise in capillary blood pressure, increased filtration, and consequently edema. Although increased venous pressure plays a part in the development of edema, the emphasis today is on the importance of retention of sodium and water in the body. The role of intrinsic renal mechanisms and hormonal or neural factors (such as reduction in glomerular filtration rate, enhanced renal tubular reabsorption of sodium, hypersecretion of aldosterone, and an increased release of antidiuretic hormone) is discussed on p. 807.

The main causes of congestive heart failure include the following conditions, which are described sequentially in the remainder of this chapter and Chapter 16.

1. Coronary artery (ischemic) heart disease
2. Inflammatory heart diseases
3. Valvular and hypertensive heart diseases
4. Cardiomyopathies and specific disorders affecting the myocardium
5. Tumors of the heart
6. Disturbances of the conducting system
7. Congenital heart disease (Chapter 16)

In addition, the techniques involved in obtaining and interpreting a cardiac biopsy specimen are presented.

CORONARY ARTERY (ISCHEMIC) HEART DISEASE
Definitions

The World Health Organization's Study Group on Atherosclerosis and Ischemic Heart Disease defined *ischemic heart disease* (IHD) as the "cardiac disability, acute and chronic, arising from reduction or arrest of blood supply to the myocardium in association with disease processes in the coronary arterial system."[4] Subsequently, the Expert Committee on Cardiovascular Diseases and Hypertension accepted the term *coronary heart disease* (CHD) as synonymous with ischemic heart disease.[5] Another term that is often used synonymously with ischemic heart disease is *arteriosclerotic* or *atherosclerotic heart disease (ASHD)*. Additional terms that are closely related are *arteriosclerotic* or *atherosclerotic cardiovascular disease (ASCVD)* and *coronary artery disease (CAD)*. ASCVD is sometimes used synonymously with CHD but is commonly considered to be a more general term, referring to death or debility because of atherosclerotic involvement of arteries to more than one organ. In the restricted sense, the term *coronary artery disease* does not indicate heart disease. The vascular disorder may exist with or without clinical or pathologic evidence of myocardial damage. Thus the terms *coronary heart disease* and *ischemic heart disease* are preferred when myocardial lesions or clinical manifestations occur as a result of disturbances of the coronary circulation. It should be recognized that coronary heart disease includes cardiac disturbances from other lesions of the coronary arteries in addition to atherosclerosis.

Incidence

As noted in the introduction to this chapter, CHD is a major cause of morbidity and mortality in the United States, accounting for 26% of all deaths in 1984. This has not always been the case. In the early part of this century, before World War I, CHD was a rarity; indeed the clinical manifestations of coronary occlusion and myocardial infarction were not described in the medical literature until 1912.[9] Thereafter, a progressive increase in mortality from coronary heart disease occurred, so that by 1940, CHD had become the leading cause of mortality in the United States, and by 1968, approximately 40% of all deaths were attributed to CHD. Thus many epidemiologists have regarded CHD as *the* epidemic of the twentieth century. Indeed, whether considered in terms of total mortality, lost output attributable to disability, or actual dollar costs of disability pensions or of direct medical and nursing home care, no other disease ranks ahead of CHD.[11]

Although CHD remains the leading cause of mortality today, a dramatic reversal in the increasing death rate from CHD has occurred. Over the past two decades, there has been a progressive decline in mortality from CHD and other cardiovascular diseases, so that the age-adjusted death rate for all cardiovascular diseases has decreased by about 40% from the peak in the 1950s and 1960s.[6] This decreased mortality has occurred in both blacks and whites and in both men and women of all age groups.[8] The explanation for this sudden reversal of the previously rising death rate from CHD has been of considerable epidemiologic interest.[6-8,10-13] Several factors may be involved though it is unclear what the relative importance of each may be. In part, the decline must be attributed to changing lifestyles of Americans, related to known risk factors for CHD including cigarette smoking and hypercholesterolemia (see later). Medical detection and treatment of hypertension may also be a contributing factor in the prevention of CHD. In addition, there have been many innovations in the treatment of chronic ischemic heart disease and acute myocardial infarction (such as coronary bypass surgery, the development of the coronary care unit, and the associated large armamentarium of monitoring devices and drugs).

Death rates from CHD increase greatly with advancing age; indeed 80% of CHD deaths occur in persons greater than 65 years of age. Even so, because CHD is so common, it ranks as the number-one cause of death for all age groups above age 35. Males are at substantially higher risk of death from CHD compared to females of any comparable age; however, CHD is particularly uncommon in women before menopause.

Etiology

A variety of disorders can affect the coronary arteries and cause partial or complete coronary obstruction. The following is a list of some of these disorders; these will be considered in more detail in the following sections of this chapter.

1. Atherosclerosis
2. Inflammatory disorders
   a. Infections—syphilis, tuberculosis, other bacteria
   b. Noninfectious inflammatory disorders—rheumatic arteritis, rheumatoid arteritis, polyarteritis nodosa, thromboangiitis obliterans, and so on
3. Embolism
4. Thrombotic disease
5. Neoplasms
6. Trauma
7. Aneurysms
8. Congenital anomalies
9. Medial calcification in infancy

Atherosclerosis

Of the aforementioned causes for coronary artery disease, at least 90% of CHD is the result of coronary atherosclerosis.

Nature of the lesion. The lesions of coronary atherosclerosis, like those of atherosclerosis elsewhere in the body, may be classified morphologically as fatty streaks, fibrous (raised) plaques, or complicated lesions.[14] The fatty streak is an intimal lesion composed of lipid-laden foam cells derived from circulating monocytes. The fatty streak is considered by most investigators to be the earliest lesion that precedes the development of the fibrous plaque. The fibrous plaque is also primarily an intimal lesion composed of increased numbers of smooth muscle cells (myointimal cells) and macrophages surrounded by an extracellular connective tissue matrix and interspersed with varying amounts of extracellular lipid. The fibrous plaque is typically composed of a cellular connective tissue layer (the "fibrous cap"), separating the arterial lumen from a deeper soft pool of primarily extracellular debris. The latter "lipid pool" often contains amorphous debris interspersed with cholesterol crystals. (Processing tissue for routine light microscopy dissolves the cholesterol crystals, leaving empty slitlike spaces on the microscopic slide known as "cholesterol clefts.") See Fig. 15-1. Complicated lesions are plaques, which include one or more of the following: necrosis and inflammation of the adjacent media of the artery, hemorrhage within the plaque, calcification, or ulceration or rupture of the endothelial surface.

Locations of coronary plaques. Atherosclerosis is much more likely to occur in some arteries than others and has a recognized predilection for specific segments of commonly involved arteries. For example, in the aorta, the ascending segment is seldom severely involved, whereas the abdominal segment is frequently extensively involved. The coronary arteries, which arise from the uninvolved aortic root, are commonly affected, whereas the renal arteries, which arise from the often-involved abdominal segment of the aorta, seldom have significant atherosclerotic disease. The carotid, iliac, and popliteal arteries often are involved, but the subclavian and axillary arteries are seldom significantly involved. The usual explanation for such selective localization is that variation in hemodynamic factors causes more or less turbulence or shear stress in some locations than in others.[15,16] The fact that atherosclerosis often is particularly severe at vascular branch points is evidence that local hemodynamic factors contribute to the development of atherosclerosis.[18]

Within the coronary vascular tree, atherosclerosis is typically a disease of the proximal segments of the major epicardial arteries, that is, the first 3 to 4 cm of each of the major arteries. Even in patients with severe

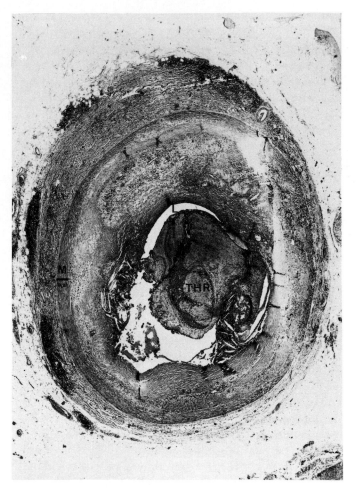

Fig. 15-1. Coronary artery showing pronounced atherosclerotic narrowing and thrombotic occlusion, *THR,* of lumen, *L,* at site of plaque rupture. The atherosclerotic plaque consists of collagen, capillaries, foci of hemorrhage, and cholesterol clefts (the needlelike clear clefts that extend into the luminal thrombus at the site of plaque rupture). The plaque and thrombus are internal to the media, *M and bar.*

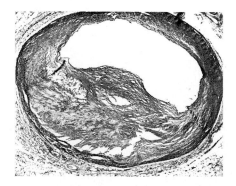

Fig. 15-2. Atherosclerosis of small branch of the anterior descending coronary artery. Notice the thick fibrous atheromatous plaque on one side, which has considerably reduced the lumen and secondarily caused thinning of the underlying media.

proximal disease, the more distal segments are often involved minimally. Intramyocardial branches of the coronary arteries are almost never involved to any significant degree. It is the proximal location of coronary atherosclerosis that makes it possible to treat ischemic heart disease by coronary bypass surgery or coronary angioplasty. Coronary atherosclerosis often involves the proximal segments of all three arteries diffusely, but lesions that are sufficiently severe to cause clinical problems (stenosis of more than 75% of the cross-sectional area) may be relatively focal. Among the three major coronary arteries, most investigators consider that significant atherosclerosis occurs most commonly in the anterior descending branch of the left coronary artery, is somewhat less common in the right coronary artery, and is least frequent in the circumflex artery.[17,19,20]

The atherosclerotic plaques are usually situated eccentrically along one side of the lumen, though occasionally there may be concentric thickening of the wall of the vessel (Fig. 15-2).

Epidemiology. There is no known specific cause of coronary atherosclerosis. Nevertheless, a large number of epidemiologic studies have established several hereditary and environmental factors and acquired disorders that are known to be associated with an increased risk of developing CHD. The American Heart Association has classified these risk factors according to the following table[120]:

> Major risk factors that *cannot* be changed
> > Heredity
> > Sex (gender)
> > Race
> > Age
> Major risk factors that *can* be changed
> > Cigarette smoking
> > Hypertension
> > Hypercholesterolemia
> > Diabetes mellitus
> Contributing factors
> > Obesity
> > Lack of physical exercise
> > Emotional stress ("type A" personality)

Evidence derived from various studies indicates a *familial or hereditary predisposition* to coronary atherosclerosis that seems to be independent of the other major risk factors; that is, the familial aggregation of CHD cannot be related to a familial clustering of other known risk factors.[35,61,62]

The influence of *gender* was mentioned previously. In brief, women are less prone to atherosclerotic coronary heart disease than men are, and it tends to develop at a later age in women.[36,47] Some reports indicate that CHD is more common in women with obesity, diabetes mellitus, hypertension, or surgical removal of the ovaries,[57,176] and that under these conditions it develops at an earlier age; others have reported that the incidence and severity of atherosclerosis are less in men treated with estrogens for carcinoma of the prostate than in nontreated men.[56] Partly because of such reports, it has been suggested that female sex hormones, especially estrogens, protect against coronary heart disease. However, some investigators have reported that they found no difference in the incidence of this disease in oophorectomized women compared to noncastrated women,[56] thus contradicting the previously mentioned reports.

The relationship between race and heart disease is less certain. Age-adjusted death rates for CHD have been similar between white and black populations in recent years.[32] In contrast, *hypertension* is more prevalent in blacks. The relative prevalences of other risk factors in blacks have not been studied extensively.[33]

The disease is more prevalent with *advancing age*[58,64] but is not limited to old age. In a post–World War II study, data on 866 cases of coronary heart disease in soldiers between 18 and 39 years of age were accumulated. Of these cases, 450 were examined at autopsy, and advanced coronary atherosclerosis with its various complications was demonstrated.[66] In a group of U.S. soldiers killed in action in Korea, averaging 22 years of age, coronary atherosclerosis was observed in 77.3%.[15] The disease process varied from fibrous thickening to large atheromatous plaques causing complete occlusion of one or more of the major vessels. In comparison to the Korean investigation, a postmortem study of American soldiers killed in action in the Vietnam conflict, also averaging 22 years of age, showed that the percentage of those affected by some degree of coronary atherosclerosis was less but still significant (45%) and that severe narrowing of the coronary arteries was less striking.[54]

Many epidemiologic, anatomic, and experimental studies provide evidence for a strong relationship between cigarette smoking and morbidity and mortality from CHD. Indeed, in part because of the increased risk of coronary atherosclerosis, but also because of the increased incidence of several types of cancer and chronic obstructive pulmonary disease, cigarette smoking is identified as the single most important cause of preventable morbidity and premature mortality in the U.S.[30,37] It has been amply demonstrated in epidemiologic studies that the risk of CHD increases with increased number and duration of cigarettes smoked and that the risk gradually declines in ex-smokers.

The mechanism through which cigarette smoking contributes to the development of atherosclerosis may be multifactorial. Endothelial injury is one possible mechanism and has been proposed to result from chronic hypoxia because of chronic carbon monoxide exposure or because of chronically increased vasomotor tone resulting from reduced PGI_2 synthesis.[45] In addition, platelets have been found to aggregate more readily in cigarette smokers, perhaps because of a direct effect of nicotine by itself or to increased circulating catecholamines, another well-known consequence of cigarette smoking.[48]

Hypertension is another recognized risk factor for CHD. In autopsy and clinical studies, atherosclerosis is more extensive and the incidence of coronary heart disease is higher among hypertensive patients than among nonhypertensive patients. The precise mechanism through which hypertension contributes to the development of atherosclerosis is unknown.[25] The increased blood pressure may accelerate the progression of atherosclerosis through increased physical stresses resulting in endothelial injury. In addition, a high intravascular pressure may accelerate infiltration of lipid through the arterial wall.[38]

Practically all the blood lipids are conjugated to proteins to form particles of varying size and composition known as the lipoproteins. There are four major classes of lipoproteins: (1) chylomicrons, the form in which ingested lipids are transported from the small intestine to the circulation and the tissues, (2) very-low-density lipoproteins (VLDL) or pre-beta-lipoproteins, which are heavily laden with triglycerides, (3) low-density lipoproteins (LDL), or beta-lipoproteins, which contain a greater proportion of cholesterol, and (4) high-density lipoproteins (HDL), or alpha-lipoproteins.

Considerable evidence in the literature indicates that abnormalities such as an increase in the serum LDL fraction, and hypercholesterolemia are associated with an increased risk for the development of atherosclerosis. Patients with coronary heart disease tend to have higher serum cholesterol and LDL values than normal subjects do.[41] Also, in several long-term follow-up studies of healthy persons in whom serum lipid levels were analyzed, the incidence of new coronary heart disease in later years was positively correlated with LDL and cholesterol levels.[41] In follow-up studies of middle-aged men in the United States, the frequency of subsequent myocardial infarction was about three times greater in men with predisease cholesterol values greater than 230 mg/100 ml of blood than in men with lower values.[44]

In contrast to the LDL fraction, the HDL fraction appears to be inversely related to the incidence of coronary heart disease.[41,55] Low concentrations of HDL in the blood are apparently associated with an increased risk of coronary heart disease. There is evidence that HDL may be important for normal clearance of cholesterol from tissues, including the arterial wall.[55]

Based on the results of several large clinical trials, there is a growing consensus that not only is serum LDL cholesterol positively correlated with the incidence of CHD, but also intervention by dietary changes or drugs that lower LDL cholesterol does reduce the morbidity and mortality from CHD.[24,50-52] There is now consensus among investigators that patients with "high-risk blood cholesterol" levels should be treated by dietary changes or, if the response is inadequate, by drugs.[22,23] Opinions differ on whether and how aggressively to treat individuals with intermediate cholesterol risk.[49]

Diet is not considered to be a risk factor by itself but is obviously important inasmuch as dietary habits, in concert with genetic metabolic traits, determine a person's circulating lipid balance. The "average" American diet, high in saturated fats and cholesterol contributes to an average ("normal") blood cholesterol level that in fact is abnormally elevated compared to cholesterol levels in the populations of countries in which the diet is low in saturated fats. Major differences in the incidence of CHD have been observed among various countries; a lower frequency of CHD in some countries has been attributed to a low fat diet. As an example, in a comparative autopsy study in a Japanese city and in a city of the United States, coronary atherosclerosis was found to be less severe in Japan, and myocardial infarction was seven times more frequent in the United States.[34] The Japanese diet has a low fat content as compared with the American diet.

Coronary heart disease also occurs more frequently and at an earlier age in patients with *diabetes* than in the general population.[42] In part, the risk of diabetes may be related to an association with the preceding two risk factors, hypertension and hyperlipidemia.[28,42] Because of the renal complications of diabetes, diabetic patients have an increased incidence of hypertension. In addition, diabetic patients tend to be more obese and are hyperlipidemic compared with the general population. On the other hand, the presence of endothelial and platelet abnormalities have been reported in diabetic patients, which may contribute to the development of atherosclerotic plaques.[26] For example, endothelial cells cultured from diabetic patients produce less prostacyclin and plasminogen activator. Platelets from diabetic patients produce more of a variety of substances including thromboxane B_2. Platelet aggregability is increased among diabetic patients.

Obesity is considered to be a minor contributor to coronary atherosclerosis, but its role is not clear.[39,63] Some investigators suggest that the increased CHD risk in obese patients is attributable to associated hyperlipidemia or hypertension. Also to be considered is the possibility that excess body weight adds an extra workload to a heart already burdened.

The possible benefits that *physical activity* may have on the likelihood of developing CHD continue to be debated.[29,43] It has been shown that physical conditioning does increase a person's serum HDL level; thus exercise does have a salutory effect on lipoprotein metabolism, which could translate into a reduced risk of CHD.[40] Physical conditioning also has been shown to augment the fibrinolytic system.[65]

Certain studies indicate that *emotional stress* may contribute to the development of atherosclerosis. For example, in a survey of physicians, it was assumed that general practitioners and anesthesiologists were subject to greater stress than dermatologists and pathologists, and coronary disease appeared to be three times more prevalent in the general practitioners and two times more prevalent in the anesthesiologists than in dermatologists and pathologists.[59]

A link between coronary heart disease and the *"type A" behavior pattern* also has been reported.[31] The type A behavior pattern is characterized by enhanced aggressiveness, ambitiousness, competitive drive, and a chronic sense of time urgency. A more relaxed "type B" behavior is associated with a lower incidence of coronary heart disease.

In epidemiologic studies in patients and in studies using experimental animal models of atherosclerosis, psychosocial stress has been associated with increased CHD or atherosclerogenesis. One postulated mechanism for the effect of behavior on atherosclerosis is that increased sympathetic tone may enhance endothelial injury.

There is substantial evidence that whereas high levels of alcohol consumption promote hypertension and can result in direct cardiac injury (alcoholic cardiomyopathy) moderate alcohol consumption (not more than two drinks a day) confers protection.[69,82] The mechanism for this protective effect is currently unknown.

Among other factors believed to be associated with coronary heart disease is the quality of *drinking water*. Several studies have shown a higher death rate from ischemic heart disease in communities with soft water than in areas with hard water.[27] It is not known why hard water seems to have a protective effect. Some investigators consider that the high content of calcium or magnesium, or both, may be responsible for this action.[53] Other studies have reported an association of coronary heart disease with a lack of various trace elements such as chromium, selenium, copper, or zinc in the water supply,[21,46,60] but the results have not been conclusive.

Pathogenesis. The steps leading to the development of the atherosclerotic plaque are not completely established though there have been developed several theories that are supported by experimental observations and explain many of the anatomic and epidemiologic observations in patients.

One of the classic theories is the *"lipid-infiltration theory."* According to this theory, infiltration of lipid from the blood into the intima is the primary event, leading to the formation of fatty streaks.[89,90] Several studies have provided evidence that LDL supplies cholesterol to tissues and HDL removes it. When the LDL cholesterol supply is excessive, lipid first accumulates within mesenchymal cells, which are believed to be multipotential smooth muscle (myointimal) cells capable of producing collagen, elastic, and muscle fibers.[88] It has been proposed that these cells are derived from cells normally present in the media, which proliferate and then migrate to the intima in response to lipid deposition.[70] In addition, some of the lipid-containing cells are macrophages derived from monocytes in the blood.[73] Cellular uptake is facilitated by specific LDL receptors on the surface of cells.[75] Later, the lipids appear extracellularly after release from the cells that have undergone necrosis.[77]

A more recent hypothesis is that some type of intimal injury precedes and causes the cellular proliferation and lipid deposition. This has been termed the *"response-to-injury" hypothesis.*[83,85] In the event of injury sufficiently severe to denude endothelial cells, platelets may adhere to the exposed basement membrane and may release one or more chemotactic or mitogenic factors. For example, platelet-derived growth factor (PDGF) is both chemotactic and mitogenic; that is, it can induce both the migration and proliferation of monocytes and smooth muscle cells in a developing plaque.[78,80,83,84] An important role of platelets has been demonstrated in experimental models in which mechanical injury (from intimal abrasion with a balloon-tipped catheter) was used as the initiating event to produce atherosclerotic lesions. These lesions could be prevented by making the animals thrombocytopenic or treating them with an agent to inhibit platelet function, such as sulfinpyrazone or dipyridamole.[72,76,86]

Alternatively, not only platelets but also monocytes, smooth muscle cells, and endothelial cells can synthesize PDGF under certain circumstances. Moreover, both endothelial cells and macrophages may produce interleukin-1, a substance that promotes endothelial adherence of neutrophils and monocytes.[68] Thus endothelial injury need not be so severe as to produce denudation. In experimental studies of hypercholesterolemia, one of the earliest changes observed is the increased adherence of monocytes to endothelium.[70,74] It is thus hypothesized[85] that hypercholesterolemia can cause sublethal injury of endothelial cells that results in endothelial synthesis of chemoattractants such as interleukin-1 or PDGF. Monocytes then adhere to the surface and can migrate to a subendothelial position. Products of monocyte/macrophage metabolism may result in further endothelial injury, with or without focal denudation, and thereby perpetuate the growth of the plaque through continued in-migration and proliferation of monocytes and smooth muscle cells. Two proposed pathways of atherogenesis according to the "response-to-injury" hypothesis are summarized in a diagram by R. Ross, reproduced in Fig. 15-3.

In addition to hypercholesterolemia, possible causes of endothelial injury include mechanical shear stress, an explanation for increased risk of CHD in patients with hypertension, carbon monoxide or other products of tobacco combustion, and ionizing radiation. Radiation therapy to the mediastinum has been associated with a risk of accelerated coronary atherosclerosis.[71,87]

A third hypothesis for the mechanism of atherogenesis is the *"monoclonal hypothesis."* This hypothesis is that the intimal cells are altered initially by mutagenic agents (such as chemicals or viruses) and that they then proliferate under the influence of certain promoting factors.[67] The implication of this hypothesis is that the proliferative lesions have properties resembling those of benign neoplasms.[91] It has been observed that when the subtype of the enzyme glucose-6-phosphate dehydrogenase is used as a marker of cell lineage, in individuals heterozygous for the X-linked gene for the enzyme, virtually all atherosclerotic plaques are monoclonal.[81] It is unclear whether this represents true neoplastic growth or is simply the result of clonal selection because of proliferation caused by repeated episodes of injury and repair. However, it is of interest that cigarette smoke contains a variety of aryl hydrocarbons, some of which are known premutagens. Also, a metabolite of cholesterol, cholesterol alpha-oxide, has been shown to induce tumors in experimental animals.

Once an atherosclerotic plaque has been formed, it may progressively encroach on the arterial lumen by the processes already described. In addition, however, such plaques may enlarge because of surface ulceration and hemorrhage into the lipid pool of the plaque, or because of the deposition of mural thrombi on the plaque, which subsequently become organized and thereby incorporated into the plaque.[92] This has been termed the *"encrustation theory"* of atherogenesis. Microscopic evaluation of arteries narrowed by atherosclerosis often does reveal plaques that appear to have developed in two or more distinct layers (Fig. 15-4).

Inflammatory disorders

Syphilis. Narrowing of the coronary ostia can occur as the result of syphilitic aortitis and is an important cause of coronary insufficiency. One or both ostia may be involved. The reported incidence of coronary stenosis in patients with syphilitic aortitis has varied from 8% to 50%.[97,111] The ostia are narrowed as a result of encroachment of intimal plaques or by extension of the aortitis to the root of the aorta from which the coronary arteries arise. Ostial involvement is more likely to occur if the coronary arteries originate above the upper level

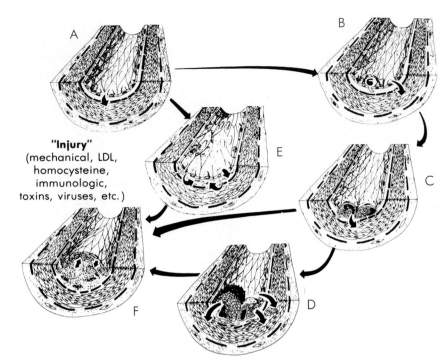

Fig. 15-3. The revised response-to-injury hypothesis. Advanced intimal proliferative lesions of atherosclerosis are proposed to occur by at least two pathways. The pathway *A-B-C-D-F* has been observed in experimentally induced hypercholesterolemia. Injury to the endothelium, *A,* may induce growth factor secretion, *short arrow.* Monocytes attach to endothelium, *B,* which may continue to secrete growth factors, *short arrow.* Subendothelial migration of monocytes, *C,* may lead to fatty-streak formation and release of growth factors such as platelet-derived growth factor (PDGF), *short arrow.* Fatty streaks may become directly converted to fibrous plaques *(long arrow* from *C* to *F)* through release of growth factors from macrophages or endothelial cells or both. Macrophages may also stimulate or injure the overlying endothelium. In some cases, macrophages may lose their endothelial cover and platelet attachment may occur, *D,* providing three possible sources of growth factors—platelets, macrophages, and endothelium, *short arrows.* Some of the smooth-muscle cells in the proliferative lesion itself, *F,* may form and secrete growth factors such as PDGF, *short arrows. LDL,* Low-density lipoproteins.
In the alternative pathway *A-E-F,* the endothelium may be injured but remain intact. Increased endothelial turnover may result in growth-factor formation by endothelial cells, *A.* This may stimulate migration of smooth-muscle cells from the media into the intima, accompanied by endogenous production of PDGF by smooth muscle as well as growth factor secretion from the "injured" endothelial cells, *E.* These interactions could then lead to fibrous-plaque formation and further lesion progression, *F.* (From Ross, R.: N. Engl. J. Med. **314:**488, 1986; reproduced with permission.)

of the sinuses of Valsalva where the aortitis tends to be prominent. The lesion seldom extends beyond the coronary orifices into the vessels, but if it does, it usually involves less than 15 mm of the proximal part of the arteries. Syphilitic coronary arteritis of the distal branches is uncommon. Coronary arterial thrombosis and aneurysm formation are rare complications. However, varying degrees of concomitant coronary ather-

osclerosis may be present. The manifestations of coronary ostial stenosis usually are seen in patients under 40 years of age and include angina pectoris and dyspnea on exertion or paroxysmal nocturnal dyspnea. A relatively prolonged terminal illness with cardiac failure is the rule, but sudden death may occur.[97] Myocardial infarction is not a common complication, probably because of the extensive collateral circulation that devel-

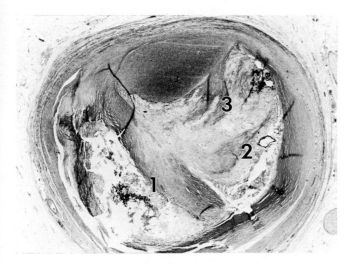

Fig. 15-4. Coronary atherosclerosis. This cross section of coronary artery shows an eccentric plaque that has narrowed the original lumen by approximately 90%. The plaque actually appears to be composed of three distinct layers, *1, 2,* and *3,* each with its own lipid pool and overlying fibrous cap. These features indicate a probable stepwise rather than continuous progession of the plaque, consistent with the "encrustation hypothesis" (see text).

ops as a result of the gradual occlusion of the coronary ostia. Myocardial fibrosis is the chief evidence of cardiac damage attributable to diminished blood supply.

Rheumatic arteritis. In active rheumatic fever, lesions occur mainly in the small intramyocardial branches of the coronary arteries and less frequently in the main coronary arteries.[102] Probably these vascular lesions contribute to myocardial damage, but in the presence of an active rheumatic myocarditis it is difficult to determine how much of the damage is caused by them. One type of lesion is an exudative and necrotizing panarteritis characterized by edema and a mild or pronounced leukocytic infiltration by lymphocytes, plasma cells, neutrophils, and sometimes basophilic cells like those found in the Aschoff bodies. Fibrinoid swelling of the collagen may be present. The more extensive lesions with prominent necrosis of the vessel wall resemble polyarteritis nodosa. Frequently, Aschoff bodies are noted in proximity to the blood vessels. Thrombi may form within the lumens of the intramyocardial vessels in association with the inflammation, followed by organization and canalization. Rare instances of thrombotic occlusion of a main coronary artery with or without myocardial infarction have been reported.

Rheumatoid arteritis. Rheumatoid arthritis is occasionally associated with cardiac manifestations including coronary arteritis. Coronary arteritis in such patients usually is confined to small arteries but in rare cases myocardial infarction attributable to arteritis of large

coronary arteries has been reported.[105,110] However, even among patients with rheumatoid arthritis who develop myocardial infarction, coexistent coronary atherosclerosis rather than rheumatoid arteritis is the more common underlying cause of the infarction.

Polyarteritis nodosa. The coronary arteries are affected in the majority of patients (approximately 70%) with polyarteritis nodosa as part of a widespread involvement of the smaller and medium-sized arteries. Rarely is the disease limited to the coronary arteries.[93] This relatively uncommon disease of unknown cause is a form of necrotizing arteritis accompanied by aneurysm formation and thrombosis in the coronary arteries. Myocardial infarction may occur.

Takayasu's arteritis. A nonspecific granulomatous type of arteritis, of unknown cause, that involves the aorta or its proximal branches is referred to as Takayasu's disease (arteritis). Although most common in the Orient, the disease has a worldwide distribution. The coronary arteries may be involved and such involvement may result in coronary thrombosis and consequent myocardial infarction.[94,107]

Thromboangiitis obliterans. Thromboangiitis obliterans (Buerger's disease) is an inflammatory disease affecting chiefly the vessels of the extremities, but occasionally it involves the visceral vessels, including the coronary arteries. The lesion may lead to coronary thrombosis and myocardial infarction.

Embolism

An infrequent cause of coronary occlusion is embolism, which most commonly involves the left coronary artery and its branches.[108] Bland emboli usually arise from vegetations of nonbacterial thrombotic endocarditis or from mural thrombi in the left ventricle, left atrium, or left atrial appendage. Atrial fibrillation is a common predisposing cause of atrial thrombi; ventricular mural thrombi can be associated with any cause of endocardial injury or turbulent flow, including congestive cardiomyopathies or previous myocardial infarction. Thrombi in the pulmonary veins caused by suppurative disease of the lungs, or as a result of invasion by tumor, also may give rise to emboli. Rarely does a coronary embolus originate from thrombi in peripheral veins (paradoxical embolism). Sometimes it is difficult to determine morphologically if a coronary occlusion is the result of thrombosis or embolism. Sudden death and myocardial infarction are possible effects of these emboli. Multiple minute emboli may be the cause of myocardial failure. Atheromatous plaques in the root of the *aorta* near the ostium of a coronary artery may rupture and give rise to more distal coronary emboli. Fat embolism and air embolism may involve the coronary circulation. The former usually produces no significant clinical manifestations, but the latter may be a cause of death. Atrial myxomas may give rise to tumor emboli, which may lodge in a coronary artery.

Thrombotic diseases

Coronary thrombosis occasionally occurs in disorders other than atherosclerosis, as in diseases associated with stasis and sludging of blood or with hypercoagulability of the blood, such as sickle cell anemia, polycythemia vera, and shock. Hyaline thrombi in the small intramyocardial vessels may be demonstrated in thrombotic thrombocytopenic purpura (Fig. 15-5).

Neoplasms

Primary or metastatic tumors of the heart may cause compression of a vessel and, in rare instances, result in coronary occlusion.

Trauma

Penetrating injuries may cause laceration of a coronary artery, with or without myocardial infarction. Occasionally, the penetrating object produces coronary thrombosis by causing contusion of an artery. It is believed that blunt trauma seldom induces coronary thrombosis in a previously normal artery but is more likely to precipitate thrombosis in an artery containing atherosclerotic plaque.[104,106]

Aneurysms

Aneurysms are not common in the coronary arteries. Fusiform or saccular aneurysms of the coronary arteries[95,99] may occur in conjunction with several of the disorders listed above; types include congenital, mycotic, atherosclerotic (Fig. 15-6), syphilitic, dissecting, rheumatic, and those caused by polyarteritis nodosa. Complications of these forms of aneurysms include thrombotic coronary occlusion and rupture with hemopericardium and cardiac tamponade. Dissecting aneurysm of a coronary artery may result from extension of a dissecting aneurysm of the aorta. In addition, dissection of the coronary arteries without involvement of the aorta may occur either spontaneously[96,98,109] or as a complication of coronary angiography or angioplasty. It may cause coronary occlusion by pressure of the blood within the wall of the vessel.

Congenital anomalies

One of the most significant abnormalities of the coronary arteries is an anomalous origin of one or both arteries from the pulmonary artery. The coronary artery most frequently involved is the left. Myocardial hypoxia caused by venous blood supplying the left ventricle may lead to severe myocardial damage and cardiac failure. Other congenital lesions of the coronary arteries include aneurysms and arteriovenous fistulas.[100]

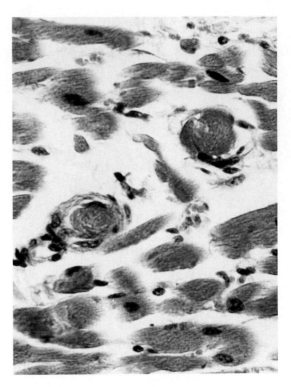

Fig. 15-5. Hyaline thrombi in small intramyocardial arterioles from a patient with thrombotic thrombocytopenic purpura.

Medial calcification in infancy

Coronary atherosclerosis as it is seen in adults rarely affects infants and children. However, there is a rare disease that occurs in infancy and occasionally in childhood and is known by several names: medial calcification with fibroblastic proliferation of the intima, coronary sclerosis of infancy, or idiopathic arterial calcification in infancy.[101,103] This is usually a generalized disease that affects many vessels throughout the body, though involvement of the coronary arteries frequently is the most prominent feature. The lesion is characterized by a fibroblastic proliferation of the intima associated with calcification that starts close to the internal elastic lamina and extends into the media and into the thickened intima, with involvement being more prominent in the media. Coronary occlusion may result, followed by infarction and calcification of the myocardium or sudden death. The occlusion is attributable chiefly to the intimal proliferation rather than to the medial calcification. Occasionally, thrombosis occurs.

Consequences of coronary artery disease

Coronary atherosclerosis by itself is asymptomatic, and as noted earlier, some degree of coronary atherosclerosis is already present by early adulthood in many

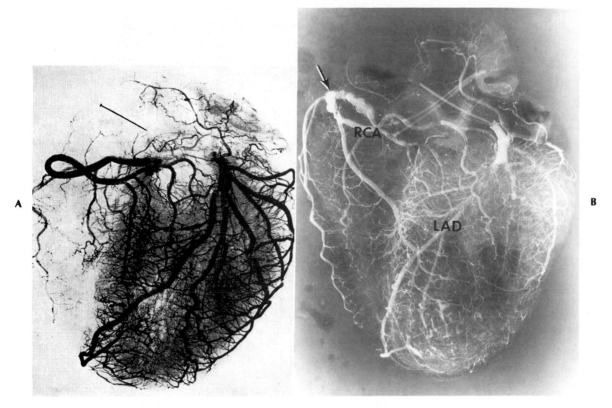

Fig. 15-6. A, Postmortem radiograph of a normal adult heart in which the coronary arteries were injected with a radiopaque suspension to illustrate the normal coronary circulation. **B,** Postmortem radiograph of another heart with similarly injected coronary arteries. In this case there is complete occlusion of the left anterior descending coronary artery, *LAD,* and an aneurysm of right coronary artery, *RCA.* Aneurysm, *arrow,* is a rare complication of coronary atherosclerosis. (**A** from Gross, L.: The blood supply to the heart, New York, 1921, Paul B. Hoeber, Inc.)

persons living in economically developed regions of the world. Coronary artery disease becomes symptomatic when it causes myocardial ischemia, defined as an imbalance between the supply of oxygenated blood to the myocardium and the myocardial requirements for oxygen.

The three major clinical consequences of acute myocardial ischemia are angina pectoris, myocardial infarction, and sudden cardiac death (Fig. 15-7). It is estimated that approximately 4.5 million Americans have known ischemic heart disease either because they have symptoms of angina pectoris or have previously suffered a nonfatal myocardial infarct.[120] Of the approximately 500,000 to 600,000 deaths per year in the United States that are attributed to ischemic heart disease, about half are attributable to one or another complication of myocardial infarction; the other half are sudden deaths caused by an arrhythmia, usually ventricular fibrillation.

Angina pectoris

Angina pectoris refers to episodic chest pain caused by transient episodes of myocardial ischemia that cause *reversible* myocyte injury, in that the duration of ischemia is insufficient to cause myocardial infarction. Chest pain may persist for a few seconds to as long as 30 minutes. Three clinical subtypes of angina are generally recognized.[115] In *chronic (stable) angina pectoris*, chest pain does not occur at rest but can be precipitated by physical exertion (exertional angina), emotional stress, or cold. Physical exertion and stress increase the hemodynamic work of the heart and thereby increase the metabolic requirements of the heart. In the presence of a fixed degree of coronary stenosis, blood flow may be adequate for the resting metabolic needs of the myocardium, but there may be no coronary reserve to permit increased perfusion for added metabolic demands. In this regard, it is known that exercise may increase myocardial oxygen require-

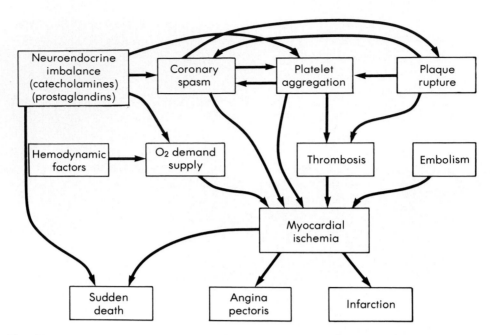

Fig. 15-7. Anatomic and pathophysiologic causes and consequences of myocardial ischemia. Myocardial ischemia has three major clinical manifestations: Transient ischemia causes angina pectoris. Sustained ischemia may result in myocardial infarction. Either a transient or sustained episode of ischemia may cause sudden cardiac death, usually attributable to a cardiac arrhythmia such as ventricular fibrillation. Transient ischemia may be caused by hemodynamic or neuroendocrine changes that cause myocardial metabolic requirements to exceed the supply of oxygenated blood through a fixed coronary stenosis; for example, physical exertion increases cardiac work and may cause exertional angina. Alternatively, a coronary thrombus may cause sustained ischemia and is considered to be the cause of up to 90% of myocardial infarcts. Ulceration or rupture of the underlying plaque is a common underlying cause of coronary thrombosis. Coronary embolism is a less common cause of myocardial infarction. A dynamic cause of ischemia, such as coronary spasm or platelet aggregation, may cause angina or may uncommonly persist sufficiently long to cause myocardial infarction. These various factors may not always occur as isolated events but may occur in concert to cause a sustained coronary occlusion; for example, a transient coronary spasm may cause deposition of platelet aggregates or might cause rupture of a plaque, or cause both. Alternatively, plaque rupture could be an initiating event leading to platelet activation; substances released from platelets can induce coronary spasm.

ments five- to tenfold over resting requirements. In the case of emotional or environmental stress (such as cold), increased sympathetic tone of coronary arteries may also contribute to restriction of blood flow and consequent onset of myocardial ischemia. *Unstable (preinfarction) angina* is another subtype of angina characterized by the new onset of angina (usually within the preceding month), precipitated by mild exertion or occurring at rest, or by progressively more severe, prolonged, or frequent symptoms (crescendo angina).

These features have been associated with an increased likelihood of myocardial infarction or sudden death (versus stable angina pectoris). *Variant (Prinzmetal's) angina* is the third subtype of angina pectoris and is characterized by chest pain occurring at rest, unrelated to physical exertion or emotional stress. This type of angina has been shown in some cases to be precipitated by coronary spasm occurring in arteries that may have underlying atherosclerosis or may be normal. Persons with this type of angina have an increased risk of sudden cardiac death.

Sudden cardiac death

Sudden cardiac death is defined as death occurring either instantaneously, without preceding symptoms, or within minutes or hours after the onset of symptoms. Definitions of sudden death vary among investigators; some use the term for deaths occurring instantaneously or within minutes, whereas other investigators have included deaths occurring up to 24 hours after the onset of symptoms. Using the former, more restrictive definition, most cases of sudden cardiac death are attributable to a cardiac arrhythmia, especially ventricular fibrillation.[114,121] In some instances, sudden death may be the first symptom of an already evolving myocardial infarct or may occur because of an acute coronary occlusion that would have been expected to cause myocardial infarction if the patient had survived. In many cases, however, neither a recent coronary occlusion nor an evolving myocardial infarct can be found at autopsy.[112,113,116,118,123,125,126,128] Moreover, clinical studies of patients successfully resuscitated from an episode of sudden cardiac "death" have revealed that less than half of such patients develop clinical evidence of myocardial infarction during subsequent follow-up study.[114] Thus it is now recognized that in a substantial number of cases, sudden cardiac death may result from a primary cardiac arrhythmia in the absence of an acute coronary occlusion or myocardial infarction. In the usual absence of any acute anatomic lesion, pathologists often attribute sudden death to the presence of chronic coronary artery disease. However, although coronary atherosclerosis is a common underlying substrate and perhaps prerequisite for sudden cardiac death, it is not, by itself, a sufficient cause.[122,127] Unfortunately, the precipitating cause or causes of sudden cardiac death are largely unknown. Several factors are known to increase the myocardial vulnerability to ventricular fibrillation; some of these are a large myocardial mass, slow heart rate, the "long QT syndrome," electrolyte abnormalities such as hypokalemia, acidosis, digitalis toxicity, sympathetic stimulation (which may be caused by emotional stress), and either myocardial ischemia or reperfusion.[124,129] Small platelet or platelet/fibrin thromboemboli have been observed in 10% to 15% of hearts of victims of sudden coronary death and are a possible cause of fatal arrhythmia.[117,119]

Myocardial infarction

Myocardial infarction refers to the death of part or all of a region of myocardial ischemia. Infarction occurs when ischemia has been sufficiently prolonged to induce *irreversible* injury of the affected cells so that necrosis occurs even if blood flow is later restored. The pathogenesis, anatomic features, and complications of myocardial infarction are described in detail below.

Causes of sudden onset of ischemia. The majority of myocardial infarcts involve myocardium supplied by a single coronary artery. When studied post mortem in the acute phase, a majority (but not all) of such infarcts can be related to recent occlusion of a coronary artery, usually by thrombosis superimposed on preexisting atherosclerotic disease.[142,162,176,182] (Other unusual causes of coronary obstruction have been discussed previously.) In many cases of coronary thrombosis, the thrombi contain fragments of atherosclerotic plaque (see Fig. 15-1). Disruption of the endothelial surface, with consequent hemorrhage into the plaque and rupture of plaque contents into the residual coronary lumen, can be found in association with nearly all coronary thrombi if serial histologic sections are examined. Based on such observations, several investigators have postulated that the immediate cause of coronary thrombosis is almost always the prior disruption of the atherosclerotic plaque[127,141,148,150,174] (Fig. 15-7).

In a significant minority of fatal cases of myocardial infarction there is no postmortem anatomic explanation for the initiation of the infarct. In such cases the coronary artery normally supplying the region of infarct either may be open or may be occluded by atherosclerotic plaque antedating the myocardial infarct.[162] In the latter situation it must be presumed that myocardial infarction was precipitated by interference with blood flow through collateral arterial anastomoses. In either case, the absence of an acute coronary event requires the postulate that the infarct was caused by a dynamic event, that is, a transient obstruction of coronary blood flow that initiated the infarct but was no longer demonstrable at the time of autopsy.[154] A likely cause of dynamic coronary occlusion is thrombosis or embolism, with subsequent spontaneous thrombolysis.[169] Alternatively, in recent years, coronary artery spasm alone, or in conjunction with platelet aggregation, has become a recognized cause of acute myocardial ischemia[149,165,168] (Fig. 15-7).

The frequency of spontaneous coronary thrombolysis is unknown. Coronary thrombi have been documented in 80% to 90% of patients with acute myocardial infarction and studied during life. For example, DeWood et al.[143] reported coronary thrombi in 87% of patients studied angiographically within 4 hours of the onset of symptoms of acute myocardial infarction. This incidence of occlusive thrombi observed in living patients, studied in an acute state, is higher than the incidence observed in most postmortem studies (range 21% to 91%).[177] Moreover, in the studies of DeWood et al.[143] the incidence of thrombi decreased with increasing duration of symptoms. These clinical studies indicate that thrombosis may be a more frequent cause of myocardial infarction than had previously been suspected. In ad-

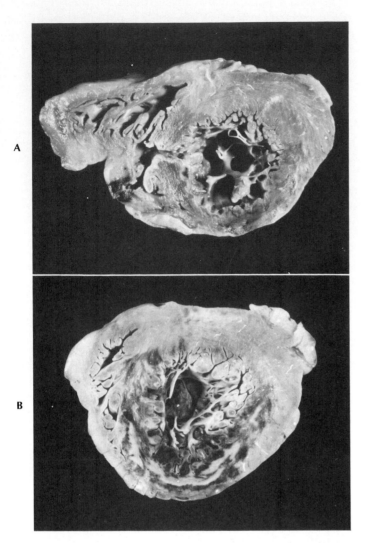

Fig. 15-8. A, Cross section of the cardiac ventricles showing a 3- to 4-day-old anteroseptal infarct of left ventricle. The view is from the base of the heart so that the anterior wall is on the bottom of the picture. The infarct is darker than the noninfarcted muscle because of congestion of the infarcted region. Notice that an anatomic complication of infarction, that is, rupture of the interventricular septum, has occurred. There is infarct expansion, evident by lateral displacement of the anterior papillary muscle and thinning of the anterior wall of the left ventricle. The medial aspect of the anterior wall of the right ventricle also is involved by the infarct. **B,** Cross section of the ventricles of the heart near the apex showing a 13-day-old (organizing) anteroseptal infarct. The infarct is characterized by a yellow-tan central zone composed of necrotic myocardium that is bordered by a dark zone composed of highly vascular granulation tissue. A mural thrombus can be seen in the left ventricular cavity.

dition, the decreasing incidence of thrombi with increasing duration of symptoms is circumstantial evidence favoring spontaneous thrombolysis.

Coronary spasm, if prolonged, might cause myocardial infarction. In addition, the possible interactions among endothelial injury, platelet microaggregation, release of prostaglandins and other vasoactive substances, and coronary spasm have sparked considerable interest.[164] However, the relative frequency of coronary vasospasm as a cause of acute myocardial infarction remains unknown.

Hemodynamic disturbances that cause increased myocardial metabolic demands or reduced coronary perfusion pressure or both also may cause myocardial infarction. Subendocardial myocardial infarcts often are unassociated with coronary thrombi and may be the consequence of hemodynamic disturbances superimposed on severe coronary atherosclerotic disease. Circumferential subendocardial infarcts may be caused by transient hypotension in the presence or absence of generalized atherosclerotic coronary disease. Anatomic causes of reduced coronary perfusion pressure include aortic stenosis or insufficiency and hypertrophic cardiomyopathy with aortic outflow obstruction.

Location of myocardial infarcts. Nearly all infarcts occur in the left ventricle. The most frequent site is the anterior region of the left ventricle, which is supplied by the anterior descending branch of the left coronary artery (Fig. 15-8). This vascular region includes the anterior two thirds of the interventricular septum and the apex of the ventricle. The next most common site is the posterior region of the left ventricle. In approximately 90% to 95% of individuals this region is supplied by the right coronary artery (right predominant coronary anatomy). This coronary vascular region includes the posterior third of the interventricular septum, and a variable portion of the posterior free wall except for the apex. Less commonly, infarcts occur in the lateral wall of the left ventricle, which is the vascular territory of the circumflex coronary artery.

Myocardial infarcts are classified as anterior, posterior (inferior or diaphragmatic), lateral, septal, and circumferential, depending on the general region of the left ventricle involved,[146] or according to combinations of these terms, such as anterolateral, posterolateral, and anteroseptal. Although the septum often is involved in infarcts of the anterior or posterior types, only rarely are infarcts limited to the ventricular septum. An infarct that is designated posterior by this classification may be referred to as either diaphragmatic or inferior in electrocardiographic terminology.

It is important to recognize that the use of these general terms to indicate infarct location does not imply that infarcts have ill-defined boundaries; the boundaries of infarcts are determined by the boundaries of the vascular territory or territories that were subjected to ischemia. For example, postmortem studies of human myocardial infarcts have shown a close relationship between the lateral boundaries of the infarct and the boundaries of the involved vascular bed, using radiographs of ventricular slices after coronary injection with radiopaque material to allow identification of the vascular bed.[162] In these studies, infarct boundaries consistently matched vascular bed boundaries. The explanation for such sharp boundaries is that the vascular territories of the major coronary arteries and their branches have sharp albeit irregular interfaces with adjacent vascular territories. Postmortem studies of the microcirculation in human hearts have shown "end-capillary loops"; that is, capillaries loop back without connecting to capillaries of adjacent vascular regions.[147]

However, widespread coronary vascular disease may make the pathophysiologic picture more complex; the area at risk of infarction is not always easily defined. For example, occlusion of one coronary artery may occur gradually, and because collateral arterial anastomoses from branches of other arteries enlarge, infarction may be prevented. As a result, two anatomic vascular regions may be dependent on flow through a single coronary artery. Occlusion of this artery not only would place its myocardial region at risk but also would jeopardize the collateral dependent vascular region[162] and thereby cause "infarction at a distance."[152] Hemodynamic disturbances also may cause ischemia in two or more vascular regions if severe coronary stenoses exist. Severe hemodynamic disturbances may place the entire ventricle in jeopardy and cause circumferential subendocardial infarction.

The right ventricle is infrequently involved, and when it is, the lesion usually is an extension of an infarct of the left ventricle.[130,157,170] Rarely is the lesion limited to the right ventricle.[178,184] Some writers have suggested that the relatively thin wall of this ventricle is sufficiently nourished by blood directly from the lumen of the heart through the luminal vessels, thus preventing infarction. Others reason that the right ventricle is less susceptible to infarction because its systolic pressure is much lower than the systolic pressure of the left ventricle. Thus the metabolic requirements of the right ventricle are not as great as those in the left ventricle. In addition, there is less interference with coronary blood flow by constriction of intramyocardial vessels during systole.

Infarcts of the atria frequently are unrecognized during life and even at autopsy. Statistics vary greatly as to the incidence of atrial infarcts, depending a great deal on the thoroughness with which one searches for them. In a study of 182 consecutive cases of myocardial infarct, 31 (17%) of the hearts examined were found to have atrial involvement.[140] Most atrial infarcts occur in the right atrium (especially in the right atrial appendage). They often are accompanied by mural thrombi and usually are associated with infarcts of the left ventricle. It is believed that the oxygenated blood of the left atrium tends to protect this chamber from infarction. In many atrial infarcts, obstructive disease of the nutrient blood vessels is not identified.

Transmural extent and course of infarction. It is now generally accepted that after coronary occlusion ischemic myocytes do not die instantaneously; mildly ischemic myocytes may survive indefinitely, and within the region that does undergo infarction, not all myocytes die simultaneously.[172,173] These concepts are crucially important; they form the basis for experimental and clinical efforts to design therapy that can limit myocardial infarct size.[156] However, the course of ischemic cell death during myocardial infarction cannot be easily established in humans. Thus the duration of time during which therapy could conceivably limit myocardial infarct size can be estimated only crudely from indirect assessments of infarct size or cardiac function in large clinical trials, or from more direct studies of the course of myocardial infarction in the experimental animal.

In dogs, the subendocardial zone of the myocardial wall is most susceptible to myocardial infarction.[172,173] This increased susceptibility may be related to a more severe degree of ischemia (lower collateral flow) in this zone after coronary occlusion or to greater metabolic requirements of the subendocardial zone, or both.[145,163] It has been consistently observed in experimental models of coronary occlusion that if there is collateral blood flow available, it is distributed disproportionately to the subepicardial zone of the ischemic region.[134,144,172,175,187]

The course of ischemic cell death has been most clearly demonstrated by studies in which various periods of temporary coronary occlusion have been followed by reperfusion. In anesthetized, open-chest dogs, even the most severely ischemic myocytes remain viable for at least 15 minutes.[158,159,199] If reperfusion is established during this interval, infarction can be prevented, and cellular metabolism, ultrastructure, and contractile function all eventually recover. Beyond 15 minutes of coronary occlusion in this experimental model, increasing numbers of ischemic myocytes become irreversibly injured, as defined by the fact that reperfusion does not prevent myocardial cell death. By 40 minutes, much of the subendocardial zone, if severely ischemic, has been irreversibly injured.[159,172] Nevertheless, much of the midepicardial and subepicardial region is still viable; reperfusion prevents infarction of these zones. With increasing duration of coronary occlusion, a transmural "wavefront" of cell death progresses from the subendocardium to the subepicardium[172,173] (Fig. 15-9). A similar temporal evolution of myocardial infarction, begin-

Myocardial infarct size after ischemia (I) and reperfusion (R)

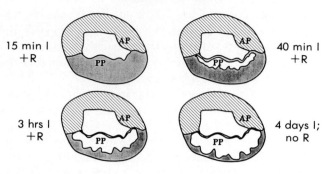

☒ Nonischemic ■ Occluded vascular bed □ Infarct
(area at risk)

Fig. 15-9. Progression of cell death versus time after circumflex coronary occlusion in dogs. Myocardial necrosis expected after various durations of ischemia, *I*, and reperfusion, *R*, is illustrated. Necrosis occurs first in the subendothelial myocardium. With longer occlusions, a wavefront of cell death moves from the subendocardial zone across the wall to involve progressively more of the transmural thickness of the ischemic zone. In contrast, the lateral margins in the subendocardial region of the infarct are established as early as 40 minutes after occlusion and are sharply defined by the anatomic boundaries of the ischemic bed. *AP,* Anterior papillary muscle; *PP,* posterior papillary muscle. (Modified from Reimer, K.A., and Jennings, R.B.: Lab. Invest. **40:**633, 1979.)

ning in the subendocardial region and only later involving the subepicardial region, has been observed in awake as well as anesthetized dogs and in other species, including rabbits, pigs, and baboons.[133,139,153,161,181] In all such experimental models of abrupt coronary occlusion, the spatial progression of infarction is complete in 3 to 6 hours. Reperfusion after 6 hours or more of myocardial ischemia does not limit infarct size.

In humans, as in experimental models, subendocardial myocardium is more susceptible to ischemic injury than subepicardial myocardium is. This concept is supported by the fact that infarcts usually are not completely transmural.[156] Most human infarcts observed at autopsy, whether or not Q waves were present in electrocardiograms obtained during life, are most extensive in the subendocardial region, with variable degrees of projection into the subepicardial region.[179,185,186] Because the subendocardial region is most susceptible to ischemic injury, it is reasonable to assume that myocardial infarction begins there and later progresses toward the epicardium, as has been demonstrated experimentally. The course of such progression in patients is unknown. It seems likely that the 3- to 6-hour course observed experimentally might apply to the subset of patients with severe myocardial ischemia, caused by sudden proximal occlusion of a major coronary artery, when no previous stimulus for collateral growth had been present. Such a worst-case scenario might result from a coronary embolus, for example. It is plausible, but not proved, that the course of ischemic cell death could be slower if the degree of ischemia is less severe or if it has a more gradual onset.[171] For example, ischemia could be less severe if the involved coronary artery is only partially obstructed, or if prior coronary disease has induced the growth of functionally important collateral interconnections. Moreover, infarction could be expected to develop relatively slowly in patients whose hemodynamic determinants of myocardial oxygen needs are low.

Recent experimental studies in dogs have shown that "preconditioning" myocardium with repetitive brief episodes of ischemia delays the onset of myocardial necrosis in a subsequent longer period of ischemia.[166] If such results are applicable to humans, infarcts either caused by or preceded by intermittent coronary spasm or intermittent thrombosis alleviated by spontaneous thrombolysis might develop over a slower course compared with the course established in experimental animals with sudden coronary occlusions.

The importance of collateral anastomoses in patients with ischemic heart disease has been the subject of much controversy in the past. It is generally accepted that coronary collaterals are present but poorly developed in normal human hearts.[132,151] On the other hand, patients with severe coronary artery disease often do have collateral anastomoses that are sufficiently well developed to be visualized by coronary angiography. The functional value of such visible collaterals has been widely debated.[138,167] From experimental studies it is known that even complete coronary occlusion, if induced gradually, may result in no myocardial infarction at all.[155,160] Moreover, it has long been recognized from postmortem studies of human hearts that complete coronary occlusion may be associated with little or no myocardial infarction.[131,135,136,183] Such observations are direct and striking evidence for the importance of coronary collateral perfusion for the prevention of infarction or limitation of infarct size. Thus it is likely that the transmural extent of a human myocardial infarct is determined at least in part by the amount of collateral blood flow to this region.[162]

Acute cellular consequences of myocardial ischemia[218,219]

Energy metabolism. Within a few seconds after occlusion of a major coronary artery, tissue oxygen content decreases and mitochondrial oxidative metabolism becomes inhibited. Flux through the respiratory chain slows, and as the net level of reduced nicotinamide adenine dinucleotide (NADH) increases, Krebs citric acid cycle and fatty acid oxidation also become inhibited. Concomitantly with the inhibition of oxidative reactions, anaerobic glycolysis becomes accelerated; in severe myocardial ischemia, sarcoplasmic glycogen is the major substrate for this pathway. Thus the early metabolic consequences of ischemia[201,220] include declining reserves of glycogen and progressive accumulation of lactate, the end product of anaerobic glycolysis. Even though contractile function, the major energy-dependent process of working myocardium, is suppressed quickly during ischemia, the basal rate of ATP use continues to outstrip the capacity of myocardium to produce ATP. Thus a major hallmark of ischemia is the progressive depletion of high-energy phosphate reserves.[200,201,210]

Accumulation of metabolic end products. Although many of the deleterious effects of ischemia may be caused by the consequences of oxygen deprivation (hypoxia) by itself, other consequences of ischemic injury may relate to the deleterious effects of catabolite accumulation. As already noted, lactate and the purine nucleosides and bases rapidly accumulate in severely ischemic tissue.[203] Acidosis increases as a consequence of several catabolic pathways, including anaerobic glycolysis, lipolysis, and ATP hydrolysis.[197] Ammonia accumulates as a result of deamination of adenosine, amino acids, and so forth, and inorganic phosphate accumulates as high-energy phosphates are degraded.

Acidosis may contribute to the inhibition of contractile functions, a potential advantage in delaying high-energy phosphate depletion. However, as noted earlier, acidosis also inhibits a variety of metabolic pathways including anaerobic glycolysis[226] and has been shown to have deleterious ultrastructural consequences including the aggregation of nuclear chromatin and the formation of mitochondrial amorphous matrix densities.[189] Lactate accumulation also has been associated with ultrastructural and functional evidence of cellular injury[188,214]; whether the observed deleterious effects are because of lactate by itself or the accompanying intracellular acidosis is difficult to differentiate.

Even in the absence of toxicity of individual catabolites, the combined effect of the aforementioned catabolic pathways is a substantial intracellular osmotic load that may contribute to cell swelling. Cell swelling has been proposed as a cause of the rupture of the sarcolemma, which occurs in irreversible ischemic damage after the sarcolemma or its cytoskeletal supports already have been weakened by other consequences of ischemia.[224]

Lipid and protein catabolism. Myocardial lipolysis is increased in ischemia, apparently through a catecholamine-dependent mechanism. Thus increased but small quantities of fatty acids, acyl coenzyme A, and acyl car-

nitine accumulate even in severely ischemic tissue.[216] In areas of mild ischemia, fatty acid uptake from the plasma also is facilitated and, coupled with the limited capacity for fatty acid oxidation and the abundant supplies of α-glycerol phosphate from glycolysis, can result in accumulation of intracellular lipid.[210]

Increased concentrations of fatty acid esters can be detrimental to myocytes in several ways.[205,209] For example, acyl coenzyme A inhibits adenine nucleotide translocase, an enzyme that is responsible for export of ATP from mitochondria to sarcoplasm. Fatty acids also inhibit mitochondrial respiration and uncouple oxidative phosphorylation. It also has been postulated that fatty acid esters such as lysophospholipids may act as detergents and disrupt cellular membranes.[214] Arachidonic acid is one of the fatty acids that accumulate in ischemic myocardium; arachidonic acid is a major component of phospholipids, and its accumulation in the tissue is indirect evidence for catabolism of cellular membranes during ischemia.[191]

Free radicals. In the last few years, much attention has focused on the idea that production of free radicals may be increased during myocardial ischemia or in the early period after reperfusion, and that free radicals such as superoxide or hydroxyl radicals could contribute to myocyte injury.[195] Free radicals are highly reactive molecular species that can cause detrimental alterations of proteins, nucleic acids, and lipids. For example, free radicals can cause lipid peroxidation and thereby alter the properties of sarcolemmal or other cellular membranes.[217] There are many potential sources for increased free-radical production in ischemia. The xanthine oxidase reaction (which converts hypoxanthine to xanthine with formation of superoxide) has been of particular interest[190] because of the known rapid catabolism of adenine nucleotides to nucleosides and bases in ischemia,[221] of which hypoxanthine and xanthine are substrates for the xanthine oxidase reaction. Neutrophils are another potential source of free-radical injury. Neutrophils participate in the inflammatory response to injured myocytes and capillaries; their beneficial role in the initial phases of infarct repair may be counterbalanced by the injurious effects of the local release of superoxide anions and lysosomal enzymes in the vicinity of myocytes that are still viable.[222]

Ion gradients. Maintenance of electrolyte gradients is energy dependent, and although the Michaelis constant (K_m) of the sodium-potassium ATPase for ATP is low, considerable ATP depletion in ischemia eventually results in its inhibition. Net sodium influx and a potassium loss occur. The loss of ion-transport activity also may contribute to net influx of water and consequent cell swelling.

Ischemia also may lead to increased cytosolic calcium because of increased influx from the extracellular space or sarcoplasmic reticulum, or because of insufficient energy for extrusion.[206,214] A cellular calcium overload could have serious consequences for the myocyte; calcium activates a variety of proteases, lipases, and phospholipases and may augment ATP depletion by activating a variety of ATPases. In addition, excess calcium inhibits mitochondrial respiration.

Neurophysiologic changes. Endogenous norepinephrine is released from adrenergic nerve terminals in ischemic myocardium within the first hour after the onset of occlusion. Simultaneously, the numbers of exposed beta-receptors detected in membrane fractions of homogenized cardiac myocytes increase.[211] The cause of excessive norepinephrine release is uncertain; however, neuronal reuptake of norepinephrine may be decreased because it is an ATP-dependent process.[212]

Ultrastructural features. Within the first few minutes after the onset of ischemia, ultrastructural changes develop and include cellular and mitochondrial swelling, progressive loss of sarcoplasmic glycogen particles, and mild margination of nuclear chromatin.[200,203,223] These early changes have been shown to be reversible in experimental studies, in that restoration of coronary blood flow after coronary occlusion up to 15 minutes in dura-

tion results in rapid recovery of myocyte ultrastructure even in the most severely ischemic zone.[203] With a longer duration of ischemia, the aforementioned changes become progressively more pronounced. In addition, two ultrastructural features of injury develop that have been associated with the transition to irreversible injury. These are the development of amorphous densities within the matrix of mitochondria and the development of breaks in the trilaminar unit membrane of the sarcolemma.[201,220] In the absence of reperfusion, these ultrastructural features persist; eventually, coagulation necrosis becomes manifest at the light-microscopic level.

Reperfusion of myocytes containing mitochondrial amorphous matrix densities and sarcolemmal breaks by electron microscopy, even though they still appear viable at the light-microscopic level, results in contraction band necrosis, which can be detected within minutes even by light microscopy[173,208] (Fig. 15-10). The development of necrosis despite reperfusion was the initial basis for defining ischemic injury as "irreversible."[159] Contraction-band necrosis is characterized at the ultrastructural level by much worse disruption of the sarcolemma, by massive calcium influx to the sarcoplasm,

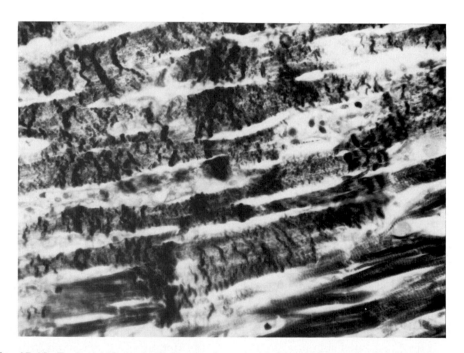

Fig. 15-10. Typical histologic features of contraction-band necrosis. A few viable myocytes are present in the lower-right corner for comparison. In contrast to coagulation necrosis, which may not become detectable for several hours after the onset of myocardial infarction, contraction-band necrosis develops almost immediately on reperfusion of irreversibly injured myocytes. This illustration is from a patient who died 2 hours after coronary bypass surgery. (Heidenhain's variant of Mallory's connective-tissue stain; 350×; reproduced with permission from Reimer, K.A., and Jennings, R.B.: In Fozzard, H.A., et al., editors: The heart and cardiovascular system, New York, 1986, Raven Press.)

and by destruction of the myofibrillar apparatus with formation of contraction bands composed of the agglutinated myofibrillar proteins of several adjacent sarcomeres.[196,208] The formation of these contraction bands probably is related to the massive calcium overload of cells that have severe damage to the sarcolemma. Additional evidence for calcium overload in these myocytes include the deposition within mitochondria of granular and crystalline deposits of calcium and phosphate (which are distinct from the amorphous densities described previously).[208]

Ultrastructural evidence of myocyte injury generally precedes ultrastructural evidence of injury to vessels.[173,194] Nevertheless, ischemia does injure blood vessels.[194,198,207,225] Mild injury may be manifest by increased capillary permeability.[198] More severe injury causes endothelial cell swelling; cytoplasmic blebs protrude into capillary lumens and may cause capillary obstruction.[207] In large infarcts, both myocytes and the microvasculature undergo necrosis, resulting in a central core of infarct that persists for weeks while infarct repair proceeds from the edge toward the center by growth of new granulation tissue.

Reperfusion of ischemic myocardium having microvascular injury may result in extensive intramyocardial hemorrhage (Plate 1, C). Moreover, in zones where capillaries have become obstructed by endothelial blebs[207] or neutrophils,[192] or compressed by microthrombi,[193] rigorous myocytes,[199] or interstitial edema, microvascular reperfusion may not be achieved despite restoration of flow through a previously occluded coronary artery. This is referred to as the "no-reflow phenomenon."[207]

Pathogenesis of irreversible ischemic cell injury. Elucidation of a specific sequence of metabolic reactions that culminate in the transition from reversible to irreversible cellular injury has proved to be difficult despite studies in many different laboratories directed toward this problem. In general, two experimental approaches have been used. The first has been to compare structural and metabolic changes in myocytes known to be in the late reversible phase of injury with changes in myocytes known to have already entered the irreversible phase of injury. A second general approach has been to intervene with a therapy designed to interrupt a metabolic reaction suspected to have critical importance in the pathogenesis of cell death, with the desired outcome being the prevention of cell death.

Several hypotheses center on disruption of the sarcolemma as the proximate cause of cell death.[201] Fig. 15-11 illustrates several intracellular processes that occur in ischemic myocytes and may contribute to sarcolemmal rupture and cell death. In general terms, two major facets of ischemia are the inadequate production of high-energy phosphates and the accumulation of potentially noxious catabolites. Declining ATP content has

many consequences, including loss of sodium and potassium gradients, calcium overload, and possible activation of endogenous phospholipases or proteases. Calcium overload may also contribute to activation of phospholipases or proteases that could damage either the sarcolemma or its cytoskeletal supports. Accumulation of catabolites such as lactate and NADH inhibit ATP production. Products of lipid degradation may act as detergents to damage cell membranes. Adenine nucleosides and bases accumulate and may be a major source of free radicals via the xanthine oxidase reaction. In addition, accumulating catabolites are an intracellular osmotic load, which may accentuate cell swelling and facilitate rupture of already weakened membranes.

In the setting of reperfusion, the prognosis of individual myocytes depends not only on their internal state at the onset of reperfusion but also on the state of the supporting microvasculature and perhaps on the manner of reperfusion, or the nature of the inflammatory response that may be elicited by damaged myocytes or capillaries.[201,202] It is possible that some myocytes that are potentially salvageable at the onset of reperfusion are killed by some aspect of reperfusion (that is, so-called "reperfusion injury").[204] It also is hypothetically possible that microvascular damage results in perpetuation of ischemia in some areas where myocytes might have been salvageable were it not for the vascular injury. However, currently available data generally support the view that severe microvascular damage is a late phenomenon in areas where myocyte death already has occurred. Finally, whereas the inflammatory response is a necessary part of the process of infarct repair, the inflammatory response also could exacerbate myocyte or microvascular injury. Under what conditions any of these or other reactions may be of seminal importance in the pathogenesis of ischemic cell death requires further elucidation.

Early diagnosis of myocardial infarction. Because the histologic features of coagulation necrosis develop slowly, much effort has been devoted to establishing methods to enable earlier anatomic recognition of the presence and extent of myocardial infarction. The ultrastructural characteristics of irreversible injury reviewed in previous paragraphs permit early recognition of infarction in experimental studies, but electron microscopy is impractical for assessment of the extent of injury. Only a few myocytes can be evaluated in any given sample of tissue; processing multiple samples is extremely time consuming. Moreover, electron-microscopic evaluation usually is of little value as an aid to early diagnosis of human myocardial infarcts because changes induced by regional ischemia in vivo soon become indistinguishable from identical changes induced by postmortem autolysis, that is, global (total) ischemia. For this reason, a variety of special histologic or histochemical staining techniques have been studied,[231] in-

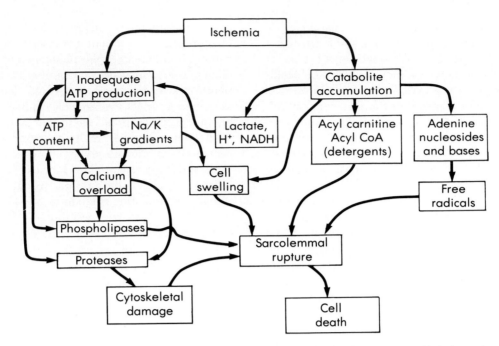

Fig. 15-11. Some potential pathways leading to sarcolemmal damage, which form the basis for various hypotheses of events leading to irreversible ischemic cell injury. In general terms, two major facets of ischemia are the inadequate production of ATP and the accumulation of potentially noxious catabolites. Declining ATP content could have many adverse consequences including loss of sodium and potassium gradients, calcium overload, and activation of endogenous phospholipases or proteases. Calcium overload also could cause activation of phospholipases or proteases; the latter could damage the sarcolemma or its cytoskeletal supports. Accumulation of catabolites such as lactate, hydrogen ion, and reduced nicotinamide adenine dinucleotide inhibit anaerobic glycolysis and thereby inhibit ATP production in ischemia. Products of lipid degradation may act as detergents and damage cell membranes. Adenine nucleosides and bases accumulate and might be a major source of free radicals through the xanthine oxidase reaction. In addition, accumulating catabolites are an intracellular osmotic load, which may accentuate cell swelling and facilitate the rupture of already weakened membranes. At present, the relative importance of these various pathways in the pathogenesis of ischemic cell death has not been established. Moreover, many reactions, which have not been studied as well and are not included on this diagram, occur in ischemic myocardium; it is not even certain that the most important pathways are illustrated. (Reproduced with permission from Reimer, K.A., and Jennings, R.B.: In Fozzard, H. A., et al., editors: The heart and cardiovascular system, New York, 1986, Raven Press.)

cluding the periodic acid–Schiff (PAS) stain for glycogen loss[227,229,233,235,241,245] or entry of PAS-positive diastase-fast plasma proteins into the myocytes,[232,245] chemical analysis of tissue potassium/sodium ratios,[239,240,246] hematoxylin–basic fuchsin–picric acid staining,[236,243] tetracycline binding,[242] and a host of stains for specific intracellular enzyme activities such as phosphorylase or succinic dehydrogenase.[227,231,233,241,244] For the most part, these staining techniques have not been widely accepted. Under controlled circumstances,

each technique may be useful. However, most of these methods are limited either by lack of specificity (failure to differentiate ischemia from postmortem autolysis) or insufficient early sensitivity.

In contrast, macroscopic methods of staining for dehydrogenase activity have become widely used. The most widely used dehydrogenase stains are *para*-nitroblue tetrazolium (pNBT) and triphenyltetrazolium chloride (TTC).[228,230,237,238] Each of these two dyes is colorless when oxidized but turns blue (pNBT) or brick red (TTC) when reduced through the transfer of hydrogen to the dyes from NADH or reduced flavoproteins, catalyzed by endogenous myocardial dehydrogenases. Viable myocardium is capable of reducing either of these dyes, but myocardium that has lost dehydrogenase activity or sufficient concentrations of the cofactors, such as NADH,[234] remains unstained after addition of the oxidized dyes. Such absence of staining is considered to indicate cell death. Of the two dyes, TTC is the more commonly employed; it is less expensive than pNBT and can be perfused throughout the ischemic region through the coronary arteries, whereas pNBT does not readily traverse the capillary and therefore must be applied to the surfaces of myocardial slices. When used with completed infarcts, or in the setting of reperfused infarcts, these histochemical stains are capable of identifying dead myocardium and demarcating the boundaries of infarcts that might otherwise be poorly differentiated from viable tissue. Some investigators hold that these histochemical staining techniques permit early diagnosis and even demarcation of the boundaries of infarcts within the first 3 hours after the onset and before histologic diagnosis is possible.[230] However, this view remains controversial. Whereas loss of dehydrogenase enzyme activity probably indicates cell death, lethal cell injury precedes loss of such activity, and the presence and extent of early infarction may be underestimated.

Inflammatory response and reparative phase. Myocardial infarction is a complex, dynamic process in which ischemic cell death is an early event. Dead cardiac myocytes do not regenerate; they must be removed and eventually replaced by scar. Whereas progression of myocardial cell death may go to completion in a matter of minutes or hours, the process of repair requires 4 to 6 weeks under optimum conditions.

Inflammatory response. Although lysosomal proteases and lipases are released and activated within dead myocytes (and may even contribute to lethality), endogenous degradative enzymes are insufficient to bring about complete dissolution of dead myocytes. Removal of necrotic myocytes depends on the influx of inflammatory cells, including polymorphonuclear neutrophils and macrophages. In the center of large infarcts, both myocytes and the microvasculature undergo necrosis; inflammatory cells initially have no access to the infarct center (Plate 1, *B*). In such areas, dead myocytes persist, retaining their basic structure for days or weeks, until inflammatory cells, initially present on the outer edge of the infarct, can invade the infarct center by direct migration or by ingrowth of new capillaries (Figs. 15-8 and 15-12).

The general characteristics of the acute inflammatory response have been studied extensively, especially in regard to infectious disease and trauma.[267] The neutro-

Fig. 15-12. Organizing myocardial infarct. Necrotic muscle is surrounded by granulation tissue, lymphocytes, and macrophages.

philic response has been characterized as a process involving margination (concentration toward the endothelial cell), emigration across the capillary wall, and chemotactic attraction to sites of injury. In general terms, chemotactic factors for polymorphonuclear neutrophils are known to include components of the complement pathway, histamine, various kinins, fibrinopeptides, and certain products of bacteria.[262,264] Macrophages are attracted by other complement components, bacterial factors, factors from degenerating neutrophils, kallikreins, lymphokines, and so on.[265]

The inflammatory response, as it relates specifically to myocardial infarction, has not been widely studied. In large myocardial infarcts, when much microvascular damage has occurred, an intense neutrophilic response often is observed. In contrast, in smaller infarcts, when most of the microvasculature has been spared, the neutrophilic response may be minimal, and macrophages will be the most notable elements of the early inflammatory response. The specific factors that attract inflammatory cells to myocardial infarcts and that determine the intensity of the inflammatory response are not completely elucidated. However, it is known that subcellular fractions of cardiac muscle can activate the complement system.[250,256] More specifically, lysosomal proteases can activate complement; components of this pathway may, in turn, attract neutrophils to the dead myocytes.[252] In addition, metabolites of arachidonic acid, such as hydroxyeicosatetraenoic acids (HETEs), are produced by the action of neutrophil lipoxygenases;

these substances also are chemotactic for neutrophils[255,264] and may serve to amplify the initial neutrophilic response.

The inflammatory response is essential for resolution and repair of an infarcted area. On the other hand, recent evidence indicates that the inflammatory response also might cause additional injury of still viable myocytes, and thereby increase infarct size. Components of the complement system as well as polymorphonuclear neutrophils accumulate in ischemic myocardium.[257,259] Polymorphonuclear neutrophils release a variety of proteases and lipases[266] as well as free radicals, such as the superoxide anion, to the myocardial interstitium.[249] Moreover, the inflammatory response begins at and is most intense at the peripheral zone of an infarct where the microvasculature permits access and where peninsulas of dead and viable myocytes interdigitate. However, whether, to what extent, and under what circumstances the inflammatory response does in fact cause additional myocyte necrosis remains open to question.[222,254,259]

Reparative phase. The general process of repair by scar formation also is known, but, again, detailed mechanisms of the reparative phase are poorly understood, and the determinants of the quantity and tensile strength of myocardial scars are unknown. The most widely held view is that necrotic myocardium, including its reticular framework,[261] is removed and replaced by granulation tissue (new capillaries and fibroblasts), with gradual deposition of both collagen and components of ground substance such as proteoglycans and glycoproteins.[248,253,263] However, in smaller infarcts, and particularly when the microvasculature has been spared, scar formation may occur by collagen deposition on the original reticular framework in the infarcted region.

Most investigators believe that the major determinant of scar size is infarct size. It also is recognized that myocardial scars may be considerably smaller than the volume of necrotic myocardium that they have replaced[247,258] (and appear even smaller because of compensatory hypertrophy of remaining viable myocardium).[247,260] However, neither the precise relationship between initial infarct size and ultimate scar size nor variables that affect this relationship are well known. Such knowledge would be of considerable value; whereas infarct size affects cardiac function through loss of contractile mass, the nature of the scar may have additional, independent effects on function. For example, an overly exuberant scar may restrict the contraction of remaining viable myocytes in an ischemic region. On the other hand, a weak scar may result in further loss of function because of aneurysmal dilatation of the infarct region, or may be fatal if cardiac rupture supervenes. It has been reported that exercise has an adverse effect on infarct repair in rats.[251]

Course of infarct repair. The speed of healing of a myocardial infarct depends first and foremost on the size of the infarct and on the extent of microvascular damage. In addition, the rate of healing depends on other less readily characterized factors, such as neutrophil competence. Nevertheless, the sequence of inflammation and repair is sufficiently predictable to permit the age of an infarct to be estimated. The precision with which infarct age can be established is inversely related to age; on the first day or so, infarct age can be established to the nearest 12 hours; the age of 10-day-old infarcts can be established plus or minus 3 or 4 days; beyond 6 months, scars of different ages often cannot be differentiated. The general sequence of events from which infarct age can be estimated has long been known from the work of Mallory et al.[271] and others[269,270] and is as follows:

Although dramatic metabolic and ultrastructural changes occur early in ischemic injury, myocardial infarction may not be detectable by routine gross or histologic techniques until 6 to 12 hours have elapsed. The earliest gross evidence of infarction often is pallor, most likely related to the development of cardiac rigor and the accompanying compression of the microvasculature and expulsion of erythrocytes. In contrast, focal areas of hemorrhage may develop because of microvascular injury. The gross changes become more prominent with time during the first 48 hours (Fig. 15-8). The classic histologic features of coagulation necrosis, consisting in increased cytoplasmic eosinophilia and nuclear karyolysis (dissolution) or pyknosis (shrinkage), may be detectable in some cases within the first 2 to 4 hours, but in some cases may not be detectable as late as 8 to 12 hours. In our experience, because staining intensity may vary, increased eosinophilia best can be recognized when the interface between dead and viable myocytes can be located. For example, because a narrow rim of myocytes below the endocardium often survives an ischemic insult (presumably by diffusion of oxygen and substrates from the left ventricular cavity), increased eosinophilia can be detected with greatest sensitivity by comparison of deeper subendocardial myocardium with this superficial layer. Increased eosinophilia is matched by increased acidophilia when connective-tissue stains such as Masson's trichrome stain are used. An additional early feature of myocardial infarction is the development of "wavy fiber change"[268] (caused by stretching of ischemic myocytes during life, with undulations developing after death when rigor contracture develops in surrounding areas). Contraction-band necrosis may be detected as early as the first hour after the onset of ischemia, if reperfusion has been established. In the absence of reperfusion, contraction-band necrosis can sometimes be seen on the edge of an infarct.[272] Although loss of sarcoplasmic cross-striations and karyolysis are often considered to be hallmarks of early necrosis according to standard textbook descriptions, these changes are not absolute; in the center of myocardial infarcts, nuclear outlines and cross-striations may be visible for days or even weeks, so long as unresorbed myocytes persist.

Polymorphonuclear neutrophils marginating within the microvasculature sometimes can be observed within the first hour or two of infarction. However, in many cases, the influx of neutrophils cannot be easily detected until 12 to 18 hours after the onset. The number of inflammatory cells increases with time, becoming most prominent by the third day after infarction (Fig. 15-13). Neutrophils that migrate to the site of infarction do not return to the circulation but undergo lysis at the site of injury. Fragments of disintegrated neutrophils are often detectable by the second day and are most prominent by the third through fifth days. By the fourth or fifth day, the influx of neutrophils has begun to subside, macrophages have become more prominent, and the removal of necrotic myocytes has begun. The progressive removal of necrotic myocytes is soon followed by ingrowth of new capillary buds and fibroblasts; by the tenth day the periphery of the infarct is bordered by a distinct rim of granulation tissue (Fig. 15-12). By gross observation, necrotic myocardium becomes yellow, as compared with the red-brown color of

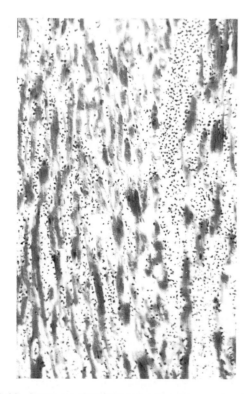

Fig. 15-13. Acute myocardial infarction (approximately 2 or 3 days old). Necrotic muscle fibers are separated by heavy neutrophilic infiltration.

normal myocardium. The peripheral rim of granulation tissue is grossly evident as a hyperemic rim around the infarct (related to the pronounced vascularity of granulation tissue) (Fig. 15-8). Between the second and fourth week, much of the necrotic muscle is removed, though the duration required for complete removal depends on the initial size of the infarct. As necrotic myocytes are removed, the rim of granulation tissue expands. This removal of necrotic muscle and ingrowth of granulation tissue is referred to as "organization" of the infarct. By about the twelfth day, thin collagen fibers begin to be deposited within the young scar. With increasing time, collagen content increases, and the cellularity of the scar gradually decreases. Grossly, the reddish-gray gelatinous character of granulation tissue is replaced by the opaque gray-white color characteristic of a dense collagen scar. Although some macrophages and mononuclear inflammatory cells may persist for as long as a year or two after infarction, the process of infarct repair is essentially complete by 3 to 6 months. Given this typical sequence of the reparative process, it is possible to estimate, from the gross character and more precisely from microscopic features, the approximate age of an acute or organizing myocardial infarct.

Early and late cardiac complications of myocardial infarction. The morbidity and mortality associated with myocardial infarction in humans can be related in most cases either to inadequate pumping capabilities of the heart (pump failure) or to cardiac arrhythmias. Severe pump failure may occur in the acute phase of myocardial infarction and result in the clinical syndrome known as "cardiogenic shock." Less severe dysfunction may persist long after an acute infarct as congestive heart failure. Usually these forms of heart failure are caused by loss of a substantial quantity of functional myocardium. Cardiac dilatation or papillary muscle dysfunction may cause mitral insufficiency, which also contributes to reduced cardiac performance. In a minority of cases, cardiac dysfunction may be attributable to specific anatomic complications such as acute infarct expansion or later formation of a ventricular aneurysm (Plate 1, *A*). Rupture of some part of the myocardium, such as the external wall, interventricular septum, or, rarely, a papillary muscle, may cause sudden and often catastrophic pump failure. Cardiac rupture is considered in more detail on the next page.

A variety of supraventricular and ventricular cardiac dysrhythmias may complicate myocardial infarction in the acute phase; a propensity for ventricular dysrhythmias may persist chronically and become manifest as recurrent ventricular tachycardia or as sudden death; the latter is believed to be usually caused by ventricular fibrillation. A specific anatomic basis for most types of acute or chronic dysrhythmias has not been identified;

however, disturbances of cardiac conduction such as complete heart block or bundle branch block[292] may be caused by necrosis of myocardium within or near a segment of the conduction pathways.[276,289]

Two additional cardiac complications of myocardial infarction are pericarditis[293,296] and left ventricular mural thrombosis.[274,278]

There also are several systemic complications of myocardial infarction or cardiac failure, such as pulmonary or systemic emboli, pulmonary edema, and acute "central hemorrhagic necrosis" or chronic "cardiac cirrhosis" of the liver. These are not considered further in this chapter.

Cardiogenic shock. The majority of deaths from myocardial infarction are caused by arrhythmias, many of which occur outside the hospital setting; the most common cause of death among hospitalized patients with myocardial infarction is "pump failure." This gives rise to the clinical syndrome of cardiogenic shock[280] and is a complication that occurs in 10% to 20% of hospitalized patients with myocardial infarction.[304] Postmortem studies of hearts of patients who died from myocardial infarction have shown that, in most cases, there are no distinctive anatomic features that permit differentiation of pump failure versus arrhythmic death.[304] However, cardiogenic shock is almost always associated with large areas of myocardial infarction involving at least 30% and often in excess of 40% of the left ventricle.[279,300] Unusually prolonged increases of plasma creatine kinase (MB fraction) have been observed in such patients; this observation is consistent with the view that cardiogenic shock by itself may cause further myocardial ischemic injury and thereby result in a vicious cycle of progressive cardiac necrosis and dysfunction.[288,300]

"Ischemic cardiomyopathy." In some patients with long-standing ischemic heart disease, often with (but sometimes without) a clinical history of one or more myocardial infarcts, impaired ventricular contractile function gives rise to the clinical features of a dilated cardiomyopathy. This entity has been termed "ischemic cardiomyopathy."[277,301] Although the term "cardiomyopathy" simply means heart muscle disease, most authorities on the cardiomyopathies restrict the definition of cardiomyopathy to heart muscle disease excluding that attributable to ischemic heart disease.[273,281] Thus "ischemic cardiomyopathy" is a contradiction in terms; the syndrome might better be referred to as "end-stage ischemic heart disease" though the latter term is admittedly more cumbersome than "ischemic cardiomyopathy." Semantics aside, the pathologic counterparts to progressive, often refractory congestive heart failure most often are diffuse, severe coronary atherosclerosis and widespread myocardial scarring attributable to one or more previous myocardial infarcts.[306,312]

Mitral regurgitation. A frequent contributing cause of pump failure in myocardial infarction is mitral regurgitation, which has been reported to occur in up to 40% of posterior (inferior) and 13% of anterior myocardial infarcts.[303] Necrosis of one of the papillary muscles as well as the adjacent free wall of the heart is the usual anatomic counterpart to this clinical problem.[297,302,307,308] However, necrosis of a papillary muscle occurs much more frequently than clinically apparent mitral insufficiency does; thus papillary muscle necrosis alone probably is not sufficient to cause mitral insufficiency.[303]

Infarct expansion and ventricular aneurysm. Pronounced thinning and lateral expansion of the infarcted region contribute to overall left ventricular dilatation, and perhaps to global left ventricular dysfunction, in one third or more of patients who die of myocardial infarction during the first 30 days.[291] Infarct expansion has been detected clinically, using serial two-dimensional echocardiography, as early as 3 days after the onset of infarction, with progression over a period of days to weeks.[284]

The incidence of ventricular aneurysms after myocardial infarction depends to a large extent on one's definition of an aneurysm; a saccular bulge with a definable neck (angiographically) or a defined external protrusion of a localized area of the left ventricular wall (by postmortem evaluation) occurs in 3% to 4% of cases of myocardial infarction.[283] On the other hand, systolic bulging (dyskinesis) of a thinned-out region of the myocardial wall (Fig. 15-8, A) undoubtedly occurs much more commonly. Of ventricular aneurysms, 65% to 80% involve the anteroapical region of the left ventricle.[283,299] Although infarct expansion occurs early, ventricular aneurysms, by the more restricted definition, are often late sequelae of myocardial infarction. For example, in a series of 40 patients described by Davis and Ebert[282] the mean time between initial infarction and detection of a ventricular aneurysm was 2.8 years. Why a small fraction of myocardial scars gradually expand to form aneurysms is unknown. Congestive heart failure is present in 30% to 85% of patients with aneurysms and is the most common cause of death.[282,283,287] Mural thrombi have been observed in more than half of cases studied post mortem, but the clinical incidence of systemic thromboemboli is less frequent (5% to 40% of cases).[282,283,287]

Cardiac rupture. Cardiac rupture is a catastrophic cause of pump failure that has a variably reported incidence of 5% to 25% of fatal cases of myocardial infarction.[275,295,298] External cardiac rupture accounts for the majority of these cases,[313] and ventricular septal (Fig. 15-8, A), papillary muscle (Fig. 15-14), or combined ruptures account for the remainder. Cardiac ruptures occur with greatest frequency during the first week of infarction, corresponding to the time when necrosis and

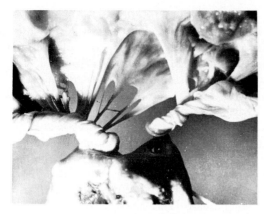

Fig. 15-14. Torsion pattern of chordae tendineae after rupture of a papillary muscle. Included in the figure is the inferior surface of mitral valve, chordae tendineae with double spiral twisting, avulsed tip of the papillary muscle, and the anterior commissure of the valve. (From Harder, H.I., and Brown, A.F.: Calif. Med. **83:**452, 1955.)

inflammation predominate; rupture is rare beyond the third week, by which time collagen deposition in the developing scar is well under way. The average duration from onset of infarction to rupture has been reported to be about 4 days in several studies of external, septal, or papillary muscle rupture[285,290,309,311,313]; however, as many as one third of external ruptures have occurred within the first 24 hours in some studies.[295] Several predisposing factors are recognized[275,290,294,295,298,310]: rupture usually requires a transmural (though not necessarily large) myocardial infarct and often occurs through first-time infarcts in hearts without a long-standing stimulus for collateral coronary growth. Systemic hypertension and cardiac hypertrophy are frequently mentioned risk factors; whether other clinical factors such as physical activity or therapy with digitalis or anticoagulants are risk factors is controversial. Cardiac rupture has been associated with preceding infarct expansion in a recent study.[305]

INFLAMMATORY HEART DISEASES
Rheumatic fever and rheumatic heart disease

Rheumatic fever is an inflammatory, nonsuppurative systemic disease that involves many different structures in the body. It is said to affect collagen or the connective tissues especially and thus has traditionally been classified with other so-called collagen or connective-tissue diseases including rheumatoid arthritis, systemic lupus erythematosus, scleroderma, dermatomyositis, and polyarteritis nodosa, but it is etiologically more closely related to acute diffuse glomerulonephritis, another disease that is caused by a hypersensitivity reaction after a beta-hemolytic streptococcal infection.

The structures involved in acute rheumatic fever include the joints, tendons, muscles, subcutaneous tissues, arteries, serous membranes, lungs, brain, and heart. However, it is the cardiac involvement that is often the cause of the morbidity and mortality that results from this disease.

Because of the protean manifestations of this disease and the lack of a specific laboratory diagnostic test, it is often difficult to differentiate it from other conditions. For this reason, T. Duckett Jones published a guide to aid in the clinical diagnosis of the acute disease. This was first published in 1944[322] and has been modified two times since then, the latest having been in 1982.[323] The criteria are divided into major and minor categories depending on their relative occurrence in rheumatic fever and the other diseases from which rheumatic fever must be differentiated. Although this system has some limitations,[320] a diagnosis of acute rheumatic fever can be made with a high probability if two major, or one major and two minor, criteria are found. In addition, it is necessary that these criteria be supported by evidence of a preceding streptococcal infection.

The major criteria are as follows:
1. Carditis
2. Polyarthritis
3. Chorea
4. Subcutaneous nodules
5. Erythema marginatum

The minor diagnostic criteria include the following:
1. Fever
2. Arthralgia
3. Longer PR interval in the ECG
4. Increased sedimentation rate, presence of C-reactive protein or leukocytosis

Rheumatic fever is thus a disease that involves many regions of the body, but it is not of serious import to the patient unless it involves the heart. It has been said that "rheumatic fever licks the joints but bites the heart."[315] The acute stage is most common in the 10- to 15-year-old group, is said to be more common and severe in blacks than in whites, and occurs more commonly under crowded and unsanitary living conditions. Rheumatic fever occasionally causes death from heart failure in the acute phase. More commonly, patients recover from the acute illness but are thereafter susceptible to recurrent attacks because of reinfection by streptococci. Such recurrences cause repeated bouts of valvulitis and may eventually result in scarred heart valves, which produce the later symptoms of heart failure and death.

Incidence

A decrease in the incidence and severity of rheumatic fever has been occurring in the United States since the beginning of the century.[321,335] The number of deaths from rheumatic fever in the United States decreased from approximately 21 per 100,000 population in 1944 to 9 per 100,000 population in 1964. In one recent study the incidence of acute rheumatic fever in white children living in the suburbs had fallen to less than one child per 200,000 population.[326]

The reasons for this striking decline are not at all clear. Improvement in socioeconomic conditions, with decreased household crowding, was a factor in the gradual decline in the incidence of rheumatic fever that began even before the advent of penicillin and other antibiotics. However, the decline in incidence and severity was probably accelerated by treatment of streptococcal infections with penicillin and other antibiotics.[314]

Despite the decline in incidence and severity in the United States, rheumatic fever is still a threat among children in many parts of the world, particularly in the "third world" or "developing" countries in which acute rheumatic fever is said to be the leading cause of death in the 5- to 15-years-of-age group.[342] For example, the incidence in schoolchildren in India is about 100 per 100,000.[339] In addition, there have been reports of scattered outbreaks and a possible return of rheumatic fever in Utah, Colorado, Pittsburgh, and New Haven, Conn.[334] In an outbreak of acute rheumatic fever that occurred in the Salt Lake City, Utah, region it was observed that there had been a recent eightfold increase in the occurrence of the disease and that the cases had occurred not in economically deprived families but in middle-class families with above-average income.[337] In addition, there was no apparent increase in streptococcal infections. However, the isolation of a particular strain of group A streptococcus (mucoid M type 18 and M type 3) indicated that there might be rheumatogenic and nonrheumatogenic types of group A streptococci, as had been suggested many years ago,[336] and that this difference could at least partly account for the altered incidence of the disease. A theoretical basis for this association has been suggested by the recent demonstration that M proteins of several rheumatogenic stereotypes share antigenic determinants with human heart tissue.[319]

Among the predisposing factors that influence the incidence of rheumatic fever are age, sex, race, climate, socioeconomic conditions, nutrition, and heredity.[338,341] The incidence in blacks has been shown to be much higher than in whites. However, the higher incidence in blacks seems to be attributable to environmental factors as was suggested by the sharper decline in blacks than in whites when a comprehensive care program was undertaken.[321]

According to many reports, the incidence of rheumatic fever is dependent on the climate. For example, earlier studies of rheumatic fever in the United States

have shown that it occurred much less frequently in southern than in northern states and that the death rate, recurrence rate, and frequency of heart damage were less in rheumatic patients in Miami, Florida, than in similar groups in some of the northern cities.[331,343-345] Also a higher incidence occurs in cold, damp regions, particularly in proximity to low-lying areas near rivers and waterways. However, other investigators have reported evidence that there are no significant differences in the occurrence and severity of rheumatic fever and rheumatic heart disease related to geographic and climatic variations.[340,346,347] Their impression is that socioeconomic factors are important in the development of the disease regardless of geography and climate. Data from Miami, Florida,[348] differed from those of the earlier investigations[331,343-345] indicating that rheumatic fever in Miami is not unlike the pattern of illness in other endemic areas of the United States.

The significance of socioeconomic factors is reflected in the observation that rheumatic fever occurs more frequently among the poor than among the affluent classes. The disease appears to coincide closely with density of population, overcrowding of living quarters (especially for sleeping), and poor nutrition. These factors tend to favor the spread of upper respiratory streptococcal infections. The observation that rheumatic fever "runs in families" has led to genetic analyses of families with this disease. As a result of such investigations, it has been suggested that susceptibility to rheumatic fever is hereditary (as a simple recessive trait), though the nature of the inherent defect is not yet clear.[349] Although the importance of heredity cannot be denied, it is probably not the only reason for a high incidence of rheumatic fever in some families. Susceptibility may be attributed to poor nutrition, group crowding, or the presence of a streptococcus carrier in the home.

Etiology and pathogenesis

The cause and pathogenesis of rheumatic fever have been the subject of controversy for a long time. Many of the theories in the past have considered several organisms as etiologic agents, such as viruses, diplococci, and nonhemolytic streptococci. But today it is generally agreed that acute rheumatic fever occurs after an infection with beta-hemolytic streptococci group A. The various manifestations of the disease in the heart and other regions of the body, excluding the initial infection (tonsillitis, nasopharyngitis), are not the result of a direct infection. The organisms characteristically are not cultured from the lesions in the heart, joints, and blood during the active phase of the disease. According to the current concept, induction of hypersensitivity or autoimmunity by products of beta-hemolytic streptococci of

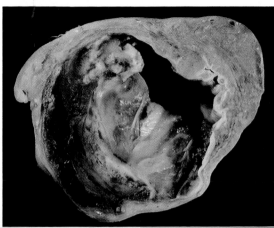

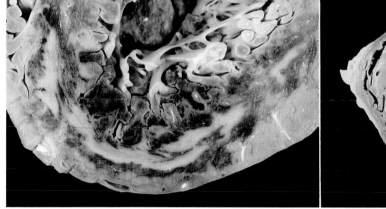

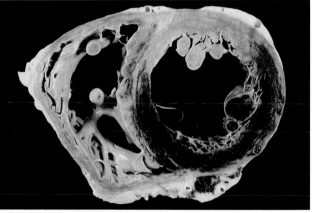

Plate 1

A, Cross section of left ventricle showing an old infarct with pronounced thinning of the wall. The infarct is the white scar, which is transmural; the wall bulges; and the resulting aneurysm is largely filled with a mural thrombus. A fragment of this thrombus had broken off and caused a cerebral infarct.

B, Cross section of the anterior wall of the left ventricle of a 51-year-old man who had chest pain 13 days before his death. Notice the yellowish tan necrotic center and the hyperemic border. This infarct microscopically showed necrosis in the central portion and organization in the periphery (that is, in the hyperemic zone).

C, This acute hemorrhagic myocardial infarct was from a 60-year-old man who had suffered from chest pain 3 days before death. A cardiac catheterization showed a complete occlusion of the left anterior descending coronary artery. Streptokinase was infused into the left coronary artery, which then opened partially. The hemorrhage is caused by the reflow into the infarcted region.

group A is responsible for the changes in rheumatic fever.

Some clinical and experimental observations that give support to the view that these organisms are the cause of rheumatic fever and that an immunologic mechanism is involved[325,332] are the following:

1. An increase in incidence of rheumatic fever has been observed after epidemics caused by beta-hemolytic streptococci of group A.[316]
2. The first attack usually occurs with a latent period of about 2 to 3 weeks after infection by this microorganism in the nasopharynx, suggestive of a period of sensitization to the bacteria.
3. Exacerbations of the disease frequently follow subsequent streptococcal infections.
4. Use of antibiotics has contributed to the reduction of the incidence and severity of rheumatic fever and has lowered the rate of recurrences.
5. In patients with rheumatic fever, elevated titers of antibodies to antigens of the beta-hemolytic group A streptococci, such as antistreptolysin, antistreptokinase, and antistreptohyaluronidase have been demonstrated.
6. Experimentally, lesions similar (but not identical) to those of rheumatic carditis have been produced by sensitization of animals to foreign protein.[330]
7. Cardiac lesions, including those resembling Aschoff bodies, have been produced in rabbits after the induction of repeated infections with group A hemolytic streptococci.[327]

It is not clear which of the streptococcal products is responsible for the pathogenesis of rheumatic fever. According to one theory, streptococcal materials have the ability to render autogenous tissue substances antigenic, so that autoantibodies are formed that react specifically with respective tissue components to cause the lesions of rheumatic fever.[317] This concept is based on experiments in which rats, immunized with mixtures of killed streptococci and emulsions of rat heart or connective tissues, were observed to form autoantibodies to the respective tissues. In these animals, changes in the valves and connective tissue of the heart that resembled those seen in rheumatic carditis in humans were identified. Such antibodies were not produced in these animals by injections of the homologous tissue emulsions alone (without streptococci). Evidence for the induction of autoantibody to heart tissue by antecedent group A streptococcal infection in humans has been provided by investigations demonstrating that the sera of patients with uncomplicated streptococcal infections, rheumatic fever, rheumatic heart disease, or glomerulonephritis often contain streptococcal antibody that is cross-reactive with heart tissue.[324]

Rheumatic fever develops in only a small number of patients with streptococcal infection. The attack rate varies from less than 1%[333] to about 3%.[329] It is difficult to account for the relatively low incidence of rheumatic fever despite the large number of streptococcal infections. However, undoubtedly the interrelationship between infection with beta-hemolytic streptococci of group A and subsequent development of rheumatic fever is dependent on other factors in addition to the presence of the organism.[331] The suggestion that a concomitant virus can enhance the effects of streptococci or vice versa[318,328] is of interest in this regard.

Cardiac manifestations

A widely accepted concept of the nature of rheumatic fever is that it is one of the so-called immune disorders of connective tissue, the principal lesions being in the connective tissues throughout the body, especially in the heart. In the early phase of development of the lesions, edema of the connective tissues is associated with an increase in acid mucopolysaccharide. The collagen fibers are pushed apart by the accumulating basophilic ground substance, and subsequently they undergo swelling, fraying, fragmentation, and disintegration. The affected areas, including the collagen fibers and the ground substance, are altered considerably and take on a deeply eosinophilic appearance resembling fibrin; thus the change is referred to as "fibrinoid" degeneration or necrosis. This fibrinoid change is a characteristic feature of many hypersensitivity reactions, but it is not a pathognomonic manifestation of hypersensitivity, since the alteration can be seen in lesions from other causes.

The early exudative and degenerative features are followed by proliferation, that is, an infiltration by lymphocytes, plasma cells, histiocytes, and fibroblasts. The most distinctive proliferative lesion is the granulomatous phase of the Aschoff body (described in the following discussion). The granulomatous lesions in the extracardiac tissues, such as the lesions in the synovial membranes of the joints, may bear a resemblance to the Aschoff bodies. As the rheumatic lesions advance in age, they undergo fibrosis and scar formation.

Aschoff bodies or nodules. Aschoff bodies occur in the interstitial tissue of the heart, especially in the myocardium and the endocardium, often in the vicinity of small blood vessels (Fig. 15-15). Occasionally, they are present in the pericardium.[358] Aschoff bodies have been described in the adventitia of the aorta,[369] but they are uncommon and usually are not present in the proximal part of the aorta. Lesions elsewhere in the body may be suggestive of, but should not be confused with, Aschoff bodies.[372] Aschoff nodules are globular, elliptic, or fusiform microscopic structures. They are seldom large enough to be detected by the unassisted eye. Three phases or stages in the development of the Aschoff body are recognized:

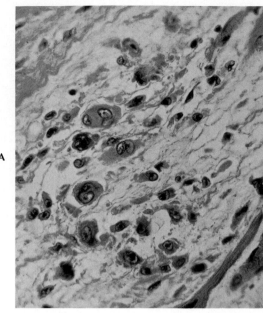

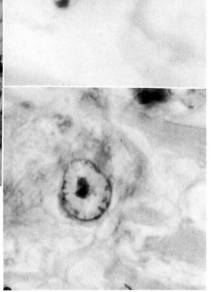

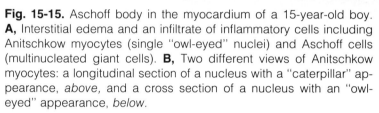

Fig. 15-15. Aschoff body in the myocardium of a 15-year-old boy. **A,** Interstitial edema and an infiltrate of inflammatory cells including Anitschkow myocytes (single "owl-eyed" nuclei) and Aschoff cells (multinucleated giant cells). **B,** Two different views of Anitschkow myocytes: a longitudinal section of a nucleus with a "caterpillar" appearance, *above,* and a cross section of a nucleus with an "owl-eyed" appearance, *below.*

1. Early (exudative, degenerative, or alterative) phase
2. Intermediate (proliferative or granulomatous) phase
3. Late (senescent, fibrous, healing, or healed) phase

It is in the granulomatous stage that the lesion is unmistakably identifiable as an Aschoff body and is regarded as pathognomonic for rheumatic carditis. This lesion, according to our present knowledge, does not occur in any other disease.

The early phase of the life cycle of the Aschoff body, said to occur up to the fourth week of acute rheumatic fever, is represented by exudative, degenerative, and fibrinoid changes in the collagenous tissue, as described in the foregoing paragraphs. There is usually a varying number of lymphocytes and plasma cells in the affected area.

In the intermediate phase, which is evident during the fourth to the thirteenth week of the disease, swelling and fragmentation of collagen fibers and fibrinoid change are present in the nodule, but cellular proliferation is the dominant feature. There is an accumulation of Anitschkow cells. These large mononuclear cells are found in normal hearts but are increased in number in the Aschoff bodies. By themselves, they do not represent a specific response to rheumatic fever.[354] These

cells have a moderate amount of faintly stained cytoplasm with vaguely defined borders. Their nuclei are large and vesicular and contain a prominent central chromatin mass that in longitudinal section is serrated (caterpillar-like). In cross section a halo is observed about the chromatin bar so that the nucleus has an "owl-eye" appearance (Fig. 15-15, *B*). Also present in the nodule are large cells with abundant basophilic cytoplasm, ragged cell borders, and one to four nuclei of the type seen in the Anitschkow cells. These characteristic mononuclear or multinucleated giant cells, known as Aschoff cells, are modified Anitschkow cells. Other cells usually seen are lymphocytes, plasma cells, and occasional neutrophils. As this phase progresses, the exudative and fibrinoid alterations gradually disappear.

In 3 to 4 months, the healing phase is reached, characterized by regression and fibrosis of the nodule. The Aschoff body is elongated or fusiform, the cytoplasm of the component cell is diminished in amount, the cells become elongated and spindle shaped, and their nuclei stain solidly. Frequently, fibrillar material appears between the cells, crowding them into rows. The collagenous fibers fuse to form dense collagenous bundles, resulting in small scars between the muscle bundles, frequently perivascularly.

The nature of the Aschoff body, particularly in regard

to the origin of the Aschoff cells, is a controversial subject. The generally accepted view, as suggested in the foregoing discussion, is that changes in the ground substance and the collagen fibers are primary and precede the formation of Aschoff cells.[378] The Anitschkow cell, from which the Aschoff cell is derived, is now widely held to be a cardiac histiocyte.[378]

In contrast to this view is the concept that Aschoff bodies originate and evolve from primary injury to muscle cells in the heart.[368] The proponents of this view claim that the seemingly interstitial Aschoff bodies are lesions of small groups of heart muscle fibers interspersed among other uninvolved bundles of heart muscle fibers. In this view, Anitschkow or Aschoff cells are considered to be derived from cardiac myocytes rather than connective tissue cells. Endocardial Aschoff bodies are considered to be lesions of smooth muscle cells, which normally occur in the zone between endothelium and myocardium. Evidence obtained from a recent study using immunofluorescence microscopy has given support to this concept.[351] In this investigation, actomyosin antigenically similar to that of normal cardiac striated muscle cells was demonstrated in the cells and cell fragments of myocardial Aschoff bodies, and actomyosin antigenically similar to that of smooth muscle cells was observed in the cells of endocardial Aschoff bodies.

According to other investigators, the Aschoff bodies are derived from diseased lymphatic vessels.[381] In this view, proliferation of the endothelial cells of the lymphatics gives rise to the characteristic Aschoff cells. The lymphedema resulting from blockage of the vessels by the proliferating endothelial cells is believed to be responsible for secondary damage to connective tissue and cardiac muscle.

Finally, according to Hutchins and Payne,[364] Aschoff bodies are derived from nerves. These authors studied serial histologic sections of Aschoff bodies and observed a close anatomic relationship between nerves and Aschoff bodies and histologic similarity of the two structures.

The development of surgical valvulotomy for mitral stenosis has made it possible to examine the left atrial appendage microscopically and to observe the rheumatic process in a part of the heart during life. The incidence of rheumatic lesions in resected atrial appendages has been reported as 16%[365] to 74%[371] even among patients with no clinical or laboratory evidence of rheumatic activity. The high incidence of Aschoff nodules in some reports may be a reflection of insufficiently strict criteria of what constitutes an Aschoff body.[357,372] Nevertheless, true Aschoff nodules have been found in a significant proportion of appendages.[367] There is a difference of opinion regarding the significance of the Aschoff bodies identified in the surgically excised atrial appendages. Some investigators regard Aschoff bodies to be evidence of active rheumatic disease despite the inability to correlate the lesions with clinical manifestations of active disease (a subclinical phase).[366,367] Another view is that the rheumatic process should be considered active only if exudative changes, alterations in collagen, and fibrinoid change are present in the Aschoff bodies.[376]

Some observers have demonstrated a significant relationship between the preoperative clinical course and the presence of Aschoff bodies in the resected atrial appendages.[355] Patients who had progressive worsening of cardiac symptoms for 18 months or less before operation had a much higher rate of occurrence of Aschoff bodies than those whose severe cardiac symptoms had remained stationary for at least 2 years before operation.[355] The authors suggest that this correlation strongly indicates that Aschoff bodies are indicative of active rheumatic heart disease, which is responsible for the progressive deterioration of the cardiac status. In another study, the postoperative course was similar in the group of patients in whom Aschoff bodies were found versus the group in whom they were absent.[367] Thus the prognostic importance of Aschoff bodies is unresolved. In one study, Aschoff bodies were found in the left atrium at necropsy in only 4% of 206 patients with chronic mitral stenosis,[370] whereas they were identified in surgically resected left atrial appendages in 21% of 191 patients.[377] The reason for this difference is not known.

• • •

The cardiac involvement in rheumatic fever is that of a pancarditis; that is, there is endocarditis, myocarditis, and pericarditis.

Endocarditis (valvulitis). The endocardial involvement can be either valvular or mural (that is, parietal). The valvular involvement is the most characteristic and clinically important and can be truly referred to as a valvulitis, since the entire valve is involved and not just the endocardial surface. In the active acute stage of the disease the valve leaflets or cusps are thickened and lose their transparency. This is followed by the appearance of characteristic wartlike nodules (verrucae) ranging from 1 to 3 mm in diameter, mainly along the line of closure of the cusps (Fig. 15-16). This lesion is referred to as *verrucous endocarditis*. The mitral valve is the most commonly involved valve, followed in descending order of frequency by the mitral and aortic valves combined, the aortic valve, and, less commonly, the tricuspid and pulmonary valves. The vegetations are located on the atrial surfaces of the atrioventricular valves and on the ventricular surfaces of the semilunar valves. Sometimes verrucae extend onto the mural endocardium of the left atrium. Lesions may also be present on the chordae tendineae, particularly at their attachment to the leaflets, and rarely on the papillary

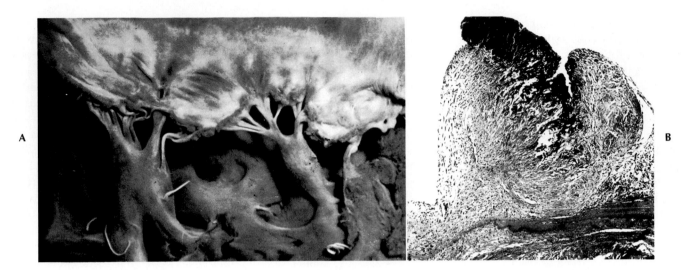

Fig. 15-16. A, Acute recurrent rheumatic endocarditis involving the tricuspid valve. Verrucae are present along the line of closure of the valve leaflets. Notice thickened chordae tendineae. **B,** Verrucous nodule. Dark cap consists of fibrin that is being organized by connective tissue cells from the valve. (**A,** Courtesy Dr. Orlyn B. Pratt, Los Angeles, Calif.)

muscles of the left ventricle. The verrucae only rarely involve the valve pockets, which are in contrast to the prominent valve pocket involvement in Libman-Sacks endocarditis (seen in systemic lupus erythematosus).[359]

The verrucae may appear in rows, in small clusters, or as isolated lesions. Since they are usually firmly attached, they are not readily dislodged to produce embolic phenomena.

Microscopically, the earliest lesion is said to occur in the valve rings (that is, the attachment of the cusps to the fibrous anulus.)[361] It then extends throughout the substance of the entire leaflet. Edema with swelling of the leaflet, an increased number of capillaries, and an infiltration by lymphocytes and occasionally by neutrophils are seen. Plasma cells and fibroblasts may be present. In some instances, this nonspecific inflammatory reaction may be all that occurs. Usually, however, there is also an increase in acid mucopolysaccharide, with alteration of collagen and a fibrinoid change near the surface of the valve and with surface deposition of fibrin from the blood in the ventricular cavity. Aschoff cells may be present, and the proliferating cells at the base of the fibrin and fibrinoid area may be lined up in a palisading fashion with their long axes at right angles to the surface. Bacteria are not present in the lesion.

The mechanism of development of the verrucae is disputed. It is probable that the degenerated fibrinoid foci within the valve substance are extruded above the surface of the valve and form the nidus for superimposed platelet thrombi. The incidence of vegetations is high in the left side of the heart, where the pressure is greatest, and their formation is along the line of closure of the valve cusps. These features indicate that a role in the pathogenesis of the vegetations may be played by mechanical trauma related to intracardiac pressure and to the impact and mutual compression of the surfaces of the valve leaflets. It is suggested that a healthy endothelium can sustain these mechanical aspects of valve function without any sign of trauma, but when there is an inflammatory lesion of the valve immediately beneath the surface, the endothelium may be disrupted.[362]

Lesions of the mural endocardium also may occur in rheumatic fever. They are seen most commonly in the posterior wall of the left atrium just above the posterior leaflet of the mitral valve. The lesion at this site is called a MacCallum patch, and it consists of a thickening of the endocardium, which has a gray, ridged and furrowed surface that, on healing, is converted to a gray-white wrinkled plaque. The microscopic picture of the acute lesion is similar to that of the valvulitis.

Healing of rheumatic valvulitis. Sometimes valvulitis is mild, and little if any fibrous thickening of the valve and chordae tendineae results. Usually, however, there is moderate to severe fibrosis with varying degrees of distortion of the valve leaflets. The following changes take place:

1. Fibroblastic proliferation and collagen formation throughout the valve with scarring, thickening, and rigidity of the leaflets
2. Organization of the vegetations, with greater thickening along the lines of closure

3. Adhesions between the lateral portions of the cusps, particularly in the region of the commissures

4. Thickening, shortening, and fusion of the chordae tendineae

5. Frequently, calcification, which contributes to the rigidity of the valve

The result is deformity of one or more valves, especially the mitral and aortic (Fig. 15-17). The incidence of deformity of the various valves, singly or in combination, has been reported to have the following descending order of frequency[353]:

1. Mitral
2. Mitral and aortic
3. Aortic
4. Mitral, aortic, and tricuspid
5. Mitral and tricuspid
6. Mitral, aortic, tricuspid, and pulmonary

However, some investigators now consider that isolated aortic deformities are rarely of rheumatic origin.[588]

The pulmonary and tricuspid valves are also rarely involved by themselves. The most characteristic type of deformity causes mitral stenosis. Another common lesion is aortic stenosis. Valvular insufficiency may result because of retraction of the scarred leaflets in the vertical direction leading to shortening of the cusps. Mitral insufficiency and stenosis are commonly combined.

Recurrences of the acute disease may occur. Thus there may be fresh verrucae adjacent to or superimposed on the healed lesions. Thrombi may be found in the chambers of the heart, particularly in the atrial appendages and especially on the left in association with mitral stenosis (Fig. 15-18). Sometimes, secondary nonspecific vegetations of the nonbacterial thrombotic type, which are not associated with active rheumatic inflammation, may be superimposed on the healed valves and may reach considerable size.[361]

The healed valves, when examined microscopically, show noticeable fibrous thickening. The presence of numerous vascular channels testifies to the fact that the normally avascular valve has been vascularized. Calcification of varying degree is often present, and metaplasia, with bone and bone marrow formation, may occur occasionally.

From the description of the valvular lesions it should be apparent that the valvulitis seen in the acute stage of the disease is functionally of little consequence to the patient and is not the basis for the murmurs that are heard clinically. The characteristic murmur of mitral insufficiency in acute rheumatic fever is usually better explained on the basis of left ventricular and valve ring dilatation secondary to heart failure caused by the myocarditis.

Myocarditis. In the acute stages, rheumatic myocarditis is characterized by the presence of (1) specific Aschoff bodies, (2) nonspecific interstitial myocarditis, and (3) parenchymal damage. The most distinctive lesions are the Aschoff bodies, or nodules, described previously. These nodules are scattered throughout the interstitial tissue of the myocardium and may also be seen in the subendocardial connective tissue. They are most common in the interventricular septum and in the upper part of the posterior left ventricular wall,[360] but they may be also found in other areas of the ventricles

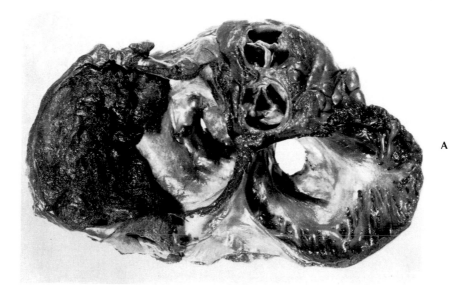

A

Fig. 15-17. A, Cross section of a heart through the atria and great vessels, showing stenosis of the mitral, tricuspid, and aortic valves caused by chronic rheumatic endocarditis. The mitral orifice is a mere slit. Also notice the large thrombus in the dilated left atrium.   *Continued.*

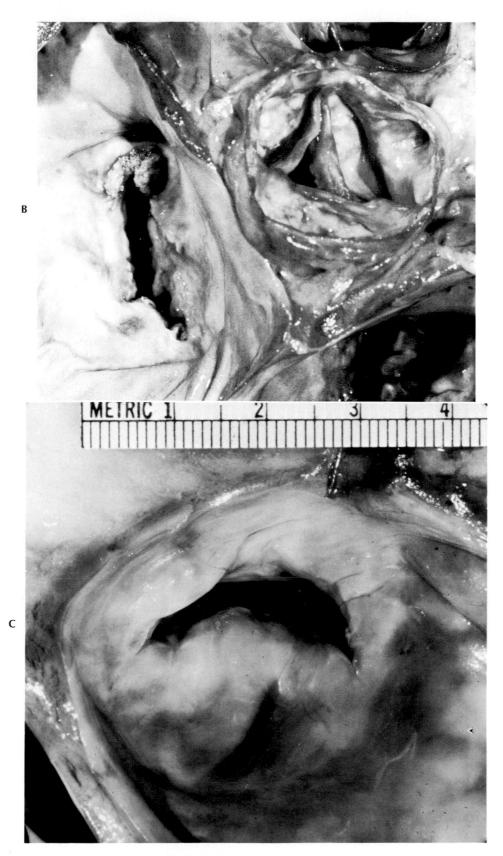

Fig. 15-17, cont'd. B, Mitral and aortic stenosis with calcification of both valves. **C,** Mitral stenosis with "fish-mouth" orifice.

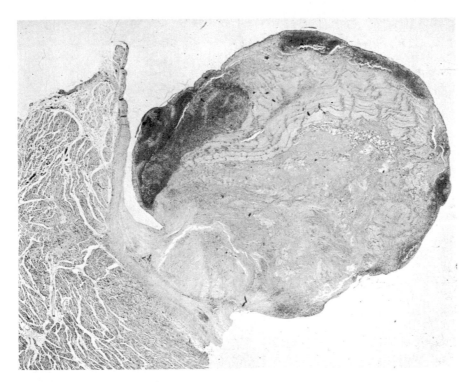

Fig. 15-18. Pedunculated mural thrombosis in the left atrium. This occurred as a complication of mitral stenosis.

and in the atria. Rheumatic myocarditis is most readily differentiated from other forms of myocarditis in its intermediate phase when Aschoff nodules are most typical. Associated with these granulomatous lesions is a nonspecific feature—the infiltration of lymphocytes, plasma cells, histiocytes, occasionally many neutrophils, and sometimes a few eosinophils throughout an edematous interstitial connective tissue. Furthermore, there is evidence of parenchymal damage varying from degenerative changes to foci of necrosis of the muscle fibers. The areas of necrosis are surrounded by various cells including cardiac histiocytes and multinucleated giant cells. The giant cells are believed to be syncytial myogenic masses that represent an attempt at regeneration. These muscle lesions resemble but are not true Aschoff bodies.[372] As mentioned previously, however, some investigators believe that Aschoff bodies originate from primary injury to myofibers.[368]

Any of the three lesions already discussed may involve the conducting system and produce various electrocardiographic changes, but it has been suggested that the nonspecific inflammation with associated muscle necrosis, rather than isolated Aschoff bodies, is more significant in this regard.[373]

In the later stages of the disease there is gradual subsidence of the inflammatory reaction, and the Aschoff bodies are converted into small scars. Myocardial fibrosis is more extensive in hearts with severe chronic val-

vular deformities, which may in part be attributable to myocardial anoxia, especially with aortic stenosis. It might also, of course, be a reflection of the more severe original and recurrent disease that produced the valvular lesions.

Pericarditis. The tendency to affect serous membranes is one of the distinctive features of rheumatic fever, and fibrinous pericarditis is a prominent part of the picture of acute rheumatic heart disease. The exudate varies from a thin film of fibrin to a shaggy coat with adhesions between the layers of the pericardium, thus the designation of *shaggy heart,* or cor villosum (Latin *villus,* 'shaggy hair'). The fibrinous exudate is sometimes referred to as a "bread-and-butter" exudate[358] because of its imagined likeness to a butter sandwich that has been pulled apart. There may be a moderate amount of serofibrinous fluid in the pericardial sac, but the exudate is rarely of the fibrinopurulent type.

Microscopically, fibrin is seen as a shaggy layer on the surface of the epicardium and an infiltrate of lymphocytes, plasma cells, histiocytes, and occasionally neutrophils is present. Also foci of fibrinoid change and Aschoff bodies may rarely be seen. Subsequently, organization of the fibrin by vascularized connective tissue may be observed. This may lead to fibrous thickening and adhesions of the visceral and parietal pericardial layers, to partial or complete obliteration of the pericardial cavity, and to a "chronic adhesive pericarditis."

The acute fibrinous pericarditis of the "bread-and-butter" variety can be diagnosed clinically by the friction rub that it produces and that can be heard with a stethoscope. Although pericarditis may be the most prominent gross manifestation of the acute disease, it is usually of little physiologic significance and does not usually affect the clinical course of the patient. Remember that the *main functionally effective lesion in the acute stage is the myocarditis,* which can produce enough myocardial damage to result in death because of congestive heart failure, with the pericardial and valvular lesions being of secondary importance. On the other hand, *in the chronic or recurrent condition, the functionally important lesions are those of the valves,* which result in heart failure because of the increased work of the heart caused by the valvular stenosis or insufficiency. The "chronic adhesive pericarditis" is only rarely severe enough to produce a true constrictive pericarditis and does not often play an important functional role compared to that of the chronic valvular lesions.

Extracardiac lesions

Subcutaneous nodules. Painless subcutaneous nodules may occur in the subcutaneous tissues of the wrist, elbows, ankles, and knees. They occur more commonly in children during the acute stage and last 4 to 6 days, unlike rheumatoid nodules, which may persist for months or years and may be painful and tender. Microscopically, the nodules could be considered to be giant Aschoff bodies and consist of a central zone of necrosis with fibrinoid change, and, bordering this, a zone of histiocytes and fibroblasts in a radial and palisading arrangement, with a surrounding zone of edematous connective tissue in which nonspecific chronic inflammation can be seen (Fig. 15-19).

Arteritis. Coronary artery inflammation (rheumatic arteritis) occurs during acute rheumatic fever and has been suggested to predispose the involved coronary artery to later atherosclerosis.

Polyarthritis. The joint changes in acute rheumatic fever are not as well known as those in the heart are. The synovial membrane and the periarticular connective tissues are the sites of hyperemia, edema, neutrophilic infiltration, fibrinoid change and necrosis, followed by granulomatous changes at a later time. Focal lesions similar to Aschoff bodies may be seen. These lesions usually subside leaving no residuum.[350]

Lungs and pleura. Pleuritis may develop in association with arthritis or carditis. Pleural effusion is usually present, and a fine fibrinous deposit may appear on the opaque pleural surface. Rheumatic pneumonia has been described, but there is some question as to its specific-

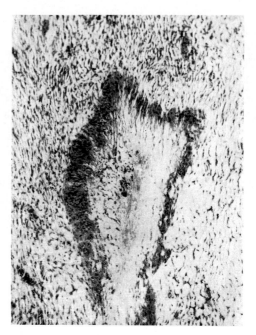

Fig. 15-19. Subcutaneous nodule from a patient with rheumatic fever. There is a central core of fibrinoid necrosis surrounded by a zone of radially palisading histiocytes and fibroblasts. (75×; AFIP.)

ity. Microscopically the lungs show mainly an interstitial inflammatory reaction not unlike a viral pneumonitis. There may be patchy fibrinous exudates in the alveoli that are often associated with monocytes.[375]

Lesions of the central nervous system. A major manifestation of rheumatic fever is chorea minor (Sydenham's chorea, St. Vitus's dance). The word "chorea" refers to the disordered and involuntary movements of the trunk and extremities that are characteristic of the disease. It is often preceded by or associated with acute rheumatic fever, is seen more commonly in girls in childhood, and is most frequently associated with a benign form of rheumatic fever.[352]

The cerebral lesions in chorea minor consist of a diffuse meningoencephalitis of mild degree, and small hemorrhages, edema, and perivascular lymphocytic collections are commonly seen.

Postmortem diagnosis of old rheumatic disease

The postmortem diagnosis of old rheumatic heart disease can be made with a variable degree of assurance depending on the anatomic features that are observable in a particular specimen. It is helpful and confirmatory, of course, to have a clinical past history of rheumatic fever; however, this should not influence the anatomic diagnosis to a great extent nor should the absence of the clinical diagnosis inhibit the anatomic interpretation. Thus, in the presence of *stigmas* of old rheumatic involvement of the heart, the anatomic diagnosis can be made with some certainty.[363,374] These signs of previous rheumatic involvement include the following:

1. Chronic adhesive pericarditis, especially circumscribed obliteration of the cardiac sac near the apex
2. Fibrous thickening of the valve leaflets, especially at the line of closure
3. Valvular deformities, especially aortic or mitral stenosis or insufficiency and, more significantly, involvement of both the aortic and mitral valves
4. Thickening, shortening, and adhesions of the chordae tendineae
5. MacCallum's patch
6. Microscopic changes, including foci of perivascular interstitial fibrosis (old healed Aschoff bodies), fibrosis, and vascularization of the valves

Causes of death in rheumatic fever and rheumatic heart disease

The chief causes of death in rheumatic fever patients are cardiac failure, infective endocarditis, and embolism.[352,379,380] Death may, however, be attributable to various other conditions such as pneumonia.

Cardiac failure is the most frequent cause of death from rheumatic heart disease. It may be caused by the myocarditis of acute rheumatic fever and is especially common in younger people. In middle-aged or older adults heart failure is more commonly attributable to the valvular lesions though an acute recurrence of the active process may occur at any age and be the cause of myocarditis and heart failure.

Bacterial endocarditis, usually of the subacute type, has become less frequent as a cause of death in more recent years, probably because of the use of antibiotics in treatment of bacterial endocarditis as well as their use in prophylactic programs in patients with old rheumatic heart disease. The peak incidence of bacterial endocarditis in patients with rheumatic heart disease occurs at about 20 to 30 years of age.[379] Older patients tend to have more of the acute than subacute type of disease.[379]

Embolism as a cause of death in patients with rheumatic heart disease has shown a substantial increase, in contrast to the downward trend in mortality caused by bacterial endocarditis.[379] The most frequently involved organ is the brain, followed by the kidneys, spleen, and lungs. Most emboli are bland, but occasionally they may be septic, the latter arising from a bacterial endocarditis. Most of the emboli arise from mural thrombi in the left atrium, particularly in association with mitral stenosis or atrial fibrillation. Another possible source of thromboemboli is a nonspecific nonbacterial thrombotic endocarditis on a valve.[379] In contrast to emboli from the atrium or its appendage, emboli from nonbacterial thrombotic endocarditis are not dependent on atrial fi-

brillation but may occur whether the rhythm is regular or not.[379,380] Sudden death may occasionally occur as a result of obstruction of the mitral valve orifice by a ball thrombus in the left atrium or as a result of coronary ischemia associated with aortic stenosis.

Another cause of death in any patient with heart disease is thrombophlebitis of leg veins and pulmonary embolism.

The heart in rheumatoid arthritis and ankylosing spondylitis
Rheumatoid arthritis

Cardiac involvement occurs in a substantial proportion of patients with rheumatoid arthritis.[382,384,388,394,402] The major manifestations are acute or chronic pericarditis, myocarditis, and arteritis involving primarily the small intramural vessels. In two large series totalling 162 patients with rheumatoid arthritis who were studied at autopsy, cardiac manifestations were reported in 62 (41%).[388,394] Active or healed pericarditis, nonspecific chronic myocarditis, and arteritis were equally common features, each occurring in approximately 20% of the patients. Another nonspecific change that occurs is valvular fibrosis. Although characteristic of rheumatoid heart disease, none of these lesions has features specific to rheumatoid disease.

Rheumatoid pericarditis illustrates a spectrum of severity.[386,392] In many patients the entity is of no clinical significance. Nevertheless, progression to an adhesive and obliterative pericarditis, with loculated pericardial effusions, occurs in a minority of patients and may require pericardiectomy to alleviate symptoms of pericardial tamponade.

Rheumatoid granulomas, histologically similar to the classical subcutaneous rheumatoid nodules, are specific for rheumatoid involvement but are found relatively infrequently; rheumatoid granulomas were observed in either the myocardium or cardiac valves of 5% of the aforementioned combined series of patients. Rheumatoid granulomas are characterized histologically by a central zone of fibrinoid necrosis surrounded by a zone of palisaded macrophages and fibroblasts accompanied by lymphocytes and plasma cells.

Although vasculitis is relatively common, it is generally confined to small intramural vessels.[388,393] Arteritis involving the large epicardial arteries, complicated by thrombosis and myocardial infarction, has been reported in a few patients but is rare.[391,396] Given that both rheumatoid arthritis and coronary heart disease are relatively common entities, myocardial infarction in patients with rheumatoid arthritis is more commonly attributable to coronary atherosclerosis than to rheumatoid coronary arteritis.[391] Rheumatoid arthritis is occasionally complicated by complete atrioventricular block or other conduction disturbances. Conduction block may result from involvement of the conduction bundle by rheumatoid granulomas but more commonly is attributable to nonspecific scarring resulting from the myocarditis or arteritis.[390,395]

Ankylosing spondylitis

Ankylosing spondylitis (Marie-Strümpell disease) was formerly referred to as rheumatoid spondylitis, but there are certain features of this disease that have influenced investigators to consider it an entity separate from peripheral rheumatoid arthritis, as follows:

1. There is a high incidence in men, whereas peripheral rheumatoid arthritis occurs mainly in women.
2. It frequently exists without peripheral arthritic manifestations.
3. The serologic reaction for the rheumatoid factor is usually negative in the absence of peripheral joint involvement, and even when peripheral joint involvement is present, the incidence of positive serologic tests is low.

The cardiac manifestations of ankylosing spondylitis are usually distinct from those of rheumatoid arthritis, characteristically consisting in aortitis and consequent aortic valve insufficiency.[385,389,403] Microscopically the aortitis is characterized by focal ischemic necrosis of the aortic media accompanied by a nonspecific inflammatory infiltration in the media and adventitia, especially around the vasa vasorum. In some instances the inflammatory process is granulomatous, and Langhans giant cells may be present. The inflammatory process may also involve the aortic valve, resulting in adhesions and partial fusion of the aortic valve commissures.

Frequently, the aortitis may result in weakening and dilatation of the aortic valve ring and consequent aortic insufficiency. Widened commissures may be present in valves in which commissural adhesion has not occurred. The valve cusps often develop thickened, rolled-free margins. These various changes in the aorta and aortic valve resemble the changes observed in syphilitic heart disease (see below). Because of the chronic volume overload imposed on the left ventricle by the aortic insufficiency, pronounced ventricular hypertrophy and dilatation may occur.

Additional cardiac manifestations of ankylosing spondylitis, as well as of rheumatoid arthritis and related conditions, are pericarditis and conduction defects.[382,401] In one study of 68 patients with ankylosing spondylitis, cardiac conduction defects were observed in 33%,[383] a frequency substantially greater than that observed in rheumatoid arthritis. Cardiac manifestations similar to those of "spondylitic heart disease" have also been reported to occur in patients with Reiter's syndrome and psoriatic arthritis with spondylitis.[397,399,400]

The distinction between the cardiac manifestations of rheumatoid heart disease and spondylitic heart disease are not absolute[404]; for example, aortic valvular deformities characteristic of ankylosing spondylitis have occasionally been observed in patients with classical clinical features of rheumatoid arthritis.[387,398]

Syphilitic (luetic) heart disease

Syphilis can affect the heart in three different ways: (1) by its involvement of the ascending aorta and aortic valve with dilatation of the aortic valve ring and valve cusps and resulting aortic insufficiency, (2) by involvement of the myocardium by gummas (a rare occurrence), and (3) by coronary ostial stenosis by extension of the aortic scarring, with resulting ischemic disease.[406]

In a compilation of statistics from several articles in the literature it was found that, in the preantibiotic era in the United States, syphilitic heart disease ranked as the third most frequent type of heart disease.[409] Syphilis still remains a public health hazard of major proportions; syphilis was the third most common communicable disease reported to the Centers for Disease Control in Atlanta in 1980.[405] However, because of early detection and antibiotic treatment, a sharp decrease in the incidence of syphilitic heart disease has occurred.

The primary lesion in the aorta is an obliterative endarteritis of the vasa vasorum of the aortic root, with perivascular lymphocytic infiltration followed by medial degeneration, necrosis, loss of elastic fibers, and fibrosis.[410] As a result, the weakened aortic valve ring may dilate. In addition, there is often an extension of the inflammatory changes into the base of the valve and the most lateral parts of the leaflets, followed by the appearance of granulation tissue and eventual fibrosis accompanied by widening of the commissures.[410] The major functional consequence of syphilitic aortitis and valvulitis is insufficiency of the aortic valve (Fig. 15-20). Aortic regurgitation may occur simply because of dilatation of the aortic valve ring.[407] However, in most cases, commissural separation is present and is believed to be a contributing factor to the regurgitation. Aortic insufficiency also has been reported in patients with commissural separation but without valve ring dilatation.[407] Thickening, eversion, and rolling of the free margins of the valve cusps also are common features of syphilitic heart disease; these changes are probably not a primary consequence of the valvulitis but the secondary result of continuous mechanical pressure of the regurgitating blood, associated with insufficiency of the aortic valve.[410] Microscopically the midportions of the valves and free margins of the cusps exhibit only fibrosis and hyalinization and no chronic inflammation or granulation tissue.

Because of the aortic insufficiency, hypertrophy and dilatation of the left ventricle occur. The trauma of the

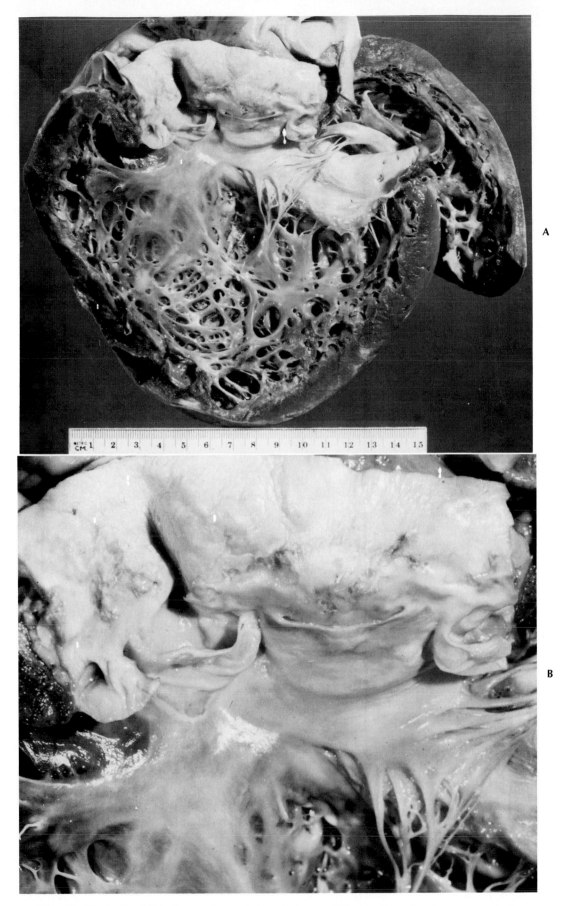

Fig. 15-20. A, Syphilitic heart disease. Insufficiency of the aortic valve has secondarily caused left ventricular hypertrophy and dilatation and endocardial fibrosis. **B,** Involvement of the aortic valve (closeup view of **A**) in syphilitic aortitis. Notice separation of the commissures of the aortic valve, deformity of cusps, and atherosclerotic plaques in the ascending aorta.

regurgitating blood causes characteristic endocardial changes, such as endocardial fibrous thickening and the formation of endocardial pockets or "bird nests" with their openings toward the aortic orifice.[408]

Endocarditis

Endocarditis can be classified as valvular, mural or parietal, chordal, trabecular, or papillary depending on the structures involved. It is the practice of many to use the word "endocarditis" without a qualifying adjective to indicate inflammation of the valvular endocardium because the valves are the structures that are most frequently involved. In some instances, such as rheumatic fever and bacterial infections, the entire valve substance is affected and the term "valvulitis" is more appropriate than "endocarditis." With few exceptions the various types of endocarditis are characterized by the presence of vegetations that are excrescences projecting from the endocardial surface at a point of damage or inflammation. They may be small and wartlike (verrucae) as in rheumatic fever, or large and sometimes massive as in infective endocarditis.

The inflammatory lesions of the endocardium may be grouped as to whether they are noninfective or infective:

1. *Noninfective*
   a. Rheumatic
   b. Atypical verrucous (Libman-Sacks)
   c. Nonbacterial thrombotic
2. *Infective*
   a. Bacterial
   b. Fungal
   c. Viral
   d. Rickettsial

Rheumatic endocarditis is discussed on p. 643.

Atypical verrucous (Libman-Sacks) endocarditis

A peculiar type of endocarditis was first recognized by Libman and Sacks.[412,413] This condition is a cardiac manifestation of systemic lupus erythematosus (see p. 1770), occurring in less than 50% of the patients. The atypical verrucae resemble those of acute rheumatic heart disease, or those of bacterial endocarditis, but they are usually larger than the former and smaller than the latter (Fig. 15-21).

The characteristic lesions of this condition are flat, granular, tawny lesions on the valve; they are not confined to the line of closure but have a tendency to spread over both valve surfaces, often occurring at the base of the valves in the valve pockets and even on the ventricular and atrial endocardium.[359] In some instances verrucae in the pockets of the mitral or tricuspid valves are very conspicuous and are the predominant or sole lesions. This is a diagnostic feature of the disease; in rheumatic endocarditis, valve pocket lesions

are either inconspicuous grossly or observed only on microscopic examination.[359] Gross ulceration or perforation of the valves are not features of Libman-Sacks endocarditis, and bacteria are not present in the lesions. Although these lesions may heal and cause fibrous thickening of the valves, they do not tend to produce valvular deformities. Verrucae commonly involve multiple valves at the same time, especially the mitral and tricuspid, but the aortic valve is not involved as frequently as in rheumatic fever. Embolic phenomena are not characteristic of Libman-Sacks endocarditis.

Microscopically, distinctive lesions may be seen even in the absence of macroscopic vegetations. There are areas of edema, fibrinoid change, and an accumulation of histiocytes, plasma cells, occasionally lymphocytes and neutrophils, and later fibroblasts. Included in the lesion are "hematoxylin bodies" of Gross,[359] which represent clumps of nuclear material that appear to be analogous to the lupus erythematous cells of the bone marrow. The verrucae consist of fibrinoid, necrotic portions of the valve substance admixed with fibrin and platelet thrombi. Associated with the vegetations is a variable degree of valvulitis, with proliferating young capillaries, between which is an infiltrate of inflammatory cells.

Frequently associated with the endocarditis are alterations in the pericardium. In early stages there may be fibrinoid changes with a serofibrinous pericarditis. This is followed by organization and by fibrosis with fibrous adhesions of the pericardium ("chronic adhesive pericarditis").

Nonbacterial thrombotic endocarditis (NBTE)

Synonyms for nonbacterial thrombotic endocarditis include terminal endocarditis, marantic endocarditis, and degenerative verrucal endocardiosis. This is an entity that usually occurs in patients who are in the terminal stages of a chronic debilitating disease.[417,418,425] The term "marantic" means "wasting away"; many patients with NBTE are cachectic. Most often, NBTE is associated with an underlying malignancy, especially adenocarcinomas such as adenocarcinomas of the lung, pancreas, and prostate. Other chronic diseases associated with NBTE include tuberculosis and uremia.

The disorder is characterized by vegetations or verrucae that occur on one or more of the cardiac valves. The valves may have underlying abnormality such as scarring from rheumatic fever; however, more commonly the valves are normal. The vegetations or verrucae may be single or multiple, are usually located on the left-sided valves (mitral or aortic), and are most often attached to the valve leaflet or cusp along the line of closure.[427] The location of the lesions is thus distinct from the verrucae of Libman-Sacks endocarditis, which involve both surfaces of the valves. The line of closure,

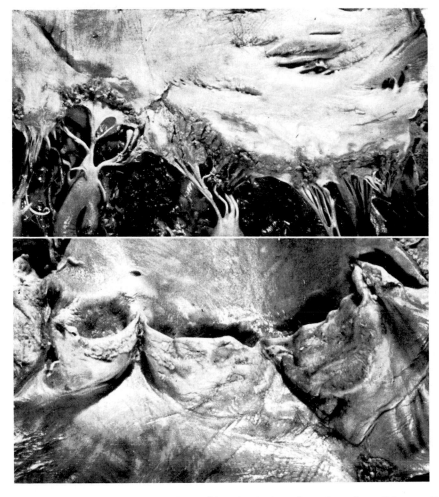

Fig. 15-21. Atypical verrucous endocarditis of mitral and aortic valves (Libman-Sacks endocarditis) from a 38-year-old woman. These lesions occurred in association with disseminated lupus erythematosus. (Courtesy Dr. Reuben Straus, Portland, Ore.)

where the vegetations of NBTE are located, is the surface of the valve, which is subject to the maximum mechanical trauma caused by the normal opening and closing of the valves. The vegetations are composed of thrombotic material and in the gross specimen appear as reddish brown nodules of variable size; in some instances they are small vegetations measuring less than 3 mm in diameter and resembling the verrucae of rheumatic valvulitis. In other cases they are large conglomerate lesions, which might be mistaken for the vegetations of infective endocarditis. Microscopically they contain fibrin, red and white blood cells, and platelets. The important difference from infective endocarditis is that there is no infection; thus infectious organisms cannot be cultured from the vegetations or observed using special histologic stains. Moreover, there is no inflammatory reaction in the underlying valve; valve ulceration or perforation, which may occur in infective endocarditis, does not occur in NBTE. Indeed, because of

the paucity of inflammation, the use of the term "endocarditis" for this condition is a misnomer and "endocardiosis" is the more accurate term.

The pathogenesis of NBTE is not entirely known. As mentioned earlier, the lesions often develop in patients who have an underlying malignancy, especially adenocarcinomas. Patients with malignancies often have an ill-defined "hypercoagulable state."[426,428] Thus NBTE occurs in the same types of patients in whom disseminated intravascular coagulation (DIC) also is common.[416,420] NBTE is particularly common in patients with mucin-secreting adenocarcinomas[424]; in this regard, it has been shown that extracts of mucin activate the coagulation system.[423] The location of vegetations on the line of closure of left-sided cardiac valves may be attributable to the greater likelihood of recurrent endothelial damage because of mechanical wear and tear at these sites.

In the past, NBTE was considered to be an insignificant entity, usually reported as an incidental postmortem observation in patients dying of cancer or some other debilitating disease. It is now recognized, however, that not all cases occur in terminally ill patients and that the vegetations may be the cause of serious clinical complications attributable to embolization and consequent infarction in organs such as the brain, heart, kidneys, or spleen.[415,419,421,422] The vegetations of NBTE may also serve as a trap for infectious organisms and may predispose to the development of infective endocarditis.[424]

Infective endocarditis

The clinical and pathologic features of infective endocarditis have changed dramatically in recent years.[436] Until recent years the term "bacterial endocarditis" was used for this general condition, most cases were fatal, and a clinical division into acute and subacute categories was useful. With the advent of antibiotic treatment, however, the clinical picture has changed so that now almost 90% of patients can be expected to recover.[460] Furthermore, various nonbacterial agents are now seen to cause a similar picture, including fungi[452,475] and rickettsias as in Q fever.[441,474] Thus the term "infective endocarditis" is preferred to refer to the overall category though "bacterial endocarditis" is still appropriate when the organism is known to be bacterial. In addition, the division into subacute and acute groups is not of much clinical valve, since the categorization no longer applies to the antibiotic-treated patient. The incidence of infective endocarditis has been relatively constant over the years, but the age distribution of the disease has changed. For example, in the period between 1913 and 1948, 10% to 25% of patients were over 50 years of age. Since 1948, 50% to 60% have been over 50 years of age.[479] Also, infection of valve prostheses has become an important setting for infective endocarditis.[445]

The primary pathologic feature of infective endocarditis is the presence of vegetations, usually on the valves, which contain microorganisms. Although the vegetations may be small, they are often massive and thus may interfere with the proper functioning of the valves.

Causative organisms. The most frequent causative agents of bacterial endocarditis are the alpha-streptococcus and staphylococci.[449] On the other hand, infection by other forms of streptococci (including enterococci), gram-negative organisms,[435] and various unusual organisms have increased in incidence. Fungal endocarditis from *Candida albicans, Histoplasma capsulatum, Coccidioides immitis, Aspergillus, Cryptococcus neoformans, Blastomyces dermatitidis,* and *Mucor* has been reported.[452] As yet, viral endocarditis has not been firmly established as a clinical entity in man, but

it has been demonstrated that viruses may produce endocarditis in experimental animals.[431,468] An occasional instance of endocarditis in patients with Q fever has been reported.[441,474]

The increase in frequency of unusual organisms, including fungi as well as bacteria, as causes of infective endocarditis may be related to the use of antimicrobial and immunosuppressive agents, unsterile techniques of self-inoculation of narcotics by drug addicts, various types of cardiovascular surgery, including placement of prosthetic valves,[429,437,445,452,476,477,478] and occasionally the presence of a transvenous pacemaker.[430]

In some patients with clinical features of infective endocarditis, premortem blood cultures are sterile despite ideal laboratory procedures.[462,473] In some of these patients, organisms can be demonstrated in vegetations at autopsy by smear or by culture.[432] Several factors have been proposed to explain negative cultures in patients with infective endocarditis.[473] These include (1) previous antibiotic therapy, (2) infection by fastidious, slow-growing bacteria, (3) infection by nonbacterial organisms, and (4) right-sided endocarditis.

Predisposing conditions. The development of infective endocarditis requires (1) the presence of infective organisms in the bloodstream and (2) preparation of the valve surface to permit adherence and subsequent proliferation of circulating organisms.[471] Transient bacteremia has been demonstrated in association with everyday procedures such as brushing of teeth or gum chewing; minor dental procedures, particularly extraction; manipulation of the genitourinary tract as in catheterization or cystoscopy; and even in normal deliveries.[439] Common initiating factors for infective endocarditis include upper respiratory infections, dental manipulation, operative genitourinary infections, and cardiac catheterization.[458] However, in many patients the source of the organisms responsible for the valvulitis is not known.

The highly pathogenic organisms that produce endocarditis commonly arise from infections elsewhere in the body (such as pneumonia, skin infections, and renal infections) or may be introduced intravenously by narcotic addicts. The organisms may also appear as a result of bacteremia initiated by procedures performed in patients of the older age group, such as extensive surgery for cancer, skin incisions for intravenous infusions (that is, cutdowns), cystoscopy, and urethral catheterization.[459]

Because of these features, it has been recommended that prophylactic antibiotics be given to patients at risk (such as those with damaged heart valves, a history of rheumatic heart disease, and the presence of prosthetic heart valves) who are to undergo procedures likely to cause bacteremia (such as dental extraction and surgical procedures to the genitourinary tract).[469]

The presence of underlying heart disease predisposes to infective endocarditis, particularly that caused by less virulent organisms, resulting in the more protracted (subacute) form of the disease. The bacteria implant on valves that are thickened and fibrotic as a result of rheumatic fever (Fig. 15-22), though the frequency of this association has decreased during the antibiotic era.[440] According to one report, the underlying heart disease in over 50% of the patients was rheumatic, and in about 20% there was congenital heart disease.[458] Congenital lesions predisposing to the infection include bicuspid aortic valves, interventricular septal defects, subaortic stenosis and pulmonary stenosis (including tetralogy of Fallot), coarctation of the aorta, and patent ductus arteriosus. Atherosclerotic aortic valvular disease and mitral valve prolapse may also predispose to infective endocarditis.[434,450,472,477] For example, one controlled study involved a group of patients who underwent echocardiographic examination and who lacked any known cardiovascular risk factors for endocarditis apart from mitral prolapse and mitral regurgitant murmurs. It was found that 25% of 51 patients with endocarditis had mitral valve prolapse as compared to 7% of the matched controls without endocarditis.[434]

Another feature that affects the occurrence of bacterial adherence is intrinsic to the bacterial organism itself. For example, it has been shown that dextran encourages adherance of bacteria. It has also been found that dextran-producing streptococci are more likely to produce endocarditis than non–dextran producing streptococci.[448]

Endocarditis from *Candida albicans* has increased as a result of widespread use of antibiotics and adrenal corticosteroids and the advent of cardiac surgery.[478] It has been noted in narcotic addicts who use unsterile procedures for intravenous injection of the drugs and occasionally has been seen in patients who have received prolonged intravenous penicillin therapy.[452,478] *Aspergillus* also has been observed as a cause of endocarditis after the insertion of pacing catheters and artificial valves (allografts and prostheses) in the heart.[429]

Pathogenesis. The microorganisms enter the bloodstream by one of the portals of entry mentioned previously. It is generally believed that the bacteria are implanted on the valves or mural endocardium directly and not through microvasculature. The infection seems to occur at sites that are under a hemodynamic strain[471]; for example, the valvular surfaces affected by mechanical trauma associated with intracardiac tension and force of contact, or an area exposed to a jetlike stream of blood such as that forced through an interventricular septal defect or a patent ductus arteriosus. Although healthy valves may be affected by hemodynamic stresses, such stresses are more pronounced on previously damaged valves.[414]

Endocardial lesions. The characteristic pathologic feature of infective endocarditis is the presence of vegetations on the valve cusps or leaflets. The valve most frequently affected is the mitral. The aortic valve is the next most commonly involved. The occurrence of vegetations on the mitral and aortic valves simultaneously is fairly common, and the valves on the right side of the heart seldom are affected. An exception to this general rule has been observed in narcotic addicts in whom infective endocarditis often involves the tricuspid valve.[463]

The vegetations vary in size from a few millimeters to a centimeter or more and are gray, tawny, reddish, or brown, fairly firm but friable, single or multiple, and flat, filiform, fungating, or polypoid (Fig. 15-22). Because the vegetations are friable, they give rise to emboli, in contrast to rheumatic lesions, which do not. The vegetations tend to localize on the atrial surface of the atrioventricular valves and on the ventricular surfaces of the semilunar valves. They arise from the contact areas of the cusps or leaflets but tend to spread along the valve surfaces onto the adjacent mural endocardium. The chordae tendineae may be involved. Ulceration and perforation of the valve leaflets or cusps may develop (Fig. 15-22, *C*).

Microscopically, the vegetations consist of fibrin, platelets, leukocytes, and the infecting organism, and in the underlying valve a nonspecific inflammatory reaction with varying degrees of necrosis is present. In

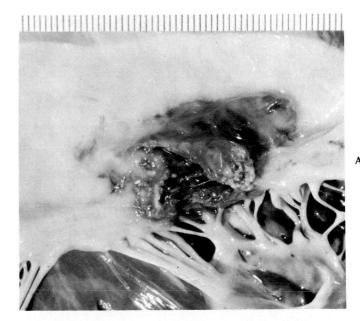

A

Fig. 15-22. Bacterial endocarditis of the mitral valve (caused by *Streptococcus viridans*). **A,** Ulcerating lesion of a valve also showing evidence of old rheumatic valvulitis (thickening, shortening, and fusion of chordae tendineae).

Continued.

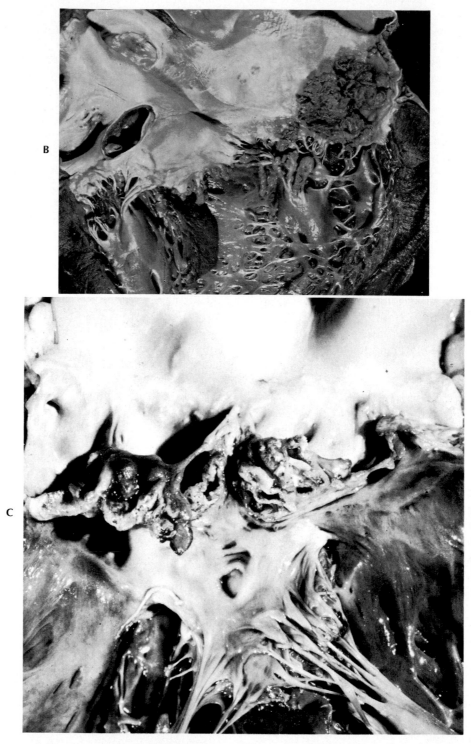

Fig. 15-22, cont'd. B, Different lesion. There is a large vegetation involving the posterior leaflet of the mitral valve and wall of left atrium. **C,** Bacterial endocarditis involving the aortic valve. Prominent vegetations are present on the aortic valve cusps, which are perforated. Smaller vegetations were present on the mitral valve but are not shown well in this view.

the acute, fulminant cases, neutrophils are prominent, and there may be extensive necrosis with abscess formation. The abscess may extend to the valve rings. In the prolonged cases, varying degrees of granulation tissue and fibroblastic proliferation with mononuclear inflammatory cells are seen (Fig. 15-23). Sometimes, foreign-body giant cells are encountered in the necrotic area.[466] Bacterial masses may be present in the periphery of the fibrin, in a position to seed the bloodstream with organisms (Fig. 15-23). Occasionally bacteria may be deeply embedded in the vegetation but not be detectable in the bloodstream.

Healing of a vegetation may take place, particularly after antibiotic therapy.[438,453] There is invasion of the fibrinous layer by granulation tissue, resulting in fibrosis. The bacteria are phagocytosed and destroyed. Hyalinization, calcification, and endothelialization of the vegetation subsequently occur. If calcification is extensive, a severely deformed nodular valve may develop.

In fungal endocarditis, vegetations that are grossly similar to those of bacterial endocarditis occur. Microscopically, many organisms are usually present in the vegetations. The inflammation of the underlying endocardium is consistent with the nature of the infecting organisms and includes granulomatous or acute and chronic nonspecific inflammation with or without suppuration.

Complications and sequelae. Complications and sequelae of bacterial endocarditis may be divided into two categories: cardiac changes and extracardiac complications.

Cardiac changes. Various degenerative changes, petechiae, and focal necrosis of the myocardium may occur as a result of the associated infection, and sometimes a focal or diffuse nonspecific myocarditis is present, with foci of myocytic necrosis and inflammation (lymphocytes and mononuclear cells) being referred to as "Bracht-Wachter bodies." Myocardial abscesses and abscesses of the valve rings may be encountered in patients with infective endocarditis. Antimicrobial agents may control the infection on the valves, but viable organisms may persist in such abscesses.[467] Embolism of the larger coronary arteries is rare, but minute embolic fragments of vegetations may be found frequently in the intramyocardial branches of the coronary arteries. Cardiac failure may result not only from the myocardial changes, but also from progressive valvular impairment. Complications produced by the destructive effects of the endocardial lesions include perforation of valve leaflets, aneurysm of valve leaflets, which may subsequently rupture, perforation of the sinuses of Valsalva, rupture of the chordae tendineae, and rupture of the interventricular septum. Despite successful therapy, a variety of serious sequelae may occur in subsequent years.[454] In particular, there may be valvular changes associated with the healing of bacterial endocarditis—aortic insufficiency, valvular perforation, and aneurysm.

Extracardiac complications. A very common and serious complication of bacterial endocarditis is embolism resulting from the breaking off of fragments of vegetations into the bloodstream. Since, in the majority of instances, vegetations are located on the mitral and aortic valves, emboli most frequently enter the systemic circulation and affect particularly the spleen, kidneys, and brain, causing infarcts, abscesses, or mycotic aneurysms. Abscesses are more likely to occur in acute than in subacute bacterial endocarditis because of the greater virulence of the causative organisms. Pulmonary abscesses may be seen in association with infective endocarditis of the right side of the heart.

Petechiae in the skin, conjunctivae, and eye grounds are common. These are now considered to be manifestations of an immune complex–mediated inflammation of the vascular walls (vasculitis). Small, raised, red, tender areas on the hands and feet and especially on the fingertips are characteristic lesions known as Osler's nodes. These also are believed to be the result of an immune complex–mediated vasculitis.[446] Janeway le-

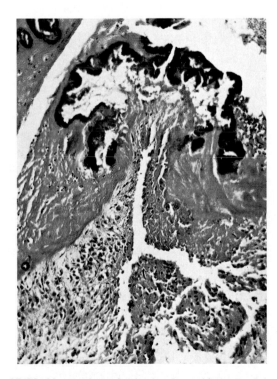

Fig. 15-23. Vegetation of mitral valve with bacterial endocarditis (same heart as that shown in Fig. 15-22, *B*). Notice dark masses of bacteria at top, partly embedded in fibrin. A few neutrophils are also present in the fibrin. The thickened valve leaflet, *below,* is diffusely infiltrated with large mononuclear cells and fibroblasts. An area at center right is necrotic.

sions are painless, hemorrhagic, slightly raised areas occurring usually in the palms and soles.

Focal necrotizing glomerulonephritis also may occur. This lesion was previously believed to be caused by small emboli that lodged in the glomeruli; the lesions were called "focal embolic glomerulonephritis." However, this complication, too, is now considered to be an immunoallergic vascular response to antigenic products of the bacteria (see p. 826).[446,456] Occasionally a diffuse glomerulonephritis occurs. The usual effects of septicemia involving many organs and tissues of the body are evident in bacterial endocarditis. These are similar to septicemia of other causes.

Clinical course. The clinical picture is that of a generalized infection with fever, cardiac manifestations (such as changing murmur), and evidences of embolism (with either septic or bland infarcts). William Osler described the clinical features of the disease that he termed "malignant endocarditis,"[457] and they have been well summarized by Hermans.[444]

In the earlier literature it was customary to use "subacute" to refer to infections that were from 6 weeks to 3 months or more in duration, and the term "acute" was applied to patients who died in less than 6 weeks.[433,442,443,477] It is apparent that current effective treatment has changed the course of the two varieties of endocarditis, and so there is now an overlapping in their clinical, bacteriologic, and pathologic features. Thus it is no longer always possible or necessary to differentiate between the two forms of the disease, since the distinction is an academic one. It would be far more useful if the name of the etiologic agent could be used, such as alpha-streptococcal endocarditis and staphylococcal endocarditis. There is no question but that the identification of the causative microorganism is most important to the clinical handling of the patient. Nevertheless, some writers still recognize a distinction between acute and subacute bacterial endocarditis. Furthermore, it is still of some value from a student's point of view to make the distinction, since several features of the disease can be thereby illustrated. The main distinctions between acute and subacute endocarditis (Table 15-1) exist in the invasive and destructive capabilities of the infecting organism. Acute bacterial endocarditis is caused by virulent and destructive organisms (such as staphylococci) that tend to produce extensive necrosis of the heart valves as well as abscesses

in the heart and elsewhere in the body. On the other hand, subacute bacterial endocarditis is the result of less virulent organisms (such as *Streptococcus viridans*) that cause little necrosis or suppuration in the host's tissues.

Prognosis and causes of death. The prognosis in bacterial endocarditis has changed decidedly in recent years. Before the advent of antimicrobial therapy, the prognosis was almost hopeless. Now with the availability of effective treatment the outlook is much better. The overall cure rates with medical therapy have been reported to range from 50% to 90%.[447,449,461,470]

Unfortunately, cure of the active phase of bacterial endocarditis is sometimes marred by the occurrence of serious sequelae such as aortic insufficiency caused by perforation of valve leaflets or valvular aneurysms, which may necessitate valve replacements.[455,470] In addition, the prognosis continues to be poor in certain subgroups of patients, including those with infection caused by virulent strains of staphylococci, gram-negative bacilli, or fungi, patients with prosthetic valve infections, and patients in whom endocarditis is complicated by cardiac failure.[470]

Since the institution of antibiotic therapy, there has been a change in the causes of death in bacterial endocarditis.[464] In the preantibiotic era, infection was the primary cause of death. Today the most common cause is usually reported to be congestive heart failure, which may occur during or after treatment.[474] Cardiac failure may be caused by valvular alterations or by an accompanying myocarditis and only rarely by coronary embolism. Other causes of death include persistent infection, embolism to major organs, rupture of mycotic aneurysms of cerebral arteries, and renal insufficiency. However, in a fairly recent autopsy study of 47 patients with infective endocarditis, infection and not congestive heart failure was found to be the major cause of death.[465] The authors of this study suggest that the increased number of deaths resulting from infection may be in part related to the fact that infective endocarditis was not recognized clinically in many of the patients, who therefore were not treated for the disease. Also, the disease in the majority of patients who did not have prosthetic valves was less than 6 weeks in duration, and so death occurred before intractable cardiac failure resulting from valve destruction had a chance to develop.

Table 15-1. Major distinguishing characteristics between acute and subacute infective endocarditis

Clinical duration	Acute (less than 6 weeks)	Subacute (more than 6 weeks)
Microorganism	*Staphylococcus aureus, Streptococcus*	*Streptococcus viridans*
Preexisting condition of valve	Usually normal	Often thickened, deformed
Damage to valve	Severe, often destruction of cusp	Cusps intact

Myocarditis

Inflammation of the muscular layer of the heart is termed *myocarditis*. The statistical incidence of this disease has undergone a profound change over the past three to four decades. Formerly, clinicians designated almost every disease of the heart muscle as myocarditis.[484] It was common to attribute death to chronic myocarditis, particularly in elderly persons, when focal or diffuse fibrosis of the myocardium was found at autopsy. Since it has been recognized that myocardial fibrosis is commonly the result of coronary artery disease, the diagnosis of chronic or fibrous myocarditis has been made less frequently.

In a survey of 5626 consecutive autopsies at Michael Reese Hospital in Chicago[511,512] 240 cases of myocarditis (4.3%) were encountered, of which 186 (approximately 78%) were nonrheumatic. In a study of autopsies accessioned at Armed Forces Institute of Pathology[491] 1402 cases of myocarditis were collected, with the estimated incidence being 3.5%. More than 90% of the 1402 cases were nonrheumatic. These incidence figures are in agreement with the statistics obtained in other investigations, such as 3.3% at Bellevue Hospital in New York[484] and 3.4% at Cincinnati General Hospital.[481]

There are various classifications of myocarditis, none of which is entirely satisfactory to both the pathologist and the clinician. The terms *specific* and *nonspecific* are sometimes applied to the morphologic pattern of an inflammatory reaction in the various forms of myocarditis. A specific inflammation is one characterized by a well-recognized histologic picture that is highly suggestive or diagnostic of a disease or group of diseases, such as the granulomatous lesions of tuberculosis and syphilis or the pathognomonic Aschoff body of rheumatic carditis. A nonspecific reaction does not conform to any distinctive pattern, as may be seen in many forms of myocarditis associated with infectious agents in which focal or diffuse collections of a variety of inflammatory cells are evident. In some forms of myocarditis, both specific and nonspecific inflammations are represented; for example, in rheumatic myocarditis the specific lesion is the Aschoff body, and commonly associated with it is a nonspecific inflammation consisting of lymphocytes, plasma cells, histiocytes, and occasionally neutrophils throughout the edematous interstitial tissue.[379] A separation of myocarditis into acute, subacute, and chronic forms is sometimes made.

Most commonly, the disease is classified according to etiologic factors. The following classification is based on that proposed by Manion[503] at the Armed Forces Institute of Pathology:

1. Caused by infectious agents
   a. Bacterial
   b. Rickettsial
   c. Viral
   d. Protozoal and parasitic
   e. Fungal
2. Idiopathic
   a. Diffuse, interstitial
   b. Granulomatous
3. In "connective tissue" diseases
   a. Rheumatic fever
   b. Rheumatoid arthritis
   c. Lupus erythematosus
   d. Polyarteritis nodosa
   e. Dermatomyositis
4. Caused by physical agents, chemical poisons, drugs, and metabolic disorders
   a. Trauma
   b. Irradiation
   c. Chemical poisons
   d. Drugs
   e. Uremia
   f. Hypokalemia
   g. Others

Myocarditis caused by infectious agents

In the myocardial lesions associated with infectious diseases, the inflammation may be attributable to an actual invasion of the myocardium by the organisms or to the action of their toxins, though it is possible that an allergic mechanism is responsible in some instances.

The gross appearance of the heart in acute myocarditis is not distinctive, but usually the myocardium is pale and flabby and the chambers are dilated. Some degree of hypertrophy may be seen, especially in those instances associated with cardiac failure. In some circumstances, abscesses may develop. These are discernible grossly as small, yellow, round, or streaky foci that sometimes become confluent. Some of the abscesses may be surrounded by a hemorrhagic zone.

The microscopic picture of acute myocarditis varies. The inflammation may be patchy (focal) or diffuse. In certain bacterial infections, degenerative changes and necrosis of the muscle are likely to be prominent, whereas interstitial inflammation is slight. In other instances a nonsuppurative inflammation of the supporting connective tissue is the predominant change, with a cellular infiltrate consisting of lymphocytes, plasma cells, eosinophils, and Anitschkow cells. Neutrophils usually are not present in great numbers and frequently are absent. The stroma may be edematous. Not uncommonly, both the parenchymal and interstitial features are prominent.

Bacterial and fungal myocarditis. Abscesses may be caused by pyogenic organisms (especially staphylococci and beta-hemolytic streptococci) either as a complication of a pyemia from a suppurative inflammation elsewhere in the body or as a consequence of bacterial en-

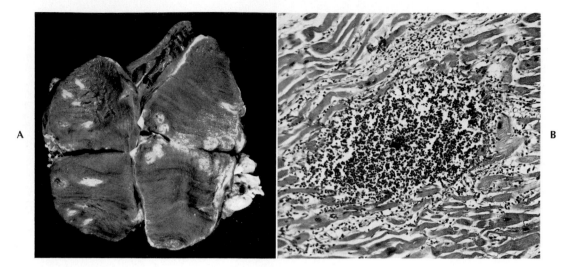

Fig. 15-24. A, Myocardial abscesses caused by *Staphylococcus aureus*. **B,** Abscess of myocardium from a patient with bacterial endocarditis (staphylococcal). The small dark mass in the center of the abscess is a cluster of organisms.

docarditis (Fig. 15-24). Abscesses also may develop in the myocardium as the result of certain fungal infections, such as candidiasis, aspergillosis, phycomycosis, actinomycosis, and blastomycosis.[480] Pyogenic organisms sometimes may produce a more diffuse suppurative myocarditis. Fibrosis is seen in the later phase of certain myocardial lesions, particularly if there has been a significant degree of parenchymal destruction (as in diphtheria).[490] In regard to the effects of diphtheria on the heart, some authors are reluctant to accept the myocardial changes as evidence of a true myocarditis because the primary lesions are degenerative and necrotic. But since a secondary inflammatory cell infiltrate occurs in response to the primary toxic injury of muscle, it seems proper to designate this as diphtheritic myocarditis.[490]

In one series of 63 patients with myocardial abscesses, the two most common causative agents were *Candida* and *Staphylococcus aureus*.[488] In approximately 20% of these patients, the myocardial abscesses occurred with infective endocarditis; nearly all were associated with disseminated sepsis. The most frequent underlying conditions preceding development of the myocardial abscesses were surgical conditions, malignancy, and alcoholic liver disease.

Granulomatous inflammation of the myocardium is produced by certain bacterial infections, such as tuberculosis, tularemia, and brucellosis. Tuberculous myocarditis is rare and occurs as nodular, miliary, and diffuse infiltrative types.[511,512] The nodular lesions also are referred to as tuberculomas. Involvement of the myocardium is mainly the result of hematogenous spread from infection elsewhere in the body but also can be

caused by extension from a tuberculous pericarditis. Foci of granulomatous inflammation and fibrosis are reported in brucellosis, though in this disease there may also be myocardial abscesses, particularly associated with *Brucella* endocarditis.[505]

Sarcoidosis is not proved to be an infectious disease, but it is mentioned at this point because of the close microscopic resemblance of its lesions to the noncaseating forms of tuberculosis. Extensive pulmonary sarcoidosis may result in cor pulmonale. In addition, but less frequently, sarcoidosis can involve the myocardium directly.[506,507] The granulomatous inflammation may be accompanied by a considerable degree of myocardial fibrosis, and myocardial dysfunction may be associated with either active or fibrotic lesions. Sarcoid lesions also occur in the endocardium and epicardium. Clinical manifestations are arrhythmias (including sudden death and conduction block), cardiac failure, papillary muscle dysfunction, and recurrent pericardial effusions.[507]

Rickettsial myocarditis. Myocarditis frequently is seen in rickettsial diseases. It is uniformly present in scrub typhus and occurs in about 50% of the cases of epidemic typhus and Rocky Mountain spotted fever.[479,482,515] Microscopic features include interstitial edema and focal or patchy infiltration by inflammatory cells—mainly lymphocytes, plasma cells, macrophages, Anitschkow cells, mast cells, and eosinophils, usually in close association with a small vessel. Neutrophils are scanty unless necrosis is present; degeneration and necrosis usually does not occur to a significant degree. A more diffuse myocarditis occurs in some instances (p. 350). Characteristically, vascular changes such as capillary and arteriolar endothelial swelling and phlebitis with thrombosis may be noted in the heart.[479] Necrotizing arteritis of the myocardium is sometimes present in epidemic typhus.[479]

Viral myocarditis. Myocarditis occurs as a consequence of a variety of viral infections[518] (Fig. 15-25). Viruses in the enterovirus group account for the majority of cases of viral myocarditis,[501] and of these, group B coxsackieviruses are believed to be the cause of one third to one half of all cases.[492,508] Group A coxsackievirus and echovirus types also have been implicated with lesser frequency. Myocarditis also has been reported as a complication of a variety of other viral diseases,[518] including poliomyelitis, varicella,[493] influenza, infectious hepatitis, mumps, infectious mononucleosis, psittacosis, and lymphocytic choriomeningitis. The microscopic features of the myocardial lesions in many of the viral infections is similar. At first, the interstitial tissue is infiltrated by lymphocytes and neutrophils, and there is necrosis of individual muscle fibers. Later, lymphocytes and histiocytes predominate and some degree of connective tissue proliferation occurs. The mechanism by which the organism produces cardiac damage is not known, but it has been postulated that the virus induces cellular damage in the heart directly by interfering with cellular metabolism or indirectly by inciting an immune response and immune-mediated injury of infected cardiac myocytes.[509]

Protozoal myocarditis. Two of the protozoal diseases in which myocarditis occurs are infection with *Trypanosoma cruzi* (Chagas' disease) and toxoplasmosis. In Chagas' disease,[487] infection is acquired from the bite of the reduviid bug, an arthropod intermediary host of the protozoon. Many organs and tissues are invaded by the organism, but the myocardium, skeletal muscle, and central nervous system are most frequently attacked. The inflammation in the myocardium usually is intense, with a cellular infiltration consisting of histiocytes, plasma cells, lymphocytes, and some polymorphonuclear leukocytes (Fig. 15-26). Degeneration and necrosis of muscle fibers may be prominent.

Toxoplasmosis is caused by an intracellular protozoon, *Toxoplasma gondii*. This organism is reported to be widespread in humans and animals.[488,494] Infection may be acquired in utero, through exposure to infected pets such as cats, or through ingestion of uncooked meat or unpasteurized milk from infected livestock.[500] Microscopic changes in the myocardium include focal necrosis, edema, and accumulation of inflammatory cells (plasma cells, macrophages, and lymphocytes). Occasional pseudocysts containing organisms are seen in the myocardium within or outside muscle fibers, often separate from the foci of inflammation.[495] Clinical manifestations include arrhythmias, embolic phenomena, and mild to moderate heart failure.[500]

Among the intestinal helminthic parasites that affect

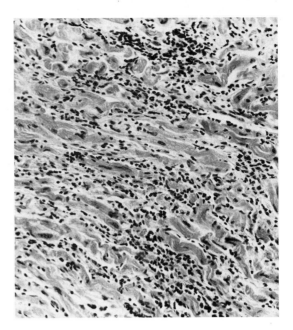

Fig. 15-25. Diffuse, nonspecific myocarditis from a child who died after an upper respiratory infection.

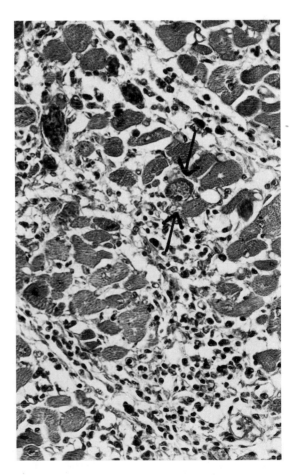

Fig. 15-26. Diffuse myocarditis in Chagas' disease. A myocyte with intracellular organisms is evident, *arrows.*

the heart are *Trichinella spiralis* and *Echinococcus granulosus*. Myocarditis is a serious complication in trichinosis and may lead to cardiac failure.[489] The inflammatory reaction is a response to the larvae, but the latter are rarely identified in the lesions. The parasites either are destroyed or pass on into the circulation and do not encyst within the myocardium. Microscopically, both muscle and interstitial tissue are involved; there is focal necrosis of the muscle fibers, along with an inflammatory infiltrate predominantly composed of lymphocytes and eosinophils. Sometimes there is an increased amount of fluid in the pericardial sac, in which few larvae may be found. *Echinococcus* disease is uncommon in the United States. However, in sheep-grazing countries such as Uruguay, Argentina, Australia, and New Zealand and in the Mediterranean area the disease is frequent.[485] Hydatid cysts occasionally occur in the myocardium. The primary hydatid cyst of the heart tends to rupture into the lumen of a cardiac chamber or into the pericardial sac. Rupture into an adjacent cardiac chamber, with release of hydatid fluid and daughter cysts into the circulation, may result in anaphylactic reactions or peripheral emboli.[496]

Idiopathic (Fiedler's) myocarditis

Idiopathic myocarditis occurs without apparent cause. As more is learned about the etiology of heart disease, it is to be expected that various conditions will be separated from this category, as has occurred in the past. Idiopathic myocarditis sometimes is termed *isolated* because typically the inflammation is limited to the myocardium and is not accompanied by endocarditis, pericarditis, or any other disease in the body that is known to cause myocarditis. There is often rapidly progressive myocardial failure or sudden death. The gross appearance of the heart is not unlike that seen in myocarditis associated with known infectious agents, the essential features being dilatation and sometimes hypertrophy. When the lesions are extensive, they appear as yellow-gray or gray foci throughout the myocardium. Mural thrombi are commonly present.

In the older literature, the classification of idiopathic

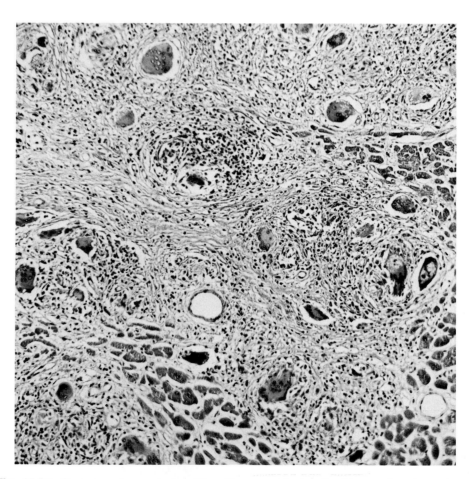

Fig. 15-27. Granulomatous myocarditis with many giant cells. Myocardium is replaced by coalescent granulomatous nodules and fibrous scar. Giant cells are of the foreign body and Langhans' types, with asteroid bodies in some cells. There are no similar lesions found in any other organs from this patient.

myocarditis has been variable and thus a source of confusion. Currently, three microscopic forms are recognized: diffuse myocarditis, granulomatous myocarditis, and giant cell myocarditis (without the formation of granulomas).[510,512,517]

Diffuse myocarditis is encountered more frequently than the granulomatous type. Microscopically it is indistinguishable from viral myocarditis and is characterized by a nonspecific inflammation consisting of lymphocytes, plasma cells, macrophages, eosinophils, and a few neutrophils throughout the interstitial tissue (Fig. 15-25). Involvement of the parenchyma with destruction of muscle fibers may be noted. Variability of the lesion is emphasized. Some are very cellular, and others culminate in fibrosis.

In the granulomatous variety, throughout the myocardium are small or large granulomas without caseation, consisting of macrophages, giant cells, other forms of leukocytes, and areas of muscle necrosis. The giant cells are of the foreign body and Langhans types, but some giant cells of myogenic origin also may be present[510] (Fig. 15-27). Acid-fast bacilli and spirochetes cannot be demonstrated. The possible relationship of granulomatous myocarditis to sarcoidosis has been questioned. Sarcoid lesions do occur in the heart as one manifestation of generalized disease, and it has been suggested that granulomatous myocarditis might represent an isolated organ form of sarcoidosis.[502] Truly isolated granulomatous myocarditis is not regarded to be sarcoidosis.[486] On the other hand, granulomatous myocarditis cannot be considered to be isolated to the heart until extracardiac sarcoidosis has been ruled out by thorough workup including histologic evaluation of lymph nodes.[507]

Several reports have appeared in the literature describing a lesion known as giant cell myocarditis,[483,486,497,513,517] the cause and nature of which are not known.

Myocarditis in connective tissue diseases

Myocarditis in rheumatic fever, rheumatoid arthritis, and lupus erythematosus is described elsewhere in the text. The lesion in the myocardium in polyarteritis nodosa is a necrotizing vasculitis with extension of the inflammatory reaction to the adjacent perivascular tissue. With formation of thrombi in the vessels, secondary ischemic changes, including infarction, may occur in the myocardium. Microscopic changes in the heart muscle reported in dermatomyositis are similar to those found in the skeletal muscle but are less severe.[514] Degeneration, loss of striations, vacuolization, and necrosis of muscle fibers may be seen. Sometimes there is interstitial edema, and in some instances an inflammatory cell infiltration (mainly lymphocytes and some histiocytes) is present interstitially or perivascularly. Hyalin-

ized thickening of the intramyocardial arterioles with narrowing of the lumens may be evident. Scleroderma is said to bear a relationship to dermatomyositis. However, the lesions in the heart consist of irregular areas of fibrous tissue replacement of the myocardium without any significant inflammatory component. Only an occasional lymphocyte and histiocyte may be present. The connective tissue appears cellular because of prominence of connective tissue cells and not because of an inflammatory cell infiltration.[516] Slight intimal or medial thickening of the arterioles may be noted.

Myocarditis caused by physical agents, chemical poisons, drugs, and metabolic disorders

The cardiac effects of trauma, ionizing radiation, chemical poisons, drugs, and metabolic disorders are considered in other sections of this chapter. In cardiac trauma a nonspecific myocarditis may be seen in association with contusions of the myocardium, with the lesion consisting of an infiltrate of neutrophils and a few eosinophils and mononuclear cells, together with focal necrosis of muscle fibers and hemorrhage.[504]

The changes in the myocardium caused by certain chemical poisons or drugs consist primarily in degeneration (parenchymatous, hydropic, or fatty) and focal necrosis of myocardial fibers. Edema and small hemorrhages also may be present. A nonspecific inflammatory reaction, consisting chiefly of lymphocytes and histiocytes, occurs in response to the necrotic tissue. Myocarditis characterized by an interstitial exudate with many eosinophils has been observed as an unusual

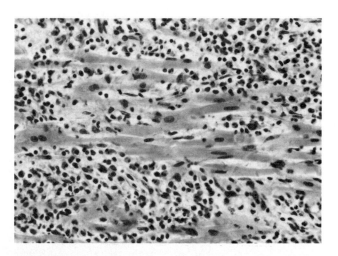

Fig. 15-28. Hypersensitivity myocarditis. Myocardial fibers are separated by a severe inflammatory infiltrate that includes numerous eosinophils (most of the inflammatory cells with segmented nuclei in this illustration are eosinophils). The patient was an 18-year-old girl who developed a severe skin rash and susequently died of heart failure after treatment of a seizure disorder with phenytoin (Dilantin) and carbamazepine (Tegretol).

complication of therapy with a variety of drugs and is generally interpreted as a manifestation of hypersensitivity (Fig. 15-28). In some instances, necrotizing arteritis accompanies the myocarditis. Myocardial changes induced by catecholamines with the production of so-called norepinephrine myocarditis are described on p. 180.

A nonspecific myocarditis has been reported in uremia,[511,512] but some investigators do not accept such an entity though they recognize the presence of fatty degeneration and edema of the myocardium attributable to uremic intoxication.[499]

Hydropericardium

Normally the pericardial cavity contains about 5 to 50 ml of clear, straw-colored fluid that includes a small amount of protein and is of low specific gravity (that is, a transudate). An excessive quantity, usually more than 100 ml, of this transudate in the pericardial sac is referred to as *hydropericardium*. This term is not applied to the effusion associated with serous or serofibrinous pericarditis, which includes the elements of an inflammatory exudate—increased protein content, higher specific gravity, and leukocytes. The color of the fluid in hydropericardium may be altered under certain conditions. It may be bile stained if jaundice is present, deep red or brown if there is hemorrhage, or red as a result of postmortem hemolysis.

The causes of hydropericardium are those conditions associated with a noninflammatory type of edema. It is seen most frequently as a part of the picture of congestive heart failure. It also occurs in the nephrotic syndrome, the hypoproteinemic state associated with malnutrition or chronic wasting diseases, myxedema, beriberi, and as a result of interference with the venous return from the pericardial circulation such as that caused by neoplastic or inflammatory lesions of the mediastinum.

The clinical significance of hydropericardium depends more on the rapidity of accumulation than on the total quantity of fluid. Large effusions up to 1000 ml or more that collect slowly in the pericardial cavity may cause no embarrassment of the heart provided that the pericardium is not thickened by disease and is permitted to stretch. On the other hand, a smaller amount (for example, 150 to 250 ml) of fluid accumulating quickly will usually cause serious disturbances by producing cardiac tamponade.

Hemopericardium

The presence of blood in the pericardial cavity is known as *hemopericardium*, or hematopericardium. Among the common causes of hemorrhage in the pericardial sac are ruptured aneurysms of the aorta, trauma of the heart and great vessels, and rupture of a recent myocardial infarct. Sometimes hemopericardium accompanies myocardial infarction in the absence of cardiac rupture as a result of bleeding from the newly formed vessels in an organizing fibrinous pericarditis (see next page). Although this complication has been

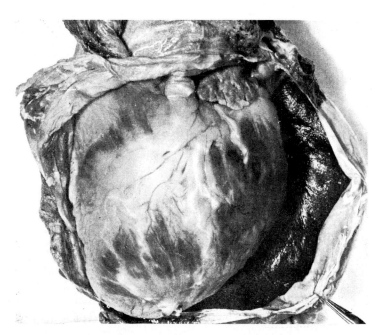

Fig. 15-29. Hemopericardium caused by rupture of an aortic aneurysm into the pericardial sac. (From Anderson, W.A.D., and Scotti, T.M.: Synopsis of pathology, ed. 10, St. Louis, 1980, The C.V. Mosby Co.)

observed in connection with anticoagulant therapy,[531,536] it can occur spontaneously in patients not treated with anticoagulants.[519,527] Leukemia, scurvy, and other diseases characterized by a hemorrhagic diathesis may cause hemopericardium. Neoplasms involving the pericardium may produce bloody effusions, particularly secondary cancers. Inflammations of the pericardium, such as tuberculosis, can cause a hemorrhagic exudate. Rare instances of hemopericardium occur after rupture of the heart in an area of the myocardium involved by an abscess or by extensive fat infiltration.

The essential morphologic feature of hemopericardium in fatal cases is distension of the pericardial sac by the blood that fills the space. The blood may be fluid or clotted (Fig. 15-29). If a small amount of fluid blood is present, it may be largely resorbed. Blood not resorbed will clot and become organized. Instances of constrictive pericarditis have been reported as a sequel to hemopericardium.[543,545]

The clinical effects of hemopericardium depend on the amount and rapidity of bleeding. As little as 150 to 250 ml of blood, rapidly filling the pericardial cavity, can cause cardiac tamponade and death. Pericardiocentesis for relief of acute tamponade may be a lifesaving procedure in some cases.

Pericarditis

Pericarditis is an inflammation of the pericardium, and it may be classified as acute, subacute, or chronic.[532] Quite frequently, it is designated according to anatomic features, such as (1) fibrinous, (2) serous, (3) serofibrinous, (4) fibrinopurulent or purulent, (5) hemorrhagic, (6) cholesterol, (7) granulomatous, (8) chronic adhesive (or obliterative), and (9) chronic constrictive. The various forms of pericarditis may be classified on the basis of etiologic factors as follows:

1. Acute nonspecific (idiopathic)
2. Infective
   a. Bacterial (acute)
   b. Viral
   c. Other infections
3. Immunologic
   a. Rheumatic fever
   b. Other connective tissue disorders
4. Neoplastic
5. Metabolic
   a. Uremic
   b. Myxedema
   c. Gout
6. Traumatic (including after cardiac surgery)
7. Associated with myocardial infarction

In the following discussion, the anatomic types of pericarditis will be considered first, followed by examples of the etiologic forms.

Anatomic types of pericarditis

Fibrinous, serous, and serofibrinous pericarditis. The most common response of the pericardium to various injurious agents, infectious and noninfectious, is an inflammation characterized by a fibrinous exudate with or without a serous effusion (Fig. 15-30). The usual known causes are uremia, acute bacterial infections, rheumatic fever, myocardial infarction, and tuberculosis. Acute nonspecific pericarditis is of unknown origin by definition, and—as in the case of idiopathic myocarditis—if an etiologic agent such as a virus can be associated with the condition, it would be separated from the "idiopathic" category.

Occasionally, acute pericarditis is of the serous type, which is characterized by an effusion of fluid that is richer in protein and of a higher specific gravity than the transudate of hydropericardium. More often, however, the reaction is a fibrinous pericarditis that may be accompanied or followed by an effusion, hence the term "serofibrinous pericarditis." The character and extent of the reaction may vary in individual cases. The exudate

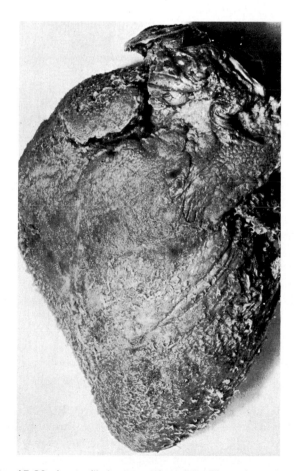

Fig. 15-30. Acute fibrinous pericarditis. There is a shaggy coat of fibrin covering the surface of the heart. (From Anderson, W.A.D., and Scotti, T.M.: Synopsis of pathology, ed. 10, St. Louis, 1980, The C.V. Mosby Co.)

may be dry or moist, thin or thick, finely granular or shaggy (like bread and butter). In the early stages the fibrin may be barely perceptible, but the pericardial surfaces lose their glistening sheen and assume a dull, opaque appearance, or the fibrin may consist of a thin film that, at times, covers only part of the pericardial surfaces. The amount of fluid accompanying the laying down of fibrin is variable.

Fibrinous pericarditis is clinically manifested by the presence of a friction rub. As fluid accumulates in the pericardial sac, the friction rub disappears. In some instances, particularly in serous pericarditis or in the less extensive forms of acute fibrinous pericarditis, the exudate is completely resorbed and the serosal surfaces return to normal. When the fibrin is more abundant, the pericarditis is likely to heal by organization; the exudate is penetrated and replaced by newly formed granulation tissue, resulting in localized or diffuse thickening of the pericardium with adhesions between the parietal and visceral pericardium. In rheumatic and tuberculous pericarditis, the distinctive inflammatory reactions of these diseases may be present in the serosal tissue in addition to the fibrinous or serofibrinous exudate.

Purulent or fibrinopurulent pericarditis. Purulent or fibrinopurulent pericarditis is caused by pyogenic organisms such as staphylococci, streptococci, and pneumococci, which reach the pericardium by way of the bloodstream from a focus of infection elsewhere, by direct extension from nearby tissues, or by direct implantation in wounds.[530] Certain nonbacterial organisms (such as fungi and rarely viruses) also may cause a suppurative inflammation of the pericardium. In the first half of this century, purulent pericarditis was a disease of young adults and usually occurred as a complication of pneumococcal pneumonia. In recent years, gramnegative bacilli and *Staphylococcus aureus* have become the most common causes of purulent pericarditis.[539] In a series of 55 patients, purulent pericarditis developed as a complication of a preexisting aseptic pericarditis, such as uremic or postsurgical in 47%.[539]

On inspection, the pericardial surfaces are seen to be covered with a yellowish or slimy gray exudate. If much fibrin is present, the exudate is thick, shaggy, and gelatinous. There are varying amounts of fluid, which at first is serous and then gradually becomes cloudy and purulent. Many organisms usually are found in the fluid. Cardiac tamponade may occur even if there is a relatively small amount of exudate present, apparently because the inflammation and thickening of the pericardial walls interfere with the usual degree of stretching. Microscopically, in addition to the fibrinopurulent or purulent exudate on the surface, there are many neutrophils throughout the serosal walls. Extension into the myocardium, pleura, or mediastinum may be noted.

Purulent pericarditis occurs less commonly than the fibrinous (or serofibrinous) type but is much more severe. Patients are acutely ill, with constitutional signs and symptoms of infection along with the manifestations of pericardial disease. As in fibrinous pericarditis, there is a friction rub. It is not likely that the purulent exudate will resorb completely. Healing by organization takes place, and the result is fibrosis, adhesions between parietal and visceral pericardium, and even calcification. The result is adhesive pericarditis or, in some instances, chronic constrictive pericarditis.

Hemorrhagic pericarditis. A hemorrhagic pericarditis is one in which blood is present in addition to the features of one of the other inflammatory exudates (serous, serofibrinous, or purulent). The causes include tuberculosis, uremia, severe acute infections, and neoplastic involvement of the pericardium. Patients with hemorrhagic diseases in whom pericarditis of any type develops are likely to have an associated hemorrhagic effusion.

Cholesterol pericarditis. A rare occurrence is pericardial effusion containing cholesterol (commonly referred to as cholesterol pericarditis). It often is associated with myxedema.[525] Another cause of this type of effusion is tuberculosis. In the latter instance, cholesterol deposits probably result from the breakdown of blood that sometimes accompanies tuberculous pericarditis. Any form of hemorrhagic pericarditis or hemopericardium may be responsible for the presence of cholesterol in the pericardial fluid. In some patients, the origin of the lipid-laden effusion is unknown. In one instance, cholesterol pericarditis of unknown cause progressed to constrictive pericarditis.[525] Microscopic examination of the pericardium removed surgically disclosed hyalinized connective tissue infiltrated by lymphocytes, plasma cells, lipid-containing foamy macrophages, foreign-body giant cells, and cholesterol crystals.

Granulomatous pericarditis. The most frequent form of granulomatous inflammation involving the pericardium is tuberculosis (described later). Gummatous (syphilitic) pericarditis is rare and usually represents an extension from myocardial gummas. Frankly granulomatous pericarditis sometimes occurs in rheumatoid arthritis.

Chronic adhesive (or obliterative) pericarditis. Fibrinous exudates exhibit a tendency to undergo organization. In the early phase of healing, vascularized granulation tissue can be seen between islands of the denser fibrinous deposits that still remain. In places where the surface layer has not been destroyed, the mesothelial cells may become cuboid and appear as proliferating masses of epithelium-like cells that sometimes form structures resembling ducts or glands. As organization progresses, fibrous adhesions develop between the pericardial surfaces. The cavity may become completely obliterated, or pockets of varying sizes may remain. At

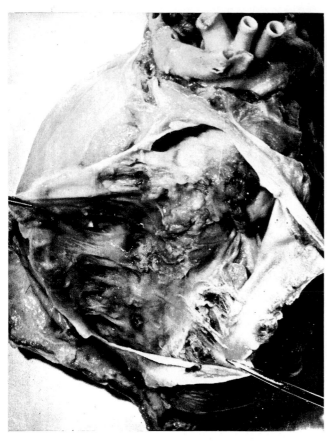

Fig. 15-31. Chronic adhesive pericarditis. The pericardial sac has been opened, displaying fibrous bands joining visceral and parietal pericardium. (From Anderson, W.A.D., and Scotti, T.M.: Synopsis of pathology, ed. 10, St. Louis, 1980, The C.V. Mosby Co.)

first, the fibrous adhesions are thin and easily separated, but later they become firmer and more difficult to tear apart (Fig. 15-31). Some authors prefer the term "adherent pericardium" to "adhesive pericarditis" because there often is no evidence of chronic inflammation. Chronic adhesive pericarditis usually causes no embarrassment of the heart, thus differing from chronic constrictive pericarditis.

Sometimes chronic adhesive pericarditis is accompanied by fibrous adhesions between the parietal pericardium and adjacent structures—mediastinum, pleura, diaphragm, and thoracic cage. This condition is referred to as mediastinopericarditis. Some observers regard the lesion as an added burden to the heart and a possible factor in the development of cardiac hypertrophy and failure in patients who have some underlying disturbance such as valvular disease.[466]

Chronic constrictive pericarditis. A most significant sequel of some types of pericarditis is chronic constrictive pericarditis, the result of healing of the inflammatory exudate (Figs. 15-32 and 15-33, *A*). It is character-ized by a pronounced fibrous thickening of the pericardium, which becomes so rigid that it mechanically interferes with the heart action and the circulation. The pericardial cavity may be completely or partially obliterated, and sometimes small collections of fluid are entrapped between adhesions. Calcification of the thickened, hyalinized pericardium may occur. Constrictive pericarditis may or may not be associated with mediastinopericarditis. When the latter is present, it usually accentuates the functional disturbances.

The main effect of the rigid pericardium is interference with diastolic relaxation of the heart. The dense fibrous tissue also may cause narrowing of the orifices of the venae cavae, but this has been demonstrated in only an occasional case.[546] The heart is usually normal or smaller than normal in size but may be enlarged.[526,538]

Pick's disease is a syndrome consisting in chronic constrictive pericarditis with severe venous congestion of the liver that may lead to fibrosis (cardiac cirrhosis) and ascites. Perihepatic and perisplenic fibrosis with hyalinization also may be associated. Polyserositis *(Concato's disease)* is characterized by large effusions into the various serous cavities: pericardial, pleural, and peritoneal. This syndrome may terminate in constrictive pericarditis and perihepatic and perisplenic fibrosis. The cause of Concato's disease is not known.

In the majority of patients with constrictive pericarditis the cause cannot be determined.[521,534,544] In years past, tuberculosis was considered to be the most common of the known causes of constrictive pericarditis[526] (Fig. 15-33, *A*). However, in recent years, tuberculosis has been observed in only a minority of cases.[521,534,544] Constrictive pericarditis also may occur as a consequence of purulent pericarditis, neoplastic involvement, and trauma.[526,545] Constrictive pericarditis also may develop after cardiac surgery, especially in patients who develop the postpericardiotomy syndrome (p. 672). Constrictive pericarditis may develop even in patients in whom the pericardium is left open after surgery.[541] Rheumatic fever is not a significant cause of constrictive pericarditis, though it has been reported to be responsible for an occasional case.[526] In one report the coexistence of rheumatic heart disease and constrictive pericarditis was observed in five cases, but the author remarked that there was no evidence that the two conditions were causally related.[538] Occasionally acute nonspecific (idiopathic) or viral pericarditis may progress to constrictive pericarditis.[534] Infrequent causes of constrictive pericarditis include rheumatoid arthritis, systemic lupus erythematosus, polyarteritis nodosa, uremia, and radiation.[534]

Pericardial plaques. Sometimes referred to as "milk spots," pericardial plaques are white, smooth, glistening, opaque, well-circumscribed areas of fibrosis of the

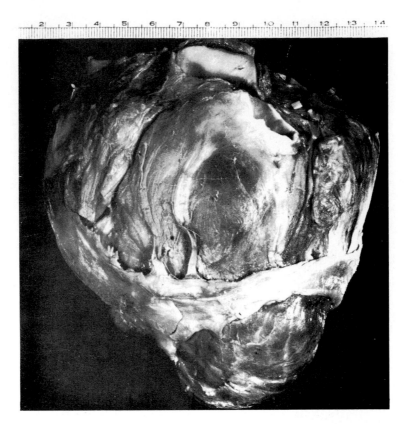

Fig. 15-32. Constrictive pericarditis. There is a band of calcified tissue that is traversing the anteroapical region and constricting the heart. There also was a generally thickened fibrous pericardium, which covered rest of heart, but has been removed. The patient was a 38-year-old white woman who had severe recurring ascites.

pericardium occurring principally on the epicardial surface of the anterior right ventricle. They are observed frequently as incidental findings at autopsy. They may be single or multiple and measure about 1 to 3 cm in diameter. The cause is not known, but they are generally believed to be the result of healed circumscribed pericarditis. In the earlier literature the term "soldier's spots" or "plaques" was used, originating in the old idea that the straps of knapsacks carried by soldiers in World War I produced pressure against the chest wall, causing chronic irritation of the visceral pericardium.

Etiologic types of pericarditis

Acute nonspecific pericarditis. Also known as acute idiopathic pericarditis and acute benign pericarditis, nonspecific pericarditis is today one of the most frequently encountered forms of pericarditis in clinical practice.[551,552] A lowering of the incidence of the former leading causes of acute pericarditis—acute bacterial infections and rheumatic fever—has been brought about apparently as a result of extensive use of antibiotics.[551] The prognosis of acute nonspecific pericarditis is usually good, though a few instances of fatal cardiac compression have been reported.[552] In most of the patients

there is a history of antecedent respiratory infection followed in 1 to 20 days by an onset of acute pericarditis, which is ushered in by severe precordial and substernal pain, pericardial friction rub, fever, chills, anorexia, and malaise. The duration of the acute illness averages 2 weeks, but there may be recurrences within 2 weeks to several months.[552]

Pericardial fibrinous inflammation and effusion are common.[533,552] Sometimes the effusion is hemorrhagic. Associated pleuritis with or without evidence of pneumonitis is common.[552] Apparently this disease may lead to a constrictive pericarditis, as judged from the occasional case histories that may indicate such a relationship.[551,552] The possibility that cases described as acute nonspecific (benign) pericarditis are of viral origin has been proposed. In a study of 34 cases of this disease, five instances were observed in which there was evidence for a viral infection (a group B coxsackievirus, echovirus type 8, adenovirus type 3, mumps, and infectious mononucleosis), but in 29 (85%) of the 34 cases, no cause was demonstrated.[537]

Bacterial (acute) pericarditis. See previous discussion of fibrinous, serous, serofibrinous, purulent, and hemorrhagic pericarditis.

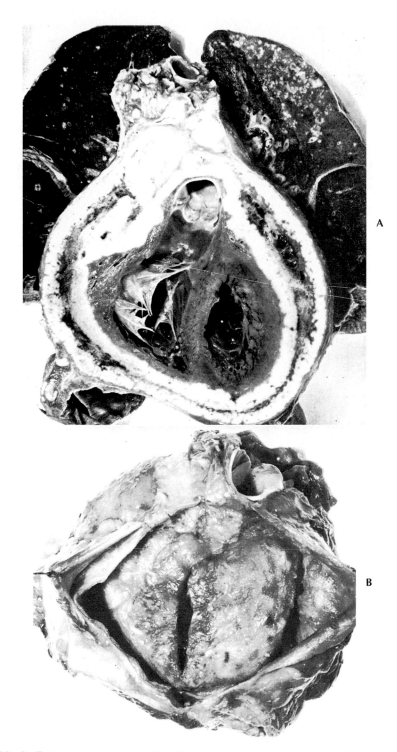

Fig. 15-33. A, Tuberculous pericarditis. There is pronounced caseous thickening of the visceral and parietal pericardium, massive caseation of mediastinal lymph nodes, and tuberculous nodules in the lung tissue. **B,** Healing tuberculous pericarditis. The roughened epicardium is covered with organizing fibrin. The parietal pericardium also is thickened. The heart and pericardium from this 51-year-old white man weighed 930 g. (**A** from Anderson, W.A.D., and Scotti, T.M.: Synopsis of pathology, ed. 10, St. Louis, 1980, The C.V. Mosby Co.)

Tuberculous pericarditis. In some cases tuberculous pericardial lesions are trivial and transient. In others they are serious and progressive.[549] In regard to its pathogenesis, tuberculous pericarditis arises either by extension from adjacent mediastinal, pulmonary, or osseous lesions or by metastatic dissemination from concurrent active tuberculosis in more distant areas.[549] Extension from adjacent structures is the most important mode of infection, and usually it is by means of retrograde lymphatic spread from lesions in the tracheobronchial lymph nodes. Occasionally a caseous lymph node adhering to the parietal pericardium ulcerates into the pericardial sac.

Anatomically there may be scattered subserosal granulomas, which arise from hematogenous spread and may be associated with small effusions. These may be difficult to identify by biopsy or at autopsy. However, the more usual form of tuberculous pericarditis is characterized by a fibrinous exudate with effusion that progresses from an acute to a chronic phase (Fig. 15-33, *B*). The epicardium is covered by thick, shaggy, blood-stained fibrin that often is arranged in ridges caused by contractions of the heart. The entire pericardium becomes thickened and leathery as a result of progressive disease and gradual fibrosis. Gray tubercles may be seen throughout the parietal and visceral pericardium, and sometimes caseous areas coalesce to form a yellowish white interrupted layer. Organization of the fibrinous exudate contributes to the fibrosis. Effusions of fluid may occur soon after fibrin formation. The amount varies from a few hundred milliliters to several liters, and so cardiac tamponade may occur occasionally. The fluid often contains fibrin and blood and sometimes liquefied caseous debris. In some instances the effusion persists for a prolonged period. In others there is abunnt fibrin with little fluid. The surfaces of both pericardial layers adhere to each other, but localized pockets of fluid or liquefied debris may be seen. The typical tuberculous granulomatous lesions can be demonstrated microscopically within the pericardial walls (Fig. 15-34). Calcification may occur in the late stages. The result may be chronic constrictive pericarditis.

Viral pericarditis. See previous discussion of acute nonspecific pericarditis.

Other infectious forms of pericarditis. Rare instances of pericardial involvement have been described in association with actinomycosis and fungal infections of the heart. Pericarditis may be caused by *Entamoeba histolytica*, usually as a result of extension of an amebic abscess of the liver into the pericardial sac. Organisms sometimes are demonstrated in the pericardial exudate.

Rheumatic pericarditis. The features of pericarditis associated with rheumatic fever are reviewed on p. 647.

Pericarditis associated with other connective tissue diseases. Pericarditis sometimes occurs in association with connective tissue disease other than rheumatic fever. Evidence of pericarditis commonly is found in patients with rheumatoid arthritis.[403] In a certain proportion of these patients the pericarditis is caused by an intercurrent disease that is not related to the arthritis. In most of the patients, evidence of healed obliterative or adhesive pericarditis of unknown cause is present. The possibility that these represent instances of previous rheumatoid granulomatous pericarditis that have completely healed has been considered.[403] Frankly granulomatous pericarditis occurs occasionally in rheumatoid arthritis. Acute fibrinous pericarditis may occur in association with the cardioaortic disease found in patients with ankylosing spondylitis and may result in fibrous adhesions of the pericardium. In systemic lupus erythematosus a fibrinous or serofibrinous pericarditis may accompany the underlying fibrinoid changes in the pericardial wall that are characteristic of this disease. Organization of the exudate leads to chronic adhesive pericarditis. Acute pericarditis occasionally is reported in other collagen diseases, including polyarteritis nodosa and thrombotic thrombocytopenic purpura.

Neoplastic pericarditis. Primary or secondary neoplasms that may involve the pericardium are discussed later in this chapter. Associated with the neoplastic infiltration, there may be a pericarditis characterized by a fibrinous or hemorrhagic exudate. Pericardial effusion is common and may be serous or bloody. The pericarditis usually is sterile, but a purulent pericarditis may occur as a result of contamination from an esophageal carcinoma extending directly into the pericardium.

Uremic pericarditis. Pericarditis has been observed at autopsy in patients who have died of uremia.[520,522,542] In addition, pericarditis is a common clinical complication of acute or chronic renal failure even in patients managed by hemodialysis.[523,550] The reported incidence has varied from 8% to 51% of patients.[540]

The pericarditis frequently consists of a diffuse fibrinous exudate. Characteristically the fibrinous pericarditis is dry. If an effusion is present, it is usually not abundant but often is hemorrhagic. This is a sterile form of pericarditis unless secondary infection supervenes. Microscopically, in addition to the fibrinous exudate, lymphocytes are present, but few if any polymorphonuclear leukocytes are seen. There is evidence of organization of the exudate in patients who survive for several days or weeks after the onset of pericarditis (Fig. 15-35). Infrequently, hemorrhagic pericarditis may result in cardiac tamponade.[550] Another uncommon complication is constrictive pericarditis.[523] The pathogenesis of uremic pericarditis is obscure. Three hypotheses have been proposed.[540] One hypothesis is

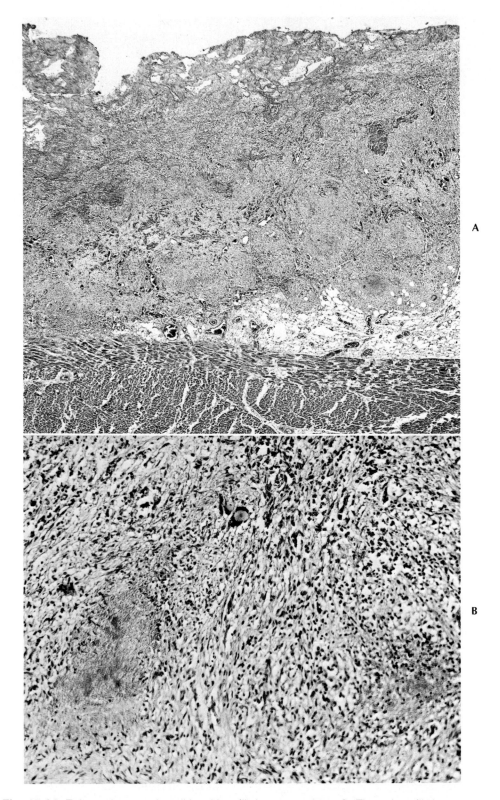

Fig. 15-34. Tuberculous pericarditis with a fibrinous exudate. **A,** There is a fibrinous exudate on overlying coalescent granulomatous nodules in the epicardium. There is caseation in the lower right part of this inflammatory mass. **B,** High-power magnification of area in **A.** Notice the coalescent tubercles with foci of caseation necrosis.

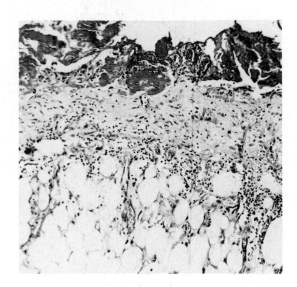

Fig. 15-35. Fibrinous pericarditis with a scanty cellular (lymphocytic) infiltration and partial organization. This pericarditis occurred in a patient who died of renal failure (uremic pericarditis).

that the pericarditis has a biochemical cause. Interestingly, among patients treated by chronic peritoneal dialysis or hemodialysis for renal failure, mean blood urea nitrogen and serum creatinine levels have not differed between those patients with and those without uremic pericarditis. In view of the observation that dialysis does not prevent pericarditis, a nondialyzable uremic toxin has been postulated as the cause of the pericarditis. Uric acid and hypercalcemia have been proposed as causative agents, but evidence supporting the role of either is lacking.[540] A second hypothesis is that uremic pericarditis has an infectious cause. However, as noted above, the pericardial exudate usually is sterile, and antimicrobial agents have not been effective means of treating the pericarditis. The third hypothesis is that hemorrhage, either occurring spontaneously or provoked by anticoagulant drugs, is the cause of the pericarditis. However, there also is little evidence favoring this hypothesis.[540] Although effusions often are hemorrhagic, bleeding is considered to be the consequence of the highly vascular granulation tissue that develops as the pericarditis organizes,[547] rather than an initiating cause of the pericarditis.

Traumatic pericarditis. Fibrinous, serofibrinous, and hemorrhagic pericarditis occur as a result of penetrating injuries. A purulent pericarditis may ensue because of contamination of a wound by bacteria. Less commonly, a fibrinous pericarditis is caused by nonpenetrating cardiac trauma, but purulent pericarditis rarely occurs with this type of injury and usually is caused by contamination from associated injuries to the esophagus or the respiratory tract.[888]

A brief episode of pericarditis with a transient friction rub often occurs in the early postoperative period after cardiac surgery.[551] In addition, a delayed pericarditis develops in 25% to 30% of patients subjected to any type of cardiac surgery. This is known as the postpericardiotomy, postcardiotomy, or postcommissurotomy syndrome.[529,535] The onset is from the first week to the sixth month after surgery, and it is characterized by pericardial pain, friction rub, and low-grade fever. A sterile pericardial effusion may be present. The cause of the pericarditis is unknown, though an autoimmune reaction has been implicated and may be triggered by a viral illness.[529] Recovery is the rule.

Pericarditis in myocardial infarction. Pericarditis associated with an infarct of the heart is characterized by a sterile fibrinous exudate. Effusions of serous or serosanguineous type occasionally occur but rarely are large enough to cause cardiac compression. In most patients the pericardial lesion is limited to the area overlying the infarct, but in some instances the entire pericardium is affected.[293] Organization of the exudate occurs, with complete healing taking place in about 4 weeks. Pericarditis with effusion, sometimes hemorrhagic, may occur after myocardial infarction (Dressler's syndrome).[296] This syndrome resembles the postpericardiotomy syndrome and may also have an immunologic basis.

VALVULAR AND HYPERTENSIVE HEART DISEASES
Acquired valvular heart disease

Acquired valvular heart disease is relatively common. In a recently reported series of 18,132 autopsies, some form of acquired valvular heart disease was diagnosed in 1136 (6.3%) patients.[591] Mitral stenosis, with or without mitral regurgitation and with or without concomitant disease of other valves, is the most commonly diagnosed deformity, occurring in 40% to 50% of cases in the aforementioned series of 1136 patients and another series of 1010 patients.[589,591] Disease of the aortic valve is next in frequency to involvement of the mitral valve, and combinations of valvular deformities, especially mitral and aortic, are common.

Among the diseases producing severe valvular deformities, rheumatic fever is the most common. Valvular deformities, regardless of the cause, commonly result in cardiac failure.

Mitral stenosis

Mitral stenosis, with or without associated insufficiency, is the result of rheumatic endocarditis in virtually all instances.[589,591] Occasional cases are caused by bacterial endocarditis, particularly if the latter is healed. Only rarely is mitral stenosis attributable to other forms of endocardial disease such as Libman-

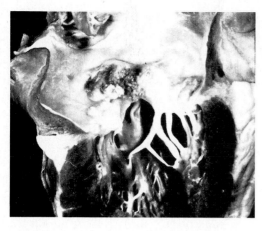

Fig. 15-36. Mitral stenosis. The mitral leaflets are thickened, fused, and ulcerated. The chordae tendineae also are greatly thickened.

Sacks endocarditis, endocardial fibroelastosis, or a congenital anomaly of the valve. Severe calcification of the mitral anulus fibrosus unassociated with mitral valvulitis has been reported as a cause of mitral stenosis, but this lesion is more often associated with mitral insufficiency.[569]

The gross appearance of the stenotic valve varies greatly according to the degree of involvement. Fibrous adhesions at the commissures may be slight or extensive. The leaflets are fibrotic and thickened, especially toward the closing edges. Contraction of scar tissue takes place, the valve leaflets become more rigid, and calcification of the mitral cusps and ring frequently is present to a greater or lesser degree (Figs. 15-17 and 15-36). Ulceration of the thickest part of the deformed valve is a common occurrence. The orifice becomes considerably narrowed. When the valves are less extensively involved and the bases of the leaflets are still somewhat pliable, the narrowed opening is surrounded by puckered, thickened tissue, so called purse-string puckering. As the entire valve becomes more rigid and nonpliable, it takes on the appearance of a fixed diaphragm with a narrow oval or curved opening, a "buttonhole" or "fish-mouth" orifice (Fig. 15-17, *C*). Thickening, shortening, and fusion of the chordae tendineae and broadening of their attachments to the valve leaflets are evident. There also may be fibrosis of the tips of the papillary muscles. In some instances the changes in the chordae tendineae and fusion of the valve leaflets may progress to such an extent that the valve becomes transformed into a funnel-shaped structure, with further narrowing of the orifice.

The effects of mitral stenosis develop as a consequence of obstruction to the outflow of blood from the left atrium and include the following:

1. Dilatation and hypertrophy of the left atrium,

which occasionally appears as a huge saclike structure (so-called giant left atrium)
2. Endocardial fibrous thickening of the left atrium
3. Pronounced chronic passive congestion of the lungs; eventual pulmonary-arteriolar thickening
4. Hypertrophy and dilatation of the right ventricle as a result of pulmonary hypertension
5. Dilatation of the right atrium as right-sided heart failure develops
6. A normal-sized left ventricle or, in prolonged mitral stenosis, atrophic left ventricle caused by reduced inflow of blood, with possible hypertrophy of this ventricle if mitral insufficiency or aortic stenosis is present

One of the complications that may occur in mitral stenosis and the consequent atrial dilatation is atrial fibrillation. Atrial fibrillation contributes to blood stasis and predisposes to development of thrombosis, especially in the left atrial appendage; systemic embolism may result (Fig. 15-18).

Mitral insufficiency

The pathophysiology of mitral regurgitation is complex. Proper closure of the mitral valve depends not only on the mitral valve leaflets by themselves but also on several additional functional components of the mitral valve apparatus, namely, the chordae tendineae, the papillary muscles, and the left ventricle.[581,582] Valvular insufficiency not only may occur as a consequence of structural damage to the valve leaflets or chordae tendineae, but also may occur because of distortion of the spatial relationships between the mitral leaflets and papillary muscles, or because of dysfunction of the papillary muscles or left ventricular myocardium in general.[581,582] Changing hemodynamic conditions may dramatically improve or worsen the degree of mitral regurgitation.[582]

Mitral insufficiency that is caused by organic disease of the valve frequently is associated with some degree of mitral stenosis but may also occur as an isolated abnormality. In Roberts' series of 1010 cases of valvular heart disease, 16% had pure mitral regurgitation (without concomitant mitral stenosis).[589] In 59% of these patients there was no concomitant disease of any other valve; the cause of mitral regurgitation was usually nonrheumatic in these instances. When mitral regurgitation was associated with aortic valve disease, it usually was caused by rheumatic disease. The most common valvular defect causing pure mitral regurgitation was rupture of one or two chordae tendineae; the most common causes of chordal rupture are mitral valve prolapse and infective endocarditis.[566,578]

Mitral insufficiency may also occur because of cardiac functional abnormalities and is commonly observed in patients with severe left ventricular failure, whether attributable to hypertensive heart disease, coronary heart disease, dilated cardiomyopathies, or any other cause. In the past it has been believed that mitral insufficiency in the setting of heart failure was caused by dilatation of the mitral valve ring. However, some authors now consider that papillary muscle contractile dysfunction is a more likely explanation for valvular insufficiency associated with heart failure.[589]

When mitral insufficiency is the main alteration, the effects are as follows:

1. Dilatation and hypertrophy of the left ventricle
2. Dilatation and hypertrophy of the left atrium, often greater than in mitral stenosis
3. Chronic passive congestion of the lungs
4. Effects on the right side of the heart as in mitral stenosis after left-sided failure

Aortic stenosis

Acquired aortic stenosis is believed to result from either postinflammatory scarring or "wear and tear," which, over time, leads to degeneration and calcification of the valve. The postinflammatory type of aortic stenosis is usually associated with scarring of the mitral valve, and almost all such cases of combined mitral and aortic disease are considered to have a rheumatic cause.[588] On the other hand, rheumatic disease is now considered to be an infrequent to rare cause of *anatomically* isolated aortic stenosis. (Rheumatic scarring of both aortic and mitral valves may result in *clinically* isolated aortic stenosis in some instances.) Anatomically isolated aortic stenosis is believed to be degenerative (calcific) disease in virtually all cases.[588] However, there is evidence that some cases of isolated aortic stenosis may be the result of previous *Brucella* endocarditis.[580]

Calcific aortic stenosis involves tricuspid aortic valves in elderly patients but more commonly occurs on valves that are congenitally bicuspid or rarely unicuspid. Congenitally bicuspid aortic valves are reported to be the most common of all congenital heart malformations[587]; a bicuspid valve is the underlying abnormality in approximately 50% of cases of isolated aortic stenosis.[587,595] The bicuspid valve is not stenotic early in life and may never develop stenosis. However, in a substantial proportion of patients with bicuspid valves, calcific aortic stenosis eventually supervenes. In one autopsy study of 152 patients with bicuspid aortic valves, stenosis had developed in 46% of all patients over 50 years of age and in 73% of patients over 70 years of age.[561] Calcific aortic stenosis among patients with bicuspid valves has a peak incidence at about 60 years of age.[595] Calcific stenosis of unicuspid valves occurs at a younger age (mean age, 48 in one study), whereas calcific aortic stenosis of tricuspid aortic valves occurs with increasing frequency among the elderly (age 75 and older).[561,595] The most likely explanation for these age

differences is that a congenital deformity of the valve enhances wear and tear on the valve and thereby accelerates degenerative changes and calcification.

There are morphologic differences between postinflammatory and degenerative causes of aortic stenosis that usually permit identification of the underlying condition.[561,586,595] Postinflammatory scarring is characterized by thickening of the valve cusps attributable to fibrosis and by partial or complete fusion of one or more commissures of the valve (Fig. 15-37). Calcification of the valve cusps occurs and may be extensive; however, calcific deposits are not confined to the base of the valve cusps but involve all parts of the cusps, extending to the free edge of the cusps. In degenerative (calcific) aortic stenosis, commissural fusion is either absent or minimal in most cases. Calcification is usually most extensive at the bases of the valve cusps and does not usually extend to the free edge of the valve.

In elderly patients with calcific aortic stenosis, the valve commonly is tricuspid. However, in patients under 75 years of age, calcific aortic stenosis will more commonly be found to involve a congenitally bicuspid valve. In some instances it may be difficult to distinguish between a congenitally bicuspid valve and a tricuspid valve that has undergone fusion of one commissure.[586,598] Bicuspid valves often have a central raphe (fibrous ridge) subdividing the larger of the two cusps

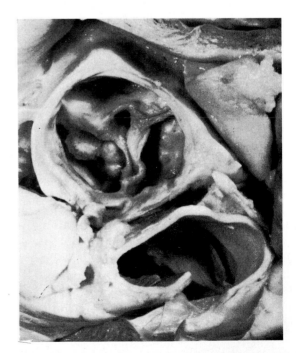

Fig. 15-37. Nodular calcific aortic stenosis. The valve orifice has been reduced to a perpendicular slit. This patient was a 60-year-old white man who had a history of rheumatic fever at 12 years of age. His heart weighed 715 g. (From Hall, E.M., and Ichioka, T.: Am. J. Pathol. **16:**761, 1940.)

of a bicuspid valve. One clue that aids differentiation is that although the cusp of a bicuspid valve that has a raphe may be larger than the other cusp and thereby will occupy more than 50% of the valve ring circumference it will occupy less than two thirds of the valve-ring circumference (in contrast to an apparently single cusp derived by commissural fusion between two of three original cusps). However, in a severely scarred valve, it may not be possible to differentiate grossly a raphe from a fused commissure. In some cases, microscopic evaluation of the valve may permit one to make this distinction.[598]

The primary effect of aortic stenosis is hypertrophy of the left ventricle as a result of an increase in the work of that chamber. When cardiac failure occurs, there is dilatation of the left ventricle as well, and there may be dilatation and hypertrophy of the other chambers later. The aorta is small as a rule, and the intima is smooth because of low intra-aortic pressure and reduced blood volume.

Clinical manifestations and complications of aortic stenosis include angina pectoris, syncope and sudden death. Angina pectoris is noted frequently in aortic stenosis. Myocardial ischemia is attributable to functional coronary insufficiency resulting from the reduced coronary blood flow reserve in the presence of pronounced ventricular hypertrophy.[571] Associated coronary ather-

osclerosis with narrowing of the lumens of the vessels may be a factor in some instances.[563] Multiple small scars in the myocardium are believed to result from this ischemia (Fig. 15-38). Clinical manifestations of the left ventricular failure may appear later and may become severe enough to cause pulmonary congestion and right-sided heart failure.

The cause of syncope is not entirely clear. In some patients it has been observed that syncope was associated with effort and followed the onset of the chest pain of angina pectoris.[564] In such patients it was postulated that the onset of myocardial ischemia reduced cardiac output; reduced cerebral perfusion then caused syncope. Alternatively it has been proposed that syncope is caused by activity of ventricular baroreceptors causing reflex vagal bradycardia.[567] In some cases syncope may result from conduction abnormalities, which may be caused by impingement on the conduction bundle of the degenerative process in the aortic root.[562] The cause of sudden death also is unclear. Sudden death could result from the same mechanisms proposed to cause syncope.[567]

Aortic insufficiency

In a recent study of a series of 225 aortic valves removed from patients undergoing valve replacement because of aortic insufficiency, the four most common causes of aortic insufficiency were reported to be postinflammatory (46%), aortic root dilatation (21%), congenitally bicuspid aortic valve (20%), and infective endocarditis (9%).[577] The postinflammatory causes of aortic insufficiency were considered to have been rheumatic in 97% and ankylosing spondylitis in 3%. Aortic root dilatation was idiopathic in 90% of the cases but was associated with Marfan's syndrome in 8% and syphilis in 2%. Other unusual or rare causes of aortic insufficiency[558,577] include ventricular septal defects, quadricuspid aortic valve, degenerative (calcific) aortic sclerosis (without stenosis),[556] Takayasu's arteritis,[553] trauma, atherosclerosis, dissecting aortic aneurysm, and myxomatous degeneration of aortic valve cusps.

The major effect of aortic insufficiency is cardiac enlargement as a result of hypertrophy and dilatation of the left ventricle, which is frequently very pronounced. Some of the largest hearts observed in autopsy studies are associated with aortic insufficiency. When left ventricular failure occurs, right-sided failure may be superimposed. Angina pectoris may result from functional coronary insufficiency attributable to diminished coronary flow (resulting from the low diastolic blood pressure) and an increased demand of the hypertrophied heart for more oxygen. However, associated coronary artery disease also may be responsible. In syphilis, the narrowing of the coronary orifices and concomitant coronary atherosclerosis are the usual causes of myocardial

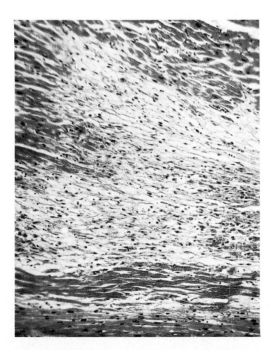

Fig. 15-38. Scarring in myocardium apparently caused by ischemia in a heart with aortic stenosis but no coronary artery disease. This patient was a 20-year-old girl who died of left ventricular failure. Her heart weight was 550 g. (From Hall, E.M., and Ichioka, T.: Am. J. Pathol. **16:**761, 1940.)

ischemia. Other characteristic clinical manifestations include the low diastolic and high pulse pressures, Corrigan's pulse with the typical waterhammer or collapsing quality, capillary pulsations, the pistol-shot sound heard over the femoral artery, and systolic and diastolic murmurs detected over the femoral artery when it is compressed (Durozier's sign).

Tricuspid stenosis

Acquired tricuspid stenosis rarely occurs in the absence of defects in other valves. Tricuspid stenosis is almost always attributable to rheumatic fever or congenital disease. It also may be caused by bacterial endocarditis. There are several other infrequent causes, including the carcinoid syndrome.

Tricuspid insufficiency

Tricuspid insufficiency is more common than stenosis and is most often functional, resulting from failure and dilatation of the right ventricle. Insufficiency may be the result of rheumatic valvulitis, rupture of the leaflets or chordae tendineae, or the unusual carcinoid syndrome.

Pulmonary stenosis

Pulmonary stenosis is, as a rule, a congenital lesion. Rheumatic endocarditis may involve the pulmonary valve but infrequently produces a deformity. Bacterial endocarditis as a cause of stenosis of the pulmonary valve is rare. Involvement of the valve is reported in the carcinoid syndrome, usually resulting in stenosis, though sometimes insufficiency occurs.

Pulmonary insufficiency

Pulmonary insufficiency may result from congenitally defective or absent pulmonic cusps and rarely from rheumatic valvulitis. More often, it is of the functional type, being associated with a general dilatation of the right side of the heart with failure. It is almost always clinically insignificant.

Mitral valve prolapse

Mitral valve prolapse (also referred to as floppy or ballooning mitral valve, mucoid degeneration of the mitral valve, blue valve syndrome, and so on) is a condition in which one or both of the mitral valve leaflets prolapse or balloon back into the left atrium during ventricular systole.[560] The posterior leaflet is nearly always involved, and the anterior leaflet is involved less frequently. This condition went largely unnoticed until the late 1960s, but after the introduction of echocardiography it is now considered to be common. It was diagnosed in approximately 1% of routine autopsies in one series. Clinically, mitral valve prolapse can be readily detected by echocardiography and is considered to occur in 5% to 10% of the general population,[560,594]

being equally frequent in all age groups. In younger age groups, it is more common in women than men.[594]

The pathologic features of mitral valve prolapse have been described by several authors.[559,572,583,600] Grossly, involved leaflets have a voluminous surface area and a domed, convex shape that projects toward the left atrium. The chordae tendineae are generally elongated though they may be shortened and thickened in a minority of cases. Microscopic examination characteristically reveals a replacement or displacement of the valve fibrosa by an expansion of the spongiosa layer of the valve in which large amounts of myxomatous or mucoid material is deposited.[559,576] The latter material stains metachromatically and is Alcian blue positive, consistent with a mucopolysaccharide composition. It should be noted that the presence of Alcian blue–positive material within a valve is a nonspecific finding, being observed in 75% of 344 mitral valves that were surgically excised for a variety of reasons.[568] However, the amount of myxomatous material is typically greater in prolapsing valves than in normal valves.[576]

The pathogenesis of the floppy mitral valve is unknown. Some authors consider that it is a hereditary, congenital lesion.[570] The increased mucopolysaccharide is believed by some to represent an underlying defect in collagen metabolism and perhaps is an incomplete expression of Marfan's syndrome in some instances.[559]

As noted earlier, mitral valve prolapse is a common condition in the general population and is asymptomatic in the vast majority of cases.[573,575] Many patients with a prolapsing mitral valve will have either a midsystolic click or a late systolic murmur of mitral insufficiency.[600] These associated findings are usually of no clinical significance. On the other hand, mitral valve prolapse is reported to be the most common cause of isolated mitral insufficiency of sufficient severity to require valve replacement.[599] Other complications of mitral valve prolapse include ruptured chordae tendineae, an increased risk of infective endocarditis, and an increased risk of embolic complications.[555,557,573] A small fraction of patients have associated arrhythmias; mitral valve prolapse is an uncommon cause of sudden cardiac death.[573,593,597] In a subset of patients composed of older men, mitral valve prolapse is considered to be a cause of congestive heart failure.

Calcification of the mitral valve anulus

Calcification of the mitral valve anulus is observed at autopsy in 8% to 10% of patients over 50 years of age.[584] The entity is reported to be about twice as common in women as in men. It is believed to be a degenerative process. Predisposing factors have been reported to be hypertension and an increased product of serum calcium and phosphate in some studies[574] and hypercholesterolemia and diabetes mellitus in others.[554]

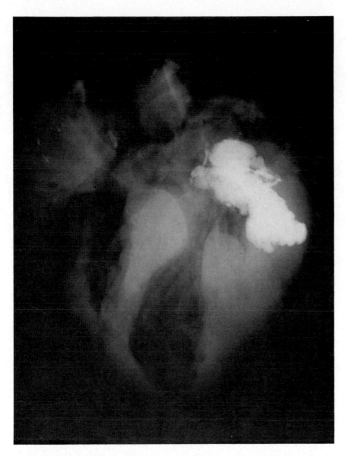

Fig. 15-39. Radiograph of a human heart showing extensive calcification of the mitral valve anulus. The calcification also has extended into the lateral free wall of the left ventricle. This calcification was an incidental finding at autopsy. The radiograph also illustrates thinning and aneurysmal dilatation of the anteroapical region of the left ventricle; the patient died from a massive anteroseptal myocardial infarct unrelated to the anular calcification.

Calcification is most likely to involve the portion of the mitral anulus to which the posterior leaflet of the valve is attached. In cases with more extensive calcification, the entire ring may be involved.[590,596] Calcium deposits may extend into the leaflets of the mitral valve, the aortic valve, or the wall of the left ventricle (Fig. 15-39).

Mitral anular calcification is usually an incidental finding at autopsy but may be clinically significant by causing mitral stenosis or insufficiency.[579] Conduction defects also may occur and are the result of extension of the calcific process to the conduction bundle.[574]

Disturbances of cardiac growth
Atrophy

The term *atrophy* indicates a reduction in the size of a heart that had previously reached full development. This is an acquired disease, in contrast to hypoplasia, which refers to a congenitally small, underdeveloped

heart. The main features of atrophy of the heart are small size, with weight being less than 200 g (in adults), resulting tortuosity of epicardial arteries, brown color of myocardium, serous atrophy of epicardial fat, and a decrease in size of myofibers.[622] The reduced size of the heart is caused chiefly by the decrease in size of the individual muscle fibers. *Brown atrophy* of the heart refers to a brownish discoloration imparted to the heart, observed grossly, because of the conspicuous accumulation of a granular, yellow-brown pigment (lipofuscin) that occurs in the sarcoplasm of the muscle fibers, usually near the poles of the nuclei. Associated microscopic changes may include cloudy swelling or fatty degeneration of myocytes. Brown atrophy is seen particularly in elderly persons, but it may occur in young adults as well. Atrophy of the heart is seen in severe inanition or starvation, in endocrine disturbances (such as Addison's disease and Simmonds' disease), and in chronic wasting disease such as pulmonary tuberculosis and cancer.

Atrophy of the epicardial fat, as well as adipose tissue in other sites of the body, also may be seen in long-standing malnutrition. Microscopically the fat cells are small and show increased density of the cytoplasm, which often contains water droplets. Edema, which is associated with fat atrophy, produces a gelatinous appearance of the fat (gelatinous or serous atrophy of fat).

Hypertrophy

General features and causes. The normal weight of the heart as a whole and of each of the ventricles is proportional to body size. Body weight is a better predictor of heart weight than body height is. In adults, normal heart weight generally ranges between 300 and 350 g in men and between 250 and 300 g in women.[640,649]

Hypertrophy refers to an increase in myocardial mass (Fig. 15-40). Hypertrophy may affect any cardiac chamber individually, or may involve all cardiac chambers. There are many different causes of hypertrophy. Hypertrophy may occur as a normal physiologic response to physical conditioning.[610] Hypertrophy of an individual chamber may also occur as a *physiologic* response to a *pathologic* condition that results in an increased workload by that chamber. Increased cardiac work may occur because of increased ventricular pressure (pressure overload) or the need to pump an increased volume of blood (volume overload) or both. Increased left ventricular pressure occurs in a variety of conditions such as systemic hypertension,[621] aortic valvular stenosis, and coarctation of the aorta. An increased volume of blood must be moved in conditions such as aortic insufficiency, mitral insufficiency, septal defects, patent ductus arteriosus, severe anemia,[635,641] and arteriovenous fistulas. Hormonal stimulation by catecholamines,[645] thyroxine,[608] or growth hormone may also induce cardiac hypertrophy.

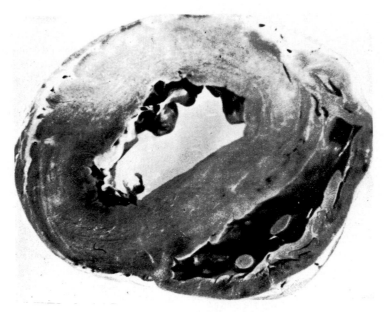

Fig. 15-40. Hypertrophy of left ventricle in chronic hypertension. Notice excessively thickened wall of left ventricle as compared with wall of right ventricle. Heart has been cut transversely through ventricles. (From Anderson, W.A.D., and Scotti, T.M.: Synopsis of pathology, ed. 10, St. Louis, 1980, The C.V. Mosby Co.)

Hypertrophy of the right ventricle results from pulmonary stenosis (isolated or in tetralogy of Fallot), pulmonary insufficiency, or tricuspid insufficiency, and especially from the various conditions producing an increased resistance to the pulmonary blood flow (pulmonary arterial hypertension). Causes of increased pulmonary vascular resistance include mitral stenosis, wide patent ductus arteriosus, lung diseases (such as chronic emphysema, long-standing bronchiectasis, and pulmonary fibrosis as in pneumoconiosis), pulmonary vascular disorders (such as multiple organizing pulmonary arterial thrombi[603] and pulmonary arteriosclerosis, which may be secondary or primary), and severe kyphoscoliosis. The incidence of primary pulmonary vascular disease is very low. The disease is described in the literature as idiopathic pulmonary hypertension.[647]

In patients with left ventricular hypertrophy, failure of the left ventricle may ensue, leading to pulmonary hypertension and right ventricular hypertrophy. Thus there is hypertrophy of both ventricles.

Other cardiac disorders that are not necessarily causes of increased cardiac work but are, nevertheless, causes of cardiac hypertrophy include coronary heart disease[602,609,612] and various types of cardiomyopathy (discussed on p. 681).

It is customary to evaluate the presence or absence and degree of hypertrophy at necropsy by obtainment of the heart weight and measurement of the thicknesses of each cardiac chamber. However, ventricular wall thickness is an insensitive measure of hypertrophy[619] because this measurement does not involve taking into account the variation in chamber volume; for example, the heart fixed in a contracted, systolic state has much thicker ventricular walls than the same heart fixed in a dilated, diastolic state.[620] Heart weight is a better index of cardiac hypertrophy, provided that excess weight is not attributable to excess epicardial fat and heart weight is interpreted in light of the patient's body size. Inasmuch as the left ventricle accounts for 50% to 60% of the weight of the entire heart, increased heart weight generally is an indication of hypertrophy of the left ventricle. Overall heart weight does not provide a reliable means of evaluating hypertrophy of the right ventricle. If precise data are desired, it becomes necessary to dissect and weigh each chamber separately.[611,615,619]

It is typical for heart weight to be increased to a range of 450 to 550 g in patients who have died from coronary heart disease. Substantially larger hearts, weighing as much as 1200 g may occur in conditions causing considerable left ventricular pressure overload, such as severe systemic hypertension or aortic stenosis. When the heart is greatly enlarged, to a weight of 800 g or more, the term *cor bovinum* ('ox heart') is sometimes used.

Hypertrophy is often classified as *concentric* when it occurs in the absence of a dilated chamber and as *eccentric* when the hypertrophy is accompanied by dilatation, that is, an increased volume capacity of the chamber. Dilatation may occur acutely, as a consequence of pulmonary embolism, cardiac arrhythmia, valvular rupture, or myocardial infarction, or may develop gradually as a manifestation of chronic cardiac failure from many different disorders. Thus eccentric hypertrophy usually implies a situation in which hypertrophy has failed to keep pace with the hemodynamic load on the ventricle, that is, "pathologic" rather than "physiologic" hypertrophy.[617]

Grossly, in addition to thickening of the walls of the chambers, the cardiac muscle is firm. When the ventricles are involved, the papillary muscles and the trabeculae carneae are rounded and enlarged, and in atrial hypertrophy the muscle fasciculi are prominent, especially the musculi pectinati of the right atrium. However, if there is also a significant degree of cardiac dilatation, the papillary muscles and the other muscular prominences of the affected chambers tend to become flattened. Microscopically, myocardial hypertrophy is characterized by an increase in size of individual muscle fibers, which is evidenced chiefly by their increased width or diameter. The nuclei often are enlarged and variable in shape.

Pathogenesis of myocardial hypertrophy. During fetal development, cardiac growth occurs by hyperplasia of cardiac myocytes, that is, by increasing numbers of mononucleated myocardial cells. This phase of hyperplastic growth continues in humans for as long as 3 months after birth.[606] It is possible that excessive cardiac size may result from myocyte hyperplasia in some cardiac disorders of infancy.[605,626] In older persons, however, both cardiac growth and hypertrophy occur by progressive enlargement of myocytes (cellular hypertrophy) and not by an increase in myocyte number.[631,633] However, myocyte hypertrophy is accompanied by a commensurate hyperplasia (increased number of cells) of capillary endothelial cells and interstitial cells. This conclusion is supported by morphometric studies in which nuclei have been counted in normal and hypertrophied hearts[631] and by experimental studies to assess the location of DNA synthesis after the induction of hypertrophy.[604,618,632]

Morphometric studies of human hearts and hearts of experimental animals have indicated that capillary luminal cross-sectional area increases during hypertrophy but the total length of capillaries does not increase.[601,646] In addition, as myocyte diameters increase, the distance oxygen must diffuse from capillary to myocyte center must increase. Thus progressive myocardial hypertrophy is believed to result in a relative loss of capillary reserve and may predispose the myocardium to hypoxic injury.[639] Loss of vascular reserve in hypertrophied hearts also has been postulated to result from insufficient enlargement of the coronary ostia and epicardial arteries.[625]

Morphometric ultrastructural studies of hypertrophied myocytes from both human patients and experimental animals has shown an increased volume fraction of myofibrils and a reduction in the ratio of mitochondrial and myofibrillar mass.[601,646] Increased myofibrillar mass is believed to be produced both by the synthesis of new myofibrils (increasing cellular width) and by the addition of new sarcomeres to existing myofibrils (cellular elongation).[607,638] Multiple intercalated discs have been frequently observed in muscle cells of hypertrophied hearts in experimental animals[624] and in human patients.[627] These structures are characterized by two, three, or four transverse segments of discs lying along the same myofibrils, each two of which are separated by one to 10 sarcomeres.[624] It has been suggested that the multiple intercalated discs may be active sites for formation of new sarcomeres.

A variety of degenerative changes have been reported in hypertrophied myocytes from hearts with a variety of underlying disorders.[628] Myocyte degeneration may occur in decompensated hypertrophy as a consequence of myocyte hypoxia; however, separating degenerative changes attributable to hypertrophy by itself from changes attributable to the underlying abnormality that initiated the hypertrophy is not a simple matter.

The biochemical basis through which an increased cardiac work load signals the induction of hypertrophy is not known but is a subject of considerable research interest. It has been observed that in various experimental models of hypertrophy the hemodynamic or hormonal stimulus for hypertrophy is quickly followed by both DNA and RNA synthesis, followed by a stimulation of protein synthesis.[614,638,649] One hypothesis is that increased metabolic requirements may cause a reduction in intracellular ATP, which in some way leads to the activation of the genetic apparatus of the cell that initiates the synthesis of nucleic acids and proteins.[630] This hypothesis is supported by the observation that a partial reduction in high-energy phosphate compounds is a common factor in several experimental models of hypertrophy.[630] However, other studies have shown no consistent correlation between the presence or absence of reduced ATP content and protein synthesis in hearts of rats subjected to isoproterenol or pressure-induced hypertrophy.[650]

Specific causes of hypertrophy

Cor pulmonale. The term *cor pulmonale* (pulmonary heart disease), in the restricted sense, refers to disease of the right side of the heart (right ventricular dilatation or hypertrophy, or both, with or without failure) that results from disorders originating in the lungs and involving the parenchyma or the pulmonary circulation. However, the term is used by some authors in a broad sense to include also the effects on the right side of the heart, of intrinsic cardiac diseases such as mitral stenosis or congenital septal defects that secondarily cause pulmonary hypertension. Cor pulmonale may be acute or chronic. Acute cor pulmonale occurs after massive pulmonary embolism and is characterized by rapid dilatation of the pulmonary trunk, conus, and right ventricle. Chronic cor pulmonale, which is more common than the acute type, is associated with diseases causing chronic pulmonary hypertension. Among the various pulmonary disorders causing chronic pulmonary hypertension are diffuse pulmonary emphysema, bronchiectasis, tuberculosis, pneumoconiosis, sarcoidosis, scleroderma, fibrosis of undetermined cause, pulmonary emboli, and hypoventilation associated with extreme obesity (pickwickian syndrome). Because the increased work load imposed on the right ventricle develops over time, the right ventricle has time to undergo compensatory hypertrophy.

Hypertensive heart disease. The etiology, pathogenesis, and clinical consequences of systemic hypertension are described in more detail on p. 841. The subject is reviewed here briefly to provide a background for consideration of hypertensive heart disease.

In a study by the National Center for Health Statistics,[616] adults between 18 and 79 years of age in the United States were classified in one of three groups in accordance with the following levels of blood pressure:

1. Nonhypertensive—systolic pressure below 140 mm Hg and diastolic pressure below 90 mm Hg
2. Definite hypertension—systolic pressure 160 mm Hg or above or diastolic pressure 95 mm Hg or above
3. Borderline hypertension—systolic and diastolic pressures between those specified in (1) and (2)

The frequency of hypertension increases steadily with age. About 20% of men between 20 and 29 years of age have a mild degree of hypertension, but only about 5% have a more severe degree. Hypertension of at least mild degree is common in middle-aged and elderly people, occurring in about 40% of both men and women between 45 and 49 years of age and in 60% of those between 60 and 64 years.[629] It is frequently stated that the disease is more common in women than in men (in a ratio of 2:1).[636] However, in one study of a representative group of the average working population, hypertension was found to occur more commonly in men up to 45 years of age and more frequently in women thereafter.[629] In the United States, more blacks than whites are found to have hypertension.[33]

Systemic hypertension is classified into two main groups according to the cause, as follows:

1. That caused by known disease of renal or extrarenal nature, referred to as secondary hypertension
2. That in which the cause is obscure, designated as idiopathic, primary, or essential hypertension

The majority of cases of hypertension (about 90%) are of the latter type, which is further subdivided into the more frequent benign and the less common malignant varieties. The principal causes of systemic hypertension may be classified as follows[634]:

1. Renal
   a. Vascular disease (arteriosclerosis, arteritis, polyarteritis nodosa, mechanical obstruction attributable to thrombosis, embolism, tumors, etc.)
   b. Parenchymal renal diseases (glomerulonephritis, pyelonephritis, hydronephrosis, polycystic disease, amyloidosis, tumors, etc.)
   c. Perinephric diseases (perinephritis, tumors, hematoma, etc.)
2. Cerebral
   a. Increased intracranial pressure (trauma, inflammation, tumors)
   b. Anxiety states
   c. Lesions of brainstem (poliomyelitis, etc.)
3. Cardiovascular
   a. Coarctation of aorta
4. Endocrine
   a. Pheochromocytoma
   b. Adrenocortical adenomas
   c. Pituitary adenomas
   d. Hyperthyroidism
   e. Arrhenoblastoma
5. Preeclampsia and eclampsia
6. Unknown causes (essential hypertension)

The pathogenesis of hypertension is discussed on p. 841. The natural history is variable. Some patients remain asymptomatic for many years, whereas others have disabling and even fatal complications.[643] There is a definite relationship between the mean age at death and the severity of hypertension. In the mildest form of the disease, the mean age is 61.7 years, and in the most severe group it is 47 years.[643] Women tolerate the disease much better than men do.[629,644] One factor that may be responsible for the more serious prognosis in men with hypertension is that coronary atherosclerosis, a complication of hypertension, is more likely to occur in men.[629,636] In the United States the death rate is higher among blacks than among whites.[636]

The morphologic effects of systemic hypertension are manifested as lesions in the heart, peripheral vessels, kidneys, and brain. The cardiac manifestations are considered here. The other lesions are described elsewhere.

Hypertensive heart disease (hypertensive cardiopathy) is an important and common form of heart disease in the United States. In one study, the causes of death among hypertensive patients were the following[643]: (1) congestive heart failure, 26%; (2) coronary artery disease, 10%; (3) cerebrovascular accidents, 15%; (4) uremia, 20%; and (5) causes unrelated to hypertension, 29%. The cardiac complications therefore account for

36% of the deaths. It should be pointed out that in other series in the literature the proportion of deaths from cardiac complications is somewhat higher.

Among the pathologic features of hypertensive cardiopathy, the most striking is hypertrophy of the heart involving chiefly the left ventricle. The average weight of the heart in hypertensive patients is 500 to 600 g, but it may be as much as 1100 g.[642] There is a rough correlation between the weight of the heart and the severity of hypertension, but there is no correlation between the weight of the heart and the duration of the disease.[642,644] The left ventricular wall is thickened (up to 20 mm or more), the papillary muscles and trabeculae carneae are rounded and prominent, and the cardiac chamber is small (concentric hypertrophy) (Fig. 15-41). When cardiac failure ensues, dilatation of the chamber also may be prominent. Endocardial fibrous thickening may be present in the left ventricle in instances of long-standing hypertension. After the onset of left ventricular failure, there may be dilatation and hypertrophy of the right side of the heart. The hypertrophy is reversible as shown by its regression when the hypertension is corrected by treatment.[613] In a significant number of patients there is associated coronary atherosclerosis, which is probably enhanced by the hypertension. Complications of coronary artery disease (such as myocardial

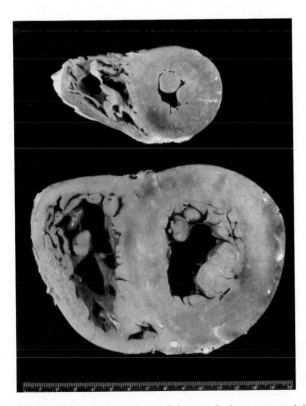

Fig. 15-41. Massively enlarged heart, *below,* caused by hypertrophy of both ventricles. The normal heart, *above,* weighed 325 g. The heart with biventricular hypertrophy weighed 1100 g. The patient had suffered from severe systemic hypertension.

infarction) can occur. Fibrinous pericarditis may be evident in patients who die as a result of uremia. Microscopically, the features include enlargement and degenerative changes of individual muscle fibers and focal myocardial fibrosis, though the latter is frequently the result of coexisting coronary atherosclerosis. Myocardial edema and foci of necrosis characterized either by intense eosinophilia or by complete dissolution of the muscle fibers occur in malignant hypertension.[623]

Cardiac hypertrophy in the cardiomyopathies. In most instances of hypertrophy or dilatation of the heart, an obvious preexisting disorder can be demonstrated. In some patients, however, cardiomegaly occurs in the absence of any known cause of heart disease and is referred to as idiopathic. Examples of this type of disorder are idiopathic congestive and hypertrophic cardiomyopathies (see later discussion).

CARDIOMYOPATHIES AND SPECIFIC DISORDERS AFFECTING THE MYOCARDIUM
Definition and classification

The term *cardiomyopathy,* in its most literal sense, means 'disease of heart muscle.' The term does not refer to a single disease but rather encompasses a miscellaneous group of diseases, with different causes. Several definitions of the term "cardiomyopathy" have been used.[651,652] In its broadest sense, "cardiomyopathy" may refer to any type of heart disease excluding the major categories of ischemic heart disease, hypertensive heart disease, and valvular heart disease. Congenital heart defects and cardiac tumors are also excluded. Using this broad definition, cardiomyopathies can be classified as primary or secondary. A *primary cardiomyopathy* is one in which the heart is the only organ involved and the cause is unknown. A *secondary cardiomyopathy* is one in which either the cause is known, or it is apparent that the cardiac involvement has occurred as a manifestation of a systemic disease.

Alternative to the aforementioned definition and classification, the World Health Organization and International Society and Federation of Cardiology more recently adopted the convention that the term "cardiomyopathy" should be reserved only for the primary cardiomyopathies.[655] Diseases that might be classified as secondary cardiomyopathies should be referred to as *specific heart muscle diseases.* For example, the antineoplastic agent adriamycin can cause cardiac damage and result in refractory heart failure. In the broad definition, this would be included among the secondary cardiomyopathies. In the restricted WHO/ISFC definition, the disease is called *adriamycin-induced heart disease* and is not classified as a "cardiomyopathy." Even using the broader definition, a discrepancy arises with the commonly used term *ischemic cardiomyopathy,*[653] discussed in the section of this chapter on coronary heart disease. The term *ischemic cardiomyopathy* refers to refractory congestive heart failure that can occur as an end stage of ischemic heart disease.

Using either the broad or restricted definitions of cardiomyopathy, the most common classification of cardiomyopathies is based on the combined clinicopathologic manifestations of the disorders. In this classification there are three major types, each of which is considered in detail below.[654] *Hypertrophic cardiomyopathy* is a specific disorder that in many cases is a hereditary disease characterized by pronounced cardiac hypertrophy, often particularly involving the interventricular septum, with or without obstruction to left ventricular outflow. *Dilated (congestive) cardiomyopathies* are a group of diseases that share the hallmark of progressive heart failure associated with considerable biventricular dilatation, with or without compensatory hypertrophy. In the broader classification scheme, dilated cardiomyopathies include end-stage cardiac diseases produced by any one of a large number of possible causes. *Restrictive (constrictive) cardiomyopathies* are a group of myocardial diseases characterized by decreased myocardial compliance, with symptoms similar

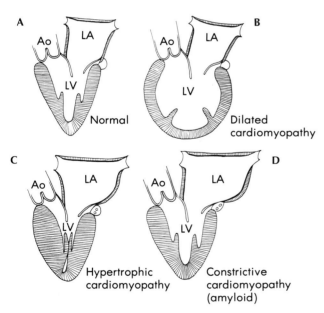

Fig. 51-42. Diagram showing the major distinguishing pathophysiologic features of the three types of cardiomyopathy. In the dilated type of cardiomyopathy, **B,** the heart has a globular shape, the largest circumference of left ventricle is not at its base but midway between apex and base. In the hypertrophic type, **C,** the wall of the left ventricle is greatly thickened; the left ventricular cavity is small but the left atrium may be dilated because of poor diastolic relaxation of the ventricle. In the restrictive (constrictive type, **D,** the left ventricular cavity is of normal size but again the left atrium is dilated because of the reduced diastolic compliance of the ventricle. (From Roberts, W.C., and Ferrans, V.J.: Pathologic anatomy of the cardiomyopathies, Hum. Pathol. **6:**289, 1975.)

to those of constrictive pericarditis. Fig. 15-42 illustrates the major distinctive features of these three types of cardiomyopathies.

Hypertrophic cardiomyopathy

Hypertrophic cardiomyopathy (HCM) is a disease that was first described by Teare in 1958.[681] Since that time, the disorder has been given many different names, a cause of considerable confusion among readers of the older literature on the subject.[679] The entity was called *idiopathic hypertrophic subaortic stenosis (IHSS)* in the United States.[658] The same disease became known as *hypertrophic obstructive cardiomyopathy (HOCM)* in Great Britain and as *muscular subaortic stenosis (MSS)* in Canada. *Asymmetric septal hypertrophy (ASH)* is a common anatomic manifestation of the disease[667,664] that can be detected clinically by echocardiography; this manifestation of the disease has sometimes been used to refer to the disease itself.[669] It is now known that not all patients with this type of cardiomyopathy have obstruction to aortic outflow[663]; the terms "obstructive" and "stenosis" have therefore been omitted from the currently preferred "hypertrophic cardiomyopathy."

Many cases of hypertrophic cardiomyopathy have been observed to be hereditary, most showing an autosomal dominant pattern of transmission, with a high degree of penetrance.[660,662] However, some cases are sporadic, and an autosomal recessive mode of transmission may exist.[657]

Major pathophysiologic features of hypertrophic cardiomyopathy include reduced diastolic compliance, pronounced hypertrophy of the interventricular septum and often of the free wall as well, systolic anterior motion (SAM) of the anterior leaflet of the mitral valve, and "myofiber disarray."

The explanation for the *reduced diastolic compliance*[678] of the myocardium is unknown. The resistance to diastolic filling of the left ventricle gives rise to another common feature of the cardiomyopathy—hypertrophy and dilatation of the left atrium.

Hypertrophy often involves the interventricular septum preferentially (Fig. 15-43, *A*). *Asymmetric septal hypertrophy* can be detected by echocardiography; a ratio of septal to posterior free wall thickness exceeding 1.3 is a hallmark of hypertrophic cardiomyopathy.[664,667] However, a ratio exceeding 1.3 is not entirely specific; such a ratio also may be present in normal fetal or newborn infant hearts, may be associated with some congenital cardiac abnormalities, and occasionally is a feature of coronary heart disease, systemic hypertension, and pulmonary hypertension.[659,671] On the other hand, not all persons with hypertrophic cardiomyopathy have asymmetric septal hypertrophy. Hypertrophy may be concentric, involving the free wall as well as the septum. It has been reported that patients without aortic outflow obstruction have asymmetric septal hypertrophy with relatively normal thickness of the posterior free wall but that patients with obstruction develop concentric hypertrophy because the increased ventricular work load causes compensatory hypertrophy of the free wall.[668]

Systolic anterior motion (SAM) of the anterior leaflet

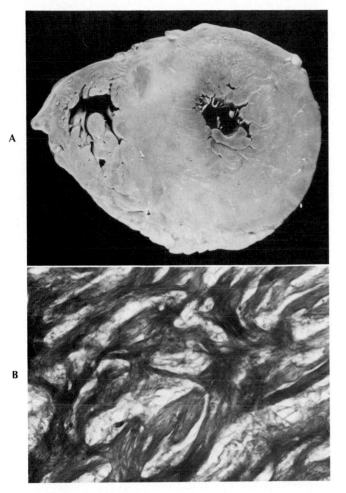

Fig. 15-43. Hypertrophic cardiomyopathy. **A,** Cross section through the ventricles is viewed from the base with the anterior surface at the bottom. Notice that the cavity of the left ventricle is unusually small, that the wall of the left ventricle is circumferentially thickened, and that the interventricular septum, especially anteriorly, is disproportionately thickened even more than the free wall (asymmetric septal hypertrophy). This patient was a 59-year-old woman who had hypertrophic cardiomyopathy complicated by mitral regurgitation and congestive heart failure; she died of ventricular fibrillation. Her heart weighed 500 g. **B,** Myofiber disarray, the characteristic microscopic feature of hypertrophic cardiomyopathy. The myocardial fibers, which normally occur in parallel bundles, are oriented in seemingly random direction within as well as perpendicular to the plane of section through the tissue.

of the mitral valve is a dynamic abnormality that also can be detected by echocardiography.[665,671,673] This abnormal movement of the mitral valve leaflet is believed to be a major contributing cause of outflow obstruction. It also may contribute to mitral insufficiency, another common manifestation of the disease. The echocardiographic observation of SAM, like ASH, is characteristic but not absolutely diagnostic of hypertrophic cardiomyopathy.[671] However, the degree of SAM is predictive of the severity of outflow obstruction.[665] At least three mechanisms have been proposed for the SAM; one or all may contribute[676,684]: (1) Because of the septal bulge into the outflow tract, the septal leaflet of the mitral valve is unusually close to the septum and may be pulled to the septum by the high-velocity flow through the narrowed outflow tract (Venturi effect).[684] (2) Because of distortion of the left ventricular architecture, contraction of the papillary muscles pull the anterior leaflet toward the septum. (3) Because of altered ventricular geometry, the leaflet may be pushed toward the septum by the increasing ventricular pressure.

Myofiber disarray is a microscopic hallmark of the disease[654,681] (Fig. 15-43, *B*). Normally, myocardial fibers are arranged in parallel, in bundles of fibers that spiral around the heart and produce synchronous shortening. Myofiber disarray is characterized by loss of this parallel organization; thus small bundles of fibers or individual fibers may course at various angles from adjacent bundles or fibers. Within a region of disarray, individual fibers may be observed to have an apparently random directional orientation. In addition, when studied by electron microscopy, there may even be a disarray of myofibrils within individual cardiac myofibers. The cause of myofiber disarray is unknown. Moreover, it is not clear whether the myofiber disarray is the underlying cause of the cardiomyopathy, or the disarray is a secondary response to a preexisting abnormal distribution of intramyocardial stresses, attributable to the underlying but as yet undefined cause of the disease. Like other manifestations of the disease, myofiber disarray was once considered to be nearly diagnostic of hypertrophic cardiomyopathy. However, myofiber disarray has subsequently been observed in other conditions, and its presence must be interpreted with caution.[656,659,682] For example, some myofiber disarray is normal at the junction where fibers of the right ventricle intersect with fibers of the interventricular septum. Myofiber disarray also has been observed in association with some congenital heart defects and adjacent to interstitial myocardial scars caused by hypertensive or ischemic heart disease. Some investigators hold the view that myofiber disarray is quantitatively more severe in hypertrophic cardiomyopathy than in the other conditions in which disarray has been reported and that *severe* disarray is virtually diagnostic of hypertrophic cardiomyopathy.[670-672]

The pathogenesis of HCM is unknown, but several hypotheses have been proposed: (1) The myofiber disarray may represent a primary disturbance leading to impaired diastolic relaxation and, because of inefficient contraction, to compensatory hypertrophy.[677] However, others consider that myofiber disarray is a consequence of an abnormal intramural distribution of stresses from any cause.[659,682] (2) Some investigators consider that HCM may result from excessive hypertrophy because of (a) an increased responsiveness to circulating catecholamines[677] or (b) abnormal atrioventricular conduction resulting in asynchronous ventricular contraction.[669] (3) Some investigators postulate that myocardial ischemia may cause interstitial scarring resulting in compensatory hypertrophy. Postulated causes of ischemia include the aforementioned thickening and narrowing of the intramural coronary arteries,[669,675] microvascular spasm,[680] and an abnormality in the adenosine-mediated autoregulation of the heart.[683] (4) Another hypothesis is that the underlying defect in HCM is an abnormality of the fibrous skeleton of the heart.[669]

Hypertrophic cardiomyopathy is usually detected in young adults. The most common clinical manifestations are arrhythmias, angina pectoris, and congestive heart failure.[658,684] Arrhythmias represent the major cause of mortality in these patients, causing sudden cardiac death. It is of interest, in this regard, that in one series of young athletic persons whose hearts were studied after sudden death the most frequent cardiac diagnosis was hypertrophic cardiomyopathy rather than ischemic heart disease.[674]

Although HCM and coronary heart disease may coexist,[666] angina also occurs in patients with normal or even dilated coronary arteries. Indeed, even transmural infarction has been reported in patients with HCM but normal coronary arteries.[672] It has been proposed that the mechanism of myocardial ischemia may be increased intramyocardial tension because of the poor diastolic relaxation.[661] Increased intramyocardial tension could compress the microvasculature and thereby impede myocardial perfusion. Alternatively, thickening and narrowing of small intramural coronary arteries have been observed in an autopsy study of patients who died of HCM, and it has been proposed that this small artery disease may cause myocardial ischemia.[675]

Obstruction to aortic outflow may be associated with syncope. As mentioned earlier, not all patients have outflow obstruction.[665,668] Some do have obstruction at rest. Others have latent obstruction that can become overt when cardiac contractility is increased. This can be demonstrated by administration of a test dose of isoproterenol. A third group of persons who may be identifiable only by clinical evaluation of family members of symptomatic patients may have neither resting nor latent obstruction. The presence and severity of obstruction has not been predictable from the degree of septal hypertrophy but does correlate with the presence and degree of SAM of the anterior leaflet of the mitral valve.[665]

Congestive cardiomyopathy

The dilated cardiomyopathies are a group of diseases characterized by cardiac enlargement attributable to biventricular dilatation and congestive heart failure. The underlying problem is poor systolic function; unlike hypertrophic and restrictive cardiomyopathies, the dilated cardiomyopathies do not have impaired diastolic ventricular filling. The diagnosis of dilated cardiomyopathy is a diagnosis of exclusion. Even when a broad definition is used (see p. 681), the term is applied to congestive heart failure only after ischemic heart disease, hypertension, acquired valvular heart disease, or congenital cardiac anomalies have been excluded from the possible causes.

Dilated cardiomyopathies (primary, idiopathic) occur with increased frequency in many recognized clinical settings. For example, a substantial fraction of patients with dilated cardiomyopathy have a history of alcohol abuse. Cardiomyopathy in such persons is generally called "alcoholic cardiomyopathy." However, only a minority of alcoholic patients develop cardiomyopathy. Moreover there are no clear pathophysiologic differences between the disease in alcoholic and nonalcoholic individuals. Thus alcohol may best be considered to be a contributory risk factor for cardiomyopathy, in the same way that cigarette smoking is considered to be a risk factor for ischemic heart disease. Dilated cardiomyopathy also has been observed to occur in women in association with pregnancy. When a cardiomyopathy develops in the last trimester of pregnancy or the first 3 months post partum, it is termed "peripartum" or "postpartum" cardiomyopathy.[691,692] Again, the cause is unknown and the pathophysiologic features of the cardiomyopathy are identical to those of other cases of dilated cardiomyopathy. Although most dilated cardiomyopathies are sporadic, a few cases have had a familial occurrence.[698]

In a substantial number of instances, dilated cardiomyopathy has followed a flu-like syndrome. This association provides circumstantial evidence for the hypothesis that dilated cardiomyopathies may occur as the late sequel to viral myocarditis. On the other hand, one must keep in mind that flu-like illnesses are quite common, occurring occasionally in everyone. Thus it would be expected that the onset of cardiomyopathy would be preceded by a flu-like illness purely by chance in some persons. More direct, albeit still circumstantial evidence favoring a viral cause of dilated cardiomyopathies comes from both prospective and retrospective studies.[697] In a prospective study of patients after group B coxsackievirus myopericarditis, 7% developed a dilated cardiomyopathy.[701] Retrospectively, several investigators have found antibody titers to enteroviruses in a substantially greater fraction of patients with dilated cardiomyopathy than in controls.[686,693,695]

The association between alcoholism and congestive heart failure, in patients with dilated flabby hearts but no coronary atherosclerosis, has been known for over a century. Several recent reviews of this "alcoholic cardiomyopathy" are available.[696,700,704] Despite many clinical and experimental studies, the pathogenesis of the cardiomyopathy among alcoholic patients remains unknown. It was first believed that alcoholic cardiomyopathy was related to nutritional deficiencies and specifically to thiamine deficiency.[685] It is known that thiamine deficiency causes beriberi, which has neuromuscular and cardiac manifestations. However, cardiac beriberi, observed among malnourished persons in third-world countries, is characterized by high-output cardiac failure associated with peripheral vasodilatation. In contrast, alcoholic cardiomyopathy may occur in persons who are seemingly well nourished. Thus the role of nutritional deficiencies in the pathogenesis of alcoholic cardiomyopathy is uncertain. In the 1960s, outbreaks of cardiomyopathy were reported among beer drinkers in Omaha and Montreal. This "beer-drinker's cardiomyopathy" was eventually linked to cobalt cardiotoxicity; cobalt had been used as an additive in the beverage.[694] Although cobalt is no longer used in beer, alcoholic cardiomyopathy persists. Most investigators now consider that the disease is related to a direct toxic effect of alcohol or its metabolites. It has been amply documented in clinical and experimental animal studies that acute or chronic ingestion of alcohol results in depressed cardiac contractile function. Moreover, a variety of metabolic and subcellular effects of alcohol have been observed. However, the link between the acute effects of alcohol, which are reversible, and the development of a dilated cardiomyopathy, in which the cardiac abnormalities persist even when alcohol is removed, has not been established. Subcellular consequences of alcohol or acetaldehyde, which hypothetically could result in permanent damage, include reduced cardiac protein synthesis,[699] damage to the sarcoplasmic reticulum resulting in impaired calcium homeostasis,[702] and myocardial lipid peroxidation.[687] Another hypothesis for the pathogenesis of alcholic cardiomyopathy is related to the hypothesis that dilated cardiomyopathies may be the result of preceding viral myocarditis: Alcoholic patients are more susceptible to viral infections; the increased incidence of cardiomyopathy in alcoholics may be related to an increased incidence of viral myocarditis. It also has been proposed that alcoholic cardiomyopathy may result from myocardial ischemia caused by small-vessel disease.[688]

Data from 104 patients with dilated cardiomyopathy at the Mayo Clinic provides some perspective regarding the relative frequency of these various associated factors.[689] Of the 104 patients, 22 had a history of excessive alcohol consumption and 20 reported a preceding influenza syndrome. Eight patients developed the cardiomyopathy after rheumatic fever. Three cases occurred in the postpartum period and two cases were familial. However, 49 cases occurred in the absence of any of these associated factors.

The anatomic features of dilated cardiomyopathy are

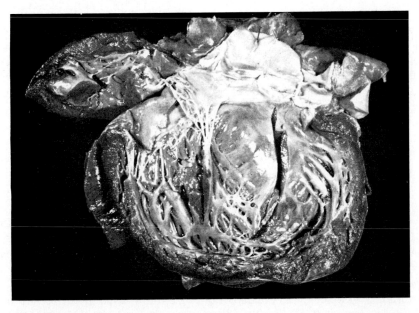

Fig. 15-44. Heart of a 46-year-old chronic alcoholic patient with a dilated cardiomyopathy (alcoholic cardiomyopathy). Notice the globular shape of the heart because of the pronounced dilatation of the left ventricle.

similar, irrespective of associated risk factors. Hearts have a distinctly rounded, globular shape because of the biventricular dilatation (Fig. 15-44). There is frequently myocardial hypertrophy, as documented by increased heart weight, but because of the considerable dilatation, ventricular wall thickness usually is not increased. The microscopic features of dilated cardiomyopathy are nonspecific and vary from virtually no detectable abnormality to pronounced interstitial fibrosis. Myocyte hypertrophy, atrophy, or degeneration, or all three, may be observed.

In general, the dilated cardiomyopathy is associated with progressively worsening heart failure. Cardiac arrhythmias and systemic embolization from mural thrombi are additional complications of dilated cardiomyopathy.[690,703] The heart failure often is refractory to therapy with digitalis; moreover, digitalis may exacerbate the cardiomyopathy. Among patients with alcoholic cardiomyopathy, abstinence from further alcohol consumption may result in gradual improvement in cardiac function.

There is a large number of miscellaneous cardiac insults or systemic diseases that have cardiac manifestations that may result in the clinicopathologic features of dilated cardiomyopathy. These include metabolic abnormalities such as hemochromatosis, endocrine disorders such as hyperthyroidism or hypothyroidism, nutritional disorders such as kwashiorkor, severe anemia, electrolyte abnormalities such as metastatic calcification, inflammatory causes including viral and rheumatic myocarditis, drugs such as catecholamines and adriamycin, and poisons such as heavy metals. Some of these specific types of heart muscle disease are considered in the following paragraphs.

Metabolic abnormalities

Hemochromatosis. The heart is almost always affected in idiopathic (primary) hemochromatosis.[707,712,716,717] In addition, cardiac iron deposits occur in secondary hemochromatosis, which occurs, for example, in patients who have received multiple blood transfusions for treatment of anemia.[707] The degree of involvement may be slight and without evidence of gross changes, but often it is sufficient to produce a brownish discoloration of the myocardium. The deposits are more prominent in the subendocardial than in the subepicardial zone.[707] Microscopically, hemosiderin granules are identified within myocardial fibers and occasionally in the connective tissue cells (Fig. 15-45). In the myocytes, the iron is deposited in sarcoplasmic siderin granules, which are distinct from lipofuscin granules.[707] Varying degrees of degeneration, edema, and fibrosis of the myocardium can be seen. Electrocardiographic changes and even cardiac failure may ensue. Arrhythmias may occur as a result of iron deposits in the fibers of the conduction system.[721]

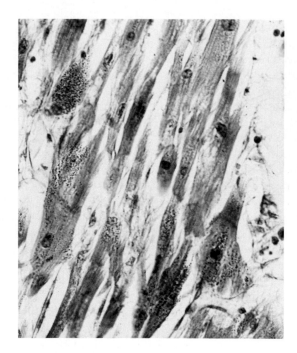

Fig. 15-45. Hemochromatosis of myocardium. Fine, granular, hemosiderin pigment is present in many muscle fibers. (Hematoxylin and eosin.)

Lipid-storage diseases. Focal collections of histiocytes, with or without lipid in the cytoplasm, may be found in the endocardium, the myocardium, or the walls of the coronary arteries in any of the lipidoses.[705] The type of lipid depends on the nature of the disease process. A low-grade inflammatory reaction may be associated with the nodular accumulation of lipid-filled cells. Although the cardiac involvement is usually part of a generalized disorder, a rare instance of lipidosis limited to the heart has been reported.[719]

Disturbances in carbohydrate metabolism

Mucopolysaccharidosis. Gargoylism, or Hurler's disease, is a rare storage disease of infancy and childhood. It was formerly classified as lipochondrodystrophy because the storage material was believed to be a lipid. Now the disease is regarded as one of the genetic mucopolysaccharidoses, in which the cellular storage substance is an acid mucopolysaccharide.[718]

The cardiac manifestations of gargoylism include the following: Aggregations of vacuolated mononuclear cells may be present in the mural or valvular endocardium, the myocardium, the pericardium, or the walls of the coronary arteries.[708,720] Varying degrees of fibrosis are associated with the lesions. Grossly, there is usually enlargement of the heart. Minute nodules on the valvular surfaces and thickening of the valve leaflets occur. Cardiac failure has been reported as a cause of death in patients with gargoylism.

Glycogen infiltration. In diabetes mellitus, there may be an increase of glycogen within the myocardial fibers

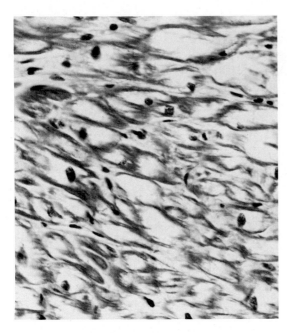

Fig. 15-46. Glycogen storage disease of myocardium. In formalin-fixed, hematoxylin and eosin–stained preparations, muscle fibers appear as clear spaces surrounded by a thin rim of sarcoplasm.

associated with the high concentration of glucose in the blood (p. 30). Glycogen infiltration also can be seen in muscle cells surrounding a healed myocardial infarct, especially in fibers near the endocardium.

Among the disorders associated with a disturbance of carbohydrate metabolism are the glycogen-storage diseases, in which the liver, kidneys, heart, and skeletal muscles may be affected. These familial diseases are caused by an inherited genetic defect. At least eight different types of glycogen-storage diseases have been described, each characterized by a deficiency of a different enzyme (p. 30). The most common is the hepatic type (the classic von Gierke's disease) with involvement primarily of the liver and the kidneys, causing enlargement of these organs.[711] The enzymatic defect is a reduction or absence of glucose-6-phosphatase, so that glycogen is not converted to glucose in the liver. The result is an abnormal accumulation of glycogen that has a normal chemical structure.

A less common form of glycogen-storage disease is the cardiac type (Pompe's disease).[709,710,714,715] This is actually a generalized glycogenosis in which the major manifestation is involvement of the heart. An intracellular enzyme localized in the lysosomes, α-1,4-glucosidase, which hydrolyzes maltose and glycogen into glucose, has been found to be absent from the tissues of children affected by this type of glycogen-storage disease. A gene mutation results in synthesis of an inactive enzyme protein.[706] The chemical structure of the gly-

cogen is normal. Clinically, the disease becomes manifest in infancy, usually at 4 months to 1 year of age and results in death from cardiac failure, usually in the first year of life. Microscopically, there is enlargement and pronounced vacuolization of almost all myocardial fibers because of the deposition of abundant glycogen; the fibers appear as clear or hollow cylinders surrounded by a thin rim of cytoplasm (Fig. 15-46), a feature which has been called a "lacework" appearance of the myocardium. Best's carmine and periodic acid–Schiff stains are useful in demonstrating the glycogen, which persists even in tissue fixed in formalin for a long time. An occasional associated feature is a thickened opaque endocardium, especially of the left ventricle—a form of secondary endocardial fibroelastosis.[722]

In addition to the diffuse form of glycogen-storage disease, there is a type characterized by a spotty or localized distribution of glycogen referred to as *circumscribed glycogen disease of the heart*.[713]

Basophilic (mucoid) degeneration of myocardium. Basophilic (mucoid) degeneration of the myocardium is a common but often overlooked alteration of the muscle fibers[870,871,873,875,877] (Fig. 15-47). The term *basophilic degeneration* is applicable because in sections stained with hematoxylin and eosin there is an accumulation of a basophilic material within the cytoplasm of the muscle cells. The lesion occurs in the muscle of all chambers, but the left ventricle is most frequently affected. Characteristically the distribution is focal or patchy, with involvement of occasional or many fibers throughout the myocardium. The change also has been observed in Purkinje fibers. The basophilic material usually accumulates at first in the perinuclear portion of the fiber, and later it extends throughout the fiber, replacing the myofibrils. It may be light blue and granular, sometimes producing a slightly vacuolated appearance of the affected area, or there may be small, irregular, homogeneous masses of deeper blue material in the degenerated myocytes. The degenerated fibers frequently also contain abundant lipofuscin pigment.

The basophilic intracytoplasmic substance has been considered to be a product of a disorder of carbohydrate (mainly glycogen) metabolism, being largely composed of a glycoprotein[875] or a glucan (polyglucosan).[870,873] Significant histochemical reactions include a positive periodic acid–Schiff reaction even after digestion with diastase, metachromasia with toluidine blue, bright blue-green stain with Alcian blue, light red stain with Mayer's mucicarmine, negative Feulgen reaction, and negative reactions with ribonuclease and hyaluronidase.[877] Since it does not stain for lipids, it probably is not a glycolipid.[868]

Basophilic degeneration occurs most frequently in persons over 40 years of age, though it is observed occasionally in younger persons. The cause is unknown. It is observed commonly in hearts from patients with

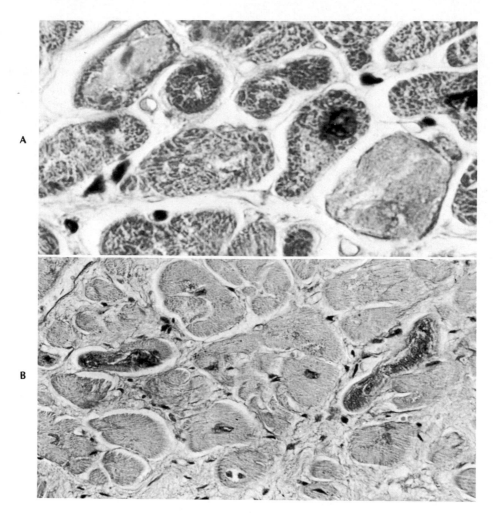

Fig. 15-47. Basophilic degeneration of myocardium. **A,** Mucoid material (blue with hematoxylin stain) is present in two muscle fibers, *upper left and lower right.* In these myocytes, only a thin rim of normal sarcoplasm remains. In the swollen fiber at the lower right, the intracytoplasmic substance is finely vacuolated. **B,** Two fibers containing mucoid material stained by periodic acid–Schiff method.

hypothyroidism,[864,867] but basophilic degeneration is not specific for this disease (see section on hypothyroidism, p. 1571). As a rule this degenerative change does not produce functional cardiac disturbances.

Fat infiltration and fatty degeneration. Fat infiltration of the heart consists in an abnormal accumulation of adipose tissue interstitially in the myocardium, usually associated with an excessive amount of adipose tissue in the stromal layer of the epicardium. It is not to be confused with fatty degeneration, in which lipid is present within the cytoplasm of the myocardial fibers (see the following discussion). Fat infiltration occurs most commonly in the anterior wall of the right ventricle. It also affects the wall of the right atrium, where it may involve the sinoatrial and the atrioventricular nodes. Sometimes it occurs in the left ventricle or interventricular septum.

Grossly, on the cut surface of the myocardium there is loss of the normally sharp demarcation of the muscle from the overlying epicardial fat. From the latter site, yellow streaks and bands extend into the myocardium. Fat deposits also may be seen beneath the endocardium. Microscopically, groups of adipocytes are interspersed between muscle bundles and individual fibers. Sometimes the adipose tissue may replace all or almost all of the muscle of a particular area (Fig. 15-48).

Fat infiltration of the heart occurs most often in patients with generalized obesity. As a rule, the lesion does not cause significant clinical manifestations even when it is severe.

Fatty degeneration of the myocardium is characterized by the presence of lipid droplets or globules within the cytoplasm of the muscle fibers as a result of injury sustained by the cells (Fig. 15-49). Fatty degeneration

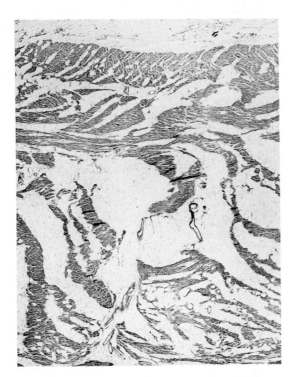

Fig. 15-48. Extensive fat infiltration of myocardium. Bundles of myocytes are separated by clusters of adipose cells.

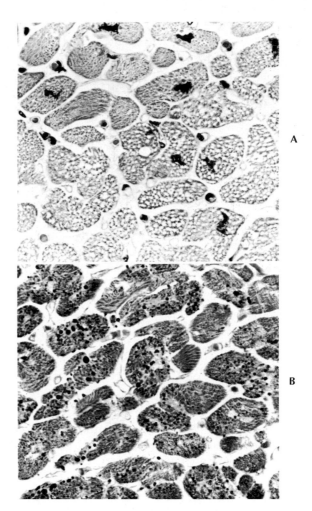

Fig. 15-49. Fatty degeneration of myocardium. **A,** Relatively uniform, fine vacuolization attributable to the presence of fat droplets in myocardial fibers. **B,** Fatty degeneration of the myocardium from a patient with phosphorus poisoning. The black droplets in the myocardial fibers are globules of fat (osmic acid stain). Occasional fat globules in the interstitial areas most likely have been expelled from fibers.

results from a variety of anoxic and toxic causes of cell injury. Anoxia may be associated with severe anemias, particularly pernicious and aplastic anemias. Sometimes leukemia is responsible. Severe loss of blood or coronary insufficiency may have a similar result. Hyaline membrane disease in newborn infants also may cause fatty degeneration.[876] Bacterial toxins (as in diphtheria), septicemias with high fever, and intoxications from chemicals, such as phosphorus, chloroform, arsenic, ether, and alcohol, also may cause fatty degeneration of the myocardium. It is thus not a primary abnormality but is a manifestation of altered myocardial metabolism from diverse causes, some of which may have significant functional consequences.

For example, in myocardial ischemia, when some oxygen is available because of significant quantities of collateral flow, fatty acids may be taken up by the ischemic myocytes from the circulating blood. Such uptake may be facilitated because the circulating level of fatty acids often is elevated during myocardial ischemia[879] attributable to systemic lipolysis induced by increased systemic sympathetic activity or reflex-mediated adrenal catecholamine release.[878] In this setting, variable rates of fatty acid oxidation may occur. However, fatty acid uptake exceeds the rate of oxidation because of the limited supply of oxygen; fatty acyl CoA and acyl carnitine accumulate in mildly ischemic myocardium.[872] Moreover, because glycerol, the backbone of triglyceride, is read-

ily available from increased quantities of α-glycerol phosphate (an intermediate product of anaerobic glycolysis),[874] triglycerides also accumulate in the mildly ischemic myocardium.[865,866,869]

Microscopically, the cytoplasm of the muscle fibers with fatty degeneration appears finely vacuolated in sections stained with hematoxylin and eosin (Fig. 15-49, *A*). The fat can be identified in frozen sections stained with Oil Red O or Sudan IV and can be seen as dense granules in tissue fixed in osmic acid[863,880] (Fig. 15-49, *B*).

Endocrine disorders

Hyperthyroidism. The association between heart disease and thyrotoxicosis is well known, but the exact relationship of hyperthyroidism to the development of the cardiac abnormalities is a subject of controversy.[747,749] The principal hemodynamic effect of hyperthyroidism is an increased cardiac output. In addition, thyroid hormone has a direct effect of increasing myocardial cellular respiration. Thus cardiac disability in thyrotoxicosis may result because of increased metabolism, superimposed on an underlying primary disturbance of the heart (such as coronary artery disease or hypertensive cardiopathy) that may or may not have been clinically evident before hyperactivity of the thyroid gland occurred. Increased adrenergic activity is a common feature in patients with hyperthyroidism,[737] and it has been suggested that thyroid hormone potentiates the effects of the adrenergic catecholamines on the heart. However, other studies have shown neither excess circulating catecholamines nor increased catecholamine responsiveness in patients with hyperthyroidism.[725,729,730] Some investigators believe that the thyrotoxicosis by itself can be a cause of heart disease and cardiac failure.[728] This view is based principally on clinical studies of thyrotoxic patients with congestive heart failure in whom no evidence of associated primary cardiac disease could be recognized.

The clinical features of a thyrotoxic heart, with or without a preexisting cardiac disorder, include tachycardia, increased cardiac output, atrial fibrillation, angina pectoris, cardiac enlargement, and cardiac failure. No constant microscopic lesions are attributable to the effects of thyrotoxicosis by itself, but foci of fatty degeneration, fibrosis, and lymphocytic infiltration of the myocardium have been described in a few cases.[738] The structural alterations characteristic of other forms of heart disease may be present. There is a lack of uniformity in the results reported in experimentally produced hyperthyroidism in animals. However, in some investigations, definite changes have been described—hypertrophy and dilatation of the heart, foci of degeneration and necrosis of myocardial fibers, myocardial fibrosis, and an infiltration by lymphocytes and a few neutrophils and eosinophils.[745]

Hypothyroidism (myxedema heart). Cardiovascular disturbances may occur in long-standing myxedema and include bradycardia, decreased cardiac output, increased heart size, reduced plasma volume, pericardial effusion, angina pectoris, and electrocardiographic changes. Whether overt congestive heart failure occurs as a consequence of uncomplicated myxedema is disputed.[731] Several explanations have been proposed for the cardiac enlargement that is observed by chest roentgenogram in the majority of patients with severe myxedema. The cardiac silhouette may be enlarged on x-ray film because of cardiac dilatation, pericardial effusion, or true increase in heart weight. Increased heart weight has been variably attributed to myocardial hypertrophy, interstitial edema, or interstitial fibrosis.[731] Pathologic data are meager, and the reported

changes are nonspecific. Grossly, the myxedematous heart is pale, flabby, and dilated. Microscopically, interstitial edema may be evident.[734,750] Other features described are hydropic vacuoles, loss of striations, small pyknotic nuclei in muscle cells,[736] and basophilic degeneration of the myocardium[724,727] (Fig. 15-47). The latter change has been observed in association with several diseases, but some investigators believe that it is more pronounced or qualitatively different in patients with thyroid disease.[727,732] Myocardial fibrosis may be present but often can be explained by coexisting coronary sclerosis.

A frequent association of coronary atherosclerosis with myxedema has been reported[723,726] and has been attributed, at least in part, to hypercholesterolemia, which is characteristic of the myxedematous state. However, there is little direct evidence that myxedema itself augments or enhances the development of atherosclerosis.[735]

Acromegaly. In acromegaly, patients often have hypertrophy of the heart. All chambers, but especially the left ventricle, are affected. In some cases, cardiomegaly may be disproportionately greater than the generalized organomegaly that occurs. Heart weights as much as 1300 g have been reported.[733,739] Hypertension is present in some patients with acromegaly and may be partly responsible for the hypertrophy, but it is not a regular feature.[741,742] Cardiomegaly usually cannot be explained by coexisting cardiac abnormalities or hypertension in acromegalic patients. Growth hormone from the pituitary adenoma is the most likely cause for the cardiac hypertrophy, but no clear relationship between the severity of hypertrophy and levels of growth hormone have been observed.[742]

Myocardial hypertrophy is the most prominent anatomic finding in patients with acromegaly. However, it is not possible to distinguish the hypertrophied heart of an acromegalic patient from a heart hypertrophied from other causes. In addition to hypertrophy of muscle fibers, there may be moderate to severe interstitial fibrosis of the myocardium.[739] Other features that have been described are small vessel disease, interstitial foci of lymphocytes and histocytes, and focal myocarditis resembling that induced by catecholamines.[739]

Clinically, acromegalic patients have a high prevalence of coronary artery disease, hypertension, and congestive heart failure.[741] In addition, conduction disturbances resulting in sudden cardiac death have been described.[746]

Carcinoid syndrome (carcinoid heart disease). The syndrome associated with metastasizing carcinoid tumors is characterized by distinctive episodic flushing of the skin, mottled cyanosis, telangiectases, asthma-like attacks, intestinal hyperperistalsis with diarrhea, an increased level of serotonin (5-hydroxytryptamine) in the blood, and an excess of 5-hydroxyindoleacetic acid in the urine.[743] Cardiac manifestations develop in some patients with this syndrome and may dominate the clinical picture. The cardiac manifestations are principally a result of tricuspid and pulmonary valve involvement (see p. 1185). Tricuspid insufficiency is the most common clinical manifestation, but pulmonary stenosis predominates in some patients. Either valvular deformity may cause congestive heart failure.

The valve lesions consist of focal or diffuse plaques on the endocardium of the valvular cusps, the mural endocardium of the cardiac chambers, and the intima of the great veins, the coronary sinus, and occasionally the great arteries.[744] They may involve both sides of the valve cusps, though when the pulmonary valve is affected the plaques are deposited almost entirely on the arterial aspect of the valve cusps. The fibrous thickening and contraction of the cusps usually cause pulmonary stenosis and tricuspid regurgitation, but some degree of pulmonary regurgitation and tricuspid stenosis also may be present. The process on the tricuspid valve may extend onto the chordae tendineae and the papillary muscles. The chordae tendineae may become thickened, shortened, and fused. Similar carcinoid lesions are known to occur in the left side of the heart but much less commonly than in the right side. Occasionally, both sides of the heart may be affected in the same patient.

These carcinoid fibrous plaques are sharply demarcated from the otherwise normal underlying endocardium of the valves and heart chambers by the elastic lamina. Likewise, the plaques in the vessels rest upon an intact inner elastic lamina. The plaques consist of a peculiar type of fibrous tissue (often referred to as cartilage-like), which is free of elastic fibers.[740] Cellular infiltration in the lesions is not pronounced, but some lymphocytes, plasma cells, and mast cells may be present, along with newly formed blood vessels.

The pathogenesis of the carcinoid heart lesions is not clearly established. Serotonin has been implicated as the substance most likely responsible for the development of the fibrous plaques, but the evidence for this assumption is not conclusive. It is not clear why cardiac disease develops in some patients with hyperserotonemia and the carcinoid syndrome but not in others. Other peptides such as bradykinin also may play a contributory role in carcinoid heart disease.[743] It is often presumed that the chemical mediator of the valve plaques is inactivated during its passage through the lungs and that left-sided lesions do not occur unless a right-to-left cardiovascular shunt exists or unless the syndrome is caused by a bronchial adenoma of the carcinoid type. However, instances of a left-sided cardiac lesions have been found in patients without such a shunt or pulmonary tumor.[744]

Practically all attempts to produce the lesions experimentally in animals have been unsuccessful. However, in one investigation,[748] intimal and endocardial proliferative lesions resembling but not identical to the carcinoid heart disease in humans have been produced in animals when a combination of the following three factors was present: hyperserotonemia (after injection of 5-hydroxytryptamine), periodic tryptophan deficiency, and hepatic injury induced by a hepatotoxic agent.

Diabetes mellitus. It was previously discussed in the section of this chapter on coronary heart disease that diabetes mellitus is considered to be a risk factor for atherogenesis, in part because of the associated increase in hypertension and hyperlipidemia and in part because of diabetes specific abnormalities. In addition, diabetes mellitus has been linked to several myocardial abnormalities that are independent of coronary atherosclerosis. Congestive heart failure is a common complication in diabetic patients even in the absence of extensive coronary atherosclerosis and is the basis for the concept of a "diabetic cardiomyopathy."[754,756,761,762] The pathogenesis of this diabetic cardiomyopathy is unknown; proposed mechanisms include a small vessel (intramural) coronary artery disease, increased interstitial and perivascular fibrosis, and a variety of metabolic alterations.[753] In addition, reduced norepinephrine content has been observed in diabetic hearts, suggestive of a reduced sympathetic responsiveness that might contribute to cardiac dysfunction.[759]

Evidence for small vessel disease comes primarily from histopathologic observations. Some investigators have observed increased thickness of the media of small arteries because of increased deposition of periodic acid Schiff (PAS)–positive material and increased cellularity in the media of small arteries.[751,757,758,766] Increased perivascular and interstitial collagen has been observed[756,761] and was accompanied by interstitial accumulation of PAS-positive material associated with degenerative changes in myofibers in one study.[761] Some investigators have found capillary changes characterized by thickening or reduplication of basement membrane material in hearts of diabetic patients.[755,763] Capillary microaneurysms have been demonstrated in diabetic hearts in one study.[753] However, other investigators have found no evidence of microvascular involvement in diabetic hearts.[758,764]

In experimental models of diabetes, both systolic and diastolic functional abnormalities have been observed. Moreover, a plethora of biochemical and subcellular defects have been described in diabetic hearts from experimental models[754] and include increased collagen and glycoprotein accumulation, altered protein synthesis, altered intracellular calcium metabolism, and alterations in several enzyme activities. Which of these numerous abnormalities is most responsible for the functional abnormalities is unknown.

Another cardiac complication of diabetes that has been described, especially among patients with peripheral neuropathies, is an autonomic cardioneuropathy.[760,765] The incidence of silent myocardial ischemia is reportedly greater in this group of diabetic patients than that in nondiabetic controls. It has been postulated that such patients may be at higher risk of sudden cardiac death.

Nutritional deficiencies

Malnutrition. Cardiac failure and associated structural changes have been observed clinically and experimentally as a consequence of protein-calorie malnutrition.[767,770,777] In severe inanition or starvation, the heart is decreased in size and often is brown as a result of accumulation of granules of yellow-brown pigment in the muscle fibers (brown atrophy). Interstitial edema and degeneration of muscle cells are associated with the atrophic fibers. Atrophy of the epicardial fat also may be evident. Paradoxically, rapid nutritional repletion may result in worsening cardiac decompensation.[774]

There is a form of heart disease in South African Bantus that is considered to be caused by chronic malnutrition and particularly with a lack of animal protein in the diet.[775] This entity is characterized clinically by cardiac failure and anatomically by the following: Grossly, the heart is usually dilated, subendocardial fibrosis may be prominent, and mural thrombi may be seen in the cardiac chambers. Microscopically, alterations in the myocardium include hydropic vacuolization of muscle fibers, interstitial edema, and fibrosis. A similar entity has been observed in infants with kwashiorkor.[781,786] Kwashiorkor is a nutritional disease caused by ingestion of a diet deficient in proteins but usually rich in carbohydrates. Coexistent vitamin deficiencies often are present.

Vitamin deficiencies

Beriberi. Among the vitamin deficiencies, the most important cause of cardiac disease is lack of vitamin B_1 (thiamine). This deficiency causes beriberi, a disease long known among peoples of the Orient. Cardiac beriberi is characterized by heart failure associated with hypoproteinemia and edema. Another important clinical feature is widespread peripheral vasodilatation leading to an elevated cardiac output. The resulting increased work required of the heart undoubtedly contributes to the cardiac failure (high-output failure).

The gross and microscopic features are not specific.[769] The heart usually is enlarged, frequently increased in weight, and often globose. The enlargement is caused chiefly by dilatation of the chambers, particularly the right ventricle, but hypertrophy also may be present. Mural thrombi are evident in some instances. The most characteristic microscopic change is interstitial edema. This is often pronounced and may be accompanied by hydropic degeneration of myocardial fibers. Slight fibrosis, especially in the subendocardial muscle and the conduction bundle, has been described.

More prominent degenerative changes have been observed in experimental studies of thiamine-deficient animals.[772] These changes include loss of striations, vacuolization, hyalinization, and focal necrosis of myocardial fibers. Infiltration by polymorphonuclear and mononuclear leukocytes occurs but is not prominent. Lesions identical to those caused by thiamine deficiency have been observed in animals on a potassium-deficient diet (see next page).

Scurvy (vitamin C deficiency). Children who exhibit severe manifestations of vitamin C deficiency in the skeleton may die suddenly.[771] These deaths have been attributed to cardiac hypertrophy, particularly of the right ventricle. Microscopic findings in the heart, however, are not significant. Myocardial degeneration has been reported in vitamin C deficiency in humans and experimentally in guinea pigs.[787]

Vitamin E deficiency. Vitamin E deficiency is not an important cause of heart disease in humans, but in experimental animals on a vitamin E–deficient diet, necrosis of myocardial fibers followed by fibrosis has been described. Fibrinoid degeneration of small myocardial vessels also has been reported.[783,784] Ultrastructural studies have shown a great proliferation of mitochondria in mildly injured myocytes but an abundance of secondary lysosomes in severely damaged fibers.[778] The proposed mechanism of injury is excess lipoperoxidation caused by the absence of vitamin E–antioxidant protection.[783,784]

Severe anemia

In the presence of advanced chronic forms of anemia, the associated myocardial anoxemia causes fatty degeneration of the myocardium. This is evident grossly as a patchy, streaking, "tigroid" or "tabby cat" pattern. The myocardium may be flabby, and frequently cardiac dilatation occurs. Cardiac hypertrophy also occurs as a manifestation of chronic anemia[779]; the overwork of the heart, because of the increased cardiac output required to compensate for the oxygen lack in the tissues, is probably the major factor causing the cardiac enlargement. Clinical manifestations include palpitations, shortness of breath on exertion, tachycardia, murmurs, cardiac enlargement, and electrocardiographic changes. Angina pectoris and congestive heart failure may occur in some patients, especially those with preexisting heart disease.

Cardiac failure associated with degenerative changes in cardiac myocytes also occurs in sickle cell anemia.[773] In this disease cardiac damage may[782] be caused by sickling-induced microvascular stasis and thrombosis as well as by the anemia itself. In some instances, pulmonary arteriolar thrombosis may lead to pulmonary heart disease (cor pulmonale).[768]

Heart failure is considered to be an important factor

in the death of newborns with hemolytic disease attributable to Rh incompatibility. In such patients, the heart is flabby, dilated, and increased in weight.[776] The nuclei of the myocardial fibers are enlarged. Other findings include epicardial hematopoietic foci and petechiae, nucleated red cell precursors in the blood vessels, and microscopic evidence of a mild degree of fibroelastosis in all chambers in the more severe cases. Sometimes one sees minute myocardial infarcts (1 to 2 mm in size) that are confined to the inner part of the myocardium, most frequently in the tips of the papillary muscles in both ventricles. Fatty degeneration also is observed.[780]

Electrolyte disturbances

Dystrophic calcification. Dystrophic calcification occurs in the absence of increased calcium levels in the blood. It occurs most frequently in valves, usually the aortic and mitral, especially those affected by old rheumatic disease. A striking example of valvular calcification is that seen in calcific aortic stenosis, in which the cusps become distorted and rigid and often are the site of massive calcified nodules. Calcification also may occur in vegetations of bacterial endocarditis. Various forms of inflammation, particularly tuberculosis, may predispose to the deposition of calcium in the pericardium. In an occasional instance, almost the entire pericardium may be involved, and so the heart becomes encased in a rigid, calcified shell that sometimes interferes with cardiac function. Dystrophic calcification occurs also in the myocardium, especially in hyalinized scars of healed myocardial infarcts. Calcification may be so extensive that it can be demonstrated in roentgenograms. Foci of myocardial necrosis from a variety of causes, such as ischemia and infections, may be the sites of calcification.[794] In these foci the calcium is deposited within encrotic muscle fibers. Calcification of the myocardium also may result from damage sustained during open-heart surgery.[788] Sometimes this postoperative calcification develops rapidly and prominently within a few days after surgery.

Osseous metaplasia in the heart is not common, but it may be present in areas of calcification, especially in the valves or pericardium and rarely in the myocardium. In the latter site the underlying lesion usually is a scar of an old, healed myocardial infarct.

Metastatic calcification. Metastatic calcification is associated with an increased serum calcium that may be the result of hyperparathyroidism, destructive bone lesions, hypervitaminosis D, or renal insufficiency. There is a tendency for localization of the mineral in the kidneys, lungs, gastric mucosae, and walls of blood vessels. In the heart, calcium is deposited in cardiac anuli, valve cusps, and media and intima of the coronary arteries.[803] If degenerated and necrotic foci are present in the myocardium, there will be an acceleration of dystrophic calcification because of the increased availability of calcium.[789,794,806]

Hypokalemia. Prolonged potassium deficiency may result in congestive heart failure associated with extensive structural changes in the myocardium.[795,796,801] The pathologic effects of hypokalemia have been elucidated in animals fed a diet deficient in potassium. Microscopically, the essential feature is a degeneration of the cardiac muscle fibers, with sarcoplasmic swelling, loss of myofibrils, and hyaline change.[792] In severe cases, necrosis of the fibers may ensue. Accompanying the myocyte degeneration and necrosis are interstitial edema, proliferation of vascular endothelium and fibroblasts, and infiltration by histiocytes. As in any necrotizing cardiac lesion, dead myocytes are removed by phagocytes, and healing is accomplished by hypertrophy of the surviving muscle and condensation of connective tissue. Electron microscopic studies have shown that even severe myocyte degeneration induced by kaliopenia[800,805] is reversible; repletion of potassium in kaliopenic rats resulted in resynthesis of myofibrils and other cytoplasmic organelles.[805]

Myocardial lesions similar to those produced experimentally in animals have been observed in potassium deficiency in humans—a neutrophilic, lymphocytic, and macrophagic infiltration associated with necrosis of muscle fibers.[802] In some patients with severe and prolonged potassium deficiency, myocardial fibrosis as well as myocardial necrosis has been reported.[799] Clinical manifestations include atrial and ventricular arrhythmias, potentiation of digitalis effects, characteristic electrocardiographic changes, and occasionally congestive heart failure.

Hyperkalemia. Hyperkalemia may produce bradycardia and other electrocardiographic changes. A very high serum potassium level can cause ventricular fibrillation or cardiac standstill. Morphologic changes in the heart caused by hyperkalemia have not been defined.

Deficiencies of miscellaneous electrolytes and trace elements. Alterations in myocardial structure or function have also been reported to result from severe deficiencies in magnesium,[790,791,804] phosphate,[793] selenium,[797] and copper.[798]

Drugs and toxic agents

Catecholamine cardiotoxicity. Excessive amounts of catecholamines including epinephrine, norepinephrine, and isoproterenol cause myocardial injury. The nature of the microscopic lesion differs somewhat among the different catecholamines. Isoproterenol toxicity causes focal contraction-band necrosis followed by an inflammatory response and repair by focal scarring. This type of injury has been termed "infarctlike."[820] This term is a misnomer in the sense that infarcts caused by persistent ischemia are characterized by coagulation necrosis; however, the contraction-band necrosis that occurs in isoproterenol poisoning is identical to contraction-band necrosis induced by temporary ischemia, followed by reperfusion (Fig. 15-10). In contrast to isoproterenol, toxic doses of norepinephrine and epinephrine produce more severe arrhythmias but relatively little necrosis. The lesions induced by norepinephrine have been termed "norepinephrine myocarditis."[824]

Catecholamine and especially isoproterenol cardiotoxicity has become a reproducible and widely studied experimental model of cardiac cell injury.[809,813,815,821] From many reports, several hypotheses of the pathogenesis of the lesion have been proposed. Initially, it was considered that the lesions were attributable to relative hypoxia caused by the greatly increased oxygen requirements of inotropically stimulated myocytes.[820] Moreover, it has been postulated that isoproterenol causes alterations in the cardiac microcirculation resulting in focal ischemia, especially of the subendocardial zone.[819,823]

Another hypothesis for the pathogenesis of catecholamine cardiotoxicity is a calcium-overload hypothesis.[807,812] It is known that the inotropic effect of stimulating beta-adrenergic receptors is mediated through increased influx of calcium from the extracellular space. The increased calcium flux and associated increased contractile work is the cause of the greatly increased oxygen requirements of the myocardium. However, calcium overload, by itself, may have a variety of deleterious consequences (see discussion of myocardial ischemia, p. 630).

Another recent hypothesis regarding catecholamine-induced injury is that oxidation products of catecholamines such as adrenochrome are toxic to various subcellular organelles, perhaps by virtue of the increased production of free radicals and resultant lipid peroxidation.[822] Both adrenochrome (the oxidation product of epinephrine) and oxidized isoproterenol are cardiotoxic.[826,827]

In clinical circumstances, it is recognized that excessive use of inotropic agents in ischemic heart disease may exacerbate the severity of ischemic injury. In addition, catecholamines may cause myocardial arrhythmias including ventricular fibrillation and myocardial necrosis in a variety of circumstances including iatrogenic catecholamine administration, pheochromocytomas,[814,825] psychologic stress,[808,811] and intracranial lesions. Catecholamine cardiotoxicity has reportedly resulted in sudden death in persons subjected to stressful situations but without actual physical injury.[808] In the case of cerebral lesions such as intracranial bleeding, increased intracranial pressure results in such a pronounced sympathetic response that arrhythmias or even focal cardiac necrosis may result.[810,816,818]

Other drugs. See section on cardiac biopsy evaluation of myocarditis, p. 706.

Carbon monoxide and heavy metals. Degeneration (parenchymatous, hydropic, or fatty) and focal necrosis of myocardial fibers may occur because of injury from a variety of toxic agents including carbon monoxide, phosphorus, cadmium, and arsenic. Edema and small hemorrhages also may be present.

Myocardial involvement in some miscellaneous systemic diseases

In *Friedreich's ataxia*, myocardial fibrosis, focal degeneration of myocardial fibers, and a scanty cellular infiltration (chiefly lymphocytes) have been described. The lesion has been referred to as a chronic, progressive myocarditis,[836] but in some instances alterations in the small intramyocardial coronary arteries have been observed (that is, medial degeneration followed by intimal proliferation and narrowing of the lumen) and have been considered to be the cause of the myocardial changes.[832] The possibility has been raised that a state of autoimmunization may exist as a result of antigens liberated by degenerating myocardium.[832] It has been postulated that there is a close relationship between the cardiac manifestations of Friedreich's ataxia and familial cardiomegaly.[833]

Myocardial degeneration and necrosis with a secondary inflammatory reaction also have been reported in the hearts of patients with *myasthenia gravis*.[834] The microscopic picture varies. There may be slight focal atrophy and vacuolization of muscle fibers with accompanying mild lymphocytic infiltration of the interstitial tissue (resembling the lymphorrhages found in the skeletal muscles), or there may be extensive myocardial necrosis associated with an abundant inflammatory cell response—neutrophils, lymphocytes, histiocytes, and occasionally multinucleated giant cells. In some instances the presence of multinucleated cells is the striking feature ("giant cell myocarditis").[829] Autoantibodies to skeletal and cardiac muscle have been demonstrated in patients with myasthenia gravis.[828]

In *progressive muscular dystrophy*, the microscopic picture is not that of a distinct inflammatory reaction, but there may be areas of muscle replacement by fibrous and adipose tissues in which a few lymphocytes and histiocytes are present.[830,835,838] The myocardial fibrosis is the most severe in the subepicardial myocardium. The myocardial fibers in and about these areas are atrophied or hypertrophied and may exhibit degenerative changes. Ultrastructurally, myocytes show loss of myofilaments, dilatation of the sarcoplasmic reticulum, and loss of sarcoplasmic glycogen particles.[837] Cardiac arrhythmias and sudden death, which sometimes occur in this disease, have been attributed to alterations in fibers of the sinus node and coronary arteries supplying both the sinus node and the atrioventricular node.[831]

Restrictive (constrictive) cardiomyopathies

Restrictive cardiomyopathy refers to a relatively small group of diseases that are characterized by decreased myocardial compliance.[840,859] The characteristic manifestations of this group of diseases resemble those of constrictive pericarditis and include increased venous pressure and a poor cardiac impulse, but no cardiac dilatation. The most common entity included in this category is cardiac amyloidosis. Other myocardial disorders that occasionally may be manifest by this restrictive pathophysiologic category include endomyocardial fibrosis, hemochromatosis, infiltrative tumors, and sarcoidosis. Interstitial fibrosis from diverse causes may rarely give rise to a restrictive rather than a congestive syndrome.[859] Endocardial fibroelastosis, though an endocardial rather than a myocardial disorder, also often causes a restrictive syndrome. Hemochromatosis and tumors are considered elsewhere in this chapter; cardiac amyloidosis, endomyocardial fibrosis, and endocardial fibroelastosis are considered below.

Amyloidosis

Amyloid deposits can be found commonly in hearts studied post mortem. The incidence increases with advanced age; amyloid deposits have been reported to occur in 30% to 70% of all patients over 60 years of age.[843] Cardiac involvement occurs in approximately 90% of cases of myeloma-associated (primary) amyloidosis.[841] This form of amyloidosis occurs in association with multiple myeloma but may also occur in the absence of associated disease. Amyloid deposits are most likely to involve the spleen, kidneys, liver, and adrenal glands. Cardiac involvement also occurs in about 55% of patients with amyloidosis associated with chronic illnesses (secondary amyloidosis) such as rheumatoid arthritis, tuberculosis, osteomyelitis, bronchiectasis, or lymphoma.[841] In this type of amyloidosis the major deposits occur in the tongue, gastrointestinal tract, lungs, skeletal muscles, skin, and other mesodermal tissues and organs in addition to the heart.

A distinctive type of amyloidosis has been described in which amyloid is restricted largely to the heart. Deposits either do not appear in other organs or are present in insignificant amounts. This is in contrast to the systemic forms of amyloidosis in which involvement of other organs is extensive. It is of considerable interest that the average age of persons with amyloid deposits confined to the heart is higher than that of those with primary systemic amyloidosis or amyloid disease complicating multiple myeloma. The disease affects elderly persons, usually in the seventh to ninth decades, and thus seems to be a manifestation of senescence. It is sometimes referred to as *senile cardiac amyloidosis*.[847,862]

In addition to the foregoing forms of amyloidosis, certain hereditary types have been reported in which the heart may become involved, and in one type it is the organ predominantly affected.[846]

Although cardiac deposits of amyloid can be found commonly, in most instances the deposits are relatively slight and produce no gross morphologic change and are clinically insignificant.[845] Less commonly, cardiac amyloidosis may be sufficiently severe to cause cardiac symptoms, and in only rare instances can death from congestive heart failure be attributed to cardiac amyloidosis.[842] The relative incidence of clinically important cardiac amyloidosis can be appreciated from data collected at the Royal Postgraduate Medical School in London.[845] Of 404 patients admitted over a 15-year period because of a cardiomyopathy, 230 had a hypertrophic cardiomyopathy, 150 had a dilated cardiomyopathy of idiopathic cause, and the remaining 24 patients had specific heart muscle disease with either congestive or restrictive pathophysiology. Of these, seven had cardiac amyloidosis. Amyloidosis was thus an uncommon cause of cardiomyopathy but, on the other hand, was the most common identifiable cause (specific heart muscle disease).

When the heart is severely involved, amyloid deposits may occur throughout the interstitium of ventricular and atrial myocardium.[843,856] Subendocardial deposits are especially common in the atria. The walls of coronary arteries and arterioles and conduction pathways also may be involved. These deposits may be readily detectable macroscopically; the ventricles may be enlarged, firm and rubbery in consistency, and tan in color. Discrete nodular deposits of amyloid may be evident on cross sections of the ventricles or under the atrial endocardium. Multiple subendocardial deposits of glistening, partially translucent amyloid deposits in the atrium have been likened to tapioca pudding. Similar nodules may occur on the epicardial surface or the parietal pericardium. Involvement of the valvular endocardium also may occur.

Microscopically, amyloid occurs as extracellular, eosinophilic, amorphous hyaline deposits (Fig. 15-50). These deposits may form rings completely surrounding and compressing individual myocytes. In severe cases atrophy, vacuolization, or even complete loss of muscle fibers may occur. Deposits may occur in the walls of small and medium-sized arteries and veins and in the interstitium of the endocardium or epicardium. Amyloid may be suspected from evaluation of hematoxylin and eosin–stained microscopic sections because of the ringlike encircling of myofibers and the lack of the wavy fibrillar character of collagen. However, amyloid can be more easily distinguished from collagen by staining

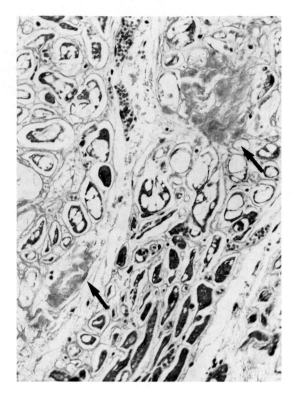

Fig. 15-50. Amyloidosis of myocardium. Myocardial fibers are separated by interstitial deposits of hyaline material (amyloid), *arrows*, which seems to surround individual fibers. Many of the myocytes show degenerative changes of vacuolation or atrophy, most likely attributable to cellular compression by the extracellular amyloid.

with Congo Red or crystal violet. With the Congo Red stain, amyloid is red orange; the protein is birefringent so that when Congo Red–stained tissue is viewed under polarized light it transmits an apple-green color. With the crystal violet stain, amyloid has a metachromatic reddish-purple cast.

Although considered here as the premier example of restrictive cardiomyopathies, amyloidosis is more often clinically manifest by congestive heart failure.[843,856] The ECG typically has low-voltage QRS complexes. Cardiac amyloidosis also may become symptomatic because of involvement of the conduction bundle, resulting in conduction defects.[854] Also, amyloid deposits in the coronary arteries can be a cause of coronary heart disease.[857]

When amyloidosis is manifest as a restrictive cardiomyopathy, it is characterized by increased venous pressure and poor cardiac impulse but, paradoxically, with minimal cardiac dilatation. These features resemble the features of constrictive pericarditis. However, amyloidosis differs from constrictive pericarditis by having slow diastolic filling of the ventricles despite elevated filling pressures and by having poor systolic function.

These features can be observed by echocardiography or angiography and have been termed the "stiff-heart syndrome."[846] Definitive diagnosis can be made by cardiac biopsy.

Endomyocardial fibrosis

Endomyocardial fibrosis is an unusual form of heart disease of uncertain cause that is particularly prevalent among East Africans.[848] In Uganda the important cardiac diseases are hypertensive, syphilitic, and rheumatic heart disease, in addition to endomyocardial fibrosis. The endomyocardial disease accounted for 15% of all cases of heart failure in autopsies at Mulage Hospital in Uganda.[849] In contrast to what is seen in the United States, coronary heart disease is an uncommon cause of cardiac disease in central Africa.

Endomyocardial fibrosis is characterized by severe scarring involving one or both ventricles.[848] The lesion is most severe in the apices and inflow tracts, extending to behind the posterior atrioventricular valve leaflets. The papillary muscles and the chordae tendineae also are affected. Chordae may be fused, and the posterior leaflet of the atrioventricular valve may be sealed to the mural endocardium. Mural thrombosis occurs, and in some instances the ventricular apex (particularly the right) may be obliterated by recent or organized thrombus. The outflow tracts are not affected except for a nonspecific jet effect resulting in slight endocardial fibroelastosis. The semilunar valves are not involved unless there is coexisting disease such as rheumatic valvulitis. Typical lesions also may be present in the atria. Dilatation of the cardiac chambers may be evident, but cardiac hypertrophy is mild or absent.

Microscopically, in the scarred areas there is destruction of the original endocardium and of the adjacent myocardium, with replacement by granulation tissue. The superficial layer of the scar is composed of hyalinized connective tissue. A few inflammatory cells of the mononuclear type are present in the lesion. Elastosis is minimal or absent in the fibrous area, and the elastic fibers of the original endocardium remain as broken irregular masses. This is in contrast to the lesion of endocardial fibroelastosis. Calcification of the scars may occur. The inner third to half of the myocardium may be invaded irregularly by fibrous tissue, though in some cases myocardial involvement is not extensive.

The clinical manifestations of endomyocardial fibrosis are somewhat similar to those of the adult form of endocardial fibroelastosis insofar as the patients present a picture of congestive heart failure of obscure origin. There may be signs of mitral or tricuspid insufficiency, rarely stenosis, and the features of constrictive pericarditis may be simulated. Embolic phenomena are uncommon.

Several hypotheses have been proposed for the cause

of endomyocardial fibrosis. In recent years, it has been observed that an endomyocardial fibrosis, resembling the African disease, occurs rarely in nontropical regions of the world and is usually associated with hypereosinophilia. The latter may occur in diverse conditions such as Löffler's eosinophilic endocarditis, eosinophilic leukemoid reaction, and parasitic infections, as with trichinosis or filariasis. There is now a growing consensus that the African form of endomyocardial fibrosis occurs as a result of an earlier microfilaria-induced eosinophilia[839] and that the nontropical and African forms of endomyocardial fibrosis are the same disease, all caused by hypereosinophilia.[839,844,853] However, the mechanism through which hypereosinophilia causes endomyocardial fibrosis is unknown. Alternative to this hypothesis, a recent study has linked endomyocardial fibrosis to increased dietary intake of thorium, perhaps accompanied by magnesium deficiency.[861]

Endocardial fibroelastosis

Endocardial fibroelastosis may be congenital (primary) or acquired (secondary). The primary type of endocardial fibroelastosis[860] is a disease of obscure origin that occurs predominantly in infants and children but is also observed in adults.

Grossly, there is usually a diffuse (but occasionally a patchy) thickening of the mural endocardium caused by overgrowth of collagenous and elastic tissues. The left ventricle is the chamber most frequently affected, and in some instances it is the only one. The endocardium of the other chambers, particularly the left atrium, also may be involved but usually with that of the left ventricle. The altered endocardium is several times thicker than normal, smooth, opaque, and white or gray-white (Fig. 15-51, *A*). The valves may be affected, usually the aortic and mitral. In some series, valvular involvement is said to occur in almost 50% of the cases. The cusps are thickened and sometimes nodular, or there may be rolling of the edges. Stenosis or insufficiency of the valve orifices may result. Mural thrombi are common in the adult form of the disease, and frequently these give rise to emboli. Thrombi are not usually seen in the infantile and childhood cases. Cardiac enlargement is present and is attributable mainly to left ventricular hypertrophy. Dilatation with flattening of the papillary muscles and trabeculae carneae may also occur.

Microscopically the most striking feature is the thickened endocardium, which results from proliferation of collagen and elastic fibers, which tend to run parallel to the surface (Fig. 15-51, *B*). The endocardial thickening usually is more severe in the infantile form of the disease. There is usually a clear line of demarcation be-

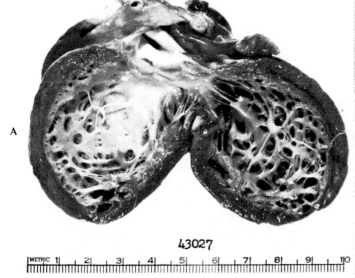

43027

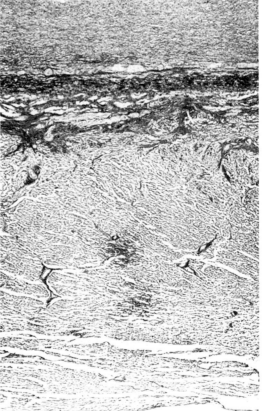

Fig. 15-51. A, Endocardial fibroelastosis in a heart from a 7-month-old black female infant. The heart weight was 77 g. Notice the associated hypertrophy and dilatation of the left ventricle. **B,** Endocardial fibroelastosis. The microscopic section was treated with an elastic tissue stain to emphasize the abundant elastic fibers in the thickened endocardium. There also is a slight degree of fibrosis in the subendocardial myocardium.

tween the altered endocardium and the adjacent myocardium. Fibrosis of the myocardium is not a prominent feature. There may be only occasional small patches of myocardial fibrosis, particularly near the endocardium.

Clinically, in infants there may be a sudden or gradual onset of cardiac failure. In some cases, death occurs within minutes or hours after birth; in others the signs of heart failure may develop weeks or months later and result in death days, weeks, or months later. In the adult form of the disease the duration of symptoms is generally longer, chronic congestive heart failure is more prominent, and embolic phenomena are a notable feature of the clinical picture. The development of cardiac hypertrophy and subsequent heart failure may be explained by the increased work of the heart as the thickened endocardium interferes with proper contraction and relaxation, mimicking the decreased diastolic filling of chronic constrictive pericarditis.

Although many hypotheses have been proposed,[858] the cause of the primary type of endocardial fibroelastosis is not known. An older hypothesis is that fibroelastosis results from intrauterine endocardial anoxia, perhaps attributable to premature closing of the foramen ovale at a crucial stage in the development of the heart.[852] In support of this hypothesis is the observation that secondary endocardial fibroelastosis occurs in association with known congenital anoxia-inducing lesions such as an anomalous origin of the left coronary artery from the pulmonary artery or one of its branches. More recently, evidence has been presented in support of a viral cause.[850,858]

The primary disease in adults is even more difficult to explain. Some writers contend that the adult form arises from the congenital infantile or childhood disease, despite the long interval between birth and the onset of symptoms. However, the majority believe that the adult lesion is etiologically different.

Primary endocardial fibroelastosis must be distinguished from endocardial thickening, which may develop secondary to a variety of cardiac disorders. Endocardial thickening may occur as a compensatory response to altered regional wall tension, as may occur after myocardial infarction[851] or valve replacement.[855] In addition, mural thrombi may undergo organization and result in a locally thickened endocardium.

Myocardial injury from mechanical causes, ionizing radiation, or hypovolemic shock
Traumatic disease

Included in the category of traumatic heart disease are injuries to the heart and the pericardium resulting from physical force.[887] The injuries are classified as penetrating and nonpenetrating.

Penetrating injuries. Penetrating injuries[889] of the heart may be caused by flying missiles (bullets, shell fragments), stab wounds from slender rigid objects (knife, ice pick, long pin or needle, splinter of glass, sharp end of broken rib, various metal or wood objects), or foreign bodies migrating from elsewhere in the body. Swallowed or aspirated foreign bodies may erode through the wall of the esophagus or bronchus and penetrate the pericardium and the myocardium. Occasionally an object such as a needle or a bullet enters the body at a distant site and migrates to the heart by way of the circulation.

A serious effect of penetrating wounds of the heart, one that is responsible for most of the early deaths, is hemopericardium with cardiac tamponade (cardiac compression). As a result of the tamponade, there is an impediment to the filling of the cardiac chambers as well as compression of the great veins, interfering with return of blood to the heart. Severe hemorrhage without tamponade, such as external hemorrhage or a hemothorax, may occur when the laceration of the pericardium is sufficiently large to allow escape of blood from the pericardial sac. It has been estimated that one out of every four persons with a penetrating heart wound will survive the immediate effects of the injury and will live long enough to receive adequate medical care.[889] Among patients whose penetrating wound is successfully repaired by emergency surgery, the incidence of secondary complications has been reported to be about 50%.[883] Causes of these later complications include the following: Infection may complicate penetrating wounds and may be followed by the development of pericarditis and abscesses of the pericardium or myocardium, or both. Valvular defects caused by direct injury or by a severing of papillary muscles are not common. Laceration of a coronary artery, with or without myocardial infarction, may be produced. Coronary thrombosis occasionally occurs as a result of contusive injury of the artery by the penetrating object. Sometimes the penetrating object is lodged within the wall of the heart and is retained as a foreign body for years without causing symptoms, but there is always the danger that it may be mobilized as an embolus in the pulmonary or systemic circulation. Embolic complications of penetrating wounds are also seen in association with a mural thrombus that results from endocardial injury or in association with a superimposed bacterial endocarditis. The development of an aneurysm at the site of myocardial injury has been reported. Arrhythmias may occur, and in some instances they may be the cause of death immediately after the cardiac trauma, for example, if ventricular fibrillation occurs.

Nonpenetrating injuries. Nonpenetrating injuries of the heart[888] are frequently caused by direct forces applied to the thorax, such as a direct blow to the precordium or a sudden compression of the heart between the sternum and the vertebrae as in the common steering-wheel accidents. Cardiac injury also may be caused by indirect forces such as sudden compression or crushing of the abdomen and extremities during a cave-in accident, unaccompanied by injury to the thoracic cage. The damage produced by these indirect forces is the result of a sudden increase in hydrostatic pressure and forcing of blood into the heart and great vessels, which already are filled with blood. Blast forces, particularly when transmitted through water, and decelerative forces as in elevator accidents are other factors that may cause nonpenetrating injuries of the heart.

Nonpenetrating cardiac trauma may produce a variety of lesions, which may be clinically evident immediately or during the subsequent week or two.[886] These lesions include rupture of the heart, myocardial contusion and laceration, pericardial laceration, pericarditis, hemopericardium, and lacerations of valves, chordae tendineae, papillary muscles,[881] and coronary arteries.[886] The latter complications are evidently rare, having not been observed in any of 546 cases of nonpenetrating cardiac trauma in the files of the Armed Forces Institute of Pathology.[888]

Myocardial *contusion* or hemorrhage, which is one of the most common traumatic heart lesions encountered clinically, may lead to serious complications or sequelae such as cardiac rupture, formation of a myocardial aneurysm,[885] calcification of the injured area, and cardiac failure. The most common complication found at autopsy in cases of nonpenetrating cardiac injuries is rupture of the heart.[888] Endocardial injury may result in mural thrombi and systemic emboli.[882] *Arrhythmias* also are significant consequences of *nonpenetrating cardiac injury* and may occur despite seemingly little myocardial damage. Occasionally, fatal ventricular arrhythmias or cardiac standstill may follow apparently minor trauma. For example, a person hit in the chest by a stick and another struck in the precordium by a pitched ball died a few minutes after the injuries.[888] No evidence of cardiac damage was found at autopsy other than a few petechiae seen especially in the pericardium; no other anatomic cause of death was discovered. Cardiac failure may occur despite minimal ECG or enzymatic evidence (such as an increase in plasma creatine kinase) of myocardial injury.[894]

At autopsy it is sometimes difficult to distinguish between contusions and certain nontraumatic causes of interstitial extravasations of blood such as those caused by anoxia and poisons. In some cases a prominent leukocytic infiltration may be associated with severe myocardial hemorrhage, consisting mainly of neutrophils but also with a few eosinophils and mononuclear cells. Focal necrosis of muscle fibers with an accompanying inflammatory response may occur and in some instances may be sufficiently extensive to simulate early infarcts.[887,888] A fibrinous pericarditis occasionally is observed in association with nonpenetrating trauma, but purulent pericarditis is rare and usually is the result of contamination from concomitant injuries to the esophagus or respiratory tract.[888]

Radiation injury

Before the mid-1960s the heart was considered to be among the most resistant organs to the effects of ionizing radiation. However, in recent years it has become recognized that the heart is often the dose-limiting organ for radiation therapy of mediastinal neoplasms such as Hodgkin's disease.[903] The degree and type of damage is related to cumulative dose. Clinical manifestations of radiation heart disease become common after cumulative mediastinal doses exceeding 3500 rad.[894] In one reported series of 48 patients with Hodgkin's disease treated by radiation therapy (total midplane dose of 3000 to 3600 rad), detailed evaluation revealed overt or subclinical cardiac disease in 96%.[892]

The most common manifestation of radiation-induced heart disease is pericarditis.[901,903] This may occur at the time of radiation therapy. However, more commonly, radiation heart disease may become manifest as delayed pericarditis, the onset of which occurs long after the radiation exposure. In one reported series of patients with delayed pericarditis, chronic constrictive pericarditis developed as long as 22 years after mediastinal radiation.[891] The explanation for such a long delay between radiation exposure and onset of symptomatic pericarditis is unknown.

Another manifestation of radiation-induced heart disease is diffuse interstitial myocardial fibrosis.[903] This may result in severe congestive heart failure, often with features of a restrictive cardiomyopathy (see p. 678) even in cases in which pericardial involvement is minimal.[902] The cause of myocardial fibrosis is unknown; however, in experimental studies it has been observed that capillary endothelial cells are the first cells to show signs of radiation injury, whereas myocytes seem to be fairly resistant to the effects of radiation.[897,898] This is in contrast to the effects of the antineoplastic drug adriamycin, which causes a dose-related injury to myocytes[897] (see pp. 183 and 708). It has been reported that the toxic effects of radiation and adriamycin are synergistic, in that patients who have received mediastinal radiation therapy develop clinical evidence of adriamycin injury after lower cumulative doses.[899,900,903]

The myocardial fibrosis also may result in functional valvular defects, believed to be caused by papillary muscle scarring, or left bundle branch block, believed to be caused by fibrosis involving the conduction system.[903]

Another well-recognized manifestation of radiation-induced heart disease is the accelerated development of coronary atherosclerosis.[894] Inasmuch as the anatomic features of coronary atherosclerosis in patients who have received radiation therapy may be indistinguishable from atherosclerosis among the general population, it is not always possible to prove radiation causation.[903] However, several cases of myocardial infarction have been reported in patients under 30 years of age,[894] one patient dying at 15 years of age,[895] after mediastinal radiation therapy. Nevertheless, the incidence of radiation-induced coronary atherosclerosis is considered to be low by some investigators and may occur primarily in subgroups of patients with other coexistent risk factors for coronary atherosclerosis[903] (see p. 618). This view is supported by observations in experimental animals that radiation alone does not produce coronary atherosclerosis,[896] but the combination of radiation and a high cholesterol diet can.[890]

Hypovolemic shock

Hypovolemic shock, whether caused by hemorrhage, trauma, or burns may result in cardiac decompensation.[909] Cardiac dysfunction results, in part because of release to the circulation of a variety of cardiodepressant polypeptides from the ischemic pancreas and other splanchnic organs. These polypeptides are referred to as "myocardial depressant factor."[905,909]

In addition, myocyte injury occurs and contributes to the cardiac dysfunction. Anatomic changes have been described in the hearts of human subjects in shock,[906] as well as in the hearts of various animals after experimental induction of hemorrhagic shock[904,907,908]; these include fatty degeneration[906,907] (Fig. 15-48), subendocardial hemorrhage, contraction-band necrosis (Fig. 15-10), and zonal lesions.[904] The zonal lesions are observed by electron microscopy and are characterized by an intense contraction of a myocyte adjacent to the intercalated disc, associated with disruption of saracomeres and displacement of mitochondria.

The etiologic basis for these myocardial lesions is not completely understood. Factors that probably are involved include cardiac ischemia, especially of the subendocardial zone caused by hypoperfusion attributable to hypotension coupled with an increased metabolic demand because of tachycardia. In addition, the left ventricular blood volume is decreased, the blood pH is decreased (metabolic acidosis), and there is a sharp increase in the concentration of circulating catecholamines. Experimental studies have suggested that the subendocardial hemorrhage and the necrotic lesions of the myocardium are caused by ischemic hypoxia, since they can be prevented when dogs in shock are treated with oxygen.[911]

TUMORS OF THE HEART
Cysts

Cysts of various types occur in the pericardium, in the myocardium, and in the heart valves.

Pericardial cysts[918,920,963] are congenital malformations characterized by a thin fibrous wall, lined by flattened mesothelial cells that are sometimes difficult to distinguish from vascular endothelial cells. These cysts occur in the anterior mediastinum and are in contact with the thoracic wall, the parietal pericardium, and sometimes the diaphragm and one of the lungs. It has been suggested that the lesions result from failure of fusion of the primitive celomic lacunae, which normally coalesce to form the pericardial cavity.[940] The cysts must be differentiated from those caused by *Echinococcus granulosus* and from other types of mediastinal cysts. Pericardial cysts frequently cause no symptoms and are identified by roentgenogram in the course of a routine examination or are found incidentally at autopsy.[920] At times they produce symptoms such as thoracic pain.

Epithelial cysts of the heart are extremely rare malformations.[942,948] There are two types: those lined by ciliated epithelium and those lined by nonciliated epithelium. The ciliated cysts (bronchogenic cysts) arise in the left ventricle and are usually solitary. The nonciliated cysts occur in the atria and often are multiple. Stratified squamous epithelium has been identified in some of the cysts. These cysts most likely are forms of heterotopia—inclusions of the more cranial endoderm or mesoderm (thyroglossal, pharyngeal, respiratory, and esophageal primordia) during embryologic development.[944] A rare tumor in the region of the atrioventricular node composed of multiple, closely grouped, nonciliated cystic structures has been described as a mesothelioma or lymphangioendothelioma (see p. 799). Conduction disturbances, including complete heart block, may result from the presence of intramyocardial epithelial cysts.

Blood cysts of the cardiac valves are small, dark red nodules, usually less than 1 or 2 mm in diameter, that are present most frequently on the atrial side of the atrioventricular leaflets and rarely on the ventricular surface of the semilunar cusps.[915] These lesions, sometimes referred to as *telangiectases*, consist of unilocular spaces lined by endothelial cells and filled with blood. These cysts produce no significant clinical manifestations.

Neoplasms

Neoplasms of the heart may be classified as primary or secondary, as benign or malignant, and as pericardial or intracardial (myocardial or endocardial). The incidence of primary neoplasms of the heart and pericardium has varied widely among published reports from 0.002% of 480,000 autopsies to 0.03% of 40,000 autopsies.[914,960] In any case, primary neoplasms of the heart and pericardium are rare. In contrast, secondary neoplasms are relatively common, occurring in 10% to 25%

of autopsies of patients dying of malignancy.[917,924,951,955] Thus, 40 to 50 secondary neoplasms of the heart may be encountered for every primary tumor observed.

Primary neoplasms

Despite the small number of total cases, the number of types of primary neoplasms that have been reported to involve the heart is large.[930,932,944,956] For example, the types of benign and malignant neoplasms found among approximately 500 primary neoplasms collected by the Armed Forces Institute of Pathology[944] are listed below in order of relative frequency:

Cardiac tumors

Benign cardiac tumors
Myxoma
Lipoma
Papillary fibroelastoma
Rhabdomyoma
Fibroma
Hemangioma
Teratoma
Mesothelioma (of AV node)
Granular cell tumor
Neurofibroma
Lymphangioma

Malignant cardiac tumors
Angiosarcoma
Rhabdomyosarcoma
Mesothelioma
Fibrosarcoma
Malignant lymphoma
Osteosarcoma
Neurogenic sarcoma
Malignant teratoma
Thymoma
Leiomyosarcoma
Liposarcoma
Synovial sarcoma

The relative frequency of primary neoplasms is dependent on the age group under study. Among adults, approximately two thirds of the neoplasms in the AFIP series were benign; myxomas accounted for half of these, and lipomas and papillary neoplasms of the valve accounted for another third. Among malignant primary neoplasms in adults, angiosarcomas, rhabdomyosarcomas, and mesotheliomas accounted for approximately 75%. Among children with primary cardiac tumors, over 90% were benign; 50% of these were rhabdomyomas. Teratomas, lipomas, and myxomas composed another 40%.

Myxoma. The most common primary tumor of the heart is the myxoma arising from the mural endocardium (Fig. 15-52). Myxomas are found almost exclusively in the atria, with about three fourths occurring in the left atrium in the region of the fossa ovalis.[943,944] This location is in contrast to that of cardiac sarcomas, which arise most frequently in the right atrium. Only occasionally do myxomas occur in the ventricles. Cardiac myxomas are usually single tumors, but they may be multiple in some patients, appearing in the same chamber or in different chambers.[962] Myxomas occur at any age, but the majority are observed in persons between 30 and 60 years of age. The sex distribution usually is reported as being equal. Grossly, the tumors are generally polypoid, frequently pedunculated, externally glistening, and smooth or slightly lobular and occasionally villous (Fig. 15-52, *A*). They may be soft or firm. On section, their cut surfaces are yellow-white or red-brown, with evidence of hemorrhage, and they are often gelatinous in appearance.

Microscopically, myxomas consist of a loose, sparsely cellular stroma with stellate, spindle, polyhedral, and multinucleated cells scattered throughout. Vessels of capillary size lined by plump endothelial cells, foci of lymphocytes, and varying amounts of collagen are present[933,925,944] (Fig. 15-52, *B*). Chondroid features also have been described.[916] Hemorrhage and granules of hemosiderin pigment commonly are seen in the stroma. Stains for mucin are usually positive. The lesions are covered by normal endothelial cells, and thrombi sometimes overlie the tumors. Occasionally, epithelial gland–like structures may be present in myxomas[925,943]; it is important to be aware of this pattern so that the lesions are not mistaken for metastatic mucin-producing adenocarcinomas.[912]

There has been some controversy concerning the nature of cardiac myxomas. Some investigators have considered them to be organizing mural thrombi,[954] but the prevalent opinion is that they are true neoplasms.[917,921,927] Organizing thrombi can have a rather myxomatous, relatively acellular appearance resembling the histologic appearance of myxomas. However, myxomas differ from organizing thrombi in several respects (Table 15-2): The characteristic location of myxomas near the left atrial side of the fossa ovalis differs from the location of thrombi, which, in the atria, often occur in the appendages. In addition, thrombi may occur in any chamber in association with underlying endocardial or myocardial injury; myxomas usually occur in otherwise normal hearts. In addition, thrombi are usually laminated whereas myxomas are not. Finally, when thrombi are grown in tissue culture, fibroblasts proliferate, whereas when myxomas are grown in culture, multipotential mesenchymal cells predominate.

Although most authors maintain that myxomas are neoplastic, there is no general agreement as to their origin. One opinion is that the tumors arise from remnants of the myxoid tissue that composes the embryonic

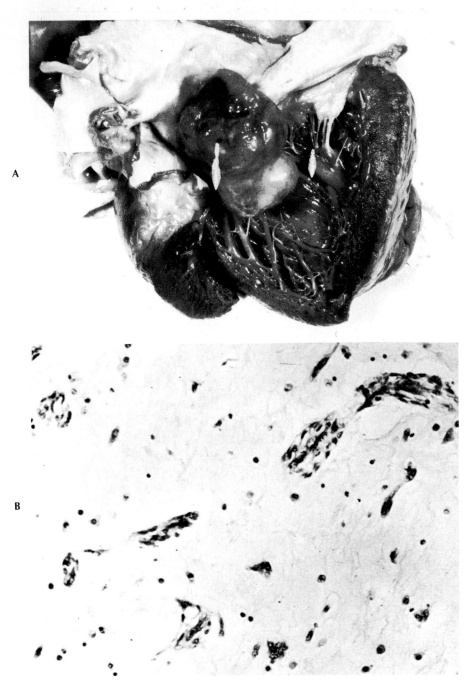

Fig. 15-52. A, Cardiac myxoma of the left atrium. This gelatinous tumor is attached to the septal wall of the left atrium. It projects into the cavity of the left atrium and is partly blocking the mitral orifice. During life, such tumors may act as ball valves, causing intermittent obstruction of the mitral valve. **B,** Cardiac myxoma. The tumor has an abundant myxomatous stroma in which the stellate mesenchymal tumor cells are embedded. The tumor cells often surround capillaries, a pattern that is illustrated here.

Table 15-2. Differences between cardiac myxomas and organizing thrombi

	Thrombus	Myxoma
Position in atria	Most common in appendages	Left atrial side of fossa ovalis
Condition of heart	Underlying injury	Normal hearts
Laminated	Yes	No
Tissue culture	Fibroblasts proliferate	Multipotential mesenchymal cells proliferate

endocardium. Another view is that they are simple connective tissue tumors in which a myxoid change occurs as a result of stresses to which they are subjected within the cardiac chamber.[951] On the basis of electron microscopic and immunocytochemical studies, various investigators have described the cell origin as smooth muscle cells derived from the subendocardium,[945,946] multipotential mesenchymal cells capable of producing various cell types,[913,923,937] or endocardial lining cells.[946,947]

Lipomas. Two types of cardiac lipomas are recognized.[944] One type occurs in the interatrial septum.[934,949,952] This type is considered to be nonneoplastic by some observers; hence the term "lipomatous hypertrophy of the atrial septum" is often used for this group. True lipomas may occur within the myocardium of any chamber. Both types of lipoma are usually asymptomatic, commonly being discovered as incidental findings at autopsy. However, the interatrial variety may be a source of cardiac arrhythmias[935,944]; sudden cardiac death has been attributed to such lipomas in a minority of cases.

Papillary tumors of the cardiac valve. Papillary tumors or papillary fibroelastomas[926,932,939,944,950] may involve cusps of either the aortic or pulmonic valves, where they usually arise from the line of closure. They generally are incidental findings at autopsy. Microscopically, these tumors consist of multiple papillary projections (said to resemble a fronded sea anemone). Individual papillae have structures similar to normal chordae tendineae, including a central fibrous core and an outer layer of looser connective tissue covered by endothelium. The true nature of these lesions also is controversial; some consider them to be exaggerated Lambl's excrescences, perhaps arising through organization of repeated microthrombi.

Rhabdomyomas. Rhabdomyomas of the myocardium appear as a single or multiple, circumscribed but not encapsulated, gray or gray-white nodules in any part of the heart. The masses often bulge into the cardiac lumen and rarely are pedunculated.

Microscopically, the nodules consist of large, swollen myocardial fibers filled with glycogen. In routine histologic preparations the cells appear as empty spaces surrounded by a rim of cytoplasm, but the characteristic feature is the presence of "spider cells." These are cells with a central nucleus that appears suspended by threads of cytoplasm separated by large, glycogen-filled vacuoles. In some cells the vacuoles are not large and the cytoplasm is abundant and granular.

Rhabdomyomas usually occur in infants and children. About a third to a half of cases occur in association with tuberous sclerosis of the brain.[928,944,958] Although the lesion is regarded as the most common primary tumor of the heart in infants and children, its neoplastic nature has been questioned. Because of the abundant glycogen deposits, some authors have considered rhabdomyomas to be a form of localized glycogen-storage disease.[936] However, in typical cases of type II glycogen-storage disease, the normal cardiac structure is preserved except for cellular distortion caused by the glycogen deposition alone. Like normal adult myocytes and Purkinje fibers, myocytes in glycogen-storage disease have intercalated discs only at the two poles of the cell. In contrast, electron-microscopic studies of the "spider cells" in rhabdomyomas have shown that these cells resemble cardiac myoblasts, in that they have multiple intercellular junctions all around the cell periphery.[916,922,957,961] Some investigators consider rhabdomyomas to be hamartomas.

Rhabdomyomas may be asymptomatic or may be symptomatic[922] because of cardiac arrhythmias or because of obstruction to blood flow through the heart. Although "benign," rhabdomyomas frequently are difficult to treat surgically because they often are multiple, often occur deep within the myocardium, and may involve the septum in proximity to the conduction system.[928]

Clinical manifestations of primary cardiac tumors. There is no single constellation of features that permit the diagnosis of a cardiac tumor.[929,944,953,956] The manifestations of a cardiac tumor depend on the nature of the tumor and its location; tumors often mimic other much more common cardiac conditions. Thus the correct diagnosis depends on inclusion of tumors among the differential diagnosis of a variety of conditions. Tumors that involve the pericardium may cause a pericardial effusion or pericarditis. Effusions occasionally develop sufficiently rapidly to cause symptoms of cardiac tamponade. Obliteration of the pericardial space and diffuse infiltration of parietal and visceral pericardium by malignant tumors may be a cause of constrictive pericarditis. Tumors that project into one of the cardiac chambers, as cardiac myxomas often do, may result in obstruction of blood flow through the chamber. Syncope, angina, pulmonary edema, and cardiac murmurs may be associated findings. Left atrial myxomas have been reported to act as ball valves, causing obstruction of the mitral valve orifice. Tumor involvement of the myocardium, by itself, or of the mitral valve orifice may impede contractile function and cause congestive heart failure. Arrhythmias and chest pain are additional nonspecific symptoms of cardiac tumors. Cardiac tumors may also give rise to noncardiac manifestations. For example, fragments of friable tumors such as myxomas, which project into a cardiac chamber, may embolize. Microscopic evaluation of peripheral emboli may result in the diagnosis of an otherwise unsuspected atrial myxoma.[919] Another manifestation of tumors projecting into the cardiac chambers is hemolytic anemia, explained by mechanical trauma to passing red blood cells. Primary malignancies of the heart may occasionally become manifest through nonlocalizing constitutional features of malignancy such as malaise or weight loss.

Angiocardiography and echocardiography have proved to be useful techniques for the diagnosis of cardiac tumors; however, angiography poses a risk of embolization of fragments of friable tumors such as myxomas. Establishing the correct diagnosis of a cardiac tumor, though difficult, can be lifesaving. As noted above, most primary cardiac tumors are benign; surgical resection often is curative.[938,956,959] Recurrence of cardiac myxoma is infrequent but may occur in circumstances of incomplete resection of unrecognized multicentric foci.[931,941]

Secondary neoplasms

The following table (Table 15-3) lists the combined incidence of cardiac and pericardial tumors from a total of approximately 8200 patients who died of cancer and were described in one of several large series.[916,924,944,955] Overall, approximately 1300 (15%) of these patients had metastatic involvement of either the heart (Fig. 15-53), pericardium, or both. The neoplasm

Table 15-3. Metastatic tumors of the heart and pericardium

	Number of patients	Metastatic involvement	%
Melanoma	135	57	42
Lung cancer	1409	457	32
Leukemia	339	108	32
Sarcomas	82	21	26
Breast cancer	930	222	24
Lymphomas	686	144	21
Esophagus cancer	273	41	15
SUBTOTAL	3854	1050	
Other	4359	250	6
TOTAL	8213	1300	

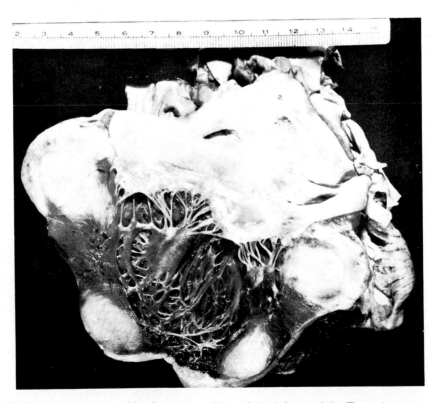

Fig. 15-53. Metastatic tumor in the myocardium of the left ventricle. The primary tumor in this case was a renal cell carcinoma.

that ranks first in frequency of cardiac metastases is malignant melanoma (42%). This observation can be explained by the fact that melanomas metastasize widely through the bloodstream and may involve virtually any organ of the body. Numerically, the most common metastatic tumor in the heart is lung cancer, a finding explained by the high frequency of lung cancer among all cancers as well as the relatively high percentage of lung cancers that involve the heart or pericardium. In general, those tumors that commonly involve the heart are those that (1) arise above the diaphragm in relative proximity to the heart (such as lung, esophageal, and breast cancer), or (2) tumors characterized by widespread systemic involvement (such as melanoma, leukemias, lymphomas, and miscellaneous sarcomas). Notable exceptions from the list of common secondary tumors of the heart are all the common subdiaphragmatic malignancies including colonic, gastric, pancreatic, prostatic, endometrial, ovarian, and uterine cervical cancers.

The clinical manifestations of metastatic tumors of the heart often are overshadowed by the systemic or noncardiac manifestations of widespread cancer. However, metastatic involvement of the heart occasionally is the principle cause of morbidity or mortality. Clinical manifestations of secondary tumors include the same range of features discussed in the preceding section on primary cardiac tumors (p. 703).

DISTURBANCES OF THE CONDUCTING SYSTEM

Normal anatomy. The cardiac impulse originates in the sinoatrial (SA) node (the "pacemaker" of the heart) and is conducted through the atrial fibers to the atrioventricular (AV) node and the common bundle (of His), which penetrates the central fibrous body and then branches into the broad left bundle and terminates in the narrow right bundle.[966,972,978]

The impulse is thus carried in the normal heart from the SA node, which has the highest intrinsic rhythmicity, to the apex of the heart. It is transmitted rapidly by all the conducting fibers except for those of the AV node. The AV node slows the conduction impulse, thereby assuring that excitation of the atria and ventricles are sequentially timed for maintenance of efficient cardiac contractile function. The common bundle is the only pathway from the atria to the ventricles in normal hearts.

Pathologic anatomy. The AV node–common bundle route can be bypassed (Fig. 15-54) by several aberrant conduction pathways[964,973]—including lateral muscle bridges that connect the atria and ventricles (bundles of Kent) and various other bypass pathways (including nodoventricular, fasciculoventricular, intranodal, and so on). These bypass pathways are composed of essentially normal myocytes, and the impulse is not slowed during its passage through them. Thus it reaches the ventricle earlier than the impulse that traverses the usual AV node–common bundle route, resulting in preexcitation. This accounts for the short PR interval and the aberration of the QRS complex and the bouts of tachycardia that are characteristic of the Wolff-Parkinson-White (WPW) syndrome.[984] The ability to correct the arrhythmia of the WPW syndrome by surgical separation of the aberrant pathway supports this as the mechanism for the arrhythmia.[969]

Lesions that interfere with normal AV conduction are of numerous origins.[966,967,972,978] They may be *congenital*, resulting from a (probably) developmental defect in the continuity of the connections between the SA node and the distal conducting bundles.[975,979] Such abnormalities may occur as an isolated entity or may occur with gross anatomic defects such as interventricular septal defect and corrected transposition of the great vessels.[971] The conducting system can be affected by the *trauma* of surgery that involves structures adjoining the common bundle region, such as repair of interventricular septal defects or tetralogy of Fallot abnormalities.[968] *Inflammatory* conditions of the heart, especially myocarditis, may result in arrhythmias or block when the conducting fibers are involved, as in viral myocarditis[981] and rheumatic fever.[970] *Circulatory* conditions can produce transient or occasionally permanent heart block, such as panarteritis nodosa or when the conducting fibers are close to or within the necrotic zone of a myocardial infarct.[974] *Neoplasms* can impinge on or transect the conducting fibers producing arrhythmias, sudden death, or heart block. These can include primary tumors of the "mesothelioma" type,[980] or sec-

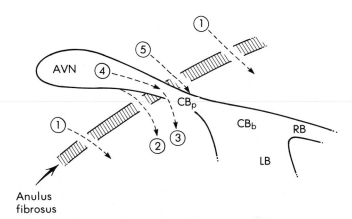

Fig. 15-54. Diagram illustrating five different pathways by which the cardiac impulse can bypass the usual atrioventricular node–common bundle–bundle branches route. *CB_b*, Branching common bundle; *CB_p*, penetrating common bundle; *LB*, left branch; *RB*, right branch. (From Benditt, D.G., and Benson, D.W.: Cardiac preexcitation syndromes, Hingham, Mass., 1986, Kluwer/Nijhoff Publishing Co.)

ondary metastatic lesions, especially from the lungs.[965] Finally, there is a *miscellaneous* category of conditions. Included is a condition said to result in wear and tear on the conducting fibers of the common bundle or bundle branch regions (so-called Lev's disease) that results in heart block in older patients[977]; somewhat similar to this is a condition in which bundle-branch fibrosis of unknown cause results in heart block in younger patients (so-called Lenègre's disease.[976] Hemochromatosis also may cause heart block associated with iron deposition in the AV node or common bundle.[983]

Heart block resulting from these conditions may sometimes be transient, as it fortunately often is in surgically induced heart block or in patients with acute posterior myocardial infarcts.[974] Transient heart block is probably attributable to local hemorrhage and edema that recedes with time, rather than to necrosis and scarring, which would cause permanent transection.

PATHOLOGY OF ENDOMYOCARDIAL BIOPSY SPECIMENS

Although the techniques for obtaining cardiac biopsy specimens were developed in the 1950s, the technique was not widely used until the present decade. The recent increase in the performance of cardiac biopsies has come about because of the diagnostic value of this method for certain conditions (see below), growing awareness that the biopsy technique can be done safely, and the fact that increasing numbers of cardiologists are learning the necessary skills required to obtain the tissue samples.[995] At present, tissue for most nonsurgical cardiac biopsies is obtained by use of a flexible catheter with a biopsy forceps at its tip. The catheter usually is passed intravenously into the right ventricle, and cardiac tissue is obtained from the right side of the interventricular septum.

Indications

Achieving a definitive diagnosis by cardiac biopsy depends on the presence of a disease process that has (1) distinctive morphologic or immunologic features and (2) a diffuse myocardial distribution so that the disease process will be represented in the very tiny pieces of cardiac tissue obtained. At the present time, the most widely accepted indications for cardiac biopsy include the following[996,1001]:

1. Diagnosis or monitoring response to therapy of cardiac allograft rejection
2. Diagnosis of active or resolving myocarditis
3. Diagnosis of adriamycin cardiotoxicity
4. Differentiation of constrictive pericarditis versus constrictive (restrictive) cardiomyopathies
5. Diagnosis of other specific myocardial diseases with distinctive pathologic features
6. Answering research questions

Specific cardiac disorders that can be diagnosed by endomyocardial biopsy include amyloidosis, sarcoidosis, hemochromatosis, Fabry's disease, carcinoid disease, irradiation injury, glycogen-storage disease, cardiac tumors, and endocardial fibrosis or fibroelastosis.[996,1001,1004,1005,1008] However, it should be recognized that the sensitivity of cardiac biopsy is low for the diagnosis of localized entities such as sarcoidosis or cardiac tumors because the lesions may not be represented in the biopsy sample.

There also are several entities in which cardiac changes are nonspecific, but their presence in biopsy tissue is confirmatory of the presence of abnormalities suspected from other indices.[1001] Thus the presence of myocardial abnormalities can be documented in congestive or hypertrophic cardiomyopathies and in cases of methysergide toxicity, hypothyroidism or hyperthyroidism, and myotonic dystrophy.

Enthusiasm for cardiac biopsy must be tempered by the recognition that the large majority of congestive cardiomyopathies are idiopathic and the likelihood that a specific disorder can be diagnosed in a given biopsy is small.[992,1001] In judging the severity of inflammation or fibrosis in cases of myocarditis or chronic cardiomyopathy, one must recognize that involvement is not uniform throughout the myocardium and that changes present in the tiny samples obtained for biopsy may not be representative of the heart as a whole. In order to optimize the chance for proper diagnosis and grading of cardiac abnormalities, many cardiac pathologists recommend that a minimum of three or four tissue samples be obtained for each biopsy.

Methods of evaluation

Despite the small amount of tissue available for biopsy, tissue samples usually are subdivided and processed for (1) routine histology, (2) immunopathology, and in some medical centers (3) electron microscopy.[991] Immunopathologic studies are of particular value for determining the presence and severity of inflammatory cell infiltration and, if present, the types of cells involved.

In the evaluation of biopsy material, the pathologist must be alert to the possibility of several artifacts that do not ordinarily cause diagnostic difficulty in the study of an entire heart at necropsy but may lead to confusion in the interpretation of changes in the small fragments of tissue obtained for biopsy.[991] Myocytes may suffer crush artifacts or develop contraction bands because of mechanical injury; the latter may be expected particularly along the cut edges of the biopsy sample. In the evaluation of acute and resolving inflammatory foci, organizing mural thrombi and ongoing repair of previous biopsy sites must not be confused with true myocarditis or allograft rejection.

Selected applications
Cardiac allograft rejection

The immunopathology of cardiac rejection is similar to that of rejection of other transplanted organs such as the kidneys (see p. 531) and is not considered in detail here. One difference between heart and kidney that should be noted is that hyperacute rejection, which may occur in renal allografts, is seldom if ever encountered in myocardial allografts. The following is a summary of the various changes in untreated acute and chronic (late) allograft rejection reactions.[986,989,990,1006,1009] In acute rejection the heart at autopsy appears dark red, swollen, firm, and edematous. Fibrinous pericarditis is a constant feature, and subendocardial and myocardial hemorrhage is usually present. The microscopic findings include swelling and disruption of the endothelium of vessels with platelet and fibrin deposition on the intimal surface, interstitial infiltration of the myocardium (especially around vessels) by mononuclear (lymphoid) cells, a similar infiltration in the thickened intima of the coronary arteries, arterial medial necrosis, edema and hemorrhages in the myocardium, and foci of myocardial degeneration and necrosis. It should be recognized that morphologic features of rejection will be influenced by the type and efficacy of immunotherapy with which a patient has been treated. The pathologic features of uninhibited allograft rejection as studied in experimental animals or as seen in early clinical experience are seldom seen in present-day cardiac allograft recipients in whom immunotherapy is being monitored by sequential endomyocardial biopsy.

In chronic or late allograft rejection, the principal morphologic features are an infiltrate of mononuclear cells (lymphocytes, plasma cells, histiocytes) in the intima of coronary arteries and in the myocardium (mainly in perivascular areas), intimal proliferation and fibrosis of coronary arteries, and foci of myocytolysis and fibrosis of the myocardium. In long-term survivors the intimal lesion may progress to an obliterative arteritis, which in the large coronary arteries mimics atherosclerosis.[1010] It has been suggested that the initiating factor in cardiac allograft atherosclerosis may be immunologic injury to the intima but that intimal platelet and fibrin microthrombi and elevated serum lipids may contribute to its development.

It has been demonstrated from experimental studies in dogs that, not only can cardiac rejection be diagnosed morphologically, but also its severity can be ascertained with considerable accuracy. Thus it is possible to use repeated cardiac biopsy samples in patients with cardiac transplants to monitor the adequacy of immunosuppressive therapy. The following grading system has been developed by Billingham[989]: Early (mild) rejection is characterized by interstitial and endocardial edema and small numbers of perivascular pyrinophilic mononuclear inflammatory cells ("immunoblasts"). Moderate rejection is characterized by focal myocyte degeneration and increased numbers of "immunoblasts" of the T-cell type. Both mild and moderate degrees of rejection are reversible with immunotherapy. Severe rejection is characterized by vascular damage (vascular necrosis, microthrombi, or interstitial hemorrhage) and focal myocardial necrosis. These changes may be associated with a neutrophilic inflammatory response. Resolving acute rejection, which follows adequate immunosuppressive therapy, can be recognized by focal interstitial scarring associated with fibroblasts and occasional plasma cells and nonpyroninophilic lymphocytes. There has been proposed a slightly modified version of this classification scheme in which an attempt is made to identify features of mild rejection that portend progression to moderate rejection.[999] Another more detailed classification scheme has been proposed by McAllister et al.[1003]

Myocarditis

The various causes and pathophysiologic features of myocarditis have been considered earlier in this chapter. From the point of view of biopsy evaluation, it is important first and foremost to diagnose the presence or absence of myocarditis. This does not always prove to be a trivial task, given that the tissue sample may contain no more than a few myocytes. Confounding this problem is the fact that until recently there were no uniform criteria (such as how many inflammatory cells need be present) on which to base a histologic diagnosis of "myocarditis." To solve this problem, a panel of cardiac pathologists have proposed what has now become known as the "Dallas criteria" for the histopathologic diagnosis of myocarditis (the name derives from the city in which the meeting of these pathologists occurred).[985]

It also is desirable to obtain information from a cardiac biopsy about the likely natural history of a given case of myocarditis. In this regard, a classification system has been proposed in which myocarditis is subclassified as acute, rapidly progressive, or chronic.[994] Whether this system will prove to have prognostic value is yet to be determined.

It also is desirable to obtain information by biopsy regarding the possible cause of myocarditis. In this regard, it is often possible to distinguish three general types of inflammatory disorders, that is, infective myocarditis, hypersensitivity (allergic) myocarditis, and toxic myocarditis.[1002] In infective (viral) myocarditis, the inflammatory infiltrate is usually characterized by a mixed population of cells including primarily lymphocytes but also plasma cells, neutrophils, and macrophages. Hypersensitivity myocarditis occurs as a complication of therapy with a growing list of drugs including sulphonamides, penicillins, streptomycin, isoniazid, amphotericin B, tetracyclines, phenylbutazone, phenytoin, and horse serum.[987,993,1002,1007] This type of myocarditis is characterized by an inflammatory infiltrate composed of eosinophils, plasma cells, and atypical lymphocytes. There usually is no myocyte necrosis in hypersensitivity myocarditis, and the inflammatory response is believed to be reversible when exposure to the offending agent is eliminated. Toxic myocarditis may result from exposure to any one of a large number of agents, including arsenicals, anthracyclines, emetine HCl, lithium carbonate, catecholamines, theophylline, quinidine, antimony, 5-fluorouracil, phenothiazines, cyclophosphamide, paraquat, amphetamines, and some antihypertensive drugs. Cardiotoxicity is often dose-related and cumulative. Myocyte necrosis, which may be associated with a neutrophilic inflammatory response, or necrotizing vasculitis may be observed in biopsy samples.[987,1002]

Adriamycin cardiotoxicity

Adriamycin is an anthracycline compound that has potent antineoplastic properties. Unfortunately, the use of this agent is limited by cardiotoxicity. The degree of cardiotoxicity has been shown to be dose dependent; a cumulative dose of 550 mg/M^2 is almost always well tolerated, but higher doses may cause diffuse myocyte damage and refractory heart failure.[998,1000,1001] The two morphologic hallmarks of adriamycin toxicity are (1) loss of myofibrillar proteins and (2) vacuolization of the sarcoplasm because of swelling of the sarcoplasmic reticulum and T tubules.[988] The severity of these changes can be evaluated by electron microscopy or by light microscopic evaluation of sections from plastic embedded tissue, stained with toluidine blue. The loss of myofibrillar material and sarcoplasmic vacuolization also can be recognized by light microscopic evaluation of paraffin-embedded tissue,[997] especially if Masson's trichrome stain is used. A system for grading the severity of myocyte injury has been developed and is employed at some medical centers on sequential cardiac biopsy specimens to achieve more precise titration of the maximum tolerated dose of adriamycin that can be used in a given person.[988]

REFERENCES
Introduction and cardiac failure
1. National Center for Health Statistics, U.S. Public Health Service, DHHS, as cited in 1987 Heart Facts, Dallas, 1986, American Heart Association.
2. Schlant, R.C., and Sonnenblick, E.M.: Pathophysiology of heart failure. In Hurst, J.W., editor: The heart, New York, 1987, McGraw-Hill Book Co.
3. Siegal, R.S., and Gravanis, M.B.: The cardiovascular system in systemic diseases. In Ahumada, G.G., editor: Cardiovascular pathophysiology, Oxford, 1987, Oxford University Press.

Coronary (ischemic) heart disease
Definition and incidence
4. Ischemic heart disease, WHO Tech. Rep. Ser. no. 117, 1957.
5. Coronary heart disease, WHO Tech. Rep. Ser. no. 168, 1959.
6. Feinleib, M.: The magnitude and nature of the decrease in coronary heart disease mortality rate, Am. J. Cardiol. **54**:2C, 1984.
7. Gillum, R.F., Folsom, A.R., and Blackburn, H.: Decline in coronary heart disease mortality: old questions and new facts, Am. J. Med. **76**:1055, 1984.
8. Goldman, L., and Cook, E.F.: The decline in ischemic heart disease mortality rates: an analysis of the comparative effects of medical interventions and changes in lifestyle, Ann. Intern. Med. **101**:825, 1984.
9. Herrick, J.B.: Clinical features of sudden obstruction of the coronary arteries, JAMA **59**:2015, 1912.
10. Kannel, W.B., and Thom, T.J.: Declining cardiovascular mortality, Circulation **70**:331, 1984.
11. Levy, R.I.: Declining mortality in coronary heart disease, Arteriosclerosis **1**:312, 1981.
12. Pyorala, K., Epstein, F.H., and Kornitzer, M.: Changing trends in coronary heart disease mortality: possible explanations, an editorial, Cardiology **72**:5, 1985.
13. Stamler, J.: The marked decline in coronary heart disease mortality rates in the United States, 1968-1981; summary of findings and possible explanations, Cardiology **72**:11, 1985.
14. Arteriosclerosis: a report by the National Heart and Lung Institute Task Force on Arteriosclerosis (DHEW Pub. no. [NIH] 72-219), vol. 2, Washington, D.C., 1971, Government Printing Office.
15. Enos, W.F., Holmes, R.H., and Beyer, J.: Coronary disease among United States soldiers killed in action in Korea: preliminary report, JAMA **152**:1090, 1953.
16. Glagov, S., Rowley, D.A., and Kohut, R.I.: Atherosclerosis of human aorta and its coronary and renal arteries: a consideration of some hemodynamic factors which may related to the marked differences in atherosclerotic involvement of the coronary and renal arteries, Arch. Pathol. **72**:558, 1961.
17. Hillis, L.D., and Winniford, M.D.: Frequency of severe (70% or more) narrowing of the right, left anterior descending, and left circumflex coronary arteries in right dominant circulations with coronary artery disease, Am. Cardiol. J. **59**:358, 1987.
18. Schwartz, C.J., and Mitchell, J.R.A.: Observations on localization of arterial plaques, Circ. Res. **11**:63, 1962.
19. Sugiura, M., Hiraoka, K., and Ohkawa, S.: Severity of coronary sclerosis in the aged: a pathological study in 968 consecutive autopsy cases, Jpn. Heart J. **17**:471, 1976.
20. Vlodaver, Z., and Edwards, J.E.: Pathology of coronary atherosclerosis, Prog. Cardiovasc. Dis. **14**:256, 1971.

Etiology
21. Abraham, A.S., Sonnenblick, M., Eni, M., Shemesh, O., and Batt, A.P.: Serum chromium in patients with recent and old myocardial infarction, Am. Heart J. **99**:604, 1980.
22. American Heart Association Special Report: Recommendations for the treatment of hyperlipidemia in adults: a joint statement of the Nutrition Committee and the Council on Arteriosclerosis of the American Heart Association, Arteriosclerosis **4**:445A, 1984.
23. National Institutes of Health Consensus Development Conference Statement: Lowering blood cholesterol, JAMA **253**:2080, 1985.
24. Brensike, J.F., Levy R.I., Kelsey, S.F., Passamani, E.R., Richardson, J.M., Loh, I.K., Stone, N.J., Aldrich, R.F., Battaglini, J.W., and Moriarty, D.J.: Effects of therapy with cholestyramine on progression of coronary arteriosclerosis: results of the NHLBI Type II Coronary Intervention Study, Circulation **69**:313, 1984.
25. Chobanian, A.V.: The influence of hypertension and other hemodynamic factors in atherogenesis, Prog. Cardiovasc. Dis. **26**:177, 1983.

26. Colwell, J.A., Winocour, P.D., Lopes-Virella, M., and Halushka, P.V.: New concepts about the pathogenesis of atherosclerosis in diabetes mellitus, Am. J. Med. Nov. 30:67, 1983.
27. Comstock, G.W.: The epidemiologic perspective: water hardness and cardiovascular disease, J. Environ. Pathol. Toxicol. 3:9, 1980.
28. Dunn, F.L.: Hyperlipidemia and diabetes, Med. Clin. North Am. 77:1347, 1982.
29. Eichner, E.R.: Exercise and heart disease: epidemiology of the "exercise hypothesis," Am. J. Med. 75:1008, 1983.
30. Fielding, J.E.: Smoking: health effects and control, N. Engl. J. Med. 313:491, and 555, 1985.
31. Friedman, M., Thoresen, C.E., Gill, J.J., Powell, L.H., Ulmer, D., Thompson, L., Price, V.A., Rabin, D.D., Breall, W.S., and Dixon, T.: Alteration of type A behavior and reduction in cardiac recurrences in postmyocardial infarction patients, Am. Heart J. 108:237, 1984.
32. Gillum, R.F.: Coronary heart disease in black populations. I. Mortality and morbidity, Am. Heart J. 104:839, 1982.
33. Gillum, R.F., and Grant, C.T.: Coronary heart disease in black populations. II. Risk factors, Am. Heart J. 104:852, 1982.
34. Gore, I., Nakashima, T., Imai, T., and White, P.D.: Coronary atherosclerosis and myocardial infarction in Kyushu, Japan, and Boston, Massachusetts, Am. J. Cardiol. 10:400, 1962.
35. Hamby, R.I.: Hereditary aspects of coronary artery disease, Am. Heart J. 101:639, 1981.
36. Heller, R.F., and Jacobs, H.S.: Coronary heart disease in relation to age, sex, and the menopause, Br. Med. J. 1:472, 1978.
37. Holbrook, J.H., Grundy, S.M., Hennekens, C.H., Kannel, W.B., and Strong, J.P.: Cigarette smoking and cardiovascular diseases: a statement for health professionals by a task force appointed by the Steering Committee of the American Heart Association, Circulation 70:1114A, 1984.
38. Hollander, W.: Role of hypertension in atherosclerosis and cardiovascular disease, Am. J. Cardiol. 38:786, 1976.
39. Hubert, H.B., Feinleib, M., McNamara, P.M., and Castelli, W.P.: Obesity as an independent risk factor for cardiovascular disease: a 26-year follow-up of participants in the Framingham Heart Study, Circulation 67:968, 1983.
40. Huttunen, J.K., Länsimies, E., Voutilainen, E., Ehnholm, C., Hietanen, E., Penttilä, I., Siitonen, O., and Rauramaa, R.: Effect of moderate physical exercise on serum lipoproteins: a controlled clinical trial with special reference to serum high-density lipoproteins, Circulation 60:1220, 1979.
41. Kannel, W.B., Castelli, W.P., and Gordon, T.: Cholesterol in the prediction of atherosclerotic disease, Ann. Intern. Med. 90:85, 1979.
42. Kannel, W.B., and McGee, D.L.: Diabetes and cardiovascular risk factors: the Framingham Study, Circulation 59:8, 1979.
43. Kannel, W.B., Wilson, P., and Blair, S.N.: Epidemiological assessment of the role of physical activity and fitness in development of cardiovascular disease, Am. Heart J. 109:876, 1985.
44. Keys, A., and Blackburn, H.: Background of the patient with coronary heart disease, Prog. Cardiovasc. Dis. 6:14, 1963.
45. Klein, L.W.: Cigarette smoking, atherosclerosis and the coronary hemodynamic response: a unifying hypothesis, J. Am. Coll. Cardiol. 4:972, 1984. (Editorial.)
46. Klevay, L.M.: The influence of copper and zinc on the occurrence of ischemic heart disease, J. Environ. Pathol. Toxicol. 4:281, 1980.
47. Lerner, D.J., and Kannel, W.B.: Patterns of coronary heart disease morbidity and mortality in the sexes: a 26-year follow-up of the Framingham population, Am. Heart J. 111:383, 1986.
48. Levine, P.H.: An acute effect of cigarette smoking on platelet function: a possible link between smoking and arterial thrombosis, Circulation 48:619, 1973.
49. Levy, R.I.: Cholesterol and cardiovascular disease: no longer whether, but rather when, in whom, and how? Circulation 72:686, 1985.
50. Levy, R.I., Brensike, J.F., Epstein, S.E., Kelsey, S.F., Passamani, E.R., Richardson, J.M., Loh, I.K., Stone, N.J., Aldrich, R.F., and Battaglini, J.W.: Influence of changes in lipid values induced by cholestyramine and diet on progression of coronary artery disease: results of the NHLBI Type II Coronary Intervention Study, Circulation 69:325, 1984.
51. Lipid Research Clinics Program: The Lipid Research Clinics Coronary Primary Prevention Trial Results. I. Reduction in incidence of coronary heart disease, JAMA 251:351, 1984.
52. Lipid Research Clinics Program: The Lipid Research Clinics Coronary Prevention Trial Results. II. The relationship of reduction in incidence of coronary heart disease to cholesterol lowering, JAMA 251:365, 1984.
53. Luoma, H., Aromaa, A., Helminen, S., Murtomaa, H., Kiviluoto, L., Punsar, S., and Knekt, P.: Risk of myocardial infarction in Finnish men in relation to fluoride, magnesium and calcium concentration in drinking water, Acta Med. Scand. 213:171, 1983.
54. McNamara, J.J., Molot, M.A., and Stremple, J.F.: Coronary artery disease in combat casualties in Vietnam, JAMA 216:1185, 1971.
55. Miller, G.J., and Miller, N.E.: Plasma–high-density-lipoprotein concentration and development of ischaemic heart-disease, Lancet 1:16, 1975.
56. Ritterband, A.B., Jaffe, I.A., and Densen, P.M.: Gonadal function and the development of coronary heart disease, Circulation 27:237, 1963.
57. Rivin, A.U., and Dimitroff, S.P.: The incidence and severity of atherosclerosis in estrogen-treated males, and in females with a hypoestrogenic or a hyperestrogenic state, Circulation 9:533, 1954.
58. Roberts, C.S., and Roberts, W.C.: Cross-sectional area of the proximal portions of the three major epicardial coronary arteries in 98 necropsy patients with different coronary events; relationship to heart weight, age and sex, Circulation 62:953, 1980.
59. Russek, H.I.: Emotional stress and coronary heart disease in American physicians, dentists and lawyers, Am. J. Med. Sci. 243:616, 1962.
60. Shamberger, R.J.: Selenium in the drinking water and cardiovascular disease, J. Environ. Pathol. Toxicol. 4:305, 1980.
61. Shea, S., Ottman, R., Grabrieli, C., Stein, Z., and Nichols, A.: Family history as an independent risk factor for coronary artery disease, J. Am. Coll. Cardiol. 4:793, 1984.
62. ten Kate, L.P., Boman, H., Daiger, S.P., and Motulsky, A.G.: Familial aggregation of coronary heart disease and its relation to known genetic risk factors, Am. J. Cardiol. 50:945, 1982.
63. Weinsier, R.L., Fuchs, R.J., and Kay, T.D., et al.: Body fat: its relationship to coronary heart disease, blood pressure, lipids and other risk factors measured in a large male population, Am. J. Med. 61:815, 1976.
64. White, N.K., Edwards, J.E., and Dry, T.J.: The relationship of the degree of coronary atherosclerosis with age, in men, Circulation 1:645, 1950.
65. Williams, R.S., Logue, E.E., Lewis, J.G., Barton, T., Stead, N.W., Wallace, A.G., and Pizzo, S.V.: Physical conditioning augments the fibrinolytic response to venous occlusion in healthy adults, N. Engl. J. Med. 302:987, 1980.
66. Yater, W.M., et al.: Coronary artery disease in men 18 to 39 years of age: report of 866 cases, 450 with necroscopy examinations, Am. Heart J. 36:334, 481, 683, 1948.

Atherosclerosis—pathology and pathogenesis

67. Benditt, E.P.: Evidence for a monoclonal origin of human atherosclerotic plaques and some implications, Circulation 50:650, 1974.
68. Bevilacqua, M.P., Pober, J.S., Wheeler, M.E., Cotran, R.S., and Gimbrone, M.A., Jr.: Interleukin 1 (IL-1) acts upon vascular endothelium to stimulate procoagulant activity and leukocyte adhesion, J. Cell. Biochem. suppl. 9A:148, 1985. (Abstract.)

69. Criqui, M.H.: Alcohol consumption, blood pressure, lipids, and cardiovascular mortality, Alcoholism **10**:564, 1986.

70. Faggiotto, A., Ross, R., and Harker, L.: Studies of hypercholesterolemia in the nonhuman primate. I. Changes that lead to fatty streak formation, Arteriosclerosis **4**:323, 1984.

71. Fajardo, L.F.: Radiation-induced coronary artery disease, Chest **71**:563, 1977. (Editorial.)

72. Friedman, R.J., Stemerman, M.B., Wenz, B., Moore, S., Gauldie, J., Gent, M., Tiell, M.L., and Spoet, H.: The effect of thrombocytopenia on experimental arteriosclerotic lesion formation in rabbits: smooth muscle cell proliferation and re-endothelialization, J. Clin. Invest. **60**:1191, 1977.

73. Gerrity, R.G.: The role of the monocyte in atherogenesis. I. Transition of blood-borne monocytes into foam cells in fatty lesions, Am. J. Pathol. **103**:181, 1981.

74. Gerrity, R.G.: The role of the monocyte in atherogenesis. II. Migration of foam cells from atherosclerotic lesions, Am. J. Pathol. **103**:191, 1981.

75. Goldstein, J.L., and Brown, M.S.: Atherosclerosis: the low-density lipoprotein receptor hypothesis, Metabolism **26**:1257, 1977.

76. Harker, L.A., Harlan, J.M., and Ross, R.: Effect of sulfinpyrazone on homocysteine-induced endothelial injury and arteriosclerosis in baboons, Circ. Res. **53**:731, 1983.

77. Haust, M.D.: The morphogenesis and fate of potential and early atherosclerotic lesions in man, Hum. Pathol. **2**:1, 1971.

78. Kinlough-Rathbone, R.L., and Mustard, J.F.: Atherosclerosis: current concepts, Am. J. Surg. **141**:638, 1981.

79. Manuck, S.B., Kaplan, J.R., and Matthews K.A.: Behavioral antecendents of coronary heart disease and atherosclerosis, Arteriosclerosis **6**:2, 1986.

80. Nilsson, J.: Growth factors and the pathogenesis of atherosclerosis, Atherosclerosis **62**:185, 1986.

81. Pearson, T.A., Kramer, E.C., and Solez, K., et al.: The human atherosclerotic plaque, Am. J. Pathol. **86**:657, 1977.

82. Rohan, T.E.: Alcohol and ischemic heart disease: a review, Aust. NZ J. Med. **14**:75, 1984.

83. Ross, R.: The pathogenesis of atherosclerosis—an update, N. Engl. J. Med. **314**:488, 1986.

84. Ross, R., Faggiotto, A., Bowen-Pape, D., and Reuines, E.: The pathogenesis of atherosclerosis, Circulation **70**(suppl. III):III-77, 1984.

85. Ross, R., and Glomset, J.A.: The pathogenesis of atherosclerosis, N. Engl. J. Med. **295**:369 and 420, 1976.

86. Rossi E.C.: Inhibitors of platelet function and atherogenesis, Artery **5**:273, 1979.

87. Simon, E.B., Ling, J., Mendizabal, R.C., and Midwall, J.: Radiation-induced coronary artery disease, Am. Heart J. **108**:1032, 1984.

88. Small, D.M.: Cellular mechanisms for lipid deposition in atherosclerosis, N. Engl. J. Med. **297**:873 and 924, 1977.

89. Spain, D.M.: Atherosclerosis, Sci. Am. **215**:48, 1966.

90. Strong, J.P., and McGill, H.C.: The natural history of coronary atherosclerosis, Am. J. Pathol. **40**:37, 1962.

91. Thomas, W.A., and Kim, D.N.: Biology of disease: atherosclerosis as a hyperplastic and/or neoplastic process, Lab. Invest. **48**:245, 1983.

92. Woolf, N.: Thrombosis and atherosclerosis, Br. Med. Bull. **34**:137, 1978.

Other causes of coronary artery disease

93. Ahronheim, J.H.: Isolated coronary periarteritis: report of a case of unexpected death in a young pregnant woman, Am. J. Cardiol. **40**:287, 1977.

94. Aufderheide, A.C., Henke, B.W., and Parker, E.H.: Granulomatous coronary arteritis (Takayasu's disease), Arch. Pathol. Lab. Med. **105**:647, 1981.

95. Befeler, B., Aranda, M.J., and Embi, A.: Coronary artery aneurysms: study of their etiology, clinical course and effect on left ventricular function and prognosis, Am. J. Med. **62**:597, 1977.

96. Bulkley, B.H., and Roberts, W.C.: Dissecting aneurysm (hematoma) limited to coronary artery: a clinicopathologic study of six patients, Am. J. Med. **55**:747, 1973.

97. Burch, G.E., and Winsor, T.: Syphilitic coronary stenosis with myocardial infarction, Am. Heart J. **24**:740, 1942.

98. Claudon, D.G., Claudon, D.B., and Edwards, J.E.: Primary dissecting aneurysm of coronary artery: a cause of acute myocardial ischemia, Circulation **45**:259, 1972.

99. Eslami, B., and Paine, T.: Coronary artery aneurysms: report of seven cases and review of the pertinent literature, Jpn. Heart J. **21**:185, 1980.

100. Gore, I., Smith, J., and Clancy, R.: Congenital aneurysms of the coronary arteries with a report of a case, Circulation **19**:221, 1959.

101. Gower, N.D., and Pinkerton, J.R.H.: Idiopathic arterial calcification in infancy, Arch. Dis. Child. **38**:408, 1963.

102. Gross, L., Dugel, M.A., and Epstein, E.Z.: Lesions of coronary arteries and their branches in rheumatic fever, Am. J. Pathol. **11**:253, 1935.

103. Moran, J.J.: Idiopathic arterial calcification of infancy: a clinicopathologic study. In Sommers, S.C., editor: Pathology annual, New York, 1975, Appleton-Century-Crofts.

104. Moritz, A.R.: Injuries of heart and pericardium by physical violence. In Gould, S.E., editor: Pathology of the heart, ed. 3, Springfield, Ill., 1968, Charles C Thomas, Publisher.

105. Morris, P.B., Imber, M.J., Heinsimer, J.A., Hlatky, M.A., and Reimer, K.A.: Rheumatoid arthritis and coronary arteritis, Am. J. Cardiol. **57**:689, 1986.

106. Parmley, L.F., Manion, W.C., and Mattingly, T.W.: Nonpenetrating wounds of the heart and aorta, Circulation **18**:371, 1958.

107. Rose, A.G., and Sinclair-Smith, C.C.: Takayasu's arteritis: a study of 16 autopsy cases, Arch. Pathol. Lab. Med. **104**:231, 1980.

108. Shrader, E.L., Bawell, M.B., and Moragues, V.: Coronary embolism, Circulation **14**:1159, 1956.

109. Smith, J.C.: Dissecting aneurysms of coronary arteries, Arch. Pathol. **99**:117, 1975.

110. Susmano, A., Muenster, J.J., Javid, H., and Carleton, R.A.: Coronary arteritis in rheumatoid arthritis, Arch. Intern. Med. **132**:241, 1973.

111. Woodruff, I.O.: Cardiovascular syphilis, Am. J. Med. **4**:248, 1948.

Consequences of coronary artery disease

112. Baba, N., Bashe, W.J., Jr., and Keller, M.D., et al.: Pathology of atherosclerotic heart disease in sudden death. I. Organizing thrombosis and acute coronary vessel lesion, Circulation **52**(6, suppl. 3):III-53, 1975.

113. Bashe, W.J., Jr., Baba, N., and Keller, M.D.: Pathology of atherosclerotic heart disease in sudden death. II. The significance of myocardial infarction, Circulation **52**(suppl. 3):III-63, 1975.

114. Cobb, L.A., Baum, R.S., Alvarez, H., III: Resuscitation from out-of-hospital ventricular fibrillation: 4 years follow up, Circulation **50**(6):123-5, 1974.

115. Cohn, P.F., and Braunwald, E.: Chronic ischemic heart disease. In Braunwald, E., editor: Heart disease: a textbook of cardiovascular medicine, Philadelphia, 1984, W.B. Saunders Co.

116. Davies, M.J., and Thomas, A.: Thrombosis and acute coronary-artery lesions in sudden cardiac ischemic death, N. Engl. J. Med. **310**:1137, 1984.

117. El-Maraghi, N., and Genton, E.: The relevance of platelet and fibrin thromboembolism of the coronary microcirculation, with special reference to sudden cardiac death, Circulation **62**:936, 1980.

118. Friedman, M., Manwaring, J.H., and Rosenman, R.H.: Instantaneous and sudden deaths: clinical and pathological differentiation in coronary artery disease, JAMA **225**:1319, 1973.

119. Fuster, V., Steele, P.M., and Chesebro, J.H.: Role of platelets and thrombosis in coronary atherosclerotic disease and sudden death, J. Am. Coll. Cardiol. **5**:175B, 1985.

120. 1987 Heart facts, Dallas, 1986, American Heart Association.

121. Hinkle, L.E., and Thaler, H.T.: Clinical classification of cardiac deaths, Circulation **65**:457, 1982.

122. James, T.N.: Chance and sudden death, J. Am. Coll. Cardiol. **1**:164, 1983.
123. Lie, J.T., and Titus, J.L.: Pathology of the myocardium and the conduction system in sudden coronary death, Circulation **51**(suppl. 3):III-41, 1975.
124. McIntosh, H.D.: The stabilizing and unstabilizing influences of neurogenic and vascular activities of the heart as related to sudden cardiac death, J. Am. Coll. Cardiol. **5**:105B, 1985.
125. Myers, A., and Dewar, H.A.: Circumstances attending 100 sudden deaths from coronary artery disease with coroner's necropsies, Br. Heart J. **37**:1133, 1975.
126. Reichenbach, D.D., Moss, N.S., and Meyer, E.: Pathology of the heart in sudden cardiac death, Am. J. Cardiol. **39**:865, 1977.
127. Roberts, W.C., and Jones, A.A.: Quantitation of coronary arterial narrowing at necropsy in sudden coronary death: analysis of 31 patients and comparison with 25 control subjects, Am. J. Cardiol. **44**:39, 1979.
128. Scott, R.F., and Briggs, T.S.: Pathologic findings in pre-hospital deaths due to coronary atherosclerosis, Am. J. Cardiol. **29**:782, 1972.
129. Surawicz, B.: Ventricular fibrillation, J. Am. Coll. Cardiol. **5**:43B, 1985.

Myocardial infarction

130. Baigrie, R.S., Haq, A., Morgan, C.D., Rakowski, H., Drobac, M., and McLaughlin, P.: The spectrum of right ventricular involvement in inferior wall myocardial infarction: a clinical, hemodynamic and noninvasive study, J. Am. Coll. Cardiol. **1**:1396, 1983.
131. Baroldi, G.: Functional morphology of the anastomotic circulation in human cardiac pathology. In Bajusz, E., and Jasmin, G., editors: Functional morphology of the heart, Basel, 1971, S. Karger AG.
132. Baroldi, G, Mantero, O., and Scomazzoni, G.: The collaterals of the coronary arteries in normal and pathologic hearts, Circ. Res. **9**:223, 1956.
133. Baughman, K.L., Maroko, P.R., and Vatner, S.F.: Effects of coronary artery reperfusion on myocardial infarct size and survival in conscious dogs, Circulation **63**:317, 1981.
134. Becker, L.C., Fortuin, N.J., and Pitt, B.: Effect of ischemia and antianginal drugs on the distribution of radioactive microspheres in the canine left ventricle, Circ. Res. **28**:263, 1971.
135. Blumgart, H., Schlesinger, M., and Davis, D.: Studies on the relationship of the clinical manifestations of angina pectoris, coronary thrombosis, and myocardial infarction to the pathologic findings, Am. Heart J. **19**:1, 1940.
136. Blumgart, H.L., Schlesinger, M.J., and Zoll, P.M.: Angina pectoris, coronary failure and acute myocardial infarction: the role of coronary occlusions and collateral circulation, JAMA **116**:91, 1941.
137. Chapman, I.: Morphogenesis of occluding coronary artery thrombosis, Arch. Pathol. **80**:256, 1965.
138. Cohen, M.W.: The functional value of coronary collaterals in myocardial ischemia and therapeutic approach to enhance collateral flow, Am. Heart J. **95**:396, 1978.
139. Connelly, C., Vogel, W.M., Hernández, Y.M., and Apstein, C.S.: Movement of necrotic wavefront after coronary artery occlusion in rabbit, Am. J. Physiol. **243**:H682, 1982.
140. Cushing, E.H., Feil, H., Stanton, E.J., and Wartman, W.B.: Infarction of cardiac auricles (atria): clinical, pathological, and experimental studies, Br. Heart J. **4**:17, 1942.
141. Davies, M.J., and Thomas, A.C.: Plaque fissuring—the cause of acute myocardial infarction, sudden ischaemic death, and crescendo angina, Br. Heart J. **53**:363, 1985.
142. Davies M.J., Woolf, N., and Robertson, W.B.: Pathology of acute myocardial infarction with particular reference to occlusive coronary thrombi, Br. Heart J. **38**:659, 1976.
143. DeWood, M.A., Spores, J., Notske, R., Mauser, L.T., Burroughs, R., Golden, M.S., and Lang, H.T.: Prevalence of total coronary occlusion during the early hours of transmural myocardial infarction, N. Engl. J. Med. **303**:897, 1980.
144. Downey, J.M.: Why the endocardium: In Hearse, D.J., and Yellon, D.M., editors: Therapeutic approaches to myocardial infarct size limitation, New York, 1984, Raven Press.
145. Dunn, R.B., and Griggs, D.M., Jr.: Transmural gradients in ventricular tissue metabolites produced by stopping coronary blood flow in the dog, Circ. Res. **37**:438, 1975.
146. Edwards, J.E.: Pathologic spectrum of occlusive coronary arterial disease, Lab. Invest. **5**:475, 1956.
147. Factor, S.M., Okun, E.M., Minase, T., and Kirk, E.S.: The microcirculation of the human heart: end-capillary loops with discrete perfusion fields, Circulation **66**:1241, 1982.
148. Falk, E.: Plaque rupture with severe pre-existing stenosis precipitating coronary thrombosis: characteristics of coronary atherosclerotic plaques underlying fatal occlusive thrombi, Br. Heart J. **50**:127, 1983.
149. Folts, J.D., Gallagher, K., and Rowe, G.G.: Blood flow reductions in stenosed canine coronary arteries: vasospasm or platelet aggregation? Circulation **65**:248, 1982.
150. Friedman, M.: The coronary thrombus: its origin and fate, Hum. Pathol. **2**:81, 1971.
151. Fulton, W.F.M.: Arterial anastomoses in the coronary circulation. I. Anatomical features in normal and diseased hearts demonstrated by stereoarteriography, Scot. Med. J. **8**:420, 1963.
152. Fulton, W.F.M.: Anastomotic enlargement and ischaemic myocardial damage, Br. Heart J. **26**:1, 1964.
153. Geary, G.G., Smith, G.T., and McNamara, J.J.: Quantitative effect of early coronary artery reperfusion in baboons: extent of salvage of the perfusion bed of an occluded artery, Circulation **66**:391, 1982.
154. Gorlin, R.: Dynamic vascular factors in the genesis of myocardial ischemia, J. Am. Coll. Cardiol. **3**:897, 1983.
155. Gregg, D.E.: The natural history of coronary collateral development, Circ. Res. **35**:335, 1974.
156. Hillis, L.D., and Braunwald, E.: Myocardial ischemia, N. Engl. J. Med. **296**:971, 1034, and 1093, 1977.
157. Isner, J.M., and Roberts, W.C.: Right ventricular infarction complicating left ventricular infarction secondary to coronary heart disease, Am. J. Cardiol. **42**:885, 1978.
158. Jennings, R.B.: Early phase of myocardial ischemic injury and infarction, Am. J. Cardiol. **24**:753, 1969.
159. Jennings, R.B., Sommers, H.M., Smyth, G.A., Flack, H.A., and Linn, H.: Myocardial necrosis induced by temporary occlusion of a coronary artery in the dog, Arch. Pathol. **70**:68, 1960.
160. Khouri, E.M., Gregg, D.E., and McGranahan, G.M.: Regression and reappearance of coronary collaterals, Am. J. Physiol. **220**:655, 1971.
161. Klein, H.H., Schubothe, M., Nebendahl, K., and Kreuzer, H.: Temporal and spatial development of infarcts in porcine hearts, Basic Res. Cardiol. **79**:440, 1984.
162. Lee, J.T., Ideker, R.E., and Reimer, K.A.: Myocardial infarct size and location in relation to the coronary-vascular bed at risk in man, Circulation **64**:526, 1981.
163. Lowe, J.E., Cummings, R.G., Adams, D.H., and Hull-Ryde, E.A.: Evidence that ischemic cell death begins in the subendocardium independent of variations in collateral flow or wall tension, Circulation **68**:190, 1983.
164. Maseri, A., and Chierchia, S.: Coronary artery spasm: demonstration, definition, diagnosis, and consequences, Prog. Cardiovasc. Dis. **25**:169, 1982.
165. Maseri, A., L'Abbate, A., Baroldi, G., Chierchia, S., Marzilli, M., Ballestra, A.M., Severi, S., Parodi, O., Biagini, A., Bistante, A., and Pesola, A.: Coronary vasospasm as a possible cause of myocardial infarction, N. Engl. J. Med. **299**:1271, 1978.
166. Murry, C.E., Jennings, R.B., and Reimer, K.A.: Preconditioning with ischemia: a delay of lethal cell injury in ischemic myocardium, Circulation **74**:1124, 1986.
167. Newman, P.E.: The coronary collateral circulation: determinants and functional significance in ischemic heart disease, Am. Heart J. **102**:431, 1981.

168. Oliva, P.B., and Breckinridge, J.C.: Arteriographic evidence of coronary arterial spasm in acute myocardial infarction, Circulation **56:**366, 1977.

169. O'Reilly, R.J., and Spellberg, R.D.: Rapid resolution of coronary arterial emboli: myocardial infarction and subsequent normal coronary arteriograms, Ann. Intern. Med. **81:**348, 1974.

170. Ratliff, N.B., and Hackel, D.B.: Combined right and left ventricular infarction: pathogenesis and clinicopathologic correlations, Am. J. Cardiol. **45:**217, 1980.

171. Reimer, K.A.: Myocardial infarct size: measurements and predictions, Arch. Pathol. Lab. Med. **104:**225, 1980.

172. Reimer, K.A., and Jennings, R.B.: The "wavefront phenomenon" of myocardial ischemic cell death. II. Transmural progression of necrosis within the framework of ischemic bed size (myocardium at risk) and collateral flow, Lab. Invest. **40:**633, 1979.

173. Reimer, K.A., Lowe, J.E., Rasmussen, M.M., and Jennings, R.B.: The wavefront phenomenon of ischemic cell death. I. Myocardial infarct size vs. duration of coronary occlusion in dogs, Circulation **56:**786, 1977.

174. Ridolfi, R.L., and Hutchins, G.M.: The relationship between coronary artery lesions and myocardial infarcts: ulceration of atherosclerotic plaques precipitating coronary thrombosis, Am. Heart J. **93:**468, 1977.

175. Rivas, F., Cobb, F.R., and Bache, R.J.: Relationship between blood flow to ischemic regions and extent of myocardial infarction: serial measurement of blood flow to ischemic regions in dogs, Circ. Res. **38:**439, 1976.

176. Roberts, W.C.: Relationship between coronary thrombosis and myocardial infarction, Mod. Concepts Cardiovasc. Dis. **41:**7, 1972.

177. Roberts, W.C., and Buja, L.M.: The frequency and significance of coronary arterial thrombi and other observations in fatal acute myocardial infarction: a study of 107 necropsy patients, Am. J. Med. **52:**425, 1972.

178. Roberts, N., Harrison, D.G., Reimer, K.A., Crain, B.S., and Wagner, G.S.: Right ventricular infarction with shock but without significant left ventricular infarction: a new clinical syndrome, Am. Heart J. **110:**1047, 1985.

179. Savage, R.M., Wagner, G.S., and Ideker, R.E.: Correlation of postmortem anatomic findings with electrocardiographic changes in patients with myocardial infarction: retrospective study of patients with typical anterior and posterior infarcts, Circulation **55:**279, 1977.

180. Schaper, W., Frenzel, H., and Hort, W.: Experimental coronary artery occlusion. I. Measurement of infarct size, Basic Res. Cardiol. **74:**46, 1979.

181. Schaper, W., Frenzel, H., Hort, W., and Winkler, B.: Experimental coronary artery occlusion. II. Spatial and temporal evolution of infarcts in the dog heart, Basic Res. Cardiol. **74:**233, 1979.

182. Silver, M.D., Baroldi, G., and Mariani, F.: The relationship between acute occlusive coronary thrombi and myocardial infarction studied in 100 consecutive patients, Circulation **61:**219, 1980.

183. Snow, P., Jones, A., and Dawber, R.: Coronary disease: a pathological study, Br. Heart J. **17:**503, 1955.

184. Vesterby, A., and Steen, M.: Isolated right ventricular myocardial infarction: a case report, Acta Med. Scand. **216:**233, 1984.

185. Wartman, W.B., and Souders, J.C.: Localization of myocardial infarcts with respect to the muscle bundles of the heart, Arch. Pathol. **50:**329, 1950.

186. Wilkinson, R.S., Schaefer, J.A., and Abildskov, J.A.: Electrocardiographic and pathologic features of myocardial infarction in man, Am. J. Cardiol. **11:**24, 1963.

187. Wusten, B., Flameng, W., and Schaper, W.: The distribution of myocardial flow. I. Effects of experimental coronary occlusion, Basic Res. Cardiol. **69:**422, 1974.

Cardiac metabolic and ultrastructural effects of ischemia

188. Armiger, L.C., Herdson, P.B., and Gavin, J.B.: Mitochondrial changes in dog myocardium induced by lactate in vivo, Lab. Invest. **32:**502, 1975.

189. Armiger, L.C., Seelye, R.N., and Phil, D.: Fine structural changes in dog myocardium exposed to lowered pH in vivo, Lab. Invest. **37:**237, 1977.

190. Chambers, D.E., Parks, D.A., Patterson, G., Roy, R., McCord, J.M., Yoshida, S., Parmley, L.F., and Downey, J.M.: Xanthine oxidase as a source of free radical damage in myocardial ischemia, J. Mol. Cell. Cardiol. **17:**145, 1985.

191. Chien, K.R., Reeves, J.P., Buja, L.M., Bonte, F., Parkey, R.W., and Willerson, J.T.: Phospholipid alterations in canine ischemic myocardium: temporal and topographical correlations with Tc-99m-PP$_i$ accumulation and an in vitro sarcolemmal Ca$_2^+$ permeability defect, Circ. Res. **48:**711, 1981.

192. Engler, R.L., Schmid-Schönbein, G.W., and Pavelec, R.S.: Leukocyte capillary plugging in myocardial ischemia and reperfusion in the dog, Am. J. Pathol. **111:**98, 1983.

193. Feinberg, H., Rosenbaum, D.S., Laritsky, S., Silverman, N.A., Kohler, J., and LeBreton, G.: Platelet deposition after surgically induced myocardial ischemia: an etiologic factor for reperfusion injury, J. Thorac. Cardiovasc. Surg. **84:**815, 1982.

194. Fishbein, M.C., Y-Rit, J., Lando, U., Kanmatsuse, K., Mercier, J.C., and Ganz, W.: The relationship of vascular injury and myocardial hemorrhage to necrosis after reperfusion, Circulation **62:**1274, 1980.

195. Freeman, B.A., and Crapo, J.D.: Biology of disease: free radicals and tissue injury, Lab. Invest. **47:**412, 1982.

196. Ganote, C.E.: Contraction band necrosis and irreversible myocardial injury, J. Mol. Cell. Cardiol. **15:**67, 1983.

197. Gevers, W.: Generation of protons by metabolic processes in heart cells, J. Mol. Cell. Cardiol. **9:**867, 1977.

198. Haack, D.W., Bush, L.R., Shlafer, M., and Lucchesi, B.R.: Lanthanum staining of coronary microvascular endothelium: effects of ischemia, reperfusion, propranolol, and atenolol, Microvasc. Res. **21:**362, 1981.

199. Humphrey, S.M., Gavin, J.B., and Herdson, P.B.: The relationship of ischemic contracture to vascular reperfusion in the isolated rat heart, J. Mol. Cell. Cardiol. **12:**1397, 1980.

200. Jennings, R.B., Hawkin, H.K., Lowe, J.E., Hill, M.L., Klotman, S., and Reimer, K.A.: Relation between high energy phosphate and lethal injury in myocardial ischemia in the dog, Am. J. Pathol. **92:**187, 1978.

201. Jennings, R.B., and Reimer, K.A.: Lethal myocardial ischemic injury, Am. J. Pathol. **102:**241, 1981.

202. Jennings, R.B., and Reimer, K.A.: Factors involved in salvaging ischemic myocardium: effect of reperfusion of arterial blood, Circulation **68:**I-25, 1983.

203. Jennings, R.B., Schaper, J., Hill, M.L., Steenbergen, C., Jr., and Reimer, K.A.: Effect of reperfusion late in the phase of reversible ischemic injury: changes in cell volume, electrolytes, metabolites, and ultrastructure, Circ. Res. **56:**262, 1985.

204. Jolly, S.R., Kane, W.J., Bailie, M.B., Abrams, G.D., and Lucchesi, B.R.: Canine myocardial reperfusion injury: its reduction by the combined administration of superoxide dismutase and catalase, Circ. Res. **54:**277, 1984.

205. Katz, A.M., and Messineo, F.C.: Lipid-membrane interactions and the pathogenesis of ischemic damage in the myocardium, Circ. Res. **48:**1, 1981.

206. Katz, A.M., and Reuter, H.: Cellular calcium and cardiac cell death, Am. J. Cardiol. **44:**188, 1979.

207. Kloner, R.A., Ganote, C.E., and Jennings, R.B.: The "no-reflow" phenomenon after temporary coronary occlusion in the dog, J. Clin. Invest. **54:**1496, 1974.

208. Kloner, R.A., Ganote, C.E., Whalen, D.A., and Jennings, R.B.: Effect of a transient period of ischemia on myocardial cells. II. Fine structure during the first few minutes of reflow, Am. J. Pathol. **74:**399, 1974.

209. Liedtke, A.J.: Alterations of carbohydrate and lipid metabolism in the acutely ischemic heart, Prog. Cardiovasc. Dis. **23:**321, 1981.

210. Moore, K.H., Radloff, J.F., Hull, F.E., and Sweeley, C.C.: Incomplete fatty acid oxidation by ischemic heart: β-hydoxy fatty acid production, Am. J. Physiol. **239:**H257, 1980.

211. Mukherjee, A., Bush, L.R., McCoy, K.E., Duke, R.J., Hagler, H., Buja, L.M., and Willerson, J.T.: Relationship between beta adrenergic receptor numbers and physiological responses during experimental canine myocardial ischemia, Circ. Res. **50:**735, 1982.

212. Muntz, K.H., Hafler, H.K., Boulas, H.J., Willerson, J.F., and Buja, L.M.: Redistribution of catecholamines in the ischemic zone of the dog heart, Am. J. Pathol. **114:**64, 1984.

213. Nayler, W.G.: The role of calcium in the ischemic myocardium, Am. J. Pathol. **102:**262, 1981.

214. Neely, J.R., and Feuvray, D.: Metabolic products and myocardial ischemia, Am. J. Pathol. **102:**282, 1981.

215. Neely, J.R., and Grootyohann, L.W.: Role of glycolytic products in damage to ischemic myocardium: dissociation of adenosine triphosphate levels and recovery of function of reperfused ischemic hearts, Circ. Res. **55:**816, 1984.

216. Prinzen, F.W., van der Vusse, G.J., Arts, T., Roemen, T.H., Coumans, W.A., and Reneman, R.S.: Accumulation of nonesterified fatty acids in ischemic canine myocardium, Am. J. Physiol. **247:**H264, 1984.

217. Rao, P.S., Cohen, M.V., and Mueller, H.S.: Production of free radicals and lipid peroxides in early experimental myocardial ischemia, J. Mol. Cell. Cardiol. **15:**713, 1983.

218. Reimer, K.A., and Ideker, R.E.: Myocardial ischemia and infarction: anatomic and biochemical substrates for ischemic cell death and ventricular arrhythmias, Hum. Pathol. **18:**462, 1987.

219. Reimer, K.A., and Jennings, R.B.: Myocardial ischemia, hypoxia, and infarction. In Fozzard, H.A., editor: The heart and cardiovascular system, New York, 1986, Raven Press.

220. Reimer, K.A., Jennings, R.B., and Tatum, A.H.: Pathobiology of acute myocardial ischemia: metabolic, functional and ultrastructural studies, Am. J. Cardiol. **52:**72A, 1983.

221. Reimer, K.A., Murry, C.E., Yamasawa, I., Hill, M.L., and Jennings, R.B.: Four brief periods of myocardial ischemic cause no cumulative ATP loss or necrosis, Am. J. Physiol. **251:**H1306, 1986.

222. Romson, J.L., Hook, B.G., Kunkel, S.L., Abrams, G.D., Schork, M.A., and Lucchesi, B.R.: Reduction of the extent of ischemic myocardial injury by neutrophil depletion in the dog, Circulation **67:**1016, 1983.

223. Schaper, J., Mulch, J., Winkler, B., and Schaper, W.: Ultrastructural, functional, and biochemical criteria for estimation of reversibility of ischemic injury: a study on the effects of global ischemia on the isolated dog heart, J. Mol. Cell. Cardiol. **11:**521, 1979.

224. Steenbergen, C., Hill, M.L., and Jennings, R.B.: Volume regulation and plasma membrane injury in aerobic, anaerobic, and ischemic myocardium in vitro: effect of osmotic cell swelling on plasma membrane integrity, Circ. Res. **57:**864, 1985.

225. West, P.N., Connors, J.P., Clark, R.E., Weldon, C.S., Ramsey, D.L., Roberts, R., Sobel, B.E., and Williamson, J.R.: Compromised microvascular integrity in ischemic myocardium, Lab. Invest. **38:**677, 1978.

226. Williamson, J.R., Schaeffer, S.W., and Ford, C.: Contribution of tissue acidosis to ischemic injury in the perfused rat heart, Circulation **53:**I-3, 1976.

Early diagnosis of myocardial infarction

227. Bajusz, E., and Jasmin, G.: Histochemical studies on the myocardium following experimental interference with coronary circulation in the rat. I. Occlusion of coronary artery, Acta Histochem. **18:**222, 1964.

228. Fallon, J.T.: Simplified method for histochemical demonstration of experimental myocardial infarct, Circulation, **60:**11-42, 1979.

229. Fine, G., Morales, A., and Scerpella, J.R.: Experimental myocardial infarction: a histochemical study, Arch. Pathol. **82:**4, 1966.

230. Fishbein, M.C., Meerbaum, S., Rit, J., Lando, U., Kanmatsuse, K., Mercier, J.C., Corday, E., and Ganz, W.: Early phase acute myocardial infarct size quantification: validation of the triphenyl tetrazolium chloride tissue enzyme staining technique, Am. Heart J. **101:**593, 1981.

231. Hecht, A.: Enzyme histochemistry of heart muscle in normal and pathologic conditions, Methods Achiev. Exp. Pathol. **5:**384, 1971.

232. Kent, S.P.: Diffusion of plasma proteins into cells: a manifestation of cell injury in human myocardial ischemia, Am. J. Pathol. **50:**623, 1967.

233. Kent, S.P., and Diseker, M.: Early myocardial ischemia: study of histochemical changes in dogs, Lab. Invest. **4:**398, 1955.

234. Klein, H.H., Puschmann, S., Schaper, J., and Schaper, W.: The mechanism of the tetrazolium reaction in identifying experimental myocardial infarction, Virchows Arch. [Pathol. Anat.] **393:**287, 1981.

235. Klionsky, B.: Myocardial ischemia and early infarction: a histochemical study, Am. J. Pathol. **36:**575, 1960.

236. Lie, J.T., Holley, K.E., and Kampa, W.R.: New histologic method for morphologic diagnosis of early stages of myocardial ischemia, Mayo Clin. Proc. **46:**319, 1971.

237. Lie, J.T., Pairolers, P.C., and Holley, K.E.: Macroscopic enzyme-mapping: verification of large homogeneous, experimental myocardial infarcts of predictable size and location in dogs, J. Thorac. Cardiovasc. Surg. **69:**599, 1975.

238. Nachlas, M.M., and Shnitka, T.K.: Macroscopic identification of early myocardial infarcts by alterations in dehydrogenase activity, Am. J. Pathol. **42:**379, 1963.

239. Rose, A.G., Opie, L.H., and Bricknell, O.L.: Early experimental myocardial infarction: evaluation of histologic criteria and comparison with biochemical and electrocardiographic measurements, Arch. Pathol. Lab. Med. **100:**516, 1976.

240. Schultz, T.C., and Skinner, J.M.: The post-mortem myocardial potassium sodium ratio in detection of infarction, Pathology **13:**313, 1981.

241. Shnitka, T.K., and Nachlas, M.M.: Histochemical alterations in ischemic heart muscle and early myocardial infarction, Am. J. Pathol. **42:**507, 1963.

242. Sybers, H.D., Ashraf, M., and Brauthwaite, J.R.: Early myocardial infarction: a fluorescent method of detection, Arch. Pathol. **93:**49, 1972.

243. Van Reempts, J., Borgers, M., and Reneman, R.S.: Early myocardial ischaemia: evaluation of the histochemical haematoxylin–basic fuchsin–picric acid (BFP) staining technique, Cardiovasc. Res. **10:**262, 1976.

244. Wachstein, M., and Meisel, E.: Succinic dehydrogenase activity in myocardial infarction and in induced myocardial necrosis, Am. J. Pathol. **31:**353, 1955.

245. Yokoyama, H.O., Jennings, R.B., Clabaugh, G.F., and Wartman, W.B.: Histochemical studies of early experimental myocardial infarction, Arch. Pathol. **59:**347, 1955.

246. Zugibe, F.T., Bell, P., Jr., and Conley, T.: Determination of myocardial alterations at autopsy in the absence of gross and microscopic changes, Arch. Pathol. **81:**409, 1966.

Inflammatory response and reparative phase

247. Anversa, P., Beghi, C., Kikkawa, Y., and Olivetti, G.: Myocardial response to infarction in the rat: morphometric measurement of infarct size and myocyte cellular hypertrophy, Am. J. Pathol. **118:**484, 1985.

248. Bing, R.J.: Reparative processes in heart muscle following myocardial infarction, Cardiology **56:**314, 1971/72.

249. Fantone, J.C., and Ward, P.A.: Role of oxygen-derived free radicals and metabolites in leukocyte-dependent inflammatory reactions, Am. J. Pathol. **107:**397, 1982.

250. Giclas, P.C., Pinckard, R.N., and Olson, M.S.: In vitro activation of complement by isolated human heart subcellular membranes, J. Immunol. **122:**146, 1979.

251. Hammerman, H., Schoen, F.J., and Kloner, R.A.: Short-term exercise has a prolonged effect on scar formation after experimental acute myocardial infarction, J. Am. Coll. Cardiol. **2:**979, 1983.

252. Hill, J.H., and Ward, P.A.: The phlogistic role of C3 leukotac-

tic fragments in myocardial infarcts of rats, J. Exp. Med. **133**:885, 1971.

253. Lerman, R.H., Apstein, C.S., Kogan, H.M., Osmer, E.L., Chichester, C.O., Vogel, W.M., Connelly, C.M., and Steffee, W.P.: Myocardial healing and repair after experimental infarction in the rabbit, Circ. Res. **53**:378, 1983.

254. Mullane, K.M., Read, N., Salmon, J.A., and Moncada, S.: Role of leukocytes in acute myocardial infarction in anesthetized dogs: relationship to myocardial salvage by anti-inflammatory drugs, J. Pharmacol. Exp. Ther. **228**:510, 1984.

255. Palmer, R.M.J., Stepney, R.J., Higgs, G.A., and Eakins, K.E.: Chemokinetic activity of arachidonic and lipoxygenase products on leukocytes of different species, Prostaglandins **20**:411, 1980.

256. Pinckard, R.N., Olson, M.S., and Giclas, P.C.: Consumption of classical complement components by heart subcellular membranes in vitro and in patients after acute myocardial infarction, J. Clin. Invest. **56**:740, 1975.

257. Pinckard, R.N., O'Rourke, R.A., Crawford, M.H., Grover, F.S., McManus, L.M., Ghidoni, J.J., Storrs, S.B., and Olson, M.S.: Complement localization and mediation of ischemic injury in baboon myocardium, J. Clin. Invest. **66**:1050, 1980.

258. Reimer, K.A., and Jennings, R.B.: The changing anatomic reference base of evolving myocardial infarction: underestimation of myocardial collateral blood flow and overestimation of experimental anatomic infarct size due to tissue edema, hemorrhage and acute inflammation, Circulation **60**:866, 1979.

259. Rossen, R.D., Swain, J.L., Michael, L.H., Weakley, S., Giannini, E., and Entman, M.L.: Selective accumulation of the first component of complement and leukocytes in ischemic canine heart muscle: a possible initiator of an extra myocardial mechanism of ischemic injury, Circ. Res. **57**:119, 1985.

260. Rubin, S.A., Fishbein, M.C., and Swan, H.J.C.: Compensatory hypertrophy in the heart after myocardial infarction in the rat, J. Am. Coll. Cardiol. **1**:1435, 1983.

261. Sato, S., Ashraf, M., Millard, R.W., Fujiwara, H., and Schwartz, A.: Connective tissue changes in early ischemia of porcine myocardium: an ultrastructural study, J. Mol. Cell. Cardiol. **15**:261, 1983.

262. Schifferman, E.: Leukocyte chemotaxis, Annu. Rev. Physiol. **44**:553, 1982.

263. Shetlar, M.R., Shetlar, C.L., and Kischer, C.W.: Healing of myocardial infarction in animal models, Tex. Rep. Biol. Med. **39**:339, 1979.

264. Snyderman, R., and Goetzl, E.: Molecular and cellular mechanisms of leukocyte chemotaxis, Science **213**:830, 1981.

265. Ward, P.A., Hugli, J.E., and Chenoweth, D.: Complement and chemotaxis. In Houck, J.C., editor: Chemical messengers of the inflammatory process, Amsterdam, 1979, Elsevier/North Holland Biomedical Press.

266. Weissman, G., Smolen, J., and Korchak, H.: Release of inflammatory mediators from stimulated neutrophils, N. Engl. J. Med. **303**:27, 1980.

267. Wilkinson, P.C.: Chemotaxis and inflammation, London, 1974, Churchill Livingstone.

Gross and microscopic patterns of infarction

268. Bouchardy, B., and Majno, G.: Histopathology of early myocardial infarcts: a new approach, Am. J. Pathol. **74**:301, 1974.

269. Fishbein, M.C., Maclean, D., and Maroko, P.R.: The histopathologic evolution of myocardial infarction, Chest **73**:843, 1978.

270. Lodge-Patch, I.: The ageing of cardiac infarcts, and its influence on cardiac rupture, Br. Heart J. **13**:37, 1951.

271. Mallory, G.K., White, P.D., and Salcedo-Salgar, J.: The speed of healing of myocardial infarction: a study of the pathologic anatomy in seventy-two cases, Am. Heart J. **18**:647, 1939.

272. Sommers, H.M., and Jennings, R.B.: Experimental acute myocardial infarction: histologic and histochemical studies of early myocardial infarcts induced by temporary or permanent occlusion of a coronary artery, Lab. Invest. **13**:1491, 1964.

Complications of infarction

273. Abelman W.H.: Classification and natural history of primary myocardial disease, Prog. Cardiovasc. Disc. **26**:73, 1984.

274. Asinger, R.W., Mikell, F.L., Elsperger, J., and Hodges, M.: Incidence of left ventricular thrombosis after acute transmural myocardial infarction, N. Engl. J. Med. **305**:297, 1981.

275. Bates, R.J., Beutler, S., and Resnekov, L.: Cardiac rupture: challenge in diagnosis and management, Am. J. Cardiol. **40**:429, 1977.

276. Becker, A.E., Lie, K.I., and Anderson, R.H.: Bundle-branch block in the setting of acute anteroseptal myocardial infarction, Br. Heart J. **40**:773, 1978.

277. Burch, G.E., Tsui, C.Y., and Harb, J.M.: Ischemic cardiomyopathy, Am. Heart J. **83**:340, 1972.

278. Cabin, H.S., and Roberts, W.C.: Left ventricular aneurysm, intraaneurysmal thrombus and systemic embolus in coronary heart disease, Chest **77**:586, 1980.

279. Caulfield, J.B., Leinbach, R., and Gold, H.: The relationship of myocardial infarct size and prognosis, Circulation **53**:141, 1976.

280. da Luz, P.L., Weil, M.H., and Shubin, H.: Current concepts on mechanisms and treatment of cardiogenic shock, Am. Heart J. **92**:103, 1976.

281. Davies, M.J.: The cardiomyopathies: a review of terminology, pathology and pathogenesis, Histopathology, **8**:363, 1984.

282. Davis, R.W., and Ebert, P.A.: Ventricular aneurysm: a clinical-pathologic correlation, Am. J. Cardiol. **29**:1, 1972.

283. Dubnow, M.H., Burchell, H.B., and Titus, J.L.: Postinfarction ventricular aneurysm: a clinicomorphologic and electrocardiographic study of 80 cases, Am. Heart J. **70**:753, 1965.

284. Eaton, L.W., Weiss, J.L., Bulkley, B.H., Garrison, J.B., and Weisfeldt, M.L.: Regional cardiac dilation after acute myocardial infarction, N. Engl. J. Med. **300**:57, 1979.

285. Edwards, B.S., Edwards, W.D., and Edwards, J.E.: Ventricular septal rupture complicating acute myocardial infarction: identification of simple and complex types in 53 autopsied hearts, Am. J. Cardiol. **54**:1201, 1984.

286. Griffith, G.C., Hegde, B., and Oblath, R.W.: Factors in myocardial rupture, Am. J. Cardiol. **8**:792, 1961.

287. Grondin, P., Kretz, J.G., Bical, O., Denzeau-Gorge, P., Petitclerc, R., and Campeau, L.: Natural history of saccular aneurysms of the left ventricle, J. Thorac. Cardiovasc. Surg. **77**:57, 1979.

288. Gutovitz, A.L., Sobel, B.E., and Roberts, R.: Progressive nature of myocardial injury in selected patients with cardiogenic shock, Am. J. Cardiol. **41**:469, 1978.

289. Hackel, D.B., Wagner, G., and Ratliff, N.B.: Anatomic studies of the cardiac conducting system in acute myocardial infarction, Am. Heart J. **97**:165, 1979.

290. Hutchins, G.M.: Rupture of the interventricular septum complicating myocardial infarction: pathological analysis of 10 patients with clinically diagnosed perforations, Am. Heart J. **97**:165, 1979.

291. Hutchins, G.M., and Bulkley, B.H.: Infarct expansion versus extension: two different complications of acute myocardial infarction, Am. J. Cardiol. **41**:1127, 1978.

292. Jones, M.E., Terry, G., and Kenmure, A.C.F.: Frequency and significance of conduction defects in acute myocardial infarction, Am. Heart J. **94**:163, 1977.

293. Khan, A.H.: Pericarditis of myocardial infarction: review of the literature with case presentation, Am. Heart J. **90**:788, 1975.

294. Kohn, R.M.: Mechanical factors in cardiac rupture, Am. J. Cardiol. **4**:279, 1959.

295. Lewis, A.J., Burchell, H.B., and Titus, J.L.: Clinical and pathologic features of postinfarction cardiac rupture, Am. J. Cardiol. **23**:43, 1969.

296. Lichstein, E., Arsura, E., Hollander, G., Greengart, A., and Sanders M.: Current incidence of postmyocardial infarction (Dressler's) syndrome, Am. J. Cardiol. **50**:1269, 1982.

297. Mittal, A.K., Langston, M., Jr., and Cohn, K.E.: Combined papillary muscle and left ventricular wall dysfunction as a cause of mitral regurgitation, Circulation **44**:174, 1971.

298. Naeim, F., Maza, L.M., and Robbins, S.L.: Cardiac rupture during myocardial infarction, Circulation 45:1231, 1972.

299. Olearchyk, A.S., Lemole, G.M., and Spagna, P.M.: Left ventricular aneurysm, J. Thorac. Cardiovasc. Surg. 88:544, 1984.

300. Page, D.L., Caulfield, J.B., and Kastor, J.A.: Myocardial changes associated with cardiogenic shock, N. Engl. J. Med. 285:133, 1971.

301. Pantely, G.A., and Bristow, J.D.: Ischemic cardiomyopathy, Prog. Cardiovasc. Dis. 27:95, 1984.

302. Perloff, J.K., and Roberts, W.C.: The mitral apparatus: functional anatomy of mitral regurgitation, Circulation 46:227, 1972.

303. Sanders, C.A., Armstrong, P.W., and Willerson, J.T.: Etiology and differential diagnosis of acute mitral regurgitation, Prog. Cardiovasc. Dis. 14:129, 1971.

304. Scheidt, S., Ascheim, R., and Killip, T., III: Shock after acute myocardial infarction: a clinical and hemodynamic profile, Am. J. Cardiol. 26:556, 1970.

305. Schuster, E.H., and Bulkley, B.H.: Expansion of transmural myocardial infarction: a pathophysiologic factor in cardiac rupture, Circulation 60:1532, 1979.

306. Schuster, E.H., and Bulkley, B.H.: Ischemic cardiomyopathy; a clinicopathologic study of fourteen patients, Am. Heart J. 100:506, 1980.

307. Shelburne, J.C., Rubenstein, D., and Gorlin, R.: A reappraisal of papillary muscle dysfunction, Am. J. Med. 46:862, 1969.

308. Tsakiris, A.G., Rastelli, G.C., Amorim, D. de S.: Effect of experimental papillary muscular damage in mitral valve closure in intact anaesthetized dogs, Mayo Clin. Proc. 45:275, 1970.

309. Wei, J.Y., Hutchins, G.M., and Bulkley, B.H.: Papillary muscle rupture in fatal acute myocardial infarction: a potentially treatable form of cardiogenic shock, Ann. Intern. Med. 90:149, 1979.

310. Wessler, S., Zoll, P.M., and Schlesinger, M.J.: The pathogenesis of spontaneous cardiac rupture, Circulation 6:334, 1952.

311. Van Tassel, R.A., and Edwards, J.E.: Rupture of heart complicating myocardial infarction: analysis of 40 cases including nine examples of left ventricular false aneurysm, Chest 61:104, 1972.

312. Virmani, R., and Roberts, W.C.: Quantification of coronary arterial narrowing and of left ventricular myocardial scarring in healed myocardial infarction with chronic, eventually fatal, congestive cardiac failure, Am. J. Med. 68:831, 1980.

313. Vlodaver, Z., and Edwards, J.E.: Rupture of ventricular septum or papillary muscle complicating myocardial infarction, Circulation 55:815, 1977.

Inflammatory heart disease
Rheumatic fever—incidence, etiology, and pathogenesis

314. Bland, E.F.: Declining severity of rheumatic fever, N. Engl. J. Med. 262:597, 1960.

315. Boyd, W.: A textbook of pathology, Philadelphia, ed. 4, 1943, Lea & Febiger.

316. Catanzaro, F.J., et al.: Symposium on rheumatic fever and rheumatic heart disease: role of streptococcus in pathogenesis of rheumatic fever, Am. J. Med. 17:749, 1954.

317. Cavelti, P.A.: Studies on pathogenesis of rheumatic fever: experimental production of autoantibodies to heart, skeletal muscle, and connective tissue, Arch. Pathol. 44:13, 1947.

318. Coburn, A.F., and Pauli, R.H.: Interaction of host and bacterium in development of communicability by Streptococcus haemolyticus, J. Exp. Med. 73:551, 1941.

319. Dale, J.B., and Beachey, E.H.: Multiple heart-cross-reactive epitopes of streptococcal M proteins, J. Exp. Med. 161:113, 1985.

320. Denny, F.W.: T. Duckett Jones and rheumatic fever in 1986, Circulation 76:963, 1987.

321. Gordis, L.: The virtual disappearance of rheumatic fever in the United States: lessons in the rise and fall of disease, Circulation 72:1155, 1985.

322. Jones, T.D.: The diagnosis of rheumatic fever, JAMA 126:481, 1944.

323. Jones, T.D.: Criteria (revised) from guidance in the diagnosis of rheumatic fever, Circulation 69:204A, 1984.

324. Kaplan, M.H., and Svec, K.H.: Immunologic relation of streptococcal and tissue antigens. III. Presence in human sera of steptococcal antibody cross-reactive with heart tissue: association with streptococcal infection, rheumatic fever, and glomerulonephritis, J. Exp. Med. 119:651, 1964.

325. Kaplan, M.H.: Rheumatic fever, rheumatic heart disease, and the streptococcal connection: the role of streptococcal antigens cross-reactive with heart tissue, Rev. Infect. Dis. 1:988, 1979.

326. Land, M.A., and Bisno, A.L.: Acute rheumatic fever: a vanishing disease in suburbia, JAMA 249:895, 1983.

327. Murphy, G.E., and Swift, H.F.: Induction of rheumatic-like cardiac lesions, closely resembling those of rheumatic fever, in rabbits following repeated skin infections with a group A streptococci, J. Exp. Med. 89:687, 1949.

328. Pearce, J.M.: Heart disease and filterable viruses, Circulation 21:448, 1960.

329. Rammelkamp, C.H., Jr., Wannamaker, L.W., and Denney, F.W.: Epidemiology and prevention of rheumatic fever, Bull. NY Acad. Med. 28:321, 1952.

330. Rich, A.R., and Gregory, J.E.: Experimental evidence that lesions with basic characteristics of rheumatic carditis can result from anaphylactic hypersensitivity, Bull. Johns Hopkins Hosp. 73:239, 1943.

331. Saslaw, M.S., and Streitfield, M.M.: Group A beta hemolytic strepococci in relation to rheumatic fever: study of school children in Miami, Florida, Am. J. Dis. Child. 92:550, 1956.

332. Senitzer, D., and Freimer, E.H.: Autoimmune mechanisms in the pathogenesis of rheumatic fever, Rev. Infect. Dis. 6:832, 1984.

333. Siegal, A.C., Johnson, E.E., and Stollerman, G.H.: Controlled studies of streptococcal pharyngitis in a pediatric population. I. Factors related to the attack rate of rheumatic fever, N. Engl. J. Med. 265:559, 1961.

334. Silberner, J.: The return of rheumatic fever, Science News 130:228, 1986.

335. Stamler, J.: Cardiovascular disease in the United States, Am. J. Cardiol. 10:319, 1962.

336. Stollerman, G.H.: Nephrogenic and rheumatogenic group A streptococci, J. Infect. Dis. 120:258, 1969.

337. Veasy, G., Weidmeier, S.E., Orsmond, G.S., Ruttenberg, H.D., Boucek, M.M., Roth, S.J., Tait, V.F., Thompson, J.A., Daly, J.A., Kaplan, E.I., and Hill, H.R.: Resurgence of acute rheumatic fever in the intermountain area of the United States, N. Engl. J. Med. 316:421, 1987.

Rheumatic fever—predisposing factors

338. Ayoub, E.M.: The search for host determinants of susceptibility to rheumatic fever: the missing link, Circulation 69:197, 1984.

339. Community control of rheumatic heart disease in developing countries: a major public health problem, WHO Chron. 34:336, 1980.

340. García-Palmieri, M.R.: Rheumatic fever and rheumatic heart disease as seen in the tropics, Am. Heart J. 64:577, 1962.

341. Maharaj, B., Hammond, M.G., Appadoo, B., Leary, W.P., and Pudifin, D.J.: HLA-A, B, DR, and DQ antigens in black patients with severe chronic rheumatic heart disease, Circulation 76:259, 1987.

342. Markowitz, M.: Observations in the epidemiology and preventability of rheumatic fever in developing countries, Clin. Ther. 4:240, 1981.

343. Saslaw, M.S.: Rheumatic fever in subtropical climate: clinical behavior and management, J. Fl. Med. Assoc. 41:357, 1954.

344. Saslaw, M.S., and Johnson, L.C.: Frequency of rheumatic heart disease in Miami, Florida: autopsy findings, Am. Heart J. 53:814, 1957.

345. Saslaw, M.S., Hernández, F.A., and Randolph, H.E.: Five and ten year follow-up study of rheumatic patients: role of climate and environment, Am. J. Cardiol. 3:754, 1959.

346. Shaper, A.G.: Cardiovascular disease in the tropics. I. Rheumatic heart, Br. Med. J. 3:683, 1972.

347. Shefferman, M.M., Goodman, J.S., Ultan, L.B., and Valdés, J.: Acute rheumatic fever in Puerto Rico, Am. J. Dis. Child. 110:239, 1965.

348. Tamer, D.M.: Acute rheumatic fever in a south Florida county hospital, Circulation 50:765, 1974.

349. Wilson, M.G.: Advances in rheumatic fever, New York, 1962, Harper & Row Publishers, Inc.

Cardiac manifestations of rheumatic fever

350. Angevine, D.M.: Pathology of rheumatic disease, Radiology 49:1, 1947.

351. Becker, C.G., and Murphy, G.E.: Demonstration of contractile protein in endothelium and cells of the heart valves, endocardium, intima, arteriosclerotic plaques, and Aschoff bodies of rheumatic heart disease, Am. J. Pathol. 55:1, 1969.

352. Bland, E.F., and Jones, T.D.: Rheumatic fever and rheumatic heart disease: 20 year report on 1000 patients since childhood, Circulation 4:836, 1951.

353. Clawson, B.J.: Rheumatic heart disease: analysis of 796 cases, Am. Heart J. 20:454, 1940.

354. Clawson, B.J.: Relation of Anitschkow "myocyte" to rheumatic inflammation, Arch. Pathol. 32:760, 1941.

355. Dalldorf, F.G., and Murphy, G.E.: Relationship of Aschoff bodies in cardiac arterial appendages to the natural history of rheumatic heart, Am. J. Pathol. 37:507, 1960.

356. Ehrlich, J.C., and Lapan, B.: Anitschkow "myocyte," Arch. Pathol. 28:361, 1938.

357. Entiknap, J.B.: Biopsy of left auricle in mitral stenosis, Br. Heart J. 15:37, 1953.

358. Friedberg, C.K., and Gross, L.: Pericardial lesions in rheumatic fever, Am. J. Pathol. 12:183, 1936.

359. Gross, L.: Cardiac lesions in Libman-Sacks disease, with consideration of its relationship to acute diffuse lupus erythematosus, Am. J. Pathol. 16:375, 1940.

360. Gross, L., and Ehrlich, J.C.: Studies on myocardial Aschoff body: descriptive classification of lesions, Am. J. Pathol. 10:467, 1934.

361. Gross, L., and Friedberg, C.K.: Lesions of cardiac valves in rheumatic fever, Am. J. Pathol. 12:855, 1936.

362. Hadfield, G., and Garrod, R.P.: Recent advances in pathology, ed. 5, Philadelphia, 1947, McGraw-Hill Book Co.

363. Hall, E.M., and Anderson, L.R.: Incidence of rheumatic stigmas in hearts which are usually considered nonrheumatic, Am. Heart J. 25:64, 1943.

364. Hutchins, G.M., and Payne, K.T.: Possible origin of myocardial Aschoff bodies of rheumatic fever from nerves, Johns Hopkins Med. J. 132:315, 1973.

365. Janton, O.H., Glover, R.P., O'Neill, T.J.E., Gregory, J.E., and Froio, G.F.: Results of surgical treatment for mitral stenosis: analysis of 100 consecutive cases, Circulation 6:321, 1952.

366. Lannigan, R.: The rheumatic process in the left auricular appendage, J. Pathol. Bacteriol. 77:49, 1959.

367. Manchester, B., Scotti, T.M., Reynolds, M.L., and Dawson, W.H.: Aschoff bodies in left auricular appendages of patients with mitral stenosis: clinicopathologic study, including postoperative follow-up, Arch. Intern. Med. 95:231, 1955.

368. Murphy, G.E.: The characteristic rheumatic lesions of striated and of nonstriated or smooth muscle cells known as Aschoff bodies and those myogenic components known as Aschoff cells or as Anitschkow cells or myocytes, Medicine 42:73, 1963.

369. Pappenheimer, A.W., and von Glahn, W.C.: Lesions of aorta associated with acute rheumatic fever, and with chronic cardiac disease of rheumatic origin, J. Med. Res. 44:489, 1924.

370. Roberts, W.C., and Virmani, R.: Aschoff bodies at necropsy in valvular heart disease, Circulation 57:803, 1978.

371. Sabiston, D.C., Jr., and Follis, R.H., Jr.: Lesions in auricular appendages removed at operations for mitral stenosis of presumed rheumatic origin, Bull. Johns Hopkins Hosp. 91:178, 1952.

372. Saphir, O.: The Aschoff nodule, Am. J. Clin. Pathol. 31:534, 1959.

373. Saphir, O., and Langendorf, R.: Nonspecific myocarditis in acute rheumatic fever, Am. Heart J. 46:432, 1953.

374. Saphir, O., and Lowenthal, M.: Changes in endocardium of pigs simulating rheumatic stigmata of man, Am. J. Pathol. 27:211, 1951.

375. Scott, R.F., Thomas, W.A., and Kissane, J.M.: Rheumatic pneumonitis: pathologic features, J. Pediatr. 54:60, 1959.

376. Tedeschi, C.G., Wagner, B.M., and Pani, K.C.: Studies in rheumatic fever: clinical significance of Aschoff body based on morphologic observations, Arch. Pathol. 60:408, 1955.

377. Virmani, R., and Roberts, W.C.: Aschoff bodies in operatively excised atrial appendages and in papillary muscles: frequency and clinical significance, Circulation 55:559, 1977.

378. Wagner, B.M., and Tedeschi, C.G.: Studies in rheumatic fever: origin of cardiac giant cells, Arch. Pathol. 60:423, 1955.

379. Wallach, J.B., Borgatta, E.F., and Angrist, A.A.: Rheumatic heart disease, Springfield, Ill., 1962, Charles C Thomas, Publisher.

380. Wallach, J.B., Lukash, L., and Angrist, A.A.: Mechanisms of death in rheumatic heart disease in different age periods, Am. J. Clin. Pathol. 26:360, 1956.

381. Wedum, B.G., and McGuire, J.W.: Origin of the Aschoff body, Ann. Rheum. Dis. 22:127, 1963.

Rheumatoid arthritis and ankylosing spondylitis

382. Baggenstoss, A.H., and Rosenberg, E.F.: Unusual cardiac lesions associated with chronic multiple rheumatoid arthritis, Arch. Pathol. 37:54, 1944.

383. Bergfeldt, L., Edhag, O., and Vallin, H.: Cardiac conduction disturbances, an underestimated manifestation in ankylosing spondylitis: a 25 year follow-up study of 68 patients, Acta Med. Scand. 212:217, 1982.

384. Bonfiglio, T., and Atwater, E.C.: Heart disease in patients with seropositive rheumatoid arthritis: a controlled autopsy study and review, Arch. Intern. Med. 124:714, 1969.

385. Bulkley, B.H., and Roberts, W.C.: Ankylosing spondylitis and aortic regurgitation: description of the characteristic cardiovascular lesion from study of eight necropsy patients, Circulation 48:1014, 1973.

386. Burney, D.P., Martin, C.E., Thomas, C.S., Fisher, R.D., and Bender, H.W., Jr.: Rheumatoid pericarditis: clinical significance and operative management, J. Thorac. Cardiovasc. Surg. 77:511, 1979.

387. Clark, W.S., Kulka, J.P., and Bauer, W.: Rheumatoid aortitis with aortic regurgitation: an unusual manifestation of rheumatoid arthritis (including spondylitis), Am. J. Med. 22:580, 1957.

388. Cruickshank, B.: Heart lesions in rheumatoid disease, J. Pathol. Bacteriol. 76:223, 1958.

389. Davidson, P., Baggenstoss, A.H., and Slocumb, C.H.: Cardiac and aortic lesions in rheumatoid spondylitis, Mayo Clin. Proc. 36:427, 1963.

390. Hoffman, F.G., and Leight, L.: Complete atrioventricular block associated with rheumatoid disease, Am. J. Cardiol. 16:585, 1965.

391. Karten, I.: Arteritis, myocardial infarction, and rheumatoid arthritis, JAMA 210:1717, 1969.

392. Kirk, J., and Cosh, J.: The pericarditis of rheumatoid arthritis, Q. J. Med. 38:397, 1969.

393. Kulka, J.P.: The vascular lesions associated with rheumatoid arthritis, Bull. Rheum. Dis. 10:201, 1959.

394. Lebowitz, W.B.: The heart in rheumatoid arthritis (rheumatoid disease): a clinical and pathological study of 62 cases, Ann. Intern. Med. 58:102, 1963.

395. Lev, M., Bharati, S., and Hoffman, F.G.: The conduction system in rheumatoid arthritis with complete atrioventricular block, Am. Heart J. 90:78, 1975.

396. Morris, P.B., Imber, M.J., Heinsimer, J.A., Hlatky, M.A., and Reimer, K.A.: Rheumatoid arthritis and coronary arteritis, Am. J. Cardiol. 57:689, 1986.

397. Reed, W.B.: Psoriatic arthritis: a complete clinical study of 86 patients, Acta Derm. Venereol. **41**:396, 1961.
398. Reimer, K.A., Rodgers, R.F., and Oyasu, R.: Rheumatoid heart disease and granulomatous aortitis, JAMA **235**:2510, 1976.
399. Rodnan, G.P., Benedek, T.G., Shaver, J.A.: Reiter's syndrome and aortic insufficiency, JAMA **189**:889, 1964.
400. Ruppert, G.B., Lindsay, J., and Barth, W.F.: Cardiac conduction abnormalities in Reiter's syndrome, Am. J. Med. **73**:335, 1982.
401. Sobin, L.H., and Hagstrom, J.W.C.: Lesions of cardiac conduction tissue in rheumatoid aortitis, JAMA **180**:1, 1962.
402. Sokoloff, L.: Cardiac involvement in rheumatoid arthritis and allied disorders: current concepts, Mod. Concepts Cardiovasc. Dis. **33**:847, 1964.
403. Toone, E.C., Pierce, E.L., and Hennigar, G.R.: Aortitis and aortic regurgitation associated with rheumatoid spondylitis, Am. J. Med. **26**:255, 1959.
404. Weintraub, A.M., and Zvaifler, N.J.: The occurrence of valvular and myocardial disease in patients with chronic joint deformity: clinical studies, Am. J. Med. **35**:145, 1963.

Syphilitic (luetic) heart disease

405. Centers for Disease Control, annual summary 1980: Morbidity and mortality in the United States, MMWR **29**:78, 1981.
406. Heggtveit, H.A.: Syphilitic aortitis: a clinicopathological autopsy study of 100 cases, Circulation **29**:346, 1964.
407. Hiraoka, K., Ohkawa, S., and Sugiura, M.: A clinicopathological study on the syphilitic aortic regurgitation in the aged, Jpn. Heart J. **14**:22, 1973.
408. Martland, H.S.: Syphilis of aorta and heart, Am. Heart J. **6**:1, 1930.
409. Phillips, J.H., Jr., and Burch, G.E.: A review of cardiovascular diseases in the white and black races, Medicine **39**:241, 1960.
410. Saphir, O., and Scott, R.W.: Involvement of aortic valve in syphilitic aortitis, Am. J. Pathol. **3**:527, 1927.

Libman-Sacks endocarditis

411. Allen, A.C., and Sirota, J.H.: Morphogenesis and significance of degenerative verrucal endocarditis (terminal endocarditis, endocarditis simplex, nonbacterial thrombotic endocarditis), Am. J. Pathol. **20**:1025, 1944.
412. Libman, E.: Characterization of various forms of endocarditis, JAMA **80**:813, 1923.
413. Libman, E., and Sacks, B.: A hitherto undescribed form of valvular and mural endocarditis, Arch. Intern. Med. **33**:701, 1924.

Nonbacterial thrombotic endocarditis (NBTE)

414. Angrist, A.A., and Oka, M.: Pathogenesis of bacterial endocarditis, JAMA **183**:249, 1963.
415. Barry, W.E., and Scarpelli, D.: Nonbacterial thrombotic endocarditis: a clinicopathologic study, Arch. Intern. Med. **109**:151, 1962.
416. Bedikian A., Valdivieso, M., Luna, M., and Bodey, G.P.: Nonbacterial thrombotic endocarditis in cancer patients: comparison of characteristics of patients with or without concomitant disseminated intravascular coagulation, Med. Pediatr. Oncol. **4**:149, 1978.
417. Bryan, C.S.: Nonbacterial thrombotic endocarditis with malignant tumors, Am. J. Med. **46**:787, 1969.
418. Deppisch, L.M., and Fayemi, A.O.: Nonbacterial thrombotic endocarditis: clinicopathologic correlations, Am. Heart J. **92**:723, 1976.
419. Fayemi, A.O., and Deppisch, L.M.: Coronary embolism and myocardial infarction associated with nonbacterial thrombotic endocarditis, Am. J. Clin. Pathol. **68**:393, 1977.
420. Kim, H.S., Suzuki, M., Lie, J.T.: Nonbacterial thrombotic endocarditis (NBTE) and disseminated intravascular coagulation (DIC): autopsy study of 36 patients, Arch. Pathol. Lab. Med. **101**:65, 1977.

421. Kooiker, J.C., MacLean, J.M., and Sumi, S.M.: Cerebral embolism, marantic endocarditis and cancer, Arch. Neurol. **33**:260, 1976.
422. MacDonald, R.A., and Robbins, S.L.: The significance of nonbacterial thrombotic endocarditis: an autopsy and clinical study of 78 cases, Ann. Intern. Med. **46**:255, 1957.
423. Pineo, G.F., Regoeczi, E., and Hatton, M.W., et al.: The activation of coagulation by extracts of mucus: a possible pathway of intravascular coagulation accompanying adenocarcinomas, J. Lab. Clin. Med. **82**:255, 1973.
424. Rohner, R.F., Prior, J.T., and Sipple, J.H.: Mucinous malignancies, venous thrombosis and terminal endocarditis with emboli: a syndrome, Cancer **19**:1805, 1966.
425. Rosen, P., and Armstrong, D.: Nonbacterial thrombotic endocarditis in patients with malignant neoplastic disease, Am. J. Med. **54**:23, 1973.
426. Sack, G.H., Jr., Levin, J., and Bell, W.R.: Trousseau's syndrome and other manifestations of chronic disseminated coagulopathy in patients with neoplasms: clinical, pathophysiologic, and therapeutic features, Medicine **56**:1, 1977.
427. Waller, B.F., Knapp, W.S., and Edwards, J.E.: Marantic valvular vegetations, Circulation **48**:644, 1973.
428. Weick, J.K.: Intravascular coagulation in cancer, Semin. Oncol. **5**:203, 1978.

Infective endocarditis

429. Braimbridge, M.V.: Cardiac surgery and bacterial endocarditis, Lancet **1**:1307, 1969.
430. Bryan, C.S., Sutton, J.P., Saunders, D.E., Jr., Longaker, D.W., and Smith, C.W.: Endocarditis related to transvenous pacemakers: syndromes and surgical implications, J. Thorac. Cardiovasc. Surg. **75**:758, 1978.
431. Burch, G.E., and De Pasquale, N.P.: Viral endocarditis, Am. Heart J. **67**:721, 1964.
432. Cates, J.E., and Christie, R.V.: Subacute bacterial endocarditis: review of 442 patients treated in 14 centers appointed by Penicillin Trials Committee of Medical Research Council, Q. J. Med. **20**:93, 1951.
433. Chase, R.M., Jr.: Infective endocarditis today, Med. Clin. North Am. **57**:1383, 1973.
434. Clemens, J.D., Horwitz, R.I., Jaffe, C.C., Feinstein, A.R., and Stanton, B.F.: A controlled evaluation of the risk of bacterial endocarditis in persons with mitral-valve prolapse, N. Engl. J. Med. **307**:776, 1982.
435. Cohen, P.S., Maguire, J.H., and Weinstein, L.: Infective endocarditis caused by gram-negative bacteria: a review of the literature, 1945-1977, Prog. Cardiovasc. Dis. **22**:205, 1980.
436. Come, P.C.: Infective endocarditis: current perspectives, Compr. Ther. **8**:57, 1982.
437. Ferrans, V.J., Boyce, S.W., Billingham, M.E., Spray, T.L., and Roberts, W.C.: Infection of glutaraldehyde-preserved porcine valve heterografts, Am J. Cardiol. **43**:1123, 1979.
438. Geiger, A.J., and Durlacker, S.H.: Fate of endocardial vegetations following penicillin treatment, Am. J. Pathol. **23**:1023, 1947.
439. Glaser, R.S., and Riskind, D.: The diagnosis and treatment of bacterial endocarditis, Med. Clin. North Am. **47**:1285, 1967.
440. Griffin, M.R., Wilson, W.R., Edwards, W.D., O'Fallon, W.M., and Kurland, L.T.: Infective endocarditis: Olmsted County, Minnesota, 1950 through 1981, JAMA **254**:1199, 1985.
441. Grist, N.R.: Rickettsial endocarditis, Br. Med. J. **53**:8, 1963.
442. Hamburger, M.: Acute and subacute bacterial endocarditis, Arch. Intern. Med. **112**:1, 1963.
443. Hayward, G.W.: Infective endocarditis: a changing disease, Br. Med. J. **2**:706, 1983.
444. Hermans, P.E.: The clinical manifestation of infective endocarditis, Mayo Clin. Proc. **57**:15, 1982.
445. Ivert, T.S.A., Dismukes, W.E., Cobbs, C.G., Blackstone, E.H., Kirklin, J.W., and Bergdahl, L.A.: Prosthetic valve endocarditis, Circulation **69**:223, 1984.
446. Kauffmann, R.H., Thompson, J., Valentijn, R.M., Daha,

M.R., and Van Es, L.A.: The clinical implications and the pathogenetic significance of circulating immune complexes in infective endocarditis, Am. J. Med. **71**:17, 1981.

447. Kaye, D.: Changes in the spectrum, diagnosis and management of bacterial and fungal endocarditis, Med. Clin. North Am. **57**:941, 1973.
448. Kaye, D.: Infective endocarditis: a review, Am. J. Med. **78**:107, 1985.
449. Lerner, P.I., and Weinstein, L.: Infective endocarditis in the antibiotic era, N. Engl. J. Med. **274**:199, 1966.
450. Marshall, C.E., and Shappell, S.D.: Sudden death and the ballooning posterior leaflet syndrome: detailed anatomic and histochemical investigation, Arch. Pathol. **98**:134, 1974.
451. McCarthy, L.J., and Wolf, P.L.: Mucoid degeneration of heart valves; "blue valve syndrome," Am. J. Clin. Pathol. **54**:852, 1970.
452. Merchant, R.K., Louria, D.B., Geisler, P.H., Edjcomb, J.H., and Litz, J.P.: Fungal endocarditis: review of the literature and report of three cases, Ann. Intern. Med. **48**:242, 1958.
453. Moore, R.A.: Cellular mechanisms of recovery after treatment with penicillin: subacute bacterial endocarditis, J. Lab. Clin. Med. **31**:1279, 1946.
454. Morgan, W.L., and Bland, E.F.: Bacterial endocarditis in the antibiotic era: with special reference to the later complications, Circulation **19**:753, 1959.
455. Nelson, R.J., Harley, D.P., French, W.J., and Boyer, A.S.: Favorable 10 year experience with valve procedures for active infective endocarditis, J. Thorac. Cardiovasc. Surg. **87**:493, 1984.
456. Neugarten, J., and Baldwin, D.S.: Glomerulonephritis in bacterial endocarditis, Am. J. Med. **77**:297, 1984.
457. Osler, W.: The Gulstonian lectures on malignant endocarditis, Br. Med. J. **1**:467, 1985.
458. Pankey, G.A.: Subacute bacterial endocarditis at the University of Minnesota Hospital, 1939 through 1959, Ann. Intern. Med. **55**:550, 1961.
459. Pankey, G.A.: Acute bacterial endocarditis at the University of Minnesota Hospital, Am. Heart J. **64**:583, 1962.
460. Pankey, G.A.: Infective endocarditis: changing concepts, Hosp. Pract. **21**:103, 1986.
461. Pelletier, L.L., Jr., and Petersdorf, R.G.: Infective endocarditis: a review of 125 cases from the University of Washington Hospitals, 1963-1972, Medicine **56**:287, 1977.
462. Pesanti, E.L., and Smith, I.M.: Infective endocarditis with negative blood cultures: an analysis of 52 cultures, Am. J. Med. **66**:43, 1979.
463. Reisberg, B.E.: Infective endocarditis in the narcotic addict, Prog. Cardiovasc. Dis. **22**:193, 1979.
464. Robinson, M.J., and Ruedy, J.: Sequelae of bacterial endocarditis, Am. J. Med. **32**:922, 1962.
465. Robinson, M.J., Greenberg, J.J., and Korn M.: Infective endocarditis at autopsy, Am. J. Med. **52**:492, 1972.
466. Saphir, O.: Nonrheumatic inflammatory diseases of the heart. In Gould, S.E., editor: Pathology of the heart, ed. 2, Springfield, Ill., 1960, Charles C Thomas, Publisher.
467. Sheldon, W.H., and Golden, A.: Abscesses of valve rings of heart, frequent but not well recognized complication of acute bacterial endocarditis, Circulation **4**:1, 1951.
468. Sohal, R.S., and Burch, G.E.: Electron microscopy study of the endocardium in coxsackie virus B4 infected mice, Am. J. Pathol. **55**:133, 1969.
469. Shulman, S.T., Amren, D.P., Bisno, A.L., Dajani, A.S., Durack, D.T., Gerber, M.A., Kaplan, E.L., Millard, H.D., Sanders, W.E., and Schwartz, R.H.: Prevention of bacterial endocarditis, Circulation **70**:1123, 1984.
470. Stinson, E.B.: Surgical treatment of infective endocarditis, Prog. Cardiovasc. Dis. **22**:145, 1979.
471. Sullam, P.M., Drake, T.A., and Sande, M.A.: Pathogenesis of endocarditis, Am. J. Med. **78**:110, 1985.
472. Uwaydah, M.M., and Weinberg, A.N.: Bacterial endocarditis: a changing pattern, N. Engl. J. Med. **273**:1231, 1965.
473. Van Scoy, R.E.: Culture-negative endocarditis, Mayo Clin. Proc. **57**:149, 1982.

474. Varma, M.P.S., McCluskey, D.R., Khan, M.M., Cleland, J., O'Kane, H.O., and Adgey, A.A.: Heart failure associated with infective endocarditis: a review of 40 cases, Br. Heart J. **55**:191, 1986.
475. Washington, J.A.: The role of the microbiology laboratory in the diagnosis and treatment of infective endocarditis, Mayo Clin. Proc. **57**:22, 1982.
476. Watanakunakorn, C.: Prosthetic valve infective endocarditis, Prog. Cardiovasc. Dis. **22**:181, 1979.
477. Weinstein, L.: "Modern" infective endocarditis, JAMA **233**:260, 1975.
478. Wilson, L.M.: Etiology of bacterial endocarditis before and since the introduction of antibiotics, Ann. Intern. Med. **53**:84, 1963.

Myocarditis

479. Allen, A.C., and Spitz, S.: Comparative study of pathology of scrub typhus (tsutsugamushi disease) and other rickettsial diseases, Am. J. Pathol. **21**:603, 1945.
480. Atkinson, J.B., Connor, D.H., Rabinowitz, M., McAllister, H.A., and Virmani, R.: Cardiac fungal infections: review of autopsy findings in 60 patients, Hum. Pathol. **15**:935, 1984.
481. Blankenhorn, M.A., and Gall, E.A.: Myocarditis and myocardosis: clinicopathologic appraisal, Circulation **13**:217, 1956.
482. Bradford, W., and Hackel, D.B.: Myocardial involvement in Rocky Mountain spotted fever, Arch. Pathol. **102**:640, 1978.
483. Burke, J.S., Medline, N.M., and Katz, A.: A giant cell myocarditis: clinicopathologic appraisal, Circulation **13**:217, 1956.
484. de la Chapelle, C.E., and Dossman, C.E.: Myocarditis, Circulation **10**:747, 1954.
485. Dighiera, J., Canabal, E.J., Aguirre, C.V., Hazen, J., and Horjales, J.O.: Echinococcus disease of the heart, Circulation **10**:127, 1958.
486. Dilling, N.V.: Giant-cell myocarditis, J. Pathol. Bacteriol. **71**:295, 1956.
487. Filho, R.I.R., and Rossi, M.B.: Chagas' disease: a medical and socioeconomic problem, Int. J. Cardiol. **9**:451, 1985. (Editorial.)
488. Frenkel, J.K.: Toxoplasma in and around us, Bio Science **23**:343, 1977.
489. Gray, D.F., Morse, B.S., and Phillips, W.F.: Trichinosis with neurologic and cardiac involvement, Ann. Intern. Med. **57**:230, 1962.
490. Gore, I.: Myocardial changes in fatal diphtheria: summary of observations in 221 cases, Am. J. Sci. **215**:257, 1948.
491. Gore, I., and Saphir, O.: Myocarditis: classification of 1402 cases, Am. Heart J. **34**:827, 1947.
492. Grist, N.R., and Bell, E.J.: A 6 year study of coxsackievirus B infections in heart disease, J. Hyg. Camb. **73**:165, 1974.
493. Hackel, D.B.: Myocarditis in association with varicella, Am. J. Pathol. **29**:369, 1953.
494. Hackel, D.B., Kinney, T.D., and Wendt, W.: Pathologic lesions in captive wild animals, Lab. Invest. **2**:154, 1953.
495. Hooper, A.D.: Acquired toxoplasmosis: report of a case with autopsy findings, including a review of previously reported cases, Arch. Pathol. **64**:1, 1957.
496. Heilbrunn, A., Kittle, C.F., and Dunn, M.: Surgical management of echinococcal cysts of the heart and pericardium, Circulation **27**:219, 1963.
497. Kean, B.H., and Hoekenga, M.T.: Giant cell myocarditis, Am. J. Pathol. **28**:1095, 1952.
498. Kim, H.S., Weilbaecher, D.G., Lie, J.T., and Titus, J.L.: Myocardial abscesses, Am. J. Clin. Pathol. **70**:18, 1978.
499. Langendorff, R., and Pirani, C.L.: Heart in uremia, Am. Heart J. **33**:28, 1947.
500. Leak, D., and Meghji, M.: Toxoplasmic infection in cardiac disease, Am. J. Cardiol. **43**:841, 1979.
501. Lerner, A.M., Wilson, F.M., and Reyes, M.P.: Enteroviruses and the heart (with special emphasis on the probable role of coxsackieviruses, group B, types 1-5). II. Observations in humans, Mod. Concepts Cardiovasc. Dis. **44**:11, 1975.
502. Long, W.J.: Granulomatous (Fiedler's) myocarditis with extra-

cardiac involvement: a case report with sudden death, JAMA **177**:184, 1961.

503. Manion, W.C.: Scientific exhibits: myocarditis; frequent complication of systemic diseases, Arch. Pathol. **61**:329, 1959.
504. Parmley, A.F., Manion, W.C., and Mattingly, T.W.: Nonpenetrating wounds of the heart and aorta, Circulation **18**:371, 1958.
505. Peery, T.M., and Belter, L.F.: Brucellosis and heart disease. II. Fatal brucellosis: a review of the literature and report of new cases, Am. J. Pathol. **36**:673, 1960.
506. Porter, G.H.: Sarcoid heart disease, N. Engl. J. Med. **263**:1350, 1960.
507. Roberts, W.C., McAllister, H.A., Jr., and Ferrans, V.J.: Sarcoidosis of the heart: a clinicopathologic study of 35 necropsy patients (group 1) and review of 78 previously described necropsy patients (group II), Am J. Med. **63**:86, 1977.
508. Sainani, G.S., Dekate, M.P., and Rao, C.P.: Heart disease caused by coxsackie virus B infection, Br. Heart J. **37**:819, 1975.
509. Sanders, V.: Viral myocarditis, Am. Heart J. **66**:707, 1963.
510. Saphir, O.: Isolated myocarditis, Am. Heart J. **24**:167, 1942.
511. Saphir, O.: Myocarditis: general review, with analysis of 240 cases, Arch. Pathol. **33**:88, 1942.
512. Saphir, O.: Myocarditis, Am. Heart J. **66**:707, 1963.
513. Tesluk, H.: Giant cell versus granulomatous myocarditis, Am. J. Clin. Pathol. **26**:1326, 1956.
514. Wainger, C.K., and Lever, W.F.: Dermatomyositis: report of 3 cases with postmortem observations, Arch. Dermatol. Syph. **59**:196, 1949.
515. Walker, D.H., Paletta, C.E., and Cain, B.G.: Pathogenesis of myocarditis in Rocky Mountain spotted fever, Arch. Pathol. Lab. Med. **104**:171, 1980.
516. Weiss, S., Stead, E.A., Jr., Warren, J.V., and Bailey, O.T.: Scleroderma heart disease, with consideration of certain other visceral manifestations of scleroderma, Arch. Intern. Med. **71**:749, 1943.
517. Wilson, M.S., Barth, R.F., Baker, P.B., Unverferth, D.V., and Kolibash, A.J.: Giant cell myocarditis, Am. J. Med. **79**:647, 1985.
518. Woodruff, J.F.: Viral myocarditis, Am. J. Pathol. **101**:427, 1980.

Hydropericardium, hemopericardium, and pericarditis

519. Anderson, M.W., Christensen, N.A., and Edwards, J.E.: Hemopericardium complicating myocardial infarction in absence of cardiac rupture: report of 3 cases, Arch. Intern. Med. **90**:634, 1952.
520. Baldwin, J.J., and Edwards, J.E.: Uremic pericarditis as a cause of cardiac tamponade, Circulation **53**:896, 1976.
521. Blake, S., Bonar, S., O'Neill, H., Hanly, P., Drury, I., Flanagan, M., and Garrett, J.: Aetiology of chronic pericarditis, Br. Heart J. **50**:273, 1983.
522. Buja, L.M., Roberts, W.C., and Friedman, C.A.: Hemorrhagic pericarditis in uremia, Arch. Pathol. **90**:325, 1970.
523. Comty, C.M., Cohen, S.L., and Shapiro, F.L.: Pericarditis in chronic uremia and its sequels, Ann. Intern. Med. **75**:173, 1971.
524. Cortes, F.M., editor: The pericardium and its disorders, Springfield, Ill., 1971, Charles C Thomas, Publisher.
525. Creech, O., Jr., Hicks, W.M., Jr., Snyder, H.B., and Erikson, E.E.: Cholesterol pericarditis: successful treatment by pericardiectomy, Circulation **12**:30, 1955.
526. Deterling, R.A., Jr., and Humphreys, G.H., II: Factors in etiology of constrictive pericarditis, Circulation **12**:30, 1955.
527. Dressler, H., Yurkofsky, J., and Starr, M.C.: Hemorrhagic pericarditis, pleurisy, and pneumonia complicating recent myocardial infarction, Am. Heart J. **54**:42, 1957.
528. Engle, M.A., Gay, W.A., Jr., McCabe, J., Longo, E., Johnson, D., Senterfit, L.B., and Zabriskie, J.B.: Postpericardiotomy syndrome in adults: incidence, autoimmunity and virology, Circulation **64**(suppl. 2):II-58, 1981.
529. Engle, M.A., McCabe, J.C., and Ebert, P.A.: The postperi-

cardiotomy syndrome and antiheart antibodies, Circulation **49**:401, 1974.
530. Fowler, N.O., and Manitsas, G.T.: Infectious pericarditis, Prog. Cardiovasc. Dis. **16**:323, 1973.
531. Goldstein, R., and Wolf, L.: Hemorrhagic pericarditis in acute myocardial infarction treated with bishydroxycoumarin, JAMA **146**:616, 1951.
532. Hackel, D.B.: Diseases of the pericardium. In Brest, A.N., and Edwards, J.E., editors: Cardiovascular clinics, 1972, R.A. Davis Co.
533. Herrmann, G.R., Marchand, E.J., Greer, G.H., and Hejtmancik, M.R.: Pericarditis: clinical and laboratory data of 130 cases, Am. Heart J. **43**:641, 1952.
534. Hirschmann, J.V.: Pericardial constriction, Am. Heart J. **96**:110, 1978.
535. Ito, T., Engle, M.A., and Goldberg, H.P.: Postpericardiotomy syndrome following surgery for nonrheumatic heart disease, Circulation **17**:549, 1958.
536. Izzo, P.A., Stevens, R.C., Tomsykoski, A.J., and Rodríguez, C.E.: Hemopericardium associated with anticoagulant therapy, Arch. Intern. Med. **92**:350, 1953.
537. Johnson, R.T., Portnay, B., Rogers, N.G., and Buescher, E.L.: Acute benign pericarditis: virologic study of 34 patients, Arch. Intern. Med. **108**:823, 1961.
538. Kaltman, A.J., Schwedel, J.B., and Strauss, B.: Chronic constrictive pericarditis and rheumatic heart disease, Am. Heart J. **45**:201, 1953.
539. Klacsmann, P.G., Bulkley, B.H., and Hutchins, G.M.: The changed spectrum of purulent pericarditis: an 86 year autopsy experience in 200 patients, Am. J. Med. **63**:666, 1977.
540. Kumar, S., and Lesch, M.: Pericarditis in renal disease, Prog. Cardiovasc. Dis. **22**:357, 1980.
541. Kutcher, M.A., King, S.B., III, Alimurung, B.N., Craver, J.M., and Logue, R.B.: Constrictive pericarditis as a complication of cardiac surgery: recognition of an entity, Am. J. Cardiol. **50**:742, 1982.
542. Langendorff, R., and Pirani, C.C.: Heart in uremia: electrocardiographic and pathologic study, Am. Heart J. **33**:282, 1947.
543. Laslo, M.H.: Constrictive pericarditis as sequel to hemopericardium: report of a case following anticoagulant therapy, Ann. Intern. Med. **46**:403, 1957.
544. Mambo, N.C.: Diseases of the pericardium: morphologic study of surgical specimens from 35 patients, Hum. Pathol. **12**:978, 1981.
545. McKusick, V.A., Kay, J.H., and Isaacs, J.P.: Constrictive pericarditis following traumatic hemopericardium, Ann. Surg. **142**:97, 1955.
546. McPhail, J.L., Sukumar, I.P., Vytilingam, K.I., Cherian, G., and John, S.: Surgical management of constrictive pericarditis, J. Thorac. Cardiovasc. Surg. **53**:360, 1961.
547. Ali Regiaba, S., White, R.P., and Gay, W.A.: Treatment of uremic pericarditis by anterior pericardectomy, Lancet **2**:12, 1974.
548. Rice, P.L., Pifarre, R., and Montoya, A.: Constrictive pericarditis following cardiac surgery, Ann. Thorac. Surg. **31**:450, 1981.
549. Schepers, G.W.H.: Tuberculous pericarditis, Am. J. Cardiol. **9**:248, 1962.
550. Silverberg, S., Oreopoulos, D.G., Wise, D.J., Uden, D.E., Meidok, H., Jones, M., Rapoport, A., and deVeber, G.: Pericarditis in patients undergoing long-term hemodialysis and peritoneal dialysis, Am. J. Med. **63**:874, 1977.
551. Sodeman, W.A., and Smith, R.H.: Re-evaluation of the diagnostic criteria for acute pericarditis, Am. J. Med. Sci. **235**:672, 1958.
552. Spodick, D.N.: Acute pericarditis, New York, 1959, Grune & Stratton.

Valvular and hypertensive heart diseases
Acquired valvular heart disease

553. Akikusa, B., Kondi, Y., and Muraki, N.: Aortic insufficiency caused by Takayasu's arteritis without usual clinical features, Arch. Pathol. Lab. Med. **105**:650, 1981.

554. Aronow, W.S., Schwartz, K.S., and Koenigsberg, M.: Correlation of serum lipids, calcium and phosphorus, diabetes mellitus, aortic valve stenosis and history of systemic hypertension with presence or absence of mitral anular calcium in persons older than 62 years in a long-term health care facility, Am. J. Cardiol. **59:**381, 1987.

555. Barnett, H.J.M., Boughner, D.R., Taylor, D.W., Cooper, P.E., Kostuk, W.J., and Nichol, P.M.: Further evidence relating mitral-valve prolapse to cerebral ischemic events, N. Engl. J. Med. **302:**139, 1980.

556. Ben-Zvi, J., Hildner, F.J., and Javier, R.P.: Calcific aortic insufficiency: a review of 26 patients, Am. Heart J. **89:**278, March 1975.

557. Clemens, J.D., Horwitz, R.I., Jaffe, C.C., Feinstein, A.R., and Stanton, B.F.: A controlled evaluation of the risk of bacterial endocarditis in persons with mitral-valve prolapse, N. Engl. J. Med. **307:**776, 1982.

558. Darvill, F.T.: Aortic insufficiency of unusual etiology, JAMA **184:**753, 1963.

559. Davies, M.J., Moore, B.P., and Braimbridge, M.V.: The floppy mitral valve, study of incidence, pathology, and complications in surgical, necropsy and forensic material, Br. Heart J. **40:**468, 1978.

560. Devereux, R.B., Perloff, J.K., and Reichek, N.: Mitral valve prolapse, Circulation **54:**3, 1976.

561. Fenoglio, J.J., Jr., McAllister, H.A., Jr., and DeCastro, C.M.: Congenital bicuspid aortic valve after age 20, Am. J. Cardiol. **39:**164, 1977.

562. Gann, D., Fernandes, H., and Samet, P.: Syncope and aortic stenosis: significance of conduction abnormalities, Eur. J. Cardiol. **9(5):**405, 1979.

563. Hakki, A., Kimbiris, D., Iskandrian, A.S., Segal, B.L., Mintz, G.S., and Bemis, C.E.: Angina pectoris and coronary artery disease in patients with severe aortic valvular disease, Am. Heart J. **100:**441, 1980.

564. Hammarsten, J.F.: Syncope in aortic stenosis, Arch. Intern Med. **87:**274, 1951.

565. Hutchins, G.M., and Maron, B.J.: Development of endocardial valvuloids with valvular insufficiency, Arch. Pathol. **93:**401, 1972.

566. Jeresaty, R.M., Edwards, J.E., and Chawla, S.K.: Mitral valve prolapse and ruptured chordae tendineae, Am. J. Cardiol. **55:**138, 1985.

567. Johnson, A.M.: Aortic stenosis, sudden death and left ventricular baroceptors, Br. Heart J. **33:**1, 1971.

568. Kern, W.H., and Tucker, B.L.: Myxoid changes in cardiac valves: pathologic, clinical, and ultrastructural studies, Am. Heart J. **84:**294, 1972.

569. Korn, D., DeSanctis, R.W., and Sell, S.: Massive calcification of the mitral annulus: a clinicopathologic study of fourteen cases, N. Engl. J. Med. **267:**900, 1962.

570. Lucas, R.V., Jr., and Edwards, J.E.: Floppy mitral valve and ventricular septal defect: an anatomic study, J. Am. Coll. Cardiol. **1:**1337, 1983.

571. Marcus, M.L., Doty, D.B., Hiratzka, L.F., Wright, C.B., and Eastham, C.L.: Decreased coronary reserve: a mechanism for angina pectoris in patients with aortic stenosis and normal coronary arteries, N. Engl. J. Med. **307:**1362, 1982.

572. McKay, R., and Yacoub, M.H.: Clinical and pathological findings in patients with "floppy" valves treated surgically, Circulation **47,48**(suppl. 3):III-63, 1973.

573. Mills, P., Rose, J., and Hollingsworth, J.: Long-term prognosis of mitral-valve prolapse, N. Engl. J. Med. **297:**13, 1977.

574. Nair, C.K., Sudhakaran, C., Aronow, W.S., Thomson, W., Woodruff, M.P., and Sketch M.H.: Clinical characteristics of patients younger than 60 years with mitral anular calcium: comparison with age- and sex-matched control subjects, Am. J. Cardiol. **54:**1286, 1984.

575. Oakley, C.M.: Mitral valve prolapse, Q. J. Med. **219:**317, 1985. (Editorial.)

576. Olsen, E.G.J., and Al-Rufaie, H.K.: The floppy mitral valve: study on pathogenesis, Br. Heart J. **44:**674, 1980.

577. Olson, L.J., Subramanian, R., and Edwards, W.D.: Surgical pathology of pure aortic insufficiency: a study of 225 cases, Mayo Clin. Proc. **59:**835, 1984.

578. Osmundson, P.J., Callahan, J.A., and Edwards, J.E.: Ruptured mitral chordae tendineae, Circulation **23:**42, 1961.

579. Osterberger, L.E., Goldstein, S., Khaja, F., and Lakier, J.B.: Functional mitral stenosis in patients with massive mitral anular calcification, Circulation **64:**472, 1981.

580. Peery, T.M.: Brucellosis and heart diseases. IV. Etiology of calcific aortic stenosis, JAMA **166:**1123, 1958.

581. Perloff, J.K., and Roberts, W.C.: The mitral apparatus: functional anatomy of mitral regurgitation, Circulation **46:**227, 1972.

582. Pierpont, G.L., and Talley, R.C.: Pathophysiology of valvular heart disease: the dynamic nature of mitral valve regurgitation, Arch. Intern Med. **142:**998-1001, 1982.

583. Pomerance, A.: Ballooning deformity (mucoid degeneration) of atrioventricular valves, Br. Heart J. **31:**343, 1969.

584. Pomerance, A.: Pathological and clinical study of calcification of the mitral ring, J. Clin. Pathol. **23:**354, 1970.

585. Pomerance, A.: The pathogenesis of aortic stenosis in the elderly, Gerontol. Clin. **14:**1, 1972.

586. Roberts, W.C.: The structure of the aortic valve in clinically isolated aortic stenosis: an autopsy study of 162 patients over 15 years of age, Circulation **42:**91, 1970.

587. Roberts, W.C.: The congenitally bicuspid aortic valve: a study of 85 autopsy cases, Am. J. Cardiol. **26:**72, 1970.

588. Roberts, W.C.: Anatomically isolated aortic valvular disease: the case against its being of rheumatic etiology, Am. J. Med. **49:**151, 1970.

589. Roberts, W.C.: Morphologic features of the normal and abnormal mitral valve, Am. J. Cardiol. **51:**1005, 1983.

590. Roberts, W.C., and Waller, B.F.: Mitral valve "anular" calcium forming a complete circle or "O" configuration: clinical and necropsy observations, Am. Heart J. **101:**619, 1981.

591. Rose, A.G.: Etiology of acquired valvular heart disease in adults: a survey of 18,132 autopsies and 100 consecutive valve-replacement operations, Arch. Pathol. Lab. Med. **110:**385, 1986.

592. Sanders, C.A., Armstrong, P.W., and Willerson, J.T.: Etiology and differential diagnosis of acute mitral regurgitation, Prog. Cardiovasc. Dis. **14:**129, 1971.

593. Savage, D.D., Levy, D., Garrison, R.J., Castelli, W.P., Kligfield, P., Devereux, R.B., Anderson, S.J., Kannel, W.B., and Feinleib, M.: Mitral valve prolapse in the general population. 3. Dysrhythmias: the Framingham Study, Am. Heart J. **106:**582, 1983.

594. Savage, D.D., Garrison, R.J., Devereux, R.B., Castelli, W.P., Anderson, S.J., Levy, D., McNamara, P.M., Stokes, J., III, Kannel, W.B., and Feinleib, M.: Mitral valve prolapse in the general population. 1. Epidemiologic features: the Framingham Study, Am. Heart J. **106:**571, 1983.

595. Subramanian, R., Olsen, L.J., and Edwards, W.D.: Surgical pathology of pure aortic stenosis: a study of 374 cases, Mayo Clin. Proc. **59:**683, 1984.

596. Sugiura, M., Uchiyama, S., and Kuwako, K.: A clinicopathological study on mitral ring calcification, Jpn. Heart J. **18:**154, 1977.

597. Swartz, M.H., Teichholz, L.E., and Donoso, E.: Mitral valve prolapse: a review of associated arrhythmias, Am. J. Med. **62:**377, 1977.

598. Waller, B.F., Carter, J.B., and Williams, H.J., Jr.: Bicuspid aortic valve: comparison of congenital and acquired types, Circulation **48:**1140, 1973.

599. Waller, B.F., Morrow, A.G., Maron, B.J., Del Negro, A.A., Kent, K.M., McGrath, F.J., Wallace, R.B., McIntosh, C.L., and Roberts, W.C.: Etiology of clinically isolated severe, chronic pure mitral regurgitation: analysis of 97 patients over 30 years of age having mitral valve replacement, Am. Heart J. **104:**276, 1982.

600. Wigle, E.D., Rakowski, H., and Ranganathan, N., et al.: Mitral valve prolapse, Annu. Rev. Med. **27:**165, 1976.

Disturbances of cardiac growth

601. Anversa, P., Loud, A.V., Giacomelli, F., and Wiener, J.: Absolute morphometric study of myocardial hypertrophy in experimental hypertension. II. Ultrastructure of myocytes and interstitium, Lab. Invest. 38(5):597-609, 1978.

602. Badeer, H.S.: Pathogenesis of cardiac hypertrophy in coronary atherosclerosis and myocardial infarction, Am. Heart J. 84:256, 1972.

603. Barnard, P.J.: The pathology of cor pulmonale, pulmonary arteriosclerosis, and pulmonary hypertension secondary to thromboembolism, Prog. Cardiovasc. Dis. 1:371, 1959.

604. Bishop, S.P., and Melsen, L.R.: Myocardial necrosis, fibrosis and DNA synthesis in experimental cardiac hypertrophy induced by sudden pressure overload, Circ. Res. 39:238, 1976.

605. Black-Schaffer, B., and Turner, M.E.: Hyperplastic infantile cardiomegaly: a form of "idiopathic hypertrophy" with or without endocardial fibroelastosis, and a comment on cardiac "atrophy," Am. J. Pathol. 34:745, 1958.

606. Brown, A.J., Jr.: Morphologic factors in cardiac hypertrophy. In Alpert, N.R., editor: Cardiac hypertrophy, New York, 1971, Academic Press, Inc.

607. Carney, J.A., and Brown, A.L., Jr.: Myofilament diameter in the normal and hypertrophic rat myocardium, Am. J. Pathol. 44:521, 1964.

608. Chilian, W.M., Wangler, R.D., Peters, K.G., Tomanek, R.J., and Marcus, M.L.: Thyroxine-induced left ventricular hypertrophy in the rat: anatomical and physiological evidence for angiogenesis, Circ. Res. 57:591, 1985.

609. Connolly, E.P., and Littman, D.: Coronary arteriosclerosis and myocardial hypertrophy, N. Engl. J. Med. 245:753, 1951.

610. Cox, M.L., Bennett, J.B., III., and Dudley, G.A.: Exercise training–induced alterations of cardiac morphology, J. Appl. Physiol. 61:926, 1986.

611. Dadgar, S.K., and Tyagi, S.P.: Importance of heart weight, weights of cardiac ventricles and left ventricle plus septum/right ventricle ratio in assessing cardiac hypertrophy, Jpn. Heart J. 20:63, 1979.

612. Dean, J.H., and Gallagher, P.J.: Cardiac ischemia and cardiac hypertrophy: an autopsy study, Arch. Pathol. Lab. Med. 104:175, 1980.

613. Dunn, F.G., Ventura, H.O., Messerli, F.H., Kobrin, I., and Frohlich, E.D.: Time course of regression of left ventricular hypertrophy in hypertensive patients treated with atenolol, Circulation 76:254, 1987.

614. Fanburg, B.L.: Experimental cardiac hypertrophy, N. Engl. J. Med. 282:723, 1970.

615. Fulton, R.M., Hutchinson, E.C., and Morgan-Jones, A.: Ventricular weight in cardiac hypertrophy, Br. Heart J. 14:413, 1952.

616. Gordon, T., and Waterhouse, A.M.: Hypertension and hypertensive heart disease, J. Chron. Dis. 19:1089, 1966.

617. Grossman, W.: Cardiac hypertrophy: useful adaptation or pathologic process?, Am. J. Med. 69:576, 1980.

618. Grove, D., Nair, K.G., and Zak, R.: Biochemical correlates of cardiac hypertrophy. IV. Observations on the cellular organization of growth during myocardial hypertrophy in the rat, Circ. Res. 25:473, 1969.

619. Hangartner, J.R.W., Marley, N.J., Whitehead, A., Thomas, A.C., and Davies, M.J.: The assessment of cardiac hypertrophy at autopsy, Histopathology 9:1295, 1985.

620. Hutchins, G.M., and Anaya, O.A.: Measurements of cardiac size, chamber volumes and valve orifices at autopsy, Johns Hopkins Med. J. 133:96, 1973.

621. Jones, R.S.: Weight of heart and its chambers in hypertensive cardiovascular disease with and without failure, Circulation 7:357, 1953.

622. Karsner, H.T., Saphir, O., and Todd, T.W.: Cardiac muscle in hypertrophy and atrophy, Am. J. Pathol. 1:351, 1925.

623. Koepsell, J.E., Kuzma, J.F., and Murphy, F.D.: Hypertensive cardiovascular disease (acute) (malignant hypertension): clinical and pathologic study of 39 cases, Arch. Intern. Med. 85:432, 1950.

624. Laks, M.M., Morady, F., and Adamian, G.E.: Presence of widened and multiple intercalated discs in the hypertrophied canine heart, Circ. Res. 27:391, 1970.

625. Linzbach, A.J.: Heart failure from the point of view of qualitative anatomy, Am. J. Cardiol. 5:370, 1960.

626. MacMahon, H.E.: Hyperplasia and regeneration of myocardium in infants and in children, Am. J. Pathol. 13:845, 1937.

627. Maron, B.J., and Ferrans, V.J.: Significance of multiple intercalated discs in hypertrophied human myocardium, Am. J. Pathol. 73:81, 1973.

628. Maron, B.J., and Ferrans, V.J.: Ultrastructural features of hypertrophied human ventricular myocardium, Prog. Cardiovasc. Dis. 21:207, 1978.

629. Master, A.M., Garfield, C.I., and Walters, M.D.: Normal blood pressure and hypertension, Philadelphia, 1952, Lea & Febiger.

630. Meerson, F.Z., and Pomoinitsky, V.D.: The role of high-energy phosphate compounds in the development of cardiac hypertrophy, J. Mol. Cell. Cardiol. 4:571, 1972.

631. Moore, G.W., Hutchins, G.M., Bulkley, B.H., Tseng, J.S., and Ki, P.F.: Constituents of the human ventricular myocardium: connective tissue hyperplasia accompanying muscular hypertrophy, Am. Heart J. 100:610, 1980.

632. Morkin, E., and Ashford, T.P.: Myocardial DNA synthesis in experimental cardiac hypertrophy, Am. J. Physiol. 215:1409, 1968.

633. Oparil, S., Bishop, S.P., and Clubb, F.J., Jr.: Myocardial cell hypertrophy or hyperplasia, Hypertension 6:III-38, 1984.

634. Page, I.H., and Corcoran, A.C.: Arterial hypertension: its diagnosis and treatment, Chicago, 1945, Year Book Medical Publishers.

635. Paplanus, S.H., Zbar, M.J., and Hays, J.W.: Chronic hypertrophy as a manifestation of chronic anemia, Am. J. Pathol. 34:149, 1958.

636. Perera, G.A.: Hypertensive vascular disease: description and natural history, J. Chron. Dis. 1:33, 1955.

637. Rabinowitz, M.: Overview on pathogenesis of cardiac hypertrophy, Circ. Res. 35:3, 1974.

638. Richter, G.W., and Kellner, A.: Hypertrophy of the human heart at the level of the fine structure: an analysis and two postulates, J. Cell. Biol. 18:195, 1963.

639. Roberts, J.T., and Wearn, J.T.: Quantitative changes in capillary-muscle relationship in human hearts during normal growth and hypertrophy, Am. Heart J. 21:617, 1941.

640. Rosahn, P.D.: Weight of normal heart in adult males, Yale J. Biol. Med. 14:209, 1941.

641. Scheel, K.W., and Williams, S.E.: Hypertrophy and coronary and collateral vascularity in dogs with severe chronic anemia, Am. J. Physiol. 249:H1031, 1985.

642. Smith, D.E., Odel, H.M., and Kernohan, J.W.: Causes of death in hypertension, Am. J. Med. 9:516, 1950.

643. Sokolow, M., and Perloff, D.: The prognosis of essential hypertension treated conservatively, Circulation 23:697, 1961.

644. Stein, B.R., and Barnes, A.R.: Severity and duration of hypertension in relation to amount of cardiac hypertrophy, Am. J. Med. Sci. 216:661, 1948.

645. Tarazi, R.C., Sen, S., Saragoca, M., and Khairallah, P.: The multifactorial role of catecholamines in hypertensive cardiac hypertrophy, Eur. Heart J. 3 suppl. A:103, 1982.

646. Warmuth, H., Fleischer, M., and Themann, H.: Ultrastructural morphometric analysis of hypertrophied human myocardial left ventricles, Virchows Arch. [Pathol. Anat.] 380:135, 1978.

647. Whitaker, W., and Heath, D.: Idiopathic pulmonary hypertension: etiology, pathogenesis, diagnosis, and treatment, Prog. Cardiovasc. Dis. 1:380, 1959.

648. Zak, R., and Rabinowitz, M.: Molecular aspects of cardiac hypertrophy, Annu. Rev. Physiol. 41:539, 1979.

649. Zeek, P.M.: Heart weight: weight of normal human heart, Arch. Pathol. 34:820, 1942.

650. Zimmer, H.G., Steinkopff, G., Ibel, H., and Koschine, H.: Is the ATP decline a signal for stimulating protein synthesis in isoproterenol-induced cardiac hypertrophy? J. Mol. Cell. Cardiol. 12:421, 1980.

Cardiomyopathies and specific disorders affecting the myocardium
Definitions and classifications

651. Abelman, W.H.: Classification and natural history of primary myocardial disease, Prog. Cardiovasc. Dis. **26:**73, 1984.
652. Davies, M.J.: The cardiomyopathies: a review of terminology, pathology and pathogenesis, Histopathology **8:**363, 1984.
653. Pantely, G.A., and Bristow, J.D.: Ischemic cardiomyopathy, Prog. Cardiovasc. Dis. **27:**95, 1984.
654. Roberts, W.C., and Ferrans, V.J.: Pathologic anatomy of the cardiomyopathies: idiopathic dilated and hypertrophic types, infiltrative types, and endomyocardial disease with and without eosinophilia, Hum. Pathol. **6:**287, 1975.
655. WHO/ISFC Task Force: Report of the WHO/ISFC Task Force on the definition and classification of cardiomyopathies, Br. Heart J. **44:**672, 1980.

Hypertrophic cardiomyopathy

656. Becker, A.E., and Caruso, G.: Myocardial disarray: a critical review, Br. Heart J. **47:**527, 1982.
657. Branzi, A., Romeo, G., Specchia, S., Lolli, C., Binetti, G., Devoto, M., Bacchi, M., and Magnani, B.: Genetic heterogeneity of hypertrophic cardiomyopathy, Int. J. Cardiol. **7:**129, 1985.
658. Braunwald, E., Lambrew, C.T., and Rockoff, S.D.: Idiopathic hypertrophic subaortic stenosis. I. A description of the disease based upon an analysis of 64 patients, Circulation **29,30**(suppl. IV):IV-3, 1964.
659. Bulkley, B.H., Weisfeldt, M.L., and Hutchins, G.M.: Asymmetric septal hypertrophy and myocardial fiber disarray: features of normal, developing, and malformed hearts, Circulation **56:**292, 1977.
660. Burn, J.: The genetics of hypertrophic cardiomyopathy, Int. J. Cardiol. **7:**135, 1985. (Editorial.)
661. Cannon, R.O., III., Rosing, D.R., Maron, B.J., Leon, M.B., Bonow, R.O., Watson, R.M., and Epstein, S.E.: Myocardial ischemia in patients with hypertrophic cardiomyopathy: contribution of inadequate vasodilator reserve and elevated left ventricular filing pressures, Circulation **71:**234, 1985.
662. Clark, C.E., Henry, W.L., and Epstein, S.E.: Familial prevalence and genetic transmission of idiopathic hypertrophic subaortic stenosis, N. Engl. J. Med. **289:**709, 1973.
663. Criley, J.M., and Siegel, R.J.: Has 'obstruction' hindered our understanding of hypertrophic cardiomyopathy? Circulation **72:**1148, 1985.
664. Epstein, S.E., Henry, W.L., Clark, C.E., Roberts, W.C., Maron, B.J., Ferrans, V.J., Redwood, D.R., and Morrow, A.G.: Asymmetric septal hypertrophy, Ann. Intern. Med. **81:**650, 1974.
665. Gilbert, B.W., Pollick, C., Adleman, A.G., and Wigle, E.D.: Hypertrophic cardiomyopathy: subclassification by M mode echocardiography, Am. J. Cardiol. **45:**861, 1980.
666. Gulotta, S.J., Hamby, R.I., and Aronson, A.L.: Coexistent idiopathic hypertrophic subaortic stenosis and coronary arterial disease, Circulation **46:**890, 1972.
667. Henry, W.L., Clark, C.E., and Epstein, S.E.: Asymmetric septal hypertrophy (ASH): echocardiographic identification of the pathognomonic anatomic abnormality of IHSS, Circulation **47:**225, 1973.
668. Henry, W.L., Clark, C.E., Roberts, W.C., Henry, W.L., Savage, D.D., and Epstein, S.E.: Differences in distribution of myocardial abnormalities in patients with obstructive and nonobstructive asymmetric septal hypertrophy (ASH): echocardiographic and gross anatomic findings, Circulation **50:**447, 1974.
669. James, T.N., and Marshall, T.K.: De subitaneis mortibus, XII. Asymmetrical hypertrophy of the heart, Circulation **51:**1149, 1975.
670. Maron, B.J.: Myocardial disorganization in hypertrophic cardiomyopathy: another point of view, Br. Heart J. **50:**1, 1983.
671. Maron, B.J., and Epstein, S.E.: Hypertrophic cardiomyopathy: recent observations regarding the specificity of three hallmarks of the disease: asymmetric septal hypertrophy, septal

disorganization and systolic anterior motion of the anterior mitral leaflet, Am. J. Cardiol. **45:**141, 1980.
672. Maron, B.J., Epstein, S.E., and Roberts, W.C.: Hypertrophic cardiomyopathy and transmural myocardial infarction without significant atherosclerosis of the extramural coronary arteries, Am. J. Cardiol. **43:**1086, 1979.
673. Maron, B.J., Gottdiener, J.S., Roberts, W.C., Henry, W.L., Savage, D.D., and Epstein, S.E.: Left ventricular outflow tract obstruction due to systolic anterior motion of the anterior mitral leaflet in patients with concentric left ventricular hypertrophy, Circulation **57:**527, 1978.
674. Maron, B.J., Roberts, W.C., McAllister, H.A., Rosing, D.R., and Epstein, S.E.: Sudden death in young athletes, Circulation **62:**218, 1980.
675. Maron, B.J., Wolfson, J.K., Epstein, S.E., and Roberts, W.C.: Intramural ("small vessel") coronary artery disease in hypertrophic cardiomyopathy, J. Am. Coll. Cardiol. **8:**545, 1986.
676. Nagata, S., Nimura, Y., Beppu, S., Park, Y.D., and Sakakibarn, H.: Mechanism of systolic anterior motion of mitral valve and site of intraventricular pressure gradient in hypertrophic obstructive cardiomyopathy, Br. Heart J. **49:**234, 1983.
677. Perloff, J.K.: Pathogenesis of hypertrophic cardiomyopathy: hypotheses and speculations, Am. Heart J. **101:**219, 1981.
678. Sanderson, J.E., Traill, T.A., Sutton, M.G., Brown, D.J., Gibson, D.G., and Goodwin, J.F.: Left ventricular relaxation and filling in hypertrophc cardiomyopathy: an echocardiographic study, Br. Heart J. **40:**596, 1978.
679. Shah, P.M.: ISHH-HOCM-MSS-ASH? Circulation **51:**577, 1975. (Editorial.)
680. Sonnenblick, E.H., Fein, F., Capasso, J.M., and Factor, S.M.: Microvascular spasm as a cause of cardiomyopathies and the calcium-blocking agent verapamil as potential primary therapy, Am. J. Cardiol. **55:**179B, 1985.
681. Teare, D.: Asymmetrical hypertrophy of the heart in young adults, Br. Heart J. **20:**1, 1958.
682. van der Bel–Kahn, J.: Muscle fiber disarray in common heart diseases, Am. J. Cardiol. **40:**355, 1977.
683. Watt, A.H.: Hypertrophic cardiomyopathy: a disease of impaired adenosine-mediated autoregulation of the heart, Lancet **1:**1271, 1984.
684. Wigle, E.D., Sasson, Z., Henderson, M.A., Ruddy, T.D., Fulop, J., Rakowski, H., and Williams, W.G.: Hypertrophic cardiomyopathy: the importance of the site and the extent of hypertrophy: a review, Prog. Cardiovasc. Res. **28:**1, 1985.

Congestive cardiomyopathy

685. Blankenhorn, M.A., Vilter, C.F., Schneinker, I.M., and Austin, R.S.: Occidental beriberi heart disease, JAMA **131:**717, 1946.
686. Cambridge, G., MacArthur, C.G., Waterson, A.P., Goodwin, J.F., and Oakley, C.M.: Antibodies to Coxsackie B viruses in congestive cardiomyopathy, Br. Heart J. **41:**692, 1979.
687. Edes, I., Tószegi, A., Csanády, M., and Bozóky, B.: Myocardial lipid peroxidation in rats after chronic alcohol ingestion and the effects of different antioxidants, Cardiovasc. Res. **20:**542, 1986.
688. Factor, S.M.: Intramyocardial small-vessel disease in chronic alcoholism, Am. Heart J. **92:**561, 1976.
689. Fuster, V., Gersh, B.J., Giuliani, E.R., Tajik, A.J., Brandeburg, R.O., and Frye, R.L.: The natural history of idiopathic dilated cardiomyopathy, Am. J. Cardiol. **47:**525, 1981.
690. Gottdiener, J.S., Gay, J.A., Van Voorhees, L., DiBianco, R., and Fletcher, R.D.: Frequency and embolic potential of left ventricular thrombus in dilated cardiomyopathy: assessment by 2-dimensional echocardiography, Am. J. Cardiol. **52:**1281, 1983.
691. Homans, D.C.: Peripartum cardiomyopathy, N. Engl. J. Med. **312:**1432, 1985.
692. Julian, D.G., and Székely, P.: Peripartum cardiomyopathy, Prog. Cardiovasc. Dis. **27:**223, 1985.
693. Kawai, C.: Idiopathic cardiomyopathy: a study on the infectious-immune theory as a cause of the disease, Jpn. Circ. J. **35:**765, 1971.

694. Kesteloot, H., Roelandt, J., and Williams, J.: An inquiry into the role of cobalt in the heart disease of chronic beer drinkers, Circulation **37**:854, 1968.

695. Kitaura, Y.: Virological study of idiopathic cardiomyopathy: serological study of virus antibodies and immunofluorescent study of myocardial biopsies, Jpn. Circ. J. **45**:279, 1981.

696. Regan, T.J.: Alcoholic cardiomyopathy, Prog. Cardiovasc. Dis. **27**:141, 1984.

697. Reyes, M.P., and Lerner, A.M.: Coxsackievirus myocarditis—with special reference to acute and chronic effects, Prog. Cardiovasc. Dis. **27**:373, 1985.

698. Schrader, W.H., Pankey, G.A., Davis, R.B., and Theologides, A.: Familial idiopathic cardiomegaly, Circulation **24**:599, 1961.

699. Schreiber, S.S., Oratz, M., and Rothschild, M.A.: Alcoholic cardiomyopathy: the effect of ethanol and acetaldehyde on cardiac protein synthesis, Rec. Adv. Studies Card. Struc. Metab. **7**:431, 1976.

700. Segal, L.D., Klausner, S.C., Gnadt, J.T., and Amsterdam, E.A.: Alcohol and the heart, Med. Clin. North Am. **68**:147, 1984.

701. Smith, W.G.: Coxsackie B myopericarditis in adults, Am. Heart J. **80**:34, 1970.

702. Thomas, G., Haider, B., Oldewurtel, H.A., Lyons, M.M., Yeh, C.K., and Regan, T.J.: Progressive myocardial abnormalities in experimental alcoholism, Am. J. Cardiol. **46**:233, 1980.

703. Unverferth, D.V., Magoien, R.D., Moeschberger, M.L., Baker, P.B., Fetters, J.K., and Leier, C.V.: Factors influencing the one-year mortality of dilated cardiomyopathy, Am. J. Cardiol. **54**:147, 1984.

704. Welch, C.C.: Alcoholic heart disease, Postgrad. Med. **61**:138, 1977.

Metabolic abnormalities

705. Batsakis, J.G.: Degenerative lesions of the heart. In Gould, S.E., editor: Pathology of the heart and blood vessels, ed. 3, Springfield, Ill., 1968, Charles C Thomas, Publisher.

706. Beratis, N.G., LaBadie, G.U., and Hirschhorn, K.: Characterization of the molecular defect in infantile and adult acid α-glucosidase deficiency fibroblasts, J. Clin. Invest. **62**:1264, 1978.

707. Buja, L.M., and Roberts, W.C.: Iron in the heart: etiology and clinical significance, Am. J. Med. **51**:209, 1971.

708. Dawson, I.M.P.: Histology and histochemistry of gargoylism, J. Pathol. Bacteriol. **67**:587, 1954.

709. di Sant'Agnese, P.A.: Diseases of glycogen storage with special reference to the cardiac type of generalized glycogenosis, Ann. NY Acad. Sci. **72**:439, 1959.

710. Ehlers, K.H., and Engle, M.A.: Glycogen storage disease of myocardium, Am. Heart J. **65**:145, 1963. (Editorial.)

711. Field, R.A.: The glycogenoses: von Gierke's disease, acid maltase deficiency, and liver glycogen phosphorylase deficiency, Am. J. Clin. Pathol. **50**:20, 1968.

712. Fitchett, D.H., Coltart, D.J., Littler, W.A., Leyland, M.J., Trueman, T., Gozzard, D.I., and Peters, T.I.: Cardiac involvement in secondary haemochromatosis: a catheter biopsy study and analysis of myocardium, Cardiovasc. Res. **14**:719, 1980.

713. Haymond, J.L., and Giordano, A.S.: Glycogen storage disease of heart, Am. J. Clin. Pathol. **16**:651, 1946.

714. Hers, H.G.: α-Glucosidase deficiency in generalized glycogen storage disease (Pompe's disease), Biochem. J. **86**:11, 1963.

715. Hsia, D.Y.Y.: The diagnosis and management of the glycogen storage diseases, Am. J. Clin. Pathol. **50**:44, 1968.

716. Keschner, H.W.: Heart in hemochromatosis, South. Med. J. **44**:927, 1951.

717. Levin, E.B., and Golum, A.: Heart in hemochromatosis, Am. Heart J. **45**:277, 1953.

718. McKusick, V.A., Kaplan, D., Wise, D., Hanley, W.B., Suddarth, S.B., Sevick, M.E., and Maumanee, A.E.: The genetic mucopolysaccharidoses, Medicine **44**:445, 1965.

719. Ross, C.F., and Belton, E.M.: A case of isolated cardiac lipidosis, Br. Heart J. **30**:726, 1968.

720. Strauss, L.: The pathology of gargoylism; report of case and review of the literature, Am. J. Pathol. **24**:855, 1948.

721. Vigorito, V.J., and Hutchins, G.M.: Cardiac conduction system in hemochromatosis, Am. J. Cardiol. **44**:418, 1979.

722. Wilson, R.A., and Clark, N.: Endocardial fibroelastosis associated with generalized glycogenosis: occurrence in siblings, Pediatrics **26**:86, 1960.

Endocrine disorders

723. Blumgart, H.I., Freedberg, A.S., and Kurland, G.S.: Hypercholesterolemia, myxedema and atherosclerosis, Am. J. Med. **11**:665, 1953.

724. Brewer, D.B.: Myxoedema: autopsy report with histochemical observations on nature of mucoid infiltrations, J. Pathol. Bacteriol. **63**:503, 1951.

725. Christensen, N.J.: Plasma noradrenaline and adrenaline in patients with thyrotoxicosis and myxoedema, Clin. Sci. Mol. Med. **42**:163, 1973.

726. Fahr, G.: Myxedema heart, report based upon study of 17 cases of myxedema, Am. Heart J. **8**:91, 1932.

727. Fisher, C.E., and Mulligan, R.M.: Quantitative study of correlation between basophilic degeneration of myocardium and atrophy of thyroid gland, Arch. Pathol. **36**:206, 1943.

728. Forfar, J.C., Muir, A.L., Sawers, S.A., and Toft, A.D.: Abnormal left ventricular function in hyperthyroidism: evidence for a possible reversible cardiomyopathy, N. Engl. J. Med. **307**:1165, 1982.

729. Forfar, J.C., Stewart, J., Sawers, A., and Toft, A.D.: Cardiovascular responses in hyperthyroidism before and during beta-adrenoceptor blockage: evidence against adrenergic hypersensitivity, Clin. Endocrinol. **16**:441, 1982.

730. Grossman, W., Robin, N.I., and Johnson, L.W.: The enhanced myocardial contractility of thyrotoxicosis: role of the beta adrenergic receptor, Ann. Intern. Med. **74**:869, 1971.

731. Hamolsky, M.W., Kurland, G.S., and Freedberg, A.S.: The heart in hypothyroidism, J. Chron. Dis. **14**:558, 1961.

732. Haust, M.D., Rowlands, D.T., Jr., Garancis, J.C., and Landing, B.H.: Histochemical studies on cardiac "colloid," Am. J. Pathol. **40**:185, 1962.

733. Hejtmancik, M.R., Bradfield, J.Y., and Herrmann, G.R.: Acromegaly and the heart: a clinical and pathologic study, Ann. Intern. Med. **34**:1445, 1951.

734. Higgins, W.H.: Heart in myxedema: correlation of physical and postmortem findings, Am. J. Med. Sci. **191**:80, 1936.

735. Kurland, G.S., and Freedberg, A.S.: Hormones, cholesterol and coronary atherosclerosis, Circulation **22**:464, 1960.

736. LaDue, J.S.: Myxedema heart: pathologic and therapeutic study, Ann. Intern. Med. **18**:332, 1943.

737. Levey, G.S.: The heart and hyperthyroidism: use of beta-adrenergic blocking drugs, Med. Clin. North Am. **59**:1193, 1975.

738. Lewis, W.: Question of specific myocardial lesion in hyperthyroidism (Basedow's disease), Am. J. Pathol. **8**:255, 1932.

739. Lie, J.T., and Grossman, S.J.: Pathology of the heart in acromegaly, Am. Heart J. **100**:41, 1980.

740. MacDonald, R.A., and Robbins, S.L.: Pathology of the heart in the carcinoid syndrome: a comparative study, Arch. Pathol. **63**:103, 1957.

741. Martins, J.B., Kerber, R.E., Sherman, B.M., Marcus, M.L., and Ehrhardt, J.C.: Cardiac size and function in acromegaly, Circulation **56**:863, 1977.

742. McGuffin, W.L., Sherman, B.M., Roth, J., Gorden, P., Kahn, C.R., Roberts, W.C., and Frommer, P.L.: Acromegaly and cardiovascular disorders: a prospective study, Ann. Intern. Med. **81**:11, 1974.

743. Mengel, C.E.: Carcinoid and the heart, Mod. Concepts Cardiovasc. Dis. **35**:75, 1966.

744. Roberts, W.C., and Sjoerdsma, A.: The cardiac disease associated with the carcinoid syndrome, Am. J. Med. **36**:5, 1964.

745. Rossen, S.H.: Goiter heart, US Armed Forces Med. J. **2**:1593, 1951.

746. Rossi, L., Thiene, G., Caragaro, L., Giordano, R., and Lauro, S.: Dysrhythmias and sudden death in acromegalic heart disease: a clinicopathologic study, Chest **72**:495, 1977.

747. Sandler, G., and Wilson, G.M.: The nature and prognosis of heart disease in thyrotoxicosis: a review of 150 patients treated with ^{131}I, Q. J. Med. **28**:347, 1959.

748. Spatz, M.: Pathogenic studies of experimentally induced heart lesions and their relation to the carcinoid syndrome, Lab. Invest. **13**:288, 1964.

749. Symons, C.: Thyroid heart disease, Br. Heart J. **41**:257, 1979.

750. Webster, B., and Cooke, C.: Morphologic changes in heart in experimental myxedema, Arch. Intern. Med. **58**:269, 1936.

Endocrine disorder—diabetes mellitus

751. Blumenthal, H.T., Alex, M., and Goldenberg, S.: A study of lesions of the intramural coronary branches in diabetes mellitus, Arch. Pathol. **70**:27, 1960.

752. Factor, S.M., Minase, T., and Sonnenblick, E.H.: Clinical and morphological features of human hypertensive-diabetic cardiomyopathy, Am. Heart J. **99**:446, 1980.

753. Factor, S.M., Okun, E.M., and Minase, T.: Capillary microaneurysms in the human diabetic heart, N. Engl. J. Med. **302**:384, 1980.

754. Fein, F.S., and Sonnenblick, E.H.: Diabetic cardiomyopathy, Prog. Cardiovasc. Dis. **27**:255, 1985.

755. Fischer, V.W., Barner, H.B., and Leskiw, L.: Capillary basal laminar thickness in diabetic human myocardium, Diabetes **28**:713, 1979.

756. Hamby, R.I., Zoneraich, S., and Sherman, S.: Diabetic cardiomyopathy, JAMA **229**:1749, 1974.

757. Ledet, T.: Histological and histochemical changes in the coronary arteries of old diabetic patients, Diabetologia **4**:268, 1968.

758. Ledet, T.: Diabetic cardiomyopathy: quantitative histological studies of the heart from young juvenile diabetics, Acta Pathol. Microbiol. Scand. [A] **84**:421, 1976.

759. Neubauer, B., and Christensen, N.J.: Norepinephrine, epinephrine, and dopamine contents of the cardiovascular system in long-term diabetics, Diabetes **25**:6, 1976.

760. Niakan, E., Harati, Y., Rolak, L.A., Comstock, J.P., and Rokey R.: Silent myocardial infarction and diabetic cardiovascular autonomic neuropathy, Arch. Intern. Med. **146**:2229, 1986.

761. Regen, T.J., Lyons, M.M., Ahmed, S.S., Levinson, G.E., Oldewartel, H.A., Ahmad, M.R., and Haider, B.: Evidence for cardiomyopathy in familial diabetes mellitus, J. Clin. Invest. **60**:885, 1977.

762. Seneviratne, B.I.B.: Diabetic cardiomyopathy: the preclinical phase, Br. Med. J. **1**:1444, 1977.

763. Silver, M.D., Huckell, V.S., and Lorber, M.: Basement membranes of small cardiac vessels in patients with diabetes and myxoedema: preliminary observations, Pathology **9**:213, 1977.

764. Sunni, S., Bishop, S.P., Kent, S.P., and Geer, J.C.: Diabetic cardiomyopathy: a morphological study of intramyocardial arteries, Arch. Pathol. Lab. Med. **110**:375, 1986.

765. Watkins, P.J., and Mackay, J.D.: Cardiac denervation in diabetic neuropathy, Ann. Intern. Med. **92**:304, 1980.

766. Zoneraich, S., and Silverman, G.: Myocardial small vessel disease in diabetic patients. In Zoneraich, S., editor: Diabetes and the heart, Springfield, Ill., 1978, Charles C Thomas, Publisher.

Nutritional deficiencies

767. Abel, R.M., Grimes, J.B., Alonso, D., Alonso, M., and Gay, W.A., Jr.: Adverse hemodynamic and ultrastructural changes in dog hearts subjected to protein-calorie malnutrition, Am. Heart J. **97**:733, 1979.

768. Akenhead, W.R., and Jaques, W.E.: Pulmonary edema, cardiomegaly, and anemia, Am. J. Clin. Pathol. **26**:926, 1956.

769. Benchimol, A.B., and Schlesinger, P.: Beriberi heart disease, Am. Heart J. **46**:245, 1953.

770. Chauhan, S., Nayak, N.C., and Ramalengaswami, V.: The heart and skeletal muscle in experimental protein malnutrition, J. Pathol. Bacteriol. **90**:301, 1965.

771. Follis, R.H., Jr.: Sudden death in infants with scurvy, J. Pediatr. **20**:347, 1942.

772. Follis, R.H., Jr.: Deficiency disease, Springfield, Ill., 1958, Charles C Thomas, Publisher.

773. Gerry, J.L., Bulkley, B.H., and Hutchins, G.M.: Clinico-pathologic analysis of cardiac dysfunction in 52 patients with sickle cell anemia, Am. J. Cardiol. **42**:211, 1978.

774. Heymsfield, S.B., Bethel, R.A., Ansley, J.D., Gibbs, D.M., Felner, J.M., and Nutter, D.O.: Cardiac abnormalities in cachectic patients before and during nutritional repletion, Am. Heart J. **95**:584, 1978.

775. Higginson, J., Gillanders, A.D., and Murray, J.F.: Heart in chronic malnutrition, Br. Heart J. **14**:213, 1952.

776. Hogg, G.R.: Cardiac lesions in hemolytic disease of the newborn, J. Pediatr. **60**:352, 1962.

777. Keys, A., Henschel, A., and Taylor, H.L.: The size and function of the human heart at rest in semi-starvation and in subsequent rehabilitation, Am. J. Physiol. **50**:153, 1947.

778. Lin, C.T., and Chen, L.H.: Ultrastructural and lysosomal enzyme studies of skeletal muscle and myocarditis in rats with long-term vitamin E deficiency, Pathology **14**:375, 1982.

779. Paplanus, S.H., Zbar, M.J., and Hays, J.W.: Cardiac hypertrophy as a manifestation of chronic anemia, Am. J. Pathol. **34**:149, 1958.

780. Scott, J.M.: Fatty change in the myocardium of newborn infants, Am. Heart J. **64**:283, 1962.

781. Swanepoel, A., Smythe, P.M., and Campbell, J.A.H.: The heart in kwashiorkor, Am. Heart J. **67**:1, 1964.

782. Uzsoy, N.K.: Cardiovascular findings in patients with sickle cell anemia, Am. J. Cardiol. **13**:320, 1964.

783. Van Vleet, J.F., Ferrans, V.J., and Ruth, G.R.: Ultrastructural alterations in nutritional cardiomyopathy of selenium–vitamin E deficient swine. I. Fiber lesions, Lab. Invest. **37**:188, 1977.

784. Van Vleet, J.F., Ferrans, V.J., and Ruth, G.R.: Ultrastructural alterations in nutritional cardiomyopathy of selenium–vitamin E deficient swine. II. Vascular lesions, Lab. Invest. **37**:201, 1977.

785. Wharton, B.A., Balmer, S.E., and Somers, K.: The myocardium in kwashiorhor, Q. J. Med. **149**:107, 1969.

786. Wharton, B.A., Balmer, S.E., Somers, K., and Templeton, A.C.: The myocardium in kwashiorkor, Q. J. Med. **149**:107, 1969.

787. Wolbach, S.B.: Pathologic changes resulting from vitamin deficiency, JAMA **108**:7, 1937.

Electrolyte disturbances

788. Bajusz, E.: Myocardial calcification and cardiac surgery, Lancet **1**:174, 1964.

789. Bonucci, E., and Sadun, R.: Experimental calcification of the myocardium, Am. J. Pathol. **71**:167, 1973.

790. Burch, G.E., and Giles, T.D.: The importance of magnesium deficiency in cardiovascular disease, Am. Heart J. **94**:649, 1977.

791. Chang, C., and Bloom, S.: Interrelationship of dietary intake and electrolyte homeostasis in hamsters. I. Severe Mg deficiency, electrolyte homeostasis, and myocardial necrosis, J. Am. Coll. Nutr. **4**:173, 1985.

792. French, J.E.: Histologic study of heart lesions in potassium-deficient rats, Arch. Pathol. **53**:485, 1952.

793. Fuller, T.J., Nichols, W.W., Brenner, B.J., and Peterson, J.C.: Reversible depression in myocardial performance in dogs with experimental phosphorus deficiency, J. Clin. Invest. **62**:1194, 1978.

794. Gore, I., and Aarons, W.: Calcification of myocardium: a pathologic study of 13 cases, Arch. Pathol. **48**:1, 1949.

795. Harrison, C.E., Jr., Cooper, G., IV, and Zijko, K.J.: Myocardial and mitochondrial function in potassium depletion cardiomyopathy, J. Mol. Cell. Cardiol. **4**:633, 1972.

796. Harrison, T.R., Pilcher, C., and Ewing, G.: Studies in congestive heart failure. IV. The potassium content of skeletal and cardiac muscle, J. Clin. Invest. **8**:325, 1930.

797. Johnson, R.A., Baker, S.S., Fallon, J.T., Maynard, E.P., III, Ruskin, J.N., Wen, Z., Ge, K., and Cohen, H.J.: An occidental case of cardiomyopathy and selenium deficiency, N. Engl. J. Med. **304**:1210, 1981.

798. Kopp, S.J., Klevay, L.M., and Feliksik, J.M.: Physiological and metabolic characterization of a cardiomyopathy induced by chronic copper deficiency, Am. J. Physiol. **245**:H855, 1983.

799. McAllen, P.M.: Myocardial changes occurring in potassium deficiency, Br. Heart J. **17**:5, 1955.
800. Molnar, Z., Larsen, K., and Spargo, B.: Cardiac changes in the potassium depleted rat, Arch. Pathol. **74**:339, 1962.
801. Olesen, K.H.: Body composition in heart disease: total exchangeable potassium, total exchangeable sodium, total exchangeable chloride and derived values for body composition in cardiac disease with and without edema, Acta Med. Scand. **175**:301, 1964.
802. Reye, J.D., Jr.: Death in potassium deficiency: report of case including morphologic findings, Circulation **5**:766, 1952.
803. Roberts, W.C., and Waller, B.F.: Effect of chronic hypercalcemia on the heart: an analysis of 18 necropsy patients, Am. J. Med. **71**:371, 1981.
804. Rude, R.K., and Singer, F.R.: Magnesium deficiency and excess, Ann. Rev. Med. **32**:245, 1981.
805. Sarkar, K., and Levine, D.Z.: Repair of the myocardial lesion during potassium repletion of kaliopenic rats: an ultrastructural study, J. Mol. Cell. Cardiol. **11**:1165, 1979.
806. Woodhouse, M.A., and Burston, J.: Metastatic calcification of the myocardium, J. Pathol. **97**:733, 1969.

Drugs and toxic agents

807. Bloom, S., and Davis, D.L.: Calcium as mediator of isoproterenol-induced myocardial necrosis, Am. J. Pathol. **69**:459, 1972.
808. Cebelin, M.S., and Hirsch, C.S.: Human stress cardiomyopathy, Hum. Pathol. **11**:123, 1980.
809. Collins, P., Billings, C.G., and Barer, G.R.: Quantitation of isoprenaline-induced changes in the ventricular myocardium, Cardiovasc. Res. **9**:797, 1975.
810. Connor, R.C.R.: Focal myocytolysis and fuchsinophilic degeneration of the myocardium of patients dying with various brain lesions, Ann. NY Acad. Sci. **156**:261, 1969.
811. Eliot, R.S., Clayton, F.C., and Pieper, G.M.: Influence of environmental stress on pathogenesis of sudden cardiac death, Fed. Proc. **36**:1719, 1977.
812. Fleckenstein, A., Janke, J., Doring, H.J., and Pachinger, O.: Ca overload as the determinant factor in the production of catecholamine-induced myocardial lesions. In Bajusz, E., et al. editors: Recent advances in studies on cardiac structure and metabolism, cardiomyopathies, vol. 2, Baltimore, 1973, University Park Press.
813. Kahn, D.S., Rona, G., and Chappel, C.I.: Isoproterenol-induced cardiac necrosis, Ann. NY Acad. Sci. **156**:285, 1969.
814. Kline, I.K.: Myocardial alterations associated with pheochromocytomas, Am. J. Pathol. **38**:539, 1961.
815. Gopinath, G., Thuring, J., and Zayed, I.: Isoprenaline-induced myocardial necrosis in dogs, Br. J. Exp. Pathol. **59**:148, 1978.
816. Kolin, A., and Norris, J.W.: Myocardial damage from acute cerebral lesions, Stroke **15**:990, 1984.
817. Mikolich, J.R., Jacobs, W.C., and Fletcher, G.F.: Cardiac arrhythmias in patients with acute cerebrovascular accidents, JAMA **246**:1314, 1981.
818. Norris, J.W., Hachinski, V.C., Myers, M.G., Callow, J., Wong, T., and Moore, R.W.: Serum cardiac enzymes in stroke, Stroke **10**:548, 1979.
819. Pieper, G.M., Clayton, F.C., Todd, G.L., and Eliot, R.S.: Transmural distribution of metabolites and blood flow in the canine left ventricle following isoproterenol infusions, J. Pharmacol. Exp. Ther. **209**:334, 1979.
820. Rona, G., Chappel, C.I., Balázs, T., and Gaudry, R.: An infarct-like myocardial lesion and other toxic manifestations produced by isoproterenol in the rat, Arch. Pathol. **67**:443, 1959.
821. Rona, G.: Catecholamine cardiotoxicity, J. Mol. Cell. Cardiol. **17**:291, 1985.
822. Singal, P.K., Beamish, R.E., and Dhalla, N.S.: Potential oxidative pathways of catecholamines in the formation of lipid peroxidase and genesis of heart disease. In Spitzer, J.J., editor: Myocardial injury, New York, 1983, Plenum Pub. Corp.
823. Somani, P., Laddu, A.R., and Hardman, H.F.: Nutritional circulation in the heart. III. Effects of isoproterenol and beta adrenergic blockage on myocardial hemodynamics and rubidium-86 extraction in the isolated supported heart preparation, J. Pharmacol. Exp. Ther. **175**:577, 1970.
824. Szakacs, J.E., and Cannon, A.: *l*-Norepinephrine myocarditis, Am. J. Clin. Pathol. **30**:425, 1958.
825. Van Vliet, P.D., Burchell, H.B., and Titus, J.L.: Focal myocarditis associated with pheochromocytoma, N. Engl. J. Med. **274**:1102, 1966.
826. Yates, J.C., Beamish, R.E., and Dhalla, N.S.: Ventricular dysfunction and necrosis produced by adrenochrome metabolite of epinephrine: relation to pathogenesis of catecholamine cardiomyopathy, Am. Heart J. **102**:210, 1981.
827. Yates, J.C., and Dhalla, N.S.: Induction of necrosis and failure in the isolated perfused rat heart with oxidized isoproterenol, J. Mol. Cell. Cardiol. **7**:807, 1975.

Myocardial involvement in some miscellaneous systemic diseases

828. Beutner, E.H., Witebsky, E., Ricken, D., and Adler, R.H.: Studies on autoantibodies in myasthenia gravis, JAMA **182**:46, 1962.
829. Burke, J.S., Medline, N.M., and Katz, A.: A giant cell myocarditis and myasthenia gravis, Arch. Pathol. **88**:359, 1969.
830. Frankel, K.A., and Rosser, R.J.: The pathology of the heart in progressive muscular dystrophy: epimyocardial fibrosis, Hum. Pathol. **7**:375, 1976.
831. James, T.N.: Observations on the cardiovascular involvement, including the cardiac conduction system, in progressive muscular dystrophy, Am. Heart J. **63**:48, 1962.
832. James, T.N., and Fisch, C.: Observations on the cardiovascular involvement in Friedreich's ataxis, Am. Heart J. **66**:164, 1963.
833. Manning, G.W.: Cardiac manifestations in Friedreich's ataxia, Am. Heart J. **39**:799, 1950.
834. Mendelow, H., and Genkins, G.: Studies in myasthenia gravis: cardiac and associated pathology, J. Mt. Sinai Hosp. **21**:218, 1954.
835. Nothacker, W.G., and Netsky, M.G.: Myocardial lesions in progressive muscular dystrophy, Arch. Pathol. **50**:578, 1950.
836. Russell, D.S.: Myocarditis in Friedreich's ataxia, J. Pathol. Bacteriol. **58**:739, 1946.
837. Sanyal, S.K., Johnson, W.W., Thapar, M.K., and Pitner, S.E.: An ultrastructural basis for electrocardiographic alterations associated with Duchenne's progressive muscular dystrophy of heart, Circulation **57**:1122, 1978.
838. Storstein, O., and Austarheim, K.: Progressive muscular dystrophy of heart, Acta Med. Scand. **150**:431, 1955.

Restrictive cardiomyopathy

839. Andy, J.J., Bishara, F.F., and Soyinka, O.O.: Relation of severe eosinophilia and microfilariasis to chronic African endomyocardial fibrosis, Br. Heart J. **45**:672, 1981.
840. Benotti, J.R.: Restrictive cardiomyopathy, Annu. Rev. Med. **35**:113, 1984.
841. Brandt, K., Cathcart, E.S., and Cohen, A.S.: A clinical analysis of the course and prognosis of 42 patients with amyloidosis, Am. J. Med. **44**:955, 1969.
842. Bridgen, W.: Cardiac amyloidosis, Prog. Cardiovasc. Dis. **7**:142, 1964.
843. Buja, L.M., Khoi, N.B., and Roberts, W.C.: Clinically significant cardiac amyloidosis: clinicopathologic findings in 15 patients, Am. J. Cardiol. **26**:394, 1970.
844. Chew, C.Y.C., Zlady, G.M., Raphael, M.J., Nellen, M., and Oakley, C.M.: Primary restrictive cardiomyopathy: non-tropical endomyocardial fibrosis and hypereosinophilic heart disease, Br. Heart J. **39**:399, 1977.
845. Chew, C.Y.C., Zlady, G.M., Raphael, M.J., and Oakley, C.M.: The functional defect in amyloid heart disease: the "stiff heart" syndrome, Am. J. Cardiol. **36**:438, 1975.
846. Cohen, A.S.: Amyloidosis, N. Engl. J. Med. **277**:522, 1967.
847. Cornwell, G.G., III, Natvig, J.B., Westermark, P., and Husby, G.: Senile cardiac amyloid: demonstration of a unique fibril protein in tissue sections, J. Immunol. **120**:1385, 1978.
848. Davies, J.N.P.: The heart of Africa: cardiac pathology in the population of Uganda, Lab. Invest. **10**:205, 1961.

849. Davies, J.N.P., and Ball, J.D.: The pathology of endomyocardial fibrosis in Uganda, Br. Heart J. **17**:337, 1955.

850. Geme, J.W.S., Davis, C.W.C., and Noren, G.R.: An overview of primary endocardial fibroelastosis and chronic viral cardiomyopathy, Perspect. Biol. Med. **17**:495, 1974.

851. Hutchins, G.M., and Bannayan, G.A.: Development of endocardial fibroelastosis following myocardial infarction, Arch. Pathol. **91**:113, 1971.

852. Johnson, F.R.: Anoxia as cause of endocardial fibroelastosis in infancy, Arch. Pathol. **54**:23, 1951.

853. Olsen, E.G.J., and Spry, C.J.F.: Relation between eosinophilia and endomyocardial disease, Prog. Cardiovasc. Dis. **27**:241, 1985.

854. Ridolfi, R.L., Bulkley, B.H., and Hutchins, G.M.: The conduction system in cardiac amyloidosis: clinical and pathologic features of 23 patients, Am. J. Med. **62**:677, 1977.

855. Roberts, W.C., and Morrow, A.G.: Secondary left ventricular endocardial fibroelastosis following mitral valve replacement: cause of cardiac failure in the late postoperatve period, Circulation 37(suppl. 2):101, 1968.

856. Roberts, W.C., and Waller, B.F.: Cardiac amyloidosis causing cardiac dysfunction: analysis of 54 necropsy patients, Am. J. Cardiol. **52**:137, 1983.

857. Saffitz, J.E., Sazama, K., and Roberts, W.C.: Amyloidosis limited to small arteries causing angina pectoris and sudden death, Am. J. Cardiol. **51**:1234, 1983.

858. Schryer, M.J.P., and Karnauchow, P.N.: Endocardial fibroelastosis: etiologic and pathogenetic considerations in children, Am. Heart J. **88**:557, 1974.

859. Siegel, R.J., Shah, P.K., and Fishbein, M.C.: Idiopathic restrictive cardiomyopathy, Circulation **70**:165, 1984.

860. Thomas, W.A., Randall, R.V., Bland, E.F., and Castleman, B.: Endocardial fibroelastosis: factor in heart disease of obscure etiology: study of 20 autopsied cases in children and adults, N. Engl. J. Med. **25**:327, 1954.

861. Valiathan, M.S., Kartha, C.C., Panday, V.K., Dang, H.S., and Sunta, C.M.: A geochemical basis for endomyocardial fibrosis, Cardiovasc. Res. **20**:679, 1986.

862. Westermark, P., Johansson, B., and Natvig, J.B.: Senile cardiac amyloidosis: evidence of two different amyloid substances in the ageing heart, Scand. J. Immunol. **10**:303, 1979.

Basophilic and fatty degeneration

863. Bilheimer, D.W.: Fatty acid accumulation and abnormal lipid deposition in peripheral and border zones of experimental myocardial infarcts, J. Nucl. Med. **19**:276, 1978.

864. Brewer, D.B.: Myxoedema: autopsy report with histochemical observations on nature of mucoid infiltrations, J. Pathol. Bacteriol. **63**:503, 1951.

865. Bruce, T.A., and Myers, J.T.: Myocardial lipid metabolism in ischemia and infarction, Recent Adv. Stud. Cardiac Struct. Metab. **3**:773, 1973.

866. Crass, M.F., III, and Sterrett, P.R.: Distribution of glycogen and lipids in the ischemic canine left ventricle: biochemical and light and electron microscopic correlates, Recent Adv. Stud. Cardiac Struct. Metab. **10**:251, 1975.

867. Fisher, C.E., and Mulligan, R.M.: Quantitative study of correlation between basophilic degeneration of myocardium and atrophy of thyroid gland, Arch. Pathol. **36**:206, 1943.

868. Haust, M.D., Rowlands, D.T., Jr., Garancis, J.C., and Landing, B.H.: Histochemical studies on cardiac "colloid," Am. J. Pathol. **40**:185, 1962.

869. Jesmok, G.J., Warltier, D.C., Gross, G.J., and Hardman, H.F.: Transmural triglycerides in acute myocardial ischaemia, Cardiovasc. Res. **12**:659, 1978.

870. Kosek, J.C., and Angell, W.: Fine structure of basophilic myocardial degeneration, Arch. Pathol. **89**:491, 1970.

871. Manion, W.C.: Basophilic mucoid degeneration of the heart, Med. Ann. DC **34**:60, 1965.

872. Moore, K.H., Radloff, J.F., Hull, F.E., and Sweeley, C.C.: Incomplete fatty acid oxidation by ischemic heart: β-hydroxy fatty acid production, Am. J. Physiol. **239**:H257, 1980.

873. Rosai, J., and Lascano, E.F.: Basophilic (mucoid) degeneration of myocardium, Am. J. Pathol. **61**:99, 1970.

874. Rovetto, M.J., Lamberton, W.F., and Neely, J.R.: Mechanisms of glycolytic inhibition in ischemic rat hearts, Circ. Res. **37**:742, 1975.

875. Roy, P.E.: Basophilic degeneration of myocardium, Lab. Invest. **32**:729, 1975.

876. Scott, J.M.: Fatty change in the myocardium of newborn infants, Am. Heart J. **64**:283, 1962.

877. Scotti, T.M.: Basophilic (mucinous) degeneration of myocardium, Am. J. Clin. Pathol. **25**:994, 1955.

878. Staszewska-Barczak, J.: The reflex stimulation of catecholamine secretion during the acute stages of myocardial infarction in the dog, Clin. Sci. **41**:419, 1971.

879. Vetter, N.J., Strange, R.C., and Adams, W.: Initial metabolic and hormonal response to acute myocardial infarction, Lancet **1**:284, 1974.

880. Wartman, W.B., Jennings, R.B., Yokoyama, H.O., and Clabaugh, G.F.: Fatty change of the myocardium in early experimental infarction, Arch. Pathol. **62**:318, 1956.

Myocardial injury from mechanical causes, ionizing radiation, or hypovolemic shock

Trauma

881. Cuadros, C.L., Hutchinson, J.E., III, and Mogtader, A.H.: Laceration of a mitral papillary muscle and the aortic root as a result of blunt trauma to the chest, J. Thorac. Cardiovasc. Surg. **88**:134, 1984.

882. Dugani, B.V., Higginson, L.A., Beanlands, D.S., and Akyurekli, Y.: Recurrent systemic emboli following myocardial contusion, Am. Heart J. **108**:1354, 1984.

883. Fallahnejad, M., Kutty, A.C.K., and Wallace, H.W.: Secondary lesions of penetrating cardiac injuries: a frequent complication, Ann. Surg. **191**:228, 1980.

884. Harley, D.P., Mena, I., Narahara, K.A., Miranda, R., and Nelson, R.J.: Traumatic myocardial dysfunction, J. Thorac. Cardiovasc. Surg. **87**:386, 1984.

885. Hellman, R.M., and Rufty, A.J., Jr.: Left ventricular aneurysms caused by blunt chest trauma, South. Med. J. **71**:652, 1978.

886. Mackintosh, A.F., and Fleming, H.A.: Cardiac damage presenting late after road accidents, Thorax **36**:811, 1981.

887. Moritz, A.R.: Injuries of heart and pericardium by physical violence. In Gould, S.E., editor: Pathology of the heart, ed. 3, Springfield, Ill., 1968, Charles C Thomas, Publisher.

888. Parmley, L.F., Manion, W.C., and Mattingly, T.W.: Nonpenetrating wounds of the heart and aorta, Circulation **18**:371, 1958.

889. Parmley, L.F., Mattingly, T.W., and Manion, W.C.: Penetrating wounds of the heart and aorta, Circulation **17**:953, 1958.

Radiation injury

890. Allenstein, B.J., Amromin, G.D., Gildenhorn, H.L., and Solomon, R.D.: The synergism of X-irradiation and cholesterol-fat feeding on the development of coronary artery lesions, J. Atherosclerosis Res. **4**:325, 1964.

891. Applefeld, M.M., Slawson, R.G., Hall-Craigs, M., Green, D.C., Singleton, R.T., and Wiernik, P.H.: Delayed pericardial disease after radiotherapy, Am. J. Cardiol. **47**:210, 1981.

892. Applefeld, M.M., and Wiernik, P.H.: Cardiac disease after radiation therapy for Hodgkin's disease: analysis of 48 patients, Am. J. Cardiol. **51**:679, 1983.

893. Billingham, M.E., Bristow, M.R., Glatstein, E., Mason, J.W., Masek, M.A., and Daniels, J.R.: Adriamycin cardiotoxicity: endomyocardial biopsy evidence of enhancement of irradiation, Am. J. Surg. Pathol. **1**:17, 1977.

894. Brosius, F.C., Waller, B.F., and Roberts, W.C.: Radiation heart disease: analysis of 16 young (aged 15 to 33 years) necropsy patients who received over 3,500 rads to the heart, Am. J. Med. **70**:519, 1981.

895. Cohn, K.E., Stewart, J.R., and Fajardo, L.F.: Heart disease following radiation, Medicine **46**:281, 1967.

896. Fajardo, L.F.: Radiation-induced coronary artery disease, Chest 71:563, 1977. (Editorial.)

897. Fajardo, L.F., Eltringham, J.R., and Stewart, J.R.: Combined cardiotoxicity of adriamycin and X-radiation, Lab. Invest. 34:86, 1976.

898. Fajardo, L.F., and Stewart, J.R.: Capillary injury preceding radiation-induced myocardial fibrosis, Radiology 101:429, 1971.

899. Kinsella, T.J., Ahmann, D.L., Giuliani, E.R., and Lie, J.T.: Adriamycin cardiotoxicity in stage IV breast cancer: possible enhancement with prior left chest radiation therapy, Int. J. Radiat. Oncol. Biol. Phys. 5:1997, 1979.

900. Merrill, J.: Adriamycin and radiation: synergistic cardiotoxicity, Ann. Intern. Med. 82:122, 1975.

901. Schneider, J.S., and Edwards, J.E.: Irradiation-induced pericarditis, Chest 75:560, 1979.

902. Stewart, J.R., and Fajardo, L.F.: Radiation-induced heart disease: clinical and experimental aspects, Radiol. Clin. North Am. 9:511, 1971.

903. Stewart, J.R., and Fajardo, L.F.: Radiation-induced heart disease: an update, Prog. Cardiovasc. Dis. 27:173, 1984.

Hypovolemic shock

904. Hackel, D.B., Ratliff, N.B., and Mikat, E.M.: The heart in shock, Circ. Res. 25:895, 1974.

905. Lefer, A.M.: Properties of cardioinhibitory factors produced in shock, Fed. Proc. 37:2734, 1978.

906. Mallory, T.B.: Systemic pathology consequent to traumatic shock, J. Mt. Sinai Hosp. 16:137, 1949.

907. Martin, A.M., Jr., and Hackel, D.B.: The myocardium of the dog in shock: a histochemical study, Lab. Invest. 12:77, 1963.

908. Melcher, G.W., and Walcott, W.W.: Myocardial changes following shock, Am. J. Physiol. 164:832, 1951.

909. Okada, K., Kosugi, I., Kitagaki, T., et al.: Pathophysiology of shock, Jpn. Circ. J. 41:346, 1977.

910. Siegel, H.W., and Downing, S.E.: Reduction of left ventricular contractility during acute hemorrhagic shock, Am. J. Physiol. 218:772, 1970.

911. Ratliff, N.B., Hackel, D.B., and Mikat, E.: Myocardial carbohydrate metabolism and lesions in hemorrhagic shock: effects of hyperbaric oxygen, Arch. Pathol. 88:470, 1969.

Tumors of the heart

912. Abenoza, P., and Sibley, R.K.: Cardiac myxoma with glandlike structures, Arch. Pathol. Lab. Med. 110:736, 1986.

913. Bell, D.A., and Greco, M.A.: Cardiac myxoma with chondroid features: a light and electron microscopic study, Hum. Pathol. 12:370, 1981.

914. Benjamin, H.S.: Primary fibromyxoma of the heart, Arch. Pathol. 27:950, 1939.

915. Boyd, T.A.B.: Blood cysts on heart valves of infants, Am. J. Pathol. 25:757, 1949.

916. Bruni, C., Prioleau, P.G., Ivey, H.H., and Nolan, S.P.: New fine structural features of cardiac rhabdomyoma: report of a case, Cancer 46:2068, 1980.

917. Davies, M.J.: Tumors of the heart and pericardium. In Pomerance, A., and Davies, M.J., editors: The pathology of the heart, Oxford, 1975, Blackwell Scientific Publications.

918. DeRoover, P.H., Maisin, J., and Lacquet, A.: Congenital pleuropericardial cysts, Thorax 18:146, 1963.

919. Diferding, J.T., Gardner, R.E., and Roe, B.B.: Intracardiac myxomas with report of two unusual cases and successful removal, Circulation 23:929, 1961.

920. Feigin, D.S., Fenoglio, J.J., McAllister, H.A., et al.: Pericardial cysts: a radiologic-pathologic correlation and review, Radiology 125:15, 1977.

921. Feldman, P.S., Horvath, E., and Kovacs, K.: An ultrastructural study of seven cardiac myxomas, Cancer 40:2216, 1977.

922. Fenoglio, J., Jr., McAllister, H.A., Jr., and Ferrans, V.J.: Cardiac rhabdomyoma: a clinicopathologic and electron microscopic study, Am. J. Cardiol. 38:241, 1976.

923. Ferrans, V.J., and Roberts, W.C.: Structural features of cardiac myxomas, Hum. Pathol. 4:111, 1973.

924. Fine, G.: Neoplasms of the pericardium and heart. In Gould, S.E., editor: Pathology of the heart and blood vessels, ed. 3, Springfield, Ill., 1968, Charles C Thomas, Publisher.

925. Fine, G., Morales, A., and Horn, R.C., Jr.: Cardiac myxoma: a morphologic and histogenetic appraisal, Cancer 22:1156, 1968.

926. Fishbein, M.C., Ferrans, V.J., and Roberts, W.C.: Endocardial papillary elastofibromas: histologic, histochemical, and electron microscopical findings, Arch. Pathol. 99:335, 1975.

927. Fisher, E.R., and Hellstrom, H.R.: Evidence in favor of the neoplastic nature of cardiac myxomas, Am. Heart J. 60:630, 1960.

928. Foster, E.D., Spooner, E.W., Farina, J.A., Shaher, R.M., and Alley, R.D.: Cardiac rhabdomyoma in the neonate: surgical management, Ann. Thorac. Surg. 37:249, 1984.

929. Goodwin, J.F.: The spectrum of cardiac tumors, Am. J. Cardiol. 31:307, 1968.

930. Griffiths, G.C.: A review of primary tumors of the heart, Prog. Cardiovasc. Dis. 7:465, 1965.

931. Hannah, H., III, Eisemann, G., Hiszczynskyj, R., Winsky, M., and Cohen, L.: Invasive atrial myxoma: documentation of malignant potential of cardiac myxomas, Am. Heart J. 104:881, 1982.

932. Heath, D.: Pathology of cardiac tumors, Am. J. Cardiol. 21:315, 1968.

933. Heath, D., Best, P.V., and Davis, B.T.: Papilliferous tumours of the heart valves, Br. Heart J. 23:20, 1961.

934. Heggtveit, H.A., Fenoglio, J.J., and McAllister, H.A.: Lipomatous hypertrophy at the interatrial septum: an assessment of 41 cases, Lab. Invest. 34:318, 1976.

935. Hutter, A.M., Jr., and Page, D.L.: Atrial arrhythmias and lipomatous hypertrophy of the cardiac interatrial septum, Am. Heart J. 82:16, 1971.

936. Kidder, L.A.: Congenital glycogenic tumor of heart, Arch. Pathol. 49:55, 1950.

937. Landon, G., Ordóñez, N.G., and Guarda, L.A.: Cardiac myxomas: an immunohistochemical study using endothelial, histiocytic, and smooth-muscle cells, Arch. Pathol. Lab. Med. 110:116, 1986.

838. Larrieu, A.J., Jamieson, W.R., Tyers, G.F., Burr, L.H., Munro, A.I., Miyagishima, R.T., Gerein, A.N., and Allen, P.: Primary cardiac tumors, J. Thorac. Cardiovasc. Surg. 83:339, 1982.

939. Lichtenstein, H.L., Lee, J.C.K., and Stewart, S.: Papillary tumor of the heart: incidental finding at surgery, Hum. Pathol. 10:473, 1979.

940. Lillie, W.I., McDonald, J.R., and Clagett, O.T.: Pericardial celomic cysts and pericardial diverticula: a concept of etiology and report of cases, J. Thorac. Cardiovasc. Surg. 20:494, 1950.

941. Markel, M.L., Armstrong, W.F., Mahoned, Y., and Waller, B.F.: Left atrial myxoma with multicentric recurrence and evidence of metastases, Am. Heart J. 111:409, 1986.

942. Marshall, F.C.: Epithelial cyst of the heart, Arch. Pathol. 64:107, 1957.

943. McAllister, H.A., Jr.: Primary tumors of the heart and pericardium, Pathol. Annu. 14:335, 1979.

944. McAllister, H.A., Jr., and Fenoglio, J.J., Jr.: Tumors of the cardiovascular system. Atlas of tumor pathology, Second Series, Fascicle 15, Washington, D.C., 1977, Armed Forces Institute of Pathology.

945. Merkow, L.P., Kooros, M.A., and Magovern, G.: Ultrastructure of a cardian myxoma, Arch. Pathol. 88:390, 1969.

946. Mikuz, G., Hofstädter, F., Hansen, A., and Hager, J.: The socalled cardiac myxoma, Virchows Arch. [A, Pathol. Anat.] 380:221, 1978.

947. Morales, A.R., Fine, G., Castro, A., and Nadji, M.: Cardiac myxoma (endocardioma), an immunochemical assessment of histogenesis, Hum. Pathol. 12:896, 1981.

948. Morris, A.W., and Johnson, I.M.: Epithelial inclusion cysts of the heart: a case report and review of literature, Arch. Pathol. 77:36, 1964.

949. Page, D.L.: Lipomatous hypertrophy of the cardiac interatrial

septum: its development and probable clinical significance, Hum. Pathol. 1:151, 1970.

950. Pomerance, A.: Papillary "tumours" of the heart valves, J. Pathol. Bacteriol. 81:135, 1961.

951. Prichard, R.W.: Tumors of heart: review of subject and report of 150 cases, Arch. Pathol. 51:98, 1951.

952. Prior, J.T.: Lipomatous hypertrophy of cardiac interatrial septum, Arch. Pathol. 78:11, 1964.

953. Reece, I.J., Cooley, D.A., Frazier, O.H., Hallman, G.L., Powers, P.L., and Montero, C.G.: Cardiac tumors: clinical spectrum and prognosis of lesions other than classical benign myxoma in 20 patients, J. Thorac. Cardiovasc. Surg. 88:439, 1984.

954. Salyer, W.R., Page, D.L., and Hutchins, G.M.: The development of cardiac myxomas and papillary endocardial lesions from mural thrombus, Am. Heart J. 89:14, 1975.

955. Scott, R.W., and Garvin, C.F.: Tumours of the heart and pericardium, Am. Heart J. 17:431, 1939.

956. Silverman, N.A.: Primary cardiac tumors, Ann. Surg. 191:127, 1980.

957. Silverman, J.F., Kay, S., and McCue, C.M.: Rhabdomyoma of the heart: ultrastructural study of three cases, Lab. Invest. 35:596, 1976.

958. Steinbiss, W.: Zur Kentniss der Rhabdomyome des Herzens und ihrer Beziehungen zur tuberosen Gehirnsklerose, Virchows Arch. 243:22, 1923.

959. Sutton, M.G.: Atrial myxomas: a review of clinical experience in 40 patients, Mayo Clin. Proc. 55:371, 1980.

960. Straus, R., and Merliss, R.: Primary tumors of the heart, Arch. Pathol. 39:74, 1945.

961. Trillo, A.A., Holleman, I.L., and White, J.T.: Presence of satellite cells in a cardiac rhabdomyoma, Histopathology 2:215, 1978.

962. Wold, L.E., and Lie, J.T.: Cardiac myxomas: a clinicopathologic profile, Am. J. Pathol. 101:217, 1980.

963. Wychulis, A.R., Connolly, D.C., and McGoon, D.C.: Pericardial cysts, tumors, and fat necrosis, J. Thorac. Cardiovasc. Surg. 62:294, 1971.

Disturbances of the conducting system

964. Anderson, R.H., Wenick, A.C.G., Losekoot, T.G., and Becker, A.E.: Congenitally complete heart block: developmental aspects, Circulation 56:90, 1977.

965. Buckberg, G.D., and Fowler, N.O.: Complete atrioventricular block due to cardiac metastasis of bronchogenic carcinoma, 24:657, 1961.

966. Davies, M.J., Anderson, R.H., and Becker, A.E.: The conduction system of the heart, London, 1983, Butterworth & Co.

967. Davies, M.J., and Harris, A.: Pathological basis of primary heart block, Br. Heart J. 31:219, 1969.

968. Fryda, R.J., Kaplan, S., and Helmsworth, J.A.: Postoperative complete heart block in children, Br. Heart J. 33:456, 1971.

969. Gallagher, J.J., Gilbert, M., and Svenson, R.H.: WPW syndrome: the problem, evaluation and surgical correction, Circulation 51:767, 1975.

970. Gross, L., and Fried, B.M.: Lesions in the auriculoventricular conduction system occurring in rheumatic fever, Am. J. Pathol. 12:31, 1936.

971. Griffiths, S.P.: Congenital complete heart block, Circulation 43:615, 1971. (Editorial.)

972. Hackel, D.B.: Anatomy and pathology of the cardiac conducting system. In Edwards, J.E., Lev, M., and Abell, M.R., editors: The heart, Int. Acad. Pathol. Monogr. no. 15, Baltimore, 1974, The Williams & Wilkins Co.

973. Hackel, D.B.: Anatomic basis for preexcitation syndromes. In Benson, D.W., and Benditt, D.G., editors: Preexcitation syndromes, Dordrecht, Netherlands, 1986, Martinus Nijhoff.

974. Hackel, D.B., and Estes, E.H.: Pathologic features of atrioventricular and interventricular conduction disturbances in acute myocardial infarction, Circulation 43:977, 1972.

975. Ho, S.Y., Esscher, E., Anderson, R.H., and Michaëlsson, M.: Anatomy of congenital heart block and relation to maternal anti-R₀ antibodies, Am. J. Cardiol. 58:291, 1986.

976. Lenègre, J.: Etiology and pathology of bilateral bundle branch block in relation to complete heart block, Prog. Cardiovasc. Dis. 6:409, 1964.

977. Lev, M.: Anatomic basis of atrioventricular block, Am. J. Med. 37:742, 1964.

978. Lev, M.: The normal anatomy of the conduction system in man and its pathology in atrioventricular block, Ann. NY Acad. Sci. 111:817, 1964.

979. Lev, M., Silverman, J., FitzMaurice, F.M., Paul, M.H., Cassels, D.E., and Miller, R.A.: Lack of connection between the atria and the more peripheral conduction system in congenital atrioventricular block, Am. J. Cardiol. 27:481, 1971.

980. Linder, J., Shelburne, J.D., Sorge, J.P., Whalen, R.E., and Hackel, D.B.: Congenital endodermal heterotopia of the atrioventricular node: evidence for the endodermal origin of so-called mesotheliomas of the atrioventricular node, Hum. Pathol. 15:1093, 1984.

981. Morales, A.R., Adelman, S., and Fine, J.: Varicella myocarditis: a case of sudden death, Arch. Pathol. 91:29, 1971.

982. Thiene, G., Valente, M., and Rossi, L.: Involvement of the cardiac conducting system in panarteritis nodosa, Am. Heart J. 95:716, 1978.

983. Vigorita, V.J., and Hutchins, G.M.: Cardiac conduction system in hemochromatosis: clinical and pathologic features of six patients, Am. J. Cardiol. 44:418, 1979.

984. Wolff, L., Parkinson, J., and White, P.D.: Bundle branch block with short P-R interval in healthy young people prone to paroxysmal tachycardia, Am. Heart J. 5:685, 1930.

Pathology of endomyocardial biopsy specimens

985. Aretz, H.T.: Myocarditis: the Dallas criteria, Hum. Pathol. 18:619, 1987.

986. Bieber, C.P., et al.: Cardiac transplantation in man. VII. Cardiac allograft pathology, Circulation 41:753, 1970.

987. Billingham, M.E.: Morphologic changes in drug-induced heart disease. In Bristow, M.R., editor: Drug-induced heart disease, Amsterdam, 1980, Elsevier/North-Holland Biomedical Press.

988. Billingham, M.E., and Bristow, M.R.: Endomyocardial biopsy for cardiac monitoring of patients receiving anthracyclines. In Fenoglio, J.J., Jr., editor: Endomyocardial biopsy: techniques and applications, Boca Raton, Fla., 1982, CRC Press.

989. Billingham, M.E., and Mason, J.W.: The role of endomyocardial biopsy in the management of acute rejection in cardiac allograft recipients. In Fenoglio, J.J., Jr., editor: Endomyocardial biopsy: techniques and applications, Boca Raton, Fla., 1982, CRC Press.

990. Chomette, G., Auriol, M., Delcourt, A., Karkouche, B., Cabrol, A., and Cabrol, C.: Human cardiac transplants: diagnosis of rejection by endomyocardial biopsy: causes of death (about 30 autopsies), Virchows Arch. [A] 407:295, 1985.

991. Fenoglio, J.J., Jr.: Diagnostic approach to the endomyocardial biopsy. In Fenoglio, J.J., Jr., editor: Endomyocardial biopsy: techniques and applications, Boca Raton, Fla., 1982, CRC Press.

992. Fenoglio, J.J., Jr.: The cardiomyopathies: diagnosis by endomyocardial biopsy. In Fenoglio, J.J., Jr., editor: Endomyocardial biopsy: techniques and applications, Boca Raton, Fla., 1982, CRC Press.

993. Fenoglio, J.J., Jr., McAllister, H.A., and Mullick, F.G.: Drug related myocarditis. I. Hypersensitivity myocarditis, Hum. Pathol. 12:900, 1981.

994. Fenoglio, J.J., Jr., Ursell, P.C., Kellogg, C.F., Drusin, R.E., and Weiss, M.B.: Diagnosis and classification of myocarditis by endomyocardial biopsy, N. Engl. J. Med. 308:12, 1983.

995. Fenoglio, J.J., Jr., and Marboe, C.C.: Endomyocardial biopsy: an overview, Hum. Pathol. 18:609, 1987.

996. Fowles, R.E., and Mason, J.W.: Role of cardiac biopsy in the diagnosis and management of cardiac disease, Prog. Cardiovasc. Dis. 27:153, 1984.

997. Isner, J.M., Ferrans, V.J., Cohen, S.R., Witkind, B.G., Virmani, R., Gottdiener, J.S., Beck, J.R., and Roberts, W.C.: Clinical and morphologic cardiac findings after anthracycline chemotherapy: analysis of 64 patients studied at necropsy, Am. J. Cardiol. 51:1167, 1983.

998. Kantrowitz, N.E., and Bristow, M.R.: Cardiotoxicity of antitumor agents, Prog. Cardiovasc. Dis. **27**:195, 1984.

999. Kemnitz, J., Cohnert, T., Schäfers, H.J., Helmke, M., Wahlers, T., Herrmann, G., Schmidt, R.M., and Haverich, A.: A classification of cardiac allograft rejection: a modification of the classification by Billingham, Am. J. Surg. Pathol. **11**:503, 1987.

1000. Lefrak, E.A., Pitha, J., and Rosenheim, S.: A clinicopathologic analysis of adriamycin cardiotoxicity, Cancer **32**:302, 1973.

1001. Mason, J.W.: Indications for endomyocardial biopsy. In Fenoglio, J.J., Jr., editor: Endomyocardial biopsy: techniques and applications, Boca Raton, Fla., 1982, CRC Press.

1002. Mason, J.W., and Billingham, M.E.: Acute inflammatory myocarditis. In Fenoglio, J.J., Jr., editor: Endomyocardial biopsy: techniques and applications, Boca Raton, Fla., 1982, CRC Press.

1003. McAllister, H.A., Schnee, M.J.M., Radovancevic, R., and Frazier, O.H.: A system for grading cardiac allograft rejection, Texas Heart Inst. J. **13**:1, 1986.

1004. O'Connell, J.B., Robinson, J.A., Subramanian, R., and Scanlon, P.J.: Endomyocardial biopsy: techniques and applications in heart disease of unknown cause, Heart Transplant. **3**:132, 1984.

1005. Olsen, E.G.J.: Special investigations of COCM: endomyocardial biopsies (morphological analysis), Postgrad. Med. J. **54**:486, 1978.

1006. Pomerance, A., and Stovin, P.G.I.: Heart transplant pathology: the British experience, J. Clin. Pathol. **38**:146, 1985.

1007. Taliercio, C.P., Olney, B.A., and Lie, J.T.: Myocarditis related to drug hypersensitivity, Mayo Clin. Proc. **60**:463, 1985.

1008. Ursell, P.C., and Fenoglio, J.J., Jr.: Spectrum of cardiac disease diagnosed by endomyocardial biopsy, Pathol. Annu. **19**:197, 1984.

1009. Uys, C.J., and Rose, A.G.: Cardiac transplantation: aspects of the pathology, Pathol. Ann. **17**:147, 1983.

1010. Uys, C.J., and Rose, A.G.: Pathologic findings in long-term cardiac transplants, Arch. Pathol. Lab. Med. **108**:112, 1984.

1011. Von Hoff, D.D., Layard, M.W., Basa, P., Davis, H.L., Jr., Von Hoff, A.L., Rozencweig, M., and Muggia, F.M.: Risk factors for doxorubicin-induced congestive heart failure, Ann. Intern. Med. **91**:710, 1979.

16 Congenital Heart Disease

MAURICE LEV
SAROJA BHARATI

Knowledge concerning congenital heart disease has increased rapidly in the past 50 years because of advanced in physiology, clinical medicine, and surgery. It is more important for students of pathology to understand mechanisms and hemodynamics than to remember detail. Intended primarily for students, the consideration herein of congenital heart disease is not exhaustive, and for more comprehensive reading the publications of Edwards,[1] Lev,[2] Lev and Bharati,[3] and Netter,[4] and their bibliographies may be consulted.

The pathology of congenital heart disease may be considered from the standpoint of the individual abnormality or from the standpoint of the complex. A *complex*, as the term is used here, is a single abnormality or a group of abnormalities that have a tendency to be associated and the effects of that individual abnormality or group of abnormalities on the economy of the heart. Effects on economy include those on the myocardium, endocardium, valves, and conduction system.

Complexes will be dealt with exclusively in this chapter. They may conveniently be divided into those associated with (1) isolated shunts, (2) isolated obstructions, and (3) obstructions combined with shunts. A few complexes that do not fit into these categories also will be discussed.

A shunt is a transfer of blood from one side of the circulation to the other through an abnormal pathway. It is self-evident that life is normally maintained only with adequate transfer of blood from the systemic to the pulmonary circulation and back again. Such transfer through an abnormal pathway may produce pathologic change. Likewise, it is clear that the entire circulation is characterized by passage of blood through narrower and wider regions. The narrower regions are not necessarily obstructions. An obstruction is one that goes beyond the limits of physiologic narrowing.

Because of the tremendous advances made in the field of congenital heart disease by physiologists, clinicians, and surgeons in the last 50 years, it is necessary to introduce certain terms not ordinarily used in discussing the pathology of heart disease. In this chapter the term *hypertrophy* of a chamber means an increase in muscle mass of that chamber. When this increase is obtained by contraction of the chamber on an increased volume, the term *volume hypertrophy* is used, but when the increase is obtained by contraction of the chamber against increased resistance, the term *pressure hypertrophy* is used. The term *atrophy* of a chamber means a decrease in the muscle mass of that chamber, which again is related to a decrease in volume or pressure. The term *enlargement* of a chamber implies an increased volume in that chamber unrelated to failure of the myocardium. When such enlargement is attributable to failure, the term *dilatation* is used. It is self-evident that volume hypertrophy is accompanied by enlargement. In pressure hypertrophy, the chamber is normal or smaller than normal. The term *endocardial hypertrophy* implies a diffuse or focal increase in thickness of the endocardium because of altered hemodynamics. When diffuse, it is considered to be related to an increase in tension. When focal, it is related to turbulent flow. Increase in tension or turbulence may be obtained either by an increase in pressure or flow or by abnormally directed flow. The histologic counterpart of endocardial hypertrophy is proliferation of the elastic tissue, collagen, and in some cases the smooth muscle components of the endocardium and sometimes also of the subendocardium. When degenerative changes have set in, the term *endocardial sclerosis* is used. The term *hemodynamic changes of valves* implies focal or diffuse thickenings at the edge, the line of closure, the ring, the anulus, or the body of the valve related to altered hemodynamics, whether of pressure or flow. Pressure produces mostly a thickening of the line of closure and edge, whereas flow produces a generalized thickening of the valve.

In the description of complexes it will be understood that changes in the endocardium and valves occur with increased pressure or flow or with turbulent flow as in jet lesions. To simplify matters, these will not always be mentioned.

Aided by Grant HL 30558-05 from the Heart, Lung and Blood Center of the National Institutes of Health, Bethesda, Md.

PATHOLOGY OF ISOLATED SHUNTS

A shunt may occur from the left to the right side or from the right to the left side of the circulation. In instances of isolated shunts (those unaccompanied by obstructive phenomena), if there is no increase in pulmonary resistance, the shunt should be left to right because pulmonary resistance is normally less than peripheral systemic resistance. Such isolated shunts, without pulmonary hypertension, are discussed first, followed by such shunts with pulmonary hypertension and then other shunts that are frequently or invariably associated with pulmonary hypertension.

Left-to-right shunt at atrial level—isolated atrial septal defect complexes

Anomaly. A defect in the atrial septum may occur in the region of the fossa ovalis—called *atrial septal defect, fossa ovalis type (or secundum type)* (Fig. 16-1). It may occur distally, in the region adjacent to the mitral and tricuspid valves—called *atrial septal defect, primum type (persistent ostium primum)* (Fig. 16-2). The latter is always associated with a cleft aortic leaflet of the mitral valve. Or a defect may occur in the proximal portion of the atrial septum—called *proximal septum (sinus venosus) type* (Fig. 16-3). This type of defect is always associated with entry of some or all of the right pulmonary veins into the right atrium, a straddling superior vena cava, a straddling inferior vena cava, or any combination of these. The fourth type of defect is the coronary sinus type. This is a defect in the atrial septum above or in the region of the coronary sinus. Thus the coronary sinus may enter both atria (straddling coronary sinus).

Complex. In the fossa ovalis type of atrial septal defect (Fig. 16-4), there is volume hypertrophy of the right atrium and right ventricle, enlargement of the tricuspid and pulmonic orifices hemodynamic changes of the tricuspid and pulmonic valves, focal or diffuse endocardial hypertrophy of the right atrium and right ventricle, and enlargement of the pulmonary trunk. The left atrium and left ventricle show volume atrophy, with the mitral and aortic orifices smaller than normal. There may be considerable hemodynamic change of the mitral valve. The mitral valve may be redundant and floppy.

These findings are related to left-to-right shunt at the atrial level with increased pulmonary flow. The shunt is in this direction because the right ventricle fills more easily than the left and the pressure in the left atrium is higher than that in the right.

In the primum type of atrial septal defect, the pathologic changes in the right side are the same as in the secundum type. However, because of the presence of the cleft in the aortic leaflet of the mitral valve and the manner of attachment of the aortic leaflet of the mitral valve to the septum, the left side of the heart may be different. The cleft aortic leaflet of the mitral valve may result in mitral insufficiency. When this condition is present, the left ventricle will show volume hypertrophy, whereas the left atrium may be normal in size or even show volume hypertrophy. The more anterior attachment of the aortic leaflet of the mitral valve uncommonly limits the outflow tract, producing subaortic stenosis, which may lead to pressure hypertrophy of the left ventricle.

The complexes formed in the sinus venosus type of atrial septal defect are variable, depending on the place of entry of the superior and inferior venae cavae. In general, there is volume hypertrophy of the right atrium and right ventricle, with the left atrium and ventricle ranging from hypertrophy to atrophy.

The coronary sinus defect is usually associated with other complexes, but occasionally it is isolated, producing a secundum type of complex.

Left-to-right shunt at ventricular level—isolated ventricular septal defect

Anomaly (Fig. 16-5). Ventricular septal defects may be present anywhere in the ventricular septum, but they have a predilection for the subaortic area. When present in the subaortic area, they may be anterior to but not involving the pars membranacea, anterior to and involving the pars membranacea, within and limited to the pars membranacea, or within the pars membranacea and involving the muscular septum both anterior and posterior to it. In any subaortic defect, the aorta may override the septum over the defect. If the defect is far anterior, it may lie beneath the pulmonary trunk. The pulmonary trunk may then override the defect. When more apical, defects may be present along the line of junction of the anterior and posterior septa, within the posterior septum at the base close to the mitral valve anulus, or in any area in the muscular ventricular septum. Depending on their position, they enter the right ventricle beneath the pulmonic orifice, adjacent to the tricuspid valve, within the lower part of the infundibulum, or in the sinus away from the tricuspid valve.

Complex (Fig. 16-6). The ventricular septal defect complex is characterized by volume hypertrophy of the right ventricle, enlargement of the pulmonic orifice, hemodynamic changes of the tricuspid and pulmonic valves, endocardial hypertrophy of the right ventricle, pressure hypertrophy of the right atrium, volume hypertrophy of the left atrium and left ventricle, enlargement of the mitral orifice, hemodynamic changes of the mitral and aortic valves, and in some cases endocardial hypertrophy of the left atrium and left ventricle. When the aorta or pulmonic trunk overrides the defect, there may be aortic or pulmonic insufficiency with increased

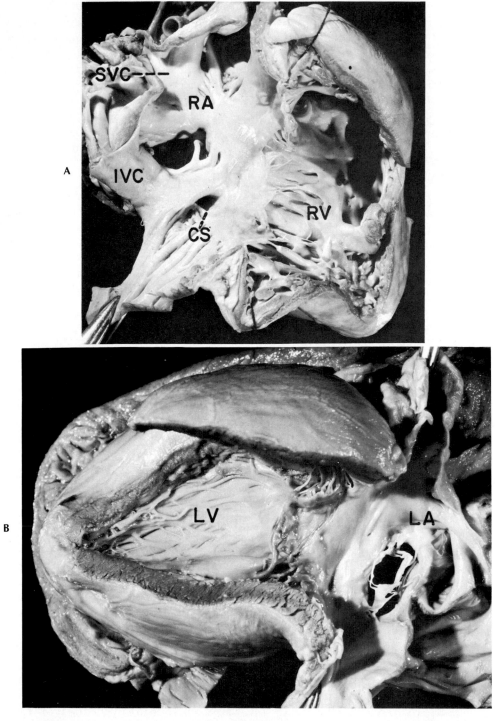

Fig. 16-1. Atrial septal defect, fossa ovalis (or secundum) type. **A,** Right atrial and ventricular view of one heart. **B,** Left atrial and ventricular view of another heart. *CS,* Coronary sinus; *IVC,* inferior vena cava; *LA,* left atrium; *LV,* left ventricle; *RA,* right atrium; *RV,* right ventricle; *SVC,* superior vena cava.

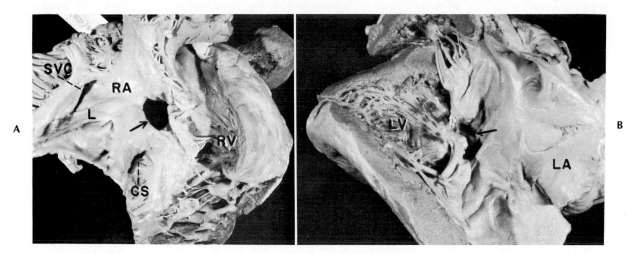

Fig. 16-2. Atrial septal defect, primum type (persistent ostium primum). **A,** Right atrial and ventricular view. **B,** Left atrial and ventricular view. Arrows point to persistent ostium primum. *CS,* Coronary sinus; *L,* limbus; *LA,* left atrium; *LV,* left ventricle; *RA,* right atrium; *RV,* right ventricle; *SVC,* mouth of superior vena cava.

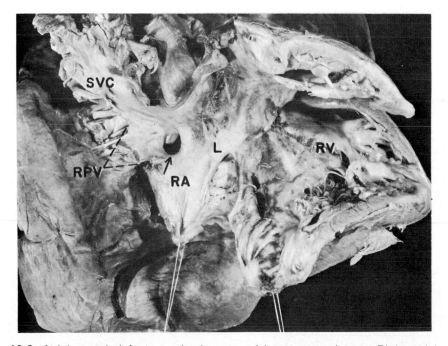

Fig. 16-3. Atrial septal defect, proximal septum (sinus venosus) type. Right atrial and right ventricular view. Arrow points to defect. *L,* Limbus; *RA,* right atrium; *RPV,* right pulmonary veins; *RV,* right ventricle; *SVC,* superior vena cava.

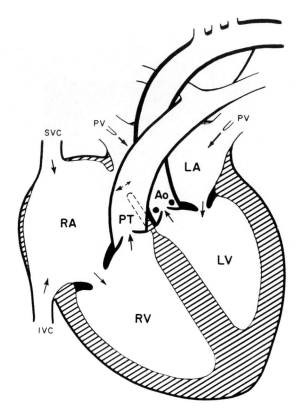

Fig. 16-4. Schema of heart in atrial septal defect, fossa ovalis type, complex. Arrows indicate direction of flow. *Ao,* Aorta; *IVC,* inferior vena cava; *LA,* left atrium; *LV,* left ventricle; *PT,* pulmonary trunk; *PV,* pulmonary veins; *RA,* right atrium; *RV,* right ventricle; *SVC,* superior vena cava.

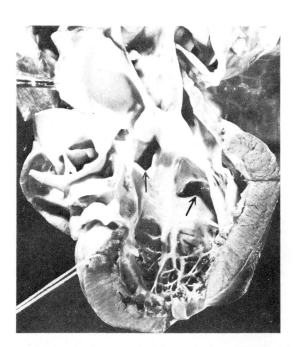

Fig. 16-5. Ventricular septal defects. Left ventricular view. Arrows point to two defects, one beneath aortic valve and one beneath mitral valve.

volume hypertrophy of the left or right ventricle respectively.

These findings are related to left-to-right shunt at the ventricular level, increased pulmonary flow, and increased volume in the left side of the heart. If left alone, many small or medium-sized ventricular septal defects may close spontaneously.

Left-to-right shunt at ductus level—isolated patent ductus arteriosus

Anomaly (Fig. 16-7). A ductus arteriosus is a muscular connection between the aorta, distal to the left subclavian artery and the left pulmonary artery at its junction with the main pulmonary trunk. A ductus arteriosus that is patent after 3 months of age is considered abnormal. A ductus may be considered abnormally large before 3 months of age, but an exact criterion of judgment is lacking today. A patent ductus may be as long as 2 cm or so brief as to constitute a windowlike structure between the aorta and the left pulmonary artery in the usual position of the ductus. Its diameter may range from 2 mm up to as much as 1 cm, and it may be a straight tube or slightly cirsoid.

Complex (Fig. 16-8). In the patent ductus arteriosus complex there is volume hypertrophy of the left atrium

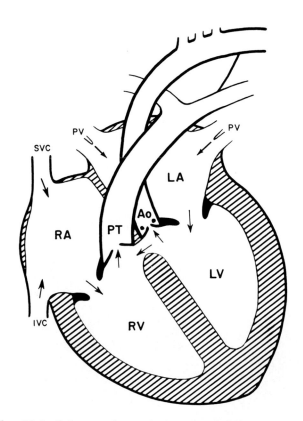

Fig. 16-6. Schema of ventricular septal defect complex. *Ao,* Aorta; *IVC,* inferior vena cava; *LA,* left atrium; *LV,* left ventricle; *PT,* pulmonary trunk; *PV,* pulmonary veins; *RA,* right atrium; *RV,* right ventricle; *SVC,* superior vena cava.

and left ventricle with or without endocardial hypertrophy, enlargement of the mitral and pulmonic orifices with hemodynamic changes of the valves, enlargement of the pulmonary trunk and the two pulmonary arteries with or without atherosclerotic changes, and enlargement of the ascending aorta.

These are the effects of left-to-right shunt at the ductus level, with increased pulmonary flow and increased volume in the left side of the heart.

Pulmonary hypertension associated with shunts

In the consideration of the shunts discussed so far, it was assumed that no pulmonary hypertension was present. Such may be the case; despite the increased pulmonary flow, the greatly distensible pulmonary vascular tree is able to accommodate it without increasing the pressure in the pulmonary circuit. However, pulmonary hypertension may develop for one or all of the following reasons:

1. A flow beyond the distensibility of the lung vasculature
2. A vasoconstriction of the pulmonary bed
3. Secondary pathologic changes in the intima or media of the muscular arteries and arterioles of the lungs, restricting the pulmonary bed.

Thus pulmonary hypertension may occur most commonly in ventricular septal defect, less commonly in patent ductus arteriosus, and least commonly in atrial septal defect.

The pathologic effects of pulmonary hypertension on the heart, developing in left-to-right shunts, are related to an increase in pressure on the right side, with or without a decrease in flow to the left side (Fig. 16-9). The former leads to pressure hypertrophy on the right side and the latter to a decrease in the previously present volume hypertrophy of the left side. This decrease may reach the point of less than normal flow, with volume atrophy on the left side. When this occurs, there is usually a reversal of shunt from left-to-right to right-to-left.

Common atrioventricular orifice

Anomaly (Fig. 16-10). In common atrioventricular (AV) orifice, there is one undivided common orifice for the mitral and tricuspid orifices, and this is guarded by a common valve consisting of four leaflets (anterior and posterior bridging and right and left lateral) or of five leaflets (there may be a fifth leaflet on the right side). This anomaly is always associated with a septal defect at the base of the heart, which consists of a persistent ostium primum combined with a basal ventricular septal defect. Also, there is often an associated secundum defect, with displacement of the atrial septum to the left.

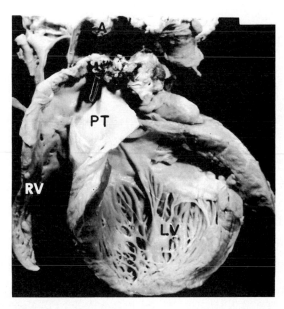

Fig. 16-7. Patent ductus arteriosus complex, without pulmonary hypertension. Probe passes through ductus. *A,* Aorta; *LV,* left ventricle; *PT,* pulmonary trunk; *RV,* right ventricle. (From Lev, M.: Autopsy diagnosis of congenitally malformed hearts, Springfield, Ill., 1953, Charles C Thomas, Publisher.)

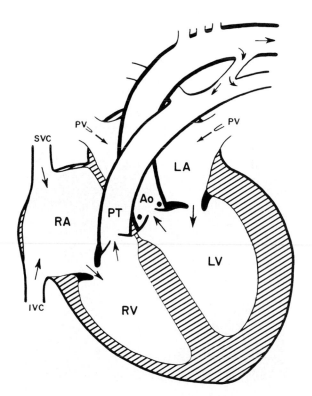

Fig. 16-8. Schema of patent ductus arteriosus complex. *Ao,* Aorta; *IVC,* inferior vena cava; *LA,* left atrium; *LV,* left ventricle; *PT,* pulmonary trunk; *PV,* pulmonary veins; *RA,* right atrium; *RV,* right ventricle; *SVC,* superior vena cava.

The common atrioventricular orifice may be divided into tricuspid and mitral portions of relatively normal size (balanced type), or either the tricuspid (right ventricular type) or mitral (left ventricular type) side may dominate.

Complex (Fig. 16-11). Thus in the balanced form both ventricles are hypertrophied and enlarged. In the dominant right form the right ventricle is hypertrophied and enlarged, whereas the left ventricle is smaller and usually thinner than normal. In the dominant left form the left ventricle is hypertrophied and enlarged, whereas the right ventricle is smaller but thicker than normal.

The pathologic changes in the balanced form are related to left-to-right shunt at the atrial and ventricular levels with pulmonary hypertension and to varying mitral or tricuspid insufficiency. The reasons for the dominant right and dominant left forms are not yet understood.

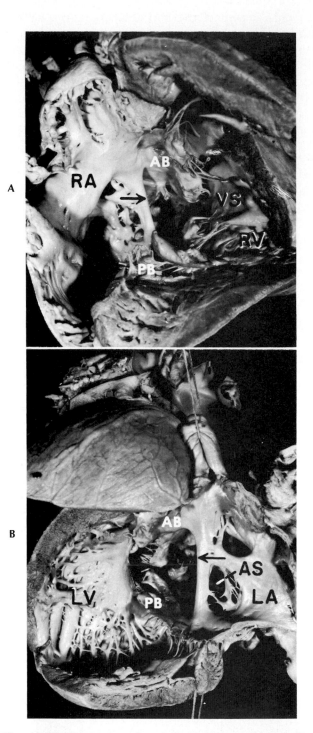

Fig. 16-10. Common atrioventricular (AV) orifice. **A,** Right atrial and right ventricular view. **B,** Left atrial and ventricular view. Arrows point to distal edge of septum primum. *AB,* Anterior bridging leaflet; *AS,* atrial septal defect, secundum type; *LA,* left atrium; *LV,* left ventricle; *PB,* posterior bridging leaflet; *RA,* right atrium; *RV,* right ventricle; *VS,* ventricular septum.

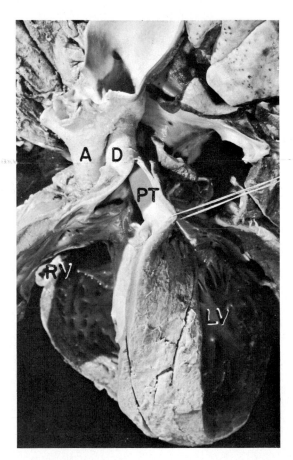

Fig. 16-9. Patent ductus arteriosus complex with left-to-right shunt, pulmonary hypertension. *A,* Aorta; *D,* ductus arteriosus; *LV,* left ventricle; *PT,* pulmonary trunk; *RV,* right ventricle.

Isolated aorticopulmonary septal defect

Anomaly (Fig. 16-12). In the aorticopulmonary septal defect an opening is present between the ascending aorta and the pulmonary trunk, usually situated above the aortic and pulmonic valves. This opening may be only a few millimeters in diameter or may be massive.

Complex. In the aorticopulmonary septal defect complex, there is pressure hypertrophy of the right atrium and right ventricle, enlargement of the pulmonary trunk and orifice, volume hypertrophy of the left atrium and left ventricle, and enlargement of the mitral and aortic orifices.

These are the effects of left-to-right shunt at the ascending aorta—pulmonary trunk level usually associated with pulmonary hypertension, with increased pulmonary flow and increased volume on the left side.

Total anomalous pulmonary venous drainage

Anomaly (Fig. 16-13). In total anomalous pulmonary venous drainage, all the pulmonary veins enter the right atrium, directly or indirectly. When they do so

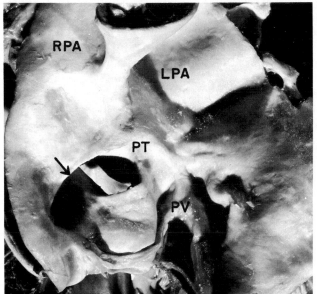

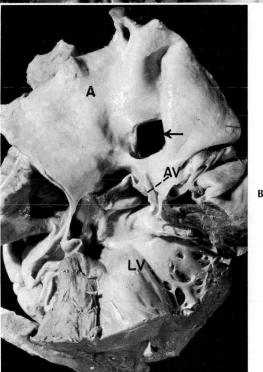

Fig. 16-12. Aorticopulmonary septal defect. **A,** Pulmonary trunk view. **B,** Aortic view. Arrows point to defect. *A,* Aorta; *AV,* aortic valve; *LPA,* left pulmonary artery; *LV,* part of left ventricle; *PT,* pulmonary trunk; *RPA,* right pulmonary artery.

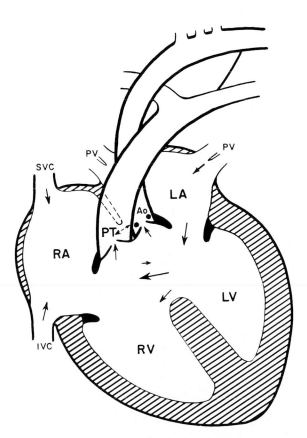

Fig. 16-11. Schema of common atrioventricular (AV) orifice complex. *Ao,* Aorta; *IVC,* inferior vena cava; *LA,* left atrium; *LV,* left ventricle; *PT,* pulmonary trunk; *PV,* pulmonary veins; *RA,* right atrium; *RV,* right ventricle; *SVC,* superior vena cava.

directly, they enter a pouchlike formation that fuses with the right atrium. When they enter indirectly, they usually form a common pulmonary vein that empties into a partial left superior vena cava, the innominate vein, the right superior vena cava, the azygos vein, the portal vein, the inferior vena cava, the coronary sinus, the left gastric vein, or the ductus venosus. There is always an atrial septal defect of the fossa ovalis type.

Complex (Fig. 16-14). In total anomalous pulmonary venous drainage there are in general two types of complexes: those without pulmonary venous obstruction and those with pulmonary venous obstruction.

Complexes without pulmonary venous obstruction. In complexes without pulmonary venous obstruction, the heart is greatly enlarged. There is volume and pressure hypertrophy of the right atrium and right ventricle, enlargement of the tricuspid and pulmonic orifices, enlargement of the pulmonary trunk, a structurally small left atrium, a normal left ventricle, or volume atrophy of the left ventricle, and a small aortic orifice, with hypoplasia of the aorta.

These changes are related to left-to-right shunt at the pulmonary venous level, increased pulmonary flow, right-to-left shunt at the atrial level, and usually pulmonary hypertension.

Complexes with pulmonary venous obstruction. When the pulmonary veins make connection with veins in the abdomen and sometimes with those in the chest, there is an obstruction of the venous return either along the course of the common pulmonary vein or along its junction with the other vein. Under these circumstances, although the heart shows the same essential characteristics as in this complex without pulmonary obstruction, the heart is smaller, being either normal in size or slightly enlarged. The size difference in this complex with pulmonary venous obstruction is considered to be attributable to a lesser volume and greater pressure hypertrophy of the right side.

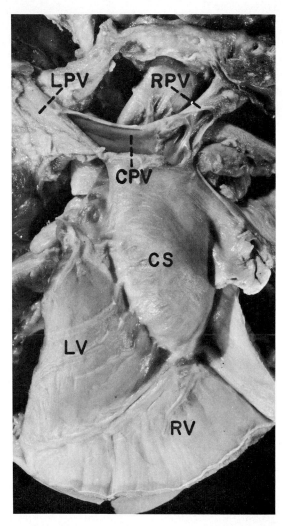

Fig. 16-13. Total anomalous pulmonary venous drainage into coronary sinus. Left posterior view. *CPV,* Common pulmonary vein; *CS,* coronary sinus; *LPV,* left pulmonary veins; *LV,* left ventricle; *RPV,* right pulmonary veins; *RV,* right ventricle. (From Lev, M.: The pathology of congenital heart disease. In Banyai, A.L., and Gordon, B.L., editors: Advances in cardiopulmonary disease; copyrighted 1964 by Year Book Medical Publishers, Inc, Chicago; used by permission.)

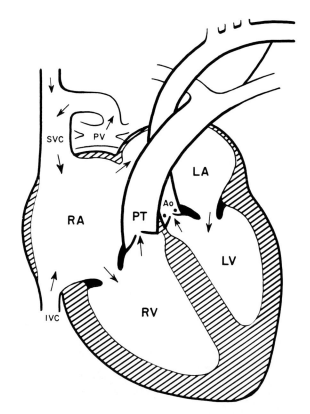

Fig. 16-14. Schema of total anomalous pulmonary venous drainage into superior vena cava complex. *Ao,* Aorta; *IVC,* inferior vena cava; *LA,* left atrium; *LV,* left ventricle; *PT,* pulmonary trunk; *PV,* pulmonary vein; *RA,* right atrium; *RV,* right ventricle; *SVC,* superior vena cava.

PATHOLOGY OF ISOLATED OBSTRUCTIONS

In this chapter only three types of obstructions are discussed: (1) obstruction to outflow from the right ventricle, (2) obstruction to outflow from the left ventricle, and (3) obstruction in the transverse aorta.

Isolated pulmonary stenosis (pulmonary stenosis with normal aortic root)

Anomaly (Fig. 16-15). The pulmonic valve usually consists of a diaphragm-like structure with only an incipient formation of cusps. This diaphragm may have a minute or larger opening. Uncommonly, the valve is fairly well formed, but its cusps are agglutinated at the commissures. Thus the obstruction is usually valvular. However, in a few cases the valve is not obstructed, but the obstruction is at the mouth of the infundibulum of the right ventricle. Here, the septal and parietal bands are greatly thickened and together form a ring of obstruction into the conus.

Complex (Fig. 16-16). In the isolated pulmonary stenosis complex there is pressure hypertrophy of the right ventricle, often poststenotic dilatation of the pulmonary trunk, hemodynamic changes in the tricuspid valve with or without mild stenosis, and endocardial hypertrophy of the right ventricle.

We are dealing here with the effects of obstruction to the outflow of the right ventricle with, however, sufficient left-sided flow to sustain life.

Isolated aortic stenosis

Anomaly (Fig. 16-17). There are three types of aortic stenosis: valvular, subvalvular (subaortic), and supravalvular.

In valvular stenosis the aortic valve consists of one, two, or three cusps that are greatly irregularly thickened often consisting of just nubbins of tissue. In the younger age groups, the anulus also is smaller than normal. Thus the stenosis is both anular and valvular in younger age groups, but chiefly valvular in older age groups.

There are several varieties of subvalvular (subaortic) stenosis. In one variety a sheet of fibroelastic tissue extends over the ventricular septum to the aortic leaflet of the mitral valve, a varying distance from the aortic valve. In a second variety a fibrous diaphragm-like structure is situated in this region. In a third variety a muscular bulge on the septum beneath the aorta narrows the subaortic area. This muscular bulge is part of a disease entity called idiopathic hypertropic subaortic stenosis (IHSS). In this disease there is more hypertrophy of the ventricular septum than of the parietal wall of the left ventricle. The architecture of the left ventri-

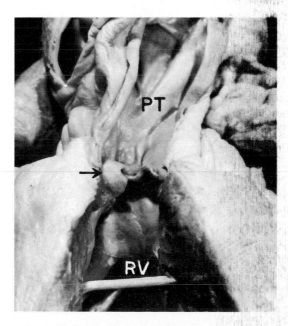

Fig. 16-15. Isolated pulmonary stenosis. Arrow points to diaphragm-like pulmonary valve. *PT*, Pulmonary trunk; *RV*, right ventricle. (From Lev, M.: Autopsy diagnosis of congenitally malformed hearts, Springfield, Ill., 1953, Charles C Thomas, Publisher.)

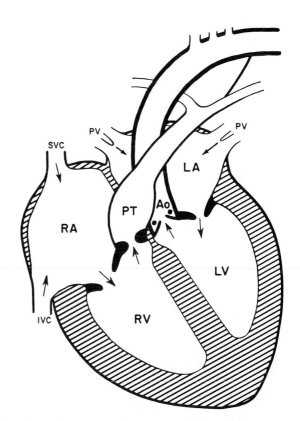

Fig. 16-16. Schema of isolated pulmonary stenosis complex. *Ao*, Aorta; *IVC*, inferior vena cava; *LA*, left atrium; *LV*, left ventricle; *PT*, pulmonary trunk; *PV*, pulmonary veins; *RA*, right atrium; *RV*, right ventricle; *SVC*, superior vena cava.

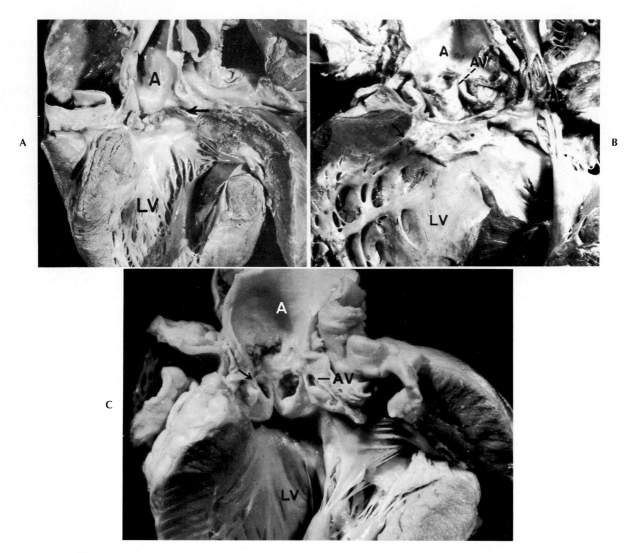

Fig. 16-17. Aortic stenosis. **A,** Valvular type. Arrow points to abnormal aortic valve with aortic stenosis. **B,** Subvalvular (subaortic) type. Notice large fibroelastic plaque producing subaortic stenosis. **C,** Supravalvular type with subacute bacterial aortitis. Arrow points to narrowing at upper margins of sinuses of Valsalva. *A,* Aorta; *AV,* aortic valve; *LV,* left ventricle. (**A** and **B** from Lev, M.: Autopsy diagnosis of congenitally malformed hearts, Springfield, Ill., 1953, Charles C Thomas, Publisher.)

cle shows a chaotic arrangement of muscle, which is congenital and often familial.

There are two varieties of the supravalvular type. One consists of a thickening and accentuation of the normal supravalvular aortic rim at the upper margins of the sinuses of Valsalva. The other consists of a ridge of thickening about 1 cm above the sinuses of Valsalva.

Complex (Fig. 16-18). The aortic stenosis complex is characterized by pressure hypertrophy of the left ventricle and often of the left atrium and hemodynamic changes at the mitral valve, in some cases with insufficiency of the valve. In the subvalvular and supravalvular types the aortic valve is always thickened. This may

be either a hemodynamic change or a structural part of the malformation. Supravalvular aortic stenosis may be associated with supravalvular or peripheral pulmonary stenoses, abnormal facies in children, and abnormalities in calcium metabolism.

Coarctation of aorta

Coarctation of the aorta means a narrowing of the aorta. As used in this chapter, the term does not necessarily imply a constrictive region. Such narrowings may occur in any part of the aorta. The only one that concerns us here is the one in the region of the isthmus.

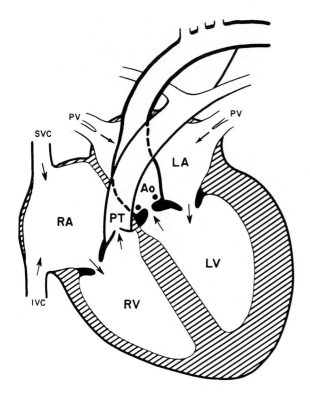

Fig. 16-18. Schema of aortic stenosis complex. *Ao*, Aorta; *IVC*, inferior vena cava; *LA*, left atrium; *LV*, left ventricle; *PT*, pulmonary trunk; *PV*, pulmonary veins; *RA*, right atrium, *RV*, right ventricle; *SVC*, superior vena cava.

The isthmus of the aorta is the segment between the origins of the left subclavian artery and the ductus or ligamentum arteriosum. In a number of newborns this region is smaller than the regions of the aorta proximal and distal to it because in fetal life the left ventricular flow passes into the brachiocephalic region, whereas the right ventricular flow passes through the ductus into the descending aorta. Thus the isthmus is a site of lessened flow and at birth may be smaller than normal. The isthmus usually attains normal size after birth. There are three types of coarctation: fetal (nonconstrictive, preductal, tubular hypoplasia of the transverse aorta), transitional, and adult (paraductal). These terms pertain chiefly to the complexes produced rather than to the topography of the narrowing of the aorta.

Fetal coarctation

Anomaly (Fig. 16-19). In fetal coarctation there is a narrowing of the transverse aorta that involves the entire isthmus or, more commonly, extends from the innominate or left common carotid artery. The left subclavian artery is given off a considerable distance from the origin of the left common carotid artery. The ascending aorta is smaller than normal.

Complex (Fig. 16-20). In the fetal coarctation complex there is always an atrial septal defect of the fossa ovalis type and a widely patent ductus arteriosus. Volume and pressure hypertrophy of the right ventricle is present, accompanied by enlargement of the tricuspid and pulmonic orifices, enlargement of the pulmonary trunk, and volume atrophy of the left atrium and left ventricle with smallness of the mitral orifice.

It is assumed that the pathogenesis of this complex is as follows: Since the complex just described is found in the newborn heart, the smallness of the left side and largeness of the right side are caused by insufficient blood reaching the left side of the heart and more blood reaching the right side. The small amount of blood entering the ascending aorta results in the small ascending aorta and, of course, even smaller isthmus. Thus the coarctation and the hypoplasia of the ascending aorta may be considered to be caused by insufficient flow. After birth there may be a left-to-right shunt at the atrial level and a right-to-left shunt at the ductus level.

Transitional coarctation

There is evidence that some cases of fetal coarctation pass through a transitional phase (transitional coarctation) and that, if the infant survives this stage, the anomaly develops to become converted adult coarctation. This is theorized to take place in the following manner.

After birth, if the child with fetal coarctation survives, the pulmonary pressure falls sufficiently to invite more blood into the left atrium and ventricle, at the same time causing the progressive closure of the ductus arteriosus and the foramen ovale. These chambers comply with this added volume and throw more blood into the aorta. The added volume in the aorta converts the narrow isthmus into a constrictive lesion. Thus the right ventricle becomes more normal in thickness, while the left ventricle takes on size and weight. When seen in the transitional phase, both chambers may be hypertrophied. If the child survives this stage, pulmonary hypertension becomes minimal and the complex takes on the physiologic features of typical adult coarctation.

Paraductal (juxtaductal, adult) coarctation

Anomaly (Fig. 16-21). In adult coarctation there is a maximum point of narrowing just proximal to, at, or just distal to the ductus arteriosus. A patent ductus may be present proximal or distal to the obstruction.

Complex (Fig. 16-22). In the adult coarctation complex, pressure hypertrophy of the left ventricle and in some cases of the left atrium is present, the mitral and aortic orifices are enlarged, and the ascending aorta is dilated.

This is a constrictive lesion in the aorta, with hypertension proximal and hypotension distal to the constric-

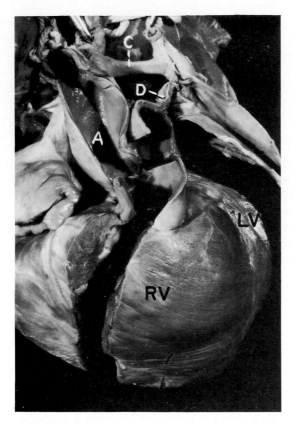

Fig. 16-19. Fetal coarctation complex. *A,* Ascending aorta; *C,* coarctation; *D,* ductus arteriosus; *LV,* left ventricle; *RV,* right ventricle.

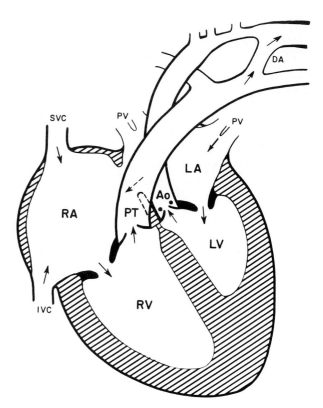

Fig. 16-20. Schema of fetal coarctation complex. *Ao,* Aorta; *DA,* ductus arteriosus; *IVC,* inferior vena cava; *LA,* left atrium; *LV,* left ventricle; *PT,* pulmonary trunk; *PV,* pulmonary veins; *RA,* right atrium; *RV,* right ventricle; *SVC,* superior vena cava.

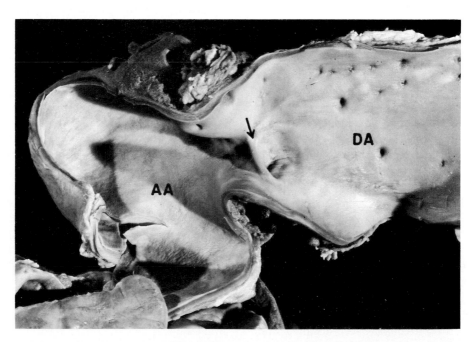

Fig. 16-21. Adult coarctation. Arrow points to coarctation. *AA,* Ascending aorta; *DA,* descending aorta. (From DeBoer, A., et al.: Arch. Surg. **82:**801, 1961.)

tion and with pressure hypertrophy of the left atrium and ventricle. Collateral anastomoses occur between the proximal and distal portions of the aorta by way of the subclavian, dorsal scapular, internal mammary, and intercostal arteries.

PATHOLOGY OF OBSTRUCTIONS COMBINED WITH SHUNTS

When an obstruction is combined with a shunt, the total effect depends on the extent of the obstruction and the direction and extent of the shunt. These principles will become evident in the discussion of the following entities: tetralogy of Fallot, double-outlet right ventricle, transposition, tricuspid atresia, and hypoplasia of the aortic tract complex.

Tetralogy of Fallot

Anomaly (Fig. 16-23). In tetralogy of Fallot the aorta overrides (straddles) the interventricular septum over a defect in this septum and emerges from both ventricles. The defect is a U-shaped excavation at the top of the ventricular septum. The pulmonary trunk emerges from the right ventricle. There is stenosis of the infundibulum somewhere along its course, and this may be associated with stenosis of the pulmonic orifice itself.

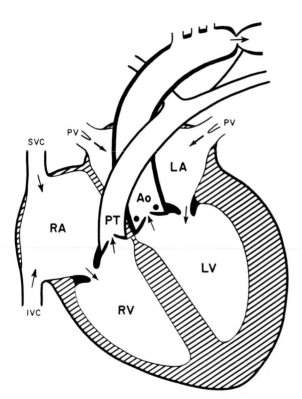

Fig. 16-22. Schema of adult coarctation complex. *Ao,* Aorta; *IVC,* inferior vena cava; *LA,* left atrium; *LV,* left ventricle; *PT,* pulmonary trunk; *PV,* pulmonary veins; *RA,* right atrium; *RV,* right ventricle; *SVC,* superior vena cava.

The stenosis of the infundibulum is produced by the deviation of the parietal band anteriorly away from the tricuspid orifice.

Depending on the extent of the stenosis and the size of the defect, there are two types of complexes—cyanotic and acyanotic. In the cyanotic type the stenosis predominates, whereas in the acyanotic type the stenosis is relatively mild and the ventricular septal defect predominates.

Complexes (Fig. 16-24). In *cyanotic tetralogy* there is pressure hypertrophy of the right atrium and right ventricle. The tricuspid orifice has a tendency to be smaller than normal, with abnormalities in structure of the valve. There often is pronounced endocardial hypertrophy (fibroelastosis) in the infundibular region. The left atrium and left ventricle have a tendency to be smaller than normal, with corresponding smallness of the mitral orifice, whereas the aortic orifice is enlarged.

We are dealing with the right ventricle contracting against systemic and infundibular resistence, decreased pulmonary flow, and the predominant right-to-left shunt at the ventricular level.

In *acyanotic tetralogy* there is pressure and volume hypertrophy of the right ventricle, pressure hypertrophy of the right atrium, volume hypertrophy of the left atrium and left ventricle, and enlargement of the mitral and aortic orifices.

We are dealing with predominant left-to-right shunt at the ventricular level, increased pulmonary flow, and increased volume on the left side of the heart.

Double-outlet right ventricle

In double-outlet right ventricle, both arterial trunks emerge completely or almost completely from the right ventricle, and there may or may not be aortic-mitral or pulmonic-mitral continuity. There are simple and complicated types. The simple types may be classified according to the position of the ventricular septal defect (VSD) in relation to the great vessels as follows: (1) with subaortic VSD (VSD related to the aorta), (2) with subpulmonic VSD (VSD related to the pulmonary trunk), (3) with doubly committed VSD (VSD related to both vessels), and (4) with noncommitted VSD (VSD related to neither vessel). Any of these types may be associated with pulmonary stenosis. The complicated types are associated with (1) mitral atresia, (2) common atrioventricular orifice, or (3) total anomalous pulmonary venous drainage. Only the simple types with subaortic and subpulmonic VSD are discussed in this chapter.

Double-outlet right ventricle with subaortic VSD and pulmonary stenosis

Anomaly (Fig. 16-25). In this anomaly both the aorta and the pulmonary trunk emerge almost completely

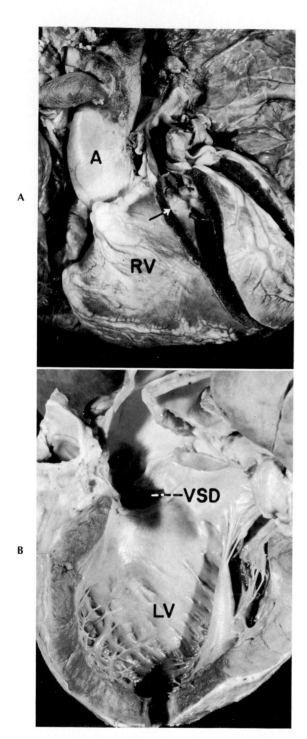

Fig. 16-23. Tetralogy of Fallot. **A,** Anterior view of one heart. **B,** Left ventricular view of another heart. *A,* Aorta; *LV,* left ventricle; *RV,* right ventricle (arrow points to infundibular stenosis); *VSD,* ventricular septal defect. (From Lev, M.: The pathology of congenital heart disease. In Banyai, A.L., and Gordon, B.L., editors: Advances in cardiopulmonary disease; copyrighted 1964 by Year Book Medical Publishers, Inc., Chicago; used by permission.)

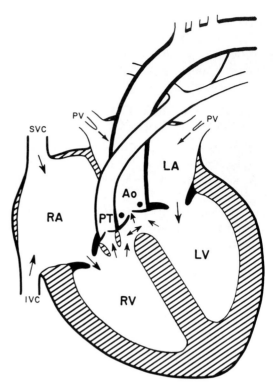

Fig. 16-24. Schema of cyanotic tetralogy of Fallot complex. *Ao,* Aorta; *IVC,* inferior vena cava; *LA,* left atrium; *LV,* left ventricle; *PT,* pulmonary trunk; *PV,* pulmonary veins; *RA,* right atrium; *RV,* right ventricle; *SVC,* superior vena cava.

from the right ventricle. The aorta lies adjacent to the defect. The infundibular stenosis resembles that in tetralogy.

Complex (Fig. 16-26). In this complex there is pressure hypertrophy of the right-sided atrium and ventricle and volume atrophy of the left atrium, whereas the left ventricle varies from atrophy to hypertrophy.

We are dealing with the right ventricle related to peripheral and infundibular resistance, right-to-left shunt at the ventricular level, decreased pulmonary flow, and decreased volume in the left side of the heart. When the left ventricle is hypertophied, this may be caused by obstruction of this chamber by an inadequately sized ventricular septal defect.

Double-outlet right ventricle with subpulmonic VSD (Taussig-Bing heart)

Anomaly (Fig. 16-27). In this anomaly the aorta emerges completely from the right ventricle removed from the defect of the ventricular septum. The pulmonary trunk is related to the defect and comes off either completely from the right ventricle (right ventricular type), comes off mostly from the right ventricle and slightly from the left (regular Taussig-Bing), comes off

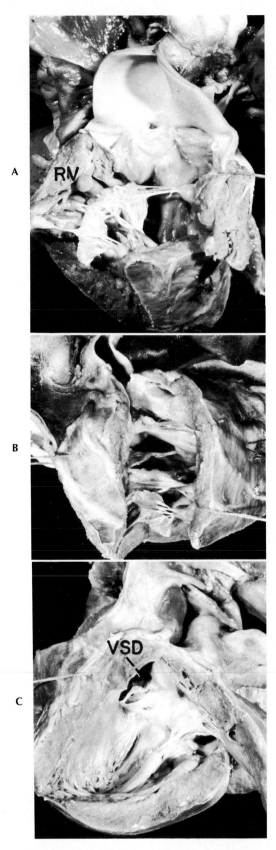

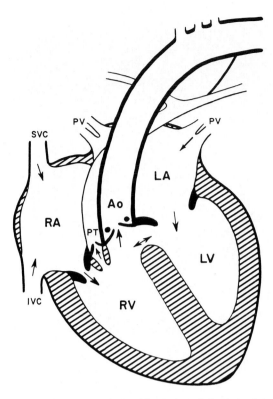

Fig. 16-26. Schema of double-outlet right ventricle with subaortic ventricular septal defect with pulmonary stenosis. *Ao,* Aorta; *IVC,* inferior vena cava; *LA,* left atrium; *LV,* left ventricle; *PT,* pulmonary trunk; *PV,* pulmonary veins; *RA,* right atrium; *RV,* right ventricle; *SVC,* superior vena cava.

Fig. 16-25. Double-outlet right ventricle with subaortic ventricular septal defect with pulmonary stenosis. **A,** Base of aorta. **B,** Base of pulmonary trunk. **C,** Left ventricle. *RV,* Right ventricle; *VSD,* ventricular septal defect.

equally from both ventricles (intermediate type), or comes off mostly from the left ventricle (left ventricle type).

Complex (Fig. 16-28). In this complex there is pressure and volume hypertrophy of the right ventricle, pressure hypertrophy of the right atrium, enlargement of the pulmonary orifice and trunk, smallness of the aortic orifice, volume hypertrophy of the left atrium and ventricle, and enlargement of the mitral orifice.

We are dealing with the right ventricle being related to systemic and pulmonary resistance, the left ventricle related to pulmonary resistance, left-to-right shunt at the ventricular level, increased pulmonary flow, pulmonary hypertension, and increased volume on the left side.

Transposition of the arterial trunks

Transposition is a controversial term with varying interpretations. It may be considered as that abnormality in which the aorta or its remnant is abnormally placed vis-à-vis the pulmonary trunk or its remnant, or one or both of these vessels emerge from the wrong chambers, or the vessels are abnormally placed vis-à-vis the atrioventricular orifices. Normally the aorta is

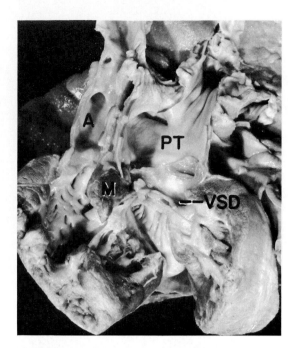

Fig. 16-27. Double-outlet right ventricle with subpulmonic VSD (Taussig-Bing heart). Right ventricular view. *A,* Aorta; *M,* muscular separation between aorta and pulmonary trunk; *PT,* pulmonary trunk; *VSD,* ventricular septal defect.

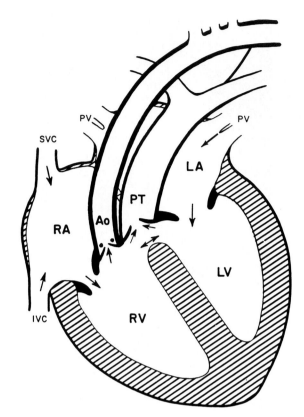

Fig. 16-28. Schema of double-outlet right ventricle with subpulmonic VSD (Taussig-Bing heart). *Ao,* Aorta; *IVC,* inferior vena cava; *LA,* left atrium; *LV,* left ventricle; *PT,* pulmonary trunk; *PV,* pulmonary veins; *RA,* right atrium; *RV,* right ventricle; *SVC,* superior vena cava.

situated to the right and posterior with the pulmonary trunk to the left and anterior. In *regular* (d-) transposition the aorta is displaced anteriorly but remains to the right. It may emerge from both ventricles or from the right ventricle. In that sense, tetralogy of Fallot and double-outlet right ventricle are mild or partial forms of transposition. When the aorta emerges from the right ventricle and the pulmonary trunk from the left ventricle, there is *regular complete* transposition. The aorta may emerge anterior but distinctly to the left of the pulmonary trunk. This is inverted (l-) transposition. In that situation the ventricles are also inverted, with the left ventricle situated to the right and anterior, giving rise to the pulmonary trunk, whereas the right ventricle is situated to the left and posterior, giving rise to the aorta. This is called *corrected transposition* because the circulation is physiologically corrected, with systemic venous blood going to the pulmonary trunk, and pulmonary venous blood going to the aorta.

There are many complexes associated with transposition of the arterial trunks. In this chapter we deal only with simple regular (d-) complete transposition.

Simple regular (d-) complete transposition

Anomaly (Fig. 16-29). In this entity the aorta emerges from the right ventricle, while the pulmonary trunk comes off the left ventricle. The aorta is in most

cases anterior and to the right, whereas the pulmonary trunk is posterior and to the left.

Complex (Fig. 16-30). In simple complete transposition complex, there may or may not be a ventricular septal defect, an atrial septal defect, or a patent ductus. There is pressure hypertrophy of the right atrium and ventricle and, in many cases, volume hypertrophy of the left side. In still other cases, where pulmonary hypertension develops, pressure hypertrophy of the left side ensues.

We are dealing with two separate circulations, systemic and pulmonic, which communicate only by shunts at the atrial, ventricular, or ductus level. The direction of shunting at the atrial level is usually left to right, at the ventricular level right to left, and at the ductus level variable.

Tricuspid stenosis or atresia complexes

There is a group of complexes that have tricuspid stenosis or atresia as their base. These may or may not be associated with transposition. In this chapter, only some of those without transposition are discussed.

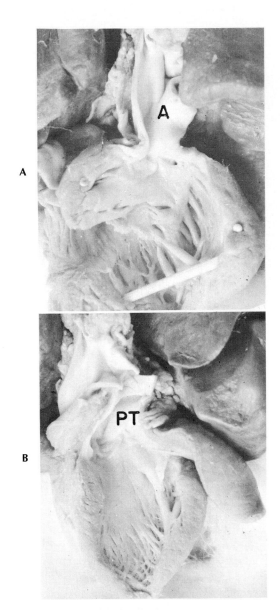

Fig. 16-29. Simple, regular complete transposition. **A,** Right ventricular view. **B,** Left ventricular view. *A,* Aorta; *PT,* pulmonary trunk. (From Lev, M.: Autopsy diagnosis of congenitally malformed hearts, Springfield, Ill., 1953, Charles C Thomas, Publisher.)

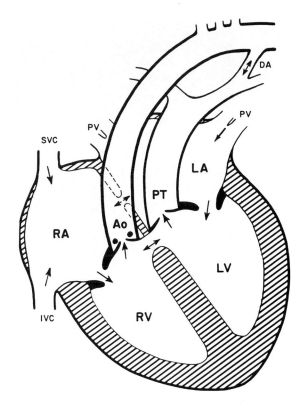

Fig. 16-30. Schema of simple, regular complete transposition complex. *Ao,* Aorta; *DA,* ductus arteriosus; *IVC,* inferior vena cava; *LA,* left atrium; *LV,* left ventricle; *PT,* pulmonary trunk; *PV,* pulmonary veins; *RA,* right atrium; *RV,* right ventricle; *SVC,* superior vena cava.

Tricuspid atresia without transposition

Anomaly (Fig. 16-31). In tricuspid atresia the tricuspid orifice is absent. In its stead there may be a slight dimple in the distal portion of the atrium where the orifice should be.

Complex (Fig. 16-32). In tricuspid atresia without transposition there is always an associated atrial septal defect of the fossa ovalis type and in most cases a small ventricular septal defect. Pressure hypertrophy of the right atrium and volume hypertrophy of the left atrium and ventricle are present. The right ventricle shows

volume atrophy, with infundibular stenosis, and small pulmonary orifice with or without a bicuspid pulmonic valve.

We are dealing with right-to-left shunt at the atrial level, left-to-right shunt at the ventricular level, decreased pulmonary flow, increased volume on the left side, and decreased volume on the right side.

Tricuspid stenosis with severe pulmonary stenosis or atresia (pulmonary atresia with intact ventricular septum)

Anomaly (Fig. 16-33). In tricuspid stenosis with pulmonary stenosis or atresia, the tricuspid anulus is small and the tricuspid valve consists of three poorly differentiated thickened leaflets, some of which may be displaced downward into the right ventricle. The right ventricle is a small chamber with a thick wall and frequently diffuse endocardial hypertrophy. The infundibular musculature is greatly thickened, and there is infundibular stenosis. The pulmonic valve, when present, may show a diaphragm-like arrangement. The pulmonary trunk is minute. There is always an atrial septal defect of the fossa ovalis type. The left atrium and left

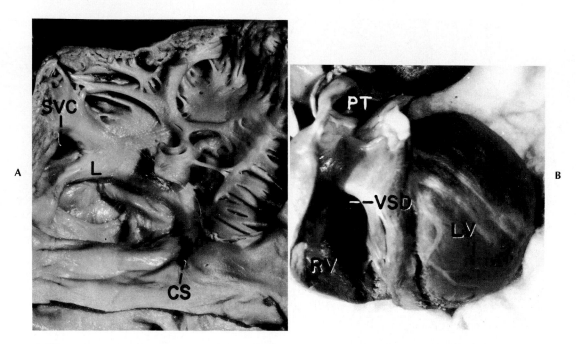

Fig. 16-31. Tricuspid atresia without transposition. **A,** Right atrial view. **B,** Anterior view. *CS,* Coronary sinus; *L,* limbus; *LV,* left ventricle; *PT,* pulmonary trunk; *RV,* right ventricle; *SVC,* superior vena cava; *VSD,* ventricular septal defect. (From Lev, M.: Autopsy diagnosis of congenitally malformed hearts, Springfield, Ill., 1953, Charles C Thomas, Publisher.)

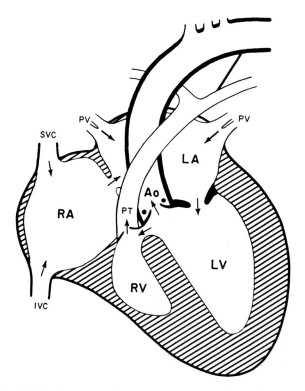

Fig. 16-32. Schema of tricuspid atresia without transposition complex. *Ao,* Aorta; *IVC,* inferior vena cava; *LA,* left atrium; *LV,* left ventricle; *PT,* pulmonary trunk; *PV,* pulmonary veins; *RA,* right atrium; *RV,* right ventricle; *SVC,* superior vena cava.

ventricle are hypertrophied and enlarged, with enlargement of the aortic and mitral orifices.

Complex (Fig. 16-34). In tricuspid stenosis with pulmonary stenosis or atresia, there is pressure hypertrophy of the right atrium and volume hypertrophy of the left atrium and ventricle, with enlargement of the aortic orifice.

We are dealing with the effects of right-to-left shunt at the atrial level, increase in volume on the left side, decreased volume but increased pressure on the right side, and decreased pulmonary flow.

Hypoplasia of aortic tract (hypoplastic left heart) complexes

Anomaly (Fig. 16-35). Hypoplasia of the aortic tract complexes is a group of complexes associated with severe aortic stenosis or atresia and with smallness of the left side of the heart. There are two types of such complexes: one with open mitral orifice and the other with mitral atresia. When the orifice is open, it is usually small. There is a small left ventricle with a relatively thick wall and diffuse endocardial hypertrophy (fibroelastosis). When it is closed, the left ventricle may be grossly absent or may be a small endocardium-lined slit.

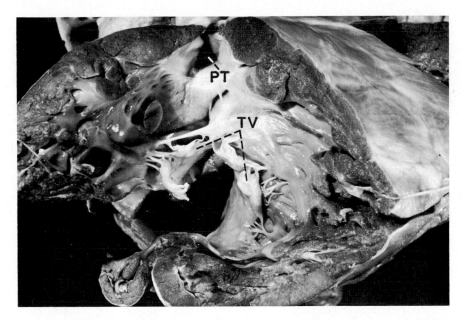

Fig. 16-33. Tricuspid stenosis with pulmonary stenosis. Right ventricular view. *PT,* Exit of pulmonary trunk; *TV,* tricuspid valve.

Complexes (Fig. 16-36). Hypoplasia of aortic tract complexes are typified by volume and perhaps pressure hypertrophy of the right atrium and right ventricle, an atrial septal defect of any type, and a widely patent ductus arteriosus. The ascending aorta is minute. The transverse aorta is larger than the ascending aorta but smaller than normal. There may or may not be a circumferential ridge at the entry of the transverse aorta into the descending aorta.

We are dealing with volume atrophy of the left side and volume hypertrophy of the right side before birth. After birth there is left-to-right shunt at the atrial level and right-to-left shunt at the ductus level. The ascending aorta and the coronary arteries are fed retrograde from the ductus arteriosus. Thus there is a ductus-dependent circulation. The reason for the peculiar left ventricle when the mitral orifice is open is not understood.

CAUSE OF DEATH

Increased pulmonary flow may lead to pneumonitis that may kill or contribute to the death of the patient. When there is decreased pulmonary flow, the patient may die from the effects of anoxia. Right or left ventricular failure, acute or chronic, may follow volume or

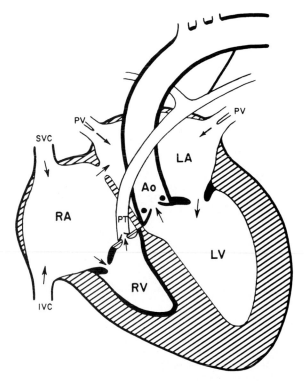

Fig. 16-34. Schema of tricuspid stenosis with pulmonary stenosis complex. *Ao,* Aorta; *IVC,* inferior vena cava; *LA,* left atrium; *LV,* left ventricle; *PT,* pulmonary trunk; *PV,* pulmonary veins; *RA,* right atrium; *RV,* right ventricle; *SVC,* superior vena cava.

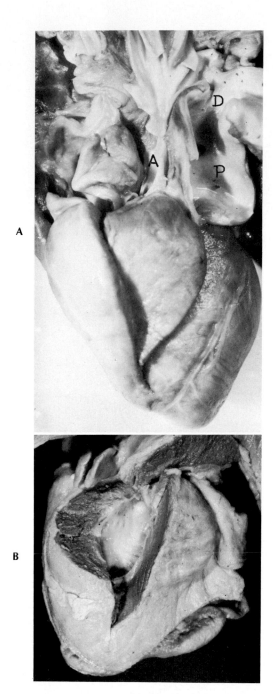

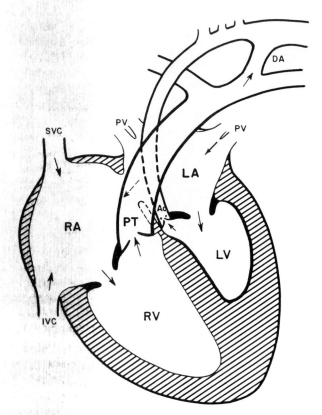

Fig. 16-36. Schema of hypoplasia of aortic tract complex. *Ao,* Aorta; *DA,* ductus arteriosus; *IVC,* inferior vena cava; *LA,* left atrium; *LV,* left ventricle, *PT,* pulmonary trunk; *PV,* pulmonary veins; *RA,* right atrium; *RV,* right ventricle; *SVC,* superior vena cava.

Fig. 16-35. Hypoplasia of aortic tract, with aortic and mitral stenosis. **A,** Anterior view of one heart. **B,** Left ventricular view of another heart. *A,* Aorta; *D,* ductus arteriosus; *P,* pulmonary trunk. In **B,** note small left ventricle, thick wall, and fibroelastosis. (**A** from Lev, M.: Autopsy diagnosis of congenitally malformed hearts, Springfield, Ill., 1953, Charles C Thomas, Publisher.)

pressure hypertrophy of either side. Subacute bacterial endocarditis may be engrafted on a bicuspid aortic valve, patent ductus arteriosus, or pulmonary stenosis and may be superimposed on persistent ostium primum and small ventricular septal defects. There is a tendency for this disease also to attack regions just distal to obstructions, as in coarctation and supravalvular aortic stenosis. Depending on the severity of the lesion, there is a wide range of longevity in some of the complexes without surgery (isolated pulmonary stenosis, tetralogy of Fallot, isolated patent ductus arteriosus, isolated aortic stenosis, and adult coarctation of the aorta), whereas other complexes do not permit long survival (tricuspid atresia, fetal coarctation, hypoplasia of the aortic tract complex, and complete transposition).

RECENT ADVANCES IN THE TREATMENT OF CONGENITAL HEART DISEASE

The great advances in the clinical and surgical treatment of congenital heart disease have resulted in most of the anomalies discussed in this chapter being amenable to surgical treatment. Those who have so been treated are in most cases able to live a normal and fruitful life.

At the same time, this has resulted in a new population who reach sexual maturity. Data are now emerging that show that these people with congenital heart disease surgically treated are producing offspring with congenital heart disease in greater numbers than the average normal population. It is estimated that 8 in 1000 births from normal parents may yield offspring with a cardiac abnormality. On the other hand, as high as 14% to 16% of births from parents with congenital heart disease have congenitally abnormal hearts.

It thus behooves students in the future to gather as much information as possible about the data of this subject.

REFERENCES

1. Edwards, J.E.: Congenital malformations of heart and great vessels. In Gould, S.E., editor: Pathology of the heart, ed. 3, Springfield, Ill., 1968, Charles C Thomas, Publisher.
2. Lev, M.: Congenital heart disease. In Saphir, O., editor: A text on systemic pathology, vol. I, New York, 1958, Grune & Stratton, Inc.
3. Lev, M., and Bharati, S.: Embryology of the heart and pathogenesis of congenital malformations of the heart. In Ravitch, M.M., et al., editors: Pediatric surgery, ed. 3, Chicago, 1979, Year Book Medical Publishers, Inc.
4. Netter, F.H., Alley, R.D., and van Mierop, L.H.S.: Diseases; congenital anomalies. In Netter, F.H.: The CIBA collection of medical illustrations, vol. 5—Heart, Summit, N.J., 1969, CIBA Pharmaceutical Co.

17 Blood Vessels and Lymphatics

JACK L. TITUS

HAN-SEOB KIM

ARTERIES
Normal structure and age changes

Arteries conventionally are divided into three types depending on their size and certain histologic features: (1) large, elastic arteries; (2) medium-sized, distributing, muscular arteries; and (3) arterioles, which connect to capillaries. The three types are not sharply divided; elastic arteries gradually merge with muscular arteries and muscular arteries with arterioles. Histologically all arteries have three layers: the tunica intima on the luminal side of the vessel, the tunica media as a middle layer, and the tunica adventitia as the outermost layer (Fig. 17-1, A and B). These three layers become less definite as the arteries diminish in size and usually are not clearly identifiable in arterioles. Arteries and veins of all sizes and types are lined by an endothelium, which is a single layer of cells (Fig. 17-1, C). The endothelial cells, basement membranes, and different amounts of connective tissues in different vessels form the tunica intima. Endothelial cells are not well demonstrated in routine histologic preparations; special techniques and electron microscopic study show them to be flattened cells with specialized junctions, intracellular organelles for transport of substances, and, in some cases, secretory organelles.

The elastic arteries include the aorta and its major branches and the major pulmonary arteries. In the first decade of life the tunica intima of these vessels is composed of endothelial cells with their basement membranes, a scanty amount of ground substance, collagen and elastic fibers, and the internal elastic lamina (lamella). The intima is bounded by the internal elastic lamina, a fenestrated sheet of elastic fibers that may be regarded both as part of the intima and as the beginning of the tunica media. The tunica media of elastic arteries constitutes the bulk of the arterial wall and consists chiefly of concentrically arranged, fenestrated laminae of elastic tissue with intervening smooth muscle cells and histologically amorphous ground substance, which biochemically is proteoglycans. An elastic lamella and the adjacent interlamellar zone is called a lamellar unit.[2] The elastic laminae become thicker and increase

in number in adulthood compared to childhood. The outermost elastic lamina of the media is the external elastic lamina. The large number of elastic laminae in the media of large elastic arteries have the capacity to absorb and transmit the pulsatile stroke of left ventricular systole and maintain intra-arterial pressure during diastole, effecting relatively constant pressure and flow of blood. The tunica adventitia consists of irregularly arranged collagen and elastic fibers. Small nutrient vessels of the arteries themselves, the vasa vasorum, are present in the adventitia together with lymphatics and nerves. In humans the outer portion of the media of the thoracic aorta also has vasa vasorum.

Muscular arteries (Fig. 17-1, A, B, D, and E) generally are branches of elastic arteries, with internal diameters ranging from 0.3 to 3 mm. The definition of a muscular artery is mainly a histologic one related to near absence of well-defined elastic laminae in the media. The intima of a muscular artery is similar to that of an elastic artery, but thinner. The internal elastic lamina in muscular arteries in usual light microscopic preparations appears to be a single, continuous, wavy line; it is not continuous, however, but fenestrated, and is not wavy in life, the waviness being a postdeath artifact. The media of the muscular arteries is thick compared with the other two layers and consists of primarily circularly disposed, spindle-shaped smooth muscle cells, fine collagen and elastic fibers, and ground substance organized in an orderly fashion. The external elastic lamina is less prominent than that of elastic arteries and is not present in cerebral arteries. The tunica adventitia is thinner than the media and consists of collagen fibers, coarse and irregular elastic fibers, vasa vasorum, lymphatics, and nerves.

In both elastic and large muscular arteries the intima and the inner part of the media derive nutrition from the vascular lumen by perfusion, whereas the nourishment of the outer media is derived from the vasa vasorum. There is therefore a nutritional boundary zone (watershed area) within the media that is especially susceptible to damage resulting from changes such as increased thickness of the intima, mural thrombosis within the arterial lumen, impaired oxygenation or oxygen release by the circulating blood, and obstruction of the vasa vasorum.

Arterioles are the smallest arteries, with an internal diameter of 0.3 mm or less. The larger arterioles have the usual three tissue layers including a poorly defined internal elastic lamina (Fig. 17-1, C). In the smaller arterioles the media is one or two smooth muscle cells in thickness. The adventitia, consisting chiefly of collagen and elastic fibers, is relatively thick in larger arterioles and less prominent in smaller ones.

Changes that are roughly proportional to age occur in arteries as a result of the constant hemodynamic stresses of intraluminal blood pressure and flow. With time the walls of all arteries become more rigid, thus the term *senile arteriosclerosis*. These age changes are reflected in dilatation (ectasia) of some large elastic arteries and in tortuosity of some large muscular arteries. The structural basis of arterial aging, which can be regarded as an inevitable physiologic process, is most conspicuous in the intima but also involves the media.

Intimal thickening. In the fetus and neonate the intima is composed almost exclusively of endothelial cells with basement membranes (Fig. 17-1, A and B). In older infants (Fig. 17-1, D and E) some splitting of the internal elastic lamina and accumulation of fine elastic fibrils between the internal elastic lamina and the basement membrane of the endothelium are found. These

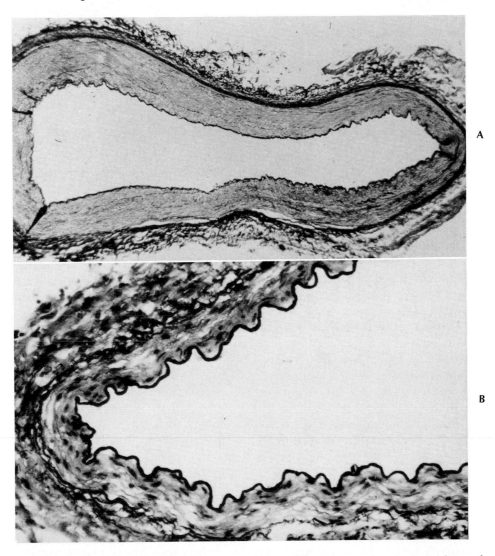

Fig. 17-1. Structure of normal muscular arteries at different ages in cross sections of coronary arteries, each stained to demonstrate elastic tissue. **A,** From a neonate. Wavy black line lining lumen is internal elastic lamina; endothelial cells and intima cannot be seen. Prominent muscular media is surrounded by black line of external elastic lamina. Adventitia is composed of loosely disposed connective tissue fibers. **B,** From a neonate. Higher-power view of a coronary artery emphasizes apparent absence of intima at this age.   *Continued.*

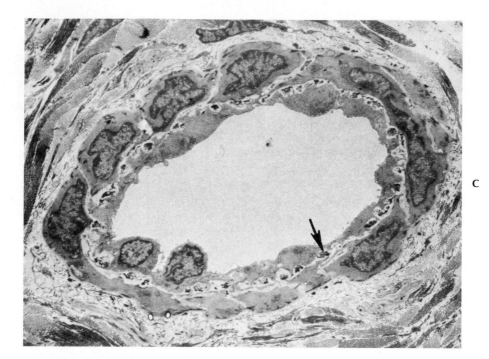

Fig. 17-1, cont'd. C, Electron micrograph of an arteriole in human skeletal muscle. Two endothelial cell nuclei *(lower left)* and endothelial cell cytoplasm line the lumen. The elastic lamina is represented by the dark material *(arrow);* the fragmented appearance of the elastic lamina is artifactual. Smooth muscle cells surround the endothelium and elastic lamina. The adventitia is collagenous tissue.

changes are the beginning of intimal thickening that is a part of normal growth and remodeling processes. By 6 to 12 months of age, smooth muscle cells are found in the intima adjacent to the internal elastic lamina, creating a musculoelastic intimal layer. These smooth muscle cells synthesize basement membrane material, collagen, elastin, and proteoglycan (ground substance) of extracellular material.[9] Throughout life, intimal thickening progresses with the addition of more elastic and collagen fibers and eventual loss of cellular elements. These changes are seen most commonly in coronary arteries, the abdominal aorta (more on the dorsal than the ventral aspect), and the larger arteries of the lower extremities, all of which tend to manifest severe atherosclerotic lesions.[4]

Medial fibrosis. Progressive increase in the amount of collagen and ground substance of the media of arteries creates medial fibrosis, which begins at an early age. Medial fibrosis is associated with loss of smooth muscle cells, and so the media is hyalinized in advanced age. In small arteries and arterioles these changes occur more commonly in the viscera and lower extremities and are similar to those of chronic hypertension. When fibrosis is severe, luminal narrowing leading to tissue ischemia may ensue, but in general, medial fibrosis has little functional effect.

Changes in chemical composition. Chemical analyses demonstrate a gradual increase in calcium salts in the arterial wall with increasing age. In addition, elastin content of the aorta increases along with changes in its amino acid composition. Aging arteries accumulate lipoproteins and glycosaminoglycans.

Arteriosclerosis

Arteriosclerosis is a generic, inclusive term that describes thickening and hardening of the arterial wall. Included in this term are four pathologic entities: arteriolosclerosis, hypertensive arteriosclerosis, Mönckeberg's medial calcific sclerosis, and atherosclerosis. Some confusion results from the use of the term *arteriosclerosis* for the more specific disease entity of *atherosclerosis*, and the use of the unqualified term to indicate the arterial changes associated with aging (senile arteriosclerosis), hypertension (hypertensive arteriosclerosis), and reparative response of the artery to injuries (reparative arteriosclerosis). The term *hyaline arteriosclerosis* usually means hyaline arteriolosclerosis.

Arteriolosclerosis

Two morphologic abnormalities of arterioles, hyaline arteriolosclerosis (arteriolar hyalinosis) and hyperplastic (proliferative) arteriolosclerosis, constitute arteriolosclerosis.

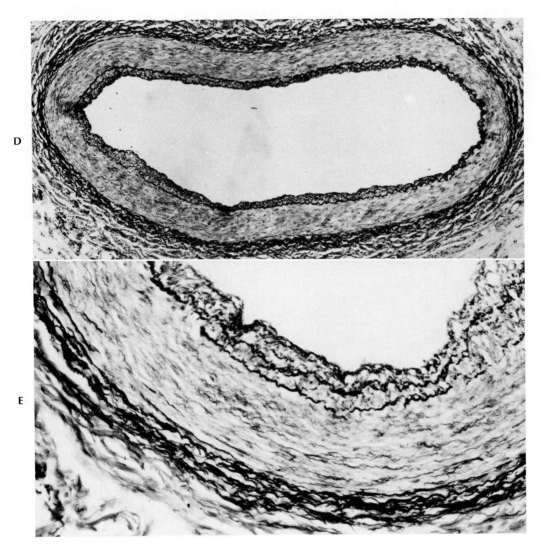

Fig. 17-1, cont'd. D, From 2-year-old child. True intima is evident. **E,** From 4 year old. Higher-power view demonstrates fibromuscular intimal layer and reduplication of internal elastic lamina.

Hyaline arteriolosclerosis. Hyaline arteriolar thickening (sclerosis) is a common pathologic lesion. Arteriolar hyalinosis (Fig. 17-2) pathologically is manifested by a subendothelial, homogeneous, glassy pink material in hematoxylin and eosin–stained sections. It may accompany hypertensive disease, be a physiologic phenomenon of aging, or occur in patients with diabetes mellitus. The usual hyalinosis of visceral arterioles begins as a focal, segmental process that spreads to involve the entire circumference of the vessel. Some of the hyaline material, which is not homogeneous chemically, appears to be derived from precipitated plasma proteins, the major component being the inactive form of complement C3b.[3] Moderate reduplication and thickening of endothelial basement membranes are usually present. The hyaline arteriolosclerosis of aging cerebral arterioles differs from that of visceral arterioles in that it appears to result from progressive fibrotic thickening of the adventitia and fibrosis of the media leading to the hyalinized vessel.

Hyperplastic (proliferative) arteriolosclerosis. Intimal thickening with consequent luminal reduction of hyperplastic arteriolosclerosis is a characteristic lesion of malignant hypertension, but identical changes may be found in patients with the hemolytic-uremic syndrome, progressive systemic sclerosis (scleroderma), homocystinemia, congenital rubella, radiation, chronic rejection, and malignant atrophic papulosis (Degos disease).[8] The process has been studied most extensively in accelerated hypertension, especially in renal interlobular arterioles and small arteries. Three main intimal morphologic patterns that can be distinguished are the "onion-skin lesion," mucinous intimal thickening, and fibrous intimal thickening.[10] The onion-skin intimal le-

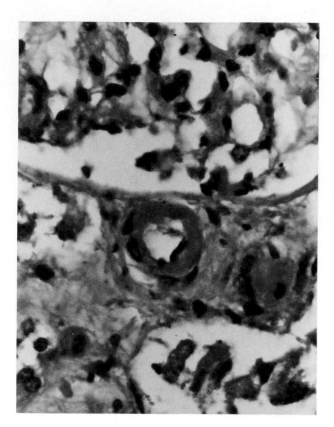

Fig. 17-2. Hyaline arteriolosclerosis of renal arteriole *(center).* Portion of glomerulus is above arteriole, and round dark mass to right of arteriole is another hyalinized arteriole cut obliquely.

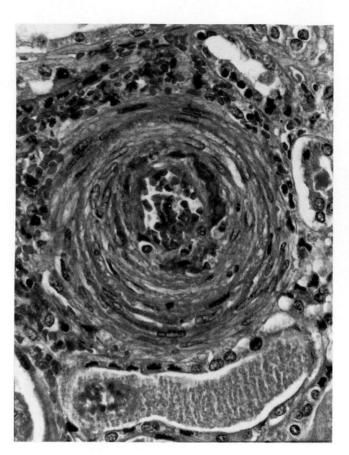

Fig. 17-3. Hyperplastic (proliferative) arteriolosclerosis of renal arteriole from patient with malignant hypertension. Concentrically arranged layers of intimal modified smooth muscle cells narrow lumen ("onion-skin" lesion). Dark amorphous material near lumen is fibrinoid necrosis.

sion consists of loosely disposed layers of modified smooth muscle cells (Fig. 17-3). The mucinous intimal thickening consists mainly of lucent amorphous material, probably proteoglycans, with few cells. Fibrous intimal thickening, which is less common, has hyaline deposits, reduplicated elastic fibers, and coarse bundles of collagen. The fine structural features of the cells of the thickened intima are those of modified smooth muscle cells, including a basement membrane, pinocytic vesicles, cytoplasmic myofilaments, and, most characteristically and constantly, spindle-shaped dense bodies or attachment devices associated with myofilaments. The pathogenesis of these intimal changes is unclear, but plasma proteins probably gain entry into the intima after endothelial injury such as increased pressure (hypertension), hypoxia, or immune damage. The common pathway is endothelial injury with increased permeability and a healing reaction of the vessel wall that involves smooth muscle cell migration from the media and proliferation of these cells with fibrosis.

Hypertensive arteriosclerosis

Regardless of its cause, hypertension may be divided clinically and to some degree pathologically into chronic ("benign") and accelerated ("malignant") types. Accelerated hypertension may occur de novo, or it may supervene in patients who are chronically hypertensive. Sustained elevation of the arterial blood pressure is associated with apparently adaptive structural changes in arteries of all sizes. The changes in the larger arteries are similar in all types of hypertension, but different processes occur in the smaller arteries and arterioles in chronic and accelerated hypertension. The possibility that the structural changes of arteriolosclerosis initiate the hypertensive state is unlikely, for such changes are sometimes absent, particularly in early cases[1]; moreover, structural changes do not develop in arterioles that are protected from hypertension by occlusive changes in the larger arteries supplying them.

The classic hypertensive arterial change of large and medium-sized arteries as found in young persons is medial hypertrophy resulting from increased numbers of smooth muscle cells and elastic fibers. The intima of these vessels may have increased numbers of longitudinally oriented smooth muscle fibers. With time, these hyperplastic and hypertrophic changes are replaced by collagenization, with the thickened arterial wall becoming less resilient and the lumen dilated and tortuous.

In benign hypertension smaller arteries may show medial thickening as in the larger arteries, but the intimal thickening is more pronounced and results in luminal narrowing. The major change is hyaline arteriolosclerosis (Fig. 17-2). In both benign and malignant forms of hypertension, reduplication of basement membranes, elastosis, fibrosis, and hyaline deposits commonly are present.

In malignant hypertension the intima of smaller arteries and arterioles is thickened by hyperplastic (proliferative) lesions described previously. In addition to the hyperplastic and hyaline changes, arterioles, especially in the kidney, may undergo fibrinoid necrosis manifested by pyknotic nuclei, polymorphonuclear leukocytes, and intramural extravasation of red blood cells (Fig. 17-3). Fibrin thrombi within the narrowed lumens may be present and may be an additional cause of ischemia.

Mönckeberg's medial calcific sclerosis

Mönckeberg's medial calcification is an age-related degenerative process of calcification of the media of large and medium-sized muscular arteries (Fig. 17-4) that is fundamentally a different process from occlusive atherosclerosis and has little or no clinical significance.[5] The vessels most commonly affected are the femoral, tibial, radial, ulnar, and uterine arteries. This calcific arteriosclerotic lesion may occur with atherosclerosis in the same vessels of an individual. Affected vessels, which are hard when palpated and are demonstrable on roentgenograms, generally are dilated and show transverse ridges of medial calcification under the intima. Sometimes medial calcification shows osseous metaplasia containing marrow elements (Fig. 17-4). The cause is unknown, but it is probably a misconception to consider Mönckeberg's medial calcification as a disease process. Similar medial calcific lesions have been produced in experimental animals by repeated infusions of vasoactive pharmacologic agents such as epinephrine or nicotine.

Medial calcification also occurs in *pseudoxanthoma elasticum* and in *idiopathic arterial calcification of infancy*. In pseudoxanthoma elasticum, a recessively inherited disease, changes occur in the elastic fibers of the skin, eyes, and vessels. The earliest detectable histologic vascular lesion is accumulation of calcium in elastic fibers, followed by fragmentation of the fibers.[7]

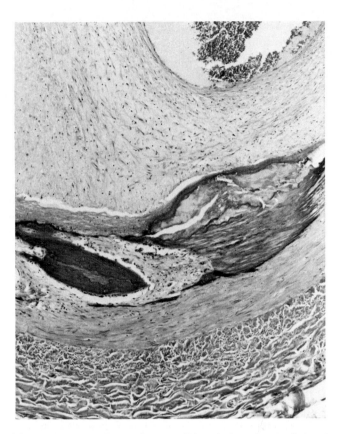

Fig. 17-4. Medial calcification (Mönckeberg's medial calcific sclerosis) of femoral artery of elderly man. Dark, irregular mass in center of photograph is calcification of inner media with osseous metaplasia; below calcific mass are normal medial muscle and adventitia. Vascular lumen containing red blood cells is in upper right of photograph. Intima is thickened by fibromuscular tissue.

Calcification is often found in the internal elastic lamina of the gastric arteries and in all medial elastic tissue of the coronary and large peripheral arteries. Coronary arterial occlusion may occur. Idiopathic arterial calcification of infancy is a rare but serious disease often involving coronary and systemic arteries[6] in babies less than 6 months old. The calcification is found in the internal elastic lamina and in the media, often associated with fibrous intimal thickening. When the coronary arteries are involved, the heart is enlarged and myocardial infarction may cause death. No pathogenic mechanism is known; results of studies of calcium and other mineral metabolism, lipid metabolism, and endocrine functions have all been normal.

Atherosclerosis

Atherosclerosis (AS), a specific form of arteriosclerosis, is primarily an intimal disease characterized by fibrous (fibrolipid, atheromatous) plaques. The most distinctive feature of AS is the localized accumulation of lipids, forming an atheroma (fibrofatty plaque) in the intima of large elastic arteries and medium-sized muscular arteries. The atheromatous plaque is a raised, localized lesion within the intima that has a central core of lipid, which is mostly cholesteryl esters complexed with proteins, and an overlying tissue plate. In addition to lipids, various cells, connective tissue fibers, and blood products accumulate in the lesions. Complications including thrombosis, calcification, hemorrhage into the plaque, and ulceration can occur. The term *atherosclerosis* derives from the combination of *athero-* ('porridge'), referring to the soft, lipid-rich material in the center of a typical intimal plaque, and *sclerosis* ('scarring'), referring to the connective tissue components.

The major clinical syndromes related to AS result from ischemia produced by narrowing of the vascular lumen (coronary heart disease, peripheral vascular disease, cerebral infarction), or from weakening of the arterial wall leading to an aneurysm. Although AS in humans begins early in life and develops progressively over years, it is rarely symptomatic in the first three decades, but thereafter the frequency of clinical atherosclerotic events increases logarithmically with age.[34]

Epidemiology. Because of its prevalence, AS can be considered epidemic in industrialized nations. In 1967, in about 50 countries on all continents, the most common causes of death (37% overall) were cardiovascular diseases, most of which were related to atherosclerosis.[45] Every year approximately 1 million persons in the United States experience either a myocardial infarct or sudden cardiac death. Nearly all of these are the result of atherosclerotic coronary artery disease (CAD). An encouraging fact is that in the United States the overall death rate for cardiovascular diseases has declined by about one third, declining 1.5% per year between 1963 and 1973 and 3.3% per year since then.[29] This decline is most evident for the major cardiovascular disease subgroup of coronary heart disease.

The geographic distribution of AS has geograpic and ethnic differences in average extent of involvement of arterial intimal surfaces at all ages, with significantly higher numbers from industrialized populations, which also had higher mortalities from CAD.[33] Geographic factors probably are more important than racial factors, supporting the belief that AS is in part an environmental disease. It has been observed repeatedly that populations that move from an area with a low incidence of atherosclerotic diseases to one with a high incidence tend gradually to acquire the higher rates of the country of adoption.

Epidemiologic investigations of living populations have disclosed risk factors that are associated with an increased likelihood of developing clinical atherosclerotic disease.[49] These risk factors, which are best defined for CAD and cerebrovascular diseases, include age, sex, genetic background, hyperlipoproteinemia, hypertension, cigarette smoking, diabetes mellitus, and obesity. These factors are not mutually exclusive, and some are irreversible, whereas others are reversible or potentially reversible.

Age. Although the natural history of AS is most often an age-related phenomenon,[51] AS is not simply the result of unmodified, intrinsic, biologic aging processes. Some populations age without showing clinical evidence of AS, and most mammalian species age without spontaneously developing AS. Although aging appears to play a role, particularly in relation to the changes in cells of the arterial wall, AS can best be considered an age-related disease that can be influenced by both environmental and genetic factors.

Sex. There is a striking difference in the incidence and severity of atherosclerosis between the two sexes. Atherosclerotic coronary heart disease is predominantly a disease of men, especially at younger ages; the prevalence in men in the fourth decade is three times that in women.[18] This difference decreases with age but remains higher at all ages in men. Possible explanations for the sex differences include levels of estrogenic hormones[35] and higher levels of high-density lipoprotein, which is known to be antiatherogenic,[24] in premenopausal women than in men.

Genetic factors. The significance of racial differences in atherogenesis may reflect the genetic background of different populations. Although such differences vary with the location of the lesions,[38] coronary atherosclerosis is generally less severe in blacks than in whites. Apparent genetic roles in familial predisposition to AS may be related to genetic effects on other risk factors, especially hyperlipoproteinemia, hypertension, and diabetes mellitus.

Hyperlipoproteinemia and diet. Atherosclerotic lesions are more severe in patients with hyperlipoproteinemia, including those with diabetes mellitus, myxedema, nephrosis, xanthomatosis, and familial hypercholesterolemia. A directly proportional relationship between the level of serum cholesterol and the risk of atherosclerotic coronary heart disease has been repeatedly established in epidemiologic, clinical, and pathologic studies.[4,39] In most animal models, elevation of the plasma cholesterol level by increased dietary cholesterol and saturated fat leads to atherosclerotic lesions similar to those in humans. The precise mechanisms by which the plasma lipoproteins contribute to the pathogenesis of AS are not known, but the lipids found in atherosclerotic lesions are believed to originate primarily from the plasma lipoproteins. Controversy exists as to the significance of elevations of serum triglyceride levels.[24] Many studies have demonstrated the specific effects of diet on lipid and lipoprotein levels, including the amount of dietary cholesterol ingested, the ratio of polyunsaturated to saturated fat, the content of *n*-3 fatty acids, the total number of calories from carbohydrates, protein, and fat, and the intake of alcohol and concentrated sweets.[25,30]

Hypertension. Hypertension has been shown to be a major risk factor for atherosclerotic CAD, cerebrovascular disease, and peripheral vascular disease.[18] Experimentally, hypertension augments the induction of atherosclerosis. The atherogenic mechanism of hypertension may be related to increased workload on arterial smooth muscle, mechanical injury to the arterial wall, or increased filtration pressure and increased permeability of the endothelium. Abnormalities of the humoral mediators of blood pressure control, including catecholamines, renin, angiotensin, kallikrein, kinin, and prostaglandins, may play a role in atherogenesis.

Cigarette smoking. The relationship between cigarette smoking and a higher risk of atherosclerotic CAD, especially sudden cardiac death, is unequivocal. Autopsy studies have shown a greater extent of coronary and aortic AS in smokers than in nonsmokers.[52] The component of cigarette smoking responsible for the acceleration of atherosclerotic events is not known. It may be related to effects of the cigarette smoking on thrombosis or to increased concentration of carboxyhemoglobin in the blood of smokers.

Diabetes mellitus. Diabetes mellitus contributes importantly to all manifestations of atherosclerotic diseases, including CAD, peripheral arterial disease, and cerebrovascular disease. Although other risk factors, particularly elevated blood cholesterol levels, high blood pressure, obesity, and low plasma levels of high-density lipoprotein, are significantly related to diabetes mellitus, these factors do not totally explain the added risk of diabetes mellitus.

Other risk factors. Other risk factors suggested to be associated with AS include obesity, physical activity, hyperglycemia, water hardness, personality type, stress, hemoglobin values, alcohol intake, coffee consumption, and nonatherosclerotic cardiac abnormalities. The role of obesity may be by virtue of its association with other risk factors for AS such as hyperlipoproteinemia, hypertension, diabetes mellitus, and hyperglycemia, but individuals 20% or more above the ideal weight have an increased risk of CAD or cerebrovascular disease. Sedentary men have approximately three times the rate of coronary heart disease of physically active men, but whether exercise has a direct effect on atherogenesis is not certain, though increased serum levels of high-density lipoprotein have been reported in the physically active. Although epidemiologic studies have identified personality attributes associated with increased risk of CAD, it has not been established that

such attributes are related to the development of AS itself. The role of the other proposed risk factors listed is controversial.

Morphology. Although the fibrous and complicated plaques are the atherosclerotic lesions associated with disturbances in blood flow that cause clinical disease states, the morphologic changes of diffuse intimal thickening and fatty streaks may be either precursors of the basic atherosclerotic lesion or stages in its development.

Diffuse intimal thickening. Diffuse fibromuscular intimal thickening of arteries that develops with age has been viewed as an integral part of the atherosclerotic process or at least a requisite change for the development of atherosclerosis.[4] The process is most rapid during the first two decades of life, occurs in all humans, and is found in most arteries, but it is not clearly related to advanced atherosclerotic lesions.

Fatty streaks. Fatty streaks are well-circumscribed, yellow (lipid-laden), flat or minimally raised foci that vary in size from barely visible dots to elongated, beaded streaks (Fig. 17-5). They begin to appear in the aorta in the first year of life just above the aortic valve

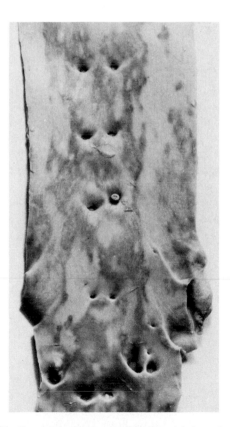

Fig. 17-5. Opened aorta of 11-year-old boy has been stained with Oil Red O to demonstrate fatty streaks, which are dark vertical streaks on wall of aorta and about orifices of branches. In the natural state these streaks are pale yellow.

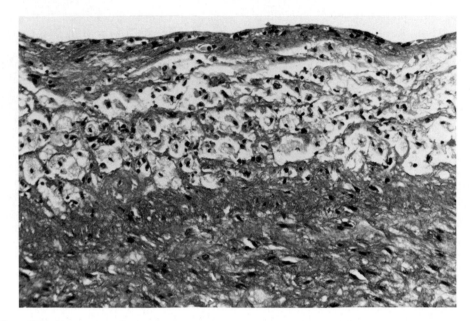

Fig. 17-6. Foam cells in intima of aorta. Lumen and endothelium are above. Media is lower third of photograph.

and at the site of the closed ductus arteriosus. In the first decade of life, fatty streaks (juvenile fatty streaks) are found near the ostia of intercostal arteries, in the aortic arch, and in the posterior wall of the thoracic and abdominal aorta. Most persons have at least some intimal fatty streaks by 3 years of age, and their extent increases in the second decade of life. These lesions are found at puberty in the proximal segments of the coronary arteries. Fatty streaks begin to develop in carotid and intracranial arteries during the third and fourth decades of life. Blacks have more extensive lesions than whites or other racial groups, and females of all racial groups have more extensive lesions than males of the same populations do.[32] Fatty streaks are not consistently associated with diet, serum lipids, geographic residence, or other risk factors for AS.

The histologic features of fatty streaks vary. All have lipids in the intima, either intracellularly or extracellularly. Most often the lipids are present in closely packed foam cells immediately beneath the endothelium or in elongated fat-containing cells scattered within the intima (Fig. 17-6). In both human and experimental models the foam cells have been shown to be derived from either smooth muscle cells[20] or macrophages.[21]

The origin and significance of fatty streaks and their relationship to atherosclerotic disease are uncertain. The location of these lesions mainly in the thoracic aorta contrasts with the more frequent location of recognized AS in the abdominal aorta. Although fatty streaks are present in the coronary arteries of most ju-

veniles, great variations exist in the incidence of atherosclerotic CAD in different adult populations. The cholesteryl esters in foam cells of fatty streaks differ chemically from those in the lipid core of atheromatous fibrous plaque.[48] These dissimilarities might be explained on the basis of two types of fatty streaks, which differ in morphology, cellular genotype, and lipid content, with one type related to the fibrous plaque and the other type not related.[40] Fatty streaks are uncommon in older persons, a finding indicating that they may be absorbed.

Fibrous (fibrolipid) plaque. The term *fibrous plaque*[28,55] refers to the gross morphologic appearance of the lesion that is the hallmark of AS. Other names include atherosclerotic plaque, atheromatous plaque, and fibrofatty plaque; the different terms reflect the relative content of lipid within the lesion. The lesions are raised, pearly white to gray, smooth-surfaced, plaque-like structures in the intima that vary in diameter from a few millimeters to over a centimeter. They usually are elongated in the direction of the long axis of the artery, and lesions may become confluent. The plaques, which are in the intima but may extend into the media, may encroach considerably on the vascular lumen, especially in muscular arteries such as the coronary arteries. On cross section (Fig. 17-7) a typical lesion has a soft, yellow central zone with gruel-like material (atheroma) covered on the luminal aspect by a layer of dense fibromuscular tissue (fibrous cap). Intact plaques do not stain with fat stains because the lipids in the center are covered by the fibrous cap. Not all grossly typical

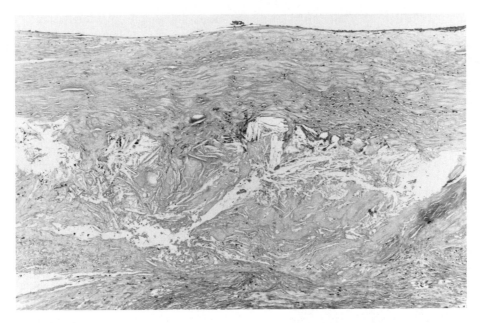

Fig. 17-7. Portion of typical fibrous plaque of aortic atheroma demonstrates fibrous cap adjacent to the lumen *(top)* over central atheromatous material with cholesterol clefts. Media *(at bottom).*

plaques contain central atheromatous material; some are made up entirely of fibrous or fibromuscular tissue.

The distribution, frequency, time of appearance, and extent of surface involvement of fibrous plaques vary in different arteries and in different segments of the same artery. In general, plaques are found most often in the abdominal aorta, large arteries of the lower limbs, carotid arteries, proximal portions of the coronary arteries, and circle of Willis. The prevalence, extent, and location of fibrous plaques parallel the frequency of clinical diseases attributable to AS.

Microscopically the central atheroma of an uncomplicated fibrous plaque consists of acellular, granular or amorphous, electron-dense material that contains lipids, especially crystals of cholesteryl esters, cellular debris, proteoglycans, fibrin, and other plasma proteins. Extracellular lipid in the lipid core originates mainly from necrosis of fat-laden cells,[13] though lipid deposition within the extracellular matrix also may contribute.[13] The fibrous cap is composed of avascular connective tissues and elongated smooth muscle cells covered by endothelium.[27] The connective tissue contains glycosaminoglycans (acidic mucopolysaccharide), elastic and collagen fibers synthesized by the smooth muscle cells,[42,44] and reticulin fibrils. Inflammatory cells, including macrophages, may be present. The histologic appearance of lesions varies considerably depending on the relative amounts of the different components. In apparently older or more advanced lesions the collagen of the fibrous cap is dense and hyalinized, and the smooth muscle cells are atrophic, though occasional fat-

laden foam cells of uncertain origin may be present near the lipid core. The smooth muscle cells in the fibrous cap[20] differ ultrastructrually in shape and cytoplasmic organelles from typical medial smooth muscle cells. In the cap they are slender, oriented in the long axis of the artery, have few cytoplasmic projections, and have few myofilaments, which are near the plasma membrane.

Complicated plaques. Complicated plaques develop from preexisting fibrous plaques as a result of one or a combination of several pathologic changes that include calcification, ulceration, thrombosis, and hemorrhage. The complicated lesion (Fig. 17-8) is the most common type of atherosclerotic lesion that produces significant circulatory change and clinical disease.

CALCIFICATION. In advanced fibrous plaques, calcification is common. The intima is brittle and cracks like an eggshell when the vessel is opened. Microscopically the dystrophic calcific process involves both the fibrous cap and the atheromatous portion of the plaque. This form of atherosclerotic intimal calcification is to be differentiated from Mönckeberg's medial calcific arteriosclerosis, which affects only the tunica media. In experimental atherosclerosis the size of calcific complicated lesions has been shown to decrease on removal of the atherosclerotic stimulus.[17]

ULCERATION AND THROMBOSIS. Advanced fibrous plaques with soft pultaceous atheromas, especially those with calcification, may ulcerate as a result of mechanical or hemodynamic forces. With ulceration, cholesterol or lipid debris from the atheroma may be dis-

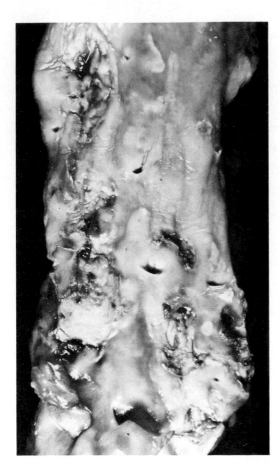

Fig. 17-8. Opened abdominal aorta shows variety of lesions of advanced atherosclerosis. White raised areas are fibrous plaques. Irregular areas along both cut edges are complicated plaques, some of which are ulcerated with superimposed thrombi *(black material).* Orifices of some branches are narrowed by atherosclerotic process.

charged and embolize. Mural thrombi may form on the ulcer or at sites of endothelial damage or mural hemorrhage. Such thrombi also may embolize, or they may become organized and incorporated within the intimal plaque. Mural thrombi in medium-sized arteries may progress to occlusive thrombi that may recanalize.

HEMORRHAGE. Hemorrhage into atherosclerotic plaques is a common finding in advanced lesions, especially in the coronary arteries (Fig. 17-9). The blood may reach the lesion from the vascular lumen through surface ulcerations or from rupture of capillaries that vascularized the atheroma from adventitial vasa vasorum. Hemosiderin pigment as evidence of prior hemorrhage is common.

Changes in the media and adventitia. Although AS is a disease of the intima, the more advanced lesions are associated with secondary changes in the media (Fig. 17-10). With encroachment of the expanding atherosclerotic lesion into the media, the internal elastic lam-

ina is attenuated and fragmented, and smooth muscle cells and elastic lamina atrophy with thinning of the media. Aneurysmal dilatation may follow, especially in elastic arteries. Fibrosis of the adventitia and foci of lymphocytes in the adventitia are common accompaniments of complicated atherosclerotic lesions.

Pathogenesis. Atherosclerosis is a multifaceted and multifactorial disease whose exact pathogenesis is not certain. Different etiologic and pathogenetic concepts have stressed one or more of the identified components of the disease and its lesions. These components include (1) the recognized risk factors of lipids, smoking, and hemodynamic stresses such as hypertension and (2) the specific contributions of various tissues, cells, and chemical products present in atherosclerotic lesions including smooth muscle cells either as a proliferative response to injury or a monoclonal proliferation, coagulation factors especially platelets, monocytes/macrophages as inflammatory cellular responses, and endothelial cells. Theories proposed in the past tended to emphasize one potential pathogenetic element leading to concepts based on aging, mechanical injury, inflammation, infection, intra-intimal hemorrhage, anoxia, insudation of blood products after endothelial injury, and encrustation (thrombosis). The insudation, imbibition, inflammation, and prefusion theories proposed that the responses to and the organization of proteins in the insudate contributed the fibrous component and the plasma lipids contributed the lipid component of advanced lesions. The encrustation (thrombogenic) theory indicated that breakdown and organization of a fibrin-platelet thrombus may lead to the atherosclerotic plaque.

Current pathogenetic concepts of AS involve most of the factors highlighted in previous theories but implicate the major rolls of arterial smooth muscle cells, endothelial cells, platelets, lipoproteins, and monocytes/macrophages. Accordingly, the pathobiology of these five that is pertinent to atherogenesis is reviewed briefly.

Arterial smooth muscle cells. Arterial smooth muscle cells can synthesize each of the three characteristic connective tissue matrix proteins—collagen, elastic fiber proteins, and proteoglycans—and are the principal source of connective tissue in the intima. Smooth muscle cells can take up and degrade some lipids, including low-density lipoprotein and can synthesize cholesterol.[12] The medial smooth muscle cells can migrate from the media to the intima to contribute to forming the fibrous (fibromuscular) plaque, the migration occurring in response to chemotactic factors.[46]

Smooth muscle cell migration and proliferation can be stimulated by platelet-derived growth factor, a macrophage factor, a possible endothelial cell factor, hyperlipidemic serum, lipoproteins, cholesterol, cholesteryl

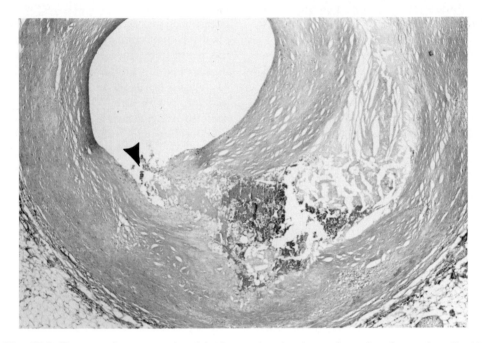

Fig. 17-9. Rupture of coronary arterial atherosclerotic plaque (at point of arrowhead) with hemorrhage into the lipid "core" lesion. Thrombosis at the rupture site usually occurs.

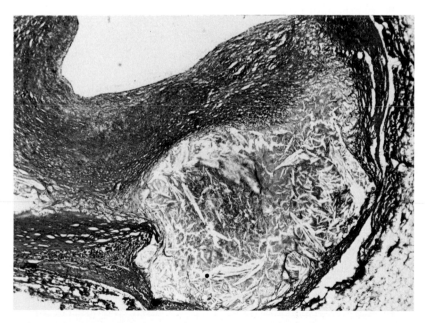

Fig. 17-10. Lumen *(above, left of center)* of coronary artery is narrowed, and media *(darkly stained tissue in lower part and right side of photograph)* are thinned by atherosclerotic process, which consists of central atheroma with cholesterol clefts, fibrin, and cellular debris covered on luminal aspect by thick fibromuscular tissue.

esters, some lipids, and insulin.[42] Smooth muscle cells in areas of increased glycosaminoglycan content are more responsive to proliferative stimuli. The proliferation or function of these cells is inhibited by prostaglandins, fatty acids, oxidative derivatives of cholesterol, high-density lipoprotein, heparin, thrombocytopenia in some models, estrogens, antirheumatic drugs, and age.[53]

For some agents one concentration may stimulate proliferation whereas another concentration causes cellular injury that may provoke inflammatory-reparative processes and thus contribute to the formation of a lesion. Although considerable information about the pathobiology of arterial smooth muscle cells is available, the combined effects of multiple factors on the behavior of these cells is less well known, particularly in intact animals and in the complex environment of a developed or developing plaque.

Endothelial cells. Structural and functional integrity of the endothelial cell layer is fundamental for maintenance of normal structure and function of the vascular system. Glycosaminoglycans of the endothelial cell plasma membrane prevent activation of blood coagulation, platelets, and leukocytes. The endothelial cell can synthesize the powerful anti–platelet aggregatory vasodilator substance prostacyclin (PGI$_2$), factor VIII (antihemophilic factor), plasminogen activator, a heparin-like anticoagulant substance, and basement membrane materials including collagen, elastin, and glycosaminoglycans.

That endothelial injury is important in atherogenesis has been known for many years. Experimentally, endothelial injury can be induced mechanically, chemically, immunologically, and by diet-induced chronic hyperlipidemia, bacterial endotoxin, viruses, hypoxia, carbon monoxide, tobacco proteins, and hemodynamic forces. An alteration in endothelial cellular function resulting from injury might not be apparent morphologically but contribute to the development of AS. The responses of the vessel to endothelial injury may be modified by insulin, vasoactive peptides, platelet and white blood cell products, and plasma lipoproteins.[15,22]

Endothelial denudation or injury permits platelet adherence, aggregation, and release of products at the site of exposed subendothelial connective tissue. Plasma constituents, such as lipoproteins, have access to the underlying arterial wall, since the permeability barrier has been altered. Endothelial cells may bind low density lipoprotein (LDL) through receptors and transcytose and modify it so that LDL is recognized and ingested by monocytes/macrophages.[50] The interaction of platelet products and plasma constituents leads to smooth muscle cell migration into and proliferation within the intima and accumulation of lipid.

Platelets. Platelets adhere to sites of endothelial in-

jury, aggregate to form platelet masses, and release granules rich in a variety of secretory products including platelet-derived growth factor (PDGF), which is both mitogenic for smooth muscle cells and also a chemoattractant for migration of smooth muscle cells from the media into the intima.[26] The most important stimulus to platelet adherence appears to be the exposure of collagen fibrils to the circulating blood. Additionally, platelets synthesize a variety of products including some prostaglandins.

Thrombin, which stimulates adherence of platelets to each other, promotes the formation of cyclic prostaglandin endoperoxides from arachidonic acid. The cyclic endoperoxides are converted into potent prostacyclin (PGI$_2$) in the endothelium and thromboxane A$_2$ in the platelets. Thromboxane is a proaggregatory, vasoconstrictive substance; prostacyclin is an antiaggregatory, vasodilatory substance.[36] Platelet aggregation also is promoted by antigen-antibody complexes, fatty acids, smoking, and hypercholesterolemia.

Lipoproteins. The plasma lipoproteins—chylomicrons, very-low-density lipoprotein (VLDL), low-density lipoportein (LDL), and high-density lipoprotein (HDL)—have a role in atherogenesis. Triglycerides of dietary and endogenous origin are transported, respectively, by the chylomicrons and VLDL. Chylomicrons are catabolized to a triglyceride-poor, cholesterol-enriched lipoprotein particle (remnant), which has been postulated to be atherogenic.[56]

LDL, which is derived from VLDL, is bound by fibroblasts, smooth muscle cells, lymphocytes, and endothelial cells by means of the receptor mechanisms of Brown and Goldstein.[14] LDL is degraded to the amino acids of the protein moiety and to the cholesterol, for cellular use, and the fatty acids of the cholesteryl ester. Intracellular accumulation of cholesterol shuts off synthesis of LDL receptors, inhibits cholesterol synthesis by enzyme inhibition, and stimulates enzymatic esterification of cholesterol.[23] Accumulation of cholesteryl esters, cholesterol, and lipoproteins is characteristic in atherosclerotic plaques, but the specific mechanisms by which hypercholesterolemia, hyperlipoproteinemia, and hyperlipemia cause AS are not known.[55] Patients with familial hypercholesterolemia develop rapidly progressing AS with elevated plasma LDL levels because of genetic absence of LDL receptors. LDL receptor–deficient rabbits of the Watanabe hereditary hyperlipoproteinemic (WHHL) strain have enormously elevated LDL and quickly develop AS and soft-tissue xanthomas.[50]

HDL has an antiatherogenic effect. This effect may be related to its role in the transport of cholesterol to the liver for breakdown and to competition of HDL with LDL for cellular binding.[24]

Monocytes/macrophages. Monocytes are known

sources of macrophages (histiocytes). In both human and experimental AS, monocyte/macrophage attachment to the arterial intima has been observed.[47] Human monocyte-derived macrophages have LDL receptors.[14] Macrophages take up lipoproteins, process them, and become foam cells.

Macrophage products with putative roles in atherogenesis include neutral and acid hydrolases, reactive oxygen derivatives, complement components, growth factors, biologically active lipids, and coagulation factors V, VII, IX, and X. Lysosomal hydrolases and superoxide anions are toxic substances that could injure the endothelium by surface or subendothelial attachment and lead to the proliferative lesions of AS. One cleavage product of complement, $C5_a$, is a powerful chemoattractant for leukocytes, including monocytes. Macrophage-derived chemoattractants, such as fibronectin, platelet-activating factor (PAF), and the leukotrienes, continuously recruit their progenitor monocytes. Macrophage-derived growth factors (MDGF) are potent mitogens for mesenchymal cells, including smooth muscle cells. In addition to being a source of foam cells in the atherosclerotic plaque with the formation of cholesteryl esters, macrophage elaboration of lipids, prostaglandins, thromboxane, leukotrienes, and PAF may promote leukocyte recruitment, platelet attachment to the endothelium, and contractile responses to the arterial wall. Among the many known, diverse capabilities of the monocyte/macrophage, at present it is difficult to identify those of major importance and specificity in atherogenesis.

Current concepts of pathogenesis. Although a single unifying concept of the pathogenesis of atherosclerosis is not yet certain, it is clear that the process has major inflammatory and proliferative aspects. These components are emphasized in the inflammatory and the response-to-injury hypotheses, respectively. Each recognizes the roles of lipids and lipoproteins, inflammatory cells (monocytes/macrophages), arterial smooth muscle cells, endothelial cells, and platelets.

The inflammatory aspect[31,37] of atherogenesis is based upon the demonstrated attachment of mononuclear cells to the endothelium (recruitment) and the accumulation of plasma constituents in the intima. As discussed previously, chemoattractants for mononuclear cells have been identified from different sources, monocyte/macrophage migration into (or out of) the intima is known, the monocyte origin of some plaque foam cells is established, and macrophages have LDL receptors and a growth factor that stimulates smooth muscle cell proliferation.

The proliferative aspect of atherogenesis is based upon the response to endothelial injury characterized by platelet adherence to the endothelium with release of PDGF, which together with plasma constituents cause intimal proliferation of smooth muscle cells.[19,42] All principal cellular components of AS—endothelium, arterial smooth muscle cells, platelets, and monocytes/macrophages—have chemoattractors and growth factors.[43]

The proliferative nature of AS also is stressed in the monoclonal (mutagenic) hypothesis proposed by Benditt.[11] Benditt suggested that each fibrous plaque begins with proliferation of a single, genetically transformed smooth muscle cell. The hypothesis is based on the finding that fibrous plaques from black females who were heterozygotes for glucose-6-phosphate dehydrogenase (G6PD) frequently contained only one of the two G6PD isoenzymes. In these women normal arterial and other tissues should be heterozygous for G6PD isoenzymes (mosaicism) because of random inactivation of one X chromosome in embryonic life. The finding of monotypism of the smooth muscle cells of the plaques indicated their probable origin from a single cell, similar to the known monoclonal nature of uterine leiomyomas, which presumably arise by mutation. Known mutagenic agents include endogenous or environmental chemical agents, radiation, some viruses, some chemicals in cigarette smoke, and some cholesterol metabolic products that are carried by the lipoproteins. Whether the monoclonal nature of the lesion is by selection processes of a certain cell line or by mutation is controversial.[41] Animal models with similar cellular markers to test the monoclonal hypothesis experimentally have not been found.

Animal models. Identification of etiologic and pathogenic factors in AS is a problem because of the difficulty in obtaining tissues at appropriate times and intervals from living persons, the limitations of materials derived from autopsy, and the long time course of the disease, which apparently begins in childhood. Accordingly, a variety of experimental animal models including pigs, nonhuman primates, rabbits, rats, mice, birds (chickens, pigeons, and turkeys), and dogs have been used for the study of AS. Since in most of these clinical atherosclerotic disease does not develop in the natural state, abnormal diets, with or without other measures, are needed to produce AS. Some common laboratory animals such as dogs and rats are relatively resistant to atherosclerotic disease induced by dietary measures alone. Certain swine and some nonhuman primates appear to be most suitable, though specific questions may be answered by use of other experimental models. Animal models are particularly suitable for regression studies, studies of the metabolism of the arterial wall, and studies of the cellular pathobiology of AS.

Experimental and some clinical studies support the possible role of viruses as injurious agents that initiate the pathogenetic mechanisms of inflammation, response to injury, and cellular proliferation that characterize the development of atherosclerosis. In chickens, infection by Marek's disease virus leads to AS by transforming arterial smooth muscle cells and altering cellular lipid metabolism.[16]

The LDL receptor–deficient rabbit, the Watanabe hereditary hyperlipoproteinemic (WHHL) strain,[54] has greatly elevated plasma cholesterol levels on a regular laboratory diet and develops severe AS at a young age. The findings in this animal and the occurrence in childhood of severe coronary artery AS and myocardial infarction in LDL receptor–deficient homozygotes indicate both a strong genetic factor in atherogenesis and the fact that hyperlipidemia alone can cause AS.[50]

Arteritis (angiitis)

Arteritis means any type of inflammatory process of an artery or arteriole. The terms *vasculitis* and *angiitis* are essentially synonyms. Veins and capillaries also may be involved synchronously or metachronously in many types of arteritis. The inflammatory process may result from invasion of the vessel by microbiologic agents or from immunologic, chemical, mechanical, or radiant energy injuries. Pathologic classification of the apparently primary, noninfective vasculitides is not entirely satisfactory because there is considerable overlap of size, type, location, and histopathologic features of involved vessels and organs among reasonably well-delineated clinical syndromes and diseases.[70,73]

Endarteritis obliterans

Although endarteritis obliterans is not a specific disease process, the condition is defined herein because it is a response of small vessels in sites of inflammation including vasculitis. Endarteritis obliterans is intimal cellular proliferation and thickening that narrows the lumen of small arteries and arterioles. The suffix "-itis" is misleading because there is minimal if any inflammatory cell infiltrate, though inflammatory processes may have been involved in the development of the lesion. The term is a descriptive pathologic designation, not a specific disease. Endarteritis obliterans is common in chronic cutaneous or gastrointestinal ulcers, tuberculous foci, chronic pulmonary abscesses, chronic meningitis, end-stage kidney disease, and functionally atrophic vessels or organs such as the ductus arteriosus, umbilical arteries, postpartum and postmenopausal uterine arteries, and arteries supplying surgically removed organs. Microscopically the lumen of the vessel is reduced or obliterated by orderly arranged, proliferated intimal fibrous tissue, which is often in a concentric pattern (Fig. 17-11). This lesion is to be distinguished from organized, recanalized thrombi.

Infective arteritis

Nonsyphilitic arteritis. Direct invasion of the artery by bacteria, fungi, parasites, rickettsias, or viruses from adjacent infected foci, by hematogenous spread includ-

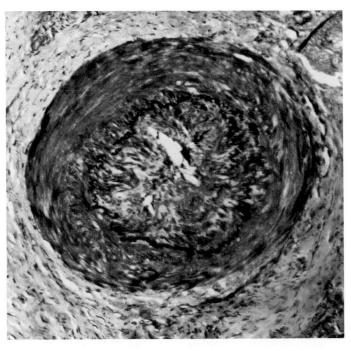

Fig. 17-11. This small artery exhibits endarteritis obliterans with vascular lumen greatly narrowed by cellular intimal proliferation. Black wavy line is internal elastic lamina.

ing infected thrombi from distant foci, or from septicemia may result in segmental inflammation (mycotic arteritis). Infective endocarditis is the most frequent condition causing infective arteritis. Weakening of the arterial wall may lead to a *mycotic aneurysm* or to rupture of the vessel. Vasa vasorum are the route of entry of organisms into large vessels such as the aorta, whereas direct invasion from the lumen occurs mainly in sites of intimal abnormality (such as ulcerated atherosclerotic plaques, mural thombi, intimal fibrosis from any cause) or in vessels small enough to entrap the infectious particles. Microscopically an inflammatory infiltrate permeates the vessel wall and causes destruction of tissues. Thrombosis with stenosis or occlusion of the vascular lumen may occur. The organ or tissue affected may suffer ischemic necrosis (infarction).[82]

Syphilitic arteritis. Syphilitic (luetic) vascular involvement occurs late in the course of luetic disease as a type of tertiary syphilis. It is relatively rare today because of improved control and treatment of syphilis, but the increase of primary syphilis in the last two decades may result in an increase of syphilitic vascular disease in the future. Cardiovascular complications occur in ap-

proximately 10% of syphilitic patients. Clinical vascular disease results mainly from aortitis, leading to an aneurysm; small arteries are frequently involved.

Syphilitic aortitis, which affects primarily the ascending aorta and aortic arch, is the most common manifestation of cardiovascular syphilis. The predilection for the proximal aorta may result from the rich vascular and lymphatic circulation in this segment and the frequent infection of mediastinal lymph nodes in the early secondary stage of syphilis. Grossly the intima of the involved aorta has pearly-white, thickened plaques separated by normal intima that is wrinkled and has small depressions so that the overall appearance vaguely resembles tree bark (Fig. 17-12). Superimposed atherosclerotic lesions may obscure the syphilitic lesions. The aortic lesions may extend to the branches of the aortic arch. Histologically the characteristic findings are adventitial thickening with endarteritis of the vasa vasorum and perivascular accumulation of plasma cells and lymphocytes, and destruction of the elastic tissue and smooth muscle cells of the media in a patchy ("moth-eaten") fashion (Fig. 17-13). Microgumma characterized by caseous necrosis with surrounding mononuclear and

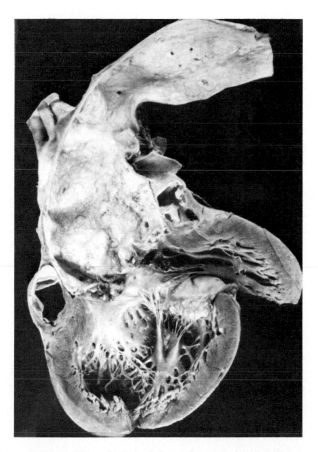

Fig. 17-12. Left ventricle, aortic valve, and thoracic aorta have been opened to demonstrate late changes of syphilitic aortitis. Intimal surface of aorta is irregularly wrinkled and thickened ("tree bark" appearance), and ascending aorta is aneurysmally dilated.

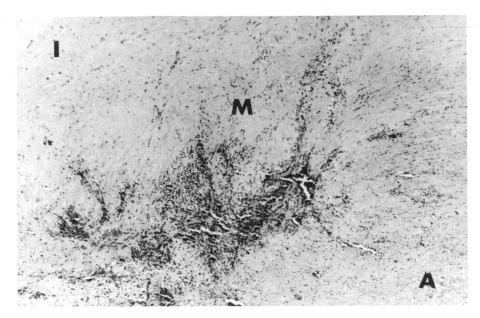

Fig. 17-13. Aortitis in a patient with tertiary syphilis has chronic inflammation, necrosis, scarring, and neovascularization of the media *(M)*. In the absence of demonstrable spirochetes, the lesion is not specifically diagnostic of syphilis. *I*, Intima; *A*, adventitia.

occasional giant cells, and polymorphonuclear leukocytes rarely may be present. Stellate medial scars result from tissue destruction and cause the wrinkling of the intima. The multiple foci of inflammatory destruction and scarring of the media weaken the aortic wall, leading to dilatation of the aorta and aneurysm formation. Often the proccess extends into the aortic valve anulus and aortic cusps, with dilatation of the anulus and fibrosis of the cusps creating aortic valvular insufficiency and narrowing of the ostia of the coronary arteries resulting in myocardial ischemia.

The histopathology of syphilitic aortitis lacks specificity except for the rare demonstration of the specific spirochetes. It may simulate other aortitides including panaortitis, inflammatory aneurysm of the aorta, Takayasu's aortitis, or the aortitis of rheumatic diseases.[86] In syphilitic aortitis, progressive sclerosis with luminal compromise, typically seen in Takayasu's disease, is rare, whereas aortic dilatation with aneurysm formation is common.

Syphilitic involvement of small arteries is most prominent in larger arterioles and arteries of the brain and meninges *(Heubner's arteritis)* characterized by striking endothelial cellular proliferation, which, however, is not specific since similar changes are seen in tuberculous disease. Cerebral ischemia results, and involved vessels may thrombose, leading to cerebral infarction. Similar changes occur rarely in other arteries, including the coronary arteries.

Noninfective vasculitides

The pathogenesis of the different types of noninfective vasculitis is not certain and probably is different for each form. Immune complexes appear to have a major role in the pathogenesis of some types, especially cutaneous hypersensitivity vascultis, mixed cryoglobulinemia vasculitis, and vasculitis associated with hepatitis B infection, systemic lupus erythematosus (SLE), and rheumatoid arthritis. The role of immune complexes in polyarteritis nodosa and Wegener's granulomatosis is more problematic,[89] but the beneficial effects of immunosuppressive therapy in these conditions indicates that an immune disorder may be a factor.

Polyarteritis nodosa. Initially described by Kussmaul and Maier[80] in 1866 as periarteritis nodosa because grossly visible nodules were seen under the skin, polyarteritis nodosa (PAN) is a necrotizing vasculitis of small and medium-sized muscular arteries. Polyarteritis is the appropriate term because the inflammatory process involves all layers of the arterial wall. Vessels in any part of the body may be affected, and multiple organs and tissues are involved. Males are more commonly affected than females by a ratio of 2.5:1. The mean age at onset of the disease is 45 years.[70]

PAN may occur in many well-defined conditions; in such circumstances it should be regarded as a pathologic lesion and not a specific disease entity.[89] When immune complexes, such as hepatitis B surface antigen-antibody, are present,[91] the necrotizing vasculitis may be regarded as a hypersensitivity vasculitis (discussed later). PAN may occur in association with or as part of connective tissue diseases that have a high incidence of circulating immune complexes, especially systemic lupus erythematosus and rheumatoid arthritis. Tumor-related antigens may be involved in the development of some cases of PAN.

The anatomic sites most commonly involved in PAN are the kidneys (85%), heart (75%), liver (60%), gastrointestinal tract (50%), muscle (40%), pancreas (35%), testes (33%), peripheral nerves (30%), central nervous system (25%), and skin (20%). The pulmonary, but not the bronchial, arteries are spared in classic PAN. Involvement of the vessel is characteristically segmental and often at branching points. Nodular, beaded indurations may be seen in larger muscular arteries.

Classically the histopathologic changes are divided into stages that are considered to be sequential.[59] These are the degenerative stage, acute inflammatory stage, granulation tissue stage, and healed or scar tissue stage. All stages may be seen simultaneously in the same vessel and in the same organ or tissue, suggestive of persistence of the inciting factors. In the acute inflammatory stage, panarteritic inflammation with neutrophilic leukocytes, eosinophils, and mononuclear cells and fibrinoid necrosis of the vessel are found (Fig. 17-14, *A*). Thrombosis with luminal obstruction occurs frequently, and aneurysms may form and possibly rupture. Repair of destruction of the degenerative and acute stages characterizes the granulation tissue stage, which leads to a scar. The healed phase of PAN (Fig. 17-14, *B*) is a vascular fibrous scar that distorts the normal architecture and often contains hemosiderin pigment and scattered round cells; an organized and recanalized thrombus may be present.

The clinical manifestations of PAN are protean, are generally nonspecific, and reflect dysfunction of multiple organ systems. Although there are no specific diagnostic laboratory findings, the erythrocyte sedimentation rate invariably is increased during the active phase of the disease, and results of serum immunologic tests are frequently abnormal.

Hypersensitivity vasculitis. Hypersensitivity vasculitis includes a heterogenous group of clinical syndromes in which inflammation of venules, capillaries, and arterioles is found. Synonyms are allergic vasculitis, microscopic polyarteritis, and leukocytoclastic vasculitis. The anatomic sites of involvement are skin, mucous membrane, lung, brain, heart, gastrointestinal tract, kidney, and muscle; skin involvement dominates the clinical picture. Hypersensitivity vasculitis is an immunologic response to antigenic material. Various agents postulated as etiologic factors are infectious agents (*Streptococcus, Staphylococcus*, hepatitis B virus, influenza virus, cytomegalovirus, malaria, mycobacterial organisms), foreign proteins (animal serum, hyposensitization

antigens), chemicals (insecticides, herbicides, petroleum products), and drugs (aspirin, phenacetin, phenothiazines, penicillin, sulfonamides, tetracycline, propylthiouracil, quinidine). The disease usually occurs 7 to 10 days after exposure to the stimulus. It is usually self-limited but can recur or become chronic.

The most common histopathologic pattern is a polymorphonuclear leukocytic infiltrate in which the cells often are fragmented (leukocytoclastic reaction), fibrinoid necrosis, endothelial cellular swelling, and extravasation of erythrocytes (Fig. 17-15). A second histopathologic pattern is a predominantly lymphocytic infiltrate of the involved vessel. The first pattern is associated with hypocomplementemia believed to be caused by deposition of immune complexes. The second pattern is believed to result from delayed hypersensitivity or cellular immune mechanisms, and the serum complement level is normal. In a given patient usually all lesions appear to be of similar duration.

Within the general group of hypersensitivity vasculitis are subgroups that have distinctive clinicopathologic characteristics but identical histopathologic features. These include *serum sickness, Henoch-Schönlein purpura, mixed cryoglobulinemia*, vasculitis associated with some collagen-vascular disease such as rheumatoid arthritis or systemic lupus erythematosus, and vasculitis associated with certain malignancies.[70] A distinctive feature of Henoch-Schönlein purpura is the predominance of IgA in the glomerular and vascular deposits.

Wegener's granulomatosis. Wegener's granulomatosis is a clinicopathologic complex of acute necrotizing granulomas of the upper and lower respiratory tracts, glomerulonephritis, and widespread small-vessel vasculitis of both arteries and veins, particularly of the lungs and upper airways. "Limited" Wegener's granulomatosis is the same entity without renal involvement.[66] Classic instances of the generalized form lead to death in months, though the use of immunosuppressive agents in recent years has given substantial remissions.[74] Males are more frequently affected than females (3:2), and the peak occurrence is in the fourth and fifth decades of life. The etiology of the disease is unknown; the findings of subepithelial immunoglobulin deposits on the glomerular basement membrane and the presence of circulating immune complexes in some patients indicate that immune-complex deposition in tissues may have a pathogenic role. The approximate frequencies of organ system involvement pathologically are lungs (100%), paranasal sinuses (95%), nasopharynx (90%), kidneys (80%), joints (60%), skin (50%), eyes (40%), ears (40%), heart (30%), and nervous system (25%).[98] The most common cardiac manifestations are pericarditis and coronary arteritis.[96]

Necrotizing granulomatous inflammation of the tissues and necrotizing vasculitis of arteries and veins with

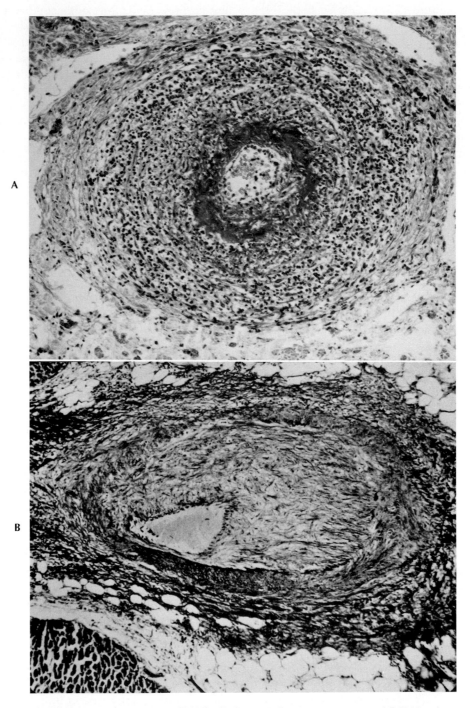

Fig. 17-14. Polyarteritis nodosa (PAN). **A,** Acute inflammatory stage of PAN is characterized by panarteritic and periarteritic inflammation and polymorphonuclear leukocytes, eosinophils, and round cells, destruction of vascular tissues, and fibrinoid necrosis *(dark, amorphous material about lumen).* **B,** In healing and healed stages of PAN, reparative fibrosis distorts vascular wall with loss of most of internal elastic lamina *(black wavy line)* and considerable narrowing of original lumen by organized thrombus and reparative fibrosis.

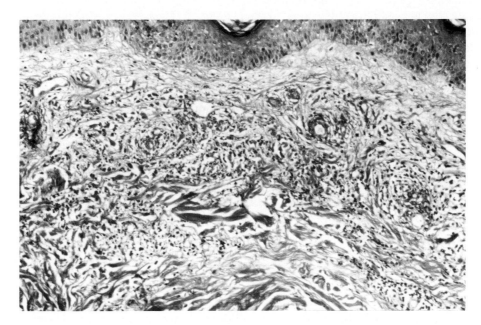

Fig. 17-15. Hypersensitivity vasculitis. The small vessels of the skin have inflammatory cellular infiltrate in and around the vascular walls of the dermis. The inflammatory cells are mainly polymorphonuclear leukocytes, some of which are fragmented. The inflammatory process extends into the immediately adjacent dermal tissue. Some vessels show fibrinoid necrosis.

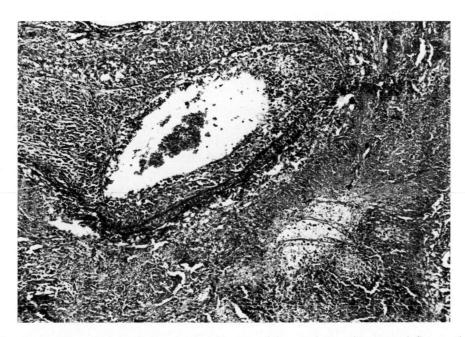

Fig. 17-16. Wegener's granulomatosis with necrotizing and granulomatous inflammation of medium-sized pulmonary artery *(center and left of photograph)* and necrotizing granulomatous inflammation of the pulmonary parenchyma *(right of pulmonary artery).*

or without granulomas are the histopathologic hallmarks of Wegener's granulomatosis (Fig. 17-16). The granulomas consist of necrotic tissue, sometimes fibrinoid necrosis, a dense infiltrate of polymorphonuclear and mononuclear cells, multinucleated giant cells, epithelioid cells, and fibroblastic proliferation. The vascular involvement may be segmental or circumferential; when it is segmental, the involved area is adjacent to a granuloma. The acute lesions heal by fibroblastic repair and scarring. Lesions in all stages may be present at the same time. The renal lesions are usually those of focal necrotizing glomerulonephritis; sometimes diffuse proliferative glomerulonephritis with crescent formation may be found, especially with rapidly progressive renal dysfunction.

Wegener's granulomatosis should be differentiated from the systemic necrotizing vasculitides polyarteritis nodosa and the Churg-Strauss syndrome, lymphomatoid granulomatosis, midline malignant reticulosis, and granulomatous diseases such as tuberculosis, sarcoidosis, and syphilis. Lymphomatoid granulomatosis may be differentiated from Wegener's granulomatosis by the absence of glomerulonephritis and the presence of atypical lymphoid cells. The relationship of the disseminated form of Wegener's granulomatosis to the limited form and of both to idiopathic (lethal) midline granuloma is controversial. Idiopathic lethal midline granuloma, a highly destructive, progressive, necrotic disease of the upper airway, may be part of a spectrum that encompasses generalized and limited forms of Wegener's granulomatosis, or it may be a separate disease that needs to be distinguished from Wegener's granulomatosis.[71]

Allergic angiitis and granulomatosis (Churg-Strauss syndrome). Churg and Strauss[68] in 1951 reported a form of disseminated necrotizing vasculitis occurring exclusively among asthmatics and characterized by tissue and blood eosinophilia and intravascular and extravascular granulomas. Characteristic findings are vasculitis of small and medium-sized arteries, veins, arterioles, and venules of the lungs with eosinophilic infiltrates. Levels of serum IgE are elevated in some cases. The pathogenesis of the disease involves an immunologic mechanism.[67]

Tissues and organs found at autopsy to be involved by the Churg-Strauss syndrome are, in order of decreasing frequency, the spleen, kidney, heart, liver, lung, gastrointestinal tract, musculoskeletal system, and central nervous system.[70] Histologically eosinophils and granulomas are seen in and around small vessels. Fibrinoid necrosis, thrombosis, infarction, and aneurysm formation may occur but are less frequent than in polyarteritis nodosa.

Although there are similarities in clinical symptoms between polyarteritis nodosa and Churg-Strauss syndrome, the latter differs in the high frequency of pulmonary findings, which usually are the initial ones, and less frequent renal and central nervous system involvement.[84] Diseases to be distinguished from the Churg-Strauss syndrome that also have pulmonary eosinophilia, granulomas, or vasculitis with or without asthma, and blood eosinophilia include eosinophilic pneumonia, allergic bronchopulmonary aspergillosis, bronchocentric granulomatosis, eosinophilic granuloma, Wegener's granulomatosis, necrotizing sarcoid-granulomatosis, and drug vasculitis.[79]

Giant cell arteries (temporal arteritis, cranial arteritis, granulomatous arteritis). Giant cell arteritis is a systemic vascular disease with granulomatous inflammation of medium-sized and large arteries. The inflammation often appears clinically to be limited to the cranial arteries, particularly the temporal. Most patients have granulomatous inflammation, but giant cells are not always found. It is a disease of protean manifestations, with fever, headache, visual symptoms, scalp tenderness, malaise, jaw claudication, anemia, and elevated erythrocyte sedimentation rate. Epidemiologic features include an average age of onset of symptoms of about 70 years (onset rarely occurs before 50 years of age),[61,81] increased prevalence with age, a female preponderance by a ratio of 2 or 3 to 1, greater frequency in northern areas and among persons of Scandinavian descent, unusual occurrence in black people, seasonal peaks in the spring and summer, and familial clusterings. An association has been observed between giant cell arteritis and polymyalgia rheumatica[72]; the two conditions may be manifestations of the same systemic disorder.

Although the cause of this arteritis is unknown, it has been suggested that damaged vascular elastic tissue, especially of the internal elastic lamina, acts as an antigen that incites vascular inflammation. Although immunoglobulin deposits have been found in affected arteries,[62] their significance and the role of cell-mediated hypersensitivity are uncertain.[76]

Preferential sites of involvement include the ophthalmic and posterior ciliary branches of the internal carotid artery and the temporal, occipital, facial, and maxillary branches of the external carotid system. Autopsy studies have shown active arteritis in many vessels including the aorta and the common carotid, axillary, brachial, femoral, and mesenteric arteries, but clinical symptoms related to these sites of involvement are uncommon or subtle.

The histologic features vary in different patients and even in the same vessel of one individual. Granulomatous arterial inflammation with or without giant cells, nonspecific inflammatory infiltrates throughout the wall with both polymorphonuclear and mononuclear cells, and intimal thickening by granulation tissue are the usual findings (Fig. 17-17). Three major histologic variants have been described: classic (typical) granuloma-

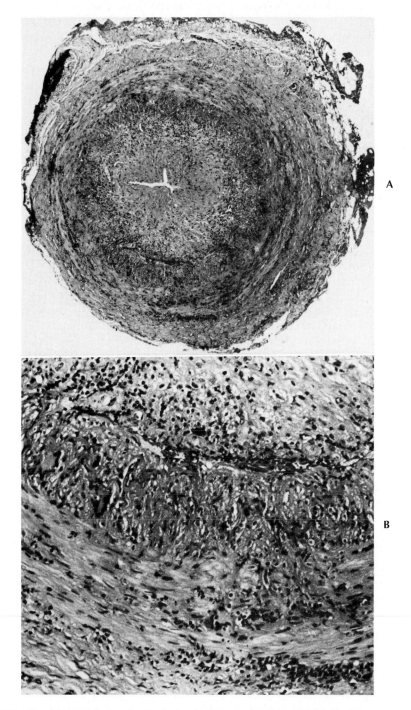

Fig. 17-17. Giant cell (temporal, cranial) arteritis. **A,** Low-power photomicrograph of biopsy specimen of temporal artery shows near occlusion of lumen (reduced to central cross-shaped slit) by granulation tissue and granulomatous inflammation of all layers of vessel. **B,** Higher-power view of portion of vessel in **A** demonstrates intimal granulation tissue *(upper one third of photograph),* giant cells in and about internal elastic lamina *(central area of photograph),* and inflammatory cells in outer media and adventitia *(lower one third of photograph).*

tous giant cell arteritis, nongranulomatous (atypical) arteritis, and predominantly intimal fibrous proliferation with focal, scanty, or no discernible inflammatory cellular infiltrate.[86] The granulomatous reaction is usually around the internal elastic lamina and typically involves the whole circumference of the vessel. Giant cells, either foreign body type or Langhans' type, are found in about half to two thirds of cases[88] and are usually close to the internal elastic lamina, which is often fragmented or focally absent. Occasionally only panarteritic inflammation or eccentric or concentric intimal cellular proliferation with considerable narrowing of the lumen is present, without disruption of the internal elastic lamina. Thrombosis of the narrowed lumen may occur. The segmental distribution of the process creates "skip lesions."

Clinically this form of granulomatous arteritis appears to be a self-limited disease, but blindness may develop rapidly as a result of involvement of the ophthalmic artery. Rarely death results, usually from systemic, especially aortic, involvement. Histopathologic diagnosis from examination of a biopsy specimen of a cranial artery, frequently the temporal, requires complete sampling because of skip lesions, as well as clinical correlations. Biopsy is important not only for confirmation of diagnosis but also for assessment of disease activity and adjustment of corticosteroid therapy.[77]

Takayasu's arteritis. Takayasu's arteritis is an inflammatory disease of large arteries, especially the aorta and its larger branches, that causes luminal stenosis and aneurysms. Synonyms include pulseless disease, primary arteritis of the aorta and its branches, idiopathic medial aortopathy and arteriopathy, obliterative brachiocephalic arteritis, panaortitis, aortic arch syndrome, aortitis syndrome, giant cell arteritis of the aorta, reverse coarctation, nonspecific aortoarteritis, and occlusive thromboaortopathy. The disease most frequently affects the young with 80% being 11 to 30 years of age; women account for 90% of cases.[87] The disease is worldwide in distribution and affects all races. The most common causes of death associated with Takayasu's disease are congestive heart failure, myocardial infarction, and sudden death.[95]

Four types of Takayasu's disease have been defined. Type I is characterized by active or chronic inflammation of the ascending aorta, the arch, and the great vessels, usually associated with the pulseless syndrome. Type II, also called atypical coarctation of the aorta, involves the descending thoracic aorta and the abdominal aorta without involving the aortic arch. Type III, which is the most common (occurring in about two thirds of reported cases), is a combination of involvement of the aortic arch, its branches, and the abdominal aorta. Type IV is a combination of one of the other three types with involvement of the pulmonary artery.

The etiology of Takayasu's arteritis has not been elucidated. It is not entirely certain whether the condition is a specific disease or a symptom complex that can result from a variety of pathologic processes. Although tuberculous infection has been suggested as a possible cause, such a relationship is doubtful in most cases of Takayasu's arteritis. An autoimmune reaction to aortic tissues[75,93] may be causative.

The aorta in Takayasu's arteritis is diffusely thickened, and the intima has a gray, pebbly appearance with localized, plaquelike elevations. Skip areas of involvement are common with focal stenoses or aneurysms of different sizes alternating with nearly normal segments. Occasionally organization of superimposed thrombi contributes to the plaque formation. Aneurysms are common in the distal thoracic and abdominal aorta, especially in older patients.[95] The histologic findings in affected vessels vary according to the stage of the disease (Fig. 17-18). Inflammation with polymorphonuclear and mononuclear cells and occasional Langhans' giant cells may be present in all layers but usually is more pronounced in the adventitia than in the media or the intima. Perivascular inflammation about vasa vasorum mimics syphilitic aortitis. Foci of medial destruction with reparative fibrosis are prone to the formation of aneurysms. In apparently late stages of the process, adventitial fibrosis and extensive intimal proliferation and fibrosis result in pronounced luminal narrowing, producing the pulseless syndrome when the subclavian arteries are involved. Segments of large arteries damaged by the inflammatory process often manifest secondary atherosclerotic changes, which may mask the basic condition. Although Takayasu's arteritis characteristically involves large arteries, medium-sized arteries, especially the coronary arteries, may be involved.

Differentiation from syphilitic aortitis may be aided by serologic tests for syphilis, by involvement of the abdominal aorta (which is uncommon in lues), and by the young age of most patients with Takayasu's arteritis. Giant cell (cranial) arteritis involving aortic segments may be indistinguishable histologically from Takayasu's arteritis, but usually medial inflammation and repair are more prominent in the former, which occurs mainly at older ages and always affects medium-sized muscular arteries. Tissue obtained for pathologic study during surgery on an affected vessel may not be diagnostic, since surgical treatment most often occurs late in the disease to treat stenotic or aneurysmal complications; nonspecific fibrotic scarring may be the main histopathologic finding.

Mucocutaneous lymph node syndrome (Kawasaki disease). Mucocutaneous lymph node syndrome (MCLS, Kawasaki disease) is an acute or subacute febrile systemic illness of unknown cause, occurring mainly in

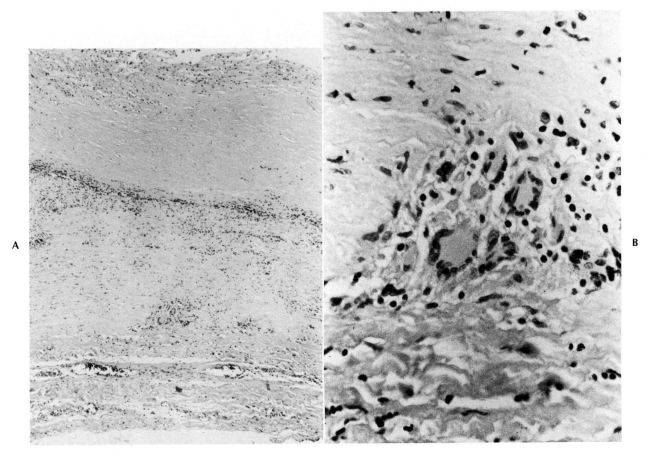

Fig. 17-18. Takayasu's arteritis involving aortic arch. **A,** Intima *(upper one third of photograph)* is thickened by fibrosis; media *(center portion of photograph)* has scattered foci of inflammatory cells, giant cells, and scarring; adventitia *(lower one fifth of photograph)* is fibrotically thickened with scattered plasma cells and lymphocytes, especially near vasa vasorum. **B,** Higher-power view of giant cells and inflammatory cells shown in **A.**

children during the first 2 years of life.[99,90] It is worldwide in distribution with a mortality of 1% to 2%. Possible causes considered are infectious, toxic, genetic, and allergic-immunologic agents.

The most striking pathologic finding at autopsy is necrotizing panarteritis of the coronary arteries with multiple aneurysms (Fig. 17-19).[58] The inflammation may be acute or chronic depending on the duration of the illness. Fibrous arterial scars with luminal stenosis are seen in later stages. Necrotizing panarteritis often is found in iliac, renal, mesenteric, hepatic, and pancreatic arteries, occasionally with aneurysms. Similar vascular lesions may be present in veins. Parenchymal, nonpurulent, nondestructive, inflammatory lesions may be seen in many tissues; these lesions heal without structural sequelae. Death from MCLS usually is the result of coronary arterial complications.

Retrospective analysis of instances of *infantile polyarteritis nodosa* (IPAN)[83] leads to the conclusion that IPAN and MCLS are essentially identical. Both differ clinically and pathologically from adult PAN.

Rheumatic vasculitis. At autopsy, fatal cases of acute rheumatic fever may have vasculitis involving the aorta, carotid and coronary arteries, and medium-sized arteries and veins of the viscera. Early aortic lesions are perivascular foci of inflammation and fibrinoid change in the adventitia and medial fibrinoid change in linear zones.[60] Although these lesions may have large basophilic histiocytes, typical Aschoff nodules in their granulomatous phase are rare. Healed lesions are perivascular fibrotic areas that, unlike those resulting from syphilis, do not involve the entire thickness of the media of the aorta. Active and healed intimal lesions analogous to those of the atrial endocardium have been reported. Involved muscular arteries, such as the coronary arteries, usually have rheumatic inflammation of all mural layers with prominent intimal lesions whose healing sometimes leads to luminal stenosis. Rheumatic vasculitis and aortitis are uncommon and generally not significant functionally. Rarely hypersensitivity vasculitis may be found in fatal acute rheumatic fever.

Rheumatoid aortitis. In the diseases rheumatoid ar-

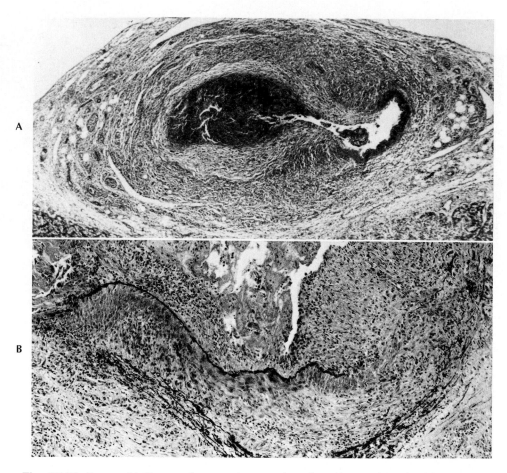

Fig. 17-19. Kawasaki disease (mucocutaneous lymph node syndrome) with panarteritis of coronary arteries. **A,** Necrotizing panarteritis of epicardial coronary artery with aneurysm that is filled with thrombus *(center of photograph).* **B,** Higher-power view of wall of coronary artery shows granulation tissue and organizing thrombus *(upper),* inflammation and necrosis of media *(lower)* with interruption of internal elastic lamina, and adventitial inflammatory tissue *(lower left and right).*

thritis and ankylosing spondylitis, aortitis or its sequelae may occur in the ascending thoracic aorta and may lead to aortic valvular insufficiency.[60] The pathologic lesions are nonspecific and primarily medial with loss of normal elements, focal scars, and scattered foci of lymphocytes and plasma cells. Mild to moderate intimal and adventitial fibrosis is present. In rheumatoid arthritis with aortitis, specific rheumatoid granulomas similar to the subcutaneous nodules of rheumatoid arthritis may be found rarely.

Ankylosing spondylitis. In ankylosing spondylitis patchy inflammation of the media with destruction of elastic fibers and smooth muscle cells followed by fibrosis may occur, primarily in the proximal ascending aorta and the sinuses of Valsalva. Dilatation of the aortic valve ring may ensue. The inflammatory process and fibrosis often extend into the aortic and mitral valves causing shortening and thickening of the valvular tissue.[64] Aortic valvular incompetence (regurgitation) is the more common functional event.

Reiter's syndrome. Aortic involvement in Reiter's syndrome is similar to that of ankylosing spondylitis. The ascending aorta is affected with disruption of elastic tissue and infiltration by inflammatory cells.[94] Rarely, the distal aorta may be involved.[92]

Relapsing polychondritis. Aortitis in relapsing polychondritis involves primarily the media with increased vascularization, perivascular infiltration of mononuclear cells, increased amount of collagen, and decreased amount of elastic tissue and acid mucopolysaccharides. Aneurysms secondary to the aortitis occur in about 10% of patients with relapsing polychondritis, usually in the ascending aorta but also may be in the abdominal segment. The aortitis of relapsing polychondritis is said to be distinct from that of syphilitic and granulomatous aortitis.[69]

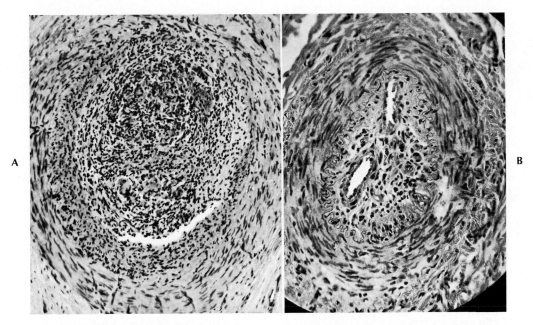

Fig. 17-20. Thromboangiitis obliterans (Buerger's disease) of small arteries of extremities. **A,** Panarteritic inflammation without mural necrosis, and beginning organization of cellular thrombus that has microabscesses and scattered giant cells. **B,** Recanalization of an organized thrombus has occurred. Internal elastic membrane *(wavy line)* is intact.

Thromboangiitis obliterans. Thromboangiitis obliterans (TAO, Buerger's disease) is an uncommon inflammatory occlusive disease involving small and medium-sized arteries and veins of the extremities in a segmental fashion. The disease affects mainly males under 35 years of age who are cigarette smokers.[63] There has been a sharp increase in the frequency to TAO in women in recent years, probably reflecting increased cigarette smoking in women in the past two decades.[85]

Although the specificity of TAO has been questioned, it is generally accepted to be a distinct clinical symptom complex[78] with reasonably characteristic pathologic features. The symptom complex consists in intermittent claudication followed by ischemic necrosis of the toes or fingers with gangrene that progresses toward the trunk. The cause of TAO is unknown, but toxic effects of cigarette smoking are important. Among other possible pathogenic mechanisms are altered immune mechanisms, hypercoagulability, and genetic factors because of the slightly greater prevalence in Orientals and Ashkenazi Jews. Increased cell-mediated sensitivity to human native collagen type I and type III, which are constituents of blood vessels, has been reported.[57]

Vessels of the lower extremities are affected more commonly than those of the upper extremities. TAO rarely has been observed in vessels of the heart, lung, brain, gastrointestinal tract, and male genitalia, almost exclusively only when the disease is severe and progressive in the extremities.

The lesions are characteristically focal or segmental, and involved segments are occluded. Microscopically, early lesions have inflammatory infiltrate of all layers of the vessel by polymorphonculear leukocytes and always are thrombosed (Fig. 17-20). The thrombi are quite cellular and frequently have microabscesses. The intima is diffusely thickened by cellular proliferation; no lipid aggregates or calcium deposits are present. The internal elastic lamina characteristically is intact. In later or more advanced stages, mononuclear cells predominate in the inflammatory infiltrates and occasional epithelioid cell granulomas with Langhans' giant cells are present in the thrombus. The architecture of the medial muscle layer is preserved. As the disease becomes more chronic, more fibrosis and fewer inflammatory cells are found and the thrombus is recanalized. Neither arterial wall necrosis nor aneurysm occurs. TAO can be distinguished from atherosclerosis and bland thrombi or emboli on the basis of the cellular thrombus, the well-preserved media, the inflammatory reaction in the intima, media, and adventitia, the size of vessels involved, and the synchronous involvement of veins as well as arteries.

Raynaud's phenomenon and disease. Raynaud's phenomenon is episodic symmetric ischemia of the fingers and rarely the hands provoked primarily by cold but also by other stimuli such as emotion, trauma, hormones, and drugs. The affected digits show pallor followed by cyanosis and then redness, reflecting underlying arterial ischemia, venostasis, and reactive hyperemia, respectively. Uncommonly, ulceration and necrosis of digits occur. Raynaud's phenomenon may be associated with many conditions, including occlusive arterial disease, trauma, neurogenic lesions, and many of the connective tissue syndromes.[97] When Raynaud's phenomenon occurs without an associated condition in an otherwise normal person, the condition may be termed Raynaud's disease or primary Raynaud's phenomenon. Although the digital arteries of patients with Raynaud's disease may not have structural abnormalities, a study of biopsy samples from the fingertips of a few patients showed segmental inflammatory and fibrinoid changes of the capillaries and regressive changes of glomus bodies.[65]

Aneurysms

An aneurysm is a permanent, abnormal dilatation of a blood vessel caused by weakening or destruction of the wall of the vessel. Aneurysms may be congenital or acquired. Most commonly elastic arteries and their major branches are involved. Larger muscular arteries are less frequently involved. Aneurysms of all types tend to enlarge with time; the enlargement and the production of clinical problems may be a slow or rapid process. Deleterious effects of aneurysms include alterations in blood flow distally, thrombosis with the potential for thromboembolism, rupture, and compression of adjacent structures.

Aneurysms can be classified by the composition of the wall of the dilatation (true, false), shape (saccular, fusiform, cylindroid, serpentine, racemose), or pathogenic mechanisms (arteriovenous, mycotic, dissecting, traumatic, atherosclerotic, syphilitic, congenital). A *true* aneurysm is composed of all layers, or parts of them, of the normal vessel. A *false* aneurysm has a fibrous wall and is the result of rupture of the vessel with the formation of a cavity contained by adventitial and perivascular tissues. *Saccular* aneurysms are more or less spherical outpouchings with reasonably well-defined origins or necks. *Fusiform* aneurysms are spindle shaped and involve more or less uniformly the entire circumference of the vascular segment. *Cylindroid* aneurysms are variants of the fusiform type. A *serpentine* aneurysm is a tortuous, dilated vessel whose enlargement usually is the result of senile ectasia, or a congenital malformation. An *arteriovenous* aneurysm refers to the dilated vessels associated with an arteriovenous fistula; *racemose (cirsoid)* aneurysms are forms of arteriovenous aneurysms in which there are masses of intercommunicating small arteries and veins. *Mycotic* aneurysms result from weakening of the arterial wall by infection with a microbiologic agent. *Dissecting* aneurysm, more appropriately termed dissecting hematoma, is the separation of the layers of the vascular wall by a column of blood from the lumen.

Aortic aneurysms

Most aneurysms of the aorta and its major elastic or musculoelastic branches are true aneuryms; false aneurysms principally result from traumatic rupture of the vessel. Medial weakness is the immediate factor leading to the development of the aneurysm. The common types are atherosclerotic, syphilitic, degenerative, and dissecting aneurysms.

Atherosclerotic aneurysm. Atherosclerosis is the most common cause of aortic aneurysms in the Western world. The abdominal aorta is the most common location. Atherosclerotic aneurysms of the abdominal aorta are more common in males and after the age of 60 with frequency increasing with age. The cause is advanced atherosclerosis, that is, complicated lesions that encroach on the media and cause thinning and destruction of medial elastic tissue with atrophy of the media resulting from pressure phenomena and from impaired nutrition of the media. In the thoracic aorta, especially the ascending and arch portions, atherosclerosis may be the basic problem, but in many cases primary medial degeneration is the underlying condition, and the atherosclerosis is a secondary and contributory factor.

Most atherosclerotic aortic aneurysms are fusiform (Fig. 17-21, *A*). In the abdominal aorta most are infrarenal, beginning 1 to 3 cm distal to the renal arteries. Many extend into one or both common iliac arteries and their external and internal branches; often separate iliac arterial aneurysms also are present. The aneurysm may involve the origins of the superior mesenteric artery and the celiac axis. The suprarenal and infrarenal portions of the abdominal aorta and the descending thoracic aorta may form one large aneurysmal structure constituting a thoracoabdominal aneurysm. Abdominal aortic aneurysms may be any size; clinically significant ones usually are greater than 5 or 6 cm in diameter, but smaller aneurysms may rupture.

Usually the aneurysm contains a mural thrombus, composed primarily of laminated fibrin that develops on the ulcerated, roughened and atherosclerotic intimal surface (Fig. 17-21, *B*). Abnormal local hemodynamic effects contribute to the thrombosis. Branches of the aorta may be obliterated by the thrombus with resultant localized ischemic effects in the region supplied by the branch. Fragments of the thrombus may embolize distally into peripheral arteries. The thrombus may build up to large size and cause aortic luminal narrowing. Large aneurysms may compress adjacent vessels and, rarely, nerves.

Abdominal aortic aneurysms may rupture into either the peritoneum or, more commonly, the retroperitoneum, and thoracic aneurysms can rupture into the mediastinum with or without intrapleural extension. Rupture may be sudden and massive with death in minutes. Generally the likelihood of rupture increases with size. Ruptures may be small and slowly progressive amount-

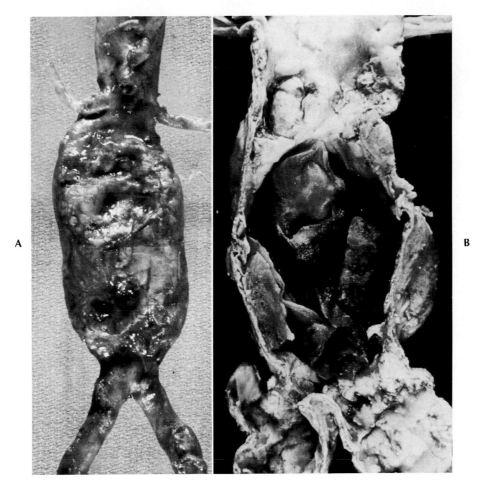

Fig. 17-21. A, Intact infrarenal atherosclerotic aneurysm of abdominal aorta viewed anteriorly. Origins of celiac axis and superior mesenteric artery, as well as the right and left renal arteries, are above aneurysm. Aortic bifurcation and common iliac arteries are below. **B,** Opened atherosclerotic aneurysm of distal abdominal aorta demonstrates laminated fibrin thrombus *(dark material)* in aneurysm. Renal arteries are at top of photograph, and aortic bifurcation with severely atherosclerotic and aneurysmal common iliac arteries is at bottom.

ing to a "leaking" aneurysm. Infection of an atherosclerotic aneurysm is uncommon and occurs more often when there is rupture.[128] Occasionally the aneurysm may impinge on vertebral bodies, in which event the posterior wall of the aneurysm is formed by the anterior spinal ligament or cancellous bone.

Microscopic examination of the wall of an atherosclerotic true aneurysm shows significant loss of normal arterial structure, and so the wall consists of fibrous tissue with only portions of normal medial components (Fig. 17-22). The adventitia is fibrotically thickened and has mild to moderate chronic inflammatory infiltration, mainly foci of lymphocytes. Remnants of medial smooth muscle and elastic tissue are present, and atheromatous materials, fibrin, and thrombus replace the normal intima and part of the media.

Inflammatory aneurysms are a distinct group of aortic aneurysms, usually of the abdominal aorta[111] that are

characterized by pronounced thickening of the wall anteriorly and laterally by fibroinflammatory processes with adhesion and extension into adjacent structures making operative dissection difficult (Fig. 17-23).

Histopathologically, the wall of the aneurysm is composed of dense, often hyalinized, fibrous tissue with large numbers of lymphocytes and plasma cells. Clinically, patients may have chronic abdominal pain, weight loss, elevated erythrocyte sedimentation rate, and partial or complete ureteral obstruction.[122]

Although some have suggested that an autoimmune reaction to transudation of blood constituents through the thinned wall of the aneurysm contributes to the formation of an inflammatory aneurysm, at this time they are best regarded as a type of atherosclerotic aneurysm.[124]

The natural course of most atherosclerotic aneurysms is gradual enlargement and eventual rupture or throm-

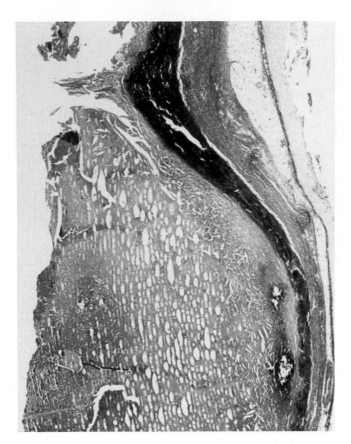

Fig. 17-22. Portion of wall of atherosclerotic aneurysm of aorta. Black tissue is medial tunica elastica. At top is non-dilated aorta with complicated atherosclerosis and fibrin thrombus. Bulge to right is wall of aneurysm, which contains fibrin thrombus on luminal side *(toward left)*, and complicated atherosclerosis with focal calcification *(irregular black masses near media)*.

bosis. Although acute rupture has a grave prognosis, the outlook with elective surgical treatment today is good.[103,104]

Syphilitic aneurysm. Syphilitic (luetic) aneurysms are complications of syphilitic aortitis that develop in the tertiary stage of syphilis. They occur predominantly in the thoracic aorta, especially in the ascending and arch portions. In the past syphilis was a common cause of aneurysms of the thoracic aorta, but today atherosclerotic and medial degenerative causes are far more common.

Syphilitic aneurysms usually become manifest after the age of 50. They are usually saccular but can be cylindroid or fusiform (see Fig. 17-12) and more often attain larger size (15 to 20 cm in diameter) than atherosclerotic aneurysms do. These aneurysms often displace, compress, or erode adjacent structures, leading to respiratory, esophageal, or skeletal complications. Rupture may occur into the mediastinum, pericardial space, pleural cavities, trachea, bronchi, or esophagus or externally through the chest wall. Although the syphilitic aneurysm itself does not necessarily cause cardiac dysfunction, commonly the aortic root and valve also have syphilitic aortitis leading to aortic valvular incompetence and cardiac failure.

The histologic features of syphilitic aneurysms, which are true aneurysms, are those of healed luetic aortitis (see Fig. 17-13). The adventitia is moderately thickened by fibrosis, and vasa vasorum manifest endarteritis obliterans with narrowing or occlusion of their lumens. The scars may extend from the adventitia through the media and into the intima. Fibrosis of the intima is common and often is continuous with that of the media. Typical atherosclerotic lesions frequently are superimposed on and may mask the underlying luetic process, especially on gross morphologic examination. Spirochetes are rarely demonstrated in typical luetic aneurysms.

Degenerative aneurysm. In some older persons, noninflammatory, medial degenerative changes of the aorta occur that are more pronounced than expected for the chronological age, leading to aneurysm formation, especially of the thoracic aorta, or to dissection.[132] Pathologically the media shows exaggerated aging changes of loss of elastic fibers and smooth muscle cells and fibrosis. The adventitia is nearly normal or is modestly fibrotic with only moderate numbers of lymphocytes. True intimal atherosclerotis may be present but is not the cause of the aneurysm. Such aneurysms tend to be diffuse in configuration.

Dissecting aneurysm. A dissecting aneurysm (DA) is a dissecting hematoma in which blood is present within the wall of the vessel and spreads (dissects) longitudinally, creating a cavity by separation of the tissues. In nearly all instances the dissection is in the media. The aorta is the most common site, but the lesion can occur in any artery. Generally the onset of the event is acute and is a dramatic clinical emergency. Modern treatment has improved the outlook for patients with acute aortic dissections with a decrease in mortality from some 90% within 3 months in untreated persons in the past to 15% to 20% with modern medical and surgical treatment.[108] DA occcurs more often in men and mainly in the age range of 50 to 70 years. Before the age of 40 there is nearly equal male to female distribution. Half of the dissections in women before the age of 40 years occurs during pregnancy.[119] In persons under 40 years of age DA occurs mainly in those with a familial predisposition, Marfan's syndrome,[127] or congenital heart disease such as coarctation of the aorta[131] and bicuspid aortic valve.[109] DA is more common in blacks,[133] perhaps because of their greater incidence of hypertension.

Morphologic and pathogenic features. The dissecting column of blood is located primarily between the outer

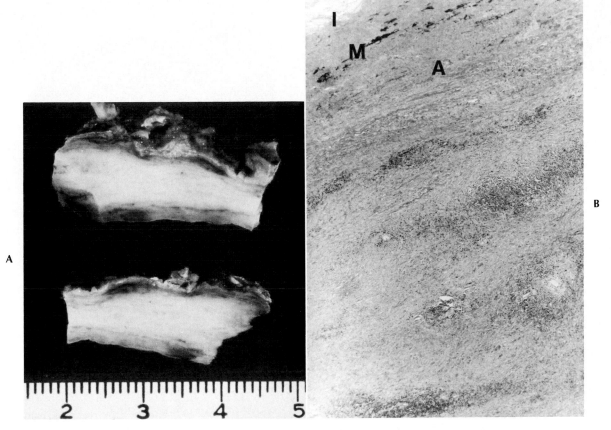

Fig. 17-23. Inflammatory aneurysm. **A,** Surgically resected portions of an inflammatory atherosclerotic aneurysm demonstrate severe atherosclerosis *(upper ragged material)* and pronounced thickening *(white)* of adventitial-periadventitial tissues. **B,** Histologic section from same specimen demonstrates portion of atherosclerotic intima *(I)*, degenerated and thinned media *(M)*, and thick layer of fibroinflammatory tissue *(A)* involving adventitia and surrounding tissues.

and middle thirds of the aortic media (Figs. 17-24 and 17-25). In more than 95% of cases an intimal tear (Fig. 17-26) that continues into the media is present and presumed to be the origin of the dissecting hematoma (Fig. 17-27), but rare instances of DA without an intimal tear have been reported. Generally the intimal tear is 4 to 6 cm in length and perpendicular to the long axis of the aorta; rarely it may be nearly circumferential in the aortic root. Most intimal tears in the ascending aorta are in its proximal portion, less than 4 cm from the aortic valve cusps near the junction of the sinus and tubular portions of the aorta[120,123] and are most often on the right lateral aspect of the aorta with the dissection following the greater curvature of the thoracic aorta. The dissection commonly extends proximally and distally from the tear. The dissecting column of blood may simply end in the media and adventitia, may rupture into adjacent tissues or body cavities, or may reenter the lumen of the aorta or one of its branches. True reentry sites occur in 10% to 20% of cases with about half com-

municating with the aorta, most often the abdominal aorta, and the other half with a major artery, most often an iliac. Often the dissecting process involves the major branches of the aortic arch, the right coronary artery, the left intercostal arteries, the left renal artery, or the left iliac artery. Muscular branches of the aorta may be completely severed from their aortic origin and originate from the dissected cavity (false lumen).

DeBakey and co-workers[107] classified DA into three types according to the apparent origin and extent of the condition. Type I (75% of cases) begins in the ascending thoracic aorta and extends distally for a variable distance; type II (5% of cases) is confined to the ascending aorta and often is found in patients with Marfan's disease; and type III (20% of the cases) begins in the descending thoracic aorta, just distal to the origin of the left subclavian artery in the aortic isthmus. The dissection extends retrograde into the ascending aorta in type IIIA but not in type IIIB. A modification of this classification also is used; type A dissections involve the as-

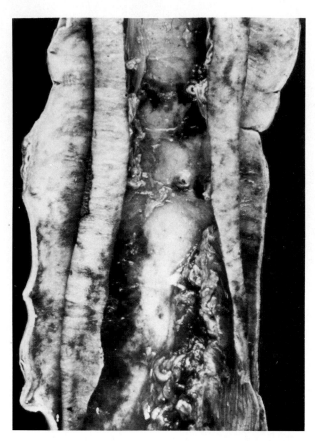

Fig. 17-24. Acute dissecting aneurysm (hematoma) of aorta. Adventitial surface of aorta is in center (notice orifices of aortic branches), and dissected channel (false lumen) that partly surrounded true aorta has been opened. Column of blood that separated medial layers to form false lumen has been removed.

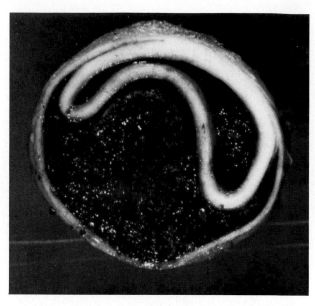

Fig. 17-25. Cross section of aorta that has acute dissecting aneurysm shows true aortic lumen *(above and right)* compressed by dissecting column of blood that separates media and creates false lumen.

cending aorta and include DeBakey types I and II; type B does not involve the ascending aorta.[105] Dissection that begins in the abdominal aorta is rare, can progress proximally (retrograde in regard to blood flow), and often is traumatic in origin, including iatrogenically produced lesions.

Occasionally the dissection is localized to just a few centimeters from the intimal tear and does not rupture or reenter, creating an "incomplete" DA; in this event the site of the tear may heal leaving a localized, sharp defect in the intima. The more common and clinically evident instances of complete DA also may heal ("healed" or "chronic" DA) with the formation of a second or even a third channel in the aorta termed the false lumen or lumens and creating a "double-barreled" or "triple-barreled" aorta. These channels become endothelialized and develop a pseudointima that rapidly may become atherosclerotic to a degree that equals or exceeds the atherosclerosis of the native channel in which the AS developed over a period of years.[114]

Death from DA most often results from rupture. Rupture sites frequently associated with rapid demise include the pericardial sac leading to acute hemopericardium, the mediastinum, the left pleural space, and the retroperitoneum. Extension of the medial dissection into the arch branches may lead to cerebral ischemia. Extension into a major coronary artery, usually the right, may cause fatal myocardial infarction. Extension to a cardiac chamber rarely may occur. DA involving the renal arteries may lead to renal failure, and involvement of intercostal arteries may cause infarction of the spinal cord. Aortic valvular insufficiency may result from loss of commissural support of the valve. Patients who survive the acute episode ("healed" or "chronic" DA) may develop a saccular aneurysm of the false channel.

About 70% of patients with DA clinically have systemic hypertension, and in autopsy studies about 90% of patients have left ventricular hypertrophy, indicating that hypertension may have been present. The frequency of DA appears greater in patients with malignant (accelerated) hypertension than in those with benign hypertension.[100] Although hypertension is the most common clinical finding associated with DA, its exact role in the production of the condition has not been defined.[116,134] Other clinical or pathologic states associated with DA include pregnancy, Marfan's syndrome, atherosclerosis, trauma, aortic valvular stenosis (especially of the congenitally bicuspid valve), and

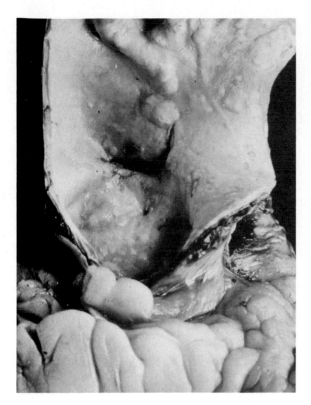

Fig. 17-26. Opened proximal ascending thoracic aorta has intimal tear *(dark hockey stick–shaped structure)* that leads to dissecting hematoma. *Below,* Unopened left ventricle.

coarctation of the aorta; in all of these conditions except Marfan's syndrome, DA is rare.[109]

The focus of study of the pathogenesis of DA is the tunica media. Histologic and electron microscopic examinations show a variety of abnormalities that may or may not be pathogenically significant, but some morphologic alteration usually is present. Cystic medial necrosis (CMN) is one such process.[110] It is characterized by focal accumulations of mucoid (myxoid) material in the aortic media in areas with loss of normal smooth muscle cells and elastic fibers, but rarely with true necrosis or inflammation (Fig. 17-28). True cysts with a limiting membrane or lining are not present; the accumulations are gel-like ground substance. Fibrosis of slight to moderate degree may exist. CMN occurs mainly in persons over 40 years of age,[102] except in Marfan's syndrome with aortic dilatation when it is found at any age. The exact relationship of CMN to DA is uncertain. In Marfan's syndrome, congenital bicuspid aortic valve, and coarctation of the aorta, the occurrence of CMN may be coincidental rather than causal for DA. Although DA is associated with hypertension, no certain correlation of hypertension and CMN exists, and a specific medial defect to explain the susceptibility of patients with hypertension to DA has not been established.[125,126]

The media of the aorta in many instances of DA does not show typical cystic medial degeneration ("necrosis") but rather manifests loss and fragmentation of elastic

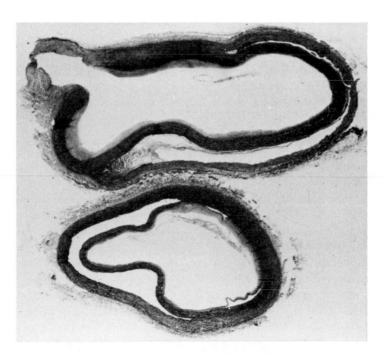

Fig. 17-27. Cross section of dissecting aneurysm of aorta. Native lumen in center is partly surrounded by false lumen that resulted from separation of media *(black tissue)* by dissecting hematoma.

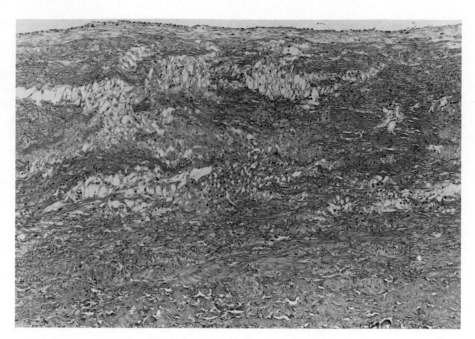

Fig. 17-28. Cytic medial degeneration in a patient with Marfan's syndrome has accumulations of acid mucopolysaccharides (cystlike areas) in media and loss and disruption of elastic fibers. *At top,* Lumen and thin intima; *lower fifth,* adventitia.

fibers and slight fibrosis, usually with some increase in ground substance. In many cases these nonspecific changes do not appear to be greater in frequency or extent in DA than in nondissected aortic media of age- and sex-matched controls. These medial changes are likely the result of the processes of injury and repair initiated by hemodynamic events as part of aging.

At this time it can be concluded that although the typical lesion of cystic medial "necrosis" and the medial degenerative changes are commonly found in DA, their pathogenesis and their precise role in DA are not yet certain. Identification of a specific biochemical abnormality, especially in Marfan's syndrome, would clarify the situation. The higher incidence of intimal-medial tears in the ascending aorta than in other aortic segments may be related to hemodynamic factors,[115] and the location of the dissection in the media might be related to the nutritional watershed zone of the media.

Atherosclerosis (AS) does not appear to be a significant factor in most instances of DA, though it may play a role by disrupting normal medial and intimal architecture. AS often is found coincidentally. The medial scarring of syphilitic aortitis seems virtually to preclude DA; at least the finding of the two conditions in the same aorta is an extreme rarity.

Aortic sinus aneurysms. Aneurysms of the aortic sinuses of Valsalva are uncommon.[106] Such aneurysms may be congenital or acquired and are to be distinguished from simple dilatation of the sinuses that occurs with aging and hypertension, and from anuloectasia associated with DA or fusiform aneurysm of the ascending

aorta. Recognized causes include congenital absence or hypoplasia of medial elements, Marfan's syndrome, syphilis, ankylosing spondylitis, and infective endocarditis. In contrast to congenital forms, acquired aortic sinus aneurysms commonly involve more than one sinus of Valsalva and also the ascending aorta.

The major clinical problems relating to aneurysms of the aortic sinuses are caused by rupture into a cardiac chamber, the pericardial cavity, or an extracardiac site. Death most commonly is the result of congestive heart failure related to arteriovenous shunting, or acute pericardial tamponade from rupture into the pericardial cavity. Surgical correction often is possible.[106]

Coronary artery aneurysms

Coronary artery aneurysms may be congenital, atherosclerotic, inflammatory, or traumatic in nature. They may be single or multiple and saccular or fusiform in shape.[121] The congenital forms have hypoplasia of the media, but secondary histopathologic changes in the wall of the aneurysm often make the distinction between congenital and atherosclerotic forms difficult. Most of the apparent congenital aneurysms occur before age 40, and atherosclerotic coronary arterial aneurysms occur at older ages. Inflammatory coronary aneurysms may be associated with syphilis, infective endocarditis, possibly rheumatic carditis or other connective tissue disorders, and Kawasaki disease and may not become apparent until after resolution of the causative disease.[117] Traumatic coronary aneurysms often are associated with fistulous communications to one of the right-sided cardiac chambers. Dissecting aneurysms of the coronary artery most often are the result of aortic DA or trauma. Death caused by coronary artery aneurysm is usually related to occlusion or embolism with myocardial ischemia, and less frequently to rupture.

Pulmonary artery aneurysms

Aneurysms of the pulmonary arterial trunk[129] or of its major branches are rare. Most involve the main trunk of the pulmonary artery, with or without involvement of its branches. Frequently aneurysms of the pulmonary artery are associated with or result from congenital cardiovascular defects. Causes of acquired pulmonary arterial aneurysms include trauma, atherosclerosis, syphilitic and tuberculous inflammation, mycotic foci from infective endocarditis, and medial degenerative changes. The clinical manifestations depend on the cause and the location and size of the aneurysm. The right ventricle frequently is enlarged. Congestive heart failure and rupture of the aneurysm are the common causes of death.

Aneurysms of other arteries

Aneurysms of systemic arteries are uncommon.[129] Aneurysms of the splenic artery may be atherosclerotic or congenital in origin, and their rupture in late stages of pregnancy is a well-recognized but rare event. Renal artery aneurysms, apart from those associated with fibromuscular dysplasia, are most commonly atherosclerotic, though congenital and traumatic types occur; renal hypertension and infarction are the most frequent complications. The most common peripheral arterial aneurysms are atherosclerotic types in the lower extremities, especially of the popliteal and femoral arteries. In the upper extremities, traumatic, mycotic, and arteritic aneurysms are more common than atherosclerotic ones.

Arteriopathy
Fibromuscular dysplasia

Fibromuscular dysplasia (FMD) is a disease of unknown cause characterized by nonatherosclerotic, noninflammatory segmental stenosing lesions with or without focal aneurysmal outpouchings of the affected artery. Clinically significant lesions are most frequent and best defined in the renal and internal carotid arteries, but the condition also has been found in the coronary, superior mesenteric, celiac, common hepatic, axillary, vertebral, subclavian, and intracerebral arteries, often in association with FMD of other vessels, especially the renal artery. The major clinical conditions resulting from FMD are hypertension, stroke, claudication, and intestinal ischemia. Renal arterial involvement is bilateral in approximately half of patients; unilateral lesions are more often on the right than on the left by a ratio of 3:1 in adults. The mean

age at diagnosis is in the fourth decade, and females predominate. Pathogenic factors considered to be important include a developmental error, hormonal effects, mechanical stress, and anatomic variations in vasa vasorum leading to mural ischemia. Pathologic lesions are found more frequently in all vessels with age but apparently often are clinically unimportant. In patients with symptoms, percutaneous transluminal angioplasty may be successful to relieve obstructions to blood flow.[118]

The general term *fibromuscular dysplasia* includes the pathologic processes of medial fibroplasia, perimedial dysplasia, medial hyperplasia, and intimal fibroplasia.[113,130] Medial fibroplasia (Fig. 17-29) is the most common type. Grossly the involved vessel has luminal ridges that narrow the lumen. Between the stenosed areas the wall is thinned and may have, or appear to have, aneurysms of the thin areas. The lesions are best demonstrated pathologically in the longitudinally opened vessel and in longitudinally oriented histologic sections. The stenosing ridges are areas of medial thickening by fibromuscular tissue in which the smooth muscle cells may show architectural disarray with loss of the normal, orderly, parallel arrangement of cells. The intervening thin areas are composed of histologically normal medial smooth muscle, which may be greatly decreased in quantity from normal. The alternating stenosed areas and thinned or aneurysmal areas give the appearance of a string of beads in arteriograms. Mild to moderate intimal fibrosis may be present; true atherosclerosis is uncommon and when present is a coincidental or complicating lesion. Perimedial dysplasia probably is the second most common form of fibromuscular dysplasia and is characterized by the accumulation of circumferential aggregations of elastic-like tissue between the media and the adventitia, creating the narrowed regions. This type is found almost exclusively in women younger than 30 years of age who have right-sided renal artery stenosis, substantial collateral circulation, and hypertension.[118] Medial hyperplasia is an uncommon form of FMD characterized by foci of apparent hyperplasia of normal medial smooth muscle with minimal architectural disorganization. Intimal fibroplasia (Fig. 17-30), a rare form of fibromuscular dysplasia, is characterized by focal eccentric or circumferential subendothelial mesenchymal cell proliferations that are somewhat similar to the histopathologic change of endarteritis obliterans, with essentially normal medial and adventitial structures.

Cystic adventitial disease of the popliteal artery

Cystic adventitial disease of the popliteal artery is a rare condition characterized by an adventitial ganglion-like cyst containing mucoid fluid that compresses the popliteal artery and causes intermittent claudication. The male-to-female ratio is 8:1, and the average ages at

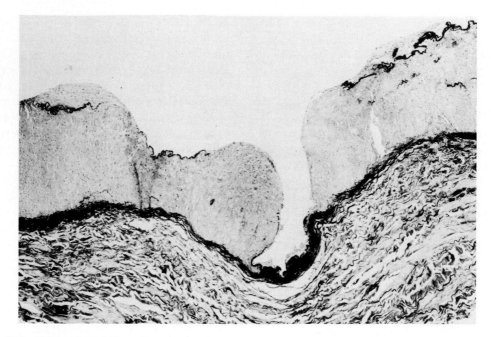

Fig. 17-29. Medial fibroplasia type of fibromuscular dysplasia of renal artery caused renovascular hypertension. In this longitudinal section of renal artery *(lumen at top)*, focal pronounced thickenings of media *(left and right halves of photograph)* caused focal stenoses. Between areas of medial thickening, media is nearly absent, permitting small aneurysmal outpouching *(center of photograph)*. Thin, wavy black line near lumen is internal elastic lamina that is absent in some areas. Heavy black lines, constituting external elastica, and adventitial tissues occupy lower part of photomicrograph. Intima is essentially normal; it can be identified in foci of slight, nonspecific thickening.

diagnosis are 36 years in men and 49 years in women. The grossly fusiform cyst is present within the adventitia (Fig. 17-31) and may or may not be lined by mucus-containing cells. Cystic adventitial disease also has been reported in the radial, ulnar, femoral, and external iliac arteries and in the saphenous and femoral veins. Theories of pathogenesis include repetitive trauma and inclusion of mucin-secreting cells within the adventitia during development.[112]

Congenital stenotic arteriopathy with medial dysplasia

Congenital stenotic arteriopathy with medial dysplasia is a uniformly stenotic arteriopathy attributable to hyperplastic and dysplastic medial elastic laminae involving the aorta and its major branches, the pulmonary trunk, and the pulmonary arteries.[101] The disease may be familial.

VEINS
Normal structure and age changes

Normal veins (Fig. 17-32) differ from arteries of the same size in that the wall of a vein is thinner, the three tunicae are less well demarcated, elastic tissue is scanty and not clearly organized into distinct internal and ex-ternal elastic laminae, and medial smooth muscle cells are relatively fewer in number, widely separated by collagen fibers, and arranged in both circular and longitudinal fashions. All veins, except the vena cavae and common iliac veins, have valves. The valves, which are best developed in the leg veins, are paired folds of intimal tissue with collagen and elastin but little smooth muscle. Valves occur every 1 to 6 cm, often just distal to the point of entry of a tributary vein, and prevent retrograde venous blood flow. The venous system is a reservoir or capacitance unit for the cardiovascular system, containing 60% to 75% of the blood volume.

The principal age change in veins is the development of a definite fibromuscular intimal layer, which often is eccentric in thickness at a given site. This intimal fibromuscular layer hyalinizes with age and may calcify focally. Although this change rarely produces luminal narrowing, the advanced forms create phlebosclerosis.

Varicosities
Varicose veins

Varicose veins are abnormally dilated and tortuous veins. Although this pathologic condition of veins may occur in any part of the body, including the lower esophagus, anal region, and spermatic cord, the most

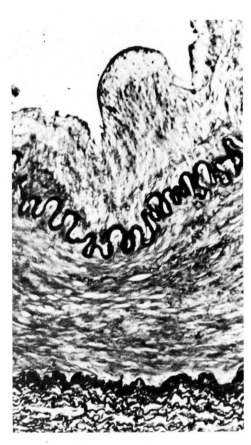

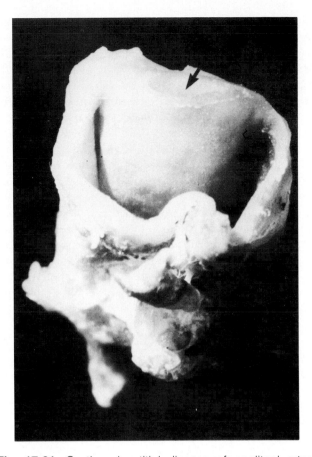

Fig. 17-30. Intimal fibroplasia form of fibromuscular dysplasia of renal artery. Focal intimal thickenings *(top)* produced focal stenoses. Upper wavy black line is internal elastic lamina; below it are normal media, external elastic lamina, and adventitia.

Fig. 17-31. Cystic adventitial disease of popliteal artery compressing arterial lumen *(arrow)*. Large cystic structure in forefront is thick-walled adventitial cyst.

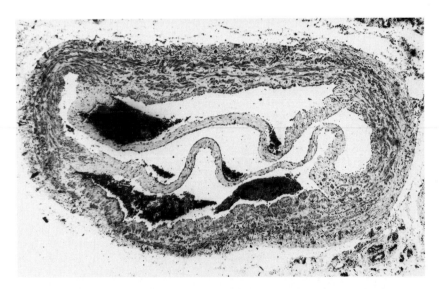

Fig. 17-32. Transverse section of normal saphenous vein shows pair of valves crossing lumen. Intima, media, and adventitia are not as well demarcated in veins as in arteries, well-defined elastic laminae are not present, and medial smooth muscle bundles are separated by collagen.

common sites are the superficial veins of the lower extremities, particularly the long saphenous vein and its tributaries. More than 20 million people in the United States are affected by varicose veins of the legs, with the peak occurrence being in the fourth and fifth decades. Women are affected three to six times more often than men. The condition appears to be more prevalent in Western countries. The etiology and pathogenesis of varicosities are multifactorial. Major considerations include hereditary (familial) weakness of the venous wall and valves, increased intraluminal pressure in leg veins from the upright posture with incompetence of the valves resulting from dilatation of the vessel, pregnancy because of compression of iliac veins and increased blood volume, and hormonal effects on smooth muscle. Less common etiologic and pathogenic factors are obesity and aging with atrophy of perivenous soft tissues. Scarring changes and thrombotic or neoplastic obstructions may be associated with varicosities distal to the involved venous segment.

Varicose veins of the legs are dilated, tortuous, elongated, and nodular. Histologic changes are similar to those of age but more pronounced. Calcific foci related to degeneration of medial elastic fibers may be present. Thrombosis is common, and organization of the thrombi may lead to intimal fibrous and hyaline plaques. All these changes are considered to be secondary, not causal. Prolonged venous stasis leads to skin changes of edema, stasis dermatitis, cellulitis, erosion, and ulceration and is a major factor in the development of thrombophlebitis in varicose veins. Pulmonary thromboembolism from varicose veins is uncommon.

Esophageal varices

Esophageal varices are tortuous and distended coronary veins of the distal esophagus and cardia of the stomach. They are almost always the result of obstruction of portal venous flow, most often caused by cirrhosis of the liver, since the coronary veins serve as collateral channels. In addition to hepatic cirrhosis, esophageal varices result from superior vena caval obstruction, portal vein thrombosis, hepatic vein thrombosis (Budd-Chiari syndrome), pylephlebitis, and tumor compression of the major portal trunk. Rupture and bleeding are the problems related to esophageal varices.

Hemorrhoids

Hemorrhoids are varicosities of the hemorrhoidal venous plexuses. External hemorrhoids are varicosities of the inferior hemorrhoidal plexus, which is located below the dentate line of the anal canal, is covered by squamous epithelium, and drains to the internal iliac veins of the systemic venous system. Internal hemorrhoids are varicose veins of the submucosal internal hemorrhoidal plexus, which is located above the dentate line, is covered by transitional and columnar epithelium, and drains to the portal venous system. Factors implicated in hemorrhoidal disease are heredity, erect posture, obstruction of venous return caused by increased intraabdominal pressure as with pregnancy, straining during bowel movement and diarrhea, and portal hypertension by virtue of the hemorrhoidal plexus serving as a collateral channel. Thrombosis, ulceration, hemorrhage, and perianal infection are frequent complications of hemorrhoids.

Varicoceles

A varicocele is a mass of varicose veins of the pampiniform plexus of the spermatic cord. This plexus is formed by the veins draining the testes and epididymis and drains by a single channel into the renal vein on the left and into the inferior vena cava on the right side of the body. Primary (idiopathic) varicocele is common on the left side but rare on the right. Secondary (symptomatic) varicocele may occur on either side and results from increased pressure on or in the spermatic veins as with hepatosplenomegaly, pronounced hydronephrosis, and abdominal tumors.

Phlebothrombosis and thrombophlebitis

In the past, two types of venous thrombosis were recognized: thrombophlebitis resulting from inflammation of the vein caused by injury or by neighboring inflammation, and phlebothrombosis as a primary condition related to hemodynamic and coagulation alterations. Today this distinction is recognized to be more theoretical than practical, since in most cases the initial problem is phlebothrombosis and the thrombus itself causes inflammatory reaction in the wall of the effected vein manifested by local and systemic signs and symptoms of an inflammatory state. The terms commonly are used synonymously.

The pathogenesis of venous thrombosis is summarized in Virchow's triad, which emphasizes the importance of changes in the vessel, particularly endothelial damage; changes in the composition of the blood; and disturbance of blood flow, especially stasis. Thrombosis is augmented if the fibrinolytic mechanism is defective or inhibited.[136] One or more of these pathogenic factors are likely to be present in certain clinical situations, including use of estrogen-containing compounds, malignancy, cardiac disease with congestive heart failure or arrhythmia, postoperative states, and inactivity or immobilization for any reason.

Phlebographic, pathologic, and radioactive tracer studies in the legs have shown that venous thrombosis develops initially in calf veins, mainly in the valvular sinuses and the related valves (Fig. 17-33). Most of these spontaneously lyse or organize. Only some en-

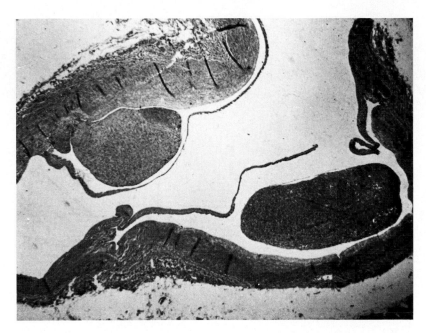

Fig. 17-33. Histologic section of leg vein with phlebothrombosis shows thrombi originating in sinuses of venous valves. Point of attachment of one thrombus *(upper left)* is shown; plane of section did not pass through attachment of other thrombus *(lower right)*.

large to form a thrombus of sufficient size to cause luminal obstruction or embolize. Thrombosis of larger veins, such as those of the iliofemoral system, which may be an extension of thrombi originating in calf veins,[142] has a higher risk of pulmonary thromboembolism. Pulmonary thromboemboli originate from veins of the legs in approximately 95% of cases. Approximately half of patients with acute venous thrombosis will have pulmonary thromboembolic episodes, but the majority of these are clinically inapparent.

The affected vein may appear normal or may be distended and firm to palpation. Internally a mural or an occlusive thrombus is present. The attachment of the thrombus to the wall may be delicate and easily separated. If the initial site of attachment of the thrombus can be determined, most often it is in the sinus of a valve. At the point of attachment an inflammatory-reparative process is present in thrombi that have been present for more than several hours (Fig. 17-34). This reaction initially consists of an ingrowth of fibroblasts into the thrombus from the venous intima, along with the deposition of scattered lymphocytes, macrophages, and a few polymorphonuclear leukocytes. Later, granulation tissue organizes the thrombus, the complete resolution may lead to a focus of fibrous intimal thickening or to an organized, recanalized thrombus.

Special types of venous thrombosis

Superficial thrombophlebitis. Superficial venous thrombosis of the legs usually results from varicose veins, whereas that of the arms usually is caused by the administration of intravenous fluids. The local inflammatory response generally is aseptic. Pulmonary thromboembolism is rare, and when it occurs, it is most often the result of extension of the thrombotic process into the common femoral vein or of the coexistence of deep vein thrombosis.

Thrombophlebitis migrans. Thrombophlebitis migrans is a clinical, but not morphologic, condition characterized by recurrent episodes of venous thrombosis of the extremities and viscera. It is most commonly associated with malignant tumors, Buerger's disease, connective tissue disorders, and blood disorders such as polycythemia rubra vera and sickle cell disease. Malignant neoplasms particularly associated with migratory thrombophlebitis are carcinomas of the lung, female reproductive tract, pancreas, gastrointestinal tract, prostate, and breast. Frequently this syndrome is accompanied by nonbacterial thrombotic endocarditis of the cardiac valves.

Phlegmasia alba dolens. The clinical finding of "white, painful leg" refers to massive swelling of the leg that is associated with some, but not all, cases of iliofemoral venous thrombosis. The massive swelling is postulated to result from blockage of veins and perivenous lymphatics by an inflammatory process. The condition is much more common in the left than in the right leg, probably because the left iliac vein is compressed by the right common iliac artery or by the aortic bifurcation. It occurs most often in women in the third trimester of pregnancy or after childbirth, or in patients who have had extensive pelvic surgery. The frequent ab-

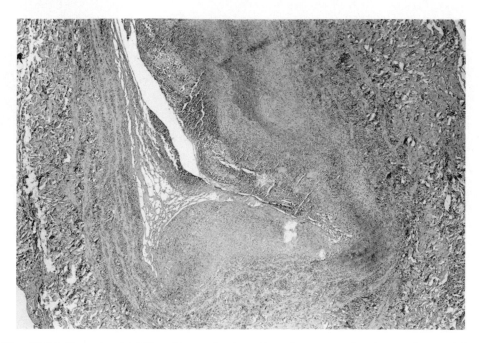

Fig. 17-34. Thrombophlebitis of leg vein show thrombus narrowing lumen *(upper left of center)* and inflammatory cells in venous wall and thrombus.

sence of valves within the iliac veins and the proximity of the iliofemoral system to the inferior vena cava may account for the development of pulmonary embolism in this condition.

Phlegmasia cerulea dolens. In some patients with massive iliofemoral venous thrombosis, the extremity is greatly swollen, the skin is blue, and bullae or superficial gangrene develops. The basis for this complication of venous thrombosis is thrombosis of collateral channels and decreased arterial blood flow. It is a serious condition with a mortality that ranges from 27% to 42%, depending on the presence or absence of venous gangrene.[135]

Superior vena caval syndrome. Obstruction of the superior vena cava (SVC) most often results from external compression. Thrombosis is present in less than half of the patients and most often results from the process that compresses or invades the wall of the SVC. Although in the past the SVC syndrome was caused by syphilitic aortic aneurysm or tuberculous mediastinitis in 40% of patients, today most instances result from malignant disease.[139] Bronchogenic carcinoma accounts for 75% of patients with the SVC syndrome, and about half of these have small-cell carcinoma, 15% have lymphoma, and 7% have metastatic neoplasms from various sites. Rare causes of the SVC syndrome include primary SVC thrombosis, pericardial constriction, idiopathic sclerosing mediastinitis, and goiter. The clinical syndrome of obstruction of the SVC consists in dilatation of veins of the upper part of the thorax and neck, edema and plethora of the face, neck, and upper part of the torso including the breasts, edema of the conjunctiva, and central nervous system symptoms of headache, visual distortion, and disturbed state of consciousness.

Inferior vena caval syndrome. The most common cause of obstruction of the inferior vena cava (IVC) is thrombosis, usually by extension from thrombosed iliac and femoral veins. Neoplastic involvement by external compression, invasion, or direct intraluminal extension is the other major cause of IVC obstruction. Renal cell carcinoma is the tumor that most commonly causes IVC obstruction (Fig. 17-35). Less frequent causes are external pressure from abdominal aortic aneurysm, ascites, pregnancy, retroperitoneal fibrosis, paravertebral lymphadenopathy, pelvic lipomatosis, pelvic inflammatory disease, and extension of hepatic and renal vein thrombi into the IVC. In childhood, IVC obstruction may result from right-sided Wilms' tumor, neuroblastoma, or multicystic kidneys. Symptoms and signs of IVC obstruction are swelling and edema of the lower extremities, distension of the superficial veins of the lower limbs, and the appearance of collateral venous channels in the lower abdomen.

Thrombosis of hepatic veins (Budd-Chiari syndrome). The Budd-Chiari syndrome is thrombotic obstruction of the major hepatic veins resulting in hepatic congestion and portal hypertension. The IVC may be involved by direct extension. Secondary slowing of blood flow in the portal vein may lead to thrombosis of the portal system. The cause can be identified in about two thirds of cases. The most frequent underlying con-

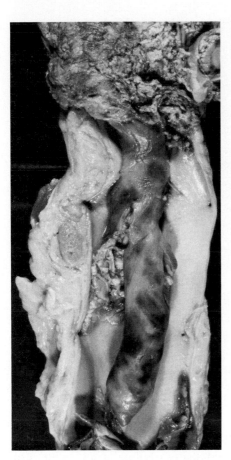

Fig. 17-35. Opened inferior vena cava shows thrombotic obstruction *(lower three fourths of photograph)* resulting from intraluminal extension *(upper one fourth of photograph)* of renal cell carcinoma.

ditions are hematologic disorders (polycythemia rubra vera, paroxysmal nocturnal hemoglobinuria, and myeloproliferative diseases) and use of oral contraceptives. Various drugs, pregnancy and the postpartum state, primary and secondary tumors of the liver, and trauma are other causes.[138] Worldwide, the most common cause of hepatic outflow obstruction is a membranous web of the inferior vena cava.[140] Intense hepatic congestion with a "nutmeg" appearance, centrilobular or panlobular necrosis and hemorrhage, and replacement fibrosis are the major pathologic features in the liver. Acute forms, characterized by abdominal pain, ascites, and acute hepatic failure, are associated with complete sudden obstruction. Subacute to chronic forms, characterized by abdominal pain, ascites, and hepatosplenomegaly, are associated with incomplete occlusion of the veins.

Portal vein obstruction. Extrahepatic obstruction of the portal vein may be caused by thrombosis (pylethrombosis), compression by intra-abdominal tumors or cysts, congenital venous atresia with cavernous malfor-

mation in childhood, and inflammation (pylephlebitis) that usually results from an intra-abdominal infection.[145] Thrombosis of the portal vein may be a complication of liver cirrhosis, visceral carcinoma, or polycythemia rubra vera. The thrombus may undergo organization and become a fibrous cord or undergo cavernous transformation to form a spongy, trabeculated venous lake involving the area of the portal vein and extending into the gastroduodenal ligament. Acute complete thrombosis of the portal vein in the absence of formed collaterals is catastrophic, leading to hemorrhagic infarction of the small bowel. Chronic forms have signs of portal hypertension with abdominal pain, ascites, splenomegaly, hematemesis, and melena.

Aortocoronary vein bypass grafts

Segments of veins, usually autologous saphenous veins, are used to bypass obstructed coronary arteries, as well as peripheral arteries, with generally good results for long periods. Changes in these venous grafts influence their long-term function. The major morphologic alteration is fibromuscular intimal proliferation (Fig. 17-36, *A* and *B*) that begins a few days after operation but is not necessarily steadily progressive with time, although it may cause severe luminal narrowing or total occlusion of the bypass graft.[141,144] Occlusion of these grafts in the early postoperative period is thrombotic and is mainly related to arterial disease distal to the coronary anastomosis or to technical surgical factors. The proliferating intimal cells are longitudinally oriented smooth muscle cells similar to those found in atherosclerotic lesions. They are capable of synthesizing collagen, elastin, and glycosaminoglycans. With time, the intimal lesion becomes less cellular and has more collagen fibers and ground substances. Factors implicated in the ubiquitous intimal proliferation in coronary artery bypass vein grafts are arterial intravascular pressure and flow, angle of anastomosis, tension on the graft, ischemic insult caused by severance of vasa vasorum of the graft, and mural deposits of fibrin that accumulate as a result of endothelial damage. True atherosclerotic changes in saphenous vein bypass grafts (Fig. 17-36, *C*) are uncommon until years after operation, though they are more common and appear earlier in patients with hyperlipidemic states.[137,143]

LYMPHATICS
Normal structure

The lymphatic system consists of lymphatic capillaries, lymphatic vessels (collecting vessels), and lymph nodes. Lymphatic capillaries are similar but not identical to blood capillaries. They consist of a single layer of endothelium with an interrupted basal lamina and scattered single smooth muscle cells. Lymphatic vessels resemble veins, and those larger than 200 to 500 μm in

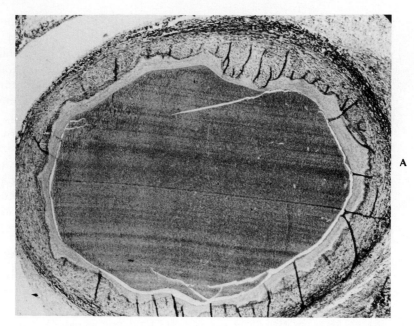

Fig. 17-36. Changes in aortocoronary artery vein bypass grafts. **A,** Saphenous vein used as coronary arterial bypass graft has slight intimal thickening 1 month after operation. Vascular lumen is filled by barium-gelatin mixture used for postmortem arteriogram. Light region surrounding lumen is thickened intima. Media and adventitia are slightly fibrotic.

external diameter have poorly defined intimal, medial, and adventitial layers whose structure quantitatively shows great variations. Virtually all lymphatic vessels have valves, which may be either bicuspid or tricuspid. The vessels often are dilated in the segments between valves. Lymphatic capillaries and vessels unite to form superficial and deep plexuses in and about many tissues and organs. The larger lymphatic vessels, such as the thoracic duct, have nerves and small blood vessels in their adventitia.

Lymphangitis

Acute lymphangitis results from the introduction of microorganisms, especially pyogenic bacteria, into the subcutaneous tissue. The superficial lymphatics are affected. Common organisms are beta-hemolytic streptococci and staphylococci. The affected lymphatics are visible as cutaneous erythematous streaks that spread up the arm or leg to the axillary or inguinal lymph nodes. Microscopically the lymphatics are dilated and contain leukocytes, cell debris, and coagulated lymph. The perilymphatic tissues are hyperemic and edematous with an inflammatory exudate. Recovery from acute lymphangitis with or without treatment usually is complete and without sequelae, but recurrent acute lymphangitis or incomplete resolution may lead to chronic lymphangitis. Chronic lymphangitis may cause permanent lymphatic obstruction by fibrosis resulting in chronic lymphedema.

Lymphedema

Lymphedema is swelling of soft tissue, especially the limbs, caused by a localized increase in the quantity of lymph.

Primary (idiopathic) lymphedema

Congenital lymphedema.[149] A familial-hereditary form *(Milroy's disease)* and a nonfamilial (simple) form of congenital lymphedema are recognized. In both forms, from birth, part or all of one extremity is diffusely swollen but is not painful or ulcerated. Milroy's disease, which also may be associated with other congenital anomalies, appears to be transmitted as an autosomal dominant trait with high penetrance, variable expression, and a predilection for males. The simple form, whose cause is unknown, may be associated with Turner's syndrome.[146] Histologic study of the involved region in either form shows dilatation of the subcutaneous lymphatics, increased interstitial fluid, and some fibrosis in long-standing cases.

Lymphedema praecox.[148] In this condition, which primarily affects females in the second or third decade of life, lymphedema begins in the foot or ankle and progresses slowly up the leg to involve the entire extremity in months or years. The skin of the extremity becomes roughened, and the edema becomes nonpitting. Other abnormalities have been observed in patients with lymphedema praecox, including yellow nails, pleural effusion, primary pulmonary hypertension, bronchiec-

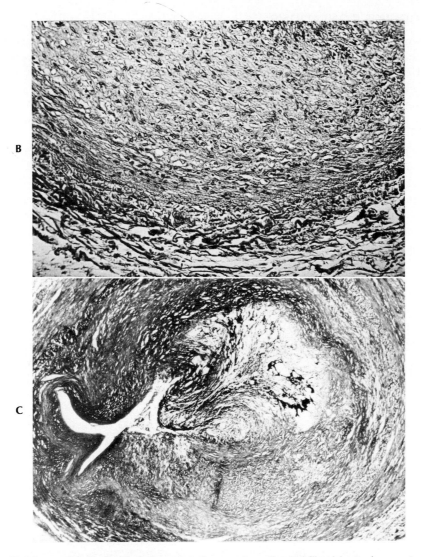

Fig. 17-36, cont'd. B, Proliferating smooth muscle cells and fibroblasts *(upper two thirds of photograph)* and their extracellular products produce intimal thickening. Fibrotic media and adventitia are in lower part of photograph. **C,** Fibromuscular intimal thickening and true atherosclerosis reduced lumen of this vein graft to cruciate slit *(left of center)* 8 years after operation.

tasis, cerebrovascular malformations, small pelvis, hypospadias, abnormal bone length, osteosclerosis, pes cavus, fused lumbar vertebrae, fixed flexion of the finger, distichiasis, hemangiomas of the feet and hands, and micrognathism.[147] The cause is unknown, but a relationship to the reproductive system is suspected because of age of onset, female preponderance, and increased swelling during menses.

Secondary (obstructive) lymphedema

The most common cause of obstructive lymphedema is a malignant tumor that occludes the lymphatic vessels or the lymph nodes. Surgical removal of lymphatics or lymph nodes and destruction of lymphatics by irradiation also are frequent causes. Less common causes include sclerosing retroperitoneal fibrosis, granulomatous processes such as sarcoidosis and tuberculosis of retroperitoneal or inguinal lymph nodes, and nematodal parasitic infestation (filariasis) of lymphatics producing elephantiasis. Because of the numerous anastomotic connections among lymphatic vessels, obstruction must be widespread or involve a critical site for draining lymph nodes, such as the axilla or the groin, for secondary lymphedema to develop. Lymphatics distal to the point of obstruction are greatly dilated, and the interstitial vessels are edematous and become fibrotic with time. Rupture of distended large lymphatics may occur, permitting the escape of milky lymphatic fluid, which may create, depending on site of drainage, chylous ascites (chyloperitoneum), chylothorax, chylopericardium, or chyluria.

TUMORS AND TUMORLIKE CONDITIONS

The distinction between true vascular neoplasms that have the potential for autonomous growth and a variety of other vasoproliferative lesions including vascular hamartomas often is not clear, leading to imprecise terminology and classification.

Arteriovenous fistula (aneurysm)

An arteriovenous (AV) fistula or aneurysm is a communication between an artery and vein without an intervening capillary bed. It may be either a congenital malformation or an acquired condition. In acquired forms, morphologic changes are found mostly in the veins, which are distended and have a thickened wall. Congenital AV fistulas have vessels that are thickened and hyalinized and a fibrotic stroma that may be calcified focally. The functional consequences of an AV communication depend on its size and include cardiomegaly and congestive heart failure, varicose veins, ulceration or gangrene of the skin, bluish red birthmarks, and increased length of an involved limb.

Hemangiomatous and telangiectatic conditions
Hemangiomas

Hemangiomas are typically of capillary origin, but they may also arise from venules and arterioles. Any organ can be affected, but the skin, especially of the face, is by far the most common site. Many are congenital; one third of all babies have a hemangioma of some type.[175] The gross appearances of hemangiomas vary depending on the size and density of the tangled vessels forming the lesion, the degree of arteriovenous shunting present, the degree of thrombosis or fibrosis, the degree of endothelial cell proliferation, and the organ involved.

Capillary hemangioma. The most common hemangiomas are of the capillary type.[161,162] In the skin they are small or large, single or multiple, flat to slightly elevated, strawberry marks that are bright red to purple, well-circumscribed, warm, soft, often lobulated lesions. The lesions are present at birth or first appear between the third and fifth weeks of life, increase in size for several months, regress spontaneously by thrombosis and fibrosis, and most often involute completely within a few years. Histopathologically, capillary hemangiomas are composed of small thin-walled vessels (Fig. 17-37) of capillary size that are lined by a single layer of flattened or plump endothelial cells that usually are surrounded by a discontinuous layer of pericytes and reticulin fibers. *Nevus flammeus* is a cutaneous telangiectatic capillary hemangioma that is a nonelevated, port wine–colored macule appearing at about 10 years of age and gradually increasing with age.

Cavernous hemangioma. Hemangiomas of the cavernous type are most common in or beneath the skin of the face, neck, and extremities, sometimes forming a subcutaneous mass with normal overlying skin. They also may be found in the oral mucosa, stomach, small intestine, liver, and bones. Lesions may be single or multiple, discrete or diffuse, red to blue, soft masses that are spongy on sectioning. Histopathologically le-

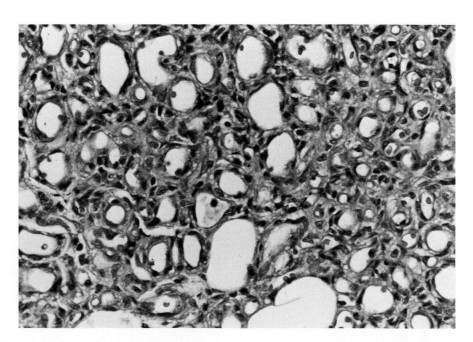

Fig. 17-37. High-power photomicrograph of capillary hemangioma of skin. Small, endothelium-lined vascular channels vary in size.

sions are composed of tangles of thin-walled, cavernous blood vessels and spaces separated by scanty connective tissue stroma that resembles erectile tissue. Cavernous hemangiomas rarely involute spontaneously. The *Kasabach-Merritt syndrome* is an extensive cavernous hemangioma, usually of the liver, and thrombocytopenic purpura with consumption coagulopathy resulting from coagulation in the hemangioma.

Combined capillary and cavernous hemangioma. Some hemangiomas histologically show a spectrum from pure capillary hemangioma through mixed capillary and cavernous types to pure cavernous structure. Clinically lesions with these histopathologic features usually resemble cavernous hemangiomas and are frequently found on the head and face in children. Such hemangiomas, especially those of skeletal muscles, may recur after incomplete resection and the histopathologic picture may cause concern because of nuclear pleomorphism, but the lesions never metastasize.[151]

Epithelioid hemangioma. Epithelioid hemangioma (angiolymphoid hyperplasia with eosinophilia) is a vascular tumor that elicits a peculiar inflammatory, often eosinophilic, response. It typically occurs during early to midadult life (20 to 40 years). Most occur in the head and neck, particularly the region around the ear. About half of the patients develop multiple lesions, usually in the same general area.[161] Histologically, the lesion is a vascular structure lined by epithelium-like endothelial cells that protrude into the lumen. A mixture of inflammatory cells including numerous eosinophils surrounds the lesion. The tumor may recur after curettage or local excision.

Hereditary hemorrhagic telangiectasia (Osler-Weber-Rendu disease)

Hereditary hemorrhagic telangiectasia (HHT, Osler-Weber-Rendu disease, Osler's disease)[154] is a genetic disorder transmitted as an autosomal dominant trait of high penetrance that is characterized by multiple telangiectases of the skin, mucous membranes, and viscera. The usual clinical presentation is recurrent bleeding from the involved site that tends to increase in frequency and severity with age. The lesions are superficial, punctate, purplish spots from 1 to 4 mm in diameter that blanch with pressure. Microscopically collections of dilated small blood vessels, lined by a single layer of endothelium and based on delicate connective tissue, are found. A pulmonary arteriovenous fistula develops in an estimated 15% of patients with HHT, and 40% to 60% of patients with pulmonary arteriovenous fistula have HHT.[163]

Angiomatosis

Angiomatosis refers to the presence of multiple, diffuse hemangiomatous lesions in association with other congenital malformations. Specific syndromes, which are probably inborn dysplastic states, are recognized. All are quite rare.

The *Klippel-Trenaunay syndrome* is a rare developmental entity comprising nevus flammeus, congenital varices, arteriovenous fistula, and hypertrophy of the soft tissue and bones.[152] The lesions may involve only a digit, a portion of a hand or a foot, or an entire extremity and may extend to the upper or lower trunk. The lesions usually continue to enlarge as the patient matures but do not progress after adulthood.

The *Sturge-Weber syndrome*[150] is a rare congenital disorder with a nevus flammeus on one side of the face in the area of the distribution of the trigeminal nerve, as well as ipsilateral retinal and leptomeningeal angiomatosis leading to ipsilateral buphthalmos and to contralateral hemiparesis or epilepsy, and mental deficiency. Calcium and iron deposits outlining the contour of cerebral gyri and sulci in a railroad-track pattern are seen on plain roentgenograms of the skull.

The *Maffucci syndrome*[153] is a congenital condition of dyschondroplasia with abnormal ossification of bone, skeletal deformities, and hemangiomas that may be capillary, cavernous, or combined types. Malignant neoplasms, especially of bones and blood vessels, occur frequently.

In the *blue rubber-bleb nevi syndrome*[154,169] bluish, rubbery, nipplelike vascular lesions of the skin and angiomas of the gastrointestinal tract are found. As a rule the skin lesions are cavernous hemangiomas, but a capillary hemangiomatous pattern with endothelial cell proliferation also may be seen.

The *von Hippel–Lindau syndrome* is a rare autosomal dominant disorder[164] in which hemangioblastomas are present in the cerebellum (Lindau's tumor) and retina (von Hippel's tumor) in association with cysts of the pancreas, kidneys, or liver. Other benign or malignant tumors of many organs may occur, including renal cell carcinoma in about 25% of patients.

Glomus tumor (glomangioma)

A glomus tumor is an uncommon, benign neoplasm usually found in the dermis, submucosal tissue, or superficial soft tissues. It arises from a neuromyoarterial body (Sucquet-Hoyer anastomosis) containing contractile glomus cells. Most glomus tumors are found in the subungual region and are typically painful, a feature that is absent in other sites.[172] These tumors are usually a few millimeters in maximum diameter and in the skin appear as rounded, red-blue, painful nodules. Histologically the tumors are composed of blood vessels lined by normal endothelial cells and surrounded by sheets of uniform, round to oval glomus cells with many nonmyelinated nerve fibers (Fig. 17-38). Although tissue culture studies identified glomus cells as pericytes, ul-

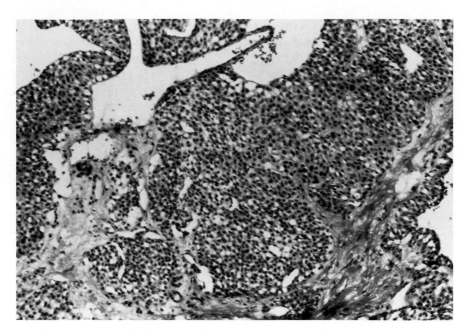

Fig. 17-38. Glomus tumor is composed of sheets of small, round to oval glomus cells surrounding vascular spaces. Nonmyelinated nerve fibers are present.

trastructural studies show them to resemble modified smooth muscle cells.[174]

Hemangioendothelioma

Most hemangioendotheliomas are true neoplasms of vascular origin with autonomous growth characteristics, in contrast to most hemangiomas, which are hamartomas.

The term "hemangioendothelioma" sometimes is used to designate tumors that are intermediate in biologic behavior between hemangioma and frankly malignant angiosarcoma[161] as well as to designate only the latter, which is also known as malignant hemangioendothelioma (see the discussion of angiosarcoma).

Benign hemangioendothelioma[157] is a cellular, hyperplastic *(juvenile) hemangioma* found in any organ but especially the skin, subcutaneous tissue, and liver of children. Grossly the lesion is a well-demarcated, grayred mass. Microscopically proliferation of uniform, endothelial cells in layers makes identification of vascular lumens difficult (Fig. 17-39). The tumor is not malignant. Juvenile hepatic hemangioendothelioma is associated with a high mortality as a result of hepatic failure or congestive heart failure.[159]

Hemangioendothelioma also has been used to designate the entity first described as *vegetant intravascular hemangioendothelioma*, which resembles a vascular malignancy. This entity is the same as *intravascular papillary endothelial hyperplasia*.[158] These lesions may be unusual organizing thrombi with florid cellular proliferation that may mimic and often are confused with angiosarcoma.

Epithelioid hemangioendothelioma. Epithelioid hemangioendothelioma is an uncommon tumor that usually arises from medium-sized or large veins of adults.[161] The tumor is composed of epithelioid or histiocytoid endothelial cells that grow in small cords or nests and only focally line well-formed vascular channels. The pattern of solid growth and the epithelioid appearance of the endothelium frequently leads to the mistaken diagnosis of metastatic carcinoma. Epithelioid hemangioendothelioma has histologic features of intravascular bronchioloalveolar tumor of lung[155] and the similar tumor of the liver.[165] Ultrastructural and immunohistochemical studies confirm the endothelial nature of the tumor cells. The tumor may have a benign or a malignant clinical course.

Hemangiopericytoma

Pericytes are perivascular cells that are found in place of smooth muscle cells in the wall of the terminal arteriole as it becomes the precapillary (metarteriole) and around capillaries, external to the basement membrane. Electron microscopic studies indicate that the tumor, hemangiopericytoma, originates from pericytes.[176]

Hemangiopericytomas[160,162] are rare tumors that can occur at any age and in any site. They vary in size from less than 1 cm up to large masses that are circumscribed or thinly encapsulated. Histologically the tumors are composed of small vessels whose lumens are surrounded by spindle-shaped pericytes in a radial arrangement outside the capillary basement membrane.

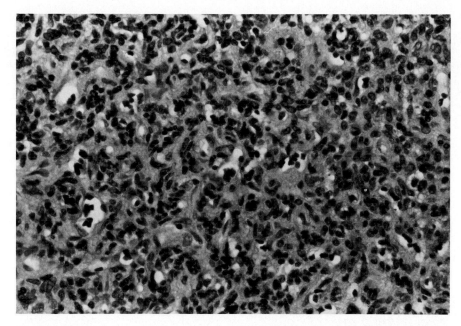

Fig. 17-39. High-power photomicrograph of benign hemangioendothelioma from skin of child. Proliferation of endothelial cells obscures scattered small vascular lumens.

Most are benign tumors, but local recurrence or distant spread eventuates in about 20% of patients.

Angiosarcoma

Angiosarcoma *(hemangiosarcoma, lymphangiosarcoma, hemangioendothelioma, malignant hemangioendothelioma)* is a malignant tumor of vascular endothelial cells. Angiosarcoma arising in the setting of chronic lymphedema has been designated lymphangiosarcoma, but a distinction between lymphangiosarcoma and hemangiosarcoma is not clear. About one third of angiosarcomas occur in the skin, particularly the area of the scalp, one fourth in the soft tissues, and another one fourth collectively in sites such as breast, liver, and bone.[161] Chronic lymphedema is the most widely recognized predisposing factor to angiosarcoma of the skin and soft tissues, often occurring after radical mastectomy for carcinoma of the breast, which situation accounts for up to one fifth of skin and soft-tissue angiosarcomas. Some hepatic angiosarcomas have been associated with prior remote exposures to arsenic, thorium dioxide (in Thorotrast), and gaseous vinyl chloride.[171]

Angiosarcomas often are dark-colored nodular masses that histologically may be well-differentiated tumors with multilayering of endothelial cells in well-formed vascular channels, or poorly differentiated lesions composed of solid clusters of cells with poorly formed vascular channels. The endothelial nature of the tumor cells can be confirmed in many cases by the use of immunohistochemical staining with antibodies to factor VIII–related antigen or a highly reliable endothelial cell marker, plant lectin (*Ulex europaeus* agglutinin I), and ultrastructural findings. The prognosis of angiosarcoma depends on the site of origin and on the tumor size but generally is grave. Angiosarcoma of the breast, for example, is a highly malignant tumor despite the relatively bland histological appearance.

Kaposi's sarcoma (KS)

KS is a multicentric malignant process of endothelial cell derivation that occurs predominantly in men. First described by Moritz Kaposi in 1872 as "idiopathic multiple pigmented sarcoma," the classic lesion is a slowly growing, indolent, dark blue to reddish plaque or nodule in the lower extremities of older men, especially those of Jewish and Italian descent. In the 1960s, an endemic form of KS was described in Africa that displayed several morphologic variants in contrast to classic KS. In tropical and southern Africa the lesions occur in younger men and involve multiple visceral organs. In these areas KS involving lymph nodes frequently affects children and has a worse prognosis. In the 1970s, KS was seen in organ-transplant recipients that were immune suppressed. Regression of the KS was observed in some of these patients after discontinuation of immunosuppressive agents. In the 1980s, KS appeared in epidemic form in patients with the acquired immune deficiency syndrome (AIDS) with a frequency of about 50% of affected homosexuals. KS in patients with AIDS is more aggressive and more widespread than classic KS with involvement of mucus membranes, lymph nodes, and virtually every organ except the brain.[178]

Histologically, the early lesion resembles granulation tissue or pyogenic granuloma with lymphocytes and plasma cells, but the diagnostic features are interweaving bands of malignant spindle cells and vascular structures forming clefts or slits between the cells, often with scattered extravasated erythrocytes or hemosiderin deposits. Three histologic variants have been described[173]: A mixed cellular form with spindle cells and vascular spaces (Fig. 17-40, *A*), a monocellular form with spindle cell proliferation predominating (Fig. 17-40, *B*), and an anaplastic type with pleomorphic cells. Electron microscopy demonstrates absence or near absence of pericytes, fragmented or absent basal lamina, discontinuity of endothelial lining cells, and scant junctional densities.[168] Tubuloreticular structures have been found by ultrastructural study only in the AIDS-associated form of KS but not in the classic, sporadically occurring tumor. Patients with classic KS lack antibody to HIV (HTLV-III) and have normal T4/T8 lymphocyte ra-

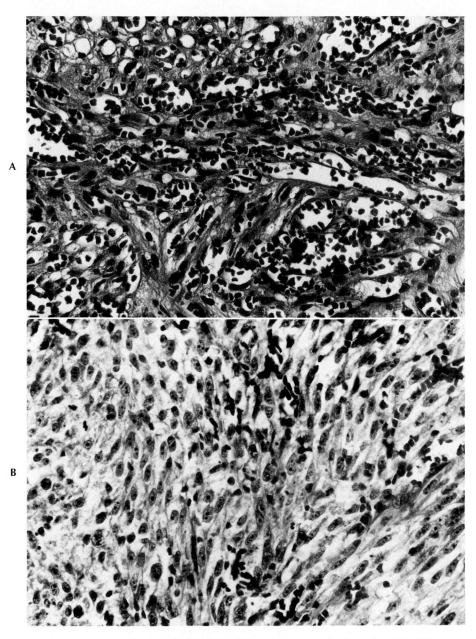

Fig. 17-40. Kaposi's sarcoma. **A,** Mixed-cellular type has spindle cells with slitlike spaces *(center)* and proliferating endothelial cells forming vascular spaces. **B,** Monocellular type is composed mainly of pleomorphic spindle cells.

tio in contrast to the patients with AIDS-associated KS. Radiotherapy is reported to be the treatment of choice for localized, nodular KS; for patients with more disseminated disease or with locally invasive tumor, chemotherapy has been effective.

Primary tumors of large veins and arteries

Primary, true tumors arising in the major blood vessels are quite rare.[166] About two thirds are in large veins in which smooth muscle tumors, especially leiomyosarcoma, are the most frequent, with more than 50% of reported cases arising in the inferior vena cava. Leiomyosarcomas of the inferior vena cava almost exclusively occur in elderly women.[170] Virtually all primary tumors of the aorta and pulmonary artery and their large branches are sarcomatous neoplasms including intimal (endothelial) sarcoma, fibrosarcoma (fibromyxoid sarcoma), leiomyosarcoma, and undifferentiated sarcoma.

Lymphangioma

Lymphangiomas are benign overgrowths of lymphatic vessels; whether these are congenital malformations, hamartomas, or true neoplasms is not certain. Lymphangiomas are classified as capillary, cavernous, or cystic (hygroma) types, and combinations are frequent.

Capillary lymphangioma (*lymphangioma simplex*) is an apparently congenital lesion of the skin or mucous membranes of the head and neck that grows slowly if at all. The small, circumscribed, pale white to pink tumors are composed of a network of endothelium-lined, thin-walled lymphatic spaces often separated by lymphoid aggregates.

Lymphangiomyoma, which can be regarded as a variant of capillary lymphangioma, has proliferating smooth muscle cells and branching, slitlike lymphatic channels.[177] It is a rare, acquired or congenital lesion most commonly involving abdominal and thoracic lymphatics of females[167] that may be associated with chylothorax.

Cavernous lymphangioma[156] is more common than the capillary variety. It also is an apparently congenital lesion that grows slowly and is composed of numerous dilated lymphatic spaces filled with lymph (chylangioma), which may be coagulated and hyalinized or calcified. The distinction from capillary lymphangioma on the basis of size of channels is somewhat arbitrary. Mixed lesions of cavernous lymphangioma and hemangioma are more common.

Cystic lymphangioma (hygroma)[156] occurs principally in the neck (*hygroma colli cysticum*) as a disfiguring congenital lesion. The cystic mass usually is multilocular and contains serous fluid or lymph. The histologic structure is similar to that of cavernous lymphangioma except for the large size of the spaces (Fig. 17-41). Large collections of lymphocytes may be present in the stroma. Total excision of large lesions may be difficult, and incomplete excision leads to recurrence. Infection of cystic hygroma is a serious problem.

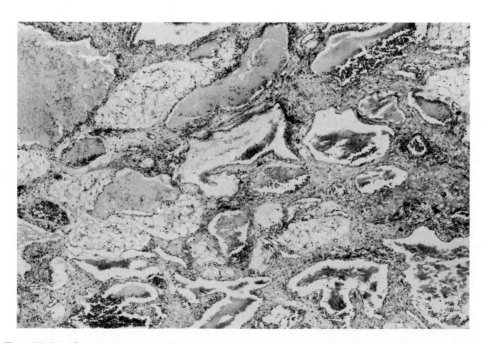

Fig. 17-41. Cystic hygroma (lymphangioma) is composed of large spaces filled with lymph and scattered collections of lymphocytes. This lesion is from neck of child.

REFERENCES
Normal structure and age changes; arteriosclerosis

1. Castleman, B., and Smithwick, R.H.: The relation of vascular disease to the hypertensive state II: the adequacy of renal biopsy as determined from a study of 500 patients, N. Engl. J. Med. **239:**729, 1948.
2. Clark, J.M., and Glagov, S.: Transmural organization of the arterial media: the lamellar unit revisited, Arteriosclerosis **5:**19, 1985.
3. Gamble, C.N.: The pathogenesis of hyaline arteriolosclerosis, Am. J. Pathol. **122:**410, 1986.
4. Haust, M.D.: Atherosclerosis in childhood. In Rosenberg, H.S., and Bolande, R.P., editors: Perspectives in pediatric pathology, vol. 4, Chicago, 1978, Year Book Medical Publishers.
5. Mönckeberg, J.G.: Über die reine Mediaverkalkung der Extremitätenarterien und ihr Verhalten zur Arteriosklerose, Virchows Arch. [Pathol. Anat.] **171:**141, 1903.
6. Moran, J.J.: Idiopathic arterial calcification of infancy: a clinicopathologic study, Pathol. Annu. **10:**393, 1975.
7. Neufeld, H.N., and Blieden, L.C.: Pediatric atherosclerosis: genetic aspects. In Strong, W.B., editor: Atherosclerosis: its pediatric aspects, New York, 1978, Grune & Stratton, Inc.
8. Rao, R.N., Hilliard, K., and Wray, C.H.: Widespread intimal hyperplasia of small arteries and arterioles, Arch. Pathol. Lab. Med. **107:**254, 1983.
9. Ross, R., Glomset, J., Kariya, B., Raines, E., and De Jong, J.B.: Cells of the artery wall and atherosclerosis. In Brinkley, B.R., and Porter, K.R., editors: International cell biology, 1976-1977, New York, 1977, Rockefeller University Press.
10. Sinclair, R.A., Antonovych, T.T., and Mostofi, F.K.: Renal proliferative arteriopathies and associated glomerular changes: a light and electron microscopic study, Hum. Pathol. **7:**565, 1976.

Atherosclerosis

11. Benditt, E.P.: The monoclonal theory of atherogenesis. In Paoletti, R., and Gotto, A.M., Jr., editors: Atherosclerosis reviews, vol. 3, New York, 1978, Raven Press.
12. Bierman, E.L., and Albers, J.J.: Lipoprotein uptake by cultured human arterial smooth muscle cells, Biochim. Biophys. Acta **388:**198, 1975.
13. Bocan, T.M.A., Schifani, T.A., and Guyton, J.R.: Ultrastructure of the human aortic fibrolipid lesion: formation of the atherosclerotic lipid-rich core, Am. J. Pathol. **123:**413, 1986.
14. Brown, M.S., and Goldstein, J.L.: Lipoprotein metabolism in the macrophage: implications for cholesterol deposition in atherosclerosis, Annu. Rev. Biochem. **52:**223, 1983.
15. Cotran, R.S.: New roles for the endothelium in inflammation and immunity, Am. J. Pathol. **129:**407, 1987.
16. Cunningham, M.J., and Pasternak, R.C.: The potential role of viruses in the pathogenesis of atherosclerosis, Circulation **77:**964, 1988.
17. Daoud, A.S., Jarmolych, J., Augustyn, J.M., Fritz, K.E., Singh, J.K., and Lee, K.T.: Regression of advanced atherosclerosis in swine, Arch. Pathol. Lab. Med. **100:**372, 1976.
18. Dawber, T.R.: The Framingham study: the epidemiology of atherosclerotic disease, Cambridge, Mass., 1980, Harvard University Press.
19. Fuster, V., Fass, D.N., and Bowie, E.J.W.: Resistance to atherosclerosis in pigs with genetic and therapeutic inhibition of platelet function, Thromb. Haemost. **42:**270, 1979.
20. Geer, J.C., and Haust, M.D.: Smooth muscle cells in atherosclerosis: monograph on atherosclerosis, vol. 2, Basel, 1972, S. Karger AG.
21. Gerrity, R.G.: The role of monocyte in atherogenesis. I. Transition of blood-borne monocytes into foam cells in fatty lesions, Am. J. Pathol. **103:**181, 1981.
22. Gimbrone, M.A., Jr.: Endothelial dysfunction and the pathogenesis of atherosclerosis. In Gotto, A.M., Jr., Smith, L.C., and Allen, B., editors: Atherosclerosis V, Proceedings of the Vth International Symposium, New York, 1980, Springer-Verlag N.Y., Inc.
23. Goldstein, J.L., and Brown, M.S.: The low density lipoprotein pathway and its relationship to atherosclerosis, Annu. Rev. Biochem. **46:**897, 1977.
24. Gotto, A.M., Jr.: Status report: plasma lipids, lipoproteins, and coronary artery disease. In Paoletti, R., and Gotto, A.M., Jr., editors: Atherosclerosis reviews, vol. 4, New York, 1979, Raven Press.
25. Gotto, A.M., Jr., Foreyt, J.P., and Scott, L.W.: Hyperlipidemia and nutrition: ongoing work. In Hegyeli, R., editor: Atherosclerosis reviews, vol. 7, New York, 1980, Raven Press.
26. Grotendorst, G.R., Chang, T., Seppä, H.E., Kleinman, H.K., and Martin, G.R.: Platelet-derived growth factor is a chemoattractant for vascular smooth muscle cells, J. Cell. Physiol. **113:**261, 1982.
27. Haust, M.D., More, R.H., and Movat, H.Z.: The role of smooth muscle cells in the fibrogenesis of arteriosclerosis, Am. J. Pathol. **37:**377, 1960.
28. Haust, M.D.: Light and electron microscopy of human atherosclerotic lesions, Adv. Exp. Med. Biol. **104:**33, 1978.
29. Kannel, W.B., and Thom, T.J.: Declining cardiovascular mortality, Circulation **70:**331, 1984.
30. Leaf, A., and Weber, P.C.: Cardiovascular effect of n-3 fatty acids, N. Engl. J. Med. **318:**549, 1988.
31. Majno, G., Joris, I., and Zand, T.: Atherosclerosis: new horizon, Hum. Pathol. **16:**3, 1985.
32. McGill, H.C., Jr.: Fatty streaks in the coronary arteries and aorta, Lab. Invest. **18:**560, 1968.
33. McGill, H.C., Jr.: Introduction to the geographic pathology of atherosclerosis, Lab. Invest. **18:**465, 1968.
34. McGill, H.C., Jr., Geer, J.C., and Strong, J.P.: Natural history of human atherosclerotic lesions. In Sandler, M., and Bourne, G.H., editors: Atherosclerosis and its origin, New York, 1963, Academic Press, Inc.
35. McGill, H.C., Jr., and Stern, M.P.: Sex and atherosclerosis. In Paoletti, R., and Gotto, A.M., Jr., editors: Atherosclerosis reviews, vol. 2, New York, 1977, Raven Press.
36. Mitchell, J.R.A.: Prostaglandins in vascular disease: a seminal approach, Br. Med. J. **282:**590, 1981.
37. Munro, J.M., and Cotran, R.S.: Biology of diseases: the pathogenesis of atherosclerosis: atherogenesis and inflammation, Lab. Invest. **58:**249, 1988.
38. National Heart and Lung Institute: Task force on genetic factors in atherosclerotic disease, DHEW Publication no. (NHH) 76-922, Washington, D.C., 1976, U.S. DHEW, Public Health Service.
39. Oalmann, M.C., Malcom, G.T., Toca, V.T., Guzman, M.A., and Strong, J.P.: Community pathology of atherosclerosis and coronary heart disease: post-mortem serum cholesterol and extent of coronary atherosclerosis. Am. J. Epidemiol. **113:**396, 1981.
40. Pearson, T.A., Dillman, J.M., Solez, K., and Heptinstall, R.H.: Evidence for two populations of fatty streaks with different roles in the atherogenic process, Lancet **2:**496, 1980.
41. Pearson, T.A., Dillman, J., Williams, K.J., Wolff, J.A., Adams, R., Solez, K., Heptinstall, R.H., Malmros, H., and Sternby, N.: Clonal characteristics of cutaneous scars and implications for atherogenesis, Am. J. Pathol. **102:**49, 1981.
42. Ross, R.: Atherosclerosis: a problem of the biology of arterial wall cells and their interactions with blood components, Arteriosclerosis **1:**293, 1981.
43. Ross, R.: The pathogenesis of atherosclerosis—an update, N. Engl. J. Med. **314:**488, 1986.
44. Ross, R., and Klebanoff, S.J.: The smooth muscle cell. I. In vivo synthesis of connective tissue proteins, J. Cell Biol. **50:**159, 1971.
45. Schettler, G., Nüssel, E., and Buchholz, L.: Epidemiological research in Western Europe. In Paoletti, R., and Gotto, A.M., Jr., editors: Atherosclerosis reviews, vol. 3, New York, 1978, Raven Press.
46. Schwartz, S.M., Reedy, M.R., and Clowes, A.: Kinetics of atherosclerosis: a stem cell model, Ann. NY Acad. Sci. **454:**292, 1985.

47. Schwartz, C.J., Valente, A.J., Sprague, E.A., Kelley, J.L., Suenram, C.A., Graves, D.T., Rozek, M.M., Edwards, E.H., and Delgado, R.: Monocyte-macrophage participation in atherogenesis: inflammatory components of pathogenesis, Semin. Thromb. Hemost. **12:**79, 1986.
48. Smith, E.B.: The relationship between plasma and tissue lipids in human atherosclerosis, Adv. Lipid Res. **12:**1, 1974.
49. Stamler, J.: Lifestyles, major risk factors, proof and public policy, Circulation **58:**3, 1978.
50. Steinberg, D.: Lipoproteins and atherosclerosis: a look back and a look ahead, Arteriosclerosis **3:**283, 1983.
51. Strong, J.P., Restrepo, C., and Guzman, M.: Coronary and aortic atherosclerosis in New Orleans. II. Comparison of lesions by age, sex, and race, Lab. Invest. **39:**364, 1978.
52. Strong, J.P., and Richards, M.L.: Cigarette smoking and atherosclerosis in autopsied men, Atherosclerosis **23:**451, 1976.
53. Titus, J.L., and Weilbaecher, D.G.: Smooth muscle cells in atherosclerosis. In Gotto, A.M., Jr., Smith, L.C., and Allen, B., editors: Atherosclerosis V, Proceedings of the Vth International Symposium. New York, 1979, Springer-Verlag N.Y., Inc.
54. Watanabe, Y.: Serial inbreeding of rabbits with hereditary hyperlipemia (WHHL-rabbit): incidence and development of atherosclerosis and xanthoma, Atherosclerosis **36:**261, 1980.
55. Wissler, R.W.: Principles of the pathogenesis of atherosclerosis. In Braunwald, E., editor: Heart disease: a textbook of cardiovascular medicine, Philadelphia, 1984, W.B. Saunders Co.
56. Zilversmit, D.B.: Atherogenesis: a postprandial phenomenon, Circulation **60:**473, 1979.

Arteritis

57. Adar, R., Papa, M.Z., Halpern, Z., Mozes, M., Shoshan, S., Sofer, B., Zinger, H., Dayan, M., and Mozes, E.: Cellular sensitivity to collagen in thromboangiitis obliterans, N. Engl. J. Med. **308:**1113, 1983.
58. Amano, S., Hazama, F., Kubagawa, H., Tasaka, K., Haebara, H., and Hamashima, Y.: General pathology of Kawasaki disease: on the morphological alterations corresponding to the clinical manifestations, Acta Pathol. Jpn. **30:**681, 1980.
59. Arkin, A.: A clinical and pathological study of periarteritis nodosa: a report of five cases, one histologically healed, Am. J. Pathol. **6:**401, 1930.
60. Baggenstoss, A.H., and Titus, J.L.: Rheumatic and collagen disorders of the heart. In Gould, S.E., editor: Pathology of the heart and blood vessels, ed. 3, Springfield, Ill., 1968, Charles C Thomas, Publisher.
61. Bengtsson, B.Å., and Malmvall, B.-E.: Giant cell arteritis, Acta Med. Scand., suppl. **658:**1, 1982.
62. Bonnetblanc, J.M., Adenis, J.P., Queroi, M., and Rammaert, B.: Immunofluorescence in temporal arteritis, N. Engl. J. Med. **298:**458, 1978.
63. Buerger, L.: Thrombo-angiitis obliterans: a study of the vascular lesions leading to presenile spontaneous gangrene, Am. J. Med. Sci. **136:**567, 1908.
64. Bulkley, B.H., and Roberts, W.C.: Ankylosing spondylitis and aortic regurgitation: description of the characteristic cardiovascular lesion from study of eight necropsy patients, Circulation **48:**1014, 1973.
65. Burch, G.E., Harb, J.M., and Sun, C.S.: Fine structure of digital vascular lesions in Raynaud's phenomenon and disease, Angiology **30:**361, 1979.
66. Carrington, C.B., and Liebow, A.A.: Limited forms of angiitis and granulomatosis of Wegener's type, Am. J. Med. **41:**497, 1966.
67. Chumbley, L.C., Harrison, E.G., and DeRemee, R.A.: Allergic granulomatosis and angiitis (Churg-Strauss syndrome): report and analysis of 30 cases, Mayo Clin. Proc. **52:**477, 1977.
68. Churg, J., and Strauss, L.: Allergic granulomatosis, allergic angiitis, and periarteritis nodosa, Am. J. Pathol. **27:**277, 1951.
69. Cipriano, P.R., Alonso, D.R., Baltaxe, H.A., Gay, W.A., and Smith, J.P.: Multiple aortic aneurysm in relapsing polychondritis, Am. J. Cardiol. **37:**1097, 1976.

70. Cupps, T.R., and Fauci, A.S.: The vasculitides, Philadelphia, 1981, W.B. Saunders Co.
71. DeRemee, R.A., McDonald, T.J., Harrison, E.G., Jr., and Coles, D.T.: Wegener's granulomatosis: anatomic correlates, a proposed classification, Mayo Clin. Proc. **51:**777, 1976.
72. Ettlinger, R.E., Hunder, G.G., and Ward, L.E.: Polymyalgia rheumatica and giant cell arteritis, Annu. Rev. Med. **29:**15, 1978.
73. Fan, P.T., Davis, J.A., Somer, T., Kaplan, L., and Bluestone, R.: A clinical approach to systemic vasculitis, Semin. Arthritis Rheum. **9:**248, 1980.
74. Fauci, A.S., Haynes, B.F., Katz, P., and Wolff, S.M.: Wegener's granulomatosis: prospective clinical and therapeutic experience with 85 patients for 21 years, Ann. Intern. Med. **98:**76, 1983.
75. Fehér, J., Horváth, M., Fehér, E., Szondy, E., Onody, K., and Gerö, S.: Changes induced by vascular antigens in the aorta of guinea-pigs: immunological and morphological studies, Br. J. Exp. Pathol. **59:**237, 1978.
76. Gallagher, P., and Jones, K.: Immunohistochemical findings in cranial arteritis, Arthritis Rheum. **25:**75, 1982.
77. Hall, S., Persellin, S., Lie, J.T., O'Brien, P.C., Kurland, L.T., and Hunder, G.G.: The therapeutic impact of temporal artery biopsy, Lancet **2:**1217, 1983.
78. Juergens, J.L.: Thromboangiitis obliterans (Buerger's disease, TAO). In Juergens, J.L., Spittell, J.A., Jr., and Fairbairn, J.F., II, editors: Allen-Barker-Hines peripheral vascular diseases, ed. 5, Philadelphia, 1980, W.B. Saunders Co.
79. Koss, M.N., Antonovych, T., and Hochholzer, L.: Allergic granulomatosis (Churg-Strauss syndrome): pulmonary and renal morphologic findings, Am. J. Surg. Pathol. **5:**21, 1981.
80. Kussmaul, A., and Maier, R.: Über eine bisher nicht beschriebene eigentümliche Arterienerkrankung (periarteritis nodosa), die mit Morbus Brightii und rapid fortschreitender allgemeiner Muskellähmung einhergeht, Dtsch. Arch. Klin. Med. **1:**484, 1866.
81. Kyle, V., and Hazelman, B.L.: Polymyalgia rheumatica/giant cell arteritis, Clin. Exp. Rheumatol. **1:**171, 1983.
82. Lande, A., Berkmen, Y.M., and McAllister, H.A., Jr., editors: Aortitis: clinical, pathologic, and radiologic aspects, New York, 1985, Raven Press.
83. Landing, B.H., and Larson, E.J.: Are infantile periarteritis nodosa with coronary involvement and fatal mucocutaneous lymph node syndrome the same? Comparison of 20 patients from North America with patients from Hawaii and Japan, Pediatrics **59:**651, 1977.
84. Lanham, J.G., Elkon, K.B., Pusey, C.D., and Hughes, G.R.: Systemic vasculitis with asthma and eosinophilia: a clinical approach to the Churg-Strauss syndrome, Medicine **63:**65, 1984.
85. Lie, J.T.: Thromboangiitis obliterans (Buerger's disease) in women, Medicine **66:**65, 1987.
86. Lie, J.T.: The classification and diagnosis of vasculitis in large and medium-sized blood vessels, Pathol. Annu. **22**(1):125, 1987.
87. Lupi-Herrera, E., Sanchez-Torres, G., Marcushamer, J., Mispireta, J., Horwitz, S., and Vela, J.E.: Takayasu's arteritis: clinical study of 107 cases, Am. Heart J. **93:**94, 1977.
88. Mambo, N.C.: Temporal (granulomatous) arteritis: a histopathological study of 32 cases, Histopathology **3:**209, 1979.
89. McCluskey, R.T., and Fienberg, R.: Vasculitis in primary vasculitides, granulomatoses, and connective tissue disease, Hum. Pathol. **14:**305, 1983.
90. Melish, M.E.: Kawasaki syndrome (the mucocutaneous lymph node syndrome), Annu. Rev. Med. **33:**569, 1982.
91. Michalak, T.: Immune complexes of hepatitis B surface antigen in the pathogenesis of periarteritis nodosa, Am. J. Pathol. **90:**619, 1978.
92. Morgan, S.H., Asherson, R.A., and Hughes, G.R.V.: Distal aortitis complicating Reiter's syndrome, Br. Heart J. **52:**115, 1984.
93. Nakao, K., Ikeda, M., Kimata, S., Niitani, H., Miyahara, M., Ishimi, Z., Hashiba, K., Takeda, Y., Ozawa, T., Matsushita, S.,

and Kuramochi, M.: Takayasu's arteritis: clinical report of eighty-four cases and immunological studies of seven cases, Circulation **35**:1141, 1967.

94. Paulus, H.E., Pearson, C.M., and Pitts, W., Jr.: Aortic insufficiency in five patients with Reiter's syndrome: a detailed clinical and pathologic study, Am. J. Med. **53**:464, 1972.

95. Rose, A.G., and Sinclair-Smith, C.C.: Takayasu's arteritis: a study of 16 autopsy cases, Arch. Pathol. Lab. Med. **104**:231, 1980.

96. Schiavone, W.A., Ahmad, M., and Ockner, S.A.: Unusual cardiac complications of Wegener's granulomatosis, Chest **88**:745, 1985.

97. Spittell, J.A., Jr.: Raynaud's phenomenon and allied vasospastic diseases. In Juergens, J.L., Spittell, J.A., Jr., and Fairbairn, J.F., II, editors: Allen-Barker-Hines peripheral vascular diseases, ed. 5, Philadelphia, 1980, W.B. Saunders Co.

98. Wolff, S.M., Fauci, A.S., Horn, R.G., and Dale, D.C.: Wegener's granulomatosis, Ann. Intern. Med. **81**:513, 1974.

99. Yanagihara, R., and Todd, J.K.: Acute febrile mucocutaneous lymph node syndrome, Am. J. Dis. Child. **134**:603, 1980.

Aneurysms; arteriopathy

100. Burchell, H.B.: Aortic dissection (dissecting hematoma: dissecting aneurysm of the aorta), Circulation **12**:1068, 1955.

101. Cagle, P.T., Kim, H.-S., and Titus, J.L.: Congenital stenotic arteriopathy with medial dysplasia, Hum. Pathol. **16**:528, 1985.

102. Carlson, R.G., Lillehei, C.W., and Edwards, J.E.: Cystic medial necrosis of the ascending aorta in relation to age and hypertension, Am. J. Cardiol. **25**:411, 1970.

103. Crawford, E.S., Walker, H.S., III, Saleh, S.A., and Normann, N.A.: Graft replacement of aneurysm in descending thoracic aorta: results without bypass or shunting, Surgery **89**:73, 1981.

104. Crawford, E.S., Saleh, S.A., Babb, J.W., III, Glaeser, D.H., Vaccaro, P.S., and Silvers, A.: Infrarenal abdominal aortic aneurysm: factors influencing survival after operation performed over 25-year period, Ann. Surg. **193**:699, 1981.

105. Daily, P.O., Trueblood, H.W., Stinson, E.B., Wuerflein, R.D., and Shumway, N.E.: Management of acute aortic dissections, Ann. Thorac. Surg. **10**:237, 1970.

106. DeBakey, M.E., and Noon, G.P.: Aneurysms of the sinuses of Valsalva. In Sabiston, D.C., and Spencer, F.C., editors: Gibbon's surgery of the chest, ed. 4, Philadelphia, 1983, W.B. Saunders Co.

107. DeBakey, M.E., Henly, W.S., Cooley, D.A., Morris, G.C., Jr., Crawford, E.S., and Beall, A.C., Jr.: Surgical management of dissecting aneurysms of the aorta, J. Thorac. Cardiovasc. Surg. **49**:130, 1965.

108. DeSanctis, R.W., Doroghazi, R.M., Austen, W.G., and Buckley, M.J.: Aortic dissection, N. Engl. J. Med. **317**:1060, 1987.

109. Edwards, W.D., Leaf, D.S., and Edwards, J.E.: Dissecting aortic aneurysm associated with congenital bicuspid aortic valve, Circulation **57**:1022, 1978.

110. Erdheim, J.: Medionecrosis aortae idiopathica cystica, Virchows Arch. [Pathol. Anat.] **276**:187, 1930.

111. Feiner, H.D., Raghavendra, B.N., Phelps, R., and Rooney, L.: Inflammatory abdominal aortic aneurysm: report of six cases, Hum. Pathol. **15**:454, 1984.

112. Flanigan, D.P., Burnham, S.J., Goodreau, J.J., and Bergan, J.J.: Summary of cases of adventitial cystic disease of the popliteal artery, Ann. Surg. **189**:165, 1979.

113. Harrison, E.G., and McCormack, L.J.: Pathologic classification of renal arterial disease in renovascular hypertension, Mayo Clin. Proc. **46**:161, 1971.

114. Hirst, A.E., and Gore, I.: The etiology and pathology of aortic dissection. In Doroghazi, R.M., and Slater, E.E., editors: Aortic dissection, New York, 1983, McGraw-Hill Book Co.

115. Klima, T., Spjut, H.J., Coelho, A., Gray, A.G., Wukasch, D.C., Reul, G.J., Jr., and Cooley, D.A.: The morphology of ascending aortic aneurysms, Hum. Pathol. **14**:810, 1983.

116. Larson, E.W., and Edwards, W.D.: Risk factors for aortic dissection: a necropsy study of 161 cases, Am. J. Cardiol. **53**:849, 1984.

117. Lie, J.T.: Coronary vasculitis: review in the current scheme of classification of vasculitis, Arch. Pathol. Lab. Med. **111**:224, 1987.

118. Luscher, T.F., Lie, J.T., Stanson, A.W., Houser, O.W., Hollier, L.H., and Shep, S.G.: Arterial fibromuscular dysplasia, Mayo Clin. Proc. **62**:931, 1987.

119. Mandel, W., Evans, E.W., and Walford, R.L.: Dissecting aortic aneurysm during pregnancy, N. Engl. J. Med. **251**:1059, 1954.

120. Murray, C.A., and Edwards, J.E.: Spontaneous laceration of ascending aorta, Circulation **47**:848, 1973.

121. Norwood, W.I., and Aretz, T.H.: Case records of the Massachusetts General Hospital (Case 35-1980), N. Engl. J. Med. **303**:571, 1980.

122. Pennell, R.C., Hollier, L.H., Lie, J.T., Bernatz, P.E., Joyce, J.W., Pairolero, P.C., Cherry, K.J., and Hallett, J.W.: Inflammatory abdominal aortic aneurysms: a thirty-year review, J. Vasc. Surg. **2**:859, 1985.

123. Roberts, W.C.: Aortic dissection: anatomy, consequences, and causes, Am. Heart J. **101**:195, 1981.

124. Rose, A.G., and Dent, D.M.: Inflammatory variant of abdominal atherosclerotic aneurysm, Arch. Pathol. Lab. Med. **105**:409, 1981.

125. Schlatmann, T.J.M., and Becker, A.E.: Histologic changes in the normal aging aorta: implication for dissection aortic aneurysm, Am. J. Cardiol. **39**:13, 1977.

126. Schlatmann, T.J.M., and Becker, A.E.: Pathogenesis of dissecting aneurysm of aorta, Am. J. Cardiol. **39**:21, 1977.

127. Sinclair, R.J.G., Kitchen, A.H., and Turner, R.W.D.: The Marfan syndrome, Q. J. Med. **29**:19, 1960.

128. Sommerville, R.L., Allen, E.V., and Edwards, J.E.: Bland and infected arteriosclerotic abdominal aortic aneurysms, Medicine **38**:207, 1959.

129. Spittell, J.A., Jr., and Wallace, R.B.: Aneurysms. In Juergens, J.L., Spittell, J.A., Jr., and Fairbairn, J.F., II, editors: Allen-Barker-Hines peripheral vascular disease, Philadelphia, 1980, W.B. Saunders Co.

130. Stanley, J.C., Gewertz, B.L., Bove, E.L., Sottiurai, V., and Fry, W.J.: Arterial fibrodysplasia: histopathologic character and current etiologic concepts, Arch. Surg. **110**:561, 1975.

131. Strauss, R.G., and McAdams, A.J.: Dissecting aneurysm in childhood, J. Pediatr. **76**:578, 1970.

132. Titus, J.L., Kim, H.-S., and Weilbaecher, D.G.: Surgical pathology of aortic diseases. In Cowgill, L.D., editor: Cardiac surgery: surgery of the aorta, Philadelphia, 1987, Hanley & Belfus, Inc.

133. Wheat, M.W., Jr., Harris P.D., Malm, J.R., Kaiser, G., Bowman, F.O., Jr., and Palmer, R.F.: Acute dissecting aneurysms of the aorta, J. Thorac. Cardiovasc. Surg. **58**:344, 1969.

134. Wilson, S.K., and Hutchins, G.M.: Aortic dissecting aneurysms, Arch. Pathol. Lab. Med. **106**:175, 1982.

Veins

135. Haimovici, H.: Ischemic forms of venous thrombosis: phlegmasia cerulea dolens and venous gangrene, Heart Bull. **16**:101, 1967.

136. Hirsh, J., Hull, R.D., and Raskob, G.E.: Epidemiology and pathogenesis of venous thrombosis, J. Am. Coll. Cardiol. **8**(6 suppl. B):104B, 1986.

137. Lie, J.T., Lawrie, G.M., and Morris, G.C., Jr.: Aortocoronary bypass saphenous vein graft atherosclerosis: anatomic study of 99 vein grafts from normal and hyperlipoproteinemic patients up to 75 months postoperatively, Am. J. Cardiol. **40**:906, 1977.

138. Mitchell, M.C., Boitnott, J.K., Kaufman, S., Cameron, J.L., and Maddrey, W.C.: Budd-Chiari syndrome: etiology, diagnosis and management, Medicine **61**:199, 1982.

139. Parish, J.M., Marschke, R.F., Jr., Dines, D.E., and Lee, R.E.: Etiologic considerations in superior vena cava syndrome, Mayo Clin. Proc. **56**:407, 1981.

140. Rector, W.G., Xu, Y.H., Goldstein, L., Peters, R.L., and Reynolds, T.B.: Membranous obstruction of the inferior vena cava in the United States, Medicine **64**:134, 1985.

141. Smith, S.H., and Geer, J.C.: Morphology of saphenous vein-

coronary artery bypass grafts: seven to 116 months after surgery, Arch. Pathol. Lab. Med. **107**:13, 1983.

142. Strandness, D.E., Jr., and Thiele, B.L.: Selected topics in venous disorders: pathology, diagnosis and treatment, New York, 1981, Futura Publishing.

143. Titus, J.L.: The heart after surgery for ischemic heart disease, Am. J. Cardiovasc. Pathol. **1**:339, 1988.

144. Unni, K.K., Kottke, B.A., Titus, J.L., Frye, R.L., Wallace, R.B., and Brown, A.L.: Pathologic changes in aortocoronary saphenous vein grafts, Am. J. Cardiol. **34**:526, 1974.

145. Webb, L.J., and Sherlock, S.: The aetiology, presentation and natural history of extrahepatic portal venous obstruction, Q. J. Med. **48**:627, 1979.

Lymphatics

146. Alvin, A., Diehl, J., Lindsten, J., and Lodin, A.: Lymph vessel hypoplasia and chromosome aberrations in six patients with Turner's syndrome, Acta Derm. Venereol. (Stock.) **47**:25, 1967.

147. Kinmonth, J.B.: The lymphatics: diseases, lymphography and surgery, Baltimore, 1972, The Williams & Wilkins Co.

148. Schirger, A., Harrison, E.G., Jr., and Janes, J.M.: Idiopathic lymphedema: review of 131 cases, JAMA **182**:14, 1962.

149. Schirger, A., and Peterson, L.F.A.: Lymphedema. In Juergens, J.L., Spittell, J.A., Jr., and Fairbairn, J.F., II, editors: Allen-Barker-Hines peripheral vascular diseases, Philadelphia, 1980, W.B. Saunders Co.

Tumors and tumorlike conditions

150. Alexander, G.L., and Norman, R.W.: The Sturge-Weber syndrome, Baltimore, 1960, The Williams & Wilkins Co.

151. Allen, P.W., and Enzinger, F.M.: Hemangioma of skeletal muscle, Cancer **29**:8, 1972.

152. Baskerville, P.A., Ackroyd, J.S., and Browse, N.L.: The etiology of the Klippel-Trenaunay syndrome, Ann. Surg. **202**:624, 1985.

153. Bean, W.B.: Dyschondroplasia and hemangiomata (Maffucci's syndrome). II., Arch. Intern. Med. **102**:544, 1958.

154. Bean, W.B.: Vascular spiders and related lesions of the skin, Springfield, Ill., 1958, Charles C Thomas, Publisher.

155. Bhagavan, B.S., Dorfman, H.D., Murthy, M.S., and Eggleston, J.C.: Intravascular bronchiolo-alveolar tumor (IVBAT): a low-grade sclerosing epithelioid angiosarcoma of lung, Am. J. Surg. Pathol. **6**:41, 1982.

156. Burbank, M.K., and Spittell, J.A., Jr.: Tumors of blood and lymph vessels. In Juergens, J.L., Spittell, J.A., Jr., and Fairbairn, J.F., II, editors: Allen-Barker-Hines peripheral vascular diseases, Philadelphia, 1980, W.B. Saunders Co.

157. Chung, E.B.: Pitfalls in diagnosing benign soft tissue tumors in infancy and childhood, Pathol. Annu. **20**(2):323, 1985.

158. Clearkin, K.P., and Enzinger, F.M.: Intravascular papillary endothelial hyperplasia, Arch. Pathol. Lab. Med. **100**:441, 1976.

159. Dehner, L.P., and Ishak, K.G.: Vascular tumors of the liver in infants and children: a study of 30 cases and review of the literature, Arch. Pathol. **92**:101, 1971.

160. Enzinger, F.M., and Smith, B.H.: Hemangiopericytoma: an analysis of 106 cases, Hum. Pathol. **7**:61, 1976.

161. Enzinger, F.M., and Weiss, S.W.: Soft tissue tumors, St. Louis, 1983, The C.V. Mosby Co.

162. Hajdu, S.I.: Pathology of soft tissue tumors, Philadelphia, 1979, Lea & Febiger.

163. Hodgson, C.H., and Kaye, R.L.: Pulmonary arteriovenous fistula and hereditary hemorrhagic telangiectasia: a review and report of 35 cases of fistula, Dis. Chest **43**:449, 1963.

164. Horton, W.A., Wong, V., and Eldridge, R.: Von Hippel-Lindau disease: clinical and pathological manifestations in nine families with 50 affected members, Arch. Intern. Med. **136**:769, 1976.

165. Ishak, K.G., Sesterhenn, I.A., Goodman, Z.D., Rabin, L., and Stromeyer, F.W.: Epithelioid hemangioendothelioma of the liver: a clinicopathologic and follow-up study of 32 cases, Hum. Pathol. **15**:839, 1984.

166. McAlister, H.A., Jr., and Fenoglio, J.J.: Tumors of the cardiovascular system: atlas of tumor pathology, second series, fascicle 15, Washington, D.C., 1978, Armed Forces Institute of Pathology.

167. McCarty, K.S., Mossler, J.A., McLelland, R., and Sieker, H.O.: Pulmonary lymphangiomyomatosis responsive to progesterone, N. Engl. J. Med. **303**:1461, 1980.

168. McNutt, N.S., Fletcher, V., and Conant, M.A.: Early lesions of Kaposi's sarcoma in homosexual men: an ultrastructural comparison with other vascular proliferations in skin, Am. J. Pathol. **111**:62, 1983.

169. Morris, S.J., Kaplan, S.R., Ballan, K., and Tedesco, F.J.: Blue rubber-bleb nevus syndrome, JAMA **239**:1887, 1978.

170. Pollanen, M., Butany, J., and Chiasson, D.: Leiomyosarcoma of the inferior vena cava, Arch. Pathol. Lab. Med. **111**:1085, 1987.

171. Popper, H., Thomas, L.B., Telles, N.C., Falk, H., and Selikoff, I.J.: Development of hepatic angiosarcoma in man induced by vinyl chloride, Thorotrast, and arsenic: comparison with cases of unknown etiology, Am. J. Pathol. **92**:349, 1978.

172. Rosai, J.: Ackerman's surgical pathology, ed. 6, St. Louis, 1981, The C.V. Mosby Co.

173. Templeton, A.C.: Kaposi's sarcoma, Pathol. Annu. **16**(pt. 2):315, 1981.

174. Venkatachalam, M.A., and Greally, J.G.: Fine structure of glomus tumor: similarity of glomus cells to smooth muscle, Cancer **23**:1176, 1969.

175. Waisman, M.: Common hemangiomas: to treat or not to treat, Postgrad. Med. **43**:183, 1968.

176. Waldo, E.D., Vuletin, J.C., and Kaye, G.I.: The ultrastructure of vascular tumors: additional observations and review of the literature, Pathol. Annu. **12**(2):279, 1977.

177. Wolff, M.: Lymphangiomyoma: clinicopathologic study and ultrastructural confirmation of its histogenesis, Cancer **31**:988, 1973.

178. Ziegler, J.L., Templeton, A.C., and Vogel, C.L.: Kaposi's sarcoma: a comparison of classical, endemic, and epidemic forms, Semin. Oncol. **11**:47, 1984.

18 The Urinary System

GEORGE F. SCHREINER
JOHN M. KISSANE

The Kidneys

STRUCTURE AND FUNCTION

The function of the kidney is to filter the plasma, selectively reabsorb solutes and water in order to maintain internal homeostasis, and secrete metabolic waste products and toxins. The form of the kidney subserves these functions with an intricate structure of vascular beds, epithelial tubules, and interstitial elements. These interdigitate in a complex, as yet incompletely understood manner to maintain the internal milieu within a narrow, precisely regulated concentration range of acids, salts, and other solutes. In addition to internal regulatory mechanisms that serve to modulate intrarenal blood flow, urine production, and epithelial reabsorption and secretion, the kidney is responsive to a host of regulatory influences, hormonal and neuronal, that permit it to respond to the metabolic needs of the entire organism. As the principal filtering unit of the body, the kidney is particularly susceptible to immunologic injury as a result of the deposition of immune complexes or its processing of immunogenic antigens. As the recipient of one fourth of the cardiac output, it is also very susceptible to vascular injury, particularly that which relates to extremes of perfusion pressures. In common with other organs, the kidney is subject to congenital, metabolic, and traumatic diseases. As a result of the heterogeneous anatomy of the kidney, there is a differential sensitivity of subregions of the kidney to various disease processes. The resulting abnormalities in renal function will thus uniquely reflect the region of kidney initially affected. Such is the interdependence of the anatomic subregions of the kidney that persistent abnormalities in one segment of the kidney tend to progressively include and distort other components of the kidney. The study of the progression of renal deterioration long after the subsidence of an initial traumatic insult is currently an area of active research.

In order to understand the current classification of renal diseases and the basis of their clinical expressions, a review of the normal structure of the kidney is in order.[60] The basic unit of the kidney is the nephron, which consists of a bed or tuft of permeable capillaries that filter into a spherical capsule that is connected to a tubule with many specialized segments for reabsorption and secretion. The nephron ends by emptying into collecting ducts that bear urine into the renal pelvis and thence to the ureter. Each nephron courses through two distinct regions of the kidney, the cortex and the medulla. The cortex surrounds the medulla and contains the glomeruli and the proximal and distal ends of the tubule. The medulla, nestled within the cortex, contains a looped segment of the tubule that connects the proximal and distal segments. This area of the kidney is dedicated to concentration of the urine by the generation of osmotic gradients.

The kidneys of normal humans each contain about 1¼ million nephrons.[60] The rich vascular network of these nephrons is perfused by roughly one fourth of the cardiac output under basal conditions. The renal arteries branch into interlobar, arcuate, and interlobular arteries. The interlobular arteries course radially from the medulla into the renal cortex, giving off a succession of afferent arterioles. After perfusing the high-pressure glomerular capillaries, the blood recollects into the smaller efferent arterioles. The efferent arterioles in the juxtamedullary region give rise to the vasa recta, which course straight down into the papilla and loop back to collect into veins. The veins of the kidney have thin walls and course with the arteries.

The afferent arteriole enters the glomerular tuft and breaks into about eight branches, each of which, in turn, branches into an anastomosing capillary network. These capillaries are lined by a unique endothelium with specialized holes or fenestrations of about 100 nm in diameter that permit free access of the plasma to the glomerular basement membrane (Fig. 18-1). The basement membrane consists of three layers: an inner subendothelial layer known as the lamina rara interna; a middle, electron-dense layer known as the lamina

In the preparation of this chapter, material has been adapted from Dr. Jones' and Dr. Pugh's chapters in the eighth edition.

densa; and an outer, subepithelial layer known as the lamina rara externa (Fig. 18-2). The glomerular epithelial cell is the principal cell synthesizing the basement membrane though the endothelium also contributes to a certain, ill-defined extent. The basement membrane is composed of several substances. A compact meshwork of type IV collagen is penetrated by a network of filaments and protein particles that form pores that restrict the passage of large-sized serum proteins and cells. The outer layers, the laminae rarae internae and externae, additionally express highly anionic glycosaminoglycans, consisting predominantly of heparan sulfate, sialic acid, and chondroitin sulfate. These negatively charged proteins serve as another important barrier to the filtration of serum proteins, most of which are negatively charged. Disruption of the anatomic integrity of the pores or removal of the anionic layer of basement membranes proteins results in the inappropriate passage of serum proteins into the urine, causing proteinuria. Additional proteins that have been localized in the basement membrane include fibronectin, entactin, and laminin.[19]

The visceral epithelial cells (podocytes) cover the external surface of each glomerular capillary basement membrane with octopus-like processes, known as foot processes, that branch and interdigitate with one another (Fig. 18-3). The foot processes are separated by a filtration slit of 20 to 50 nm in width, but a thin film of plasma membrane connects the foot processes (the filtration-slit membrane)[60] (Fig. 18-1). The barrier to leakage of plasma macromolecules apparently depends on maintenance of the charge barrier of the laminae rarae, a normal lamina densa, and a healthy covering of glomerular epithelial cells.

Where the capillaries adjoin in the central portion of the lobule, the basement membrane thickens and encloses the mesangium (Fig. 18-3). The mesangium is composed of a spongelike meshwork of basement membrane (mesangial matrix) that encloses mesangial cells.[61] The mesangial region provides support to the capillary tufts. Like the trunk of a tree, the mesangium runs in the axis of the glomerulus and connects with the interstitial region around the proximal tubule and the portion of the distal tubule that loops back toward its glomerular origin after rising out of the medulla. The mesangial cells resemble smooth muscle cells and are contractile. The state of their contractility appears to regulate the surface area of the glomerulus available for filtration. Thus the state of activation of the mesangial region is an important determinant of glomerular filtration. In addition, the mesangial cells synthesize the extracellular mesangial matrix. Several diseases are associated with mesangial cell proliferation or synthesis of too much matrix, either of which can ultimately result in occlusion of the glomerulus, rendering it nonfunctional.[54] The mesangial region is particularly susceptible to infiltration by mononuclear leukocytes, which can reside in the mesangium for extended periods of

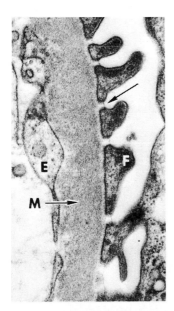

Fig. 18-1. Glomerular capillary wall showing foot processes of podocytes, *F;* filtration slit membrane, *arrow;* basement membrane, *M;* and fenestrated endothelium, *E.* (40,000×.)

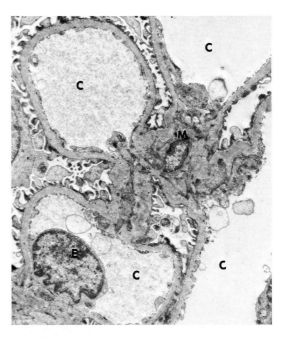

Fig. 18-2. Portion of human glomerulus showing endothelial cell, *E;* mesangial cell, *M;* and capillaries, *C.* Basement membrane is somewhat thickened by hypertension. (3600×.)

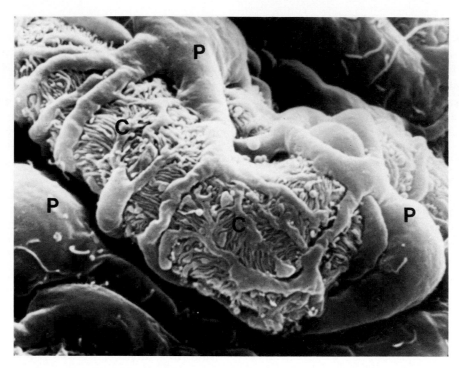

Fig. 18-3. Scanning electron micrograph of normal glomerular capillary, *C*, enclosed by podocytes, *P*, with primary processes and interdigitating foot processes. (5200×.)

time. Both intrinsic mesangial cells and invading mononuclear cells are phagocytic. Deposits within the mesangium of materials such as immune complexes can cause activation of mesangial cells and eventual scarring of the mesangial region.

The glomerular tuft is enclosed by Bowman's capsule, which opens into the proximal tubule. The proximal tubules with their complex cytologic specialization are highly adapted to the resorption of nutrients (amino acids, glucose) and electrolyte transport. Welling and Welling[114] have shown that the brush-border microvilli of the proximal tubules increase the luminal surface area thirtyfold; the complex interdigitations of the basal antiluminal surface increases that area twentyfold. Such a large surface is critical for the resorptive and electrolyte-transporting functions of the epithelium. The proximal tubule leads into the medullary portion of the kidney, forming the loops of Henle. The loops of Henle and the loops of the vasa recta form the anatomic basis for the countercurrent multiplier system whereby a high osmotic gradient is produced in the renal papilla, permitting water resorption and the formation of urine that is hyperosmolar to plasma.

The tubule returns from the medulla toward its glomerulus of origin to form the distal tubule, several of which unite to become the cortical collecting ducts. The distal tubule is responsible for the final adjustments in sodium and water reabsorption and potassium

and hydrogen secretion. This segment of the nephron is particularly sensitive to systemic hormonal regulation of salt and water balance, particularly that mediated by aldosterone and antidiuretic hormone. As the distal tubule returns closest to the glomerulus, a specialized area known as the "macula densa" is found. In the macula densa, the distal tubular cells form a compact plaque of highly specialized cells that are in intimate contact with the juxtaglomerular cells. The cells of the juxtaglomerular apparatus form a collar of granulated and ungranulated cells that replace the smooth muscle cells of the afferent arteriole at the hilum of the glomerulus. Nonmyelinated, sympathetic nerve fibers are found amid these cells. There is much evidence that this region monitors pulse pressure and the sodium content of the distal tubule and is concerned with its control, perhaps through the synthesis of renin.

PRINCIPLES OF RENAL PATHOPHYSIOLOGY

Renal injury can be temporally characterized as either acute or chronic. Each has a distinctive clinical expression.

Acute renal insufficiency

Acute renal insufficiency typically presents with the symptoms of volume overload secondary to impaired urine formation or excretion.[35] The consequent retention of sodium and therefore of water can cause an expansion of the intravascular space and extravasation of fluid into the interstitial spaces throughout the body. The resulting volume expansion can therefore present as peripheral edema, pulmonary edema, or congestive heart failure. The acute inability of the kidney either to excrete or to buffer the endogenous metabolic production of acids results in acute acidemia. This is often accompanied by hyperkalemia resulting from the lack of excretion of dietary potassium, the displacement of intracellular potassium to the extracellular space as a result of acidemia, and the release of endogenous potassium as a result of the breakdown of blood and the heightened catabolism of acute uremia. Both acidemia and hyperkalemia can result in cardiac arrhythmias and sudden death. Acute uremia, the toxic state arising from the failure to eliminate a wide range of metabolic waste products, has a particularly inhibitory effect on platelet function. The resulting tendency to bleed may be manifest as an acute pericarditis or as bloody diarrhea attributable to colitis. There may be a particular tendency toward bleeding from acute ulcers anywhere along the gastrointestinal tract.

Chronic renal failure

In chronic renal failure the metabolic consequences of uremia are slowly progressive in nature, in part because the body has had some time to adapt to the metabolic derangements of impaired renal function.[35,75] Chronic acidosis arises both from an inability to excrete all the metabolic acids that are generated as waste products, including phosphates and sulfates, and from incapacity of the scarred kidney to secrete ammonia to buffer urinary hydrogen and to generate bicarbonate to accompany reabsorbed cations such as sodium. Chronic acidosis can affect myocardial contractility, contribute to central nervous system toxicity, and induce persistent bone reabsorption secondary to the bone serving as a buffer for hydrogen ions. When water and salt intake persistently exceeds excretory capacity, edema formation occurs, typically accumulating in the face, eyelids, and feet. Chronic sodium retention can be manifest as persistent arterial hypertension, which can become more severe with progression of renal insufficiency. The chronically damaged kidney also fails to convert 25-hydroxyvitamin D to the metabolically active 1,25-dihydroxy vitamin D, resulting in the defective absorption of calcium from the intestinal tract. The secondary hypocalcemia induces secondary parathyroid hyperplasia with concomitant demineralization and resorption of bone, known as "osteomalacia." Bone pain and bony deformities may develop, particularly in children, as a result of long-standing chronic renal disease; this process is exacerbated by acidosis.

Chronic renal failure is a multisystem disease. It is associated with central nervous system toxicity, which can manifest as tremor, lethargy, and even convulsions and coma. This can be the result of accumulated uremic poisons, hyperosmolarity, acidosis, and hyponatremia. In addition, peripheral nerve degeneration occurs in uremia, often causing both a sensory and a motor neuropathy that can be disabling. Chronic renal failure is also associated with a tendency toward pericarditis, often fibrinous in nature, a fibrin-rich edema and congestion of the lungs ("uremic pneumonia"), and pancreatitis. Chronic uremia can be associated with gastroenteritis; intestinal obstruction can result from uremic, paralytic ileus.

The anemia of chronic renal failure is often striking and may in fact be the feature bringing the patient to the physician for evaluation. It appears to result from both decreased production of red blood cells and shortened red cell life. Depression of red cell production is the consequence of decreased renal production of the hormone erythropoietin. Recently, recombinant erythropoietin has been highly successful in restoring the hematocrit to normal levels when it is administered to patients on chronic hemodialysis.[27] The effects of impaired production of red cells are exacerbated by the increased red blood cell destruction resulting from uremic toxins as well as the mechanical damage to red cells observed in a variety of glomerular diseases. Finally, patients with chronic renal failure experience had depressed cellular immunity and humoral immunity, making them more susceptible to a variety of bacterial and viral infections that can contribute to the increased mortality observed in this patient population.

THE ANATOMY OF RENAL FAILURE

The causes of renal failure, whether acute or chronic, can be conveniently compartmentalized as prerenal, renal, or postrenal. Prerenal causes of uremia center upon the renal vasculature and its perfusion. Impaired cardiac contractility or severe vasoconstriction of the arteries can result in a decrease or even a cessation of glomerular filtration and urine formation. Persistent poor renal perfusion because of hypovolemia, vasoconstriction, or low cardiac output may result in oliguria and azotemia. Acute pathosis of the renal vasculature includes embolism or thrombosis with subsequent renal infarction. Chronic arteriolar obstruction is seen in arteriolosclerosis, with progressive narrowing and eventual obliteration of arteriolar lumens by hyperplastic or hyaline changes in the vessel walls. Chronic arteriolar obstruction results in a progressive ischemia of the part of the kidney supplied by those vessels. This results in eventual collapse and sclerosis of glomeruli, tubular atrophy, and interstitial fibrosis. When a sufficiently large proportion of nephrons is involved by this process, the glomerular filtration rate falls to critical levels, and renal function fails. This arteriolosclerotic disease of the kidney, nephrosclerosis, may be a primary process and may be a renal manifestation of diffuse atherosclerosis occurring elsewhere in the body. However, obliteration of the renal vascular bed because of primary glomerular or interstitial disease may also result in arteriolosclerotic changes in the renal vasculature as a secondary process. Acute and chronic arteriolar disease is discussed later in this chapter.

Postrenal causes of kidney failure involve occlusion of the urinary tract beyond the distal nephron. Obstruction can occur in the renal pelvis, throughout the course of the ureter, in the bladder, or in the urethra. As is described later, obstruction may be intrinsic and consist in tumors arising anywhere along the genitourinary tract, cysts, clots, or stones. Alternatively, obstruction can be induced by extrinsic compression of the urinary tract by metastatic tumor, vascular structures, abscess, or scarring. Persistent obstruction of the urinary tract results in chronic tubular atrophy and interstitial scarring as a result of persistently elevated pressures within the nephron.

Renal azotemia

Numerous diseases cause renal insufficiency as a result of injury to either glomeruli or tubules. Classification systems for renal disease distinguish between diseases that affect primarily glomeruli and those that affect primarily the tubules and interstitium. Insults to either glomeruli or interstitium are heterogeneous in nature and can involve multiple mechanisms of injury ranging from antibody-mediated lesions to toxins. However, certain generalizations can be made about glomerular and tubular injury. It is useful to summarize these before discussion of specific disease entities.

Glomerular disease

Glomerular diseases are classified by distribution and by intraglomerular localization of either histologic abnormalities or etiologic agents. As adapted from Spargo and co-workers,[103] classification by distribution involves the use of specific terms. Focal glomerular diseases affect some but not all glomeruli, whereas diffuse glomerular diseases affect nearly all glomeruli. Segmental glomerular diseases involve only a portion of a glomerulus, whereas global lesions involve the entire glomerulus. Localization-dependent schemes of classification of glomerular injury may emphasize extraglomerular distribution of histologic changes, as in crescentic glomerulonephritis, or particularly affected glomerular regions. Thus, in mesangioproliferative glomerulonephritis, proliferating cells or immune complexes, or both, are found primarily in the mesangial region. Glomerular pathosis can consist of acute inflammatory lesions,

Table 18-1. Syndromes of glomerular injury

Renal abnormality	Effect
NEPHRITIC SYNDROME	
Decreased glomerular filtration	Oliguria
Sodium retention	Hypertension, edema
Basement membrane trauma	Hematuria
NEPHROTIC SYNDROME	
Excessive urinary loss of:	
Albumin	Decreased plasma oncotic pressure: edema, ascites, hyperlipidemia
Transferrin	Microcytic anemia
Antithrombin III	Thrombosis
Factor B	Impaired opsonization of bacteria
IgG	Increased infections
Lipoprotein lipase	Altered lipoprotein metabolism
Zinc-binding proteins	Dysgeusia, impotence, impaired wound healing

whose clinical expression is the nephritic syndrome as noted in Table 18-1. The clinical expressions of the nephritic syndrome—oliguria, hypertension, edema, and hematuria—reflect glomerular trauma and diminished function. Alternatively there may be primary alterations in the integrity of the basement membrane without the presence of inflammatory cells. Impairment of the glomerular basement membrane barrier function causes proteinuria. This can be sufficiently severe to cause the nephrotic syndrome, a clinical clustering of proteinuria exceeding 3 g/day, hypoalbuminemia, and hyperlipemia. Glomerular function itself is not necessarily diminished. The symptoms of the nephrotic syndrome are primarily attributable to the effects of the loss of specific proteins, summarized in Table 18-1.

Acute glomerulonephritis

When glomeruli are involved with acute inflammation, there is increased capillary permeability and sometimes actual discontinuity of capillary basement membranes. The increased permeability permits plasma proteins (proteinuria), red blood cells (hematuria), and white blood cells (pyuria) to leak into the urine. Tamm-Horsfall glycoprotein may precipitate in the tubular lumen and entrap these components, forming cylindrical casts. The identification of casts, protein, and red blood cells in the urine is important in the diagnosis of glomerular inflammation.

With acute inflammation, the glomeruli become swollen and hypercellular because of infiltration with neutrophils and monocytes and because of proliferation and hydropic swelling of mesangial and endothelial cells.[91] There may result impaired blood flow through most of the glomerular capillary loops, so that only a few capillaries shunt blood to the efferent arteriole. This may lead to oliguria ('little urine formation') or anuria ('no urine formation'). In more severe injury to the basement membrane, particularly that associated with the activated deposition of fibrin in the urinary space, glomerular epithelial cells may proliferate, filling the urinary space together with invading monocytes. The circumferential accumulation of cells in the urinary space is termed a "crescent."

As inflammation subsides, hydropic swelling decreases, and inflammatory cells leave. Resolution to near-normal function can occur. Crescentic forms of glomerulonephritis, however, tend to form permanent scar tissue in Bowman's space and are less amenable to recovery.

In contrast, glomerular diseases causing the nephrotic syndrome may involve little or no inflammation. Instead, as noted above, there is a primary alteration in the ability of the basement membrane to serve as a barrier to the filtration of plasma proteins. Such glomerular disease, though dissimilar in pathogenesis and many clinical features, may share the nephrotic symptoms of massive proteinuria, hypoproteinemia, edema or anasarca, hyperlipemia, and lipiduria.[13] Although the exact mechanism of hyperlipemia is not known, most investigators believe that the liver, stressed by the need for massive synthesis of plasma protein in response to urinary loss of albumin, concurrently overproduces lipoproteins. The low plasma albumin level results in a fall in plasma volume because of the loss of its osmotic effect. This leads to increased aldosterone release with conservation of sodium and water, resulting in edema formation.

In both nephritic and nephrotic states, glomeruli can eventually develop chronic injury if the inciting insult is persistent. Chronic glomerular injury is expressed as progressive scarring.[47] Scar tissue in the glomerular tuft is composed of new formations of basement membrane resulting in obliteration of capillary channels and eventual obliteration of the entire glomerulus. New types of inflammatory collagen appear and may be synthesized by interstitial cells migrating into the injured glomerulus. Scarring causes a progressive decrease in glomerular filtration rate, and renal plasma flow decreases because of obstruction of the arteriolar bed. A sharp fall in glomerular filtration rate eventually results in renal failure and death. Since the tubular blood supply depends on postglomerular blood flow, chronic obliterative glomerular lesions are accompanied by progressive tubular atrophy and deranged tubular function (see below).

Acute tubular injury

Ischemia, immunologic insults, and a variety of toxic substances may result in acute tubular injury or necrosis, which may produce oliguria or anuria if most or all nephrons are involved. The failure of urine formation in the presence of morphologically normal arteries and glomeruli may be explained by the following[104]:

1. Arterial vasoconstriction
2. Mechanical plugging of tubules by necrotic tubular debris and precipitated protein (casts)
3. Backdiffusion of glomerular filtrate into the interstitium through gaps in the walls of necrotic tubules and ruptured peritubular basement membranes
4. A rise in tissue turgor pressure from filtrate backdiffusion, resulting in decreased glomerular filtration

In the great variety of acute tubular injuries, many or all of these factors may play a role.

If oliguria persists, azotemia (a sharp rise in nitrogenous waste products in the blood) and acute renal failure may result. If the patient survives for 14 to 21 days, the remarkable regenerative capacity of the tubules permits a return to normal or near-normal function.

Chronic tubular loss or atrophy

In chronic renal disease, whether caused by chronic glomerular disease, chronic vascular renal insufficiency, or chronic interstitial inflammatory disease, the tubules may be destroyed or may develop irregular atrophy with interstitial fibrosis and thickened peritubular basement membranes.[47] Such chronic tubular changes are associated with decreased ability to pump sodium, synthesize ammonium ions, exchange hydrogen ions, and form a concentrated urine. The large reserve of proximal tubular function in resorbing many substances such as amino acids and glucose usually prevents their appearance in the urine even in advanced tubular atrophy. The formation of urine of fixed osmolality, nearly isotonic with plasma, is attributable in part to the structural and functional impairment of the countercurrent multiplier system and in part to the solute load of accumulated waste products (urea) that forces an osmotic diuresis in the few remaining functioning nephrons.

CLASSIFICATION OF RENAL DISEASES

Prerenal and postrenal diseases are most typically diagnosed by functional tests addressed toward either the vasculature (angiography, renal flow scans, and so on) or toward the urinary tract (intravenous or retrograde pyelography, ultrasonography, and so on). Intrarenal diseases can generally be safely diagnosed only by use of the percutaneous renal biopsy. This procedure, in which a specialized needle is inserted into the kidney through the back in order to remove a small core of tissue, has been in wide use only in the last 30 years. As a result, the classification of renal diseases is still in a state of flux, with terminology reflecting either the kinetics of the disease ("rapidly progressive glomerulonephritis"), the cause ("IgA nephropathy"), or the histologic abnormality ("membranoproliferative glomerulonephritis"). This section addresses glomerular and then interstitial syndromes, grouped by pathologic appearance whenever possible. We will make a distinction between primary and secondary syndromes. Primary diseases, particularly of the glomerulus, are diseases arising within the kidney, usually of unknown cause, in which all the affected structures are uniformly involved. Secondary diseases are those in which the kidneys are affected as a result of a systemic or extrarenal disorder. Diabetes, for example, affects not only glomeruli but also small blood vessels throughout the body. Secondary renal syndromes tend to be variable in their effects on the kidney with a resulting overlapping of histologic classifications. Thus heterogeneity of glomerular pathologic lesions is quite characteristic of systemic lupus erythematosus (SLE). Discussion of primary disease entities is followed by a presentation of secondary syndromes most likely related by histologic classification. A review of glomerular inflammation, in which the glomerulus is traumatized by components of either cellular or humoral immunity, precedes the discussion of glomerular diseases in which the injury is vascular or metabolic.

GLOMERULAR DISEASE
Pathogenesis of immune glomerular injury

Glomeruli may be injured by immunologic, metabolic, vascular, thrombotic, hereditary, or toxic mechanisms. Immunologic mechanisms are of particular importance in both experimental and human glomerular diseases. Immunoglobulins IgG, IgM, and IgA can be demonstrated in both human and experimental glomerulonephritis.[45] In addition, components of the classical and alternative pathways of complement may be demonstrated in such lesions and at times appear as the principal deposits, with little immunoglobulin being demonstrable. Three important mechanisms of glomerular immunologic injury are anti–glomerular basement membrane disease, immune complex disease, and complement-mediated injury.

Anti–glomerular basement membrane disease

Lindeman[63] first demonstrated that antibodies develop when a kidney of one species is injected into another species and that when such antibodies (nephrotoxic serum) are reinjected into the original species, acute glomerular inflammation results. This experimental mechanism was extensively explored by Masugi and is often referred to as "Masugi nephritis." Subsequent

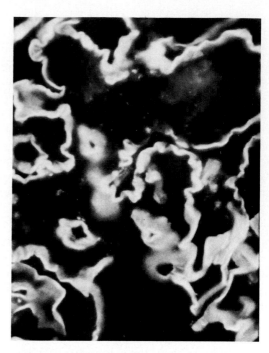

Fig. 18-4. Rapidly progressive glomerulonephritis of anti-glomerular basement membrane type showing linear staining of glomerular basement membrane with fluorescent antihuman IgG. (Courtesy Dr. Claude Cornwall, Syracuse, N.Y.)

research has shown that the critical antigens involved are in the glomerular basement membrane. In some cases of human glomerulonephritis it has been possible to isolate anti–glomerular basement membrane antibody from the serum or to elute it from the glomeruli.[22]

One can couple fluorescein to antibodies against immunoglobulins or complement components (fluorescent antibodies) and react these reagents with frozen sections of either experimental or human glomeruli afflicted by anti–glomerular basement membrane disease. Fluorescence microscopy reveals a linear deposition of anti–glomerular basement membrane antibody and complement along the glomerular basement membrane (Fig. 18-4). Electron microscopy may show a thin, fluffy, linear layer of material between the capillary endothelium and the basement membrane in such cases.[22]

Studies indicate that anti–glomerular basement membrane disease is the basis for all cases of Goodpasture's syndrome and about one third the cases of rapidly progressive glomerulonephritis. The mechanism by which one develops antibodies against one's own glomerular basement membrane is not known, but it is possible that one develops antibodies initially against endogenous or exogenous antigens that cross-react with glomerular basement membrane.

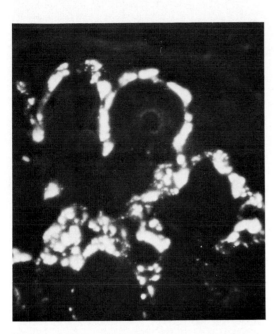

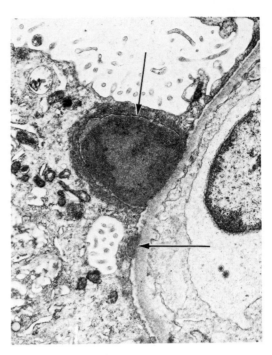

Fig. 18-5. Acute poststreptococcal glomerulonephritis. "Humps" of immune complex stained with fluorescent anti-human complement (C3). (1000×; courtesy Dr. Claude Cornwall, Syracuse, N.Y.)

Fig. 18-6. Acute poststreptococcal glomerulonephritis. "Humps" of immune complex outside basement membrane are indicated by arrows. (6000×.)

Immune complex disease

The experimental injection of certain foreign, non-glomerular antigens into animals stimulates antibody formation. The antibody then combines with still-circulating antigen, and the complex is deposited in glomeruli along with complement. This complex of antigens, antibody, and complement, plus chemotactically attracted neutrophils and monocytes, causes glomerular injury.[16,22] Fluorescent antibody reagents show that the immune complexes are deposited as lumpy deposits just outside the basement membrane and in the mesangium (Fig. 18-5). Electron microscopy confirms the presence of deposits between the podocytes and the glomerular basement membrane and in the mesangium (Fig. 18-6). This type of glomerular deposit occurs when there is moderate antigen excess to antibody because small aggregates are trapped in the glomerular filter. With antibody equivalence or excess, large aggregates are formed and are taken up by the reticuloendothelial system. With great antigen excess, only small, soluble aggregates form and remain in the circulation or are filtered.

Human diseases that appear to be of this immune complex type include acute glomerulonephritis, membranous glomerulonephritis (see Fig. 18-25), some cases of rapidly progressive and chronic glomerulonephritis, systemic lupus erythematosus (SLE), and some cases of mesangiopathic glomerulonephritis. The experimental analog is the glomerulonephritis of experimental serum sickness.

Complement-mediated injury

Certain patients with membranoproliferative glomerulonephritis have greatly depressed serum complement component C3 levels but normal levels of C1, C2, and C4.[43] The glomeruli of such patients show little immunoglobulin deposition by immunofluorescence studies but heavy deposits of complement C3 and also deposits of properdin of the alternative pathway of the complement system. A circulating nephritic anticomplementary factor, C3NeF, has been found in such patients. This factor has been found to be an immunoglobulin that acts to stabilize C3 convertase and enhance alternative pathway activity. With electron microscopy these sites of complement and properdin deposition are shown to be very electron dense. Such glomerular lesions have been called "dense-deposit disease." Alternative pathway disease also occurs in some patients with rapidly progressive glomerulonephritis. Acute poststreptococcal glomerulonephritis usually shows striking activation of the alternative pathway of complement, and to a lesser extent SLE shows activation of this pathway as a supplement to the classical complement pathway activation by immune complex deposition.[115] Focal glomerulonephritis induced by IgA deposits appears also to implicate the alternative pathway.

Diffuse glomerulonephritis

Acute diffuse glomerulonephritis is characterized by an acute inflammatory process involving all the glomeruli of both kidneys. Involvement of the glomeruli is usually global and uniform. This inflammation results in blockage of many of the glomerular capillaries with infiltrating cells and swollen endothelium, thus decreasing glomerular filtration. The inflammation also results in increased capillary permeability so that plasma proteins, red blood cells, and white blood cells appear in the urine, often as casts. Diffuse glomerulonephritis is characterized by the acute, massive deposition of immune complexes within the glomerulus, typically in the peripheral capillary loops in a subepithelial distribution. The antigens may be endogenous, as is the DNA antigen of systemic lupus erythematosus (see below). However, most commonly, the appearance of such complexes follows an acute infection, often bacterial, especially streptococcal.

Acute poststreptococcal or postinfectious glomerulonephritis[30]

Careful epidemiologic, bacteriologic, and serologic studies indicate that at least two thirds of the cases of acute diffuse glomerulonephritis follow hemolytic streptococcal infections after about a 10-day latent period. Only certain strains of hemolytic streptococci seem to be nephritogenic. Although most of these infections are of the upper respiratory tract, skin and wound infections may be responsible. The streptococcal infection may be identified by culture, or it may be inferred later by a rising titer of antibodies against streptococcal antigens, such as antistreptolysin O (ASO). The inflammation is clearly not attributable to the local presence of streptococci in the glomeruli, since bacteria cannot be demonstrated in the kidney; and treatment of the extrarenal infection with antibiotics does not prevent the development of nephritis. Immunofluorescent and electron microscopic studies indicate that poststreptococcal diffuse glomerulonephritis is an immune complex disease because antibody aggregates compose the deposits. Recently streptococcal antigens have been localized to deposits in some patients, but no single antigen has been unequivocally defined for most patients.

Acute poststreptococcal glomerulonephritis is seen mostly in children, particularly from 3 to 7 years of age, and in young adults. The disease affects males with about twice the frequency of females. It is common and occurs throughout the world. Characteristically the patient experiences hematuria, olguria, and edema. Hy-

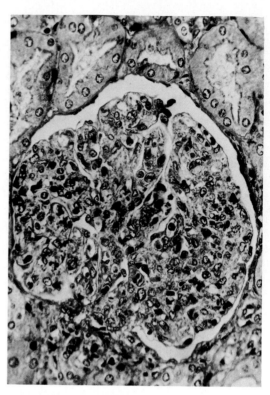

Fig 18-7. Acute poststreptococcal glomerulonephritis. Swollen, hypercellular glomerular lobules with few open capillaries. (250×.)

pertension occurs in about half of patients sufficiently ill to enter the hospital. In 5% to 10% the hypertension may be sufficiently severe to cause cerebrovascular damage and cerebral edema (hypertensive encephalopathy).

After a few days the hematuria, proteinuria, and hypertension diminish, and in the favorable cases all findings have usually returned to normal in 6 months, though sometimes up to 3 years is required. Resolution of the illness may pass through a nephrotic stage. About 80% to 90% of children have a good outcome, whereas only 50% to 70% of adults do as well. About 2% to 5% of patients die in the acute phase as a result of uremia, infection, or cardiovascular problems.[23] Some patients surviving the acute phase may have persistent, active, progressive disease, which heals with a large loss of nephrons, or they may have a slow, smoldering, downhill course.[7]

The kidneys in acute diffuse glomerulonephritis are moderately swollen and may be either pale or congested. Microscopically the changes are mainly in the glomeruli. All glomeruli are involved and to about the same extent. The glomeruli are swollen and distend Bowman's capsule. There is a sharp increase in the number of cells within the glomerular tuft. The individ-

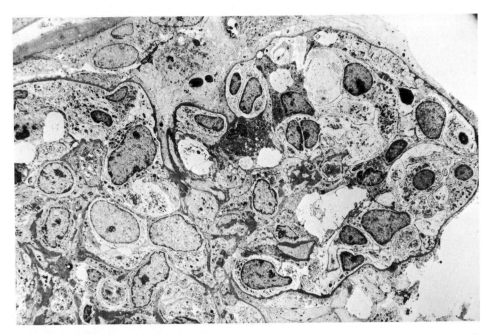

Fig. 18-8. Acute poststreptococcal glomerulonephritis. Electron micrograph showing swollen, hypercellular glomerular lobules. (1600×.)

ual glomerular tuft lobules often are club shaped because of the ballooning of the tuft (Figs. 18-7 and 18-8). Electron microscopy and immunofluorescence microscopy show varying-sized "humps" of immune complex deposit between the basement membrane and podocytes (Fig. 18-8). Typically IgG is present in a "lumpy-bumpy" pattern.

The increased cellularity is caused by proliferation of mesangial and endothelial cells and the infiltration of the tuft by neutrophils and monocytes. When there are many neutrophils in most of the glomeruli, the disease is called "acute exudative glomerulonephritis"; whereas when the cellularity is predominantly caused by mesangial cells, endothelial cells, and monocytes,[16] the term "acute proliferative glomerulonephritis" is used. When damage is more serious, rupture and thrombosis of capillaries may occur with pronounced red blood cell leakage and fibrin clot formation in Bowman's space. A proliferation of Bowman's capsular cells in this exudate may result in a loose epithelial crescent partially or completely filling Bowman's space. Such a condition is called "acute necrotizing glomerulonephritis." The severity of the clinical picture and the eventual outcome correlate well with the degree of glomerular inflammation and destruction as seen in renal biopsy. Whereas acute exudative or proliferative lesions may resolve with only a minor increase in mesangial thickening and cellularity, acute necrotizing lesions are intrinsically irreversible and, if widespread, cause permanent loss of function.

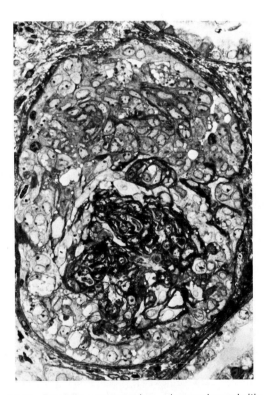

Fig. 18-9. Rapidly progressive glomerulonephritis, anti-glomerular basement membrane type. Notice crescent of epithelial cells encircling compressed glomerular tuft.

Acute nonstreptococcal glomerulonephritis

About one third of the cases of acute diffuse glomerulonephritis are apparently not related to infection by hemolytic streptococci. Pneumococcal infections, viral infections, bacterial endocarditis, and other infections have been associated with acute diffuse glomerulonephritis, whereas other cases have no evidence of a preceding infection. Some cases of diffuse glomerulonephritis are associated with the deposit of immune complexes in which the antigen is an endogenous protein. They include thyroiditis (thyroglobulin), tumor antigens, and cryoglobulinemia (IgM).[30]

Rapidly progressive glomerulonephritis[34,91]

Rapidly progressive glomerulonephritis, an unusually severe form of glomerulonephritis, is characterized by proliferation of glomerular cells and invasion by inflammatory mononuclear cells in which the primary localization of proliferation is outside the glomerular basement membrane (extracapillary) but within Bowman's capsule, that is, within the urinary space. Patients with this form experience an extremely rapid deterioration of kidney function occurring over a few weeks to 1 to 2 months. Hypertension and edema are common; urinalysis is characterized by hematuria, proteinuria, and pyuria. The characteristic lesion is a "crescent," a complex mixture of proliferating epithelial cells and infiltrating monocytes that form concentric layers of cells around the capillary tufts, which become compressed under the encirclement (Fig. 18-9). A particular feature of crescentic glomerulonephritis is the presence of fibrin, which is a potent stimulant of epithelial cell proliferation (Fig. 18-10). The fibrin appears to be derived in part from extravasated fibrinogen. Recently, however, it has been observed that the infiltrating monocytes carry a procoagulatory activity on their membranes, resembling a tissue factor, which can generate large amounts of fibrin.[93] Adhesions of glomerular tufts to the capsule and obliteration of Bowman's space are common. Thus these patients are typically oliguric or anuric. Scarring of the glomerular tufts proceeds rapidly, with few patent capillaries remaining. As a result of postglomerular ischemia, the tubules become atrophic and the interstitium ultimately becomes fibrotic. Arteries typically show little evidence of change, though rare cases evince an acute fibrinoid arteritis confined to the kidney.

Approximately one third of such patients show immune complexes deposited in a heterogeneous pattern throughout the glomerulus. The inciting antigen is not known, though often such patients report a viral-like syndrome occurring weeks to months before the onset of acute renal failure.[35] Another one third of patients have crescents in the absence of any immunoglobulin

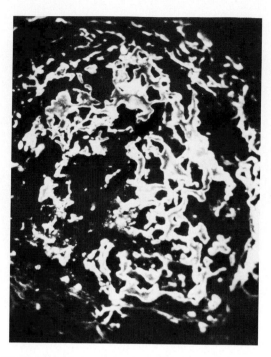

Fig. 18-10. Rapidly progressive glomerulonephritis stained with fluorescent antihuman fibrin. Both tuft and crescent contain fibrin. (Courtesy Dr. Claude Cornwall, Syracuse, N.Y.)

deposition in the glomerulus. The mechanisms underlying this variant are completely unknown. A subset of these patients have symptoms suggestive of systemic vasculitis; they are less responsive to therapy. Finally, approximately one third of such patients display linear antibody staining of the glomerular basement membrane. These patients have autoantibodies directed against antigens found on the glomerular basement membrane. Although fluorescent staining for antibody deposited on the glomerular basement membrane is florid, immune complexes are not demonstrable by ultrastructural analysis because the antigen-antibody union is of molecular dimensions. This expression of autoimmune kidney disease is most commonly known as "Goodpasture's syndrome." In Goodpasture's syndrome, acute necrotizing, rapidly progressive glomerulonephritis is associated with pulmonary hemorrhage and hemoptysis. This is believed to be caused by cross-reactivity between pulmonary basement membrane and renal basement membrane because antibody can be demonstrated in both locations. The disease can progress rapidly, with renal failure occurring in weeks to months. The lungs can show alveolar hemorrhage, hemosiderin-filled macrophages, and thickening of the alveolar walls. Anti–glomerular basement membrane disease without lung involvement is termed "nonpulmonary Goodpasture's syndrome."

The therapy of rapidly progressive glomerulonephritis has involved the use of high-dose, pulse steroids, with or without the addition of cytotoxic agents. There may be a particular role for plasmaphoresis to acutely remove circulating anti–basement membrane antibody. Although many patients can respond dramatically to immunosuppressive therapy, the majority progress to renal failure within 1 to 2 years even after initial response to therapy.[93]

Focal glomerulonephritis

Focal glomerulonephritis is the pathologic name applied to an inflammatory process involving some glomeruli while sparing others.[103] Most cases of focal glomerulonephritis affect only portions of a glomerulus and thus can be regarded as segmental rather than global. The pattern of partial involvement of glomeruli may be an expression of systemic diseases as well as diseases affecting only the kidney (Fig. 18-11).

Focal glomerulonephritis can occur in a setting of several types of vasculitides, including polyarteritis nodosa, Wegener's granulomatosis, and systemic lupus erythematosus. These are discussed more extensively below.

Focal glomerulonephritis with systemic bacterial infection

For many years physicians have recognized that patients may have hematuria and proteinuria at the peak of bacterial infection. When death occurs at this time, some glomeruli show hypercellularity, focal necrosis, thrombosis of glomerular lobules, or even focal capsular epithelial proliferation, producing epithelial crescents or adhesions (Fig. 18-11). Since this involves only a small proportion of glomeruli, it is not surprising that survivors generally show no abnormalities of renal function. The term "glomerulitis" has been used by some for such changes.

A striking lesion of this type, known as "focal embolic glomerulonephritis," is seen in patients with subacute bacterial endocarditis. Of patients having endocarditis for at least 6 weeks, approximately two thirds develop thrombonecrosis of individual glomerular lobules with leakage of red cells from ruptured capillaries into Bowman's space, producing hematuria. A small epithelial crescent often develops at the site of this necrotic lobule. Red blood cells in the proximal and the distal convoluted tubules, leaking from a damaged glomerulus, produce small reddish spots on the capsular or cut surface. This produces the so-called flea-bitten kidney of subacute bacterial endocarditis. In patients whose endocarditis is of longer duration, scarring of the glomerular lobule and adjacent crescent is seen.

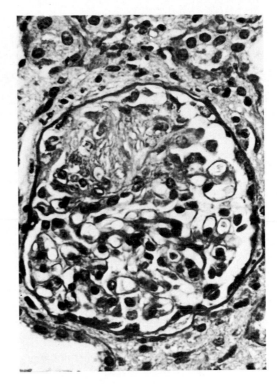

Fig. 18-11. Focal glomerulonephritis with focal crescent and scarring.

The term "focal embolic glomerulonephritis" implies that the necroses are the result of small emboli from the valvular vegetations. Although microemboli might produce such a lesion, bacteria rarely are seen in the lesions. The disease may occur with valvular lesions of the right side of the heart in association with cardiac malformations producing right-to-left shunting of blood, or with surgically implanted, infected shunts. Immunofluorescence and electron microscopy study of renal specimens from patients with bacterial endocarditis has revealed immune complex deposits in the glomerular lesions, an indication that bacterial antigenemia contributes to the disease.[41]

Mesangioproliferative glomerulonephritis

The subset of glomerular diseases called "mesangioproliferative glomerulonephritis" is characterized by the presence of an abnormally large number of cells or deposits within the mesangial region of the glomerulus. The cells may be intrinsic, that is, resident, proliferating mesangial cells. Alternatively, they may be monocytes or macrophages, which appear to have a predilection for migrating into the mesangium. The mesangial hypercellularity may be focal, and it may be accompanied by evidence of acute necrosis. The most common type of mesangioproliferative glomerulonephritis is

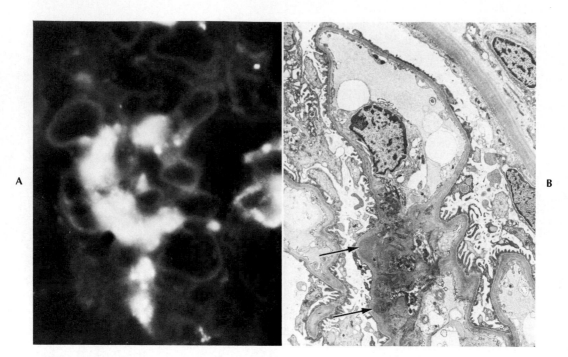

Fig. 18-12. Berger's IgA focal glomerulonephritis. **A,** Stained fluorescent with antihuman IgA. IgA is limited to mesangium. **B,** Deposits in mesangium, *arrows.* (**A,** Courtesy Dr. Claude Cornwall, Syracuse, N.Y.; **B,** 3000×.)

known as "IgA nephropathy,"[15,21] also called "Berger's disease" after its discoverer. These patients typically present with gross hematuria, often temporally related to a concurrent upper respiratory tract infection. Most patients are older adolescents or young adults; there is a slight preponderance of males. They usually have a normal glomerular filtration rate and blood pressure. Immunofluorescence and electron microscopy demonstrate prominant immunoglobulin deposits of IgA and IgM and traces of IgG in the glomerular mesangium (Fig. 18-12). The antigen or antigens contributing to the mesangial deposits of immune complexes have not been identified. The majority of such patients recover with no clinical residua, often after months to years of intermittent hematuria. However, as many as 10% to 20% of such patients may manifest progressive destruction of the nephrons until chronic renal failure develops. These patients may not be diagnosed until years after the onset of their disease, at which point they become part of a large group of cases of end-stage chronic glomerulonephritis, characterized by glomerular sclerosis and interstitial fibrosis. There is no available therapy. IgA nephropathy, which typically occurs in young adults, is part of a continuum of glomerular lesions whose childhood expression is a syndrome known as "Schönlein-Henoch purpura" (anaphylactoid purpura). Children with this syndrome present with purpuric lesions in their skin, arthritis, and gastroenteritis, all at-

tributable to the acute deposition of IgA immune complexes. The lesion has a rapid onset, often accompanied by gross hematuria, and often resolves within weeks to a few months. Resolution is spontaneous and occurs more completely in the pediatric population than in the adult counterpart, which lacks the systemic manifestations of IgA deposition in the periphery.

Another variant of mesangioproliferative glomerulonephritis is known as "IgM nephropathy," in which the immune deposits within the mesangium are predominantly IgM.[15] This syndrome is rare and, unlike IgA nephropathy, often associated with nephrotic-range proteinuria. These patients are believed to respond to immunosuppressive therapy, including prednisone and cytotoxic agents.

Membranoproliferative glomerulonephritis

The group of glomerular diseases called "membranoproliferative glomerulonephritis" is characterized by infiltration of inflammatory cells, by proliferation of intrinsic glomerular cells, and by altered structure and function of the glomerular basement membrane. The membranoproliferative syndromes have both an inflammatory component, causing a nephritic clinical expression, and an altered basement membrane component, causing abnormal loss of protein and often a nephrotic syndrome.

Membranoproliferative glomerulonephritis,[15] also

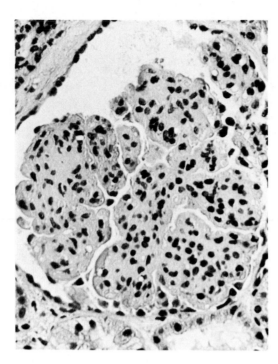

Fig. 18-13. Membranoproliferative glomerulonephritis. Notice cellular, swollen lobules.

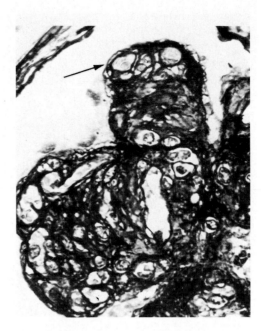

Fig. 18-14. Membranoproliferative glomerulonephritis. Notice duplication of capillary basement membrane, *arrow.* (Silver methenamine stain.)

known as "mesangiocapillary glomerulonephritis," occurs in 10% to 15% of patients with nephrotic syndrome and is most common in the second decade. The glomeruli by light microscopy are large and hypercellular and show distinctive club-shaped glomerular lobules (Fig. 18-13). There is a striking increase in mesangial cells and mesangial basement membrane substance. The glomerular capillary walls are often double contoured from splitting of the basement membrane (Fig. 18-14). Neutrophils are seen in these tufts during peaks of clinical activity. Electron microscopy and immunofluorescence have revealed that there are two types of this disease. Type I is an immune complex disease with lumpy immunoglobulin deposits in the mesangium and in the capillary walls of the tuft (Figs. 18-14 to 18-16). Occasionally one observes subepithelial humps of electron-dense material. The splitting of the capillary basement membrane results from the enlarged mesangium extending out to encircle the capillary.

Type II (hypocomplementemic glomerulonephritis) is an alternative pathway disease. Although immunoglobulin deposits are slight or absent, there is a striking deposit of complement in the capillary walls. This complement deposit is associated with peculiar lamellar "dense deposits" in the capillary walls in the position of the lamina densa[15,43] (Figs. 18-17 and 18-18). Such patients have very low serum complement levels and often have a circulating anticomplementary gamma globulin,

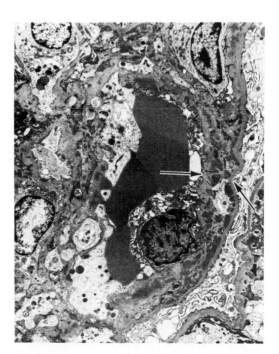

Fig. 18-15. Membranoproliferative glomerulonephritis, immune complex type. Notice double layer of basement membrane, *arrows,* and immune complex deposits. (3000×.)

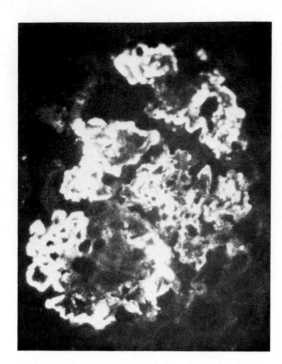

Fig. 18-16. Membranoproliferative glomerulonephritis, immune complex type, stained with fluorescent antihuman complement (C3). (Courtesy Dr. Claude Cornwall, Syracuse, N.Y.)

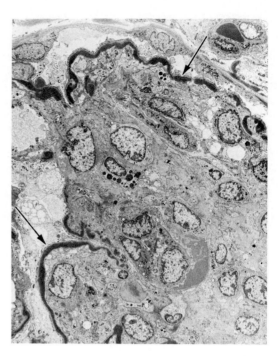

Fig. 18-17. Membranoproliferative glomerulonephritis, dense deposit type. Notice dense linear deposits about periphery of lobules, *arrows*. (3000×.)

C3NeF (nephritic factor).[98] Some patients develop segmental lipodystrophy, a progressive atrophy of fat deposits in different parts of the body. The basis for this association is not known.

These two types of membranoproliferative glomerulonephritis may be indistinguishable clinically. In acute exacerbations of disease the clinical picture of membranoproliferative glomerulonephritis may resemble acute diffuse glomerulonephritis. The nephrotic syndrome is resistant to steroid therapy, and the disease tends to progress to renal failure in a few months or years. Recently therapy designed to inhibit platelet function, employing aspirin and dipyramidole, has been found to be effective in slowing the progression of the disease in a significant subset of patients. Both variants have a striking tendency to recur in renal allografts.

Strife and co-workers[106] have described a variant of this lesion in which there are massive deposits disrupting the glomerular basement membranes, so-called type III membranoproliferative glomerulonephritis.

The following glomerular diseases are not characterized by an inflammatory cell infiltrate. Some, such as minimal change disease and membranous nephropathy, are associated with humoral immunity, with injury arising from immune complexes or immune factors. Others are associated with the synthesis of excessive or altered components of the basement membrane or deposits of exogenous material in the basement membrane. They share in common an excessive filtration of protein attributable to impaired functional integrity of the basement membrane. They thus are associated with the nephrotic syndrome.

Minimal change disease

Minimal change disease is a major cause of the nephrotic syndrome. It is a disease primarily of young children (2 to 4 years of age) but may occur in older children and occasionally in adults. Clinically it is characterized by the insidious onset of a gross nephrotic syndrome without significant hypertension, hematuria, or azotemia, except late in the course of patients with unremitting disease. Remissions and exacerbations of the nephrotic syndrome are common in this disease with or without treatment. Renal biopsy specimens studied with the light microscope characteristically reveal normal or near-normal glomeruli. Many studies have failed to show deposits of immunoglobulins or complement in these glomeruli. Electron microscopy shows no abnormality of glomerular basement membranes of mesangium and no immune deposits. The foot processes of the glomerular epithelial cells or podocytes show flattening, loss of filtration slit pores, and development of tight junctions between adjacent epithelial cell processes[42] (Figs. 18-19 and 18-20). The tubular epithelium may show hyaline droplets as evidence of proteinuria and fatty droplets, reflecting hyperlipemia and

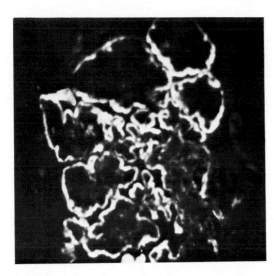

Fig. 18-18. Membranoproliferative glomerulonephritis, dense deposit type, stained with fluorescent antihuman complement (C3). (Courtesy Dr. Claude Cornwall, Syracuse, N.Y.)

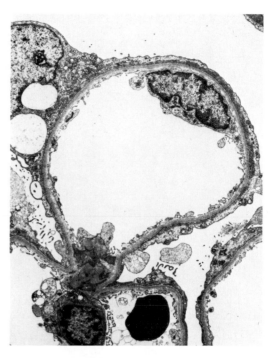

Fig. 18-19. Lipoid nephrosis (minimal change disease). Notice foot-process flattening. (4000×.)

lipiduria. Accumulated lipid produces the pale yellow renal cortex seen at autopsy. The kidneys usually are enlarged or of normal size.

In the preantibiotic era, death from intercurrent bacterial infection, particularly pneumococcal peritonitis, was common. Approximately 60% of the patients died within 5 years. With antibiotic therapy the mortality at 5 years fell to about 25%. With steroid therapy, sometimes combined with immunosuppressive drugs, complete remission or control occurs in most cases, and the mortality is less than 10%.[12]

The cause of minimal change disease, or lipoid nephrosis as it was once termed, remains obscure. Clinical evidence supports the contribution of a circulating immune-derived factor. Children with nephrotic syndrome tend to have a history of atopy. The disease is responsive to steroids, suggestive of an immune cause. In adults with minimal change disease, there is a strong clinical association with lymphoproliferative disease, particularly lymphoma. Finally, the urine and plasma of steroid-responsive patients with this disorder contain a factor that derives from suppressor lymphocytes.[94] Nonetheless, no factor causing increased glomerular permeability has been unequivocally identified. The origins of this disease remains unknown.

Membranous nephropathy

Idiopathic membranous glomerulonephritis (membranous nephropathy) is the most important cause of nephrotic syndrome in adults, though occasional cases occur in children. The disease is characterized by the

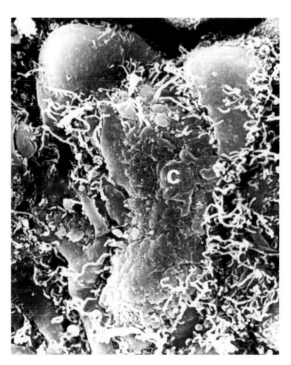

Fig. 18-20. Scanning electron micrograph of glomerular capillary, C, in minimal change disease. Notice loss of foot processes and many microvilli. Similar appearance is seen in membranous nephropathy. (1800×.)

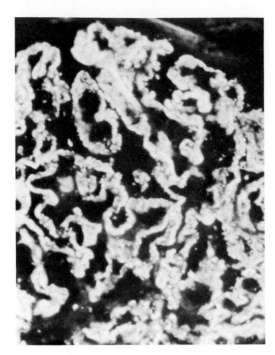

Fig. 18-21. Idiopathic membranous nephropathy, an immune complex disease, showing lumpy staining of glomerular immune complex deposits with fluorescent antihuman IgG. (Courtesy Dr. Claude Cornwall, Syracuse, N.Y.)

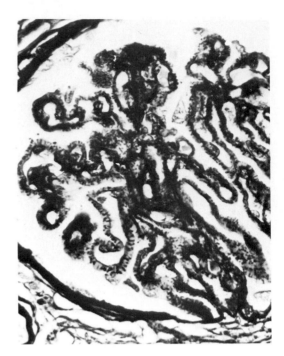

Fig. 18-22. Membranous nephropathy. Notice spikes of basement membrane between deposits. (Silver methenamine stain.)

insidious onset of proteinuria and the nephrotic syndrome. The process tends to have a long course somewhat modified by steroid or cytotoxic therapy. Even with clinical improvement there may be little morphologic change in the glomerular lesions. This disease may progress to pronounced glomerular scarring, tubular atrophy, and uremia after a period of years. Immunologic and structural evidence indicates that this is an immune complex disease[79,90] (Figs. 18-21 to 18-23).

Grossly the kidneys may be of normal size or slightly enlarged early in the disease but somewhat shrunken and granular in the late stages. The yellowish cast of the cut surface is attributed to lipid in the tubules. Light microscopy reveals normal glomeruli in early lesions, but later a uniform thickening of the glomerular capillary wall is seen. With the periodic acid–silver methenamine stain, thin clublike projections of the basement membrane may be seen extending out between minute, beadlike, hyaline droplets (Fig. 18-22). These droplets are shown to be immunoglobulin deposits by immunofluorescence. Electron microscopy in early lesions reveals granular protein deposits outside the basement membrane under the flattened podocytic foot processes (stage I). As the disease progresses, the basement membrane thickens, and clublike processes of new basement membrane form between the protein deposits (stage II). In advanced stages of the disease, basement membranes, including the deposits, may be-

come 5 to 10 times the usual thickness (stage III). In stage IV, the membrane looks moth-eaten; deposits become smaller, denser, and irregular. Fibrin caps in Bowman's space can be noted late in the course. The mesangium is often mildly hypercellular, perhaps reflecting a moderate infiltration of leukocytes. There is often an associated, mild interstitial nephritis.

The antigens in the immune complexes have been infrequently identified.[108] They can be viral (as in hepatitis B) or related to other infectious agents such as *Treponema pallidum* or *Plasmodium malariae*, or endogenous proteins (thyroglobulin in thyroiditis), or can be neoantigens created by therapeutic agents (gold and pencillamine are two prominent examples). There is a well-documented association between membranous nephropathy and solid tumors, particularly those of lung, breast, and intestines. In some of these cases, the antigen or antigens appear to be tumor derived. More commonly, the antigen of membranous nephropathy is not known. The glomerular disease pursues an indolent and unpredictable course. Only 25% progress to renal failure, with the remainder experiencing full or partial remissions, often spontaneously.

Focal segmental glomerulosclerosis

Focal sclerosis is a progressive, obliterative disease of glomeruli associated with pronounced proteinuria.[44] It

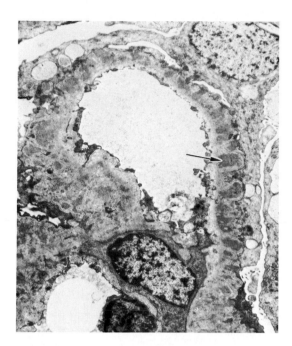

Fig. 18-23. Membranous nephropathy. *Arrow,* Nodular deposits in outer part of thickened basement membrane. (6000×.)

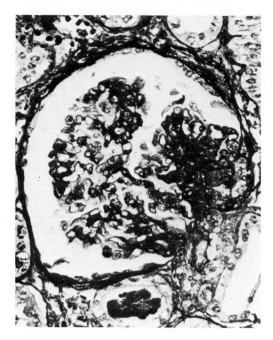

Fig. 18-24. Focal glomerular sclerosis. (Silver methenamine stain.)

afflicts young and middle-aged adults, in contrast to the predominance of minimal change disease among nephrotic patients who are adolescents or children. In addition to the diffuse foot-process changes in all the glomeruli, focal sclerosis of glomerular lobules with thick basement membranes, adhesions, and fibrinoid nodules develops first in the juxtamedullary glomeruli (Fig. 18-24). Early in the course of the disease such lesions may be missed by biopsy, and the erroneous diagnosis of minimal change disease is made. As in minimal change disease, immunofluorescence studies show no immunoglobulin or complement deposits in focal glomerulosclerosis except for nonspecific traces of IgM in old scars. Periglomerular accumulation of mononuclear leukocytes is commonly observed. Lesions resembling focal sclerosis have been observed in patients with acquired immunodeficiency syndrome and in intravenous heroin abusers.

Focal segmental glomerulosclerosis tends to be resistant to steroid therapy and to progress to renal failure. There is a significant rate of recurrence in transplanted kidneys.

Systemic amyloidosis

The syndrome of systemic amyloidosis is characterized by the deposition of fibrillary proteins in multiple organs, particularly the kidney.[36,37] Patients with amyloidosis can be divided into two distinct groups. In the first group, the protein is a segment of a light chain of immunoglobulin (AL, amyloid light chain). This disease can occur as a primary form or in association with multiple myeloma or other plasma cell dyscrasias. The second group of patients (AA, or secondary amyloid) develop amyloid in association with chronic inflammatory disease such as infections or rheumatoid arthritis. The fibrillary protein in this group is protein A, synthesized by the liver as an apoprotein and acute phase reactant. Amyloid has a predilection for deposition in the heart, liver, spleen, kidneys, skin, and gastrointestinal tract. Clinical manifestations depend on the organ involved; many tissues can be affected.

The kidneys are usually pale and enlarged. Glomeruli are typically involved, with amyloid deposits appearing first in the mesangium. The deposits are nodular and expansive, ultimately compressing and then collapsing the capillaries. The deposits are acidophilic with hematoxylin and eosin stain and are metachromatic on crystal violet stain. More specific is the appearance of green-yellow birefringence in Congo Red–stained sections examined under polarized light. On electron microscopic examination, amyloid deposits consist of nonbranching fibrils, approximately 10 nm in diameter, randomly tangled (Figs. 18-25 and 18-26). Tubular vacuolization caused by formation of glycogen secondary to massive glycosuria ("Drummart-Ebstein lesion") is now rarely seen.

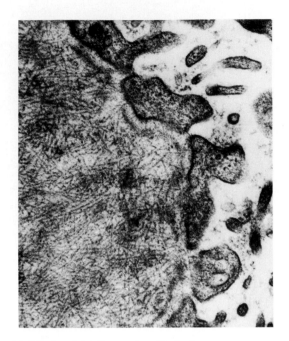

Fig. 18-25. Amyloid filaments with foot processes covering them. (40,000×.)

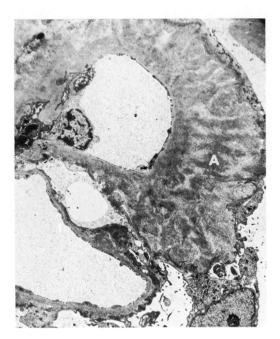

Fig. 18-26. Amyloidosis. Capillary wall thickened by amyloid filaments, *A.* (3400×.)

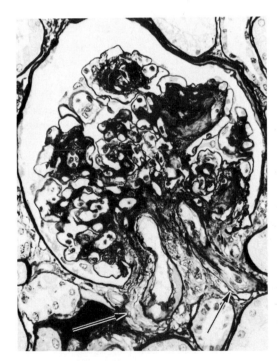

Fig. 18-27. Diabetic glomerulosclerosis. Notice nodules in glomerular lobules, basement membrane thickening, and hyaline arteriolar sclerosis involving both afferent and efferent arterioles, *arrows.* (Silver methenamine stain.)

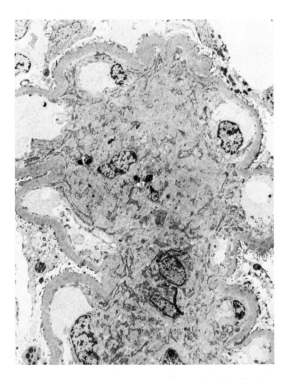

Fig. 18-28. Diabetic glomerulosclerosis. Capillaries with thick basement membranes surrounding mesangium enlarged by thick strands of mesangial matrix. (1300×.)

Amyloid deposits are commonly found in the interstitium, particularly adjacent to the distal tubules. Amyloid will surround the medullary tubules and vasa recta, eventually causing atrophy and fibrosis of the parenchyma. The cortex similarly progresses to tubular atrophy and interstitial fibrosis.

Amyloid AA and AL both involve the kidney. Proteinuria, typically in the nephrotic range, is a classic symptom of amyloidosis; it is attributable to the glomerular deposits. Approximately 50% of patients have significant proteinuria. The majority progress to chronic renal failure within a few years, often in a few months. There is no effective therapy.

Diabetic nephropathy

Nephropathy, a common complication of diabetes, is composed of three entities: severe arteriolar nephrosclerosis, glomerulosclerosis (Kimmelstiel-Wilson disease),[56] and often acute or chronic pyelonephritis. The most severe form of hyaline arteriolar sclerosis occurs in diabetes mellitus, and a unique hyaline involvement of both afferent and efferent arterioles is often seen. Hypertension accompanies this severe vascular change. In about 25% of diabetics, a peculiar massive deposition of basement membrane matrix occurs in the mesangium of some or many glomeruli (nodular intercapillary glomerulosclerosis, or Kimmelstiel-Wilson disease).[20,56] This deposition produces a typical globular hyaline ball in the center of a glomerular lobule with the capillaries displaced to the periphery (Fig. 18-27). Mesangial cells are increased but are peripherally displaced by the hyaline matrix. The basement membranes of the glomerular capillaries may be normal or thickened. Bright red deposits of fibrinoid material may block some of these capillaries. More commonly the glomeruli show a diffuse moderate thickening of capillary basement membranes and increased mesangial cellularity and matrix (diffuse diabetic glomerulosclerosis).[20] This diffuse process may or may not accompany the nodular form of Kimmelstiel-Wilson disease. The diffuse glomerular change mirrors the vascular membrane thickening of many small vessels in the body (diabetic angiopathy).

Electron microscopy of renal biopsy specimens reveals diffuse basement membrane thickening of capillaries and mesangium even in diabetes of relatively short duration, though this may not be discernible by light microscopy (Fig. 18-28). Chemical analysis of diabetic glomeruli indicates increased carbohydrate content in the basement membrane. This finding may explain the increased permeability and proteinuria noted in these patients. Hyaline nodular deposits in Bowman's capsule are said to be quite specific for diabetes.[56]

Foci of acute or chronic inflammation from pyelonephritis are common in the diabetic kidney and reflect the continuing problem diabetics have with bacterial infections. Tubular atrophy and interstitial fibrosis parallel vascular, glomerular, and pyelonephritic involvement. Clinically, proteinuria and hypertension reflect the development of diabetic nephropathy, which may progress slowly, resulting in renal or heart failure. Proteinuria is heavy enough to produce a nephrotic syndrome in about 5% of diabetics. A renal biopsy sample typically shows diffuse diabetic glomerulosclerosis in these nephrotic diabetics.

Congenital glomerular diseases

Inherited glomerular diseases are associated with altered basement membrane function. Congenital nephrotic syndrome[48] is characterized by the onset of severe nephrotic syndrome within the first few days or weeks of life. Death usually occurs within the first year. Some cases are familial, though most arise spontaneously. On biopsy, patients have either minimal change disease or a peculiar variant in which glomerular scarring is associated with microcystic dilatation of proximal tubules.

The most common hereditary glomerular disease is Alport's syndrome. Alport's syndrome can be inherited as either an autosomal dominant or an X-linked dominant disorder with variable penetrance.[39] In 30% to 50% of patients, it is associated with neurosensory deafness, particularly in the high-frequency range. Associated eye disorders include anterior lenticonus and perimacular deterioration. The glomerular basement membrane displays thinning and splitting of the lamina densa at irregularly scattered sites. This is observed only on ultrastructural examination. Routine histologic lesions are nonspecific and include mesangial widening, segmental sclerosis, and an associated interstitial infiltrate. Proteinuria is usually present, though not usually severe. Hematuria is very common. The disease usually progresses to diffuse glomerular sclerosis, tubar atrophy, and interstitial fibrosis, particularly in males. Females with the lesion show a much milder form of the disease. Recently an association between Alport's disease and lack of a noncollagenous basement membrane protein has been noted.[59] This protein serves to link and lock collagen fibrils into a semirigid membrane. Its absence or paucity may result in fragility of the basement membrane. Whether this association holds for all patients with Alport's remains to be seen.

Thin–basement membrane nephropathy associated with recurring hematuria has recently been described.[107] These patients exhibit a normal histologic appearance with light microscopy. Morphometric analysis of electron micrographs, however, reveals glomerular basement membranes approximately half the thickness of normal basement membranes. Except for recurrent hematuria, such patients are not known to develop additional evidence of renal pathosis.

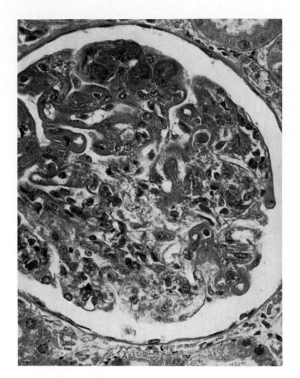

Fig. 18-29. Diffuse lupus glomerulonephritis with "wire loop" lesions and immune deposits.

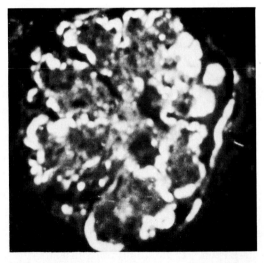

Fig. 18-30. Diffuse lupus glomerulonephritis stained with fluorescent antihuman IgG. Notice coarse loops and lumps of deposits. (Courtesy Dr. Claude Cornwall, Syracuse, N.Y.)

Systemic disease and glomerular injury

Glomeruli are susceptible to injury as a result of disease processes affecting the rest of the body. Two examples of this, diabetes and amyloid, were more conveniently discussed in the section dealing with glomerular proteinuria arising from structural abnormalities of the basement membrane. This section addresses secondary glomerular injury arising from systemic disease affecting the vascular system. We will start with the vasculitides and then proceed to paraproteinemias and systemic thrombotic disorders.

Glomerular vasculitides

Inflammatory diseases of the vascular tree frequently involve the kidney, reflecting not only the organ's vascularity but also the high pressures, potentially traumatic, unique to the glomerular capillary tuft. The most common of the glomerular vasculitides is systemic lupus erythematosus (SLE). It is also the most variable in its morphologic presentation and clinical course.

Systemic lupus erythematosus

SLE involves the kidney in 60% to 70% of cases. The renal glomeruli are the prime sites of injury in this disease. The mechanism of injury appears to be the trauma induced by the deposition of immune complexes, consisting of DNA–anti-DNA antibodies or, in some series, Ig–anti-Ig antibodies. The disease is intermittent, with episodes of flaring exacerbation interspersed with periods of remission. Acute renal injury tends to correlate with systemic evidence of clinical activation: fever, hypertension, increasing titers of circulating immune complexes and associated hypocomplementemia (secondary to activation), and increases in the erythrocyte sedimentation rate. Curiously, as renal function becomes increasingly insufficient, the systemic symptoms of SLE—the rash, arthritis, and fevers, for example—tend to become clinically less significant. Examination of the urine reveals proteinuria, hematuria, white and red blood cell casts, and oval fat bodies. The nephrotic syndrome develops in 20% to 30% of patients, a development carrying a poor prognosis.

The characteristic glomerular lesions of SLE include irregular hypercellularity of glomerular lobules associated with "fibrinoid" necrosis and nuclear karyorrhexis. The fibrinoid immune complex material is deposited as a thick coat in the mesangium and inside the glomerular basement membranes. This produces thick-walled capillary loops, the so-called "wire-loop lesion" (Figs. 18-29 and 18-30).

Electron microscopy demonstrates deposits of electron-dense protein between the endothelium and the lamina densa of the basement membrane. The deposits also accumulate in the mesangium adjacent to the basement membrane (Fig. 18-31). In reaction to this inflam-

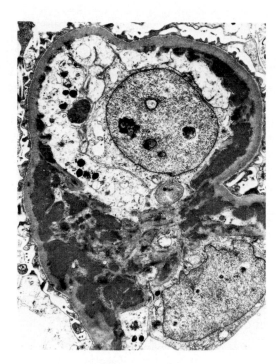

Fig. 18-31. Systemic lupus erythematosus with subendothelial and mesangial deposits. (6000×.)

mation, epithelial crescents, adhesions to Bowman's capsule, and glomerular scarring occur. Occasional hyaline thrombi are seen in glomerular capillary lumens. Fuzzy basophilic aggregates of nuclear material (hematoxylin bodies) occasionally may be seen in zones of necrosis. In more severe cases a lymphoid and plasma cell intertubular infiltrate is present.

Although the ultrastructural hallmark of SLE is the presence of immune complexes in the basement membrane, in subendothelial and in subepithelial distribution, as well as in the mesangium, morphologically the disease can manifest itself in one of six different patterns,[70,99] summarized below:

Minimal disease. A small number of patients have no significant histologic abnormality when biopsied, despite the presence of small amounts of immune complexes upon ultrastructural analysis.

Mesangial glomerulonephritis. There is mesangial hypercellularity, consisting of proliferating mesangial cells and infiltrating monocytes. By electron microscopy and immunofluorescence, immune complexes are concentrated in the mesangium. They are typically IgG or IgG/IgA. C3 is also detectable.

Focal proliferative glomerulonephritis. There is focal endothelial and mesangial cell proliferation and leukocyte infiltration. Some glomeruli may be relatively unaffected. Granular IgG and complement is found in the mesangium and capillaries. There are moderate subendothelial and mesangial deposits on electron microscopy.

Diffuse proliferative glomerulonephritis. All glomeruli are hypercellular with extensive immune complexes in the capillaries and the mesangium. These may be focal areas of necrotizing inflammation with fibrin deposition. Epithelial crescents are frequently observed.

Membranous lupus glomerulonephritis. This type resembles idiopathic membranous nephropathy with proteinuria, thickened basement membranes, extensive subepithelial deposits, and relatively little inflammatory infiltrate.

Sclerosing nephropathy. Sclerosing nephropathy is a steadily progressing sclerotic process in which glomerular structures are segmentally and then globally replaced by hyaline material, resulting in diffusely scarred, atrophic glomeruli.

• • •

Prognosis is related to histologic pattern.[8,62] Mesangial and focal glomerulonephritis have the slowest progression of renal injury. Current therapy consists in an immunosuppressive regimen of corticosteroids, frequently coupled with cytotoxic agents such as cyclophosphamide. Recently a combination of prednisone and intermittent, intravenous cyclophosphamide has been shown to be highly efficacious with relatively few side effects. If patients progress to renal transplantation, recurrence of SLE in the renal allograft is quite rare.

It has recently been observed that the degree of interstitial inflammation correlates with the severity of progression of renal disease. It has further been appreciated that the responsiveness of the patient to therapy correlates with the degree of activity or chronicity of the lupus histologic pattern.[8] Active lesions, more amenable to immunosuppression, are characterized by the presence of (1) proliferation, (2) necrosis with karyorrhexis, (3) hyaline thrombi, (4) cellular crescents, and (5) cellular, interstitial inflammation. Relatively resistent to therapeutic intervention are those cases of lupus nephritis with the attributes of chronicity: (1) glomerular sclerosis, (2) fibrous crescents, (3) tubular atrophy, and (4) interstitial fibrosis.

Polyarteritis nodosa[28]

The kidneys are affected in 70% to 80% of patients with polyarteritis nodosa, an acute inflammatory disease of arteries, and renal failure is common.

This disorder is divided into a classic form with predominant involvement of larger muscular arteries often producing aneurysms and infarcts and a microscopic form with predominantly small artery and glomerular involvement. Immunofluorescence studies fail to show evidence of immune complexes in most cases; however, some cases do show immunoglobulin deposits in both arteries and glomeruli. Hypertension is common with polyarteritis, and renal failure is often the mode of death, particularly in the microscopic form. The glomeruli may show ischemic wrinkling, focal glomerulitis with necrosis and epithelial crescents, or diffuse proliferative glomerulonephritis. There may be considerable morphologic heterogeneity within the same biopsy specimen. Corticosteroids are used for therapy, but the disease tends to progress.

Wegener's granulomatosis[28]

Wegener's granulomatosis is characterized by necrotizing granulomas typically affecting the nasal sinuses, the lungs, and the kidneys. Granulomas are occasionally seen on renal biopsy; more typical is the presence of diffuse proliferative glomerulonephritis with acute necrosis. Immunofluorescence is not helpful, and deposits are rare by ultrastructural analysis. Combination therapy of corticosteroids and cyclophosphamide has greatly improved the formerly grim prognosis.

Scleroderma (progressive systemic sclerosis)[14]

About 40% of patients dying of scleroderma show severe renal involvement and renal failure. The striking changes are intimal proliferation of arcuate arteries and afferent arterioles. Severe hypertension may develop with severe renal involvement, contributing to the changes. Acute thrombonecrotic changes in arterioles and glomeruli closely resemble those in malignant nephrosclerosis but may develop before severe hypertension. Severe interstitial fibrosis and tubular atrophy accompany the vascular involvement.

Paraproteinemia and secondary glomerular disease

Cryoimmunoglobulinemia and light-chain disease are two classical examples of systemic paraproteinemias causing inflammatory glomerular injury.

The glomerular lesion of mixed cryoimmunoglobulinemia resembles membranoproliferative glomerulonephritis.[10] There is considerable monocyte infiltration, mesangial proliferation with new basement membrane synthesis associated with mesangial interposition, and subendothelial and mesangial deposits of IgG and IgM. There is often associated arteriolar vasculitis. Such patients present with hematuria, red blood cell casts, and proteinuria, often in the nephrotic range. The immediate cause of injury is the deposition of cryoimmunoglobulins, immune complexes consisting of IgM antibody directed against another immunoglobulin, usually IgG. The IgM component of the complexes tends to precipitate at temperatures below 37° C and gives the syndrome its name. High circulating levels of cryoimmunoglobulins are associated with B-cell proliferative disorders and systemic vasculitides or can present as a primary, idiopathic disorder.

Although multiple myeloma preferentially affects the interstitium, a distinct subset of patients with multiple myeloma present with a glomerular lesion consisting of nodular deposits within the mesangium associated with mesangial hypercellularity. By light microscopy, the lesion resembles diabetic nodular glomerulosclerosis. When it was appreciated that the deposits consisted of monoclonal light chains of immunoglobulin, the disease was termed "light-chain nephropathy."[84] This lesion is also seen in association with lymphoma and benign monoclonal gammopathies. The disease is associated with the synthesis of free immunoglobulin light chains that are not necessarily associated with abnormal levels of intact monoclonal immunoglobulins. Patients with light-chain nephropathy usually present with significant proteinuria and moderate renal insufficiency. The clinical course reflects the prognosis of the underlying systemic disorder.

Thrombotic renal disease

A group of diseases characterized by fibrin and platelet thrombus formation in arterioles and glomeruli of the kidney can cause acute renal failure. These cases may result from initiation of disseminated intravascular coagulation triggered by bacteremia (gram-negative endotoxic shock, gram-positive bacterial sepsis) and accidents of childbirth (abruptio placentae, amniotic fluid embolism, toxemia of pregnancy).[72] Often the renal involvement in these states is overshadowed by other systemic symptoms. When arterial and capillary fibrinous thrombosis is massive and associated with shock, as in abruptio placentae or endotoxic shock, bilateral renocortical necrosis may develop.[40] Even if the patient survives the primary disease, the renal lesion is often lethal. Bilateral renocortical necrosis exhibits symmetric infarction of the renal cortex and columns of Bertin and thrombotic occlusion of small arteries adjacent to the infarction.

If vascular obstruction is less extreme, even with acute impairment of renal function, permanent loss of renal function is not to be expected. Apparently, most of the thrombi are rapidly lysed and only focal scars result.

Hemolytic uremic syndrome is closely related to the aforementioned diseases. It usually occurs in children but is seen in adults.[32,110] An acute arteriolar and glomerular thrombotic process associated with thrombocytopenia occurs often after an acute gastroenteritis, with anatomic damage limited to the kidney (Figs. 18-32 and 18-33). Viral infections and infections with some strains of *Escherichia coli* have been clinically associated with onset of the disease. The thrombi cause acute renal failure; in addition, extensive fragmentation of red blood cells results from blood perfusing the damaged vessels. The fragmented cells hemolyze, and ane-

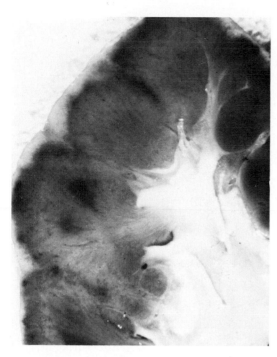

Fig. 18-32. Hemolytic uremic syndrome with cortical necrosis. Notice white infarcted outer cortex.

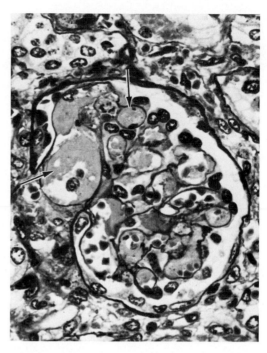

Fig. 18-33. Hemolytic uremic syndrome. Notice thrombi in entering arteriole and glomerular capillaries, *arrows*. (Silver methenamine stain.)

mia results. Most patients recover, but with severe involvement there may be fatal bilateral cortical necrosis or residual severe damage to arterioles and glomeruli.

Thrombotic thrombocytopenic purpura closely resembles the hemolytic uremic syndrome, but it involves various organs such as the central nervous system and has prolonged or recurrent activity usually ending in death.[86] Corticosteroids and plasmapheresis have been employed in the therapy of hemolytic uremic syndrome and thrombotic, thrombocytopenic purpura. More recently, a syndrome resembling hemolytic uremia has been observed in patients with renal allografts who are taking cyclosporine. The only effective therapy is to stop the drug. However, once intravascular thrombosis has started, the allograft is frequently lost even in the absence of additional cyclosporine. A morphologically similar disorder may follow pregnancy or prolonged use of oral contraceptive agents.[96]

Toxemia of pregnancy (preeclampsia and eclampsia)

In the third trimester of pregnancy, proteinuria, edema, and hypertension may develop. This clinical syndrome is called "preeclampsia." If the condition becomes more severe with decreased renal function, convulsions, and perhaps death, it is called "eclampsia." Women whose mothers had toxemia have a high risk of the condition. This syndrome may be simulated by es-

sential hypertension or chronic glomerulonephritis or other chronic renal disease in a pregnant woman. The clinical syndrome is therefore pathophysiologically heterogeneous, and statements regarding natural history or clinical course must be interpreted with caution.

In true toxemia of pregnancy the glomeruli are the main site of involvement. By light microscopy the glomeruli are revealed to be swollen without increased cellularity but are relatively bloodless because of narrowed or collapsed capillary channels. The mesangium is swollen, and the capillary walls often appear thickened as a result of deposition of a thin layer of pink fibrinoid material and as a result of endothelial cell swelling. Electron microscopy reveals hydropic swellings of endothelial and mesangial cell cytoplasm and electron-dense protein deposits between the endothelium and glomerular basement membrane and in the mesangium[40,80] (Fig. 18-34). Fluorescent antibody studies have shown that the glomerular protein deposits are predominantly fibrin.[109] It appears that circulating, partially polymerized fibrinogen is present as a result of activation of the clotting mechanism and is trapped in the glomerulus. This apparently leads to the increased glomerular permeability and proteinuria. The tubular changes seen in toxemia of pregnancy (hyaline droplets, fatty droplets, and cloudy swelling) are believed to be the result of glomerular disease.

After delivery of the baby and if the hypertension has been appropriately treated, a remarkable resolution of

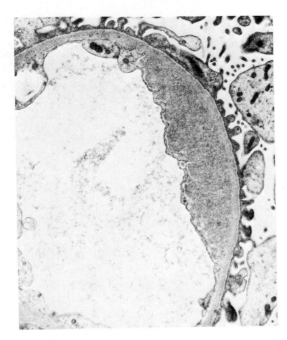

Fig. 18-34. Toxemia of pregnancy. Fibrin between endothelium and basement membrane of glomerular capillary. (7000×.)

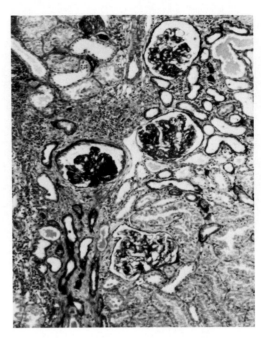

Fig. 18-35. Chronic progressive glomerulonephritis. Notice glomeruli in various stages of scarring and patchy tubular atrophy.

glomerular morphology to normal may be expected, and urinary findings return to normal.[40] Hypertension occurs after toxemia of pregnancy in 40% to 50% of patients. It is not clear whether toxemia causes this hypertension, merely hastens its onset, or is a nonspecific complication of preexisting renal disease unrelated to pregnancy.

Chronic glomerular injury

The injured glomerulus has a limited response to injury, regardless of whether the etiologic agent was immunologic, metabolic, or vascular in origin. A small, contracted, scarred kidney appears to be the final common pathway.[47] It is difficult in this late stage to recognize the nature of the preceding process because of the extensive scarring. Such a kidney may be formed from the progression of acute glomerulonephritis, poststreptococcal or nonstreptococcal, rapidly progressive glomerulonephritis, hereditary nephritis, lipoid nephrosis, membranous glomerulonephritis, or focal glomerulonephritis. A large group is first recognized in terminal renal failure with no antecedent history. This group is diagnosed on biopsy, for want of a better term, as chronic, progressive glomerulonephritis.

Chronic progressive glomerulonephritis is characterized by smoldering activity over a period of years. Proteinuria and microscopic hematuria may be the only signs for a long time. Some cases occur after a clinical attack of acute glomerulonephritis, but most appear insidiously with no preceding history of renal problems. In some patients, early or late in the disease, such severe proteinuria occurs that hypoproteinemia and a nephrotic syndrome develop. As the scarring progresses in the kidneys, hypertension is often seen. Renal failure slowly develops as the number of functioning nephrons is depleted.

Renal biopsy during the smoldering active phase of the disease shows two types of reaction: a chronic proliferative pattern in which most glomeruli show at least some degree of scarring or the focal pattern in which normal glomeruli are associated with scattered glomeruli in various stages of scarring (Fig. 18-35). Tubular atrophy, interstitial fibrosis, and arteriosclerosis increase with the degree of glomerular involvement and loss.

At the end stage of all forms of glomerular disease the kidneys are small and firm with a granular, pebbly surface to which the renal capsule is adherent (Fig. 18-36). The renal cortices are irregularly thinned and scarred with loss of normal architectural markings. Microscopically the majority of the glomeruli are the site of intense scarring and hyalinization (Figs. 18-35 and 18-37). Many old glomerular scars have been resorbed, and so the number of glomeruli is decreased. Tubular atrophy is pronounced, with irregular dilated tubules interspersed with small shrunken tubules. There is a

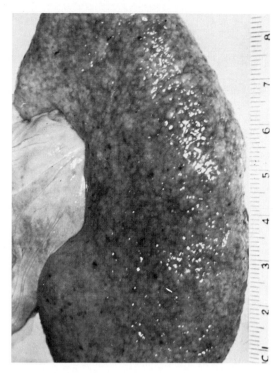

Fig. 18-36. End-stage chronic glomerulonephritis. Pebbly surface corresponds to surviving hypertrophied nephrons amid atrophy.

high degree of interstitial fibrosis, and a mild infiltrate of lymphocytes and histiocytes is seen in the stroma. A few, less severely damaged nephrons remain with enlarged, partially scarred glomeruli and hypertrophied tubules. Medium-sized and small arteries commonly show pronounced intimal and medial proliferation. The hyperplastic arteriosclerosis is a reaction both to the obliterated renal vascular bed and to the hypertension that is usually present. In some cases in which the hypertension has become severe, there may be evidence of fibrinoid necrosis and hemorrhage in the vessel walls.

In our experience, the anatomic nature of the underlying renal lesion is unknown in more than half of patients with chronic progressive renal disease coming to chronic hemodialysis or renal transplantation.

TUBULOINTERSTITIAL DISEASE

Tubulointerstitial diseases are a diverse group of disorders that directly involve the tubules and interstitium to a greater degree than the glomeruli and vasculature.

The variety of histologic lesions associated with any one disease and the heterogeneity of involvement of different segments of the tubules has made pathologic classifications exceedingly difficult. Thus interstitial diseases tend to be classified by etiologic agents rather than by histologic pattern. Furthermore, the response of the tubules to a wide range of mechanical injury is even more limited than that of the glomerulus. Thus highly diverse disease states may share remarkably similar pathologic findings.

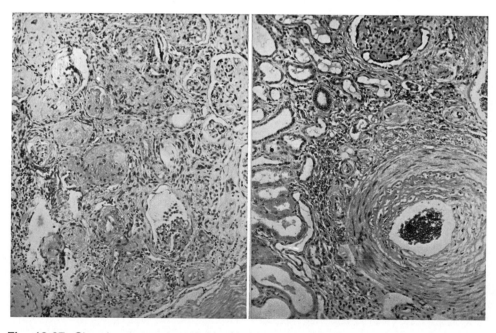

Fig. 18-37. Chronic glomerulonephritis. Notice glomerular capsular adhesions and hyalinization and thickening of blood vessels.

One fundamental classification that is helpful is the distinction between acute and chronic injury. Acute interstitial injury is characterized by tubular cell swelling, vacuolization, and necrosis if sufficiently severe. Interstitial edema separating the normally closely opposed tubules is readily apparent. There is often an inflammatory cell infiltrate even in the setting of nonimmunologic diseases. Chronic interstitial disease is characterized by interstitial fibrosis, mononuclear cell infiltrates, and tubular atrophy and dilatation. As tubules atrophy, they undergo a process known as tubular simplification in which the different segments of the nephron come to resemble each other. There is a considerable loss of cytoplasm, the disappearance of specialized membrane features such as the brush border of the proximal tubule cells, and, in areas of scar or severe fibrosis, a thickening of the tubular basement membrane. The result is an array of homogeneous, tubular structures with dilated lumens and flattened epithelium.

Functional disturbances

Tubular injury is expressed in a bewildering variety of ways. The heterogeneity of clinical symptoms reflects variations in both time and place of injury along the length of nephrons.[26] Most forms of tubular injury are associated with a decrease in glomerular filtration that is known to be a reflex of some type but whose mechanism is not yet understood. This is why the clinical severity of inflammatory diseases of the kidney tends to correlate better with the intensity of the interstitial lesions rather than with that of the glomeruli. Injury to proximal tubules is associated with impaired bicarbonate reabsorption and hydrogen excretion (proximal renal tubular acidosis) and proteinuria secondary to impaired reabsorption of low molecular weight proteins filtered by the glomerulus (proteinuria is usually not within the nephrotic range, that is, exceeding 3 g/day). Proximal tubule dysfunction may also be manifest by urine excretion of glucose, phosphate, amino acids, and other solutes and sodium wasting. Medullary injury causes urinary excretion of both salt and water. Distal tubule injury can be associated with impaired potassium and hydrogen excretion (distal renal tubular acidosis), sodium wasting, and nephrogenic diabetes insipidus. Some disorders preferentially affect a segment of the nephron; more typically, however, some or all segments are involved, producing an array of renal deficiencies.

The causes of tubulointerstitial disease are usually diverse. They reflect the specialized role of the kidney as a principal transporter of wastes and toxins, its unique environment of a highly hypertonic interstitium, and its vulnerability as a network of capillary plexuses, first intraglomerular and then peritubular, in which the vas-

Table 18-2. Common causes of tubulointerstitial injury

Acute ischemia	Acute tubular necrosis, emboli
Chronic ischemia	Hypertensive nephrosclerosis Sickle cell anemia
Toxic	Endogenous Calcium Oxalate Myoglobulin Exogenous Lead and other heavy metals Analgesics Contrast media Radiation
Infectious	Acute pyelonephritis Tuberculosis
Immunologic	Allergic interstitial nephritis Sarcoidosis Systemic lupus erythematosus Sjögren's syndrome
Metabolic	Diabetes
Abnormal protein deposition	Multiple myeloma Amyloid Light-chain disease
Genetic	Polycystic disease Medullary cystic disease
Pressure and flow abnormalities	Urinary tract obstruction Reflux nephropathy

cular compartment is exposed to high pressures and extreme fluxes of water and solutes.

Table 18-2 provides a partial list, categorized by etiology, of interstitial disorders. There is only space to discuss a limited number, selected for their exemplifying characteristic attributes of unique types of injury.

Acute tubular necrosis

Acute tubular necrosis resulting from a variety of mechanisms is the most important and common cause of acute renal failure.[65] Because of the reparative and regenerative capability of renal tubules, if the patient can survive the initial period of renal failure and concurrent disease, excellent recovery of renal function can be expected.

The onset of the acute renal failure may be abrupt when associated with severe injury or may be gradual if the injury develops slowly. Pronounced oliguria develops, with a progressive rise in nitrogenous waste products in the blood. Complete anuria is rarely seen. This oliguric phase may last from 4 days to a month but usually is about 10 to 12 days. It is during this stage that water and salt overload and hyperkalemia are dangerous problems. The small amount of urine formed is of low osmolality and may contain tubular cell casts, red blood cells, and some protein. When hemolysis has been a feature of the disease, hemoglobin also is present in the urine.

After 10 to 12 days the urinary volume in such a patient will typically be increased to over 1 liter per 24 hours. In this early diuretic phase the urine is still of low osmolality, and considerable sodium, potassium, and chloride may be lost in the urine. Up to 25% of deaths occur during this critical period. There may be little lowering of blood urea and creatinine levels despite the diuresis. As tubular regeneration is completed, about day 17, renal concentrating ability improves, and there is a rapid fall in blood urea levels.

Prognosis of acute tubular necrosis depends, to a considerable extent, on the causative agents. In patients with associated severe lesions, such as peritonitis, extensive burns, or severe surgical trauma, which are life threatening in themselves, there is a high mortality. Patients with acute tubular necrosis uncomplicated by severe systemic disease, as is seen in a hemolytic transfusion reaction or a toxic injury, have an excellent prognosis with modern therapy, which includes water and electrolyte control and peritoneal dialysis or hemodialysis.

Acute tubular necrosis may be associated with a large variety of diseases, but the immediate causes may be divided into (1) those of toxic origin (toxic nephropathy) and (2) those related to pronounced hypovolemia, shock, and renal vasoconstriction (ischemic acute tubular necrosis). Often, toxic and ischemic factors complement each other in producing the tubular injury.

Toxic nephropathy. Toxic nephropathy may result from general poisons damaging tubular epithelium such as mercuric chloride, carbon tetrachloride, ethylene glycol (antifreeze), insecticides, antibiotics such as polymyxin and amphotericin B, and iodinated organic compounds used as contrast materials in roentgenographic studies.[97]

Acute mercury nephropathy is a characteristic example of this type of injury. Mercuric chloride is sometimes taken in a suicide attempt. Those patients who do not die of shock within the first day develop acute renal failure with pronounced oliguria. If the kidneys are examined between the fifth and tenth days, they are found to be swollen and pale. Microscopically the epithelium of the proximal convoluted tubules is necrotic and desquamated into the lumen and may undergo striking dystrophic calcification (Fig. 18-38). The regenerating epithelium is seen lining the tubular basement membrane and is flat and thin and contains occasional mitoses.

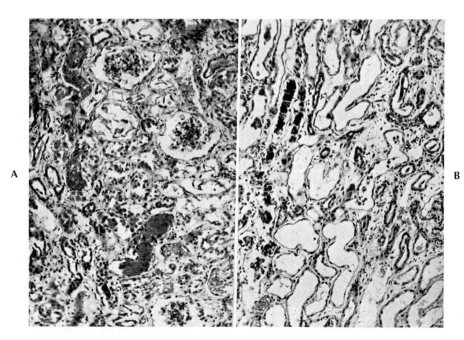

Fig. 18-38. Mercury bichloride poisoning in kidney. **A,** Kidney on seventh day after ingestion of mercury. Notice desquamation and destruction of tubular epithelium. **B,** Kidney on eleventh day. Notice loss of tubular epithelium, flattened tubular lining, and dark calcium masses in tubular lumens.

Other poisons may produce relatively characteristic appearances. Ethylene glycol (antifreeze) induces tubular necrosis with innumerable calcium oxalate crystals in the tubular lumens. A few round, slightly greenish concretions of calcium oxalate may be seen in a variety of cases of acute tubular necrosis, particularly those associated with liver damage. Dioxane and diethylene glycol produce a distinctive ballooning, hydropic degeneration of proximal convoluted tubules, progressing to focal hemorrhagic cortical necrosis. The tubular necrosis of carbon tetrachloride poisoning is characterized by large amounts of neutral fat in the basal portions of proximal convoluted tubules. Although it has no characteristic pathosis, lead nephropathy should be mentioned as one of the more common forms of heavy metal toxicity.[112] Initially described in workers in lead mines, it is increasingly seen in areas associated with lead contamination of the air, secondary to vehicle exhaust, and with ingestion of lead-based paint, as occurs in children in economically depressed urban areas. Lead nephropathy is a chronic interstitial lesion manifested by interstitial fibrosis and tubular atrophy. Dense basophilic intranuclear inclusions may be found in renal tubular epithelial cells. Hypertension and gouty arthritis may occur clinically.

Tubular lesions secondary to therapeutic agents

Tubular injury lesions associated with therapeutic agents include analgesic nephropathy, contrast nephropathy, radiation nephritis, and acute tubular necrosis secondary to drugs such as the aminoglycoside antibiotics. The pathology of drug-induced acute tubular necrosis is not unique and will not be discussed further.

Analgesic abuse nephropathy

Analgesic abuse (phenacetin nephropathy) is a major cause of papillary necrosis and chronic renal failure. These patients tend to be middle-aged women in warm climates who have consumed several kilograms of phenacetin-aspirin mixtures over several years. Recurrent pyelonephritis, hypertension, and renal colic from passing necrotic papillae are common clinical manifestations. Analgesic nephropathy, one of the principal causes of renal failure in Australia, is particularly associated with necrosis of the renal papillae of one or both kidneys. Acutely sloughed papillae can cause acute obstruction, with symptoms of back pain, hematuria, and ureteral colic. Experimental data are confusing but indicate that aspirin as well as phenacetin may contribute to the process. The prognosis of analgesic abuse nephropathy is better than the other papillary necrosis processes, and about two thirds remain stable or improve after drug abuse is stopped.[58]

Pathologically the appearance of the kidney with analgesic abuse is variable in that the process often extends over a long time.[11] At first only yellow necrotic tips of papillae are seen. Later the papillae become dark, shrunken, sloughed, or even calcified. The surface of the renal cortex overlying these necrotic papillae is depressed whereas the intervening cortex between papillae is raised so that nodules or ridges are produced. Microscopically the necrotic papillae are structureless and sclerotic. The renal cortex shows tubular atrophy, interstitial fibrosis, and varying amounts of chronic inflammatory reaction.

It has been reported that analgesic abuse patients appear to have an increased incidence of renal transitional cell carcinomas.

Contrast nephropathy

Contrast nephropathy is a form of acute renal failure occurring after the use of iodinated contrast agents intravenously for radiologic visualization. It typically occurs in the setting of cerebral, cardiac, or renal angiography. The cause is obscure, but predisposing risk factors have been identified. In order of importance they include preceding renal insufficiency, diabetes mellitus, multiple myeloma, volume depletion, and age. Pathologic features include tubular cell vacuolization and interstitial inflammation. The mechanism appears to be a combination of direct tubular toxicity and renal ischemia (causing increased concentration of the agent in the tubular lumen). The renal failure is slowly reversible, less so in those with precontrast insufficiency. It is best prevented by use of contrast dye only when strictly indicated, volume repletion, and vigorous diuresis while the dye is being administered.

Radiation nephritis

Treatment of the abdomen with high doses of ionizing radiation may result in renal damage, hypertension, and renal failure after a latent period of 6 to 12 months.[66] Thrombonecrotic (fibrinoid) changes develop in the particularly susceptible glomeruli and in arterioles. Tubular atrophy is moderate early in the disease but may become severe. Changes resulting from severe or malignant hypertension may be superimposed.

Ischemic acute tubular necrosis

The many clinical states predisposing to ischemic acute tubular necrosis share the underlying feature of intense renal vasoconstriction, initiating an irreversible sequence of tubular damage.

The factors that provide the background for development of ischemic acute tubular injury are dehydration, hypovolemia, shock, renal arterial vasoconstriction, and often the presence of hemoglobinuria, myoglobinuria, jaundice, or toxins from bacterial infections. Typical clinical situations in which such tubular injury occurs are as follows:

1. Mismatched blood transfusion, or other circumstances with massive hemolysis, such as infection with *Plasmodium malariae*.
2. Massive crushing injury in which myoglobin is released from damaged muscle in the presence of shock
3. Massive cutaneous burns with hemolysis of red blood cells and inadequate fluid replacement
4. Severe bacterial infection, such as generalized peritonitis
5. Massive hemorrhage with inadequate replacement

The mechanisms contributing to oliguria after acute tubular necrosis are outlined in the previous section on acute tubular injury. Experimental and clinical data indicate that renocortical ischemia occurs in either toxic or ischemic tubular necrosis. A massive increase in epithelial intracellular calcium may be a common, toxic pathway of injury.[113]

The kidneys of patients dying after 10 days of renal failure are grossly swollen and show a pale cortex separated from a darker medulla by a "sooty halo." Microscopically the kidney of ischemic tubular necrosis frequently shows somewhat dilated proximal convoluted tubules lined by a low epithelium (Fig. 18-39). The distal tubules characteristically are dilated with flattened cells having basophilic cytoplasm. Granular reddish or brownish casts (heme casts) may be seen in the distal tubules or collecting ducts, particularly at the juxtamedullary zone. The tubular epithelium adjacent to the cast is often degenerating, and the basement membrane may be disrupted (tubulorrhexis). The casts that rupture into the interstitial tissues may result in small granulomas and in thrombosis of adjacent venules. Solez, Morel-Maroger, and Sraer[112] have demonstrated that reduction of the brush borders of proximal tubules is particularly characteristic of acute tubular necrosis. The tremendous normal luminal and antiluminal surface areas necessary for pumping electrolytes are severely decreased. This may result in a sodium- and chloride-rich fluid reaching the juxtaglomerular complex, which may produce vasoconstriction (tubuloglomerular feedback) and sustained oliguria.[77] The glomeruli characteristically show no lesions. Interstitial edema separating the tubules often is seen.

Reversible tubular lesions

Osmotic (sucrose) nephrosis. When hypertonic solutions of sucrose or mannitol or similar substances are given intravenously, as in the treatment of cerebral edema, a hydropic swelling of the proximal tubules of the kidney results (Fig. 18-40). This change is caused by the filling of the cytoplasm of these cells with innumerable, small pinocytic vesicles. This is generally an

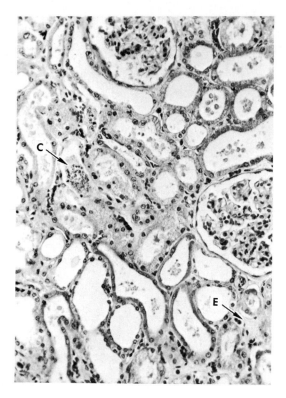

Fig. 18-39. Ischemic acute tubular necrosis with low regenerating tubular epithelium, dilated lumens, casts, *C,* and intertubular edema, *E.* (120×.)

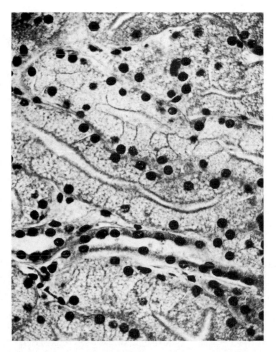

Fig. 18-40. Osmotic nephrosis. Notice proximal tubular cells laden with pinocytic vesicles.

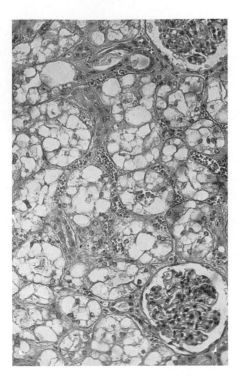

Fig. 18-41. Hypokalemic (vacuolar) nephropathy of potassium deficiency from case of regional enteritis. (Courtesy Dr. Joseph F. Kuzma; from Anderson, W.A.D.: Synopsis of pathology, ed. 10, St. Louis, 1980, The C.V. Mosby Co.)

asymptomatic and promptly reversible lesion.

Hypokalemic (vacuolar) nephropathy. In severe chronic potassium depletion such as that seen in chronic diarrhea, impairment of the renal concentrating mechanism may result, with the development of large vacuoles at the basal portion of the cytoplasm of mainly the proximal convoluted tubules (Fig. 18-41). Electron microscopy shows these vacuoles to be the result of pronounced distension of the basal infoldings of these cells. These distended infoldings are believed to be caused by a disturbance of electrolyte transport. With potassium therapy the functional and structural changes revert to normal.

PYELONEPHRITIS[5]

The etiology and pathogenesis of lower as well as upper urinary tract infection are interrelated. Most cases of acute pyelonephritis occur after infection of the lower tract.

Escherichia coli is the cause of 85% of urinary tract infections. Other common pathogens are *Proteus, Enterococcus, Pseudomonas, Klebsiella,* and *Staphylococcus.* With recurrent acute attacks the latter organisms are more common and may be more resistant to antibiotics. All the organisms excluding *Staphylococcus* are

inhabitants of the colon and normally colonize the perineal skin about the urethral orifices, awaiting an opportunity for invasion, which can occur spontaneously or by inoculation by catheterization.

The pathogenesis of lower urinary tract infection depends on introduction of the organism and depression of normal antibacterial mechanisms. Organisms may more readily gain access to the female bladder because of the shorter urethra and urethrovesical reflux in which straining forces bladder urine into the contaminated upper urethra. This urine may then passively reflux into the bladder. These features help explain the high incidence in females. Sexual activity and childbearing are additional contributing factors.

Catheterization of the bladder is of profound significance in urinary infection. The combination of carrying in organisms and mechanical damage is important. Indwelling catheters routinely cause cystitis. Normal antibacterial mechanisms in the lower urinary tract may be depressed by mechanical obstruction and stasis of urine. Infection of the urinary tract is common therefore in congenital urinary tract anomalies, prostatic hyperplasia, spinal cord injury with cord bladder, and pregnancy. Diabetes mellitus also predisposes to infection. By contrast, voluminous hypotonic urine and frequent micturition aid local antibacterial factors.

Once acute cystitis is established, the pathogenesis of infection of the kidney is not so clear. Although lymphogenous spread to the kidney is generally discounted, hematogenous and direct ascending intraluminal spread may occur. Animal experiments indicate that both mechanisms may induce bacterial infection of the kidney and renal pelvis, though at least transient obstruction is needed to lower resistance in a normal kidney to permit infection except with highly virulent organisms such as staphylococci. In humans there is little evidence that bacteremia precedes nonstaphylococcal acute pyelonephritis. Yet in acute pyelonephritis, characteristically, with absence of obstruction one sees a wedge-shaped zone of inflammation involving papilla and cortex with the remaining kidney free of disease, a condition suggestive of vascular inoculation. Ureterovesical reflux is demonstrable in some patients and so indicates a direct manner of carrying organisms to the kidney.[55] The problem of hematogenous versus the ascending route of infection remains unsettled. Once the kidney is infected, the papilla in particular is susceptible to colonization because its high stromal osmolality interferes with white blood cell and complement function. Intrarenal scarring in the healing process causes intrarenal obstruction, which also lowers resistance and aids intrarenal spread of infection.

Clinically, lower tract infection is characterized by dysuria, frequency, and bacteriuria. A bacterial colony count on cultured urine over 100,000 colonies per mil-

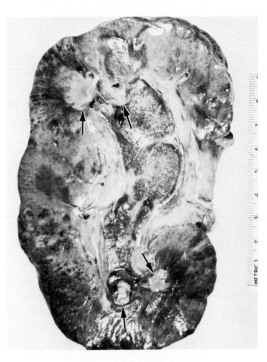

Fig. 18-42. Papillary necrosis resulting from acute pyelo-nephritis and obstruction. Notice necrotic papillae *(arrows)*, mottled patchy cortical infiltrate of acute pyelone-phritis, and congested, dilated renal pelvis.

liliter indicates an established infection. Patients with acute pyelonephritis clinically exhibit fever, chills, flank pain, and costovertebral angle tenderness. Urinalysis will show mild proteinuria, red blood cells, many white blood cells, and white cell inclusion casts. In absence of bilateral obstruction, the blood urea nitrogen is not elevated. Acute pyelonephritis in the absence of obstruction is characterized grossly by a swollen wedge-shaped area involving the papilla and adjacent cortex, infiltrated by gray-white foci of inflammatory reaction. Microscopically there are neutrophils in the tubules and in the edematous stroma. Microabscesses may be present. The glomeruli are relatively spared. The adjacent, uninvolved kidney is without lesions.

With acute obstruction the process may spread to extensively involve the kidney and even produce necrosis of the renal papillae (Fig. 18-42).

Hematogenous pyelonephritis caused by *Staphylococcus* differs in that multiple cortical abscesses may be seen occurring after bacteremia. Sometimes these produce a large, localized, tumorlike, multilocular abscess—carbuncle of the kidney—which may be confounding clinically. A serious complication of staphylococcal acute pyelonephritis is extrarenal rupture of a cortical abscess and development of a huge perinephric abscess.

If obstruction is absent or corrected, acute pyelonephritis responds well to treatment, leaving one or more depressed wedge-shaped zones of fibrosis, tubular atrophy, and collapsed atrophic glomeruli.

Recurrent and chronic pyelonephritis

Unfortunately the very features that resulted in the first episode of acute pyelonephritis are inclined to result in recurrent episodes. Thus ensues the problem of recurrent and chronic pyelonephritis in which multiple foci of bacterial infection gradually destroy renal function until the reserve of normal kidney is consumed, and chronic renal failure supervenes. When the process is unilateral, extreme destruction, scarring, and contraction may occur, and so the end-stage scar may be misinterpreted as a congenital hypoplasia.

Pathologically the kidney in chronic pyelonephritis[29] may be recognized by multiple wedge-shaped scars involving cortex and papillae. The surface of the kidney exhibits a U-shaped depression over these scars in contrast to the sharply depressed V-shaped scars of vascular disease. The corresponding minor calyx is dilated. Intervening zones of relatively normal kidney lie between the scars. Microscopically one sees in the kidney chronic interstitial inflammatory reaction with lymphocytes and plasma cells, often with foci of neutrophils. The interstitium shows varying degrees of dilated or atrophic tubules, often containing many colloidlike casts. There is pronounced interstitial fibrosis. The glomeruli, though relatively spared, may exhibit varying degrees of periglomerular fibrosis and may collapse, becoming converted to hyaline pellets. Secondary intimal hyperplasia of small muscular arteries is present, but severe vascular changes are usually associated with concomitant hypertension (Fig. 18-43).

In the literature there is a great discrepancy in the supposed incidence of chronic pyelonephritis seen at autopsy, varying from 1.4% to 33%. Using rigid criteria to eliminate other causes of chronic interstitial inflammation, most authors believe that the incidence is only about 1.5% to 3%.[57] It appears that cases of chronic renal failure that may have been loosely called chronic pyelonephritis in the past were actually nonbacterial reflux nephropathy or other tubulointerstitial lesions.

Tuberculous pyelonephritis

Hematogenous spread to the kidneys occurs from pulmonary or other foci of infection. Progressive renal tuberculosis results from hematogenous seeding of the renal cortex to form small caseous foci that spread to the medulla, where a progressive caseous ulcerative lesion develops. Involvement of the pelvis and other adjacent renal papillae follows, with caseous ulceration of the papillae and extensive intrarenal spread of tuberculous inflammation eventually causing loss of function,

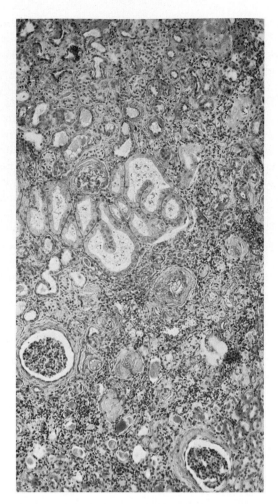

Fig. 18-43. Chronic pyelonephritis. Capsular thickening of glomeruli, interstitial fibrosis and cellular infiltrate, hyaline casts in some tubules, and enlargement of other tubules. (AFIP 76640.)

hydronephrosis, and spread to the lower urinary tract. In miliary tuberculosis (tuberculous sepsis) the kidney may be as involved as other organs with many miliary tubercles, but renal dysfunction is not a prominent feature.

PRESSURE AND FLOW ABNORMALITIES
Reflux nephropathy

It is now known that many cases that were formerly diagnosed as chronic pyelonephritis are more appropriately attributable to reflux nephropathy. This disorder is characterized by gross areas of cortical scarring alternating with relatively normal areas.[6,88] The poles of the kidneys have the greatest amount of scarring. There is massive atrophy of the papillae and outer medulla. Tubules become atrophic and may display cystic dilatation. They frequently contain casts of colloid material. Arterioles may show obliterative changes. Glomeruli are typically surrounded by fibrotic changes and classi-

cally exhibit focal and segmental glomerulosclerosis with hyalinosis, even when present in an unscarred area.[18]

As the name implies, reflux nephropathy occurs only in the presence of vesicoureteric reflux. This can occur as a result of congenital defects in the valvelike anatomy of the vesicoureteric junction or can occur as a sequel to bladder neck obstruction, infection, surgery, or neurogenic bladder defects secondary to spinal cord malformation or injury. Sterile, high-pressure reflux alone appears to cause the lesion described above, but the disorder is commonly associated with urinary tract infection, which probably exacerbates the progression of renal insufficiency. Susceptibility of the kidney to scarring in response to reflux appears to be highest in infancy and early childhood. Reflux nephropathy may account for 10% to 20% of renal failure in patients less than 15 years old. Proteinuria is a bad prognostic sign. Currently antireflux surgery is undertaken only if gross reflux is present. If the patient has hypertension, renal insufficiency, or significant proteinuria, surgery is usually too late to confer significant benefit.

Obstruction of urinary tract[118]

Mechanical obstruction to urinary outflow causes a rise in luminal pressure and proximal dilatation of the ureter (hydroureter) and renal pelvis (hydronephrosis). The cause of the obstruction may be congenital anomalies (particularly in children), neuromuscular defects such as cord bladder, benign and malignant tumors, renal and bladder calculi, infection and subsequent fibrosis, pregnancy, or anomalous arteries at the ureteropelvic junction. This is only a partial list.

Pathogenesis of the progressive dilatation of the ureter and renal pelvis depends on the pressure of continued glomerular filtration to replace urine that is resorbed by the lymphatics, vasa recta of the papilla, capillaries of the pelvic mucosa, or a hypothesized direct pyelovenous outflow.

The progression of the process is determined by the degree and location of obstruction. Unilateral, rapidly developing, complete ureteral obstruction without infection results in moderate proximal dilatation of the ureter and renal pelvis. Renal blood flow rapidly falls, and intimal vascular hyperplasia and eventual atrophy of tubules and glomeruli follow. Partial obstruction with maintenance of more renal function results in a slow but progressive dilatation of the renal pelvis, often to extreme degrees when unilateral. With advanced hydronephrosis the renal parenchyma is stretched over the dilated caliceal system and undergoes intense fibrous atrophy of all components. When hydronephrosis is bilateral and early, the kidney may show only moderate tubular dilatation and flattening and mild chronic interstitial inflammatory infiltrate. When renal biopsy is performed on such a patient with unexplained renal failure as a result of unrecognized bilateral ureteral obstruction, the pathologic diagnosis can be difficult.

Clinical manifestations of obstruction are pain, renal enlargement, polyuria, or anuria. Recurrent pyelonephritis or refractory urinary tract infections may be an important problem. When a hydronephrotic kidney becomes infected, it may become a sac filled with purulent exudate (pyonephrosis) usually requiring surgery. With relief of the cause of mechanical obstruction the recovery of renal function depends on the duration of the obstruction and the degree of vascular change and tubular atrophy. After relief of the obstruction, renal concentrating power is reduced but usually improves with time. Occasionally relief of severe obstruction is followed by massive polyuria with electrolyte loss, which may be life threatening.

Renal papillary or medullary necrosis (necrotizing renal papillitis)

Acute or chronic necrosis of the renal papilla of one or both kidneys results in extreme impairment of renal function. Although it was first recognized chiefly in diabetics with pyelonephritis, investigators now recognize that acute pyelonephritis with acute obstruction, analgesic abuse (discussed previously), and sickle cell disease or other hematologic disturbances may induce papillary necrosis. The incidence has increased greatly in the last few years, and this is attributed mainly to analgesic abuse and better recognition.

Diabetic patients with pyelonephritis, even in the absence of obstruction, may exhibit fever, back pain, pyuria or hematuria, and perhaps ureteral colic from sloughed necrotic papillae passing down the ureter. Oliguria and renal failure follow. It is believed that the diabetic vascular disease results in ischemic papillae that are sensitized to further injury by pyelonephritis.

Papillary necrosis also occurs in nondiabetic patients with acute pyelonephritis and acute obstruction of the drainage of one or both kidneys. It occurs in older men and is often clinically overshadowed by the problems of the accompanying obstruction and infection. Papillary ischemia induced by the acute obstruction is believed to be an important pathogenic mechanism.

Pathologic examination of the kidney with acute necrotizing papillitis reveals yellow or opaque grayish papillae, some of which may have sloughed away. The necrosis generally involves the distal two thirds and is sharply defined from the often congested surviving medulla. The renal cortex may show whitish streaks and mottled areas of inflammatory reaction and small abscesses. Microscopically the papilla usually shows an acellular necrotic remnant of stroma with some acute inflammation at the junction with the medulla. Bacte-

rial colonies may sometimes be seen in the necrotic zone with obstructive necrosis.

Sickle cell nephropathy

Patients with sickle cell disease are prone to papillary necrosis as a result of the ischemic and obstructive effects of sickling red blood cells. Occlusion of the vasa recta results in calicectasis (improperly caliectasis) and papillary necrosis.[74] This autosomal codominant disorder is expressed as a single substitution of valine for glutamic acid in the beta chain of the hemaglobin molecule. As a result, the hemaglobin is prone to form molecular aggregates within the red blood cell, particularly under the conditions of acidosis, hypoxia, or hyperosmolality. The renal interstitium, particularly the medulla, is characterized by hyperosmolality and relative hypoxia. Thus the kidney of patients with sickle cell disease is usually affected. As the sickled red cell becomes elongated, it becomes leaky and eventually lyses. The concurrent changes in blood viscosity attributable to the conformational change further contribute to vascular occlusion and eventual infarction.

Although the kidneys of patients with sickle cell disease are near normal in size, at autopsy calicectasis is observed in more than 50% of cases. In addition to papillary necrosis, renal medullary infarcts are common. The medulla typically exhibits a loss of the vasa recta. In contrast, cortical infarcts are rare. Microscopically, the glomeruli are enlarged and usually distended with blood, particularly in the juxtamedullary area. The medulla displays scarring, fibrosis, edema, tubular atrophy, and mononuclear cell infiltrates. A small number of patients develop the nephrotic syndrome. This is associated either with focal sclerosis or glomerulonephritis associated with electron-dense deposits in the mesangium. This latter finding has been attributed to an autologous immune complex nephritis after renal tubular antigens were found deposited with immunoglobulins along the glomerular basement membrane.[105] It has been postulated that such antigens are released by damaged tubular cells and initiate an immune antibody response.

Renal insufficiency tends to progress once it has begun and is not responsive to any particular therapy. Patients with sickle cell disease do as well with dialysis or with renal allografting as other patients. A fibrinolytic inhibitor, epsilon-aminocaproic acid, has been effective in the treatment of the life-threatening hematuria that can develop in these patients.

Interstitial nephritis

The term "interstitial nephritis" is used for the variety of acute and chronic inflammatory processes that predominantly involve the renal interstitial tissue. The diagnosis of primary interstitial nephritis is made difficult by the fact that glomerular, vascular, and obstructive disease may all result in secondary interstitial inflammation. Primary interstitial nephritis may be divided into nonbacterial interstitial nephritis and pyelonephritis. The latter has been discussed previously. This section focuses on the immunologically based interstitial nephritides.

Allergic interstitial nephritis

Often unrecognized, allergic interstitial nephritis is one of the more common forms of iatrogenic renal disease.[64] It is almost always attributable to drug sensitivity. Although almost any drug can cause this syndrome, the most commonly implicated drugs are the sulfonamides, phenytoin, the penicillin derivatives (particularly methicillin), allopurinol, and the nonsteroidal anti-inflammatory drugs. Such patients typically present with fever, skin rash, eosinophilia and eosinophiluria, and azotemia. Renal biopsy reveals patchy infiltrates consisting of eosinophils, macrophages, plasma cells, and lymphocytes in an edematous interstitial stroma. The nephritis induced by nonsteroidal anti-inflammatory agents is distinctive for its paucity of eosinophils and its association with nephrotic-range proteinuria.[31] Otherwise proteinuria is usually moderate, and the urinary sediment is characterized by hematuria and sterile pyuria. Staining the urine sediment for eosinophils is a valuable diagnostic assay. If the process proceeds unchecked, tubular necrosis and atrophy ensues, and end-stage renal failure develops.

The most effective therapy is to recognize the syndrome and withdraw the offending agent. Resolution of allergic interstitial nephritis can be quite slow, and corticosteroids have been shown to hasten improvement in renal function. It should be emphasized that this syndrome can occur in the absence of systemic signs of hypersensitivity. The susceptibility of the kidney to this complication of drug therapy reflects the tubular epithelium's role in concentrating and transporting a wide range of solutes, including potentially immunogenic compounds.

A similar interstitial nephritis can occur in certain infectious diseases in which the pathogen does not directly infect the kidney. This indicates that hypersensitivity may play a role in the pathogenesis of the lesion. Two classic examples are diphtheria and scarlet fever. An allergic type of interstitial nephritis can also occur in leptospirosis (Weil's disease), but in this instance organisms may be seen in the lesion.[100]

Vasculitis and interstitial nephritis

Several systemic vasculitides are noted for involvement of both glomeruli and the interstitium. Systemic lupus erythematosus (SLE) is the best example of this. As noted earlier, the degree and activity of the interstitial inflammation in SLE is employed by pathologists to provide both prognosis and predict responsiveness to therapy. The interstitial infiltrate can heterogeneously involve both cortex and medulla. Lymphocytes, monocytes, histiocytes, and plasma cells contribute in varying proportions to the leukocyte infiltration.

Two vasculitides that manifest themselves *primarily* in the interstitium are sarcoidosis and Sjögren's syndrome.

Sarcoidosis is an idiopathic disease in which noncaseating granulomas appear in the lungs, skin, liver, kidney, eyes, and parotid glands.[76] It typically occurs in young adults and is more common in blacks. It is associated with hypercalcemia secondary to enhanced synthesis of 1,25-dihydroxyvitamin D by the granulomas. The renal cortex is involved more commonly with lymphocytic infiltrates and less commonly with noncaseating epithelioid granulomas. Giant cells can be present. There can be a variety of associated glomerulopathies including focal glomerulosclerosis, membranous glomerulopathy, and crescentic glomerulonephritis. The disease is responsive to glucocorticoids.

Sjögren's syndrome is an uncommon, autoimmune disease predominantly of adult females in which the lacrimal and salivary glands are invaded by lymphocytes, resulting in the "sicca complex" of xerophthalmia and xerostomia. It can occur with rheumatoid arthritis or occasionally in patients with other collagen-vascular diseases. The kidney can be involved by an interstitial nephritis composed predominantly of lymphocytes and plasma cells.[71] The nephritis can be quite severe, leading to tubular atrophy and interstitial fibrosis. A variety of secondary glomerular lesions, including mesangial proliferation and focal sclerosis, has been described. In most patients renal involvement tends not to progress to failure. In severe cases, glucocorticoids and cytotoxic agents can be effective.

Chronic interstitial nephritis

Chronic, diffuse, nonbacterial, interstitial nephritis is usually caused by other processes such as the papillary necrosis of analgesic abuse, sarcoidosis, and ischemia. After chronic pyelonephritis and other causes are excluded, the cause of many cases of diffuse chronic interstitial nephritis remains unknown.

Balkan nephritis is a remarkable chronic interstitial nephritis that occurs commonly in certain areas of Yugoslavia and Bulgaria. It progresses to uremia and is characterized by chronic interstitial inflammation, intense fibrosis, and tubular atrophy. A nephrotoxin is suspected but has not been identified.[67]

Interstitial disease and paraproteins

Amyloid and multiple myeloma are two examples of tubulointerstitial injury induced and sustained by the deposition of paraproteins produced outside the kidney. Amyloid preferentially affects glomeruli and was dis-

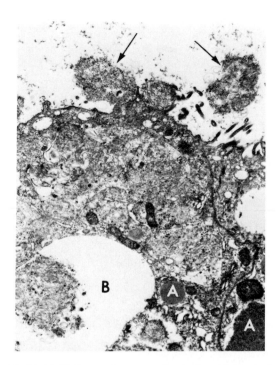

Fig. 18-44. Multiple myeloma nephropathy. Light-chain protein is absorbed in proximal tubular cells, *A,* polymerizes in lysosomes, *B,* and is extruded in lumen as amyloid fibrils, *arrows.*

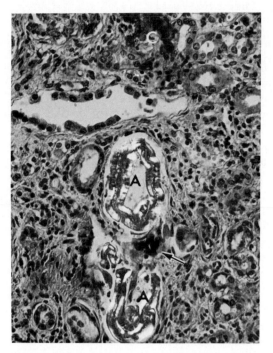

Fig. 18-45. Multiple myeloma nephropathy. Congo Red stain under polarized light. Notice laminar casts showing bright green dichroism characteristic of amyloid, *A,* foreign-body giant cell *(arrow),* tubular atrophy, and renal calcinosis, *C.*

cussed earlier. Multiple myeloma, which often coexists with amyloid, is primarily an interstitial disease.

MULTIPLE MYELOMA

Renal insufficiency develops in multiple myeloma in 30% to 50% of cases.[69] Amyloidosis, renal calcinosis, and pyelonephritis contribute to this failure, but the basic lesion is a chronic interstitial nephritis with tubular atrophy and laminar "hard" casts showing a multinucleated giant cell reaction. Bence Jones proteinuria (light-chain excretion) appears to induce tubular injury by overloading of proximal tubules with light chains, which may form intracytoplasmic crystalloids or may be converted into insoluble amyloid in giant lysosomes (Fig. 18-44). Exocytosis of the amyloid into the tubular lumen results in amyloid-containing casts, which are commonly seen in myeloma (Fig. 18-45). The often massive formation of casts may result in obstruction and contribute to the tubular atrophy and renal failure. Actual neoplastic involvement of the renal interstitium by myeloma cells is uncommon.

METABOLIC TUBULOINTERSTITIAL TOXICITY

Several altered metabolic states produce characteristic pathologic alterations in the renal parenchyma. The

most prevalent is diabetes, discussed earlier in the context of proteinuric glomerular lesions. Two other examples are the hyperuricemia of gout and hypercalcemia with renal calcinosis.

Gout nephropathy

Renal disease in gout results from hypertension, renal stones, and formation of gouty tophi in the renal medulla.[25] These tophi show the usually histiocytic inflammatory reaction to the crystalline urates. When renal insufficiency develops in about 20% to 25% of gouty patients, interstitial inflammation, fibrosis, tubular atrophy, arterionephrosclerotic changes, and gouty tophi are characteristically seen.

Amorphous urates within tubules may be seen in neonatal kidneys as yellow streaks in the medulla, the so-called uric acid infarcts. These arise from the normal striking breakdown of blood cells in the neonatal period and are of no clinical significance.

Hypercalcemia and renal calcinosis

Hypercalcemia and hypercalciuria may cause calcium deposition in the kidney (renal calcinosis), renal injury, dysfunction, or failure, and may commonly result in formation of renal calculi.[101] Hypercalcemia results from excessive bone resorption attributable to hyperparathyroidism, vitamin D intoxication, extensive bone destruction by cancer, hyperthyroidism, excessive calcium intake as in milk-alkali syndrome, sarcoidosis, and the rare, idiopathic infantile hypercalcemia.

Clinically hypercalcemia may result in renal stones and renal colic, band keratopathy (calcium deposits of the cornea), calcified conjunctival deposits, polyuria from loss of concentrating ability, and renal failure. Pronounced hypercalcemia (over 15 mg/dl) may produce a crisis with polyuria changing to oliguria and severe central nervous system symptoms. Massive visceral metastatic calcification may occur, with a poor prognosis.

Renal calcinosis results either from dystrophic calcification of necrotic tissue, as may be seen in calcified necrotic tubular cells in acute mercury chloride poisoning, or from hypercalcemia. In calcinosis attributable to hypercalcemia the major site is in the basement membranes of Henle's loop and collecting ducts, particularly in the medulla near the cortex, but in severe disease, extensive cortical deposition is also seen. The calcium tends to be deposited in concretions on the inner aspect of the tubular basement membrane. These concretions enlarge, damage cells, and obstruct the lumen. When renal calcinosis is very severe, there may be linear deposition along many tubular basement membranes. Secondary tubular atrophy, interstitial fibrosis, and nonspecific chronic inflammation then occur.

RENAL LITHIASIS

Renal stones have been recognized since antiquity, and renal colic resulting from ureteral passage of a stone is legend because of the characteristic pain produced.

Pathogenesis. Renal stone formation is believed to be the result of both excessive concentration of the stone constituents and conducive physicochemical situations. Important factors are excess concentration of urinary excretory products because of highly concentrated urine resulting from environmental or habitual chronic dehydration. Hypercalciuria from various causes, excessive oxalate, or uric acid production on an acquired or genetic basis, and hereditary cystinuria are important causes. Of equal if not greater importance are those factors conducive to precipitation of the crystalloid. An alkaline pH favors calcium phosphate stone formation, whereas an acid pH encourages stone formation in a child with cystinuria.[100]

Stabilization of the solution supersaturated with phosphates and other constituents in the urine is of great importance. Failure of stabilization mechanisms results in deposition onto a nidus of an endogenous or exogenous foreign body such as necrotic tissue, fibrin, a true foreign body in the bladder, or a Randall plaque.

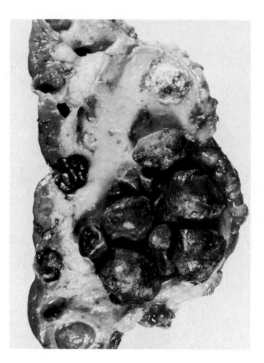

Fig. 18-46. Hydronephrosis with renal stones in renal pelvis and calyces.

A Randall plaque is a minute focus of stromal calcification at the tip of the papilla.[83] When the epithelium is eroded, it acts as a nidus for stone formation of considerable size before the stone tears free from its attachment and becomes free in the pelvis. Stasis of urine induced by partial obstruction tends to facilitate stone formation.

Types of stones.[82,101] Calcium stones are the most common (50% to 70%) and may be pure or mixtures of oxalate, phosphate, and hydroxyapatite. Massive phosphate stones called "staghorn calculi" may form a cast of the entire renal pelvis and calyces.

Magnesium ammonium phosphate pure or mixed stones are common in infection with urea-splitting bacteria such as *Proteus*. Uric acid stones compose from 5% to 10% and cystine stones from 2% to 3% of renal stones.

Phosphate stones are white, smooth, and soft, whereas oxalate stones are hard, crystalline with sharp edges, and dark brownish. Uric acid stones are dark brown when pure. On fracture most stones show a concentric laminar structure.

Effects of stones are obstruction of the outflow of urine and production of hydronephrosis, the promotion of infection, and the production of renal colic by the passage of small stones down the ureter. Stones and infection often combine to destroy renal function in the involved kidney (Fig. 18-46).

VASCULAR RENAL DISEASE

The enormous renal blood flow and the contribution of the kidney to the homeostasis and pathophysiology of the circulation make renal vascular disease of utmost importance. This renal blood flow is modulated by systemic and local hydrodynamic and hormonal factors and incompletely understood intrinsic intrarenal control. In disease, these flow-control mechanisms are modified and may contribute to renal dysfunction and damage, by arterial hypertension, shock, or vascular obstruction. Vascular insufficiency affects glomeruli and interstitium, cortex and medulla. Thus it is appropriate to consider vascular disorders as a separate category from those concerning primarily one renal compartment.

Renal infarction

The most dramatic form of vascular insufficiency is renal infarction. Typically, renal infarction involves only a segment of the kidney and is embolic in origin. Renal infarctions are common, are often multiple, and usually result from emboli arising from cardiac vegetations or mural thrombi. Less commonly atheromatous emboli from the aorta, usually associated with the atheromatous aortic aneurysm or aortography or operative manipulation of the severly atherosclerotic aorta, may cause renal infarction, hypertension, and renal failure.[50] Intrinsic renal artery occlusion from dissecting aneurysm, arteritis, or thrombosis also causes infarction. Although the infarcts may cause back pain and hematuria, acute renal failure is seen only with extensive bilateral occlusion as with dissecting aneurysm of the aorta. Ischemic renal tissue adjacent to infarcts may be a source of excessive renin production and hypertension.

Hypertensive vascular disease

In medically advanced countries, hypertension is the most common serious chronic disease, affecting about half the population over 50 years of age. Arterial hypertension is defined clinically as borderline when it reaches 140/90 mm Hg and hypertensive when 165/95 mm Hg. Whether there is elevation of systolic pressure alone (systolic hypertension) or elevation of both systolic and diastolic pressure (diastolic hypertension), both have an increased risk of serious complications, but diastolic hypertension is more dangerous.[51,52] The arterial changes and vascular complications increase with the severity and duration of the hypertension but are modified by genetic factors, environmental factors, sex (females tolerate hypertension better), and associated diseases.

The increased peripheral resistance resulting in sustained hypertension may arise from (1) increased sympathetic tone, (2) increased release of renin and generation of angiotensin II, (3) the presence of vasoconstrictive substances in the circulation, (4) increased sodium load and extracellular fluid load, and finally (5) a postulated excessive responsiveness to the other factors. In a given individual hypertension may be attributable to a combination of these factors.

Role of renin.[78] The juxtaglomerular cells at the hilum of the glomerulus synthesize renin. These cells release renin when stimulated by baroreceptors in the afferent arteriole, by sympathetic nervous system stimulation, or after detection of changes of sodium or other electrolyte levels in the distal tubule. Released renin hydrolyzes plasma substrate into angiotensin I. Convertase in the lung causes conversion of angiotensin I to the potent octapeptide angiotensin II, which both causes arteriolar smooth muscle contraction and triggers the release of aldosterone, in turn facilitating renal sodium conservation. This physiologic homeostatic mechanism may be disrupted in pathologic states. The juxtaglomerular apparatus may misinterpret chronic renal cortical ischemia as inadequate blood volume. This results in increased renin release and increased sodium load. In severe cases hyperplasia of juxtaglomerular cells (see Fig. 18-50) and an excessive release of renin occur, and hyperrenin hypertension results.

Essential hypertension: nature and pathogenesis. Essential hypertension occurs in about 90% of hypertensive persons. Although the cause of essential hypertension is unknown, several factors are related to its development. Genetic factors are indicated by a strong family history of essential hypertension and the inordinately high incidence in the black population, about double that of the white population. The absence of any sharp separation between normal, mild hypertension and severe hypertension is an indication that a mosaic of factors causes hypertension, including electrolyte control, nervous system reactivity, arterial reactivity, vasoactive chemical substances, and other environmental factors.

Renal hypertension. The kidney can be an important cause of secondary hypertension. Renal arterial obstruction results in decreased renal blood flow when it exceeds 50%. When arterial obstruction is severe, there is striking activation of the renin-angiotensin system, and juxtaglomerular hyperplasia and hypertension from excessive renin may result. Important causes of renal artery stenosis producing hypertension are atheroma near the renal artery ostia and thromboemboli of the renal artery or main branches. Atheromatous emboli produce ischemia and hypertension, but the obstructions are in small intrarenal arteries.[50] Fibromuscular dysplasia causing stenosis of renal arteries may lead to severe hypertension in children or young women. Surgery repairing these congenital dysplasias or acquired arterial stenosis may be curative.[46]

Many chronic parenchymatous renal diseases may result in hypertension—chronic glomerulonephritis, chronic pyelonephritis, polycystic kidneys, radiation nephritis, diabetic nephropathy, or hydronephrosis, to name a few. When unilateral disease is present, as in hydronephrosis, nephrectomy may be curative. The mechanisms of hypertension induction by parenchymal disease are sodium and water load increase attributable to chronic renal failure and in some cases to renin and aldosterone. In many cases of chronic renal disease there is an endarterial intimal proliferation, termed "endarteritis obliterans," which is induced by a shrunken vascular bed in the scarred kidney and intimal hyperplasia induced by hypertension. This may exaggerate the hypertension and even induce malignant hypertension.

Effect of hypertension upon the kidney. The most commonly affected organs in systemic hypertension are the heart, which is susceptible to myopathy and the progression of atherosclerosis with its own set of life-threatening complications, and the central nervous system, in which vascular disease is manifest as thromboses and hemorrhage.[51,52] Except for malignant hypertension, less than 5% of patients with significant hypertension die of renal failure. Nonetheless, the kidney is very commonly affected by systemic hypertension. The ensuing moderate renal insufficiency may exacerbate the effects of hypertension elsewhere in the body.

Benign nephrosclerosis (arterionephrosclerosis)

Benign nephrosclerosis is the most common form of renal disease and is seen in most persons over 60 years of age. Long-standing moderate arterial hypertension induces arteriosclerotic proliferative and hyaline changes in small muscular branches of the renal arteries and renal arterioles.[53] These changes result in focal atrophy of tubules and sclerosis of glomeruli. The intervening kidney is relatively uninvolved; thus renal function is usually fairly well maintained. Even when it is severe, benign nephrosclerosis causes chronic renal failure in less than 5% of patients. Mild arteriosclerotic intimal thickening may occur in the elderly without hypertension, but extensive nephrosclerosis is consistently associated with hypertension. Clinical problems of the patient are usually related to hypertensive complications in other organs. The vessels of the human retina mirror the visceral arteriolar changes, and an ophthalmoscopic estimation of the severity of vascular involvement is of great clinical value.

With increasing severity of the nephrosclerosis, mild shrinking of the kidneys results because of a loss of tubular mass. The renal cortex is thinned, and the surface of the kidney develops a punctate scarring resembling grained leather. The fibrosis in the minute foci of isch-

emic atrophy makes the kidney firmer and slightly paler than normal. Muscular arteries with thickened walls may be seen.

Microscopically the small muscular arteries show intimal thickening because of proliferation of intimal smooth muscle cells, which deposit new elastic fibers, the lamina of basement membrane, and collagen fibrils. Under the light microscope this material has a pink hyaline appearance. Although some intimal thickening occurs with age, it is most striking when associated with hypertension.

Hyaline arteriolar sclerosis is a characteristic lesion of benign nephrosclerosis. A pink, homogeneous protein is deposited in the intima, narrowing the lumen. The electron microscope shows this vascular hyaline as a finely granular protein deposit often containing minute lipid inclusions. It is believed to be the result of insudation of plasma proteins into the arteriolar wall where the proteins are denatured into insoluble residues. With more severe hypertension, hypertrophy of the smooth muscle cells and some intimal proliferation of smooth muscle cells occur[74] (Fig. 18-47).

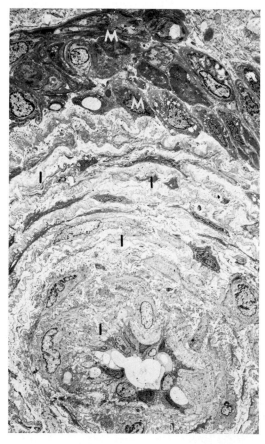

Fig. 18-47. Hyperplastic changes in small artery with hypertension. Hypertrophied medial cells, *M,* and "onion-skin" layers of intimal cells and basement membrane, *I.* (1200×.)

The glomeruli in benign nephrosclerosis may appear normal by light microscopy except for old sclerosed scars in foci of ischemic atrophy. With more severe hypertension, mild thickening of the basement membranes may be seen in most glomeruli, but some show various stages of ischemic wrinkling of capillaries and collagenous scarring (glomerular ischemic obsolescence).

Malignant nephrosclerosis

A vicious complication called "malignant or accelerated hypertension" develops in about 5% of patients with hypertension of whatever cause. This is characterized by very high systolic and diastolic blood pressure, papilledema, hypertensive encephalopathy, and rapidly developing renal failure (malignant nephrosclerosis). High renin and angiotensin blood levels are present. Life expectancy without adequate treatment is less than 2 years. Only rarely does malignant nephrosclerosis develop anew in a normal kidney. Most commonly malignant hypertension arises in a patient with benign hypertension whose kidneys manifest the changes of benign nephrosclerosis. Thus the acute renal changes of malignant nephrosclerosis are superimposed on benign nephrosclerosis. The acute changes in arteries and arterioles[49] are (1) striking intimal proliferation of smooth muscle cells with loose laminae of collagen and basement membrane (onion-skin proliferation) and (2)

arteriolar necrosis. The necrotic arterioles show extravasation of red blood cells and proteins through incompetent endothelium into the vessel wall (fibrinoid deposits) and often show thrombosis of the lumen. This process is distinguished from arteritis by the presence of few or no inflammatory cells. Immunofluorescence studies of these lesions show fibrinogen, gamma globulins, complement, and albumin (Figs. 18-48 and 18-49). Even though gamma globulin and complement may be seen in these lesions, many believe that this is a passive trapping of these plasma proteins rather than an immunologic process. Glomerular changes in malignant nephrosclerosis are an exaggeration of the glomerular basement membrane thickening and ischemic wrinkling seen in benign nephrosclerosis. In addition, thrombonecrotic and hemorrhagic lesions develop in some glomeruli, analogous to the arteriolar necrosis. These acute glomerulitic lesions heal with scarring. Hypertrophy of the juxtaglomerular apparatus and hypergranularity of these cells correlate well with the hyperreninism of these patients (Fig. 18-50). With the progression of the obstruction of the vascular bed by arterial and glomerular lesions, tubular atrophy and interstitial fibrosis develop.

The gross appearance of the kidney in malignant nephrosclerosis reflects the processes just described (Fig. 18-51). The kidney is usually somewhat reduced in size, has a finely granular cortex with tiny hemor-

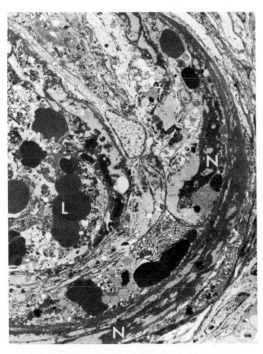

Fig. 18-48. Malignant nephrosclerosis with necrotic arteriole showing laminar insudation of plasma proteins and red cells into necrotic wall, *N,* and cell debris and red cells in lumen, *L.* (2500×.)

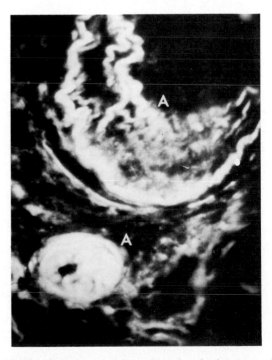

Fig. 18-49. Malignant nephrosclerosis. *A,* Artery and necrotic arteriole stained with fluorescent antihuman fibrin. (Courtesy Dr. Claude Cornwall, Syracuse, N.Y.)

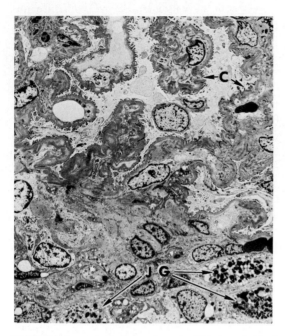

Fig. 18-50. Malignant nephrosclerosis. Thick, wrinkled capillary basement membranes, *C,* and heavily granulated juxtaglomerular cells, *JG.* (1000×.)

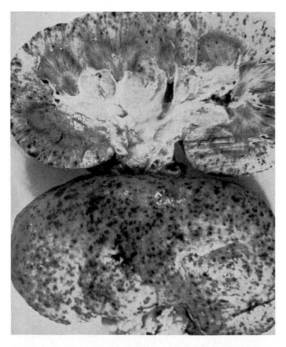

Fig. 18-51. Malignant nephrosclerosis with focal hemorrhages caused by thrombonecrosis of arterioles and glomeruli.

rhages (flea-bitten kidney), and may show tiny cortical infarcts.

When malignant hypertension is superimposed on other diseases such as chronic glomerulonephritis, a composite of the acute hyperplastic and thrombonecrotic lesions is added to the primary disease changes.

CONGENITAL ANOMALIES
Agenesis

Bilateral renal agenesis is uncommon. It is often associated with somatic features of wide-set eyes, parrot-beak nose, receding chin, and floppy low-set ears as described by Potter (actually somatic features of oligohydramnios).

Unilateral renal agenesis is more common (about 1 per 1000 births). The disorder is more common in males than in females, more commonly involves the left kidney, and may be associated with extrarenal anomalies such as esophageal atresia or congenital heart disease. If an isolated malformation, unilateral renal agenesis is compatible with normal life expectancy. The congenitally solitary kidney is usually compensatively hypertrophied.

Hypoplasia

True renal hypoplasia is rare. Most diminutive kidneys result from acquired disease, often arteriosclerotic renal artery stenosis or chronic pyelonephritis. True renal hypoplasia is usually bilateral, and the kidneys have diminished numbers of lobes and calices. A variant is termed "oligomeganephrony" in which the decreased numbers of nephrons in the hypoplastic kidney are hypertrophied with very large glomeruli.

Anomalies of renal position or form

One or both kidneys may remain in the embryonic pelvic location rather than ascending to the normal lumbar position. Pelvic ectopic kidneys usually derive their blood supply from contiguous large arteries.

Because of inefficient ureteral drainage, pelvic ectopic kidneys are prone to infection or stone formation. Bilateral pelvic ectopic kidneys are usually fused as "lump," "clump," or "cake" kidneys.

Crossed renal ectopy describes the rare situation in which both renal masses lie on the same side of the retroperitoneum. From one renal mass, usually the caudal one, the ureter crosses the midline to enter the lower urinary tract. Crossed ectopic kidneys are often fused, producing a clinically or radiographically detectible mass.

The familiar horseshoe kidney results from fusion of both renal masses by an isthmus of renal tissue between their lower poles. Fusion across cephalic poles is much less common. Horseshoe kidneys are usually mildly caudally ectopic. The isthmus that con-

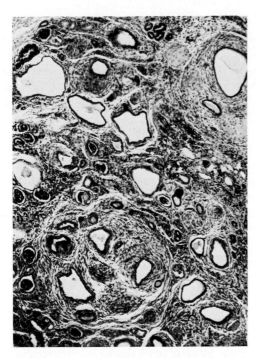

Fig. 18-52. Dysplasia of kidney. Notice disorganized renal structure with embryonic type of peritubular stromal proliferation.

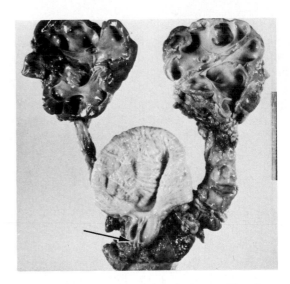

Fig. 18-53. Obstructive renal dysplasia resulting from congenital valves in the posterior urethra, *arrow*.

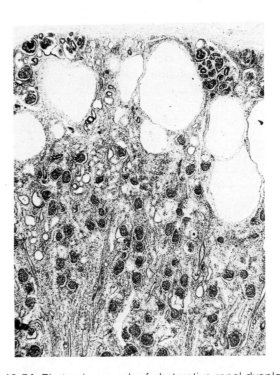

Fig. 18-54. Photomicrograph of obstructive renal dysplasia.

nects the two renal masses is subject to obstruction and infection.

Defective renal differentiation (renal dysplasia)

Defective differentiation of all or portions of one or both renal masses is termed "renal dysplasia." In the most common form, an irregular aggregate of thin-walled cysts presents in one or another (rarely both) renal fossae, often in the presence of congenital discontinuity of the ureter. The unilateral condition constitutes the commonest abdominal mass detected in newborn infants and is usually sporadic. The cystic mass consists of epithelium-lined cystically dilated structures, aggregates of tubular structures, and dysontogenic tissues, often with spicules of hyaline cartilage (Fig. 18-52). Foci with microscopic features of dysplasia occur in the kidneys in a variety of multifaceted teratologic syndromes, many of them hereditary.

Obstructive renal dysplasia (Potter type IV)

Congenital obstruction of the drainage of all or part of one or both kidneys may be associated with microscopic features as renal dysplasia. Usually the obstructing lesion—urethral valve or atresia or an ectopic ureterocele—is the major clinical lesion, and dysplastic features in the relevant renal parenchyma remain as etiologically provocative findings (Figs. 18-53 and 18-54).

Polycystic renal disease
Autosomal recessive (infantile) polycystic kidney (Potter type I)

Autosomal recessive (infantile) polycystic renal disease presents as the homozygous phenotype of a recessive trait. The disorder is usually fatal in the perinatal period. Rare patients may survive into childhood, adolescence, or even early adulthood. Proliferation of portal biliary ducts in the liver is always present but is clinicopathologically silent except in patients who survive infancy.

The kidneys are large and smooth in contour. The renal parenchyma is distorted by innumerable fusiform or cylindrical ectatic structures that extend from the renal cortex to the medulla. Microscopically, these can be recognized as enormously dilated collecting ducts. There is no obstructing lesion (Fig. 18-55).

Autosomal dominant polycystic renal disease

Considerably more common than autosomal recessive polycystic renal disease is autosomal dominant polycystic renal disease. Although usually clinically silent until middle adulthood, hence the designation "adult polycystic renal disease," this cystic renal lesion has come to be increasingly recognized by modern imaging techniques, chiefly renal ultrasonography, in young asymptomatic individuals in pedigrees at risk, even infants, and even in utero. The disease is inherited as an autosomal dominant with high penetrance associated with a locus on autosome 16. Some phenotypically indistinguishable lesions have specifically not been attributable to a mutant locus on autosome 16.

Grossly the kidneys are often huge, weighing more than 1500 g apiece. The innumerable cysts, varying

from barely visible to 5 cm in size, produce a cobblestone-like external surface (Fig. 18-56). On cross section the cysts contain straw-yellow, hemorrhagic, or even gelatinous fluid. The renal pelvis and calyces are stretched, compressed, and distorted by the cysts, and this results in a characteristic roentgenographic appearance. The intervening islands of renal parenchyma may be normal in appearance or may show secondary compression, atrophy, and fibrous arterionephrosclerosis, or pyelonephritis, resulting in eventual renal failure. Dissections of the nephrons and collecting ducts in such cases have shown that the cystic dilatations and proliferations occur in any part of the nephron but have a special predilection for the angle of Henle's loop and Bowman's capsule.

Associated with adult polycystic disease are multiple liver cysts in about one third of cases and, much less commonly, cysts of the pancreas and spleen. About 15% of cases are associated with berry aneurysms of cerebral arteries.

Medullary cystic diseases

Unrelated to either autosomal recessive (infantile) or autosomal dominant (adult) polycystic renal diseases are familial renal disorders that are often associated with epithelium-lined cysts in the renal medullae. Some patients in pedigrees at risk suffer from renal insufficiency without the presence of renal cysts. The inheritance is complex, most commonly characterized as autosomal recessive, but there are exceptions. Renal insufficiency in adolescence or early adulthood is the usual clinical feature. Pathologic features are those of essentially nonspecific renal cortical contraction by interstitial fibrosis,

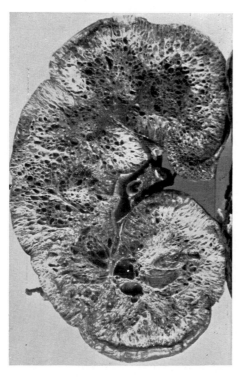

Fig. 18-55. Autosomal recessive ("infantile") polycystic disease in a newborn infant.

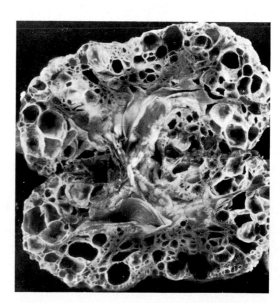

Fig. 18-56. Autosomal dominant ("adult") polycystic renal disease.

mild nonspecific mononuclear cell infiltration, tubular basement membrane thickening, and compensatory glomerulomegaly with or (rarely) without small to medium-sized epithelium-lined cysts usually localized at the corticomedullary junction (Fig. 18-57). The disease has a controversial relationship to "familial juvenile nephronophthisis."

An anatomically somewhat similar but probably unrelated lesion, medullary sponge kidney features multiple epithelium-lined cysts in the tips of renal papillae. These cysts may harbor calculi, and ureteral calculous disease or its complications are the major clinical manifestations of the lesion usually in adulthood. Evidence of a familial tendency is controversial.

RENAL NEOPLASMS
Benign tumors

Benign renal tumors are usually small and are seen at nephrectomy or autopsy. They include ectopic adrenocortical nodules, hamartomas, benign mesenchymal neoplasms, and cortical tubular adenomas.

Adrenocortical nodules are small yellow nodules of microscopically typical adrenocortical cells found in the subcapsular portion of the renal cortex or elsewhere along the urogenital ridge.

Hamartomas. Angiomyolipomas are a common form of hamartoma found in the kidney. They consist of circumscribed but nonencapsulated masses of blood vessels, smooth muscle, and fat cells in varying proportions. They are usually clinically insignificant but constitute the commonest renal lesion of the hereditary disease tuberous sclerosis, which includes hamartomatous masses or true tumors in the kidneys, brain, heart, skin, and other organs.

Mesenchymal neoplasms. Medullary fibromas are common small white nodules seen incidentally at autopsy in the renal medulla. They consist of swirls of stellate interstitial connective tissue cells and collagen that encase renal tubules. The cells contain lipid droplets and are believed to arise from medullary instial cells that they resemble histologically. Renal fibromas, lipomas, and leiomyomas are rare and resemble their counterparts seen elsewhere. Hemangiomas are rare but may be responsible for hematuria.

Cortical tubular adenomas. Cortical tubular adenomas vary from minute lesions to white or yellow spherical masses up to 3 cm in diameter. They are more common in kidneys contracted by acquired disease than in the normal organ. Microscopically they consist of cords and papillary strands of uniform cuboid cells and may be cystic. Since these nodules are often indistinguishable microscopically from renal adenocarcinomas, Bennington and others believe them to be either precancerous or small carcinomas. Those smaller than 3 cm are rarely associated with metastases. Both tubular adenomas and renal adenocarcinomas have ultrastructural and immunologic features consistent with origin from renal proximal tubular cells.

Malignant tumors

Adenocarcinoma of kidney. This tumor comprises 70% to 80% of renal cancers. The designation "hypernephroma" reflects an outmoded concept that they arise from ectopic adrenocortical cells. Renal adenocarcinoma usually occurs between 50 and 70 years of age and is twice as common in men as in women. Hematuria, either painless or accompanied by flank pain, or crampy ureteral colic is a common presenting feature along with the presence of a flank mass, but the presentation may be extremely bizarre. Polycythemia may occur and is attributed to erythropoietin produced by the tumor or the compressed contiguous renal tissue. Peculiar paraneoplastic syndromes such as a hyperparathyroid-like condition or hepatic dysfunction may occur. Metastases may occur early in a variety of sites. The diagnosis depends on radiographic studies of the kidney or other imaging techniques. Cytologic study of the urine may indicate the diagnosis. Nephrectomy is the basis of therapy because the tumors generally respond poorly to chemotherapy or irradiation.

Prognosis depends on the extent of spread and the presence or absence of vascular invasion. McDonald and Priestly found vascular invasion in 54% of cases.[71a] Kaufman and Mimms found a 60% 5-year and 50% 10-

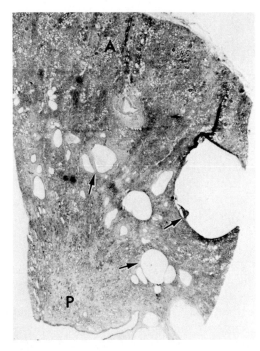

Fig. 18-57. Uremic medullary cystic disease. Macrophotograph of tissue section. Renal cortex with atrophy, *A,* papilla, *P,* and medullary cysts, *arrows.*

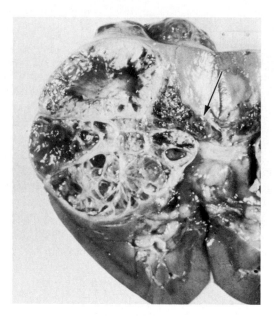

Fig. 18-58. Adenocarcinoma of kidney. *Arrow,* Tumor thrombus in renal vein branch.

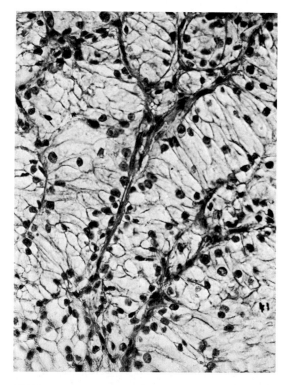

Fig. 18-59. Adenocarcinoma of kidney of clear cell type showing papillary structure. (350×; courtesy Dr. S.E. Gould.)

year survival when the lesion was confined to the kidney. These figures were halved if extrarenal extension had occurred. Overall cure rates at 10 years vary from 17% to 28%.[54a]

Grossly renal adenocarcinoma may arise from any portion of the renal cortex. The tumors are roughly spherical and are often large. They are often conspicuously yellow in color and show central areas of hemorrhage, coagulative necrosis, and cystic excavation (Fig. 18-58). Tumor thrombi in renal veins may extend into the inferior vena cava and even as far centrally as the heart. In fatal cases, metastases are usually widespread in lymph nodes, lungs, and bones.

Microscopically renal adenocarcinoma is very variable. Most commonly, these tumors consist of sheets, cords, or tubular arrays of cuboidal cells with prominent cell walls and conspicuously vacuolated or foamy cytoplasm rich in glycogen and lipids (Fig. 18-59). Occasionally a stellate or spindle-cell pattern indicates a possible sarcoma. Prognosis in such cases is poor.

A variant of renal adenocarcinoma termed "oncocytoma" consists of sheets or papillary arrangements of large polyhedral cells with abundant coarsely granular eosinophilic cytoplasm. Most authorities regard these tumors as malignant tumors, variants of the more usual renal adenocarcinoma.

Nephroblastoma (Wilms' tumor). Nephroblastoma, a malignant tumor that arises from metanephrogenic tissue, is the commonest solid abdominal tumor in children. Truly congenital nephroblastoma is, however, quite uncommon. Although this tumor may occur in adults, even older adults, it is distinctly rare in patients older than 10 years. Both sexes are approximately equally involved. Some cases occur in children with teratologic syndromes such as aniridia or the Wiedemann-Beckwith syndrome of macroglossia, somatic disproportions, and umbilical defects. A mass detected by a parent or a physician is usually the first manifestation. Fever and hypertension are present in about half the cases. Hematuria is uncommon.

Grossly nephroblastomas are bulky, spherical, deceptively circumscribed white or gray-white masses usually without hemorrhage, necrosis, or cyst formation. Microscopically the commonest pattern is a dimorphic distribution of sheets of undifferentiated immature cells resembling metanephric blastema and variously differentiated elements, tubules, abortive glomeruli, or even dysontogenetic tissue such as skeletal muscle with cytoplasmic cross-striations (Fig. 18-60). Rapid local invasion and distant metastases, importantly to the lungs, are seen. Surgery is the foundation of therapy, and these tumors are radiosensitive. The application of multiagent chemotherapy has in recent years conspicuously improved the prognosis to about 80%, or even higher

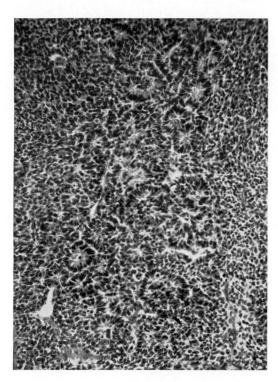

Fig. 18-60. Wilms' tumor of kidney. Notice tubular or rosettelike structures amid tissue of sarcomatous appearance.

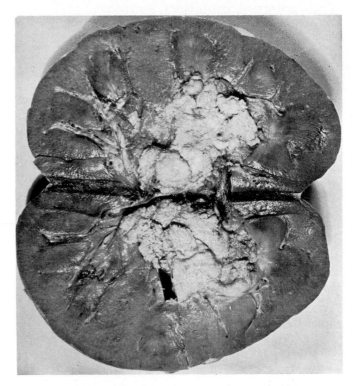

Fig. 18-61. Papillary carcinoma of renal pelvis.

in favorable cases. The prognosis is conspicuously better in lesions that become apparent in the first 2 years of life.

A bizarre large cell "rhabdoid tumor" of the kidney and a monotonously sarcomatoid "clear cell" tumor with a tendency to metastasize to bone clinically imitate nephroblastoma but are regarded by authorities as distinctive neoplasms rather than variants.

Two interesting lesions, perhaps not unrelated, have recently been recognized as occurring in the kidneys of young persons. These are "congenital mesoblastic nephroma," a bulky mass composed of fascicles of spindle cells and associated with an almost invariably good prognosis, and "multilocular cystic nephroma," an encapulated mass of nonconnecting spherical epithelium-lined locules, again with practically always an excellent prognosis.

Leukemic or lymphomatous infiltration. Leukemic infiltration of the kidney often occurs during the course of acute lymphocytic leukemia in children or chronic lymphocytic leukemia in older adults. Such lesions are ordinarily radiosensitive and so are currently rarely available for pathologic examination. The infiltrate may be unilateral or bilateral, nodular or diffuse, and consists of monotonous sheets of malignant cells arrayed in the renal interstitium with surprisingly little alteration

in renal parenchymal elements. Functional renal disturbances are surprisingly infrequent.

Tumors of renal pelvis. These cancers arise from the urothelium, the transitional epithelium (Fig. 18-61). Tumors of the renal pelvis are twice as common in males as in females and comprise about 8% of renal cancers. The presenting clinical picture is usually of hematuria, either painless or painful if blood clots are passed. The tumor cells may be shed in the urine and recognized in cytologic smears, affording an opportunity for early diagnosis. Radiographic demonstration of the tumor in the renal pelvis is the usual diagnostic tool. The cancers vary from very low-grade transitional carcinoma or "papilloma" composed of cells resembling transitional epithelium all the way to solid, infiltrating, anaplastic carcinoma. Multicentric new foci of in situ or invasive transitional cell carcinoma may be present in the ureter in 70% of cases at the time of surgery or later. Of renal pelvic cancers, 15% are keratinizing squamous cell carcinomas arising from metaplasia of the urothelium, and they have a poor prognosis. Riches[87] found that all patients with so-called papillomas survived; 57% of patients with low-grade papillomas survived 5 years, 38% of those with high-grade papillary tumors survived 5 years, and none of those with various solid, infiltrating cancers survived after 5 years.

The Urinary Collecting System

CALYCES, PELVES, AND URETERS
Congenital abnormalities

The calyces, pelves, and ureters develop from the ureteric buds, paired tubular endodermal protrusions from the urogenital sinus that branch dichotomously and extend cephalodorsally. Ultimately the ureteric buds enter and arborize in retroperitoneal metanephrogenic mesenchyme where they induce the formation of nephrons of the definitive (metanephric) kidney. In microdissection studies, Potter and Osathanondh have elicited the selective fusion of branches of the ureteric buds that eventuate in formation of calyces, pelves, and ureters.

Caliceal diverticulum. A caliceal diverticulum (congenital hydrocalycosis, megacalycosis, or caliceal cyst) is a spherical extension of a calyx lined by urothelium and possessing a muscular tunic continuous with that of the upper collecting system. Most are solitary and unilateral. Caliceal diverticula may harbor infection, serve as sites of stone formation, or distort radiographic studies of the kidney.

Ureteropelvic stenosis. Ureteropelvic stenosis, congenital narrowing of the ureteropelvic junction, is most frequently diagnosed in male infants younger than 6 months of age. Infection of the upper urinary tract is the usual presenting feature. Less commonly dilatation of the system is detected in radiographic study. The left side is more commonly affected than the right; about 25% of cases are bilateral. In about 25% of cases, a mechanical cause of obstruction as by an anomalous or normal renal vessel is demonstrated. The disorder may be familial.

Duplications. Duplication of the ureter is the commonest malformation of the urinary collective system. Triplication is rare. The abnormality is usually unilateral. In about half the cases, duplicated ureters join in their lower third to enter the bladder together at the vesical trigone. In complete duplication, the two ureters enter the bladder separately, that from the upper role of the relevant kidney almost always caudal to that from the lower pole (Fig. 18-62), often in an ectopic location, that is, distal to the vesical trigone.

Congenital ureteral valves. Congenital ureteral valves are rare. The resultant hydroureter is often accompanied by infection. It is necessary to distinguish true valves from valves that result from tortuosity of otherwise dilated ureters.

Ureterocele. A ureterocele is a globular expansion of the distal orifice of a ureter at its point of discharge. Simple (obstructive) and ectopic ureteroceles are described. Simple ureteroceles surmount the orthotopic orifice of one or both ureters at the base of the vesical trigone as globular thin-walled structures with a central

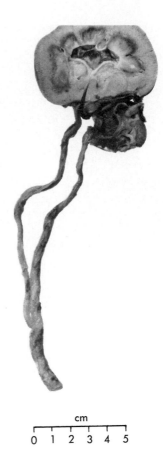

cm

0   1   2   3   4   5

Fig. 18-62. Incomplete duplication of ureter. Kidney has been rotated, and small upper (dysplastic) part lies to right and inferiorly.

minute orifice. Obstructive features, of course, predominate clinically. Simple ureteroceles are attributed to abnormal persistence of Chwalla's membrane, an epithelial lamina that transiently occludes the ureterovesical junction and normally becomes resorbed. Ectopic ureteroceles terminate the point of discharge of a proximally duplicated ureter distal to the vesical trigone: the membranous urethra or perineum in boys or the fourchette, vaginal fornix, or perineum in girls. More exotic terminations have been described. The disorder is overwhelmingly more common in girls. The upper pole of a kidney drained by an ectopic ureterocele is often dysplastic. Obstructive features and continuous wetness dominate the clinical picture.

Trauma

Ureteral damage caused by external violence is rare, usually results from road traffic accidents, and is more common in children than in adults. Rupture or avulsion may occur at or just below the pelviureteral junction, and clinically the condition is often masked by the severity of other injuries. Penetrating wounds of the abdomen do not usually involve the ureters, but on rare occasions they may be damaged during gynecologic operations, by the passage of a stone, by the use of a Dormia basket, or by overvigorous attempts at retrograde pyelography. Pelvic irradiation sometimes leads to ureteral fibrosis and obstruction.

Obstruction and dilatation

The ureter may be obstructed by pressure from without (as in retroperitoneal fibrosis, retroperitoneal tumors, and pelvic lipomatosis), by changes in its wall (caused by amyloidosis, endometriosis, bilharzial fibrosis, and neoplasms), by intraluminal lesions (such as polyps), or by the impaction of calculi, tumor fragments, blood clots, or fungus balls. There may be actual stricturing, or the obstruction can be caused by kinking of the ureter and, depending on the completeness of the obstruction and the length of time that obstruction of whatever cause has been present, there will be a variable amount of proximal myohypertrophy and luminal dilatation. Temporary obstruction often occurs when the ureteral orifice becomes edematous during an episode of acute cystitis. Dilatation is also seen when there is bladder outflow obstruction, as with the enlarged prostate, and in pregnancy when there is loss of tone, possibly caused by hormonal influences, or actual pressure on the ureter at the pelvic brim.

Vesicoureteral reflux

The urine secreted by the kidney passes down the ureter by peristaltic action. When the peristaltic wave reaches the lower end, the ureterovesical opening relaxes to allow the urine to enter the bladder and then closes again and remains closed until the next wave arrives. Peristalsis is essentially myogenic, and musculomuscular junctions allow transmission of the contractions. There is also adrenergic and cholinergic innervation of the ureter with scanty neuromuscular junctions, and ganglion cells are found only in its terminal parts.

The prevention of reflux depends on the integrity of the ureterovesical junction, which in turn depends on compression of the submucosal portion of the ureter against the underlying detrusor muscles and the active contraction of the trigonal muscles. Any interference with either of these components will result in reflux, allowing bladder pressures, which always rise during micturition and may be abnormally high at other times, to be transmitted to the kidney. Any rise in intracaliceal pressure above the filtration pressure will inevitably alter intrarenal hemodynamics. Reflux itself is not necessarily harmful, but when it is accompanied by intrarenal reflux, parenchymal scarring (reflux nephropathy) is likely to develop, especially if the urine is infected.

The mechanism of scarring is not yet known, but experimental evidence indicates that the configuration of the renal papillae may determine whether intrarenal reflux is likely. There may also be alterations in concentrations of antibody against Tamm-Horsfall protein.

Reflux may be primary, when the intramural portion of the ureter is unduly short or there is lack of the firm muscular backing at the ureteral hiatus in the bladder, or secondary as a result of, for example, urethral valves, neuropathic bladder, or a diverticulum. There is evidence of racial differences in incidence and possibly of a familial predisposition to the condition. Reflux in children may be reversible.

Local lesions of acquired type that cause damage to and dilatation of the ureter are not infrequently accompanied by reflux. Cystitis, if localized to the region of the ureteral orifice, is liable to cause rigidity of the periureteral tissues, which allows reflux to occur.

Calculous disease

Ureteral stones are rarely primary and have usually migrated from the renal pelvis. They are of several types—endemic uric acid, oxalate, or ammonium acid urate stones occurring in certain specific localities throughout the world and usually associated with a high proportion of cereal in the diet; infective stones composed of magnesium ammonium phosphate or calcium phosphate, occurring in association with urinary tract infection (most commonly with *Proteus* organisms), and, in about a fourth of the cases, complicating a local urologic abnormality; and metabolic stones associated with disorders of calcium, oxalate, purine, or amino acid metabolism. In the presence of infection, endemic or metabolic stones may acquire a coating of phosphates. The majority of ureteral stones occur in men between 20 and 50 years of age. The stones may become impacted anywhere in the lumen of the ureter, the sites of predilection being the pelviureteral junction, the pelvic brim, the point where the ureter enters the bladder, and the ureteral orifice itself. Stone impaction usually leads to proximal dilatation of the ureter or of the renal pelvis and calices with pyelonephritis or pyonephrosis if infection is present. At the site of impaction there may be local inflammation, sometimes leading to ulceration and periureteritis. Very occasionally the ureteral orifice prolapses into the bladder, producing an intravesical mass that has to be distinguished from a ureterocele.

Inflammation

Nonspecific inflammation of the ureter is usually part of a more generalized inflammatory process, also affecting the renal pelvis or the bladder, and frequently is associated with and results from vesicoureteral reflux. Trauma to the mucosal surface by the passage of a calculus or by instrumentation may be an aggravating factor. The gross and microscopic features do not call for particular comment. Sometimes the mucosal surface has a granular appearance because of subepithelial collections of lymphoid cells (ureteritis follicularis). Malacoplakia sometimes affects the ureter.

Tuberculosis is the most common specific inflammation. The ureter is almost always involved by downward spread of the disease from the kidney, occurring either by continuity of tissue or by lymphatics. When healing occurs, there is often dense fibrosis that may completely obliterate the lumen or occlude its lower end and cause obstructive hydronephrosis and hydroureter.

Proliferative mucosal lesions

In response to inflammation and often adjacent to urothelial tumors, the lesions of ureteritis cystica and von Brunn's nests are sometimes seen. Essentially similar lesions are seen in both the renal pelvis and bladder, and the mode of their production and significance are considered in more detail later. The lesions of ureteritis cystica may be so large as to produce a curious cobblestone appearance on the intravenous urogram. The condition occurs especially in elderly patients and is most often seen in the upper third of the ureter.

Tumors

The benign tumors most often seen in the ureter are the fibroepithelial polyps, which have a central core of loose connective tissue and a covering of transitional epithelium (Fig. 18-63). The lesions are usually single, but occasionally multiple, and are commonly found in the upper ureter but are sometimes seen lower down and may protrude through the ureteral orifice. On rare occasions fibromas, myomas, and angiomas involve the ureter.

The most common primary malignant tumors arise from the transitional epithelium, usually as a part of generalized urothelial neoplasia. About 5% of all urothelial tumors are primary within the ureter and occur with about equal frequency on the right and left sides. Males are more commonly affected than females, and patients are usually in their sixth or seventh decade though no age is exempt. Macroscopically the lesions are papillary (or, less often, sessile) and may be single or multiple. The majority are situated in the lower part of the ureter. Invasion of the ureteral wall is not often seen. The etiology and general characteristics of ureteral tumors are similar to those of the urothelial tumors of the bladder and are considered later. Uncommon forms are the so-called stump tumors arising in the residual ureter months or years after simple nephrectomy, often for benign disease. Tumors occasionally arise at the site of a ureterocolic anastomosis.

The ureter is sometimes involved in metastatic disease with deposits in the ureteral wall itself or in adja-

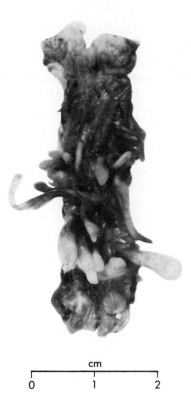

cm
0   1   2

Fig. 18-63. Excised segment of ureter with multiple fibroepithelial polyps.

cent retroperitoneal nodes from primary tumors in the testis, prostate, breast, colon, lung, or lymphoid system.

THE URINARY BLADDER
Congenital malformations

The urinary bladder originates in two stages. Early the embryonic cloaca, the caudal termination of the archenteron, the primitive gut, is divided by proliferation of a frontal urorectal septum into a dorsal intestinal channel, the rectum, and a ventral urogenital sinus continuous rostrally with the allantois that terminates at the umbilicus. Subsequently the urogenital sinus will be again divided by a second frontal septum, which serves differently in the two sexes to separate excretory from reproductive components of the genitourinary system.

Congenital malformations of the bladder are very rare. Absence, duplications, hourglass deformity, and diverticula have been described.

Exstrophy of the bladder is persistence of a vesiculocutaneous fistula resulting from incomplete closure of the anterior wall of the urogenital sinus and anterior abdominal wall (Fig. 18-64). Associated abnormalities include epispadias, failure of fusion of the labia, and lack of fusion of the symphysis pubis. The frequency is estimated at 1 per 50,000 births. Males predominate. The exstrophic bladder is subject to infection, metapla-

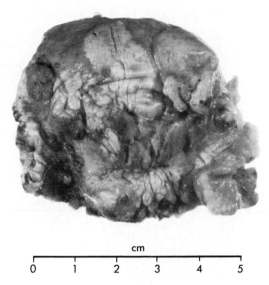

Fig. 18-64. Exstrophied bladder excised from middle-aged man (in whom transitional cell carcinoma subsequently developed at site of ureterocolic anastomosis). Notice pale smooth areas of squamous metaplasia.

sia, and ultimately often neoplastic change. Adenocarcinoma, less commonly squamous cell carcinoma, and least frequently transitional cell carcinoma are complications.

The urachus is a tapered sinus continuous with the allantois, which normally terminates at the umbilicus. Late in gestation, the urachus normally undergoes progressive fibrous obliteration, ultimately to form the median umbilical ligament. Discontinuous epithelium-lined structures can be found in 30% to 70% of dissections. Complete patency as a vesicoumbilical sinus may rarely persist in cases of congenital lower urinary tract obstruction. Persistence of discontinuous remnants may give rise to midline or periumbilical cysts. The least common but most important complication is neoplastic transformation, usually to adenocarcinoma.

Diverticulum

Bladder diverticula are relatively common but require surgical treatment rarely. Most are acquired results of urinary tract obstruction, usually in men older than 50 years with prostatic obstruction. Acquired diverticula are usually in a paraureteral location. Diverticula of congenital origin are rare.

Trauma

The bladder may be damaged by gunshot wounds and in other penetrating injuries, and occasionally it is inadvertently opened during surgical operations (such as those on large sliding hernias), or in the course of transurethral procedures, or is damaged by attempts to procure abortion. Rupture of the bladder may result from direct violence to the lower abdomen, as with a kick, and is commonly seen in those who have been in road traffic accidents, especially when there is a fractured pelvis. When the bladder is full at the time of the accident, the rupture may be intraperitoneal, but much more commonly it is extraperitoneal, with the wall being either torn open or penetrated by a spicule of bone. The mucosal surface is sometimes damaged by an indwelling catheter or a foreign body, producing an area of ulceration or polypoid cystitis, often with a heavy local eosinophil infiltration.

Dilatation

The bladder dilates to a varying degree in the presence of organic outflow obstruction caused by congenital lesions, such as urethral valves, or by acquired conditions, such as prostatic enlargement or urethral stricture, or when there are neurologic disorders. These conditions may be congenital (such as spina bifida) or may occur after trauma, inflammation, other disease (tabes dorsalis or disseminated sclerosis), or neoplasms—all of which can interfere with the normally smooth interaction of the sphincters, which are under cerebral control through the somatic nerves, and the detrusors controlled by the autonomic system. The effects produced depend on the level of the lesion and the extent to which local conditions within the bladder are modified by urinary infection. In cauda equina and conus lesions there is partial or complete interruption of the sacral reflex arc, which affects detrusor action. Initially the bladder distends painlessly, but later irregular detrusor activity returns and the bladder hypertrophies and becomes coarsely trabeculated (hypertonic or autonomic bladder). Reflux and ascending infection are common. When the cord lesion is above the sacral level, the initial stage of spinal shock and retention with overflow is followed by reflex micturition mediated through the spinal reflex arc (reflex or automatic bladder). If there is urinary infection, the bladder capacity may become greatly reduced. The uninhibited neurogenic bladder occurs when there is loss of higher cortical control, as with a cerebral tumor, and the large atonic neurogenic bladder, with a thin wall and atrophied muscle, develops when there is overdistension from lack of sensation because of interruption of the sensory limb of the reflex arc.

Simple obstruction of short duration will result in dilatation that is usually recoverable when the cause is removed, but when it is of long standing, the bladder wall gradually hypertrophies because of the rise in intravesical pressure and becomes trabeculated, and diverticula may appear. Eventually decompensation occurs and the bladder wall then thins and dilates, usually with reflux and hydroureter. Evidence indicates that the abnormality in bladder neck obstruction without prostatic enlargement (Marion's disease) may be a disorder of function rather than a mechanical obstruction attributable to local fibrosis.

Diverticula of the bladder are occasionally congenital but are much more commonly seen in patients with acquired outflow obstruction, being especially frequent in elderly patients with an enlarged prostate and a trabeculated bladder. They are particularly common in the posterolateral wall and are often large and multiple. They usually fail to empty completely on micturition, leading to urinary stasis within their lumens. Their walls consist of fibrous tissue and a variable amount of smooth muscle with an inner lining of transitional epithelium, which often undergoes squamous metaplasia. Complications include ulceration, stone formation, and neoplastic change in the lining mucosa.

Calculous disease

Many of the calculi seen in the bladder are secondary, since they originate in the upper urinary tract or form on a nucleus of dead tissue or a foreign body, especially when the urine is infected with urea-splitting organisms. Urinary stasis is often an added factor and predisposes to the "recumbency" calculi occurring in bedridden patients. Endemic calculi—once frequently seen, but now rare, in parts of England—are rare in blacks but are common in certain nonindustrialized Mediterranean and Far Eastern countries where there is a high cereal content in the diet. In children these endemic stones are more common in boys than in girls, occur more frequently in the bladder and urethra than in the upper urinary tract, and usually consist of ammonium acid urate and calcium oxalate. Endemic stones in adults in these countries usually consist of uric acid, calcium oxalate, and ammonium acid urate. In westernized areas of the world, bladder stones in children are infection stones, whereas in adults they are composed of pure calcium oxalate or a mixture of calcium oxalate and phosphate or are infection stones. Metabolic stones, similar to those seen in the ureter, also occur in the bladder and in the presence of infection may become coated with phosphates.

Calculi composed of phosphates are gray or gray-white and may be hard, or soft and friable. Oxalate stones are usually hard and either are smooth, rounded or nodular, resembling mulberries, or are irregularly spiculated; if there has been much local bleeding, they are frequently black or a very dark brown. Uric acid and urate stones are smooth, yellow or brown, and round or oval. Cystine stones are hard, smooth, and yellow and have a somewhat waxy appearance.

Fistulas

A vesicovaginal fistula between the posterior wall of the bladder and the upper anterior wall of the vagina may occur after obstetric injuries or irradiation damage

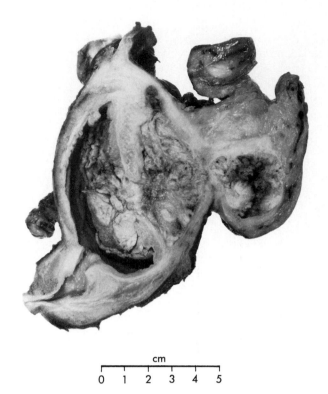

Fig. 18-65. Vesicointestinal fistula. Adenocarcinoma of colon invading posterior wall of bladder.

or is attributable to direct extension of tumor from one viscus to another. A vesicointestinal fistula between the bladder and either the rectum or sigmoid colon or small intestine occurs most commonly in diverticulitis or malignant disease of the large bowel and is seen only infrequently in regional ileitis (Fig. 18-65).

Inflammation

A variety of bacterial and fungal infections can cause inflammatory changes in the bladder, which may also occur with parasitic infestation or direct exposure to chemical irritants, with foreign bodies, or after local trauma. Any congenital or acquired lesion causing obstruction and stasis is liable to exacerbate an inflammatory process.

Since the normal bladder epithelium is very resistant to bacterial infection, primary cystitis is rare. Most cases are caused by spread of infection from the upper urinary tract, as occurs with tuberculosis, or from the urethra as when cystitis follows instrumentation. Cystitis occurs much more commonly in females than in males because of the short urethra, which is liable to fecal contamination and to mechanical trauma during intercourse. Prostatic obstruction is a very frequent cause in males.

It is often difficult to correlate symptoms with the presence or absence of bacteria in the urine, and patients with clinical cystitis may at various times be asymptomatic with or without bacteriuria or symptomatic either way. Asymptomatic bacteriuria is a common disorder in childhood, occurring, according to different estimates, between 5 and 30 times more frequently in girls than in boys. It is also seen in both nonpregnant and pregnant women, and in a significant number of the latter asymptomatic bacteriuria in early pregnancy may be followed by symptomatic urinary tract infection—and in particular by acute pyelonephritis—the nearer it is to term. The particular danger of infection is the frequency with which it is complicated by vesicoureteral reflux and residual urine, which may lead to chronic renal disease, hypertension, and renal failure. In children with urinary infection there is probably little if any permanent structural damage to the urinary tract in the absence of reflux.

For treatment to be effective, it is important to localize the infection and, in particular, to distinguish between upper and lower tract infection. This is often difficult. In addition to microbiologic examinations of midstream and clean-catch specimens of urine, many techniques, including ureteral catheterization, suprapubic bladder aspiration, bladder washouts, detection of antibody-coated bacteria, and determinations of nonspecific C-reactive protein concentrations and serum antibodies to O antigens of *Escherichia coli* may have to be employed.

The most common causative organisms are *E. coli*, *Staphylococcus aureus*, and *Streptococcus faecalis*. In hospital practice, infection with *Proteus* and *Pseudomonas aeruginosa* occurs quite commonly. Specific cystitis caused by tuberculosis is not uncommon, and several viruses, including herpesvirus and adenovirus, and fungi such as *Actinomyces* and *Candida* are sometimes responsible. Urinary tract infection is usually accompanied by an immune response with a rise in antibody titer to the somatic antigens of the infecting organisms, but it is generally believed that specific antibodies play little or no part in protecting against or eradicating urinary infection. During the course of an infection there may be rises in IgA, IgG, and IgM levels in the urine, and secretory IgA (half of which is derived from urethral secretions) is also found in increased amounts, which may be partly responsible for protecting the urethra against infection and may also explain the relative infrequency of cystitis as a complication of urethritis.

The variable severity of urinary tract infection from patient to patient may be related to the virulence of the responsible organism because of the presence of bacterial capsules or the ability to produce an endotoxin. The tendency for certain organisms to colonize different parts of the tract preferentially is believed to be attributable to their "adhesiveness" (capacity to attach to a particular type of epithelium and not to others).

Acute cystitis, or an acute exacerbation of chronic cystitis, may be of variable severity. In mild cases there is mucosal congestion with some local edema and polymorphonuclear leukocyte infiltration. With severe infection the congestion and edema are pronounced and the epithelium is either hyperplastic or ulcerated; there is widespread inflammatory cell infiltration, principally by polymorphonuclear leukocytes, which affects the lamina propria and may spread into the muscle coat. The vessels are thick walled, and their lining endothelium is often prominent. Abscesses may occur. Chronic nonspecific cystitis occurs after persistent or repeated attacks of acute cystitis. The epithelium may be deficient, irregularly hyperplastic, or sometimes polypoid, and in long-standing cases there is often squamous metaplasia. The lamina propria is usually broadened, contains more fibrous tissue than is usual, and is congested and diffusely or focally infiltrated with inflammatory cells. These are mainly lymphocytes and plasma cells, with a few eosinophils here and there, and the lymphoid cells may be collected into follicles. The process spreads into the muscle coat to a varying depth, and the blood vessels throughout the bladder wall are usually thickened. In the later stages of the disease the fibrous tissue contracts and the bladder capacity is greatly reduced.

Descriptive adjectives are sometimes used to indicate the predominant change (for example, hemorrhagic cystitis or ulcerative cystitis), and the term "follicular cystitis" describes the accumulation of lymphoid cells that is often seen deep to the mucosa in many types of chronic cystitis and can be recognized as pale granular lesions when viewed through the cystoscope or in the fixed specimen. Bullous cystitis is a rare form in which there is localized edema of the lamina propria resulting in a folded or polypoid mucosa that appears cystic. There may be local hemorrhages, and macroscopically the lesion may simulate the grapelike masses of embryonal sarcoma. Emphysematous cystitis, seen in diabetics or in association with infection with gas-forming organisms, is a very rare condition in which the bladder wall is studded with gas-filled cysts lying in the lamina propria.

Special forms of cystitis

In abacterial cystitis inflammatory changes are often severe and accompanied by mucosal ulceration, though the urine is persistently sterile. The cause is not known, but some of the patients have Reiter's disease characterized by conjunctivitis, arthritis, and nonspecific urethritis, cystitis, or prostatitis, and attributable possibly to *Mycoplasma hominis* or *Chlamydia*. In Britain and North America Reiter's disease frequently complicates nongonococcal genital infections, whereas in Scandinavia and on the European continent it is more likely to occur after a dysenteric type of illness.

Gangrenous cystitis (also described as croupous, diphtheritic, membranous, or pseudomembranous cystitis) has a wide variety of causes, such as chemical irritants, physical damage by excess heat or irradiation, infections, overdistension, extravesical pressure from an impacted gravid uterus, damage to blood vessels, and thrombosis or embolism, which either interfere with the blood supply of the bladder or produce severe inflammation. Very rarely gangrene occurs after transurethral resection of the prostate. Cystoscopically, gray sloughing areas are seen and the mucosa and parts of the lamina propria may be passed as a cast of the bladder. The mucosa is often covered with a layer of fibrin, pus, degenerated epithelium, and organisms.

In encrusted cystitis, when the urine is infected with urea-splitting organisms, and especially when the bladder wall has been damaged (for example, by local irradiation or repeated diathermy), deposits of calcium phosphate or calcium magnesium phosphate occur on the damaged area. Macroscopically there are grayish white gritty plaques or crusts on the mucosal surface, and microscopically there is irregular ulceration or hyperplasia of the epithelium with adherent calculous material, which sometimes elicits a local foreign-body giant cell reaction.

In irradiation cystitis the bladder is damaged by local or external irradiation of the bladder wall itself or of adjacent organs. The first changes to be noted are mucosal congestion and a variable amount of local edema, sometimes progressing to the formation of bullae. More prolonged exposure results in mucosal ulceration, edema of the lamina propria with acute necrotizing arteriolitis, and some inflammatory cell infiltration. In the later stages mucosal ulceration persists, but there are often epithelial proliferation and hyperplasia, with or without squamous metaplasia, as well as considerable fibrosis of the lamina propria and muscle coat, leading to contraction of the bladder. There are varying degrees of endarteritis, and if tissue damage is severe, fistulas are liable to form.

Interstitial cystitis characteristically occurs in middle-aged or elderly women, who complain of distressing and disabling frequency, dysuria, and suprapubic pain and are found on cystoscopy to have a hyperemic, usually contracted, bladder that bleeds easily when distended. Most of the changes are seen on the posterior wall or at the vault. Microscopically the mucosa may or may not be ulcerated, but the most striking changes are seen in the lamina propria, which is broadened and more fibrous than normal and is diffusely infiltrated with lymphocytes, plasma cells, and some eosinophils and polymorphonuclear leukocytes. The fibrous septa in the muscle coat are also widened and infiltrated with inflammatory cells, and there may be fibrous tissue re-

placement of muscle fibers and spread of the inflammatory process through the full thickness of the bladder wall. The capillaries in the lamina propria are usually very prominent, and the arterioles are frequently thick walled. The cause is not known. Although hormonal changes, infection, and lymphatic obstruction have been believed to play a part, recent work has suggested that the disease has an autoimmune basis. Interstitial cystitis is essentially a disease of women; any male patient with symptoms that in a female would immediately suggest the diagnosis is much more likely to have malignant disease in his bladder. He should be thoroughly investigated and kept under regular surveillance with cytologic examinations of the urine and, if necessary, repeated bladder biopsies.

Cyclophosphamide, when administered as a cytotoxic agent, may produce a hemorrhagic cystitis that can eventually lead to bladder contracture. The changes are caused by the breakdown products of cyclophosphamide rather than by the drug itself and are not dose dependent. Tumor formation is a very rare complication.

The local infiltration of the bladder wall with eosinophils commonly seen in the base of ulcers caused by indwelling catheters and during the reparative stages after bladder biopsy, and as a constant feature of the acute stages of bilharzial infestation, needs to be distinguished from eosinophilic cystitis. This is a rare condition believed to be attributable to infection or to food or drug allergy occurring in young patients (sometimes children) and often accompanied by blood eosinophilia. Cystoscopically the bladder mucosa is usually polypoid and the appearances may resemble a tumor, but microscopically the bladder wall, especially the lamina propria, is diffusely and heavily infiltrated with eosinophils and there is no suggestion of neoplasia. Granulomatous cystitis has been reported in the rare syndrome of chronic granulomatous disease of childhood in which the bactericidal activity of the leukocytes is depressed, probably because of a genetically determined enzyme deficiency.

Malakoplakia is a rare condition that was first described in the urinary tract and has subsequently been found in the testes, epididymides, prostate, and, very occasionally, the gut. In the bladder yellowish, round or oval, plaquelike or occasionally polypoid lesions are scattered over the mucosal surface, and the lamina propria contains dense collections of large histiocytes with granular cytoplasm (von Hansemann cells). These contain small, rounded, sometimes apparently laminated bodies (Michaelis-Gutmann bodies, Fig. 18-66) that stain for iron and with the von Kossa and periodic acid–Schiff techniques and are believed to be altered bacteria or breakdown products of bacteria that have become mineralized. There is often a clinical history of urinary

Proliferative and metaplastic mucosal lesions

Von Brunn's nests, cystitis cystica, and cystitis glandularis are three related conditions commonly seen in the inflamed bladder or around the stalk of papillary tumors and the margins of sessile or invasive tumors, both in experimental animals and in humans. To consider the cystic and glandular lesions as types of cystitis is both unfortunate and inaccurate, since (in common with von Brunn's nests) they are really reactive in nature and would be better designated as examples of cystic or glandular metaplasia. For the present, however, they will continue to be referred to as "cystitis." It is sometimes stated that these lesions are precancerous, but, although undoubtedly they sometimes have a malignant potential, the association with neoplasia is by no means invariable and all three are better regarded as being indicative of mucosal instability, which is often capable of complete resolution.

Von Brunn's nests are formed by buds or sprouts of transitional epithelium that grow down from the surface into the underlying lamina propria and later become surrounded by a condensed layer of connective tissue that eventually separates them from the overlying cells. Central cavitation of the cysts or infolding of the surface epithelium, with the formation of crypts that become obstructed, will lead to the formation of cystitis cystica (Fig. 18-67). In the fully formed cysts there is a lining of flattened or low cuboid cells, and if the cysts are of sufficient size, the mucosal surface becomes irregular and has a granular appearance. Cystitis glandularis is produced when the cells lining the cysts differentiate into columnar epithelium.

Squamous metaplasia of the transitional epithelium of the bladder is commonly seen in inflammatory disease and is not necessarily precancerous. The same cannot be said with certainty when the change occurs in cells lining a diverticulum, where there is a much higher incidence of both squamous metaplasia and squamous carcinoma than in the bladder. The type of squamous change in which, because of estrogen stimulation, the cell cytoplasm becomes vacuolated (and is therefore often referred to as vaginal metaplasia), is frequently seen as a white patch with clear-cut edges on the trigone of young women with the urethral syndrome. It has no association with neoplastic disease. Leukoplakia, a rare condition more common in men than in women, is distinguished from squamous metaplasia by surface keratinization with or without parakeratosis and the presence of a stratum granulosum and intercellular bridges. It is frequently associated with chronic or recurrent urinary tract infection, and malignancy (commonly squamous carcinoma) occurs in about one fourth of cases.

Polypoid cystitis commonly occurs with incipient or established vesicointestinal fistula or when the bladder

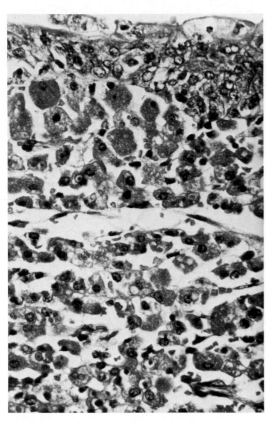

Fig. 18-66. Malakoplakia. Lamina propria contains many large macrophages with granular cytoplasm. Notice round, targetlike, Michaelis-Gutmann bodies. (Hematoxylin and eosin; 600×.)

tract infection, and the condition is considered to be an atypical form of granulomatous response to coliform infection. The lesions should not be mistaken for neoplasms.

The bladder is involved in most cases of renal tuberculosis, and in tuberculous cystitis the changes are usually first seen near the ureteral orifices. The early lesions are hyperemic and granular but soon progress to ulceration, whereas fibrosis occurs in the later stages of the disease and may result in very gross contracture of the bladder. The histologic appearance is in no way different from that seen in tuberculous lesions elsewhere in the body.

The bladder is very occasionally affected in fungal infections, especially actinomycosis and candidiasis, sometimes by direct spread from adjacent organs or more commonly through the bloodstream in generalized systemic disease, which may complicate the prolonged use of antibiotics, steroids, or immunosuppressive drugs.

The bladder is frequently involved in bilharzial disease and is occasionally affected in infestation with *Echinococcus* and *Strongyloides stercoralis.*

is stimulated locally, for example, by the tip of an indwelling catheter. It is distinguished from a papillary tumor by the shape of the papillae, which taper from a broad base to a narrow tip (Fig. 18-68).

Epithelial (urothelial) tumors

More than 90% of all bladder tumors arise from the transitional epithelium, which is continuous with a sim-

ilar epithelium that lines the renal pelves, the ureters, and the greater part of the urethra. Many workers object to the term "urothelium" to describe this common cell lining, but its use has the distinct advantage of emphasizing the basic fact that the various parts of the urinary tract form a coherent whole and that tumor formation in any one area, such as the bladder, must be considered and treated in the light of the changes else-

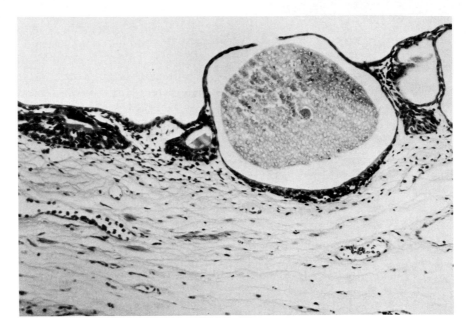

Fig. 18-67. Cystitis cystica. (Hematoxylin and eosin; 240×.)

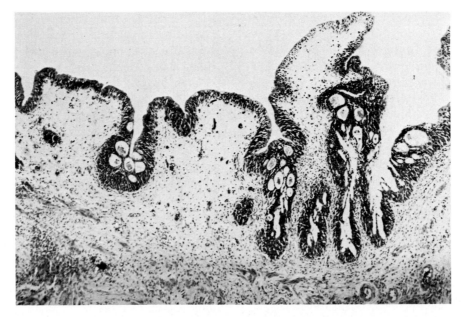

Fig. 18-68. Polypoid cystitis. Notice broad-based mucosal projections. (Hematoxylin and eosin; 96×.)

where in the urinary system. Urothelial neoplasia is therefore a single, potentially multifocal disease that may affect any part of the urothelium. That several areas may be involved is simultaneously suggestive of a single common cause, but in many cases the disease pattern becomes evident only over a period of years. For example, a renal pelvic tumor on one side may be followed by a bladder tumor, with a urethral tumor developing later (Fig. 18-69). Common causes may again be operative, but other factors, such as implantation of cells in the lower tract from a lesion higher up, lymphatic spread, or direct surface spread of tumor by continuity along an epithelial surface, may be responsible for the multicentricity of the tumors. Local conditions may be important in determining where neoplastic change will occur.

Etiology

The association between bladder cancer and industrial occupation was first recognized in aniline dye workers in Germany at the turn of the century, and the list of occupations in which there is risk now includes the chemical, rubber, and cable industries, gas retort house workers, rat catchers, sewage workers, and laboratory technicians. The toxic substances responsible for neoplasia are the metabolic products of α- and β-

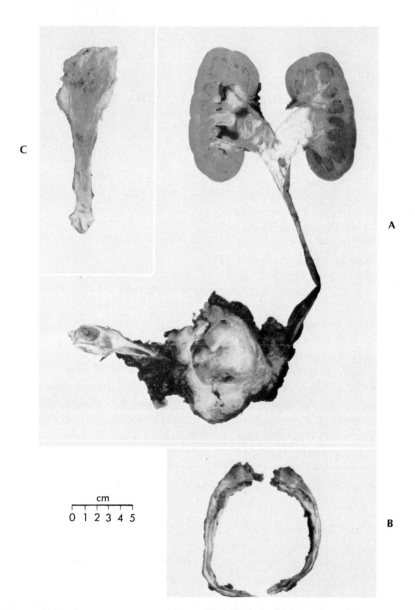

Fig. 18-69. Multiple urothelial tumors in middle-aged man. **A,** Nephroureterocystoprostatectomy (in 1969) for tumors in left renal pelvis, lower end of left ureter, region of internal meatus, and right ureter. **B,** Urethrectomy (early 1972) for tumor. **C,** Right ureterectomy (late 1972) for multiple urothelial tumors.

naphthylamine, benzidine, and 4-aminodiphenyl, some of which are carcinogenic in experimental animals. Occupational tumors occur at an earlier age than spontaneous ones do, after an induction period, sometimes as long as 20 or more years, between contact with the chemical and the clinical appearance of tumor. Histologically, industrial bladder tumors are similar to spontaneous lesions. It has been estimated that in heavily industrialized areas of the United States and United Kingdom between 20% and 30% of bladder tumors in men are associated with occupation. Cigarette smoke, phenacetin-containing analgesics, and antineoplastic drugs such as cyclophosphamide and chlornaphazin can act as carcinogens, but coffee and the artificial sweeteners saccharin and cyclamate are no longer considered to be harmful.

Local lesions in the urinary tract itself may also be important. Within a short time of birth, areas of squamous and glandular metaplasia develop in the mucosa of the exstrophied bladder as a result of repeated infection and trauma, and in very rare cases malignancy supervenes. The tumors occur at a younger age than those in patients with normally developed bladders, and adenocarcinomas are particularly common though they rarely metastasize. The proliferative changes in the mucosa may persist after the exstrophy is corrected surgically, with a continued risk of tumor formation. The same considerations apply in the defunctionalized bladder after urinary diversion, since pyocystis is not uncommon and tumors occasionally develop. A vesical diverticulum also predisposes to tumor formation; squamous metaplasia frequently occurs in the epithelial lining and there is a higher incidence of squamous carcinoma within a diverticulum than in the bladder itself. The significance of leukoplakia and the mucosal proliferative lesions has already been discussed. The association between bladder cancer and schistosomiasis is frequently reported, and there is a high incidence of squamous carcinoma in some parts of the world where infestation is common. The belief that there is a direct causal relationship between the two is yielding place to the concept that neoplasia might be initiated by urine-borne carcinogens, possibly nitrosamines formed during attacks of urinary tract infection, and accelerated by irritation from the presence of ova.

Incidence and frequency

In the United States, bladder cancer accounts for about 4% of all cancers in males and about 2% of cancers in females, the comparable figures for England and Wales being 7% for males and 2.5% for females. In both countries tumors occur more commonly in males than in females, in ratios of between 2 and 4 males to 1 female. Although tumors may occur at any age, neoplasia is rare in the first five decades but thereafter shows a sharp rise in incidence.

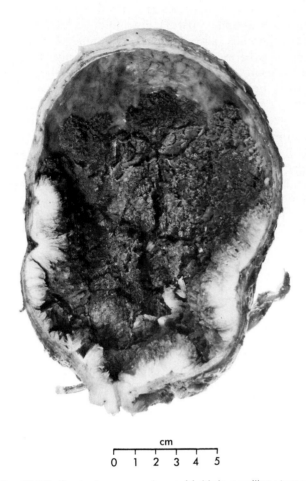

cm
0 1 2 3 4 5

Fig. 18-70. Cystectomy specimen. Multiple papillary tumors cover greater part of bladder wall. There was no histologic evidence of invasion of lamina propria or muscle.

Gross appearance

Urothelial tumors may be single or multiple (Fig. 18-70), finely or coarsely fronded, papillary, sessile (Fig. 18-71), nodular, or ulcerated or, in the in situ disease, recognizable only as areas of mucosal reddening or granularity. When a tumor extends into the bladder wall, there is a variable amount of thickening in and around its base. Tumors may occur anywhere in the bladder but have a predilection for the trigone, the region of the ureteral orifices, and the posterolateral walls.

Microscopic appearance

The recognition of neoplastic change in urothelium using only the light microscope is often difficult, subjective, and dependent in no small measure on the experience of the observer. Recent work correlating transmission and scanning electron microscope studies with light microscopic findings is beginning to introduce some degree of objectivity and helping to estab-

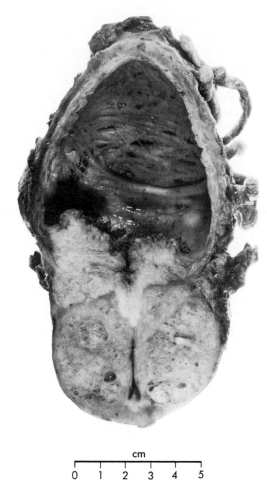

cm

0 1 2 3 4 5

Fig. 18-71. Cystoprostatectomy specimen. There is sessile invasive tumor at bladder base and in prostatic urethra. Notice enlarged prostate and vesical trabeculation.

The pattern is determined by examination of histologic sections with a hand lens or the low power of the microscope and can be described as papillary, solid (infiltrating), papillary and solid, or noninvasive (in situ). In the first, tumor growth is into the lumen of the bladder and the tumor can be seen to have a finely fronded pattern with delicate papillary processes. In the solid tumors, growth occurs mostly into the bladder wall, and in a papillary and solid tumor, both types of growth pattern are seen. In the noninvasive tumor there may be very little to see other than, possibly, some localized thickening of the epithelium.

The cell type may be transitional, squamous, or glandular, and it is important to distinguish between squamous metaplasia and squamous carcinoma and between glandular metaplasia and adenocarcinoma. The most practical distinction is that if the squamous or glandular areas are focal within a tumor that is otherwise transitional in type, the correct designation is metaplasia, whereas an overall change indicates a squamous or glandular carcinoma. Another feature of the pure squamous carcinoma is that the infiltrating processes of tumor cells sometimes have a somewhat spiky or angular outline and are surrounded by a fibroblastic or fibrous stroma (Fig. 18-72). The incidence of squamous carcinoma is difficult to assess. Figures of 1% to 7% of all bladder tumors are quoted, with the differences being attributable to failure to distinguish between tumor and metaplasia. Pure adenocarcinoma of the bladder is another rare type of primary tumor and, indeed, most of the grandular tumors seen in the bladder are extravesical tumors arising, for example, in the bowel and growing into the contiguous bladder wall. Glandular tumors arising at the apex of the bladder may originate in the urachus, and the extremely rare examples occurring at the bladder base are believed to arise either from endodermal remnants or from areas of cystitis glandularis arising by a process of metaplasia in the trigonal epithelium. Pure adenocarcinomas comprise less than 1% of all bladder tumors.

Before the grades of transitional cell carcinoma are described, it is first necessary to define the papilloma and establish the means of distinguishing it from a carcinoma. The papilloma is a papillary lesion with a central core of loose, rather delicate, connective tissue and a covering of transitional epithelium up to four or five layers in thickness. The individual cells vary little, if at all, from normal bladder epithelial cells and are of regular size and shape; they lie at right angles to the basement membrane except for the most superficial layer, which often lies parallel to it. Mitoses are absent. Characteristically the papilloma is a cylindrical structure and, when seen in longitudinal section, has parallel sides, which distinguishes it from polypoid cystitis in which there are tapering fingerlike processes broader at their bases than at their tips. With these criteria the

lish more firmly the diagnostic characteristics of normal, premalignant, and malignant epithelium. Pleomorphic microvilli, seen with the scanning electron microscope, are reported in premalignant and malignant epithelia but are not specific features, since they sometimes occur in inflammatory lesions. The luminal membrane of normal urothelium seen with transmission electron microscopy has a unique appearance, and the superficial cells are seen to be joined by tight junctions and desmosomes. The deeper cells similarly are joined by desmosomes whose numbers may be increased in noninvasive tumors and decreased when invasion has occurred. The electron microscope can also reveal discontinuities in the basal lamina that are not seen with the light microscope.

To fully assess a bladder tumor, one needs to determine four specific features: the pattern of its growth, the cell type, the degree of tumor differentiation (or grade), and the depth of invasion of the bladder wall (pathologic stage).

papilloma will be diagnosed only rarely. All other papillary lesions should be considered as carcinomas, provided that polypoid cystitis has been excluded. In many carcinomas there is evidence of penetration of the basement membrane and invasion of the bladder wall, but the diagnosis of carcinoma can and should be made in their absence if the changes in the epithelium justify it.

Transitional cell carcinomas can be divided into three grades depending on their degree of dedifferentiation.

In the differentiated (grade I) tumor the cells are clearly of transitional type, but the criteria of papilloma are not fulfilled (Fig. 18-73). The most noticeable difference is a significant increase in the number of layers of cells, usually accompanied by some loss of polarity and minor degrees of hyperchromicity. Occasional mitoses are often seen. The intermediate (grade II) tumor is still recognizable as being of transitional origin (Fig. 18-74). There are more cell layers than in the normal epithe-

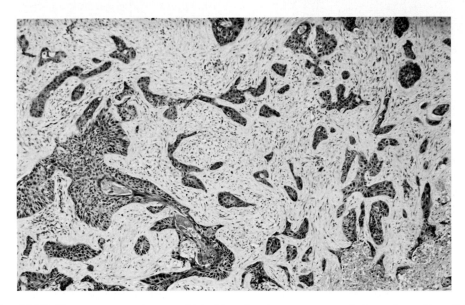

Fig. 18-72. Squamous carcinoma of bladder showing pronounced stromal reaction. (Hematoxylin and eosin; 96×.)

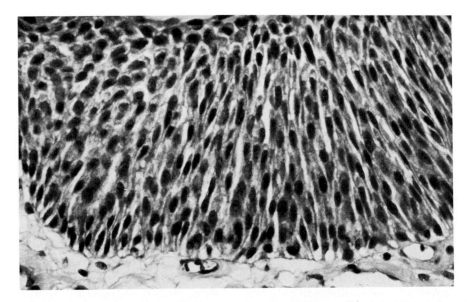

Fig. 18-73. Differentiated (grade I) transitional cell carcinoma. (Hematoxylin and eosin; 600×.)

lium or papilloma, and this is associated with a greater loss of polarity and more pronounced nuclear hyperchromicity and mitotic activity than is seen in the differentiated tumor. There may also be some irregularity of the luminal aspect of the epithelium. The anaplastic or undifferentiated (grade III) tumor (Fig. 18-75) is no longer clearly recognizable as having originated in transitional epithelium. All the features noted in the previous grades are much more pronounced, and the su-

perficial layers of cells have often become loosened and been shed into the lumen of the bladder. Squamous and glandular metaplasia may occur in any type of transitional cell tumor, but both are much more common in the less well-differentiated ones.

The squamous carcinomas and adenocarcinomas can each be graded similarly according to their degree of differentiation.

From the prognostic point of view it is important to

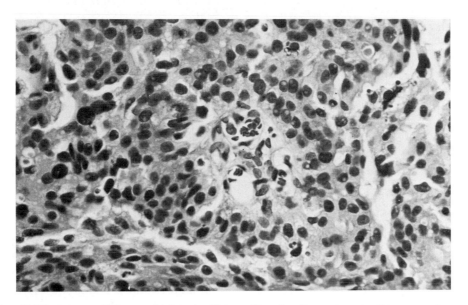

Fig. 18-74. Intermediate grade (grade II) transitional cell carcinoma. (Hematoxylin and eosin; 600×.)

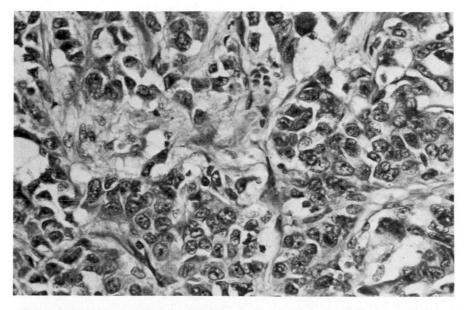

Fig. 18-75. Anaplastic (grade III) carcinoma. (Hematoxylin and eosin; 600×.)

assess the depth to which the bladder wall is invaded by a tumor, that is, to determine the pathologic stage. The greater the amount of tissue available to the pathologist, the more comprehensive and accurate the staging is likely to be, but even in very small specimens the amount of infiltration should always be assessed. The following pathologic stages are recognized in the 1978 edition of the International Union against Cancer (UICC) booklet:

pTis Preinvasive (in situ) carcinoma
pTa   Papillary noninvasive carcinoma
pT1   Tumor not extending beyond lamina propria
pT2   Invasion of superficial muscle
pT3   Invasion of deep muscle or perivesical tissue
pT4   Invasion of prostate or other extravesical structures
pTO   No tumor found
pTX   Extent of invasion cannot be assessed

It is important to stage a tumor according to the greatest depth reached by its advancing edge. Lymphatic or vascular invasion ahead of the main tumor mass should not increase the stage, though it should be noted.

Proliferative changes, consisting in epithelial hyperplasia, von Brunn's nests, cystitis cystica, and sometimes polypoid cystitis, are commonly seen in the bladder mucosa around the base of the tumor and between multiple tumors even when there is little or no obvious abnormality on unassisted-eye or cystoscopic examination. The specific red cell adherence test, which needs to be further refined before it can be recommended un-reservedly, has been used to assess the invasive potential of bladder tumors.

Carcinoma in situ

Carcinoma in situ, or noninvasive bladder cancer, is an important type of tumor whose natural history is not yet fully known. In some patients it progresses within a relatively short time to papillary or invasive tumor, but in others it remains latent for several years and constitutes an extremely difficult therapeutic problem. It can be defined simply as diffuse or localized histologic change in the epithelium resembling carcinoma, but without evidence of invasion, and characterized by some or all of the following features: an increase in the number of cell layers, crowding of the nuclei, loss of the regular arrangement and polarity of the cells, hyperchromatic nuclei, increased mitotic activity, presence of mitoses above the basal layer of cells, and frequently lack of cohesion of the superficial layers of cells, which desquamate into the lumen of the bladder. In fully developed examples one should have no problem in making the diagnosis but may sometimes have difficulty in distinguishing carcinoma in situ from reactive hyperplasia. In some patients monitored with serial biopsies it is possible to see the in situ disease evolve through the stages of hyperplasia and hyperplasia with atypia, but the precise point at which the diagnosis of carcinoma will be made is likely to vary from observer to observer. Regularly repeated cytologic examinations of the urine are essential for diagnosis and for monitoring therapy.

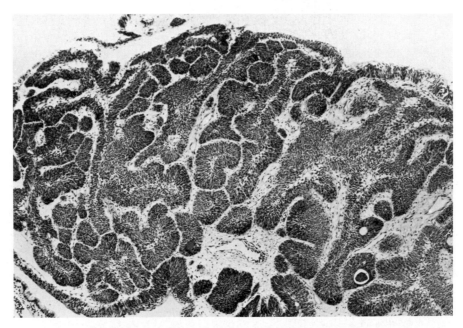

Fig. 18-76. Inverted papilloma of bladder. There is thin surface layer of epithelium, continuous with solid, and occasionally cystic, transitional epithelial masses in lamina propria. (Hematoxylin and eosin; 96×.)

Differential diagnosis

Care should be taken to distinguish between polypoid cystitis and papilloma or papillary carcinoma and not to confuse von Brunn's nests with invasive tumor. There should be no difficulty when the nests are in continuity with the surface, but one should remember that in a late stage of their development they may become separated from the overlying epithelium by a layer of connective tissue. The inverted papilloma (Fig. 18-76), in which there is a localized subepithelial proliferation of epithelium producing a rounded or oval nodule that histologically combines the features of von Brunn's nests and cystitis cystica, is sometimes seen at the bladder base and may be mistaken for a tumor. In the nephrogenic adenoma (Fig. 18-77), which is almost certainly a reparative lesion occurring after previous mucosal damage, the transitional epithelium is usually replaced by a single layer of cuboid cells from which small acini and tubular structures extend into the underlying lamina propria. This lesion may be mistaken for an adenocarcinoma.

Inflammatory lesions such as eosinophilic cystitis and malakoplakia may simulate a tumor on gross examination, though there should be no difficulty when they are examined microscopically. Problems may also arise with certain types of chronic cystitis, and the practical difficulties that may occur in patients with the clinical picture of interstitial cystitis have already been mentioned. Primary amyloidosis of the bladder may cause profuse hematuria. Histologic examination will reveal deposits of amyloid in the lamina propria, bladder muscle, or blood vessels. The overlying epithelium is frequently thickened and hyperplastic, and if it is unduly polypoid, there may be some resemblance to an epithelial tumor. Endometriosis occasionally involves the bladder and causes hematuria.

Specimens of epithelial tumors at the bladder base obtained by transurethral biopsy are often a problem in histologic diagnosis, and one should remember that a bladder tumor may invade the superficial prostate, that a prostatic carcinoma occasionally spreads upward into the lamina propria of the bladder and masquerades as a bladder tumor, and that very occasionally carcinoma of the bladder and prostate may coexist. The bladder is commonly invaded by gastrointestinal adenocarcinomas, with incipient or actual vesicointestinal fistula and preceding or accompanying polypoid cystitis, and cervical tumors may spread into the bladder base. Other forms of metastasis are uncommon and include transcelomic spread from upper abdominal malignancies, hematogenous spread in malignant melanoma, and implantation of renal parenchymal carcinomas that have invaded the pelvicalicine system and spread down the ureter.

Spread of urothelial tumors

The most important method of spread is by direct extension into and eventually through the bladder wall and the subsequent invasion of adjacent organs and tethering of the bladder to the pelvic wall. Involvement of one or another ureteral orifice or intramural ureter sometimes occurs relatively early and has an important bearing on prognosis.

The tendency for vesical tumors to be associated with tumors elsewhere in the urothelium has already been emphasized. A tumor may recur at its original site after local treatment, but it is difficult if not impossible for the urologist always to make a clear distinction between

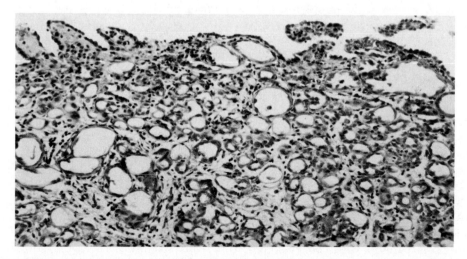

Fig. 18-77. Nephrogenic adenoma. Surface epithelium is cuboid, and lamina propria contains many acini and tubules lined by flattened cells. (Hematoxylin and eosin; 96×.)

a true recurrence and new multicentric tumor formation. Spread by lymphatics occurs commonly; when the superficial lymphatics in the bladder wall are invaded, there may be centrifugal spread deep to the surface mucosa producing a subepithelial plaque-like mass of tumor, whereas spread by the deeper lymphatics, which is particularly liable to occur with the anaplastic types of tumor, leads to involvement of the regional lymph nodes in the pelvis and abdomen. Blood-borne metastases often occur in the later stages of the disease with deposits in the liver, lungs, bone, and adrenals. Other sites include the heart, brain, and kidney.

Cytologic diagnosis of urothelial tumors

Exfoliative cytology is playing an increasingly important part in the diagnosis of urothelial tumors and is of special value in screening asymptomatic individuals who are at industrial risk. It is also useful as an additional diagnostic aid in patients with hematuria, but the technique has serious limitations if it is used as a method of routine follow-up examination of patients who have already been treated for a bladder tumor. The accuracy of the technique varies from observer to observer, and false-positive results may occur with urinary tract infections and in patients with urinary calculi, and false negatives with low-grade tumors, which in general tend to exfoliate less readily than do high-grade ones. To obtain reproducible results and improve accuracy, it is essential that the techniques of collection and preparation of the specimens be standardized.

Immunologic aspects

Genitourinary malignancy may be associated with changes in both cell-mediated and humoral immunity. Although there is a high incidence of neoplasia in the elderly, and it is known that tumors sometimes occur in patients receiving immunosuppressive therapy, there is as yet no proof that depression of the immune system always precedes or is associated with the early stages of malignancy. The evidence indicates that only in disseminated neoplastic disease is there serious immunodeficiency.

Other tumors

Connective tissue tumors of all types, some benign and some malignant, and taking origin from fibrous tissue, smooth muscle, nerves, and blood vessels, account for only about 5% of all bladder tumors. Some are symptomless and are incidental findings at autopsy or operation, whereas others cause hematuria or, much less commonly, produce hormonal effects such as those occurring with pheochromocytomas. Some neurofibromatous tumors develop in patients with von Recklinghausen's disease. Lymphomas of the bladder are rare tumors, occurring particularly in middle-aged and el-

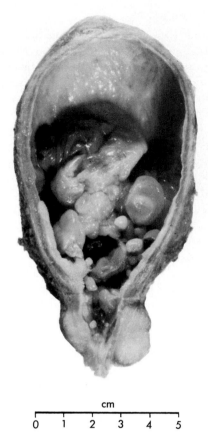

cm
0 1 2 3 4 5

Fig. 18-78. Embryonal sarcoma ("grapelike sarcoma") of bladder base and prostate in young boy.

derly patients, producing rounded masses in the lamina propria that have a characteristic appearance when seen with the cystoscope.

The most common bladder tumor in infants and young children is the embryonal sarcoma (Fig. 18-78), which produces pale, fleshy, polypoid, grapelike masses that typically arise over a large area at the base of the bladder. Microscopically the bladder epithelium is usually thinned but is otherwise normal, and the lamina propria is occupied by embryonic mesenchyme consisting of masses of pleomorphic, darkly stained, often stellate cells in a loose, almost myxomatous background. In about half the cases the tumor cells have eosinophilic cytoplasm in which cross-striations can be identified (rhabdomyoblasts). The tumor may also involve the lower ends of the ureters, the prostate, and the seminal vesicles, and in females polypoid masses may be present at the introitus.

THE URACHUS

The urachus is the remains of the narrow allantoic canal, which in fetal life runs between the apex of the bladder and the umbilicus and in adults is not infrequently found incidentally in histologic sections taken from the fundus of the bladder. The central lumen is usually small, and the wall consists of a layer of cuboid, low columnar, or transitional epithelium, a small amount of connective tissue, and a smooth muscle sheath, which is distinct from the surrounding bladder muscle. Part or all of the urachus may remain patent after birth. If the entire canal is open (urachal fistula), urine is discharged at the umbilicus. Patency at the vesical end only leads to the formation of a urachal diverticulum, and if the other end is patent at the umbilicus, there is a urachal sinus. A urachal cyst forms if the two ends are closed off and the central portion becomes distended. The tumors arising in the urachus are derived from its epithelial lining or, less commonly, from the surrounding fibrous tissue and muscle. The most frequent type is an adenocarcinoma, which only rarely involves the mucosal surface of the bladder and grows either in the deeper part of the bladder wall or outside it in the supravesical area, where it may form a mass of considerable size. The prognosis is not good, and the tumors must be excised widely to prevent local recurrence.

REFERENCES
Kidney
General

1. Heptinstall, R.: Pathology of the kidney, ed. 3, Boston, 1983, Little, Brown & Co.
2. Rosen, S.: Pathology of glomerular disease, New York, 1983, Churchill Livingstone.
3. Schrier, R., and Gottschalk, C.: Disease of the kidney, ed. 4, Boston, 1988, Little, Brown & Co.
4. Spargo, B., Seymour, A., and Ordonez, N.: Renal biopsy pathology with diagnostic and therapeutic implications, New York, 1980, John Wiley & Sons, Inc.

Specific

5. Andriole, V.: Urinary tract infections: recent developments, J. Infect. Dis. **156**:865, 1987.
6. Bailey, R.: End-stage reflux nephropathy, Nephron **27**:302, 1981.
7. Baldwin, D.S.: Poststreptococcal glomerulonephritis: a progressive disease? Am. J. Med. **62**:1 1977.
8. Balow, J., Austin, H., Tsokos, G., Antonovych, T., and Klippel, J.: Lupus nephritis, Ann. Intern. Med. **106**:79, 1987.
9. Bolande, R.P., Brough, I.J., and Izant, Jr., R.J.: Congenital mesoblastic nephroblastoma of infancy, Pediatrics **40**:272, 1967.
10. Brovet, J., Clauvel, J., Danon, F., et al.: Biologic and clinical significance of cryoglobulins: a report of 86 cases, Am. J. Med. **57**:775, 1974.
11. Burry, A.: Pathology of analgesic nephropathy: Australian experience, Kidney Int. **13**:34, 1978.
12. Cameron, J., Turner, D., and Ugg, C.: The nephrotic syndrome in adults with minimal change glomerular lesions, Q. J. Med. **43**:461, 1974.
13. Cameron, J.: The nephrotic syndrome and its complications, Am. J. Kidney Dis. **10**:157, 1987.
14. Cannon, P.J., Hassar, M., Case, D.B., et al.: The relationship of hypertension and renal failure in scleroderma (progressive systemic sclerosis) to structural and functional abnormalities of the renal cortical circulation, Medicine **53**:1, 1974.
15. Cohen, A., and Border, W.: Mesangial proliferative glomerulonephritis, Semin. Nephrol. **2**:228, 1982.
16. Cotran, R.S.: Monocytes, proliferation and glomerulonephritis, J. Lab. Clin. Med. **92**:837, 1978.
17. Cotran, R.S.: Interstitial nephritis. In Churg, J., et al., editors: Kidney disease: present status, Baltimore, 1979, The Williams & Wilkins Co.
18. Cotran, R.S.: Glomerulosclerosis in reflux nephropathy, Kidney Int. **21**:528, 1982.
19. Cotran, R., and Rennke, H.: Anionic sites and the mechanisms of proteinuria, N. Engl. J. Med. **309**:1050, 1983.
20. Dachs, S., Churg, J., Mautner, W., et al.: Diabetic nephropathy, Am. J. Pathol. **44**:155, 1964.
21. D'Amico, G.: The commonest glomerulonephritis in the world: IgA nephropathy, J. Med. **64**:709, 1987.
22. Dixon, F.J.: The pathogenesis of glomerulonephritis, Am. J. Med. **44**:493, 1968.
23. Dodge, W.F., Spargo, B.H., Travis, L.B., et al.: Poststreptococcal glomerulonephritis: a prospective study in children, N. Engl. J. Med. **286**:273, 1972.
24. Downing, V., and Levine, S.: Erythrocytosis and renal cell carcinoma with pulmonary metastases: case report with 18-year followup and brief discussion of literature, Cancer **35**:1701, 1975.
25. Dykman, D., Simon, E., and Avioli, L.: Hyperuricemia and uric acid nephropathy, Arch. Intern. Med. **147**:1341, 1987.
26. Eknoyan, G.: Chronic tubulointerstitial nephropathies. In Schrier, R., and Gottschalk, C., editors: Diseases of the kidney, Boston, 1988, Little, Brown, & Co.
27. Erslev, A.: Erythropoietin coming of age, N. Engl. J. Med. **316**:101, 1987.
28. Fauci, A.S., Haynes, B.F., and Katz, P.: The spectrum of vasculitis: clinical, pathologic, immunologic, and therapeutic considerations, Ann. Intern. Med. **89**:660, 1978.
29. Freedman, L.: Chronic pyelonephritis at autopsy, Ann. Intern. Med. **66**:697, 1967.
30. Gallo, G., and Emancipator, S.: Postinfectious glomerulonephritis. In Rosen, S., editor: Pathology of glomerular disease, New York, 1983, Churchill Livingstone.
31. Garella, S., and Matasese, R.: Renal effects of prostaglandins and clinical adverse effects of nonsteroidal anti-inflammatory agents, Medicine **63**:165, 1984.
32. Gianantonio, C., Vitacco, M., Mendilaharzu, F., et al.: The hemolytic-uremic syndrome, J. Pediatr. **61**:478, 1964.
33. Gilbert, E., and Opitz, J.: Renal involvement in genetic hereditary malformation syndromes. In Hamburger, J., Crosnier, J., and Gruenfeld, J.P., editors: Nephrology, New York and Paris, 1979, Wiley-Flammarion.
34. Glassock, R.: A clinical and immunopathologic dissection of rapidly progressive glomerulonephritis, Nephron **22**:253, 1978.
35. Glassock, R.: Clinical aspects of glomerular diseases, Am. J. Kidney Dis. **10**:181, 1987.
36. Glenner, G.: Amyloid deposits and amyloidosis: the B fibrilloses, I, N. Engl. J. Med. **302**:1283, 1980.
37. Glenner, G.: Amyloid deposits and amyloidosis: the B fibrilloses, II, N. Engl. J. Med. **302**:1333, 1980.
38. González-Crussi, F., Sotelo-Avila, C., and Kidd, J.M.: Malignant mesenchymal nephroma of infancy: report of a case with pulmonary metastases, Am. J. Surg. Pathol. **4**:185, 1980.
39. Grünfeld, J.P.: The clinical spectrum of hereditary nephritis, Kidney Int. **27**:83, 1985.
40. Grünfeld, J.P., and Pertuiset, N.: Acute renal failure in pregnancy, Am. J. Kidney Dis. **9**:359, 1987.
41. Gutman, R.A., Striker, G., Gilliland, B., and Cutler, R.: The immune complex glomerulonephritis of bacterial endocarditis, Medicine **51**:1, 1972.
42. Habib, R., and Kleinkneckt, C.: The primary nephrotic syndrome of childhood: classification and clinicopathologic study of 406 cases. In Sommers, S.C., editor: Pathology Annual, New York, 1971, Appleton-Century-Crofts.
43. Habib, R., Gubler, M.C., Loirat, C., et al.: Dense deposit disease: a variant of membranoproliferative glomerulonephritis, Kidney Int. **7**:204, 1975.
44. Habib, R.: Focal glomerular sclerosis, Kidney Int. **4**:355, 1973.
45. Habib, R., and Levy, M.: Contribution of immunofluorescent microscopy to classification of glomerular diseases. In Kincaid-Smith, P., D'Apice, A., and Atkins, R., editors: Progress in glomerulonephritis, New York, 1979, John Wiley & Sons, Inc.
46. Harrison, E.G., and McCormack, L.J.: Pathologic classification

of renal arterial disease in renovascular hypertension, Mayo Clin. Proc. **46**:161, 1971.

47. Heptinstall, R.H.: Pathology of end stage renal disease, Am. J. Med. **44**:656, 1968.
48. Huttenen, N.P.: Congenital nephrotic syndrome: a study of 75 patients, Arch. Dis. Child. **51**:344, 1973.
49. Jones, D.B.: Arterial and glomerular lesions associated with severe hypertension: light and electron microscopic studies, Lab. Invest. **31**:303, 1974.
50. Jones, D.B., and Iannaccone, P.M.: Atheromatous emboli in renal biopsies: an ultrastructural study, Am. J. Pathol. **78**:261, 1975.
51. Kannel, W.B., Schwartz, M.J., and McNamara, P.M.: Blood pressure and risk of coronary heart disease: the Framingham study, Dis. Chest **56**:43, 1969.
52. Kannel, W.B., Wolf, P.A., Verter, J., et al.: Epidemiologic assessment of the role of blood pressure in stroke: the Framingham study, JAMA **214**:301, 1970.
53. Kashgarian, M.: Pathology of small blood vessel disease in hypertension, Am. J. Kidney Dis. **5**:A104, 1985.
54. Kashgarian, M.: Mesangium and glomerular disease, Lab. Invest. **52**:569, 1985.
54a. Kaufman, J.J., and Mims, M.M.: Tumors of the kidney, Curr. Probl. Surg. **1**:1, 1966.
55. Kim, Y., and Michael, A.: Idiopathic membranoproliferative glomerulonephritis, Annu. Rev. Med. **31**:273, 1980.
56. Kimmelstiel, P., and Wilson, C.: Intercapillary lesions in glomeruli of kidney, Am. J. Pathol. **12**:83, 1936.
57. Kimmelstiel, P., Kim, O.J., Beres, J.A., and Wellman, K.: Chronic pyelonephritis, Am. J. Med. **30**:589, 1961.
58. Kincaid-Smith, P.: Analgesic nephropathy, Ann. Intern. Med. **68**:949, 1968.
59. Kleppel, M., Kashtass, C., Butkowski, R., Fish, A., and Michael, A.F.: Alport familial nephritis: absence of 28 kilodalton non-collagenous monomers of type IV collagen in glomerular basement membrane, J. Clin. Invest. **80**:263, 1987.
60. Kriz, W., and Kaissling, B.: Structural organization of the mammalian kidney. In Seldin, D., and Giebisch, G., editors: The kidney: physiology and pathophysiology, New York, 1985, Raven Press.
61. Latta, H., Maunsbach, A., and Madden, S.: The centrolobular region of the renal glomerulus studied by electron microscopy, J. Ultrastruct. Res. **4**:455, 1960.
62. Lewis, E., Kawala, K., and Schwartz, M.: Histologic features that correlate with the prognosis of patients with lupus nephritis, Am. J. Kidney Dis. **10**:192, 1987.
63. Lindeman, W.: Sur la mode d'action de certains poisons rénaux, Ann. Inst. Pasteur **14**:49, 1900.
64. Linton, A.L., Clark, W.F., and Driedger, A.A., Turnbull, D.I., and Lindsay, R.M.: Acute interstitial nephritis due to drugs, Ann. Intern. Med. **93**:735, 1980.
65. Linton, A.L., Eliahou, H., and Solez, K.: Acute renal failure: a continuing enigma, Renal Failure **10**:3, 1987.
66. Luxton, R.W.: Radiation nephritis: a long-term study of 54 patients, Lancet **2**:1221, 1961.
67. Mandal, A., Sindjic, M., and Sommers, S.: Kidney pathology in endemic nephropathy, Clin. Nephrol. **27**:304, 1987.
68. Marsden, H.B., Lawler, W., and Kumar, P.M.: Bone metastasizing renal tumor of childhood: morphological and clinical features, and differences from Wilms' tumor, Cancer **42**:1922, 1978.
69. Martínez-Maldonado, M., Yium, J., Suki, W.N., et al.: Renal complications in multiple myeloma: pathophysiology and some aspects of clinical management, J. Chronic Dis. **24**:221, 1971.
70. McCluskey, R.T.: Lupus nephritis. In Sommers, S., editor: Kidney pathology decennial 1965-1975, New York, 1975, Appleton-Century Crofts.
71. McCluskey, R., and Colvin, R.: Immunological aspects of renal tubular and interstitial diseases, Annu. Rev. Med. **29**:191, 1978.
71a. McDonald, J.R., and Priestly, J.T.: Malignant tumors of kidney: surgical and prognostic significance of tumor thrombosis of renal vein, Surg. Gynecol. Obstet. **77**:295, 1943.

72. McKay, D.G.: Disseminated intravascular coagulation: an intermediary mechanism of disease, New York, 1965, Harper & Row, Publishers, Inc.
73. Morales, A., Wasan, S., and Bryniak, S.: Renal oncocytomas: clinical, radiological and histological features, J. Urol. **123**:261, 1980.
74. Mostofi, F., Brugge, C., and Diggs, L.: Lesions in kidneys removed for unilateral hematuria in sickle cell disease, Arch. Pathol. **63**:336, 1957.
75. Mujais, S.: Renal metabolic absence, Int. J. Artif. Organs **10**:20, 1987.
76. Muther, R., McCarron, D., and Bennett, W.: Renal manifestations of sarcoidosis, Arch. Intern. Med. **141**:643, 1981.
77. Oliver, J., MacDowell, M., and Tracey, A.: The pathogenesis of acute renal failure associated with traumatic and toxic injury: renal ischemia, nephrotoxic damage and the ischemic episode, J. Clin. Invest. **30**:1307, 1951.
78. Oparil, S., and Haber, E.: The renin-angiotensin system, N. Engl. J. Med. **291**:389, 1974.
79. Pirani, C.L., and Salinas-Madrigal, L.: Evaluation of percutaneous renal biopsy, Pathol. Annu. **3**:249, 1968.
80. Pirani, C.L., Pollak, V.E., Lannigan, R., et al.: The renal glomerular lesions of pre-eclampsia: electron microscopic studies, Am. J. Obstet. Gynecol. **87**:1047, 1963.
81. Potter, E.L.: Facial characteristics of infants with bilateral renal agenesis, Am. J. Obstet. Gynecol. **51**:885, 1946.
82. Prien, E.L., and Frondel, C.: Studies in urolithiasis: composition of urinary calculi, J. Urol. **57**:949, 1947.
83. Randall, A.: Etiology of primary renal calculus, Surg. Gynecol. Obstet. **71**:209, 1940.
84. Randall, R., Williamson, W., Mullinax, F., et al.: Manifestations of systemic light chain deposition, Am. J. Med. **60**:293, 1976.
85. Reeders, S.T., Breuning, M.H., Corney, G., Jeremiah, S.J., Merra Khan, P., Davies, K.E., Hopkinson, D.A., Pearson, P.L., and Weatherall, D.J.: Two genetic markers closely linked to adult polycystic kidney disease on chromosome 16, Br. Med. J. **292**:851, 1986.
86. Remuzzi, G.: HUS and TTP: variable expression of a single entity, Kidney Int. **32**:292, 1987.
87. Riches, E.: Tumors of the kidney and ureter, Edinburgh, 1964, E. & S. Livingstone, Ltd.
88. Rolleston, G., Maling, T., and Hodson, C.: Intrarenal reflux and the scarred kidney, Arch. Dis. Child. **49**:531, 1974.
89. Romeo, G., De voto, M., Costa, G., Roncuzzi, L., Catizone, L., Zuchelli, P., Germino, G.G., Keith, T., Weatherall, D.J., and Reeders, S.T.: A second genetic locus for autosomal dominant polycystic kidney disease, Lancet **2**:8, 1988.
90. Rosen, S.: Membranous glomerulonephritis: current status, Hum. Pathol. **2**:209, 1971.
91. Rosen, S.: Crescentic glomerulonephritis: occurrence, mechanisms, and prognosis, Pathol. Annu. **10**:37, 1975.
92. Rosen, S.: Classification of glomerular disease. In Rosen, S., editor: Pathology of glomerular disease, New York, 1983, Churchill Livingstone.
93. Salant, D.: Immunopathogenesis of crescentic glomerulonephritis and lung purpura, Kidney Int. **32**:408, 1987.
94. Schmidt, D., Harms, D., and Zieger, G.: Malignant rhabdoid tumor of the kidney: histopathology, ultrastructure, and comments on differential diagnosis, Virchows Arch. [Pathol. Anat.] **398**:101, 1982.
95. Schnaper, H.W., and Aune, T.: Steroid-sensitive mechanism of soluble immune response suppressor production in steroid-responsive nephrotic syndrome, J. Clin. Invest. **79**:257, 1987.
96. Schoolworth, A., Sandler, R., Klahr, S., and Kissane, J.: Nephrosclerosis post partum and in women taking oral contraceptives, Arch. Intern. Med. **136**:178, 1976.
97. Schreiner, G.E., and Maher, J.F.: Toxic nephropathy, Am. J. Med. **38**:409, 1965.
98. Scott, D.M., Amos, N., Sissons, J.G., Lachmann, P.J., and Peters, D.K.: The immunoglobulin nature of nephrotic factor (NeF), Clin. Exp. Immunol. **32**:12, 1978.

99. Silva, F.: The nephropathies of systemic lupus erythematosus. In Rosen, S., editor: Pathology of glomerular disease, New York, 1983, Churchill Livingstone.

100. Sitprija, V., Pipatanagul, V., Mertowidjojo, K., et al.: Pathogenesis of renal disease in leptospirosis: clinical and experimental studies, Kidney Int. **17**:827, 1980.

101. Smith, L.: Urolithiasis. In Schrier, R., and Gottschalk, C., editors: Diseases of the kidney, ed. 4, Boston, 1988, Little, Brown & Co.

102. Solez, K., Morel-Maroger, L., and Sraer, J.D.: The morphology of "acute tubular necrosis" in man: analysis of 57 renal biopsies and a comparison with the glycerol model, Medicine **58**:362, 1979.

103. Spargo, B., Seymour, A., and Ordonez, N.: Renal biopsy pathology with diagnostic and therapeutic implications, New York, 1980, John Wiley & Sons, Inc.

104. Stein, J.H., Lifschitz, M.D., and Barnes, L.D.: Current concepts on the pathophysiology of acute renal failure, Am. J. Phys. **234**:F171, 1978.

105. Strauss, J., Pardo, V., and Koss, M.: Nephropathy associated with sickle cell anemia: an autologous immune complex nephritis, Am. J. Med. **58**:382, 1975.

106. Strife, C.F., McEnery, P., McAdams, A., and West, C.: Membranoproliferative glomerulonephritis with disruption of the glomerular basement membrane, Clin. Nephrol. **7**:65, 1977.

107. Tiebosch, A., Frederik, P., van Breda-Vriesman, P., et al.: Thin-basement-membrane nephropathy in adults with persistent hematuria, N. Engl. J. Med. **320**:14, 1989.

108. Törnroth, T.: Membranous glomerulonephritis. In Rosen, S., editor: Pathology of glomerular disease, New York, 1983, Churchill Livingstone.

109. Vassalli, P., Morris, R.H., and McCluskey, R.T.: The pathogenic role of fibrin deposition in the glomerular lesions of toxemia of pregnancy, J. Exp. Med. **118**:467, 1963.

110. Vitsky, B.H., Suzuki, Y., Strauss, L., et al.: The hemolytic-uremic syndrome: a study of renal pathologic alterations, Am. J. Pathol. **57**:627, 1969.

111. Walsh, P.N., and Kissane, J.M.: Nonmetastatic hypernephroma with reversible hepatic dysfunction, Arch. Intern. Med. **122**:214, 1968.

112. Wedeen, R., D'Haese, P., deVyver, V., Verpooten, G., and DeBroe, M.: Lead nephropathy, Am. J. Kidney Dis. **8**:380, 1986.

113. Weinberg, J.M.: The role of cell calcium overload in nephrotoxic renal tubular cell injury, Am. J. Kidney Dis. **8**:284, 1986.

114. Welling, L.W., and Welling, D.J.: Surface areas of brush border and lateral cell walls in the rabbit proximal nephron, Kidney Int. **8**:343, 1975.

115. Wilson, C.B., and Dixon, F.J.: The renal response to immunological injury. In Brenner, B.M., and Rector, F.C., editors: The kidney, ed. 2, Philadelphia, 1981, W.B. Saunders Co.

116. Wilson, D.: Urinary tract obstruction. In Schrier, R., and Gottschalk, C., editors: Diseases of the kidney, ed. 4, Boston, 1988, Little, Brown & Co.

The urinary collecting system

117. Alroy, J., Pauli, D.U., and Weinstein, R.S.: Correlation between numbers of desmosomes and the aggressiveness of transitional cell carcinoma in human urinary bladder, Cancer **47**:104, 1981.

118. Andersen, D.A.: Historical and geographical differences in the pattern of incidence of urinary stones considered in relation to possible aetiological factors. In Hodgkinson, A., and Nordin, B.E.C., editors: Renal Stone Research Symposium, London, 1969, J. & A. Churchill, Ltd.

119. Andersen, J.A., and Hansen, B.F.: The incidence of cell nests, cystitis cystica and cystitis glandularis in the lower urinary tract revealed by autopsies, J. Urol. **108**:421, 1972.

120. Aquilina, J.N., and Bugeja, T.J.: Primary malignant lymphoma of the bladder: case report and review of the literature, J. Urol. **112**:64, 1974.

121. Babaian, R.J., Johnson, D.E., Llamas, L., and Ayala, A.G.: Metastases from transitional cell carcinoma of the urinary bladder, Urology **16**:142, 1980.

122. Barlebo, H., Sorensen, B.L., and Ohlsen, A.S.: Carcinoma in situ of urinary bladder—flat intraepithelial neoplasia, Scand. J. Urol. Nephrol. **6**:213, 1972.

123. Barrett, J.C.: Gangrenous cystitis, Br. J. Urol. **34**:312, 1962.

124. Booth, C.M., Cameron, K.M., and Pugh, R.C.B.: Urothelial carcinoma of the kidney and ureter, Br. J. Urol. **52**:430, 1980.

125. Brannan, W., Lucas, T.A., and Mitchell, W.T., Jr.: Accuracy of cytologic examination of urinary sediment in the detection of urothelial tumors, J. Urol. **109**:483, 1973.

126. Brumfitt, W., and Asscher, A.W.: Urinary tract infection, Proc. Second National Symposium held in London, 1972, London, 1973, Oxford University Press.

127. Carpenter, A.A.: Pelvic lipomatosis: successful surgical treatment, J. Urol. **110**:397, 1973.

128. Carswell, J.W.: Intraperitoneal rupture of the bladder, Br. J. Urol. **46**:425, 1974.

129. Catalona, W.J.: Practical utility of specific red cell adherence test in bladder cancer, Urology **18**:113, 1981.

130. Clayson, D.B.: Recent research into occupational bladder cancer. In Connolly, J.G., editor: Carcinoma of the bladder, New York, 1981, Raven Press.

131. Cohen, G.H.: Obstructive uropathy caused by ureteral candidiasis, J. Urol. **110**:285, 1973.

132. Cole, P.: Coffee drinking and cancer of the lower urinary tract, Lancet **1**:1335, 1971.

133. Cole, P., Monson, R.R., Haning, H., et al.: Smoking and cancer of the lower urinary tract, N. Engl. J. Med. **284**:129, 1971.

134. Cullen, T.H., Popham, R.R., and Voss, H.J.: An evaluation of routine cytological examination of the urine, Br. J. Urol. **39**:615, 1967.

135. Cyr, W.L., Johnson, H., and Balfour, J.: Granulomatous cystitis as a manifestation of chronic granulomatous disease of childhood, J. Urol. **110**:357, 1973.

136. Dale, G.A., and Smith, R.B.: Transitional cell carcinoma of the bladder associated with cyclophosphamide, J. Urol. **112**:603, 1974.

137. Davies, R., and Hunt, A.C.: Surface topography of the female bladder trigone, J. Clin. Pathol. **34**:308, 1981.

138. de Klotz, R.J., and Young, B.W.: Conservative surgery in the management of benign ureteral polyps, Br. J. Urol. **36**:375, 1964.

139. Doctor, V.M., Phadke, A.G., and Sirsat, M.V.: Pheochromocytoma of the urinary bladder, Br. J. Urol. **44**:351, 1972.

140. Finlay-Jones, L.R., Blackwell, J.B., and Papadimitriou, J.M.: Malakoplakia of the colon, Am. J. Clin. Pathol. **50**:320, 1968.

141. Friedman, N.B., and Ash, J.E.: Tumors of the urinary bladder. In Atlas of tumor pathology, sect. VIII—sect. 31a, Washington, D.C., 1959, Armed Forces Institute of Pathology.

142. Friedman, N.B., and Kuhlenbeck, H.: Adenomatoid tumors of the bladder reproducing renal structures (nephrogenic adenomas), J. Urol. **64**:657, 1950.

143. Gettel, R.R., Lee, F., and Ratliff, R.K.: Ureteral diverticula, J. Urol. **108**:392, 1972.

144. Gordon, H.L., Rossen, R.D., Hersh, E.M., et al.: Immunologic aspects of interstitial cystitis, J. Urol. **109**:228, 1973.

145. Halawani, A., Al-Waidh, M., and Said, S.M.: Serology in the study of the relationship between *S. haematobium* infestation and cancer of the urinary bladder, Br. J. Urol. **42**:580, 1970.

146. Hanna, M.K.: Bilateral retroiliac-artery ureters, Br. J. Urol. **44**:339, 1972.

147. Hanson, L.A., Fasth, A., Jodal, U., Kaijser, B., and Svanborg Edén, C.: Biology and pathology of urinary tract infections, J. Clin. Pathol. **34**:695, 1981.

148. Harmer, M.H., editor: TNM classification of malignant tumours, ed. 3, Geneva, 1979, International Union against Cancer.

149. Hicks, R.M.: Carcinogenesis in the urinary bladder: a multistage process. In Connolly, J.G., editor: Carcinoma of the bladder, New York, 1981, Raven Press.

150. Hicks, R.M., Walters, C.L., Elsebai, I., et al.: Demonstration of N-nitrosamines in human urine: preliminary observations on a possible aetiology for bladder cancer in association with

chronic urinary tract infections, Proc. R. Soc. Med. **70:**413, 1977.

151. Highman, W., and Wilson, E.: Urine cytology in patients with calculi, J. Clin. Pathol. **35:**350, 1982.
152. Hodge, J.: Avulsion of a long segment of ureter with Dormia basket, Br. J. Urol. **45:**328, 1973.
153. Jacobs, J.B., Cohen, S.M., Farrow, G.M., and Friedell, G.H.: Scanning electron microscopic features of human urinary bladder cancer, Cancer **48:**1399, 1981.
154. Javadpour, N., Solomon, T., and Bush, I.M.: Obstruction of the lower ureter by aberrant vessels in children, J. Urol. **108:**340, 1972.
155. Johansson, S., Angervall, L., Bengtsson, U., et al.: Uroepithelial tumors of the renal pelvis associated with abuse of phenacetin-containing analgesics, Cancer **33:**743, 1974.
156. Johnson, F.R.: Some proliferative and metaplastic changes in transitional epithelium, Br. J. Urol. **29:**112, 1957.
157. Lambird, P.A., and Yardley, J.H.: Malakoplakia: report of a fatal case with ultrastructural observations on Michaelis-Gutmann bodies, Johns Hopkins Med. J. **126:**1, 1970.
158. Malek, R.S., Greene, L.F., and Farrow, G.M.: Amyloidosis of the urinary bladder, Br. J. Urol. **43:**189, 1971.
159. Marshall, F.F., and Middleton, A.W., Jr.: Eosinophilic cystitis, J. Urol. **112:**335, 1974.
160. Morgan, R.J., and Cameron, K.M.: Vesical leukoplakia, Br. J. Urol. **52:**96, 1980.
161. Marshall, V.F., and Keuhnelian, J.G.: Crossed ureteral ectopia with solitary kidney, J. Urol. **110:**176, 1973.
162. Mostofi, F.K., Sobin, L.H., and Torloni, H.: W.H.O. international histological classification of tumours, no. 10—Histological typing of urinary bladder tumours, Geneva, 1973, World Health Organization.
163. Newman, J., and Hicks, R.M.: Detection of neoplastic and preneoplastic urothelia by combined scanning and transmission electron microscopy of urinary surface of human bladders, Histopathology **1:**125, 1977.
164. O'Flynn, J.D., and Mullaney, J.: Vesical leukoplakia progressing to carcinoma, Br. J. Urol. **46:**31, 1974.
165. O'Grady, F., and Brumfitt, W.: Urinary tract infection, Proc. First National Symposium held in London, 1968, London, 1968, Oxford University Press.
166. O'Kane, H.O.J., and Megaw, J. McI.: Carcinoma of the exstrophic bladder, Br. J. Surg. **55:**631, 1968.
167. Ormond, J.K.: Idiopathic retroperitoneal fibrosis: an established clinical entity, JAMA **174:**1561, 1960.
168. Packham, D.A.: The epithelial lining of the female trigone and urethra, Br. J. Urol. **43:**201, 1971.
169. Peterson, L.J., Paulson, D.F., and Bonar, R.A.: Response of human urothelium to chemical carcinogens in vitro, J. Urol. **111:**154, 1974.
170. Peterson, L.J., Paulson, D.F., and Glenn, J.F.: The histopathology of vesical diverticula, J. Urol. **110:**62, 1973.
171. Potts, I.F., and Hirst, E.: Inverted papilloma of the bladder, J. Urol. **90:**175, 1963.
172. Prall, R.H., Wernett, C., and Mims, M.M.: Diagnostic cytology in urinary tract malignancy, Cancer **29:**1084, 1972.
173. Price, D.A., Morley, A.R., and Hall, R.R.: Scanning electron microscopy in the study of normal inflamed and neoplastic human urothelium, Br. J. Urol. **52:**370, 1980.
174. Ransley, P.G.: Vesico-ureteric reflux. In Hendry, W.F., editor:

Recent advances in urology/andrology, ed. 3, New York, 1981, Churchill Livingstone.
175. Reiter's disease, Br. Med. J. **4:**576, 1969.
176. Rose, G.A., and Wallace, D.M.: Observations on urinary chemiluminescence of normal smokers and non-smokers and of patients with bladder cancer, Br. J. Urol. **45:**520, 1973.
177. Rubin, L., and Pincus, M.B.: Eosinophilic cystitis: the relationship of allergy in the urinary tract to eosinophilic cystitis and the pathophysiology of eosinophilia, J. Urol. **112:**457, 1974.
178. Schulman, C.C.: Electron microscopy of the human ureteric innervation, Br. J. Urol. **46:**609, 1974.
179. Slater, R.B., and Kirkpatrick, J.R.: A case of closed injury of the upper ureter, Br. J. Urol. **43:**591, 1971.
180. Smith, A.F.: An ultrastructural and morphometric study of bladder tumours, Virchows Arch. [Pathol. Anat.] **390:**11, 1981.
181. Stamey, T.A.: Pathogenesis and treatment of urinary tract infections, Baltimore, 1980, The Williams & Williams Co.
182. Stanton, M.J., and Maxted, W.: Malacoplakia: a study of the literature and current concepts of pathogenesis, diagnosis and treatment, J. Urol. **125:**139, 1981.
183. Sutor, D.J., Wooley, S.E., and Illingworth, J.J.: A geographical and historical survey of the composition of urinary stones, Br. J. Urol. **46:**393, 1974.
184. Tannenbaum, M., Tannenbaum, S., and Romas, N.A.: Conformational membrane changes in early bladder cancer. In Connolly, J.G., editor: Carcinoma of the bladder, New York, 1981, Raven Press.
185. Turner-Warwick, R., Whiteside, C.G., Worth, P.H., et al.: A urodynamic view of the clinical problems associated with bladder neck dysfunction and its treatment by endoscopic incision and trans-trigonal posterior prostatectomy, Br. J. Urol. **45:**44, 1973.
186. Union Internationale contre le Cancer: Cancer incidence in five continents, vol. 2, Geneva, 1970, Springer-Verlag.
187. Utz, D.C., Hanash, K.A., and Farrow, G.M.: The plight of the patient with carcinoma in situ of the bladder, Trans. Am. Assoc. Genitourin. Surg. **61:**90, 1969.
188. Utz, D.C., Farrow, G.M., Rife, C.C., Segura, J.W., and Zincke, H.: Carcinoma in situ of the bladder, Cancer **45:**1842, 1980.
189. Wallace, D.M.: Urothelial neoplasia: causes, assessment and treatment, Ann. R. Coll. Surg. Eng. **51:**91, 1972.
190. Wallace, D.M., Chisholm, G.D., and Hendry, W.F.: T.N.M. classification of urological tumours (U.I.C.C.), 1974, Br. J. Urol. **47:**1, 1975.
191. Watson, N.A., and Notley, R.G.: Urological complications of cyclophosphamide, Br. J. Urol. **45:**606, 1973.
192. Wesolowski, S.: Bilateral ureteral injuries in gynaecology, Br. J. Urol. **41:**666, 1969.
193. Whitaker, R.H., Pugh, R.C.B., and Dow, D.: Colonic tumours following uretero-sigmoidostomy, Br. J. Urol. **43:**562, 1971.
194. Whitehead, E.D., and Tessler, A.N.: Carcinoma of the urachus, Br. J. Urol. **43:**468, 1971.
195. Williams, D.I.: Urology in childhood. Handbuch der Urologie [Encyclopedia of urology], vol. XV, supplement, New York, 1974, Springer-Verlag.
196. Wisheart, J.D.: Primary tumours of the ureteric stump following nephrectomy, Br. J. Urol. **40:**344, 1968.
197. Zincke, H., Furlow, W.L., and Farrow, G.M.: *Candida albicans* cystitis: report of a case with special emphasis on diagnosis and treatment, J. Urol. **109:**612, 1973.

19 Male Reproductive System and Prostate

F. KASH MOSTOFI
CHARLES J. DAVIS, JR.

TESTES

Normally the adult testicle is located in the scrotum. Its main components are the seminiferous tubules. Germ cells in various stages of maturation are the major population of adult normal seminiferous tubules, and their sole function is to produce spermatozoa. In addition to these cells, the seminiferous tubules also contain the sustentacular cells of Sertoli, which have three functions: (1) they support the germ cells; (2) they produce estrogens and some androgens; and (3) they form the basement membrane of the seminiferous tubules. The seminiferous tubules drain into collecting ducts, which join to form the rete testis, thence vasa efferentia, and finally the epididymis; these serve to transmit the spermatozoa out of the gonad. The seminiferous tubules are surrounded by a delicate basement membrane (tunica propria) and are supported by a delicate fibrovascular stroma in which varying numbers of interstitial cells of Leydig are seen. The main functions of Leydig cells are to constitute part of the supporting stroma of the gonad and to produce hormones; they are the main source of testosterone and other androgenic hormones in men, and they produce estrogens and possibly progesterone and corticosteroids. Sertoli and Leydig cells are thus the hormone-producing cells of the male gonad and, along with their homologs in the ovary (granulosa-theca cell), are designated the specialized stromal cells of the gonad to differentiate them from the usual fibrovascular stroma that the gonads have in common with all other organs. The entire structure is covered by tunica, which contains the smooth muscle layer of Dartos. The outer layer is covered by mesothelium. Thus, in addition to the testicle, the scrotum contains the testicular adnexa.

Anomalies

Excluding malposition of the testicle, anomalies are very rare. Anorchidism (congenitala absence) and monorchidism (one testicle) have been reported. Synorchidism (fusion of testicles) occurs intra-abdominally. Polyorchidism has been found at operation and necropsy.

Ectopic testis

Ectopic testis is a congenital malposition of the testicle outside the normal channel of descent. This ectopia, according to its location, is classified as interstitial, pubopenile, femoral, crural, transverse, or perineal.

Cryptorchidism

When the congenital malposition results in retention of the testicle anywhere along the route of descent, it is known as cryptorchidism. The cause of cryptorchidism is not always evident. The various apparent causes are short spermatic vessels of vas deferens, adhesions to the peritoneum, poorly developed inguinal canal or superficial abdominal ring, maldevelopment of the scrotum or cremaster muscles, and hormonal influences. Incomplete descent is found quite frequently during the first few months of infancy. The incidence is about 4% in boys under 15 years of age and about 0.2% in adults. Histologically the cryptorchid testis before puberty does not differ from the normally descended organ (Fig. 19-1). After puberty, however, it is always smaller than normal. The capsule is somewhat thickened and wrinkled. The epididymis is separated from the mesorchium. There is progressive loss of germ cell elements. The tubules may be lined only with spermatogonia and spermatids, but occasionally there is spermatogenesis. In fact, foci of spermatogenesis are found in 10% of undescended testes. This condition has also been reported in abdominal testis. It is estimated that 10% of men with untreated cryptorchidism remain fertile. The basement membrane of the tubules thickens and hyalinizes. In later stages spermatogenesis is rare or absent and the tubules are lined only with Sertoli cells. Tubules with completely occluded lumens are not uncommon. The collecting tubules and rete may be quite prominent, a condition that indicates possible hyperplasia and even adenoma. The intertubular tissue is sparsely cellular and becomes more dense with age. The interstitial cells of Leydig are conspicuous and vary in number. In some cases the Leydig cells are decreased in number, and in other cases they are in-

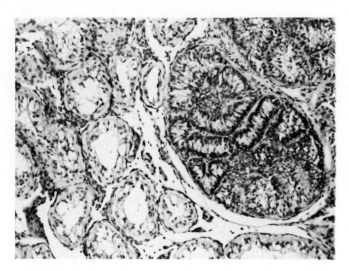

Fig. 19-1. Cryptorchid testis. Notice the two islands of immature tubules. (100×.)

creased both in size and in number. They are found singly, in small groups, and occasionally in large masses. In some cryptorchid testicles most of the atrophied organ is composed of large groups of polyhedral Leydig cells, between which may be found scanty fibrous tissue and a few fibrosed tubules. In rare instances very few cellular elements are encountered, and the entire testis becomes completely fibrosed.

The cause of atrophy of undescended and ectopic testes is not known. There is convincing evidence that an optimum temperature is necessary for spermatogenesis and that temperatures higher than that within the scrotum suppress spermatogenesis. When aspermia or hypospermia exists, the testicle atrophies. The chief function of the scrotum is to regulate the temperature for the testes. Ischemia caused by pressure, stressed by some authors, is definitely a minor factor in causing suppression of spermatogenesis in cryptorchidism.

Cryptorchid testis may be the seat of malignancy, and such testes should be biopsied if orchiopexy is contemplated. There is a high incidence of tumors of testes in cryptorchidism especially in abdominal testes. A pelvic mass in a patient with an absent testis should arouse suspicion of germ cell malignancy in an abdominal testis. The tumor is usually a seminoma.

Intersexuality

A true hermaphrodite or ambisexual is one who possesses an ovary and a testicle or true ovotestes with or without external genitalia of both sexes. A pseudohermaphrodite possesses gonads of one sex and genitalia of either both sexes or the opposite sex. In the male pseudohermaphrodite the testes are present but the internal genitalia are of both sexes, and the penis and scrotum are poorly developed. In the female pseudoherma-

phrodite the ovaries are present, usually in their normal position, the vagina is rudimentary and opens into the urethra, and the clitoris is hypertrophied.

Testis in male infertility

About 15 of every 100 marriages in the United States are barren, and male infertility accounts for about half of the cases. In all such patients quantitative determination of urinary 17-ketosteroids, estrogens, and gonadotropins, karyotyping, and testicular biopsy are essential to determine the specific cause of the male infertility and whether it is curable. Wong, Straus, and Warner[77-79] have proposed a simple classification of male infertility: pretesticular, testicular, and posttesticular.

Pretesticular causes of infertility are mainly hypopituitarism, endogenous or exogenous estrogen or androgen excess, hypothyroidism, diabetes mellitus, and glucocorticoid excess.

Hypopituitarism may be prepubertal or postpubertal. Prepubertal causes include lesions in or adjacent to the pituitary, for example, craniopharyngiomas, trauma, and cysts. Such patients eventually manifest sexual infantilism, failure of somatic growth, and varying degrees of adrenal and thyroid hypofunction. Testicular biopsy shows small immature seminiferous tubules and immature Leydig cells similar to those in prepubertal testis.

Postpubertal hypopituitarism results from tumors, trauma, or infarction. Testicular biopsy shows maturation arrest, loss of germ cells, reduced diameter of tubules, and progressive thickening and hyalinization of tunica propria. The Leydig cells are small and shriveled.

Hypopituitarism may be the result of genetic defects in gonadotropin secretion. There are no demonstrable lesions of the pituitary or deficiencies of adrenal and thyroid function or growth. The patients may show deficiency of both follicle-stimulating hormone (FSH) and luteinizing hormone (LH), or the FSH may be normal but the LH deficient. Testicular biopsy in the former shows small and immature seminiferous tubules resembling prepubertal testis. In the latter the seminiferous tubules show a greater degree of development than the Leydig cells do. In both cases the patients are generally tall and eunuchoid.

Estrogen excess may be endogenous (hepatic cirrhosis, adrenal tumor, Sertoli or Leydig cell tumor) or exogenous (administered to patients with cancer of prostrate). Initially the biopsy sample shows failure of maturation, progressive decrease of germinal elements, diminished diameter of seminiferous tubules, and thickening and hyalinization of tunicapropria. Eventually there are complete sclerosis of tubules and atrophy of Leydig cells. The findings are identical to those in postpubertal hypopituitarism.

Androgen excess may be endogenous (adrenogenital syndrome or androgen-producing adrenocortical or testicular tumors) or exogenous (oral administration). Pathologic findings depend on whether the condition developed before or after puberty. If prepubertal, the result is virilism and failure of the testis to mature. If postpubertal, there is progressive loss of germ cells and, unless recognized and remedied, tubular sclerosis.

Glucocorticoid excess, whether endogenous (Cushing's syndrome) or exogenous (administered for treatment of ulcerative colitis, rheumatoid arthritis, or bronchial asthma) can result in oligospermia and maturation arrest or hypospermatogenesis.

Hypothyroidism and diabetes mellitus may result in decreased fertility. Hypospermatogenesis is followed by thickening of tunica propria. In uncontrolled diabetes autonomic neuropathy may result in impotence.

Testicular causes of infertility are agonadism, cryptorchidism, maturation arrest, hypospermatogenesis, absence of germ cells (Sertoli cell–only syndrome), Klinefelter's syndrome, mumps orthitis, and irradiation damage.

Agonadism

Congenital agonadism is extremely rare and is the total absence of the testes. If this occurs in early embryonic life, the infant will be female. Occasionally in cryptorchid boys the epididymis ends blindly, but careful search fails to show any gonadal tissue (vanishing testis syndrome). The chromosomal pattern is XY. Because testes must have been present in fetal life to initiate development, they must have been resorbed after that period.

Bilateral anorchia may be associated with incomplete differentiation of male genitalia. The gonads and the internal genital structures may be absent or rudimentary. These findings indicate that the testes must have been present to initiate male sex development but vanished before maturity.

Jost[75] showed that fetal testis plays an important role in the early development of the wolffian structures and regression of müllerian elements. The development of wolffian structures is related to the local androgen production, whereas regresssion of müllerian elements seems to be influenced by additional nonandrogenic factors. Federman's[70] excellent discussion of the situation may be summarized as follows: If the male fetus begins life with dysgenetic testis, varying degrees of pseudohermaphroditism may ensue; if gonadal failure occurs before organization of the gential tract, female external genitalia will result; if gonadal failure occurs during the period of male sexual differentiation, ambiguous genitalia may result; if, however, testicular failure occurs after the sixteenth week of gestation, the male structures are established and the fetus will develop as a male but without testes.

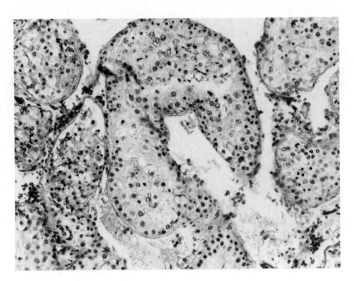

Fig. 19-2. Maturation arrest. (160×.)

Cryptorchidism

The histology of cryptorchidism is described on p. 871.

Maturation arrest

Maturation arrest is manifested in a testicular biopsy by the failure of normal spermatogenesis at some stage. Complete maturation arrest appears as failure of spermatogenesis beyond one of the immature phases of the process (Fig. 19-2). No secondary spermatocytes, spermatids, or spermatozoa are present. Incomplete maturation arrest is similar except that in some areas maturation has progressed to the spermatid stage and in some areas even to spermatozoa. The Sertoli cells, tunica propria, and Leydig cells are normal, as is the diameter of the seminiferous tubules. Oligospermia or azoospermia is present. Levels of urinary FSH, LH, and 17-ketosteroids are normal.

Hypospermatogenesis

Hypospermatogenesis is more difficult to detect (Fig. 19-3, A). All cells of spermatogenic series are present in the same proportions as normal, but the number of each variety is decreased. The seminiferous tubules are of normal size. Sertoli and Leydig cells and the tunica of the tubules are normal. Patients have oligospermia with normal urinary FSH, LH, and 17-ketosteroid levels.

Absence of germ cells (Sertoli cell–only syndrome)

Two categories of germ cell absence are recognized: the congenital (Del Castillo syndrome) and the acquired. In the former the seminiferous tubules are usually small, germ cells are absent, the tunica propria is

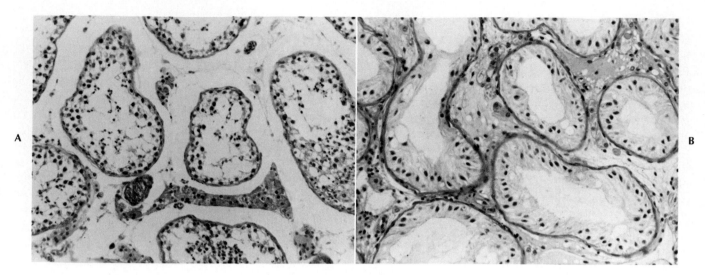

Fig. 19-3. A, Hypospermatogenesis. **B,** Sertoli cell–only syndrome. (**A,** 160×; **B,** 100×.)

thin, and Leydig cells are normal. In the acquired form, the seminiferous tubules are large (Fig. 19-3, *B*), the tunica propria is thickened, some of the tubules may show persistent germ cell elements, the Leydig cells may be hyperplastic, and there may be inflammatory cell infiltration. The secondary sex characteristics are well developed: the patients are potent but infertile. The serum testosterone levels are normal, but urinary FSH and LH levels are invariably high.

Klinefelter's syndrome

About 3% of male sterility is attributable to primary hypogonadism. This syndrome is characterized by testicular hypoplasia, azoospermia, gynecomastia, eunuchoid build, increase in urinary gonadotropin, and, not infrequently, subnormal intelligence (Fig. 19-4). The diagnosis is seldom made before puberty. Chromosome studies reveal an XXY intersexuality caused by fertilization of an ovum in which the divided X chromosome failed to separate. Such individuals have a sex-chromatin pattern similar to that of genetic females. However, other individuals with a similar or nearly similar syndrome are genetically males. There is increased urinary excretion of pituitary gonadotropic hormones.

The testes are usually small (1.5 × 0.5 cm). The histologic findings vary widely. The tubules are sclerosed and hyalinized, and there is an apparent increase in the number of interstitial cells. Tubular fibrosis is progressve and is associated with retardation of spermatogenesis. Spermatogenic activity varies greatly. Careful examination of a biopsy specimen may fail to show any activity whatsoever, but it may be found on examination of the entire testis. Maturation as far as primary spermtogenesis, even to the stage of secondary spermatogenesis and spermatids and, in rare instances,

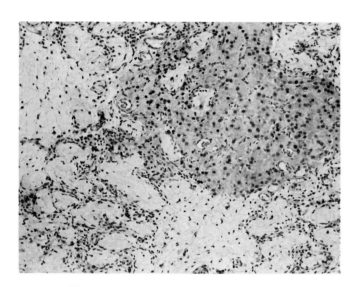

Fig. 19-4. Klinefelter's syndrome. (70×.)

spermatozoa, has been reported. The release of sperm from the testis to the ejaculate is uncommon, but a few have been observed.

Kallman's syndrome

Kallman's syndrome is a form of hypogonadotropic hypogonadism also referred to as olfactory-genital syndrome. It is characterized by anosmia, occasional color blindness, and congenital absence of Leydig cells, resulting in eunuchoidism and infantile testes, scrotum, and penis (Fig. 19-5).

Immature testes

As the name indicates, immature testes are morphologically identical to those of prepubertal individuals

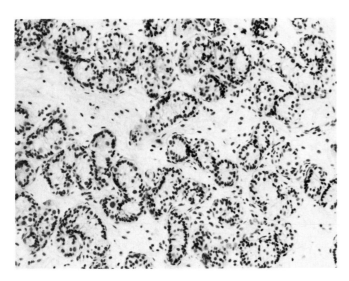

Fig. 19-5. Kallman's syndrome. (100×.)

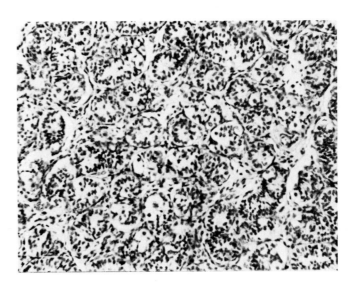

Fig. 19-6. Immature testes. (100×.)

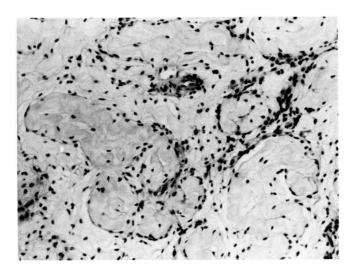

Fig. 19-7. Tubular interstitial sclerosis. (100×.)

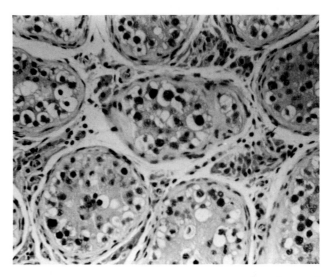

Fig. 19-8. Intratubular malignant germ cell (carcinoma in situ). (150×.)

(Fig. 19-6). The condition is seen in prepubertal gonadotropin deficiency (isolated gonadotropin deficiency and Kallman's syndrome).

Tubular and interstitial sclerosis

Tubular and interstitial fibrosis is an end stage in which all the seminiferous tubules are sclerotic and the interstitium is fibrotic (Fig. 19-7). The testes are small, and there is total absence of spermatogenesis.

Excurrent duct obstruction

Obstruction at any point from the epididymis to the ejaculatory ducts results in zero sperm count (azoospermia), but the testes are of normal size and testicular

biopsy specimens show active but not necessarily normal spermatogenesis.

Unsuspected malignancy in infertility biopsies

In about 1% of biopsies for infertility the seminiferous tubules show an unusual picture. They are lined not only by Sertoli cells but also by large cells with vacuolated cytoplasm surrounding hyperchromaticc nuclei with irregular nuclear borders (Fig. 19-8). These cells contain glycogen and placental alkaline phosphatase. They are usually situated along the base or intermingled with Sertoli cells. We have designated them as "intratubular malignant germ cells," since they represent the earliest undifferentiated pluripotential malignant germ cell. They have also been called "carcinoma in situ."

Mumps orchitis

The histologic findings in mumps orchitis are described on p. 877. Ten to 20 years after the initial infection, depending on the extent of testicular involvement, there may be oligospermia or azoospermia. The 17-ketosteroid and LH levels are normal, but the level of FSH is elevated.

Irradiation damage

Permanent germ cell destruction results from exposure to radiation, and so in time the tubules are lined by Sertoli cells only. The diameter of seminiferous tubules is progressively smaller, and the tunica is thicker, terminating in sclerosis. Leydig cells are preserved. The patient is azoospermic or oligospermic. The urinary FSH level is elevated, but the 17-ketosteroid and LH levels are normal.

Posttesticular causes of infertility

Posttesticular causes of infertility are mainly block, which may be congenital (absence or atresia of vas deferens or epididymis) or acquired. Acquired is more frequent and may result from infection (such as gonorrhea) or surgical intervention (voluntary or iatrogenic). The clinical manifestation is azoospermia. The testicular biopsy specimen in such patients shows active spermatogenesis. The seminiferous tubules may be dilated, and there may be hypospermatogenesis or cellulaar sloughing or both.

Another cause of posttesticular infertility is impaired sperm mobility. Wong and associates[77-79] reserve this term specifically for those patients in whom sperm counts are adequate and testicular biopsy specimens are normal yet the mobility of spermatozoa in the semen is either greatly impaired or absent.

In all men with infertility, testicular biopsy is necessary for proper categorization and prognosis.

Acquired atrophy

Excluding undescended testicles, acquired atrophy occurs in senility, prolonged hyperpyrexia, debility, avitaminosis, cirrhosis of the liver, hypothyroidism, schizophrenia, estrogen medication for carcinoma of the prostate, chemotherapy, and diseases of the pituitary gland and hypothalamus. Faulty or suppressed spermatogenesis without other changes may questionably be considered mild atrophy. The early findings in atrophy are degenerative changes of the spermatogonia cells. As atrophy progresses, the germinal cells disappear, leaving only Sertoli cells resting on a thickened basement membrane. The seminiferous tubules become small and farther apart, and the interstitial cells of Leydig appear prominent (Fig. 19-9).

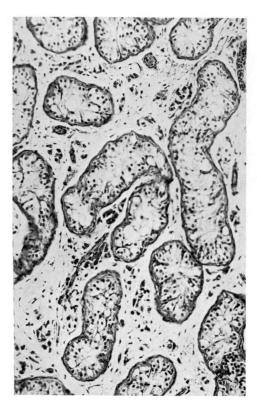

Fig. 19-9. Atrophy of testicle. Thickened tubular basement membranes are lined with degenerated spermatogonia and Sertoli cells. Leydig cells are prominent in interstitial tissue. (100×.)

Thrombosis and infarction

Hemorrhage, thrombosis, and infarction of the testicle occur in trauma, torsion, leukemias, bacterial endocarditis, and polyarteritis nodosa (Fig. 19-10). Birth trauma may cause hemorrhage of the testicle. Many such hemorrhages are small hematomas that resorb rapidly.

Torsion

A sudden twisting of the spermatic cord results in strangulation of the blood vessels serving the testicle and epididymis. The predisposing causes of torsion are free mobility and high attachment of the testicle. These anatomic features are found in such conditions as failure of the tunica vaginalis to close, large tunica vaginalis, absence of scrotal ligaments, gubernaculum testis or posterior mesorchium, or elongation of the globus minor. Abnormal attachment of the common mesentery and vessels to the globus minor and lower pole of the testicle provides attachment of the testicle by a narrow stalk instead of a wide band. The exciting cause may be violent exercise or straining. The majority of the cases of torsion involve undescended testicles. Torsion may occur at any age; cases have been reported in newborn infants and in very elderly persons. The twist is com-

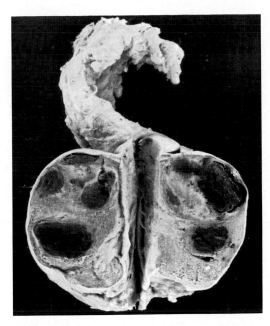

Fig. 19-10. Multiple infarcts of testicle in polyarteritis nodosa.

monly located in the free intravaginal portion of the cord. It may be a half turn to two full turns in either direction. The gross and microscopic findings depend on the degree of strangulation. Usually the picture is that of congestion and hemorrhage followed by necrosis of the testicle. The interstitial tissue may or may not be infiltrated with leukocytes. The tubules suffer varying degrees of degeneration and necrosis. At times the entire testicle is found to be necrotic and acellular, and "ghost" tubules remain as conspicuous components in the histologic picture.

Inflammation: orchitis

Acute orchitis. Acute orchitis is (1) an infection via the vas deferens and epididymis, (2) a combination epididymo-orchitis, or (3) a metastatic lymphogenous or hematogenous infection. Epididymo-orchitis is predominantly caused by urethritis, cystitis, and seminal vesiculitis. Acute orchitis may be a complication of mumps, smallpox, scarlet fever, diphtheria, typhoid fever, glanders, dengue fever, influenza, typhus fever, pneumonia, malaria, filariasis, and Mediterranean fever. Acute orchitis also has been encountered as a complication in focal infections such as sinusitis, osteomyelitis, cholecystitis, and appendicitis.

In acute orchitis the testicle becomes firm, tense, and swollen. In gonorrheal orchitis, which is usually an extension from the epididymis, single or multiple abscesses develop or the testicle may be diffusely infiltrated with neutrophilic leukocytes, lymphocytes, and plasma cells.

Mumps orchitis. The incidence of orchitis as a com-

plication of parotitis is between 20% and 30%. This complication occurs mostly in adults. Grossly the testicle is enlarged, and the tunica albuginea contains punctate hemorrhages. In the early stages the parenchyma appears edematous. Microscopically the acute inflammatory process is characterized by diffuse interstitial infiltration with polymorphonuclear neutrophils, lymphocytes, and histiocytes. Similar cellular elements fill the lumens and distend the tubules. Very few tubules suffer necrosis, but in severe cases the germinal cells and spermatogonia undergo degeneration with subsequent loss of spermatogenesis. In subacute and chronic phases of mumps orchitis, the interstitial tissue is infiltrated with lymphocytes. When degeneration has been extensive, the testicle becomes smaller and the thickened tubules are lined with a few Sertoli cells. The incidence of testicular atrophy and consequent sterility in this type of orchitis is not known.

Chronic orchitis. Acute inflammation of the testicle may completely resolve, or the inflammatory may continue in a chronic form. The inflammation may be focal or diffuse, unilateral or bilateral. In some cases fibrosis may be seen grossly. There is a varying degree of degeneration and disappearance of the tubular cells, and the basement membranes of the tubules become thickened and hyalinized. Many patients with testicular tumors give a history of some form of orchitis.

Granulomatous orchitis. The etiology and pathogenesis of a rather characteristic type of nonspecific granulomatous orchitis that may be misinterpreted as tuberculosis have not been entirely clarified despite excellent research and studies of the lesion. It occurs predominantly among middle-aged men and frequently is associated with trauma. Grossly the testis is enlarged, and the tunica albuginea may be normal or thickened. The tissue is usually grayish, white, tan, or brownish. Histologically there is a striking tuberculoid pattern. The relatively circumscribed microscopic tubercles originate from and within the tubules. They are composed of epithelioid cells, lymphocytes, plasma cells, some polymorphonuclear neutrophils, and multinucleated giant cells. The walls of the tubules are thickened by fibrous proliferation and, with the inflammatory cellular infiltrate, blend with the contiguous interstitial tissue. The interstitial tissue shows fibrosis and is predominantly infiltrated with lymphocytes and plasma cells. The origin of the epithelioid cells is Sertoli cells lining the tubules. The transformation of the Sertoli cells to epithelioid or histocytic cells is the result of the effect of a lipid fraction of spermatozoa. Berg[2] has produced granulomas in hamsters with an acid-fast staining lipid fraction of human spermatozoa.

Malakoplakia. One type of granulomatous orchitis, often with abscess formation, is characterized by infiltration with large histiocytes with small round or oval nuclei and "ground-glass" granular cytoplasm containing Michaelis-Gutmann bodies. The lesion is described on p. 856.

Tuberculosis of testicle and epididymis

Tuberculosis of the testicle without involvement of the epididymis is rare. Discrete tubercles in the testicle may be encountered in generalized miliary tuberculosis. Tuberculosis of the epididymis is usually unilateral, may occur at any age, and frequently is associated with tuberculosis of the lungs and genitourinary tract. The location of the primary focus of genital tuberculosis has stimulated considerable controversy among many investigators. Young's extensive surgical experience[49] has convinced him that, in most of the cases of genital tuberculosis, the primary site is in the seminal vesicles. Walker[46] lends support to advocates of the theory that the prostate gland or siminal vesicles harbor the primary focus.

The earliest lesions are seen as discrete or conglomerated, yellowish, necrotic areas in the globus minor. Microscopically these reveal either characteristic tubercules or disorganized inflammatory cellular reaction consisting of polymorphonuclear leukocytes, plasma cells, desquamated epithelial cells, some large monocytes, occasional multinucleated giant cells, and many acid-fast bacilli. The early lesion may regress and become calcified. Usually, however, there is progressive invasion until the entire epididymis becomes involved. When the tunica vaginalis is invaded, a considerable amount of serofibrinous or purulent exudate develops. Usually the tunica vaginalis serves as a barrier against extension into the testicle, and it is often surprising to find complete destruction of the epididymis with no invasion of the testicle.

Syphilis

The testicles are involved in almost every syphilitic patient. Syphilitic orchitis occurs either as a diffuse interstitial inflammation with fibrosis or as single or multiple gummas. Either of these types of lesion may be found in the acquired or congenital forms of syphilis. In contrast to tuberculosis, acquired syphilitic orchitis affects the testicle before the epididymis.

Grossly in the diffuse interstitial type the testis is enlarged, the cut surface is bulging grayish to yellowish white, and there is loss of normal architecture. The gummatous testicle is enlarged, firm, globular, smooth, and, rarely, nodular. When sectioned, the yellowish white or grayish white gummas bulge from the surrounding parenchyma. Extension of the gumma into the tunica vaginalis causes adhesion to the scrotum, and secondary infection induces ulceration of the scrotum with herniation of the testicle. In fibrous syphilitic orchitis the testicle is small and hard. When fibrosis is not pronounced, however, the testicle is of normal size and somewhat indurated.

Microscopically in secondary syphilis both the interstitial tissue and the seminiferous tubules are involved. The inflammatory reaction is similar to that seen in other orgams. There is heavy infiltration with plasma cells, lymphocytes, and monocytes. The inflammatory reaction often surrounds small and large blood vessels that show hyperplasia of their walls. Angiitis of small arteries is characteristic. The involved seminiferous tubules resemble those of granulomatous orchitis with replacement of normal cell population with histiocytes, lipophages, and proliferating Sertoli cells. Spirochetes are readily demonstrable with Levaditi or Warthin-Starry stains.

Microscopically the gummas of the testicle are similar to those found elsewhere. The gumma is composed of a central area of necrosis surrounded by a zone of edematous fibrous tissue infiltrated with plasma cells, lymphocytes, and occasional multinucleated giant cells. There is decreased spermatogenesis and thickening of the basement membrane of the tubules. Spirochetes are readily demonstrable in this stage. In later stages there is diffuse fibrosis, peritubular and basal hyalinization with necrosis of the tubular cells, and shrinking of the tubules. The interstitial cells usually are well preserved and often are hypertrophied. Spirochetes are rarely found in the fibrotic state.

Chronic vaginalitis (chronic proliferative periorchitis, pseudofibromatous periorchitis)

Chronic proliferative periorchitis frequently has been designated as multiple fibromas of the tunica vaginalis. The cause of this peculiar inflammatory lesion is unknown. Some cases are definitely associated with trauma. The age incidence is between 20 and 40 years.

Grossly the tunica vaginalis is found to be greatly thickened and nodular (Fig. 19-11). The surface is smooth and glistening. The nodules are multiple, scattered irregularly throughout the tunica vaginalis, and more numerous along the epididymis. They range from 1 mm to 2 cm in diameter. On sectioning, some of the nodules are found to be circumscribed and resemble uterine fibroids, whereas other are ill defined or confluent. Occasionally some nodules become calcified.

Microscopically the sections reveal a scanty cellular collagenous fibrous tissue, often interlacing or having a whorling architecture, infiltrated with lymphocytes and plasma cells. In other cases there is very little inflammatory cellular reaction.

Spermatic granuloma

Invasion of spermatozoa into the stroma of the epididymis provokes an inflammatory reaction designated as spermatic granuloma. The lesions are not uncommon, and similar lesions occur within the testes. Trauma or inflammation injures the wall of the tubule, and spermatozoa are spilled into the stroma. In some

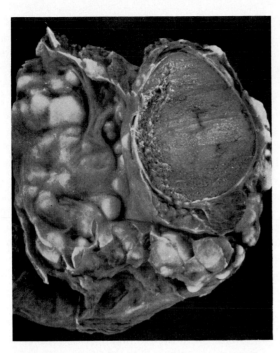

Fig. 19-11. Nodular vaginalitis (pseudofibromatous periorchitis). (Courtesy Dr. Robert S. Haukohl, Tampa, Fla.)

patients who have had vasectomies, loss of ligature from the proximal (testicular) end of the vas allows extravasation of spermatozoa resulting in sperm granuloma. Such loss of ligature may also result in reestablishing communication between severed ends of the vas. The lesions range from 3 mm to 3 cm in diameter. They are firm and white and may contain soft yellow or yellowish brown areas. They may be located in any part of the epididymis, but the majority occur in the upper pole.

Histologically the early reaction is infiltration with neutrophilic leukocytes and phagocytes, followed by various mononuclear cells, among which are histiocytes and epithelioid cells. At this stage the lesions is tuberculoid in character, with a center containing spermatozoa and debris. Lymphocytes appear among the epithelioid cells, and a mild fibroblastic proliferation replaces the epithelioid cells. The late lesions consist of hyalinized fibrous tissue, spermatozoa, granules of calcium, and very few inflammatory cells. Lipochrome pigment may be present in some lesions.

Tumors

Intrascrotal tumors may be divided into nine categories. The most common of these are germ cell tumors, and the least common are various benign and malignant tumors of fibrovascular stroma and the adnexa. Unless otherwise designated, "testicular tumors" refers to those of germ cell origin.

Categories of intrascrotal tumors:
   Germ cell tumors
   Gonadal stromal tumors
   Tumors and tumorlike lesions containing both germ cells and gonadal stromal tumors
   Miscellaneous tumors
   Lymphoid and hematopoietic tumors
   Secondary tumors
   Adnexal tumors
   Unclassified tumors
   Tumorlike lesions

One of the products of World War II was the realization that germ cell tumors of the testis, though rare among the general population, are common in young men. The work of U.S. Army clinicians and pathologists who studied these tumors initiated an unusual interest in the biology and pathology of these neoplasms and the management of the patients. In the last decade tremendous advances have been made, justifying the claim that progress in treating testicular germ cell tumors is among the greatest developments in cancer research in this century.

It has been learned that a malignant germ cell tumor is capable of producing markers that can be used to diagnose a tumor accurately and monitor its progression reliably, that the neoplastic germ cell capable of responding to the influence of organizers, and that some malignant germ cell tumors can undergo transformation into a benign phenotype. More important, the introduction of multimodal treatment, using various chemotherapeutic agents with or without radiotherapy, has brought about a miraculous improvement in the prognosis of these tumors. Complete elimination of malignancy in these patients is still a great challenge to the imagination of the biologic scientist.

Incidence and prevalence

The incidence of germ cell tumors is 2 to 3 per 100,000 white male population. They are rare among blacks in the United States and among Africans and Asians.

In the 20- to 39-year age group the incidence of germ cell testis tumors is 5.8 to 7.2 per 100,000. In this group they are the most common solid tumors and the most common cause of death from malignancy. In the white male popultion in the United States about 90% of germ cell tumors occur before 45 years of age, but the tumors have a trimodal age distribution with peaks during infancy, in late adolescence and early adulthood, and after 60 years of age. The histologic findings and behavior of the tumors vary with age. A doubling of mortality from these testicular tumors was reported between the mid-1940s (1943-1947) and the late 1950s and early 1960s (1958-1962).

Etiology

The cause of testicular germ cell tumors is unknown, but several factors are suspect. Genetic factors apparently play a role in the high incidence of testicular tumors in brothers, identical twins, monozygous twins, and members of the same family. Muller[34] has reported a history of malignant disease of the testis in the next of kin in 16% of cases. Patients with one testis tumor have a high incidence of another tumor in the opposite testis. Tumors commonly develop in dysgenetic gonads. There is a high incidence of testicular tumor in certain strains of mice, and this can be genetically manipulated.

It is generally said that the probability of a tumor developing in a undescended testis is 33 times greater than in a normally descended testis. Of 2200 testis tumors we have seen, 72 were in undescended testes. Because cryptorchidism after 21 years of age affects only 1 in 250 men, this would indicate an incidence of 2.6% of maldescent in this group. The high incidence is attributed to the higher temperature to which undescended testis is subjected in the groin or abdomen. Other possible factors are abnormal structure of the undescended testis and interference with blood supply. In humans there is a slightly higher incidence of tumors on the right side (52% versus 48% on the left).

Many patients with testicular germ cell tumors give a history of mumps or other form of orchitis. Many patients give a history of trauma, but whether trauma initiates the process or simply brings to focus an abnormal testis has not been settled. In connection with trauma it may be mentioned that induction of teratomas in fowl by intratesticular injection of zinc salts, alone or with pituitary gonadotropic hormones, is attributed to the necrotizing effects of the injection.

In recent years testicular germ cell tumors have been reported in two men after the use of lysergic acid diethylamide (LSD), in patients who have received certain drugs for long periods, and in those exposed to microwave radiation.

Endocrine abnormalities may play a role in development of testicular tumors. As mentioned previously, there is a high incidence of testicular germ cell tumors in young adulthood, when sexual activity is at its highest. Levels of pituitary gonadotropins, chorionic gonadotropins, and estrogens may be elevated in some patients with testicular tumors, and this may play a role in the genesis of testicular tumors. A seminoma was reported in a man who had received hormone therapy for sterility. Experimentally germ cell tumors have been induced in fowl by injection of zinc or copper; zinc-induced fowl teratomas occur only during the period of maximal pituitary gonadotropin secretion. In strain 129 mice, which have a high incidence of spontaneous testicular germ cell tumors, transplantation of genital ridge of 12½- to 13½-day-old embryos to the testes of adult mice of the same strain induced large numbers of testicular teratomas and embryonal carcinomas.

In summary, maldescent, mumps orchitis, and trauma to the testes are the three most important factors in the genesis of testicular germ cell tumors in humans, but most testicular tumors occur in individuals who appear to be otherwise normal.

Symptoms

There are no early symptoms of testicular tumor other than gradual enlargement of the testis, pain, and a heavy or dragging sensation. Presence of a nodule or hardness with or without pain may be detected incidentally by a patient, his physician, or sexual partner. Gynecomastia is seen in 2% to 10% of patients, indicating the desirability of examining the testes in all patients with gynecomastia. In about 10% the symptoms are acute, simulating epididymitis, torsion, or infarction of the testis. About 25% of patients are found to have generalized metastases. Rarely the initial symptom may be infertility.

Diagnosis

A complete physical examination should be done. The testis may be enlarged and have a rubbery consistency. There may be one or more nodules. The shape of the testis is often maintained. The tumor is usually distinct from the epididymis and not attached to the overlying scrotal tunica or the skin. The epididymis and the spermatic cord are usually uninvolved. In boys a painful, tender intrascrotal mass may be caused by torsion. With an associated abdominal mass, care should be taken in the examination to avoid rupture of the mass.

Discussion of specific diagnostic procedures used in suspected cases of testicular tumors is beyond the scope of this presentation, but mention should be made that these are directed toward the determination of (1) whether the tumor is confined to the testis, has extended beyond but is still confined to the scrotum, or has already metastasized and how extensively and (2) whether the tumor is producing any hormones or markers and the serum level of such markers.

For many years it has been known that patients with testicular tumor may show positive pregnancy test results. The crude bioassays of Ascheim-Zondek and Friedman's tests have now been superseded by more specific and more sensitive tests.

At present two tumor markers are widely used in diagnosis, staging, and follow-up monitoring of patients with testicular tumors: beta fraction of human chorionic gonadotropin (HCG) and alpha-fetoprotein (AFP). After some initial confusion the cell of origin of these markers has now been established. In testicular tumors HCG is synthesized by syncytiotrophoblasts either alone or as choriocarcinoma. Any preorchiectomy elevation of HCG or its presistence after orchiectomy indicates the presence of one of these elements in the primary tumor or in the metastasis. Ectopic production of HCG has been demonstrated in about 8% of patients with a variety of nontesticular, non–germ cell tumors; thus the presence of elevated HCG level or its demonstration in a nongerminal tumor cell does not itself indicate choriocarcinoma or syncytiotrophoblasts.

The situation is a little more complex with AFP. This fetoprotein was initially demonstrated in human fetal serum and in mice with hepatomas. In the human embryo it is produced first by the yolk sac and later by the liver. Thus in adults pregnancy is the only normal state in which AFP is elevated. In testicular tumors AFP is most often associated with yolk sac elements, whose epithelium usually demonstrates this fetal albumin. Rarely, embryonal carcinoma cells and some columnar mucus-containing epithelial cells of mature and immature teratomas also contain AFP.

One or both of these markers are present in about 70% of testicular germ cell tumors. The half-life of HCG is 24 hours; that of AFP is 5 days. Persistence of one or both of these markers 1 week after the removal of the tumor-bearing testis indicates the presence of metastasis.

Follicle-stimulating hormone (FSH) levels are also frequently elevated, but this has no clinical significance. In addition to these three markers, carcinoembryonic antigen (CEA), human placental lactogen (HPL), pregnancy-specific antigen 1 (SP1), testosterone, estrogens, luteinizing hormone, placental alkaline phosphatase (PLAP), and human chorionic somatomammotropin may also be elevated.

There is no satisfactory clinical classification of testicular germ cell tumors beyond distinguishing those that are confined to the parenchyma of the testis from those that have extended to the adnexa, metastasized below the diaphragm, or spread above the diaphragm.

Testicular biopsy is contraindicated in patients with suspected testicular tumor because biopsy has been associated with a high incidence of local recurrence, which is otherwise rare. Orchiectomy is done in all such patients. Wide sampling of the tumor and the nontumorous testicular tissue is indicated because sometimes a small focus of more malignant cell types is found in a tumor that is predominantly of a different histologic type. The application of stains for tumor markers is the only reliable means to find their specific site of origin.

Because almost all deaths from nonseminomatous germ cell tumors are caused by metastases and because most testicular germ cell tumors have the potentiality for metastasis, most patients are given some form of postorchiectomy treatment—radiation, surgery, or chemotherapy, or all three. The decision to give further treatment and the choice of specific type of therapy are based on three factors: (1) the clinical evidence of metastasis, (2) the histology of the primary tumor, and (3) the persistence of tumor markers after orchiectomy. Most patients who will die of germ cell tumors of the testis do so within 2 years after orchiectomy.

The rarity of testicular germ cell tumors, the heterogeneity of their structure, ranging from simple to complex neoplasms, and the absence of readily available experimental models have resulted in considerable confusion about the histogenesis, pathology, natural history, and behavior of these tumors. The classic work of Friedman and Moore[13] and Dixon and Moore,[10] who reported their observations on 1000 cases of testicular tumors collected at the Army Institute of Pathology (now the Armed Forces Institute of Pathology) in Washington during World War II, followed by Mostofi's studies[20] of an additional 10,000 testicular tumor cases collected in the American Testicular Tumor Registry, housed at the institute, and Sesterhenn's work[42] with tumor markers have clarified many of the problems. The discussion of pathology of these neoplasms is based on these studies, the work of the World Health Organization Scientific Advisory Group on Testicular Tumors, and the experimental research of Stevens[44] and Pierce and Beals.[35]

Histogenesis

Willis[48] advocated two distinct sites of origin of testicular tumors: seminomas arise from cells in the seminiferous tubules, and all other tumors arise from foci of pluripotential embryonic tissue that escaped the influence of the primary organizer during embryonic development. Based on this, he proposed a classification of these tumors into seminoma and teratoma. Because the latter category included tumors of different structure and behavior, the classification has not been accepted, though it has been somewhat modified in recent years by some English investigators. The American writers, on the other hand, have maintained that all these tumors originate from the germ or sex cell (Fig. 19-12). This position has now been conclusively confirmed. Stevens[44] demonstrated experimentally the origin of murine embryonal carcinoma and teratoma from the germ cells. Pierce and Beals[35] showed that, ultrastructurally, embryonal carcinoma cells resemble the primitive germ cells. Mostofi[19,20] has conclusively demonstrated that all human testicular germ cell tumors, except teratomas, originate directly from malignant transformation of intratubular germ cells.

To understand the pathology and the modern pathologic classification of germ cell tumors of the testis, one must remember the potentialities of the fertilized germ cell. Almost immediately this cell divides into two groups: the precursors of embryonic (somatic) elements and of extraembryonic (trophoblastic) elements. The progression of these precursors is in an orderly, organized, controlled manner to result in the embryo and

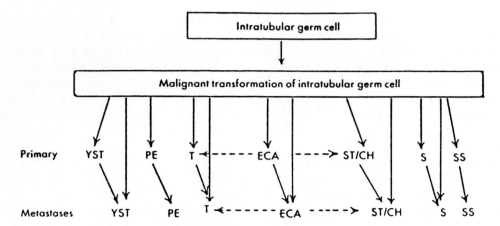

Fig. 19-12. Schematic relationship of testicular germ cell tumors. Neoplastic germ cell may remain intratubular and undifferentiated, or it may invade testicular parenchyma, vascular spaces, and rete testis. In adults embryonal carcinoma may progress to teratoma or choriocarcinoma, or both, either in primary tumor or in metastases, as indicated by broken lines. *CH,* Choriocarcinoma; *ECA,* embryonal carcinoma; *PE,* polyembryomia; *S,* seminoma; *SS,* spermatocytic seminoma; *ST,* syncytiotrophoblast; *T,* teratoma; *YST,* yolk sac tumors, infantile embryonal carcinoma, endodermal sinus tumor.

the placenta, respectively. Very early in embryogenesis one cell is destined to become the germ cell and eventually develop into the gonads.

The malignant germ cell has the same potentialities except that the growth is disorganized, haphazard, and uncontrolled. Stevens has demonstrated that teratomas in mice originate from malignant transformation of germ cells. Mostofi has demonstrated that malignant transformation of intratubular germ cell may progress, while the cells are still intratubular, to form one or more of the following basic histologic types: seminoma, spermatic seminoma, embryonal carcinoma, yolk sac tumor, syncytiotrophoblast, and, by implication, choriocarcinoma (Fig. 19-12). He also demonstrated that the malignant germ cell can invade the stroma and the lymphatics and metastasize. The undifferentiated intratubular malignant germ cells or any of the basic cell tyes may be seen in the seminiferous tubules adjoining the main tumor. These undifferentiated intratubular malignant germ cells have also been called carcinoma in situ.

Histopathologic classification of germ cell tumors

Modern histopathologic classification of testicular germ cell tumors initially separates them into two main categories: tumors of one histologic type, which constitute about 38% of testicular germ cell tumors, and tumors of more than one histologic type, which are seen in 62% of cases:

A. Tumors of one histologic type
   1. Seminoma
   2. Spermatocytic seminoma
   3. Embryonal carcinoma
   4. Yolk sac tumor, infantile embryonal carcinoma, endodermal sinus tumor
   5. Polyembryoma
   6. Choriocarcinoma/syncytiotrophoblasts
   7. Teratoma

B. Tumors of more than one histologic type
Any combination of the seven basic types may occur. The specific types and the relative proportions of each should be mentioned.

Tumors of one histologic type

Seminoma. Compared with the incidence of other germ cell tumors, seminoma occurs in the older age group and is relatively less malignant. Undescended testes harbor this tumor more frequently than other forms of germinal tumors. Seminoma constitutes 31% of all germ cell tumors and 72% of germ cell tumors of one histologic type. Clinically in pure seminoma no elevation of AFP or beta fraction of HCG is seen; if either of these is detected in the serum, the tumor contains other elements.

The involved testis may be only slightly enlarged or may be 10 times larger than normal, yet it usually maintains almost its normal contour. This gross feature is attributable to the fact that the tunical covering is rarely invaded. The neoplasm is opaque grayish white or yellowish white and sometimes contains a yellowish and yellowish brown areas of necrosis (Fig. 19-13). Some tumors are homogeneous, whereas others are distinctly lobulated. The large tumors replace the entire testis, whereas small tumors are circumscribed but not encapsulated. Hemorrhagic necrosis is rare, and cysts

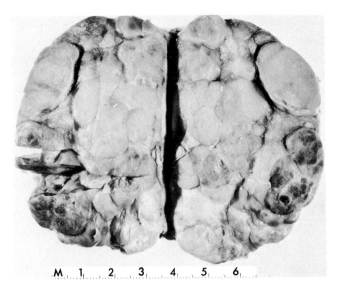

Fig. 19-13. Seminoma of testis.

are never found in pure seminomas.

Microscopically seminomas are readily recognized because of their monocellularity. The cells are moderately large, round, cuboid, or polyhedral and quite uniform in size, and most reveal distinct cell borders. The cytoplasm usually is quite clear, containing glycogen, but occasionally it is slightly stained. Placental alkaline phosphatase (PLAP) is a positive finding in over 90% of tumors. The relatively large, round, centrally located nucleus may occupy one third to one half of the cell. The nucleolus is prominent and slightly eosinophilic, and some nuclei have two nucleoli (Fig. 19-14).

The cells are quite regular, and mitotic figures are infrequent. In about 10%, however, there is increased mitotic activity (high mitotic seminoma), indicating a more aggressive tumor. The seminoma cells occur in cords, columns, or sheets; they may be infiltrating or intratubular. The stroma is usually delicate but almost invariably shows varying degrees of lymphocytic infiltration that may sometimes be quite prominent. In some the stroma may be granulomatous and in a few, very fibrous. The stroma divides the tumor into lobules. The reaction of the stroma is interpreted as an immunologic response of the body to the tumor. The tumors are very radiosensitive, and the 5-year mortality is less than 5% in tumors confined to the testis and 20% to 60% in those that have already metastasized at the time of orchiectomy. Most deaths from germ cell tumors occur in 2 years and almost all in 5 years since discovery.

Spermatocytic seminoma. Spermatocytic seminoma (Fig. 19-15) usually occurs in older patients. Grossly it is softer and more yellowish and mucoid than is seminoma and has small or large spaces containing pinkish fluid. Microscopically, although the major cell popula-

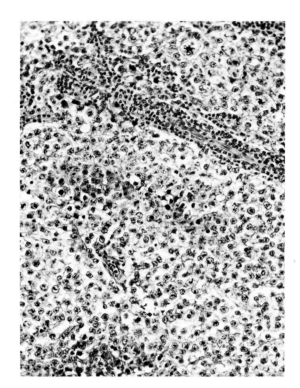

Fig. 19-14. Seminoma of testis. (145×.)

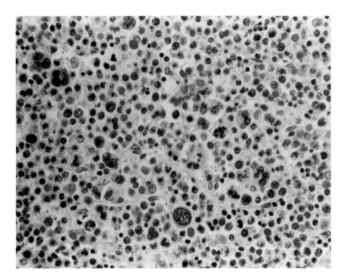

Fig. 19-15. Spermatocytic seminoma. (250×.)

tion is of intermediate size as in seminoma, there are many cells resembling secondary spermatocytes and huge mononucleate or multinucleate giant cells. The cytoplasm has no glycogen. A few cells give a positive reaction for PLAP. The nuclei of the intermediate and large cells have a distinct chromatin distribution, which resembles the meiotic phase of normal primary spermatocytes and is described as filamentous or spireme.

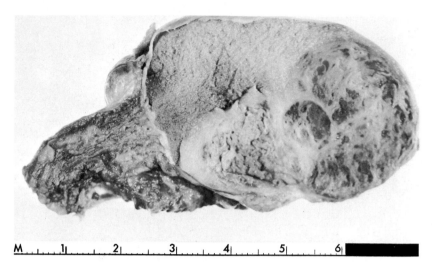

Fig. 19-16. Embryonal carcinoma of testis.

Lymphocytic and granulomatous reactions are absent. The tumors are believed to be radiosensitive, and the prognosis is very good. Up to now, spermatocytic seminomas have not been reported in any site other than the testis. We have seen it in a rat and an albino African lungfish. Rarely spermatocytic seminoma may be associated with an undifferentiated sarcoma that may metastasize and terminate fatally.

Embryonal carcinoma. Pure embryonal carcinoma constitutes 3% of germ cell tumors, but areas of embryonal carcinoma are found in 47% of all tumors. HCG levels are not elevated in pure embryonal carcinoma, but some elevation of AFP may be found. Grossly the tumors are among the smallest. They distort the contour of the testicle more than the seminoma because of their invasion of the capsule and epididymis. The cut surfaces reveal a soft gray or grayish red tissue with areas of hemorrhage and necrosis (Fig. 19-16). The tumors are rarely cystic.

Microscopically the characteristic feature of these tumors is that the are made up of definitely carcinomatous cells—large, highly anaplastic with amphophilic cytoplasm, often with indistinct cell borders (Fig. 19-17). The nuclei are prominent and eosinophilic and may be quite large. Mitotic figures are always present and often numerous. The cells usually form glandular, tubular, papillary, or pseudocystic structures or rarely solid sheets. Hemorrhage and necrosis are not uncommon. The stroma does not have the distinct pattern of the seminoma. It may be imperceptible or abundant, fibrous, primitive, or even sarcomatous. The tumors are less sensitive to radiation than seminomas are. Chemotherapy has miraculously reduced the mortality.

Thirteen percent of tumor cells contain AFP, but none of the cells of pure embryonal carcinoma contains

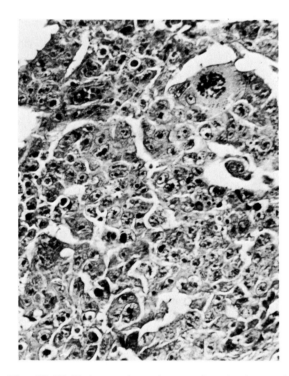

Fig. 19-17. Embryonal carcinoma of testis. (230×.)

HCG. Ultrastructural studies have shown that embryonal carcinoma consists of primitive cells intermingled with more mature cells. Some investigators believe that the primitive cells have the capability of differentiating into embryonic or trophoblastic tissue.

For many years retroperitoneal lymph node dissection (RPLND) was carried out in all patients with embryonal carcinoma. If results were positive, the patients were further treated by radiation or chemotherapy or both. This regimen is under scrutiny, and it is possible that RPLND will be eliminated.

One of the most dramatic results of current treatment of cancer has occurred in testicular embryonal carcinoma. In the 1970s, 75% of patients with embryonal carcinoma died with 5 years; 1989, through chemotherapy, over 80% of those whose tumor is confined to the testis survive after orchiectomy. If metastases have occurred, 70% may survive.

Yolk sac tumors (infantile embryonal carcinoma). These tumors have also been designated as "endodermal sinus tumors" because they resemble the yolk sac or the endodermal sinus. They are the most common testicular tumor in infants and children. AFP levels are usually high. Grossly the testis is usually enlarged, and the cut surface is yellowish gray, mucinous, and greasy. Microscopically the tumor has a reticular pattern with epithelial cells that range from flattened to cuboid and even low columnar cells forming anastomosing tubular structure (Fig. 19-18).

AFP is demonstrable in many tumor cells. The survival in infants and children is over 80%. A pure yolk sac tumor is rarely seen in adults and has a poor prognosis, but yolk sac tumor areas are found in over 40% of adult testicular tumors of more than one cell type.

Polyembryoma. This very rare tumor is composed predominantly of embryoid bodies. These are structures containig a disc and cavities surrounded by loose mesenchyme simulating an embryo of about 2 weeks' gestation. Tubular structures resembling endoderm and syncytiotrophoblastic elements may be present. Polyembryoma as defined is very rare, but embryoid bodies are found frequently with embryonal carcinoma and teratoma.

Choriocarcinoma. Pure choriocarcinomas are the most malignant of germ cell tumors, but fortunately they are extremely rare (18 in 6000). They are usually small and always hemorrhagic and necrotic with a small rim of viable tissue at periphery. Frequently the patients, who are usually in their early twenties, initially have symptoms of metastasis. Sometimes, because of its small size, the primary lesion is completely missed until autopsy. The level of chorionic gonadotropins is greatly elevated, and there is gynecomastia.

To diagnose choriocarcinoma, one must recognize two types of cells, the cytotrophoblast and the syncytiotrophoblast (Fig. 19-19). The cytotrophoblasts are polyhedral cells having a clear or pinkish cytoplasm with relatively large hyperchromatic nuclei. They lie in sheets or make up the major portion of the villuslike structures, which are usually boardered by syncytiotrophoblasts. The syncytiotrophoblasts are large, often huge, irregular, bizarre cells with pseudopodia extending between other cells. Their cell wall is indistinct. They possess a large amount of azurophilic cytoplasm, which frequently is vacuolated. Their deeply staining

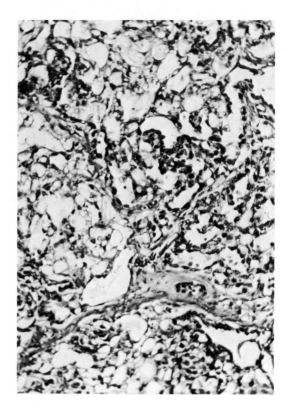

Fig. 19-18. Yolk sac tumor (infantile embryonal carcinoma) of testis. (130×.)

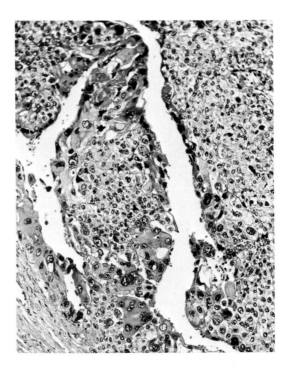

Fig. 19-19. Choriocarcinoma of testis. (100×.)

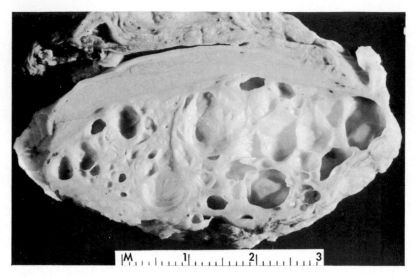

Fig. 19-20. Teratoma of testis.

nuclei are large, irregular, and pyknotic. Some of the cells are multinucleated.

The syncytiotrophoblasts are usually located (as in choriocarcinoma of the uterus) in the advancing edge of the tumor, but distinct villus formation is very rare. None of the current markers is demonstrable in cytotrophoblasts. Syncytiotrophoblasts contain HCG, human placental lactogen (HPL), and pregnancy-specific antigen 1 (SP1). All of our patients with pure choriocarcinoma of the testes were dead within 35 weeks of the diagnosis.

In contrast to the rarity of pure choriocarcinoma, syncytiotrophoblasts or areas of choriocarcinoma are not infrequently seen in association with other testicular tumors. This is discussed under tumors of more than one histologic type. In some cases in which the primary tumor has no demonstrable chorionic elements, the metastasis may show choriocarcinoma.

Teratoma. Teratoma in the testis is defined as a complex tumor with recognizable elements of more than one germ layer. It constitutes about 3% of all germ cell tumors, 7% of tumors of one histologic type in adults, and about 40% of infantile testicular tumors. Teratomatous areas are found in 47% of tumors of more than one histologic type. The AFP level may be slightly elevated. Grossly the tumors are of moderate size, grayish white, cystic, and honeycombed with areas of cartilage and bone (Fig. 19-20). The cysts mostly contain keratohyaline matter but may contain mucin. In contrast to the ovaries, dermoid tumors are rare in the testes.

Microscopically the testicular teratoma is a complex tumor revealing a disorderly arrangement of a great variety of fetal and adult structures originating from the three germ layers: ectoderm, mesoderm, and entoderm.

Three categories of teratoma are recognized: mature teratoma, immature teratoma, and teratoma with malignant areas. Mature teratoma is the most common. It is characterized by well-differentiated structures such as cartilage, smooth muscle, mucous glands, respiratory and gastrointestinal structures, squamous and transitional epithelium-lined cysts (Fig. 19-21). In infants and children nerve tissue may be seen. Immature teratoma shows primitive neuroectodermal elements, primitive cartilage, mesenchyme, abortive eye, and intestinal and respiratory elements. AFP is demonstrable in columnar mucus containing epithelial cells of mature and immature teratoma. Teratoma with malignant areas consists of teratoma and a definite malignant tissue, such as rhabdomyosarcoma, neuroblastoma, squamous cell carcinoma, mucinous adenocarcinoma, and carcinoid. Mature and immature teratomas have been demonstrated to invade blood vessels and lymphatics and to metastasize. Teratomas with malignant areas may show both teratoma and the malignant tumor in the metastases. In infants and children the prognosis of teratoma is much better.

Tumors of more than one histologic type. In 62% of patients with testiculaar germ cell neoplasms the tumor consists of more than one histologic type. Except for spermatocytic seminoma, which tends to occur in pure form, all other cell types may occur in combination. The detection of the various types that may be present and the designation of the mixtures have been the source of considerable confusion. The application of tumor markers to the tissue has clarified the presence of various elements and provided the proper explanation

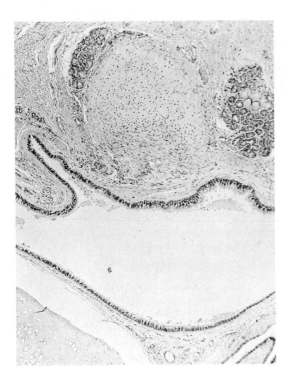

Fig. 19-21. Teratoma of testis. (48×.)

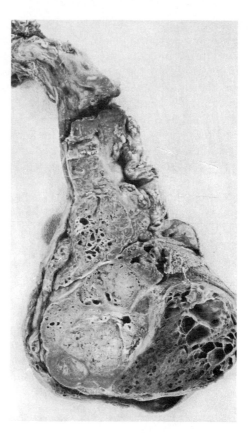

Fig. 19-22. Teratoma and embryonal carcinoma (teratocarcinoma) of testicle infiltrating spermatic cord.

for the bizarre clinical behavior of this group of tumors and the divergence between the histologic findings in primary tumor and the metastasis. For a long time the prevalent concept was that the most frequent combination was embryonal carcinoma and teratoma, to which the term *teratocarcinoma* was applied; it has now been demonstated that, in fact, the most frequent combination is embryonal carcinoma, teratoma, yolk sac tumor, and syncytiotrophoblasts. Thus one or both HCG and AFP may be present in the serum.

Grossly these tumors are usually quite large and solid with cystic areas. They may have areas of hemorrhage and necrosis (Fig. 19-22). Histologically the embryonal carcinoma segment is readily identifiable. The teratomatous component may consist of mature or immature teratoma. The yolk sac elements and the syncytiotrophoblasts are often overlooked and are likely to be missed unless the sections are stained for tumor markers. The second most frequent combination is seminoma and syncytiotrophoblasts. Any one or more of the elements that are present in the primary tumor may metastasize.

In these tumors of more than one histologic type, one clinical finding causes considerable consternation— serum elevation of HCG in the range of below 2000 units, particularly in patients with seminoma. Such a finding raises the suspicion of choriocarcinoma. Sometimes a focus of choriocarcinoma is readily detected and the problem is resolved. More often, either some syn-

cytiotrophoblasts are seen, or nothing is found that can explain the elevated HCG. In such cases staining for tumor markers and torough examination of the tumor and the testis will reveal the presence of syncytiotrophoblasts in the tumor, in the supporting stroma, or in the adjacent seminiferous tubules. Syncytiotrophoblasts may recapitulate any of the forms that they show in various stages of placenta. Where no explanation can be found in the testis for the elevated HCG levels, the existence of HCG-producing cells in metastasis should be ruled out; this can be done by postorchiectomy determination of HCG levels. Elevation 1 week after orchiectomy indicates the existence of metastasis. A normal tumor marker level, however, does not exclude metastasis of components that do not produce markers.

One of the fascinating features of testicular germ cell tumors is that, although the histology of the metastases reflects the histology of the primry tumor in over 90%, occasionally the metastases are entirely different histologically from the primary tumor, or metastatic foci may have different histologic types. A primary tumor that may consist of embryonal carcinoma, teratoma, or a mixture of these may show the same or choriocarcinoma in the secondary, or the metastases in the lymph nodes may be different histologically from those in the liver, lung, or kidney. A primary lesion may consist of a small mature teratoma or seminoma, either alone or in association with an area of scarring and calcific and hemosiderin deposition, but the widespread metastases may consist of choriocarcinoma, embryonal carcinoma, or teratocarcinoma. In many testicular tumors of all types it is not unusual to find intratubular undifferentiated malignant germ cells, intratubular seminoma, embryonal carcinoma, yolk sac tumor, or syncytiotrophoblasts. Any of these may invade the parenchyma and metastasize.

The observed histologic discrepancies between the primary lesion and the metastasis may be explainable on one of several bases: a small focus of the cell type present in the metastasis may have been missed in the primary; the totipotential malignant germ cell or the primitive embryonal carcinoma cell may have been carried away to develop into another cell type in the metastasis; or the location may have influenced the histologic type of the metastasis.

In recent years chemotherapy has dramatically reduced death rates in nonseminomatous germ cell tumors from 70% to 20%. About 40% of residual metastases consist of mature cystic teratoma, and 14% consist of sarcomas of various types. As far as cystic teratoma in the metatases is concerned it was initially postulated that chemotherapy transformed embryonal carcinoma to mature teratoma; as far as sarcomas are concerned it was believed that chemotherapy transformed embryonal carcinoma to sarcoma or it induced sarcoma in the host tissue. Mostofi and associates have demonstrated that when adequate tissue was available for study in every case when either teratoma or sarcoma was present in the metastases it was also present in the primary; that such elements could be found in the metastases before the patient had received any treatment; and mature or immature teratoma and teratoma with malignant areas are all capable of vascular and lymphatic invasion and metastases. These authors believe that treatment destroyed the sensitive elements, that is, seminoma, embryonal carcinoma, yolk sac tumor, and choriocarcinoma, allowing the resistant elements, that is, teratoma and sarcoma, to propagate.

Metastasis

Extratesticular spread of germ cell tumors constitutes the ominous progression of these neoplasms. It can be lymphogenous or directly or indirectly hematogenous. Lymphogenous metastasis occurs much more frequently than hematogenous except in choriocarcinoma. The lymph nodes predominantly involved are the iliac, periaortic, mediastinal and supraclavicular groups. Eventually hematogenous spread occurs either directly through testicular vascular channels or indirectly through lymphatic drainage into superior vena cava.

The organs most frequently harboring metastases are the lungs, liver, and kidneys, but no organ is immune.

Burned-out testicular tumors

Discovery of an apparent extragonadal germ cell tumor—choriocarcinoma, embryonal carcinoma, seminoma, or teratocarcinoma—should lead to careful and thorough examination of the testes before the tumor is accepted as extragonadal. Not infrequently one of the testes of patients with such tumors shows a well-defined, acellular, rather dense scar with or without hemosiderin deposition and with or without dark blue–staining masses (hematoxyphilic bodies). A small focus of mature teratoma, seminoma, or embryonal carcinoma may be seen, or there may be intratubular malignant germ cells.

Tumors derived from specialized gonadal stroma

To understand the hormonal and morphologic features of tumors derived from specialized gonadal stroma, remember that the primitive mesenchyme of the genital ridge forms the whole gonad of each sex except for the germ cells that migrate from their site of origin in the yolk sac entoderm. These primitive mesenchymal cells constitute the supporting stromal elements for the germ cells. In the female they give rise to theca, granulosa, and lutein cells and in the male, to the sustentacular cells of Sertoli and the interstitial cells of Leydig. The cells of origin of the testis and ovary are identical, and in neoplastic proliferation one might suppose that the strict control that directs the differentiation of these two dissimilar structures might be deranged and structures reminiscent of either ovary or testis may develop. Thus Sertoli and Leydig cell tumors may be found in the ovary (in addition to granulosa cell, theca cell, and lutein cell tumors), and the latter three tumors may be seen in the testis (in addition to Sertoli cell and Leydig cell tumors).

Nodules consisting of Sertoli cell–lined or immature tubules are not infrequent in the undescended testis, and although sometimes erroneously designated as adenomas, they are persistent or hyperplastic nodules. Unless there is a distinct grossly visible tumor, the lesion should not be so designated. Sertoli, granulosa, or theca cell tumors or those showing admixtures occur in all ages but more commonly in infants and children. They correspond to arrhenoblastoma of the ovary and androblastomas of the testis. About one third of adult patients show gynecomastia. Grossly the tumors are usually fairly large, well circumscribed, round or oval, firm, and yellowish or yellowish gray. The cut surfaces are bulging and somewhat greasy.

Microscopically three basic patterns of Sertoli cell tumors may be recognized: tubular, stroma, or mixed. In the tubular type, tubules are lined by high or low co-

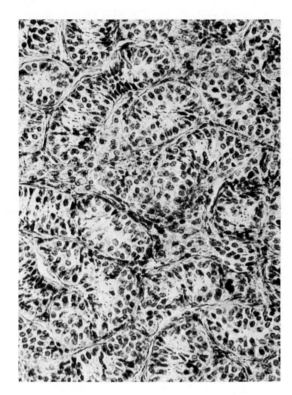

Fig. 19-23. Sertoli cell tumor of testis. (250×.)

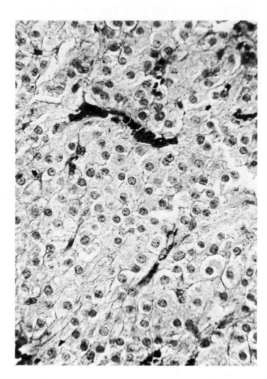

Fig. 19-24. Leydig cell tumor of testis. (250×.)

lumnar Sertoli-like cells (Fig. 19-23) or cuboid cells resembling granulosa cells. The stromal type shows closely packed rounded or spindle-shaped cells with dark-staining nuclei and a small amount of cytoplasm, which resemble theca cells. The mixed type contains all cell types and even Leydig cells. The cells contain estrogens. These tumors have been designated as "androblastoma" by Teilum,[45] who reported three cases with gynecomastia. Mostofi, Theiss, and Ashley[33] have reported a series of 23 cases and suggested the designation "tumors of specialized gonadal stroma." These tumors are mostly benign—only about 10% are malignant and those that metastasize do so within 1 year.

The manifestations of Leydig cell tumors are extremely interesting. Normally Leydig cells produce mostly testostereone but some estorgens and other hormones as well. They undergo morphologic and endocrine involutional changes beginning in fetal and newborn life when they are stimulated by gonadotropins to appear as large epithelium-like cells; in infancy and childhood they resemble fibroblastic cells; in adulthood they are large and granular; and in old age they are small and vacuolated, have a dark-staining nucleus, and are often again spindly.

Clinically all boys with Leydig cell tumors manifest macrogenitosomia, with voice changes, enlargement of the penis, pubic and axillary hair, and precocious body development. If the condition is not recognized and the

tumor-bearing testis is not removed, premature closure of the epiphysis may occur, resulting in dwarfism. In others, gynecomastia develops as the child approaches adolescence. In adult patients no supermasculinizing features are observed but about half show gynecomastia and other feminizing features. Gynecomastia may be attributable to estrogen production or to metabolism of increased or altered androgens. The tumors produce testosterone, estrogens, progesterone, and even corticosteroids.

Grossly the testis usually is enlarged, though this may not be detected. About half of the patients consult a physician because of gynecomastia, with the breasts about two times larger than normal. The testicular tumors are lobulated, well circumscribed, and homogeneously yellowish to mahogany brown. Areas of necrosis and hemorrhage are extremely rare, but calcification may be encountered.

Microscopically the most common cell type is large polyhedral cells with vacuolated or eosinophilic cytoplasm, a round or oval vesicular nucleus, and a single or double nucleolus (Fig. 19-24). Binuclear and trinuclear cells are not uncommon. In addition to lipids, testosterone and other hormones, and brown pigment, the cytoplasm and the nucleus may contain Reinke's crystals, which are characteristic of interstitial cells but seem to have no function. The tumors may recapitulate the various types of interstitial cells encountered in the normal testis in its involution. The cells are arranged in columns and cords separated by well-vascularized fibrous tissue, frequently giving the tumors an endocrine pattern of vascularity.

Differentiation between hyperplasia and tumor (adenoma or carcinoma) is sometimes difficult, especially in children and in patients with adrenogenital syndrome. In tumors there is a distinct mass, and there usually are no entrapped seminiferous tubules, except at the periphery. Differentiation between a benign and a malignant interstitial cell tumor is difficult on a histologic basis, but cellular anaplasia, increased mitoses, and vascular invasion are disturbing features. Fortunately 90% of the tumors are benign. The only criterion for malignancy is metastasis, and this usually is late in development. It is important to do hormone assays in such patients because a rise in or a persistently elevated androgen level after orchiectomy may indicate the development of metastasis. Differentiation from a tumor derived from an adrenal rest is sometimes difficult, but adrenal rests occur almost entirely outside the tunica of the testis, and tumors in the substances of the testis must be regarded as interstitial cell tumors. Histologically and endocrinologically the two tumors frequently are indistinguishable.

Tumors and tumorlike conditions containing both germ cell and gonadal stromal elements

These tumors are usually seen in dysgenetic gonads but rarely also in undescended testis and, more rarely, in normally located testis. The tumors, designated as gonadoblastomas, show large cells resembling seminoma and rarely embryonal carcinoma and small cells resembling immature Sertoli-granulosa cells and occasionally Leydig cells (Fig. 19-25). The tumors are usually benign, but the germ cell element may metastasize.

Lymphoid tumors initially manifested as testicular tumors

These tumors, which may occur at any age, are more frequent in older patients and are often the initial manifestation of the systemic disease. In recent years, with the control of generalized lymphoma by chemotherapeutic agents, some patients have shown involvement of the testis, which is usually enlarged. The cut surface is grayish or yellowish, and areas of necrosis are frequent.

Microscopically there is massive infiltration of the testicular parenchyma with one or more types of reticuloendothelial cells and compression and atrophy of seminiferous tubules. In such infiltrates, infiltration of vascular walls and invasion of seminiferous tubules are pathognomonic of lymphoma. Generalized lymphoma develops in many patients within 2 years.

Secondary tumors

The testis may be a site of metastases from the lungs, prostate, stomach, kidney, colon, pancreas, bladder, and rectum. Although in most cases these are autopsy

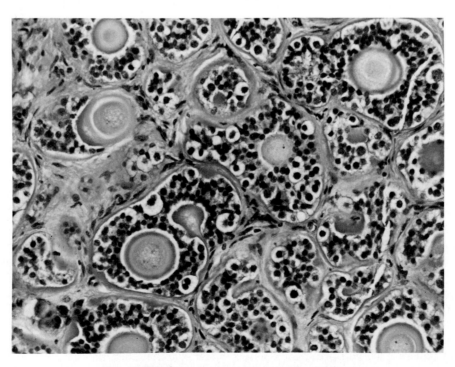

Fig. 19-25. Gonadoblastoma of testis. (160×.)

findings, occasionally they may simulate a primary tumor. Characteristically the infiltrate does not resemble a germ cell or stromal tumor, and it is interstitial and intravascular.

EPIDIDYMIS

Anomalies. Absence of the epididymis is rare. The testis in such instances may or may not be present. Duplication of the epiodidymis is usually associated with polyorchidism. Abnormal descent is associated with abnormal descent of the testis. On occasion the epididymis may be located anterior to the testis, which further complicates the often difficult problem of distinguishing between lesions in the epididymis and those in the testis. Anomalies of fusion are rare. In this situation there is a lack of fusion between the ducts and the seminiferous tubules.

Inflammation. Epididymitis is the most common intrascrotal inflammatory process and usually results from the spread of organisms from the prostatic urethra, prostate, or seminal vesicle. Less often the process is hematogenous. The usual causative agents are the common pyogenic organisms, though in patients under 35 years of age, gonococci and chlamydias are more common. Histologically epididymitis may be acute or chronic, with or without abscesses and ductal destruction. Not infrequently the epididymal epithelium undergoes squamous metaplasia to produce a picture that has been confused with squamous carcinoma. The so-called traumatic epididymitis has been a subject of controversy for many years. The problem is whether straining or heavy lifting can cause retrograde passage of sterile urine down the vas to produce irritation and inflammation. Tuberculous epididymitis generally occurs in patients with renal tuberculosis, and frequently the disease also exists in the prostate and seminal vesi-cle. Tuberculous epididymitis is more likely to be bilateral than other types of inflammation; in the well-developed disease, nodules may be found along the spermatic cord. Inflammation of the epididymis frequently extends into the adjacent parenchyma of the testis, and a diagnosis of epididymo-orchitis is applicable.

Tumors. Exception for the adenomatoid tumor, tumors of the epididymis are uncommon. Longo and associates[56] collected 134 cases of primary tumors of the epididymis from the world literature. The adenomatoid tumor (Fig. 19-26) has been reported under a variety of names such as mesothelioma, lymphangioma, and adenomyoma. Similar tumors are encountered in the tunica vaginalis, spermatic cord, posterior aspect of the uterus, fallopian tube, and ovary.

Adenomatoid tumors are believed to originate from mesothelial cells. Most of the tumors occur in persons between 20 and 40 years of age. About 80% are attached to the epididymis, usually the globus minor, and the remainder are located on the tunica of the testis and in the cord. They are painless, single, firm, round or ovoid nodules ranging from less than 1 cm to 5 cm in greatest diameter. The cut surfaces are homogeneous, grayish white, and fibrous, having a whorled appearance; they occasionally reveal yellow areas. Histologically they have glandlike structures and irregular spaces, and some contain cords of epithelium-like cells (Fig. 19-27). The stroma varies in amount and is com-

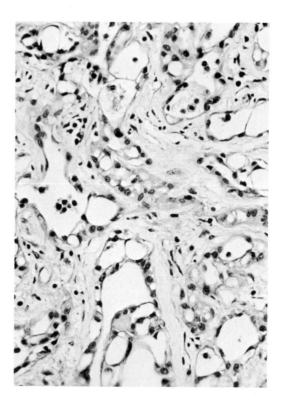

Fig. 19-27. Adenomatoid tumor of epididymis. (225 ×.)

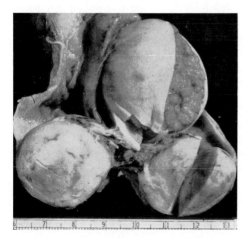

Fig. 19-26. Large adenomatoid tumor of lower pole of epididymis. Tumor is bisected and almost as large as testis above. (Courtesy Dr. Paul C. Dietz, La Crosse, Wis.)

posed of a loose or dense fibrous connective tissue in which broad smooth muscle fibers are recognized. The glandlike structures may be lined with flat, cuboid, or low columnar cells. Many of the cells, particularly those arranged in cords, are vacuolated.

Leiomyoma, the second most common tumor of the epididymis, may be associated with a hydrocele. Other benign tumors that have been reported are angiomas, fibromas, and lipomas. Adrenocortical rests are rather common but are seldom large enough to be detected clinically. Splenic rests may also descend with the testis (gonadal-splenic fusion). Papillary cystadenoma of the epididymis occurs as a small nodule in the head of the organ. The size range is from 1 to 5 cm (mean 2.3 cm). They may have a solid, cystic, or multicystic appearance and are well circumscribed. Histologically the ducts are dilated and lined by clear or vacuolated cells that protrude into the lumen as papillations. The appearance is similar to a low-grade, clear-cell carcinoma of the kidney, but they are apparently benign. Price[62] found that these lesions represent the epididymal component of Lindau's disease. Patients with bilateral lesions showed manifestations of the syndrome in other organs, whereas unilateral cystadenomas were interpreted as a forme fruste of the disease. Carcinomas of the epididymis and adjacent structures (appendix testis, appendix epididymidis, and rete testis) occur but are rare, and it is often difficult to be certain one is not dealing with metastatic carcinoma or mesothelioma of tunica vaginalis. Up to now, epididymal carcinoma has not been established as a distinct clinicopathologic entity.

RETE TESTIS

Tumors and tumorlike lesions. The rete testis often becomes prominent when there is noticeable atrophy of the testis. At times, this appears to represent a true hyperplasia of rete epithelium but is often misinterpreted as a neoplasm. However, this is a microscopic observation only and is not associated with a tumorlike lesion on gross examination. A second point of confusion is the invasion of rete by a germ cell tumor where it is often regarded as an element of mature teratoma or yolk sac tumor. Third, malignant germ cells often invade the subepithelial zone of rete testis and are misinterpreted as carcinoma of the rete. Primary carcinoma of rete is rare and is seen usually in patients over 50 years of age. Grossly there is a dominant mass at the hilum of the testis, which may be solid or cystic. Microscopically the lesion tends to recapitulate the structure of the rete, and in some fields it is difficult to distinguish the two. There are both solid and tubulopapillary areas. Large or small cystic spaces, probably representing ectatic rete, are often filled with a colloidlike material. An excellent review of the light-microscopic and

ultrastructural features of rete adenocarcinoma is that of Nochomovitz and Orenstein.[60] The most common pitfall with respect to the rete testis is the misinterpretation of malignant mesotheliomas of the tunica vaginalis with primary rete carcinoma. The former is considerably more common, and it would be most unusual for a primary rete tumor to present with diffuse thickening of the tunica or with multiple excrescences of the tunica.

SPERMATIC CORD

Anomalies. Anomalies of the spermatic cord are congenital absence and congenital atresia of the vas deferens. Sterility is present when either of these conditions is bilateral. Complete or incomplete duplication of the vas deferens has been reported.

Inflammation. Inflammation of the vas deferens is known as vasitis or deferentitis, whereas inflammation of the entire spermatic cord is termed funiculitis. Lymphangitis, phlebitis, and thromboangiitis may be attributed to a variety of causes. Vasitis may be caused by extension of epididymitis or lymphogenous transportation from urethritis and cystitis. The causes of some cases of both vasitis and funiculitis are not definitely known, but trauma and focal and general infections are suspected. Tuberculosis of the spermatic cord results from tuberculous epididymitis and seminal vesiculitis. Filarial funiculitis is associated with elephantiasis of the penis and scrotum. There is lymphangiectasia and fibrosis of the interstitial tissue. The walls of the lymph vessels become thickened and frequently reveal obliterative lymphangitis, with calcific and crystalline deposits. Calcified filarias may be found in whorls of hyalinized fibrous tissue. The various inflammatory cells encountered in filarial funiculitis are lymphocytes, plasma cells, eosinophils, and, in some cases, multinucleated giant cells.

Cysts. Cysts of the epididymis (spermatocele) or the testicular appendix (hydatid of Morgagni) or epididymal appendices are quite common. The most important are spermatoceles, which may be unilateral or bilateral, unilocular or multilocular. The epithelium is flattened or cuboidal or may be ciliated and surrounded by various amounts of hyalinized fibrovascular tissue and occasionally cholesterol crystals. The lumen is filled with fluid that is either neutral or slightly alkaline. The sediment contains lymphocytes, cellular debris, fat globules, and sometimes cholesterol. The presence of spermatozoa distinguishes these cysts from hydrocele.

Varicocele. Varicocele is a common condition in which the veins of the pampiniform plexus are dilated and elongated and their tortuosity is increased. The cause of primary or idiopathic varicocele is not definitely known. Secondary or symptomatic varicocele is the result of pressure on the spermatic veins or its trib-

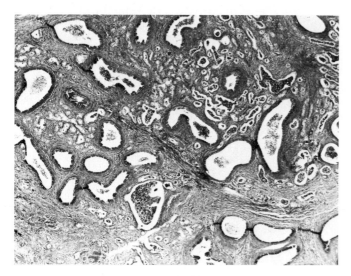

Fig. 19-28. Vasitis nodosa of epididymis. (25×.)

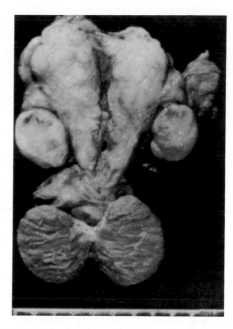

Fig. 19-29. Testis and spermatic cord. Fibrosarcoma of spermatic cord. (Courtesy Dr. Joseph L. Teresi, Brookfield, Wis.)

utaries by an enlarged liver and spleen, pronounced hydronephrosis, muscle strain, and abdominal tumors. Primary varicocele usually involves the left spermatic cord and occurs predominantly in young boys.

Tumors. Lipoma is the most common tumor of the spermatic cord. Leiomyomas and neurofibromas occur less frequently. Vasitis nodosa is a benign tumorlike lesion of the vas that is more frequently seen as more men resort to vasectomy as a means of contraception. Several years after vasectomy a nodule may appear near the surgical site. Histologically it is composed of numerous tubular structures lined by cuboidal or columnar epithelium. The tubules usually contain spermatozoa. These structures occur in and adjacent to the wall of the vas and are usually associated with sperm granulomas. Less frequently the lesion occurs in the epididymis (Fig. 19-28) without a history of ligation, but obstruction is the most likely causative factor. Malignant tumors of the spermatic cord are chiefly sarcomas. In the first three decades of life this is almost invariably embryonal rhabdomyosarcoma. The bulk of such lesions are generally found in the spermatic cord, but there may be extension into the epididymis and even into adjacent areas of the testis. The parietal tunica vaginalis may also be invaded. Other sarcomas occur chiefly between 50 and 80 years of age as liposarcoma, malignant fibrous histiocytoma, fibrosarcoma, and leiomyosarcoma (Fig. 19-29). Liposarcomas are usually the well-differentiated sclerosing variety. These and most of the histiocytomas tend to be of low-grade malignancy; they are prone to local recurrence, but metastases are uncommon.

SCROTUM

Anomalies. Arrest of development may result in the formation of a separate pouch for each testicle. Half of the scrotum corresponding to undescended testicle may be rudimentary. A cleft scrotum resembling labia majora is encountered in pseudohermaphroditism. Partial cleft scrotum may accompany other congenital defects of the genitourinary system.

Dermatologic lesions. The common skin diseases of the scrotum are scabies *(Sarcoptes scabiei)*, pediculosis, prurigo, eczema, erysipelas, psoriasis, and, not infrequently, syphilitic lesions. Sebaceous and epidermal cysts are common and are frequently multiple and calcified.

Gangrene. Gangrene of the scrotum may be caused by trauma or may be a complication of infectious diseases, phimosis, chancroid, balanitis, or periurethritis. Idiopathic or spontaneous gangrene is unassociated with trauma or infection. There is often associated gangrene of the penis.

Hematoma. Hematoma of the scrotum is an effusion of blood within the tissue of the scrotal wall. The blood may collect beneath the tunica dartos, between the tunica vaginalis and the fibrous coat (paravaginal hematoma), or in the scrotal septum. Hematomas are usually of traumatic origin.

Elephantiasis. Elephantiasis of the scrotum is characterized by diffuse increase and fibrosis of the subcutaneous tissue and obvious thickening of the skin resembling elephant's hide and resulting in enlargement of the scrotum. The disease is the result of lymph stasis either from blocking of the lymphatics by microfilarias *(Wuchereria bancrofti)* or from cicatricial closure of the lymph channels caused by chronic inflammation after trauma, excision of lymph nodes, or chronic lymphadenitis. In filariasis the adult worm obstructs the lymph channels. Secondary infection, according to some investigators, is necessary to produce elephantiasis. The live worm apparently provokes little or no inflammation. The dead and disintegrating forms stimulate proliferation of the intima, followed by thrombosis and organization.

Tumors. The most common tumor of the scrotum, squamous cell carcinoma, has been declining in frequency, probably because of its recognized association many years ago with environmental carcinogens. The well-known and almost legendary "chimney-sweep's cancer" has been replaced by that arising among workers with tar, paraffin, and mineral oil, as well as in mule spinners in cotton mills. Squamous cell carcinomas of the scrotum do not differ appreciably from similar lesions of the penis, including the age of prevalence. They appear initially as a nodular, ulcerative, or exophytic lesion and may be multiple. Most are well or moderately differentiated and grow slowly. Metastases involve the inguinal nodes, and distant spread is uncommon. Death usually results from extensive local disease. According to Dean,[82] there is an increased incidence of multiple primary malignancies in patients with scrotal carcinoma. A variety of soft tissue tumors, benign and malignant, occur in the scrotal wall, but none is particularly common.

TUNICA VAGINALIS

Hydrocele. A hydrocele is an abnormal accumulation of serous fluid in the sac of the tunica vaginalis (Fig. 19-30). Normally there are a few drops of serous fluid between the visceral and parietal layers.

In the congenital type of hydrocele, there is a direct communication with the abdominal cavity as a result of failure of closure of the funicular process. In infantile hydrocele there is an accumulation of fluid in the partly closed funicular process and the sac of the tunica vaginalis, but there is no communication with the abdominal cavity. Acute hydrocele may be a complication of gonorrhea, tuberculosis, syphilis, erysipelas, rheumatism, typhoid, or neoplasms. Between 25% and 50% of acute hydroceles are the result of trauma.

The fluid of the hydrocele is odorless, viscid, and straw to amber colored. The usual amount varies from 10 to 300 ml but in one case was 4.5 liters. It has a neutral reaction, and its specific gravity varies from 1.020 to 1.026. It contains about 6% protein (serum albumin, cholesterol, serum globulin, and fibrinogen), alkaline carbonates, and sodium chloride. Occasionally fibrous bodies coated with fibrin are found floating in the fluid. The bodies originate from detached villous projections of the tunica vaginalis. If the hydrocele is in-

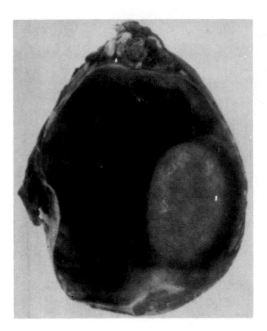

Fig. 19-30. Hydrocele. Normal testicle.

fected, the fluid may be cloudy, or it may be brownish red if slight hemorrhage has occurred. Microscopic examination of comparatively clear hydrocele fluid reveals a few mesothelial cells, lymphocytes, cholesterin crystals, and lecithin bodies.

The sac of the hydrocele may be a single- or multiple-chambered structure. The inner surface of the tunica vaginalis is usually smooth, but there may be adhesions and fibrous projections. The wall is variously thickened, composed of scanty cellular fibrous tissue infiltrated with lymphocytes and some plasma cells. Calcific deposits occasionally are encountered after meconium peritonitis, extensive deposits of calcification and mucin may be found over the tunica.

Hematocele. Hemorrhage in the sac of the tunica vaginalis is known as hematocele. Spontaneous hematocele is slow and insidious in its development, whereas a rapidly developing hematocele is invariably the result of trauma. The blood coagulates, fibrin settles out and organizes, and the wall becomes thick and rough. In long-standing hematocele the tunica vaginalis becomes enormously thickened with dense fibrous tissue, which occasionally becomes partly calcified. Trauma may result in the formation of both hematoma and hematocele.

Tumors. Fibrous pseudotumor (nodular periorchitis) is a tumorlike lesion that typically occurs as well-circumscribed, round, ovoid, or localized plaquelike nodules over the tunica. It is very firm in consistency and is white. It consists almost entirely of mature collagen, though it may contain foci of calcific deposits, scattered inflammatory cells, and mesothelial cell inclusions. The cause is unknown. About one third of the patients have a history of trauma or epididymo-orchitis. Many such tumors are associated with hydrocele; they appear as asymptomatic nodules from the third through the sixth decades and are benign.[59]

Mesothelial lesions of the tunica. Hyperplasia of the mesothelial cells lining the tunica vaginalis and tunica albuginea is common and may be found in association with any inflammatory process that involves the tunica. Histologically, small acinar, tubular, or papillary structures lined by small mesothelial cells are found within the zone of inflammation. This process typically rather sharply outlines the deep margin of this zone. The presence of solid sheets of such cells or their extension into normal tissue such as epididymis or normal adipose tissues of the cord should raise the question of malignancy. A second form of benign mesothelial proliferation has been referred to as nodular mesothelial hyperplasia.[61] This occurs as small nodules of tissue within the fluid of hydroceles or hernia sacs, particularly in infants and children. Microscopically the nodules are composed of viable sheets of mesothelial cells enmeshed in fibrin. Malignant mesothelioma of tunica is a tumor usually associated with hydrocele. Multiple, friable excrescences are found studding the visceral and parietal tunica vaginalis and the tunica albuginea. The tumor grows into the structures of the cord and testicular adnexa and invades the periphery of the testis. It should be noted that invasion of rete testis by mesothelioma is frequently confused with a primary tumor of rete testis. Spread is to the regional lymph nodes. Not infrequently these tumors represent the early manifestation of generalized mesothelioma of peritoneum or pleura; the latent period may be as long as 4 years.

PENIS

Anomalies

Phimosis. Phimosis is a condition in which the preputial orifice is too small to permit retraction of the prepuce behind the glans. It is independent of inflammation of the foreskin. An acquired phimosis may result from inflammation, trauma, or edema that narrows the preputial opening so that the prepuce cannot be retracted. Congenital phimosis predisposes to development of preputial calculi and squamous cell carcinoma. Paraphimosis is a condition in which the retracted prepuce cannot be reduced, with swelling of the prepuce and ulceration of the constricting tissue. It is usually a complication of gonorrhea, chancre, chancroid, balanitis, or trauma.

Hypospadias. Hypospadias is a developmental arrest in which the urethral meatus is present on the undersurface of the penis. It is probably a result of disturbance of sex differentiation, causing imperfect closure of the urethral groove. The arrest may take place any-where along the urethral groove, thus resulting in hypospadias with location from the glans penis to the perineum. Hypospadias is associated with a rather high incidence of genital anomalies such as cryptorchidism, enlarged prostatic utricle, and bifid scrotum. In about 25% of the cases hypospadias is inherited as a recessive trait.

Epispadias is a rare form of congenital defect in which the urethral meatus is located at the upper surface of the penis. Its incidence in newborn infants is 1 in 50,000, and it frequently is associated with cryptorchidism, exstrophy of the urinary bladder, or absence of the prostate gland. In fact, it is a mild form of exstrophy.

Inflammation

Syphilis. The common site of a hard chancre is on the glans near the frenum or on the inner surface of the prepuce. It also may occur within or at the site of the urethral meatus, or rarely, on the shaft (see p. 325).

Chancroid. An acute venereal disease caused by *Haemophilus ducreyi* and usually transmitted by sexual intercourse, chancroid produces a painful ulcer on the corona, prepuce, or shaft of the penis. This ulcer is necrotic and suppurative and bleeds readily. It is not as indurated as the syphilitic chancre and is therefore termed "soft chancre" (see p. 310).

Herpes progenitalis. Herpes progenitalis is characterized by development of a group of vesicles on the glans or prepuce. The surrounding tissue is inflamed. The vesicles rupture, and small discrete or confluent ulcers develop but heal with a short time.

Granuloma inguinale. Granuloma inguinale usually begins in the inguinal region and spreads to the perineum, scrotum, and penis. Nodules and serpiginous ulcers develop on the prepuce, and these spread to the glans and the shaft (see p. 324).

Lymphopathia venereum. Lymphopathia venereum is often confused with granuloma inguinale, but it is a specific venereal disease caused by a filterable agent (see p. 357).

Fusospirochetosis. Erosive and gangrenous balanitis is a disease comparable to Vincent's angina and is caused by a fusiform bacillus *(Vibrio)* and a spirochete (see p. 329).

Plastic induration. Plastic induration (Peyronie's disease) is a fibrositis of the penis involving Buck's fascia and the sheath of one or both corpora cavernosa. The cause is unknown. It resembles Dupuytren's contracture and keloids, and 25% of patients do show Dupuytren's contracture. The disease is more common than reports in the literature indicate. About 5% to 10% of cases reveal mild lesions. Two types are described: (1) thickening and contracture of the median septum and (2) localized nodules or indurated thickened areas involving the sides and underportion of the sheath of the

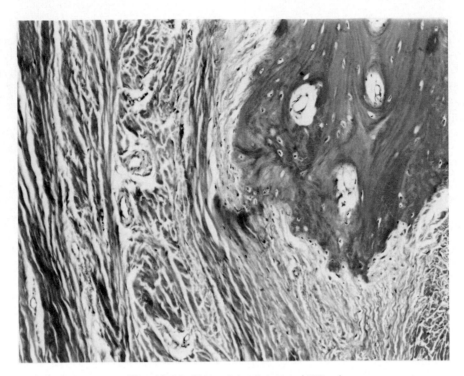

Fig. 19-31. Peyronie's disease. (150×.)

corpus cavernosum. There is curvature of the penis and pain on erection and difficult or impossible intromission. Microscopically there is a scanty cellular fibrous tissue in which there are few blood vessels and mild evidence of inflammation. The lesion often resembles scar tissue. Occasionally the fibrous tissue undergoes ossification (Fig. 19-31).

Sclerosing lipogranuloma (paraffinoma). Sclerosing lipogranuloma is a subcutaneous granulomatous reaction seen most often in the penis and scrotum. It appears as painful or painless nodules, plaques, or fistulas and can be demonstrated by infrared absorption spectrophotometry to result from the presence of exogenous lipid (paraffin hydrocarbons). Microscopically the involved area exhibits diffuse hyalinized tissue with variable numbers of inflammatory cells and numerous vacuoles. The latter vary in size from several micrometers to those that are grossly visible. Some vacuoles have no lining, whereas others may be partially outlined by flattened multinucleated, foreign-body type of giant cells (Fig. 19-32). A history of lipid injection is rarely volunteered, but the lesion is believed to result from an effort to facilitate erection or increase potency.

Tumors

Benign tumors. Squamous cell papillomas occur on the glans and shaft under various names, the most common being the condyloma. Hemangioma is the most common mesodermal lesion of the glans. Neurofibromas and leiomyomas occur rarely as small nodules of the glans, frenulum, prepuce, or shaft.

CONDYLOMA ACUMINATUM. Incorrectly termed venereal wart, condyloma acuminatum is a raspberry- or cauliflower-shaped tumor usually located on the coronal sulcus. The tumor may be a single papilloma, or there may be multiple or conglomerated papillomas. These tumors frequently are associated with or occur after various inflammatory diseases of the penis. A viral cause cannot be excluded. Microscopically these are essentially squamous papillomas characterized by pronounced acanthosis and hyperplasia of the prickle cell layer. Parakeratosis is present. The rete ridges are elongated and may be branching, but they all extend to about the same level. The growth is characteristically upward toward the surface and not downward into the tissue. Sometimes the tumor is quite extensive. A histologically similar lesion has received attention. It has been designated giant condyloma, Buschke-Lowenstein tumor, or verrucous carcinoma. It forms grotesque cauliflower-like warty masses of large size with a strong tendency to extend, perforate the prepuce, destroy the underlying tissue, ulcerate, become infected, and produce many fistulas. Clinically the masses behave as cancer, and recurrence is the rule, but histologically they are benign. In contrast to the usual condylomas, the stratum corneum is thicker, parakeratosis is present, and there is pronounced acanthosis and papillation, as well as pronounced hyperplasia of the prickle cell layer. The papillae extend much deeper. Mitoses are limited to the basal layers, and stratification is normal. The tumors rarely metastasize.

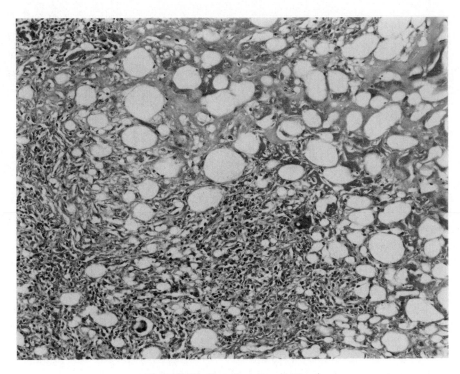

Fig. 19-32. Paraffinoma. (150×.)

VERRUCA. Verruca is an ordinary squamous cell papilloma revealing hyperkeratosis and thus differing from simple condyloma, in which the epithelium is piled up in the middle layer (acanthosis).

BOWENOID PAPULOSIS. The benign lesions of bowenoid papulosis occur chiefly on the penile shaft and adjacent perigenital skin of men between 20 and 45 years of age. Mucosal lesions may also occur but seldom without involvement of adjacent skin. The lesions may be solitary but usually are multiple and typically vary from 1 to 10 mm in size. The appearance is that of a shiny, flesh-colored, pink to red-brown, black, or violaceous papular or verrucoid lesion. Histologically there may be hyperkeratosis, frequently parakeratosis, focal hypergranulosis, vacuolated keratinocytes, irregular acanthosis, and occasional papillomatosis. There is orderly maturation with scattered hyperchromatic nuclei, dysplastic cells, and mitoses. Many of the last are in the same stage of development, chiefly metaphase. The most important feature that distinguishes bowenoid papulosis from erythroplasia and Bowen's disease is the absence of full-thickness involvement by atypical keratinocytes. Recent evidence points to the human papilloma virus and herpes simplex virus (type 2) as the etiologic agents. Treatment should be conservative.

Premalignant lesions

ERYTHROPLASIA OF QUEYRAT. Erythroplasia of Queyrat is a pinkish pagetoid lesion that usually involves the glans but occasionally may occur on the coronal sulcus or prepuce. It is shiny, pinkish red, flat, faintly elevated, and sharply marginated. The surface is smooth, slightly eroded, "velvety," more firm than the surrounding normal tissue, quite pliable, and with definite evidence of fixation to the underlying tissue. Histologically erythroplasia of Queyrat shows an area of irregular acanthosis in which the keratin layer is decreased and there is parakeratosis. The epidermis is thickened and composed of atypical cells with loss of normal polarity and of normal maturation. Many of the cells are vacuolated, and numerous mitotic figures are seen at all levels. The rete ridges are elongated and extend into the underlying stroma and sometimes are attached to each other. The subepithelial layer of dermis is edematous and shows infiltration that is predominately plasmacytic. One distinguishes between erythroplasia, which occurs on the penile mucosa, and Bowen's disease, which occurs on penile skin.

BOWEN'S DISEASE. In contrast to erythroplasia of Queyrat, which is located on the glans, an essentially similar lesion is encountered on the shaft of the penis. Aside from the differences in histology between the two occasioned by the fact that Bowen's disease is derived from the keratinizing epithelium of the skin and the skin appendages may be involved and the role of arsenic in Bowen's disease, there is controversy as to whether Bowen's disease is associated with high incidence of internal malignancy or such occurrence is entirely accidental (see p. 1797).

Malignant tumors

SQUAMOUS CELL CARCINOMA. In the United States less than 2% of all cancers in men arise in the penis. The incidence on other parts of the world is as follows: China, 18.3%; continental Europe, 4.9%; Great Britain, 1.27%. In the United States, penile cancer occurs about three or four times more frequently in blacks than in whites. The greatest incidence is between 45 and 60 years. Rare cases in childhood and early adult life have been reported.

It would not be an exaggeration to state that the presence of a foreskin is a predisposing cause of squamous cell carcinoma of the penis, since without this structure the incidence is insignificant. In India carcinoma of the penis rarely develops in Muslims, who practice circumcision in infancy as a religious rite, whereas Hindus, who do not circumcise, have about a 10% incidence. Among Jews, who are also regularly circumcised in infancy, the disease is almost unknown. The exciting causes of this neoplasm are irritation by retained smegma, phimosis, and trauma. Smegma has been shown to be possibly carcinogenic. Some patients give a history of previous venereal disease.

The location of the neoplasm, in order of frequency, is the (1) frenum and prepuce, (2) glans, and (3) coronal sulcus. The tumors may be papillary or flat and ulcerating. They grow slowly. Histologically they are of low malignancy. Metastasis to the inguinal lymph nodes occurs in about 50% of the cases. Visceral metastasis is extremely rare.

SARCOMA. Fibrosarcoma, leiomyosarcoma, Kaposi's sarcoma, endothelioma, and malignant melanoma are seen rarely. Kaposi's sarcoma occurs on the glans penis as a nodular or multinodular lesion. This is discussed on p. 1092. Metastatic carcinoma to the penis usually is a terminal event in the course of carcinomatosis. The tumor characteristically fills the vascular spaces of erectile tissue to produce a rather generalized induration of the organ. The primary lesions are most commonly in the prostate, bladder, kidney, or gastrointestinal tract.

URETHRA

Mechanical disturbances

Diverticula. Urethral diverticula are fairly common in females but rare in males. They may be congenital or acquired. Congenital true diverticula, arising from the periurethral glands, always occur on the ventral wall of the anterior portion of the urethra, whereas acquired diverticula develop in the posterior portion. The acquired diverticula are caused by inflammation, trauma, or, in the male obstruction of the urethra.

Prolapse. Prolapse of the urethra occurs almost exclusively in females. It usually involves the entire circumference, and the lumen is located in the center.

Unless reduced promptly, pressure and infection produce vascular engorgement and acute inflammation.

Obstruction. Strictures of the urethra may be congenital or acquired. The former occurs usually in male infants at either the corona or the membranous urethra. Infant girls also may manifest congenital stricture of the distal portion of the urethra. Acquired strictures are the most common, and at one time most of them were complications of gonorrheal urethritis. This will probably be the case again with the recent increase in the incidence of venereal disease. About 10% are the result of trauma, but tuberculosis, other venereal diseases, periurethral abscesses, and caruncles also may cause urethral strictures. In women, obstetric trauma is the chief cause. Whatever the cause, the urethra heals by proliferation of fibroblasts and scarring, resulting in contraction. If left untreated, eventually there is back pressure, dilatation of the urethra, hypertrophy of the vesical musculature, vesical dilatation, and finally hydroureter and hydronephrosis.

Inflammation

Gonococcal urethritis. Acute urethritis may be attributed to a variety of bacteria. Gonococcal urethritis in the male, as a rule, involves the portion of urethra anterior to the triangular ligament (p. 309).

Nonspecific urethritis. Trauma, injection of chemical irritants, masturbation, coitus (in which the female partner may suffer a nonspecific vaginitis), redundant foreskin, and pinhole meatus are causes of nonspecific urethritis. The same conditions that predispose to cystitis act similarly in the urethra. Various bacteria have been isolated, among which staphylococci, streptococci, and colon bacilli predominate. In recent years nongonococcal urethritis has been recognized with increasing frequency; it is most commonly caused by *Chlamydia trachomatis*. Gonococci and chlamydias produce similar symptoms and often coexist. Thus treatment of gonococcal urethritis with penicillin is often followed by recurrent symptoms (postgonococcal urethritis) because of the resistant *Chlamydia* organisms. Because laboratory procedures have now progressed to the point that both organisms can be readily identified, tetracycline has been advocated when both are present.

Abscesses. Abscesses within and continuous with the urethra are infrequent. They are usually complications of gonorrhea, but they may be complications of nonspecific infections. These abscesses develop when the urethral glands are infected and their ducts occluded.

Reiter's disease. Urethritis, conjunctivitis, and arthritis form a clinical triad known as Reiter's disease. The cause of this disease is not known, and tissue changes have not been investigated. Several workers have recovered viruslike agents by inoculating embryonated eggs with filtered urethral and conjunctival exudates. Spontaneous recovery is the rule, but relapses occur in about 25%, sometimes after a considerable silent period.

Urethrolithiasis. Calculi are rarely formed in the urethra. They either are dislodged bladder calculi or, when primary, originate in a urethral diverticulum.

Tumors

Benign tumors. The most common benign tumors and tumorlike lesions of the urethra are caruncles, cysts, leiomyomas, and condylomas. The last is the most common lesion in young adult males, in whom it is frequently multifocal and recurrent. A lesion that has been designated ectopic prostate occurs in the prostatic urethra. The latter, including the verumontanum, are normally lined in part by prostatic acinar epithelium. When this tissue projects into the urethral lumen as a result of either hyperplasia or mucosal redundancy, it is said to be ectopic. Such a lesion can cause hematuria or hematospermia, if in proximity to the orifices of the ejaculatory ducts.

CARUNCLES. Urethral caruncles are confined almost entirely to the female urethra. Their cause is unknown. There are several theories: regional or circumscribed prolapse of urethral mucosa caused primarily by postmenopausal shrinkage of vaginal tissue with secondary trauma and infection, infection and chronic irritation resulting from lack of proper hygiene, and trauma consequent to coitus or childbirth.

Histologically there are three somewhat arbitrary types. The papillomatous type is frequently grossly lobulated as a result of clefts or crypts. The surface is covered by transitional and stratified squamous epithelium in various places. The epithelium continues along the crypts, from which sprouts extend deep into the stroma. Some of the epithelium-lined crypts on cross section appear as deep-seated nests of epithelial cells. Such areas may be confused with carcinoma. The stroma is usually infiltrated with inflammatory cellular elements.

The telangiectatic caruncle is highly vascular. The vessels are so numerous that the lesion has an appearance similar to the papillomatous type.

The granulomatous type lacks epithelial hyperplasia and is almost entirely composed of granulation tissue.

CYSTS. Cysts of the urethra may be congenital or acquired. Acquired cysts are more common and result from inflammatory occlusion of the urethral glands. The cysts of the posterior urethra arise from occlusion of the periurethral and subcervical ducts. Polyps are usually encountered in the folds of the urethra. Some of the polyps are difficult to differentiate from fibromas and papillomas. Papillomas occur in any part of the urethra, but the majority are encountered about the vesicle neck at or near the meatus.

Malignant tumors. Malignant tumors of the urethra include squamous cell carcinoma, transitional cell carcinoma, adenocarcinoma, mesonephric carcinoma, and, rarely, melanoma. Squamous cell carcinoma of either male or female urethra is uncommon, but vulvourethral carcinoma is not infrequent. Transitional cell carcinomas occur chiefly in the posterior urethra and most often are associated with similar lesions in the bladder. Some of the urethral adenocarcinomas probably originate from periurethral glands, but others clearly arise by glandular metaplasia of the transitional cell epithelial lining of the mucosa. Some urethral carcinomas have a tubular pattern composed of cells with clear or granular cytoplasm, reminiscent of renal cell carcinoma. These are designated as tubular or clear-cell carcinomas. Their origin is uncertain.[134] Urethral melanomas are usually seen in older women. Malignant tumors of Cowper's gland are rare. They occur as ulcerative, nodular, or fungating lesions in the perineum and histologically show a mucinous or adenoid cystic appearance.

PROSTATE GLAND

The prostate gland, the largest accessory sex organ in males, is situated immediately blow the internal urethral orifice. In embryonic life the prostate is formed by several evaginations from the posterior and lateral walls of the posterior urethra. At about the twelfth week of embryonic development, the prostate reveals five lobes—anterior, middle, posterior, and two lateral lobes. These lobes fuse during the last half of fetal life so that at birth the divisions are imperceptible. During the third trimester of fetal life, the prostate enlarges as a result of gonadal and gonadotropic hormones of the mother. The hyperplasia persists for a few days after birth, and then the organ atrophies and does not fully develop until puberty.

From 15 to 30 branching tubular glands embedded in fibromuscular tissue make up the adult prostate. The glandular epithelium consists of two layers: tall columnar luminal cells and flattened cuboidal basal cells. The epithelium rests on a thin basement membrane. The supporting stroma consists of equal amounts of smooth muscle and fibrous tissue.

Functionally, three different types of glands are recognized (Fig. 19-33):

1. The smallest, the mucosal glands, lie in the periurethral tissue and open at various points around the urethra.
2. The submucosal glands are situated in the tissue around the periurethral area. Their ducts are longer and open into the urethral sinuses. The mucosal and submucosal glands together form the inner gland group, which is of mixed embryologic origin and develops from the dorsal wall of the urethra above the mesonephric ducts. They are partially separated from the main mass of prostatic glands by an indefinite capsule.

3. The external or main glands are derived entirely from the endodermal epithelium of the urogenital sinus and form the outer and largest portion of the prostate. Their ducts also open into the urethral sinuses. The inner group of glands, commonly referred to as the "female prostate," give rise to benign nodular hyperplasia. For this reason benign enlargement mainly produces urinary symptoms. Prostatic cancer almost invariably begins in the

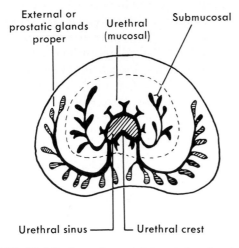

Fig. 19-33. Distribution of normal prostatic glands slightly modified. Urethral (mucosal) and submucosal glands together form inner group, which is separated from outer gland group by an inconstant capsule. (From Grant, J.C.B.: A method of anatomy, ed. 5, Baltimore, 1952, The Williams & Wilkins Co.)

outer groups of glands, commonly referred to as the "male prostate."

Although it has been customary to divide the adult prostate gland into five lobes (two lateral lobes, a median lobe, a posterior lobe, and an anterior lobe), there are no sharp lines of demarcation between the lobes (Fig. 19-34). Based on embryologic, ultrastructural, and arterial injection studies, the prostate is now regarded as essentially two separate organs: (1) the periurethral, female portion, which is sensitive to estrogens and androgens, and (2) the subcapsular true male prostate, which is sensitive to androgens; the latter forms a horseshoelike sheath around the former.

The normal development and maintenance of the prostate depend on testicular androgens. The prostate undergoes certain involutional changes with age. It atrophies after orchiectomy or administration of estrogens.

Nontumorous conditions

Acute prostatitis. Acute inflammation usually results from ascent of bacteria from the urethra or descent from the upper urinary tract or bladder. It may be spontaneous, but it is a fairly frequent complication of urethral manipulation by catheterization, urethral dilatation, and cystoscopy, especially if the patient has had a quiescent (chronic) prostatitis. Infection also may occur by hematogenous and lymphogenous spread. The most common bacteria are gonococci, staphylococci, streptococci, and the coliform bacilli. Not infrequently, smears and cultures are negative, but both must always be examined.

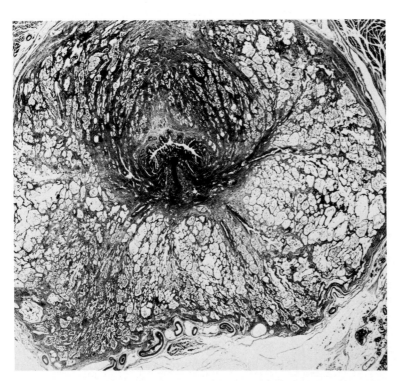

Fig. 19-34. Transverse section of prostate showing main mass of outer glands, submucosal glands, and urethral (mucosal) glands. There is no sharp line of separation between submucosal and outer glands in this section. Age unknown. (Approximately 3×.)

Grossly the prostate gland is enlarged, boggy, and edematous and contains multiple abscesses and foci of necrosis. Microscopic sections reveal multiple circumscribed collections of polymorphonuclear leukocytes, the glands being distended with a purulent exudate, or the inflammatory process may be diffuse. Edema, hyperemia, and foci of necrosis are frequent concomitant histologic findings.

Chronic prostatitis. Chronic inflammation of the prostate gland is common, and as with teeth and tonsils, the prostate has been considered to harbor foci of infection, causing arthritis, myositis, neuritis, and iritis. Allergic manifestations also have attributed to chronic prostatitis. Asthma, dermatitis, and pseudoangina pectoris have been reported to be relieved by adequate treatment of prostatitis. At necropsy the prostate gland of about 70% of men past 50 years of age reveals inflammatory changes.

The etiologic agents of chronic prostatitis are the same as those causing acute prostatitis, though in some types of chronic prostatitis the cause is unknown. Corpora amylacea, or prostatic calculi, may cause obstruction and stasis of secretion, leading to secondary inflammatory changes. A great number of cocci and bacilli are isolated from the chronically inflamed prostate. Frequently, however, the cultures are entirely negative.

Several forms of chronic prostatitis may be seen. The most common reveals diffuse, patchy, or very discrete foci of lymphocytic and plasma cell infiltration with or without changes in the acini and ducts. Some of these may be intact with the lumens empty and others with the lumens filled with debris and desquamated epithelial cells. Still others may show transformation to squamous epithelium. Some acini may become dilated as a result of intraluminal occlusion of ducts by various cellular elements and corpora amylacea, with loss of the epithelial lining and abscess formation.

Granulomatous prostatitis. An interesting chronic inflammatory lesion is nonspecific granulomatous prostatitis, the cause of which is unknown but is believed to be related to prostatic secretions. It is postulated that, as a result of inflammation, the integrity of ductal epithelial lining is lost and the secretions escape into the adjacent prostatic tissue. The resulting inflammatory reaction consists of many macrophages and lipophages as well as lymphocytes, plasma cells, and monocytes. Occasionally eosinophils, epithelioid cells, and Langhans type of giant cells also are seen. Sometimes fragments of corpora amylacea are present amid the inflammatory reaction.

The significance of this type of reaction is twofold: (1) it may be confused with tuberculosis, and (2) it may be mistaken clinically and pathologically for carcinoma. In such patients rectal examination may reveal stony hardness of the prostate gland and lead to a clinical diagnosis of carcinoma. The biopsy specimen may be misinterpreted as clear-cell carcinoma of the prostate.

Specific granulomas. Primary tuberculosis of the prostate gland is rare, and tuberculous involvement is almost always the result of either direct spread from the urethra, vas deferens, or bladder or spread by hematogenous or lymphatic routes. It occurs in younger people. Granulomatous and fibrocaseous forms are the most common types. Syphilitic, blastomycotic, and coccidiomycotic granulomas are rare.

Parasitic infection. Echinococcal cyst of the prostate gland is quite rare, and its occurrence is limited to the regions in which the parasite is endemic. Bilharzial involvement of the prostate is common among men in endemic regions and is considered a possible contributing factor to the obstruction of the bladder neck that occurs in these patients. *Trichomonas vaginalis* also may infect the prostate gland.

Cavitary or diverticular prostatitis. Diverticula or cavities may develop in any type of prostatitis in which there is stagnation of exudate in ducts and acini. Prolonged stagnation causes reactive fibrous tissue proliferation, which constricts the ducts. Acini dilate, and intra-acinar septa become thin and break down, resulting in formation of cavities. Prostatic diverticula may develop in cases of urethral stricture because of dilatation of prostatic ducts opening into the posterior urethra as a result of back pressure. Urine may enter the cavities, and salts may precipitate to form calculi. The end stage of various types of chronic prostatitis is fibrosis and scarring.

Corpora amylacea and calculi. Corpora amylacea are found in increasing numbers with age. They are formed from desquamated epithelial cells producing concentric lamellae around inspissated prostatic secretions that accumulate because of partial ductal obstruction. They are composed largely of protein and nucleic acid. Cyclic growth of corpora amylacea results from addition of concentric layers. Corpora amylacea may block the ducts with dilatation and further inspissation of secretions. Inflammatory reaction of the ducts may result in deposition of calcium salts (phosphate and carbonate) to form calculi.

Prostatic calculi are quite common, occurring in 20% to 30% of all men over 50 years of age, but they are rarely of clinical importance. Two types are identified: true (endogenous) and false (exogenous). Endogenous calculi are formed around the nuclei of corpora amylacea as already described. Other calculi may form from a nucleus of compact cellular debris, blood clots, or necrotic tissue. The number may vary from a few to hundreds and the size from 1 mm to 5 cm or larger. There may be one in a dilated acinus or duct or several packed in a cavity. They may be round, ovoid, or triangular and, when grouped together, may have faceted surfaces. Their color varies from white or grayish white to various shades of brown. Some are very firm and brittle, whereas others are somewhat plastic. Exogenous calculi occur less frequently. They arise from urine and are always brittle and rough.

The type of calculus may be determined by chemical examination of the nucleus. The nucleus of an exogenous calculus contains urates and phosphates, whereas the nucleus of an endogenous calculus is composed of organic material. Prostatic calculi may lead to the erroneous diagnosis of carcinoma of the prostate gland on rectal examination of the prostate because of its hardness. They are easily identified by roentgenographic examination unless they are radiolucent.

Thrombosis and infarction. A common necropsy finding, especially in bedridden patients, is thrombosis of the periprostatic venous plexus. Some investigators doubt that thrombi of these veins are an important source of pulmonary embolism. The thrombosed areas usually organize and form phleboliths, which often are seen on roentgenograms. Infarcts may be caused by vascular changes associated with arteriosclerosis, hypertension, or polyarteritis and occasionally may be of embolic origin, as in bacterial endocarditis. Local changes resulting from trauma caused by the passage of sounds, catheters, and cystoscopes, by massage of the prostate gland, and by transurethral prostatic resection have initiated infarction. The glands around the infarcts frequently undergo squamous cell metaplasia.

Recent investigations indicate the possible role of estrogens of testicular or adrenal origin in stimulating squamous cell metaplasia. Squamous cell nests may persist in the zone of a healed infarct and occasionally be misinterpreted as carcinoma.

Tumorlike lesions

Cysts. Cysts of the prostate gland may be congenital or acquired. Congenital cysts are symmetric and are associated with other abnormalities, such as patent urachus and spina bifida. The müllerian duct cyst is usually retroprostatic. The müllerian duct, if it were patent, would extend from the appendix testis in a groove between the testicle and epididymis and up the spermatic cord and lie between the vas deferens and bladder, where it would join the duct from the opposite side. It would then become incorporated in the musculature of the bladder wall, pass through the prostate gland, and end in the utricle. Thus it is understandable that such cysts, forming from abnormal remnants of the müllerian duct, may form anywhere along its course. Müllerian duct cysts vary in size from a small dilatation of the utricle to huge masses containing several liters of clear, straw- to chocolate-colored fluid. The wall of the cyst is composed of a laminated collagenous fibrous tissue lined by flat or low cuboidal epithelial cells. Acquired forms are retention, echinococcal, and bilharzial cysts.

Amyloid deposits. Amyloid deposits may form in the prostate. They may be part of primary amyloidosis or may be confined to the prostate. They occur around the blood vessels and in periglandular areas. Amyloidosis of the prostate is asymptomatic but may be responsible for postprostatectomy bleeding.

Hyperplasia. Nonneoplastic nodular enlargement of the prostate—nodular hyperplasia, benign prostatic hypertrophy—is the most common symptomatic tumorlike condition in humans. It seldom occurs before 50 years of age, but the incidence increases with age, and it can be found at autopsy in 75% to 80% of men over age 80. It is rare in Orientals.

Prostatic hyperplasia appears a decade earlier in American blacks than in whites, and it is rare among Koreans, Indians, Japanese, and Bantus. It is common in the dog and the *Mastomys*. Prostatic hyperplasia occurs more frequently in men of the digestive, pyknic, or endomorphic type. The normal prostate in an adult weighs about 20 g. The enlarged prostate can be two to four times larger but seldom weighs more than 200 g, though one weighing 820 g has been reported.

Despite extensive clinical and laboratory research, the cause of hyperplasia has not been fully established. Clinical research at various times has pointed to inflammation, arteriosclerosis, and sexual indulgence or perversion as etiologic factors or has suggested that the nodules in hyperplastic prostate glands are akin to adenomas and leiomyomas of the uterus. Laboratory investigations, both anatomic and endocrinologic, have presented considerable evidence to indicate an endocrine basis for hyperplasia.

Prostatic hyperplasia occurs in the inner zone of the prostate, whereas carcinoma is usually found in the outer portion (Fig. 19-35). It occurs at a time in a man's life when there are disturbances of sex hormones. Although males possess a high level of androgens and females a high level of estrogens, both sexes harbor both sex hormones. In the female the ovaries are the major source of estrogens and some androgens, and the adrenal glands are the major source of androgens and probably some estrogens. In the male the testes produce most of the androgens, but some also are produced in the adrenal glands, and both organs contribute to the estrogen pool in the male. With advancing age there is a distinct fall in the level of androgens in the male and of estrogens in the female and a corresponding increase in the other sex hormones—estrogens in the male and androgens in the female. Whether this is a relative or absolute increase has not been settled. Both hormones have a tropic, stimulating effect on the reproductive organs that possess homologous tissues. The periurethral inner prostate and certain other sex organs and the breasts are responsive to the estrogens, whereas the

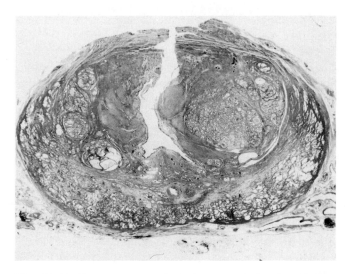

Fig. 19-35. Transverse section of prostate showing distinct nodules of stromal hyperplasia in periurethral zone. Large nodules consist of glandular and cystic structures. Tissues of outer prostate are compressed around edges. (3×.)

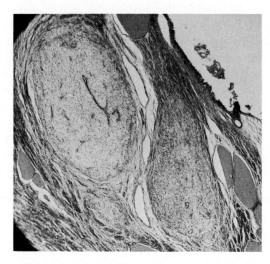

Fig. 19-36. Two small stromal nodules near urethra. Lower nodule has ill-defined margin and merges with surrounding tissues above and below. Well-formed blood vessels can be seen in nodules. (40×.)

outer prostate and the secondary sex organs of men are responsive to the androgens. Several possibilities may be considered in the endocrine relationship of prostatic hyperplasia:

1. A relative increase in the production of androgens by the active interstitial cells of Leydig associated with decreased function of tubules and decreased estrogen production
2. A relative increase in the production of estrogens by the increased Sertoli cells seen in old age and associated with decreased androgenic production by the interstitial cells of Leydig
3. A simultaneous stimulation of the prostate by both hormones, the action being, however, on different cells—the androgens acting on the epithelium and the estrogens on the fibromuscular stroma
4. A change in the structure of androgens or estrogens or both or some other hormone
5. A synergistic stimulation of the prostate by both the hormones and one or more endogenous or exogenous compounds
6. A change in the response of the endocrine-sensitive target organ, the prostate, brought about by environmental, circulatory, or genetic disturbances
7. A nonhormonal stimulation of the prostate, endogenous or exogenous, acting independently of the endocrine system

Any one or a combination of these factors could result in hyperplasia of the prostate gland.

Evidence based on histologic examination indicates that the etiologic agent of this disease may begin to produce changes in the prostate after 40 years of age, reach its maximum intensity at about 60 years of age, and continue to be present in sufficient amounts to cause changes during the remainder of life. The majority of investigators in the field believe that in the senile or presenile age groups a shift in the androgen/estrogen ratio results in the dominance of estrogen, and this, acting on the ambisexual estrogen-sensitive tissue of the prostatic area, produces nodular hyperplasia.

The anatomic location of the prostate readily explains the symptoms of hyperplasia. There is interference with and obstruction to the flow of urine. Rectal examination shows a soft, boggy, nodular prostate.

Grossly the enlarged prostate gland is smooth of nodular, firm, and somewhat elastic or rubbery. The appearance of the surfaces made by sectioning depends on whether the greatest amount of hyperplasia involves the glands or the fibromuscular tissue. If the hyperplasia is more glandular, the cut surface reveals many various-sized nodules, some of which are well circumscribed and surrounded by pearl-white fibromuscular tissue. Some of the nodules have a honeycombed architecture. The cut surface of an enlarged prostate is yellowish and moist with a milky fluid. Cysts are common, and some of these may contain white or amber-colored corpora amylacea or calculi. If the hyperplasia is predominantly of fibromuscular tissue, the cut surfaces are pallid, glossy, and homogeneous, and very little milky fluid can be expressed. In contrast to the lobular architecture of the normal prostate gland, the rather spongy hyperplastic nodules form a mass that compresses the surrounding tissues into a false capsule, enabling the nodular masses to be shelled out with ease.

The initial lesion has been demonstrated to be a multicentric aglandular fibromuscular nodule (Figs. 19-36 and 19-37) originating in the submucous portion of the prostatic urethra. This stimulates the proliferation of nearby glands, with early invasion of the nodules by the epithelial elements to produce the usual stromal glandular mixture. The acini are increased in number and size. Many undergo dilatation and invagination, forming villous projections (Fig. 19-38).

Some of the acini are lined by active cells and others by inactive cells (Fig. 19-39). The active cells are tall columnar cells with poorly defined borders, abundant finely granular or homogeneous cytoplasm, and basal nuclei often forming a double layer. The papillary infoldings are numerous and elongated, and the intralobular trabeculas are thin and delicate. The inactive cells that line many of the cystic acini are cuboidal or low columnar with well-defined cell walls, scanty vesiculated cytoplasm, and single layered basal nuclei. The papillae are few and relatively small and the intralobular septa thick and coarse. The lumens contain desquamated epithelial cells, granular secretory material, and occasional corpora amylacea. Lymphocytic infiltration is a frequent accompaniment, but this is probably not an indication of chronic inflammation.

Depending on the relative amounts of stromal and glandular elements. Franks[145] has recognized the following types of hyperplasia: stromal (fibrous or fibrovascular) nodule, fibromuscular nodule, muscular nodule, fibroadenomatous nodule, and fibromyoadenomatous nodule. To these may be added the purely glandular adenomatous nodule. The true stromal nodules are found only in subepithelial tissues around the urethra above the verumontanum. The smaller nodules are made up of a meshwork of fine fibrils with groups of elongated spindle cells or flat stellate cells arranged around small vascular spaces. No elastic tissues are present in the nodules. The fibromuscular and muscular nodules are similar except that there is more fibrous tissue in the former. Fibroadenomatous and fibromyoadenomatous nodules are also similar except for the presence of smooth muscle elements in the latter.

The purely glandular adenomatous nodule is rare in humans, but it is seen in dogs. It may be so pronounced as to be suggestive of an adenoma.

Secondary changes in the nodule. Areas of chronic and occasionally acute inflammation are seen in almost all nodules. Areas of chronic inflammation often surround distended ducts filled with inspissated secretion.

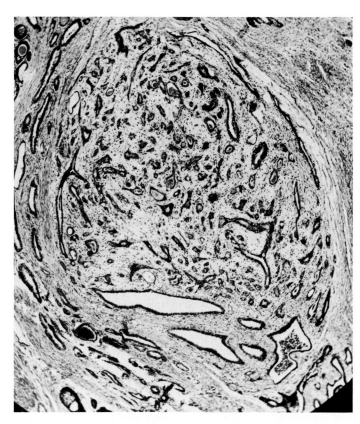

Fig. 19-37. Fibroadenomatous nodule. Epithelium lining the glands is low, cuboidal, and inactive. (65×.)

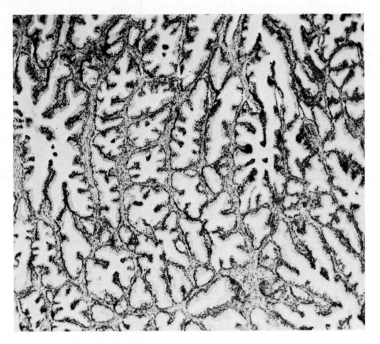

Fig. 19-38. Area of intra-acinar papillary hyperplasia. (65×.)

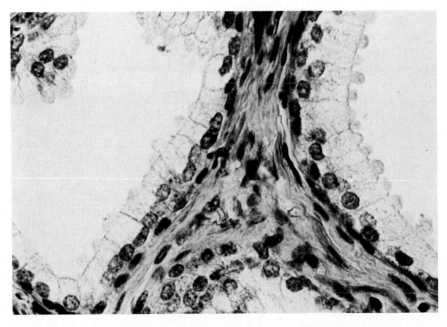

Fig. 19-39. Epithelium in intra-acinar papillary hyperplasia showing inconspicuous layer of flattened basal cells beneath surface epithelium. (870×.)

The mechanical effect of the expanding hyperplastic nodules within the relatively confined prostate is manifested in another important change—prostatic infarction—which occurs in 25% of hyperplastic glands.

The genesis of these infarcts is readily explained by the fact that all the blood supply of the hyperplastic nodules comes from the periphery, and sometimes it is stretched over the nodule. As the nodules expand, they sometimes compress the blood vessels at the periphery, with resultant ischemia in the center of the nodule and a hemorrhagic infarction.

Clinically this may be manifested as hematuria or complete urinary shutdown. The prostate may feel hard, and there may be elevation of prostatic acid phosphatase levels. The infarcted area consists of a lobule with a central hemorrhagic area and necrosis of the tissue. Prostatic infarction is invariably associated with squamous metaplasia of tubuloacinar structures. With healing there are fibrosis of the stroma and development of compact transitional or squamous cell nests. Scattered hemosiderin deposits are seen.

The chief complication of the enlarged prostate is urethral obstruction with secondary effects on the bladder, ureters, and kidneys (Fig. 19-40). The enlarging prostate causes elongation, tortuosity, and compression of the posterior portion of the urethra, and the urinary outlet is elevated above the floor of the bladder. These changes result in retention of urine, and with retention there is usually secondary infection. The enlarged median lobe stretches the sphincter vesicae muscles, resulting in incompetence of the sphincter and constant dribbling. In its efforts to overcome the obstruction, the crisscrossing vesical musculature undergoes compensatory hypertrophy, which produces the characteristic ribbed appearance of the muscle (trabeculation). The bladder wall may be twice its normal thickness. Contractions of the vesical musculature to increase the intravesical pressure in order to overcome bladder neck obstruction lead to outpocketings of the mucosa through the thinner portions of the wall to form diverticula. If not treated, decompensation results in dilatation of the bladder and thinning of the wall.

Normally the ureters enter the bladder at an angle and traverse intramurally before opening into the bladder lumen. This arrangement tends to provide an effective valve action so that as the bladder becomes temporarily filled normally, the elevated intravesical pressure closes off the ureteral orifices to prevent reflux of the urine up the ureters. As soon as the bladder is emptied, pressure on the wall is released and the ureteral orifices open. When dilatation and thinning of the bladder occur after obstruction at the bladder neck, the normal sphincter action of the vesical musculature at the ureteral orifices is removed. The increased intravesical pressure is thus transmitted to the ureters

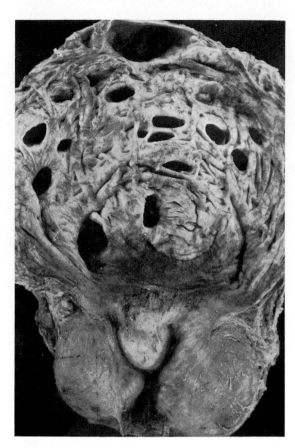

Fig. 19-40. Hyperplasia of prostate gland. Obstruction of urethra by large middle lobe and hypertrophied bladder with cellules and diverticula.

and the renal pelvis, and they also undergo compensatory hypertrophy and dilatation (hydroureter and hydronephrosis). There is usually infection and pyelonephritis. The increased intrapelvic pressure leads to hydronephrotic atrophy of the renal parenchyma as a result of ischemia. If this is bilateral, hypertension may develop. The renal lesions are the most important sequelae of prostatic enlargement.

Benign tumors. If the nodules of nodular hyperplasia of the prostate gland are considered tumors (as some believe they should be), adenomas, fibroadenomas, fibromas, or leiomyomas are very common. Differentiation of stromal hyperplasia from neoplasia is sometimes difficult. Although some of the circumscribed nodules of the enlarged prostate gland are similar to tumors, they should not be designated as neoplasms. Some of the reported adenomas are actually circumscribed areas of glandular hyperplasia. Likewise, many of the recorded leiomyomas are instances of fibromuscular hyperplasia.

Excluding prostatic hyperplasia, benign tumors of the prostate are rare. Kaufman and Berneike[156] recorded 38 cases of leiomyomas. The average age of the patients was about 60 years. The tumors weighed from about 15 to 1450 g. They were firm, rubbery, yellowish white, and homogeneous. Microscopically the tumors revealed interlacing whorls of smooth muscle with little intervening fibrous tissue. Neurofibromas occasionally involve the prostate gland.

Other benign epithelial abnormalities. These are described on p. 902.

Malignant tumors

Carcinoma. Although the large majority of prostatic cancers are glandular and usually referred to as adenocarcinoma, the term "carcinoma" is generally preferred. Carcinoma of the prostate gland is the second most frequent cause of death from cancer in the male population in the United States. The incidence of carcinoma of the prostate is highest among the black population in the United States (blacks, 23 per 100,000; whites, 14.3 per 100,000), whereas the incidence in Israel is 7.3 and in Japan 1.1. In the United States the incidence of prostatic carcinoma is lowest among Jews, intermediate among Catholics, and highest among Protestants. It is high among married men and those with children and among persons living in metropolitan and urban areas; it has a familial incidence. Four categories of carcinoma of the prostate are recognized.

LATENT CARCINOMA. In autopsies of men after dying of other causes, carcinoma of the prostate is found unexpectedly in 26% to 37% of prostates. In a worldwide study conducted by the International Agency for Cancer Research,[139] the frequency of such carcinomas was determined from autopsies performed in Hong Kong, Singapore, Israel, Uganda, Germany, Sweden, and Jamaica. It was found that the incidence of small carcinomas was the same; however, the incidence of larger latent carcinomas varied. It was lowest in Hong Kong and Singapore, intermediate in Israel and Uganda, and high in Germany, Sweden, and Jamaica. These figures corresponded to deaths from carcinoma of the prostate, indicating that environmental factors may play a role in incidence and prevalence of carcinoma of prostate; they also mean that, although many of these carcinomas remain dormant during the lifetime of the host, environmental factors must play a role in inciting latent carcinomas into clinical carcinoma in some men.

INCIDENTAL CARCINOMA. In 6% to 20% of tissues removed surgically for clinically benign prostatic hyperplasia, histologic examination shows carcinoma of the prostate. The discovery of incidental carcinoma in a patient who has no symptoms referable to his carcinoma raises many questions. Are these accidental discoveries of carcinomas that would have remained dormant? Should these carcinomas be left alone, or are they the group in which surgical extirpation may be lifesaving?

OCCULT CARCINOMA. Some patients who have no symptoms of prostatic carcinoma show evidence of metastases on clinical examination, such as roentgenographic changes in the site of a fracture or an enlarged lymph node. Biopsy of the metastatic lesion may reveal carcinoma, the prostatic origin of which is demonstrated by stains by prostatic acid phosphatase and prostate-specific antigen and is then confirmed by biopsy examination of the prostate. It would seem that at least some, if not most, occult carcinomas originate from latent carcinomas.

CLINICAL CARCINOMA. The category of clinical carcinoma includes all cases in which rectal examination, by either digital or ultrasonographic or other imaging techniques, has aroused suspicion of carcinoma of the prostate and the diagnosis is confirmed by pathologic examination of the tissue removed from the prostate.

ETIOLOGY. Although the cause of carcinoma of the prostate is unknown, androgens have been suspect. Androgens are essential for the development and maintenance of the prostate. Carcinoma of the prostate is extremely rare in eunuchs and in patients with Klinefelter's syndrome. Testosterone accelerates the activity of carcinoma cells, whereas orchiectomy or estrogen therapy causes regression of tumor. Ultrastructurally cancer cells resemble testosterone-treated rabbit prostate cells. These observations have led to the theory that androgens are in some way responsible for carcinoma of the prostate. But prolonged administration of androgens has not produced any tumors, and cancer of the prostate occurs at the time of life when the level of androgens is normally low. The most prevalent hypothesis is that carcinoma of the prostate, which is a slow-growing tumor, may begin at the stage of life when androgen levels are high and may remain quiescent in most men whose androgen levels decline with advancing age. In many cases, some disturbance of the hypothalamic-pituitary-adrenal-testicular-prostatic axis may stimulate the dormant malignant cells to develop clinical cancer.

Viral inclusions have been observed in carcinoma of the prostate; Paulson, Rabson, and Fraley[167] reported that cultures of hamster prostate tissue infected with simian virus 40 underwent transformation 5 to 8 days after injection. These transformed cells developed into carcinoma when they were injected into the homologous hosts. Histologically the tumor resembled carcinoma of the prostate and gave the chemical and histochemical properties of carcinoma.

Exposure to cadmium has also been suspected.

SYMPTOMS. There are no distinct symptoms of early carcinoma of the prostate, and the symptoms, when present, are indistinguishable from those of benign hyperplasia of the prostate. Late cancers usually manifest themselves through back pain and anemia, which indicate bone metastases. Rectal examination is the only way carcinoma of the prostate can be detected and is indicated in every patient over 50 years of age. A hard nodule or an area of induration in the prostate gland should be considered cancerous unless proved otherwise.

DIAGNOSIS. Cytologic, biochemical, roentgenographic, and pathologic methods are employed in the diagnosis of cancer of the prostate. The neoplastic cells in the smears are pleomorphic and hyperchromatic. The nuclear/cytoplasmic and the nucleolar/nuclear ratios are disturbed. The cells occur in clusters, and cell borders are indistinct, but nuclear borders are definite. Prostatic massage is contraindicated because neoplastic cells have been found in the bloodstream of 15% of patients with carcinoma of the prostate who had prostatic massage. Recently fine-needle aspiration has been employed with good results.

Two tumor markers have been used in diagnosis and monitoring of prostatic carcinoma: prostatic acid phosphatase (PAP) and prostate-specific antigen (PSA). In a recent study Stamey and co-workers[169] evaluated the clinical usefulness of these by serum radioimmunoassay. Two thousand two hundred serum samples of 699 patients were examined, and 378 had prostatic carcinoma. PAP concentration was elevated in only 57 of patients with cancer and correlated less closely with tumor volume. PSA was elevated in 122 of 127 patients with newly diagnosed untreated prostatic cancer, including 7 of 12 patients with unsuspected early disease and all of 115 with more advanced disease. The PSA level increased with more advanced disease and with clinical stage. It was proportional to the estimated volume. After radical prostatectomy for cancer, PSA, with a biologic half-life of 2.2 days, routinely fell to undetectable levels. If initially elevated, PAP fell to normal levels within 24 hours but always remained detectable. In a small number of patients followed postoperatively by means of repeated measurements, PSA but not PAP appeared to be useful in detecting residual and early recurrence of the tumor and in monitoring response to radiation therapy. Prostatic massage increased the levels of both approximately 1.5 to 2 times. Needle biopsy and transurethral resection increased both considerably. These authors concluded that PSA is more sensitive than PAP in the detection of prostatic cancer and will probably be more useful in monitoring responses and recurrence after therapy. But since both may be elevated in benign prostatic hyperplasia, neither marker was regarded as specific.

Both prostatic acid phosphatase (PAP) and prostate-specific antigen (PSA) are demonstrable in tissue. In well-differentiated carcinomas the distribution of these enzymes is essentially similar. In moderately and poorly differentiated carcinomas some cells may react strongly to one or the other or both or neither; the reaction may involve all the cells, clones of cells, or none

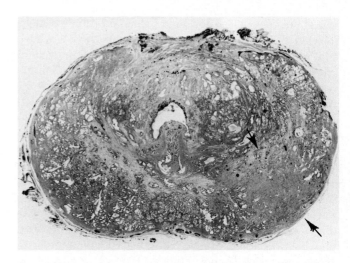

Fig. 19-41. Transverse section of prostate showing large area of carcinoma involving subcapsular zone *(arrows)*. (15×.)

of the cells. In suspected prostatic carcinoma, if one test is negative, the other should be done.

Roentgenographic examination, including pyelography, chest x-ray examination, CT scan, bone scan, ultrasonography, and nuclear magnetic resonance, is essential for diagnosis and staging of carcinoma of the prostate. Most often the metastatic lesions of bone are osteoblastic, but osteolytic and mixed osteoblastic and osteolytic lesions also may be seen. A biopsy of bone lesions is necessary for diagnosis of metastatic carcinoma.

CLINICAL CLASSIFICATION. Clinical classification takes into consideration whether the lesion is incidentally found in clinically benign but pathologically cancer-containing prostate or discovered on rectal examination. If the latter, classification depends on whether it is a single nodule or multiple nodules, unilateral or bilateral, in the prostate, whether the tumor is confined to the prostate or has extended beyond the confines of the prostate to the seminal vesicles, periprostatic tissue, or adjacent structures, and whether there is evidence of metastasis. Such categorization, combined with pathologic findings, determines the specific mode of therapy.

PATHOLOGIC FINDINGS. Grossly the malignant prostate may be large, of normal size, or smaller than normal. Approximately 15% to 20% of nodular hyperplastic prostates harbor carcinoma. Carcinoma may originate in any part of the gland; however, in about 75% it is located mainly in the posterior lobe. About 95% begin in the subcapsular zone (Fig. 19-41). As a rule, the malignant prostate is very firm in consistency, but occasionally it may be soft. The cut surface is dry, fibrous, and homogeneously pallid and often contains irregular yellowish areas.

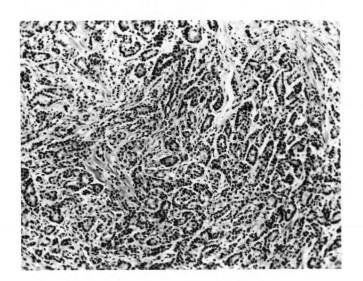

Fig. 19-42. Carcinoma of prostate, small acinar type. (145×.)

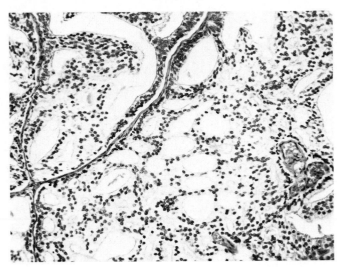

Fig. 19-43. Carcinoma of prostate, cribriform pattern. (63×.)

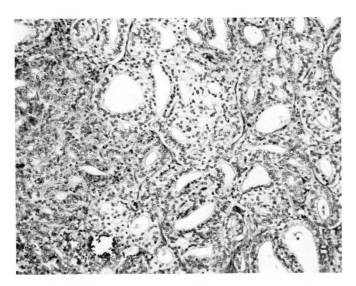

Fig. 19-44. Carcinoma of prostate. Mixed pattern of small and large acini and cribriform patterns. Notice that some cells have pale cytoplasm whereas others have darker cytoplasm. (150×.)

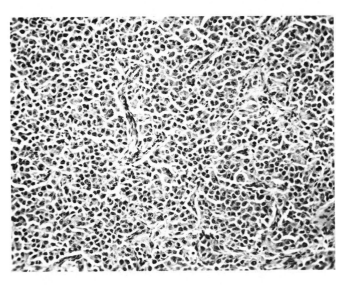

Fig. 19-45. Carcinoma of prostate, undifferentiated pattern. (160×.)

Microscopically about 96% of malignant neoplasms of the prostate are adenocarcinomas, but they are generally referred to as carcinoma (Fig. 19-42). The tumor may consist of tiny, small, or simple large glands, fused glands, glands within glands, papillary structures, columns and cords, or solid sheets with little or no gland formation (Figs. 19-43 to 19-45). Often a combination of two or more of these is seen. Usually the glands are closely packed with little or no stroma between them, but in some cases the glands may be haphazardly distributed in the stroma. The cells may vary from cuboidal to columnar; they may form a single layer or be piled up. The cytoplasm varies a great deal. It may be pale or dark staining, vacuolated, amphophilic, granular, or eosinophilic. It contains varying amounts of prostatic acid phosphatase, prostate-specific antigen, and other tumor markers.

In many cases the individual cells lack the usual distinct morphologic criteria for malignancy. Cellular anaplasia is slight, and giant cells and mitotic figures are often absent (Fig. 19-46). The nuclei may be small, fairly uniform, and pale or dark staining, the nuclear membranes may be delicate, and the chromatin distribution may be fairly homogeneous. Other carcinomas

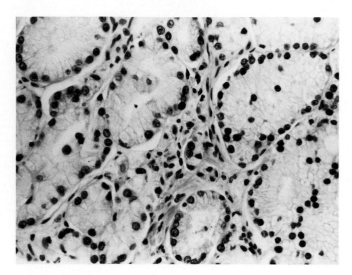

Fig. 19-46. Carcinoma of prostate showing slight anaplasia with fairly uniform nuclei. (160×.)

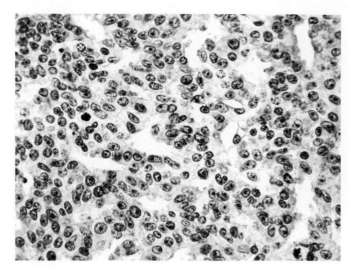

Fig. 19-47. Carcinoma of prostate showing moderate anaplasia, intermediate degree of variation in shape, and staining of nuclei. (160×.)

may show moderate or pronounced anaplasia (Figs. 19-47 and 19-48). The characteristic features of nuclei of carcinoma of prostate are coarse chromatin distribution, vacuolization, and a large but ill-defined nucleolus.

In contrast to normal or benign prostatic hyperplasia, in which the distribution of prostatic acid phosphatase and prostate-specific antigen is fairly uniform and luminal in location, considerable variation is seen in the distribution of these markers in carcinoma of the prostate. Individual cells or clones of cells may contain one marker, both markers, or neither; this is seen in both tumors that form glands and those that do not. Thus carcinomas of the prostate tend to be heterogeneous in regard to pattern of growth, cell population, functional state of the cell, and degree of anaplasia. DNA analyses have also demonstrated a heterogeneous cell population.

Tumors forming regular small or large glands populated by cells that show little or no anaplasia are often diagnostic problems. In examining such tumors one must focus attention on disturbances of architecture, evidence of invasion, arrangement and structure of nuclei, and distribution of enzymes. Tiny and small glands, glands back to back, glands inside glands, large glands without convolutions, and haphazard distribution of glands are diagnostic of carcinoma of prostate. Acini lined by a single layer of nuclei that are homogeneously pale or dark staining or vacuolated and contain an irregularly outlined nucleolus are carcinoma. Uneven distribution of prostatic acid phosphatase or prostate-specific antigen in cell cytoplasm is indicative of carcinoma. Distortion and disruption of the delicate periacinar basement membrane and invasion of the stroma are other helpful criteria. Invasion of the stroma

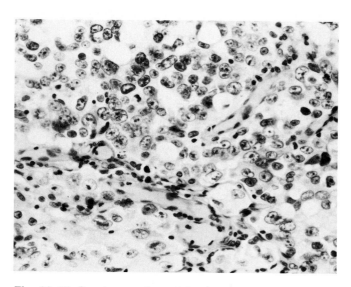

Fig. 19-48. Carcinoma of prostate showing pronounced anaplasia. Many nuclei are vacuolated and contain large irregular nucleoli. (160×.)

is best detected by finding acini situated directly on muscle bundles or infiltrating them. The most reliable pathologic criterion for diagnosis of carcinoma of the prostate is perineural invasion. We have found this in over 85% of patients with prostate carcinoma (Fig. 19-49). The spaces are not lymphatics, and the finding has no prognostic significance.

It can be assumed that all carcinomas of prostate start as clinically inapparent carcinomas that are eventually detected either during a physical examination or because of symptoms of metastases. Carcinoma of the prostate is usually a slowly growing tumor. In its earliest stages the neoplastic transformation may be unifo-

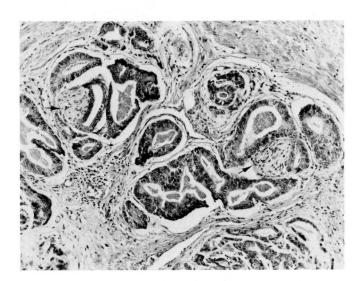

Fig. 19-49. Carcinoma of prostate showing perineural invasion *(arrows).*

cal, but Byar and Mostofi[140] have shown that prostatic carcinoma is multifocal. Whether pathologic examination of the removed tissue shows a unifocal or multifocal lesion is of clinical significance, as is whether the tumor is confined to the prostate, has extended locally, or has metastasized via lymphatics or the bloodstream.

LOCAL EXTENSION. The subcapsular location of the prostate predisposes to early invasion and penetration of the capsule and extension beyond the capsule with resultant anchoring of the prostate. In later stages the tumor may extend to the bladder neck, the seminal vesicles, the trigone, and, not infrequently, one or both ureteral orifices.

METASTASES. Lymphatic metastases have been reported in 7% to 25% of prostatic carcinomas that are confined to the prostate; the incidence increases with local extension. The pelvic, inguinal, periaortic, mediastinal, and supraclavicular lymph nodes are often involved, the earliest and most frequent involvement being in the pelvic nodes.

Hematogenous spread is manifested most frequently by osseous metastases, which occur in 70% in cases. The pelvis and the lumbar spine are the most frequent sites, but the ribs, femur, clavicle, or any other bone may be involved. The route of metastases to the spine has been extensively studied, and considerable disagreement prevails. According to some investigators, the route of metastasis to the spine is by way of the lymphatics. However, it has been demonstrated that metastasis also occurs along the vertebral venous plexus. Willis[170] maintained that carcinoma of the prostate invades the systemic circulation in the same manner as other tumors do. By careful necropsy studies, he was able to demonstrate pulmonary metastasis in the majority of his cases.

EFFECTS OF THERAPY. The mode of therapy for prostate carcinoma is controversial especially for carcinomas that are small, confined to the prostate, incidentally discovered, or of low histologic or cytologic grade. In these patients, it is assumed that the tumor constitutes the early and presumably curable stage of disease. Complete surgical removal would seem to be the treatment of choice, but there is serious question as to whether patients should be treated at all because some of these patients live a long time without treatment and die of other causes, or whether they should be irradiated.

The pathologists challenge is to distinguish between tumors that will remain silent and those that will progress to kill the patient. If treatment is contemplated, controversy exists as to whether it should be radical prostatectomy or radiation therapy. Until recently radical prostatectomy was associated with 90% impotence and 10% incontinence. The introduction of "nerve-sparing" procedure has reduced impotence to 10% or 15% and incontinence has essentially disappeared. But about 25% of such tumors have already metastasized to regional nodes by the time they are discovered. To rule out such metastases regional lymph nodes are examined microscopically. If there are no metastases, radical prostatectomy is carried out; if there are, radiation therapy is advocated. However, even this is controversial. Some centers depend on DNA analysis for a decision. Radiation therapy in one form or another is also used in patients who because of age (65 years or over) or some other reason are not candidates for surgery. Up to now, there are no adequate data that compare long-term results of radical prostatectomy versus radiation therapy for prostate carcinoma.

Less controversial is the treatment of patients in whom the carcinoma has extended beyond the prostate or has metastasized. Such patients are given one of several types of internal or external irradiation and antiandrogen therapy.

Because androgens are essential for the development and maintenance of the prostate gland, which undergoes atrophy after castration, and because androgens are known to stimulate the growth of carcinoma of the prostate, Huggins and Hodges[154] demonstrated that removal of the main source of androgen (testes) and treatment with estrogens are beneficial in the control of carcinoma of the prostate. In 80% of cases the tumors respond. The cells show vacuolization of cytoplasm and "ballooning." In such a cell the nucleus is pushed to the periphery (Fig. 19-50). The chromatin of the nucleus becomes condensed, the nucleolus disappears, and the nucleus becomes pyknotic. The swollen cells ultimately rupture and fuse with the stroma, which becomes vacuolated, pale staining, and fibrillar. This stromal change is followed by fibrosis. In some cases estrogen therapy

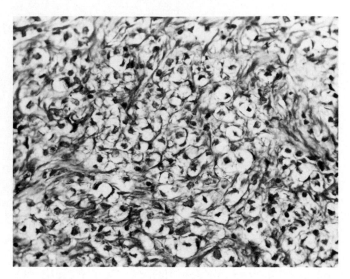

Fig. 19-50. Carcinoma of prostate showing estrogen effect. (300×.)

causes inactivity of the neoplastic cells and disappearance of acid phosphatase from the cytoplasm. Squamous cell metaplasia following estrogenic effect may occur in the prostate and in the metastatic areas of the bones. The process may progress to squamous cell carcinoma. Orchiectomy and estrogen therapy do not cure carcinoma of the prostate; the only successful method is early and complete renewal of the tumor. The neoplasm may be and usually is controlled by antiandrogen therapy, but eventually the tumor cells fail to respond to such therapy. Massive increase in estrogen levels, adrenalectomy, and hypophysectomy have been tried with temporary beneficial results. Evidence has been presented that the incidence of cardiovascular deaths is increased in the first 9 months after initiation of estrogen therapy in patients with nonmetastatic carcinoma of the prostate, and there is general agreement to limit antiandrogen therapy to patients with biochemical or x-ray evidence of metastasis. Considerable research is in progress exploring pituitary hormone blocking and other agents and chemotherapy.

Lesions that simulate prostatic carcinoma. Mention has already been made that granulomatous prostatitis may simulate prostatic carcinoma. Several epithelial changes may do the same: atypical hyperplasia, secondary hyperplasia, basal cell hyperplasia, cribriform (intra-acinar) hyperplasia, squamous metaplasia secondary to infarction, and involutional changes in the seminal vesicles. Typical hyperplasia is easily distinguished from carcinoma. Atypical hyperplasia may have one of several forms: Lobular hyperplasia is characterized by proliferation of small normal-appearing acini around a central duct. Another pattern is a group of small glands lined by a single layer of cells, the nuclei of which may vary somewhat in size but show no anaplasia. These are frequently at the periphery of a hyperplastic nodule. Another type is a group of glands, some of which are lined with piled-up but benign-appearing cells. The term "adenosis" has been used to designate "dysplastic" glandular proliferation containing either mild nuclear pleomorphism or atypia of growth pattern. Thus two categories of adenosis have been claimed: (1) those with mild nuclear pleomorphism confined to circumscribed collections of glands in which the nucleoli are small, and (2) those in which the infiltrating glands are lined by columnar cells with benign nuclei. The concept and definition of adenosis are confusing, and we believe the term is superfluous. Secondary hyperplasia is characterized by the presence of large acini lined partly by a single layer of cells and partly by papillary projections covered by similar epithelium (Fig. 19-51). No anaplasia is seen. Basal cell hyperplasia consisting of intra-acinar proliferation of small basophilic cells with ovoid nuclei often capped by a secretory cell layer may be focal, diffuse, or lobular. The cells have a primitive appearance (Fig. 19-52). Progression of basal cell hyperplasia may lead to intra-acinar or cribriform hyperplasia or adenoid cystic hyperplasia. Cribriform hyperplasia consisting of glands in glands is distinguished from intra-acinar or cribriform carcinoma by the presence of delicate fibrovascular stroma between the glands, a distinct basal cell layer, and uniform-appearing nuclei. In all types of basal cell hyperplasia there is hyperplasia of the fibromuscular stroma and the epithelium is benign. In atrophy the acini are small and lined by small cuboid cells with somewhat dark staining nuclei and little or no cytoplasm. The entire lobule is involved, with small acini surrounding a collapsed duct, and the stroma may or may not show sclerotic changes. The cells show no PAP and PSA but do show keratin. Atrophy-associated hyperplasia, also designated as postatrophic hyperplasia, is a proliferation of small irregularly shaped and distributed acini but still oriented in lobular configuration toward a central duct. This type of hyperplasia is seen in the peripheral zone of the prostate and has been associated with small acinar carcinoma. In squamous or transitional cell metaplasia secondary to infarction, the acinar and ductal epithelium is replaced by flattened or transitional epithelium (Fig. 19-53), which may be three to five layers thick. The cells are well differentiated without any anaplasia but with nuclear pleomorphism and mitotic activity. Involutional changes in the seminal vesicles appear as closely packed complex ductal structures lined by two or more layers of cells in which the superficial luminal cells have large or even giant-sized hyperchromatic nuclei. When viewed by themselves the nuclei seem to show malignancy, but there is no vacuolization of nuclei and no nucleoli, the nucleocytoplasmic ratio is maintained, and the cells usually contain brown pigment.

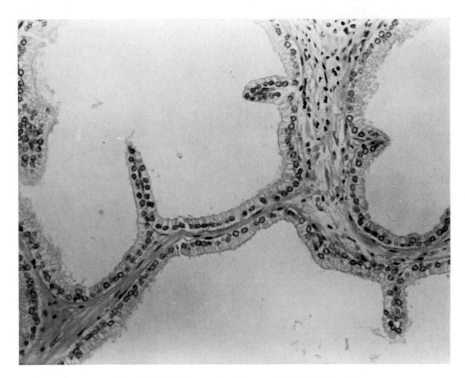

Fig. 19-51. Secondary hyperplasia. (150×.)

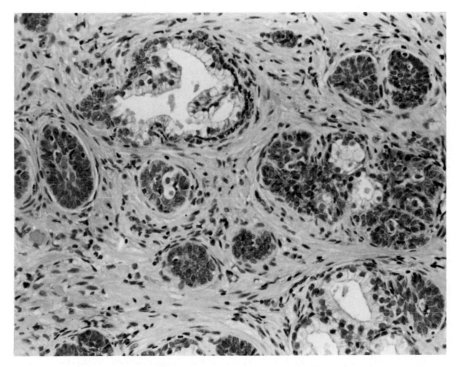

Fig. 19-52. Basal cell hyperplasia. (150×.)

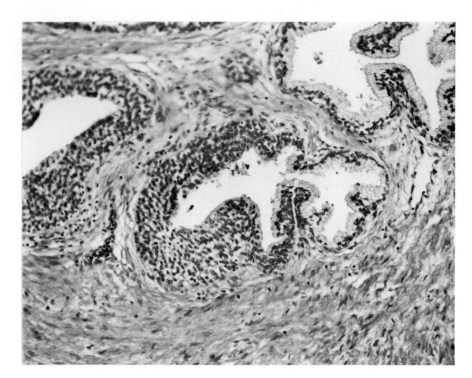

Fig. 19-53. Transitional cell metaplasia. (150×.)

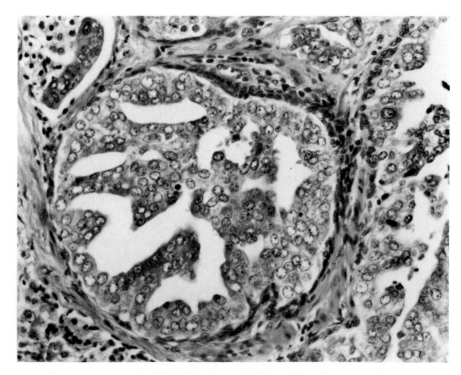

Fig. 19-54. Hyperplasia with malignant change (carcinoma in situ). (150×.)

Hyperplasia with malignant change. In many prostates removed for carcinoma, one may see clones of glands that retain the hyperplastic pattern but are lined by obviously neoplastic epithelial cells characterized by pleomorphism, nuclear vacuolization and prominent large ill-defined nucleoli (Fig. 19-54). In a sense these represent carcinoma in situ, and this term is an acceptable diagnosis provided that the term is restricted to this category. The progression of the lesion to infiltrating carcinoma would seem to be unquestionable, but this has not been demonstrated. It is probable that in most cases there is a long lag period between the lesion and frank carcinoma. The terms "prostatic ductal dysplasia" and "intraepithelial neoplasia of prostatic ducts" have been recently introduced for several lesions ranging from atypia to carcinoma. With the problems and confusion created by these terms in the cervix and bladder their use for a prostatic lesion is regrettable. We prefer the terms "malignant change" or "carcinoma in situ" for lesions that show definite nuclear anaplasia and refer to the others as "atypia."

Other carcinomas. A papillary adenocarcinoma initially believed to be confined to the utricle and to be of müllerian origin, has been designated endometrioid carcinoma. However, it has been demonstrated that the tumor is of prostatic acinar origin, that it may occur in other locations (in the substance of the prostate rather than in the utricle), that the tumor in the utricle is usually associated with a typical carcinoma in the prostate, and that the cells contain both prostatic acid phosphatase (PAP) and prostate-specific antigen (PSA).

TRANSITIONAL CELL CARCINOMA. Prostatic ducts are lined for the most part with transitional epithelium and partly with acinar epithelium. Thus it is conceivable that the transitional epithelium of the ducts may become malignant. However, in such cases before the diagnosis of primary transitional cell carcinoma of prostatic ductal origin is made, it is essential to rule out a carcinoma of the bladder or posterior urethra because carcinomas in these locations frequently grow into the prostate and replace prostatic ductal epithelium. Occasionally a transitional cell carcinoma is discovered in the bladder, but there is no apparent connection with the prostatic transitional cell carcinoma. In such cases it is probable that the carcinogenic agents that have induced malignant transformation of vesical or urethral epithelium have also acted on the prostatic ductal epithelium to induce neoplasia.

SQUAMOUS CELL CARCINOMA. Squamous cell carcinoma of prostate is also extremely rare; the comments made in reference to transitional cell carcinoma are equally applicable for this tumor. We have seen several cases of adenocarcinoma of prostate that, after prolonged administration of estrogens, have been transformed into squamous cell carcinoma.

MUCINOUS ADENOCARCINOMA. Many carcinomas of the prostate have mucin-containing cells, but rarely the tumor is predominantly or entirely mucinous adenocarcinoma. In all such cases PAP and PSA will reveal whether the tumor is prostatic acinar or extraprostatic in origin.

UNDIFFERENTIATED CARCINOMAS. Undifferentiated carcinoma of the prostate is another rarity, but it is more common than transitional or squamous cell carcinoma. In such cases it is essential to stain the tissue for PAP and PSA. This reveals one of several patterns: sheets of positive cells side by side with negative cells or more often scattered PAP/PSA–positive clones among cells that are negative.

DUCTAL CARCINOMA. Prostatic ducts and prostatic urethra are lined by three types of epithelium: the secretory, the basal, and the transitional. The three cell types are found in various amounts in prostatic ducts and prostatic urethra. All three types may undergo benign or malignant proliferation. The hyperplasia of secretory cells is usually associated with cribriform or papillary configuration. These react positively with PAP and PSA. Proliferation of ductal transitional epithelium, benign or malignant, obliterates the lumen in part or in toto. These are negative for PAP and PSA. Transitional cell carcinoma involving the ducts and the urethra are almost always associated with an unrecognized or unexpected bladder carcinoma. In basal cell hyperplasia involving ducts, the proliferating cells often assume a spindled configuration and show differentiation to either squamous or secretory epithelium. The term "ductal carcinoma" is an incomplete diagnosis because the various cell types require different treatment.

ADENOID CYSTIC CARCINOMA. Adenoid cystic carcinoma has been described in the prostate. Most of the reported cases are basal cell hyperplasia with adenoid cyst–like areas. These can be readily distinguished from adenoid cystic carcinoma by the presence of typical basal cell hyperplasia adjacent to the lesion, by the lack of anaplasia of the cells, and by hyperplastic stroma. True adenoid cystic carcinoma is extremely rare.

CARCINOID OF THE PROSTATE. Neurosecretory cells as demonstrated by chromogranin and Cherukian-Schenk stains and ultrastructurally are present in normal prostates. Frequently they are demonstrated in prostatic carcinomas. The cells may also react with PAP and PSA. As in other organs this category should be distinguished from the rare pure carcinoid of the prostate.

Sarcoma. Sarcoma of the prostate gland is rare. It occurs at any age but is much more frequent in the young. We have seen rhabdomyosarcomas, leiomyosarcomas, fibrosarcomas, lymphosarcomas, angiosarcomas, malignant fibrous histiocytoma, and carcinosarcomas of the prostate. In recent years dramatic results have been reported in treatment of rhabdomyosarcoma in children.

SEMINAL VESICLES

The seminal vesicles are bilateral saclike outpouchings from the vas deferens at its termination in the ejaculatory duct. They have irregular, branching lumens with numerous outpocketings lined by pseudostratified epithelium, which often contains yellow pigment and secretory granules. The walls are composed of smooth muscle similar to but thinner than that of the vas.

Congenital anomalies of seminal vesicles are rare. Entrance of ectopic ureter to seminal vesicle may form cysts. Two types have been recognized: congenital and acquired. The former are regarded as malformations of either müllerian or wolffian ducts; the latter result from secondary inflammation, causing stenosis of the terminal portion of the duct and cystic dilatation in the proximal portion.

Grossly the cut surface shows a thin-walled structure filled with gray mucoid material. Histologically the inner surface is covered with a single layer of flattened and attenuated cuboid epithelial cells. The cytoplasm is scant and contains occasional brownish granules and relatively large, irregularly shaped hyperchromatic nuclei. The lamina propria is usually thick and fibrotic.

Inflammation. Inflammation may be categorized as nonspecific seminal vesiculitis (acute or chronic), abscess, or specific vesiculitis such as tuberculosis, trichomoniasis, and schistosomiasis. Inflammatory reaction of the seminal vesicles usually results from urethral or prostatic infection.

Tumors and tumorlike lesions. Two tumorlike lesions merit mention: amyloid deposition and calcification.

Amyloidosis of seminal vesicle is similar to amyloid deposition elsewhere. It consists of deposits of a pale, pinkish, homogeneous substance in the connective tissue, in muscle, and in blood vessels. Some lymphocytic or granulomatous reaction may be seen.

Calcification of seminal vesicles is rare. It may follow chronic infection, such as tuberculosis in older patients, especially those with diabetes. It may be unilateral or bilateral. Its clinical significance is that it may be misinterpreted on rectal examination as prostatic carcinoma. The calcific masses are irregular and are surrounded by fibrous tissue. The epithelial lining is intact in early stages but may be destroyed in later stages.

Tumors of seminal vesicles are very rare—fewer than 100 have been described. They may be benign or malignant, epithelial or mesenchymal. The most common tumors are papillary adenomas, fibromas, and leiomyomas. Most malignant tumors of seminal vesicles are secondary, coming usually from the prostate.

Malignant tumors. Primary carcinomas are rare. They usually occur in patients over 50 years of age, but we have seen one in a young patient. Urinary retention, dysuria, and hematuria are the usual symptoms. A high level of serum fructose has been reported in some cases.

For diagnosis of carcinoma of the seminal vesicles it is mandatory that involvement of seminal vesicles be

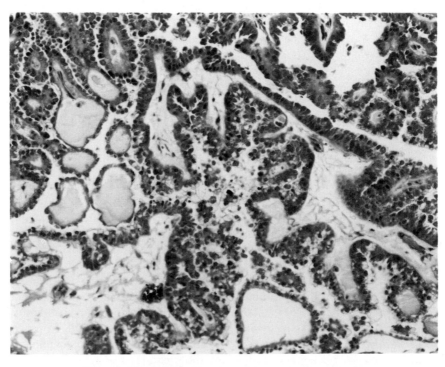

Fig. 19-55. Carcinoma of seminal vesicles. (150×.)

anatomically proved. Histologically the tumors are usually papillary adenocarcinomas, but undifferentiated areas may be seen in some. The tumor consists of clear columnar cells, often with brown lipofuscin pigment forming acinar and papillary structures (Fig. 19-55).

Because many reported carcinomas of the seminal vesicles are extensions from the prostate or are papillary carcinomas of the prostate that are misdiagnosed as carcinomas of the seminal vesicles, it is essential to rule out a primary carcinoma of the prostate; this can be done by stains for PAP and PSA.

Sarcomas are usually of prostatic and vesicle origin but may originate in the seminal vesicles.

REFERENCES
Testes

1. Atkin, N.B.: Y bodies and similar fluorescent chromocentres in human tumours including teratomata, Br. J. Cancer **28**:275, 1973.
2. Berg. J.W.: Acid-fast lipid from spermatozoa, Arch. Pathol. (Chicago) **57**:115, 1954.
3. Brown, R.C., and Smith, B.H.: Malakoplakia of the testis, Am. J. Clin. Pathol. **47**:135, 1967.
4. Burke, A.P., and Mostofi, F.K.: Placental alkaline phosphatase immunohistochemistry of intratubular malignant germ cells and associated testicular germ cell tumors, Hum. Pathol. **19**:663, 1988.
5. Campbell, C.M., and Middleton, A.W., Jr.: Malignant gonadal stromal tumor: case report and review of literature, J. Urol. **125**:257, 1981.
6. Capers, T.H.: Granulomatous orchitis, Am. J. Clin. Pathol. **34**:139, 1960.
7. Carr, B.I.: The variable transformation of metastases from testicular germ cell tumors: the need for selective biopsy, J. Urol. **126**:52, 1981.
8. Cohn, B.D.: Histology of the cryptorchid testes, Surgery **62**:536, 1967.
9. Dickinson, S.J.: Structural abnormalities in the undescended testis, J. Pediatr. Surg. **8**:523, 1973.
10. Dixon, F.J., and Moore, R.A.: In Atlas of tumor pathology, section VIII, fascicle 32, Washington, D.C., 1952, Armed Forces Institute of Pathology.
11. Dow, J.A., and Mostofi, F.K.: Testicular tumors following orchiopexy, South. Med. J. **60**:193, 1967.
12. Friedman, N.B., and Garske, G.L.: Inflammatory reactions involving sperm and the seminiferous tubules, Urology **62**:363, 1949.
13. Friedman, N.B., and Moore, R.A.: Tumors of the testis: a report on 922 cases, Milit. Surg. **99**:573, 1943.
14. Givler, R.L.: Testicular involvement in leukemia lymphoma, Cancer **23**:1290, 1969.
15. Levin, H.S., and Mostofi, F.K.: Symptomatic plasmacytoma of the testes, Cancer **25**:1193, 1970.
16. Li, F.P., Connelly, R.R., and Myers, M.: Improved survival rates among testis cancer patients in the U.S.A., JAMA **247**:825, 1982.
17. Maier, J., et al.: An evolution of lymphadenectomy in the treatment of malignant testicular germ cell neoplasms, Trans. Am. Assoc. Genitourinary Surgeons **60**:71, 1962.
18. Merrin, C., Sarcione, E., Bohne, M., et al.: Alpha fetoprotein in testicular tumors, J. Surg. Res. **15**:309, 1973.
19. Mostofi, F.K.: Testicular tumors: epidemiologic, etiologic and pathologic features, Cancer **32**:1186, 1973.
20. Mostofi, F.K.: Pathology of germ cell tumors of testis: progress report, Cancer **45**:1735, 1980.
21. Mostofi, F.K.: Histological changes ostensibly produced by therapy in the metastases of germ cell tumors of testis, Prog. Clin. Biol. Res. **203**:47, 1985.
22. Mostofi, F.K., and Davis, C.J., Jr.: Rare tumors of testis and adnexal tumors. In Pavone-Macaluso, M., Smith, P.H., and Bagshaw, M.A., editors: Testicular and other tumors, New York, 1985, Plenum Press.
23. Mostofi, F.K., and Davis, C.D., Jr.: Pathology of scrotal tumors. In Javadpour, N., editor: Principles of management of testicular cancer, ed. 2, New York, 1986, Thieme-Stratton, Inc.
24. Mostofi, K., Davis, C.J., Jr., and Sesterhenn, I.A.: Pathologist's view of testicular germ cell tumor management, American Urological Association Update Series **7**:137-148, Baltimore, 1988.
25. Mostofi, F.K., and Price, E.B., Jr.: Tumors of male genital system. In Atlas of tumor pathology, series 2, fascicle 7, Washington, D.C., 1973, Armed Forces Institute of Pathology.
26. Mostofi, F.K., and Sesterhenn, I.A.: Testicular germ cell tumors: pathology and tumor markers, Prog. Clin. Biol. Res. **153**:68, 1984.
27. Mostofi, F.K., and Sesterhenn, I.A.: Factors that affect the histology of metastasis in germ cell tumors of the testis, Adv. Biosci. **55**:351, 1986.
28. Mostofi, F.K., and Sesterhenn, I.A.: Pathology of germ cell tumors of testes: current status, Prog. Clin. Biol. Res. **203**:1, 1985.
29. Mostofi, F.K., and Sesterhenn, I.A.: World Health Organization: International histological classification of germ cell tumors of testes, Adv. Biosci. **55**:1, 1986.
30. Mostofi, F.K., and Sesterhenn, I.A.: The diagnosis of choriocarcinoma in the male, Adv. Biosci. **55**:187, 1986.
31. Mostofi, F.K., Sesterhenn, I.A., and Davis, C.J.: Immunopathology of germ cell tumors of the testes, Semin. Diagn. Pathol. **4**:320, 1987.
32. Mostofi, F.K., and Sobin, L.H.: International histological classification of tumors of testes, Geneva, 1977, World Health Organization.
33. Mostofi, F.K., Theiss, E.A., and Ashley, D.J.B.: Tumors of specialized gonadal stroma in human male patients (androblastoma, Sertoli cell tumor, granulosa-theca cell tumor of the testis, and gonadal stromal tumor), Cancer **12**:944, 1959.
34. Müller, K.: Cancer testis, Copenhagen, 1962, Munksgaard.
35. Pierce, G.B., Jr., and Beals, T.F.: The ultrastructure of primordial germinal cells of the fetal testes and of embryonal carcinoma cells of mice, Cancer Res. **24**:1533, 1964.
36. Price, E.B., Jr.: Epidermoid cysts of the testis, J. Urol. **102**:708, 1969.
37. Price, E.B., Jr., and Mostofi, F.K.: Secondary carcinomas of the testis, Cancer **10**:592, 1957.
38. Reyes, F.I., and Faiman, C.: Development of testicular tumor during *cis*-clomiphene therapy, Can. Med. Assoc. J. **109**:502, 1973.
39. Rosai, J., Khodadoust, K., and Silber, I.: Spermatocytic seminoma. II. Ultrastructural study, Cancer **24**:103, 1969.
40. Rosai, J., Silber, I., and Khodadoust, K.: Spermatocytic seminoma. I. Clinicopathologic study of six cases and review of the literature, Cancer **24**:92, 1969.
41. Scorer, C.G.: The anatomy of testicular descent: normal and incomplete, Br. J. Surg. **49**:357, 1962.
42. Sesterhenn, I.A., Mostofi, F.K., and Davis, C.J., Jr.: Testicular tumors in infants and children, Adv. Biosci. **55**:173, 1986.
43. Shiffman, M.A.: Androblastoma (Sertoli cell tumor): case report, J. Urol. **98**:493, 1967.
44. Stevens, L.C.: Embryonic potency of embryoid bodies derived from a transplantable testicular teratoma of the mouse, Dev. Biol. **2**:285, 1960.
45. Teilum, G.: Special tumors of ovary and testis, Copenhagen, 1971, Munksgaard.
46. Walker, K.M.: Hunterian lecture of the paths of infection in genitourinary tuberculosis, Lancet **1**:435, 1913.
47. Westcott, J.W.: Reticulum sarcoma with primary manifestation in the testis, J. Urol. **96**:243, 1966.
48. Willis, R.A.: Pathology of tumors, ed. 4, London, 1967, Butterworth & Co. (Publishers) Ltd.
49. Young, H.H.: Radical cure of tuberculosis of seminal tract, Arch. Surg. (Chicago) **4**:334, 1922.

Epididymis; spermatic cord

50. Brossman, S.A., Cohen, A., and Fay, R.: Rhabdomyosarcoma of testis and spermatic cord in children, Urology 3:568, 1974.
51. Broth, G., Bullock, W.K., and Morrow, J.: Epididymal tumors, J. Urol. 100:530, 1968.
52. Glassy, F.J., and Mostofi, F.K.: Spermatic granulomas of the epididymis, Am. J. Clin. Pathol. 26:1303, 1956.
53. Jackson, J.R.: The histogenesis of the adenomatoid tumor of the genital tract, Cancer 11:337, 1958.
54. Klingerman, J.J., and Nourse, M.H.: Torsion of the spermatic cord, JAMA 200:673, 1967.
55. Kyle, V.N.: Leiomyosarcoma of the spermatic cord: a review of the literature and report of an additional case, J. Urol. 96:795, 1966.
56. Longo, V.J., McDonald, J.R., and Thompson, G.J.: Primary neoplasms of epididymis: special reference to adenomatoid tumors, JAMA 147:937, 1951.
57. Lundblad, R.R., Mellinger, G.T., and Gleason, D.F.: Spermatic cord malignancies, J. Urol. 98:393, 1967.
58. Mostofi, F.K., and Davis, C.J.: Pathology of urologic cancer. In Javadpour, N., editor: Principles and management of urologic cancer, Baltimore, 1979, The Williams & Wilkins Co.
59. Mostofi, F.K., and Price, E.B.: Tumors of the male genital system. In Atlas of tumor pathology, series 2, fascicle 8, Washington, D.C., 1973, Armed Forces Institute of Pathology.
60. Nochomovitz, L.E., and Orenstein, J.M.: Adenocarcinoma of the rete testis: case report, ultrastructural observations, and clinicopathologic correlates, Am. J. Surg. Pathol. 8:625, 1984.
61. Rosai, J., and Dehner, L.P.: Nodular mesothelial hyperplasia in hernia sacs, Cancer 35:165, 1975.
62. Price, E.B.: Papillary cystadenomas of the epididymis, Arch. Pathol. 91:456, 1971.
63. Remzi, D.: Tumors of the tunica vaginalis, South. Med. J. 66:1295, 1973.
64. Silverblatt, J.M., and Gellman, S.Z.: Mesotheliomas of spermatic cord, epididymis, and tunica vaginalis, Urology 3:235, 1974.
65. Smith, B.A., Jr., Webb, E.A., and Price, W.E.: Carcinoma of the seminal vesicle, J. Urol. 98:743, 1967.
66. Williams, G., and Banerjee, R.: Paratesticular tumours, Br. J. Urol. 41:332, 1969.

Intersexuality; infertility; agonadism

67. Amelar, R.D.: Infertility in men, Philadelphia, 1966, F.A. Davis Co.
68. Ashley, D.J.B.: Human intersex, Edinburgh, 1962, Churchill Livingstone.
69. Charny, C.W.: The treatment of male infertility. In Behrman, S.J., and Kistner, R.W., editors: Progress in infertility, Boston, 1968, Little, Brown & Co.
70. Federman, D.D.: Abnormal sexual development: a generic and endocrine approach to differential diagnosis, Philadelphia, 1967, W.B. Saunders Co.
71. Goldberg, L.M., Skaist, L.B., and Morrow, J.W.: Congenital absence of testis: anorchism and monorchism, J. Urol. 11:84, 1974.
72. Inhorn, S.L., and Opitz, J.M.: Abnormalities of sex development. In Bloodworth, J.M.B., editor: Endocrine pathology, Baltimore, 1968, Williams & Wilkins Co.
73. Jirasek, J.E.: Development of the genital system and male pseudohermaphroditism, Baltimore, 1971, The Johns Hopkins Press.
74. Jones, H.W., Jr., and Scott, W.W.: Hermaphroditism, genital anomalies, and related endocrine disorders, ed. 2, Baltimore, 1971, The Williams & Wilkins Co.
75. Jost, A.: Problems of fetal endocrinology: the gonadal and hypophyseal hormones, Recent Prog. Horm. Res. 8:379, 1953.
76. Paulsen, C.A. In Williams, R.H., editor: Textbook of endocrinology, ed. 4, Philadelphia, 1968, W.B. Saunders Co.
77. Wong, T.W., Straus, F.H., and Warner, N.E.: Testicular biopsy in the study of male infertility. I. Testicular causes of infertility, Arch. Pathol. 95:151, 1973.
78. Wong, T.W., Straus, F.H., and Warner, N.E.: Testicular biopsy in the study of male infertility. II. Posttesticular causes of infertility, Arch. Pathol. 95:160, 1973.
79. Wong, T.W., Straus, F.H., and Warner, N.E.: Testicular biopsy in the study of male infertility. III. Pretesticular causes of infertility, Arch. Pathol. 98:1, 1974.

Scrotum

80. Borden, T.A., Rosen, R.T., and Schwartz, G.R.: Massive scrotal hematoma developing after transfemoral cardiac catheterization, Am. Surg. 40:193, 1974.
81. Burpee, J.F., and Edwards, P.: Fournier's gangrene, J. Urol. 107:812, 1972.
82. Dean, A.L.: Epitheliomas of scrotum, J. Urol. 60:508, 1948.
83. Fardon, D.W., Wingo, C.W., Robinson, D.W., et al.: The treatment of brown spider bite, Plast. Reconstr. Surg. 40:482, 1967.
84. Exelby, P.R.: Malignant scrotal masses in children, Cancer 24:163, 1974.
85. Himal, H.S., McLean, A.P., and Duff, J.H.: Gas gangrene of scrotum and perineum, Surg. Gynecol. Obstet. 139:176-178, 1974.
86. Keeler, L.L., and Harrer, W.V.: Chronic lymphedema of the scrotum and penis, J. Med. Soc. NJ 71:575, 1974.
87. Kickham, C.J., and DuFresne, M.: Assessment of carcinoma of the scrotum, J. Urol. 98:108, 1967.
88. Lee, W.R., and McCann, J.K.: Mule spinners' cancer and the wool industry, Br. J. Industr. Med. 24:149, 1967.
89. Smulewicz, J.J., and Donner, D.: Gas gangrene of the scrotum, J. Urol. 111:621, 1974.
90. Vermillion, C.D., and Page, D.L.: Puget's disease of the scrotum: a case report with local lymph node invasion, J. Urol. 107:281, 1972.

Penis

91. Bivens, C.H., Marecek, R.L., and Feldman, J.M.: Peyronie's disease: a presenting complaint of the carcinoid syndrome, N. Engl. J. Med. 289:844, 1973.
92. Campbell, M.: Epispadias: report of 15 cases, J. Urol. 67:988, 1952.
93. Dehner, L.P., and Smith, B.H.: Soft tissue tumors of the penis, Cancer 25:1431, 1970.
94. Editorial: Med. J. Aust. 2:1035, 1973.
95. Frew, I.D.O., Jefferies, J.D., and Swinney, T.: Carcinoma of penis, Br. J. Urol. 39:398, 1967.
96. Graham, J.H., and Helwig, E.B.: Bowen's disease and its relationship to systemic cancer, Arch. Dermatol. 80:133, 1959.
97. Graham, J.H., and Helwig, E.B.: Erythroplasia of Queyrat, Cancer 32:1396, 1973.
98. Grossberg, P., and Hardy, K.J.: Carcinoma of the penis, Med. J. Aust. 2:1050, 1973.
99. Gursel, E.O., Georgountzos, C., Uson, A.C., et al.: Penile cancer, Urology 1:569, 1973.
100. Hagerty, R.F., and Taber, E.: Hypospadias, Am. Surg. 24:244, 1958.
101. Horton, G.E., and Devine, C.J., Jr.: Plast. Reconstr. Surg. 52:503, 1973.
102. Johnson, D.E., Fuerst, D.E., and Ayala, A.G.: Carcinoma of the penis: experience with 153 cases, Urology 1:104, 1973.
103. Kao, G.F., and Graham, J.H.: Bowenoid papulosis, Int. J. Dermatol. 21:445, 1982.
104. Kaplan, C., and Katoh, A.: Erythroplasia of Queyrat (Bowen's disease of the glans penis), J. Surg. Oncol. 5:281, 1973.
105. Masih, B.K., and Brosman, S.A.: Webbed penis, J. Urol. 111:690, 1974.
106. Melicow, M.M., and Ganem, E.J.: Cancerous and precancerous lesions of penis, J. Urol. 55:486, 1946.
107. Moulder, J.W.: The psittacosis group as bacteria (Ciba lectures in microbial biochemistry, 1963), New York, 1964, John Wiley & Sons, Inc.
108. Najjar, S.S.: Webbing of the penis, Clin. Pediatr. 13:377, 1974.
109. Ngai, S.K.: Etiological and pathological aspects of squamous cell carcinoma of penis among Chinese, Am. J. Cancer 19:259, 1933.
110. Oertel, Y.C., and Johnson, F.B.: Sclerosing lipogranuloma of male genitalia, Arch. Pathol. Lab. Med. 101:321, 1977.
111. Poutasse, E.F.: Peyronie's disease, J. Urol. 107:419, 1972.
112. Powley, J.M.: Buschke-Loewenstein tumor of the penis, Br. J. Surg. 51:76, 1964.

113. Rege, P.R., and Evans, A.T.: Erythroplasia of Queyrat, J. Urol. **111**:784, 1974.
114. Smith, B.H.: Peyronie's disease, Am. J. Clin. Pathol. **45**:670, 1966.
115. Tan, R.E.: Fournier's gangrene of the scrotum and the penis, J. Urol. **92**:508, 1964.

Urethra

116. Agusta, V.E., and Howards, S.S.: Posterior urethral valves, J. Urol. **112**:280, 1974.
117. Bissada, N.K., Cole, A.T., and Fried, F.A.: Condylomata acuminata of male urethra and bladder, J. Urol. **112**:201, 1974.
118. Chambers, R.M.: Proceedings: the anatomy of the urethral structure, Br. J. Urol. **46**:123, 1974.
119. Cobb, B.G., Wolf, J.A., Jr., and Ansell, J.S.: Congenital stricture of the proximal urethral bulb, J. Urol. **99**:629, 1968.
120. Grewal, R.S., and Francis, J.: Foreign body of the urethra, Int. Surg. **48**:591, 1967.
121. Hills, B.H.: Gonorrhea and nonspecific urethritis, NZ Med. J. **69**:198, 1969.
122. Huvos, A.G., and Grabstald, H.: Urethreal meatal and parameatal tumors in young men, J. Urol. **110**:688, 1973.
123. Kaplan, G.W., Buckley, G.J., and Grayhack, J.T.: Carcinoma of the male urethra, J. Urol. **98**:365, 1967.
124. Klaus, H., and Stein, R.T.: Urethral prolapse in young girls, Pediatrics **52**:645, 1973.
125. Knoblich, R.: Primary adenocarcinoma of female urethra, Am. J. Obstet. Gynecol. **80**:353, 1960.
126. Malhoski, W.E., and Frank, I.N.: Anterior urethral valves, Urology **2**:382, 1973.
127. Marshall, F.C., Uson, A.C., and Melicow, M.M.: Neoplasma and caruncles of the female urethra, Surg. Gynecol. Obstet. **110**:723, 1960.
128. McEwen, C.: Reiter's disease: its nature and relationship to other diseases, Trans. Coll. Physicians Phila. **34**:39, 1966.
129. Meadows, J.A., Jr., and Quattlebaum, R.B.: Polyps of the posterior urethra in children, J. Urol. **100**:317, 1968.
130. Mitchell, J.P.: Injuries to the urethra, Br. J. Urol. **40**:649, 1968.
131. Mogg, R.A.: Congenital anomalies of the urethra, Br. J. Urol. **40**:638, 1968.
132. Morrison, A.I.: Treatment of relapses and re-infections in nonspecific urethritis, Br. J. Vener. Dis. **43**:170, 1967.
133. Smith, T.F., Weed, L.A., Pettersen, G.R., and O'Brien, P.C.: A comparison of genital infections caused by *Chlamydia trachomatis* and by *Neisseria gonorrhoeae*, Am. J. Clin. Pathol. **70**:333, 1978.
134. Young, R.H., and Scully, R.E.: Clear cell adenocarcinoma of the bladder and urethra: a report of three cases and review of the literature, Am. J. Surg. Pathol. **9**:816, 1985.

Prostate

135. Baker, W.J., and Graf, E.C.: Tuberculosis in obstructive prostate gland, J. Urol. **66**:254, 1951.
136. Batson, O.V.: Vertebral veins, Ann. Surg. **112**:138, 1940.
137. Bostwick, D.G., and Brawer, M.K.: Prostatic intraepithelial neoplasia and early invasion in prostate cancer, Cancer **59**:788, 1987.
138. Brawn, P.N.: Adenosis of the prostate: a dysplastic lesion that can be confused with prostatic adenocarcinoma, Cancer **49**:826, 1982.
139. Breslow, N.: Latent carcinoma of prostate at autopsy in seven areas, Int. J. Cancer **20**:680, 1977.
140. Byar, D.P., and Mostofi, F.K.: Carcinoma of the prostate: prognostic evaluation of certain pathological features in 208 radical prostatectomies, Cancer **30**:5, 1972.
141. Catalona, W.J., and Scott, W.W.: Carcinoma of the prostate. In Walsh, P., et al., editors: Campbell's urology, ed. 5, Philadelphia, 1986, W.B. Saunders Co.
142. Delaney, W.E., Burros, H.M., and Bhisitikul, I.: Eosinophilic granulomatous prostatitis simulating carcinoma, J. Urol. **87**:169, 1962.
143. Ferro, M.A., Barnes, I., Roberts, J.B., and Smith, P.J.: Tumor markers in prostatic carcinoma: a comparison of prostate specific antigen with acid phosphatase, Br. J. Urol. **60**:69, 1987.

144. Fisher, E.R., and Sieracki, J.C.: Ultrastructure of human normal and neoplastic prostate. In Sommers, S.C., editor: Pathology Annual, vol. 5, New York, 1970, Appleton-Century-Crofts.
145. Franks, L.M.: Benign nodular hyperplasia of prostate: a review, Ann. R. Coll. Surg. Engl. **14**:92, 1954.
146. Franks, L.M.: Latent carcinoma of prostate, J. Pathol. Bacteriol. **68**:617, 1954.
147. Franks, L.M.: The spread of prostatic cancer, J. Pathol. Bacteriol. **72**:603, 1956.
148. Franks, L.M.: The incidence of carcinoma of prostate: an epidemiological survey, Recent Results Cancer Res. **39**:149, 1972.
149. Franks, L.M.: Etiology, epidemiology and pathology of prostatic cancer, Cancer **32**:1092, 1973.
150. Franks, L.M.: Recent research on prostatic pathology. In Sommers, S.C., editor: Pathology Annual, vol. 5, New York, 1975, Appleton-Century-Crofts.
151. Grayhack, J.T., Wilson, J.D., and Scherbenske, M.J., editors: Benign prostatic hyperplasia, NIAMDD (National Institute of Arthritis, Metabolism, and Digestive Diseases) Workshop Proceedings, p. 63, 1975.
152. Hill, P., Wynder, E.L., Garnes, H., and Walker, A.R.: Environmental factors, hormone status, prostatic cancer, Prev. Med. **9**:657, 1980.
153. Hoffmann, E., and Garrido, M.: Malakoplakia of the prostate: report of a case, J. Urol. **92**:311, 1964.
154. Huggins, C., and Hodges, C.V.: Studies on prostatic cancer, the effect of castration, of estrogen and of androgen injection on serum phosphatases in metastatic carcinoma of prostate, Cancer Res. **1**:293, 1941.
155. Kadmon, D., Heston, W.D., and Fair, W.R.: Treatment of a metastatic prostate derived tumor with surgery and chemotherapy, J. Urol. **127**:1238, 1982.
156. Kaufman, J.J., and Berneike, R.R.: Leiomyoma of the prostate, J. Urol. **65**:297, 1951.
157. Kovi, J., Jackson M.A., Rao, M.S., Heshmat, M.D., Akberzie, M.E., Williams, A.O., and Christian, E.C.: Cancer of the prostate and aging: an autopsy study in black men from Washington, D.C., and selected African cities. Prostate **3**:73, 1982.
158. Kovi, J., Mostofi, F.K., Heshmat, M.Y., and Enterline, J.P.: Large acinar atypical hyperplasia and carcinoma of the prostate, Cancer **61**:555, 1988.
159. Lupovitch, A.: The prostate and amyloidosis, J. Urol. **108**:301, 1972.
160. McNeal, J.E., and Bostwick, D.G.: Intraductal dysplasia: a premalignant lesion of the prostate, Hum. Pathol. **17**:64, 1986.
161. Mostofi, F.K.: Precancerous lesions of the prostate. In Carter, R.L., editor: Precancerous states, Oxford, 1984, Oxford University Press.
162. Mostofi, F.K.: Grading of prostatic carcinoma: current status. In Bruce, A.W., and Trachenberg, J., editors: Adenocarcinoma of the prostate, Berlin, 1987, Springer-Verlag.
163. Mostofi, F.K., and Morse, W.H.: Epithelial metaplasia in "prostatic infarction," Arch Pathol. (Chicago) **51**:340, 1951.
164. Mostofi, F.K., Sesterhenn, I., and Sobin, L.H.: International histological classification of tumors of prostate, Geneva, 1981, World Health Organization.
165. Mostofi, F.K., Sesterhenn, I.A., and Davis, C.J., Jr.: Progress in pathology of carcinoma of prostate, Prog. Clin. Biol. Res. **243A**:439, 1987.
166. Murphy, G.P., Natarajan, N., Pontes, J.E., Schmitz, R.L., Smart, C.R., Schmidt, J.D., and Mettlin, C.: The National Survey of Prostatic Cancer in the United States, J. Urol. **127**:928, 1982.
167. Paulson, D.F., Rabson, A.S., and Fraley, E.E.: Viral neoplastic transformation of hamster prostate tissue in vitro, Science **159**:200, 1968.
168. Sesterhenn, I.A., Mostofi, F.K., and Davis, C.J., Jr.: Immunopathology of prostate and bladder tumors. In Russo, J., editor: Immunocytochemistry in tumor diagnosis, Boston/Dordrecht/Lancaster, 1985, Martinus Nijhoff Publishing.
169. Stamey, T.A., Yang, N., Hay, A.R., McNeal, J.E., and Freiha, F.S.: Prostatic specific antigen as a serum marker for adenocarcinoma of the prostate, N. Engl. J. Med. **317**:906, 1987.
170. Willis, R.A.: Carcinoma of prostate. In Pathology of tumours, London, 1948, Butterworth & Co., Ltd.

20 Lung and Mediastinum

CHARLES KUHN III
FREDERIC B. ASKIN

PEDIATRIC LUNG DISEASE
Lung development

The lung is a foregut derivative and appears at about the twenty-sixth postovulatory day as a bud from the caudal end of the laryngotracheal sulcus.[3,19] Lung development in humans can be roughly separated into four phases: embryonic, pseudoglandular, canalicular, and terminal sac.[14,19] In the embryonic period (first 6 weeks) the lung buds form the lobar bronchi and the major segmental branches. The entire epithelial lining of lung airways and air spaces is of endodermal origin, but branching is apparently controlled by the mesenchymal tissues into which the lung buds grow.[7,10,18] In the pseudoglandular period (sixth to sixteenth weeks), bronchial branching continues and cartilage is formed. The distal lung-lining epithelium is composed of large cuboid cells closely apposed around a potential space. During the canalicular period (sixteenth to twenty-fourth weeks) the pulmonary mesenchyme becomes richly vascular; septa appear in the lung and the epithelium of the distal air spaces begins to flatten. Capillaries protrude into the areas of epithelium, and the glycogen-filled cuboid cells lining the distal air spaces begin to differentiate into recognizable type I (squamous) and type II (surfactant-producing) cells.[8,12] Progressive flattening of epithelium and intrusion of capillaries lead to a thin air-blood barrier, and by the end of the twenty-eighth week it should theoretically be possible to maintain respiration.[19] Lamellar intracytoplasmic inclusions representing pulmonary surface-active material begin to appear in type II cells after the twentieth week but are present in an amount sufficient to provide lung stability only after the twenty-fourth to twenty-sixth weeks of gestation.[9,16] The lung in utero is not collapsed but is distended by a distinctive fluid produced by lymphatic leakage and contributed to by the alveolar type II lung cells.[3,7,16] The final phase of intrauterine lung development, the terminal sac period (twenty-sixth week to term), is characterized by the development of shallow distal air spaces that have been variably termed "saccules," or true but immature alveoli.[19] Alveoli continue to form and multiply after birth.[19] With a wide range of individual variability alveoli increase approximately tenfold in number, from 30×10^6 at birth to 300×10^6 at 8 years of age.[19] Most of the increase in numbers occurs in the first 4 years of life. After age 8, alveoli increase primarily in size until the growth of the chest wall is complete. There is some evidence that total alveolar number is related to body height.[19]

Airway branching is complete by birth, and the major cartilaginous airways have formed by the sixteenth week of intrauterine life.[14,17,19] Pulmonary artery development in the preacinar (airway) region parallels that of the bronchial tree and is complete by birth.[14] A pulmonary artery gives off more branches along its length than its neighboring airway does. "Conventional" branches accompany airways. "Spurious" or "supernumerary" branches pass into the adjacent alveolar region and supply the capillary bed. In the acinar (respiratory) region conventional and spurious pulmonary arteries proliferate after birth to accompany alveolar multiplication. The structure of the pulmonary arteries in infants differs greatly from that of adults in the amount and distribution of muscle in the media.[14] The difference is most apparent if one takes into account the location of the artery in the lung parenchyma. In children a complete muscle layer is present in the small arteries of the alveolar region by the end of the second decade of life. In terms of thickness, fetal arteries of all sizes contain more muscle than those of adults. By 4 months after birth this difference disappears. In the smaller arteries (less than 250 μm) the fall in thickness is much more rapid. The wall size of veins and the pattern of muscle distribution appear to be the same in adults and infants.[14] Lymphatic channels can be seen in the lungs of fetuses of 20 weeks' gestational age, and lymph nodes are seen in the peribronchial regions at birth and increase in prominence with advancing age.[15] Loose lymphoreticular aggregates appear after birth and are seen among alveoli, in peribronchiolar sites, and underneath the epithelium of bronchi, presumably representing a response to environmental antigenic stimuli.[11]

920

Congenital anomalies

Pulmonary agenesis may be unilateral or bilateral.[20,36,41] The former is compatible with long survival in the absence of severe infection or coexistent malformations. Tracheal agenesis has been described as well.[27,44] Abnormal pulmonary fissures and lobations and bronchial anomalies are probably the most common pulmonary malformations.[24,28,31,36,38,39] The azygous lobe, for example, is produced by pressure of the azygous vein on the apex of the right lung and is of little clinical significance. The relationship, however, of mirror image lobation (pulmonary isomerism) to a variety of cardiovascular anomalies has been well documented.[35-37] The horseshoe lung is fused behind the heart but anterior to the esophagus and may have abnormal venous drainage.[29,36] Abnormal bronchi may be either supernumerary or displaced. The most common is the tracheal bronchus, which supplies an upper lobe, usually the right, directly from the trachea.[26,36,38] The rare bridging bronchus joins right lower lobe airways to those of the left lung.[31] Congenital or acquired bronchial stenosis may cause either atelectasis or overinflation depending on whether the obstruction is complete or partial.[24,40]

Heterotopic tissues including adrenal cortex, striated muscle, liver, and glial tissues have been reported in the lung.[21,22,25,33,34,36] Glial heterotopia in the lung parenchyma is usually found in anencephalic newborns and must be distinguished from cases in which traumatic central nervous system tissue emboli are found in pulmonary arteries.[30]

Congenital alveolar capillary dysplasia is a developmental anomaly in which anomalous veins accompany the bronchi and bronchioles and blood vessels fail to become established in the distal air spaces.[32] Extrauterine oxygen diffusion in the lung is inadequate to support life. The lesion is a rare cause of perinatal pulmonary hypertension. Complete acinar dysplasia has also been described.[42]

Hypoplasia and diaphragmatic hernia

Hypoplasia of the lung can be defined as a decrease in relative volume or weight of lung tissue appropriately mature for the patient's age. A representative group of standards is available from the work of Langston[19] and Thurlbeck and associates.[19] Page and Stocker and others[54,59] have found the lung weight/body weight ratio to be a reliable indicator of hypoplasia. The diminution in lung tissue may be unilateral or bilateral and may be related to a deficit of airways, acini, or alveoli, to diminished alveolar size, or to any combination of these factors. Primary pulmonary hypoplasia is a rare entity, occasionally familial, and of unknown cause. Etiologic factors causing secondary hypoplasia can be identified and classified (Table 20-1) as

Table 20-1. Etiology of pulmonary hypoplasia

Category	Example
Unexplained	Idiopathic (isolated or familial), Down's syndrome
Compression of the lungs Inadequate or abnormal thoracic space	Diaphragmatic hernia, scoliosis, thoracic mass lesions, asphyxiating thoracic dystrophy, various types of dwarfism
Large extrathoracic mass	Polycystic kidneys, large bladder, abdominal masses
Decreased fetal respiratory movement	Amniotic fluid deficit (renal agenesis/dysplasia, bladder outlet obstruction), amniotic fluid leak, neuromuscular disorders affecting diaphragm and other respiratory muscles, anencephaly
Metabolic defect	Renal agenesis, anencephaly, Rh incompatibility, (?) other immune disorders

related to direct intrathoracic or extrathoracic compression of the lung or lungs, deformities of the chest wall, a variety of renal, urinary tract, and placental abnormalities that lead to oligohydramnios, or one of a seemingly unrelated mixture of disorders.[45-55,59] More than one mechanism may be responsible in some instances. Direct compression of pulmonary parenchyma seems a straightforward cause of lung hypoplasia. It is more difficult to explain hypoplasia related to either oligohydramnios or the other factors mentioned above. Formerly it was suggested that oligohydramnios caused pulmonary hypoplasia by allowing the uterus to compress the underlying lung through the malleable chest wall. It now seems clear that other factors, especially loss of lung fluid and interference with fetal respiratory movements, can better explain the hypoplasia of the lungs associated with oligohydramnios or polyhydramnios, neuromuscular disorders, and anencephaly. It is also possible that renal agenesis may contribute to lung hypoplasia by interference with collagen metabolism.[19] The mechanism of pulmonary hypoplasia in infants with Down's syndrome is unknown.[46]

Pulmonary hypoplasia is frequently found in association with herniation of abdominal contents through a congenital, usually left-sided, diaphragmatic defect called Bochdalek hernia (Fig. 20-1). The ipsilateral lung

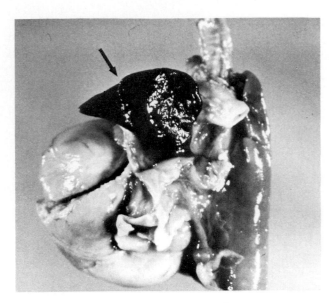

Fig. 20-1. Posterior view of hypoplastic left lung *(arrow)* from patient who had antenatal herniation of bowel loops into left side of chest through posterior diaphragmatic hernia. Compressed lung is hypoplastic because of diminished numbers of airways and alveoli.

is distorted and hypoplastic with a reduction in airways and in alveolar number and size.[19,58] The contralateral lung is hypoplastic as well but is not as dramatically distorted. Infants with diaphragmatic hernia appear to be particularly susceptible to the development of persistent pulmonary hypertension (see p. 954), which may be fatal. Infants who survive after surgical repair of the hernia have pulmonary function that may be close to normal. Morphologic studies in a few cases have shown a persistent deficit in alveolar multiplications and the development of compensatory emphysema.[58]

Pulmonary hyperplasia has been described in patients with laryngeal atresia.[56,59]

Pulmonary vascular anomalies

Several general reviews covering pulmonary vascular anomalies are available.[2,6,36,63,65] Arterial malformations include origin of one or both main pulmonary vessels from the aorta.[64,73] Absence (actually interruption) of a main artery with vascular supply to the lung through bronchial artery collaterals has been noted as well.[63,65] A pulmonary arterial system is present within the lung proper in these patients. In aberrant origin of the left pulmonary artery from the right pulmonary artery ("pulmonary artery sling"),[61,67,78] the anomalous vessel courses behind the trachea and may partially obstruct the airways (see discussion of congenital lobar overinflation, p. 923). Isolated or multiple discrete areas of stenosis may be found in the pulmonary artery. Some of these patients have other cardiovascular malformations.[69,72] Children with the Alagille syndrome of cho-

lestasis and a peculiar facies often have peripheral stenoses of the pulmonary arteries.[62] Diffuse hypoplasia of pulmonary arteries has been described in patients with congenital rubella.[77]

Venous anomalies include anomalous pulmonary venous return to the heart, stenosis or atresia, and the "scimitar" syndrome. A complete review is available elsewhere.[36,60,63,65,70] In total anomalous venous return all four main pulmonary veins converge and then drain into the innominate vein, coronary sinus, or right atrium or they run below the diaphragm and enter the inferior vena cava or portal vein. Pulmonary lymphangiectasis (see p. 923) may be a prominent feature. Partial anomalous venous return has been reported as well.[70]

Isolated or multiple stenosis or even atresias may be found in the pulmonary veins and are also associated with diffuse or localized lymphangiectasis or hemorrhage and hemosiderin deposition in the lung.[68,74,76]

The "scimitar" syndrome is a multifaceted malformation characterized by a large anomalous pulmonary vein that drains from one lung, usually the right, into the inferior vena cava.[65,66] The broad roentgenographic shadow of this vein forms the scimitar. The ipsilateral lung is hypoplastic and has at least partial anomalous systemic arterial blood supply. There may be overlap in this syndrome with pulmonary sequestration (see below) or horseshoe lung (see p. 921).

Pulmonary arteriovenous fistulas may be congenital or acquired. Congenital lesions may be solitary or multiple, and between one third and one half of the patients have the Osler-Weber-Rendu syndrome with similar lesions in other organs. The blood supply of the fistula usually comes from the pulmonary artery but is occasionally derived from systemic vessels.[62,75]

Bronchopulmonary sequestration

Sequestered pulmonary lobes or segments are not connected to the airway system of the associated normal pulmonary parenchyma.[1,2,81,88-91] The blood supply of the sequestered area is usually through systemic vessels arising from the aorta or its branches. Two major types of sequestration occur: intralobar and extralobar.

Intralobar sequestrations occur almost equally in adults and children. The usual but not invariable location is in the posterior segment of the left lower lobe, and the sequestered area is incorporated within the pleural investment of that lobe. The disorder may be discovered when a mass lesion is seen on a routine chest roentgenogram or because of recurrent infection in the same area of the lung. Pathologically the features are frequently those of obstructive pneumonitis. Grossly the lesion may be solid or cystic, depending on the degree of inflammatory change. One or more elastic arteries supply blood to the affected area; venous drainage is usually through the pulmonary system.[1,2,5,88]

Extralobar sequestrations have also been termed accessory lobes. They are completely separate from the pleural covering of the normal lung. The usual location of extralobar sequestrations is in the left lower hemithorax, but they may occur near the esophagus or within or even below the diaphragm. Both the arterial supply and venous drainage are usually of systemic origin. In contrast to intralobar sequestration, the extralobar lesion occurs predominantly in infants and children and is frequently associated with coexisting malformations, especially diaphragmatic hernia and pectus excavatum.[36,88-90] Secondary infection and obstruction are not common features, but the basic architecture resembles that of immature lung or dysplastic bronchiolar structures.

It is likely that both types of lesion arise from an accessory lung bud from the foregut, though many intralobar "sequestrations" may actually represent lesions acquired as a result of recurrent infection or as a response to the presence of abnormal systemic arterial supply to the lung.[80,91] The accessory lung bud may persist in some instances and may connect the sequestration with the esophagus, stomach, or biliary tract—the so-called bronchopulmonary foregut malformation.[36,82,84,88]

Certain vascular anomalies may mimic or actually belong in the spectrum of intralobar sequestration: isolated supply of a portion of otherwise normal pulmonary parenchyma by a systemic artery may occur and produce a large vascular shunt.[1,2,92] The scimitar syndrome (see p. 922) may also overlap with pulmonary sequestration.[79]

Bronchogenic cyst

Bronchogenic cysts also arise from accessory lung buds from the foregut. Although they usually lack any formation of pulmonary parenchyma, transitional forms between this lesion and sequestration have been found. Bronchogenic cysts usually appear in the anterior mediastinum but can occur within the lung substance or chest wall as well.[83,86,87] They are characterized by a lining of a bronchial epithelium and the presence of cartilage in their wall. These cysts are unilocular and may contain watery fluid, mucus, or, rarely, purulent material. They must be differentiated from enteric cysts lined with gastric or intestinal epithelium and, when they occur within the lung parenchyma, from a lung abscess.[86,87] The abscess has multiple airways connecting with its lumen, whereas a bronchogenic cyst does not. Bronchiectasis in young children is often misinterpreted as representing a congenital cystic disease of the lung.

Congenital adenomatoid malformation

The congenital adenomatoid malformation (Fig. 20-2, A) is an unusual lesion combining features of a hamartoma, dysplasia, and a true neoplasm in the lung.[89,93-102] The adenomatoid malformation usually affects a single lobe and is an expanding mass that compresses the adjacent lung and may cause severe respiratory distress and even death. Grossly a spectrum of solid to multilocular cystic lesions has been described. Multiple or bilateral lesions are rare. The malformation lacks bronchi but does appear to communicate with the airway system of the normal lung. Microscopically the cysts are lined by bronchial or cuboid epithelium; prominent clusters of mucinous cells may be interspersed among the septa (Fig. 20-2, B or C). More solid lesions are composed of multiple curving, branched structures that resemble dysplastic or immature bronchioles. Clinically and roentgenographically, but not histologically, the differential diagnosis of adenomatoid malformation includes congenital lobar overinflation and sequestration. A recently described infiltrative congenital spindle cell lesion may or may not be related to adenomatoid malformation.[103]

Congenital pulmonary lymphangiectasis

Congenital pulmonary lymphangiectasis is a rare lesion characterized by pronounced distension of subpleural and septal lymphatic spaces.[104-110] Usually the disorder results from pulmonary venous obstruction, predominantly total anomalous pulmonary venous return (p. 922) and other cardiac anomalies. Rarely it may be primary in the lung or may be part of a generalized syndrome of lymphangiectasis including chylous effusions and bone destruction. Pulmonary lymphangiectasis, as a specific disorder, must be distinguished from pulmonary interstitial emphysema (see the following discussion) and from the dilated lymphatic vessels often seen in hyaline membrane disease (see p. 925).

Congenital pulmonary overinflation (lobar or segmental "emphysema")

Congenital lobar overinflation occurs in infants as a lobar disorder and in older children or adults as a segmental area of pulmonary hyperinflation without tissue destruction.[111-121] The popular term "emphysema" is not strictly correct for this entity, since the lung parenchyma is not destroyed. In infants the lesion is a rapidly enlarging mass, usually in an upper or middle lobe, causing mediastinal shift and respiratory distress. Multiple causes have been identified, the most common being partial intrinsic or extrinsic bronchial obstruction. Deficiency of bronchial cartilage in the large bronchi of the affected lobe has been identified in many cases, and in others extrinsic pressure from engorged or aberrant pulmonary vessels is presumed to be the cause.[111,116,119,120] Endobronchial trauma resulting from therapeutic suctioning has been implicated to some patients.[114,117] In a few cases the primary lesion appears to be an increased number of alveoli in the affected

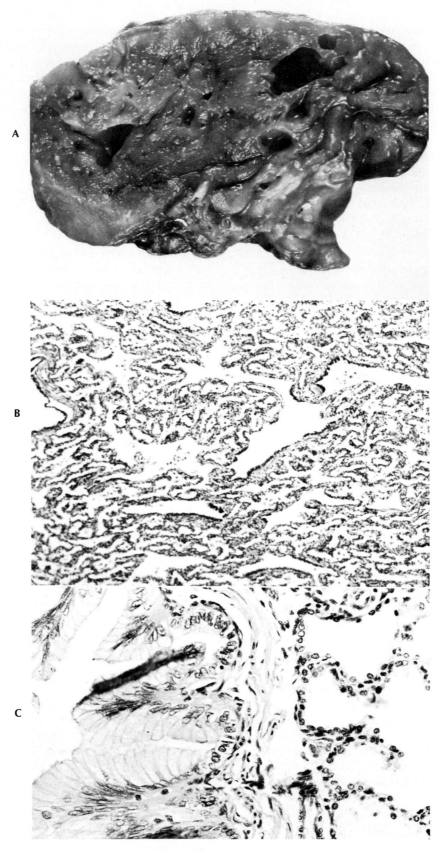

Fig. 20-2. A, Congenital adenomatoid malformation. Central portion of this upper lobe is replaced by multiple cysts. Rim of normal lung tissue is present. **B,** Low-power photomicrograph showing irregularly branching spaces lined with cuboidal epithelium. **C,** Mucigenic cells *(left)* are characteristic but are not always present in adenomatoid malformations.

lobe.[112] Although emergency surgery may be necessary in some cases of lobar overinflation, conservative management has been possible in others.[115]

Segmental overinflation usually is diagnosed in an older child or adult and is related to segmental bronchial atresia.[113] The involved segment appears to enlarge because of air trapping.

In either lobar or segmental overinflation the microscopic pattern is usually simply that of normal-appearing but overinflated alveoli. Bronchial cartilage deficiency can ordinarily be demonstrated only by special dissection and staining techniques.

Adaptation to extrauterine life

The successful transition from intrauterine to extrauterine life requires some major changes in lung physiology.[3,7,16,59,122] The liquid that expanded alveoli in utero must be replaced by air, and surfactant must be discharged into alveoli from type II pneumocytes so that a stable residual volume can develop in the lung. The presence of surfactant ensures that alveoli do not collapse completely with each expiration.[9] In addition, the pulmonary vasculature in the newborn must change rapidly from a low-flow, high-resistance system to a low-resistance, high-flow circulation with closure of the ductus arteriosus.

Failure of one or more of these physiologic changes to occur may be associated with a variety of diseases seen only in neonates. These disorders include hyaline membrane disease and its complications (bronchopulmonary dysplasia and interstitial emphysema), meconium aspiration, massive pulmonary hemorrhage, and persistent unexplained pulmonary hypertension in the newborn (persistent fetal circulation).

Perinatal lung disease

Transient tachypnea of the newborn ("neonatal wet lung"). During the first several breaths of life, lung fluid is removed by pulmonary lymphatics and through the airways. On occasion the removal of this fluid is delayed and transient tachypnea may be seen. The chest roentgenogram shows increased interstitial vascular markings, but the condition of the infant stabilizes rapidly as parenchymal and alveolar edema fluid is resorbed. No fatalities from this condition have been reported.[122-125]

Hyaline membrane disease. Hyaline membrane disease (HMD, idiopathic respiratory disease syndrome of the newborn) is a clinical, biochemical, and pathologic entity characteristically seen in a semispecific population.[3,143-145,147,148] Infants at greater risk for HMD include the following:

1. Appropriate for gestational age premature infants
2. Males
3. Whites

4. Infants of mothers with a history of previously affected premature infants
5. Infants born by cesarean section before 38 weeks' gestation, mother not in labor
6. Infants of diabetic mothers
7. Infants with asphyxia or whose delivery was precipitous
8. Second born of twins

The basic cause appears to be a deficiency of pulmonary surface-active material and consequent lung instability. Whether this deficit is related to type II cell immaturity, to inhibition of production, to release or function of surfactant, or to all three or additional factors in varying proportion is not resolved. There is probably variation in the cause of individual cases.[134]

Microscopically the most important feature is the abnormal expansion pattern. The distal air spaces are collapsed and the distal airways are dilated and lined by the characteristic eosinophilic ("hyaline") membranes (Fig. 20-3). Septal lymphatics are often dilated, and focal hemorrhage and edema fluid may be seen.[138,147] These features correlate with the roentgenographic "ground-glass" appearance and air-bronchogram effect seen on the chest film in HMD. The histologic features may be altered by the fixative employed, the time between death and autopsy, and the method of fixation.[138,143,146,147]

For the practical examination of the infant's lung at autopsy, it is generally wise to perfuse one lung with intrabronchial fixative and sample the other lung in the uninflated state. In this way both the interstitium and the expansion pattern can be examined. Fixative inflation of the lung removes the air-liquid barrier and obscures the effects of abnormally high surface tension on the lung.

Morphologic variations include the peculiar large, round air spaces described by Gruenwald[135] as "exaggerated atelectasis"; yellow staining of the membranes,[132] apparently by bilirubin; and sloughing of bronchial or alveolar epithelium to form a pseudoglandular or even giant cell pattern. The morphologic diagnosis of HMD in very small infants may be difficult because they may die before the hyaline membranes form or because the very immature lung may not be able to collapse in the recognizable HMD pattern. In a tiny infant the distinction between a lung too immature to sustain respiration and HMD may be impossible to make.

It seems logical that the hyaline membranes in HMD simply represent a characteristic manifestation of diffuse alveolar damage and that the abnormal expansion pattern is attributable to lung instability.

Methods for prenatal detection of lung maturity and pharmacologic methods for possible prevention of HMD are discussed elsewhere.[7,16,143,144]

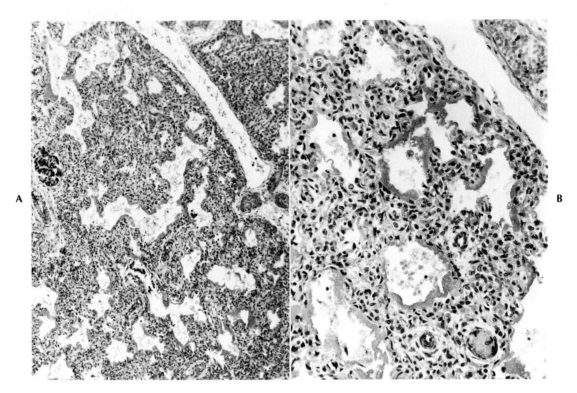

Fig. 20-3. Hyaline membrane disease. **A,** Lower-power photomicrograph shows dilated airways lined with eosinophilic ("hyaline") membranes. Distal air spaces are collapsed. Dilated lymphatics *(top)* are commonly seen. **B,** High-power view shows membranes and collapsed distal air spaces.

Physiologic derangements in HMD include hypoxia, acidosis, pulmonary hypertension, and large right-to-left shunts through the lung and through failure of closure of the ductus arteriosus.[140,141,148] Complications include bronchopulmonary dysplasia and interstitial emphysema (see the following discussion). Problems related to therapy for HMD include subglottic stenosis and hypopharyngeal or tracheal perforation.[131,137,139,148,151]

Bronchopulmonary dysplasia. Bronchopulmonary dysplasia (BPD) is a clinical and pathologic syndrome usually found in infants treated for HMD with oxygen and artificial ventilation.[126-129,131,133,140,141] The relative importance of these two factors has been vigorously debated, but the immaturity of the lung exposed to these injurious agents may be more important than either. The alveolar septa in the immature lung are wide and cellular and seem to contain a greater potential space in which vessels and fibroblasts can proliferate. In patients who die within the first month of life the histologic features are those of diffuse alveolar damage and its repair, with the added insult of bronchiolar necrosis and florid bronchiolitis obliterans (Fig. 20-4). The question of how BPD differs from resolving untreated HMD is difficult to approach because before the use of oxygen or mechanical ventilation patients usually died within 72

hours or survived without further difficulty. Several older studies have suggested that in resolving HMD the membranes are fragmented and are phagocytosed by macrophages.[16] Why such florid bronchiolitis obliterans and interstitial fibrosis occur in treated infants is unclear. High-frequency ventilation appears to produce a characteristic pattern of necrotizing tracheobronchitis.[130]

Complications of BPD include the development of pulmonary interstitial emphysema, pneumothorax, and pneumomediastinum. Patent ductus arteriosus and intrapulmonary shunting may lead to impressive right ventricular hypertrophy. Autopsy study of long-term survivors of BPD who required continuous ventilation usually shows a pattern of chronic bronchitis and patchy interstitial fibrosis (Fig. 20-5). Areas of collapsed lung alternate with enlarged simplified air spaces that represent coalescence of groups of alveoli whose walls have been destroyed and remodeled. Interstitial vascularity is increased as well. This "late-stage healed" BPD may be the same as or at least related to the so-called Wilson-Mikity syndrome.[136,140,141,149]

Complete follow-up studies of patients who survive HMD and BPD are not available. Such studies are complicated by the inability to separate deleterious effects of premature birth and therapy in general from

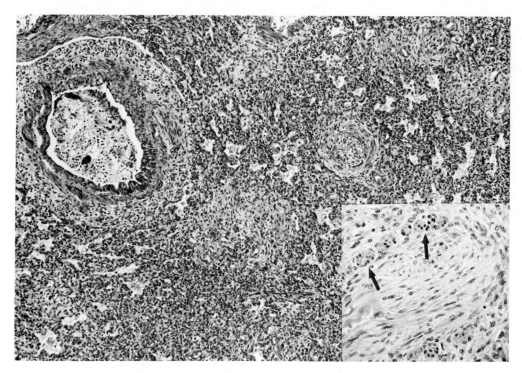

Fig. 20-4. Bronchopulmonary dysplasia in acute phase. Some bronchioles *(upper left)* show epithelial necrosis and squamous metaplasia. Lighter nodules in lung represent bronchioles whose lumen is obliterated by fibrous tissue. Inset shows such a lesion. Residual smooth muscle wall of bronchiole is outlined by arrows.

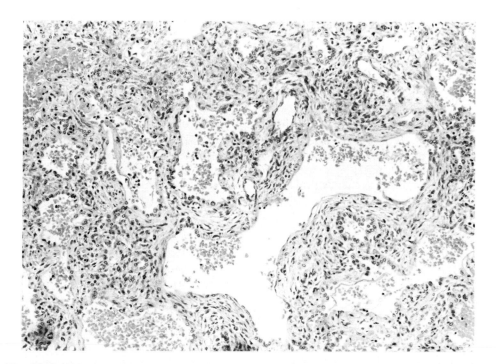

Fig. 20-5. Bronchopulmonary dysplasia, late phase. There has been extensive rearrangement of lung architecture. Interalveolar septa are fibrotic, and residual air spaces are relatively avascular. This interface does not provide efficient ventilation and perfusion matching in lung.

the specific effects of lung disease at an early age. Several investigators have reported an increased incidence of subsequent pulmonary infection and of persistently abnormal chest roentgenograms with patchy fibrosis.[140,141] The presence of small airway disease has recently been documented.[140,141] Developmental and other central nervous system abnormalities are found with variable incidence in recent studies.[128,131,133,140,141]

Pulmonary interstitial emphysema and its complications. Although small pneumothoraces are not uncommon in newborn full-term infants, the development of significant pulmonary interstitial air with subsequent pneumomediastinum, pneumopericardium, and even pneumoperitoneum is most often seen in the premature newborn infant treated with artificial ventilation.[152-161] Most such infants also have bronchopulmonary dysplasia, and systemic air embolism has been reported as well.[152,156] Other clinical situations in which pulmonary interstitial emphysema (PIE) and its sequelae occur are the meconium aspiration syndrome; the pulmonary hypoplasias, especially those associated with severe renal abnormalities and oligohydramnios; and as a complication of amniocentesis. The pathogenesis of PIE involves dissection of air into the pulmonary interstitial space and probably into lymphatics as well.[152,154,157,160] Subpleural blebs rupture causing pneumothorax, or air dissects into the hilum of the lung with subsequent extension to the mediastinum, pericardium, or subcutaneous tissues. Grossly and microscopically, cystic spaces are seen around bronchovascular bundles and in the septa of the lung (Fig. 20-6), and the morphologic features may be misinterpreted as representing a cystic malformation. Extensive dissection of air around the pulmonary vessels at the hilum may cause air block and circulatory compromise.[152] The large potential space available in the interalveolar (intersaccular) septa in the premature infant's lung probably contributes greatly to the more extensive PIE found in premature infants. Giant cells may be seen in the air-filled spaces and represent a response to air as an irritant.

PIE is usually a diffuse process but may occur as a predominantly localized but expanding lesion in a single lobe or lung.[152,153,158-161] Localized PIE often presents a surgical emergency. Although pneumoperitoneum may be a complication of PIE, a more likely cause of pneumoperitoneum is a gastric or bowel perforation and that consideration should not be overlooked. Lung perforation can occur as a complication of treatment of pneumothorax with chest tubes.[151]

Meconium aspiration syndrome. Massive meconium aspiration is generally associated with hypoxia and fetal distress in the full-term or postmature infant.[3,163,164,168-170,173] Pulmonary interstitial emphysema and pneumothorax are frequent complications. On gross examination the lungs may have silvery green dis-

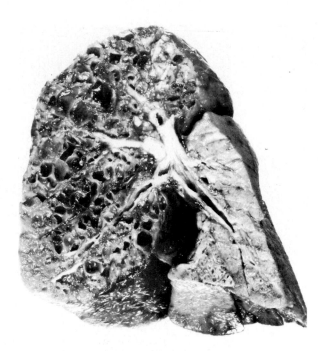

Fig. 20-6. Interstitial pulmonary emphysema. Upper lobe shows multiple coalescent cysts representing interstitial air dissecting along interlobar septa and around small and large airways. The lower lobe *(right)* shows the solid appearance associated with the collapsed air spaces of hyaline membrane disease.

coloration, and tenacious mucoid material may be expressed from the tracheobronchial tree. Microscopically, distended distal airways filled with mucus, bile pigments, and squames are the characteristic features. Since squames alone are routinely found in the distal air spaces of stillborn infants and infants dying in the neonatal period, the presence of mucin obstructing the bronchioles provides a more definitive diagnosis of meconium aspiration. Polymorphonuclear cells may be present in the alveoli. Morphologic evidence of neonatal pulmonary hypertension is present in some cases.[175] Whether meconium can cause "chemical pneumonitis" is controversial.[178] Meconium does seem to enhance the development of bacterial pneumonia.[168,172]

Although the amniotic fluid and placenta are usually deeply stained in cases of meconium aspiration, some reports suggest that a clinically similar syndrome can occur without external evidence of meconium staining. Although most investigators believe that meconium aspiration occurs at or after delivery, an intrauterine aspiration syndrome has been reported.[174,176,177]

Massive pulmonary hemorrhage in the newborn. Focal pulmonary hemorrhages can be seen in the lungs of neonates dying of a variety of causes.[162,165-167] Larger interstitial hemorrhages are not uncommon in the pulmonary parenchyma of stillborn infants. The term *mas-*

sive pulmonary hemorrhage (MPH) is usually employed in reference to a clinical syndrome of respiratory distress with acute collapse. Often hemorrhagic fluid pours from the nose and mouth. These infants at autopsy have pulmonary hemorrhage, predominantly intra-alveolar, involving more than one third of the total lung parenchyma. The syndrome characteristically appears in premature, small for gestational age, male infants. Infants with congenital cardiovascular disease should probably be considered as a separate population.

The cause of MPH is unknown. Major theories advanced up to now include infection (unlikely), cold injury, hemorrhagic pulmonary edema, a terminal manifestation of intracerebral damage or increased intracerebral pressure, pulmonary capillary fragility, and oxygen damage.[165,171] Most cases in the British Perinatal Study occurred between the third and seventeenth days of life.[167] MPH is not simply a severe manifestation of HMD; MPH occurs in growth-retarded infants, whereas HMD occurs in premature infants with appropriate development for their gestational age.

Persistent fetal circulation. Persistent fetal circulation (PFC, unexplained persistent pulmonary hypertension of the newborn) is a clinical syndrome in which the pulmonary circulation fails to be transformed into a high-flow, low-resistance system after birth.[180,181,183-190] Infants with PFC are cyanotic and hypoxic after birth, and there is evidence of significant pulmonary hypertension with a large right-to-left shunt in the absence of a cardiovascular malformation. Some of these infants have associated hyaline membrane disease or meconium aspiration, but others have no evidence of other underlying pulmonary disorders. If the ductus arteriosus closes, right ventricular hypertrophy and heart failure may supervene.

At autopsy, morphologic evidence of pulmonary hypertension as seen in adults (see p. 954) is usually not demonstrable. Geggel and associates[182] and others have demonstrated, however, that striking abnormalities may be present in the small pulmonary arteries. In patients with PFC there is an abnormal smooth muscle coat in the media of the pulmonary arteries (arterioles) in that part of the lung acinus distal to respiratory bronchioles. Ordinarily muscle is present in these vessels only after adolescence or during adult life. Less commonly, small thrombi may be seen in the pulmonary arteries of affected infants.[187,188] Other findings may reflect associated pulmonary disease and the effects of therapy. Some infants with bilateral pulmonary hypoplasia and especially infants with hypoplastic lungs related to diaphragmatic hernia also have a clinical syndrome resembling PFC.[179,182] Infants whose mothers have taken large doses of prostaglandin inhibitors have had a similar disorder.[186]

All of these findings suggest that intrauterine and perinatal events may initiate and perpetuate PFC. Rudolph[189] has proposed a valuable clinical etiologic classification distinguishing three groups of patients with PFC. In patients with normal pulmonary vascular development, acute vasoconstriction or abnormally high blood viscosity may impede flow. In another group of patients, increased pulmonary vascular smooth muscle is present, presumably reflecting a variety of intrauterine insults. In the final group a decreased cross-sectional area of pulmonary vessels is found. These infants have pulmonary hypoplasia of varying degree. Other intrauterine events such as infection or drug exposure may also adversely affect pulmonary vascular development.

The presence of pulmonary hypertension early in the clinical course and of severity out of proportion to any associated pulmonary parenchyma changes seen on chest roentgenogram is a feature that can help to differentiate PFC from other respiratory disorders of the newborn.

Infectious disorders in the infant lung

Neonatal pulmonary infection (congenital and perinatal pneumonia) is a common finding in neonatal necropsies.[190-213] Pneumonia, as a primary or complicating phenomenon, was found in 36% of the cases in the British Perinatal Mortality Survey in 1958 and, including the amniotic fluid infection syndrome, accounted for approximately 20% of neonatal deaths in the U.S. Collaborative Perinatal Projects.[198,203,205] The organisms implicated vary with the clinical features. Pneumonias in the perinatal period may be classified as the following:

1. Transplacental—part of a systemic congenital disease
2. Congenital (intrauterine)—amniotic fluid infection syndrome; usually found in stillborns, abortuses, or early postnatal deaths in full-term infants
3. Acquired during birth—signs appear in the first week; usually caused by organisms in maternal birth canal; affects premature infants especially
4. Acquired after birth—appears during the first months; caused by organisms acquired from environment

Congenital pneumonia usually accompanies the amniotic fluid infection syndrome (AFIS). The placental membranes and amniotic fluid are infected by organisms ascending from the vagina, and concomitantly clusters of polymorphonuclear cells are aspirated in utero and appear in bronchi and alveoli. The isolation of bacteria or other infective agents depends on the care with which routine and special cultures are performed. The placental membranes may have ruptured before birth but may have been intact. Maternal urinary tract infection appears to be important in the pathogenesis of infection when membranes are intact.[202] Racial and socioeconomic factors appear associated with AFIS; perhaps the usual bacteriostatic activity of amniotic fluid is adversely affected in certain populations.[203-205] The presence of pulmonary vessels filled with polymorphonuclear cells has been used to differentiate true congenital pneumonia from the infant who "drowned in pus" from aspiration of infected amniotic fluid, but basically the findings seem to represent different portions of a spectrum. Whether the pulmonary disease is the cause or an accompanying phenomenon of events causing abortion, stillbirth, or neonatal death is not clear. Lung tissue or aspirated heart blood should be submitted for culture when pneumonia is suspected.

Pneumonia acquired during birth is usually caused by organisms acquired from the birth canal. Group B streptococcal infection has attracted major attention because of its rapidly fatal course if untreated and the histologic feature of hyaline membranes, which may obscure the true diagnosis.[191,195,212] The membranes are not present in all cases, and the lung in very early cases may show only polymorphonuclear leukocytes, gram-positive cocci, and edema. When membranes are present, the expansion pattern differs from that in HMD, and more polymorphonuclear leukocytes are seen. Pleural effusion may be seen in group B streptococcal infection and would be unusual in HMD or even other neonatal pulmonary infections.

Late-onset pneumonia is usually caused by organisms, such as staphylococci, *Pseudomonas*, or *Serratia*, acquired from human or environmental contacts.[192,194,212] Chlamydial pneumonitis is a distinctive pneumonitis of infants, usually appearing at 3 weeks of age with tachypnea and a staccato cough.[190,199,200,207,209,213] Associated conjunctivitis is seen in 50% of the infants. An absolute blood eosinophilia may be present. The course may be protracted, but recovery is the rule. Interstitial pneumonitis and florid bronchiolitis have been described as histologic features.[190] In most neonatal cases, maternal genital infection is suspected as the source.

Transplacental pneumonia appears as a part of the generalized disease associated with cytomegalovirus, herpesvirus, or other "TORCH" agents or with syphilis or certain bacterial infections such as listeriosis.[203,208,212] Evaluation of the placenta, special culture or fluorescent antibody techniques, or serum studies in mother and infant are helpful.

Bronchiolitis and bronchiolitis obliterans

In the older pediatric age groups, viral infection (adenovirus and respiratory syncytial virus) is a frequent cause of bronchiolitis.[214,222-224] Toxic inhalants can produce a similar picture, and both types of injury may be followed by progressive obliteration of the small airways. This bronchiolitis obliterans is essentially a syndrome caused by many reactive processes in the lung and is a descriptive term for a pattern of injury, not a specific diagnosis. Cases with apparent antenatal origin are reported.[221] Gastroesophageal reflux with aspiration of gastric acid can also produce severe bronchiolar damage in infants.[215,216,218]

Microscopically the acute phase consists in bronchiolar necrosis and peribronchial cuffing by inflammatory cells. Severe damage may be followed by obliteration of bronchiolar lumens by fibrous plugs.[214,219] In rare instances extensive obliteration of the small airways has produced the unilateral hyperlucent lung, a small lung with evidence of air trapping and generally with a small pulmonary artery (Swyer-James syndrome).[217,220,222,224] The small pulmonary artery is generally considered to be an acquired phenomenon. The bronchioles in the affected lobe are often reduced to small scars, and the lesion may be overlooked unless one makes a specific attempt to identify a bronchiole accompanying most of the small pulmonary arteries. Focal hyperlucency of the lung related to bronchial atresia is discussed on p. 921.

INFECTIONS OF THE LUNGS AND BRONCHI
Incidence

According to the U.S. vital statistics, pneumonia and influenza together account for 3% of all deaths and are the fifth leading cause of death, exceeded only by heart disease, cancer, cerebrovascular disease, and accidents. Respiratory infections are responsible for 8.5% of hospitalizations in the United States. Nosocomial pneumonias develop in 0.7% of all hospitalized patients but in as much as 13% of the critically ill patients admitted to intensive care units. With the use of potent therapies that deliberately or incidentally produce immunosuppression, there is every prospect that respiratory infections will remain a serious clinical problem. For example, pneumonia develops in one third of patients receiving chemotherapy for leukemia.

Routes of infection

Pathogenic organisms gain access to the lung through the airways, through the bloodstream, by traumatic implantation, or by direct spread across the diaphragm from a subphrenic source, probably through the lymphatics. The most common route is the airways. Airway spread can result from inhalation of the organism as an aerosol on droplet nuclei. This is the major mechanism of spread of many viral infections and of tuberculosis. Often, however, the development of overt infection begins with colonization of the upper respiratory tract by potential pathogens followed by aspiration into the lower respiratory tract.[228,229] This is a major mechanism for many of the gram-negative organisms. Two important determinants of the ability of a bacterium to colonize are bacterial interference by the existing flora and the binding of the bacterium to the epithelial surface, believed to be mediated by specific molecules on the epithelial cell membrane. Antibiotic therapy, by eliminating interference by the normal flora, promotes colonization by resistant organisms. Serious illness increases the ability of nasopharyngeal epithelium to bind gram-negative bacteria because of proteolytic changes in the cell surface.[230,233]

Pulmonary defenses

The respiratory tract has several protective mechanisms that dispatch most organisms deposited in the respiratory tract before they can set up an infection.[225,227,231] The trachea and bronchi are coated with a layer of mucus produced by the goblet cells of the bronchial mucosa and the glands in the lamina propria. This layer provides a physical barrier to organisms deposited in the airways and is swept upward to the oropharynx by ciliary action, removing deposited microbes. The mucus contains specific antibody, mainly IgA, produced by plasma cells in the lamina propria of the bronchus, as well as other antibacterial substances such as lysozyme and lactoferrin produced in the serous cells of the glands. At the alveolar level the main defense under ordinary circumstances is the alveolar macrophage. Most organisms that reach the alveoli are engulfed by macrophages and killed long before they are physically cleared from the lung.[226] The rate of killing varies among species of bacteria and indeed among strains of the same species. Clinically important factors that have been shown to depress macrophage function include starvation, ethanol ingestion, hypoxia, uremia, air pollutants, cigarette smoke, and antecedent viral infection.[231] The alveolar lining layer contains some antibody (mainly IgG) as well as complement components. The alveolar macrophages when stimulated can also produce a variety of chemotactic substances that recruit neutrophils and more mononuclear phagocytes. With lymphoid nodules located at the branch points of small airways and in the pleura and with complete lymph nodes in the hila, the lungs are also one of the major lymphoid organs of the body.[232]

Viral infections

Viral infections are discussed in Chapter 9. The most important in terms of both morbidity and mortality is influenza, which is discussed in detail on p. 363. Viral infections early in life may also be important as a predisposing factor for the development of chronic lung disease in adulthood.

In children lethal viral infections take one of two pathologic forms, bronchiolitis or pneumonia.[234] The majority of cases of bronchiolitis are caused by respiratory syncytial virus (RSV), but parainfluenza virus, ad-

enovirus, and *Mycoplasma pneumoniae* can also cause this syndrome.[246] Bronchiolitis is exceedingly common, comprising more than one fifth of lower respiratory infections seen in pediatric practice. Epidemics of the disease occur usually in winter, with the highest incidence in children under 2 years of age.[239] Most cases are mild, and only 1% to 2% of children require hospitalization. Among these hospitalized the mortality is only 1% to 2%. The onset of symptoms is acute with tachypnea, dyspnea, cough, and wheezing. Sternal retractions may be present. Most patients are afebrile. When patients with the rare severe cases are seen at autopsy, the lungs are well expanded and may be considered normal on gross examination. Close inspection reveals thickening of the small airways, which appear on the cut surface of the lung as 2 to 4 mm gray nodules with a pinpoint lumen barely visible. Microscopically the walls of the bronchioles are densely infiltrated with mononuclear inflammatory cells (Fig. 20-7). Early, there is necrosis of the ciliated epithelium with the formation of plugs of necrotic material and leukocytes in the bronchiolar lumen. Regeneration of the epithelium begins after 3 to 4 days and is complete by 15 days with the regeneration of cilia. The alveoli are expanded and have a round contour indicative of air trapping. There may be limited extension of the inflammatory infiltrate into the walls of alveoli abutting the bronchioles. Bron-

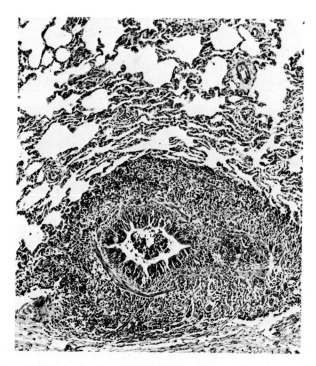

Fig. 20-7. Viral bronchiolitis. Wall of bronchiole is greatly infiltrated with mononuclear inflammatory cells, and lumen also contains exudate. Focally, alveoli are collapsed but noninflamed.

chiolitis caused by adenovirus tends to be more severe. Necrosis of the bronchiolar epithelium is extensive and may extend into the bronchiolar wall. This probably accounts for the higher mortality of adenoviral bronchiolitis (5% to 7%) and for the high frequency of sequelae.

Viral pneumonias may occur at any age. The specific infecting virus determines the cytologic features of the infected cells, including the presence and morphology of inclusions and the tendency to form syncytia and giant cells.[235,236,243,244] However, one can make generalizations concerning the morphologic response of the lung to viruses. Most viruses that produce pneumonia infect the epithelial cells, either exclusively or in addition to infecting other cell types. The predominant tissue response is an acute interstitial pneumonia. The walls of the air spaces are thickened by congestion, edema, and an interstitial infiltrate predominantly of mononuclear cells. Hyaline membranes form in respiratory bronchioles and alveolar ducts, and many of the alveoli are collapsed (microatelectasis). The air spaces contain edema, fibrin, and a scanty cellular exudate of monocytes, macrophages, occasional neutrophils, and sloughed epithelial cells. There are usually focal hemorrhages. Foci of necrosis may be present, particularly with herpesviruses and adenovirus, but often are absent even in lethal infections. The alveolar epithelial cells are enlarged and hyperplastic. In some areas they may be seen overlying or beneath hyaline membranes. Patients who have been ill for more than a few days usually have foci of epithelial regeneration and metaplastic epithelium of squamous or bronchiolar type, even in alveoli.

Bronchioles are often inflamed and may show viral inclusions in the epithelium. Occlusive plugs of necrotic material, which are common in bronchiolitis, are seen only infrequently in viral pneumonia.

Mycoplasmal pneumonia

Mycoplasmas are simple organisms, 150 nm in diameter, that occupy a taxonomic place between the large viruses and bacteria. Unlike viruses, they can be cultured on simple media in vitro. They are enclosed by a membrane but lack cell walls and therefore are difficult to demonstrate in tissue sections except by immunohistochemical methods. *Mycoplasma pneumoniae* is a common cause of upper respiratory infections. It appears that pneumonia develops in less than 10% of infected subjects.[238,242]

In large ambulatory civilian populations, 15% to 20% of pneumonias are caused by mycoplasmas. In certain closed military populations the proportion may be higher. *M. pneumoniae* is a cause of both endemic and epidemic pneumonia. The infection rate varies little with season, unlike other pneumonias. The peak age is between 5 and 15 years, and infection is relatively in-frequent in those over 45 years.[270] Clinically, mycoplasmal pneumonia is a benign, self-limited disease with few complications. Usually only one lung is involved, and the process is patchy or segmental in distribution.[238]

A characteristic feature is the presence of cold agglutinins, IgM antibodies that do not react at 37° C but cause agglutination of the patient's erythrocytes at 4° C. They develop in almost all cases of mycoplasmal pneumonia but are not specific and can be seen in pneumonias caused by a variety of other organisms.[238] Occasionally they may be the cause of Raynaud's phenomenon by producing agglutination of erythrocytes in chilled extremities, and they are occasionally responsible for hemolytic anemia.[242,245]

Extrapulmonary spread of mycoplasmas has only recently been recognized. Almost any tissue can be involved; gastrointestinal disease, myocarditis, and a variety of neurologic manifestations have been described.[242]

Because of the benign course of mycoplasmal pneumonia, pathologic features of only a few cases have been described.[237,241] Grossly the lungs show a fibrinous pleurisy and patchy consolidation. Microscopically there are bronchiolitis and interstitial pneumonia. The walls of bronchioles are congested, edematous, and infiltrated with mononuclear cells. Epithelial cells degenerate and are sloughed. The parenchyma shows edema and interstitial pneumonia with hyaline membranes and mononuclear cell infiltration of the alveolar walls. The gross and histologic changes are indistinguishable from those of viral pneumonia. Culture or immunohistochemical demonstration of the organism is necessary to differentiate the diseases.

Bacterial infections
Acute tracheobronchitis

Diphtheria is discussed elsewhere. Acute bacterial infections of the large airways are a frequent complication of viral infection. In small children, because of the small caliber of the airways, bacterial infection can cause severe obstruction. The syndrome acute tracheitis is an acute bacterial infection of the airways seen in children usually below 6 years of age. The clinical picture resembles croup but also includes stridor, high fever, and toxicity. Epiglottitis is not present. Most cases are caused by *Staphylococcus aureus*, but *Haemophilus influenzae* and other bacteria may also be responsible. Subglottic edema and thick mucopurulent exudate can cause tracheal obstruction.[258]

Bacterial pneumonia

Pneumococcal pneumonia. *Streptococcus pneumoniae* is a gram-positive facultative anaerobe that produces alpha hemolysis when cultured on blood agar. It is recognized in smears and histologic sections as a lancet-shaped diplococcus, but it can also appear in chains and clumps. The more than 80 strains that have been identified differ in the antigenic structure of their capsular polysaccharide.

The pneumococcus continues to be responsible for 30% to 80% or more of community-acquired pneumonias.[259,260] Groups at particular risk include the very young and the very old, alcoholics, diabetics, splenectomized subjects, and patients with multiple myeloma or sickle cell disease.[260] Pneumococci also cause nosocomial infections, in which case the clinical picture is often atypical. The mortality of pneumococcal pneumonia before modern therapy was 30%, but a considerable improvement was obtained with the introduction of type-specific antisera and antibiotics.[250] Even with modern antibiotic therapy, however, the mortality is 20% in those with bacteremic infection.[247,250,255]

Pathology. Pneumococcal pneumonia typically presents the picture of lobar pneumonia. One or occasionally several lobes of the lung are involved.[248] The individual involved lobes are relatively uniform in appearance, the process being rapidly spread through the lobe, and limited by the lobar fissures. Occasionally a few lobules are uninvolved or at a different stage, indicating some restraint of the spread by the lobular septa. Traditionally the progress of the disease is divided into four stages: edema, red hepatization, gray hepatization, and resolution or organization.

The organisms colonize the upper respiratory tract and gain access to the lung by aspiration. Not uncommonly this follows a viral respiratory infection by several days, the way being paved by viral damage to the ciliated epithelium.[260] The initial response to the organism is an outpouring of edema fluid, which provides a rich broth in which the organisms proliferate and which spreads them throughout the lobe through pores of Kohn and bronchioles (Fig. 20-8). At this stage an involved lobe appears distended, moist, and deep red or purple. The pleura is shiny, and fluid exudes from the cut surface. With the passage of time progressively more fibrin and neutrophils enter the alveoli. Phagocytosis of bacteria begins, and within 24 hours most organisms are found within neutrophils. At first the alveolar capillaries are distended with erythrocytes and there is diapedesis of erythrocytes into the alveoli, giving the lobe a red color, while the filling of the air spaces with fibrin and leukocytes gives it a firm, liverlike consistency. Classically the lobe at this phase is described as red hepatization. With the further evolution of the process, increasing amounts of fibrin and leukocytes enter the air spaces, the alveolar capillaries appear compressed, and the lobe becomes progressively grayer in appearance, evolving into the stage of gray hepatization (Figs. 20-9 and 20-10). In untreated persons, organisms

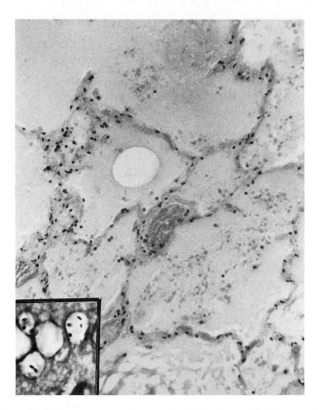

Fig. 20-8. Pneumococcal pneumonia in stage of edema. Air spaces are filled with fluid and a few erythrocytes. *Inset,* With Gram's stain, edema fluid teems with gram-positive diplococci. Halo surrounding organisms represents unstained capsular material.

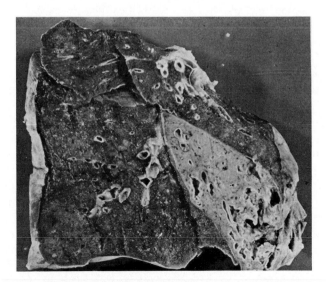

Fig. 20-9. Gray hepatization in pneumococcal pneumonia. Lobe shows beginning abscess formation.

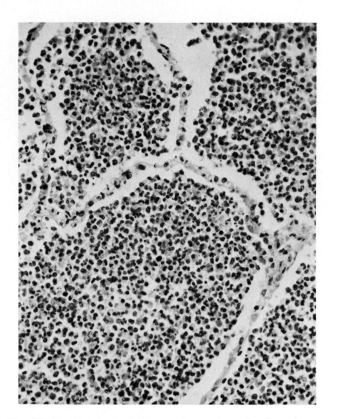

Fig. 20-10. Histologic features of gray hepatization. Alveolar spaces are filled with neutrophils and fibrin. Alveolar walls are comparatively normal.

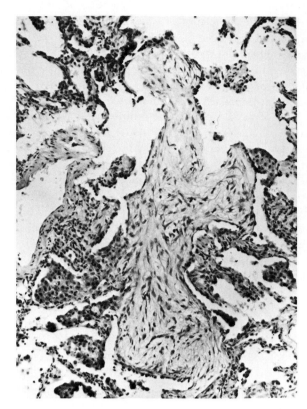

Fig. 20-11. Organizing pneumonia. Alveolar duct is filled by plug of young connective tissue containing fibroblasts and proteoglycan-rich matrix, which has replaced inflammatory exudate.

decrease in number progressively after approximately 5 days.

In the usual course of events the final stage is resolution. As a rule necrosis of alveolar walls is not a feature of pneumococcal pneumonia except with serotype III. Since the exudation is intra-alveolar, it can be cleared through the bronchial tree, restoring the lung to normal. Macrophages are the predominant cells during this process.[257]

Beginning as early as 48 hours after onset, a few monocytes can be found in the alveolar exudate. With time they increase in number and differentiate into macrophages at a time that varies from case to case. Usually between 5 and 12 days after onset monocytes and macrophages become the predominant types of inflammatory cell. The neutrophils degenerate, and the fibrin network breaks down under the influence of proteases released from the neutrophils and newly arriving macrophages. Macrophages containing both degenerating neutrophils and organisms can be observed. Over the ensuing several days organisms disappear and empty space begins to appear progressively in the exudate, which gradually is removed by the phagocytes or is expectorated. Alveolar architecture ultimately returns to normal.

In a small proportion of cases, resolution fails to take place or is incomplete and the unresolved areas undergo organization (Fig. 20-11). The remaining exudate is invaded by fibroblasts and converted to fibrous tissue. Masses of fibroblasts invading the air spaces lay down a matrix of myxoid connective tissue rich in proteoglycan, which is gradually converted to collagenous tissue. In some areas alveolar epithelium migrates over organizing exudate within the air spaces, incorporating it into the alveolar walls and giving rise to an appearance indistinguishable from interstitial fibrosis. In other areas the air spaces remain filled, and the lung is converted to fleshy, gray, glistening, solid tissue whose meaty consistency accounts for the old term for this process, carnification. Factors that predispose to organization rather than resolution include bronchial obstruction and necrosis of alveolar walls.

Although the typical pathologic pattern of pneumococcal pneumonia is lobar consolidation, a pattern of bronchopneumonia is by no means rare. Even in preantibiotic series, bronchopneumonia accounted for more than 40% of fatal pneumococcal pneumonias.[251] Patients tend to be either very young or over 50 years of age and usually have underlying disease, either chronic obstructive lung disease or serious extrathoracic disease. The pneumonia is commonly bilateral and has an appearance similar to other bronchopneumonias, notably multiple foci of consolidation centered on terminal airways.

Complications. Pleural involvement occurs commonly in lobar pneumonia. In two thirds of patients there is a fibrinous pleuritis without infection of the pleural space. Pleural fluid if present has a relatively low white cell content and glucose concentration. In 15% to 25% of patients, infection of the pleural space (empyema) develops and the pleural surface becomes covered with shaggy white layers of fibrin and neutrophils. Pleural fluid becomes turbid and then frankly purulent with loculated pockets of pus. Unlike purulent exudate in the alveoli, that in the pleural cavity is not in communication with the exterior and cannot be readily cleared; instead of resolving, empyema heals by organization. This can lead to encasement of the lung by a thick fibrous peel that is several millimeters thick and ultimately may restrict lung expansion.

Bacteremia occurs in 20% to 35% of patients with lobar pneumonia and a much smaller proportion of those with bronchopneumonia. It is a serious complication that continues to have a mortality of 20% to 30% despite antibiotics. Bacteremic spread leads to meningitis, bacterial endocarditis, arthritis, or pericarditis in a small proportion of patients.

Lung abscess results from the breakdown of alveolar walls. The frequency of this complication is twice as great with type III pneumococcus as with other types,[251,262] probably because the type III organism is protected from phagocytosis by its abundant production of capsular material.

Clinical correlations. The onset of pneumococcal pneumonia is usually abrupt with a shaking chill followed by high fever and systemic symptoms such as malaise, nausea, myalgias, and weakness. Pleuritic chest pain is common. Most patients cough up rusty or purulent sputum. Leukocytosis (up to 20,000/cu mm) is common; leukopenia is a grave prognostic sign. Before antibiotic therapy patients remained acutely ill for 5 to 6 days and then often went through a dramatic clinical change known as a crisis with profuse sweating and fall in the fever, after which they greatly improved. This change corresponded to the appearance of circulating antibodies. It did not correlate with any abrupt alteration in the morphology of the lung, which might be in the stage of red or gray hepatization. Less often clinical recovery was gradual (by lysis). The response to antibiotics is rapid, with improvement usually within 24 hours.

Beta-hemolytic streptococcal pneumonia. Beta-hemolytic streptococci are an uncommon cause of pneumonia at the present time. Lancefield group A streptococci were formerly the most prominent strains, but recently group B organisms have been assuming greater importance.[261] Infections caused by beta-hemolytic streptococci in the newborn are discussed elsewhere. Formerly many streptococcal pneumonias in older children followed the childhood viral exanthema; they are now decreasing in incidence because the use of vaccines against the viruses.[253] In adults, streptococcal pneumonia like other pneumonias usually occurs in elderly, severely debilitated patients.[261] Diabetes is also a risk factor.

The lower lobes are usually the site of major involvement. The airways appear thickened and are filled with a bloody or purulent exudate. The pneumonia is lobular with consolidated patches clearly centered on terminal bronchioles. The distinctive microscopic feature of streptococcal pneumonia is greater interstitial involvement than in other bacterial pneumonias. There is necrosis of the epithelium of distal airways with infiltration of the bronchial walls by neutrophils and mononuclear cells. The interstitial infiltrate also extends into the adjacent alveolar walls. The lung surrounding the pneumonic foci is edematous. The interlobular septa are swollen with edema, and the lymphatics are distended and sometimes plugged with fibrin strands. Effusions and empyema can develop with great rapidity.[253]

Staphylococcal pneumonia. *Staphylococcus aureus* commonly colonizes the nose and skin. Staphylococcal pneumonia usually occurs either in the presence of a source of bacteremia or after a viral infection. Hematogenous pneumonia is seen in those with soft-tissue infections,[256] in patients undergoing long-term dialysis, because of infected shunts, and in parenteral narcotic users, especially those with right-sided bacterial endocarditis. Hematogenous staphylococcal pneumonia most often produces multiple rounded lesions that are more numerous in the lower lung zones where blood flow is greatest. The lesions may appear as septic infarcts that are yellow and purulent but preserve to some degree the wedge-shaped configuration of infarcts and are associated with thrombosed vessels, or they may be rounded patches of necrotizing pneumonia that break down, giving rise to abscesses.

Staphylococcal pneumonia also results from spread of organisms from the colonized nasopharynx. This often follows damage to the mucociliary apparatus by viral infection, notably in influenza epidemics.[252,254] The lesions are those of a bronchopneumonia accompanied by a hemorrhagic and necrotizing bronchitis. Purulent exudate fills the bronchioles and spreads into the adjacent acini. Colonies of bacteria can usually be found without difficulty. Necrosis and breakdown of alveolar walls are early features and may result in hemorrhage in the surrounding lung.

Staphylococcal bronchopneumonia is not rare in children less than 6 months of age. A notable feature of staphylococcal pneumonia in small children is development of pneumatoceles, air-containing lesions that are seen roentgenographically within areas of confluent pneumonia and that enlarge very rapidly, often over hours. It is unlikely that they are simple abscesses because they are thin walled and can disappear over several weeks without residua. Although their morphology has rarely been described since patients commonly recover, most radiologists assume that they arise from the trapping of air distal to partial obstruction to a bronchus, which acts as a check valve.[249]

Local complications of staphylococcal pneumonia include empyema and bronchopleural fistula.

Pneumonia caused by gram-negative aerobic bacteria. In the preantibiotic era, gram-negative pneumonias accounted for only 0.5% to 5% of pneumonias, usually attributable to *Klebsiella* and *Enterobacter* species. The incidence of gram-negative pneumonia has increased until currently between 5% and 30% of community-acquired bacterial pneumonias and up to 50% of nosocomial bacterial pneumonias are attributable to gram-negative organisms. Even when community acquired, gram-negative pneumonias are virtually limited to persons with underlying chronic illness.[271,274]

The routes of infection vary with the species.[276] *Escherichia coli*, *Enterobacter*, and *Pseudomonas* often reach the lung through the bloodstream. The other gram-negative bacilli usually colonize the upper airways. The spread of infection in the hospital by the use of contaminated inhalation therapy equipment has been well documented,[272] but with improvements in sterilization techniques and increased awareness of the problem it is diminishing in frequency.

Pneumonia caused by *Klebsiella pneumoniae* is classically a disease of alcoholic men, but it also occurs in other debilitated patients.[274] The organism colonizes the upper respiratory tract or oral cavity and gains access to the lung by aspiration. This undoubtedly accounts for its predilection for the right upper lobe.[263]

The onset of the disease is sudden with rigors, fever, and severe prostration and toxicity. Cough and hemoptysis are common, and the sputum is typically (though not invariably) gelatinous and brick red.

The anatomic distribution of pneumonia is typically lobar and in the right lung in the majority of cases. The involved lung is bulging and gray-red and exudes slimy material. In cases of more than a few days' duration, abscesses are found. Microscopically the exudate consists of both neutrophils and macrophages, and organisms may be abundant (Fig. 20-12). Necrosis of alveolar walls appears early, and by 4 to 5 days after onset granulation tissue is forming at the margins of abscesses. The infection is more destructive than pneumococcal pneumonia, and the frequency of fibrosis in the involved tissue in survivors is much higher. The organism can be cultured from the blood in 20% to 60% of pa-

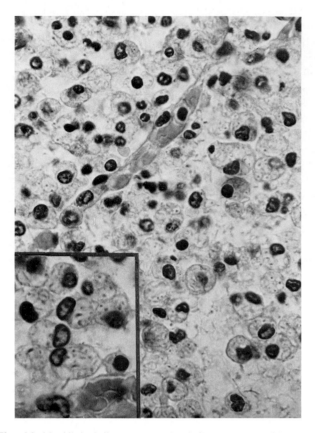

Fig. 20-12. *Klebsiella* pneumonia. Inflammatory infiltrate in air spaces consists almost entirely of macrophages containing organisms. *Inset,* Higher power showing encapsulated bacilli within macrophages.

tients in the acute phase of the illness, but extrathoracic spread is unusual.

Pneumonias produced by the various species of *Proteus* are less common than *Klebsiella-Enterobacter* pneumonias but have many similar features.[279] Most patients are alcoholics with underlying chronic pulmonary disease. Pneumonia follows aspiration during a period of stupor or delirium tremens. The pneumonia most often produces consolidations of the involved lobe with multiple abscesses. Cases of bacteremic spread to the lung have also been reported.

Infections of a variety of tissues by *Haemophilus influenzae* are common in children below 3 years of age. Pneumonia caused by *H. influenzae*, however, seems to occur mainly in adults with chronic lung disease. *H. influenzae* is part of the normal flora of the upper respiratory tract and commonly colonizes the lower respiratory tract of those with chronic bronchitis. Some data have indicated that the frequency of *H. influenzae* pneumonia may be increasing, but the increased rates of recovery of the organism from patients with pneumonia may also be explained by recent improvements in culture technique.[266,281]

Pneumonia caused by *H. influenzae* follows viral respiratory infection in approximately half the patients.[268] The symptoms are similar to those of other pneumonias. Two roentgenographic patterns are recognized: a lobar consolidation, which is often associated with bacteremia, and a diffuse bronchopneumonia, often miliary in appearance, which usually is not bacteremic.[268,280] Parapneumonic (sterile) pleural effusions are common. Empyema and abscess occur in the lobar form. The prognosis of treated *Haemophilus* pneumonia is good with a mortality of less than 10%, though a mortality of 33% has been reported in septicemic cases.[268,281]

Pseudomonas aeruginosa is infrequently a cause of community-acquired pneumonia but is a major agent of nosocomial infections. *Pseudomonas* pneumonia takes two rather distinct forms depending on whether infection follow colonization of the airways or reaches the lung through the bloodstream. Colonization of the airways is common in patients in intensive care units and appears to increase in frequency with duration of hospitalization and severity of illness.[229] The pneumonia that follows colonization is a bronchopneumonia, frequently confluent and accompanied by abscesses. Pleural effusions are characteristically small, and empyema is rare.[273,278] Patients at particular risk for bacteremic *Pseudomonas* pneumonia are those with hematologic malignancy, granulocytopenia, or burns.[265,270]

The bacteremic form of pneumonia is characterized by severe hemorrhage and necrosis.[264,269,273] Early lesions consist mainly of subpleural hemorrhages with a small, firm, necrotic center. Microscopically the hemorrhage is accompanied by necrosis of alveolar walls and contains numerous organisms. Established lesions are discrete yellow nodules a few millimeters to centimeters in size and surrounded by hemorrhage. Microscopically these lesions consist of eosinophilic coagulative necrosis in which the outlines of the underlying tissue structure remain and inflammatory cells are few (Fig. 20-13). The walls of arteries and veins are faintly basophilic and hazy, and Gram's stain shows that they are teeming with bacilli.[264,265,269,273] In an experimental model of *Pseudomonas* septicemia Teplitz found that the bacteria lodged in alveolar capillaries initially and then spread to involve larger vessels.[275] It might be thought that the infarctlike necrosis results from arterial occlusion, but in neither human cases nor the experimental model is thrombosis of the infarcted vessels conspicuous, and it is more likely that the necrosis is the result of the local effects of exotoxins and proteases produced by the *Pseudomonas*.

The prognosis for pseudomonal pneumonia is dire. Even with modern antibiotics, the current mortality is close to 50%. The septicemic form remains almost invariably fatal.

Escherichia coli usually reaches the lung through the

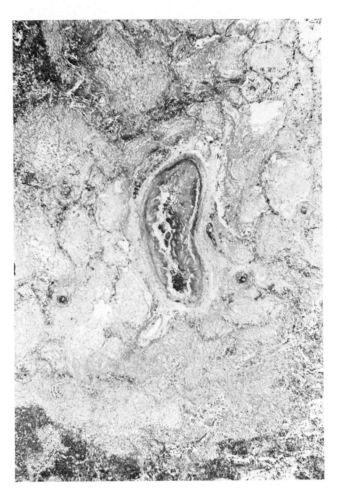

Fig. 20-13. Hematogenous *Pseudomonas* pneumonia. Nodule of infarctlike necrosis surrounded by hemorrhage. Dark haze in wall of necrotic artery *(center)* is bacteria.

bloodstream from a site of infection in the urinary or gastrointestinal tract.[267,277] Often pneumonia follows surgery. The lungs are involved by a patchy, bilateral, lower lobe pneumonia. Initially the pneumonia is hemorrhagic with pronounced edema and a scanty mononuclear exudate in alveoli. In patients surviving more than a few days, the intra-alveolar cellular exudate is more pronounced but still predominantly mononuclear. Epithelial regeneration is present focally. Typical abscess with necrosis of alveolar walls and purulent exudate develops in some cases. Empyema is common in patients surviving more than 48 hours.[277]

Legionella and related pneumonias. In the 1970s a previously unknown genus of bacteria was discovered. The first member of the genus, *Legionella pneumophila*, was recognized as the result of investigation into a highly publicized epidemic of pneumonia that struck those attending an American Legion convention in Philadelphia in July 1976 and produced 29 fatalities among the 182 persons affected.[286] The causative bacterium had previously escaped detection because of its fastidious growth requirements and failure to stain by Gram's method.[283] The Legionellaceae are slowly growing, motile bacteria, 2 to 4 μm in length, that resemble other gram-negative bacteria ultastructurally. All have a single flagellum and a high content of branched-chain fatty acids.[284] There are currently six known species, which differ in antigenicity and have a DNA sequence homology of less than 30%. Each species may have several serotypes. *L. pneumophila* causes two epidemic clinical syndromes, a pneumonia with a fairly low attack rate and significant mortality and Pontiac fever, a self-limited, influenza-like, febrile illness with a high attack rate and no mortality. *L. pneumophila* also causes sporadic community-acquired and nosocomial pneumonias.[285,289,294] Other *Legionella* species also can cause nosocomial infections but are much less frequent. Data from the Centers for Disease Control indicate that *L. pneumophila* accounts for 90% of *Legionella* infections.

Epidemics usually occur in the summer months. The organism is commonly spread by aerosols of contaminated water from showerheads, air-conditioning cooling towers, and evaporative condensers.[287] As with other infections, impaired host defenses have an important role. In the original epidemic most of those affected were cigarette smokers over 50 years of age. In hospital epidemics patients with chronic disease and especially those receiving corticosteroid therapy have been affected, whereas the members of the hospital staff who were also exposed to the source rarely became ill.[289]

Although pathologic changes are usually limited to the lungs, the onset of the disease often is that of systemic illness with high fever and constitutional symptoms accompanied by diarrhea, leukopenia, and hyponatremia. Cough, sputum production, and signs of pneumonia may not appear until the fifth to seventh days. Whether systemic manifestations are attributable to a toxin or to bacteremia is unknown.

The gross findings in the lung are those of a confluent bronchopneumonia, usually with involvement of multiple lobes.[282-284,293] Entire lobes may be consolidated, but areas of early involvement usually show a lobular distribution. Small pleural effusions and a fibrinous pleuritis are commonly present. Abscesses are unusual but may occur.[290] The histologic findings are not distinctive. The alveoli are filled with an exudate of fibrin, neutrophils, and mononuclear phagocytes in varying proportions. Most alveolar septa show only minor changes, consisting mainly of foci of hyperplasia in the alveolar lining epithelium. Thrombosis of vessels and necrosis of alveolar walls are present in some cases. In cases of long duration, organization of the intra-alveolar exudate occurs.

The organisms are weakly gram-negative bacilli or coccobacilli that are usually invisible in sections stained by the commonly used variants of Gram's stain. With Dieterle's silver stain, however, organisms are usually numerous, appearing mainly but not exclusively in the cytoplasm of phagocytes. Dieterle's stain is nonspecific, and the diagnosis should be confirmed by immunohistochemical staining with type-specific antisera. Formalin-fixed tissue is usually satisfactory.

The relentless progression and resistance to therapy of *Legionella* pneumonia is probably a consequence of the organism's ability to survive and proliferate within phagocytes. In vitro studies indicate that the organisms can reproduce within the cytoplasm of macrophages. Specific antibodies and complement promote phagocytosis but not intracellular killing. The fusion of lysosomes with phagosomes containing the bacilli is inhibited. Antibiotics such as erythromycin and rifampicin, which are effective in vivo, suppress intracellular proliferation but do not kill the organisms, which are only slowly eliminated by cellular mechanisms that are not understood.[288]

Tatlockia mcdadei, also known as the Pittsburgh pneumonia agent, is a bacterium related to *Legionella*, although serologically distinct and sharing less than 10% DNA sequence homology. The organism was originally recovered from renal transplant patients who were severely immunosuppressed and had acquired nosocomial pneumonia,[291] but it appears to be able to produce pneumonia in patients with a variety of chronic illness not specifically involving the immune system.[292] The pathologic features are similar to those of *Legionella* pneumonia, though there may be a greater tendency to abscess formation.[293] The organism is weakly acid fast and can be stained with modifications of the acid-fast stain in which 1% sulfuric acid is used to decolorize the carbol fuchsin.

Lung lesions caused by anaerobic bacteria. Anaerobic bacteria are plentiful in the oral cavity where they colonize the tissues beneath the gum margins and the tonsillar crypts.[296,298] They gain access to the lung by aspiration. Consequently the usual clinical context for anaerobic pulmonary infections is a combination of severe gingival disease (pyorrhea) and an altered state of consciousness such as occurs with alcohol intoxication, anesthesia, or a seizure disorder or other neurologic disease. In the past, anaerobic infections were seen after tonsillectomy in children, but with modern anesthetic techniques this complication is rare.

Aspiration introduces a mixed flora into the lung. In a large series of pulmonary infections by anaerobes, an average of 3.2 different species of bacteria was recovered per case.[296] Although many infections involved only anaerobes, in a nearly equal number of cases both aerobic and anaerobic bacteria were found. The most frequent organisms were anaerobic and microaerophilic streptococci, *Fusobacterium nucleatum*, and various species of *Bacteroides*.

Anaerobes cause four types of lesion: abscess, necrotizing pneumonia, pneumonitis, and empyema.[296] Aspirational lung abscesses are often called primary or simple lung abscesses to distinguish them from abscesses developing as a complication of another disease such as an obstructing lesion in a bronchus or pneumonia caused by one of the usual pathogens.[299,300] They occur most often in the posterior segments of the upper lobes, which are dependent when one is supine, and next most often in the basal segments of the lower lobes, which are dependent when one is erect. The right lung is involved more often than the left because of the straighter course of the right main-stem bronchus. The lesions are usually solitary with a cavity 2 cm to several centimeters in diameter and a shaggy, irregular lining. Often they have a dirty brown appearance and fetid odor. Occasionally the cavity may contain sloughed necrotic tissue. Microscopically the cavity is lined by a pyogenic membrane and enclosed by granulation tissue. In chronic cases there may be a well-developed fibrous capsule. Partial reepithelialization of the cavity, usually by metaplastic squamous epithelium, may occur. Large arteries and veins in the wall usually show fibrous intimal thickening and even complete obliteration of the lumen. Occasionally they may be thrombosed or necrotic.

Sequential roentgenographic observations indicate that abscesses may begin as areas of pneumonia that undergo necrosis and cavitate over a period of 1 to 3 weeks or even longer. Patients often show signs of chronicity such as weight loss or anemia. The prognosis for primary lung abscess is good, and more than 95% of patients are cured, though one or more relapses may occur before healing is finally effected. Deaths occur rarely and result either from massive hemoptysis or occasionally from extrathoracic spread of infection. The course of secondary lung abscesses is strongly influenced by the underlying disease, and the mortality is much greater than that of primary abscesses.[299]

Like primary lung abscess, necrotizing pneumonia (chronic destructive pneumonia) occurs in those with severe gingivodental disease and a predisposition to aspiration and probably represents a severe form of aspiration disease.[296] Typically more than one lobe is involved, and the process includes areas of differing age or activity. The pleura is thickened and fibrotic but highly vascularized. The lung parenchyma is consolidated with multiple cavities containing pus or sloughed necrotic tissue. Histologically there is a combination of exudative and organizing pneumonia with alveolar necrosis. The bronchi show changes ranging from acute bronchitis with ulceration to bronchiectasis.[297] The organisms responsible are the same as those causing lung abscess. The clinical picture is highly variable, ranging from asymptomatic to chronic disease with fever, anemia, and weight loss to acute fulminant pneumonia. In a large series from Africa the mortality was 7.8%, a fig-

ure comparable to contemporary North American experience.[297]

Acute pneumonitis caused by anaerobes can be difficult to distinguish from other forms of bacterial pneumonia, since the characteristic fetid sputum is absent.[295] The disease is usually of short duration and responds well to antibiotic therapy. If untreated, it would probably evolve into abscesses.

Empyema is usually associated with underlying lung abscess or pneumonia and may be associated with bronchopleural fistula. Occasionally an empyema can result from spread of anaerobes from a subphrenic abscess in the absence of lung disease.

Mycobacterial infections

The mycobacteria include *Mycobacterium tuberculosis*, the causative organism of tuberculosis; *M. leprae*, which causes leprosy; and a variety of organisms found in the environment that are normally saprophytic, though many of them are potential pathogens.[303] Of these, *M. tuberculosis* and certain of the saprophytic mycobacteria cause pulmonary disease. The term *tuberculosis* should be reserved for infections with the species *M. tuberculosis*, since infections by other mycobacteria differ from tuberculosis in their epidemiology, clinical setting, and response to therapy.

Tuberculosis. Tuberculosis is a disease of great antiquity, having been identified in mummies from the fourth millenium BC. Since it is preeminently a disease of crowded conditions, it was probably unimportant in hunter-gatherer cultures but began to appear with the development of agriculture.[325] With the Industrial Revolution it assumed epidemic importance as a cause of death and disability.[314] In 1900 at least 90% of adults in Western populations had been infected with the organism as indicated by skin test reactivity to tuberculin, though many had no clinical illness. It has been estimated that 20% of all deaths in Victorian England were attributable to tuberculosis.

With improvement of hygiene, nutrition, and social conditions, the incidence of tuberculosis fell steadily, a trend that accelerated with the development of chemotherapy in the late 1940s. The current United States annual incidence of the 9 new cases per 100,000 population is less than a third that of 25 years earlier. In 1985, however, the decline leveled off, and in 1986, for the first time, a rise was noted.[334] One factor in this sudden change in the trend is infection with the human immunodeficiency virus. AIDS patients have as much as 100 times greater risk of acquiring tuberculosis than the general population has.

Tuberculosis remains a major public health problem in the developing nations of Asia, Africa, and South America.[310] In parts of Southeast Asia and Oceania case rates of 300 to 500 per 100,000 are reported, 20 to 40 times the United States rate. In the Philippines 10% of deaths are attributable to tuberculosis.

Even in technically advanced countries tuberculosis remains a public health problem in certain populations. In the United States the incidence in nonwhites is five times that in whites, and in Britain the incidence in immigrants from India and Pakistan is 38 times that in native Britons.[323] In the United States tuberculosis remains the most common reportable disease, with an incidence greater than that of all other reportable diseases combined.

Causative organism. The mycobacteria occupy a taxonomic niche between the eubacteria and the actinomycetes.[303,337] The two principal species responsible for tuberculosis in humans are *M. tuberculosis* and *M. bovis.* They differ from each other in pathogenicity in different species of mammals, cultural requirements for optimum growth, and response to certain biochemical tests. A species isolated from patients in East Africa, *M. africanus*, has properties intermediate between the human and bovine strains.

The tubercle bacillus is a straight or curved rod, 0.2 to 0.5 by 2 to 5 μm, that is acid fast in Ziehl-Neelsen stains. It may stain uniformly but often takes on a beaded appearance. There are no free-living or saprophytic forms of *M. tuberculosis* in nature. In the laboratory the organism can be cultured on simple media. Growth is slow; the doubling time in culture is more than 12 hours, compared with 20 minutes for a typical pyogenic organism such as *E. coli.* Tubercle bacilli are strictly aerobic. Their dependence on molecular oxygen probably accounts in part for their propensity for growth in the lung and for the tendency for reactivation of infection in the apical regions where the alveolar Po_2 is highest. Biochemically *M. tuberculosis* is remarkable for the high lipid content of its cell wall, which accounts for its resistance to staining and, once stained, its resistance to decolorization with dilute acids or alkali. The complex chemistry of the cell wall lipids has been extensively investigated because several lipids have been implicated in important biologic activities of the organism. The lipids include the mycolic acids, α-alkyl-β-hydroxy fatty acids found only in the mycobacteria, corynebacteria, and nocardias. One of the mycosides, trehalose 6,6′-dimycolate, or "cord factor," is responsible for the tendency of certain strains to grow in serpiginous cords and for the antitumor activity of the organism. Other mycosides are implicated in the resistance of the organism to destruction by lysosomal enzymes. A mixture of chloroform-soluble lipids, wax D, contains the materials responsible for the immunologic adjuvant activity of *M. tuberculosis.* The immunologic activity is particularly associated with the peptidoglycan components of wax D, however, and the simplest material with adjuvant activity is the peptide *N*-acyl muramyl-L-alanyl-D-isoglutamine.

Preparations of antigens from *M. tuberculosis* are known as tuberculins.[305] After the discovery of the tubercle bacillus in 1882, Koch observed that guinea pigs exposed to killed organisms were protected against the lethal effects of a subsequent infection by living organisms. In an effort to treat tuberculous patients, he injected them with concentrates of boiled liquid cultures of tubercle bacilli, which he called "old tuberculin" (OT). Although OT was never proved to be of therapeutic benefit, Koch's observation that patients responded to injections of OT with a greater inflammatory reaction than uninfected subjects did has been of great diagnostic usefulness and is the basis for the tuberculin skin test.

A positive response to the tuberculin skin test demonstrates the presence of delayed hypersensitivity to one or more antigens in an extract of proteins from a culture of tubercle bacilli and reflects past or present infection with an organism bearing those antigens. It does not necessarily indicate the presence of disease, since the hypersensitivity persists after the healing of all active lesions. Although the tuberculins most often used currently are more refined than OT, they are still mixtures of many antigens, some of which are shared by saprophytic mycobacteria.[305] Consequently exposure to these mycobacteria can lead to false-positive reactions.

Eleven major antigens and several minor antigens are present in tuberculins. One aim of current research is to purify these antigens from tuberculins prepared from various species of mycobacteria in hopes that some will prove species specific.[305]

Transmission. The organism can be transmitted by inhalation, by ingestion, or rarely by direct implantation. A fetus can be infected in utero transplacentally. Patients with active pulmonary disease are the major source of human infection, and inhalation is overwhelmingly the most frequent route.[313,326] Droplets containing one or a few organisms become airborne during coughing, speaking, or even singing; the fluid phase evaporates, leaving particles called droplet nuclei that range from 1 to 5 μm in diameter, small enough to remain suspended in room air for hours. This size produces maximum retention in the acini of the lung. Indeed, single organisms have been demonstrated experimentally to produce infection in rabbits if inhaled on 1 to 5 μm particles, whereas aggregates of several hundred organisms may be noninfectious because they form particles larger than 10 μm, which impact on the mucus coating the walls of the large bronchi and are cleared by ciliary activity.[315]

Both the human and the bovine varieties of *Mycobacterium* can be spread by ingestion, and in the past the ingestion of raw milk from cows with tuberculosis mastitis was the usual mode of transmission of the bovine type. Although bovine tuberculosis was responsible for approximately 20% of tuberculosis in 1917, it has ceased to be a public health problem because of tuberculin testing of cattle and pasteurization of milk. Entry was either through the tonsils or more commonly through the small intestine, with spread to the cervical or mesenteric lymph nodes respectively. The gastrointestinal tract is more resistant to infection than the lung as evidenced both by animal studies and by the rarity with which tuberculous enteritis develops in patients who swallow large numbers of organisms in their sputum.

Transplacental infection of a fetus is rare, occurring when the mother has the miliary type of tuberculosis. The fetus is surprisingly resistant to infection and may remain free of lesions even in the presence of severe placental disease.

Susceptibility. Tuberculosis is a disease of the economically disadvantaged. Crowded living conditions and poor nutrition are predisposing factors.[313,314] In addition, breeding experiments with rabbits have shown that there is a genetic influence on susceptibility to the disease.[316] Racial differences in the incidence of tuberculosis are no doubt attributable largely to socioeconomic factors though inherent, presumably genetic, influences are involved. Jews appear to have a high natural resistance, probably because of natural selection over the centuries in the crowded urban ghettos of Europe. However, blacks, Native Americans, and Eskimos are particularly susceptible because crowded living conditions are relatively recent in their histories and they were spared the selective influence of extensive exposure to the organism. Resistance is also lowered by certain diseases, notably silicosis and diabetes mellitus, and by gastrectomy and corticosteroid therapy.

Immunity and hypersensitivity. Tubercle bacilli produce no known toxins.[313] The tissue changes caused by infection result from the host response to the organisms.[304] It has been known since the time of Koch that the tissue response varies in its severity and tempo of development between an animal with no prior contact with tubercle bacilli and an animal that was previously infected. When Koch injected bacilli into naïve guinea pigs, a localized nodule appeared at the injection site 10 days to 2 weeks later, ulcerated, and healed poorly. Tubercles appeared in the draining lymph nodes. When tubercle bacilli were injected into the skin of an animal that had been infected with tuberculosis 4 to 6 weeks earlier, an area of induration appeared at the inoculation site and grew to a diameter of 1 cm or more within 2 to 4 days. The skin over the site underwent necrosis and ulcerated but then went on to heal. Spread to the regional nodes failed to occur. In short, the previously infected animal has altered responsiveness or hypersensitivity: the altered response is more rapid and

vigorous and is accompanied by necrosis. On the other hand, growth of organisms is restrained, and the spread of infection is prevented. The animals have acquired relative resistance. Koch also showed that tuberculin (OT) could be used instead of living organisms to elicit the hypersensitivity response. The relationship between hypersensitivity and resistance has long been a matter of contention.[315] They are closely related. Antibodies play little role in either process. Lymphoid cells from a tuberculin-sensitive animal will transfer both hypersensitivity and resistance to a normal animal. It is now well established that both properties are transferred with specifically sensitized T-lymphocytes. These T-cells respond to the specific antigens in tuberculin with the elaboration of lymphokines that bring about an enhanced ability of the macrophages to kill intracellular parasites, including tubercle bacilli. The macrophages enlarge and develop increased levels of lysosomal enzymes, enhanced spreading activity on surfaces, and increased production of H_2O_2 and other oxidants that possess antimicrobial activity. The T-lymphocyte responds only to the specific sensitizing antigen. The induced change in the macrophage is nonspecific. Tubercle bacilli are only one of a number of microbes whose killing by the macrophages is enhanced.[318]

Some authors regard hypersensitivity as inseparable from resistance. According to this view, the presence of sensitized T-cells is beneficial when the dose of organisms is modest as with a new airborne infection or when small numbers of organisms are released from a tuberculous focus in the body. Under these conditions the macrophages are activated to engulf and dispatch the organisms with an enhanced release of oxidants and lysosomal enzymes. With massive stimulation when a very large dose of organisms is encountered, there is an overproduction of these same oxidants and hydrolases with resultant tissue damage, exudation, and necrosis. Other authors have shown that animals can be desensitized locally to the tuberculin skin test without destroying systemic resistance to infection. They argue that this militates against the view that hypersensitivity and resistance are inseparable phenomena. The answer will become clearer when it is known whether the same T-cell subsets and mediators are responsible for both hypersensitivity and resistance.[315]

As a rule hypersensitivity and enhanced resistance to infection persist for many years after a clinical infection and not uncommonly they last lifelong. This may be attributable to the persistence of small numbers of organisms in apparently healed lesions. Hypersensitivity to tuberculin may disappear after many years, perhaps because of slow attrition among specifically sensitized T-cells if organisms have disappeared. In the presence of overwhelming infection or in the terminal stages of a chronic tuberculous infection, there may also be loss of tuberculin skin reactivity, or anergy. Several mechanisms have been invoked to explain this relatively infrequent phenomenon: that very large doses of tuberculoprotein activitate suppressor cell populations, that sensitized T-cells may be recruited from the skin to sites of active lesions in the viscera, or that high endogenous antigen burdens may saturate or downregulate the available receptors.[305]

Tissue response to tubercle bacilli. The characteristic tissue response to tuberculosis is the granuloma, a compact organized collection of macrophages.[304] In a previously uninfected animal or human the earliest response to the presence of bacilli in the tissue is an influx of inflammatory cells, both polymorphonuclear leukocytes and mononuclear phagocytes that engulf the organisms. The organisms are resistant to killing by the phagocytes, attributable in part to their ability to inhibit lysosome-phagosome fusion. They proliferate intracellularly, eventually killing the phagocytes. In time, mononuclear cells come to predominate in the inflammatory infiltrate and begin to form aggregates. The organisms continue to proliferate, and as macrophages containing organisms degenerate and die, new mononuclear phagocytes enter the tissue and take up the liberated organisms. Thus there is a continuous and high turnover of mononuclear phagocytes. Some of the replacement of phagocytes takes place by proliferation of local tissue macrophages, but the majority are monocytes that enter the tissue from the circulation and divide once or twice locally as they differentiate into mature macrophages. The monocytes enlarge, their nucleus becomes eccentric, their cytoplasm more abundant, and they tend to aggregate first into loose sheets of cells and then more tightly into spherical aggregates. The cells composing these aggregates or granulomas develop eccentric vesicular nuclei and abundant pale cytoplasm. Although the cells initially remain distinct, later their cytoplasm borders become indistinct when viewed with the light microscope; with the electron microscope this is seen to be attributable to the close interlocking of the pseudopodia of neighboring cells. These characteristic mononuclear cells are called epithelioid cells because they are closely packed like epithelium without interposed connective tissue. They are not joined by junctional complexes, do not closely resemble epithelium morphologically, and of course are the progeny of monocytes, not epithelium. Epithelioid cells are characterized by their well-developed granular endoplasmic reticulum, as well as numerous lysosomes and high levels of lysosomal enzyme activity. They are less actively phagocytic than typical macrophages, and it has been suggested that they are macrophages specialized for secretory functions as well as for the degradation and destruction of microbes. A striking feature of the granulomas of tuberculosis and many other granulomas is the presence of multinucleated cells. Some

multinucleated cells have their nuclei evenly dispersed in the cytoplasm. These cells are called foreign body giant cells, since they are similar in appearance to the giant cells that frequently enclose foreign material in tissues. Other giant cells called Langhans' giant cells have their nuclei disposed in a ring surrounding an eosinophilic cytocenter. Both types of giant cells, formed by the fusion of several epithelioid cells, are commonly found in epithelioid granulomas irrespective of their cause.

As the granuloma matures, it becomes surrounded by lymphocytes, plasma cells, capillaries, and fibroblasts (Fig. 20-14). Between 4 and 6 weeks after infection, necrosis begins to appear in the granulomas, the surrounding tissue may become edematous, and the number of organisms begins to diminish. The necrosis is termed caseation because its dry crumbly appearance resembles cheese. Microscopically the necrosis is granular and eosinophilic and contains nuclear debris. The outlines of the cells are usually not evident, in contrast to the coagulation necrosis of infarcts. The reticulin and

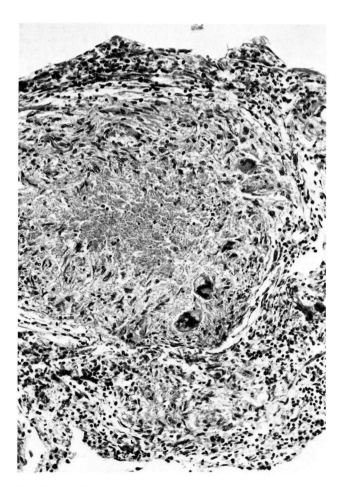

Fig. 20-14. Well-developed tubercle with caseous center surrounded by epithelioid histiocytes and giant cells. Mantle of lymphocytes, plasma cells, and monocytes surrounds epithelioid cell zone.

elastic fibers in the tissue initially remain intact, however, and can be demonstrated with appropriate stains. The appearance of necrosis and edema and the decrease in organisms correspond temporally with the development of a positive reaction to the tuberculin skin test and reflect the host's acquisition of delayed hypersensitivity.

The granuloma can follow several possible courses. The low pH and oxygen tension in the necrotic caseous center are not favorable for the rapid proliferation of bacilli. Usually the number of organisms continues to decrease and a fibrous capsule forms in the surrounding zone of nonspecific inflammation. The encapsulated granuloma becomes quiescent, the inflammatory cells decrease in number, and calcium salts are usually deposited in the caseous material. Sometimes the calcium is deposited in concentric laminations known as Liesegang rings. After several years, organisms completely disappear and the contents of the granuloma are no longer infective if injected into a guinea pig.

If the organisms are particularly virulent or resistance

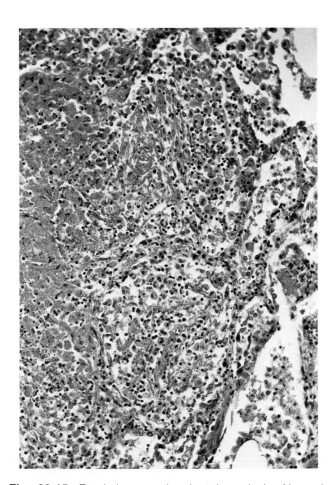

Fig. 20-15. Exudative reaction in tuberculosis. Necrosis and exudation of monocytes and macrophages without development of encapsulated granuloma.

is low, the granuloma may continue to enlarge by centrifugal growth. Satellite granulomas may form, grow, and coalesce with the original granuloma. At any time this process may cease and the lesions become arrested. Occasionally in one or more granulomas the caseous center liquefies, acquiring a more fluid, puslike consistency, mainly through the agency of proteases and other hydrolases produced by the epithelioid cells and macrophages of the granuloma.[306] When the contents of the granuloma liquefy, rapid extracellular growth of organisms ensues and the stage is set for the dissemination of disease.

The events after the introduction of a large dose of tubercle bacilli into the tissue of a highly sensitized person differ from the proliferative granuloma just described. The reaction is greatly accelerated, with a rapid outpouring of fibrin and edema, an increased influx of neutrophils and monocytes, and the more rapid and extensive development of necrosis. This is termed the "exudative response" (Fig. 20-15).

Natural history[302,307,321,337]

PRIMARY COMPLEX. The initial tissue response in the nonimmune host is similar regardless of the site of infection and involves the development of granulomas at the portal of entry and the formation of a secondary focus in the draining lymph nodes, the combination being known as the primary complex. In the majority of instances the primary complex involves foci in the lung and hilar lymph nodes, but it may involve tonsil and cervical nodes or intestine and mesenteric nodes in the case of ingested bacilli.

The initial infection in the lung is caused by the deposition of organisms in the acini at one or more sites. The primary, or Ghon's, focus may develop anywhere in the lung, though usually it is within 1 cm of the pleura and not infrequently in a lower lobe where the ventilation is greater and deposition is more likely. The process probably begins as a focus of tuberculous pneumonia with some edema, fibrin, and an influx of neutrophils and mononuclear phagocytes. Some organisms or perhaps phagocytes containing engulfed bacilli reach the lymphatics and are transported to the hilar lymph nodes where they set up a secondary focus. Additional lesions may be present along the pathway of the lymphatic drainage in the lung. The primary focus in the lung usually remains less than a centimeter in size and evolves into a typical granuloma with caseation. Over several weeks or months the lesion becomes encapsulated with fibrous tissue and the necrotic contents calcify. After many years ossification may occur. The lymph node focus generally follows a parallel course. The lymph node focus is almost invariably larger than the primary parenchymal focus and heals more slowly, but it too usually undergoes eventual encapsulation and calcification.

During the early evolution of the primary complex,

spread may occur to adjacent nodes, even reaching the superior mediastinal nodes or the nodes of the upper abdomen. A few bacilli commonly escape through the lymphatics to the venous system whence they are taken up in the reticuloendothelial organs, liver, spleen, or bone marrow where small granulomas are established and subsequently heal. Hematogenous seeding of the lungs can result in the establishment of a new caseous focus (Simon's focus), which is distinct from the primary complex and is usually near the apex where the oxygen tension is high.

Despite the acquisition of resistance in the form of improved bacterial killing by macrophages, bacilli may remain in the acellular caseous centers of pulmonary or systemic granulomas. Such bacilli may remain dormant for months, years, or decades, becoming activated at any time by a breakdown in local immunity.

PROGRESSIVE PRIMARY TUBERCULOSIS. The pattern of transient growth, spread to lymph nodes, and subsequent encapsulation and healing of lesions is the natural history of primary tuberculous infection followed by more than 90% of patients. Symptoms are mild and nonspecific, and most primary infections pass unrecognized. In a few patients, because of some combination of increased virulence of the organism, increased hypersensitivity, and low resistance, the primary infection is progressive. In some cases the primary focus in the lung continues to grow, and caseation outstrips the rate of epithelioid cell formation and encapsulation. The caseous material may liquefy, and the liquefied material containing bacilli may become disseminated through the bronchi to other regions of the same lung and op-

posite lung. The dissemination of large numbers of bacteria produces a reaction of exudation of fibrin, neutrophils, and monocytes followed by the appearance of necrosis. More commonly dissemination occurs when the enlarged hilar lymph nodes undergoing necrosis and liquefaction erode a bronchus resulting in the discharge of caseous material containing organisms. If the number of organisms is large and hypersensitivity is pronounced, the ensuing exudative reaction may further spread the organisms, resulting in caseous pneumonia (Fig. 20-16). Finally, if erosion of a blood vessel occurs, the dissemination of large numbers of bacteria hematogenously can result in the establishment of numerous tiny foci of tuberculosis in many organs, a form of the disease known as miliary tuberculosis (after millet

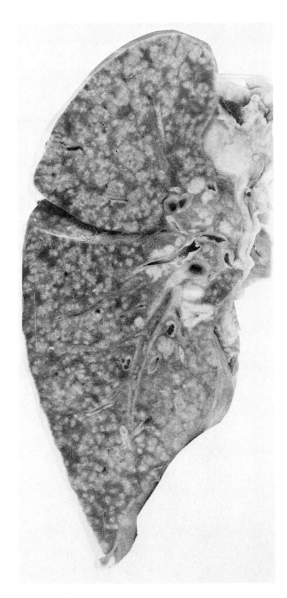

Fig. 20-17. Miliary tuberculosis. (From pathological museum of University of Manchester, U.K.)

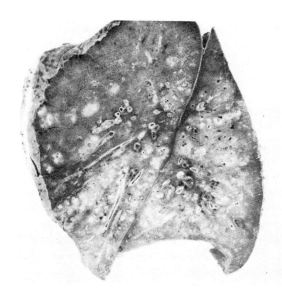

Fig. 20-16. Lung of child with a few tubercles in upper lobe and confluent areas of tuberculous pneumonia in middle and lower lobes. (From pathological museum of University of Manchester, U.K.)

seeds, which like the granulomas of severe hematogenously spread tuberculosis are 1 to 2 mm in diameter). Miliary granulomas can occur in any site but are most numerous in the liver, spleen, kidneys, bone marrow, brain, and lungs (Fig. 20-17). Although the various forms of progressive primary tuberculosis are serious and indeed life threatening, they may become arrested, undergo encapsulation, and heal as a result of therapy or the spontaneous development of resistance.

POSTPRIMARY TUBERCULOSIS. It is not unusual for tuberculosis to develop in adults who have been tuberculin positive for many years without evidence of clinical disease. Phthisiologists have long argued whether the new active disease is the result of a new exogenous infection or recrudescence of dormant foci. There is no reason to doubt that both occur. Stead[331] has argued persuasively on the basis of epidemiologic evidence that

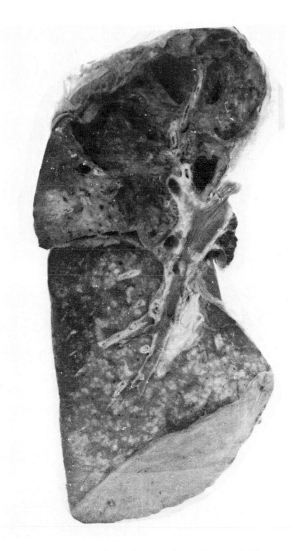

Fig. 20-18. Advanced cavitary tuberculosis. Entire upper lobe is destroyed. There are foci of acinous spread in lower lobe. (From pathological museum of University of Manchester, U.K.)

endogenous reactivation is the more important mechanism. In a retrospective review of published data on more than 14,000 subjects, he found only a slightly higher incidence of disease in tuberculin-positive persons (medical and nursing students) who had frequent contact with patients with active lesions than in tuberculin-positive controls with only sporadic exposure. Among tuberculin-negative persons, the highly exposed group had five times the incidence of their controls. However, when phage typing has been used to determine whether postprimary disease is attributable to a new strain, a new strain has been detected in 10% to 20% of cases, depending on the population studied.[319,327]

In most cases, postprimary tuberculosis is first detected in the subapical region of one or both lungs, perhaps caused by spread of viable bacteria from a Simon's focus.

The disease starts as a small area of lobular tuberculous pneumonia characterized by intra-alveolar exudate of fibrin, neutrophils, and monocytes. This area can undergo one of several courses. At this stage while the lesion is still intra-alveolar, it may resolve completely. It may progress slowly to the development of epithelioid granulomas, which gradually caseate in the center but remain encapsulated by epithelioid cells and capillaries and proliferating fibrous tissue. The granulomas may follow an irregular course, some healing and calcifying whereas others grow for a while, stimulating continuing fibrosis. If the original area of pneumonia undergoes necrosis, the entire area may become encapsulated or it may undergo liquefaction and slough through a patent bronchus, giving rise to a cavity (Fig. 20-18).

The formation of a cavity is an important development. The bacteria in the lining of the cavity proliferate, probably because of the higher PO_2 than in necrotic tissue. The cavity's communication with the bronchial tree makes it an important source for spread of organisms elsewhere in the lung. When small amounts of caseous material are released from a cavity, they may be cleared harmlessly by the mucociliary mechanism and swallowed or may be aspirated into alveoli in the more dependent areas of the lung. If the dose of organisms is small, organisms reaching the alveoli set up minute new foci of tuberculous pneumonia, filling air spaces clustered about terminal bronchioles and called "acinous lesions" (Fig. 20-18). If the number of organisms is large and the degree of hypersensitivity great, aspiration of infected debris produces a severe exudative reaction with an outpouring of edema, fibrin, polymorphonuclear cells, and monocytes. This rapidly progresses to necrosis, a condition known as caseous pneumonia.

Cavities in tuberculosis are generally spherical and may have a thick wall or very little encapsulation depending on their age and rate of growth. The lining appears trabeculated because of the persistence of obliterated cordlike blood vessels. If only part of the original necrotic focus becomes liquefied, remnants of necrotic lung may also be present. Microscopically the lining of cavities typically is heterogeneous with areas of caseous necrosis with nuclear debris and organisms, pyogenic membrane of fibrin and inflammatory exudate, and granulation tissue where epithelioid cells in variable numbers are accompanied by capillaries and fibroblasts. A capsule of nonspecific fibrous tissue of variable thickness encloses the cavity. The cavity can grow by continuing necrosis or the incorporation of surrounding granulomas. Should the bronchial opening become plugged or obliterated, the necrotic contents of the cavity become inspissated, the air is absorbed, and the necrotic material remains encapsulated or eventually becomes organized into a stellate scar. Cavities that remained open rarely healed before the availability of specific antibacterial therapy. Because of this, interventions such as artificial pneumothorax or thoracoplasty were used in the past to bring about closure of the cavity. With adequate chemotherapy, open healing can occur. The cavity remains open, but the necrotic tissue, pyogenic membrane, and granulation tissue organize, leaving a fibrous wall that becomes partly or completely reepithelialized.[333]

The complications of cavities are aneurysms of the arteries that cross the cavity and extension to the pleura. Although most of the vessels in the cavity wall are obliterated, the lumen of a few may persist. Destruction of the vessel wall leads to aneurysm formation, which can cause hemoptysis and even lethal hemorrhage. Extension to the pleura can lead to bronchopleural fistula. The seeding of caseous material onto the pleural surface in a hypersensitive person leads to an acute exudative reaction with effusion or tuberculous empyema.

Just as late reactivation of primary tuberculosis occurs in the lung, activation can occur in any site in which seeding of organisms has occurred during the initial infection.[329] The pathologic features of tuberculosis in other organs are discussed in chapters dealing with those organs. Nonetheless, the lung remains the most common site of reactivation, a fact usually attributed to its higher oxygen tension. Generalized or miliary tuberculosis resulting from hematogenous spread of the organism can occur from a pulmonary or extrapulmonary source. Whereas formerly miliary tuberculosis occurred mainly in children, it is now being seen increasingly in the elderly as a manifestation of postprimary disease.

Clinical considerations. Given the potential variation in organ distribution, pathologic forms, and rate of evolution of tuberculosis, it is not surprising that the clinical manifestations are protean. In one recent series involving only 41 cases, patients were admitted to seven different clinical services and in nearly half the disease was initially misdiagnosed.[317]

Tuberculosis is now seen in an older population than formerly, most patients being over 40 years of age.[311,317] Symptoms are usually referable to the lungs (cough) or are systemic (fatigue, sweats, weight loss, fever). The initial chest roentgenogram shows classical apical changes in only two thirds of cases of pulmonary tuberculosis; in the remaining cases the roentgenographic manifestations are atypical, including such nonspecific changes as pleural effusion, solitary nodule, infiltrates in unusual locations, and miliary infiltrates.[311] As the disease becomes less common, the proportion of patients with primary tuberculosis can be expected to increase and the proportion of atypical presentations will also increase.

The course of active tuberculosis is extremely variable and in fatal cases ranges from weeks to years. Auerbach,[302] writing of the preantibiotic and early antibiotic era, gives the average duration as 1 to 2 years with wide variations. Death is usually from pulmonary insufficiency, or general sepsis in the case of miliary tuberculosis.

Disease caused by nontuberculous mycobacteria. Mycobacteria other than *M. tuberculosis* are widely distributed in nature and infrequently cause disease though several species are potentially pathogenic. The widely used classification of Runyon based on pigment production and growth rate has been superseded by classifications in which the organisms are grouped according to biochemical and antigenic similarities.[336] The major pathogenic groups include the following:

1. Slow-growing potential pathogens
   a. *M. avium-intracellulare*
   b. *M. scrofulaceum*
   c. *M. kansasii*
   d. *M. marinum*
2. Rapidly growing potential pathogens
   a. *M. fortuitum*
   b. *M. chelonei*

The nontuberculous or "atypical" mycobacteria are less fastidious than *M. tuberculosis* in their requirements for growth, which accounts for their ability to survive in such environments as soil, swimming pools, milk, and water taps, as well as in animals. Humans appear to acquire the organisms from the environment, and person-to-person transmission rarely if ever occurs. Familial cases can usually be explained by exposure to a common source. The organisms often colonize humans as saprophytes, and unlike the situation with *M. tuberculosis*, isolation of an atypical mycobacterium from a clinical specimen is not presumptive evidence of a pathogenic process. Disease should be attributed to nontuberculous mycobacteria when there are moderate or large numbers of organisms, multiple isolations of the same strain of mycobacterium over an extended period, a compatible clinical and roentgenographic picture, and the absence of another pathogen that would account for the condition. Isolation of atypical mycobacteria from cultures of tissue obtained under sterile conditions is also significant if the tissue contains lesions consistent with infection.

Infection with the atypical mycobacteria usually involves the lung in adults or the cervical lymph nodes in young children.[336] *M. ulcerans* and *M. marinum* produce skin infections. Osseous, renal, and meningeal disease also occur, and in the immunosuppressed patient a picture similar to miliary tuberculosis may develop.

Pulmonary infection commonly occurs in subjects with underlying chronic lung disease such as pneumoconiosis, chronic airflow limitation, bronchiectasis, or healed tuberculosis.[328] In one third of cases there is no predisposing lung disease. Men are affected three times as often as women. The majority of cases are associated with *M. kansasii*, *M. avium-intracellulare*, and *M. scrofulaceum*. Other organisms are much less common.

The pathogenesis of atypical mycobacterial infections is not well understood. Whether there is a phase analogous to the primary complex in tuberculosis has not been established. Common clinical presentations are with a solitary nodule or with upper lobe infiltrates that are frequently cavitary. It has been suggested that thin-walled cavities are more characteristic of atypical infection than of tuberculosis, but this difference is not a reliable way to distinguish the diseases.

The histologic response to the atypical mycobacteria in the lung is indistinguishable from that of tuberculosis.[320,322,330] The granulomas are similar, and caseation occurs commonly in infection with atypical mycobacteria despite their low virulence. In sections stained with the acid-fast stain the presence of large (20 μm), beaded, curved bacilli probably indicates *M. kansasii*,[330] but etiologic diagnosis ultimately rests on the results of culture. The histologic features of the cavities are similar to those of tuberculosis. Endobronchial granulomas are observed more commonly in infection by atypical mycobacteria than in tuberculosis, but the difference is not absolute. Atypical mycobacteria have been isolated from lungs that histologically showed only organizing pneumonia, without granulomas, but their etiologic role is unproved.

Although *M. kansasii* is sensitive to rifampin, the other mycobacteria are relatively resistant to antibiotics. Because of this, organisms may persist for years even when therapy is continued. Nevertheless, the lesions often remain of constant size or progress only very slowly. Death can result from pulmonary insufficiency but often is a consequence of underlying chronic disease.

Mycobacterial infections in acquired immunodeficiency syndrome

M. tuberculosis frequently produces infection in AIDS. The manifestations are severe and atypical. Of tubercular AIDS patients, 50% to 70% have predominantly extrapulmonary infection compared to 15% in tuberculosis in the population at large. Mediastinal and hilar lymph node enlargement are conspicuous and pulmonary lesions occur in atypical locations such as the lower lung fields. Because of the depressed cell-mediated immunity, the tuberculin skin test is usually nonreactive, and some patients fail to form granulomas.[332]

Infection with *Mycobacterium avium-intracellulare* is so common in AIDS that it is used by the Centers for Disease Control as a diagnostic criterion for AIDS. It occurs late in the course of the disease usually as a disseminated infection with involvement of lymph nodes, bone marrow, and reticuloendothelial organs.[335] Blood cultures are often positive. Because pulmonary involvement is unusual, the portal of entry may be the gastrointestinal tract rather than the respiratory tract.[312] Affected organs are enlarged, and either show no obvious gross lesions or contain miliary nodules.[312] Histologically affected tissues are infiltrated with foamy histiocytes with weakly basophilic cytoplasm (Fig. 20-19). Intracellular organisms are often numerous. Epithelioid cells and necrosis are rare. When the lung is affected, the lesions are usually interstitial infiltrates in perivascular spaces and the walls of airways.

Fungal infections

See Chapter 10.

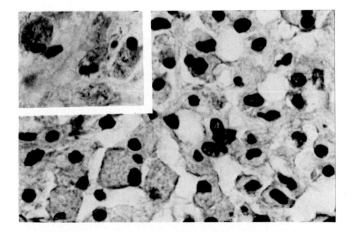

Fig. 20-19. *Mycobacterium avium* infection in AIDS. Mediastinal lymph node infiltrated with foamy macrophages, which have failed to develop into epithelioid cells or to form granulomas. *Inset,* Acid-fast stain shows bacilli in macrophages.

Pneumocystis carinii pneumonia

Pneumocystis carinii is an organism, usually classified as a sporozoon, that causes pneumonia in children and adults who are debilitated or immunosuppressed.[349,351] The biologic features of the organism are not well understood. It is probably widespread in the environment, since more than two thirds of normal children develop antibodies to the organism by 4 years of age.[347] *Pneumocystis* may be able to colonize the lung without causing disease. In rabbits and rats treated with corticosteroids, interstitial pneumonia containing *Pneumocystis* organisms occur, indicating widespread latent infection in these species.

Infection with *Pneumocystis* was recognized during World War II in Europe, where it caused a characteristic pneumonia in infants who had been born prematurely.[350] The pneumonia was characterized by a heavy infiltration of the interstitium of the lung with plasma cells and a frothy intra-alveolar exudate.[350] This form of infection, known as "interstitial plasma cell pneumonia," is now rarely seen in developed countries, and the wartime cases can probably be explained by malnutrition rampant at the time.

Currently *Pneumocystis* pneumonia is seen mainly in the immunosuppressed patients, either as an isolated infection or in combination with disease caused by other agents such as cytomegalovirus. A variety of immune defects predispose to *Pneumocystis* pneumonia, including agammaglobulinemia, malnutrition, and the complex immunosuppression produced by steroids, antineoplastic drugs, or regimens used in transplantation.[349,351] *Pneumocystis* pneumonia has been recognized as one of the characteristic infections of the acquired immunodeficiency syndrome (AIDS).[337,338] Infection is limited to the lungs in most cases, but rare instances of systemic dissemination have been documented.[340]

The development of *Pneumocystis* pneumonia is manifested clinically by the rapid onset of dyspnea, tachypnea, and cyanosis, sometimes accompanied by mild nonproductive cough. There are few physical signs, but the chest roentgenogram usually shows diffuse alveolar and interstitial infiltrates. Less often, localized densities are seen. The lungs in typical cases are firm and heavy. The pleura is blue-gray and without exudate. Interlobular septa are edematous. The cut surface of the lung is dusky and uniform. The typical histologic picture is an interstitial pneumonitis with thickening and mononuclear infiltration of the alveolar walls and hyperplasia of the epithelium.[348,352] The alveolar spaces are filled with a characteristic frothy exudate, which is eosinophilic or amphophilic with round holes up to 6 or 8 μm in diameter. Some of the holes contain one or a few weakly basophilic dots no more than 1 μm in diameter. The histologic findings may be atypical in up to half the cases, showing diffuse alveolar damage with hyaline membranes, nonspecific interstitial pneumonia, or even granulomas.[352] Organisms can most easily be seen in sections stained with Gomori's methenamine-silver or sulfonated toluidine blue, which stain the cysts. Giemsa or Gram's stain demonstrates the intracystic bodies in imprints or clinical fluids but is difficult to interpret on sections. In sections the cysts are 4 to 6 μm in diameter and often appear collapsed or cup shaped. The absence of budding helps distinguish the organisms from fungi.

A tentative life cycle for the organism has been suggested by electron microscopy[338,339,342,343] and observations of cells cultured on chick embryo epithelium in vitro.[346] Organisms occur as free trophozoites and as cysts containing up to eight intracystic bodies. The vegetative trophozoites are ameboid organisms 1.5 to 2 μm in diameter. In culture they attach to the epithelial cells by short filopodia through which they are apparently obtain nutrients. They grow to form large 2 to 5 μm trophozoites that cantain abundant glycogen. Large trophozoites begin to encyst by laying down a cyst wall. After fission of the nucleus the cytoplasm divides, giving rise to the eight sporozoites or intracystic bodies. These are then liberated from the cyst through one or more pores as small trophozoites. In culture the entire life cycle requires 4 to 6 hours. The characteristic frothy exudate seen with light microscopy consists of organisms enmeshed in pellicular material, fibrin, and alveolar secretions, including a form of surfactant.

BRONCHIECTASIS

Bronchiectasis is irreversible dilatation of the bronchi. It is accompanied by infection of the bronchial wall and frequently by obliteration of distal airways. It occurs in several clinical settings: (1) after damage to the bronchi by acute infection, especially early in life, (2) distal to a lesion that produces occlusion of a major bronchus, such as a tumor, foreign body, or lymph node involved by granulomas, (3) in a heterogeneous group of conditions in which bronchial antibacterial defense mechanisms are defective, such as agammaglobulinemia, immotile cilia syndrome, and cystic fibrosis, (4) as a manifestation of allergy to certain molds (see p. 964), and (5) after inhalation of certain toxic gases.

Commonly postinfectious bronchiectasis has its onset in childhood or early adult life.[358] In over half the patients the onset follows an overt episode of infection, but in some 30% of cases the onset is insidious. In the past, pertussis, measles, and scarlet fever were prominent as antecedent infections, but as these have become rare, adenovirus infection has assumed importance. Although bronchiectasis may be asymptomatic, most patients seek medical attention because of cough, expectoration of fetid sputum, recurrent bouts of chest infection, or hemoptysis. The majority of patients have sinusitis, and many have clubbing of the fingers.

The distribution of bronchiectasis after infection has never been satisfactorily explained. Characteristically one or a few segments are involved, whereas the rest are normal. The left lung is involved in three fourths of cases. The posterior basal segment is almost invariably involved, and the remaining two basal segments and the two lingular segments all have a high frequency of disease. Right lung involvement is relatively uncommon.[358]

The disease characteristically affects the first three generations of bronchi beyond the segmental bronchi; it is usually impossible to trace the bronchi past the fourth to sixth generations.[355,358] The more distal airways are obliterated. The affected bronchi are dilated nearly to the pleura, irregular in contour, and filled with mucus or more commonly mucopus (Fig. 20-20). The walls may be thickened or, in dilated saccules, abnormally thinned. The normal longitudinal ridges are replaced by transverse mucosal folds. Some authors have subclassified bronchiectasis as saccular or cylindrical according to its gross or bronchographic configura-

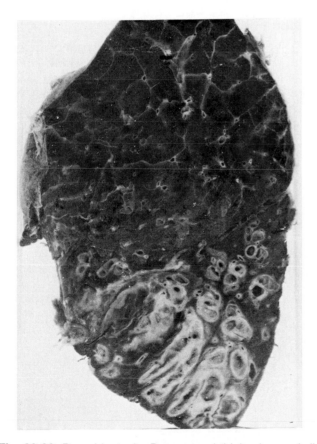

Fig. 20-20. Bronchiectasis. Pronounced thickening and dilatation of lower lobe bronchi. (From pathological museum of University of Manchester, U.K.)

tion, and others by a combination of histologic and gross features,[358] but the value of such subclasses is still not established.

Microscopically the bronchial epithelium may be normal or ulcerated or show mucous hyperplasia or squamous metaplasia. In the wall are varying degrees of chronic inflammation, fibrosis, and destruction of normal elements. The muscle and elastic tissue are destroyed and replaced by fibrosis, and often the cartilage is also replaced. Sometimes lymphocytic infiltrate is conspicuous and germinal centers are present. Whitwell[358] has termed this "variant follicular bronchiectasis." The lung adjacent to the ectatic bronchus usually shows fibrosis.

The distribution of bronchiectasis distal to an obstruction varies depending on the cause of the obstruction. Bronchiectasis caused by compression of the bronchus by granulomatous lymph nodes is most common in the right middle lobe because the right middle lobe bronchus is relatively long and its origin is surrounded by nodes that are wedged against it by the lower lobe bronchi. The nodes at this location receive drainage from both the lower and the middle lobes, contributing to the frequency with which they are involved as part of a primary tuberculous complex. In addition to extrinsic compression, the bronchus may be obstructed by erosion of a calcified granuloma into the bronchus to form a broncholith.

Pathogenesis

Bronchiectasis results from damage to the bronchial wall, which permits the establishment of smoldering infection with destruction of the muscle and elastic tissue, and from increased traction on the bronchial wall caused by changes in the surrounding parenchyma. Varying combinations of collapse, organizing pneumonia, and obliteration of small airways result in poorly compliant lung parenchyma that efficiently transmits the negative pleural pressure to the peribronchial tissue while at the same time the inflammation and resultant destruction of muscle and elastic tissue render the bronchial wall vulnerable to the increased mechanical forces. Once dilated and distorted, the bronchi tend to retain secretions that serve as a nidus of continuing infection. A variety of organisms can be recovered from bronchiectatic secretions, including various species of streptococci, *Haemophilus influenzae*, *Staphylococcus aureus*, and anaerobic mycoplasmas.[357]

Natural history

The introduction of antibiotics has not only lowered the incidence of bronchiectasis but also dramatically changed its natural history. In the preantibiotic era almost all patients with bronchiectasis died of suppurative infections or rarely complications thereof such as amyloidosis, the majority of deaths occurring before 40 years of age. Currently, bronchiectatic patients die at an average of 55 years, as often from a condition unrelated to bronchiectasis as one related to it. Respiratory failure caused by chronic airflow obstruction and cor pulmonale, rather than suppurative infection, are currently the important related causes of death.[356] However, 80% of patients with bronchiectasis have no greater annual loss of pulmonary function than normal controls do.[354] Accelerated decline in pulmonary function appears to be related to long bouts of lower respiratory infection.[353]

Immotile cilia syndrome

In the immotile cilia syndrome, airway clearance mechanisms are defective because of any of a variety of structural defects in the axoneme, the internal machinery of the cilium. The axoneme is formed by nine peripheral doublet microtubules surrounding two central single microtubules together with several accessory structures. Arranged in rows along each doublet are paired side arms that contain dynein, an ATPase. The beating of the cilia is powered by ATP and produced by sliding shear generated by the dynein arms, which is converted into bending waves by rows of radial spokes that project from each doublet toward projections attached to the central microtubule pair.[362]

In the immotile cilia syndrome the cilia are either completely inactive or beat slowly and ineffectively. Clearance of radiolabeled aerosols from airways is absent except during coughing. The following abnormalities of axonemes have been reported to cause the syndrome:

1. Absent dynein arms
2. Selective absence of inner or outer arms
3. Absent radial spokes
4. Microtubule transposition
5. Combined absence of inner dynein arm and spoke head
6. Complete axonemal agenesis

The most common abnormality is absence of one or both dynein arms (Fig. 20-21). The disease appears to be hereditary, and within any one family the structural abnormality of the axoneme breeds true.[359,360]

The onset of symptoms in immotile cilia syndrome occurs soon after birth. Patients have repeated bouts of otitis, sinusitis, and chest infection. In 50% of patients there is situs inversus. Kartagener's triad of sinusitis, bronchiectasis, and situs inversus thus is a subset of immotile cilia syndrome. Bronchiectasis is present in one third of affected children but may be more common in adults.[361] Often it is of the follicular type. Since sperm flagella are powered by the same mechanism as cilia, male infertility is the rule.[359] Curiously, affected women are able to conceive despite the fact that the fallopian tube is lined with ciliated epithelium.

The diagnosis of immotile cilia syndrome can conveniently be based on phase microscopy of living ciliated cells obtained from the nasal cavity by curetting or brushing, followed by electron microscopy.

Cystic fibrosis

Cystic fibrosis (CF) is a systemic disease with widespread organ involvement and an intriguing array of metabolic derangements.[364,366,382] The pulmonary involvement dominates the clinical picture in those who survive the neonatal period. Improved therapy has led to survival of many patients into late childhood and adulthood. Lung involvement occurs in virtually all patients and is the cause of death in over 95%.[367,377] The

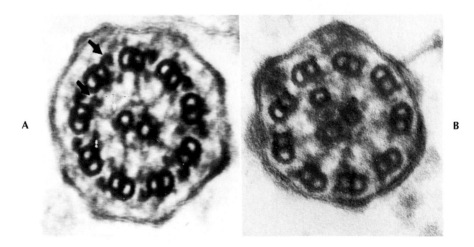

Fig. 20-21. A, Cross section of normal cilium. Arrows indicate dynein arms. **B,** Immotile cilia syndrome. Dynein arms are missing. In addition, there is an extra single microtubule. Extra microtubules were present in approximately one third of the cilia. (150,000 ×.)

pathologic features of the pulmonary disease are well documented.[365,368,369,381,383] Although the lungs appear normal at birth, hypertrophy of the mucous glands can be demonstrated by an increase in the gland/wall ratio (Reid index).[365] In patients dying after the first month of life, progressively severe changes develop with metaplasia of bronchiolar epithelium to a mucus-secreting type followed by mucous plugging, bronchitis, and bronchopneumonia. After 4 months of age mucopurulent plugging of the large and small airways is universal at autopsy, and bronchiectasis is the rule. The bronchiectasis is widespread, occurring in all lobes without any particular predilection. As much as 30% to 40% of the total volume of the lung is occupied by dilated bronchi, compared with a normal value of 5%.[380] Mild emphysema is found in the lungs of older children and adults when adequate morphologic methods are used,[365,381] but it is rarely if ever of clinical significance. Physiologically the lungs show severe airflow obstruction and abnormal distribution of ventilation but do not show the changes in lung mechanics characteristic of emphysema.[372]

The underlying basis for the pulmonary disease is a defect in anion transport by airway epithelium. The normal rheologic properties of the mucus blanket depend on the degree of hydration of the mucus and on the composition and quantity of fluid bathing the cilia. These properties in turn are believed to be regulated by chloride secretion by the airway epithelium. Chloride in the epithelial cells is secreted into the airway lumen through chloride channels open in the apical plasma membrane. In normal subjects the chloride channels open in response to several stimuli that act by raising the intracellular levels of cyclic AMP. The airway epithelium in cystic fibrosis is abnormally impermeable to chloride because the chloride channels fail to open in response to cyclic AMP.[373,376] This defect is ultimately expressed as abnormal microbial clearance, with chronic relentless colonization of airways and repeated episodes of bronchopneumonia.

A curious feature of infections in patients with CF is the propensity for specific infectious agents to be involved, notably staphylococci and *Pseudomonas aeruginosa*.[371,375] As much as 50% to 90% of CF patients are colonized by mucoid variants of *Pseudomonas*. The reason for the selection of these organisms is unexplained. The immune response to *Pseudomonas* is grossly normal, though there is evidence that the IgG produced is ineffective in promoting the phagocytosis and killing of the *Pseudomonas* by macrophages.[370]

Cor pulmonale is a late complication of the lung disease in CF and affects approximately one third of all patients and half of those over 15 years of age.[378] Hypoxia is a major factor producing cor pulmonale. All the patients with clinical right-sided heart failure studied by Stern and associates[378] were severely hypoxemic, and most were hypercarbic. Morphologic muscular hypertrophy of small pulmonary arteries and arterioles occurs in the lungs of CF patients and is similar to that found in other conditions producing hypoxia.[379] Shunts between the bronchial and pulmonary arteries in the walls of ectatic bronchi[380] may also be a factor promoting pulmonary hypertension.

PULMONARY VASCULAR DISEASE
Histologic features of normal pulmonary vasculature

The main pulmonary artery and its branches down to a diameter of 1 to 0.5 mm are classified as elastic pulmonary arteries.[384] Their media consists of concentric elastic lamellae separated by smooth muscle and other connective tissue matrix components. At birth the main pulmonary artery is similar to the aorta in thickness and elastic pattern, but by 2 years of age it is only half as thick as the aorta, and the elastic lamellae are fewer and appear fragmented. In the intrapulmonary branches the elastic lamellae remain intact and concentrically arranged. The number of lamellae decreases with decreasing size from 16 to 20 lamellae in lobar arteries to 3 or 4 lamellae in arteries less than 1 mm in diameter. Arteries that accompany the membranous and respiratory bronchioles and extend long proximal alveolar ducts in adults are classified as muscular arteries. They are less than 500 μm in diameter with a media defined by well-developed internal and external elastic laminae and composed mainly of smooth muscle. The arterioles less than 100 μm arise as either side branches or extensions of the muscular arteries. During their course they undergo a change in structure. Close to their origin they have a thin but complete muscular media two or three cells thick. In their terminal section, muscle is absent and the endothelium is supported only by a single elastic lamina. In the transition zone the initially complete muscle coat becomes a spiral that appears in cross section as a discontinuous muscle layer. Thus cross sections of normal arterioles can appear muscular, partially muscular, or nonmuscular depending on the level of section. The level of the respiratory tract at which transitions occur in varies with both age and disease.[385]

The arterioles give rise to a network of capillaries in the alveolar walls, which are gathered into venules similar in appearance to the nonmuscular arterioles. One can distinguish an arteriole from a venule only by serial sectioning to determine its connections to larger vessels. The venules drain into veins that lie between acini at some distance from the bronchi and bronchioles and occupy perilobular septa. Their walls consist of muscle and connective tissue with several elastic fibers that are not organized into distinct lamellae and are concentrated in the media adjacent to the adventitial connective tissue. In children there is little intima, but with aging a distinct zone of hyalinized of collagen appears.

The bronchial arteries that supply the cartilage-containing airways and portions of the pleura are easily distinguished from pulmonary arteries by their smaller diameter, their thick wall characteristic of systemic vessels, and their elastic pattern. Their internal elastic lamina is well formed, but the external elastic lamina is absent or poorly developed. In addition they often have a prominent longitudinal muscle coat in the intima.

Pulmonary thromboembolism

The embolism of thrombi to the lung is considered to be both underdiagnosed[397] and overdiagnosed[395] by clinicians. Thrombi can be found in pulmonary arteries in 20% to 60% of adult autopsies, though many of these are small and probably not of clinical consequence. The general mechanisms of thrombosis and embolism are discussed on p. 788.

In principle, thrombi forming anywhere in the venous circulation can embolize to the lung. In practice more than 90% of clinically significant emboli arise in the deep veins of the legs and thighs and are associated with venous stasis.[390,392,396]

The clinical effects of thromboembolism vary depending on the volume of emboli and on the condition of both the pulmonary and systemic circulations.[386] Emboli may cause no symptoms, acute transient dyspnea, pulmonary infarcts, pulmonary hypertension, cardiac failure, or even sudden death. Some but not all of the physiologic consequences of thromboembolism can be explained by mechanical obstruction of the vascular bed. The effects of embolism on gas exchange are (1) increased dead space ventilation, (2) pneumoconstriction, and (3) impaired synthesis of pulmonary surfactant.[392] The ventilation of unprefused lung adds to the work of breathing and produces tachypnea and a sense of dyspnea. Transient constriction of smooth muscle in airways and alveolar ducts occurs in response to vagal reflexes and humoral mediators such as serotonin, adenosine diphosphate, and thromboxane released from platelets. The hypoxemia that commonly follows pulmonary embolism is attributable to the production of areas of low ventilation/perfusion ratio by the constriction of small airways in well-perfused lung tissue surrounding an occluded area. Some patients manifest asthma-like wheezing. Impaired surfactant production is a delayed effect that produces edema and atelectasis, which may account for reversible roentgenographic changes in areas of embolism.[387] The hemodynamic effects of embolism are slight unless more than 50% of the vascular bed is occluded. They include a rise in pulmonary artery pressure and in severe cases congestive heart failure and shock.

Massive pulmonary embolism is a well-recognized cause of sudden death, which may be virtually instantaneous or extend over a period of a few minutes. The major pulmonary arteries are distended with clots that are often coiled or twisted and bear the imprint of venous valves. The lung parenchyma shows little change except congestion, which presumably comes by way of the bronchial circulation. Sublethal thromboemboli are often recurrent. Consequently it is common to find emboli of varied age at autopsy. Fresh emboli are poorly adherent to the vessel wall but can be distinguished from postmortem closts because they distend the artery, have a drier, more granular surface, and seem less elastic. Lines of Zahn and imprints of valves are diagnostic. Older thrombi are adherent and retracted to varying degrees.

The fate of nonfatal emboli is variable. Fibrinolytic mechanisms produce dissolution of the embolus within a few days, as demonstrated by serial angiograms and lung scans.[388,398] Organization of emboli and recanalization restore the vascular lumen more slowly, within weeks. The embolus becomes invaded by myofibroblasts from the vascular intima, while endothelial cells migrate out over the surface of the clot and invade the thrombotic material to form new vascular channels within it. Gradually the clot is transformed into a ridge or into a web with multiple points of attachment to the intima (Fig. 20-22).[389,391,393] The core of the web is fibrous tissue, perhaps containing a few siderophages, and the surface is endothelialized. Occasionally such webs can be detected angiographically.[394]

Pulmonary emboli as a cause of hypertension are discussed later in the chapter.

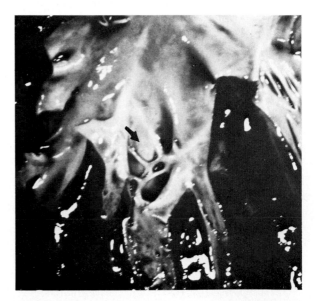

Fig. 20-22. Web in pulmonary artery *(arrow)*. Such webs result from organization of pulmonary thromboemboli.

Pulmonary infarcts

Ordinarily, emboli to the pulmonary arteries do not produce infarcts. Since the lung can obtain its oxygen from the alveolar gas and has a second blood supply through the bronchial arteries, occlusion of a pulmonary artery does not usually produce tissue necrosis. Tissue distal to the obstructed artery may be normal or merely show congestion, hemorrhage, and intra-alveolar fibrin with intact alveolar walls. These changes may be visible roentgenographically but are reversible. In the presence of congestive heart failure or chronic pulmonary disease, however, emboli often produce tissue infarcts. This happens most often with occlusion of segmental or subsegmental arteries. Very large and microscopic occlusions are rarely associated with infarcts. Pulmonary infarcts are typically wedge-shaped, pleural-based, hemorrhagic foci, usually in the lower lung zones. Fibrinous exudate is present on the overlying pleura after several hours. With time the center of the infarct becomes brown and eventually pale as the hemorrhage breaks down and is removed. Alveolar walls undergo necrosis, and small numbers of neutrophils may be present. Over the next few weeks granulation tissue appears surrounding the necrotic tissue, which becomes encapsulated, gradually organizes, and is converted to a linear fibrous scar. During the first few weeks when granulation is taking place, there are often nests of metaplastic squamous epithelium associated with the granulation tissue, which should not be mistaken for squamous carcinoma.

Other forms of embolism

Fat emboli are discussed under the adult respiratory distress syndrome (p. 962).

Bone marrow emboli commonly follow vigorous cardiopulmonary resuscitation. Like thrombotic emboli they become adherent, endothelialized, and eventually organized.[405]

Amniotic fluid emboli are a rare complication of pregnancy. Infusion of amniotic fluid occurs during tumultuous uterine contractions when the head is in the birth canal. The amniotic fluid is forced through a rupture in the chorion into the maternal veins, precipitating severe dyspnea, tachypnea, and hypotension. Disseminated intravascular coagulation is a common consequence. At autopsy the lungs are hemorrhagic. Squamous cells are lodged in the arterioles. Amniotic debris also contains lipid and mucin, which can be identified with appropriate stains.[399] Reportedly the clinical diagnosis can be confirmed by demonstration of squamous cells in blood withdrawn by a pulmonary artery catheter.

Air embolism can be produced during inspiration if negative intrathoracic pressure draws air into an open vein, an event most likely to happen during a neurosurgical or ear, nose, and throat procedure in which the patient sits upright and the operative wound is above the level of the heart. Air bubbles become trapped in pulmonary arteries and right ventricle where they mechanically impede blood flow. Reactions at the gas-fluid interface trigger blood clotting and the accumulation and activation of neutrophils. Small fibrin and platelet thrombi are found in pulmonary arteries. The physiologic consequences include transient airway constriction and vasoconstriction with great increases in pulmonary vascular resistance and pulmonary artery pressure. With large emboli pulmonary edema, hypoxemia, systemic hypotension and myocardial ischemia are seen. Fatalities have been reported with embolism of 100 ml of air.[403]

Foreign-body embolism can result from introduction of foreign material into the veins during medical procedures[404,406] but is also common among intravenous narcotic users. Particles of insoluble material added as "fillers" to drugs intended for oral use embolize to the lung and impact in arterioles and small muscular arteries where they cause thrombosis and proliferation of intimal cells.[401,402,407] Often they migrate into the perivascular space or interstitium where they give rise to foreign-body granulomas composed of macrophages, multinucleated giant cells, and a few lymphocytes (Fig. 20-23). The process of migration appears to involve the production of a granulomatous response in the vascular wall with disintegration of muscle and elastic tissue. In cases where lesions are not numerous, their detection

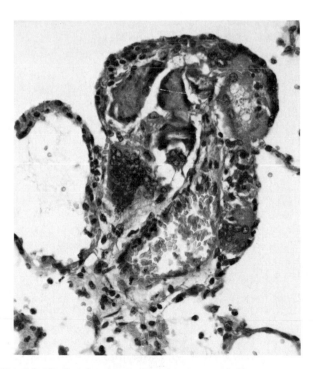

Fig. 20-23. Foreign-body giant cells containing talc particles in adventitial space around small pulmonary artery. Patient had history of intravenous drug abuse.

is aided by the use of polarizing filters, since cornstarch and talc, two of the materials commonly used as fillers, are strongly birefringent. When vascular thrombosis is widespread, pulmonary hypertension results. Lesions may resemble those of primary pulmonary hypertension, particularly in view of the cellular proliferation induced by the foreign material, but Tomashefski and Hirsch[407] could find scant morphologic evidence for an important vasoconstrictive element of the pulmonary hypertension. Extensive interstitial granulomas can produce roentgenographic nodularity and a restrictive ventilatory defect.[400]

Pulmonary hypertension

The pressure drop across the pulmonary vascular bed equals the product of the pulmonary vascular resistance and the pulmonary blood flow.[412] This relationship can be expressed as:

$$P_{pa} = QR + P_{LA}$$

where P_{pa} is the mean pressure in the pulmonary artery, Q and R are the pulmonary blood flow and resistance respectively, and P_{LA} is left atrial mean pressure, measurable in practice as pulmonary wedge pressure. From this relationship it is evident that pulmonary hypertension can be associated with increased flow as occurs with left-to-right shunt, with a process elevating pulmonary vascular resistance, or with increased wedge pressure as occurs with mitral stenosis, left-sided heart failure, left atrial myxoma, or diseases obstructing the pulmonary veins. Many disease processes change more than one of these variables.

In congenital heart disease with left-to-right shunt, the extent of vascular disease depends on interaction of several factors. With ventricular septal defect or patent ductus arteriosus there is increased flow because of the shunt accompanied by increased pulmonary arterial pressure because of the direct transmission of systemic pressure to the lesser circulation through the anatomic defect. The combination of elevated pressure and flow produces vascular damage by the time the child is several years of age, and the pulmonary vascular resistance becomes elevated and eventually fixed. In atrial septal defect a large increase in pulmonary blood flow may occur with little increase in pulmonary artery pressure. Pulmonary vascular damage with the attendant rise in pulmonary vascular resistance develops only over several decades. With either type of shunt the eventual vascular damage may be severe enough to cause reversal of the shunt. Changes caused by abnormal hemodynamics have become a source of dysfunction in their own right.

The vascular changes in congenital heart disease have been of particular interest since the development of cardiac surgery, because the nature and extent of the

lesions in the muscular arteries determines whether correction of the cardiac defect will relieve pulmonary hypertension. In 1958 Heath and Edwards[415] divided the vascular changes into the six grades listed below. The first three grades are reversible, but grades IV to VI generally are not.

Grade I   Muscular extension into arterioles, medial hypertrophy of muscular arteries
Grade II   Medial hypertrophy with intimal proliferation
Grade III   Progressive intimal fibrosis and occlusion
Grade IV   Plexiform lesions
Grade V   Chronic dilatation lesions with veinlike arteries
Grade VI   Arterial necrosis

The earliest changes in this scheme are muscle hypertrophy evident as distal extension of muscle in the arterioles and an increased thickness of the media of muscular arteries. Grade II changes include the preceding, but in addition some arteries show reduplication of the internal elastic lamina and proliferation of smooth muscle or myofibroblasts in the intima (Fig. 20-24). The intimal thickening of grade III changes is much more severe with considerable narrowing or complete obliteration of the lumen (Fig. 20-25). The intimal proliferation often takes the form of concentrically arrayed intimal cells in a proteoglycan-rich stroma, a pattern described as onion-skin thickening. In some vessels with severe intimal thickening the media is

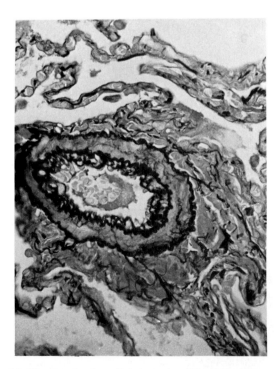

Fig. 20-24. Grade II pulmonary hypertensive change in muscular artery. Reduplication of internal elastic lamina and intimal thickening of minimal degree.

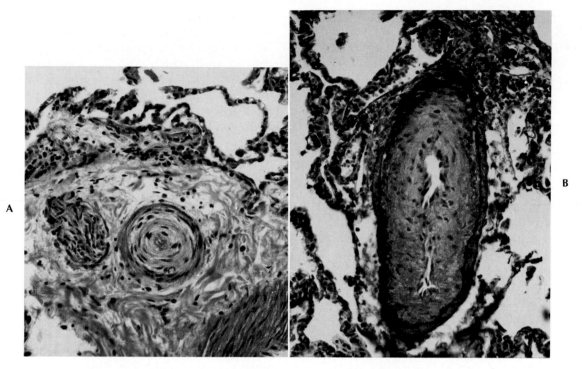

Fig. 20-25. Grade III pulmonary hypertensive change. **A,** Onion-skin hyperplasia of intima of small pulmonary artery. **B,** Severe intimal thickening with mild atrophy of media.

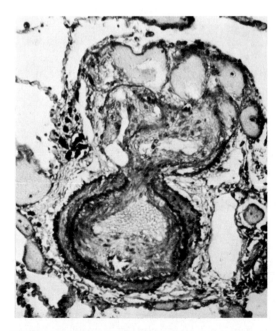

Fig. 20-26. Plexiform lesion. Muscular pulmonary artery with pronounced intimal fibrosis. Side branch *(top)* is filled with proliferating cells separated by anastamosing vascular channels that communicate with dilated veinlike branches.

relatively thin, indicating beginning evolution into the next stage. Grade IV changes include plexiform arterial lesions (Fig. 20-26). These are complex structures that often occur just distal to the point of branching of a muscular artery. The proximal segment of the lesion consists of an artery with a distinct muscular media and severe intimal thickening and fibrosis. The segment of artery downstream is thin walled and tortuous and has little tunica media. At the junction between these segments there is pronounced cellular proliferation with complex anastomosing channels between groups of proliferated cells and often deposits of fibrin in the intercellular spaces or within the channels. The elastic laminae are often destroyed in the proliferative zone. In grade V there are numerous dilated, thin-walled, tortuous vessels that resemble veins at first glance, though serial sections show their position to be on the arterial side of the circulation and in close relation to severely thickened arteries. Overt fibrinoid necrosis is the hallmark of grade VI hypertensive changes. The fiery red "fibrinoid" staining is the result of severe endothelial damage with the entry of fibrin into the media and its deposition between medial muscle cells.[417] There may or may not be an associated inflammatory reaction (Fig. 20-27). The Heath-Edwards grading scheme has been criticized by Wagenvoort[426] on three grounds. First, grades IV to VI imply a progression that may be the

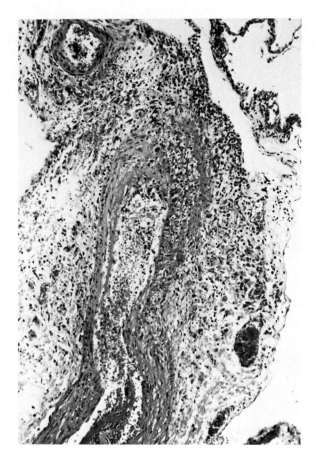

Fig. 20-27. Necrosis of muscular artery in patient with ventricular septal defect.

reverse of the actual pathogenic sequence. Plexiform lesions probably do not precede necrosis; on the contrary, there is experimental evidence that they arise after the necrosis. Arterial necrosis gives rise to medial degeneration, leading to the dilated, thin-walled vessels that are in part poststenotic dilatation of the damaged pulmonary artery and in part bronchial vessels involved in organizing the necrosis. The very cellular zone of transition with its many endothelium-lined channels may arise as an attempt at organization of the damaged vessel wall.[424] Thus grades IV to VI in Wagenvoort's view should be combined. Second, the grading is based on identification of the most severe type of lesions and takes no account of the proportion of arteries affected. Third, Reid[385] has identified loss of arteries or failure of their development that can be detected only by careful quantitative studies. The ratio of arterioles less than 10 μm diameter to alveoli counted in sections can be used to estimate the extent of arteriolar development. Subnormal arteriolar development is an additional determinant of reversibility of the elevated vascular resistance in congenital heart disease. Thus Heath-Edwards grading must be regarded as an incomplete but rapid and convenient first estimate of prognosis.

Hypoxic vasoconstriction is one of the most common causes of pulmonary hypertension accompanied by increased vascular resistance. In contrast to the systemic circulation, in which hypoxia causes vasodilatation, alveolar hypoxia from any cause produces constriction of the small pulmonary arteries.[412,413] Physiologically this is an important mechanism for directing blood flow to well-ventilated parts of the lung, but if widespread and sustained, hypoxic vasoconstriction can lead to pulmonary hypertension and cor pulmonale. Conditions in which hypoxia is the major mechanism of pulmonary hypertension include residence at high altitude,[408] chronic hypoventilation either as a primary disease or resulting from neuromuscular disease, pathologic obesity (pickwickian syndrome), or rarely upper airway disease such as tonsillar hypertrophy. In severe kyphoscoliosis, hypoventilation is aggravated by distortion of the arteries and areas of collapse of alveoli in which capillary resistance is elevated. In many forms of chronic lung disease hypoxic vasoconstriction is combined with destruction of the vascular bed. The histologic changes of chronic hypoxia are distal extension of smooth muscle along the arterioles and the development of a longitudinal muscle layer in the intima. Electron microscopic study of experimental hypoxia indicates that the muscle in the distal regions of arterioles arises by the differentiation of pericytes, which ordinarily are inconspicuous when viewed with the light microscope.[385] Hypertrophy of the tunica media of muscular arteries is characteristically mild.

Pulmonary hypertension of unknown cause is a clinical syndrome that can be produced by three distinct pathologic processes: multiple occult pulmonary emboli, primary pulmonary hypertension (primary-plexogenic pulmonary arteriopathy), and pulmonary veno-occlusive disease.[382,383,427]

Despite the high frequency of pulmonary emboli, they rarely present the clinical picture of slowly progressive pulmonary hypertension. Owen and associates[422] found only 12 cases in 8000 autopsies over a 20-year span. Although the chest roentgenograms had shown no abnormalities, five of the patients had small infarcts at autopsy. This histologic features of the vessels in thromboembolic pulmonary hypertension include a variable degree of muscular hypertrophy, intimal thickening that is characteristically eccentric (Fig. 20-28), and recanalized arteries.[393,427] The recanalized arteries may have multiple lumens ("collander" type) or a single fibrous septum giving it two lumens. Plexiform lesions and onion-skin intimal proliferation are not found. At autopsy most patients have some macroscopic thromboemboli in central arteries, which are rarely included in biopsies.[393,422]

Primary pulmonary hypertension affects persons of all ages including young children, but a large majority of patients are young women.[429] The manifestations are

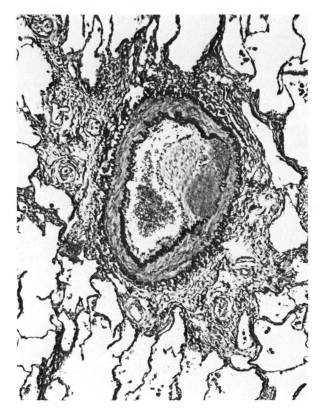

Fig. 20-28. Eccentric intimal thickening resulting from organization of thromboembolus. (Verhoef–Van Giesen stain for elastic tissue.)

usually the insidious onset of dyspnea or symptoms attributable to low cardiac output such as heart failure, syncope, or angina. One third of patients experience Raynaud's phenomenon. The chest roentgenogram shows right ventricular hypertrophy and enlarged central pulmonary arteries. Pulmonary arterial pressure can reach systemic values, but the wedge pressure is normal. Pathologic findings in the lungs cannot be distinguished from those in patients with congenital cardiac shunts. The characteristic features include onion-skin intimal proliferation in small muscular arteries, plexiform lesions, and dilatation lesions. Arterial necrosis is present in some cases. Morphometric studies of a small number of cases, conducted by Reid,[385] showed no abnormal muscular extension along arterioles but did demonstrate loss of arterioles less than 40 μm in diameter.

The cause of primary pulmonary hypertension is unknown. Familial cases have been reported. Its association with Raynaud's phenomenon suggests a hyperreactivity of the vascular system that is not limited to the lungs. Since identical histopathologic changes occur rarely in systemic lupus erythematosus, primary pulmonary hypertension may be related to the collagen-vascular diseases. This idea is supported by the occurrence of arthritis and autoantibodies in some pa-

tients.[429] Aminorex, an anorexigenic drug, caused a European epidemic of pulmonary hypertension in which the course and histopathologic changes were similar to those of primary pulmonary hypertension.[430] Some cases are associated with cirrhosis or portal hypertension, though the mechanism is unknown.[419,420]

The natural history of primary pulmonary hypertension is one of relentless progression despite the use of a number of vasodilatory drugs. Death is often sudden, attributable to low cardiac ouput. The rate of disease progression is variable. More than half of the patients die within 3 years of the onset of symptoms, but some live more than a decade.

In pulmonary veno-occlusive disease, fibrous obliteration of small veins is believed to be the cause of pulmonary hypertension, and changes in the arteries and parenchyma are secondary. There is widespread obliteration of veins and venules by eccentric or concentric fibrosis.[416,425,428] Often fibrous septa divide the lumen into one or several channels. In some cases recent and organizing thrombi were present in the veins, and it is likely that organization of thrombi is responsible for the fibrosis in many, perhaps most, cases. On the other hand, cases have been recorded in which granulomatous or other types of inflammation are responsible for the obliteration of veins.[411] The arteries show muscular hypertrophy and mild intimal fibrosis. Arterial thrombi have been reported in several cases, but whether they are in situ thrombi or emboli is uncertain. The lung parenchyma shows nodular areas of hemosiderosis and fibrosis or occasionally venous infarcts that are typically based on perilobular septa. Basophilic elastic fibers encrusted with iron and calcium are a striking feature in some cases, since affected elastic fibers act as foreign bodies, stimulating giant cell formation.

The clinical features are difficult to distinguish from those of primary pulmonary hypertension. Patients tend to be younger (most are children), and the sex incidence is equal. The chest roentgenogram may allow one to suggest the diagnosis. There are signs of interstitial edema with Kerley-B lines, but the pulmonary veins are not visible and there is no left atrial enlargement. Vascular marking is no more prominent in the upper than in the lower lobes.[425]

The cause of veno-occlusive disease is unknown. A few features indicate that it may be triggered by infection. In many patients clinical onset has followed an influenza-like episode, and some patients have shown pathologic or serologic evidence of a preceding infection. In one case evidence of immune complex deposition in the alveolar capillaries was found by electron microscopy and immunofluorescence.[410]

In addition to the aforementioned histologic changes, which vary from disease to disease, certain morphologic features accompany chronic pulmonary hypertension irrespective of its cause. Right ventricular hypertrophy is present in almost all cases, and one can evaluate it at autopsy by dissecting away the atria and epicardial fat and separating the free wall of the right ventricle from the left ventricle and septum.[409,414] In adult men a weight of the free wall of the right ventricle greater than 75 g indicates hypertrophy. In children or those in whom a cause of independent left ventricular hypertrophy can reasonably be excluded, the ratio of the weight of the left ventricle and septum to the right ventricle can be used. A value less than 2 is abnormal. Measurement of the thickness of the ventricular wall is not reliable. If significant hypertension is present from birth, the elastic tissue of the pulmonary trunk does not undergo the normal fragmentation and regression, and the aorta-like elastic pattern seen in the neonate is retained.[418] If pulmonary hypertension develops after regression, the pulmonary trunk hypertrophies and may even approach the aorta in thickness if the hypertension is sufficiently severe, but the elastic lamellae continue to appear fragmented as in the normal adult. The elastic arteries also hypertrophy and develop accelerated atherosclerosis of the usual type.

PULMONARY EDEMA
General mechanisms of edema

There are few organs in which the development of edema causes greater functional impairment than in the lung. The late stages of edema with alveolar flooding are accompanied by severe disorders of gas exchange. Fortunately, involvement of the alveolar space usually develops late, after a series of sequential changes in fluid filtration in which interstitial involvement precedes air-space involvement.

The alveolar epithelium is relatively impermeable both to proteins and to small solutes.[442] The alveolar epithelial cells, which are the barrier between the air and the interstitium, are joined by tight junctions (zonulae occludentes). In freeze-fracture replicas the junctions are composed of three to five complete junctional strands. Although the endothelium of the pulmonary capillaries is nonfenestrated, the type seen in vascular beds of low permeability, the zonulae occludentes between endothelial cells are less tight than those of the epithelium. Usually they consist of two to three junctional strands, but sometimes only a single discontinuous strand is seen.[437] In consequence the capillary endothelium is more permeable than the epithelium.

The forces governing fluid filtration in the lungs, as in other tissues, are expressed in the Starling equation[436,441]:

$$Q_f = K_f(P_{mv} - P_i) - \sigma(\pi_{mv} - \pi_i)$$

where Q_f is the fluid filtration rate, K_f is the filtration coefficient of the microvessels, P_{mv} is the hydrostatic pressure in the microvessels, P_i is the hydrostatic pressure of the interstitial tissue, σ is a coefficient measur-

ing the resistance of the microvascular to the flow of protein, π_{mv} is the colloid osmotic pressure of the plasma, and π_i is the colloid osmotic pressure of the interstitial fluid surrounding the microvessels. Thus the main force favoring filtration of fluid and protein out of the pulmonary vascular bed is the hydrostatic pressure across the vessel wall, and that restraining it is the colloid osmotic gradient between the vessel lumen and the perivascular space.

Filtered interstitial fluid is cleared by the lymphatics. The alveolar walls themselves have no lymphatics, but there are lymphatics in the loose connective tissue spaces surrounding the bronchioles, small muscular arteries, and veins. Consequently no alveolar wall is more than 1 to 2 mm from a lymphatic. The interstitial pressures in the lung are lower in the junctions between alveoli, which helps to drain the interstitial fluid from the alveolar walls first to the junctions and thence to the perivascular and peribronchial connective tissue spaces.

The development of edema thus is a dynamic process.[440] As the filtration of fluid across the pulmonary vascular bed increases, initially the fluid is efficiently conducted to the lymphatics and removed. As the capacity of the lymphatics is exceeded, excess fluid accumulates first in the loose connective tissue spaces surrounding the bronchioles and arteries and in the lobular connective tissue septa. At this stage clinical manifestations are usually mild, but early closure of small airways because of the peribronchiolar edema can be detected by sensitive physiologic tests of small airway function. Only occasionally is overt expiratory airflow obstruction present.

Thickening of the alveolar walls because of interstitial edema is a late manifestation of increased fluid filtration but is accompanied by little impairment of gas exchange, since the excess fluid in the interstitial connective tissue of the alveolar wall does not materially widen the barrier for gaseous diffusion. In a section through normal alveolar wall the capillaries lie eccentrically with a space containing collagen and elastic fibers and cells on one side of the capillary but only a basement membrane shared with the alveolar epithelium on the opposite side (Fig. 20-29). When excess fluid builds up in the alveolar walls, it accumulates in the connective tissue space while the capillary remains attached to the alveolar epitheluim through their shared basement membrane.

When flooding of the alveolar air spaces occurs, it tends to involve alveoli in an all-or-none manner. As fluid builds up in the corners of alveoli, the radius of the air-containing volume is reduced. In accordance with the Laplace equation the air pressure required to maintain its expansion rises, and at a critical point the air is driven out of the alveolus. Consequently, the air spaces in a lung developing edema are either at normal

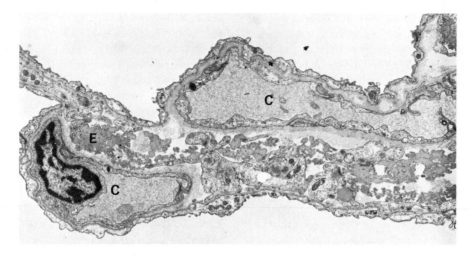

Fig. 20-29. Electron micrograph of alveolar septum of human lung. Capillaries *(C)* lie to side of septum, sharing basal lamina with alveolar epithelium. Connective tissue core contains elastic *(E)* and collagenous fibers. Interstitial edema accumulating within connective tissue space will not produce significant widening of diffusion barrier, since capillaries remain associated with shared basal lamina.

volume with only a minimal amount of intra-alveolar fluid or are filled with edema fluid and are at a reduced volume.

Lung in left-sided heart failure

Elevation of the pulmonary venous pressure from any cause can provoke pulmonary edema. Among its causes are left ventricular failure, disease of the mitral valve, or even mediastinal fibrosis. The lungs are heavy and moist, and frothy fluid may exude from the cut surface. Microscopically the alveolar capillaries are congested, and the perivascular spaces and interlobular septa are dilated with distended lymphatics. The alveolar spaces contain an eosinophilic coagulum of protein often with erythrocytes and macrophages in variable numbers.

Chronically elevated venous pressure produces the condition known as chronic passive congestion of the lung or brown induration. The lungs are heavy and firm, and the sectioned surface has a brown hue. Microscopically the alveolar septa are thickened and often lined with cuboid epithelial cells, identifiable as hyperplastic type II pneumocytes by electron microscopy. The alveolar spaces contain clusters of hemosiderin-laden macrophages. The interlobular septa are thickened and the lymphatics dilated.[433]

Particularly severe cases of chronic passive congestion are commonly seen in association with rheumatic mitral stenosis. Because the stenosis develops gradually over many years, the pressure in the left atrium and pulmonary veins rises slowly. There is time for the lymphatics to hypertrophy, providing a measure of compensation for accelerated fluid filtration and permitting high venous pressures to develop without severe intra-alveolar edema. The chronic interstitial edema leads to

fibrosis of the alveolar and interlobular septa and thickening of the basement membranes, which have been observed with electron microscopy.[438] Changes occurring in the pulmonary veins include fibrous thickening of the intima and hypertrophy of the medial smooth muscle. Sometimes the smooth muscle becomes organized into a distinct circumferential band separating elastic lamellae and resembling the tunica media of the muscular arteries.[433]

Among the consequences of venous distension is reflex constriction of the pulmonary arteries. This increase in precapillary resistance may give a small measure of protection to the pulmonary capillary bed but produces pulmonary hypertension with concomitant changes in the pulmonary arteries. The muscular pulmonary arteries develop medial hypertrophy and intimal fibrosis, whereas the precapillary arterioles develop a muscular media. Higher-grade hypertensive vascular changes such as those seen in congenital heart disease with left-to-right shunt, notably dilated arteries and plexiform lesions, do not occur with mitral stenosis.

Secondary changes are sometimes found in the lungs of patients with mitral stenosis or other causes of severe chronic pulmonary congestion. The elastic tissue in and around small arteries may become encrusted with calcium and ferric iron salts as a consequence of perivascular hemorrhages. The encrusted elastin fibers act as foreign bodies leading to the formation of giant cells. Small trabeculas of bone may be formed in alveolar spaces, though mechanisms for this change is not clear.[433]

Certain of the histologic changes in the chronically congested lung can be detected on the chest roentgenogram. The accumulated iron-laden macrophages give a fine nodularity to the lung fields. The thickened interlobular septa with their dilated lymphatics can be seen as fine linear shadows perpendicular to the pleura, known as septal, or Kerley, lines. Those lines in the depths of the lung near the hilum are the A lines. Subpleural lines are called B lines and are most clearly seen in the costophrenic angles.

Other causes of edema with a hemodynamic component

High-altitude pulmonary edema is an acute form of edema that develops in the first 48 hours after reaching high altitude in some persons with neither heart nor lung disease. The disease affects both those who live at sea level and travel for the first time at altitudes higher than 10,000 feet and dwellers at high altitude who descend to sea level for a period of time and then return to high altitude. Even in normal individuals the hypoxia of high altitude produces arteriolar constriction and pulmonary arterial hypertension, but in those with high-altitude pulmonary edema this response is greatly exaggerated.[439] Although the arterial pressure is high, pulmonary wedge and left atrial pressures are normal. These hemodynamic measurements indicate that overall capillary pressure may not be elevated, and some authorities have suggested that leakage of fluid takes place only in the arteries. The few autopsy cases reported had not only edema of the perivascular connective tissue septa and alveolar spaces but also hyaline membranes, indicating that the alveolar walls themselves were damaged.[431] Electron microscopic studies of animals exposed to simulated high altitude have also shown damage to alveolar capillaries.[434] To reconcile the evidence of alveolar damage with the hemodynamic findings, it has been proposed that the intense vasoconstriction responsible for the raised arterial pressure is not uniform. Those unconstricted arterioles permit transmission of the raised pressure to the capillary bed focally, producing fluid leak and capillary damage at the alveolar level.

Massive pulmonary edema develops after head injury of a wide variety of types. This neurogenic pulmonary edema can develop within seconds. In the early phase of the edema there is intense systemic and pulmonary vasoconstriction with a shift in blood volume to the pulmonary circulation. The intravascular pressures soon return to normal, but the edema may persist. The high protein content of the edema fluid indicates that microvascular permeability is increased. Evidence indicates that after head injury there may be massive sympathetic discharge, resulting in the intense vasoconstriction. The consequent elevated pulmonary microvascular pressures initiate hemodynamic edema and produce capillary damage that increases microvascular permeability and maintains the leak after the pressures return to normal.

Pulmonary edema of extremely rapid onset and fatal outcome occasionally develops in users of heroin and other narcotics. The mechanism is not understood, but the high protein content of the edema fluid indicates altered permeability.

In patients with renal failure, edema may develop with a characteristic perihilar distribution seen roentgenographically. Histologic features are hemorrhagic and fibrin-rich edema in the air spaces and hyaline membranes focally lining alveolar ducts. In chronic cases the fibrinous exudate may organize. Although this disorder is commonly known as uremic pneumonia, the pneumonia is not closely related to the degree of azotemia, and a variety of hemodynamic factors must contribute in individual cases. These include hypertension with left ventricular failure, fluid overload, cerebral edema in some patients, and decreased plasma colloid osmotic pressure in those with the nephrotic syndrome and hypoproteinemia.[432,435]

Altered capillary permeability

Acute injury to the alveolar capillary endothelium and epithelium leads to edema rich in proteins. The edema tends to be more prolonged than simple hemodynamic edema, in part because of the decrease in the osmotic forces favoring reabsorption and the precipitation of insoluble fibrin in the air spaces. Whether the lesions resolve, progress, or organize depends on the intensity and duration of the injury. Since the morphologic changes and pathophysiology are similar regardless of the etiology, the anatomic pattern has been called diffuse alveolar damage to emphasize its nonspecificity.[457] The early effects of injury are congestion and edema with widening of the peribronchial and perivascular spaces and filling of air spaces with proteinaceous edema and focal hemorrhages.[446,462] The alveolar walls become thickened by interstitial edema, and after 1 to 2 days hyaline membranes begin to appear, initially as deeply eosinophilic smudgy bands at the tips of alveolar septa where they protrude into the alveolar ducts.[446,457,461] With the passage of time the membranes extend to line alveolar ducts and respiratory bronchioles (Fig. 20-30). Electron microscopic study of hyaline membranes shows that they occur at sites where the alveolar basement membranes are denuded by necrosis of the type I epithelial cells.[445,453] As in infants, they consist of cellular debris, membranelike fragments, and serum proteins but only rarely contain fibrin. Beneath the hyaline membranes in alveolar ducts, the alveoli are often collapsed. Inflammatory cells including small numbers of mononuclear cells and neutrophils infiltrate the alveolar septa and appear in the air spaces. In the second week reparative changes become prominent.[445,457,459,466] The alveolar epithelial cells enlarge and proliferate. Air spaces become lined with prominent cuboidal or elongated epithelial cells

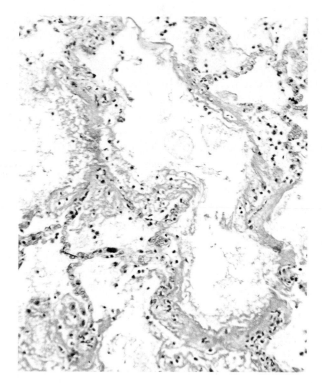

Fig. 20-30. Diffuse alveolar damage. Hyaline membrane in alveolar duct, accompanied by a few inflammatory cells. The principal cause in this instance was hyperoxia, but similar morphologic changes could be produced by a variety of agents.

with atypical nuclei and abundant basophilic cytoplasm, sometimes vacuolated in appearance. Where there are hyaline membranes, these cells either cover their surface or extend along the basement membrane beneath the hyaline membranes. These epithelial changes are the general response to necrosis of type I epithelial cells. Type II cells first undergo hyperplasia to form a cuboid lining over the denuded basement membrane, and then some of the proliferated cells spread out and differentiate into type I cells. During the transition they appear as elongated atypical epithelium.[445,453]

Fibroblastic organization occurs in two forms.[445,466] Fibroblasts proliferate and collagen is laid down within the interstitium of the lung, and fibroblasts invade the fibrinous exudate and hyaline membranes in the airspaces. In the early stages the organizing exudate is clearly within the air spaces where it appears as polypoid collections of parallel fibroblasts in a myxoid stroma. As the organizing intra-alveolar masses become collagenized and covered with regenerating epithelium, they are incorporated into the air-space walls, giving the appearance of interstitial fibrosis.

Clinically, patients with diffuse alveolar damage are tachypneic, short of breath, and cyanotic.[450,464,467] Severe hypoxemia is present, and high pressures are required to ventilate the poorly compliant lungs. The chest roentgenogram shows patchy or diffuse infiltrates. Together this group of clinical features has been called the adult respiratory distress syndrome (ARDS).[444] Although nonspecific, it is highly characteristic of patients with diffuse alveolar damage. The pathologic basis for the physiologic changes is complex and probably varies with the stage of the disease.[459] Hypoxemia is a consequence of physiologic shunting, ventilation-perfusion imbalance, and thickening of the diffusion barrier. Shunting occurs through perfusion of unventilated, edema-filled, or atelectatic air spaces. Premature closure of bronchioles cuffed by edema or directly damaged by the primary process, and unequal compliance of diseased tissue lead to ventilation-perfusion inequality. Direct morphometric measurements of the thickness of the tissues to be traversed by oxygen have shown that the diffusion barrier is thickened. Early in the process, compliance is lost because of edema, abnormal surfactant synthesis, and interference with surfactant function by the serum components leaking from the damaged capillaries.[454,465] In the late phase of the process, diminished compliance is attributable to fibrosis.

Approximately half the patients whose disorder is clinically diagnosed as ARDS survive with modern therapy. Some survivors have residual pulmonary dysfunction. Some of these have a restrictive ventilatory pattern as one would expect with pulmonary fibrosis. Others have expiratory airflow obstruction with hyperreactive airways for which the explanation is not obvious.[468]

The pathogenesis of the lung damage varies with the cause. Several of the major causes of diffuse alveolar damage follow:

1. Shock
2. Infection
   a. Viral pneumonia
   b. Extrathoracic sepsis
3. Trauma
   a. Fat embolism
   b. Lung contusion
4. Aspiration
   a. Gastric acid
   b. Near drowning
   c. Hydrocarbon fluids
5. Toxic inhalants
   a. Oxygen
   b. Smoke
   c. War gases
   d. Oxides of nitrogen
   e. Metal fumes (cadmium, mercury)
   f. Other
6. Pancreatitis
7. Radiation
8. Narcotics
   a. Heroin

b. Methadone
c. Propoxyphene
9. Drugs
  a. Salicylates
  b. Ethchlorvynol
  c. Colchicine

Hyperoxia

The toxic effects of high concentrations of oxygen have been demonstrated repeatedly in a variety of species. When oxygen is used therapeutically, the exact level at which lung damage will occur depends on the underlying condition of the patient, but no concentrations above 50% can be regarded as entirely safe. The toxic effects of oxygen are mediated by its reduction products.[449,460] Even during normal metabolism the reduction of oxygen leads to the production of some highly reactive, short-lived intermediates such as superoxide (O_2^-), hydrogen peroxide, and hydroxyl radicals (—OH). During exposure to oxygen the production of these radicals is increased, and they can overwhelm the endogenous antioxidant defenses. The effects of oxidants that cause tissue damage include oxidation of sulfhydryl groups, DNA damage, and peroxidation of membrane lipids. Circulating neutrophils are powerful producers of oxygen radicals, which may explain why the earliest effect of hyperoxia detectable by electron microscopy is damage to endothelium rather than to epithelium.[458]

Lung damage associated with extrathoracic injuries

ARDS is often associated with severe extrathoracic trauma, shock, intra-abdominal sepsis, burns, and pancreatitis.[450,467] Often the histopathologic changes correspond to diffuse alveolar damage. The mechanisms in such a complex clinical setting are not entirely clear. In the early phase of the process the lungs may contain thrombi in small arterioles or alveolar capillaries in addition to edema, hemorrhage, and hyaline membranes.[446] Activation of complement, agglutination of platelets, and adhesion of leukocytes in the lung with the release of oxygen radicals, vasoactive mediators, and enzymes are probably involved.[447,448,461,467] With major trauma, particularly if there are fractures of the long bones, fat emboli are a further factor producing lung injury. Fat embolism is the result of abrupt pressure changes in the long bones, which rupture thin-walled venous sinuses and force marrow fat into them, whence it embolizes to the lung. In addition, levels of plasma triglycerides, free fatty acids, and lipase rise as part of the stress response. Endothelial damage is caused by fatty acids released from embolized fat and by mediators released during associated blood coagulation. Fat emboli can be recognized in ordinary histo-

logic sections as sharply delimited, empty-appearing capillary loops or arterioles, but frozen sections stained for fat are required for confirmation.[451]

Inhalation of toxic gases is another cause of diffuse alveolar damage. A variety of gases can produce the syndrome, including war gases, smoke, oxides of nitrogen as in silo-filler's disease, and others. Inhalation injury also involves conducting airways, and organizing exudates are often found in the respiratory bronchioles, a change known as bronchiolitis obliterans.

IMMUNOLOGIC LUNG DISEASE

Immunologic mechanisms play a role in a wide variety of lung diseases.[485] The diseases discussed in this section are believed in most instances to be induced by immune reactions to identifiable antigens that are not themselves directly pathogenic, Asthma has been included, though evidence indicates that immunologic reactions may be only one of many inciting agents.

Asthma

Asthma is a disorder characterized by increased responsiveness of the airways to various stimuli, as manifested by episodes of wheezing and increased resistance to expiratory airflow. The stimuli vary widely and include antigens, infection, air pollutants, respiratory tract irritants, exercise, and emotional factors. Stimuli that cause slowing of expiration in nonasthmatic persons are effective in asthmatics at far lower concentrations. Methacholine and histamine, drugs commonly used in inhalation studies, caused bronchoconstriction in asthmatics at 1% of the normal dose.

Asthma is a common condition with an incidence in the U.S. population of approximately 4%. Clinically it has been divided into two types, extrinsic and intrinsic,[481] though the distinction is not sharp, and cases with mixed features occur commonly. In extrinsic (allergic) asthma the attacks are triggered by specific identifiable allergens. The patients are usually children or young adults with an atopic history; that is, they or members of their families have histories of multiple allergies such as allergic rhinitis or urticaria. Many of these patients have elevated serum concentrations of IgE and peripheral blood eosinophilia. Asthmatic attacks typically become less frequent with time, often disappearing in adulthood.[480,482]

Most asthmatics whose symptoms develop in middle age or later do not give a history of atopy and have no identifiable allergens. The serum IgE level and white blood cell count are normal. The patient may have a history of chronic bronchitis, in which case the term "asthmatic bronchitis" is appropriate. This nonallergic or intrinsic asthma may become worse with time.[480] Deaths occur in approximately 1% of asthmatics.[469] Death may be sudden allowing insufficient time for hospitalization, or may occur during status asthmaticus, a severe unremitting asthmatic episode that fails to give the usual prompt response to therapy. At autopsy the lungs of patients dying of status asthmaticus appear grossly distended with air and fail to collapse as the thorax is opened. On the sectioned surface the parenchyma appears normal and the lesions of destructive emphysema are generally absent. The bronchi of segmental size and smaller are filled with ropy mucus, which may be clear and gelatinous or may have a laminated yellow appearance. On microscopic examination the bronchi and bronchioles are filled with laminated mucus that may appear eosinophilic or faintly basophilic (Fig. 20-31). The mucus is continuous with that in the cytoplasm of goblet cells and ducts of the mucous glands. The intraluminal mucus may contain sloughed epithelium, eosinophils, and crystals derived from eosinophil phospholipase (Charcot-Leyden crystals), especially in allergic asthma. The epithelium lining the bronchi usually shows an increase in goblet cells at the expense of ciliated cells. Often there is extensive sloughing of columnar epithelium, leaving the bronchi lined only by basal cells (Fig. 20-32). This sloughing is unlikely to be an artifact, since it has been since in biopsy specimens[473,484] and expectorated sputum,[479] as well as at autopsy.[478] The epithelium rests on an eosinophilic basement membrane that is usually 5 to 20 μm thick, compared with 1 to 2 μm normally. Electron microscopy shows that this structure consists of a basal lamina of normal thickness just beneath the epithelium and a deeper zone of cross-banded collagen fibers, which accounts for the abnormal thickening. The mucous glands show hypertrophy, dilated ducts, and an increased proportion of mucous cells. The bronchial muscle is hypertrophied, with all layers of the bronchial wall are infiltrated with inflammatory cells.[471] The inflammatory infiltrate may contain many eosinophils, but often eosinophils are few and plasma cells predominate. Where mast cell counts have been performed, the number of recognizable mast cells was reduced, and many of these present appeared to be degranulating.[470,484]

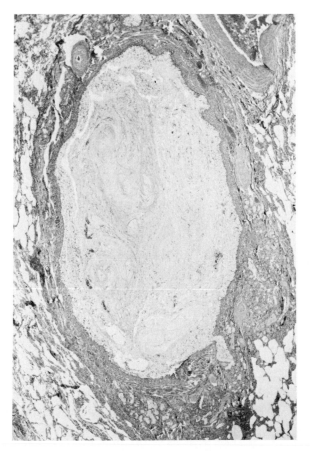

Fig. 20-31. Asthma. Laminated mucus filling small bronchus.

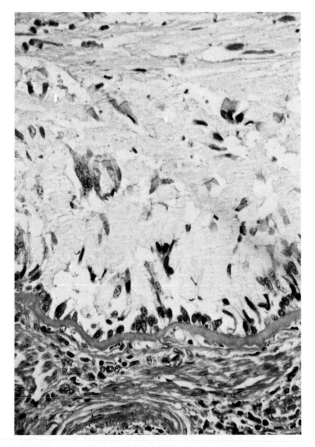

Fig. 20-32. Asthma. Higher magnification of bronchus shown in Fig. 20-31. There is sloughing of mucus-secreting and-ciliated cells, leaving mainly basal cells attached to thickened basement membrane.

The pathologic changes in nonfatal asthma are less well known. The rapidity with which airflow obstruction can be reversed in an acute asthmatic episode indicates that bronchospasm may be an important cause of the obstruction. Biopsy specimens taken during or soon after attacks, however, show changes similar to those described in fatal status asthmaticus, mucus hypersecretion, epithelial damage, and inflammatory infiltrate. It appears therefore that inflammation and mucus hypersecretion, as well as bronchospasm, contribute to the airflow obstruction in many ordinary asthmatic episodes.

The mechanisms that account for the altered airway responsiveness probably vary.[472,483,485] Many asthmatic patients, especially those with extrinsic asthma, form antibodies capable of binding to and sensitizing lung tissue, mast cells, and blood basophils so that they promptly release mediators in response to the specific antigens.[485] These antibodies are usually of the IgE class but may be of an IgG$_4$ subclass. The sensitized tissue releases histamine, leukotriene C and D (slow-reacting substance of anaphylaxis), and platelet-activating factor (PAF; 1-*O*-alkyl 2-acetyl-*sn*-glyceryl phosphoryl choline), all potent bronchoconstrictors and stimulators of mucus secretion, as well as tetrapeptides with chemotactic activity for eosinophils (eosinophil chemotactic factor of anaphylaxis). Thus the reaction of specific inhaled allergens with cytophilic antibody on the surface of mast cells leads to the release of mediators and the generation of the asthmatic attack.

Evidence indicates that the modulation of the neural regulation of bronchial muscle tone and mucus secretion may be abnormal in asthma.[474,476] The sensory innervation of the bronchus includes small, nonmyelinated afferent nerves that terminate within the bronchial epithelium between the columnar epithelial cells. They contain physiologically active peptides including substance P, neurokinin A, and calcitonin gene-related peptide which can be released by an axon reflex when the nerves are stimulated.[476] These fibers serve as irritant receptors, triggering cough and bronchospasm. The main motor innervation of the bronchi is via the vagus nerve. Presynaptic vagal fibers synapse on ganglion cells in the connective tissue sheaths around the bronchi. The ganglion cells give rise to cholinergic fibers that end on the mucous glands and bronchial smooth muscle. Acetylcholine is both a bronchoconstrictor and a stimulant of mucus secretion through its effect on muscarinic receptors. Its stimulatory activity is modulated by adrenergic influences, with alpha-adrenergic agonists such as norepinephrine enhancing bronchoconstriction and mucus secretion and beta-adrenergic agonists such as epinephrine inhibiting them. Asthmatics show increased responsiveness to cholinergic and alpha-adrenergic agonists and diminished response to beta-adrenergic agonists, but it is uncertain that any of these abnormalities is the primary defect of asthma.[474,483]

Epithelial injury from a variety of causes such as viral infections or air pollutants triggers airway hyperresponsiveness. Several mechanisms may be involved. Sloughing of the epithelium exposes the sensory nerve endings.[472,475] There is evidence that epithelial cells produce mediators that cause relaxation of the bronchial smooth muscle and that would be lost when the epithelial cells slough. Finally, enzymes in the apical plasma membrane of bronchial epithelial cells catabolize sensory neurotransmitter peptides such as substance P. Loss of this catabolic function because of epithelial damage may prolonge the effective half-life of the transmitters.

Other pathophysiologic mechanisms may be important in particular asthmatics. Some asthmatics have symptoms when exercising or exposed to cold. In these patients cooling of the airway mucosa triggers the attack.[477] Some patients have asthmatic attacks after ingesting aspirin. Commonly this type of asthma is associated with nasal polyps. An explanation for the influence of aspirin may be that it inhibits the cyclooxygenase pathway to prostaglandins, increasing the metabolism of arachidonic acid by the competing lipoxygenase pathway that leads to the leukotrienes, including leukotriene C$_4$ and D$_4$ (slow-reacting substance), potent bronchoconstrictors and stimulants of mucus secretion.

Asthmatic symptoms can develop in sensitized persons in some industries or occupations. Fumes released during the cutting of polyvinylchloride films with a hot electric wire while wrapping produce, fumes emanating during the curing of urea-formaldehyde–based particle board, proteolytic enzymes added to detergents, and toluene diisocyanate fumes are examples of materials that can induce asthma in exposed workers.

Allergic bronchopulmonary mycosis (aspergillosis)

Colonization of the airways by certain fungi can lead to sensitization and the development of asthma complicated by disease of the parenchyma.[492,501,502,505] In most cases the colonizing fungus is *Aspergillus fumigatus* or one of the other *Aspergillus* species, though in some cases other fungi such as *Candida* or *Helminthosporium* have been isolated. Allergic aspergillosis is to be distinguished from *Aspergillus* fungus ball, or mycetoma, and from invasive aspergillosis. Mycetomas are aggregates of matted fungal hyphae in the lumen of a cavity such as that caused by chronic tuberculosis, histoplasmosis, or even a cavitary carcinoma. The fungi do not invade tissue and usually do not themselves cause symptoms. Invasive aspergillosis occurs in the chronically ill and especially in immunosuppressed patients and is a true infection in which organisms invade tissue and can disseminate.

Allergic bronchopulmonary aspergillosis develops in atopic persons. Signs are asthmatic episodes accompanied by eosinophilia, an elevated serum IgE level, and the appearance of parenchymal infiltrates on the chest roentgenogram. Bronchial casts containing organisms, mucus, and fibrin may be expectorated. Early in the course of the disease, roentgenograms show plugging of the bronchi and bronchiectasis involving segmental and subsegmental bronchi but sparing those more peripheral. In the late stages with severe involvement the bronchiectasis may be indistinguishable from ordinary bronchiectasis in which peripheral airways are obliterated.

Resected tissue shows severe bronchiectasis with plugging of bronchi by brown to yellow casts. The plugs consist of mucus and fibrin, and usually organisms can be stained in the intraluminal mucus but do not invade the bronchial wall. Mucus plugs usually contain large numbers of eosinophils, sloughed epithelium, and Charcot-Leyden crystals. The bronchi show mucus hypersecretion and infiltration with inflammatory cells. The lung may show obstructive pneumonia with fibrosis and lipid-laden macrophages, or infiltration with eosinophils and macrophages. Small granulomas are not unusual and consist of nodular collections of foreign body giant cells surrounding degenerated material, which includes products of cell breakdown and perhaps degenerated eosinophils.

Immunologic mechanisms involve an immediate hypersensitivity, an immune complex–mediated Arthus type of reaction, or both. Patients typically have specific IgE antibodies to *Aspergillus* extracts, as well as IgG-precipitating antibody. They respond to skin tests with an immediate wheal and flare followed in many cases by second reaction 4 to 6 hours later. When exposed to *Aspergillus* antigen by inhalation, patients show an immediate fall in vital capacity from which they recover, often followed by a second fall 4 to 6 hours later.

Bronchocentric granulomatosis

Bronchocentric granulomatosis is a response of the lung in which small airways are the site of necrotizing granulomatous inflammation.[494,496] Roughly one third to one half the patients with this histologic picture have asthmatic episodes, eosinophilia, and evidence of sensitization to *Aspergillus*. In the remainder the cause is unknown and eosinophilia absent. The tissue reaction consists in the development of necrotizing granulomas in small bronchi and bronchioles. Initially the lining of the bronchi is replaced by palisading epithelioid cells. Later the bronchi themselves are destroyed and the lo-

calization of the granulomas can be recognized only by their proximity to a pulmonry artery that is either normal or involved only by contiguity with the bronchial granuloma. The center of the granuloma may contain necrotic neutrophils, eosinophils, or simply amorphous debris surrounded by palisaded histiocytes. Rarely fungal hyphae can be found in the center of the necrotic material. Central airways are relatively spared. In addition to a nonspecific chronic inflammatory infiltrate in large bronchi, thre may be small granulomas in the mucous glands and invasion and destruction of cartilage by a mononuclear inflammatory infiltrate.

Hypersensitivity pneumonitis (extrinsic allergic alveolitis)

The clinical picture of hypersensitivity pneumonitis varies depending on the nature of the exposure to antigen. An isolated exposure to a high dose of antigen produces an acute onset, whereas repetitive low-dose exposure may result in the insidious development of illness that is much more difficult for the clinician to associate with exposure. Farmer's lung is the archetype of hypersensitivity pneumonitis. The disease typically develops in a farmer who has been working in moldy hay. Four to 8 hours after exposure there is an acute onset of malaise, fever, myalgia, dyspnea, and cough. The chest roentgenogram shows patchy or miliary parenchymal shadows bilaterally. Manifestations gradually subside if further exposure is avoided. In some patients, however, the onset of disease is more insidious and a physician may not be consulted until the patient has had several attacks or chronic dyspnea has already developed.[491]

The lesions seen in biopsy specimens taken relatively early in the disease tend to be localized around terminal and respiratory bronchioles (Fig. 20-33). Alveolar walls are diffusely infiltrated with lymphocytes, plasma cells, and macrophages. In at least two thirds of cases there are granulomas consisting of aggregates of histiocytes and giant cells, which may be of foreign body or Langhans' type (Fig. 20-34). Necrosis is not a feature of the granulomas of hypersensitivity pneumonitis, and as a rule the granulomas are less compact than those of sarcoidosis. Loose organizing fibrous tissue often fills respiratory bronchioles or alveolar ducts. Alveoli may contain macrophages filled with lipid, a nonspecific change seen in association with obstruction of air passages. Eosinophils and polymorphonuclear cells are relatively few. Fragments of foreign material are present in some cases, but organisms are rarely identified.[489,499,504] Vasculitis is rarely seen, though it was described in one patient dying less than 2 weeks after the onset of symptoms.[486]

In chronic cases the lungs show fibrosis with or without honeycombing. Involvement is most severe in the

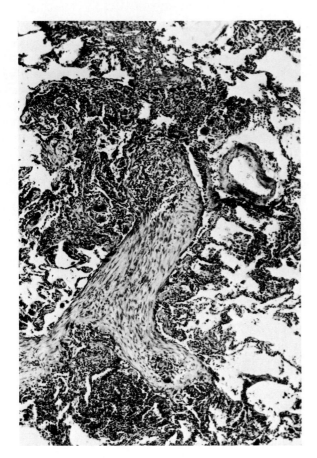

Fig. 20-33. Hypersensitivity pneumonitis. Lesion is centered on terminal airway. Respiratory bronchiole is filled in part with inflammatory cells and in part with proliferating fibrous tissue.

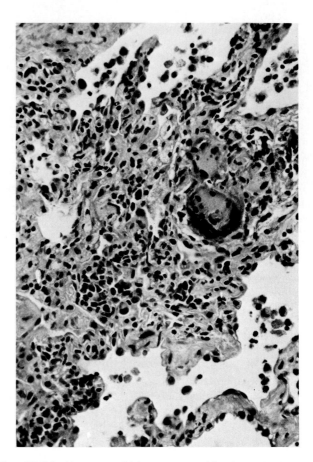

Fig. 20-34. Hypersensitivity pneumonitis. Loosely formed granuloma with giant cells.

Table 20-2. Some causes of hypersensitivity pneumonitis

Syndrome	Source of antigen	Antigen
Farmer's lung	Moldy hay	*Thermoactinomyces vulgaris, Micropolyspora faeni*
Bagassosis	Moldy sugar cane	*T. vulgaris, M. faeni*
Mushroom-worker's disease	Mushroom compost	*T. vulgaris, M. faeni*
Maple bark stripper's disease	Maple bark	*Cryptostroma corticale*
Sequoiosis	Redwood dust	*Graphium* sp.
Malt-worker's lung	Malt dust	*Aspergillus clavatus*
Bird-fancier's lung	Avian serum droppings	Avian proteins
Pituitary snuff user's lung	Pituitary powder	Bovine or porcine proteins

upper lobes. The histologic changes may be entirely nonspecific with interstitial fibrosis and some inflammatory infiltrate, though frequently a few granulomas are still found.[504]

The physiologic abnormalities are those common to interstitial lung disease, including reductions in total lung capacity and its subdivisions, a low diffusing capacity, hypoxemia, and reduced compliance. A minority of patients also have evidence of airflow obstruction[491] because of inflammation, organizing fibrous exudate in small airways, or more rarely granulomas in their walls.

A variety of antigens can give rise to hypersensitivity pneumonitis (Table 20-2). In farmer's lung the antigens are the spores of thermophilic actinomycetes, *Thermoactinomyces vulgaris* and *Micropolyspora faeni*, which thrive in wet hay. Thermophilic actinomycetes can also grow in the fibrous residues from the processing of sugar cane (bagasse) and in mushroom compost, giving rise to the clinical syndromes of bagassosis and mushroom-worker's lung, respectively. Hypersensitivity pneumonitis caused by thermophilic actinomycetes contaminating furnace filters or domestic humidifiers causes hypersensitivity pneumonitis of insidious onset, which is often chronic by the time of clinical examinations.[490] Antigens from avian serum or droppings are responsible for bird-fancier's disease, and molds, wood dust, or animal antigens produce other clinical syndromes (Table 20-2). Despite the variety of antigens and types of environmental exposure involved, the clinical syndromes and histopathologic findings vary more with the intensity and duration of exposure than with the inciting antigen.[487,499,504]

The immunologic mechanisms responsible for hypersensitivity pneumonitis are incompletely understood.[485] The lag of 4 to 6 hours between exposure to antigen and the onset of symptoms is appropriate for an Arthus reaction, and patients have precipitating antibodies to the causative antigens. Since biopsies are not performed in patients ill for only hours, the earliest histologic changes are unknown. The histologic hallmarks of an Arthus reaction, vasculitis and infiltration with polymorphonuclear leukocytes, are usually absent at the time tissues are obtained, however, and immunofluorescence has usually failed to demonstrate, deposition of immunoglobulin or complement. However, vasculitis was described in the lungs of a single patient dying less than 12 days after the onset of farmer's lung disease.[468]

The microscopic characteristics of hypersensitivity pneumonitis, granulomas and mononuclear inflammatory cells, are more in keeping with delayed type of hypersensitivity than an Arthus reaction. The cells retrieved from the alveoli by bronchoalveolar lavage through a fiberoptic bronchoscope characteristically include an increased proportion of T-lymphocytes.[500] Studies of persons who raise pigeons as a hobby show that most have precipitating antibodies to pigeon antigens though few have respiratory symptoms. A better correlation with respiratory symptoms was obtained when peripheral blood lymphocytes were studied to determine their ability to produce migration-inhibitory factor in response to pigeon antigen.[498] In sum, these observations indicate that the pathogenesis may involve both an Arthus reaction and delayed hypersensitivity. A defect in T-suppressor cell function in symptomatic persons offers a plausible explanation for their abnormal immune response.[495]

Pulmonary infiltration and eosinophilia

The combination of elevated eosinophil counts in the peripheral blood and infiltration of the lungs seen on the chest roentgenogram constitutes the clinical syndrome of pulmonary infiltration and eosinophilia (PIE syndrome).[503] The syndrome has numerous causes, as follow:

A. Illnesses in which PIE is a major component
1. Allergic bronchopulmonary aspergillosis
2. Chronic eosinophilic pneumonia

3. Drug reaction
4. Helminth infestation
   a. Tropical eosinophilia
   b. Others
5. Vasculitis (Churg-Strauss syndrome)

B. Illness infrequently associated with PIE
1. Infections (bacterial and fungal)
2. Tumors
3. Sarcoidosis
4. Other

When PIE syndrome is attributable to infestation with worms such as *Ascaris*, *Toxicara canis*, or *Strongyloides*, the infiltrates are seen roentgenographically during the phase of larval migration through the lung en route to the intestine. At that time stool examination may not show ova. To make a diagnosis, it is necessary to reexamine the stool several weeks later, after the larvae have matured to adults that shed ova. Among the lesions of the lung that can be responsible for the infiltrates in PIE syndrome is eosinophilic pneumonia.[493,497] In eosinophilic pneumonia the predominant morphologic feature is exudate of edema fluid, monocytes, macrophages, and eosinophils into the air spaces. Infiltration of the alveolar walls takes place to a variable extent, but the predominant exudation is intra-alveolar. Collections of degenerating eosinophils known as eosinophilic abscesses are a characteristic feature. Organizing fibrous exudate infiltrated with eosinophils may be present in respiratory bronchioles.

Eosinophilic pneumonia is more common in women than in men. Patients often have a history of asthma or atopy. Symptoms include cough, fever, sweats, dyspnea, and weight loss. Occasionally blood eosinophilia is absent.[488] The most characteristic radiographic pattern is the presence of infiltrates with a strikingly subpleural distribution. The response to treatment with corticosteroids is so prompt and dramatic that a trial of therapy is accepted as a diagnostic maneuver.[493]

TRANSPLANTATION

The introduction of cyclosporin into clinical medicine has made it possible to transplant lungs either for the treatment of end-stage lung disease or in combination with the heart for diseases of the pulmonary circulation. The immunosuppression required to prevent immunologic rejection of the graft places the transplanted lung at risk for infection and drug-induced lesions. In addition, the graft is subject to specific processes as a result of the transplantation process.

The reimplantation response is a form of high-permeability pulmonary edema seen in the first few days after transplantation, resulting from surgical trauma, ischemic injury to the graft, denervation, and disruption of lymphatic drainage.[507] The pathology resembles diffuse alveolar damage from other causes. In classical allograft rejection, a previously functioning transplanted lung becomes opacified radiographically, and ventilation and perfusion decrease. Histologically there are alveolar exudates containing fibrin and a mixture of inflammatory cells. Perivascular lymphocytic cuffs are prominent. Less frequent variants of allograft rejection include the alveolar form of rejection in which perivascular lymphocytes are absent and a vascular form in which the blood vessels are infiltrated with lymphocytes but the alveoli are spared.[507]

The late complications of heart-lung transplantation include alveolar wall fibrosis and vascular thickening. A particularly serious late complication in patients who have undergone successful heart-lung transplantation is the development of severe and progressive airflow obstruction attributable to obliterative bronchiolitis.[508] In this process, the parenchyma usually shows only mild abnormalities. The bronchioles are the seat of an acute bronchiolitis that begins with sloughing of the bronchiolar epithelium and infiltration of inflammatory cells and proceeds to concentric fibrosis of the lamina propria and often complete filling of the lumen of the bronchiole with granulation tissue. The cause of this lesion is unclear. Although it is difficult to exclude an infectious or drug-induced cause, evidence is in favor of the idea that it is a consequence of chronic rejection.

Patients who have undergone bone-marrow transplantation for hematologic diseases often manifest an identical type of obliterative bronchiolitis (Fig. 20-35). Donor lymphocytes transplanted with the grafted marrow can recognize recipient tissues as foreign and react against them producing a condition called "graft versus host disease" (GVHD), which affects skin, salivary gland, esophagus, liver, and other tissues. Marrow-transplant patients with bronchiolitis obliterans almost invariably have a history of chronic GVHD, an indication that GVHD may be the cause of the bronchiolitis, but as is the case with heart-lung transplant patients, it has not been possible to exclude infection, drugs, or aspiration as contributing causes.[506]

ACQUIRED IMMUNODEFICIENCY SYNDROME

The lung is one of the major target organs in AIDS and becomes involved in at least 40% of patients.[509] The most common form of involvement is infection, directly traceable to the impaired cell-mediated immunity. Eighty-five percent of lung infections are caused by *Pneumocystis carinii*, alone or in combination with other organisms. Cytomegalovirus and mycobacterial infections are also common. Other agents sometimes infect AIDS patients, ranging from the common pyogenic bacteria to exotic organisms like *Toxoplasma* and *Cryptosporidium*.

AIDS also predisposes to neoplastic involvement of the lung, most often by Kaposi's sarcoma, or malignant lymphoma. Interstitial pneumonias with nonspecific histologic appearance are also common and may represent viral infection or the healing of other types of lung damage. Lymphoid interstitial pneumonia occurs in children or adults infected with HIV either manifesting AIDS-related complex (ARC) or full-fledged AIDS.[510,511] The lung is infiltrated with small lymphocytes and a variable proportion of plasma cells and sometimes contains germinal centers. Most of the lymphocytes are T_8 suppressor T-cells, and the few B-cells

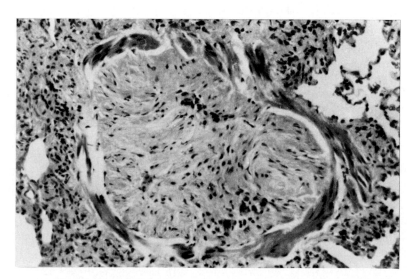

Fig. 20-35. Obliterative bronchiolitis after bone marrow transplantation. Smooth muscle outlines the bronchial wall. The lumen is occluded by fibrous tissue. (Courtesy Dr. Robert C. Hackman, Seattle, Wash.)

are polyclonal.[510] In some patients, lymphoid infiltrates have also been found in organs other than in the lungs.[511]

INTERSTITIAL PNEUMONIA (DIFFUSE INTERSTITIAL FIBROSIS)

Fibrosis of the lung can result from many types of lung injury. The general pathologic processes that lead to fibrosis include the organization of intra-alveolar exudates and hyaline membranes, the healing of granulomatous inflammation, and the response to chronic interstitial edema or inflammation.[520] The specific causes are too diverse and numerous to list. Despite the huge number of known causes of fibrosis, no cause is evident in half the patients who consult a physician because of diffuse interstitial pulmonary fibrosis. The diagnostic labels applied in such cases include idiopathic interstitial pneumonia or chronic idiopathic interstitial fibrosis in the United States and cryptogenic fibrosing alveolitis in Britain.

Clinical features

Persons of any age can be affected, though most cases develop in middle age or later.[523] The onset of symptoms is usually gradual with dry cough and increasing dyspnea, which initially is noticeable only on vigorous exercise but later appears on mild exertion or at rest. In some cases, however, the process begins with a febrile illness, suggestive of a viral pneumonia from which the patient never fully recovers. Clubbing of the fingers is observed in over half of the patients, and a few basilar crackles can be heard on chest auscultation. The chest roentgenogram usually shows bilateral infiltrates but may be normal early in the course. The rate of progression of the process is variable. The average survival is 5 years, but the course may be more acute or much longer, even without therapy.[526] Hamman and Rich[519] were the first to record an acute course leading to death in 6 weeks to 6 months, and the term *Hamman-Rich syndrome* is sometimes used to describe the rapidly progressive form of the disease.

Pathology

The lungs are heavier than normal but reduced in volume, and the pleural surface often has a hobnail appearance. The tissue is firmer than normal and tends to retain its shape during slicing. The process is variable in character, even within a given lung. Normal areas are interspersed with foci of scarring in which the air spaces are obliterated, whereas in other areas the air spaces are abnormally large and thick walled (Fig. 20-36). Honeycombing, the term used to describe areas in which enlarged thick-walled air spaces predominate, can be recognized roentgenographically.

The microscopic changes vary considerably from case

to case, at different stages during the course of the disease, and even from area to area in the same lung. In the early phase of the process the alveolar septa are widened by edema and a cellular infiltrate that is predominantly mononuclear but often also contains neutrophils and sometimes eosinophils. The epithelium covering the alveolar walls is easily seen, some areas being covered by cuboid epithelium identifiable as type II cells by electron microscopy (Fig. 20-37). Other epithelial cells are hypertrophied but partly spread over the alveolar wall and are probably transitional between type I and type II cells. They can be atypical with large nucleoli and basophilic cytoplasm.

The alveolar spaces contain an exudate that may be purely cellular—macrophages, lymphocytes, and neutrophils—or may also contain fibrin and hyaline membranes in varying stages of organization.[523] During organization, fibrin and hyaline membranes are invaded by fibroblasts, usually arrayed parallel or concentrically, and are converted to an edematous matrix initially consisting mainly of proteoglycan but gradually becoming more collagenous. Epithelial cells from the alveolar walls migrate over the surface of the organizing buds of fibrous tissue and become incorporated into the alveolar wall, contributing to the septal thickening.[512]

In the later stages of interstitial pneumonitis, air-

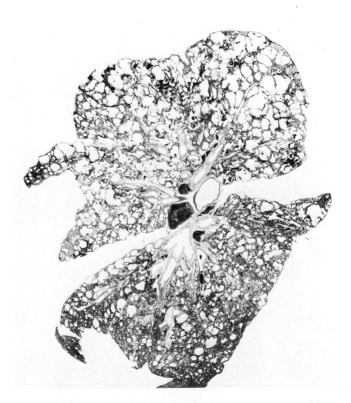

Fig. 20-36. Paper-mounted lung showing honeycombing. Air spaces are greatly enlarged and abnormal with thick fibrous walls. (Courtesy Dr. A.A. Liebow.)

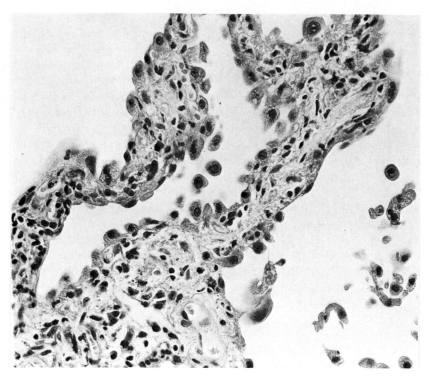

Fig. 20-37. Chronic interstitial pneumonia. Alveolar walls are fibrotic and contain predominantly mononuclear inflammatory cells. Alveolar epithelium is hyperplastic. Loss of capillaries in fibrotic septa is one factor contributing to abnormal gas exchange in this process.

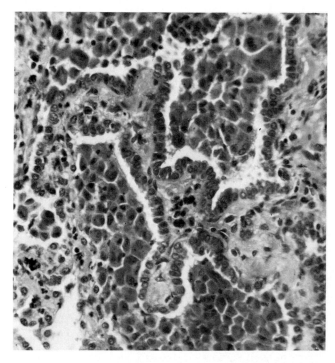

Fig. 20-38. Chronic interstitial pneumonia. This is morphologic pattern called desquamative interstitial pneumonia, in which appearance of biopsy specimen is uniform and alveoli are filled with macrophages.

space walls become increasingly fibrous and alveolar capillaries disappear and are replaced by scar.[520] The number of inflammatory cells is variable but tends to decrease. The epithelium lining the fibrotic air spaces may become bronchiolar in type either by extension from bronchioles or by metaplasia of the alveolar epithelium. Foci of squamous metaplasia can also be found. Arteries are thickened by a combination of medial hypertrophy and the development of an intimal layer of longitudinal muscle. Smooth muscle hyperplasia can also be striking in the interstitium, where it probably arises mainly from hyperplasia of the smooth muscle of alveolar ducts and respiratory bronchioles but possibly also from vessels or by differentiation of septa connective tissue cells.

Histologic classification

In 1965 Liebow, Steer, and Billingsley[522] classified the interstitial pneumonias into several morphologic types. They used the term *desquamative interstitial pneumonia* (DIP) to describe cases in which biopsy specimens showed an apparently uniform pattern, with only modest interstitial fibrosis accompanied by hyperplasia of the alveolar lining epithelium and filling of the alveolar spaces with large mononuclear cells (Fig. 20-38). They believed the mononuclear cells to be

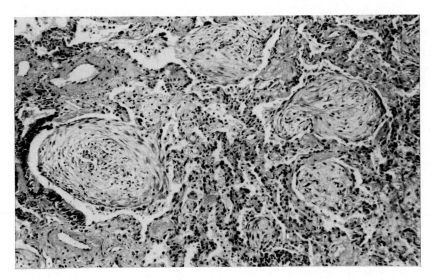

Fig. 20-39. Cryptogenic organizing pneumonitis. Buds of fibroblasts in young connective tissue (Masson bodies) project into respiratory bronchiole and alveolar ducts.

sloughed type II epithelial cells (hence "desquamative"), but subsequent studies by electron microscopy have proved that these cells are mostly macrophages. Some interstitial lymphoid nodules and vascular thickening were present in most cases, but diffuse interstitial inflammation was not striking. They contrasted this appearance with the more heterogeneous appearance in the majority of cases of interstitial pneumonia, with greater inflammation, intra-alveolar organization, and fibrosis (usual interstitial pneumonia, UIP). Subsequent observations indicate that the DIP pattern is probably one end of a spectrum of morphologic changes.[524] There is no evidence that cases with the histologic features of DIP are separable on the basis of etiology or pathogenesis from other cases of interstitial pneumonia. The clinical course of patients with biopsy-proved DIP is more benign, however, and they respond more favorably to therapy with corticosteroids than do patients with UIP.[513]

Another morphologic variant, which Liebow and coworkers called "bronchiolitis obliterans and interstitial pneumonia" (BIP) is now generally known as "bronchiolitis obliterans with organizing pneumonia,"[517] or "cryptogenic organizing pneumonitis."[515] The tissue response in cryptogenic organizing pneumonia is indistinguishable from organizing infectious or chemical pneumonia, being characterized histologically by organizing buds of connective tissue (Masson bodies) projecting into the lumens of respiratory bronchioles, alveolar ducts, and even alveoli (Fig. 20-39). Not infrequently obstruction by the Masson bodies results in collections of lipid-laden macrophages in more distal alveoli. The alveolar septa are usually slightly thickened by inflammatory infiltrate and covered by hyperplastic epithe-

lium which migrates onto the surface of the Masson bodies. The onset of clinical illness in this form of pulmonary fibrosis is often abrupt with a flu-like febrile episode followed by cough and dyspnea that fail to fail to resolve even after several weeks. The chest roentgenogram shows irregular patchy infiltrates or ground-glass opacities.[517] Although the clinical and pathologic pictures seem to show an infectious cause, none is demonstrable, and the process does not respond to antibiotics but usually resolves with treatment by corticosteroids.

Physiologic abnormalities

The major physiologic abnormalities of lungs with interstitial pneumonia are decreased lung volumes, decreased compliance, and impaired gas exchange.[514,518] In advanced disease, reduced lung volumes and compliance are readily explained by obliteration of air spaces by fibrous tissue and by the decreased distensibility of the tissue because of its excess collagen content. Early in the course, edema and exudation of fibrin may also alter the surface-tension properties of the lung. The irregular disposition of connective tissue produces uneven tissue compliance that, combined with inflammation around small airways, produces abnormal distribution of the inhaled air. Destruction of capillary bed in scarred alveolar septa decreases perfusion of diseased areas and probably increases flow in less-affected regions. The result of these functional changes is poor matching of ventilation to perfusion, which is measurable in the pulmonary function laboratory as widening of the gradient of oxygen tension between alveolus and arterial blood and a decreased diffusion capacity; these ultimately result in a low arterial oxygen pressure.

Pathogenesis

The pathogenesis of idiopathic interstitial pneumonia is unknown, but several lines of evidence point to an immunologic mechanism. These include the high incidence of circulating autoantibodies such as rheumatoid factor and antinuclear antibodies[527]; the occurrence of a similar interstitial pneumonia in diseases such as rheumatic fever, rheumatoid arthritis, scleroderma, polymyositis, and mixed connective tissue disease in which an immune pathogenesis is strongly suspected; the presence of elevated titers of circulating immune complexes in some patients, especially those with active disease[516]; and the immunofluorescent demonstration of the deposition of immunoglobulin and complement in some biopsy specimens.[521,525,528] The deposition of immune complexes in the lungs of experimental animals leads to tissue damage and inflammation.[529] The frequency with which elevated levels of circulating immune complexes or immunofluorescent deposits can be detected is much greater early in the disease than in its late fibrotic stage. Even in studies of patients with active disease, however, medical centers vary greatly in the frequency with which these evidences of immune activity are found,[515,521,525,528] and no inciting antigen has been identified. It seems likely that immune complexes are responsible for some cases of idiopathic interstitial pneumonia, but this is by no means proved in all cases.

PULMONARY INVOLVEMENT IN COLLAGEN-VASCULAR DISEASE
Acute rheumatic fever

Pulmonary involvement in acute rheumatic fever is not uncommon, though reported figures vary greatly. Clinically it may be difficult to distinguish heart failure, bacterial infection, and involvement by the primary disease. In the pathologic series reviewed by Brown, Goldring, and Behrer[533] the incidence of rheumatic pneumonia varied from 12% to 50% of patients with acute rheumatic fever. Patients show tachypnea, hypoxemia, and a patchy migratory infiltrate on the chest roentgenogram. Pathologic changes are nonspecific but resemble those in other acute interstitial pneumonias with evidence of fibrous repair. The alveolar walls are thickened by edema and a mixed mononuclear infiltrate. Many alveoli and alveolar ducts are lined with hyaline membranes. Fibrin in various stages of organization is present in alveoli. Thrombosis of arterioles, alveolar septal necrosis, vasculitis, and patchy areas of infarctlike necrosis are found in a minority of cases.[549,566]

Rheumatoid disease

Pulmonary involvement in rheumatoid disease takes several forms including pleural effusion, infiltrative lung disease, bronchiolitis, necrobiotic nodules, vasculitis, and rheumatoid pneumoconiosis. Pleural effusions commonly occur in male patients with high titers of rheumatoid factor. Pleural fluid glucose is reduced to below 30 mg/dl in most cases, and the pH is low.[557,563] The very low glucose concentration has been attributed to a selective block to transport of glucose from plasma into the pleural fluid. Rheumatoid arthritis (RA) cells (leukocytes containing ingested rheumatoid factor–IgG complex) have been seen in the pleural fluid in several cases.[543,558] The histologic changes in the pleura are often those of a nonspecific pleuritis, but in some cases rheumatoid granulomas similar to the subcutaneous nodules have been observed in the pleura.[543]

The frequency of interstitial fibrosis in rheumatoid arthritis is difficult to gauge. Only 1.6% have been reported to have roentgenographic changes, whereas 30% to 40% of patients have been reported to have abnormalities of diffusion, often without symptoms.[544]

The pathologic features of parenchymal infiltrates associated with rheumatoid disease are variable and nonspecific. Biopsy samples may show lymphoid hyperplasia, organizing pneumonia, or usual interstitial pneumonia and fibrosis.[571] At necropsy, there is often honeycomb-like change, most noticeable subpleurally.

The pathogenesis of the interstitial pneumonia is not clear. IgM rheumatoid factor deposits have been demonstrated in the alveolar walls by immunofluorescence,[538] and experimental studies point to a role for such complexes in accentuating inflammation.[537]

In some cases of rheumatoid disease during treatment, the drugs rather than the primary disease may be the cause of pulmonary infiltrates.[545,548] Severe progressive obstructive lung disease caused by bronchiolitis obliterans is a recognized complication of rheumatoid arthritis.[546] Although a relationship to penicillamine therapy has been suggested,[541] not all patients with bronchiolitis obliterans have received this drug. Minor degrees of bronchiolitis probably are not a rare complication of RA, since many patients with RA have small airway dysfunction detectable by sensitive physiologic tests.[547]

Necrobiotic nodules are pathologically the most specific manifestation of rheumatoid disease.[569] They closely resemble the more common subcutaneous nodules. They occur in patients with active disease and high titers of rheumatoid factor, may be single or multiple, and may occur as an isolated form of lung disease or against a background of pulmonary fibrosis. The center of the nodules may consist of fibrinoid necrosis or degenerating neutrophils. A band of palisading histiocytes surrounds the necrotic center. External to the palisaded cells is a zone of fibrous tissue infiltrated with lymphocytes and plasma cells (Fig. 20-40). Necrobiotic nodules developing in patients with pneumoconiosis are discussed later in the chapter (p. 1002).

Necrotizing vasculitis is rare in rheumatoid disease.

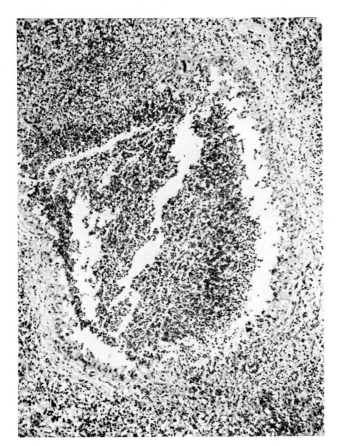

Fig. 20-40. Necrobiotic subpleural nodule in patient with systemic rheumatoid disease. Center is filled with debris of necrotic inflammatory cells and is surrounded by palisading histiocytes.

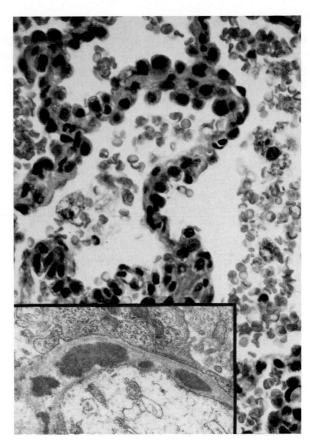

Fig. 20-41. Pulmonary hemorrhage in systemic lupus erythematosus. Alveolar walls show minimal inflammation and epithelial hyperplasia. *Inset,* Electron micrograph shows dense deposits, presumably immune complexes, in basal lamina.

Pulmonary involvement usually occurs with systemic vasculitis, but it has also been described as a localized process.[531]

Systemic lupus erythematosus

Patients with systemic lupus erythematosus (SLE) commonly have lung disease during the course. Often this is attributable to bacterial infection, which was a well-recognized problem even before modern intensive immunosuppressive therapy.[550,554] Presumably hypocomplementemia and general debility were predisposing factors. The most common manifestation of SLE in the thorax is pleurisy that may be painful and is accompanied by small effusions.[550,552] The fluid has properties of an exudate and may contain LE cells. The histopathologic findings in the pleura are those of a nonspecific fibrous or fibrinous pleurisy. The major parenchymal manifestations of SLE are pulmonary hemorrhage, interstitial pneumonitis, and vasculitis. Pulmonary hemorrhage of varying degrees is common in the lungs of patients with SLE at autopsy. As a clinical problem it is a rare, potentially lethal manifestation that occasion-

ally is the earliest sign of SLE.[539] Histologically the lungs show extensive intra-alveolar hemorrhage accompanied by minimal light microscopic changes in the alveolar walls, small arteries, or veins. The alveolar walls may be subtly hypercellular because of an increase of neutrophils and mononuclear cells (Fig. 20-41). Kapanci and Chamay have described wire loop lesions in alveolar capillaries.[555] The alveolar epithelium is focally hyperplastic. Inflammatory cells can be found in or around small arterioles and venules.

Immunohistochemical examination reveals granular deposits of IgG in the alveolar walls, and electron microscopy shows dense deposits (Fig. 20-41) compatible with immune complexes in a subendothelial location and in the interstitium.[534,539]

Interstitial pneumonia occurs in less than 10% of patients with SLE and can be acute[559] or chronic.[540] Biopsies have been performed in relatively few cases of acute lupus pneumonitis. In retrospective autopsy studies of SLE the changes of diffuse alveolar damage are common and include inflammatory cell infiltration and edema of alveolar septa, hyaline membranes, and an intra-alveolar exudate of fibrin in various stages of organization.[550] These changes are nonspecific, and the importance of associated uremia or changes resulting from therapy has not always been critically assessed. Biopsy examination in a few cases of acute lupus pneumonitis has shown mononuclear infiltration of alveolar walls and intra-alveolar organization.[559] Immunohistochemical examination has shown the presence of DNA and immune complexes in the alveolar walls.[553] Eluted antibody had anti-DNA activity. Chronic interstitial fibrosis in SLE may have more than one pathogenesis. Usually it is caused by low-grade interstitial pneumonia, but some cases may result from the healing of infarcts.[540]

Vasculitis involves the lung in some cases of acute SLE and may be responsible for pulmonary hypertension.[542,560] Necrobiotic nodules have been described but are very rare.[568]

Sjögren's syndrome

Sjögren's syndrome combines lymphoid infiltration of lacrimal and salivary glands with other manifestations of collagen-vascular disease, most commonly arthritis and hyperglobulinemia. Involvement of the bronchial mucous glands by a process similar to that in the salivary glands can lead to inadequate bronchial clearance and repeated infections.[567] Chronic airflow obstruction associated with bronchiolitis is common and can be disabling.[561] Whether the explanation is damage from infection or is a manifestation of a rheumatoid process is unknown. In the lung periphery, nonspecific interstitial pneumonia is present in approximately 3% to 4% of patients.[552,569] A variety of lymphoproliferative lesions also occur in the lungs in Sjögren's syndrome.[530,556] These range from lymphoid interstitial pneumonia in which the lung interstitium is heavily infiltrated by lymphocytes and plasma cells, to pseudolymphoma with nodules and masses of benign lymphoid tissue with germinal centers and a well-differentiated lymphoplasmacytic infiltrate, to frankly malignant lymphoma usually of the large cell ("histiocytic") type. In one patient with Sjögren's syndrome, lymphomatoid granulomatosis developed, and amyloidosis has developed in several.[532]

Progressive systemic sclerosis

Progressive systemic sclerosis (PSS) is a systemic disease that frequently involves the skin, kidney, gastrointestinal tract, and skeletal muscle, as well as the lung.[551] The lung is abnormal in 80% of cases both clinically and at autopsy.[536] The most characteristic pathologic change is a myxoid thickening with concentric cellular hyperplasia of the intima of muscular arteries, which is found in 30% to 50% of patients with classical scleroderma.[536,571] In the relatively benign variant of

PSS known as the CREST syndrome (calcinosis, Raynaud's phenomenon, esophageal dysfunction, sclerodactyly, telangiectasia) it occurs much less commonly.[564] In either clinical setting it can be associated with severe and progressive pulmonary hypertension. Pulmonary fibrosis, the most common form of pulmonary involvement in PSS, evolves slowly compared with the idiopathic form.[535] It usually involves the lower lobes and subpleural regions of the lung, and honeycombing is common. The vascular change and parenchymal fibrosis can occur together (Fig. 20-42) or separately. The prevalence of pneumonia is also increased in PSS, which is not surprising, since esophageal dysfunction is common and predisposes to aspiration.

Polymyositis and dermatomyositis

Interstitial pneumonitis and fibrosis may accompany polymyositis and dermatomyositis.[552,565] When the interstitial pneumonitis precedes the myopathic symptoms, the diagnosis of polymyositis may be missed and the muscular manifestations may be attributed to restricted activity and chronic illness. Involvement of the muscles of deglutition promotes aspiration.

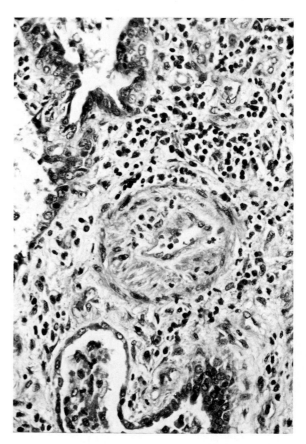

Fig. 20-42. Progressive systemic sclerosis. There is pronounced intimal thickening of small muscular artery. Lung shows severe interstitial fibrosis.

Wegener's granulomatosis

The four components of Wegener's granulomatosis are granulomas of the upper respiratory tract, granulomas of the lung, systemic vasculitis, and a focal, usually necrotizing, glomerulonephritis.[584,585,590] Granulomas occasionally are present in other organs as well. Not all components may be present in a given patient. The term *limited Wegener's granulomatosis* has been used to describe those who do not have glomerulitis.[578] Lesions in some cases of so-called lethal midline granuloma of the upper respiratory tract are histologically identical to Wegener's lesions and probably represent Wegener's granulomatosis without involvement of other sites.[577]

The clinical manifestations vary according to the site of involvement. Persons of any age may be affected, but most patients are middle aged. Men outnumber women by a small margin. Upper respiratory tract symptoms may be referable to the sinuses, nose, nasopharynx, or middle ear, whereas pulmonary symptoms are quite nonspecific and include cough, dyspnea, or pleurisy. Systemic manifestations such as fever, weight loss, anemia, and leukocytosis are common when multiple sites are involved but infrequent when disease is limited to one or a few sites.[581] The chest roentgenogram shows single or multiple, large, rounded densities that may cavitate and that occur predominantly in the lower lobes.

Grossly the pulmonary lesions may have the appearance of pale infarcts or vary from small to bulky necrotic nodules (Fig. 20-43).[578,589] The histologic features of upper and lower respiratory tract lesions are similar, consisting of necrotizing granulomas with an associated vasculitis. Granulomatous inflammation including macrophages, lymphocytes, plasma cells, and fibroblasts encloses geographic zones of necrosis that are often infarctlike, bland, and with preservation of the outlines of the underlying tissue, but that may be softer and contain an abundance of debris. Giant cells vary from scanty to numerous and are usually of the foreign body type. Discrete compact epithelioid granulomas like those of sarcoidosis or tuberculosis are distinctly unusual.[578,585,586,589]

Vasculitis involves both veins and arteries and vessels from millimeters to tens of micrometers in size. In some cases fibrinoid necrosis may predominate and the involved vessels closely resemble those in polyarteritis nodosa, but more often there is cellular invasion of the vessel wall by mononuclear cells that thicken the intima, replace the media, and focally destroy the elastic tissue. In larger vessels the granulomatous quality of the inflammation may be obvious with palisading histiocytes and giant cells (Fig. 20-44).[578,585,586,589]

The association of vasculitis with necrotizing granulomatous inflammation is required for the diagnosis of Wegener's granulomatosis, but it is by no means specific. Special stains and cultures are needed to rule out infection, since vasculitis is not rare in contiguity with infectious granulomas. Vasculitis in vessels remote from the actual granulomas is helpful in making the diagnosis but is not always found, especially when biopsy specimens are of limited size.

Extrapulmonary lesions, usually consisting of vasculitis and sometimes of granulomas, can be found in a

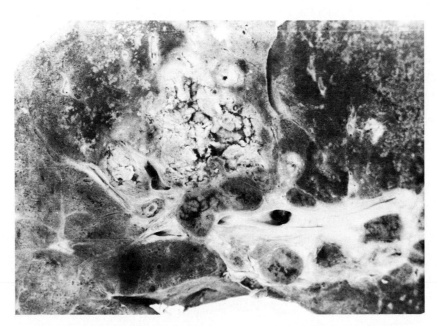

Fig. 20-43. Necrotic pulmonary lesion in Wegener's granulomatosis.

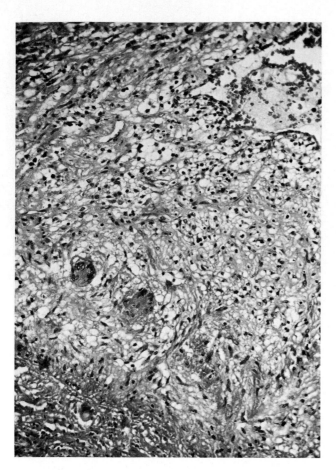

Fig. 20-44. Granulomatous vasculitis in Wegener's granulomatosis. Lumen of vessel is at upper right.

variety of organs. Necrosis of the spleen was mentioned in Wegener's original report, and granulomatous trabeculitis can be striking. The usual renal lesions are a segmental necrotizing glomerulitis, but cases have been described in which necrotizing granulomas were present in the kidney without glomerulitis.[578]

The pathogenesis of Wegener's granulomatosis is unknown, but as with many other forms of vasculitis, an immunologically mediated injury is likely. Elevated levels of circulating immune complexes have been detected in some cases. Immunofluorescence of the glomerular lesions gives variable results, but granular staining of immunoglobulin and complement have often been reported.[552] Therapy based on a presumption of immunologic injury has been remarkably successful. Persons with untreated, full-blown Wegener's granulomatosis with glomerulitis had a median survival of only 5 months, and 80% of patients died in the first year.[590] With vigorous immunosuppressive therapy remissions occur in as much as 80% to 90% and long-term survival is common.[584]

Allergic granulomatosis and angiitis

Like Wegener's disease, the entity allergic granulomatosis and angiitis (Churg-Strauss syndrome) involves a combination of vasculitis and respiratory tract granulomas.[580] Asthma is usually present for several years before there develops a systemic illness that resembles polyarteritis nodosa accompanied by eosinophilia of the peripheral blood and in most cases infiltrates or nodules on the chest roentgenogram. Clinical renal involvement is uncommon, but skin eruptions or subcutaneous nodules have been reported in two thirds of patients.[579] The pulmonary lesions include infiltrates of eosinophils and necrotizing granulomas with central fibrinoid necrosis surrounded by palisading histiocytes and giant cells.[580] Vasculitis involving small arteries and veins may be present in any organ. As a rule the vasculitis is manifest by fibrinoid necrosis and an eosinophil-rich inflammatory infiltrate, but when larger muscular arteries are involved, inflammation can be frankly granulomatous. Chumbley, Harrison, and DeRemee[579] reported a mortality of 50%. The average survival was 4½ years after the onset of symptoms.

Hypersensitivity angiitis

In 1953 Zeek[591] reviewed the vasculitides and differentiated polyarteritis nodosa, a disease affecting muscular arteries near their branch points, from hypersensitive angiitis, which involved smaller vessels, arterioles, and venules. Polyarteritis nodosa was characterized by lesions of varying ages and had no identifiable cause, whereas hypersensitivity pneumonitis often began after exposure to a definite allergen, usually a drug or serum, and lesions were of the same histologic age. The two conditions differed in their patterns of organ involvement: the lung and spleen were rarely involved in classic polyarteritis nodosa but were frequent targets of hypersensitivity pneumonitis. Subsequent series put the frequency of lung involvement in hypersensitivity angiitis at about 40%. Although recent writers have divided this small vessel vasculitis into subtypes,[552] the pathologic features are similar in all, consisting in fibrinoid necrosis and leukocytic infiltration of the walls of arterioles, venules, and capillaries. In the lung these usually result in hemorrhage, which may be difficult to distinguish from Goodpasture's syndrome, though antibodies to basal lamina are not found.

Goodpasture's syndrome

The development of antibodies to antigens in the basal lamina can produce either glomerulonephritis alone or pulmonary hemorrhage and glomerulonephritis, a combination known as Goodpasture's syndrome. Goodpasture's syndrome usually occurs in men between the ages of 16 and 30 years.[574] The majority of cases have been reported to be of the HLA-DRW2 haplotype. The pulmonary manifestations usually precede the renal disease.[574] Hemoptysis is the initial symptom in 95% of patients and is often accompanied by exertional dyspnea, fatigue, and weakness. Iron-deficiency anemia, hematuria, and proteinuria follow. Without therapy the disease is usually lethal within a year, but spontaneous remissions can occur.

In acute cases light microscopy shows little alteration of the lung parenchyma, whereas in more chronic cases there is interstitial fibrosis accompanied by filling of air spaces with hemosiderin-laden macrophages. Elastic fibers in the walls of small arteries and veins may be encrusted with iron salts accompanied by foreign-body giant cells. Immunofluorescence shows linear deposition of immunoglobulin and complement in the basal lamina regions.[575,588] Deposition is uniform in the kidney, but focal in the lung, and can be missed if only a small lung biopsy specimen is available for staining. Electron microscopy shows swelling, irregular lucency, and overt breaks in the basal lamina.[576,582] Gaps are present between endothelial cells, and occasional neutrophils or monocytes have been described passing through discontinuities in the alveolar-capillary membrane.

The antibodies responsible for Goodpasture's syndrome are usually IgG, rarely IgA or IgM.[575] They most often recognize a globular domain in basement membrane (type IV) collagen.[587] The stimulus to antibody formation is unknown. The increased incidence of Goodpasture's syndrome during the year of an influenza pandemic indicates that viral injury to the alveolar basal lamina could be one stimulus.[574] Investigators have encountered a history of exposure to volatile solvents or smoke inhalation,[572] suggestive of chemical injury as a stimulus.

OTHER NONINFECTIOUS GRANULOMAS
Pulmonary histiocytosis X

Histiocytosis X (well-differentiated histiocytosis) is a proliferative disease involving a subset of mononuclear phagocytes similar to the Langerhans' cells of the skin.[598] The lung can be involved either as part of disseminated histiocytosis or in a localized process limited to the lung. Disseminated histiocytosis has been described in detail by Newton and Hamoudi.[597] The lung involvement is typically widespread and diffuse in acute disseminated histiocytosis (Letterer-Siwe type), whereas in chronic disseminated histiocytosis the lesions are focal and nodular. On healing they can result in striking honeycomb change (Fig. 20-45). The prognosis of disseminated histiocytosis depends largely on the extent and activity of the systemic process.[593,597]

Histiocytosis limited to the lung (pulmonary eosino-

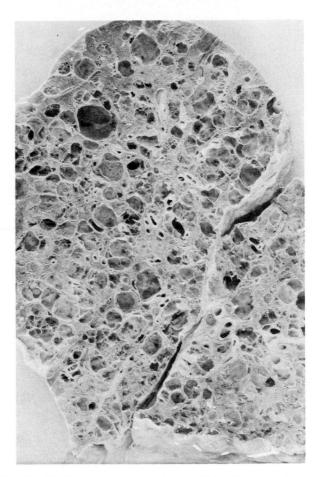

Fig. 20-45. Honeycomb lung from child with disseminated histiocytosis X.

philic granuloma) is a disease mainly of young adults, with an average age of 30 years. Men have predominated in most series. Symptoms are variable. Some patients are asymptomatic, and the process is discovered accidentally by chest roentgenography. Some patients are first seen for pneumothorax, whereas others have cough and gradually worsening dyspnea as a result of interstitial involvement.[593] Early chest roentgenograms show bilateral nodular infiltrates that may resolve or may become reticular with the subsequent appearance of bullae or honeycombing. Sparing of the costophrenic angles is characteristic but nonspecific.[596]

The pathologic features were well described by Auld,[592] as well as subsequent observers.[593-595] At low power a striking feature is the nodular pattern with intervening normal or near-normal lung. Many lesions are centered on bronchioles or small vessels. Within the nodules the interstitium is infiltrated by a mixed cell population including lymphocytes, plasma cells, eosinophils, and some typical macrophages, as well as the characteristic histiocytosis X (Hx) cells. These cells have

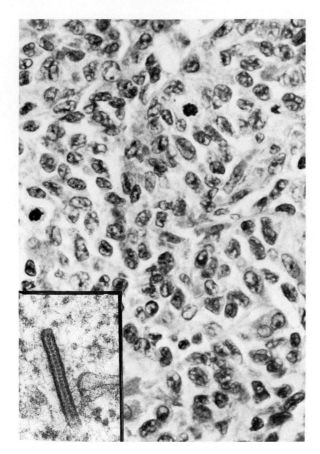

Fig. 20-46. Localized pulmonary histiocytosis X. Many nuclei have characteristic notched or folded appearance. Notice mitotic figures. *Inset,* Electron micrograph of characteristic cytoplasmic organelle of Langerhans type of histiocyte.

an indistinct pale pink or amphophilic cytoplasm and an elongated or reniform nucleus that is folded or notched (Fig. 20-46).

They have characteristic cytoplasmic organelles, known as "Birbeck granules," that can be identified by electron microscopy (Fig. 20-46), and they stain with antibodies to S-100 protein and with OKT-6 monoclonal antibody. Although these cells can be found in small numbers in other lung conditions, their presence in abundance is diagnostic of histiocytosis.[594]

The early nodular lesions are highly cellular with a predominance of Hx cells. Mitotic figures are present in some cells. Rarely invasion and obliteration of vessels by the Hx cells lead to necrosis or cavitation of the nodules, but necrosis is usually absent. With healing the center of the lesion becomes more fibrous, but at the periphery an infiltrate of Hx cells extends into the interstitium of neighboring alveolar walls, giving the lesion a stellate configuration. Ultimately the lesions heal, leaving a stellate scar. The pathologic differential

diagnosis is discussed elsewhere.[5] The principal consideration is usually eosinophilic pneumonia. In eosinophilic pneumonia the low-power pattern is not nodular and the cellular infiltrate is predominantly intra-alveolar, whereas in histiocytosis it is interstitial. The eosinophilic abscesses characteristic of eosinophilic pneumonia are not found in histiocytosis. The nuclear characteristics of the mononuclear phagocytes in the two conditions differ, but in difficult cases electron microscopy and immunohistochemistry may be used to confirm the nature of the mononuclear phagocytes.

The course of localized pulmonary histiocytosis is extremely variable. The majority of patients undergo spontaneous or induced arrest or remission. In some cases cysts or bullae develop leading to recurrent pneumothorax. A few, probably less than 10%, progress to disabling interstitial fibrosis and death from respiratory failure or cor pulmonale.[596]

Sarcoidosis

Sarcoidosis is a systemic disease that involves the thoracic organs in 90% of cases.[615] Scadding has defined it as a disease "characterized by the presence in all of several affected organs and tissues of noncaseating epithelioid-cell granulomas proceeding either to resolution or to conversion into featureless hyaline connective tissue."[612] This definition does not mention causation, about which nothing is known, nor an underlying alteration in immunologic reactivity, about which much remains to be learned. It is not clear whether sarcoidosis is a syndrome of many causes or a single entity.

Sarcoidosis most commonly affects adults between 20 and 40 years of age and is rare below 10 years of age. Its distribution is worldwide. In the United States the prevalence is more than 10 times higher in blacks than in whites and greater in women than in men.[609] In South Africa the prevalence is also higher in blacks.[610] In Europe the prevalence is highest in Scandinavians and there is no distinct sex predilection.

Pathology

The diagnostic feature of sarcoidosis is the noncaseating granuloma, a compact nodule of epithelioid cells with a few lymphocytes, monocytes, and macrophages (Fig. 20-47).[599,612,614] As a rule necrosis is absent, but even in cases that are clinically typical and from which infection is excluded, a few granulomas may have a small amount of granular eosinophilic necrosis in the center.[614] The epithelioid cells are generally similar to those in tuberculosis when viewed by light and electron microscopy.[611] By electron microscopy two types of epithelioid cells have been described,[611] one with extensively developed endoplasmic reticulum and few granules or vacuoles and the other with many vacuoles containing finely granular material. They may represent

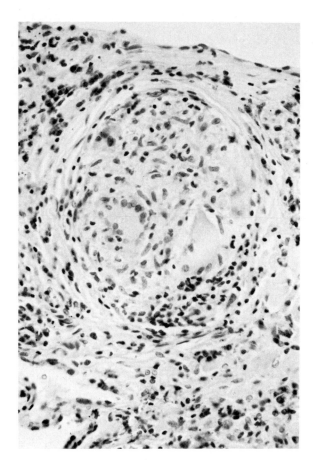

Fig. 20-47. Noncaseating granuloma in sarcoidosis. Compact epithelioid granuloma with giant cells. Early fibrous capsule has formed.

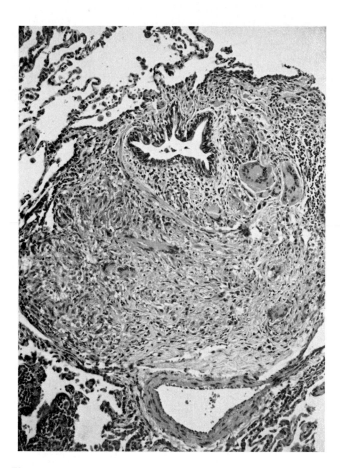

Fig. 20-48. Sarcoidosis. Involvement of bronchiole by granulomas.

different phases in the life cycle of a single cell line, since cells with transitional ultrastructural features were seen. The epithelioid cells appear to be derived from the mononuclear phagocyte series, but because of their paucity of phagosomes and well-developed endoplasmic reticulum, they have been interpreted as a poorly phagocytic secretory form.

Giant cells of either foreign body or Langhans' type are common. Their ultrastructure and the results of thymidine-labeling studies suggest that they form by fusion of epithelioid cells.[600] They may contain a variety of inclusions, none of which can be considered specific for sarcoidosis.[614] Asteroid bodies are stellate, strongly eosinophilic bodies that are seen in giant cells in a variety of diseases. The few ultrastructural studies indicate that they are derived from the cytosphere.[601] Schaumann or conchoid bodies are concentric lamellae of iron- and calcium-containing material associated often with birefringent crystals that lie between the lamellae. They vary in size from 10 to 30 μm and may be either in the cytoplasm of an individual giant cell or apparently extracellular in close association with several giant cells. Some giant cells contain colorless birefrin-

gent crystals 1 to 25 μm in size. Electron probe microanalysis has shown only elements that are compatible with an endogenous origin for the crystals. Some, at least, are calcium oxalate.

The earliest stages of the sarcoid granuloma are not well known. Rosen and associates[613] observed a nongranulomatous interstitial infiltrate of mononuclear cells accompanying nonfibrotic granulomas in early sarcoidosis. They propose that the granulomas evolve from a nonspecific alveolitis.

The healing of a granuloma begins with the appearance of a thin fibrous capsule enclosing the granuloma. In cases of longer duration the capsule is thicker and formed of coarser lamellae of hyalinized connective tissue. In old and quiescent lesions the periphery of the granuloma is replaced by hyalinized connective tissue, often leaving only a few macrophages or a giant cell or two in the center. Eventually these too are replaced by fibrous tissue.

Sarcoid granulomas can involve any of the structures of the lung.[602,614] They can be found in airways of any size (Fig. 20-48), in walls of blood vessels, and in the pleura. Parenchymal granulomas are commonly inter-

Table 20-3. Frequency of major organ involvement in sarcoidosis

Organ system	United States (%)	Worldwide (%)
Thoracic	92	87
Reticuloendothelial	50	28
Ocular	15	15
Skin	23	9
Erythema nodosum	10	17
Salivary gland	7	4
Nervous system	3	4
Osseous	6	3

From James, G.D., and Neville, E.: Pathobiol. Annu. 7:31, 1977.

stitial, but some appear to develop within alveolar spaces. Conglomeration of granulomas matted together by fibrosis can give rise to large nodules. The healing and scarring late in the process can produce honeycombing, bullae, or upper lobe cavities that lack the caseous or liquefied contents of tuberculous cavities. Other organs are also involved (Table 20-3), and involvement of some, notably the heart and nervous system, may determine the outcome of the disease.

Natural history

The natural history of sarcoidosis can be followed sequentially from study of the chest roentgenogram.[606,607] The stages are as follows:

Stage 1   Bilateral hilar lymphadenopathy
Stage 2   Hilar adenopathy with pulmonary infiltrates
Stage 3   Pulmonary infiltrates

The earliest manifestation of sarcoidosis is bilateral hilar lymph node enlargement without roentgenographic changes in the parenchyma. Some patients at this stage have the cutaneous lesions of erythema nodosum. This combination is particularly common in Scandinavia, where it is known as Löfgren's syndrome. Although the parenchyma appears normal roentgenographically, transbronchial biopsy specimens show the presence of either nonspecific alveolitis or granulomas in a high proportion of patients. Pulmonary function is abnormal in only 20% to 30% of patients however, and the degree of abnormality is mild.

The disease in 50% of patients at this stage will regress spontaneously within a year. In others it will take longer. In only 10% does pulmonary parenchymal disease of sufficient severity to be roentgenographically detectable develop. Patients with parenchymal infiltrates and hilar adenopathy seen on the roentgenogram usually have pulmonary dysfunction. In only half will the chest roentgenogram return to normal. Patients with parenchymal disease without hilar adenopathy (stage 3) rarely improve and usually have dysfunction. Reduced diffusion capacity and restriction of ventilation are the rule, but concomitant airflow obstruction is also

common. The airflow obstruction probably results from direct involvement of bronchi and bronchioles by granulomas.

Diagnosis

The diagnosis of sarcoidosis can be based on the clinical findings and the demonstration of noncaseating granulomas in any involved tissue.[612] Transbronchial biopsy has proved to be a valuable tool, disclosing granulomas in more than 90% of patients with roentgenographic lung involvement and roughly half of those with stage 1 disease.[614] It should be emphasized that the histologic findings are not distinguishable from those in the infectious granulomas. Staining for tubercle bacilli and fungi should always be done, and even when no organisms are seen, the pathologist would be foolish to make a stronger statement than that the lesions are "compatible with sarcoidosis."

The Kveim-Siltzbach reaction is a potentially useful diagnostic test.[610,612] An antigen prepared from involved lymph node or spleen is injected intradermally. Three to 6 weeks later if a nodule has appeared, biopsy is performed and the specimen is observed microscopically. The presence of noncaseating granulomas constitutes a positive result. With carefully prepared and standardized antigen there are very few false-positive reactions. False-negative results usually occur in those with chronic inactive disease. The antigen is not approved by the U.S. Food and Drug Administration and is not generally available.

There are abnormalities in the serum of sarcoid patients, but none are specific. Hyperglobulinemia is common; hypercalcemia less so. Response of the hypercalcemia to corticosteroids is a helpful diagnostic feature. Elevation in angiotensin-converting enzyme (ACE) occurs in 40% to 80% of patients with sarcoidosis, more often in those with active disease. However, it also occurs in a small proportion of patients with diseases such as miliary tuberculosis, histoplasmosis, hypersensitivity pneumonitis, or idiopathic interstitial fibrosis, which can easily be confused with sarcoidosis. Consequently ACE elevation should be interpreted in the light of other clinical data. The ACE level decreases with corticosteroid therapy and is a valuable tool for following disease activity and effect of therapy.

Etiology and pathogenesis

The cause of sarcoidosis remains unknown. The possibility of involvement by the tubercle bacillus has been raised but is unlikely. Granules of acid-fast material are occasionally stainable in epithelioid cells, but these may be lipid sequestered in lysosomes and need not be derived from bacilli.

The presence of granulomas indicates the possible involvement of a cell-mediated immune response. Cells lavaged from the lung include increased numbers of helper T-lymphocytes, which proliferate spontaneously and secrete interleukin-2, gamma interferon, and chemoattractants for monocytes. The immature mononuclear phagocytes in lavage fluid are efficient antigen-presenting cells compared to typical alveolar macrophages. This behavior supports the hypothesis of a cell-mediated immune reaction in the lung.[604,605,608,616] The antigen, if any, is unknown, but the fact that reactivity to Kveim antigen is shared by patients worldwide indicates that a single antigen could be involved.

Necrotizing sarcoid granulomatosis

The relationship between the condition that Liebow designated "necrotizing sarcoid granulomatosis" and ordinary sarcoidosis is unclear.[589] Kveim testing has not been reported in the former condition. Some clinical differences have been noted. Roughly half of the patients with necrotizing sarcoid granulomatosis have systemic symptoms such as fever, sweating, malaise, and weight loss. Chest pain is common, usually described as a dull ache and rarely pleuritic. A few patients are asymptomatic. The chest roentgenogram shows bilateral nodular densities or less often a miliary pattern or ill-defined infiltrates. In a few cases lesions appear to be solitary. Pathologically the lesions consist of a collection of epithelioid granulomas united in a background of fibrous tissue and nonspecific inflammatory cells. The granulomas are less discrete or encapsulated than those of typical sarcoidosis. Irregular, sometimes extensive patches of fibrinoid or coagulative necrosis are present. Central necrosis of individual granulomas, as occurs in tuberculosis, is not a feature. Vasculitis, which can take several morphologic forms, involves both veins and arteries. Vessels can be invaded or obliterated by granulomas or can be involved by an inflammatory process resembling giant cell arteritis with a preponderance of the giant cell reaction associated with the external elastic lamina, or the vasculitis can be a nonspecific mononuclear inflammatory infiltration of vessel walls. Extrapulmonary manifestations are rare. The hilar lymph nodes have been enlarged in roentgenograms of the chest in only a few patients though small granulomas in hilar lymph nodes are sometimes seen microscopically. A few patients have had hepatic granulomas or uveitis.[603] Cultures and stains have not demonstrated organisms. Although only a few patients have had adequate follow-up monitoring, the course of the disease generally has been favorable. Patients have either remained stable or have had regression of lesions with steroid or cytotoxic therapy. Recrudescences have been reported in a few instances.

The generally benign course, occurrence of epithelioid granulomas, and failure to recover an infectious agent are all properties shared with sarcoidosis. Granulomatous vasculitis is not uncommon in sarcoidosis, and nodules of confluent granulomas also occur. Necrosis is infrequent and mild in sarcoidosis but appears to be explicable in necrotizing sarcoid granulomatosis as infarction resulting from the vasculitis rather than as a characteristic of the granulomas. On the other hand, the absence of roentgenographic hilar adenopathy and the rarity with which extrapulmonary lesions have been described in necrotizing sarcoid granulomatosis are arguments against the identity of the two diseases.

MISCELLANEOUS LUNG DISEASES
Alveolar proteinosis

In 1958 Rosen, Castleman, and Liebow[628] described 27 patients with a new disease in which the distal air spaces of the lung become filled with a curious exudate consisting of granular eosinophilic material containing cholesterol clefts, occasional naked nuclei, and eosinophilic globules that are 5 to 20 μm in size and appear to be the ghosts of cells, an impression verified by electron microscopy.[622] In some areas there are numerous lipid-filled macrophages, whereas in other regions the exudate is nearly acellular (Fig. 20-49). The exudate stains strongly with the periodic acid–Schiff reaction, which led Rosen and associates to conclude that the in-

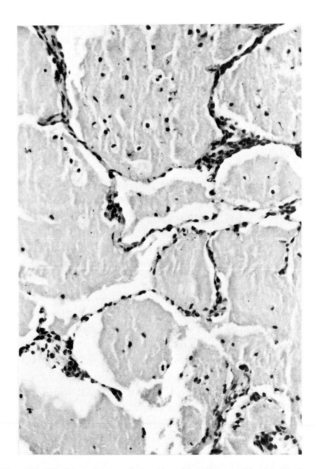

Fig. 20-49. Alveolar proteinosis. Alveoli are filled with flocculent exudate with a few nuclei, remnants of degenerated cells. Alveolar walls are normal.

tra-alveolar material is glycoprotein. They also had biochemical analyses that indicated a high lipid content.[628] The alveolar septa are only minimally abnormal with focal regions of type II cell hyperplasia and a few collections of lipid-filled interstitial macrophages but little inflammation. The nature of the intra-alveolar material has been studied extensively by electron microscopy and histochemical and biochemical analyses of specimens obtained by bronchoalveolar lavage.[618,621-623,625,629] The exudate contains serum protein, some cell debris, and large amounts of alveolar surfactant including both the characteristic saturated phospholipids and specific surfactant proteins. The serum proteins present are of low molecular weight. The absence of high–molecular weight components militates against a major alteration in the permeability of the alveolar capillary membrane.

The reason for the accumulation of this material is unknown. Because other materials are present, it is probably not a simple primary overproduction of surfactant.[619] The material composing the exudate is not itself surface active, probably because of the presence of other components that are inhibitory.[622,623] There is evidence that the intra-alveolar material turns over very slowly, a finding suggestive of a primary defect in alveolar clearance.[626] The cause of the disease is unknown. Persons of any age can be affected including young children. Increased numbers of birefringent crystals are found in the lungs of many patients, which might indicate an occupational cause or impaired alveolar clearance.[624] The occurrence of proteinosis in patients heavily exposed to silica (p. 997) is evidence in favor of the former interpretation. An association of proteinosis with hematologic malignancy has also been observed.[617]

The clinical manifestations of alveolar proteinosis are variable, ranging from nearly asymptomatic to life-threatening hypoxemia. The chest roentgenogram in uncomplicated cases shows an alveolar filling pattern with a variable distribution but often resembling the butterfly distribution of the pulmonary edema of heart failure without cardiomegaly or effusions. As a rule disability is surprisingly mild considering the degree of roentgenographic change. Infections with fungi, nocardias, or mycobacteria are a common and serious complication, explainable in part by the presence of a nutritious broth within the air spaces[627] and in part by an acquired defect in the function of the alveolar macrophages, which are already burdened with a heavy load of lipid and debris.[620] The course of the disease is unpredictable, with some patients having spontaneous clearing whereas others deteriorate.

Alveolar microlithiasis

Alveolar microlithiasis is a rare disease occurring in sporadic form and in familial groupings.[633,636,637] Persons of all ages can be affected, the youngest recorded being a premature infant of 29 weeks' gestational age and the oldest an octogenarian at the time of death. The largest number of patients become symptomatic between 30 and 60 years of age, but roughly 25% of all patients are children. The disease is characterized by the deposition of concentrically laminated calcified bodies (calcospheritis) within the alveoli. Grossly the lungs are heavy, firm, and difficult to slice. They are said to feel like sandpaper. The calcospherites, which consist mainly of calcium phosphate, range up to several hundred micrometers in size and by light microscopy are found predominantly within alveolar spaces. The alveolar walls are usually little affected. In some cases interstitial fibrosis is present and some of the calcospherites are in an interstitial location. Electron microscopy shows that the calcospherites seem to form in relation to collagen by a process initiated by the shedding of matrix vesicles from connective tissue cells much like other forms of ectopic mineralization. Rarely calcospherites have also been found in the submucosa of the bronchi or extrathoracic sites.

Clinically the mild dyspnea contrasts with the dramatic miliary roentgenographic shadowing, which spares only the apices. Many patients are asymptomatic when the disease is discovered. After many years restrictive lung disease and cor pulmonale may develop.

The calcospherites should be distinguished from other forms of pulmonary concretions. Corpora amylacea are strongly periodic acid–Schiff–positive bodies with a dense central nidus surrounded by a cortex with fine radial striations.[632] They are indistinguishable morphologically from the corpora amylacea that are common in the brain and prostate. Their cause is unknown, and they are found in both normal and diseased lungs, usually in small numbers. So-called blue bodies are laminated basophilic concretions, 12 to 25 μm in diameter, that contain calcium carbonate and small amounts of iron deposited in a mucopolysaccharide matrix. They are found in association with macrophages, usually in lungs with interstitial pneumonias of the DIP type.[631] They never attain the size of the calcospherites of microlithiasis and are not detectable as calcific density on chest roentgenograms.

Metastatic calcification and ossification

Metastatic calcification is the result of elevation of the product of ionized calcium and phosphate. It is a common finding at autopsy in patients with chronic renal disease,[630] destructive bone metastases, or multiple myeloma and has also been reported in milk-alkali syndrome and primary hyperparathyroidism. The calcific deposits are interstitial, initially localizing in basement membranes and on the elastic fibers of alveolar walls. Eventually the whole interstitial compartment and the walls of blood vessels become encrusted. The deposits are basophilic, initially appearing as fine stippling of the connective tissue fibers and eventually growing into broad bands of homogeneous brittle basophilic material. Frequently the involved alveolar septa are thickened by the presence of loose fibrillar connective tissue, and at times there is intra-alveolar fibrosis as well. It is not clear whether the fibrosis is a reaction to the calcium or conditions in tissue undergoing fibrosis favor deposition of calcium salts, but the former seems more likely.

Most cases of metastatic calcifications are clinically inapparent and are not detected roentgenographically. When severe, metastatic calcification can lead to restrictive lung disease with impaired gas exchange. The roentgenograms show nonspecific infiltrates that are usually not recognizable as calcium. The clinical diagnosis can be made by demonstrating the uptake of bone-seeking radionuclides.

Bone forms in the lung under several circumstances. Ossification of the bronchial cartilages is common in the aged. In tracheobronchopathia osteoplastica, nodules of cartilage and bone form in the submucosal connective tissue of the trachea and major bronchi. The affected airways are stiff, and the mucosal surface is rough and knobby. The nodules of bone and cartilage may be entirely within the submucosa or fixed to the perichondrium of the bronchial cartilages. The bone may have fatty or hemopoietic marrow. Diffuse pulmonary ossification has two forms: granular and branched.[634,635] The granular form usually occurs in the context of chronic congestion, especially that caused by mitral stenosis. Spicules of lamellar bone are found in the alveolar spaces attached to alveolar septa. The spicules are irregularly shaped and do not contain marrow. Ossification occurs in the interstitium of chronically fibrotic lung in a racemose or branched pattern. Marrow may be present but frequently is not.

Amyloidosis of the lung

Amyloidosis affecting the lung usually takes one of three forms.[643] Tracheobronchial amyloidosis is usually limited to the respiratory tract and causes bronchial obstruction manifest by wheezing, stridor, or recurrent infection distal to the obstruction.[640] A single bronchus or multiple bronchi may be affected. The gross amyloid deposits may be plaquelike, circumferential, or polypoid. The amyloid is deposited in the submucosa and may surround and compress mucous glands, which then atrophy. Nodules of amyloid occurring in the lung periphery usually appear clinically as single or multiple masses with few symptoms.[642] Multiple nodules usually appear synchronously, though in one patient two amyloid nodules developed 9 years apart.[639] Microscopically amyloid nodules are composed of deposits of brittle-appearing, homogeneous eosinophilic material, usually embedded in fibrous tissue containing an infiltrate of

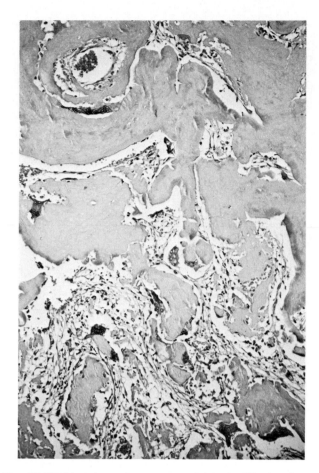

Fig. 20-50. Nodular pulmonary amyloidosis. Giant cells associated with amorphous deposits of amyloid.

plasma cells. Multinucleated giant cells applied to the surface of the amyloid deposits are often conspicuous (Fig. 20-50). Areas of cartilage and ossification are not unusual.

Diffuse septal amyloidosis is usually a manifestation of generalized primary amyloidosis, though in a few case reports it was limited to the lungs or part of generalized secondary amyloidosis.[638] The amyloid is deposited as homogeneous eosinophilic material in alveolar septa and vessels. The clinical manifestations in the lung are usually overshadowed by associated heart disease when septal amyloidosis is part of generalized primary amyloidosis. Because the amyloid is deposited in the interstitium displacing the capillaries, diffusion of oxygen is little affected until late when there is obliteration of capillaries.[641] The tinctorial and ultrastructural properties of amyloid are discussed elsewhere.

Lymphangiomyomatosis

Lymphangiomyomatosis is a diffuse proliferative disease of smooth muscle involving the lung and in some cases neighboring lymphatic structures including the thoracic duct.[644-646] Grossly the lungs are large but show widespread, severe honeycombing. Microscopic sections show widespread smooth muscle proliferation along the course of lymphatics in the perivenous and bronchoarterial connective tissue spaces and pleura, as well as within alveolar septa.[646] The absence of inflammation distinguishes lymphangiomyomatosis from other interstitial lung diseases, and the distribution of the smooth muscle proliferation, conforming after a fashion to anatomic structures, distinguishes it from benign metastasizing leiomyoma in which the muscle forms distinct nodules.

The clinical features of lymphangiomyomatosis are as distinctive as its morbid anatomy. The disease almost exclusively affects women of childbearing age.[646] Compression of veins by the perivenous smooth muscle proliferation leads to hemoptysis; compression of small airways results in severe expiratory airflow obstruction, air trapping, and in some cases repeated pneumothoraces. When there is involvement of neighboring lymphatics, chylous pleural effusion may develop. The chest roentgenogram shows the unique combination of severe linear reticulation, indicative of advanced interstitial lung disease, with greatly enlarged lungs and low diaphragms, indicative of severe air trapping.[645] Similar features are seen in the lungs of some patients with tuberous sclerosis.

Drug- and radiation-induced pulmonary disease

Pulmonary disease is estimated to account for only 1% to 5% of drug-induced disease. With the development of multiple drug and radiation regimens for the treatment of malignancy, it appears to be increasing in importance. Too many drugs have been implicated as pulmonary toxins to discuss individually. Recent reviews have discussed drug-induced pulmonary reactions according to drug implicated[654] and type of tissue response.[647] Some drug-induced effects on the respiratory system, such as bronchospasm or depressed ventilation, are not visible to the pathologist. The reactions that the pathologist can detect include pulmonary edema, diffuse alveolar damage, chronic interstitial pneumonia, eosinophilic pneumonia, hypersensitivity pneumonitis, phospholipidosis, lupuslike reactions, vasculitis, and primary pulmonary hypertension.[647,647a] As with drug reactions in other organs, some pulmonary drug reactions are toxic effects that are dose related and reproduceable in experimental animals, whereas others are idiosyncratic, occurring in only a few of the patients who receive the drug and at highly variable doses. Idiosyncratic reactions may result from either metabolic differences between individuals or immunologic (allergic) reactions. The situation is complicated by the observation that a given drug may cause disease on either a toxic or an allergic basis. For example, bleomycin, a valuable antitumor drug, causes direct dose-related tox-

icity that can be reproduced in a variety of animals. Ordinarily toxicity is not seen until doses of 300 to 400 mg have been given, and the histopathologic picture is that of an organizing interstitial pneumonia.[653] In an occasional patient, respiratory disease develops at much lower doses[650] or may have an atypical histologic picture suggestive of hypersensitivity, such as eosinophilic pneumonia.[649] Methotrexate is implicated in both hypersensivity pneumonitis and toxic interstitial fibrosis. Interactions between drugs or between radiation and drugs may occur.[657] Prior irradiation may predispose patients to drug reactions at doses lower than expected. Oxygen therapy also modifies the response to drugs. In experimental animals, doses of oxygen that are nontoxic in themselves can convert self-limited bleomycin-induced fibrosis to progressive fibrosis. It is now common to encounter patients with diffuse lung disease who have received multiple cytotoxic drugs and often thoracic radiation as well. Biopsy examination shows either diffuse alveolar damage or nonspecific interstitial pneumonia, and no infectious organism can be found. Although no single therapeutic agent has been given to toxic levels, lung injury probably reflects the cumulative damage produced by several agents.[655,657]

The most common morphologic response to cytotoxic drugs is diffuse alveolar damage evolving into chronic interstitial pneumonia. The pathologic sequence has been described in detail with electron microscopy in the case of busulfan[652] and bleomycin.[647] Other alkylating agents produce similar changes. Early the alveolar spaces contain cellular debris and fibrin. Hyaline membranes line many air spaces. Organization of the intra-alveolar fibrin and hyaline membranes with migration of alveolar epithelium over the surface of the hyaline membranes leads to a picture of mixed interstitial and intra-alveolar fibrosis. Pronounced atypism of the regenerating alveolar epithelium is characteristic of the pulmonary fibrosis seen with alkylating agents. The epithelial cells are large with irregular outlines. The cytoplasm is abundant, and the nuclei are large with prominent nucleoli. Squamous metaplasia and atypism may be found in the airways as well and can be recognized in exfoliated cells in the sputum.

The acute phase of radiation pneumonitis is difficult to distinguish histologically from other forms of acute lung injury.[651,656] The hyaline membranes, enlarged hyperplastic epithelial cells, alveolar septal edema, and sparse inflammation are nonspecific. The chronic phase is characterized by a poorly cellular fibrillar eosinophilic fibrosis affecting alveolar walls and blood vessels.[651,656] The vascular lumens are shrunken and irregular. The subendothelial space of many larger vessels is edematous with an occasional inflammatory cell. Absence of inflammatory cells other than an occasional plasma cell, fibrillar quality of the fibrosis, and atypical nuclei of the interstitial fibroblasts are all features that help distinguish radiation fibrosis from fibrosis of other causes.

The relation between dose, time, and histologic reaction is complex.[648] Jennings and Arden[651] found chronic radiation fibrosis as early as 6 months after high-dose irradiation, whereas in other cases acute radiation pneumonitis was still present 2 years after irradiation.

Pulmonary hemorrhage

Bleeding from pulmonary capillaries occurs in many settings. As noted previously, immunologic injury from either antibasal lamina antibodies or immune complex deposition can produce capillary bleeding.[665] Pulmonary hemorrhage can also occur in association with glomerulonephritis in the absence of detectable immunologic reactions in the lung. Hemorrhage is common at autopsy in severe heart failure where it probably results from a combination of hemodynamic factors and alveolar injury.[658] In thrombocytopenic patients minor alveolar injury can result in hemorrhage. This explains the occasional life-threatening hemorrhages in leukemic patients.[660,666] There remains a small group of patients in whom repeated episodes of pulmonary hemorrhage occur in the absence of any discernible predisposing illness. To this group the diagnosis of idiopathic pulmonary hemosiderosis applies. Eighty percent of patients with idiopathic pulmonary hemosiderosis are children, and most of the remainder are young adults.[667] The illness usually begins with mild episodes of intrapulmonary bleeding associated with cough and dyspnea. Occasionally the first episode is one of brisk hemoptysis. The respiratory bleeding is usually accompanied by the development of iron-deficiency anemia. Whether the anemia is entirely explicable on the basis of blood loss and sequestration of iron in the lung is controversial, but there is no evidence of hemolysis. When blood is injected into the lungs of experimental animals, they can mobilize the iron,[663] leading some to question whether there is some additional defect that prevents patients with pulmonary hemosiderosis from mobilizing their iron.

Repeated hemorrhages lead to the development of pulmonary fibrosis, the accumulation of large numbers of hemosiderin-filled macrophages (siderophages) in the alveoli, and iron deposition on the vascular elastic fibers. The basis for the bleeding is not clear, and neither auto-antibodies nor immune complexes have been demonstrable in the circulation. In a few cases abnormalities of capillary basement membranes have been seen with electron microscopy, but they have been of different types in each report.[661,663] Many investigators have failed to detect any abnormalities by electron microscopy or immunofluorescence.[659,664] The course of idiopathic pulmonary hemosiderosis is variable. Pa-

tients can die during an initial episode or survive for many years with recurring episodes leading to fibrosis and pulmonary insufficiency. Remissions of many years' duration may occur. In the cases reviewed by Soergel and Sommers[667] the average survival was 3 years.

Aspiration pneumonia

The term "aspiration pneumonia" is used to cover several quite different clinicopathologic processes caused by different agents that have a common means of entry to the lung.[675] The aspiration of infected material from the oral cavity can lead to bacterial pneumonia often caused by anaerobic organisms as discussed previously. The aspiration of gastric contents with a pH below 2.5 produces hemorrhagic edema in the involved region of lung and, if extensive, is rapidly fatal. The bronchi are hemorrhagic, and the lung exudes frothy fluid.[675] In patients dying rapidly there is massive pulmonary edema. Survivors for 2 or 3 days show infiltration of neutrophils, hyaline membranes, and sloughing of the bronchial epithelium. The clinical picture is that of the adult respiratory distress syndrome.

Quite different is the response to food-particle aspiration that occurs in those who have difficulty swallowing because of neurologic or esophageal disease or who have undergone certain types of radical head and neck surgery.[675] Small food particles that are aspirated lodge in respiratory bronchioles. In the first few hours there is hemorrhage into the air spaces accompanied by infiltration of neutrophils and monocytes. Between 24 and 48 hours after aspiration a monocyte-macrophage response predominates, and by 48 to 72 hours distinct granulomas with conspicuous foreign-body giant cells form about the food particles. Food particles (vegetable cells or skeletal muscle) and squamous cells can be recognized within the granulomas. The granulomas heal by fibrosis, and in the late phase the appearance of fibrous nodules with giant cells closely simulates an infectious granuloma. The clinical setting and localization strictly at the termination of the bronchial tree are helpful clues to the pathologic diagnosis. Repeated small aspirations can lead to fibrosis of the lower lung zones.

Aspiration of large particles is common in young children but also occurs in adults. Particles blocking the trachea can cause suffocation, and those lodging in major bronchi can cause air trapping or obstructive pneumonia and bronchiectasis.

Lipid pneumonia

Aspiration of lipid is the principal cause of exogenous lipid pneumonia. The lipid is usually mineral oil taken as a laxative, as a vehicle for medication, or as nose drops.[669,674] Lipid can also be inhaled while burning[672] or when added to smoking tobacco as a humectant.[675]

Although relatively inert, mineral oil stimulates a chronic inflammatory response with scarring. Clinically exogenous lipid pneumonia can occur as a diffuse infiltrative process involving the lower lobes or can form a localized mass (paraffinoma) that closely simulates a neoplasm.[669] Grossly the lesions appear as a yellow, doughy area of consolidation or as a discrete, yellow, hard mass. Retraction of the pleura over the mass enhances the resemblance to carcinoma. Microscopically much lipid is within macrophages in both the air spaces and interstitium, but in cases of long duration with severe fibrosis large extracellular lipid globules are trapped within fibrous tissue. Lipid vacuoles vary from micrometers to tens of micrometers in diameter, the largest being extracellular where they may be partly enclosed by multinucleated giant cells. Nodular aggregates of lymphocytes are almost invariably present (Fig. 20-51). The diagnosis can be made without biopsy by identification of lipid-laden macrophages in the sputum.

Lipid pneumonia arising from the retention of lipids released during the breakdown of tissue is known as endogenous lipid pneumonia. It occurs in the parenchyma distal to an obstructed bronchus or on a microscopic scale distal to blocked bronchioles and alveolar ducts. The affected tissue is consolidated and speckled bright yellow. The lipid is found in the form of uniform droplets 1 μm or less in diameter in the cytoplasm of macrophages, which are aggregated within the air spaces. Extracellular cholesterol clefts with giant cells are not unusual.

The histologic features of the two types of lipid pneumonia are distinctive, and it is rarely necessary to resort to histochemical examination to distinguish them. In frozen sections both types of lipid stain with a Sudan type of stain, but only the endogenous type blackens with OsO_4 (osmium tetroxide).

Lung collapse and pneumothorax

The expansion of the lung is maintained by the pressure difference between the alveoli, which are normally in free communication with the atmosphere, and the subatmospheric pressure of the pleural space. The causes of collapse (atelectasis) of the lung are pleural filling, bronchial obstruction with absorption of the intra-alveolar gas, and changes in surfactant function. The lung collapses when compressed by pleural effusions, tumors, other space-occupying intrathoracic lesions, or elevation of the diaphragm. Lung collapsed because of entrapment by thick pleural fibrosis can have a tumor-like roentgenographic image called rounded atelectasis. In pneumothorax the lung collapses because air gains access to the pleural space, permitting the negative pleural pressure to rise. This can occur as the result of thoracic trauma, perforation of the esophagus, extension of lung abscess or other infections through the pleura with formation of a bronchopleural fistula, or rupture of air-containing cysts or bullae associated with emphysema or other forms of diffuse or localized lung disease. In young adults without generalized underlying pulmonary disease, pneumothorax develops most often in tall slender persons who have a few localized bullae, usually in the upper lung fields.[670] The histologic changes in the walls of the bullae are nonspecific, consisting in fibrosis, chronic inflammation, focal alveolar epithelial hyperplasia, and a few hemosiderin-laden macrophages.[670] Neither the underlying cause of the bullae nor the reason for their rupture is known, but it seems doubtful that they can be explained by the greater vertical gradient in transpulmonary pressure that exists in taller persons because of gravity. A few such persons have abnormalities of connective tissue such as Marfan's syndrome or Ehlers-Danlos syndrome.

Both the parietal and visceral pleura respond to pneumothorax by the exudation of fibrin associated with a proliferation of macrophages, giant cells, mesothelial cells, and eosinophils known as reactive eosinophilic pleuritis.[668] It is important not to confuse this nonspecific reaction to pneumothorax with the lesions of eosin-

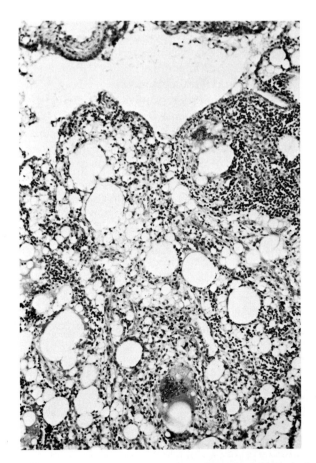

Fig. 20-51. Lipid pneumonia. Vacuoles are sites of dissolved lipid. Nodules of lymphocytes are common.

ophilic granuloma, which is one underlying cause of pneumothorax.

Behind a totally occluded bronchus, the absorption of alveolar gas can produce collapse of the lung. This happens rapidly in patients breathing 100% oxygen when, for example, mucus plugs an airway. In persons breathing room air, however, relatively minor volume loss follows bronchial obstruction because the nitrogen in the air spaces is absorbed only slowly and is replaced by edema fluid. Gradual occlusion of a bronchus leads to lipid pneumonia, chronic organizing pneumonia, and bronchiectasis, rather than simple collapse.

Shallow respiration also leads to alveolar collapse as a result of rising surface tension in the alveolar lining. The process is incompletely understood, but deep ventilation acts as a stimulus to surfactant secretion by type II epithelial cells and is required for the formation of a stable surface film. Collapse because of shallow ventilation is particularly likely to occur in postoperative patients whose respiration is depressed because of anesthetics and who have a shallow pattern of ventilation because of incisional pain.[673] The administration of oxygen only compounds the problem.

If a small volume of lung is collapsed, the pleura is dark and sunken below the level of the pink, well-expanded lung. When an entire lobe or lung is affected, the pleura is wrinkled. The involved parenchyma is dark, firm, and without crepitance. Microscopically the alveolar walls are compressed, giving the tissue a solid appearance. The vascularity of the alveolar walls helps distinguish normal airless lung from fibrosis.

After collapse there is a progressive rise in pulmonary vascular resistance in the involved better-ventilated tissue. Several mechanisms are probably involved, including hypoxia, tortuosity and distortion of the vascular bed, and reflex vasoconstriction.

CHRONIC AIRFLOW LIMITATION
Definitions

The term "chronic obstructive pulmonary disease" (COPD) is an unfortunate one, since it logically should describe lesions, such as tumors, foreign bodies, and impacted secretion, that obstruct the airways to portions of the lung. However, it is too firmly embedded in clinical jargon to dislodge. The syndrome that is described as COPD or better, as chronic airflow limitation, is a functional condition in which the rate of expiratory airflow is reduced to a degree that produces disability. The entities usually associated with COPD are chronic bronchitis, emphysema, and inflammation of small bronchi and bronchioles variously called bronchiolitis, or small-airways disease. These three conditions commonly occur together, since they are the responses of different anatomic levels of the respiratory tract to similar irritants, and they are not always sepa-

rable clinically. Asthmatic patients and many patients with bronchiectasis also manifest chronic airflow limitation, as described elsewhere. By international agreement chronic bronchitis has been defined as chronic cough and sputum production not attributable to some specific disease (such as tuberculosis or carcinoma).[698] In epidemiologic studies sputum production on most days during at least 3 months of the year in 2 consecutive years is sufficient basis for a diagnosis of chronic bronchitis. Practitioners generally make the diagnosis in patients who not only have chronic cough with sputum but also have repeated chest infections or COPD, or both. Emphysema is defined in anatomic rather than clinical terms, being an anatomic change in the acini of the lung characterized by abnormal enlargeemnt of air spaces accompanied by destruction of air space walls without significant fibrosis.[726] Small-airways disease has only recently been documented physiologically and pathologically but is not generally used as a diagnosis in clinical practice. The term is used here to describe a group of nonspecific inflammatory changes in bronchioles and small bronchi that correlate with physiologic airflow obstruction.

Chronic bronchitis and emphysema are extremely common. They often occur together, but each can occur without the other. Small-airways disease has been described accompanying each, but its prevalence has not been studied directly.

Incidence

COPD is the fifth leading cause of death in the United States and is responsible for about 2.5% of all deaths annually. Combining all deaths certified as resulting from chronic bronchitis, emphysema, and COPD, the mortality has nearly trebled since 1950. Although COPD is more common in Britain than in the United States, the mortality in Britain appears to be falling. COPD is a chronic process that progresses slowly over a period of years. It causes or contributes to 100,000 deaths each year, and more than 1.5 million new cases are diagnosed annually. The amount of disability it causes is enormous, with estimates running as high as 250 million hours lost from work annually.

Chronic bronchitis

Chronic bronchitis is a common condition that increases in prevalence at least until 40 years of age and affects men more often than women. Roughly 20% of men have cough and sputum production, but only a fraction of these have recurrent chest infections and fewer still have disabling COPD.

The microscopic finding that most consistently correlates with hypersecretion of mucus is enlargement of the mucous glands. This can be conveniently appraised using the gland/wall ratio or Reid index,[722] the ratio of

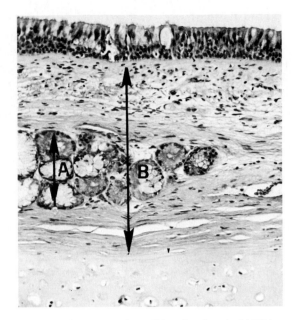

Fig. 20-52. Normal bronchus. Gland/wall ratio *(A/B)* is quick measure of mucous gland volume. It increases in chronic bronchitis.

the thickness of the lobules of mucous glands to the distance between the perichondrium and the basal lamina of the bronchial lining epithelium (Fig. 20-52). For normal individuals Reid obtained values of 0.14 to 0.36, whereas a group of bronchitic subjects averaged 0.59. A value of 0.4 was taken as the upper limit of normal. Subsequent work has shown that the gland/wall ratio is unimodally distributed; that is, there is a continuous distribution of gland/wall ratios rather than two distinct populations, one normal and one diseased. More accurate but laborious methods for measuring mucous gland volumes lead to the same conclusion: there is a bell-shaped distribution of mucous gland volumes, with asymptomatic subjects tending to have smaller glands and those with overt clinical bronchitis tending toward the higher end of the curve, but without a sharp separation between normal persons and those with disease.[724,730]

Another common abnormality in chronic bronchitis is an increase in the ratio of mucous cells to serous cells in the mucous glands. Normally, relatively equal numbers of mucous and serous cells make up the secretory tubules, but in many bronchitic patients serous cells are rare and mucous cells make up the great majority of glandular epithelium. The ducts of the glands become dilated and plugged with mucus. These dilated ducts can often be demonstrated clinically in bronchograms and have been called diverticula.

Inflammatory edema or cellular infiltration may be present in chronic bronchitis but are not constant or

diagnostic features. Changes in the bronchial lining epithelium are variable. Hyperplasia of the basal cells, increased numbers of goblet cells, and foci of squamous metaplasia can all be found. The basement membrane can be thickened, and focal atrophy of the connective tissue leads to irregularity of the bronchial caliber visible on the opened bronchi as shallow depressions with transverse ridges. Increased smooth muscle has been observed in bronchitic patients who have wheezing.[729]

Patients with clinical bronchitis are often subject to repeated chest infections, probably because excessive amounts of mucus result in inefficient bronchial clearance and colonization of airways with nasopharyngeal flora. Normally the airways are sterile, but in a large proportion of bronchitic patients bacteria can be cultured from the airways. The most frequent organism to be recovered is *Haemophilus influenzae*, followed by *Streptococcus pneumoniae*. Acute infections are often associated with these organisms but also may be caused by viruses or *Mycoplasma pneumoniae*.[697,713,728] During acute infections there is often deterioration of lung function, but it is reversible, and surprisingly the long-term development of chronic airflow limitation is unaffected by intercurrent infections.[679,694,695]

Chronic airflow limitation can develop in patients with little or no emphysema and can even be lethal. Such patients usually have mucus hypersecretion of some degree, and their disability is commonly attributed to chronic bronchitis, but the relationship between the process causing chronic airflow limitation and simple chronic bronchitis is not clear. Mucous gland hyperplasia produces thickening of the bronchial wall, which narrows the bronchus and could in principal increase airway resistance, but in practice there is not a strong relationship between morphologic mucous gland hypertrophy or indices of mucus expectoration, on the one hand, and clinical outcome or results of pulmonary function tests, on the other.[730] Reid observed that in patients with chronic bronchitis dying of COPD there was mucus plugging, acute obliteration of bronchioles by purulent exudate, and organizing pneumonia.[723] These observations served to focus attention on the small airways, though some of the changes she described were the result of terminal infection. Subsequent studies have shown narrowing of airways in chronic bronchitis without emphysema,[712] as well as some morphologic features of small airways that correlate with physiologic chronic airflow limitation, notably goblet cell metaplasia, inflammatory cell infiltration, and narrowing of the airway.[681,682,688] It should be stressed that these changes are often subtle and may be missed during inspection of histologic slides. Their importance emerges when quantitative analysis is applied to series of cases. Nevertheless, it is likely that the changes in the airways less than 2 mm in diameter are the important ones in determining airflow limitation.

The factors implicated in causing chronic bronchitis are cigarette smoking, air pollution, infection early in childhood, and a poorly defined familial tendency.[718] The most important of these is cigarette smoke. In epidemiologic studies cigarette smoking is associated with cough and phlegm, increased frequency of respiratory infections, and decreased pulmonary function. In pathologic studies it is correlated with mucous gland hyperplasia and small-airways inflammation.[688,733] Exposure of experimental animals to cigarette smoke produces hyperplasia of the mucus-secreting apparatus. Many effects of cigarette smoke help to account for the increased tendency to infections, including impaired mucociliary clearance because of squamous metaplasia of the bronchial epithelium and hypersecretion of mucus and decreased antibacterial function of alveolar macrophages.

The importance of community air pollution is difficult to evaluate because the powerful influence of cigarette smoking tends to overwhelm other influences. Holland and Reid[701] showed that residents of several small communities in Britain had less cough and sputum production and slightly better ventilatory function than similar occupational groups in London. Their study was controlled for smoking. Effects of air pollution are more easily demonstrable in schoolchildren, since smoking is not a factor, but the significance of changes in respiratory symptoms in children in relation to the development of COPD in middle age is not established. Studies in both Britain and the United States have shown an increased incidence of lower respiratory infections in schoolchildren living in areas of higher pollution.[693] Experimental exposure of animals to pollutants supports a possible role for common air pollutants in chronic bronchitis. Sulfur dioxide, a major product of burning coal, causes mucus hypersecretion in animals, and nitrogen dioxide and ozone, products of the photochemical oxidation of automobile exhaust, produce inflammation in small airways. In most instances the concentrations used in animal experiments are higher than those observed in even heavily polluted atmospheres, but it may be unreasonable to expect low concentrations of any single pollutant used in the laboratory to reproduce the effect of the complicated mixtures found in urban atmospheres.

Although chest infections in adults have little lasting influence on pulmonary function, some studies have found that patients with bronchitis or impaired pulmonary function more commonly have a history of lung infections early in life than normal persons do. Follow-up monitoring of young children with infections has shown poorer performance on pulmonary function testing persisting even into adolescence. Perhaps damage to the growing lung predisposes to COPD later in life.

Emphysema

With the passage of years the lung gradually loses elastic recoil, alveolar ducts dilate, and the fraction of the lung parenchyma that is composed of alveolar ducts (rather than alveoli) increases.[725,730] These changes are part of the normal process of aging and are not emphysema, which is by definition an abnormal enlargement of air spaces.

Since emphysema is defined morphologically, it is most reliably diagnosed pathologically. Mild degrees are difficult to recognize in the fresh lung. Fixation by distending the lung with fixative through the bronchi greatly improves its recognition and is adequate for routine purposes, but for optimum study and photography barium sulfate impregnation improves the recognition of emphysema and requires only a few extra minutes. In the inflation-fixed lung the alveolar ducts are at the limit of resolution for the unaided eye, though in the aged they can often be recognized as holes of up to 0.5 mm in diameter. Spaces in the parenchyma over 1 mm in size are abnormal.

Emphysema is common at autopsy, but its reported prevalence varies from 20% to 100% depending on the population studied and the technique and criteria used.[730] The prevalence and severity increase with age and are greater in men than in women. Minor degrees of emphysema are clinically inapparent, however, and as a rule subjects with less than 20% of lung involved have no symptoms.

Classification

On the sectioned surface of an inflated lung, connective tissue septa extend inward from the pleura and outline units of parenchyma, termed secondary lobules, that are 1 to 2 cm in diameter and contain two to five acini. The acini are the functional gas-exchanging units of the lung and consist of three to five generations of respiratory bronchioles and a variable number of alveolar ducts and alveolar sacs, each with their alveoli. Emphysema is classified according to the portion of the acinus it involves.[699,730]

Centriacinar emphysema. Emphysema that initially involves the respiratory bronchioles is termed centriacinar or centrilobular emphysema (CLE). The lesions of CLE appear grossly as roughly spherical holes 1 to 5 mm in diameter near the center of the lobules and separated from the perilobular septa by a rim of normal tissue (Fig. 20-53). Usually dark pigment is associated with the lesions and in advanced lesions strands of tissue, containing vessels remaining after destruction of the alveolar walls, cross the emphysematous space (Fig. 20-54). Usually the upper lobes are involved more severely than the lower and the superior segments more than the basilar ones. The bronchioles supplying centrilobular emphysema often are inflamed, distorted,

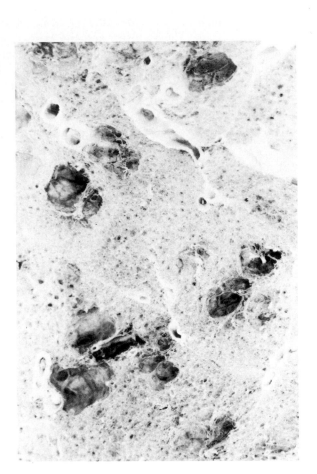

Fig. 20-53. Centriacinar emphysema. Barium sulfate–impregnated lung. Enlarged, abnormal air spaces in center of lobules are surrounded by normal tissue.

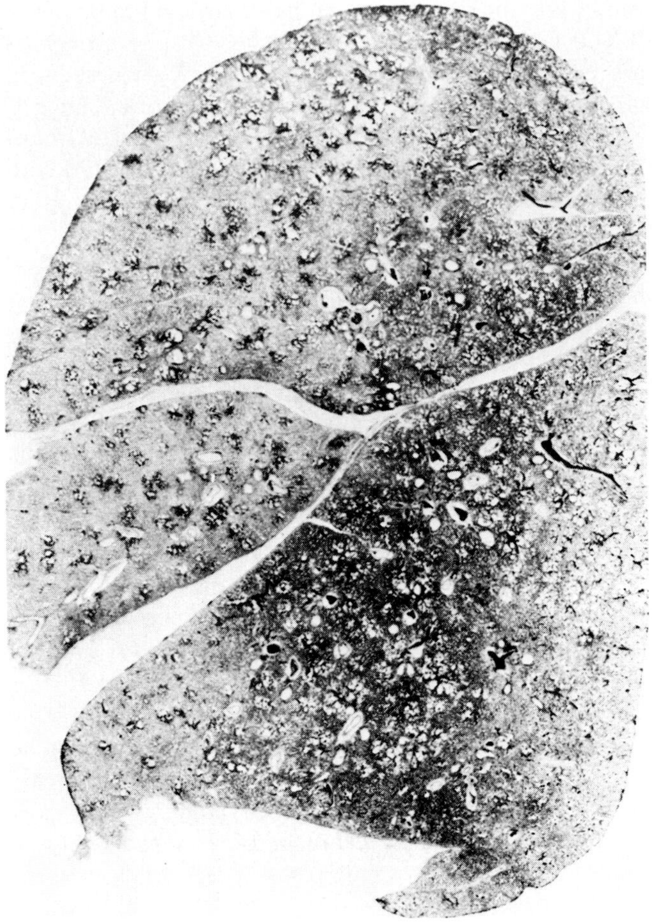

Fig. 20-54. Centriacinar emphysema. Paper-mounted lung section. (Courtesy Dr. A.A. Liebow.)

and stenotic. CLE is usually the type of emphysema found when chronic bronchitis and emphysema coexist, and patients with CLE are almost invariably smokers.

Panacinar emphysema. In panacinar emphysema all portions of the acinus are affected, but usually the alveolar ducts are involved more severely than the respiratory bronchioles. Individual lobules are variably involved, but even in minimally involved lobules abnormally enlarged air spaces reach the perilobular septa (Fig. 20-55). Both upper and lower lobes are usually involved to a comparable degree (Fig. 22-56) but the lower zones may have the more severe lesions. Panacinar emphysema occurs most often in middle-aged cigarette smokers,[730] but it is also the characteristic form of emphysema in rare familial cases occurring in young adults, whose serum antritrypsin levels may be normal[710] or reduced.[692]

Distal acinar (paraseptal) emphysema. Distal acinar emphysema is a form that is localized along the pleura and perilobular septa. As an isolated finding it is not

associated with COPD but does predispose to pneumothorax. It can be associated with CLE.

Irregular (paracicatricial) emphysema. Enlarged and distorted abnormal air spaces are often seen surrounding scars from any cause. Since the process giving rise to the scarring may not respect acinar architecture, the lesions may be irregular in distribution within the acinus as well as within the lung as a whole.

Mixed and unclassified emphysema. It is not unusual to find emphysema of more than one type in a given lung, for example, centriacinar emphysema in the upper lobes and panacinar in the lower lobes. Many cases of emphysema do not fit unambiguously into one of the above types, either because the lesions are atypical or because they are so severe that it is impossible to recognize the portion of the acinus that was initially involved (Fig. 20-57). In one study only 27 of 122 emphysematous lungs examined by three expert pathologists unequivocally showed panacinar or centriacinar emphysema, the remainder being either mixed or unclassifia-

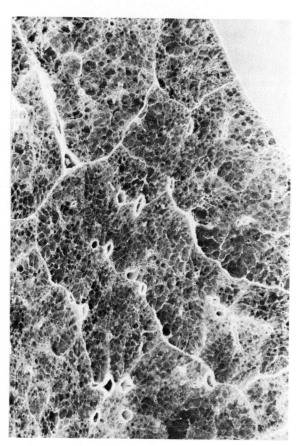

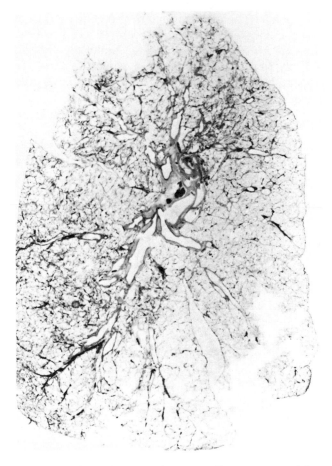

Fig. 20-55. Panacinar emphysema. Enlarged air spaces involve lobule uniformly. Barium sulfate–impregnated lung.

Fig. 20-56. Panacinar emphysema. Paper-mounted lung section. (Courtesy Dr. A.A. Liebow.)

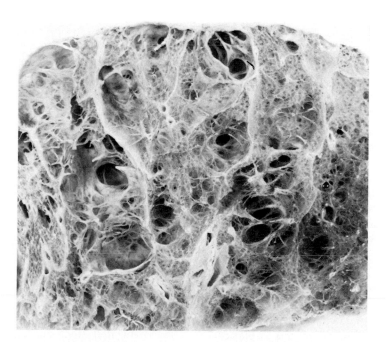

Fig. 20-57. Severe emphysema. It is difficult to discern what portion of acinus was involved initially.

ble.[714] There is general agreement that centriacinar emphysema is most severe in the upper lobes whereas panacinar emphysema is more uniformly distributed,[676,714] but there are no other clinical features that consistently distinguish them and whether they have a similar pathogenesis has not been established.

Bullae

Bullae are subpleural, air-filled, cystlike structures, greater than 1 cm in diameter, that are found most frequently along the sharp margins of the lung anteriorly and near the apices. In pathologic specimens they bulge outward from the surface of the lung, but during life they are confined by the chest wall and indent and compress the lung. They are found in association with each of the other forms of emphysema and sometimes, especially in young people, in otherwise normal lungs. Some bullae appear essentially empty, but often they contain strands or remnants of tissue, indicating that they represent severely damaged lung tissue that has lost its elastic recoil. Microscopically the walls show fibrosis and chronic inflammation. The most common cause of spontaneous pneumothorax in young people is apical bullae,[670] but rupture is fortunately rare in generalized emphysema. Large bullae can also cause pulmonary dysfuction by compression of the remaining lung.

Morphogenesis of emphysematous lesions

There seem to be at least two mechanisms by which destruction of alveolar walls takes place. One mechanism, first described by Waters in 1862, is through departition of air spaces, which takes place by the enlargement and coalescence of the interalveolar pores.[706,720,721] It now is well established from observations in both humans and animals that there are small holes (pores of Kohn) in normal alveolar septa. These generally lie in the spaces between capillaries. Some enlargement of pores takes place with aging, even in nonemphysematous lungs,[721] but the process is exaggerated in emphysema. The pores encroach on and obliterate alveolar capillaries and coalesce, and gradually alveolar walls disappear leaving behind strands of tissue that often contain more resistant arteries. The abnormally large pores, called fenestrae, can be observed directly in slices of barium sulfate–impregnated lung with a stereomicroscope or in histologic sections 50 μm or more thick; their presence can be recognized in routine sections because the airspace walls between fenestrae appear to be detached from the rest of the lung parenchyma where the plane of the section passes through the fenestrae. Thus the appearance of "floating" segments of alveolar wall in ordinary sections is one reliable indicator of destruction of air-space walls.

The second mechanism, which is more difficult to understand, is a simplification of lung structure. For example, in early panacinar emphysema, Heppleston and Leopold[699] observed dilatation of alveolar ducts with shortening and effacement of the interalveolar septa, and similar morphologic changes occur in an animal model of emphysema.[706] The surface area of the lung is diminished, indicating tissue loss, but fenestration is not prominent. The mechanisms by which this rearrangement of lung structure takes place are still unclear.

Pathophysiology

Emphysema differs from other causes of chronic airflow limitation by the presence of destruction in the acinar region. The loss of gas-exchanging surface and associated vascular bed results in a decreased diffusion capacity. There are many other causes of decreased diffusion capacity, but in a patient with COPD, magnitude of the decrease correlates well with extent of emphysema.[719] The most specific physiologic abnormality of the emphysematous lung is its loss of elastic recoil.[683,719] Two factors determine the retractive force (elastic recoil) of the lung: forces derived from surface tension in the fluid lining of small air spaces and forces derived from the stretching of connective tissue elements. In emphysema the enlarged air spaces and decreased surface area, which are a consequence of destruction of alveolar walls, tend to decrease the surface tension component of elastic recoil. Abnormalities of connective tissue are also important. Elastin is responsible for lung compliance at low and intermediate lung volumes. Collagen has little influence on lung compliance in the physiologic range but does determine the tensile strength of the tissue and provides the "mechanical stop" that limits lung expansion at total lung capacity. In the emphysematous lung the increased compliance is attributable in part to disruption of the elastic network, which can be seen in histologic sections.[734] Total lung capacity is increased, indicating that the collagen also is remodeled.

The basis for the airflow obstruction in emphysema has been studied intensively. Hogg and co-workers[700] showed that the major site of obstruction is in small airways. They compared the distribution of airway resistance between central airways (larger than 2 mm) and peripheral airways (smaller than 2 mm) in normal lungs and in seven emphysematous lungs. In the emphysematous lungs the resistance of the central airways was no more than twice normal but the resistance of the peripheral airways increased ten- to fortyfold. Anatomic studies point to two factors that correlate with airflow obstruction, the severity of the emphysema itself and the associated small-airways disease.[715] Emphysema is associated with airway obstruction because of decreased elastic recoil. The bronchioles have thin muscular walls, and their caliber varies with lung volume. The force that holds them open during expiration is the retractive force of the surrounding lung, which of course is greater the more the lung is expanded. In emphysema the retractive force is much reduced. Physiologic studies of carefully selected emphysematous patients have shown that the conductance of their airways (the reciprocal of the resistance) is normal for the elastic recoil of their lungs, but to generate a given elastic recoil their lungs must be at higher volume than normal. In contrast, asthmatic patients with intrinsic bronchial disease had reduced conductance for a given elastic recoil. Morphologic studies showing that there are fewer alveolar walls attached to the bronchioles of emphysematous lungs provide an anatomic basis for the diminished support of small airways in emphysema.

Emphysematous patients also are likely to have associated small-airways disease as a major contributor to airflow limitation. This has been especially well documented in centriacinar emphysema and has been elegantly illustrated by French investigators using casts (Fig. 20-58).[690] A variety of lesions can be found, including loss of small airways, stenosis and distortion of airways, inflammation, goblet cell metaplasia, and mu-

cus plugging.[690,700,708,711,715,730] These factors cause obstruction in various ways. Narrowing of airways increases resistance in accordance with Poiseuille's law even when flow is laminar, but distortion and abrupt stenosis convert laminar to turbulent flow. Mucus plugs may totally obstruct the airways, but goblet cell metaplasia may also impair airway function by replacing the normal bronchiolar lining of surfactant and Clara cell secretions with sticky mucus. Physiologists believe that airways close in dependent regions of the lung at the end of expiration, and the abnormal secretions in goblet cell metaplasia would be expected to impair their reopening. The diminished support of small airways resulting from the loss of elastic recoil in emphysema and the intrinsic changes in small airways reinforce each other in producing airway dysfunction when both are present in the same lung.

Etiology

The evidence that cigarette smoking is the major cause of emphysema is overwhelming. A variety of autopsy populations from hospitals and coroners' offices have been studied, and the relationship held true.[677,678,727,730] Severity of emphysema is roughly dose related. In nonsmokers emphysema is infrequent and almost always of low grade. In smokers over 40 years of age normal lungs are unusual, and heavy smokers have more severe and extensive emphysema than light smokers do. Between 20% and 40% of those who smoke more than a pack a day have disease of relatively high grade. The activities of tobacco smoke that promote emphysema are discussed later in the chapter. In all studies, however, there are some heavy smokers who escape emphysema. This indicates that there are other factors that also determine individual susceptibility to emphysema or that cigarette smoke acts additively with other agents in the environment.

Air pollution is often mentioned as a cause of emphysema. Ishikawa and associates[702] compared paper-mounted whole lung sections from autopsies in St. Louis, Missouri, a relatively industrialized city, with a similar series from Winnipeg, Manitoba, where the pollution is less. When matched according to age, sex, and smoking history, the St. Louis patients had more severe emphysema.

There are genetic influences in emphysema. A poorly understood familial factor in COPD acts independently of any known specific disease. In addition, emphysema is a complication in several rare heritable diseases of connective tissue such as cutis laxa, Marfan's syndrome, and Menkes' syndrome.[705] Emphysema is also closely linked to deficiency of the serum protein alpha$_1$-antitrypsin or alpha-1-protease inhibitor (alpha-1-PI).[717] Although deficiency of alpha-1-PI is responsible for only about 1% of cases of emphysema, the recognition of al-

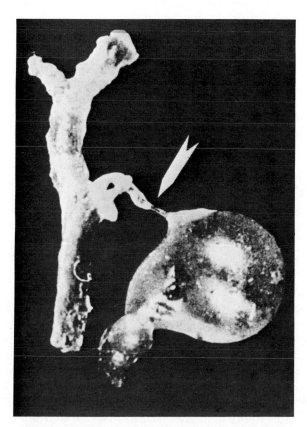

Fig. 20-58. Cast of centriacinar emphysematous space. *Arrow,* Area of stenosis in bronchiole leading into space. (From Depierre, A., et al.: Chest **62:**699, 1972.)

pha-1-PI deficiency has had such a pivotal role in shaping the modern theory of the pathogenesis of emphysema that it is described in some detail below.

Alpha-1-protease inhibitor deficiency. Alpha-1-PI is the major protein responsible for the alpha-1 band in the conventional serum electrophoretogram. A glycoprotein of 51,000 daltons, alpha-1-PI is synthesized in the liver and distributed in the circulating blood and other body fluids including that of the lower respiratory tract. Its function is to inhibit proteases with serine at the active proteolytic site, including leukocyte elastase, chymotrypsin, cathepsin G, plasmin, and thrombin, as well as trypsin. Alpha-1-PI deficiency was first discovered in 1963 by Swedish investigators who observed a series of patients whose serum apparently lacked the alpha-1-globulin band on electrophoresis. Of the original 36 patients, 27 had chronic airflow limitation, mainly as a result of emphysema.[692] The emphysema of alpha-1-PI deficiency is of the panacinar type and predominately involves the basilar portion of the lung.[692,696] Emphysema in alpha-1-PI deficiency develops early in adult life, with an equal sex incidence, and in nonsmokers as well as smokers, though on the average smokers become symptomatic 15 years earlier than nonsmokers. COPD develops in as much as 85% of deficient subjects.

The other organ affected clinically is the liver. One half of newborn infants with the deficiency have minor abnormalities of liver function, and in 1 in 10 obstructive jaundice develops in the first few months of life but usually clears before the end of the first year.[717] In a small fraction of children cirrhosis develops during childhood or adolescence. The distinctive pathologic feature of the livers of these children is the presence in the cytoplasm of hepatocytes of periodic acid–Schiff–positive globules, which react with antibodies to alpha-1-PI. Electron microscopy shows the globules to be accumulations of alpha-1-PI within dilated sacs of endoplasmic reticulum in the hepatocytes. Similar globules are present in the livers of adult carriers of the gene for the deficiency even without cirrhosis. In addition, the incidence of both cirrhosis and hepatoma is increased in deficient adults, though both these complications are rare in comparison with emphysema.

The basis for the defect is now well understood.[686] Alpha-1-PI is the product of two alleles, one from each parent, located on chromosome 14. Both alleles are expressed, resulting in a codominant pattern of inheritance. The more common molecular form of alpha-1-PI found in 90% of the population has been designated M, and so the protease inhibitor (Pi) phenotype of a normal individual with two M alleles is written Pi MM. Over 20 abnormal variants of the alpha-1-PI molecule are known, but the one associated with most cases of clinical deficiency is designated Z. In the classic deficiency, the phenotype is Pi ZZ; that is, both genes code for the Z variant. The concentration of alpha-1-PI is the plasma is reduced to only 10% to 15% of normal, and its electrophoretic mobility is greatly reduced. The heterozygotes Pi MZ have a level of alpha-1-PI that is 60% of normal, a reduction in alpha-1-PI that is not of sufficient degree to be of major clinical importance, though there may be a small increase in the risk of emphysema in Pi MZ heterozygotes who smoke heavily.[717]

The basic abnormality in the Z protein is a point mutation that results in the substitution of a lysine in the Z protein for a glutamic acid residue in the M protein. This reduces the negative charge on the Z molecule by two charge units, accounting for its slow electrophoretic mobility. The Z protein is slightly less efficient as a protease inhibitor than an equal amount of M protein, but the main reason for the deficient inhibitory activity of plasma is the low concentration of inhibitor protein in Pi ZZ individuals. Although the Z gene is transcribed normally, intracellular processing of the protein is defective, and it accumulates in the endoplasmic reticulum of the hepatocyte instead of being released.

The pathogenesis of the liver disease is not well understood. The accumulation of alpha-1-PI in the endoplasmic reticulum of hepatocytes may predispose the liver to injury by exogenous agents, since the presence of globules themselves does not cause hepatic dysfunction. The lung disease is the result of the low level of protease inhibitory activity in the plasma and lung, which permits proteases released from phagocytes by the inflammatory stimuli to which the lung is inevitably exposed to act unopposed on lung connective tissue. The degradation of connective tissue triggers the remodeling of lung architecture, ultimately producing emphysema.

Pathogenesis

At the same time that the association of emphysema with deficiency of alpha-1-protease inhibitor was recognized, Gross[704] reported the production of emphysema in rats by the intratracheal injection of the protease papain. These two observations indicate that the maintenance of normal lung structure requires a balance between proteases and their inhibitors and that excessive proteolytic activity in the lung because of increased protease release or decreased inhibition results in emphysema. Only proteases that degrade elastin can produce emphysema in experimental animals; attempts to use nonelastolytic proteases including bacterial collagenase have been uniformly unsuccessful.[704] Alpha-1-PI is only one of at least seven known serum protease inhibitors, but it is the major inhibitor of granulocyte elastase. Disruption of the elastic fiber network is a morphologic feature of emphysema.[734] Thus the evidence is strong that degradation of elastic fibers is a critical event in the development of emphysema.

There is evidence that cigarette smoke promotes emphysema both by increasing the amount of elastolytic protease brought to the lung and by decreasing the amount of functioning inhibitor. Cigarette smokers have four to 10 times more phagocytes in their lungs than nonsmokers. The majority of these phagocytes are macrophages, but 1% to 3% are neutrophils. There is controversy regarding which cell is the main source of the elastase that is hypothesized to initiate emphysema. Neutrophils are few in the lung but have high levels of elastase activity and turn over rapidly. Macrophages, however, are the cells associated pathologically with the earliest lesions of emphysema and can degrade elastin efficiently in culture.[687] The macrophages obtained by bronchoalveolar lavage from the lungs of smokers have several other properties that are germane to protease balance in the lung. They secrete a factor chemotactic for neutrophils that might indirectly increase the elastase burden in the lung, but they also can take up and sequester neutrophil proteases, both free and complexed to inhibitors, and they synthesize small amounts of protease inhibitors.[705] Consequently their presence in early emphysematous lesions may be either a cause of injury or a protective response.

The active inhibitory site on the alpha-1-PI molecule is a methionyl-seryl bond near the carboxy terminus of the molecule. In vitro oxidation of the methionine destroys the inhibitory activity of alpha-1-PI for elastase.[686,705]

Cigarette smoke inactivates alpha-1-PI in vitro, but whether it does so in vivo is controversial.[680,703,707] Finally, damaged elastic fibers are replaced by synthesis of new elastin. Cigarette smoke interferes with this repair and may thereby promote emphysema.[703] Together, these mechanisms offer possible explanations of how a relatively mild inflammatory stimulus, cigarette smoke, promotes emphysema whereas more formidable inflammatory stimuli do not.

Natural history of chronic airflow limitation

In normal persons there is a decline in pulmonary function that begins around 20 years of age and continues lifelong. For the majority of cigarette smokers with cough and phlegm and even for many with recurrent chest infections, the annual rate of decline is no greater than normal. In a small number of more sensitive smokers, however, the rate of decline is accelerated. The accelerated loss of function may be detectable by spirometry by 30 or 40 years of age, long before overt COPD develops. If the smoker stops smoking, the cough may disappear and the rate of decline in pulmo-

nary function returns to normal but the lost function is not regained and the subject functions at a lower level than normal for his or her age. With a normal rate of decline the decrease in ventilatory function does not reach clinical significance, even in advanced age. Chronic airflow limitation develops only in that minority who are unusually susceptible to cigarette smoke and whose loss of function is accelerated.[679,694,695]

By the time symptoms develop, the abnormal decline in lung function and by implication the pathologic process have been going on for many years. Survival after the development of symptoms is variable but often is for many years. Respiratory failure heralds the terminal phase of the disease, and although many patients survive their first episode of respiratory failure, two thirds will be dead within 2 years.

The pathophysiologic features of patients with COPD and bronchitis differ in some respects from those of patients with severe emphysema. Patients with COPD but little emphysema tend to produce more sputum, to have more severe hypoxemia and carbon dioxide retention for a given degree of ventilatory impairment, and to have repeated episodes of heart failure.[684] This is because bronchitic patients whose COPD is caused by intrinsic disease of the conducting airways with intact lung parenchyma have many areas of lung with a low ventilation/perfusion ratio, that is, blood flow going through areas of underventilated lung, which results in hypoxemia.[732] Patients with severe emphysema have compliant lungs with loss of parenchyma and capillary bed; their ventilation/perfusion ratios are actually higher than normal, which produces wasted ventilation.[732] With increased effort they can maintain their oxygenation for many years until progression of the disease, increasing rigidity of the chest wall, and weakening of the respiratory muscles finally result in respiratory failure.

Hypertrophy and eventual failure of the right ventricle are terminal events in some COPD patients. Factors that raise pulmonary vascular resistance in COPD and contribute to cor pulmonale include hpoxic vasoconstriction, loss of capillary bed because of emphysema, increased viscosity of the blood as a result of secondary polycythemia and elevated alveolar pressures that may compress the alveolar capillaries during expiration against high airway resistance. Of these factors, the most important is hypoxic vasoconstriction. A large number of studies have failed to show a high degree of correlation between right ventricular weight and extent of emphysema,[689,691,716] a measure of capillary destruction, and in clinical practice the administration of oxygen usually has a rapid effect in lowering pulmonary artery pressure and improving right ventricular function.

Small airways obstruction in the absence of atypical chronic bronchitis and emphysema

Although the majority of patients with COPD are middle-aged or older cigarette smokers with slowly evolving disease, a few patients differ considerably from this epidemiologic pattern. They are younger, their disease evolves more rapidly, and in some cases it seems to be traceable to episodes of chest infection in childhood. In other cases the onset seems to follow a pneumonic episode in adult life, though sometimes no history of infective onset is obtained. The chest roentgenogram often has a miliary pattern, and bronchiectasis may also be present. The bronchioles show a spectrum of changes including fibrosis, obliteration, inflammation, and mucus plugging.[709]

Byssinosis

Byssinosis is an occupational disorder of workers exposed to cotton, flax, or hemp dust. In workers returning to work on Monday after the weekend, dyspnea and a feeling of chest tightness develop during the course of the workday. Physiologic studies have documented the development of airflow obstruction during the work shift. The severity of disease in a given individual can be gauged by the number of days into the week on which symptoms recur. In more severely affected individuals airflow obstruction recurs on successive working days and after many years may become permanent.

The mechanisms underlying the bronchial reaction have not been determined and may not be uniform in all patients. There is evidence for allergy to cotton dust antigens, for the presence of pharmacologically active substances in cotton dust that directly cause histamine release, and for bacterial endotoxin contaminating the cotton dust. There are no specific pathologic changes in byssinosis. At autopsy, lungs of former workers with disability resulting from obstructive lung disease show nonspecific chronic bronchitis and emphysema. Both the smooth muscle and the mucous glands of central airways are hypertrophied.[744] However, when studies are controlled for the influence of cigarette smoking, incidence of emphysema in textile workers is not excessive, though there is an excess of mucous hyperplasia.[744] Thus it appears that the mill dust exerts its main and perhaps sole effect on airways.

PNEUMOCONIOSIS

The term "pneumoconiosis" refers to the nonneoplastic tissue responses of the lung to the presence of deposits of inorganic dusts. The dusts of concern are of limited solubility in body fluids and remain largely in the lung and draining lymph nodes. The tissue responses are of three general types: fibrous nodules exemplified by silicosis or coal worker's pneumoconiosis, interstitial fibrosis exemplified by asbestosis or aluminosis, and hypersensitivity reactions such as chronic berylliosis.

Dust deposition and clearance

The tissue response to inhaled dust depends on the chemical composition, crystalline form, and quantity of the dust and on host factors including the efficiency of the clearance mechanism, immune status of the host, and associated diseases. Some mineral dusts, such as iron oxide, produce little fibrosis, whereas others such as silica are potentially highly fibrogenic, depending on their crystalline structure. Amorphous silica and silica with an octagonal crystal lattice are usually not fibrogenic, whereas tetrahedral crystalline silicas such as quartz dust do produce fibrosis. The amount of dust deposited in the lung depends not only on the quantity of dust in the atmosphere but also on the ventilatory pattern of the subject and on the physical properties of the particles, including shape, density, electrostatic charge, hygroscopic properties, and, most important, size.[737] Particles greater than 10 μm in diameter impact on airway bifurcations and fail to reach the acini. Particles smaller than this but larger than 0.1 μm remain suspended in rapidly flowing air but settle quickly under the influence of gravity when flow is slow. Consequently they are deposited in respiratory bronchioles and proximal alveolar ducts as airflow slows at the end of inspiration. Particles less than 0.1 μm behave essentially as gases, reaching the most distal alveoli by diffusion even though these alveoli are not ventilated in normal tidal breathing. Most particles of interest to the pathologist are in the range of 0.5 to 5 μm; deposition in the acini is most efficient at about 1 μm. Particles deposited in large airways are removed within hours by mucociliary clearance to the oropharynx to be swallowed. The clearance from the acini takes place mainly within alveolar macrophages. The uptake by alveolar macrophages also takes place within hours, but the macrophages are removed from the lung so slowly that the net half-time for particles deposited in the acini is measurable in weeks. A tiny fraction of the deposited duct, typically about 1%, escapes phagocytosis by the macrophages and is transported across the alveolar epithelium to the interstitium, mainly through the cytoplasm of type I epithelial cells. Much of the dust that escapes clearance ends up either in macrophages aggregated in the connective tissue around muscular arteries, respiratory bronchioles, and pleura where the lymphatic system begins or in the regional lymph nodes. Whether it is transported to these sites within the interstitial fluid or within macrophages is still uncertain.

Dusts in normal lungs

Small amounts of pigment are found in virtually all lungs after infancy. The amount increases with age and tends to be greater in persons from urban areas than in those from less polluted rural areas. The dust is found within macrophages in the adventitia of muscular arteries and bronchioles and in the pleura at the junctions with the interlobular septa. It is amorphous and contains carbon, silicon, iron, aluminum, phosphorus, and titanium, associated with a poorly characterized organic pigment.[766,774] The material incites little inflammation or fibrosis. In cigarette smokers the alveolar macrophages contain tobacco residues, including kaolinite.

Silicosis

Silicon comprises approximately 28% of the earth's crust. It occurs combined with oxygen as free silica (SiO_2) and with additional elements as silicates. Because of its ubiquitous occurrence in the earth's crust and usefulness as an abrasive, miners, quarry workers, tunnelers, sandblasters, grinders, and workers in many other trades are exposed to airborne silica. The ability of mineral dusts to cause lung disease has been recognized since the time of Hippocrates. Agricola (1556) in his treatise on mining called attention to the ability of mine dust of "corrode the lungs," and Ramazzini(1700) in his treatise on the diseases of various occupations described small "stones" in the lungs of quarrymen and stonecutters. The importance of silica in the production of disease was realized in the late nineteenth century, and the term "silicosis" was introduced by Visconte in 1870. The introduction of high-speed drills and efficient energy sources in the early twentieth century greatly compounded the problem.

Unfortunately, the effects of silica are insidious and the process often continues to progress after exposure has ended.[767,784] Usually 20 years of more of exposure is required for the development of classic chronic silicosis, but with high levels of exposure disease can be produced more rapidly. The most acute form of silicosis, acute silicoproteinosis, is seen in persons exposed to very high concentrations of free silica of small particle size. Silicoproteinosis is rare and was recognized as an entity only in 1969,[738] though disease described in the 1930s among those engaged in the production of scouring powders probaby represented earlier cases. The patients in the 1969 report were sandblasters who had been employed for 3 to 6 years. The onset of symptoms was acute, with dyspnea, cough, and fever, and the course was progressive deterioration with weight loss of 20 to 30 pounds, respiratory failure, and death in an average 7½ months. The lungs at autopsy showed interstitial pneumonitis with focal alveolar septal fibrosis and interstitial collections of dust-containing macrophages but only few small fibrous nodules. The alveolar spaces were filled with a flocculent or granular periodic acid–Schiff–positive exudate indistinguishable from that of alveolar proteinosis.[738] The exudate can readily be distinguished from edema fluid by the presence of cholesterol clefts and homogeneous eosinophilic blobs, 5 to 20 μm in diameter, which are remnants of necrotic cells. The lymph nodes show little fibrosis, but pleural adhesions may be present. Since the lesions of acute silicoproteinosis have been reproduced in experimental animals, the human cases do not represent the chance occurrence of alveolar proteinosis in a patient with silicosis.

Chronic silicosis usually becomes evident roentgenographically 20 to 40 years after first exposure. Many of those with fine nodularity on chest roentgenograms have no symptoms; as in other fibrosing lung diseases, exertional dyspnea develops in symptomatic patients. In accelerated silicosis the disease becomes manifest within 5 to 10 years, but the pathologic features are similar to those of chronic silicosis.[773,784]

The chronic silicotic lung is studded with well-circumscribed, dark, hard nodules, 1 to 5 mm in size, scattered through the parenchyma and in the pleura. The nodules are round to oval with a pale center and a more heavily pigmented periphery and sometimes a laminated appearance. They are more numerous in the upper lung zones than at the bases. The hilar lymph nodes are enlarged and fibrotic and may reach sufficient size to distort the bronchi. They may contain peripheral calcium deposits, giving rise to a characteristic appearance known as "eggshell" calcifications on the chest roentgenogram.

Microscopically the nodules consist of a central zone of hyalinized fibrous tissue containing only few cells and a variable amount of dust (Fig. 20-59). Concentric bundles of collagen surround and merge with the hyaline center. A mantle of more cellular connective tissue encloses the central acellular zone and contains fibroblasts, dust-filled macrophages, and lesser numbers of lymphocytes and plasma cells. Stellate projections of fibrous tissue extend a short distance into the adjacent alveolar walls. Calcium is deposited in some hyaline nodules.

Initially the hyaline nodules form in the regions of the respiratory bronchioles and muscular arteries and in the pleura where the dust is concentrated. As the nodules grow and increase in number, their distribution within the acinus becomes widespread.

In some patients with severe disease individual nodules grow rapidly and coalesce to form large conglomerate masses of fibrous tissue. This process is termed complicated pneumonconiosis with the implication that some additional stimulus "complicates" the simple pneumoconiosis. In some instances the stimulus is tuberculosis and in others some other disease may produce altered immunologic responsiveness, but most often the stimulus is unknown. Conglomerate masses form predominantly in the upper lobes and can grow to considerable size, cross lobar fissures, and occupy a large portion of the lung volume. Blood vessels and even bronchi can be obliterated by the process, and slitlike cavities form by ischemic degeneration. Large, ragged cavities usually indicate tuberculosis.

The functional effects of silicosis are as varied as its

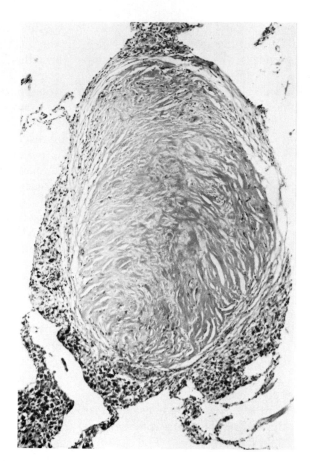

Fig. 20-59. Hyaline nodule in silicosis. Center of hyalinized collagen is enclosed by mantle of dust.

pathologic features. Many patients with simple pneumoconiosis detected by chest roentgenography have normal function. Symptomatic patients may have either an obstructive or a restrictive ventilatory pattern.[784] The airflow obstruction may result from involvement of bronchioles by the pneumoconiosis, an associated industrial or cigarette-induced bronchitis, or distortion of airways by larger conglomerate masses. Complicated pneumoconiosis presents a restrictive ventilatory pattern and reduced diffusing capacity because of the replacement of lung tissue by the fibrous mass, but obstruction may also be present.

Pathogenesis

Silicosis is seen in humans in the form of established lesions. The early tissue response is inferred from animal studies, which usually involve a large single dose given by either inhalation or injection. The majority of the silica is taken up by macrophages that undergo necrosis, and new macrophages engulf the debris and released silica in a repetitive cycle of phagocytosis and necrosis. Gradually macrophages migrate or are carried to the region of respiratory bronchioles where they ag-

gregate in alveoli and in the interstitial tissues around blood vessels. Mast cells, plasma cells, and fibroblasts become associated with the cellular aggregates, and gradually reticulin fibers and eventually mature collagen fibers are laid down. The resultant lesions resemble human hyaline nodules to a degree depending on species, technique of administration, size of particles, and dose of silica.

The mechanisms involved in the formation of these lesions are incompletely understood. There is a high correlation between the cytotoxicity of different types of silica for macrophages and their ability to produce fibrosis. This indicates that the repetitive necrosis of macrophages, release of silica, reuptake, and new cycle of necrosis may be an important part of the self-perpetuating nature of the lesions. The available evidence indicates that the mechanism of cytotoxicity is related to the ability of silica to damage cellular membranes. The uptake of siica into phagosomes and phagolysosomes is followed by membrane damage, leakage of acid hydrolases from the lysosomes into the cytosol, and the loss of the ability of the plasma membrane to exclude extracellular calcium.[755] These events in turn lead to depletion of ATP and cell death.

A substantial body of experimental data indicates that stimulated or necrotic macrophages may provide a stimulus for fibroblast proliferation and collagen synthesis.[768] In 1967 Heppleston and Styles[753] reported that extracts of rat alveolar macrophages that had ingested silica stimulated collagen synthesis by chick fibroblasts. Silica induces macrophages to produce interleukin-1 and perhaps other mediators, which induce fibroblasts to proliferate and synthesize collagen.[770]

Silicosis produces changes in the immune response, but the role of immunologic factors in the pathogenesis of silicosis is unknown.[777] Hyperglobulinemia and autoantibodies occur frequently in silicotic subjects. The prevalence of rheumatoid factor and antinuclear antibodies is approximately 30% in silicotic patients and is higher still in those with complicated pneumoconiosis. Immunoglobulin has been identified in silicotic hyalin, and lung reactive antibodies have been detected in the serum of silicotic patients, but whether the antibodies are the cause or the result of the tissue damage is unknown. Limited studies of cell-mediated immunity have been carried out in silicosis. No decrease in circulating T-cells has been found, and patients do not have anergy to most common skin test antigens. Diminished responsiveness of the peripheral blood lymphocytes to the T-cell mitogen concanavalin A has been observed, however, and in silica-treated animals defective cellular immunity is shown by prolongation of skin-graft survival.[777] The increased susceptibiity of silicotic persons to tuberculosis probably indicates that a significant defect in cell-mediated immunity exists.

Tuberculosis and silicosis

Clinical and epidemiologic studies have repeatedly shown an increased risk of tuberculosis and other mycobacterial infections in silicotic persons.[775] The prevalence of tuberculosis varies depending on the prevalence of tuberculosis in the surrounding population but is always severalfold higher in those with silicosis. The relative risk is greater in those with classic silicosis than in those with mixed-dust pneumoconiosis.

Typical lesions of silicosis and ordinary caseous granulomas can coexist in the lungs of silicotic persons, but the combination of silicosis and tuberculosis may also produce atypical morphologic lesions. In one form of silicotuberculosis, lesions closely resemble siicotic hyaline nodules with an outer mantle of dust-filled macrophages and fibroblasts enclosing a hyaline core that centrally appears softer and more granular than usual, reminiscent of caseous necrosis. The most dramatic form of siicotuberculosis has already been mentioned: the large conglomerate fibrous masses that form in the upper lobe of some patients. Extensive cavitation developing within massive fibrosis is presumptive evidence of tuberculosis (Fig. 20-60). Organisms are difficult to culture from sputum and even from tissue, presumably because they are trapped within the fibrous scar. Characteristically cavities are round, shaggy, and filled with black fluid that is noticeably purulent. Unlike the usual tubercular cavity, those in complicated silicosis are not trabeculated. Microscopic examination shows a thin zone of necrosis, with a few inflammatory cells and capillaries, that makes up at least a portion of the lining of the cavity.[778]

The effect of silica in modifying the response to *Mycobacterium tuberculosis* is readily demonstrable in animal experiments. Exposure of guinea pigs to silica causes enhanced growth of tubercle bacilli, reactivates healing lesions, and leads to progressive infection by ordinarily avirulent strains, including bacillus Calmette-Guérin (BCG), a strain widey used for vaccination. Interestingly the overproduction of connective tissue characteristic of progressive massive fibrosis is also reproduceable in animals. Gross, Westrick, and McNerney[750] administered nonfibrogenic quartz dust, accompanied by living or dead tubercle bacilli or tuberculin purified protein derivative (PPD), to tuberculin-sensitive guinea pigs. Fibrotic lesions were most extensive with living organisms, less so with dead ones. Even the addition of soluble PPD increased the amount of fibrosis compared with quartz alone. Necrosis and calcification were seen only with organisms.

One reason for the increased susceptibility to tubercle bacilli is the direct action of silica on macrophages. Allison and D'Arcy Hart[735] found that cultured macrophages that had ingested sublethal amounts of silica permitted more rapid growth of tubercle bacilli and re-

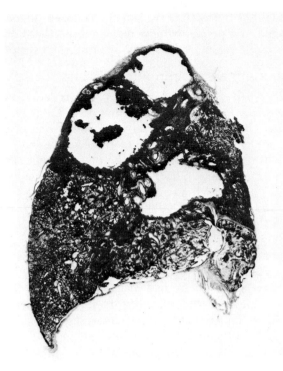

Fig. 20-60. Paper-mounted whole lung section from coal miner with tuberculosis shows massive fibrosis with extensive cavitation. (Preparation by Prof. J. Gough.)

leased more organisms into the culture medium than normal macrophages did.

Other diseases

There is no evidence that silica increases the risk of lung cancer, nor does it enhance tobacco-induced carcinogenesis. The incidence of progressive systemic sclerosis (scleroderma) has been reported to be increased in miners. Perhaps silicosis predisposes to the development of scleroderma.

Mixed-dust pneumoconiosis

The tissue response to silica is modified by the presence of other components of a dust. When the dust contains more than approximately 18% free silica, a typical hyaline nodule is produced, but with lesser amounts of silica the tissue response is modified. Modified reactions are seen in foundry workers, hematite miners, and those engaged in removing boiler scale. The lesions are firm nodules, 2 to 5 mm in diameter, that are uniformly pigmented. Large conglomerate masses develop in some cases. As with other pneumoconioses the lesions are concentrated around respiratory bronchioles and muscular arteries and consist of a mixture of dust-laden macrophages and collagen fibers. In contrast to hyaline nodules, the dust is uniformly distributed through the nodule rather than being concentrated at the periphery, and the collagen fibers are arranged in a stellate pattern radiating into the walls of neighboring alveoli, rather than in a concentric pattern.

Pulmonary disease in coal workers

Coal worker's pneumoconiosis (CWP) is the focus of current medical and political controversy. Although few medical authorities would deny that inhalation of coal dust produces characteristics morphologic lesions, the relationship of these lesions to the development of disability is in dispute. This issue is of great economic importance. Although the coal mining population currently numbers only 120,000 miners who are at risk for CWP, the annual outlay for black lung benefits is over 1 billion dollars.[761]

For many years coal dust was considered innocuous. When disease occurred in miners, it was attributed to silicosis. Coal trimmers load coal and distribute it in the holds of ships; the identification of lesions in their lungs that were similar to those of miners established that coal itself without silica could cause lesions.[747] The subsequent description of pneumoconiosis in groups working with pure carbon, electrotypers, carbon electrode workers, and graphite workers confirms the pathologic potential of carbonaceous dusts.[780] Currently three conditions are associated directly with coal mine dust: silicosis, coal worker's pneumonconiosis, and industrial bronchitis.[762,767]

Silicosis most commonly develops in anthracite miners and in certain occupational specialties among bituminous miners. Anthracite in eastern Pennsylvania occurs in narrow undulating seams, and so miners frequently are obliged to tunnel horizontally from one seam to another through hard rock, which exposes them to silica. Roof bolters and transportation workers have a high rate of silicosis, the former because they drill into hard rock and the latter because they inhale sand dusted on the tracks to provide traction for the shuttle cars.[762]

Coal worker's pneumoconiosis

CWP was first described in Britain by Gough and Heppleston[752] in the 1940s. The spectrum of morphologic changes found in the lungs of coal workers has been reviewed recently.[749,757,763] The process known as simple CWP begins with the accumulation of dust-laden macrophages in the alveoli evaginating from the respiratory bronchioles, but with time the alveoli become filled and dust and macrophages also accumulate in the adventitia of the respiratory bronchioles and arteries. Small amounts of reticulin fibers are laid down, and the respiratory bronchioles become thickened and encased by solid dust-filled tissue. The alveolar ducts gradually dilate. Initially there is little overt destruction of air-space walls, but in more advanced cases emphy-

sema develops in association with dust foci, the so-called focal emphysema. Heppleston and Leopold[699] consider it a distinctive type of emphysema separable from other centriacinar emphysema by the absence of inflammation, but this opinion is not uniformly accepted in the United States.[783]

The typical dust accumulations in the respiratory bronchiolar region of miners appear grossly as dust macules, nonpalpable pigmented spots, 1 to 3 mm in diameter, in the centers of lobules (Figs. 20-61 and 20-62). Miners' lungs also may have palpable black nodules 1 to 7 mm in diameter. These are more heavily collagenized than the typical macules and may have a higher silica content.[757]

In complicated CWP or progressive massive fibrosis (PMF), masses 2 cm to several centimeters in diameter form usually in the upper zones of the lung (Fig. 20-63). Rubbery and black, they may have foci of degeneration and cavitation filled with inky fluid. When associated with CWP, the lesions of progressive massive fibrosis usually grow as a single mass, whereas in silicosis they arise by the fusion of several nodules bound together in a fibrous mass.[743] The collagen in complicated CWP is laid down haphazardly, whereas in silicosis the concentric organization of the hyaline nodules is discernible.

The cause of complicated CWP is unknown in most cases. The incidence of roentgenographically diagnosed PMF varies considerably from area to area, from a high of 14% in some anthracite mines to none in Colorado

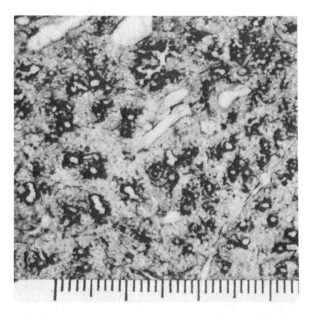

Fig. 20-61. Simple coal worker's pneumoconiosis. Paper-mounted lung section shows black dust deposits outlining respiratory bronchioles. (Preparation by Prof. J. Gough.)

bituminous miners. Tuberculosis was once held to be the major cause, but despite the dramatic fall in the prevalence of tuberculosis, no comparable fall in the frequency of PMF has occurred. Silica may play a role; PMF tends to be more frequent in lungs having a high silica content, but the correlation in individual cases is not good. PMF has been reported in carbon-electrode workers exposed to little silica. The prevalence of auto-antibodies such as rheumatoid and antinuclear antibodies is higher in patients with complicated CWP than in those with simple CWP, an indication that immunologic factors may be involved. However, PMF has not been associated with any specific human lymphocyte histocompatibility antigen, as might be expected if there were a genetic basis for abnormal immunologic response.

The diagnosis of CWP is based on a compatible occupational history and the presence of rounded opacities on the chest roentgenogram. The International Labor Organization (ILO) has devised a system of grading pneumoconiosis roentgenographically based on the size of the opacities (p, q, r in increasing size) and their profusion (increasing from 1 to 3). Complicated pneumoconiosis is diagnosed if opacities exceed 1 cm in size

and is graded A, B, or C depending on size of lesions. When Naeye and Dellinger[764] correlated the roentgenographic grading of simple CWP with the pathologic features in the tissue, the best correlations were with dust and collagen content of the tissue.

Disability in coal workers

Disability in coal workers has been discussed in detail by Morgan.[762] The mortality in coal miners is greater than in other occupational groups, largely because of trauma and accidents. Mortality from respiratory disease is not demonstrably higher. A higher than expected number of deaths from COPD is balanced by a lower frequency of lung cancer than in comparable occupational groups. The lower frequency of lung cancer, if real, is attributable to lower levels of cigarette consumption by miners, who are prohibited from smoking underground.

Breathlessness and cough are more prevalent among miners than in controls. These symptoms show little correlation with roentgenographic category, or, in pathologic studies, with the dust, the collagen content, or the volume of macules in the lung. Most patients with grade 1 or 2 CWP on the chest roentgenogram

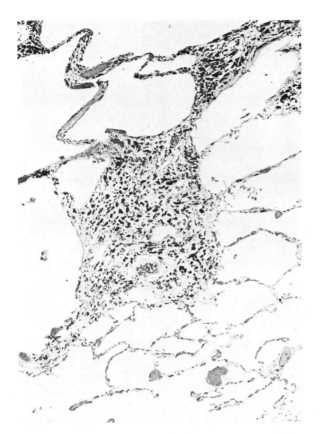

Fig. 20-62. Microscopic appearance of dust macule in coal worker.

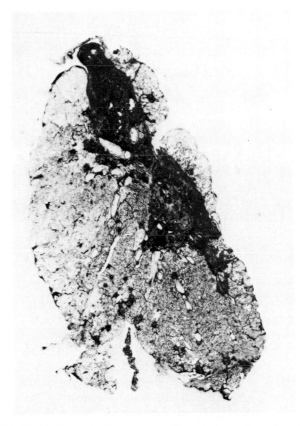

Fig. 20-63. Progressive massive fibrosis in coal worker. Paper-mounted whole lung section. (Preparation by Prof. J. Gough.)

have no impairment of ventilation. It is unlikely that simple CWP by itself causes disability.

Coal workers who complain of dyspnea and have impaired ventilation usually have an obstructive pattern.[762] Whether they can have hypoxemia without a reduction in expiratory flow is controversial. Currently either an $FEV_{1.0}$ below 80% of that predicted for normals or a decrease in the arterial oxygen tension can qualify a worker for compensation. Impaired ventilation is a consequence of emphysema and bronchitis as it is in the nonmining population. Right ventricular thickening, an indirect measure of hypoxemia, is also related to emphysema and unrelated to pathologic measures of CWP.[764] Although there is no doubt that cigarette smoking plays a role (some would say a predominant role) in the production of emphysema and bronchitis in most disabled miners, data indicate that coal workers have more emphysema than others who smoke a comparable amount and some nonsmoking miners have emphysema sufficient to impair lung function.[740,765,769] Whether the causative agent is coal dust or some other element of the mine environment such as fumes from lamps or gases from diesel exhaust or shotfiring is uncertain.

Cough and sputum production (bronchitis) are more prevalent in miners than in nonminers and correlate with level of dust exposure, being highest in workers at the coal face where dust levels are highest and lowest in surface workers where dust is least. Slight impairment of ventilation is seen after many years of exposure.[762] Since airflows are reduced at high lung volumes but not at low lung volumes, the abnormalities appear to be in the large airways, but the mechanisms are unknown.

Whereas simple CWP does not affect life span or directly cause disability, complicated pneumoconiosis is clearly associated with airflow obstruction, reduced diffusion capacity, and restriction of ventilation. With higher grades of PMF cor pulmonale often develops. The process can progress after exposure has ceased (indeed it can first manifest itself long after exposure has ended) and life span is shortened.

Association with other diseases

Bronchogenic carcinoma does not appear to be more common in coal workers than in other groups. Some studies from both Britain and the United States point to a lesser incidence in coal workers. Tuberculosis is more common in coal workers than in the general population but less common than in patients with silicosis.

The combination of rheumatoid arthritis with CWP produces a characteristic lesion known as rheumatoid pneumoconiosis, or Caplan's syndrome, after the British radiologist who first recognized it.[739] Over a few months round opacities from 0.3 cm to several centi-

meters in diameter develop, mainly in the peripheral lung fields. The lesions evolve more rapidly than those of PMF and may finally cavitate or develop calcifications. The pathologic changes were described by Gough, Rivers, and Seal.[748] The lesions may be solitary, or several may fuse to form a large conglomerate mass. They are pale gray-yellow with concentric darker layers of pigment. The pale areas tend to liquefy, leaving clefts. Histologically the center is necrotic and often contains foci of calcium. Concentric bands of dust are found in the necrotic material. A zone of palisading fibroblasts or histocytes surrounds the necrotic center. The outer layer consists of a capsule of circumferential collagen fibers with lymphocytes and plasma cells. Thus the lesions have characteristics of a rheumatoid necrobiotic nodule modified by the setting of pneumonconiosis.

Rheumatoid pneumoconiosis can appear in miners without articular disease, but circulating rheumatoid factor is invariably present. Arthritis subsequently develops in at least some such patients.

Diseases related to asbestos

Asbestos is a general term denoting any naturally occurring silicate mineral whose crystals are in the form of fibers. The major commercial types, chrysotile, crocidolite, amosite, and anthophyllite, differ in their elemental composition, fiber morphology, physical properties, and certain of their effects on cells. They probably differ also in their capacity to produce each of the various lesions associated with asbestos exposure, but since based on current knowledge none can be exonerated as a cause of any of the lesions to be discussed, no effort is made to distinguish among them in the following discussion.

Asbestos is a ubiquitous contaminant of the urban environment and has been identified in urban air.[772] Asbestos bodies, fibers coated with iron and protein, can be found in virtually 100% of adult lungs if gram amounts of tissue are digested and the residue collected on a filter and examined with a microscope. The number of uncoated fibers is approximately 10^5 fibers per gram. The significance of this relatively low-level asbestos exposure is uncertain, but there is no evidence at present linking it to disease.

The lesions associated with exposure to elevated levels of asbestos include pulmonary fibrosis, tumors, pleural plaques, and pleural effusions.[736] Pulmonary fibrosis requires the highest levels of exposure and is practically limited to those with direct industrial exposure. Tumors and pleural plaques are induced by lower levels of exposure and can be found in those whose exposure is indirect, such as family members who handle a worker's dusty clothes or those who dwell near asbestos mines, mills, or dump sites.

Asbestosis

The term "asbestosis" should be reserved for pulmonary fibrosis caused by asbestos. Asbestosis is seen in shipyard and construction workers, insulation workers, and those engaged in the manufacture of asbestos cement, tiles, or brake linings. Disease first appears at least 10 and usualy 20 or more years after first exposure.[736]

The symptoms of asbestosis are insidious and are similar to those of interstitial fibrosis of any cause: breathlessness, initially associated only with exertion, accompanied by a nonproductive cough. Physical examination usually shows basilar crackles and may show clubbing. Early in the disease the chest roentgenogram may be normal, though physiologic measurements such as vital capacity or diffusing capacity may show abnormalities. Later dyspnea becomes more severe, hyperventilation is apparent, and cor pulmonale may develop. The chest roentgenogram, which initially shows small irregular opacities at the bases, later shows honeycombing.

The lungs are small and firm with a thickened pleura.[741,742] On the sectioned surface gray zones of fibrosis enclose abnormally enlarged air spaces a few millimeters to a centimeter in size. Lesions are most prominent in the bases and the subpleural areas (Fig. 20-64).

The microscopic changes are those of a nonspecific interstitial fibrosis accompanied by the presence of characteristic structures known as asbestos or ferruginous bodies.[741,742]

Ferruginous bodies vary in length from 10 to 50 μm or more and consist of a straight or curved translucent core of asbestos coated with globules of brown refractile material, which give the body a beaded, dumbbell, or drumstick shape (Fig. 20-65).[782] The coating stains strongly with the Prussian blue reaction for ferric iron and by electron microscopy is shown to consist of ferritin. The formation of these bodies has been observed with electron microscopy in experimental animals. Only the largest fibers give rise to ferruginous bodies; small fibers remain uncoated. The fibers are phagocytosed or,

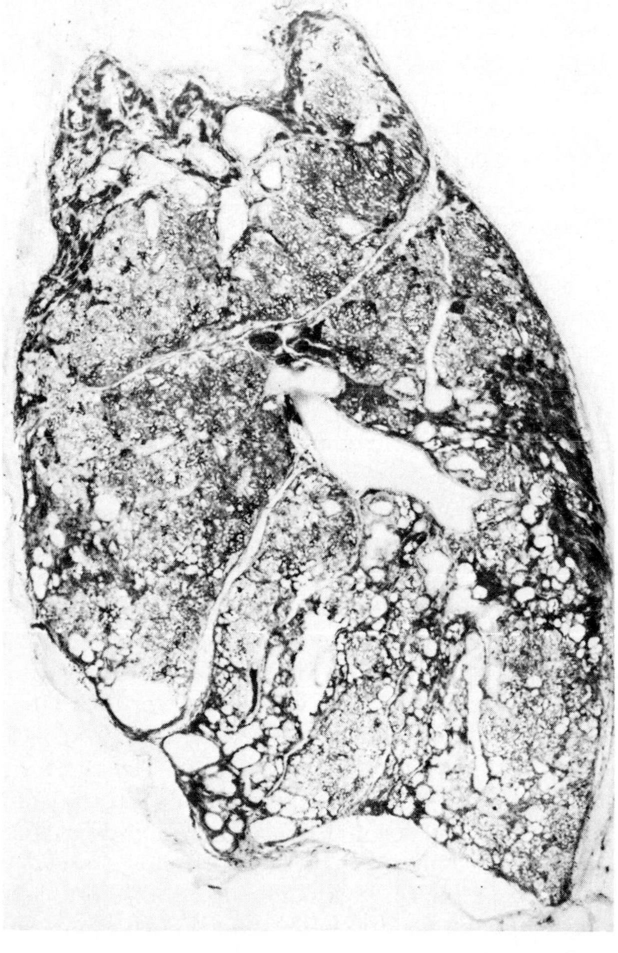

Fig. 20-64. Paper-mounted whole lung section from patient with asbestosis shows areas of honeycombing, especially in subpleural zones. (From pathological museum of University of Manchester, U.K.)

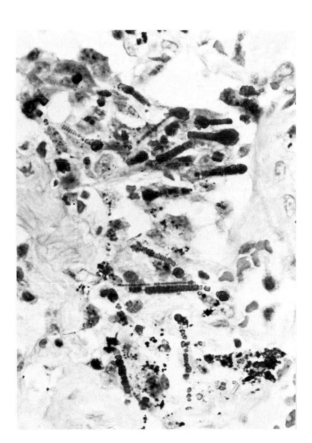

Fig. 20-65. Asbestosis. Interstitial fibrous tissue contains dust and asbestos bodies.

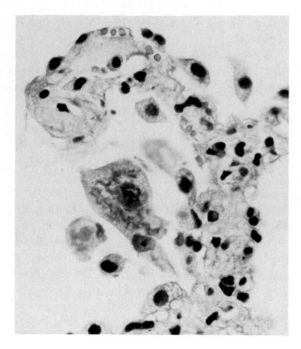

Fig. 20-66. Asbestosis.

if too large to be completely phagocytosed, are enclosed by macrophage cytoplasm, forming an incomplete phagosome. Vacuoles, probably lysosomes, containing ferritin discharge onto the surface of the fiber, leading to the buildup of coating material.[776]

The disease begins in the respiratory bronchioles, and early cases show only interstitial fibrosis in some respiratory bronchioles, accompanied by prominent hyperplastic alveolar epithelium and the accumulation of macrophages in the air-space lumens.[741] Asbestos bodies may be present either in the air-space or in the interstitium, usually in association with macrophages. With time the process extends to involve alveolar ducts, and fibrosis in neighboring lobules links up, resulting in the picture of diffuse interstitial fibrosis. The thickened alveolar walls are often infiltrated with lymphocytes and rarely with neutrophils. The alveolar epithelium is hyperplastic with areas of metaplasia to squamous or mucin-secreting epithelium. Commonly a few of the hyperplastic alveolar epithelial cells contain hyaline inclusions reminiscent of hepatic Mallory bodies, and occasionally this phenomenon is prominent (Fig. 20-66).[759] It is not specific for asbestosis, being seen occasionally in other forms of lung injury. Large numbers of macrophages, sometimes with multinucleated giant cells, are commonly present in the air spaces. Asbestos bodies are often plentiful but may be rare. One case has been reported in which no asbestos bodies were present but electron microscopy showed large numbers of uncoated fibers. In contrast to silicosis, the hilar lymph nodes show little involvement in asbestosis though a few asbestos bodies may be present.

Pleural disease

Pleural effusions develop in as much as 5% of asbestos workers, but most are small and asymptomatic.[745] Occasionally they cause pain or fever. Pleural plaques are the most common lesion associated with asbestos.[736] They are circumscribed, usually bilateral lesions that develop on the pleural surface of the diaphragm and the parietal pleura of the chest wall. Grossly they appear as flat, ivory-colored deposits 1 mm to several millimeters thick with a smooth or knobby surface. They often calcify, which aids their roentgenographic recognition. Microscopically they consist of hyalinized collagenous tissue with few cells. Asbestos bodies are not generally found within the plaques, even when digestion techniques are used.

Plaques take many years to develop. They are infrequent in the first 20 years after exposure, but by 30 to 40 years as much as 50% of workers have calcified plaques that are seen roentgenographically. Plaques rarely cause symptoms and apparently do not restrict ventilation unless very extensive. There is no evidence that they predispose to mesotheliomas. Their importance is as a marker for exposure to asbestos.

Tumors

The association of mesothelioma with asbestos exposure was reported by Wagner, Sleggs, and Marchand[779] in 1960, and many additional cases have since been reported.[736,741,742] The asbestos exposure need not be intense, and indirect (nonoccupational) exposure is responsible for some cases. The latent period is generally more than 20 years. Either the pleura or the peritoneum may be the primary site. The pathologic features and natural history of mesothelioma are discussed elsewhere (p. 1018), but it is appropriate here to reiterate that approximately 50% of mesotheliomas in men in the United States are associated with exposure to asbestos.

Bronchogenic carcinoma is the greatest single cause of excess mortality in asbestos workers.[771] The risk of bronchogenic carcinoma is slightly increased by asbestos in nonsmokers, but in smokers tobacco smoke and asbestos are synergistic. Hammond, Selikoff, and Seidman[751] found the relative risks of bronchogenic carcinoma to be 10 times greater in smokers than in nonsmokers and five times greater in asbestos-exposed nonsmokers that in other nonsmokers. The risk for asbestos workers who smoke was an appalling 50 times greater than that for nonsmoking, unexposed subjects. The bronchogenic carcinomas in asbestos exposed patients occur more commonly in the lower lobes, whereas in the general population bronchogenic carcinoma occurs predominantly in the upper lobes. Some observers have reported adenocarcinomas to be the predominant histologic type,[781] but others have not found a preponderance of any particular histologic type.[756]

Carcinomas in other sites may also be more common in asbestos workers. The risk of carcinoma of the larynx and large intestine is greater in asbestos workers, and there are unconfirmed reports of an increase in renal cell carcinoma and hematologic malignancies.

Beryllium disease

Beryllium disease was first recognized in Europe in the 1930s. Epidemics occurred in the United States in the 1940s, particularly in the fluorescent light industry. These disappeared once the hazard was recognized and the use of beryllium in fluorescent lights was abandoned. Although the use of beryllium is increasing again because of its use in aerospace industries, the disease remains rare and is of interest principally for contrast with conventional pneumoconioses.

In the past, acute berylliosis was seen in the extraction industry, typically in workers who had been exposed to high concentrations for 2 to 4 weeks. The onset is acute with dyspnea, hyperpnea, and in some cases substernal pain. Most patients recover, though this may take as long as 12 weeks. The few patients examined at autopsy showed an acute chemical pneumonitis. The alveolar walls were thickened by interstitial edema and mononuclear cell infiltration. The air spaces contained edema and hyaline membranes in various stages of organization. Bronchiolitis obliterans was present in a few patients. Tissue beryllium levels were usually high.[746]

Chronic beryllium disease is a systemic disorder, though the lung, being the port of entry, is usually the major site of clinical involvement. The symptoms may begin at any time during exposure or up to 20 years after exposure, but the majority of patients become ill in the first 5 years. Typically patients have a gradual onset of dyspnea and nonproductive cough that progress to cyanosis. Weight loss is common and may be dramatic. Other systemic manifestations incude hyperglobulinemia, hypercalcemia, and occasionally renal stones.

The disease is probably not merely a manifestation of toxicity but a hypersensitivity reaction of cell-mediated type in which beryllium acts as a hapten and as an immunologic adjuvant.[758] The histologic changes are similar to those in other types of hypersensitivity pneumonitis. Changes range from diffuse interstitial pneumonitis with nonspecific infiltration of air space walls by histiocytes, lymphocytes, and plasma cells, to mononuclear infiltration accompanied by loose or well-formed granulomas, to tightly organized noncaseating epithelioid granulomas like those of sarcoid with little interstitial infiltrate.[746] Giant cells are present with each type and frequently contain inclusions, either asteroid bodies or the concentric laminated hematoxyphilic bodies known as conchoid or Schaumann bodies. First described in sarcoid, in which they are rare,

Schaumann bodies are present in 50% to 70% of patients with berylliosis, especially those with interstitial pneumonitis. Although they are by no means specific, their presence in abundance suggests a diagnosis of beryllium disease. Discrete hyalinized nodules surrounded by a fibrous capsule are present in 40% of cases and may occasionally be the predominant lesion. The center of the nodules may show infarctlike necrosis, calcification, or cholesterol clefts.

The experience of the U.S. Beryllium Disease Case Registry indicates that the course and prognosis of the disease are strongly correlated with histologic findings.[746] Among patients with diffuse interstitial pneumonia with or without granulomas, the mortality was 75% with an average survival of 8 years. Those with a sarcoidlike reaction with little interstitial infiltrate had a much better prognosis, with only a 4% mortality during an average follow-up period of 11 years.

LUNG TUMORS
Carcinomas of the lung
Incidence

The incidence of carcinoma of the lung in industrialized countries has been increasing at a phenomenal rate during the twentieth century (Fig. 20-67). Infrequent early in the century, lung cancer is now the second most common carcinoma (after skin cancer) in American men, accounting for 22% of all cancers and one third of all deaths resulting from malignancy. The incidence in women is rising 5% annually, and lung cancer is expected shortly to become the leading cause of cancer

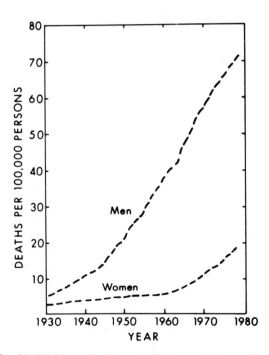

Fig. 20-67. Mortality from carcinoma of lung, 1930 to 1980.

mortality in women, surpassing carcinoma of the breast before the end of the 1980s. In Britain lung cancer accounts for nearly 40% of cancer deaths in men and 13% in women.

In 1983, for the first time, the lung cancer incidence failed to rise in men. In women it continues to rise, and if the present trend persists as expected, the incidence rates for men and women will be equal by the year 2000.

Cancer of the lung is a disease of middle and late life. The incidence is low in those below 35 years of age, rises to a peak at age 60, and declines slowly thereafter.

Classification

Lung tumors are classified on the basis of histologic findings. The various histologic types of lung cancer differ in clinical presentation, natural history, and response to treatment. Evidence of more than one type of differentiation can be found in many lung carcinomas if special techniques such as electron microscopy are used,[789,847] but the practical value of standard histologic classifications based on the predominant cell type is amply justified on clinical grounds. The following is the classification recommended by an expert panel convened by the World Health Organization[884]:

1. Squamous cell carcinoma (epidermoid carcinoma)
   a. Spindle cell squamous carcinoma (variant)
2. Small cell carcinoma
   a. Oat cell carcinoma
   b. Intermediate cell type
   c. Combined oat cell carcinoma
3. Adenocarcinoma
   a. Acinar adenocarcinoma
   b. Papillary adenocarcinoma
   c. Bronchioloalveolar carcinoma
   d. Solid carcinoma with mucus formation
4. Large cell carcinoma
   a. Giant cell carcinoma (variant)
   b. Clear cell carcinoma (variant)
5. Adenosquamous carcinoma
6. Carcinoid tumor
7. Bronchial gland carcinomas
   a. Adenoid cystic carcinoma
   b. Mucoepidermoid carcinoma
   c. Others
8. Others

In common clinical usage the first four categories, squamous cell carcinoma, small cell carcinoma, adenocarcinoma, and large cell carcinoma, are grouped as "bronchogenic carcinoma." A strict histogenetic classification would group small cell carcinoma and carcinoid together as tumors with neuroendocrine differentiation, but in clinical presentation small cell carcinomas resemble the other "bronchogenic" carcinomas more closely than they do carcinoid.

The diagnostic differentiation of the histologic classes of bronchogenic carcinoma can be made using either exfoliated cells or tissue sections. Both are reliable when the tumors are well differentiated. When a tumor is poorly differentiated, even expert pathologists using multiple sections may disagree.[868] In one study three experienced pathologists could agree on the classification of only 50% of poorly differentiated tumors.[887]

Bronchogenic carcinomas

Squamous cell carcinoma. Squamous cell carcinoma is probaby the most common type of bronchogenic carcinoma, comprising 30% to 35% of autopsy series and 35% to 60% of surgical series,[786,855,876] though some recent studies indicate that adenocarcinoma may have overtaken it in incidence.[874] Squamous carcinomas are more common in men than in women, usually develop in middle or later life, and are strongly associated with cigarette smoking.[786] The relative risk of contracting squamous cell carcinoma was 25 times greater for smokers than nonsmokers in Kreyberg's study.[838] Roughly two thirds of squamous carcinomas are central tumors, involving the main or lobar bronchi, whereas one third

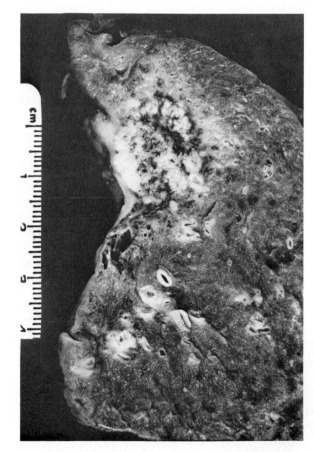

Fig. 20-68. Epidermoid carcinoma of lung. This is peripheral tumor not associated with major bronchus. Overlying pleura is thickened and retracted.

arise in the lung periphery, either in small bronchi or in association with scars (Fig. 20-68).[802,877] However, in some patients with large bronchi involved at the time of diagnosis, serial roentgenographic observations indicate that the tumor actually arose in a more peripheral location and grew to involve the central bronchi late in its course.[857] Bronchial involvement may take the form of a warty endobronchial protrusion, or the tumor may ulcerate the bronchus and grow outward.[844] If the tumor obstructs a large bronchus, the lung distal to the tumor will often be the site of obstructive pneumonia and bronchiectasis. The gross appearance of most squamous carcinomas is not distinctive, but large, well-differentiated tumors may have shiny caseous yellow foci where heavily keratinized. The expectoration of keratinous or necrotic material may produce cavities within the tumor. Indeed, the majority of cavitary lung carcinomas are of the squamous cell type.

The microscopic diagnosis of squamous carcinoma depends on the identification of either intercellular bridges or keratinization (Fig. 20-69). Keratinized cells can be recognized in sections by their brightly eosinophilic refractile cytoplasm and pyknotic nuclei. Squa-

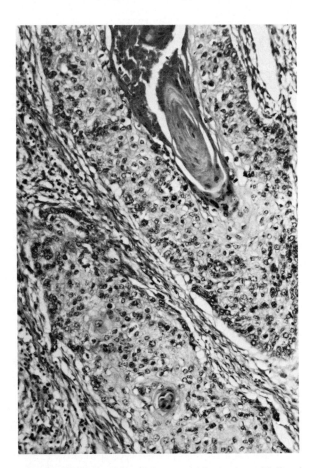

Fig. 20-69. Epidermoid carcinoma of bronchus. Notice keratin nests.

mous carcinomas of the lung tend to be poorly differentiated and often vary from area to area. Typically they are composed of nests of cells that palisade at the periphery of the lobules and become enlarged and flattened centrally. Whorls or eddies of cells may be keratinized (epidermoid pearls); the whole center of the lobule may be filled with keratin, or at the other extreme only a few single cells may be keratinized.

Although most squamous cell carcinomas have at least some areas of large cells with plentiful cytoplasm, some tumors consist ony of relatively small basophilic cells resembling those of basal cell carcinoma in the skin. The distinction from small cell carcinoma is difficult in such cases. Electron microscopy and immunohistochemical studies may be helpful. The electron microscope shows that the cells of squamous carcinoma are joined by desmosomes on short projections of cytoplasm, which correspond to the intercellular bridges seen with light microscopy.[846] Secretory granules are absent, and the endoplasmic reticulum is poorly developed. Immunohistochemistry shows that keratin is invariably present and carcinoembryonic antigen is usual.[862]

Squamous cell carcinomas tend to grow more rapidly than other histologic types, with doubling times of 2 to 4 months and relatively high mitotic indices.[878,880] Despite this, they have a more favorable prognosis than other types of bronchogenic carcinoma, with a 5-year survival of 20% to 35%.[837,860,871,882]

Squamous carcinoma is believed to arise through a series of changes in the epithelium of the bronchi that includes hyperplasia of the basal cells, loss of cilia, metaplasia of the epithelium, development of a squamous type of epithelium, increasing atypism, squamous carcinoma in situ, and eventually invasion (Fig. 20-70).[788] The squamous cells derive either from abnormal differentiation of the basal cells or from metaplasia of mucous cells.[872] The time required for the various stages in the proposed sequence is unknown, but many patients have been observed to have cytologically malignant cells in their sputum for several years before any tumor could be detected roentgenologically.

Adenocarcinoma. Between 20% and 30% of carcinomas of the lung are adenocarcinomas, and the proportion has risen at the last 15 years.[786,855,874,876] Adenocarcinoma is the most common histologic type of bronchogenic carcinoma in women,[875] and the increasing proportion of women in the lung carcinoma population is undoubtedly a factor in the relative increase in adenocarcinomas. Although adenocarcinoma is the most common type of bronchogenic carcinoma in nonsmokers,[881,885] the great majority of patients with adenocarcinoma are smokers.[871] Even in Kreyberg's study,[838] which established the strong association of small cell and squamous cell carcinomas with cigarette

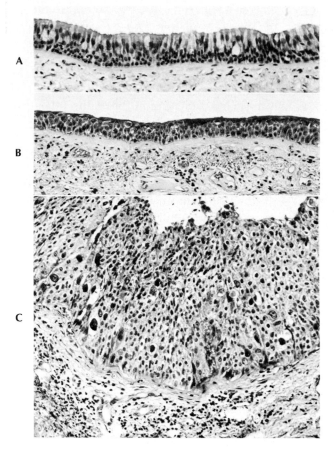

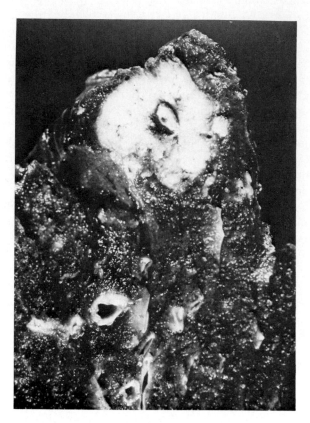

Fig. 20-70. Presumptive stages in histogenesis of epidermoid carcinoma. **A,** Normal bronchus. **B,** Squamous metaplasia. **C,** In situ carcinoma. Malignant-appearing epithelium without invasion. (130×.)

Fig. 20-71. Adenocarcinoma of lung. This tumor presumably arose in a scar. Ring of pigment in center outlines edge of calcified granuloma that occupied center of tumor.

smoking, the relative risk of adenocarcinoma was three times greater in smokers than in nonsmokers.

The majority of adenocarcinomas arise in the periphery of the lung.[786,796,876] As much as 50% may arise in scars,[858] though recent investigations indicate that the fibrosis associated with some adenocarcinomas is stroma laid down in the tumor rather than preexisting scar.[845] The association of adenocarcinoma with diffuse interstitial fibrosis[816,849] and the many instances in which a sudden change in a previously roentgenographically stable lesion turned out to be cancer leave little doubt that scarring with associated epithelial hyperplasia predisposed to carcinoma.

Adenocarcinomas appear as discrete masses, usually at the lung periphery where they often cause retraction of the overlying pleura (Fig. 20-71).[844] The borders of the tumor may be smooth, or stellate protrusions may extend into the surrounding lung. Irregular pigmentation of the tumor is not unusual, since inhaled dust and soot are not easily cleared from areas of tumor and the lymphatics are often obstructed. Microscopically adenocarcinomas are highly variable in appearance. As evi-

dence of secretory differentiation the tumor cells may form distinct acini or have intracellular mucin (Fig. 20-72). When fibrosis is pronounced because of the presence of preexisting scar or excessive production of stroma, the glands and columns of tumor cells may be distorted and difficult to recognize. Papillary patterns do occur, but more often the spread of tumor through the alveolar spaces merely gives the appearance of a papillary pattern as tumor cells cover the alveolar septa where they protrude into alveolar ducts. Solid sheets of tumor cells may fill alveolar spaces.

When studied with electron microscopy, lung adenocarcinomas show moderately well-developed endoplasmic reticulum, secretory granules or vacuoles, and sometimes intracytoplasmic lumen formation.[799,846] Cells are often polarized with a microvillous apex where neighboring cells are joined by tight junctions, defining a lumen that may be invisible under the light microscope. Immunohistochemistry typically shows the presence of carcinoembryonic antigen and cytokeratin.

Adenocarcinomas are relatively slow growing, with doubling times of 4 to 10 months and low mitotic

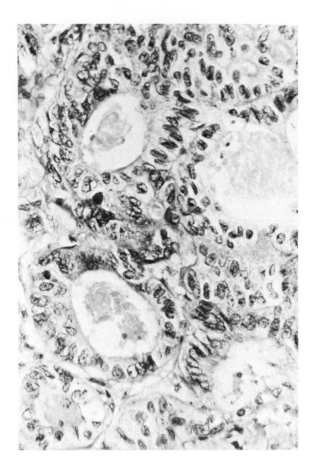

Fig. 20-72. Adenocarcinoma of lung showing well-formed glands.

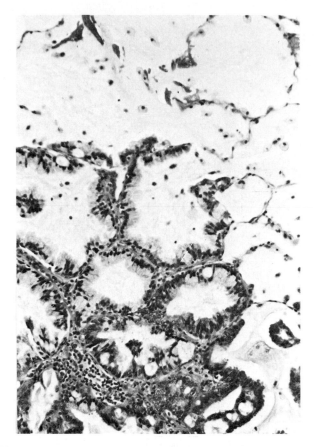

Fig. 20-73. Bronchioloalveolar carcinoma. Tall mucin-secreting epithelium spreading along alveolar septa. Air spaces are filled with mucus.

indices.[878,880] Because of their peripheral location they have a high resectability rate. Despite these seemingly favorable properties, the prognosis for primary adenocarcinoma of the lung is poor, with a 5-year survival of only 5% overall.[796,837,871,882] Treatment failure is attributable to the presence of metastases. Evidently because of their peripheral location, adenocarcinomas do not cause symptoms by obstructing bronchi, and the diagnosis is not made until late in the course.

Bronchioloalveolar carcinoma is a morphologic variant of adenocarcinoma in which the sole or predominant pattern of growth is spread along the existing airspace walls, which serve as the stroma for the tumor.[840] The walls of alveoli, alveolar ducts, and to a variable extent bronchioles are lined by malignant epithelial cells that vary in shape from cuboidal to columnar. The alveolar walls over which the tumor cells spread may be normal or may be thickened by fibrosis. When they are thickened, an abrupt transition to normal thickness usually occurs precisely where the neoplastic epithelium ends, an indication that the thickening is reaction to the tumor rather than preexisting fibrosis. The ma-

lignant epithelium may be highly atypical or closely resemble normal bronchiolar or alveolar lining cells. Some bronchioloalveolar carcinomas are composed of tall mucin-producing cells that fill the involved air spaces with mucus (Fig. 20-73). In rare instances this can lead to the clinical syndrome of bronchorrhea with electrolyte depletion.[843]

Electron microscopic studies of bronchioloalveolar carcinomas have shown differentiation along several lines. Tumors with ultrastructural features of type II alveolar epithelial cells have been described and the cells of some tumors have been shown to contain the antigens of the protein portion (apoprotein) of alveolar surfactant.[864] Other tumors are composed mainly of cells with granules like those of Clara cells or produce mainly mucin.[824,839]

Grossly and roentgenographically bronchioloalveolar carcinoma can appear as a discrete solitary peripheral mass, as multiple small nodules in one or both lungs, or as an ill-defined area of infiltrate resembling pneumonia (Fig. 20-74).[840,843] Whether the multiple nodular form develops from multiple independent foci of origin

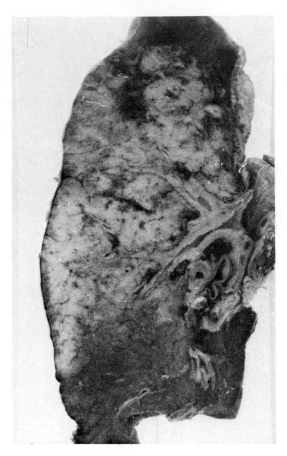

Fig. 20-74. Bronchioloalveolar carcinoma. Tumor is spreading through lung like pneumonia rather than remaining as discrete mass. (From pathological museum of University of Manchester, U.K.)

or by metastasis of tumor cells through the air spaces is not established. The infrequent, highly secretory mucinous tumors appear shiny and gelatinous.

Whether bronchioloalveolar carcinoma is a distinct entity has engendered much controversy. Metastatic carcinoma can spread in the lung with a histologic pattern identical to that of bronchoalveolar carcinoma. However, even before markers for lung-specific differentiation such as surfactant-apoprotein were available, autopsies had established the absence of an extrapulmonary primary lesion in many cases. The differentiation of bronchioloalveolar carcinoma from other pulmonary adenocarcinomas is often difficult. Tumors occur with various proportions of solid growth and growth along alveolar walls, and the decision of where to make the separation is subjective.[795] This is one of the areas in which disagreement among pathologists is common.[887] Electron microscopy indicates that both solid or acinar adenocarcinoma and bronchioloalveolar carcinoma differentiate along similar lines toward mucinous, Clara, or type II cells.[799] Two features support-

ing the idea that bronchioloalveolar carcinoma is distinct are its lack of association with cigarette smoking in some studies and that according to some reports it has a better prognosis than other adenocarcinomas when it appears as a solitary nodule.[843] The diffuse pneumonic and multinodular forms, on the other hand, are rapidly fatal.[843] In recent reports survival has been the same for bronchioloalveolar carcinoma and other adenocarcinomas.[860]

Large cell undifferentiated carcinoma. Large cell undifferentiated carcinoma is a diagnosis by default. When viewed with the light microscope between 7% and 15% of carcinomas of the lung are composed of relatively large cells (greater than 12 μm in diameter) that lack specific features by which they could be assigned to either the squamous or the adenocarcinoma group. The tumors vary in microscopic appearance from lobules of well-formed epithelium lacking evidence of gland formation, secretion, or keratin to anaplastic tumors formed of poorly cohesive cells scarcely recognizable as epithelium. These tumors are considered undifferentiated, but if electron microscopy or other special techniques are used, the majority of such tumors show some evidence of differentiation, indicating that they are really poorly differentiated variants of adenocarcinoma, squamous cell carcinoma, combined adenosquamous carcinoma, or neuroendocrine carcinoma.[804,820,831,847]

Large cell undifferentiated carcinomas are more common in men than in women, have a peak age of onset near 60 years, and are associated with tobacco smoking in 95% of cases. They can arise either at the lung periphery[801,851] or centrally.[785] They grow rapidly and are usually large tumors by the time of diagnosis. The prognosis is poor, with a median survival time of only 6 months and a 5-year survival overall of 6%.[851] Tumors with ultrastructural evidence of squamous differentiation seem to have a somewhat better prognosis than those with glandular differentiation.[831]

Giant cell carcinoma is a highly malignant form of undifferentiated carcinoma composed of huge, poorly cohesive cells with eosinophilic cytoplasm and one or several large convoluted nuclei (Fig. 20-75). The tumors are often infiltrated with polymorphonuclear leukocytes, and collections of neutrophils appear within the cytoplasm of the tumor cells as if phagocytosed. Typically they are bulky, rapidly growing tumors that often involve a major bronchus. Metastases are usually evident by the time of diagnosis, and the course is rapid, with survival for more than 1 year of exception.[815,853,856]

In the preceding discussion the category of clear cell carcinoma was omitted. Although clear cell carcinoma was included as a subtype of large cell undifferentiated carcinoma in the WHO classification, adenocarcinomas,

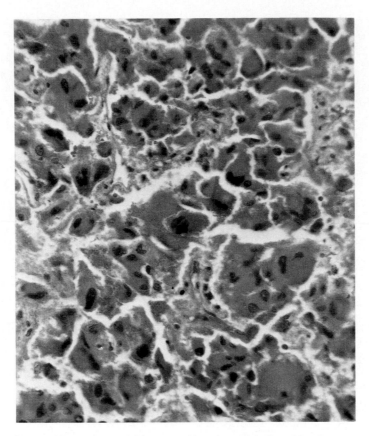

Fig. 20-75. Giant cell carcinoma. Large multinucleated cells with abundant cytoplasm. Cells are so poorly cohesive that their epithelial nature is difficult to appreciate.

squamous carcinomas, and undifferentiated carcinomas can all be composed predominantly of cells with clear cytoplasm. The appearance of a clear cytoplasm reflects, for the most part, a high glycogen content but is also influenced by the lipid content, intracellular edema, and the type and efficiency of fixation. It does not form a useful basis for classifying bronchogenic carcinomas, since it is not known to influence the biology of the tumor.

Adenosquamous carcinoma. By light microscopy 1% to 3% of lung carcinomas have clear evidence of both keratinization and glandular or secretory differentiation.[855] Most are peripheral tumors associated with scars. Adenosquamous carcinomas should be distinguished from mucoepidermoid carcinoma of the mucous glands.

Small cell carcinoma. In the normal lung, cells containing small, electron-dense, membrane-bound granules are found at all levels of the tracheobronchial tree including the bronchi, mucous glands, and bronchioles. These cells contain serotonin and several biologically active peptides including bombesin, calcitonin, calcitonin gene–related peptide, and met-enkephalin.[834] They appear to give rise to several tumors, including the highly malignant small cell carcinoma, the less malignant carcinoid, and small tumorlike proliferations known as tumorlets.

Small cell carcinomas comprise 20% to 25% of bronchogenic carcinomas.[822,834,836,854] They occur predominantly in middle-aged men and are strongly associated with tobacco smoking.[839] They rarely if ever occur among nonsmokers in the general population[885] but are found in some occupational groups, including uranium miners[861] and workers exposed to chloromethyl methyl ether.[814]

Small cell carcinomas appear as fleshy encephaloid tumors infiltrating and destroying the wall of a major bronchus (Fig. 20-76). Hilar and mediastinal lymph node involvement is usually extensive in untreated patients and is often more conspicuous than the primary tumor. Microscopically several patterns are recognized.[844,884] The oat cell type consists of round or elongated poorly cohesive cells 10 to 12 μm in length or slightly larger than lymphocytes (Fig. 20-77). The tumor cells have dark clumped chromatin and little recognizable cytoplasm. Nucleoli are absent or inconspicuous. Necrosis is usually present and is widespread in larger tumors. Blood vessels in necrotic areas become

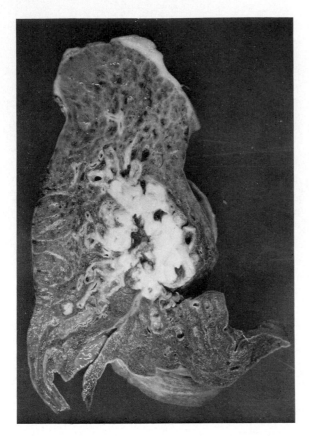

Fig. 20-76. Small cell carcinoma. This is central tumor growing within large bronchus and extending through its wall.

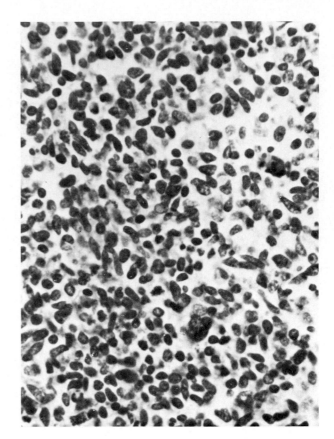

Fig. 20-77. Small-cell carcinoma, oat cell type. Slightly elongated, poorly cohesive cells with scarcely any cytoplasm.

encrusted with DNA, staining blue with hematoxylin in routine sections. The pattern of tumor growth is diffuse but with some division into lobules by vessels and stroma, which helps to distinguish oat cell carcinoma from lymphoma. The intermediate cell type of small cell carcinoma is composed of cells slightly larger than those of the oat cell type and with somewhat better intercellular cohesion and organization into lobules. Some tumors are composed of spindle-shaped cells, and some are organized into ribbons of cells or pseudorosettes closely associated with vessels, making their endocrine origin easy to recognize.[790]

By electron microscopy, 70% to 80% of small cell carcinomas contain small secretory granules of neuroendocrine type.[797,829] The characteristic granules are membrane bound, with an electron-lucent gap between the membrane and the dense granule matrix. The granules are not present in every cell, and sometimes extensive search is required for granules on which to base the diagnosis. Immunohistochemistry is helpful for diagnosis, since many small cell carcinomas contain serotonin, NSE (neuron-specific enolase), peptides such as bombesin or ACTH, and synaptophysin.[812,820] Cytokeratin is usually present, sometimes along with neuro-

filament protein. Carcinoembryonic antigen on the other hand is unusual. However, the interpretation of these markers requires correlation with light microscopy. The same markers can be present in non–small cell carcinomas.[847]

Small cell carcinoma is highly malignant and almost invariably has metastasized by the time of diagnosis. Median survival is only 4 months, and the 5-year survival with surgery is a dismal 1%, with at most only a marginal influence of histologic subtype.[803,809,854] Since these tumors are sensitive to chemotherapy and radiation, they are generally not treated surgically.[822] Therefore accurate diagnosis is mandatory to avoid unnecessary surgery, and electron microscopy or immunologic markers should be used in doubtful cases.

Spread of bronchogenic carcinoma. Carcinoma of the lung can invade contiguous structures directly and metastasize by the lymphatics and bloodstream. Lymphatic metastasis usually takes place in the hilar lymph nodes initially with spread to contiguous groups leading to mediastinal, cervical, and para-aortic involvement. When pleural adhesions are present, spread to the lymphatic plexus of the parietal pleura can lead to the appearance of tumor in axillary or supraclavicular nodes.

The brain, liver, bone, and adrenal glands are the most common sites of vascular dissemination. Adrenal involvement may also develop via lymphatic connections across the diaphragm. With small cell carcinoma bone marrow involvement is common even in the absence of overt bone destruction; therefore bone scanning and marrow aspiration are useful as staging procedures.[830]

Clinical manifestations

Symptoms of lung cancer are widely variable and result from local effects of the tumor, occlusion of a bronchus, or local and distant metastases.[833] Since most patients are smokers, cough and sputum production have often been present for years. Local irritation by the tumor results in a change in the cough or sputum. Other local effects of the tumor include wheezing, hemoptysis, dyspnea, and chest pain. Infections distal to bronchial obstructions tend to resolve slowly or recur in the same location, leading to bronchiectasis and chronic pneumonia with their attendant symptoms. Pleural effusions can develop as a result of metastasis to the pleura, infection, or lymphatic obstruction. All too often the first symptoms of lung cancer are caused by distant spread: superior vena caval obstruction, recurrent nerve paralysis, painful bone lesions, neurologic symptoms resulting from brain metastases, and so forth. Indeed, in 75% of patients spread beyond the lung has occurred by the time of diagnosis.

Several rare, so-called paraneoplastic syndromes are associated with lung cancer:
1. Endocrine
    a. Cushing's syndrome
    b. Inappropriate antidiuretic hormone (ADH) secretion
    c. Hypercalcemia
    d. Carcinoid syndrome
    e. Gynecomastia
2. Neuromuscular
    a. Polymyositis
    b. Carcinomatous myopathy
    c. Eaton-Lambert (myasthenic) syndrome
    d. Peripheral neuropathy
    e. Subacute cerebellar degeneration
3. Skeletal
    a. Clubbing
    b. Hypertrophic osteoarthropathy
4. Cutaneous
    a. Acanthosis nigricans
    b. Dermatomyositis
5. Cardiovascular
    a. Migratory thrombophlebitis
    b. Nonbacterial thrombotic endocarditis

Although some are associated with malignant tumors in many sites, others such as the Eaton-Lambert (myasthenic) syndrome and hypertrophic osteoarthropathy are particularly associated with lung cancer. Ectopic hormone production is a rare clinical problem but one that affects lung cancer patients more often than patients with cancer of other sites. Different hormonal syndromes are characteristic of different histologic types of lung cancer. Ectopic adrenocorticotropic hormone (ACTH) production, inappropriate ADH secretion, and the carcinoid syndrome are most often associated with small cell carcinoma.[791,800,827,841] Between 3% and 19% of patients with small cell carcinoma have the clinical syndrome of ectopic ACTH production,[841] which is dominated by hypokalemic alkalosis, hypertension, and signs of mineralocorticoid excess and frequently lacks the classic features of Cushing's syndrome. Up to 50% of patients with small cell carcinoma have abnormalities of adrenal function such as loss of diurnal fluctuation in plasma cortisol concentration and loss of dexamethasone suppression, but only a fraction of these have the full clinical syndrome.[800] The second most frequent endocrine abnormality with small cell carcinoma is the syndrome of inappropriate ADH secretion, characterized by low plasma sodium concentration and osmolality with a high urine osmolality.[800] Plasma ADH activity is inappropriately high for the low plasma osmolality, and if a water load is given, it is not excreted as rapidly as would be expected. Although calcitonin levels in tumor and plasma are elevated in many patients with small cell carcinoma, this does not cause symptoms.[826,827] Evidently parathyroid or other compensatory mechanisms are adequate to prevent hypocalcemia. Nevertheless, some observers have found calcitonin the most reliable of several hormones studied in following the clinical progress of small cell carcinoma. Although there is strong evidence that tumor is the source of the calcitonin in many cases,[826,827] in some instances of lung cancer the thyroid has been the apparent source of increased calcitonin production.

Parathormone production by lung tumors explains the rare occurrence of hypercalcemia in the absence of bone metastasis.[794] It is usually associated with squamous cell or large cell carcinomas. Chorionic gonadotropin production occurs with all histologic types of bronchial cancer.[807,883] Although it can be associated with gynecomastia, it is often asymptomatic. The presence of growth hormone has also been reported.[792]

Staging and prognosis

Although the overall prognosis of bronchogenic carcinoma is grim, with a cure rate of only 5% to 8%, there are some factors that influence prognosis in individual cases. The initial choice of therapy depends on histologic type of tumor and clinical stage, a grouping of patients according to tumor size, extent of apparent dissemination, and proximity of tumor to potential surgical margins.[852] The clinical staging of lung cancer is:

Occult carcinoma	Malignant cells in bronchopulmonary secretions without evidence of primary tumor or metastases
Stage 0	Carcinoma in situ
Stage I	Tumor without metastasis or extrapulmonary invasion
Stage II	Tumor without extrapulmonary invasion; metastases to peribronchial or ipsilateral hilar lymph nodes only
Stage IIIa	Tumor extending into the chest wall, mediastinal pleura, or pericardium or within 2 cm of the carina but not involving the heart, great vessels, diaphragm, trachea, esophagus, or vertebral bodies
	Tumor of lesser extent, but with metastasis to ipsilateral mediastinal or subcarinal lymph nodes
Stage IIIb	Tumor with invasion of vital mediastinal structures or metastasis to nonresectable lymph nodes but without spread beyond the thorax.
Stage IV	A tumor with metastatic spread beyond the thorax and its regional lymph nodes (that is, beyond scalene or supraclavicular nodes)

Except for patients with small cell carcinoma, those with stage I or II disease are potentially curable. For small cell carcinoma irrespective of stage, the probability of surgical cure is less than the operative mortality.

The study of the resected tissue gives additional prognostic information. Hilar lymph node metastasis has little effect on the prognosis of squamous carcinoma but has a strong deleterious effect when it occurs with the other histologic types.[837] Tumor size greater than 5 cm has a deleterious effect on prognosis that is independent of the status of the lymph nodes.[866] Mitotic rates, however, have little correlation with prognosis.[850,880]

In general, for any stage of disease, symptomatic patients fare worse than those without symptoms,[813] and systemic symptoms such as fever or weight loss are particularly bad omens.[813] Performance status refers to the ability of patients to carry out their customary activities. Scales for evaluating performance, ranging from those able to carry out normal work, to disability permitting restricted activity at home, to severe disability leaving the patient bedridden, are strong predictors of survival time.[867] Age, sex, and smoking status also influence prognosis.[823,867]

Etiology

It has been clear at least since the mid-1950s that the major cause of the epidemic increase in the incidence of lung cancer is cigarette smoking. The evidence has been summarized in the Surgeon General's reports[873] and in a report by the Royal College of Physicians.[865] Epidemiologic studies of both case-control and retrospective and prospective cohort types have documented a strong relationship between the amount of smoking and the incidence of lung cancer. Pipe and cigar smokers have a greater risk than nonsmokers but a lesser risk than cigarette smokers. The relative risk of developing lung cancer for regular cigarette smokers is 10 times greater than for nonsmokers, and the risk for smokers of more than 25 cigarettes a day is 20 times greater. The relationship with smoking is strongest for squamous and small cell carcinoma, but large cell carcinoma and adenocarcinoma are also associated with smoking. Cigarette smoke contains the following classes of known carcinogens:

1. Nitrosamines
   a. Dimethyl nitrosamine
   b. Diethyl nitrosamine
   c. Nitrosopyrolidine
   d. N-Nitrosonornicotine
   e. N'-Nitrosoanatabine
2. Polycyclic aromatic hydrocarbons
   a. Benzo[a]pyrene
   b. Benzanthracene
   c. Methylfluoranthenes
   d. Chrysenes
   e. Benzophenanthrene
3. Heterocyclic hydrocarbons
   a. Dibenzacridines
   b. Dibenzocarbazole
4. Aromatic amines
   a. Beta-naphthylamine
5. Alpha particle–emitting radionuclides
   a. ^{210}Pb
   b. ^{210}Po

Each of these is present in low concentration but has the potential for interactions. Smoke also contains many irritants, some of which have been shown to act as tumor promoters. Smoke condensate is carcinogenic for animals in standard skin-painting assays. It has been difficult to reproduce patterns of human respiratory tract cancer in animals, however, probably because of the difficulty of reproducing human smoking methods. In addition to the increased incidence of overt tumors, the bronchi of smokers have an increased prevalence of ciliary loss, epithelial hyperplasia, squamous metaplasia, and nuclear atypism, lesions believed to be precursors of carcinoma.[788] Perhaps the most compelling epidemiologic evidence comes from the effect of stopping smoking. In Doll and Peto's 20-year study of 34,000 British physicians, which began in 1951, the use of tobacco declined during the study period as physicians became convinced of the risks of smoking.[810] During this time the lung cancer mortality in the physician population fell from roughly 60% of the rate for all British men to only 40% of that for all British men. Among those who gave up smoking, the relative risk of contracting lung cancer fell with time after quitting from an initial lung cancer risk 16 times that of a nonsmoker to only twice that of a nonsmoker after 15 years. Similarly, in the United States, among those who gave up smoking the relative risk gradually declined over 13 years to the level in those who never smoked.[821] The use of filters and smoking cigarettes with a lower tar content also decrease the relative risk.[886]

The risk of cancer to nonsmokers from inhaling the smoke of other people's cigarettes (passive smoking) is small compared to the risk of active smoking. Non-smoking spouses of smokers have a 1.5-fold increased risk compared to those married to nonsmokers. This extrapolates to a risk comparable to smoking 0.1 to 1 cigarette per day.[870]

Epidemiologic studies have shown a small urban-rural gradient in lung cancer rates that cannot be entirely explained on the basis of smoking habits. This indicates that air pollution may play a role in the causation of lung cancer. High local rates for lung cancer in neighborhoods near petrochemical industries indicate that specific industrial pollutants may be at fault.[819] Lung cancer rates are also inversely related to income level. Although this too may be related to a tendency for the more wealthy to live in areas of lesser pollution, other explanations such as dietary patterns could also explain the trend.

If 10% of smokers will die of lung cancer, 90% will not. One factor that seems to influence susceptibility to respiratory carcinogenesis in experimental systems is vitamin A intake. Smokers with low vitamin A, or beta-carotene, intake have a greater risk of lung cancer than those with a vitamin A–rich diet.[798,805,848] There is also a familial influence in lung cancer; the risk of relatives of lung cancer patients is 2½ times greater than that of the general population. Some studies have suggested that the ability to metabolize carcinogenic polycyclic aromatic hydrocarbons is under genetic control, but the observations have been difficult to reproduce, and currently the nature of the familial influence is uncertain.

There are several well-established occupational causes of lung cancer, as follows[817,835]:

1. Radioisotopes (radon gas)
2. Mustard gas
3. Asbestos
4. Coal tar distillates
5. Bis(chloromethyl) ether
6. Nickel
7. Chromium
8. Arsenic

Some industrial carcinogens act synergistically with tobacco smoke. Occupational lung cancers do not always follow the usual distribution of histologic types.[835] Exposure to bis(chloromethyl) ether,[814] radon gas,[861] and perhaps chromates is associated with the development of small cell carcinoma, whereas exposure to asbestos may produce relatively more adenocarcinomas.[781]

Molecular biology

Abnormalities of growth regulation and gene expression are common in lung cancer and often correlate with histologic type of differentiation. Epidermoid carcinomas express high levels of the receptor for transforming growth factor–alpha and epidermal growth factor. This receptor is the product of the c-*erb* B oncogene. K-*ras* oncogenes are activated in many adenocarcinomas as a result of a point mutation in codon 12 of the gene.[859] Small cell carcinomas have a rich variety of abnormalities. A deletion in the short arm of chromosome 3 is almost universal, and several other deletions are common. Abnormalities of the retinoblastoma antioncogenes are common in both small cell carcinoma and atypical carcinoid and lead to failure to express its protective message.[828] Bombesin-like peptides synthesized in small cell carcinoma have autocrine growth factor activity. Finally, amplification of c-*myc* oncogene occurs in a subset of small cell carcinomas with particularly aggressive clinical behavior.[863]

Carcinoids

Bronchial carcinoids are tumors of low-grade malignancy with neuroendocrine differentiation. They tend to occur at a younger age than bronchogenic carcinomas, often appearing below 40 years of age and sometimes in childhood. Bronchial carcinoids are not related to cigarette smoking and have an equal sex incidence.[955] The majority of carcinoids arise in central bronchi where they form a smooth-surfaced endobronchial polypoid growth. However, the major portion of the tumor lies outside the bronchial wall, the so-called iceberg pattern of growth (Fig. 20-78). The tumor tissue often has a yellow-tan color, especially after fixation with formaldehyde. Microscopically carcinoids are formed of uniform cells with a fairly abundant, finely granular cytoplasm and oval, centrally located nuclei with clumped chromatin. The outstanding feature is that the tumor cells are grouped in relation to regularly disposed capillaries. The grouping may be in spherical aggregates (*Zellballen*), trabeculas, or ribbons (Fig. 20-79). The stroma is usually scant but may be plentiful and may contain hyalinized connective tissue or more rarely amyloid or bone. Mitoses are rare, and necrosis is usually absent.

Twenty percent of carcinoids arise in small bronchi or bronchioles and occur as peripheral lung nodules.[900] Often the peripheral carcinoids are composed of spindle-shaped cells with little cytoplasm. Such tumors can be mistaken for small cell carcinoma but are distinguishable by the uniformity of the cells and the absence of necrosis or mitosis.

The secretory granules of bronchial carcinoids resemble those of other foregut carcinoids.[961] They do not reduce silver in the argentaffin reaction and stain only erratically with argyrophil stains in which the reducing

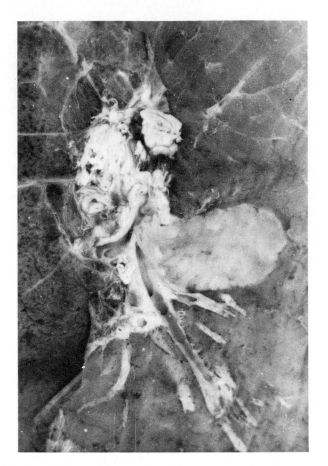

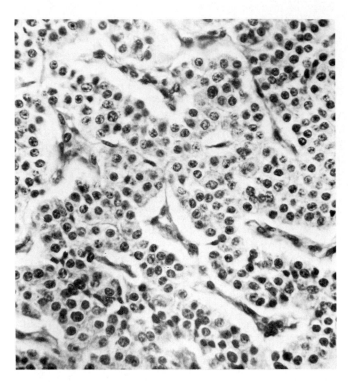

Fig. 20-78. Bronchial carcinoid. Tumor protrudes into bronchus, but its bulk lies outside bronchus.

Fig. 20-79. Bronchial carcinoid. Regular ribbons of benign-appearing epithelial cells closely associated with capillaries.

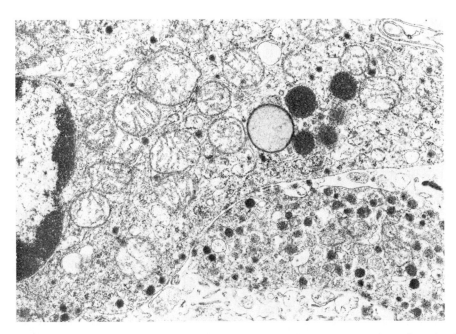

Fig. 20-80. Bronchial carcinoid. Electron micrograph illustrates granules of endocrine type.

agent is added. Electron microscopy, however, usually shows abundant, electron-dense, spherical granules with an average diameter of 200 nm (Fig. 20-80). Bronchial carcinoids express cytokeratin and sometimes neurofilament protein. They stain immunologically for the neural markers NSE (neuron-specific enolase), synaptophysin, and serotonin and often contain bombesin and calcitonin.[820]

As a rule, bronchial carcinoids produce symptoms as a result of bronchial obstruction. Only exceptionally are symptoms the result of endocrine function of the tumor, usually in the presence of distant metastases. The most characteristic endocrine syndrome resulting from bronchial carcinoids is one of severe and prolonged flushing accompanied by diarrhea, edema, lacrimation, and hypotension. Urinary excretion of the serotonin metabolite 5-hydroxyindoleacetic acid is elevated, but whether peptide hormones or serotonin is responsible for these symptoms is unknown.[836] Carcinoids can also cause ectopic ACTH syndrome.[955]

The prognosis for bronchial carcinoids is in stark contrast to that of small cell carcinoma. Of 108 patients treated at military hospitals for carcinoid tumors, more than 90% survived 10 years.[860]

A small number of tumors combine an architectural pattern similar to the usual carcinoid with greater cytologic atypism and more mitotic activity or necrosis. Such tumors are known as atypical carcinoids or well-differentiated neuroendocrine carcinomas. They stain for similar immunohistochemical markers to ordinary carcinoids but more often express ectopic peptide hormones. Their behavior is more aggressive than that of ordinary carcinoids but less than that of small cell carcinoma.[820]

Tumors of the mucous glands

The mucous glands give rise to a variety of tumors that mimic the morphology and biologic behavior of tumors of the salivary glands. The most common is the adenoid cystic carcinoma,[955] followed by mucoepidermoid carcinoma,[956] pleomorphic adenoma,[905,941] and rare tumors such as oncocytoma, mucous gland adenoma,[916] and acinic cell carcinoma.[908] Adenoid cystic carcinomas arise at any level of the respiratory tract where there are mucous glands, from paranasal sinus to bronchi. They are the most common tumors in the upper third of the trachea. They grow as a smooth-surfaced submucosal endobronchial polypoid mass that invades the airway wall. In the trachea this produces stridor and airflow obstructions; in the bronchi it leads to obstructive pneumonia. Microscopically the characteristic appearance of the uniform small, slightly elongated cells arranged in a cribriform pattern is indistinguishable from that of the salivary gland tumors (Fig.

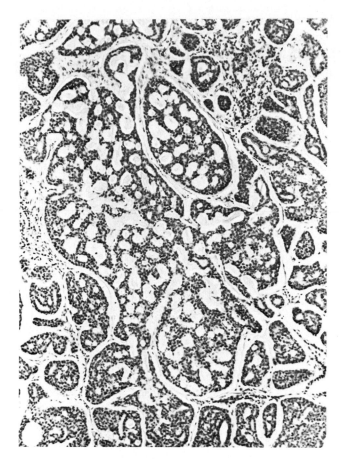

Fig. 20-81. Adenoid cystic adenocarcinoma of trachea. Lobules of epithelium are perforated by deposits of hyaline matrix in cribriform pattern.

20-81). The "holes" in the cribriform sheets of cells are occupied by an eosinophilic hyaline or basophilic mucoid material, which electron microscopy has shown to be extracellular matrix separated from the tumor cells by basal lamina rather than a glandular secretion. Small ductular lumens with microvilli can be identified between tumor cells by electron microscopy but are too small to be seen with the light microscope. The evolution of adenoid cystic carcinomas is usually slow. Although they are malignant, survival for many years is not unusual, even with metastases.

Mucoepidermoid tumors of the bronchi also form smooth submucosal endobronchial masses.[891,944,956] Microscopically they are composed of three types of cells: well-differentiated squamous cells, mucous cells, and intermediate cells with a clear cytoplasm and distinct plasma membrane. Controversy surrounds their natural history. Some authors consider them slow growing and rarely metastasizing[891,944]; others have found them aggressive and rapidly fatal.[956]

Mesothelial tumors

The biologic behavior of primary pleural mesotheliomas can usually be predicted by their gross appearance.[929] Those that form a solitary discrete mass are usually benign, can be removed surgically, and rarely recur, whereas those that grow diffusely are malignant. Histologically mesotheliomas of either type may be predominantly epithelial, fibroblastic, or mixed.

Solitary mesotheliomas form circumscribed, rounded masses that are usually attached to either the parietal or the visceral pleura (Fig. 20-82).[910,939] Those arising from the pleura of the interlobar fissures may appear roentgenographically to be within the lung parenchyma, and rarey solitary mesotheliomas seem to arise entirely within the lung with at most a tenuous pedicle reaching the pleura. Solitary mesotheliomas are tough and rubbery with whorls and streaks of fibrous tissue evident on the cut surface. Microscopically they tend to be predominantly fibroblastic, with interlacing bundles of fibroblastic cells and varying amounts of extracellular matrix. Clefts lined by mesothelial cells may extend into the tumor, but only rarely are mesothelial cells predominant.

Solitary mesotheliomas cause few symptoms and usually are incidental findings on chest roentgenograms. Some patients complain of a shifting weight in the chest. Solitary mesotheliomas may be associated with either osteoarthropathy or hypoglycemia. Removal of the tumor is curative in both syndromes. Asbestos exposure plays no role in the cause of solitary mesotheliomas.

Diffuse mesotheliomas are highly malignant tumors producing death in the majority of cases within a year of the onset of symptoms.[929] They appear as a nodular or homogeneous coating of white fleshy tissue over parietal and visceral pleura and diaphragm usually extending into the interlobular fissures (Fig. 20-83). Involvement of regional lymph nodes and pericardium is common at autopsy, and distant metastases sometimes occur. Clinical manifestations include chest pain, pleural effusion, and infection caused by entrapment of the lung.

Considerable variation is found histologically in the proportion of fibroblastic and mesothelial elements.[934] Mesothelial cells may form solid sheets but more often line slitlike spaces, tubules, or papillary projections (Fig. 20-84). Fibroblastic tissue varies from poorly cellular fibrous scar to frankly fibrosarcomatous.

Metastatic adenocarcinomas may closely resemble mesothelioma, grossly and microscopically, but a variety of techniques can help the pathologist make the distinction. Mesotheliomas produce hyaluronic acid, which can be identified histochemically or biochemically.[957] Adenocarcinomas often contain mucin and carcinoembryonic antigen, whereas mesothelium contains neither.[940] Cytokeratin staining is present in both.

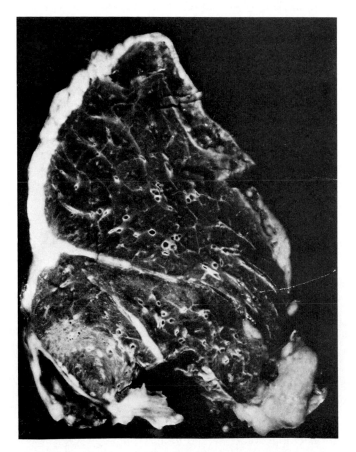

Fig. 20-83. Diffuse mesothelioma. Visceral pleura is encased by tumor, which extends into lobar fissures and to a limited extent invades interlobular septa.

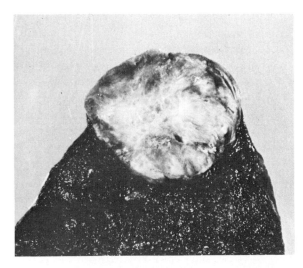

Fig. 20-82. Solitary mesothelioma. Well-circumscribed mass is adherent to visceral pleura. Sectioned surface has streaky pattern of fibrous lesion.

When viewed with the electron microscope, mesothelial cells can be recognized by their unusually long microvilli, absence of secretory vacuoles, and extensive endoplasmic reticulum and tonofilament bundles.[953,958]

The association of pleural and peritoneal mesothelioma with exposure to asbestos is now well recognized.[736,741,742] The period between exposure and the development of tumor varies greatly but is usually 20 to 40 years. Exposure need not be heavy; the occurrence of mesothelioma is documented in family members exposed only indirectly via the dusty clothing of workers. The evidence from both epidemiology and asbestos body counts made on lungs obtained at autopsy indicates that neary half of the diffuse mesotheliomas in North American men are attributable to occupational exposure to asbestos.[935] There is no evidence that cigarette smoke is a factor.

Carcinosarcoma and pulmonary blastoma

There are two types of rare tumor in which both the epithelial and mesenchymal components are malignant. Carcinosarcomas are, as the name imples, tumors composed of a mixture of carcinomatous and sarcomatous elements.[897,905,906,943] The most common epithelial component is squamous carcinoma and usually the stroma fibrosarcoma, but the stroma may have osteoid or cartilaginous tissue as well. Carcinosarcomas are usually polypoid endobronchial tumors that occur in the middle aged and elderly. The prognosis is somewhat better than for bronchogenic carcinomas.

Pulmonary blastomas are peripheral lung tumors that derive their name from a resemblance to fetal lung.[912,924,942,949] The sarcomatous component resembles embryonic mesenchyme, and the epithelial component consists of primitive columnar epithelium lining branching slits and tubules (Fig. 20-85). Because of its high glycogen content, this epithelium often appears vacuolated like embryonic respiratory epithelium.[912] Although the analogy to Wilms' tumor of the kidney is sometimes made, pulmonary blastoma is not primarily a childhood tumor. It occurs at any age from childhood to old age, with the peak incidence in the fifth decade. The tumors evolve rapidly, and many patients die within a year of diagnosis. On the other hand, the 30% to 40% cure rate is much better than for bronchogenic carcinoma.

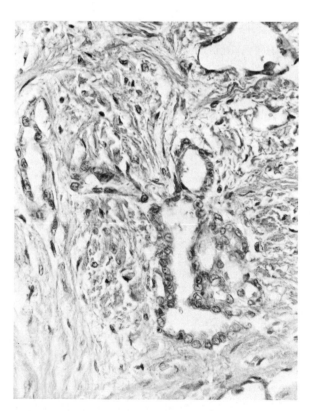

Fig. 20-84. One histologic pattern in diffuse mesothelioma. Tubules lined by flattened type of epithelium in abundant fibrous stroma. Microscopic appearance of mesotheliomas varies greatly.

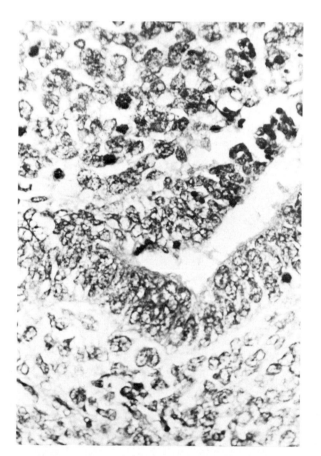

Fig. 20-85. Pulmonary blastoma. Tubule is lined by primitive epithelium in highly cellular malignant stroma.

Sarcomas

The connective tissues of the lung give rise to a variety of tumors that are similar pathologically to their counterparts in the soft tissues.[937] There is one curious sarcoma of vascular origin that usually originates in the lung. This is the lesion originally named "intravascular bronchoalveolar tumor" but better called "sclerosing angiogenic tumor." Sclerosing angiogenic tumor is a multifocal lesion manifested clinically as slowly progressive dyspnea and multiple nodules on the chest roentgenogram. Histologically the nodules result from a process involving the filling of the alveolar spaces with accumulations of myxoid matrix containing aggregates and small chains of irregularly shaped mesenchymal cells (Fig. 20-86). In the center of the nodules the matrix becomes sclerotic and eosinophilic and the cells appear to fade out and disappear, leaving ghosts of alveoli filled with dense hyalinized matrix. At the expanding margins of the lesions where the alveoli are only partially filled with matrix, the tumor cells grow over the surface of the matrix, looking like epithelium. However, despite this appearance and a predominantly intra-alveolar pattern of growth, electron microscopy and immunohistochemical staining for the endothelial

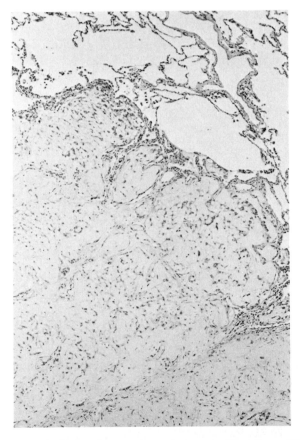

Fig. 20-86. Sclerosing angiogenic tumor. Alveoli are filled with myxoid stroma containing short rows of tumor cells.

marker, clotting factor VIII antigen, have shown that the tumor cells have properties of endothelium.[898,960] The myxoid matric contains abundant proteoglycan and a few disorganized collagenous and elastic fibers. The lesions are slowly progressive, but the tumor has the capacity to invade vessels and metastasize. Survival for many years is not unusual.

Small cell tumors involving the chest wall pleura and adjacent lung have been described in children and young adults. They are aggressive tumors composed of round or oval cells, 10 to 14 μm in diameter, arranged in compact sheets or nests.[890] They appear to be of neural origin.[933]

Metastatic tumors

The variety of tumors that metastasize to the lungs is too great to list. Metastases usually are easily diagnosed clinically if solitary or multiple nodules appear in a patient known to have a malignancy, but lymphangitic spread of carcinoma can mimic interstitial lung disease clinically and roentgenographically. The tumor is seen pathologically as a delicate vermiform tracery on the surface of the pleura and a thickening around airways and bronchi. Microscopically tumor distends lymphatics and usually infiltrates the loose connective tissue around vessels and airways where the lymphatics are located. Patients with multiple small tumor emboli may have severe dyspnea but a normal chest roentgenogram.

Multiple nodules of well-differentiated smooth muscle sometimes appear in the lungs of women who have had a hysterectomy recently or up to several years earlier for fibromyomas. The term "benign metastasizing leiomyomas" has been applied to such lesions. Mitoses, the usual criterion for malignancy in smooth muscle tumors, are few in the lung lesions, and even on restudy the uterine lesions may not fulfill the criteria for malignancy. Nevertheless, the lung lesions probably represent metastases of a very low-grade uterine leiomyosarcoma whose malignancy is unrecognizable microscopically.[923] In some cases the pulmonary nodules have decreased in size during pregnancy and reappeared after delivery.[918] This retention of hormonal sensitivity is evidence of the müllerian origin of such smooth muscle nodules in the lung.

Benign tumors

Laryngeal papillomas seen in children and young adults sometimes spread to involve the trachea. If after multiple excisions spread extends to involve the small bronchi, usually the prognosis is grim and obstruction and pneumonia develop.[947]

In older adults solitary squamous papillomas of the bronchi occur. They consist of a branching fibrovascular stroma covered by a thick squamous epithelium that varies greatly in its degree of differentiation in different cases. Although most appear benign, atypism of some degree is present in others and some show frankly carcinomatous cytologic features.[948,951] Less commonly glandular or transitional epithelium may be found.[951]

Inflammatory polyps are rare in bronchi. Like those occurring commonly in the nose, they consist of an edematous stroma infiltrated with inflammatory cells and covered by ciliated epithelium. Symptoms result from bronchial obstruction.[889,954]

Hamartomas are the most common benign tumors of the lung.[901] Despite their name, which implies a developmental defect, they appear to be acquired lesions, since they are not found in infancy and their maximum incidence is not until 60 years of age.[893] They produce no symptoms but are often discovered incidentally on chest roentgenograms and removed. They form well-circumscribed nodules, 1 to 4 cm in diameter, that shell out readily and are easily recognized grossly by their translucent cartilage-like appearance, cauliflower-like clefts, and rubbery consistency. They consist of lobules of connective tissue, usually containing cartilage, often with fat or fibrous tissue. The lobules are separated by clefts or tubules lined with columnar or cuboidal epithelium growing in from the surface of the tumor. The epithelium is probably entrapped respiratory epithelium and the connective tissue the neoplastic component.[893]

The so-called sclerosing hemangioma also causes few symptoms and is usually discovered accidentally as a rounded nodule on the chest roentgenogram.[932] Rarely it is a cause of hemoptysis. These lesions are of controversial histogenesis. They consist of a circumscribed unencapsulated nodule formed by the proliferation in the interstitium of epithelium-like cells with an oval central nucleus and a clear or pale eosinophilic cytoplasm with distinct cytoplasmic margins. Individual cells may be surrounded by fibrous tissue that in some areas compresses and replaces the tumor cells, resulting in foci of sclerosis. Where cellular or sclerotic tumor abuts air spaces, it is covered with hyperplastic alveolar epithelium composed mainly of type II cells. In some areas involved alveolar walls protruding into alveolar ducts give the tumor a papillary appearance; hemorrhage into alveolar spaces remaining in the tumor may mimic vascular spaces, hence the original name "hemangioma."[932]

Electron microscopy shows that the characteristic tumor cells are partly enclosed by basal lamina and are partly separated by spaces into which peculiar branching microvilli extend.[914,926,938] Although these features are consistent with either an epithelial or mesothelial origin, the antigens displayed by the tumor cells favor an epithelial origin.[962]

A third tumor that occurs as an asymptomatic solitary nodule in middle-aged persons is the benign clear cell tumor, known informally as the "sugar tumor" because of its high glycogen content.[951] These lesions are circumscribed masses in the lung parenchyma formed of cords or nests of large cells with a cytoplasm sometimes entirely clear and sometimes empty but with wispy eosinophilic strands radiating from the nucleus (spider cells). The cords and nests are separated by delicate capillaries that lead into characteristic dilated sinusoids. At first glance the lesions resemble metastatic renal cell carcinoma, but extended follow-up observation has proved their benign nature. The cytoplasm of renal cell carcinoma is clear, mainly because of fat, whereas that of benign clear cell tumor is filled with glycogen.[931] Electron microscopy characteristically shows glycogen-filled lysosomes as well as free cytoplasmic glycogen but has shown no specific feature that unambiguously establishes the histogenesis of the tumors.[894,917]

Inflammatory pseudotumors (plasma cell granulomas, fibrous xanthomas) are tumorlike lesions that are usually entirely intraparenchymal but may be attached to the pleura or are even endobronchial.[892,950] They occur at any age but are most common in adolescents and children. They are morphologically heterogeneous, usually consisting of a background of edematous or hyalinized fibrous tissue infiltrated with varying numbers of plasma cells, Russell bodies, and lymphocytes (Fig. 20-87). Although the plasma cells are mature and well differentiated, they are often greatly distorted by fibrous tissue. Histiocytes with or without fat may be part of the solid lesions or fill adjacent obstructed air spaces. There is uncertainty whether these lesions are neoplasms or tumorlike inflammatory reactions. The isolation of the organism of Q fever from one such lesion favors the inflammatory origin.[921]

Lymphoproliferative diseases

Since the lung is a major lymphoid organ and nodules of lymphoid tissue are present normally at bronchiolar bifurcations and in the pleura and perilobular septa, it is not surprising that the lung is commonly involved at some time during the course of leukemia, lymphoma, and other lymphoproliferative diseases such as angioimmunoblastic lymphadenopathy. Generally infiltrates are concentrated in the perivascular and peribronchial sheaths, and the clinical presentation resembles that of interstitial disease. In multiple myeloma, pulmonary interstitial disease may be attributed to malignant plasma cell infiltrates, amyloidosis, or metastatic calcification. At times lymphomatous involvement takes the form of large masses or areas of consolidation. Cavitation is not unusual in Hodgkin's disease.

Sometimes malignant lymphomas arise initially in the lung. Care must be taken to distinguish malignant lymphomas from localized inflammatory masses composed

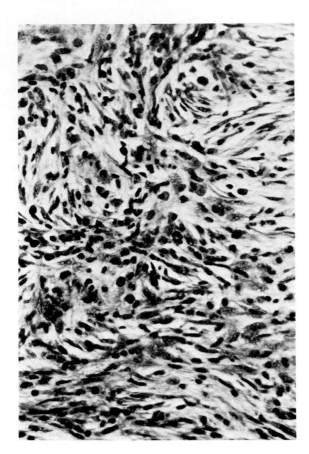

Fig. 20-87. Plasma cell granuloma. There is mixture of spindle-shaped fibroblasts and inflammatory cells, mainly plasma cells.

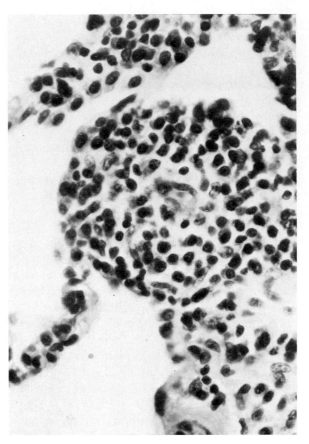

Fig. 20-88. Lymphoid interstitial pneumonia. Interstitium of alveolar walls and connective tissue surrounding a small vessel are heavily infiltrated by lymphocytes and plasma cells.

mainly of lymphocytes, so-called pseudolymphomas.[904,913,945,946] The pseudolymphomas are characterized by a mixed population of mature lymphocytes, plasma cells, and some histiocytes. Germinal centers are often numerous against a background of fibrosis. In one case, lymphocyte markers documented polyclonal B- and T-cell populations.[909] In contrast, in non-Hodgkins lymphoma, the lymphocyte population is uniform, follows the distribution of lymphatics, and invades the pleura. Germinal centers may be present in some well-differentiated lymphomas.[904] The course of well-differentiated pulmonary lymphomas can be very indolent, a feature that further blurs the distinction from pseudolymphoma.[904]

In lymphoid interstitial pneumonia the lung is more or less diffusely infiltrated by mature lymphocytes and plasma cells with or without germinal centers (Fig. 20-88).[556,904] The cellular populations are similar to those of pseudolymphoma, but instead of forming discrete nodules the infiltrate is exclusively interstitial and widespread. Abnormalities of serum immunoglobulins are common, taking the form of either monoclonal or polyclonal hyperglobulinemia or hypoglobulinemia.[556] Lung involvement in some patients with Sjögren's syndrome, Waldenström's macroglobulinemia, and angioimmunoblastic lymphadenopathy[919,959] fits the morphologic picture of lymphoid interstitial pneumonia.

Lymphomatoid granulomatosis describes a lymphoproliferative process with a strong propensity for invading blood vessels.[925,930] Invariaby the lung and frequently the skin and brain are involved. Nodular infiltrative lesions occur in the kidney and occasionally other viscera. Lethal midline reticulosis is a similar process involving the nose.

Grossly the pulmonary lesions appear as discrete unencapsulated nodules of pinkish tan tissue. Necrosis may be visible grossly. Microscopically the nodules consist of a variegated infiltrate with lymphocytes, plasma cells, histiocytes, and large atypical lymphoid cells with prominent nucleoli and a heavy rim of chromatin at the nuclear membrane. Some of the atypical cells show peripheral clumping of the chromatin reminiscent of plasma cell differentiation, suggestive of these cells being lymphoblasts. The atypical cells tend

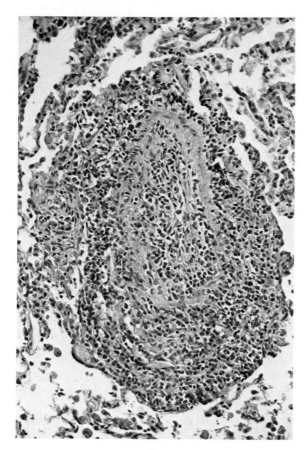

Fig. 20-89. Lymphomatoid granulomatosis. Muscular artery has been invaded by atypical lymphoid cells, which have infiltrated intima, reducing lumen.

to invade small arteries and veins and expand the intima with severe reduction or obliteration of the lumen (Fig. 20-89). Although this vascular infiltration is described as a vasculitis, fibrinoid necrosis of vessels is not a feature. Large geographic areas of coagulative necrosis are common in large lesions, probably as a result of ischemia.

Patients may be of any age but are usually adults in their fourth to seventh decades. Initial symptoms are either referable to the lung, such as cough, dyspnea, hemoptysis, or chest pain, or systemic, such as fever or weight loss. Occasionally symptoms of involvement of other organs may precede pulmonary manifestations. The overall prognosis is poor; the majority of patients die of the disease with a median survival of only slightly more than 1 year. Many patients die of respiratory insufficiency; others die with obvious malignant lymphoma.

The nature and pathogenesis of the disease are controversial.[920] Many authorities believe that it is a form of malignant lymphoma from the start.[904] Although some cases have terminated as monoclonal B-cell lym-

phomas, most resemble peripheral T-cell lymphomas.[920]

Tumorlike proliferations

Whitwell introduced the whimsical term *tumorlet* to describe microscopic proliferations of epithelium either associated with inflammatory lung disease or occurring in nearly normal lung. Tumorlets are nests of small, slightly elongated epithelial cells in the walls of bronchiectatic bronchi or proliferating in the lumen of bronchioles, invading the wall or extending into adjacent alveoli. The epithelial cell nuclei have the slightly clumped regular chromatin seen in carcinoids, and electron microscopy has shown the presence of neurosecretory granules. Thus these lesions arise from the neuroendocrine cells.[889,902] Although it might be thought that these lesions are an early stage of small cell carcinoma, there is no direct evidence that this is the case, and their peripheral location and frequent multicentricity militate against such a relationship. In rare cases lymph node metastases from tumorlets have been noted but were not of clinical consequence.

Strands and whorls of epithelium-like cells are sometimes found in the connective tissue around small veins or extending into the walls of perivenous air spaces. Generally they are separated from air spaces by the alveolar capillaries. These clusters of cells have abundant cytoplasm with indistinct cell margins. They were originally designated minute pulmonary chemodectomas,[927] but with the application of electron microscopy their relation to chemoreceptor tissue became doubtful. The epithelial cells form whorls like those of meningiomas in the brain, and by electron microscopy the cells are indistinguishable from meningiomas and lack the secretory granules characteristic of chemodectomas.[902,928] No plausible explanation has been offered for the appearance of meningothelial cell nests around pulmonary veins.

The differential diagnosis between tumorlet and "minute chemodectoma" can be based on location of the abnormal cells. Tumorlets are related to airways and contact the lumens of air spaces; "minute chemodectomas" are perivenous interstitial, and separated from air space lumens.

MEDIASTINUM
Anatomic divisions

The central thoracic space lying between the two pleural cavities is called the mediastinum. It contains the heart, great vessels, esophagus, and trachea. The mediastinum is divided into three compartments by the pericardium. The space bounded posteriorly by the pericardium and first four thoracic vertebral bodies extending from the diaphragm to the thoracic inlet is known as the anterior mediastinum and includes the thymus, the aortic arch and its branches, the innominate veins, the vagus and phrenic nerves, and the cardiac plexus, as well as the trachea, paratracheal lymph nodes, and upper esophagus. The middle mediastinum is bounded by the fibrous pericardium and includes the heart, the ascending aorta, the pulmonary trunk, and the roots of the lungs including the tracheobronchial lymph nodes. The posterior mediastinum, between the pericardium and lower thoracic vertebrae, contains the descending aorta, the esophagus, the para-aortic lymph nodes, the paravertebral sympathetic ganglia, the azygous veins, and the thoracic duct.

Mediastinitis

Acute mediastinitis is caused by spread of infection from the neck or by perforations of the esophagus. The pretracheal fascia in the neck extends into the mediastinum to blend with the adventitia of the aortic arch. Cervical infections in front of the pretracheal fascia spread into the anterior mediastinum, whereas those behind the pretracheal fascia localize to the posterior mediastinum. Infections are usually suppurative and result in abscess formation.

Granulomatous mediastinitis is the result of spread of granulomatous infections to the mediastinal lymph nodes, usually from a primary tuberculous or histoplasmal focus in the lung.[964] This results in a mass of matted enlarged lymph nodes with caseous necrosis and fibrous encapsulation varying from a thin capsule separating the necrotic focus from the neighboring structures to an exuberant fibrous reaction up to 1 cm thick that encroaches on and compresses or invades neighboring structures. At its extreme the fibrous reaction predominates and a fibroma-like mass is produced in which the original granuloma may be overlooked.[964] This is the origin of many if not all cases of sclerosing mediastinitis.

In sclerosing mediastinitis a poorly circumscribed mass of woody white tissue surrounds and binds together mediastinal structures. Histologically, few cells are present in the tissue, which is composed of wavy thick bands of hyaline collagen separated by narrow spaces containing scattered lymphocytes and plasma cells. Foci of calcification or even ossification may be present in long-standing cases. The collagen bundles are arranged concentrically surrounding granulomas, but elsewhere the arrangement is more haphazard. The fibrous tissue entraps nerves and arteries, invades veins and bronchi, and obliterates lymphatics.[963] The clinical manifestations are highly variable depending on the structures involved but tend to fall into two groups depending on whether the paratracheal or hilar and subcarinal lymph nodes are the origin of the process.[963] Paratracheal lesions usually produce caval or innominate vein obstruction. Some patients complain of cough, hoarseness, or ill-defined discomfort. The prog-

nosis is relatively favorable; although involvement of vital structures precludes resection, patients usually survive for years despite persistent disease. When the involvement occurs around the subcarinal lymph nodes or in the hila of lung, pulmonary veins, bronchi, or arteries may be compromised. Patients may have hemoptysis, pulmonary hypertension, and venous infarcts because of pulmonary vein obstruction.[963,965] The arterioles and muscular arteries show pronounced intimal thickening and recanalization, and dilatation of perivascular lymphatics can be striking. When one pulmonary artery is compressed, volume loss occurs in the affected side.[967] With bilateral arterial compression, cor pulmonale may result.

Although many patients with sclerosing mediastinitis also have granulomatous lymphadenitis, in some cases granulomas are never found. This plausibly could be attributed to oversight, but the occasional association of sclerosing mediastinitis with retroperitoneal fibrosis or Riedel's struma points to some sort of systemic sclerosing process.[966] Retroperitoneal and mediastinal fibrosis has also been reported as a complication of therapy with methysergide.

Pneumomediastinum

The soft tissues of the mediastinum are in communication with those of the neck through the thoracic inlet, with the peritoneum and retroperitoneum through the diaphragmatic hiatuses, and with the interstitium of the lung through the pulmonary ligaments. Interstitial emphysema of the mediastinium, or so-called pneumomediastinum, can develop as the result of perforation of a mediastinal structure or extension of air from one of these communicating compartments. Its causes include not only esophageal perforations or traumatic tears of the trachea or bronchi but also perforation of abdominal viscera, extension of subcutaneous emphysema around tracheostomy sites and dissection of pulmonary interstitial emphysema.

Developmental cysts

A variety of developmental cystic lesions occur in the mediastinum, including cystic hygromas (lymphangiomas), meningomyeloceles, and cysts of bronchial, enteric, and pericardial origin. Pericardial cysts are usually solitary cysts adjacent to the pericardium, but 20% communicate with the pericardium.[979] Most are seen roentgenographically as smooth densities in the right cardiophrenic angle. Although they are considered to be developmental, most are detected in adult life. They consist of a fibrous wall with a thin mesothelial lining.

Bronchogenic cysts occur in the middle mediastinum behind the heart, usually below the carina. Their origin and structure are discussed on p. 923.

Enteric cysts (reduplications) occur in the posterior

mediastinum along the course of the esophagus or less commonly embedded in its wall. Their wall is composed of smooth muscle, and their mucosa may recapitulate the esophageal gastric or intestinal lining. Cysts with a gastric type of lining can ulcerate and bleed or perforate.

Occasional thoracic cysts have a wall only of fibrous tissue or inflammatory tissue with no lining. Such cysts are called nonspecific, and their origin is uncertain.[979]

Tumors

Tumors and cysts arise from many of the structures of the mediastinum and have characteristic locations among the different anatomic compartments. The tumors found in each of the mediastinal compartments are listed in the following:

A. Anterior
   1. Thymoma
   2. Malignant lymphoma
   3. Intrathoracic goiter
   4. Parathyroid adenoma
   5. Germ cell tumors
   6. Paraganglioma
   7. Lymphangioma
B. Middle
   1. Malignant lymphoma
   2. Developmental cysts
      a. Pericardial
      b. Bronchogenic
C. Posterior
   1. Neurogenic
      a. Schwann cell
      b. Sympathetic
      c. Paraganglioma
   2. Gastroenteric cyst

Table 20-4 contrasts the frequency of tumors and cysts in adults and children. In general the histopath-

Table 20-4. Relative frequency of mediastinal cysts and tumors

Type of lesion	Frequency (%)	
	Children	Adults
Neurogenic tumor	40	21
Lymphoma	18	13
Thymoma	—	19
Germ cell tumor	11	11
Mesenchymal tumor	9	7
Endocrine tumor	—	6
Cysts (pericardial, bronchogenic, enteric, and others)	18	20
Other malignancies	4	3

Data from Silverman, N.A., and Sabiston, D.C.: Surg. Clin. North Am. **60:**757, 1980.

ologic features and age distribution of mediastinal tumors mirror those of similarly named tumors in other parts of the body. Their natural history, however, can be influenced by their location.[968,972,979,981] Lesions of thymic origin are discussed in Chapter 29.

Lymphoproliferative disorders

Since all three compartments of the mediastinum contain numerous lymph node groups, they may be involved by malignant lymphomas and other lymphoproliferative diseases. Primary appearance of malignant lymphomas in the mediastinum is not uncommon and can run the gamut of histologic types. Non-Hodgkin's lymphomas are usually diffuse in pattern with convoluted nuclei in both adults and children.[977] Early dissemination is common. Mediastinal Hodgkin's disease is often of the nodular sclerosing type, particulary in young people, and is responsive to therapy.

A lymphoproliferative lesion that should not be mistaken for malignant lymphoma or thymoma is angiofollicular lymph node hyperplasia, or Castleman's disease. Castleman originally encountered this lesion during a review of thymic tumors in 1954. He and his colleagues subsequently recognized two types, which differ in their clinical implications.[976] The more common, 80% to 90% of the total, is the hyaline-vascular type. In order of frequency, the locations for this lesion are the anterior mediastinum, the hila of the lungs, and the posterior mediastinum. Extrathoracic locations are rare. The lesion is a mass with a mean diameter of 7 cm and is composed of abnormal germinal centers in a background of vascularized and fibrous lymphoid tissue. Sinusoids are rarey retained. The germinal centers are small, composed of slightly flattened and concentrically arranged lymphoreticular cells that give a superficial resemblance to Hassal's corpuscles. They are invaded by fine capillaries or arterioles cuffed with hyaline connective tissue. The interfollicular zones are well vascularized and contain lymphocytes, polyclonal plasma cells, and activated lymphoid cells including immunoblasts and suppressor T-cells.[975] The hyaline-vascular type of angiofollicular lymph node hyperplasia is usually discovered accidentally on routine chest roentgenography and is asymptomatic. Patients with symptomatic disease complain of cough or a sensation of pressure. Surgery is curative.

In the less common plasma cell type of angiofollicular lymph node hyperplasia, germinal centers are larger but more typical.[976] They may be of irregular shape or confluent. The interfollicular zones contain sheets of plasma cells. Extrathoracic sites are involved more frequently than with the hyaline-vascular type, and a variety of systemic manifestations can be seen, including anemia, hyperglobulinemia, fever, growth failure, nephrotic syndrome, and peripheral neuropathy.[970,971,973,982]

Transitions between the two types of Castleman's disease have been recorded.

Castleman's disease appears to be a severe form of reactive lymph node hyperplasia in response to either local or systemic stimuli, as those cases that have been studied with lymphocyte markers are polyclonal.[975] Evolution of multifocal angiofollicular hyperplasia to malignant lymphoma and an association with Kaposi's sarcoma have both been recorded.

Neurogenic tumors

Neurogenic tumors arise from the peripheral nerves, the sympathetic ganglia, or the aortic and pulmonary chemoreceptive glomera. Peripheral nerve tumors are unilateral paravertebral masses that usually occur in adults. Most are neurilemomas or neurofibromas. Malignant schwannomas are rare, and most occur in patients with von Recklinghausen's neurofibromatosis.[979,981] In children the majority of neural tumors are of sympathetic origin: neuroblastoma, ganglioneuroblastoma, or ganglioneuroma.[972,974] The degree of differentiation tends to vary with age: almost all tumors in patients less than 1 year of age are neuroblastomas, whereas in teenagers most are ganglioneuromas. The prognosis for malignant sympathetic nerve tumors in the mediastinum is better than for those in other locations. The cure rate is 50% for patients over 1 year of age, and the majority of those below 1 year of age can be cured with modern therapy even when metastases are present.

Paragangliomas are most common in the anterior mediastinum but can also be found in the paravertebral area. Few metastasize, but local invasion can make extirpation difficult. Most are hormonally inactive, but catecholamine-secreting thoracic paragangliomas can cause hypertension.[974]

Germ cell tumors

Extragonadal germ cell tumors arise in a variety of midline structures from the retroperitoneum to the pineal gland. Those in the thorax are found in the anterior mediastinum and are similar in distribution to thymomas. Germ cell tumors are more likely than thymomas to contain calcification, however. Ninety percent are benign cystic teratomas, which are similar morphologically to the common ovarian teratomas. The sex incidence of cystic teratomas is equal, whereas malignant germ cell tumors occur almost exclusively in young men. Seminomas are locally invasive and often metastasize to the regional lymph nodes, but with well-planned management the prognosis is excellent.[980] Unfortunately, the same cannot be said for the other malignant germ cell tumors. Cures are sometimes obtained with embryonal carcinomas but are extremely rare with choriocarcinomas and solid or immature teratomas.[969,978]

Since the histologic features of mediastinal germ cell tumors are indistinguishable from those of testicular germ cell tumors, it is important to exclude the possibility of a testicular primary tumor when a mediastinal germ cell tumor is found. A mediastinal germ cell tumor may be accepted as primary if no mass has been found during careful palpation of the testis and a lymphangiogram of the retroperitoneum shows no abnormalities.

Thoracic thyroid and parathyroids

Parathyroid tissue can migrate into the chest with the thymus, with which it shares a common origin in the third and fourth branchial pouches. Consequently parathyroid adenomas occasionally occur within the anterior mediastinum or within the thymus proper. An enlarged thyroid can extend inferiorly through the thoracic inlet. Less commonly, thyroid tissue is present as a discrete mass in the anterior mediastinum.

REFERENCES
Pediatric lung disease

1. Askin, F.B.: Pulmonary disorders in the neonate, infant and child. In Thurlbeck, W.M., editor: Pathology of the lung, New York, 1988, Thieme Medical Publishers, Inc.
2. Askin, F.B.: Respiratory tract disorders in the fetus and neonate. In Wigglesworth, J.S., and Singer, D.B., editors: A textbook of perinatal pathology, Oxford, 1989, Blackwell.
3. Avery, M.E., Fletcher, B.A., and Williams, R.G.: The lung and its disorders in the newborn infant, ed. 4, Philadelphia, 1981, W.B. Saunders Co.
4. Dehner, L.P.: Pediatric surgical pathology, ed. 2, Baltimore, 1987, The Williams & Wilkins Co.
5. Katzenstein, A.-L., and Askin, F.B.: The surgical pathology of nonneoplastic lung disease, ed. 2, Philadelphia, 1989, W.B. Saunders Co.
6. Spencer, H.: Pathology of the lung, ed. 4, Oxford, 1984, Pergamon Press, Inc.

Lung development

7. Ballard, P.L.: Hormones and lung maturation, Berlin, 1986, Springer-Verlag.
8. Campiche, M.A., Gautier, A., Hernández, E.I., et al.: An electron microscope study of the fetal development of human lung, Pediatrics 32:976, 1963.
9. Comroe, J.H., Jr.: Premature science and immature lungs (in three parts), Am. Rev. Respir. Dis. 116:127, 311, 497, 1977.
10. D'Ercole, A.J., and Underwood, L.E.: Somatomedin in fetal growth, Pediatr. Pulmonol. 1(suppl.):599, 1985.
11. Emery, J.L., and Dinsdale, F.: The postnatal development of lymphoreticular aggregates and lymph nodes in infants' lungs, J. Clin. Pathol. 26:539, 1973.
12. Hage, E.: The morphological development of the pulmonary epithelium of human foetuses studied by light and electron microscopy, Z. Anat. Entwicklungsgesch. 140:271, 1973.
13. Hislop, A., and Reid, L.: Fetal and childhood development of the intrapulmonary veins in man: branching pattern and structure, Thorax 28:313, 1973.
14. Reid, L.M.: Lung growth in health and disease, Br. J. Dis. Chest 78:113, 1984.
15. Reid, L.M., and Rubino, M.: The connective tissue septa in the foetal human lung, Thorax 14:3, 1959.

16. Robertson, B., von Golde, L.M.G., and Batenburg, J.J., editors: Pulmonary surfactant, Amsterdam, 1984, Elsevier Science Publishers.
17. Sinclair-Smith, C.C., Emery, J.L., Gadsdon, D., et al.: Cartilage in children's lungs: a quantitative assessment using the right middle lobe, Thorax 31:40, 1976.
18. Spooner, B.S., and Wessels, N.K.: Mammalian lung development: interactions in formation and bronchial morphogenesis, J. Exp. Zool. 175:445, 1970.
19. Thurlbeck, W.M.: Lung growth. In Thurlbeck, W.M., editor: Pathology of the lung, New York, 1988, Thieme Medical Publishers, Inc.

Congenital anomalies

20. Booth, J.B., and Berry, C.L.: Unilateral pulmonary agenesis, Arch. Dis. Child. 42:361, 1967.
21. Bozic, C.: Ectopic fetal adrenal cortex in the lung of a newborn, Virchows Arch. [Pathol. Anat.] 363:371, 1974.
22. Campo, E., and Bombi, J.A.: Central nervous system heterotopia in the lung of a fetus with cranial malformation, Virchows Arch. [Pathol. Anat.] 391:117, 1981.
23. Chan, Y.T., Ng, W.D., Mak, W.P., Kwong, M.L., and Chow, C.B.: Congenital bronchobiliary fistula associated with biliary atresia, Br. J. Surg. 73:240, 1984.
24. Chang, N., Hertzler, J.H., Gregg, R.H., et al.: Congenital stenosis of the right mainstem bronchus: a case report, Pediatrics 41:739, 1968.
25. Chi, J.G., and Shong, Y.K.: Diffuse striated muscle heteroplasia of the lung, Arch. Pathol. Lab. Med. 106:641, 1982.
26. Cope, R., Campbell, J.R., and Wall, M.: Bilateral tracheal bronchi, J. Pediatr. Surg. 21:443, 1986.
27. Faro, R.S., Goodwin, C.D., Organ, C.H., Jr., et al.: Tracheal agenesis, Ann. Thorac. Surg. 28:295, 1979.
28. Foster-Carter, A.F.: Broncho-pulmonary anomalies, Br. J. Dis. Chest 40:111, 1946.
29. Freedom, R.M., Burrows, P.E., and Moes, C.A.G.: "Horseshoe" lung: report of five new cases, AJR 146:211, 1986.
30. Gariepy, G., and Fugere, P.: Pulmonary embolization of cerebellar tissue in a newborn child, Obstet. Gynecol. 42:118, 1973.
31. González-Crussi, F., Padilla, L.M., Miller, J.K., et al.: "Bridging bronchus": a previously undescribed airway anomaly, Am. J. Dis. Child. 130:1015, 1976.
32. Janney, C.G., Askin, F.B., and Kuhn, C., III.: Congenital alveolar capillary dysplasia: an unusual cause of respiratory distress in the newborn, Am. J. Clin. Pathol. 76:772, 1981.
33. Kanbour, A.I., Barmada, M.A., Klionsky, B., and Moosey, J.: Anencephaly and heterotopic central nervous tissue in lungs, Arch. Pathol. Lab. Med. 103:116, 1979.
34. Mendoza, A., Voland, J., Wolf, P., and Benirschke, K.: Supradiaphragmatic liver in the lung, Arch. Pathol. Lab. Med. 110:1085, 1986.
35. Landing, B.H.: Syndromes of congenital heart disease with tracheobronchial anomalies, AJR 123:679, 1975.
36. Landing, B.H., and Dixon, L.G.: Congenital malformations and genetic disorders of the respiratory tract (larynx, trachea, bronchi and lungs), Am. Rev. Respir. Dis. 120:151, 1979.
37. Landing, B.H., and Wells, T.R.: Tracheobronchial anomalies in children, Perspect. Pediatr. Pathol. 1:1, 1973.
38. Maisel, R.H., Fried, M.P., Swain, R., et al.: Anomalous tracheal bronchus with tracheal hypoplasia, Arch. Otolaryngol. 100:69, 1974.
39. Mangiulea, V.G., and Stinghe, R.V.: The accessory cardiac bronchus: bronchologic aspects and review of the literature, Chest 54:433, 1968.
40. Nagaraj, H.S., Shott, R., Fellows, R., and Yacoub, U.: Recurrent lobar atelectasis due to acquired bronchial stenosis in neonates, J. Pediatr. Surg. 15:411, 1980.
41. Ostor, A.-G., Stillwell, R., and Fortune, D.W.: Bilateral pulmonary agenesis, Pathology 10:243, 1978.
42. Rutledge, J.C., and Jensen, P.: Acinar dysplasia: a new form of pulmonary maldevelopment, Hum. Pathol. 17:1290, 1986.
43. Wagenvoort, C.A.: Misalignment of lung vessels: a syndrome causing persistent neonatal pulmonary hypertension, Hum. Pathol. 17:727, 1986.

44. Warfel, K.A., and Schulz, D.M.: Agenesis of the trachea: report of a case and review of the literature, Arch. Pathol. Lab. Med. 100:357, 1976.

Hypoplasia and diaphragmatic hernia

45. Chamberlain, D., Hislop, A., Hey, E., et al.: Pulmonary hypoplasia in babies with severe rhesus isoimmunisation: a quantitative study, J. Pathol. 122:43, 1977.
46. Cooney, T.P., and Thurlbeck, W.M.: Pulmonary hypoplasia in Down's syndrome, N. Engl. J. Med. 307:1170, 1982.
47. Cooney, T.P., Dimmick, J.E., and Thurlbeck, W.M.: Increased acinar complexity with polyhydramnios, Pediatr. Pathol. 5:183, 1986.
48. Cullen, M.L., Clein, M.D., and Philippart, A.I.: Congenital diaphragmatic hernia, Surg. Clin. North Am. 65:1115, 1985.
49. Currarino, G., and Williams, B.: Causes of congenital unilateral pulmonary hypoplasia, Pediatr. Radiol. 15:15, 1985.
50. Geggel, R.L., Murphy, J.D., Langleben, D., Crone, R.K., Vacanti, J.P., and Reid, L.M.: Congenital diaphragmatic hernia: arterial structural changes and persistent pulmonary hypertension after surgical repair, J. Pediatr. 107:457, 1985.
51. Goldstein, J.D., and Reid, L.: Pulmonary hypoplasia resulting from phrenic nerve agenesis and diaphragmatic amyoplasia, J. Pediatr. 97:282, 1980.
52. Hislop, A., Hey, E., and Reid, L.: The lungs in congenital bilateral renal agenesis and dysplasia, Arch. Dis. Child. 54:323, 1979.
53. Langer, R., and Kaufman, H.J.: Primary (isolated) bilateral pulmonary hypoplasia: a comparative study of radiologic findings and autopsy results, Pediatr. Radiol. 16:175, 1986.
54. Page, D.V., and Stocker, J.T.: Anomalies associated with pulmonary hypoplasia, Am. Rev. Respir. Dis. 125:216, 1982.
55. Thibeault, D.W., Beatty, E.C., Jr., Hall, R.T., Bowen, S.K., and O'Neill, D.H.: Neonatal pulmonary hypoplasia with premature rupture of fetal membranes and oligohydramnios, J. Pediatr. 107:273, 1985.
56. Silver, M.M., Thurston, W.A., and Patrick, J.E.: Perinatal pulmonary hyperplasia due to laryngeal atresia, Hum. Pathol. 19:110, 1988.
57. Stahl, G.E., Warren, W.S., Rosenberg, H., Spackman, T.J., and Schnaufer, L.: Congenital right diaphragmatic hernia: a case report and review of the literature, Clin. Pediatr. 20:422, 1981.
58. Thurlbeck, W.M., Kida, K., Langston, C., Cowan, M.J., Kitterman, J.A., Tooley, W., and Bryan, H.: Postnatal lung growth after repair of diaphragmatic hernia, Thorax 34:338, 1979.
59. Wigglesworth, J.S.: Pathology of the lung in the fetus and neonate, with particular reference to problems of growth and maturation, Histopathology 11:671, 1987.

Pulmonary vascular anomalies

60. Ben-Menachem, Y., et al.: The various forms of pulmonary varices: report of three new cases and review of the literature, Am. J. Roentgenol. Radium Ther. Nucl. Med. 125:881, 1975.
61. Berdon, W.E., and Baker, D.H.: Vascular anomalies and the infant lung: rings, slings, and other things, Sem. Roentgenol. 7:39, 1972.
62. Burke, C.M., Safai, C., Nelson, D.P., and Raffin, T.A.: Pulmonary arteriovenous malformations: a critical update, Am. Rev. Respir. Dis. 134:334, 1986.
63. Edwards, J.E.: Congenital pulmonary vascular disorders. In Moser, K.M., editor: Pulmonary vascular disease, New York, 1979, Marcel Dekker, Inc.
64. Edwards, J.E., and McGoon, D.C.: Absence of anatomic origin from heart of pulmonary arterial supply, Circulation 47:393, 1973.
65. Freedman, R.M., Culhan, J.A.G., and Moes, C.A.F.: Angiocardiography of congenital heart disease, New York, 1984, The McMillan Publishing Co.
66. Godwin, J.D., and Tarver, R.D.: Scimitar syndrome: four new cases examined with CT, Radiology 159:15, 1986.
67. Grote, W.R., and Tenholder, M.F.: Pulmonary artery malformation syndrome, South. Med. J. 77:1139, 1984.

68. Hawker, R.E., Celermajer, J.M., Gengos, D.C., et al.: Common pulmonary vein atresia: premortem diagnosis in two infants, Circulation 46:368, 1972.

69. Kamio, A., Fukushima, K., Takebayashi, S., and Toshima, H.: Isolated stenosis of the pulmonary artery branches: an autopsy case with review of the literatures, Jpn. Circ. J. 42:1289, 1978.

70. Lucas, R.V., Jr.: Anomalous venous connections, pulmonary, and systemic. In Adams, F.H., and Emmanouilides, G.C., editors: Moss' heart disease in infants, children, and adolescents, ed. 3, Baltimore, 1983, The Williams & Wilkins Co.

71. Mardini, M.K., Sakati, N.A., Lewall, D.B., Christie, R., and Nyhan, W.L.: Scimitar syndrome, Clin. Pediatr. 21:350, 1982.

72. McCue, C.M., Robertson, L.W., Lester, R.G., et al.: Pulmonary artery coarctations: a report of 20 cases with a review of 319 cases from the literature, J. Pediatr. 67:222, 1965.

73. Penkoske, P.A., Castañeda, A.R., Fyler, D.C., and Van Praagh, R.: Origin of pulmonary artery branch from ascending aorta: primary surgical repair in infancy, J. Thorac. Cardiovasc. Surg. 85:537, 1983.

74. Presbitero, P., Bull, C., and Macartney, F.J.: Stenosis of pulmonary veins with ventricular septal defect: a cause of premature pulmonary hypertension in infancy, Br. Heart J. 49:600, 1983.

75. Przybojewski, J.E., and Maritz, F.: Pulmonary arteriovenous fistulas: a case presentation and review of the literature, S. Afr. Med. J. 57:366, 1980.

76. Swischuk, L.E., and L'Heureux, P.: Unilateral pulmonary vein atresia, AJR 135:667, 1980.

77. Tang, J.S., Kauffman, S.L., and Lynfield, J.: Hypoplasia of the pulmonary arteries in infants with congenital rubella, Am. J. Cardiol. 27:491, 1977.

78. Tesler, U.F., Balsara, R.H., and Niguidula, F.N.: Aberrant left pulmonary artery (vascular sling): report of five cases, Chest 66:402, 1974.

Bronchopulmonary sequestration; bronchogenic cyst

79. Alivizatos, P., Cheatle, T., de Leval, M., and Stark, J.: Pulmonary sequestration complicated by anomalies of pulmonary venous return, J. Pediatr. Surg. 20:76, 1985.

80. Case reports of the Massachusetts General Hospital: Case 48-1983), N. Engl. J. Med. 309:1347, 1983.

81. Clements, B.S., and Warner, J.O.: Pulmonary sequestration and related congenital bronchopulmonary vascular malformations: nomenclature and classification based on anatomical and embryological considerations, Thorax 42:401, 1987.

82. Corrin, B., Danel, C., Allaway, A., Warner, J., and Lenney, W.: Intralobar pulmonary sequestration of ectopic pancreatic tissue with gastropancreatic duplication, Thorax 40:637, 1985.

83. Dubois, P., Belanger, R., and Wellington, J.L.: Bronchogenic cyst presenting as a supraclavicular mass, Can. J. Surg. 24:530, 1981.

84. Heithoff, K.B., Sane, S.M., Williams, H.J., et al.: Bronchopulmonary foregut malformations, Am. J. Roentgenol. Radium Ther. Nucl. Med. 126:46, 1976.

85. Lucaya, J., García-Conesa, J.A., and Bernadó, L.: Pulmonary sequestration associated with unilateral pulmonary hypoplasia and massive pleural effusion: a case report and review of the literature, Pediatr. Radiol. 14:228, 1984.

86. Reed, J.C., and Sobonya, R.E.: Morphologic analysis of foregut cysts in the thorax, Am. J. Roentgenol. Radium Ther. Nucl. Med. 120:851, 1974.

87. Salyer, D.C., Salyer, W.R., and Eggleston, J.C.: Benign developmental cysts of the mediastinum, Arch. Pathol. Lab. Med. 101:136, 1977.

88. Savic, B., Birtel, F.J., Knoche, R., Tholen, W., and Schild, H.: Pulmonary sequestration, Ergeb. Inn. Med. Kinderheilkd. 43:57, 1979.

89. Stocker, J.T., Drake, R.M., and Madewell, J.E.: Cystic and congenital lung disease in the newborn, Perspect. Pediatr. Pathol. 4:93, 1978.

90. Stocker, J.T., and Kagan-Hallet, K.: Extralobar pulmonary sequestration: analysis of 15 cases, Am. J. Clin. Pathol. 72:917, 1979.

91. Stocker, J.T., and Malczak, H.T.: A study of pulmonary ligament arteries: relationship to intralobar pulmonary sequestration, Chest 86:611, 1984.

92. Yabek, S., Burstein, J., Berman, W., Jr., and Dillon, T.: Aberrant systemic arterial supply to the left lung with congestive heart failure, Chest 80:636, 1981.

Congenital adenomatoid malformation

93. Adzick, N.S., Harrison, M.R., and Glick, P.R.: Fetal cystic adenomatoid malformation: prenatal diagnosis and natural history, J. Pediatr. Surg. 20:483, 1985.

94. Alt, B., Shikes, R.H., Stanford, R.E., and Silverberg, S.G.: Ultrastructure of congenital cystic adenomatoid malformation of lung, Ultrastruct. Pathol. 3:217, 1982.

95. Avitabile, A.M., Greco, M.A., Hulnick, D.H., and Feiner, H.D.: Congenital cystic adenomatoid malformation of the lung in adults, Am. J. Surg. Pathol. 8:193, 1984.

96. Benning, T.L., Godwin, J.D., Roggli, V.L., and Askin, F.B.: Cartilaginous variant of congenital adenomatoid malformation of the lung, Chest 92:514, 1987.

97. Cachia, R., and Sobonya, R.E.: Congenital cystic adenomatoid malformation of the lung with bronchial atresia, Hum. Pathol. 12:947, 1981.

98. Holland-Moritz, R.M., and Heyn, R.: Pulmonary blastoma associated with cystic lesions in children, Med. Pediatr. Oncol. 12:85, 1984.

99. Mendoza, A., Wolf, P., Edwards, D.K., Leopold, G.R., Voland, J.R., and Benirschke, K.: Prenatal ultrasonographic diagnosis of congenital adenomatoid malformation of the lung: correlation with pathology and implications for pregnancy management, Arch. Pathol. Lab. Med. 110:402, 1986.

100. Miller, R.K., Sieber, W.K., and Yunis, E.J.: Congenital adenomatoid malformation of the lung: a report of 17 cases and review of the literature, Pathol. Annu. 15(pt. 1):387, 1980.

101. Petit, P., Bossens, M., Thomas, D., Moerman, P., Fryns, J.P., and Van den Berghe, H.: Type III congenital cystic adenomatoid malformation of the lung: another cause of elevated alpha fetoprotein? Clin. Genet. 32:172, 1987.

102. Stocker, J.T.: Congenital and developmental diseases. In Dail, D.H., and Hammar, S.P., editors: Pulmonary pathology, Berlin, 1988, Springer-Verlag.

103. Warren, J.S., Seo, I.S., and Mirkin, L.D.: Massive congenital mesenchymal malformation of the lung: a case report with ultrastructural study, Pediatr. Pathol. 3:321, 1985.

Congenital pulmonary lymphangiectasis

104. Bhatti, M.A.K., Ferrante, J.W., Gielchinsky, I., and Norman, J.C.: Pleuropulmonary and skeletal lymphangiomatosis with chylothorax and chylopericardium, Ann. Thorac. Surg. 40:398, 1985.

105. Case records of the Massachusetts General Hospital: Case 30-1980, N. Engl. J. Med. 303:270, 1980.

106. Esterly, J.R., and Oppenheimer, E.H.: Lymphangiectasis and other lesions in the asplenia syndrome, Arch. Pathol. 90:553, 1970.

107. Gardner, T.W., Domm, A.C., Brock, C.E, and Pruitt, A.W.: Congenital pulmonary lymphangiectasis: a case complicated by chylothorax, Clin. Pediatr. 22:75, 1983.

108. Hernández, R.J.: Pulmonary lymphangiectasis in Noonan syndrome, AJR 134:75, 1980.

109. Morphis, L.G., Arcinue, E.L., and Krause, J.R.: Generalized lymphangiectasis in infancy with chylothorax, Pediatrics 46:566, 1970.

110. Shannon, M.P., et al.: Congenital pulmonary lymphangiectasis: report of two cases, Pediatr. Radiol. 2:235, 1974.

Congenital pulmonary overinflation

111. Buckner, D.M.: Congenital lobar emphysema, Clin. Perinatol. **5**:105, 1978.
112. Case records of the Massachusetts General Hospital: Case 41-1979, N. Engl. J. Med. **301**:829, 1979.
113. Jederlinic, P.J., Sicilian, L.S., Baigelman, W., and Gaensler, E.A.: Congenital bronchial atresia: a report of 4 cases and a review of the literature, Medicine **66**:73, 1987.
114. Miller, K.E., Edwards, D.K., Hilton, S., Collins, D., Lynch, F., and Williams, R.: Acquired lobar emphysema in premature infants with bronchopulmonary dysplasia: an iatrogenic disease? Radiology **138**:589, 1981.
115. Morgan, W.J., Lemen, R.J., and Rojas, R.: Acute worsening of congenital lobar emphysema and subsequent spontaneous improvement, Pediatrics **71**:844, 1983.
116. Murray, G.F.: Congenital lobar emphysema, Surg. Gynecol. Obstet. **124**:611, 1967.
117. Nagaraj, H.S., Shott, R., Fellows, R., and Yacoub, U.: Recurrent lobar atelectasis due to acquired bronchial stenosis in neonates, J. Pediatr. Surg. **15**:411, 1980.
118. Powell, H.C., and Elliot, M.L.: Congenital lobar emphysema, Virchows Arch. [Pathol. Anat.] **374**:197, 1977.
119. Rabinovitch, M., Grady, S., David, I., Van Praagh, R., Sauer, U., Buhlmeyer, K., Castaneda, A.R., and Reid, L.: Compression of intrapulmonary bronchi by abnormally branching pulmonary arteries associated with absent pulmonary valves, Am. J. Cardiol. **50**:804, 1982.
120. Stanger, P., Lucas, R.V., Jr., and Edwards, J.E.: Anatomic factors causing respiratory distress in acyanotic congenital cardiac disease: special reference to bronchial obstruction, Pediatrics **43**:760, 1969.
121. Wall, M.A., Eisenberg, J.D., and Campbell, J.R.: Congenital lobar emphysema in a mother and daughter, Pediatrics **70**:131, 1982.

Adaptation to extrauterine life
Perinatal lung disease
TRANSIENT TACHYPNEA OF THE NEWBORN

122. Chernick, V.: Mechanics of the first inspiration, Semin. Perinatol. **1**:347, 1977.
123. Halliday, H.L., McCleve, G., and Reid, M.McC.: Transient tachypnea of the newborn: two distinct clinical entities, Arch. Dis. Child. **56**:332, 1981.
124. Swischuck, L.E., Hayden, C.K., Jr., and Richardson, C.J.: Neonatal opaque right lung: delayed fluid resorption, Radiology **41**:671, 1981.
125. Yeh, T.F., Tilien, L.D., and Pildes, R.S.: Diffuse radiographic infiltrates in a neonate, Chest **74**:291, 1978.

HYALINE MEMBRANE DISEASE; BRONCHOPULMONARY DYSPLASIA

126. Ahlström, H., Mortenson, W., and Robertson, B.: Alveolar lesions in bronchopulmonary dysplasia, OPMEAR (Opuscula Medica) **29**:102, 1984.
127. Anderson, W.R., and Engel, R.R.: Cardiopulmonary sequelae of reparative stages of bronchopulmonary dysplasia, Arch. Pathol. Lab. Med. **107**:603, 1983.
128. Berman, W., Jr., Katz, R., Yabek, S.M., Dillon, T., Fripp, R.R., and Papile, L.A.: Long-term follow-up of bronchopulmonary dysplasia, J. Pediatr. **109**:45, 1986.
129. Bonikos, D.S., Bensch, K.G., Northway, W.H., Jr., et al.: Bronchopulmonary dysplasia: the pulmonary pathologic sequel of necrotizing bronchiolitis and pulmonary fibrosis, Hum. Pathol. **7**:643, 1976.
130. Boros, S.J., Mammel, M.C., Lewallen, P.K., Coleman, J.M., Gordon, M.J., and Ophoven, J.: Necrotizing tracheobronchitis: a complication of high-frequency ventilation, J. Pediatr. **109**:95, 1986.
131. Coates, A.L., et al.: Long-term pulmonary sequelae of premature birth with and without idiopathic respiratory distress syndrome, J. Pediatr. **90**:611, 1979.
132. Doshi, N., Klionsky, B., Fujikura, T., and MacDonald, H.: Pulmonary yellow hyaline membranes in neonates, Hum. Pathol. **11**:520, 1980.

133. Escobedo, M.B., and González, A.: Bronchopulmonary dysplasia in the tiny infant, Clin. Perinatol. **13**:315, 1986.
134. Esterly, J.R., Langegger, F., and Gruenwald, P.: Hyaline membranes in full-size infants, Virchows Arch. [Pathol. Anat.] **341**:259, 1966.
135. Gruenwald, P.: Exaggerated atelectasis of prematurity: a complication of recovery from the respiratory distress syndrome, Arch. Pathol. **86**:81, 1968.
136. Hodgman, J.E., Mikity, V.G., Tatter, D., et al.: Chronic respiratory distress in the premature infant: Wilson-Mikity syndrome, Pediatrics **44**:179, 1969.
137. Jones, R., Bodnar, A., Roan, Y., and Johnson, D.: Subglottic stenosis in newborn intensive care unit graduates, Am. J. Dis. Child. **135**:367, 1981.
138. Lauweryns, J.: "Hyaline membrane disease" in newborn infants: macroscopic, radiographic, and light and electron microscope studies, Hum. Pathol. **1**:175, 1970.
139. Myers, A.D., Lillydahl, P., and Brown, G.: Hypopharyngeal perforations in neonates, Arch. Otolaryngol. **104**:51, 1978.
140. Nickerson, B.G.: Bronchopulmonary dysplasia: chronic pulmonary disease following neonatal respiratory failure, Chest **87**:528, 1984.
141. O'Brodovich, H.M., and Mellins, R.B.: Bronchopulmonary dysplasia: unresolved neonatal acute injury, Am. Rev. Respir. Dis. **132**:694, 1985.
142. Perelman, R.H., Palta, M., Kirby, R., and Farrell, P.M.: Discordance between male and female deaths due to the respiratory distress syndrome, Pediatrics **78**:238, 1986.
143. Raivio, K.O., Hallman, N., Kouvalainen, K., and Valimaki, I., editors: Respiratory distress syndrome, London, 1984, Academic Press, Inc.
144. Rooney, S.A.: The surfactant system and lung phospholipid biochemistry, Am. Rev. Respir. Dis. **131**:439, 1985.
145. Rosan, R.C.: Hyaline membrane disease and a related spectrum of neonatal pneumonopathies, Perspect. Pediatr. Pathol. **2**:15, 1975.
146. Shanklin, D.R.: The influence of fixation on the histologic features of hyaline membrane disease, Am. J. Pathol. **44**:823, 1964.
147. Singer, D.B.: Morphology of hyaline membrane disease and its pulmonary sequelae. In Stern, L., editor: Hyaline membrane disease: pathogenesis and pathophysiology, Orlando, Fla., 1984, Grune & Stratton, Inc.
148. Stark, A.R., and Frantz, I.D., III: Respiratory distress syndrome, Pediatr. Clin. North Am. **38**:533, 1986.
149. Stocker, J.T.: Pathologic features of long-standing "healed" bronchopulmonary dysplasia: a study of 28 3- to 40-month old infants, Hum. Pathol. **17**:943, 1986.
150. Tou, S.S., et al.: Clinical and roentgenographic scoring systems for assessing bronchopulmonary dysplasia, Am. J. Dis. Child. **138**:581, 1984.
151. Váldes-Dapena, M.: Iatrogenic disease in the perinatal period as seen by the pathologist. In Naeye, R.L., Kissane, J.M., and Kaufman, N., editors: Perinatal disorders, Baltimore, 1981, The Williams & Wilkins Co.

PULMONARY INTERSTITIAL EMPHYSEMA

152. Askin, F.B.: Pulmonary interstitial air and pneumothorax in the neonate. In Stocker, J.T., editor: Pediatric pulmonary pathology, vol. 2, Aspen Seminars on Pediatric Disease, Washington, D.C., 1988, Hemisphere Publishing Corp.
153. Levine, D.H., Trump, D.S., and Waterkotte, G.: Unilateral pulmonary interstitial emphysema: a surgical approach to treatment, Pediatrics **68**:510, 1981.
154. Madansky, D.L., Lawson, E.E., Chernick, V., and Taeusch, H.W., Jr.: Pneumothorax and other forms of pulmonary air leak in newborns, Am. Rev. Respir. Dis. **120**:729, 1979.
155. Mayo, P., and Saha, S.P.: Spontaneous pneumothorax in the newborn, Am. Surg. **49**:192, 1983.
156. Oppermann, H.C., Willie, L., Obladen, M., and Richter, E.: Systemic air embolism in the respiratory distress syndrome of the newborn, Pediatr. Radiol. **8**:139, 1979.

157. Plénat, F., Vert, P., Didier, F., and André, M.: Pulmonary interstitial emphysema, Clin. Perinatol. **5:**315, 1978.

158. Smith, T.H., Currarino, G., and Rutledge, J.C.: Spontaneous occurrence of localized pulmonary interstitial and endolymphatic emphysema in infancy, Pediatr. Radiol. **14:**142, 1984.

159. Stocker, J.T., and Madewell, J.E.: Persistent interstitial pulmonary emphysema: another complication of the respiratory distress syndrome, Pediatrics **59:**847, 1977.

160. Wood, B.P., Anderson, V.M., Mauk, J.E., and Merritt, T.A.: Pulmonary lymphatic air: locating "pulmonary interstitial emphysema" of the premature infant, AJR **138:**809, 1982.

161. Zimmerman, H.: Progressive interstitial pulmonary lobar emphysema, Eur. J. Pediatr. **138:**258, 1982.

MECONIUM ASPIRATION SYNDROME; MASSIVE PULMONARY HEMORRHAGE

162. Ahvenainen, E.K., and Call, J.D.: Pulmonary hemorrhage in infants: a descriptive study, Am. J. Pathol. **28:**1, 1952.

163. Bacski, R.D.: Meconium aspiration syndrome, Pediatr. Clin. North Am. **24:**463, 1977.

164. Bancalari, E., and Berlin, J.A.: Meconium aspiration and other asphyxial disorders, Clin. Perinatol. **5:**317, 1978.

165. Cole, V.A., Normand, I.C., Reynolds, E.O., et al.: Pathogenesis of hemorrhagic pulmonary edema and massive pulmonary hemorrhage in the newborn, Pediatrics **51:**175, 1973.

166. Esterly, J.R., and Oppenheimer, E.H.: Massive pulmonary hemorrhage in the newborn. I. Pathologic considerations, J. Pediatr. **69:**3, 1966.

167. Fedrick, J., and Butler, N.R.: Certain causes of neonatal death. IV. Massive pulmonary hemorrhage, Biol. Neonate **18:**243, 1971.

168. Gregory, G.A., Gooding, C.A., Phibbs, R.H., et al.: Meconium aspiration in infants: a prospective study, J. Pediatr. **85:**858, 1974.

169. Hoffman, R.R., Jr., Campbell, R.E., and Decker, J.P.: Fetal aspiration syndrome: clinical, roentgenographic and pathologic features, Am. J. Roentgenol. **122:**90, 1974.

170. Jose, J.H., Schreiner, R.L., Lemons, J.A., Gresham, E.L., Mirkin, L.D., Siddiqui, A., and Cohen, M.: The effect of amniotic fluid aspiration on pulmonary function in the adult and newborn rabbit, Pediatr. Res. **17:**976, 1983.

171. Kotas, R.V., Wells, T.J., Mims, L.C., et al.: A new model for neonatal pulmonary hemorrhage research, Pediatr. Res. **9:**161, 1975.

172. Lauweryns, J., Bernat, R., Lerut, A., et al.: Intrauterine pneumonia: an experimental study, Biol. Neonate **22:**301, 1973.

173. Leake, R.D., Gunther, R., and Sunshine, P.: Perinatal aspiration syndrome: its association with perinatal events and anesthesia, Am. J. Obstet. Gynecol. **118:**271, 1975.

174. Manning, F.A., Schreiber, J., and Turkel, S.B.: Fatal meconium aspiration "in utero": a case report, Am. J. Obstet. Gynecol. **132:**111, 1978.

175. Murphy, J.D., Vawter, G.F., and Reid, L.M.: Pulmonary vascular disease in fetal meconium aspiration, J. Pediatr. **104:**758, 1984.

176. Ohlsson, A., Cumming, W.A., and Najjar, H.: Neonatal aspiration syndrome due to vernix caseosa, Pediatr. Radiol. **15:**193, 1985.

177. Turbeville, D.F., McCaffree, M.A., Block, M.F., and Krous, H.F.: In utero distal pulmonary meconium aspiration, South. Med. J. **72:**535, 1979.

178. Tyler, D.C., Murphy, J., and Cheney, F.W.: Mechanical and chemical damage to lung tissue caused by meconium aspiration, Pediatrics **62:**454, 1978.

PERSISTENT FETAL CIRCULATION

179. Bloss, R.S., Aranda, J.V., and Beardmore, H.E.: Congenital diaphragmatic hernia: pathophysiology and pharmacologic support, Surgery **89:**518, 1981.

180. Fos, W.W., and Duara, S.: Persistent pulmonary hypertension in the neonate: diagnosis and management, J. Pediatr. **103:**505, 1983.

181. Geggel, R.L., and Reid, L.M.: The structural basis of PPHN, Clin. Perinatol. **11:**525, 1984.

182. Geggel, R.L., Murphy, J.D., Langleben, D., Crone, R.K., Vacanti, J.P., and Reid, L.M.: Congenital diaphragmatic hernia: arterial structural changes and persistent pulmonary hypertension after surgical repair, J. Pediatr. **107:**457, 1985.

183. Gersony, W.M.: Neonatal pulmonary hypertension: pathophysiology, classification and etiology, Clin. Perinatol. **11:**517, 1984.

184. Haworth, S.G.: Primary and secondary pulmonary hypertension in childhood: a clinicopathological reappraisal, Curr. Top. Pathol. **73:**92, 1983.

185. Levin, D.L., Weinberg, A.G., and Perkins, R.M.: Pulmonary microthrombi syndrome in newborn infants with unresponsive persistent pulmonary hypertension, J. Pediatr. **102:**229, 1983.

186. Levin, D.L., Fixler, D.E., Moriss, F.C., and Tyson, J.: Morphologic analysis of the pulmonary vascular bed in infants exposed in utero to prostaglandin synthetase inhibitors, J. Pediatr. **92:**478, 1978.

187. Morrow, W.R., Haas, J.E., and Benjamin, D.E.: Nonbacterial endocardial thrombosis in neonates: relationship to persistent fetal circulation, J. Pediatr. **100:**117, 1982.

188. Oelberg, D.G., Fisher, D.J., Gross, D.M., Denson, S.E., and Adcock, E.W.: Endocarditis in high-risk neonates, Pediatrics **71:**392, 1983.

189. Rudolph, A.M.: High pulmonary vascular resistance after birth. I. Pathophysiologic considerations and etiologic classification, Clin. Pediatr. **19:**585, 1980.

Infectious disorders in the infant lung

190. Arth, C., von Schmidt, B., Grossman, M., and Schachter, J.: Chlamydial pneumonitis, J. Pediatr. **93:**447, 1978.

191. Baker, C.J.: Group B streptococcal infections, Adv. Intern. Med. **25:**475, 1980.

192. Barter, R.A., and Hudson, J.A.: Bacteriological findings in perinatal pneumonia, Pathology **6:**223, 1974.

193. Bernstein, J., and Wang, J.: The pathology of perinatal pneumonia, Am. J. Dis. Child. **101:**350, 1961.

194. Boyer, K.M., and Cherry, J.D.: Pneumonias in children. In Moss, A.J., editor: Pediatrics update, 1979, New York, 1979, American Elsevier Publishing Co.

195. Craig, J.M.: Group B beta hemolytic streptococcal sepsis in the newborn, Perspect. Pediatr. Pathol. **6:**139, 1982.

196. Dudgeon, J.A.: Intrauterine infection, Proc. R. Soc. Med. **68:**365, 1975.

197. Fedrick, J.: Neonatal deaths: time of death, maturity and lesion, Biol. Neonate **18:**369, 1971.

198. Fedrick, J., and Butler, N.R.: Certain causes of neonatal death: III. Pulmonary infection (A.) Clinical factors (B.) Pregnancy and delivery, Biol. Neonate **17:**458; **18:**45, 1971.

199. Gilbert, G.L.: Chlamydial infections in infancy, Aust. Paediatr. J. **22:**13, 1986.

200. Hobson, D., Rees, E., and Viswalingam, N.D.: Chlamydial infections in neonates and older children, Br. Med. Bull. **39:**128, 1983.

201. Langley, F.A., and Smith, J.A.M.: Perinatal pneumonia: a retrospective study, J. Obstet. Gynecol. Br. Cmwlth. **66:**12, 1959.

202. Naeye, R.L.: Causes of excessive rates of perinatal mortality and prematurity in pregnancies complicated by maternal urinary-tract infections, N. Engl. J. Med. **200:**819, 1979.

203. Naeye, R.L., Kissane, J.M., and Kaufman, N., editors: Perinatal diseases, Baltimore, 1981, The Williams & Wilkins Co.

204. Naeye, R.L., and Peters, E.C.: Amniotic fluid infections with intact membranes leading to perinatal death: a prospective study, Pediatrics **61:**171, 1978.

205. Naeye, R.L., and Tafari, N.: Risk factors in pregnancy and diseases of the fetus and newborn, Baltimore, 1983, The Williams & Wilkins Co.

206. Paisley, J.W., Lauer, B.A., McIntosh, K., Glode, M.P., Schachter, J., and Rumack, C.: Pathogens associated with acute lower respiratory tract infection in young children, Pediatr. Infect. Dis. **3:**14, 1984.

207. Radkowski, M.A., Kranzler, J.K., Beem, M.O., and Tipple, M.A.: *Chlamydia* pneumonia in infants: radiography in 125 cases, AJR **137**:703, 1981.
208. Remington, J.S., and Klein, J.O.: editors: Infectious disease of the fetus and newborn infant, ed. 2, Philadelphia, 1983, W.B. Saunders Co.
209. Rettig, P.J.: Perinatal infections with *Chlamydia trachomatis,* Clin. Perinatol. **15**:321, 1988.
210. Rhine, W.D., Arvin, A.M., and Stevenson, D.K.: Neonatal aspergillosis: a case report and review of the literature, Clin. Pediatr. **25**:400, 1986.
211. Sun, C.-C.J., and Duara, S.: Fatal adenovirus pneumonia in two newborn infants, one case caused by adenovirus type 30, Pediatr. Pathol. **4**:247, 1985.
212. Wigglesworth, J.S.: Perinatal pathology, Philadelphia, 1982, W.B. Saunders Co.
213. Wilfert, C.M., and Gutman, L.T.: *Chlamydia trachomatis* infections of infants and children, Adv. Pediatr. **33**:49, 1986.

Bronchiolitis and bronchiolitis obliterans
214. Azizirad, H., Polgar, G., Borns, P.F., et al.: Bronchiolitis obliterans, Clin. Pediatr. **14**:572, 1975.
215. Berquist, W.E., Rachelefsky, G.S., Kadden, M., Siegel, S.C., Katz, R.M., Fonkalsrud, E.W., and Ament, M.E.: Gastroesophageal reflux–associated recurrent pneumonia and chronic asthma in children, Pediatrics **68**:29, 1981.
216. Buts, J.P., Barudi, C., Moulin, D., Claus, D., Cornu, G., and Otte, J.B.: Prevalence and treatment of silent gastroesophageal reflux in children with recurrent respiratory disorders, Eur. J. Pediatr. **145**:396, 1986.
217. Daniel, T.L., Woodring, J.H., Vandiviere, H.M., and Wilson, H.D.: Swyer-James syndrome—unilateral hyperlucent lung syndrome: a case report and review, Clin. Pediatr. **23**:393, 1984.
218. Herbst, J.J.: Gastroesophageal reflux, J. Pediatr. **98**:859, 1981.
219. Kargi, H.A., and Kuhn, C.K., III: Bronchiolitis obliterans: unilateral fibrous obliteration of the lumen of bronchi with atelectasis, Chest **93**:1107, 1988.
220. McKenzie, S.A., Allison, D.J., Singh, M.P., and Godrey, S.: Unilateral hyperlucent lung: the case for investigation, Thorax **35**:745, 1980.
221. Rosen, N., and Gaton, E.: Congenital bronchiolitis obliterans, Beitr. Pathol. **155**:309, 1975.
222. Spigelblatt, L., and Rosenfeld, R.: Hyperlucent lung: long-term complication of adenovirus type 7 pneumonia, Can. Med. Assoc. J. **128**:47, 1983.
223. Wenman, W.M., Pagtakhan, R.D., Reed, M.H., Chernick, V., and Albritton, W.: Adenovirus bronchiolitis in Manitoba: epidemiologic, clinical and radiographic features, Chest **81**:605, 1982.
224. Wohl, M.E.B., and Chernick, V.: Bronchiolitis, Am. Rev. Respir. Dis. **118**:759, 1978.

Infections of the lungs and bronchi
Routes of infection; pulmonary defenses
225. Dunnill, M.S.: Some aspects of pulmonary defense, J. Pathol. **128**:221, 1979.
226. Green, G.M., and Kass, E.H.: The role of the alveolar macrophage in the clearance of bacteria from the lung, J. Exp. Med. **119**:167, 1964.
227. Green, G.M., Jakab, G.J., Low, R.B., et al.: Defense mechanisms of the respiratory membrane, Am. Rev. Respir. Dis. **115**:479, 1977.
228. Higuchi, J.H., and Johanson, W.G.: Colonization and bronchopulmonary infection, Clin. Chest Med. **3**:133, 1982.
229. Johanson, W.G., Jr., Pierce, A.K., Sanford, J.P., et al.: Nosocomial respiratory infections with gram-negative bacilli: the significance of colonization of the respiratory tract, Ann. Intern. Med. **77**:701, 1972.
230. Johanson, W.G., Jr., Higuchi, J.H., Chaudhuri, T.R., and Woods, D.E.: Bacterial adherence to epithelial cells in bacillary colonization of the respiratory tract, Am. Rev. Respir. Dis. **121**:55, 1980.

231. Kass, E.H., Green, G.M., and Goldstein, E.: Mechanisms of antibacterial action in the respiratory system, Bacteriol. Rev. **30**:488, 1966.
232. McDermott, M.R., Befus, A.D., and Bienenstock, J.: The structural basis for immunity in the respiratory tract, Int. Rev. Exp. Pathol. **23**:48, 1982.
233. Woods, D.E., Straus, D.C., Johanson, W.G., Jr., and Bass, J.A.: Role of salivary protease activity in adherence of gram negative bacilli to mammalian buccal epithelial cells in vivo, J. Clin. Invest. **68**:1435, 1981.

Viral infections; mycoplasmal pneumonia
234. Aherne, W., Bird, T., Court, S.D., et al.: Pathological changes in virus infections of the lower respiratory tract in children, J. Clin. Pathol. **23**:7, 1970.
235. Archibald, R.W.R., Weller, R.O., and Meadow, S.R.: Measles pneumonia and the nature of the inclusion-bearing giant cells: a light and electron microscopy study, J. Pathol. **103**:27, 1971.
236. Becroft, D.M.O.: Histopathology of fatal adenovirus infection of the respiratory tract in young children, J. Clin. Pathol. **20**:561, 1967.
237. Benisch, B.M., Fayemi, A., Gerber, M.A., et al.: Mycoplasmal pneumonia in a patient with rheumatic heart disease, Am. J. Clin. Pathol. **58**:343, 1972.
238. Clinical conferences at the Johns Hopkins Hospital, mycoplasma pneumonia, Johns Hopkins Med. J. **139**:181, 1976.
239. Denny, F.W., Collier, A.M., Henderson, F.W., et al.: The epidemiology of bronchiolitis, Pediatr. Res. **11**:234, 1977.
240. Foy, H.M., Kenny, G.E., McMahan, R., et al.: *Mycoplasma pneumoniae* pneumonia in an urban area: five years of surveillance, JAMA **214**:1666, 1970.
241. Maisel, J.C., Babbett, L.H., and John, T.J.: Fatal *Mycoplasma pneumoniae* infection with isolation of organisms from lung, JAMA **202**:139, 1967.
242. Murray, H. Masur, H., Senterfit, L.B., et al.: The protean manifestations of *Mycoplasma pneumoniae* infection in adults, Am. J. Med. **58**:229, 1975.
243. Nash, G., and Foley, F.D.: Herpetic infection of the middle and lower respiratory tract, Am. J. Clin. Pathol. **54**:857, 1970.
244. Triebwasser, J.H., Harris, R.E., Bryant, R.E., et al.: Varicella pneumonia in adults, Medicine **46**:409, 1967.
245. Turtzo, D.F., and Ghatak, P.K.: Acute hemolytic anemia with *Mycoplasma pneumoniae* pneumonia, JAMA **236**:1140, 1976.
246. Wohl, M.E., and Chernick, V.: Bronchiolitis, Am. Rev. Respir. Dis. **118**:759, 1978.

Bacterial infections
247. Austrian, R., and Gold, J.: Pneumococcal bacteremia with special reference to bacteremic pneumococcal pneumonia, Ann. Intern. Med. **60**:759, 1964.
248. Berry, F.B.: Lobar pneumonia: analysis of 400 autopsies, Med. Clin. North Am. **4**:571, 1920.
249. Dines, D.E.: Diagnostic significance of pneumatocele of the lung, JAMA **204**:79, 1968.
250. Finland, M.: Pneumonia and pneumococcal infections with special reference to pneumococcal pneumonia, Am. Rev. Respir. Dis. **120**:481, 1979.
251. Finland, M., Brown, J.W., and Ruegsegger, J.M.: Anatomic and bacteriologic findings in infections with specific types of pneumococci including types I to XXXII, Arch. Pathol. **23**:801, 1937.
252. Hers, J.F., Masarel, N., and Mulder, J.: Bacteriology and histopathology of the respiratory tract and lungs in fatal Asian influenza, Lancet **2**:1141, 1958.
253. Kevy, S., and Lowe, B.A.: Streptococcal pneumonia and empyema in childhood, N. Engl. J. Med. **264**:738, 1961.
254. Miller, W.R., and Jay, A.R.: Staphylococcal pneumonia in influenza: 5 cases, Arch. Intern. Med. **109**:76, 1962.
255. Mufson, M.A., Kruss, D.M., Wasil, R.E., et al.: Capsular types and outcome of bacteremic pneumococcal disease in the antibiotic era, Arch. Intern. Med. **134**:505, 1974.

256. Naraqui, S., and McDonnell, G.: Hematogenous staphylococcal pneumonia secondary to soft tissue infection, Chest **79**:173, 1981.
257. Robertson, O.H., and Uhley, C.G.: Changes occurring in the macrophage system of the lungs in pneumococcus lobar pneumonia, J. Clin. Invest. **15**:115, 1936.
258. Sofer, S., Dundan, P., and Chernick, V.: Bacterial tracheitis: an old disease rediscovered, Clin. Pediatr. **22**:407, 1983.
259. Sullivan, R.J., Dowdie, W.R., Marine, W.M., et al.: Adult pneumonia in a general hospital, Arch. Intern. Med. **129**:935, 1972.
260. Tuazon, C.U.: Gram-positive pneumonias, Med. Clin. North Am. **64**:343, 1980.
261. Verghese, A., Berk, S.L., Boelen, L.J., and Smith, J.K.: Group B streptococcal pneumonia in the elderly, Arch. Intern. Med. **142**:1642, 1982.
262. Yangco, B.G., and Deresinski, S.C.: Necrotizing or cavitating pneumonia due to *Streptococcus pneumoniae*, Medicine **59**:449, 1980.

Bacterial pneumonia
PNEUMONIA CAUSED BY GRAM-NEGATIVE AEROBIC BACTERIA

263. Erasmus, L.D.: Friedländer bacillus infection of the lung: with special reference to classification and pathogenesis, Q. J. Med. **25**:507, 1956.
264. Fetzer, A.F., Werner, A.S., and Hagstrom, J.W.C.: Pathology features of pseudomonal pneumonia, Am. Rev. Respir. Dis. **96**:1121, 1967.
265. Forkner, C.E., et al.: *Pseudomonas* septicemia: observations on twenty-three cases, Am. J. Med. **25**:877, 1958.
266. Hirschman, J.V., and Everett, E.D.: *Haemophilus influenzae* infections in adults: report of nine cases and a review of the literature, Medicine **58**:80, 1979.
267. Jonas, M., and Cunha, B.A.: Bacteremic *Escherichia coli* pneumonia, Arch. Intern. Med. **142**:2157, 1982.
268. Levin, D.C., Schwarz, M.I., and Matthay, R.A.: Bacteremic *Haemophilus influenzae* pneumonia in adults, Am. J. Med. **62**:219, 1977.
269. McHenry, M.C., Baggenstoss, A.R., and Martin, W.J.: Bacteremia due to gram-negative bacilli: clinical and autopsy findings in 33 cases, Am. J. Pathol. **59**:160, 1968.
270. Pennington, J.E., Reynolds, H.Y., and Carbone, P.P.: *Pseudomonas* pneumonia, Am. J. Med. **55**:155, 1973.
271. Pierce, A.K., and Sanford, J.P.: Aerobic gram-negative bacillary pneumonias, Am. Rev. Respir. Dis. **110**:647, 1974.
272. Pierce, A.K., Edmondson, E.B., McGee, G., et al.: An analysis of factors predisposing to gram-negative bacillary necrotizing pneumonia, Am. Rev. Respir. Dis. **94**:309, 1966.
273. Renner, R.R., Coccaro, A.P., Heitzman, E.R., et al.: *Pseudomonas* pneumonia: a prototype of hospital-based infection, Radiology **105**:555, 1972.
274. Reyes, M.P.: The aerobic gram-negative bacillary pneumonias, Med. Clin. North Am. **64**:363, 1980.
275. Teplitz, C.: Pathogenesis of *Pseudomonas* vasculitis and septic lesions, Arch. Pathol. **80**:297, 1965.
276. Tillotson, J.R., and Lerner, A.M.: Pneumonias caused by gram-negative bacilli, Medicine **45**:65, 1966.
277. Tillotson, J.R., and Lerner, A.M.: Characteristics of pneumonias caused by *Escherichia coli*, N. Engl. J. Med. **277**:115, 1967.
278. Tillotson, J.R., and Lerner, A.M.: Characteristics of nonbacteremic *Pseudomonas* pneumonia, Ann. Intern. Med. **68**:295, 1968.
279. Tillotson, J.R., and Lerner, A.M.: Characteristics of pneumonias caused by *Bacillus proteus*, Ann. Intern. Med. **68**:287, 1968.
280. Tillotson, J.R., and Lerner, A.M.: *Haemophilus influenzae* bronchopneumonia in adults, Arch. Intern. Med. **121**:428, 1968.
281. Wallace, R.J., Musher, D.M., and Martin, R.R.: *Haemophilus influenzae* pneumonia in adults, Am. J. Med. **64**:87, 1978.

LEGIONELLA AND RELATED PNEUMONIAS

282. Blackmon, J.A., Chandler, F.W., and Hicklin, M.D.: Legionnaires' disease—a review for pathologists, Pathol. Annu. **2**:383, 1979.
283. Blackmon, J.A., Hicklin, M.D., and Chandler, F.W.: Legionnaires' disease: pathologic and historical aspects of a "new" disease, Arch. Pathol. Lab. Med. **102**:337, 1978.
284. Blackmon, J.A., Chandler, F.W., Cherry, W.B., England, A.C., III, Feeley, J.C., Hicklin, M.P., McKinney, R.M., and Wilkinson, H.W.: Review article: legionellosis, Am. J. Pathol. **103**:428, 1981.
285. England, A.C., III, Fraser, D.W., Plikaytis, B.D., Tsai, T.F., Storch, G., and Broome, C.V.: Sporadic legionellosis in the United States: the first thousand cases, Ann. Intern. Med. **94**:164, 1981.
286. Fraser, D.W., Tsai, T.R., Orenstein, W., Parkin, W.E., Beecham, H.J., Sharrar, R.G., Harris, J., Mallison, G.F., Martin, S.M., McDade, J.E., Shepard, C.C., and Brachman, P.S.: Legionnaires' disease: description of an epidemic of pneumonia, N. Engl. J. Med. **297**:1189, 1977.
287. Helms, C.M., Massanari, R.M., Zeitler, R., Streed, S., Gilchrist, M.J., Hall, N., Hausler, W.J., Jr., Sywassink, J., Johnson, W., Wintermeyer, L., and Hierholzer, W.J., Jr.: Legionnaires' disease associated with a hospital water system: a cluster of 24 nosocomial cases, Ann. Intern. Med. **99**:172, 1983.
288. Horowitz, M.A., and Silverstein, S.C.: Intracellular multiplication of Legionnaires' disease bacteria (*Legionella pneumophila*) in human monocytes is reversibly inhibited by erythromycin and rifampicin, J. Clin. Invest. **71**:15, 1983.
289. Kirby, B.D., Snyder, K.M., Meyer, R.D., and Finegold, S.M.: Legionnaires' disease: report of sixty-five nosocomially acquired cases and review of the literature, Medicine **59**:188, 1980.
290. Lewin, S., Brettman, L.R., Goldstein, E.J., Holzman, R.S., Devila, H., Taubman, F., Sierra, M.F., and Edelstein, P.H.: Legionnaires' disease: a cause of severe abscess-forming pneumonia, Am. J. Med. **67**:339, 1979.
291. Meyerowitz, R.L., et al.: Opportunistic lung infection due to "Pittsburgh pneumonia agent," N. Engl. J. Med. **301**:953, 1979.
292. Muder, R.R., Yu, V.L., and Zuravleff, J.J.: Pneumonia due to the Pittsburgh pneumonia agent: new clinical perspective with a review of the literature, Medicine **62**:120, 1983.
293. Winn, W.C., and Meyerowitz, R.L.: The pathology of *Legionella* pneumonias, Hum. Pathol. **12**:401, 1981.
294. Yu, V.L., Krobath, F.J., Shonnard, J., Brown, A., McDearman, S., and Magnussen, M.: Legionnaires' disease: new clinical perspective from a prospective pneumonia study, Am. J. Med. **73**:357, 1982.

LUNG LESIONS CAUSED BY ANAEROBIC BACTERIA

295. Bartlett, J.G.: Anaerobic bacterial pneumonitis, Am. Rev. Respir. Dis. **119**:19, 1979.
296. Bartlett, J.G., and Finegold, S.M.: Anaerobic infections of the lung and pleural space, Am. Rev. Respir. Dis. **110**:56, 1974.
297. Cameron, E.W.J., Appelbaum, P.C., Pudifin, D., Hutton, W.S., Chatterton, S.A., and Duursma, J.: Characteristics and management of chronic destructive pneumonia, Thorax **35**:340, 1980.
298. Johanson, W.G., and Harris, G.D.: Aspiration pneumonia, anaerobic infections and lung abscess, Med. Clin. North Am. **64**:385, 1980.
299. Perlman, L.V., Lerner, E., and D'Esopo, N.: Clinical classification and analysis of 97 cases of lung abscess, Am. Rev. Respir. Dis. **99**:390, 1969.
300. Safron, R.D., and Tate, C.F.: Lung abscesses: a five year evaluation, Dis. Chest **53**:12, 1968.
301. Tillotson, J.R., and Lerner, A.M.: *Bacteroides* pneumonias: characteristics of cases with empyema, Ann. Intern. Med. **68**:308, 1968.

Mycobacterial infections

302. Auerbach, O.: The natural history of the tuberculous pulmonary lesion, Med. Clin. North Am. **43**:239, 1959.

303. Barkisdal, L., and Kim, K.S.: *Mycobacterium,* Bacteriol. Rev. **41:**217, 1977.
304. Boros, D.: Granulomatous inflammations, Prog. Allergy **24:**183, 1978.
305. Daniel, T.M.: The immunology of tuberculosis, Clin. Chest Med. **1:**189, 1980.
306. Dannenberg, A.M.: Liquefaction of caseous foci in tuberculosis, Am. Rev. Respir. Dis. **113:**257, 1976.
307. Dannenberg, A.M.: Pathogenesis of pulmonary tuberculosis, Am. Rev. Respir. Dis. **125:**25, 1982.
308. Dubos, R., and Dubos, J.: The white plague: tuberculosis, man and society, Boston, 1952, Little, Brown & Co.
309. Green, G.M., Daniel, T.M., and Ball, W.C., editors: Koch Centennial supplement, Am. Rev. Respir. Dis. **125:**1, 1982.
310. Hershfield, E.S.: Tuberculosis in the world, Chest **176**(suppl.):805, 1979.
311. Khan, M.A., Kovnat, D.M., Bachus, B., et al.: Clinical and roentgenographic spectrum of pulmonary tuberculosis in the adult, Am. J. Med. **62:**31, 1977.
312. Klatt, E.C., Jensen, D.F., and Meyer, P.R.: Pathology of *Mycobacterium avium-intracellulare* infection in acquired immunodeficiency syndrome, Hum. Pathol. **18:**709, 1987.
313. Leff, A., and Geppert, E.F.: Public health and preventive aspects of pulmonary tuberculosis, Arch. Intern. Med. **139:**1405, 1979.
314. Leff, A., Lester, T.W., and Addington, W.W.: Tuberculosis: a chemotherapeutic triumph but a persistent socioeconomic problem, Arch. Intern. Med. **139:**1375, 1979.
315. Lefford, M.J.: Delayed hypersensitivity and immunity in tuberculosis, Am. Rev. Respir. Dis. **111:**243, 1975.
316. Lurie, M.B.: Resistance to tuberculosis: experimental studies in native and acquired defensive mechanisms, Cambridge, Mass., 1964, Harvard University Press.
317. MacGregor, R.R.: A year's experience with tuberculosis in a private urban teaching hospital in the postsanatorium era, Am. J. Med. **58:**221, 1975.
318. Mackaness, G.B.: The induction and expression of cell mediated hypersensitivity in the lung, Am. Rev. Respir. Dis. **104:**813, 1971.
319. Mankiewicz, E., and Liivak, M.: Phage types of *Mycobacterium tuberculosis* in cultures isolated from Eskimo patients, Am. Rev. Respir. Dis. **111:**307, 1975.
320. Marchevsky, A., Damsker, B., Gribetz, A., Teppen, S., and Geller, S.A.: The spectrum of pathology of non-tuberculous mycobacterial infections in open-lung biopsy specimens, Am. J. Clin. Pathol. **78:**695, 1982.
321. Medlar, E.M.: The behavior of pulmonary tuberculous lesions: a pathological study, Am. Rev. Tuberc. **71:**1, 1955.
322. Merckx, J.J., Soule, E.H., and Karlson, A.G.: The histopathology of lesions caused by infection with unclassified acid-fast bacteria in man, Am. J. Clin. Pathol. **41:**244, 1964.
323. National survey of tuberculosis notifications in England and Wales, 1978-9: Report from the Medical Research Council Tuberculosis and Chest Diseases Unit, Br. Med. J. **281:**895, 1980.
324. Pagel, W., et al.: Pulmonary tuberculosis, ed. 4, London, 1964, Oxford University Press.
325. Perzigian, A.J., and Widmer, L.: Evidence for tuberculosis in a prehistoric population, JAMA **241:**2643, 1979.
326. Riley, R.L.: Disease transmission and contagion control, Am. Rev. Respir. Dis. **125:**8, 1982.
327. Romeyn, J.A.: Exogenous reinfection in tuberculosis, Am. Rev. Respir. Dis. **101:**923, 1970.
328. Rosenzweig, D.Y.: Pulmonary mycobacterial infections due to *Mycobacterium intracellulare-avium* complex: clinical features and course in 100 consecutive cases, Chest **75:**115, 1979.
329. Slavin, R.E.: Late generalized tuberculosis: a clinical and pathologic analysis of a diagnostic puzzle and a changing pattern, Pathol. Annu. **16:**81, 1981.
330. Snijder, J.: Histopathology of pulmonary lesions caused by atypical mycobacteria, J. Pathol. Bacteriol. **90:**65, 1965.
331. Stead, W.W.: Pathogenesis of a first episode of chronic pulmonary tuberculosis in man: recrudescence of residuals of the primary infection or exogenous reinfection? Am. Rev. Respir. Dis. **95:**729, 1967.
332. Sunderam, G., et al.: Tuberculosis as a manifestation of the acquired immunodeficiency syndrome (AIDS), JAMA **256:**362, 1986.
333. Sutinen, S.: Evaluation of activity in tuberculous cavities of the lung, Scand. J. Respir. Dis. **67**(suppl):1, 1968.
334. Tuberculosis—United States, 1985, MMWR **35:**699, 1986.
335. Wallace, J.M., and Hannah, J.B.: *Mycobacterium avium* complex infection in patients with the acquired immunodeficiency syndrome: a clinicopathologic study, Chest **93:**926, 1988.
336. Wolinsky, E.: Non-tuberculous mycobacteria and associated diseases, Am. Rev. Respir. Dis. **119:**107, 1979.
337. Youmans, G.P.: Tuberculosis, Philadelphia, 1979, W.B. Saunders Co.

Pneumocystis carinii pneumonia

338. Campbell, W.G., Jr.: Ultrastructure of pneumocystis in human lung: life cycle in human *Pneumocystis,* Arch. Pathol. **93:**312, 1972.
339. Cushion, M.T., Ruffolo, J.J., and Walzer, P.D.: Analysis of the developmental stages of *Pneumocystis carinii* in vitro, Lab. Invest. **58:**324, 1988.
340. Follansbee, S.E., Busch, D.F., Wofsy, C.B., Coleman, D.L., Gullet, J., Aurigemma, G.P., Ross, T., Hadley, W.K., and Drew, W.L.: An outbreak of *Pneumocystis carinii* pneumonia in homosexual men, Ann. Intern. Med. **96:**705, 1982.
341. Gottlieb, M.S., Schroff, R., Schanker, H.M., Weisman, J.D., Fan, P.T., Wolf, R.A., and Saxon, A.: *Pneumocystis carinii* pneumonia and mucosal candidiasis in previously healthy homosexual men: evidence of a new acquired cellular immunodeficiency, N. Engl. J. Med. **305:**1425, 1981.
342. Ham, E.K., Greenberg, D., Reynolds, R.C., et al.: Ultrastructure of *Pneumocystis carinii,* Exp. Mol. Pathol. **14:**362, 1971.
343. Huang, S.-N., and Marshall, K.G.: *Pneumocystis carinii* infection: a cytologic, histologic, and electron microscopic study of the organism, Am. Rev. Respir. Dis. **102:**623, 1970.
344. LeGolvan, D.P., and Heidelberg, K.P.: Disseminated, granulomatous *Pneumocystis carinii* pneumonia, Arch. Pathol. **95:**344, 1973.
345. Masur, H., Michelis, M.A., Greene, J.B., Onorato, I., Stouwe, R.A., Holzman, R.S., Wormser, G., Brettman, L., Lange, M., Murray, H.W., and Cunningham-Rundles, S.: An outbreak of community acquired *Pneumocystis carinii* pneumonia: initial manifestations of cellular immune dysfunction, N. Engl. J. Med. **305:**1931, 1981.
346. Pifer, L.L., Hughes, W.T., and Murphy, M.J.: Propagation of *Pneumocystis carinii* in vitro, Pediatr. Res. **11:**305, 1977.
347. Pifer, L.L., et al.: *Pneumocystis carinii* infection: evidence for high prevalence in normal and immunosuppressed children, Pediatrics **61:**35, 1978.
348. Price, R.A., and Hughes, W.T.: Histopathology of *Pneumocystis carinii* infestation and infection in malignant disease in childhood, Hum. Pathol. **5:**737, 1974.
349. Robbins, J.B.: *Pneumocystis carinii* pneumonitis: a review, Pediatr. Res. **1:**131, 1967.
350. Vanek, J., Jirovec, O., and Lukes, J.: Interstitial plasma cell pneumonia in infants, Ann. Pediatr. **180:**1, 1953.
351. Walzer, P.D., Pevi, D.P., Krogstad, D.J., et al.: *Pneumocystis carinii* pneumonia in United States, Ann. Intern. Med. **80:**83, 1974.
352. Weber, W.R., Askin, F.B., and Dehner, L.P.: Lung biopsy in *Pneumocystis carinii* pneumonia: a histopathologic study of typical and atypical features, Am. J. Clin. Pathol. **67:**11, 1967.

Bronchiectasis

353. Cherniack, N.S., Dowling, H.F., Carton, R.W., et al.: The role of acute lower respiratory infection in causing pulmonary insufficiency in bronchiectasis, Ann. Intern. Med. **66:**489,1967.

354. Ellis, D.A., Thornley, P.E., Wightman, A.J., Walker, M., Chalmers, J., and Crofton, J.W.: Present outlook in bronchiectasis: clinical and social study and review of factors influencing prognosis, Thorax **36**:659, 1981.
355. Hayward, J., and Reid, L.M.: The cartilage of the intrapulmonary bronchi in normal lungs, in bronchiectasis, and in massive collapse, Thorax **7**:98, 1952.
356. Konietzko, N.F.J., Carton, R.W., and Leroy, E.P.: Causes of death in patients with bronchiectasis, Am. Rev. Respir. Dis. **100**:852, 1969.
357. Rytel, M.W., Conner, G.H., Welch, C.C., et al.: Infectious agents associated with cylindrical bronchiectasis, Dis. Chest **46**:23, 1964.
358. Whitwell, F.: A study of the pathology and pathogenesis of bronchiectasis, Thorax **7**:213, 1952.

Immotile cilia syndrome
359. Afzelius, B.A.: Immotile cilia syndrome and ciliary abnormalities induced by infection and injury, Am. Rev. Respir. Dis. **124**:107, 1981.
360. Chao, J., Turner, J.A.P., and Sturgess, J.M.: Genetic heterogeneity of dynein-deficiency in cilia from patients with respiratory disease, Am. Rev. Respir. Dis. **126**:302, 1982.
361. Corkey, C.W.B., Levison, H., and Turner, J.A.P.: The immotile cilia syndrome: a longitudinal study, Am. Rev. Respir. Dis. **124**:544, 1981.
362. Gibbons, I.R.: Cilia and flagella of eukaryotes, J. Cell. Biol. **91**:1075, 1981.
363. Rutland, J., and Cole, P.J.: Non-invasive sampling of nasal cilia for measurement of beat frequency and study of ultrastructure, Lancet **2**:564, 1980.

Cystic fibrosis
364. Anderson, D.H.: Cystic fibrosis of the pancreas and its relations to celiac disease, Am. J. Dis. Child. **56**:344, 1938.
365. Bedrossian, C.W.M., Greenberg, S.D., Singer, D.B., et al.: The lung in cystic fibrosis: a quantitative study including the prevalence of pathologic findings among different age groups, Hum. Pathol. **7**:195, 1976.
366. diSant'Agnese, P.A., and Davis, P.B.: Research in cystic fibrosis, N. Engl. J. Med. **295**:481, 534, 597, 1976.
367. diSant'Agnese, P.A., and Davis, P.B.: Cystic fibrosis in adults: 75 cases and a review of 232 cases in the literature, Am. J. Med. **66**:121, 1979.
368. Esterly, J.R., and Oppenheimer, E.H.: Cystic fibrosis of the pancreas: structural changes in peripheral airways, Thorax **23**:670, 1968.
369. Esterly, J.R., and Oppenheimer, E.H.: Observations in cystic fibrosis of the pancreas. III. Pulmonary lesions, Johns Hopkins Med. J.**122**:93, 1968.
370. Fick, R.B., Jr., Naegel, G.P., Matthay, R.A., and Reynolds, H.Y.: Cystic fibrosis *Pseudomonas* opsonins: inhibitory nature in an in vitro phagocytic assay, J. Clin. Invest. **68**:899, 1981.
371. Kulczycki, L.L., Murphy, T.M., and Bellanti, J.A.: *Pseudomonas* colonization in cystic fibrosis, JAMA **240**:30, 1978.
372. Landan, L.I., and Phelan, P.D.: The spectrum of cystic fibrosis: a study of pulmonary mechanics in 46 patients, Am. Rev. Respir. Dis. **108**:593, 1973.
373. Li, M., McCann, J.D., Liedtke, C.M., Nairn, A.C., Greengard, P., and Welsh, M.J.: Cyclic AMP dependent protein kinase opens chloride channels in normal but not cystic fibrosis airway epithelium, Nature **331**:358, 1988.
374. Oppenheimer, E.H., and Esterly, J.R.: Pathology of cystic fibrosis: review of the literature and comparison with 146 autopsied cases, Perspect. Pediatr. Pathol. **2**:241, 1975.
375. Reynolds, H.Y., diSant'Agnese, P.D., and Zierdt, C.H.: Mucoid *Pseudomonas aeruginosa*: a sign of cystic fibrosis in young adults with chronic pulmonary disease, JAMA **236**:2190, 1976.
376. Shoumacher, R.A., Shoemaker, R.L., Halm, D.R., Tallant, E.A., Wallace, R.W., and Frizzell, R.A.: Phosphorylation fails to activate choride channels from cystic fibrosis airway cells, Nature **330**:752, 1987.
377. Shwachman, H., Kowalski, M., and Khaw, K.T.: Cystic fibrosis: a new outlook: 70 patients above 25 years of age, Medicine **56**:129, 1977.
378. Stern, R.C., Borkat, G., Hirschfeld, S.S., Boat, T.F., Matthews, L.W., Liebman, J., and Doershuk, C.F.: Heart failure to cystic fibrosis, Am. J. Dis. Child. **134**:267, 1980.
379. Symchych, P.S.: Pulmonary hypertension in cystic fibrosis, Arch. Pathol. **92**:409, 1971.
380. Vawter, G.F., and Shwachman, H.: Cystic fibrosis in adults: an autopsy study, Pathol. Annu. **14**:357, 1979.
381. Wentworth, P., Gough, J., and Wentworth, J.E.: Pulmonary changes and cor pulmonale in mucoviscidosis, Thorax **23**:582, 1968.
382. Wood, R.E., Boat, T.F., and Doershuk, C.F.: State of the art: cystic fibrosis, Am. Rev. Respir. Dis. **113**:833, 1976.
383. Zuelger, W.W., and Newton, W.A.: The pathogenesis of fibrocystic disease of the pancreas: a study of 36 cases with special references to the pulmonary lesions, Pediatrics **4**:53, 1949.

Pulmonary vascular disease
Histologic features of normal pulmonary vasculature
384. Brenner, O.: Pathology of the vessels of the pulmonary circulation, Arch. Intern. Med. **56**:211, 1935.
385. Reid, L.M.: Structure and function in pulmonary hypertension, Chest **89**:279, 1986.

Pulmonary thromboembolism; pulmonary infarcts
386. Bell, W.R., Simon, T.L., and DeMels, D.L.: The clinical features of submassive and massive pulmonary emboli, Am. J. Med. **62**:355, 1977.
387. Dalen, J.E., Haffajee, C.I., Alpert, J.S., III, et al.: Pulmonary embolism, pulmonary hemorrhage and pulmonary infarction, N. Engl. J. Med. **296**:1431, 1977.
388. Fred, H.L., Axelrad, M.A., Lewis, J.M., et al.: Rapid resolution of pulmonary thromboemboli in man, JAMA **196**:1137, 1966.
389. Korn, D., Gore, I., Blenke, A., and Collins, D.P.: Pulmonary arterial bands and webs: a previously unrecognized manifestation of organized pulmonary emboli, Am. J. Pathol. **40**:129, 1962.
390. LeQuesne, L.P.: Relation between deep vein thrombosis and pulmonary embolism in surgical patients, N. Engl. J. Med. **291**:1292, 1974.
391. Morell, T.M., and Dunnill, M.S.: Fibrous bands in conducting pulmonary arteries, J. Clin. Pathol. **20**:39, 1967.
392. Moser, V.M.: Pulmonary embolism, Am. Rev. Respir. Dis. **115**:829, 1977.
393. Orell, S.R.: The fate and late effects of non-fatal pulmonary emboli, Acta Med. Scand. **172**:473, 1962.
394. Peterson, K.L., Fred, H.L., and Alexander, J.K.: Pulmonary arterial webs: a new angiographic sign of previous pulmonary thromboembolism, N. Engl. J. Med. **277**:33, 1967.
395. Robin, E.D.: Overdiagnosis and overtreatment of pulmonary embolism: the emperor may have no clothes, Ann. Intern. Med. **87**:775, 1977.
396. Rosenow, E.C., Osmundson, P.J., and Brown, M.L.: Pulmonary embolism, Mayo Clin. Proc. **56**:161, 1981.
397. Rossman, I.: True incidence of pulmonary embolization and vital statistics, JAMA **230**:1677, 1974.
398. Walker, R.H.S., Jackson, J.A., and Goodwin, J.: Resolution of pulmonary embolism, Br. Med. J. **4**:135, 1970.

Other forms of embolism
399. Attwood, H.D.: The histological diagnosis of amniotic-fluid embolism, J. Pathol. Bacteriol. **76**:211, 1958.
400. Douglas, F.G., Kafilmout, K.J., and Patt, N.L.: Foreign particle embolism in drug addicts: respiratory pathophysiology, Ann. Intern. Med. **75**:865, 1971.
401. Hopkins, G.B.: Pulmonary angiothrombotic granulomatosis in drug offenders, JAMA **221**:909, 1972.
402. Johnston, W.H., and Waisman, J.: Pulmonary cornstarch granulomas in a drug user, Arch. Pathol. **92**:196, 1971.

403. O'Quin, R.J., and Lakshminarayan, S.: Venous air embolism, Arch. Intern. Med. **142**:2173, 1982.
404. Robinson, M.J., Nestor, M., and Rywlin, A.M.: Pulmonary granulomas secondary to embolic prosthetic valve material, Hum. Pathol. **12**:759, 1981.
405. Schinella, R.A.: Bone marrow emboli, Arch. Pathol. **95**:386, 1973.
406. Tang, T.T., Chambers, G.H., Gallen, W.J., and McCreadie, S.R.: Pulmonary fiber embolism and granuloma, JAMA **239**:948, 1978.
407. Tomashefski, J.F., and Hirsch, C.S.: The pulmonary vascular lesions of intravenous drug abuse, Hum. Pathol. **11**:133, 1980.

Pulmonary hypertension

408. Arias-Stella, J., Kruger, H., and Recavarren, S.: Pathology of chronic mountain sickness, Thorax **28**:701, 1973.
409. Bove, K.E., and Scott, R.C.: The anatomy of chronic cor pulmonale secondary to intrinsic lung disease, Prog. Cardiovasc. Dis. **9**:227, 1966.
410. Corrin, B., Spencer, H., Turner-Warwick, M., et al.: Pulmonary veno-occlusion: an immune complex disease, Virchows Arch. [Pathol. Anat.] **364**:81, 1974.
411. Crissman, J.D., Koss, M., and Carson, R.P.: Pulmonary veno-occlusive disease secondary to granulomatous venulitis, Am. J. Surg. Pathol. **4**:93, 1980.
412. Edwards, J.E.: Pathology of chronic pulmonary hypertension, Pathol. Annu. **9**:1, 1974.
413. Fishman, A.P.: Hypoxia on the pulmonary circulation: how and where it acts, Circ. Res. **38**:331, 1976.
414. Fulton, R.M., Hutchinson, E.C., and Jones, A.M.: Ventricular weight in cardiac hypertrophy, Br. Heart J. **14**:413, 1952.
415. Heath, D., and Edwards, J.E.: The pathology of hypertensive pulmonary vascular disease, Circulation **18**:533, 1958.
416. Heath, D., Scott, O., and Lynch, J.: Pulmonary veno-occlusive disease, Thorax **26**:663, 1971.
417. Heath, D., and Smith, P.: Electron microscopy of hypertensive pulmonary vascular disease, Br. J. Dis. Chest **77**:1, 1983.
418. Heath, D., et al.: The structure of the pulmonary trunk at different ages and in cases of pulmonary hypertension and pulmonary stenosis, J. Pathol. Bacteriol. **77**:443, 1959.
419. Molden, D., and Abraham, J.L.: Pulmonary hypertension: its association with hepatic cirrhosis and iron accumulation, Arch. Pathol. Lab. Med. **106**:382, 1982.
420. Morrison, E.B., Gaffney, F.A., Eigenbrodt, E.H., Reynolds, R.C., and Buja, L.M.: Severe pulmonary hypertension associated with macronodular (postnecrotic) cirrhosis and autoimmune phenomena, Am. J. Med. **69**:513, 1980.
421. Naeye, R.I.: Hypoxemia and pulmonary hypertension: a study of the pulmonary vasculature, Arch. Pathol. **71**:447, 1961.
422. Owen, W.R., Thomas, W.A., Castleman, B., and Bland, E.F.: Unrecognized emboli to the lungs with subsequent cor pulmonale, N. Engl. J. Med. **249**:919, 1953.
423. Rochester, D.F., and Enson, Y.: Current concepts in the pathogenesis of the obesity-hypoventilation syndrome: mechanical and circulatory factors, Am. J. Med. **57**:402, 1974.
424. Saldana, M.E., Harley, R.A., Liebow, A.A., et al.: Experimental extreme pulmonary hypertension and vascular disease in relation to polycythemia, Am. J. Pathol. **52**:935, 1968.
425. Thadani, U., Burrow, C., Whitaker, W., et al.: Pulmonary veno-occlusive disease, Q. J. Med. **44**:133, 1975.
426. Wagenvoort, C.A.: Grading of pulmonary vascular lesions in a reappraisal, Histopathology **5**:595, 1981.
427. Wagenvoort, C.A., and Wagenvoort, N.: Primary pulmonary hypertension: a pathologic study of the lung vessels in 156 clinically diagnosed cases, Circulation **42**:1163, 1970.
428. Wagenvoort, C.A., Wagenvoort, N., and Takahashi, T.: Pulmonary veno-occlusive disease, Hum. Pathol. **16**:1033, 1985.
429. Walcott, G., Burchell, H.B., and Brown, A.L.: Primary pulmonary hypertension, Am. J. Med. **49**:70, 1970.
430. Widgren, S.: Pulmonary hypertension related to aminorex intake: histologic ultrastructural and morphometric studies of 37 cases in Switzerland, Curr. Top. Pathol. **64**:2, 1977.

Pulmonary edema

431. Arias-Stella, J., and Kruger, H.: Pathology of high altitude pulmonary edema, Arch. Pathol. **76**:147, 1963.
432. Bleyl, U., Sandler, E., and Schindler, T.: The pathology and biology of uremic pneumonitis, Intensive Care Med. **7**:193, 1981.
433. Heath, D., and Edwards, J.E.: Histological changes in the lung in diseases associated with pulmonary venous hypertension, Br. J. Dis. Chest **53**:8, 1959.
434. Heath, D., Moosavi, H., and Smith, P.: Ultrastructure of high altitude pulmonary edema, Thorax **28**:694, 1973.
435. Hughes, R.T.: The pathology of butterfly densities in uremia, Thorax **22**:97, 1967.
436. Hurley, J.V.: Current views on the mechanisms of pulmonary edema, J. Pathol. **125**:59, 1978.
437. Inoue, S., Michel, R.P., and Hogg, J.C.: Zonulae occludentes in alveolar epithelium and capillary endothelium of dog lungs studied with the freeze-fracture technique, J. Ultrastruct. Res. **56**:215, 1976.
438. Kay, J.M., and Edwards, R.: Ultrastructure of the alveolar-capillary wall in mitral stenosis, J. Pathol. **111**:239, 1975.
439. Kleiner, J., and Nelson, W.P.: High altitude pulmonary edema: a rare disease? JAMA **234**:491, 1975.
440. Staub, N.C.: The pathophysiology of pulmonary edema, Hum. Pathol. **1**:419, 1970.
441. Staub, N.C.: Pulmonary edema, Physiol. Rev. **54**:678, 1974.
442. Taylor, A.E., and Gaar, K.A.: Estimation of equivalent pore radii of pulmonary capillary and alveolar membranes, Am. J. Physiol. **218**:1133, 1970.
443. Theodore, J., and Robin, E.D.: Speculations on neurogenic pulmonary edema, Am. Rev. Respir. Dis. **113**:405, 1976.

Altered capillary permeability

444. Ashbaugh, D.G., Bigelow, D.B., Petty, T.L., et al.: Acute respiratory distress in adults, Lancet **2**:319, 1967.
445. Bachofen, M., and Weibel, E.R.: Structural alterations of lung parenchyma in the adult respiratory distress syndrome, Clin. Chest Med. **3**:35, 1982.
446. Blaisdell, F.W.: Respiratory distress syndrome, Surgery **74**:251, 1973.
447. Bone, R.C., Francis, P.B., and Pierce, A.K.: Intravascular coagulation associated with the adult respiratory distress syndrome, Am. J. Med. **61**:585, 1976.
448. Cochrane, C.C., Spragg, R., and Revak, S.D.: Pathogenesis of the adult respiratory distress syndrome: evidence of oxidant activity in bronchoalveolar lavage fluid, J. Clin. Invest. **71**:754, 1983.
449. Deneke, S.M., and Fanburg, B.L.: Normobaric oxygen toxicity of the lung, N. Engl. J. Med. **303**:76, 1980.
450. Divertie, M.D.: The adult respiratory distress syndrome, Mayo Clin. Proc. **57**:371, 1982.
451. Emson, H.E.: Fat embolism studied in one hundred patients dying after injury, J. Clin. Pathol. **11**:28, 1958.
452. Gossling, H.R., and Donohue, T.A.: The fat embolism syndrome, JAMA **241**:740, 1979.
453. Gould, V.E., Tosco, R., Wheelis, R.F., et al.: Oxygen pneumonitis in man: ultrastructural observations on the development of alveolar lesions, Lab. Invest. **26**:499, 1972.
454. Hallman, M.: Evidence of lung surfactant abnormality in respiratory failure, J. Clin. Invest. **70**:673, 1982.
455. Jacob, H.S., Craddock, P.R., Hammerschmidt, D.E., and Moldow, C.F.: Complement-induced granulocyte aggregation: an unsuspected mechanism of disease, N. Engl. J. Med. **302**:789, 1980.
456. Kapanci, Y., Tosco, R., Eggermann, J., et al.: Oxygen pneumonitis in man: light and electron microscopic morphometric studies, Chest **62**:162, 1972.
457. Katzenstein, A.A., Bloor, C.M., and Liebow, A.A.: Diffuse alveolar damage: the role of oxygen, shock and related factors, Am. J. Pathol. **85**:210, 1976.
458. Kistler, G.S., Caldwell, P.R., and Weibel, E.R.: Development

of fine structural damage to alveolar and capillary lining cells in oxygen-poisoned rat lungs, J. Cell Biol. **32**:605, 1967.

459. Lamy, M., Fallat, R.J., Koeniger, E., et al.: Pathologic features and mechanisms of hypoxemia in adult respiratory distress syndrome, Am. Rev. Respir. Dis. **114**:267, 1976.

460. McCord, J.M., and Fridovich, I.: The biology and pathology of oxygen radicals, Ann. Intern. Med. **89**:122, 1978.

461. McGuire, W.W., Spragg, R.G., Cohen, A.B., and Cochrane, C.G.: Studies on the pathogenesis of the adult respiratory distress syndrome, J. Clin. Invest. **69**:543, 1982.

462. Moon, V.H.: The pathology of secondary shock, Am. J. Pathol. **24**:235, 1948.

463. Nash, G., Blennerhassett, J.B., and Pontoppidan, H.: Pulmonary lesions associated with oxygen therapy and artificial ventilation, N. Engl. J. Med. **276**:368, 1967.

464. Petty, T.L., and Ashbaugh, D.G.: The adult respiratory distress syndrome: clinical features, factors influencing prognosis and principles of management, Chest **60**:233, 1971.

465. Petty, T.L., et al.: Characteristics of pulmonary surfactant in adult respiratory distress syndrome associated with trauma and shock, Am. Rev. Respir. Dis. **115**:531, 1971.

466. Pratt, P.C., Vollmer, R.T., Shelburne, J.D., and Crapo, J.D.: Pulmonary morphology in a multihospital collaborative extracorporeal membrane oxygenation project, Am. J. Pathol. **95**:191, 1979.

467. Rinaldo, J.E., and Rogers, R.M.: Adult respiratory distress syndrome, N. Engl. J. Med. **306**:900, 1982.

468. Simpson, D.L., Goodman, M., Spector, S.L., and Petty, T.L.: Long term follow up of adult respiratory distress syndrome survivors, Am. Rev. Respir. Dis. **117**:449, 1978.

Immunologic lung disease
Asthma

469. Banatar, S.R.: Fatal asthma, N. Engl. J. Med. **314**:423, 1986.

470. Connell, J.T.: Asthmatic deaths: role of the mast cell, JAMA **215**:769, 1971.

471. Dunnill, M.S., Massarella, G.R., and Anderson, J.A.: A comparison of the quantitative anatomy of the bronchi in status asthmaticus in chronic bronchitis and in emphysema, Thorax **24**:176, 1969.

472. Empey, D.: Mechanisms of bronchial hyperreactivity, Eur. J. Respir. Dis. **63**(suppl. 117):33, 1982.

473. Glynn, A.A., and Michaels, L.: Bronchial biopsy in chronic bronchitis and asthma, Thorax **15**:142, 1960.

474. Kaliner, M., Shelhamer, J.H., Davis, P.B., Smith, L.J., and Venter, J.C.: Autonomic nervous system abnormalities and allergy, Ann. Intern. Med. **96**:349, 1982.

475. Laitinen, L.A., Meino, M., Laitinen, A., Kava, T., and Haahtela, T.: Damage of the airway epithelium and bronchial reactivity in patients with asthma, Am. Rev. Respir. Dis. **131**:599, 1985.

476. Leff, A.R.: Endogenous regulation of bronchomotor tone, Am. Rev. Respir. Dis. **137**:1198, 1988.

477. McFadden, E.R., and Ingram, R.H.: Exercise-induced asthma: observations on initiating stimulus, N. Engl. J. Med. **301**:763, 1979.

478. Messer, J.W., Peters, G.A., and Bennett, W.A.: Causes of death and pathologic findings in 304 cases of bronchial asthma, Dis. Chest **38**:616, 1960.

479. Naylor, B.: The shedding of the mucosa of the bronchial tree in asthma, Thorax **17**:69, 1962.

480. Ogilvie, A.G.: Asthma: a study in prognosis of 1,000 patients, Thorax **17**:183, 1962.

481. Rackemann, F.M.: Other factors besides allergy in asthma, JAMA **142**:534, 1950.

482. Rackemann, F.M., and Edwards, M.C.: Asthma in children: a follow-up study of 688 patients after an interval of twenty years, N. Engl. J. Med. **246**:815, 858, 1952.

483. Reed, C.E.: Mechanisms of hyperreactivity of airways in asthma, Eur. J. Respir. Dis. **63**(suppl. 117):88, 1982.

484. Salvato, G.: Some histological changes in chronic bronchitis and asthma, Thorax **23**:168, 1968.

485. Schatz, M., Patterson, R., and Fink, J.: Immunologic lung disease, N. Engl. J. Med. **300**:1310, 1979.

Other allergic lung diseases

486. Barrowcliff, D.F., and Arblaster, P.G.: Farmer's lung: a study of an early acute fatal case, Thorax **23**:490, 1968.

487. Boonpucknavig, V., Bhamarapravati, N., Kamtorn, P., et al.: Bagassosis: a histopathologic study of pulmonary biopsies from six cases, Am. J. Clin. Pathol. **59**:461, 1973.

488. Carrington, C.B., Addington, W.W., Goff, A.M., et al.: Chronic eosinophilic pneumonia, N. Engl. J. Med. **280**:786, 1969.

489. Colemen, A., and Colby, T.V.: Histologic diagnosis of extrinsic allergic alveolitis, Am. J. Surg. Pathol. **12**:514, 1988.

490. Fink, J.N.: Interstitial lung disease due to contamination of forced air systems, Ann. Intern. Med. **84**:406, 1976.

491. Hapke, E.J., Seal, R.M., Thomas, G.O., et al.: Farmer's lung, Thorax **23**:451, 1968.

492. Hinson, K.F.W., Moon, A.J., and Plummer, N.S.: Bronchopulmonary aspergillosis: a review and a report of eight new cases, Thorax **7**:317, 1952.

493. Jederlinic, P.J., Sicilian, L., and Gaesler, E.A.: Chronic eosinophilic pneumonia, Medicine **67**:154, 1988.

494. Katzenstein, A.-L., Liebow, A.A., and Friedman, P.J.: Bronchocentric granulomatosis, mucoid impaction and hypersensitivity reactions to fungi, Am. Rev. Respir. Dis. **111**:497, 1975.

495. Keller, B.H., et al.: Immunoregulation in hypersensitivity pneumonitis. I. Differences in T-cell and macrophage suppressor activity in symptomatic and asymptomatic pigeon breeders, J. Clin. Immunol. **2**:46, 1982.

496. Koss, M.N., Robinson, R.G., and Hochholzer, L.: Bronchocentric granulomatosis, Hum. Pathol. **12**:632, 1981.

497. Liebow, A.A., and Carrington, C.B.: The eosinophilic pneumonias, Medicine **48**:251, 1969.

498. Moore, V.L., Fink, J.N., Barboriak, J.J., et al.: Immunologic events in pigeon breeder's disease, J. Allergy Clin. Immunol. **53**:319, 1974.

499. Reyes, C.N., Wenzel, F.J., Lawton, B.R., and Emanuel, D.A.: The pulmonary pathology of farmer's lung disease, Chest **81**:142, 1982.

500. Reynolds, H.Y., Fulmer, J.D., Kazmierowski, J.A., et al.: Analysis of cellular and protein-content of bronchoalveolar lavage fluid from patients with idiopathic pulmonary fibrosis and chronic hypersensitivity pneumonitis, J. Clin. Invest. **59**:165, 1977.

501. Richetti, A.J., et al.: Allergic bronchopulmonary aspergillosis, Arch. Intern. Med. **143**:1553, 1983.

502. Rosenberg, M., Patterson, R., Mintzer, R., et al.: Clinical and immunologic criteria for the diagnosis of allergic bronchopulmonary aspergillosis, Ann. Intern. Med. **86**:405, 1977.

503. Schatz, M., Wasserman, S., and Patterson, R.: The eosinophil and the lung, Arch. Intern. Med. **142**:1515, 1982.

504. Seal, R.M.E., Hapke, E.J., Thomas, G.O., et al.: The pathology of the acute and chronic stages of farmer's lung, Thorax **23**:469, 1968.

505. Slavin, R.G., Gottlieb, C.C., and Avioli, L.V.: Allergic bronchopulmonary aspergillosis, Arch. Intern. Med. **146**:1799, 1986.

Transplantation

506. Chan, C.K., Hyland, R.H., Hutcheon, M.A., Minden, M.D., Alexander, M.A., and Kossakowska, A.E., Urbanski, S.J., Fyles, G.M., Fraser, I.M., Curtis, J.E., et al.: Small-airways disease in recipients of allogeneic bone marrow transplants, Medicine **66**:327, 1987.

507. Veith, F.S., Kamholz, S.L., Mollenkopf, F.P., and Montefusco, C.M.: Lung transplantation 1983, Transplantation **35**:271, 1983.

508. Yousem, S.A., Burke, C.M., and Billingham, M.E.: Pathologic pulmonary alterations in long-term human heart-lung transplantation, Hum. Pathol. **16**:911, 1985.

AIDS

509. Joshi, V.V., Oleske, J.M., Minnefor, A.B., Saad, S., Klein, K.M., Singh, R., Zabala, M., Dadzie, C., Simpser, M., and Rapkin, R.H.: Pathologic pulmonary findings in children with

the acquired immunodeficiency syndromes: a study of ten cases, Hum. Pathol. **16**:241, 1985.

510. Kornstein, M.S., Pietra, G.G., Hoxie, S.A., and Conley, M.E.: The pathology and treatment of interstitial pneumonitis in two infants with AIDS, Am. Rev. Respir. Dis. **133**:1196, 1988.

511. Solal-Celigny, P., Couderc, L.J., Herman, D., Herve, P., Schaffar-Deshayes, L., Brun-Vezinet, F., Tricot, G., and Clauvel, J.P.: Lymphoid interstitial pneumonitis in acquired immunodeficiency syndrome–related complex, Am. Rev. Respir. Dis. **131**:956, 1985.

Interstitial pneumonia

512. Basset, F., Ferrans, V.J., Soler, P., Takemura, T., Fukuda, Y., and Crystal, R.G.: Intraluminal fibrosis in interstitial lung disorders, Am. J. Pathol. **122**:443, 1986.

513. Carrington, C.B., Gaensler, E.A., Coutu, R.E., FitzGerald, M.X., and Gupta, R.G.: Natural history and treated course of usual and desquamative interstitial pneumonia, N. Engl. J. Med. **298**:801, 1978.

514. Crystal, R.G., Bitterman, P.B., Rennard, S.I., Hance, A.J., and Keogh, B.A.: Interstitial lung disease of unknown cause. Part I, N. Engl. J. Med. **310**:154, 1984.

515. Davison, A.G., Heard, B.E., McAllister, W.A.C., et al.: Cryptogenic organizing pneumonitis, Q. J. Med. **52**:382, 1983.

516. Dreisin, R.B., Schwarz, M.I., Theofilopoulos, A.N., and Stanford, R.E.: Circulating immune complexes in the idiopathic interstitial pneumonias, N. Engl. J. Med. **298**:353, 1978.

517. Epler, G.R., Colby, T.V., McLeod, T.C., et al.: Bronchiolitis obliterans organizing pneumonia, N. Engl. J. Med. **312**:152, 1985.

518. Fulmer, J.D., Roberts, W.C., von Gal, E.R., and Crystal, R.G.: Morphologic-physiologic correlates of the severity of fibrosis and degree of cellularity in idiopathic pulmonary fibrosis, J. Clin. Invest. **63**:665, 1979.

519. Hamman, L., and Rich, A.R.: Acute diffuse interstitial fibrosis of the lungs, Bull. Johns Hopkins Hosp. **74**:177, 1944.

520. Heppleston, A.G.: The pathology of honeycomb lung, Thorax **11**:77, 1956.

521. Hogan, P.G., Donald, K.J., and McEvoy, J.D.S.: Immunofluorescence studies of lung biopsy tissue, Am. Rev. Respir. Dis. **118**:537, 1978.

522. Liebow, A.A., Steer, A., and Billingsley, J.G.: Desquamative interstitial pneumonia, Am. J. Med. **39**:369, 1965.

523. Scadding, J.G.: Chronic diffuse interstitial fibrosis of the lungs, Br. Med. J. **1**:443, 1960.

524. Scadding, J.G., and Hinson, K.F.W.: Diffuse fibrosing alveolitis (diffuse interstitial fibrosis of the lungs): correlation of histology at biopsy with prognosis, Thorax **22**:291, 1967.

525. Schwarz, M.I., Dreisin, R.B., Pratt, D.S., and Stanford, R.E.: Immunofluorescent patterns in the idiopathic interstitial pneumonias, J. Lab. Clin. Med. **91**:929, 1978.

526. Stock, B.H.R., Choo-Kang, Y.F.J., and Heard, B.E.: The prognosis of cryptogenic fibrosing alveolitis, Thorax **27**:535, 1972.

527. Turner-Warwick, M., and Haslam, P.: Antibodies in some chronic fibrosing lung diseases. I. Non-organ specific autoantibodies, Clin. Allergy **1**:83, 1971.

528. Turner-Warwick, M., Haslam, P., and Weeks, J.: Antibodies in some chronic fibrosing lung diseases. II. Immunofluorescent studies, Clin. Allergy **1**:209, 1971.

529. Ward, P.A.: Immune complex injury of the lung, Am. J. Pathol. **97**:85, 1979.

Pulmonary involvement in collagen-vascular disease

530. Anderson, L.G., and Talal, N.: The spectrum of the benign to malignant lymphoproliferation in Sjögren's syndrome, Clin. Exp. Immunol. **9**:199, 1971.

531. Armstrong, J.G., and Steele, R.H.: Localized pulmonary arteritis in rheumatoid disease, Thorax **37**:313, 1982.

532. Bonner, H., Jr., Ennis, R.S., Geelhoed, G.W., et al.: Lymphoid infiltration and amyloidosis of lung in Sjögren's syndrome, Arch. Pathol. **95**:42, 1973.

533. Brown, G., Goldring, D., and Behrer, R.: Rheumatic pneumonia, J. Pediatr. **52**:508, 1958.

534. Churg, A., Franklin, W., Chan, K.L., Kopp, E., and Carrington, C.B.: Pulmonary hemorrhage and immune-complex deposition in the lung, Arch. Pathol. Lab. Med. **104**:388, 1980.

535. Colp, C.R., Riker, J., and Williams, M.H., Jr.: Serial changes in scleroderma and idiopathic interstitial lung disease, Arch. Intern. Med. **132**:506, 1973.

536. D'Angelo, W.A., Fries, J.F., Masi, A.T., et al.: Pathologic observations in systemic sclerosis (scleroderma), Am. J. Med. **46**:488, 1969.

537. DeHoratius, R.J., and Williams, R.C.: Rheumatoid factor accentuation of pulmonary lesions associated with experimental diffuse proliferative lung disease, Arthritis Rheum. **15**:293, 1972.

538. DeHoratius, R.J., Abruzzo, J.L., and Williams, R.C., Jr.: Immunofluorescent and immunologic studies of rheumatoid lung, Arch. Intern. Med. **129**:441, 1972.

539. Eagen, J.W., Memoli, V.A., Roberts, J.L., Matthew, G.R., Schwartz, M.M., and Lewis, E.J.: Pulmonary hemorrhage in systemic lupus erythematosus, Medicine **57**:545, 1978.

540. Eisenberg, H., Dubois, E.L., Sherwin, R.P., et al.: Diffuse interstitial lung disease in lupus erythematosus, Ann. Intern. Med. **79**:37, 1973.

541. Elper, G.R., et al.: Bronchiolitis and bronchitis in connective tissue disease: a possible relationship to the use of penicillamine, JAMA **242**:528, 1979.

542. Fayemi, A.O.: Pulmonary vascular disease in systemic lupus erythematosus, Am. J. Clin. Pathol. **65**:284, 1976.

543. Feagler, J.R., Sorenson, G.D., Rosenfeld, M.G., et al.: Rheumatoid pleural effusion, Arch. Pathol. **92**:257, 1971.

544. Frank, S.T., Weg, J.G., Harkleroad, L.E., et al.: Pulmonary dysfunction in rheumatoid disease, Chest **63**:27, 1973.

545. Geddes, D.M., and Brostoff, J.: Pulmonary fibrosis associated with hypersensitivity to gold salts, Br. Med. J. **1**:1444, 1976.

546. Geddes, D.M., Corrin, B., Brewerton, D.A., Davies, R.J., and Turner-Warwick, M.: Progressive airway obliteration in adults and its association with rheumatoid disease, Q. J. Med. **46**:427, 1977.

547. Geddes, D.M., Webley, M., and Emerson, P.A.: Airways obstruction in rheumatoid arthritis, Ann. Rheum. Dis. **38**:222, 1979.

548. Gould, P.W., McCormack, P.L., and Palmer, D.G.: Pulmonary damage associated with sodium aurothiomalate therapy, J. Rheumatol. **4**:252, 1977.

549. Grunow, W.A., and Esterby, J.R.: Rheumatic pneumonitis, Chest **61**:298, 1972.

550. Harvey, A.M.G., et al.: Systemic lupus erythematosus: review of the literature and clinical analysis of 138 cases, Medicine **33**:291, 1954.

551. Hochberg, M.C.: The spectrum of systemic sclerosis—current concepts, Hosp. Pract. **16**:61, 1981.

552. Hunninghake, G.W., and Fauci, A.S.: Pulmonary involvement in the collagen vascular diseases, Am. Rev. Respir. Dis. **119**:471, 1979.

553. Inoue, T., Kanayama, Y., Ohe, A., Kato, N., Horiguchi, T., Ishii, M., and Shiota, K.: Immunopathologic studies of pneumonitis in systemic lupus erythematosus, Ann. Intern. Med. **91**:30, 1979.

554. Israel, H.L.: The pulmonary manifestations of disseminated lupus erythematosus, Am. J. Med. Sci. **266**:387, 1953.

555. Kapanci, Y., and Chamay, A.: Lésions en anse de fil de fer des capillaires pulmonaires dans le lupus erythémateux disséminé (LED), Virchows Arch. [Pathol. Anat.] **342**:236, 1967.

556. Liebow, A.A., and Carrington, C.B.: Diffuse pulmonary lymphoreticular infiltrations associated with dysproteinemia, Med. Clin. North Am. **57**:809, 1973.

557. Lillington, G.A., Carr, D.T., and Mayne, J.G.: Rheumatoid pleurisy with effusion, Arch. Intern. Med. **128**:764, 1971.

558. Mandl, M.A.J., Watson, J.I., Henderson, J.A., et al.: Pleural fluid in rheumatoid pleuritis, Arch. Intern. Med. **124**:373, 1969.

559. Matthay, R.A., et al.: Pulmonary manifestations of systemic lupus erythematosus: review of twelve cases of acute lupus pneumonitis, Medicine **54**:397, 1974.

560. Nair, S.S., Askari, A.D., Popelka, C.G., and Kleinerman, J.F.: Pulmonary hypertension and systemic lupus erythematosus, Arch. Intern. Med. **140:**109, 1980.

561. Newball, H.H., and Brahim, S.A.: Chronic obstructive airway disease in patients with Sjögren's syndrome, Am. Rev. Respir. Dis. **115:**295, 1977.

562. Popper, M.S., Bogdonoff, M.L., and Hughes, R.L.: Interstitial rheumatoid lung disease, Chest **62:**243, 1972.

563. Sahn, S.A., Kaplan, R.L., Maulitz, R.M., and Good, J.T., Jr.: Rheumatoid pleurisy: observations on the development of low pleural fluid pH and glucose level, JAMA **140:**1237, 1980.

564. Salerni, R., Rodnan, G.P., Leon, D.F., et al.: Pulmonary hypertension in the CREST syndrome variant of progressive systemic sclerosis (scleroderma), Ann. Intern. Med. **86:**394, 1977.

565. Salmeron, G., Greenberg, D., and Lidsky, M.D.: Polymyositis and diffuse interstitial lung disease: a review of the pulmonary histopathologic findings, Arch. Intern. Med. **141:**1005, 1981.

566. Scott, R.F., Thomas, W.A., and Kissane, J.M.: Rheumatic pneumonitis: pathologic features, J. Pediatr. **54:**60, 1959.

567. Strimlan, C.V., Rosenow, E.C., III, Divertie, M.B., et al.: Pulmonary manifestations of Sjögren's syndrome, Chest **70:**354, 1976.

568. Teilum, G., and Paulsen, H.E.: Disseminated lupus erythematosus: histopathology, morphogenesis and relation to allergy, Arch. Pathol. **64:**414, 1957.

569. Walker, W.C., and Wright, V.: Pulmonary lesion and rheumatoid arthritis, Medicine **47:**501, 1968.

570. Young, R.H., and Mark, G.J.: Pulmonary vascular changes in scleroderma, Am. J. Med. **64:**998, 1978.

571. Yousem, S.A., Colby, T.V., and Carrington, C.B.: Lung biopsy in rheumatoid arthritis, Am. Rev. Respir. Dis. **131:**770, 1985.

Goodpasture's syndrome and vasculitis

572. Abboud, R.T., Chase, W.H., Ballon, H.S., Grzybowski, S., and Magil, A.: Goodpasture's syndrome: diagnosis by transbronchial lung biopsy, Ann. Intern. Med. **89:**635, 1978.

573. Beirne, A.J., Octaviano, G.N., Kopp, W.L., et al.: Immunohistology of the lung in Goodpasture's syndrome, Ann. Intern. Med. **69:**1207, 1968.

574. Benoit, F.L., Rulon, D.B., Theil, G.B., et al.: Goodpasture's syndrome: a clinicopathologic entity, Am. J. Med. **37:**424, 1964.

575. Border, W.A., Baehler, R.W., Bhathena, D., and Glassock, R.J.: IgA antibasement membrane nephritis with pulmonary hemorrhage, Ann. Intern. Med. **91:**21, 1979.

576. Botting, A.J., Brown, A.L., and Divertie, M.D.: The pulmonary lesion in a patient with Goodpasture's syndrome as studied with the electron microscope, Am. J. Clin. Pathol. **42:**387, 1964.

577. Byrd, L.J., Shearn, M.A., and Tu, W.H.: Relationship of lethal midline granuloma to Wegener's granulomatosis, Arthritis Rheum. **12:**247, 1969.

578. Carrington, C.B., and Liebow, A.A.: Limited forms of angiitis and granulomatosus of the Wegener's type, Am. J. Med. **41:**497, 1966.

579. Chumbley, L.C., Harrison, E.G., and DeRemee, R.A.: Allergic granulomatosis and angiitis (Churg-Strauss syndrome): report and analysis of 30 cases, Mayo Clin. Proc. **52:**477, 1977.

580. Churg, J., and Strauss, L.: Allergic granulomatosis, allergic angiitis and periarteritis nodosa, Am. J. Pathol. **24:**277, 1956.

581. DeRemee, R.A., Weiland, L.H., and McDonald, T.J.: Respiratory vasculitis, Mayo Clin. Proc. **55:**492, 1980.

582. Donald, K.J., Edwards, R.L., and McEvoy, J.D.S.: Alveolar capillary basement membrane lesions in Goodpasture's syndrome and idiopathic pulmonary hemosiderosis, Am. J. Med. **59:**642, 1975.

583. Fauci, A.S., Haynes, B.F., and Katz, P.: The spectrum of vasculitis: clinical pathologic, immunologic, and therapeutic considerations, Ann. Intern. Med. **89:**660, 1978.

584. Fauci, A.S., and Wolff, S.M.: Wegener's granulomatosis: studies in eighteen patients and a review of the literature, Medicine **52:**535, 1973.

585. Godman, G., and Churg, J.: Wegener's granulomatosis: pathology and review of the literature, Arch. Pathol. **58:**533, 1954.

586. Katzenstein, A.L.: The histologic spectrum and differential diagnosis of necrotizing granulomatous inflammation of the lung, Prog. Surg. Pathol. **1:**41, 1980.

587. Kefalides, N.A.: The Goodpasture antigen and basement membranes: the search must go on, Lab. Invest. **56:**1, 1987.

588. Koffler, D., Sandson, J., Carr, R., et al.: Immunologic studies concerning the pulmonary lesions in Goodpasture's syndrome, Am. J. Pathol. **54:**293, 1969.

589. Liebow, A.A.: Pulmonary angiitis and granulomatosis, Am. Rev. Respir. Dis. **108:**1, 1973.

590. Walton, E.W.: Giant cell granuloma of the respiratory tract (Wegener's granulomatosis), Br. Med. J. **2:**265, 1958.

591. Zeek, P.: Polyarteritis nodosa and other forms of necrotizing angiitis, N. Engl. J. Med. **248:**764, 1953.

Other noninfectious granulomas
Pulmonary histiocytosis X

592. Auld, D.: Pathology of eosinophilic granuloma of the lung, Arch. Pathol. **63:**113, 1957.

593. Basset, F., Corrin, B., Spencer, H., Lacronique, J., Roth, C., Soler, P., Battesti, J.P., Georges, R., and Chrétien, J.: Pulmonary histiocytosis X, Am. Rev. Respir. Dis. **118:**811, 1978.

594. Basset, F., Soler, P., Wyllie, L., et al.: Langerhans' cells and lung interstitium, Ann. NY Acad. Sci. **278:**599, 1976.

595. Corrin, B., and Basset, F.: A review of histiocytosis X with particular reference to eosinophilic granuloma of the lung, Invest. Cell Pathol. **2:**137, 1979.

596. Friedman, P.J., Liebow, A.A., and Sokoloff, J.: Eosinophilic granuloma of the lung, Medicine **60:**385, 1981.

597. Newton, W.A., and Hamoudi, A.B.: Histiocytosis: a histologic classification with clinical correlation, Perspect. Pediatr. Pathol. **1:**251, 1973.

598. Silberberg-Sinakin, I., Baer, R.L., and Thorbecke, G.J.: Langerhans cells: a review of their nature with emphasis on their immunologic functions, Prog. Allergy **24:**268, 1978.

Sarcoidosis

599. Azar, H.A., Moscovic, E.A., Abu-Nassar, S.G., et al.: Some aspects of sarcoidosis, Curr. Top. Pathol. **57:**49, 1973.

600. Black, M.M., and Epstein, W.L.: Formation of multinucleate giant cells in organized epithelioid cell granulomas, Am. J. Pathol. **74:**263, 1974.

601. Cain, H., and Kraus, B.: Asteroid bodies: derivatives of the cytosphere, Virchows Arch. [Cell Pathol.] **26:**119, 1977.

602. Carrington, C.B.: Structure and function in sarcoidosis, Ann. NY Acad. Sci. **278:**265, 1976.

603. Churg, A., Carrington, C.B., and Gupta, R.: Necrotizing sarcoid granulomatosis, Chest **76:**406, 1979.

604. Crystal, R.G., Bitterman, P.B., Rennard, S.I., Hance, A.J., and Keogh, B.A.: Interstitial lung diseases of unknown cause: disorders characterized by chronic inflammation of the lower respiratory tract, N. Engl. J. Med. **310:**235, 1984.

605. Dauber, J.H., Rossman, M.D., and Daniele, R.P.: Bronchoalveolar cell populations in acute sarcoidosis, J. Lab. Clin. Med. **94:**862, 1979.

606. DeRemee, R.A.: The roentgen staging of sarcoidosis: historic and contemporary perspectives, Chest **83:**128, 1981.

607. Huang, C.T., Heurich, A.E., Rosen, Y., Moon, S., and Lyons, H.A.: Pulmonary sarcoidosis: roentgenographic, functional, and pathologic correlations, Respiration **37:**337, 1979.

608. Hunninghake, G.W., and Crystal, R.G.: Pulmonary sarcoidosis: a disorder mediated by excess helper T-lymphocyte activity at sites of disease activity, N. Engl. J. Med. **305:**429, 1981.

609. Israel, H.L.: Influence of race and geographical origin on sarcoidosis, Arch. Environ. Health **20:**608, 1970.

610. James, G.D., and Neville, E.: Pathology of sarcoidosis, Pathobiol. Annu. **7:**31, 1977.

611. Jones-Williams, W., et al.: The fine structure of sarcoid and tuberculous granulomas, Postgrad. Med. J. **46:**496, 1970.

612. Mitchell, D.N., and Scadding, J.G.: State of the art, Sarcoidosis **110:**774, 1974.

613. Rosen, Y., Athanassides, T.J., Moon, S., and Lyons, H.A.: Nongranulomatous interstitial pneumonitis in sarcoidosis, Chest **74**:122, 1978.

614. Rosen, Y., Vuletin, J.C., Pertschuk, L.P., and Silverstein, E.: Sarcoidosis from the pathologist's vantage point, Pathol. Annu. **14**:405, 1979.

615. Scadding, J.G.: Sarcoidosis, London, 1967, Eyre & Spotiswoode.

616. Thomas, P.D., and Hunninghake, G.W.: Current concepts of the pathogenesis of sarcoidosis, Am. Rev. Respir. Dis. **135**:747, 1987.

Miscellaneous lung diseases
Alveolar proteinosis

617. Bedrossian, C.W., Luna, M.A., Conklin, R.H., and Miller, W.C.: Alveolar proteinosis as a consequence of immunosuppression: a hypothesis based on clinical and pathologic observations, Hum. Pathol. **11**:527, 1980.

618. Bell, D.Y., and Hook, G.E.R.: Pulmonary alveolar proteinosis: analysis of airway and alveolar proteins, Am. Rev. Respir. Dis. **119**:979, 1979.

619. Carson, R.K., and Gordinier, R.: Pulmonary alveolar proteinosis: report of six cases, review of the literature and formulation of a new theory, Ann. Intern. Med. **62**:292, 1965.

620. Golde, D.W., Territo, M., Finley, T.N., et al.: Defective lung macrophages in pulmonary alveolar proteinosis, Ann. Intern. Med. **85**:304, 1976.

621. Hook, G.E.R., Bell, D.Y., Gilmore, L.B., Nadeau, D., Reasor, M.J., and Talley, F.A.: Composition of bronchoalveolar lavage effluents from patients with pulmonary alveolar proteinosis, Lab. Invest. **39**:342, 1978.

622. Kuhn, C., Györkey, F., Levine, B.E., et al.: Pulmonary alveolar proteinosis, Lab. Invest. **15**:492, 1966.

623. McClenahan, J.B., and Mussenden, R.: Pulmonary alveolar proteinosis, Arch. Intern. Med. **133**:284, 1974.

624. McEuen, D.D., and Abraham, J.L.: Particulate concentrations in pulmonary alveolar proteinosis, Environ. Res. **17**:334, 1978.

625. Ramírez-R., J., and Harlan, W.R.: Pulmonary alveolar proteinosis: nature and origin of alveolar lipid, Am. J. Med. **45**:502, 1968.

626. Ramírez-R., J., Nuka, W., and McLaughlin, J.: Pulmonary alveolar proteinosis: diagnostic technique and observations, N. Engl. J. Med. **268**:165, 1963.

627. Ramírez-R., J., Savard, E.V., and Hawkins, J.E.: Biological effect of pulmonary washings from cases of alveolar proteinosis, Am. Rev. Respir. Dis. **94**:244, 1966.

628. Rosen, S.H., Castleman, B., and Liebow, A.A.: Pulmonary alveolar proteinosis, N. Engl. J. Med. **258**:1123, 1958.

629. Singh, G., Katyal, S.L., Bedrossian, C.W., and Rogers, R.M.: Pulmonary alveolar proteinosis: staining for surfactant apoprotein in alveolar proteinosis and in conditions simulating it, Chest **83**:82, 1983.

Alveolar microlithiasis; metastatic calcification and ossification

630. Conger, J.D., Hammond, W.S., Alfrey, A.C., et al.: Pulmonary calcifications in chronic dialysis patients: clinical and pathologic studies, Ann. Intern. Med. **83**:330, 1975.

631. Koss, M.N., Johnson, F.B., and Hochholzer, L.: Pulmonary blue bodies, Hum. Pathol. **12**:258, 1981.

632. Michaels, L., and Levene, C.: Corpora amylacea of lung, J. Pathol. Bacteriol. **74**:49, 1957.

633. O'Neill, R.P., Cohn, J.E., and Pellegrino, E.D.: Pulmonary alveolar microlithiasis—a family study, Ann. Intern. Med. **67**:957, 1967.

634. Pear, B.L.: Idiopathic disseminated pulmonary ossification, Radiology **91**:746, 1968.

635. Popelka, C.G., and Kleinerman, J.: Diffuse pulmonary ossification, Arch. Intern. Med. 523, 1977.

636. Prakash, U.B., Barham, S.S., Rosenow, E.C., III, Brown, M.L., and Payne, W.S.: Pulmonary alveolar microlithiasis: a review including ultrastructural and pulmonary function studies, Mayo Clin. Proc. **58**:290, 1983.

637. Sears, M.R., Chang, A.R., and Taylor, A.J.: Pulmonary alveolar microlithiasis, Thorax **26**:704, 1971.

Amyloidosis of the lung

638. Celli, B.R., Rubinow, A., Cohen, A.S., and Brody, J.S.: Patterns of pulmonary involvement in systemic amyloidosis, Chest **74**:543, 1978.

639. Dyke, P.C., Demaray, M.J., Delavan, J.W., et al.: Pulmonary amyloidoma, Am. J. Clin. Pathol. **61**:301, 1974.

640. Prowse, C.B.: Amyloidosis of the lower respiratory tract, Thorax **13**:308, 1958.

641. Rajan, V.T., and Kikkawa, Y.: Alveolar septal amyloidosis in primary amyloidosis, Arch. Pathol. **89**:521, 1970.

642. Rubinow, A., Celli, B.R., Cohen, A.S., Rigden, B.G., and Brody, J.S.: Localized amyloidosis of the lower respiratory tract, Am. Rev. Respir. Dis. **118**:603, 1978.

643. Thompson, P.J., and Citron, K.M.: Amyloid and the lower respiratory tract, Thorax **38**:84, 1983.

Lymphangiomyomatosis

644. Basset, F., Soler, P., Marsac, J., et al.: Pulmonary lymphangiomyomatosis: three new cases studied with electron microscopy, Cancer **38**:2357, 1976.

645. Carrington, C.B., Cugell, D.W., Gaensler, E.A., Marks, A., Redding, R.A., Schaaf, J.T., and Tomasian, A.: Lymphangioleiomyomatosis: physiologic-pathologic-radiologic correlations, Am. Rev. Respir. Dis. **116**:977, 1977.

646. Corrin, B., Liebow, A.A., and Friedman, P.J.: Pulmonary lymphangiomyomatosis: a review, Am. J. Pathol. **79**:347, 1975.

Drug- and radiation-induced pulmonary disease

647. Bedrossian, C.M.W.: Pathology of drug-induced lung diseases, Semin. Respir. Med. **4**:98, 1982.

647a. Cooper, A.C., et al.: Drug-induced pulmonary disease, Am. Rev. Respir. Dis. **133**:321, 340, 1986.

648. Gross, N.J.: Pulmonary effects of radiation therapy, Ann. Intern. Med. **86**:81, 1977.

649. Holoye, P.Y., Luna, M.A., MacKay, B., and Bedrossian, C.W.: Bleomycin hypersensitivity pneumonitis, Ann. Intern. Med. **88**:47, 1978.

650. Iacovino, J.R., Leitner, J., Abbas, A.K., et al.: Fatal pulmonary reaction from low doses of bleomycin: an idiosyncratic tissue response, JAMA **235**:1253, 1976.

651. Jennings, F.L., and Arden, A.: Development of radiation pneumonitis: time and dose factors, Arch. Pathol. **74**:351, 1962.

652. Littler, W.A., Kay, J.M., Hasleton, P.S., et al.: Busulphan lung, Thorax **24**:639, 1969.

653. Luna, M.A., Bedrossian, C.W., Lichtiger, B., et al.: Interstitial pneumonitis associated with bleomycin therapy, Am. J. Clin. Pathol. **58**:501, 1972.

654. Rosenow, E.C.: The spectrum of drug-induced pulmonary disease, Ann. Intern. Med. **77**:977, 1972.

655. Sostman, H.D., Matthay, R.A., and Putman, C.E.: Cytotoxic drug-induced lung disease, Am. J. Med. **62**:608, 1977.

656. Warren, S., and Spencer, J.: Radiation reaction in the lung, AJR **43**:682, 1940.

657. Weiss, R.B., and Muggia, F.M.: Cytotoxic drug-induced pulmonary disease: update 1980, Am. J. Med. **68**:259, 1980.

Pulmonary hemorrhage

658. Buja, L.M., Freed, T.A., Berman, M.A., et al.: Pulmonary alveolar hemorrhage: a common finding in patients with severe cardiac disease, Am. J. Cardiol. **27**:168, 1971.

659. Dordan, C.J., Srodes, C.H., and Duffy, F.D.: Idiopathic pulmonary hemosiderosis: electron microscopic, immunofluorescent and iron kinetic studies, Chest **68**:577, 1975.

660. Golde, D.W., et al.: Occult pulmonary hemorrhage in leukemia, Br. Med. J. **2**:166, 1975.

661. González-Crussi, F., Hull, M.T., and Grossfeld, J.L.: Idiopathic pulmonary hemosiderosis: evidence of capillary basement membrane abnormality, Am. Rev. Respir. Dis. **114**:689, 1976.

662. Hukill, P.B.: Experimental pulmonary hemosiderosis: the liability of pulmonary iron deposits, Lab. Invest. **12**:577, 1963.

663. Hyatt, R.W., Adelstein, E.R., Halazun, J.F., et al.: Ultrastructure of the lung in idiopathic pulmonary hemosiderosis, Am. J. Med. **58**:822, 1972.

664. Irwin, R.S., Cottrell, T.S., Hsu, K.C., et al.: Idiopathic pulmonary hemosiderosis: an electron microscopic and immunofluorescent study, Chest **65**:41, 1974.

665. Morgan, P.G.M., and Turner-Warwick, M.: Pulmonary haemosiderosis and pulmonary haemorrhage, Br. J. Dis. Chest **75**:225, 1981.

666. Smith, L.J., and Katzenstein, A.L.A.: Pathogenesis of massive pulmonary hemorrhage in acute leukemia, Arch. Intern. Med. **142**:2149, 1982.

667. Soergel, K.H., and Sommers, S.C.: Idiopathic pulmonary hemosiderosis and related syndromes, Am. J. Med. **32**:499, 1962.

Aspiration pneumonia; lipid pneumonia; lung collapse and pneumothorax

668. Askin, F.B.: McCann, B.G., and Kuhn, C.: Reactive eosinophilic pleuritis: a lesion to be distinguished from pulmonary eosinophilic granuloma, Arch. Pathol. Lab. Med. **101**:187, 1977.

669. Borrie, J., and Gwynne, J.F.: Paraffinoma of lung: lipid, pneumonia, Thorax **28**:214, 1973.

670. Licter, I., and Gwynne, J.F.: Spontaneous pneumothorax in young subjects: a clinical and pathological study, Thorax **26**:409, 1971.

671. Miller, G.J., Ashcroft, M.T., Beadnell, H.M., et al.: The lipoid pneumonia of Blackfat tobacco smokers in Guyana, Q. J. Med. **40**:457, 1971.

672. Oldenburger, D., Mauer, W.J., Beltaos, E., et al.: Inhalation lipoid pneumonia from burning fats, JAMA **222**:1288, 1972.

673. Rigg, J.R.A.: Pulmonary atelectasis after anesthesia: pathophysiology and management, Can. Anaesth. Soc. J. **28**:305, 1981.

674. Timmerman, B.J., and Schroer, J.A.: Lipid pneumonia caused by methenamine mandelate suspension, JAMA **225**:1524, 1973.

675. Wynne, J.W., and Modell, J.H.: Respiratory aspiration of stomach contents, Ann. Intern. Med. **87**:466, 1977.

Chronic airflow limitation

676. Anderson, A.E., and Foraker, A.G.: Centrilobular emphysema and panlobular emphysema: two different diseases, Thorax **28**:547, 1973.

677. Anderson, J.A., Dunnill, M.S., and Ryder, R.C.: Dependence of the incidence of emphysema on smoking history, age and sex, Thorax **27**:547, 1972.

678. Auerbach, O., Hammond, E.C., Garfinkel, L., et al.: Relation of smoking and age to emphysema: whole lung section study, N. Engl. J. Med. **286**:853, 1972.

679. Bates, D.V.: The fate of the chronic bronchitic: a report of the ten-year follow-up in the Canadian Department of Veteran's Affairs coordinated study of chronic bronchitis, Am. Rev. Respir. Dis. **108**:1043, 1973.

680. Beatty, K., Robertie, P., Senior, R.M., and Travis, J.: Determination of oxidized alpha-1-proteinase inhibitor in serum, J. Lab. Clin. Med. **100**:186, 1982.

681. Berend, N., Woolcock, A.J., and Marlin, G.E.: Correlation between the function and structure of the lung in smokers, Am. Rev. Respir. Dis. **119**:695, 1979.

682. Berend, N., Wright, J.L., Thurlbeck, W.M., Marlin, G.E., and Woolcock, A.J.: Small airways disease: reproduceability of measurements and correlation with lung function, Chest **79**:263, 1981.

683. Boushy, S.F., Aboumrad, M.H., North, L.B., et al.: Lung recoil pressure, airway resistance and forced flows related to morphologic emphysema, Am. Rev. Respir. Dis. **104**:551, 1971.

684. Burrows, B., Fletcher, C.M., Heard, B.E., et al.: The emphysematous and bronchial types of chronic airways obstruction: a clinicopathologic study of patients in London and Chicago, Lancet **1**:830, 1966.

685. Burrows, B., Knudson, R.J., Cline, M.G., et al.: Quantitative relationship between cigarette smoking and ventilatory function, Am. Rev. Respir. Dis. **115**:195, 1977.

686. Carrell, R.W.: Alpha-1-antitrypsin: molecular pathology, leucocytes and tissue damage, J. Cin. Invest. **78**:1427, 1986.

687. Chapman, H.A., and Stone, O.L.: Comparison of live human neutrophil and alveolar macrophage elastolytic activity in vitro, J. Clin. Invest. **74**:1693, 1984.

688. Cosio, M.G., Hale, K.A., and Niewoehner, D.E.: Morphologic and morphometric effects of prolonged cigarette smoking on the small airways, Am. Rev. Respir. Dis. **122**:265, 1980.

689. Cromie, J.B.: Correlation of anatomic pulmonary emphysema and right ventricular hypertrophy, Am. Rev. Respir. Dis. **84**:657, 1961.

690. Depierre, A., Bignon, J., Lebeau, A., et al.: Quantitative study of parenchyma and small conductive airways in chronic non-specific lung disease, Chest **62**:699, 1972.

691. Dunnill, M.S.: An assessment of the anatomical factor in cor pulmonale in emphysema, J. Clin. Pathol. **14**:246, 1961.

692. Eriksson, S.: Studies in alpha-1-antitrypsin deficiency, Acta Med. Scand. **177**(suppl. 432):1, 1965.

693. Ferris, B.G.: Air pollution. In Macklen, P.T., and Permutt, S., editors: The lung in transition between health and disease, New York, 1979, Marcel Dekker.

694. Fletcher, C., and Peto, R.: The natural history of chronic airflow obstruction, Br. Med. J. **1**:1645, 1977.

695. Fletcher, C., et al.: The natural history of chronic bronchitis and emphysema, Oxford, Engl., 1976, Oxford University Press.

696. Greenberg, S.D., Jenkins, D.E., Stevens, P.M., et al.: The lungs in homozygous alpha$_1$-antitrypsin deficiency, Am. J. Clin. Pathol. **60**:581, 1973.

697. Haas, H., et al.: Bacterial flora of the respiratory tract in chronic bronchitis: comparison of transtracheal, fiberbronchoscopic, and oropharyngeal sampling methods, Am. Rev. Respir. Dis. **116**:41, 1977.

698. Heard, B.E., Khatchatourov, V., Otto, H., Putov, N.V., and Sobin, L.: The morphology of emphysema, chronic bronchitis and bronchiectasis: definition, nomenclature and classification, J. Clin. Pathol. **32**:882, 1979.

699. Heppleston, A.G., and Leopold, J.G.: Chronic pulmonary emphysema: anatomy and pathogenesis, Am. J. Med. **31**:279, 1961.

700. Hogg, J.C., Macklem, P.T., and Thurlbeck, W.M.: Site and nature of airway obstruction in chronic obstructive lung disease, N. Engl. J. Med. **278**:1355, 1968.

701. Holland, W.W., and Reid, D.D.: The urban factor in chronic bronchitis, Lancet **1**:445, 1965.

702. Ishikawa, S., Bowden, D.H., Fisher, V., et al.: The "emphysema profile" in two midwestern cities in North America, Arch. Environ. Health **18**:660, 1969.

703. Janoff, A.: Elastases and emphysema: current assessment of the protease-antiprotease hypothesis, Am. Rev. Respir. Dis. **132**:417, 1985.

704. Karlinksy, J.B., and Snider, G.I.: Animal models of emphysema, Am. Rev. Respir. Dis. **117**:1109, 1978.

705. Kuhn, C., Senior, R.M., and Pierce, J.A.: The pathogenesis of emphysema. In Witschi, H.P., and Nettesheim, P., editors: Mechanisms in respiratory toxicology, Boca Raton, Fla., 1982, CRC Press.

706. Kuhn, C., and Tavassoli, F.: Scanning electron microscopy of elastase-induced emphysema: a comparison with emphysema in man, Lab. Invest. **34**:2, 1976.

707. Lellouch, J., Claude, J.R., Martin, J.P., Orssaud, G., Zaoui, D., and Bieth, J.G.: Smoking does not reduce the functional activity of serum alpha-1-proteinase inhibitor, Am. Rev. Respir. Dis. **132**:818, 1985.

708. Linhartova, A., Anderson, A.E., and Foraker, A.G.: Further observations on luminal deformity and stenosis of non-respiratory bronchioles in pulmonary emphysema, Thorax **32**:53, 1977.

709. Macklem, P.T., Thurlbeck, W.M., and Fraser, R.G.: Chronic obstructive disease of small airways, Ann. Intern. Med. **74**:167, 1971.

710. Martelli, N.A.: Lower-zone emphysema in young patients without α_1-antitrypsin deficiency, Thorax **29**:237, 1974.

711. Matsuba, K., and Thurlbeck, W.M.: The number and dimensions of small airways in emphysematous lungs, Am. J. Pathol. **67**:265, 1972.

712. Matsuba, K., and Thurlbeck, W.M.: Disease of small airways in chronic bronchitis, Am. Rev. Respir. Dis. **107**:552, 1973.

713. McNamara, M.J., Philips, I.A., and Williams, O.B.: Viral and *Mycoplasma pneumoniae* infections in excerbations of chronic lung disease, Am. Rev. Respir. Dis. **100**:19, 1969.

714. Mitchell, R.S., et al.: Are centrilobular emphysema and panlobular emphysema two different diseases? Hum. Pathol. **1**:433, 1970.

715. Mitchell, R.S., Stanford, R.E., Johnson, J.M., et al.: The morphologic features of the bronchi, bronchioles, and alveoli in chronic airway obstruction: a clinicopathologic study, Am. Rev. Respir. Dis. **114**:137, 1976.

716. Mitchell, R.S., Stanford, R.E., Silvers, G.W., et al.: The right ventricle in chronic airway obstruction: a clinicopathologic study, Am. Rev. Respir. Dis. **114**:147, 1976.

717. Morse, J.O.: Alpha-1-antitrypsin deficiency, N. Engl. J. Med. **299**:1045, 1099, 1978.

718. Oswald, N.C.: Chronic bronchitis: factors in pathogenesis and their clinical application, Lancet **1**:271, 1954.

719. Park, S.S., Janis, M., Shim, C.S., et al.: Relationship of bronchitis and emphysema to altered pulmonary function, Am. Rev. Respir. Dis. **102**:927, 1970.

720. Pump, K.K.: Fenestrae in the alveolar membrane of the human lung, Chest **65**:431, 1974.

721. Pump, K.K.: Emphysema and its relation to age, Am. Rev. Respir. Dis. **114**:5, 1976.

722. Reid, L.: Measurement of the bronchial mucous gland layer: a diagnostic yardstick in chronic bronchitis, Thorax **15**:132, 1960.

723. Reid, L.M.: Pathology of chronic bronchitis, Lancet **1**:275, 1954.

724. Restrepo, G., and Heard, B.E.: The size of the bronchial glands in chronic bronchitis, J. Pathol. Bacteriol. **85**:305, 1963.

725. Ryan, S.F., Vincent, T.N., Mitchell, R.S., et al.: Ductectasia: an asymptomatic pulmonary change related to age, Med. Thorac. **22**:181, 1965.

726. Snider, G.L., et al.: The definition of emphysema: report of a National Heart Lung and Blood Institute, Division of Lung Disease workshop, Am. Rev. Respir. Dis. **132**:182, 1985.

727. Spain, D.M., Siegel, H., and Bradess, V.A.: Emphysema in apparently healthy adults: smoking, age, and sex, JAMA **224**:322, 1973.

728. Tager, I., and Speizer, F.E.: Role of infection in chronic bronchitis, N. Engl. J. Med. **292**:563, 1975.

729. Takizawa, T., and Thurlbeck, W.M.: Muscle and mucous gland size in the major bronchi of patients with chronic bronchitis, asthma, and asthmatic bronchitis, Am. Rev. Respir. Dis. **104**:331, 1971.

730. Thurlbeck, W.M.: Chronic airflow obstruction in lung disease, Philadelphia, 1976, W.B. Saunders Co.

731. Thurlbeck, W.M., Ryder, R.C., and Sternby, N.: A comparative study of the severity of emphysema in necropsy populations in three different countries, Am. Rev. Respir. Dis. **109**:239, 1974.

732. Wagner, P.D., Dantzker, D.R., Dueck, R., et al.: Ventilation-perfusion inequality in chronic obstructive pulmonary disease, J. Clin. Invest. **59**:203, 1977.

733. Wright, J.L., Hobson, J., Wiggs, B.R., Pare, P.D., and Hogg, J.C.: Effect of cigarette smoking on structure of the small airways, Lung **165**:91, 1987.

734. Wright, R.R.: Elastic tissue of normal and emphysematous lungs: a tridimensional histologic study, Am. J. Pathol. **39**:355, 1961.

Pneumoconiosis

735. Allison, A.C., and D'Arcy Hart, P.: Potentiation by silica of the growth of *Mycobacterium tuberculosis* in macrophage cultures, Br. J. Exp. Pathol. **49**:465, 1968.

736. Becklake, M.R.: Asbestos-related diseases of the lung and other organs: their epidemiology and implications for clinical practice, Am. Rev. Respir. Dis. **114**:187, 1976.

737. Brain, J.D., and Valberg, P.A.: Deposition of aerosol in the respiratory tract, Am. Rev. Respir. Dis. **120**:1325, 1979.

738. Buechner, H.A., and Ansari, A.: Acute silico-proteinosis: a new pathologic variant of acute silicosis in sandblasters characterized by histologic features resembing alveolar proteinosis, Dis. Chest **55**:247, 1969.

739. Caplan, A.: Certain radiological appearances in the chest of coalminers suffering from rheumatoid arthritis, Thorax **8**:29, 1953.

740. Cockcroft, A., Seal, R.M., Wagner, J.C., Lyons, J.P., Ryder, R., and Andersson, N.: Postmortem study of emphysema in coalworkers and non-coalworkers, Lancet **2**:600, 1982.

741. Churg, A., and Golden, J.: Current problems in the pathology of asbestos-related disease, Pathol. Annu. **17**:33, 1982.

742. Craighead, J.E., Abraham, J.L., Churg, A., Green, F.H., Kleinerman, J., Pratt, P.C., Seemayer, T.A., Vallyathan, V., and Weill, H.: The pathology of asbestos-assisted diseases of the lungs and pleural cavities: diagnostic criteria and proposed grading schema, Arch. Pathol. Lab. Med. **106**:544, 1982.

743. Davis, J.M.G., Chapman, J., Collings, P., Douglas, A.N., Fernie, J., Lamb, D., and Ruckley, V.A.: Variations in the histological patterns of the lesions of coal workers' pneumoconiosis in Britain and their relationship to lung dust content, Am. Rev. Respir. Dis. **128**:118, 1983.

744. Edwards, C., Macartney, J., Rooke, G., et al.: The pathology of the lung in byssinotics, Thorax **30**:612, 1975.

745. Epler, G.R., McLoud, T.C., and Gaensler, E.A.: Prevalence and incidence of benign asbestos pleural effusion in a working population, JAMA **247**:617, 1982.

746. Freiman, D.G., and Hardy, H.L.: Beryllium disease, Hum. Pathol. **1**:25, 1970.

747. Gough, J.: Pneumoconiosis in coal trimmers, J. Pathol. Bacteriol. **51**:277, 1940.

748. Gough, J., Rivers, D., and Seal, R.M.E.: Pathological studies of modified pneumoconiosis in coal miners with rheumatoid arthritis (Caplan's syndrome), Thorax **10**:9, 1955.

749. Green, F.H.Y., and Laqueur, W.A.: Coal workers pneumoconiosis, Pathol. Annu. **15**:333, 1980.

750. Gross, P., Westrick, M.L., and McNerney, J.M.: Experimental tuberculosilicosis: a comparison of the effects produced by some of its various pathogenic components, Am. Rev. Respir. Dis. **83**:510, 1961.

751. Hammond, E.C., Selikoff, I.J., and Seidman, H.: Asbestos exposure, cigarette smoking and death rates, Ann. NY Acad. Sci. **330**:473, 1979.

752. Heppleston, A.G.: The pathogenesis of simple pneumokoniosis in coal workers, J. Pathol. Bacteriol. **67**:51, 1954.

753. Heppleston, A.G., and Styles, J.A.: Activity of a macrophage factor in collagen formation by silica, Nature **214**:521, 1967.

754. Holt, P.C., and Keast, D.: Environmentally induced changes in immunological function: acute and chronic effects of inhalation of tobacco smoke and other atmospheric contaminants in man and experimental animals, Bacteriol. Rev. **41**:205, 1977.

755. Kane, A.B., Stanton, R.P., Raymond, E.G., Dobson, M.E., Knafelc, M.E., and Farber, J.L.: Dissociation of intracellular lysosomal rupture from the cell death caused by silica, J. Cell Biol. **87**:643, 1980.

756. Kannerstein, M., and Churg, J.: Pathology of carcinoma of the lung associated with asbestos exposure, Cancer **30**:14, 1972.

757. Kleinerman, J., et al.: Pathology standards for coal workers pneumoconiosis, Arch. Pathol. Lab. Med. **103**:375, 1979.

758. Kriebel, D., et al.: The pulmonary toxicity of beryllium, Am. Rev. Respir. Dis. **137**:464, 1988.

759. Kuhn, C., and Kuo, T.: Cytoplasmic hyalin in asbestosis, Arch. Pathol. **95**:189, 1973.

760. Lyons, J.P., Ryder, R., Campbell, H., et al.: Pulmonary disability in coalworkers' pneumoconiosis, Br. Med. J. **1**:713, 1972.

761. Morgan, W.K.C.: Respiratory disease in coal miners, JAMA **231**:1347, 1975.

762. Morgan, W.K.C., and Lapp, N.L.: Respiratory disease in coal miners, Am. Rev. Respir. Dis. **113**:531, 1976.

763. Naeye, R.L.: Black lung disease, the anthracotic pneumoconiosis, Pathol. Annu. **8**:349, 1973.

764. Naeye, R.L., and Dellinger, W.S.: Coal workers' pneumoconiosis: correlation of roentgenographic and postmortem findings, JAMA **220**:223, 1972.

765. Naeye, R.L., Mahon, J.K., and Dellinger, W.: Effects of smoking on lung structure of Appalachian coal workers, Arch. Environ. Health **22**:190, 1971.

766. Newman, J.K., Vatter, A.E., and Reiss, O.K.: Chemical and electron microscopic studies of the black pigment of the human lung, Arch. Environ. Health 5:420, 1967.

767. Parkes, W.R.: Occupational lung disorders, London, 1982, Butterworth & Co., Ltd.

768. Reiser, K.M., and Last, J.A.: Silicosis and fibrogenesis: fact and artifact, Toxicology 17:51, 1979.

769. Ryder, R., Lyons, J.P., Campbell, H., et al.: Emphysema in coal workers' pneumoconiosis, Br. Med. J. 3:481, 1970.

770. Schmidt, J.A., Oliver, C.N., Lepe-Zuniga, J.L., Green, I., and Gery, I.: Silica-stimulated monocytes release fibroblast proliferation factors identical to interleukin 1: a potential role for interleukin 1 in the pathogenesis of silicosis, J. Clin. Invest. 73:1462, 1984.

771. Selikoff, I.J., Hammond, E.C., and Seidman, H.: Mortality experience of insulation workers in the United States and Canada, Ann. NY Acad. Sci. 330:91, 1979.

772. Selikoff, I.J., Micholson, W.J., and Langer, A.M.: Asbestos air pollution, Arch. Environ. Health 25:1, 1972.

773. Silicosis and Silicate Disease Committee: Diseases associated with exposure to silica and non-fibrous silicate materials, Arch. Pathol. Lab. Med. 112:673, 1988.

774. Slatkin, D.N., Friedman, L., Irsa, A.P., and Gaffney, J.S.: The $^{13}C/^{12}C$ ratio in black pulmonary pigment: a mass spectrometric study, Hum. Pathol. 9:259, 1978.

775. Snider, D.E.: The relationship between tuberculosis and silicosis, Am. Rev. Respir. Dis. 118:455, 1978.

776. Suzuki, Y., and Churg, J.: Formation of the asbestos body: a comparative study with three types of asbestos, Environ. Res. 3:107, 1969.

777. Uber, C.L., and McReynolds, R.A.: Immunotoxicology of silica, CRC Crit. Rev. Toxicol. 303, 1982.

778. Vorwald, A.F.: Cavities in the silicotic lung: a pathological study with clinical correlation, Am. J. Pathol. 17:709, 1941.

779. Wagner, J.C., Sleggs, C.A., and Marchand, P.: Diffuse pleural mesothelioma and asbestos exposure in the North Western Cape Province, Br. J. Ind. Med. 17:260, 1960.

780. Watson, A.J., et al.: Pneumoconiosis in carbon electrode makers, Br. J. Ind. Med. 16:274, 1959.

781. Whitwell, F., Newhouse, M.L., and Bennett, D.R.: A study of the histological cell types of lung cancer in workers suffering from asbestosis in the United Kingdom, Br. J. Ind. Med. 31:298, 1974.

782. Wood, W.B., and Gloyne, S.R.: Pulmonary asbestosis, Lancet 1:445, 1930.

783. Wyatt, J.P.: Morphogenesis of pneumoconiosis occurring in southern Illinois bituminous workers, Arch. Indust. Health 21:445, 1961.

784. Ziskind, M., Jones, R.N., and Weill, H.: State of the art: silicosis, Am. Rev. Respir. Dis. 113:643, 1976.

Lung tumors
Carcinomas of the lung

785. Albain, K.S., True, L.D., Golomb, H.M., Hoffman, P.C., and Little, A.G.: Large cell carcinoma of the lung, Cancer 56:1618, 1985.

786. Ashley, D.J.B., and Davies, H.D.: Cancer of the lung: histology and biological behavior, Cancer 20:165, 1967.

787. Auerbach, O., Hammond, E.C., and Garfinkel, L.: Changes in bronchial epithelium in relation to cigarette smoking, 1955-1960 vs. 1970-1977, N. Engl. J. Med. 300:381, 1979.

788. Auerbach, O., et al.: Changes in bronchial epithelium in relation to cigarette smoking and in relation to lung cancer, N. Engl. J. Med. 265:253, 1961.

789. Auerbach, O., Frasca, J.M., Parks, V.R., and Carter, H.W.: Comparison of World Health Organization (WHO) classification of lung tumors by light and electron microscopy, Cancer 50:2079, 1982.

790. Azzopardi, J.G.: Oat cell carcinoma of the bronchus, J. Pathol. Bacteriol. 78:513, 1959.

791. Azzopardi, J.G., and Bellau, A.R.: Carcinoid syndrome and oat cell carcinoma of the bronchus, Thorax 20:393, 1965.

792. Beck, C., and Burger, H.G.: Evidence for presence of immunoreactive growth hormone in cancers of lung and stomach, Cancer 30:75, 1972.

793. Bedrossian, C.W., Weilbaecher, D.G., Bentinck, D.C., et al.: Ultrastructure of human bronchioloalveolar cell carcinoma, Cancer 36:1399, 1975.

794. Bender, R.A., and Hansen, H.: Hypercalcemia in bronchogenic carcinoma: a prospective study of 200 patients, Ann. Intern. Med. 80:205, 1974.

795. Bennett, D.E., and Sasser, W.F.: Bronchiolar carcinoma: a valid clinicopathologic entity? A study of 30 cases, Cancer 24:876, 1969.

796. Bennett, D.E., Sasser, W.F., and Ferguson, T.B.: Adenocarcinoma of the lung in men: a clinicopathologic study of 100 cases, Cancer 23:431, 1969.

797. Bensch, K.G., Corrin, B., Pariente, R., et al.: Oat-cell carcinoma of the lung: its origin and relationship to the bronchial carcinoid, Cancer 22:1163, 1968.

798. Bjelke, E.: Dietary vitamin A and human lung cancer, Int. J. Cancer 15:561, 1975.

799. Bolen, J.W., and Thorning, D.: Histogenetic classification of pulmonary carcinomas: peripheral adenocarcinomas studied by light microscopy, histochemistry and electron microscopy, Pathol. Annu. 17:77, 1982.

800. Bondy, P.K., and Gilby, E.D.: Endocrine function in small cell undifferentiated carcinoma of the lung, Cancer 50:2147, 1982.

801. Byrd, R.B., Miller, W.E., Carr, D.T., et al.: The roentgenographic appearance of large cell carcinoma of the bronchus, Mayo Clin. Proc. 43:333, 1968.

802. Byrd, R.B., Miller, W.E., Carr, D.T., et al.: The roentgenographic appearance of squamous cell carcinoma of the bronchus, Mayo Clin. Proc. 43:327, 1968.

803. Carney, D.N., Matthews, M.J., Ihde, D.C., Bunn, P.A., Jr., Cohen, M.H., Makuch, R.W., Gazdar, A.F., and Minna, J.D.: Influence of histologic subtype of small cell carcinoma of the lung on clinical presentation, response to therapy and survival, J. Natl. Cancer Inst. 65:1225, 1980.

804. Churg, A.: The fine structure of large cell undifferentiated carcinoma of the lung: evidence for its relation to squamous cell carcinomas and adenocarcinomas, Hum. Pathol. 9:143, 1978.

805. Colditz, G.A., Stampfer, M.J., and Willett, W.C.: Diet and lung cancer: a review of the epidemiologic evidence in humans, Arch. Intern. Med. 147:157, 1987.

806. Corson, J.M., and Pinkus, G.S.: Mesothelioma: profile of keratin proteins and carcinoembryonic antigen: an immunoperoxidase study of 20 cases and comparison with pulmonary adenocarcinomas, Am. J. Pathol. 108:80, 1982.

807. Cottrell, J.C., Becker, K.L., and Moore, C.: Immunofluorescent studies in gonadotropin-secreting bronchogenic carcinoma, Am. J. Clin. Pathol. 59:422, 1968.

808. Cuttita, F., Carney, D.N., Mulshine, J., Moody, T.W., Fedorko, J., Fischler, A., and Minna, J.D.: Bombesin-like peptides can function as autocrine growth factors in human small cell lung cancer, Nature 316:823, 1985.

809. Davis, S., Stanley, K.E., Yesner, R., Kuang, D.T., and Morris, J.F.: Small-cell carcinoma of the lung: survival according to histologic subtype, Cancer 47:1863, 1981.

810. Doll, R., and Peto, R.: Mortality in relation to smoking: 20 years' observations on male British doctors, Br. Med. J. 2:1525, 1976.

811. Doll, R., and Peto, R.: The cause of cancer: quantitative estimates of avoidable risks of cancer in the United States today, J. Natl. Cancer Inst. 66:1191, 1981.

812. Erisman, M.D., Linnoila, R.I., Hernandez, O., DiAugustine, R.P., and Lazarus, L.H.: Human lung small-cell carcinoma contains bombesin, Proc. Natl. Acad. Sci. USA 79:2379, 1982.

813. Feinstein, A.R.: Symptoms as an index of biological behavior and prognosis in human cancer, Nature 209:241, 1966.

814. Figueroa, W.G., Raszkowski, R., and Weiss, W.: Lung cancer in chloromethyl methyl ether workers, N. Engl. J. Med. 288:1096, 1973.

815. Flanagan, P., and Roeckel, I.E.: Giant cell carcinoma of the lung: anatomic and clinical correlation, Am. J. Med. 36:214, 1964.

816. Fraire, A.E., and Greenberg, S.D.: Carcinoma and diffuse interstitial fibrosis of lung, Cancer 31:1078, 1973.
817. Fraumeni, J.F.: Respiratory carcinogenesis: an epidemiologic appraisal, J. Natl. Cancer Inst. 55:1039, 1975.
818. Garfinkel, L.: Time trends in lung cancer mortality among nonsmokers and a note on passive smoking, J. Natl. Cancer Inst. 66:1061, 1981.
819. Gottlieb, M.S., Shear, C.L., and Seale, D.B.: Lung cancer mortality and residential proximity to industry, Environ. Health Perspect. 45:157, 1982.
820. Gould, V.E., Lee, I., and Warren, W.H.: Immunohistochemical evaluation of neuroendocrine cells and neoplasm of the lung, Pathol. Res. Pract. 183:200, 1988.
821. Graham, S., and Levin, M.L.: Smoking withdrawal and the reduction of risk of lung cancer, Cancer 27:865, 1971.
822. Greco, F.A., and Oldham, R.K.: Current concepts of cancer: small cell lung cancer, N. Engl. J. Med. 301:355, 1979.
823. Green, N., Kurohara, S.S., and George, F.W.: Cancer of the lung: in-depth analysis of prognostic factors, Cancer 25:1229, 1971.
824. Greenberg, S.D., Smith, M.N., and Spjut, H.J.: Bronchioloalveolar carcinoma: cell of origin, Am. J. Clin. Pathol. 63:153, 1975.
825. Hammond, E.C., and Horn, D.: The relationship between human smoking habits and death rates, JAMA 155:1316, 1954.
826. Hansen, M., Hammer, M., and Hammer, L.: ACTH, ADH and calcitonin concentrations as markers of response and relapse in small cell carcinoma of the lung, Cancer 46:2062, 1980.
827. Hansen, M., Hansen, H.H., Hirsch, F.R., Arends, J., Christensen, J.D., Christensen, J.M., Hummer, L., and Kühl, C.: Hormonal polypeptides and amine metabolites in small cell carcinoma of the lung with special reference to stage and subtypes, Cancer 45:1432, 1980.
828. Harbour, J.W., et al.: Abnormalities in structure and expression of the human retinoblastoma gene in SCLC, Science 241:353, 1988.
829. Hattori, S., Matsuda, M., Tateishi, R., et al.: Oat cell carcinoma of the lung: clinical and morphological studies in relation to its histogenesis, Cancer 30:1014, 1972.
830. Hirsch, F., Hansen, H.H., Dombernowsky, P., et al.: Bone-marrow examination of the staging of small-cell anaplastic carcinoma of the lung with special reference to subtyping: an evaluation of 203 consecutive patients, Cancer 39:2563, 1977.
831. Horie, A., and Ohta, M.: Ultrastructural features of large cell carcinoma of the lung with reference to the prognosis of patients, Hum. Pathol. 12:423, 1981.
832. Horne, J.W., and Asire, A.J.: Changes in lung cancer incidence and mortality rates among Americans: 1969-78, J. Natl. Cancer Inst. 69:833, 1982.
833. Hyde, L., and Hyde, C.I.: Clinical manifestations of lung cancer, Chest 65:299, 1974.
834. Iannuzzi, M.C., and Scoggin, C.H.: Small cell lung cancer, Am. Rev. Respir. Dis. 134:593, 1986.
835. Ives, J.C., Buffler, P.A., and Greenberg, S.D.: Environmental associations and histopathologic patterns of carcinoma of the lung: the challenge and dilemma in epidemiologic studies, Am. Rev. Respir. Dis. 128:195, 1983.
836. Kato, Y., Ferguson, T.B., Bennett, D.E., et al.: Oat cell carcinoma of the lung: a review of 138 cases, Cancer 23:517, 1969.
837. Kirsch, M.M., et al.: Effect of histological cell type of prognosis of patients with bronchogenic carcinoma, Ann. Thorac. Surg. 13:303, 1972.
838. Kreyberg, L.: Histological lung cancer types: a morphological and histological correlation, Oslo, 1962, Norwegian Universities Press.
839. Kuhn, C.: Fine structure of bronchioloalveolar cell carcinoma, Cancer 30:1107, 1972.
840. Liebow, A.A.: Bronchiolo-alveolar carcinoma, Adv. Intern. Med. 10:329, 1960.
841. Lokich, J.J.: The frequency and clinical biology of the ectopic hormone syndromes of small cell carcinoma, Cancer 50:2111, 1982.
842. Lukeman, J.M.: Reliability of cytologic diagnosis in cancer of the lung, Cancer Chemother. Rep. 4:79, 1973.
843. Marcq, M., and Galy, P.: Bronchioloalveolar carcinoma: clinical relationships, natural history, and prognosis in 29 cases, Am. Rev. Respir. Dis. 107:621, 1973.
844. Matthews, M.J.: Morphology of lung cancer, Semin. Oncol. 1:175, 1974.
845. McDonnell, L., and Long, J.P.: Lung scar cancer: a reappraisal, J. Clin. Pathol. 34:996, 1981.
846. McDowell, E.M., McLaughlin, J.S., Merenyl, D.K., Kieffer, R.F., Harris, C.C., and Trump, B.F.: The respiratory epithelium. V. Histogenesis of lung carcinomas in the human, J. Natl. Cancer Inst. 61:587, 1978.
847. Mendelsohn, G., et al.: Histopathologic, immunohistochemical and ultrastructural studies of lung carcinomas, Prog. Surg. Pathol. 6:127, 1986.
848. Mettlin, C., Graham, S., and Swanson, M.: Vitamin A and lung cancer, J. Natl. Cancer Inst. 62:1435, 1979.
849. Meyer, E.C., and Liebow, A.A.: Relationship of interstitial pneumonia, honey combing and atypical epithelial proliferation to cancer of the lung, Cancer 18:322, 1965.
850. Meyer, J.A.: The concept and significance of growth rates in human pulmonary tumors, Ann. Thorac. Surg. 14:309, 1972.
851. Mitchell, D.M., Morgan, P.G.M., and Ball, J.B.: Prognostic features of large cell anaplastic carcinoma of the bronchus, Thorax 35:118, 1980.
852. Mountain, C.F.: A new international staging system for lung cancer, Chest 89:2253, 1986.
853. Nash, A.D., and Stout, A.P.: Giant cell carcinoma of the lung: report of 5 cases, Cancer 11:369, 1958.
854. Nixon, D.W., Murphy, G.F., Sewell, C.W., Kutner, M., and Lynn, M.J.: Relationship between survival and histologic type in small cell anaplastic carcinoma of the lung, Cancer 44:1045, 1979.
855. Percy, C., and Sobin, L.: Surveillance, epidemiology and end results: lung cancer data applied to the World Health Organization's classification of lung tumors, J. Natl. Cancer Inst. 70:633, 1983.
856. Ruzzuk, M.A., et al.: Giant cell carcinoma of lung, J. Thorac. Cardiovasc. Surg. 59:574, 1970.
857. Rigler, L.G.: The Health Memorial Lecture: Peripheral carcinoma of the lung: incidence, possibilities for survival, methods of detection, identification, radiologic and other biophysical methods in tumor diagnosis, Chicago, 1975, Year Book Medical Publishers.
858. Ripstein, C.B., Spain, D.M., and Bluth, I.: Scar cancer of the lung, J. Thorac. Cardiovasc. Surg. 56:362, 1968.
859. Rodenhuis, S., van de Wetering, M.L., Mooi, W.J., Evers, S.G., van Zandwijk, N., and Bos, J.L.: Mutational activation of the K-ras oncogene: a possible pathogenetic factor in adenocarcinoma of the lung, N. Engl. J. Med. 317:929, 1987.
860. Rossing, T.H., and Rossing, R.G.: Survival in lung cancer: an analysis of the effects of age, sex, resectability and histopathologic type, Am. Rev. Respir. Dis. 126:771, 1982.
861. Saccomanno, G., Archer, V.E., Auerbach, O., et al.: Histologic types of lung cancer among uranium miners, Cancer 27:515, 1971.
862. Said, J.W., Nash, G., Tepper, G., and Banks-Schlegel, S.: Keratin proteins and carcinoembryonic antigen in lung carcinoma: an immunoperoxidase study of 54 cases with ultrastructural correlations, Hum. Pathol. 14:70, 1983.
863. Saksela, K., Bergh, J., Lehto, V.P., Nilsson, K., and Alitalo, K.: Amplification of the c-myc oncogene in a subpopulation of human small cell lung cancer, Cancer Res. 45:1823, 1985.
864. Singh, G., Katyal, S.L., and Torikata, C.: Carcinoma of type II pneumocytes: immunodiagnosis of a subtype of "bronchioloalveolar carcinomas," Am. J. Pathol. 102:195, 1981.
865. Smoking and health: a report of the Royal College of Physicians of London on smoking in relation to cancer of the lung and other diseases, New York, 1962, Pitman Publishing Corp.
866. Soorae, A.S., and Smith, R.A.: Tumour size as a prognostic factor after resection of lung carcinoma, Thorax 32:19, 1977.

867. Stanley, K.E.: Prognostic factors for survival in patients with inoperable lung cancer, J. Natl. Cancer Inst. **65**:25, 1980.

868. Stanley, K.E., and Matthews, M.J.: Analysis of a pathology review of patients with lung tumors, J. Natl. Cancer Inst. **66**:989, 1981.

869. Straus, M.J., editor: Lung cancer: clinical diagnosis and treatment, New York, 1983, Grune & Stratton, Inc.

870. Surgeon General: The health consequences of involuntary smoking, Rockville, Md., 1986, US Dept. of Health and Human Services.

871. Taylor, A.B., Shinton, N.H., and Waterhouse, J.A.H.: Histology of bronchial carcinoma in relation to prognosis, Thorax **18**:178, 1963.

872. Trump, B.F., McDowell, E.M., Glavin, F., Barrett, L.A., Becci, P.J., Schürch, W., Kaiser, H.E., and Harris, C.C.: The respiratory epithelium. III. The histogenesis of epidermoid metaplasia and carcinoma in situ in the human, J. Natl. Cancer Inst. **61**:563, 1978.

873. U.S. Department of Health, Education and Welfare: Smoking and health: report of the advisory committee to the Surgeon General of the Public Health Service, Washington, D.C., 1964, the Department.

874. Valaitis, J., Warren, S., and Gamble, D.: Increasing incidence of adenocarcinoma of the lung, Cancer **47**:1042, 1981.

875. Vincent, T.N., Satterfield, J.V., and Ackerman, L.V.: Carcinoma of the lung in women, Cancer **18**:559, 1965.

876. Walter, J.B., and Pryce, D.M.: The histology of lung cancer, Thorax **10**:107, 1955.

877. Walter, J.B., and Pryce, D.M.: The site of origin of lung cancer and its relation to histological type, Thorax **10**:117, 1955.

878. Weiss, W.: The mitotic index in bronchogenic carcinoma, Am. Rev. Respir. Dis. **104**:536, 1971.

879. Weiss, W.: Cigarette smoke as a carcinogen, Am. Rev. Respir. Dis. **108**:364, 1973.

880. Weiss, W., Boucot, K.R., and Cooper, D.A.: The histopathology of bronchogenic carcinoma and its relation to growth rate, metastasis, and prognosis, Cancer **26**:965, 1970.

881. Weiss, W., Altan, S., Rosenzweig, M., et al.: Lung cancer type in relation to cigarette dosage, Cancer **39**:2568, 1977.

882. Wellons, H.A., Jr., Johnson, G., Jr., Benson, W.R., et al.: Prognostic factors in malignant tumors of the lung: analysis of 582 cases, Ann. Thorac. Surg. **5**:228, 1968.

883. Wilson, T.S., McDowell, E.M., McIntire, K.R., and Trump, B.F.: Elaboration of human chorionic gonadotropin by lung tumors, Arch. Pathol. Lab. Med. **105**:169, 1981.

884. World Health Organization: Histological typing of lung tumors. In International histological classification of tumors, no. 1, ed. 2, Geneva, 1981, World Health Organization.

885. Wynder, E.L., and Berg, J.W.: Cancer of the lung among non-smokers: special reference to histologic patterns, Cancer **20**:1161, 1967.

886. Wynder, E.L., Mabuchi, K., and Beattie, E.J.: The epidemiology of lung cancer: recent trends, JAMA **213**:2221, 1970.

887. Yesner, R.: Observer variability and reliability in lung cancer diagnosis, Cancer Chemother. Rep. **4**:55, 1973.

888. Yesner, R., Gelfman, N.A., and Feinstein, A.R.: Reappraisal of histopathology in lung cancer and correlation of cell types with antecedent cigarette smoking, Am. Rev. Respir. Dis. **107**:790, 1973.

Other lung tumors

889. Ashley, D.J.B., Dinino, E.A., and Davies, H.D.: Bronchial polyps, Thorax **18**:45, 1963.

890. Askin, F.B., Rosai, J., Sibley, R.K., Dehner, L.P., and McAlister, W.H.: Malignant small cell tumor of the thoracopulmonary region in childhood: a distinctive clinicopathologic entity of uncertain histogenesis, Cancer **43**:2438, 1979.

891. Axelsson, C., Burcharth, F., and Johansen, A.: Mucoepidermoid lung tumors, J. Thorac. Cardiovasc. Surg. **65**:902, 1973.

892. Bahadori, M., and Liebow, A.A.: Plasma cell granulomas of the lung, Cancer **31**:191, 1973.

893. Bateson, E.M.: So called hamartoma of the lung: a true neoplasm of fibrous connective tissue of the bronchi, Cancer **31**:1458, 1973.

894. Becker, N.H., and Soifer, I.: Benign clear cell tumor ("sugar tumor") of the lung, Cancer **27**:712, 1971.

895. Bender, B.L., and Jaffe, R.: Immunoglobulin production in lymphomatoid granulomatous and relation to other "benign" lymphoproliferative disorders, Am. J. Clin. Pathol. **73**:41, 1980.

896. Bensch, K.G., Gordon, G., and Miller, L.: Electron microscopic and biochemical studies on the bronchial carcinoid tumor, Cancer **18**:592, 1965.

897. Bergmann, M., Ackerman, L.V., and Kemler, R.L.: Carcinosarcoma of the lung: review of the literature and report of two cases treated by pneumonectomy, Cancer **4**:919, 1951.

898. Bhagavan, B.S., Dorfman, H.D., Murthy, M.S., and Eggleston, J.C.: Intravascular bronchiolo-alveolar tumor (IVBAT): a low grade sclerosing epithelioid angiosarcoma of lung, Am. J. Surg. Pathol. **6**:41, 1982.

899. Bonikos, D.S., Archibald, R., and Bensch, K.G.: On the origin of the so-called tumorlets of the lung, Hum. Pathol. **7**:461, 1976.

900. Bonikos, D.S., Bensch, K.G., and Jamplis, R.W.: Peripheral pulmonary carcinoid tumors, Cancer **37**:1977, 1976.

901. Butler, C., and Kleinerman, J.: Pulmonary hamartoma, Arch. Pathol. **88**:584, 1969.

902. Churg, A., and Warnock, M.L.: Pulmonary tumorlet: a form of peripheral carcinoid, Cancer **37**:1469, 1976.

903. Churg, A.M., and Warnock, M.L.: So-called "minute pulmonary chemodectoma": a tumor not related to paraganglioma, Cancer **37**:1759, 1976.

904. Colby, T.V., and Yousem, S.A.: Pulmonary lymphoid neoplasms, Semin. Diagn. Pathol. **2**:183, 1985.

905. Davis, P.W., Briggs, J.C., Seal, R.M., et al.: Benign and malignant mixed tumours of the lung, Thorax **27**:657, 1972.

906. Drury, R.A.B., and Stirland, R.M.: Carcinosarcomatous tumours of the respiratory tract, J. Pathol. Bacteriol. **77**:543, 1959.

907. Fechner, R.E., and Bentinck, B.R.: Ultrastructure of bronchial oncocytoma, Cancer **3**:1451, 1973.

908. Fechner, R.E., Bentinck, B.R., and Askew, J.B.: Acinic cell tumor of the lung: a histologic and ultrastructural study, Cancer **29**:501, 1972.

909. Feoli, F., Carbone, A., Dina, M.A., Lauriola, L., Musiani, P., and Piantelli, M.: Pseudolymphoma of the lung: lymphoid subsets in the lung mass and in peripheral blood, Cancer **48**:2218, 1981.

910. Foster, E.A., and Ackerman, L.V.: Localized mesotheliomas of the pleura: the pathologic evaluation of 18 cases, Am. J. Clin. Pathol. **34**:349, 1960.

911. Freeman, C., Berg, J.W., and Cutler, S.J.: Occurrence and prognosis of extranodal lymphomas, Cancer **29**:252, 1972.

912. Fung, C.H., Lo, J.W., Yonan, T.N., et al.: Pumonary blastoma: an ultrastructural study with a brief review of literature and a discussion of pathogenesis, Cancer **39**:153, 1977.

913. Gibbs, A.R., and Seal, R.M.E.: Primary lymphoproliferative conditions of lung, Thorax **33**:140, 1978.

914. Haas, J.E., Yunis, E.J., and Totten, R.S.: Ultrastructure of a sclerosing hemangioma of the lung, Cancer **30**:512, 1972.

915. Hage, E.: Histochemistry and fine structure of bronchial carcinoid tumors, Virchows Arch. [Pathol. Anat.] **361**:121, 1973.

916. Heard, B.E., Corrin, B., and Dewar, A.: Pathology of seven mucous cell adenomas of the bronchial glands with particular reference to ultrastructure, Histopathology **9**:687, 1985.

917. Hoch, W.S., Patchefsky, A.S., Takeda, M., et al.: Benign clear cell tumor of the lung: an ultrastructural study, Cancer **33**:1328, 1974.

918. Horstmann, J.P., Pietra, G.G., Harman, J.A., et al.: Spontaneous regression of pulmonary leiomyomas during pregnancy, Cancer **39**:314, 1977.

919. Iseman, M.D., Schwarz, M.I., and Stanford, R.E.: Interstitial pneumonia in angio-immunoblastic lymphadenopathy with dysproteinemia: a case report with special histopathologic studies, Ann. Intern. Med. **85**:752, 1976.

920. Jaffe, E.: Pulmonary lymphocytic angiitis: a nosologic quandry, Mayo Clin. Proc. **63**:411, 1988.

921. Janigan, D.T., and Marrie, T.J.: An inflammatory pseudotumor of the lung and Q fever, N. Engl. J. Med. **308**:86, 1983.

922. Kapanci, Y., and Toccanier, M.F.: Lymphomatoid granulomatosis of the lung: an immunohistochemical study, Appl. Pathol. 1:97, 1983.
923. Kaplan, C., Katoh, A., Shamoto, M., et al.: Multiple leiomyomas of the lung: benign or malignant? Am. Rev. Respir. Dis. 108:656, 1973.
924. Karcioglu, Z.A., and Someren, A.O.: Pulmonary blastoma: a case report and review of the literature, Am. J. Clin. Pathol. 61:287, 1974.
925. Katzenstein, A.-L.A., Carrington, C.B., and Liebow, A.A.: Lymphomatoid granulomatosis: a clinicopathologic study of 152 cases, Cancer 43:360, 1979.
926. Katzenstein, A.L., Weise, D.L., Fulling, K., and Battifora, H.: So-called sclerosing hemangioma of the lung: evidence for mesothelial origin, Am. J. Surg. Pathol. 7:3, 1983.
927. Korn, D., et al.: Multiple minute pulmonary tumors resembling chemodectomas, Am. J. Pathol. 37:641, 1960.
928. Kuhn, C., and Askin, F.B.: The fine structure of so-called minute pulmonary chemodectomas, Hum. Pathol. 6:681, 1975.
929. Legha, S.S., and Muggia, F.M.: Pleural mesothelioma: clinical features and therapeutic implications, Ann. Intern. Med. 87:613, 1977.
930. Liebow, A.A., Carrington, C.R.B., and Friedman, P.J.: Lymphomatoid granulomatosis, Hum. Pathol. 3:457, 1972.
931. Liebow, A.A., and Castleman, B.: Benign clear cell ("sugar") tumors of the lung, Yale J. Biol. Med. 43:213, 1971.
932. Liebow, A.A., and Hubbell, D.S.: Sclerosing hemangioma (histiocytoma, xanthoma) of the lung, Cancer 9:35, 1956.
933. Linnoila, R.I., Tsokos, M., Triche, T.J., Marangos, P.J., and Chandra, R.S.: Evidence for neural origin and PAS-positive variants of the malignant small cell tumor of thoracopulmonary region ("Askin tumor"), Am. J. Surg. Pathol. 102:124, 1986.
934. McCaughey, W.T.E.: Criteria for the diagnosis of diffuse mesothelial tumors, Ann. NY Acad. Sci. 132:603, 1965.
935. McDonald, A.D., and McDonald, J.C.: Malignant mesothelioma in North America, Cancer 46:1650, 1980.
936. Melmon, K.L., Sjoerdsma, A., and Mason, D.T.: Distinctive clinical and therapeutic aspects of the syndrome associated with bronchial carcinoid tumors, Am. J. Med. 39:568, 1965.
937. Nascimento, A.G., Unni, K.K., and Bernatz, P.E.: Sarcomas of the lung, Mayo Clin. Proc. 57:355, 1982.
938. Navas Palacios, J.J., Escribano, P.M., Toledo, J., Garzon, A., Larrú, E., and Palomera, J.: Sclerosing hemangioma of the lung: an ultrastructural study, Cancer 44:949, 1979.
939. Okike, N., Bernatz, P.E., and Woolner, L.B.: Localized mesothelioma of the pleura: benign and malignant variants, J. Thorac. Cardiovasc. Surg. 75:363, 1978.
940. Otis, C.N., Carter, D., Cole, S., and Battifora, H.: Immunohistochemical evaluation of pleural mesothelioma and pulmonary adenocarcinoma, Am. J. Surg. Pathol. 11:445, 1987.
941. Payne, W.S., Schier, J., and Woolner, L.B.: Mixed tumors of the bronchus/salivary gland type 1, J. Thorac. Cardiovasc. Surg. 49:663, 1965.
942. Peacock, M.J., and Whitwell, F.: Pulmonary blastoma, Thorax 31:197, 1976.
943. Prive, L., Tellem, M., Meranze, D.R., and Chodoff, R.D.: Carcinosarcoma of the lung, Arch. Pathol. 72:351, 1961.
944. Reichle, F.A., and Rosemond, G.P.: Mucoepidermoid tumors of the bronchus, J. Thorac. Cardiovasc. Surg. 51:443, 1966.
945. Saltzstein, S.L.: Pulmonary lymphomas and pseudolymphomas: classification, therapy, and prognosis, Cancer 16:928, 1963.
946. Saltzstein, S.L.: Extranodal malignant lymphomas and pseudolymphomas. In Sommers, S.C., editor: Pathology Annual, 1969, New York, 1969, Appleton-Century-Crofts.
947. Singer, D.B., Greenberg, S.D., and Harrison, G.M.: Papillomatosis of the lung, Am. Rev. Respir. Dis. 94:677, 1966.
948. Smith, J.F., and Dexter, D.: Papillary neoplasms of the bronchus of low grade malignancy, Thorax 18:340, 1963.
949. Spencer, H.: Pulmonary blastomas, J. Pathol. Bacteriol. 82:161, 1961.
950. Spencer, H.: The pulmonary plasma cell/histiocytoma complex, Histopathology 8:903, 1984.

951. Spencer, H., Dail, D.H., and Arneaud, J.: Non-invasive bronchial epithelial papillary tumors, Cancer 45:1486, 1980.
952. Strott, C.A., Nugent, C.A., and Tyler, F.H.: Cushing's syndrome caused by bronchial adenomas, Am. J. Med. 44:97,1968.
953. Suzuki, Y., Churg, J., and Kannerstein, M.: Ultrastructure of human malignant diffuse mesothelioma, Am. J. Pathol. 85:241, 1976.
954. Tedeschi, L.G., Libertini, R., and Conte, B.: Endobronchial polyp, Chest 63:110, 1973.
955. Toole, A.L., and Stern, H.: Carcinoid and adenoid cystic carcinoma of the bronchus, Ann. Thorac. Surg. 13:63, 1972.
956. Turnbull, A.D., Huvos, A.G., Goodner, J.T., et al.: Mucoepidermoid tumors of the bronchial glands, Cancer 28:539, 1971.
957. Wagner, J.C., Munday, D.E., and Harington, J.S.: Histochemical demonstration of hyaluronic acid in pleural mesotheliomas, J. Pathol. Bacteriol. 84:73, 1962.
958. Wang, N.-S.: Electron microscopy in the diagnosis of pleural mesotheliomas, Cancer 31:1046, 1973.
959. Weisenburger, D., Armitage, J., and Dick, F.: Immunoblastic lymphadenopathy with pulmonary infiltrates, hypocomplementia and vasculitis: a hyperimmune syndrome, Am. J. Med. 63:849, 1977.
960. Weldon-Linne, C.M., Victor, T.A., Christ, M.L., and Fry, W.A.: Angiogenic nature of the "intravascular bronchoalveolar tumor" of the lung, Arch. Pathol. Lab. Med. 105:174, 1981.
961. Williams, E.D., and Sandler, M.: The classification of carcinoid tumours, Lancet 1:238, 1963.
962. Youssem, S.A., et al.: So-called sclerosing hemangiomas of lung: an immunohistochemical study supporting respiratory epithelial origin, Am. J. Surg. Pathol. 12:582, 1988.

Mediastinum
Mediastinitis

963. Eggleston, J.G.: Sclerosing mediastinitis, Prog. Surg. Pathol. 2:1, 1980.
964. Goodwin, R.A., Nickell, J.A., and DesPrez, R.M.: Mediastinal fibrosis complicating healed primary histoplasmosis and tuberculosis, Medicine 51:227, 1972.
965. Katzenstein, A.L.A., and Mazur, M.T.: Pulmonary infarct: an unusual manifestation of fibrosing mediastinitis, Chest 77:521, 1980.
966. Light, A.M.: Idiopathic fibrosis of mediastinum: a discussion of three cases and review of the literature, J. Clin. Pathol. 31:78, 1978.
967. Yacoub, M.H., and Thompson, V.C.: Chronic idiopathic pulmonary hilar fibrosis, Thorax 26:365, 1971.

Tumors and cysts of the mediastinum

968. Benjamin, S.P., McCormack, L.J., Effler, D.B., et al.: Primary tumors of the mediastinum, Chest 62:297, 1972.
969. Cox, J.D.: Primary malignant germinal tumors of the mediastinum: a study of 24 cases, Cancer 36:1162, 1975.
970. DePaepe, M., Van der Straeten, M., and Roels, H.: Mediastinal angiofollicular lymph node hyperplasia with systemic manifestations, Eur. J. Respir. Dis. 64:134, 1983.
971. Fizzera, G., et al.: A systemic lymphoproliferative disorder with morphologic features of Castleman's disease, Am. J. Surg. Pathol. 7:211, 1983.
972. Grosfeld, J.L., Weinberger, M., Kilman, J.W., et al.: Primary mediastinal neoplasms in infants and children, Ann. Thorac. Surg. 12:179, 1971.
973. Hineman, V.L., Phyliky, R.L., and Banks, P.M.: Angiofollicular lymph node hyperplasia and peripheral neuropathy, Mayo Clin. Proc. 57:379, 1982.
974. Hodgkinson, D.L., Telander, R.L., Sheps, S.G., Gilchrist, G.S., and Crowe, J.K.: Extra-adrenal intrathoracic functioning paraganglioma (pheochromocytoma) in childhood, Mayo Clin. Proc. 55:271, 1980.
975. Jones, E.L., Crocker, J., Gregory, J., Guibarra, M., and Curran, R.C.: Angiofollicular lymph node hyperplasia (Castleman's disease): an immunohistochemical and enzyme histochemical study of the hyaline-vascular form of the lesion, J. Pathol. 144:131, 1984.

976. Keller, A.R., Hochholzer, L., and Castleman, B.: Hyaline-vascular and plasma cell types of giant lymph node hyperplasia of the mediastinum and other locations, Cancer **29:**670, 1972.

977. Lichtenstein, A.K., Levine, A., Taylor, C.R., Boswell, W., Rossman, S., Feinstein, D.I., and Lukes, R.J.: Primary mediastinal lymphoma in adults, Am. J. Med. **68:**509, 1980.

978. Oberman, H.A., and Libcke, J.H.: Malignant germinal neoplasms of the mediastinum, Cancer **17:**498, 1964.

979. Oldham, H.N., and Sabiston, D.C.: Primary tumors and cysts of the mediastinum, Monogr. Surg. Sci. **4:**243, 1967.

980. Schantz, A., Sewall, W., and Castleman, B.: Mediastinal germinoma: a study of 21 cases with an excellent prognosis, Cancer **30:**1189, 1972.

981. Silverman, N.A., and Sabiston, D.C.: Mediastinal masses, Surg. Clin. North Am. **60:**757, 1980.

982. Weissenberger, D.D., et al.: Multicentric angiofollicular lymph node hyperplasia, Hum. Pathol. **16:**162, 1985.

21 Ophthalmic Pathology

MORTON E. SMITH

ADNEXAL STRUCTURES
Lids

Most of the pathologic processes involving the eyelids are those that involve the skin in general; these are discussed in detail in Chapter 36. Consideration is given here to lesions that present particular problems.

Chalazia (lipogranulomas) (Figs. 21-1 to 21-3) and sebaceous gland carcinomas of the lid are often discussed together, though chalazia are common and carcinomas are rare. The important clinical point is that a sebaceous gland carcinoma of the lid may masquerade as a "recurrent" chalazion (Fig. 21-4).

Sebaceous gland carcinomas arise from either the meibomian glands within the tarsus (Fig. 21-5) or from Zeis glands closer to the skin surface. Small sebaceous gland carcinomas are usually cured with local excision. Larger ones may eventually metastasize to the preauricular, anterior cervical, or submandibular chain of lymph nodes. Distant metastasis is not common but may include the lungs.

Many localized lesions are found on the lids; these include seborrheic keratosis, papillomas, nevi, amyloid deposits, and xanthelasma. Basal cell carcinoma is more common than squamous cell carcinoma.

Orbit

The usual clinical hallmark of orbital disease is exophthalmos, though there may not be a neoplasm involved. For example, the most common cause of exophthalmos is dysthyroid ophthalmopathy (Graves' disease); rarely is a histopathologic specimen obtained in these cases.

In dysthyroid ophthalmopathy there is a dysfunction between the pituitary-thyroid axis. When examined for the ocular problem, the patient may be hyperthyroid, hypothyroid, or euthyroid by clinical and chemical manifestations. There is edema, accumulation of acid mucopolysaccharide, and chronic inflammatory cell infiltration of the extraocular muscles. In fact, the noticeable thickening of the extraocular muscles is easily recognized on computerized tomographic (CT) scan and ultrasound examination and is an important diagnostic sign. Eventually muscle fibers degenerate and become hyalinized.

Other systemic diseases that may involve the orbit include leukemia and malignant lymphoma, the histiocytoses, juvenile xanthogranuloma, sinus histiocytosis, metastatic carcinoma, connective tissue disorders, and Wegener's granulomatosis (Fig. 21-6).

The orbit may be secondarily invaded by lesions originating in adjacent structures such as mucoceles (Fig. 21-7) and carcinomas from the paranasal sinuses or intraocular melanomas that have broken through the sclera. The phycomycoses may spread from the sinuses to the orbit, especially in debilitated patients and in diabetics in acidosis. Localized lesions of the orbit include hemangiomas, lymphangiomas, dermoid cysts, peripheral nerve tumors, perioptic meningiomas, optic nerve gliomas, fibrous histiocytomas, inflammmatory pseudotumors, and the rhabdomyosarcomas seen in children. The lacrimal gland may give rise to benign mixed cell tumors (pleomorphic adenomas), adenoid

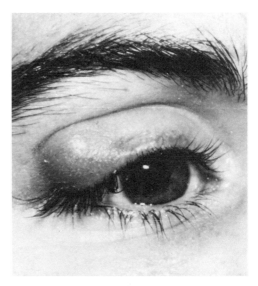

Fig. 21-1. Chalazion of right upper eyelid. (WU 79-1631; from Rosai, J.: Ackerman's surgical pathology, ed. 6, St. Louis, 1981, The C.V. Mosby Co.)

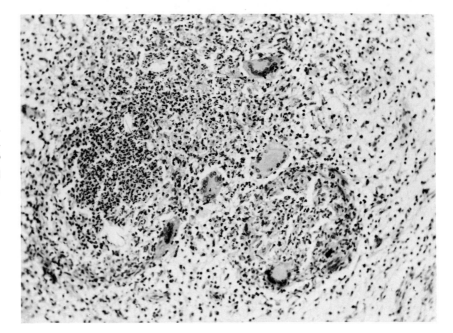

Fig. 21-2. Multiple foci of granulomatous inflammation with microabscesses and Langhans' giant cells in chalazion. (137×; AFIP 91218; from Rosai, J.: Ackerman's surgical pathology, ed. 6, St. Louis, 1981, The C.V. Mosby Co.)

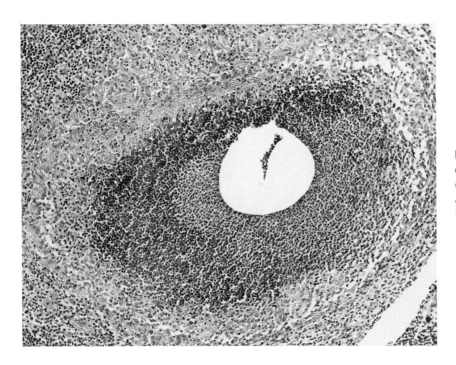

Fig. 21-3. Presence of pools of fat in center of many of granulomas is characteristic of chalazia. (115×; AFIP 732397; from Rosai, J.: Ackerman's surgical pathology, ed. 6, St. Louis, 1981, The C.V. Mosby Co.)

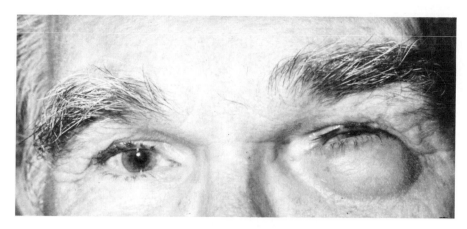

Fig. 21-4 Sebaceous gland carcinoma of left lower lid.

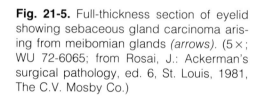

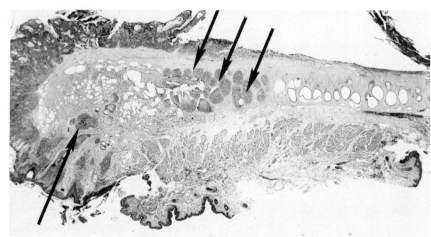

Fig. 21-5. Full-thickness section of eyelid showing sebaceous gland carcinoma arising from meibomian glands *(arrows)*. (5×; WU 72-6065; from Rosai, J.: Ackerman's surgical pathology, ed. 6, St. Louis, 1981, The C.V. Mosby Co.)

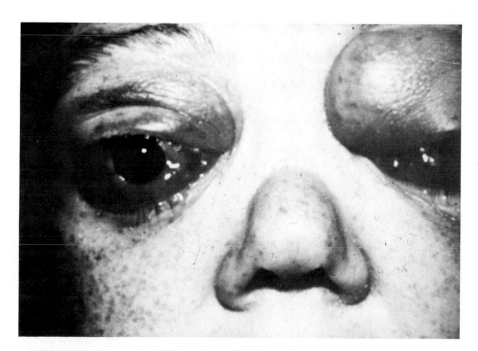

Fig. 21-6. Pronounced bilateral exophthalmos in Wegener's granulomatosis.

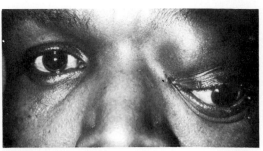

Fig. 21-7. Mucocele producing downward and lateral displacement of left eye. (WU 69-7637; from del Regato, J.A., and Spjut, H.J.: Ackerman and del Regato's cancer, ed. 5, St. Louis, 1977, The C.V. Mosby Co.)

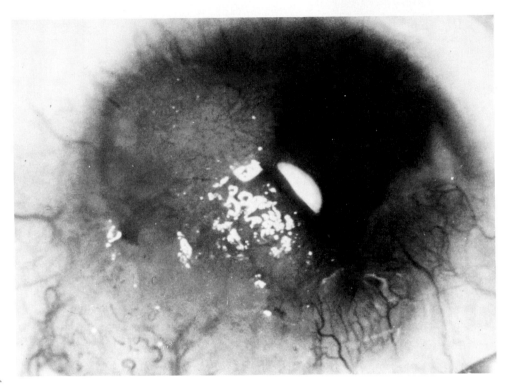

Fig. 21-8. Carcinoma in situ of conjunctiva and cornea (WU 79-1633; from Rosai, J.: Ackerman's surgical pathology, ed. 6, St. Louis, 1981, The C.V. Mosby Co.)

Fig. 21-9. Epidermoid carcinoma of conjunctiva. Tumor grew rapidly over 4-month period. (WU 64-3837; from Rosai, J.: Ackerman's surgical pathology, ed. 6, St. Louis, 1981, The C.V. Mosby Co.)

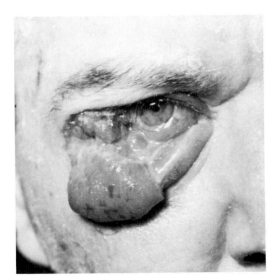

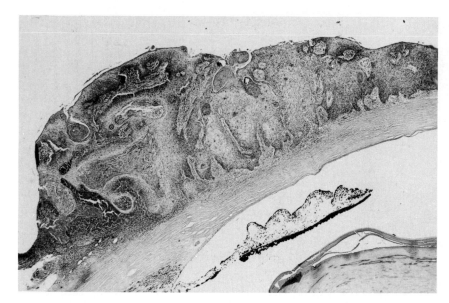

Fig. 21-10. Carcinoma of limbus. Exophytic growth pattern with formation of papillomatous mass is typical of more advanced limbal carcinomas. Even in such large tumors, corneoscleral stroma tends to prevent neoplasm from invading intraocular tissues. (18×; AFIP 785865; from Rosai, J.: Ackerman's surgical pathology, ed. 6, St. Louis, 1981, The C.V. Mosby Co.)

cystic carcinomas, and undifferentiated carcinomas. The benign lymphoepithelial lesion of Sjögren's syndrome may be seen in the lacrimal gland.

Conjunctiva

Most of the pathologic processes involving the conjunctiva are localized and not associated with any systemic process. The surgical pathologist would see common lesions such as cysts, pterygia, papillomas, and nevi. Localized amyloid lesions are rare.

Carcinoma in situ of the bulbar conjunctiva usually is manifested as a leukoplakic lesion at the limbus (Fig. 21-8). The histopathologic characteristics of the lesion are similar to those observed elsewhere in mucous membranes.

Invasive squamous cell carcinoma (Figs. 21-9 and 21-10) of the conjunctiva is rare. It is usually cured with simple excision, though an exenteration of all orbital contents may be necessary for extensive lesions. Metastases are rare but may include regional lymph nodes (preauricular, anterior cervical, and submandibular).

Benign nevi of the conjunctiva are common and melanomas are rare. Melanomas may arise de novo, from a preexisting nevus, or from acquired melanosis. Local excision may be curative, but recurrences are common and there may be eventual metastasis to regional lymph nodes.

INTRAOCULAR LESIONS
Congenital and developmental lesions
Phacomatoses

The phacomatoses are a heredofamilial group of congenital syndromes having in common the presence of disseminated, benign hamartomas. The eyes are usually involved.

In angiomatosis retinae (von Hippel's disease) hemangioblastomas may occur in any part of the retina. These are often multiple and bilateral. Severe or untreated cases may lead to retinal detachment. The combination of retinal plus central nervous system hemangioblastomas is referred to as von Hippel-Lindau disease.

Along with meningeal calcification and facial nevus flammeus (port-wine stain) (Fig. 21-11), patients with encephalotrigeminal angiomatosis (Sturge-Weber syndrome) also have congenital glaucoma and a diffuse cavernous hemangioma of the choroid (Fig. 21-12). The choroidal hemangioma often leads to microcystoid degeneration of the overlying retina and leakage of serous fluid into the subretinal space.

Neurofibromatosis (von Recklinghausen's disease) is characterized by plexiform neurofibromas in the lid and orbit (Fig. 21-13), congenital glaucoma, multiple nevi of the iris, diffuse neurofibroma of the uveal tract, optic nerve gliomas, or absence of orbital bones leading to a pulsating exophthalmos.

In tuberous sclerosis (Bourneville's disease) there are glial hamartomas of the retina (Fig. 21-14), which are usually multiple and bilateral.

The two least frequently encountered phacomatoses are ataxia telangiectasia (Louis-Bar syndrome) and Wyburn-Mason syndrome. Telangiectasis of the conjunctiva occurs in the former and retinal arteriovenous communications in the latter.

Chromosomal aberrations

In trisomy 13 the eyes are microphthalmic. There is usually a colobomatous defect, as well as persistence and hyperplasia of the primary vitreous. Cartilage is often seen within the coloboma, and the retina is usually dysplastic. A multitude of major and minor ocular de-

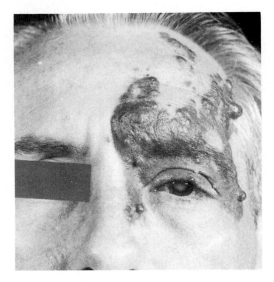

Fig. 21-11. Sturge-Weber syndrome. Patient, 42-year-old white man, had had facial hemangioma all his life and was blind in ipsilateral eye because of retinal degeneration, glaucoma, and cataract. Choroidal hemangioma was found in enucleated eye, but clinical study failed to disclose evidence of intracranial lesion. (AFIP 761707; courtesy Veterans Administration Hospital, Hines, Ill.; from Rosai, J.: Ackerman's surgical pathology, ed. 6, St. Louis, 1981, The C.V. Mosby Co.)

fects can occur in trisomy 18, trisomy 21, chromosome 5 deletion defect, chromosome 18 deletion defect, and mosaicism.

Retinopathy of prematurity

Retinopathy of prematurity, previously referred to as "retrolental fibroplasia," is an acquired developmental disorder resulting from the unique sensitivity of blood vessels of the premature retina to oxygen. There is incomplete vascularization of the peripheral retina, and the exposure to oxygen inhibits the normal vascularization process. On withdrawal of oxygen, pathologic neovascularization occurs, often with leakage of blood and serum, organization, and eventual retinal detachment.

Retinitis pigmentosa

Retinitis pigmentosa is a group of diseases in which there is a generalized degeneration of the retinal pigment epithelium and photoreceptor cells, especially the rods; they are of unknown cause and exhibit a variety of inheritance patterns. These patients have night blindness and a decreased or absent electroretinographic response. Retinitis pigmentosa may be an associated finding in the following systemic diseases: Usher's syndrome, Laurence-Moon-Berdet-Biedl syndrome, syringomyelia, Bassen-Kornzweig syndrome, Friedreich's ataxia, Refsum's disease, and myotonic dystrophy.

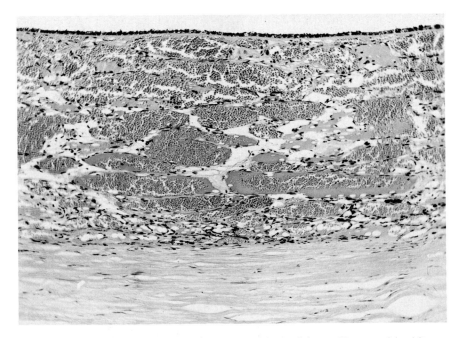

Fig. 21-12. Hemangioma of choroid in eye enucleated from 42-year-old white woman who had had a port-wine facial hemangioma since birth and ipsilateral glaucoma since early childhood. (115×; AFIP 759801; from Rosai, J.: Ackerman's surgical pathology, ed. 6, St. Louis, 1981, The C.V. Mosby Co.)

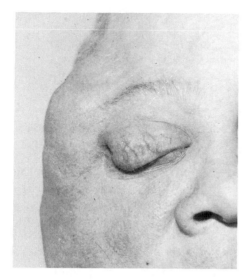

Fig. 21-13. Severe unilateral deformity of face in patient with von Recklinghausen's neurofibromatosis. (AFIP 55-17512; courtesy Dr. L.L. Calkins, Kansas City, Kan.; from Rosai, J.: Ackerman's surgical pathology, ed. 6, St. Louis, 1981, The C.V. Mosby Co.)

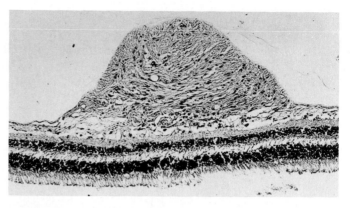

Fig. 21-14. Tuberous sclerosis showing glial nodule or hamartoma projecting against vitreous from nerve fiber layer of retina. (90×; AFIP 511046; from Rosai, J.: Ackerman's surgical pathology, ed. 6, St. Louis, 1981, The C.V. Mosby Co.)

Other congenital anomalies

In Marfan's syndrome, in homocystinurea, and in Weil-Marchesani syndrome, the lens of the eye is prone to dislocation.

Complete albinism involves skin, hair, and eyes, whereas incomplete albinism occurs in the ocular tissues with a deficiency but rarely a complete lack of melanin in pigment epithelium and uveal melanocytes. Poor vision, nystagmus, and photophobia are the clinical manifestations.

Other congenital anomalies include Lowe's syndrome, in which there are cataracts and glaucoma, and aniridia, in which nonfamilial cases may be associated with Wilms' tumor.

Infections and inflammations
Infections

Acute suppurative intraocular inflammation, clinically referred to as endophthalmitis or panophthalmitis, is usually infectious in origin; it results from a bacterium or fungus introduced through an accidental or surgical perforating wound (Fig. 21-15). This disease is confined to the eye and rarely includes systemic manifestations.

Occasionally endophthalmitis is endogenous, that is, by hematogenous spread. The most important lesions in this category are the "opportunistic" infections. A typical example is the patient who has received hyperalimentation after bowel surgery and in whom candidemia develops. The fungus may reach the eye and produce endophthalmitis. Other organisms that can cause opportunistic infections and produce a similar picture include *Toxoplasma, Nocardia, Aspergillus,* and *Cryptococcus* organisms.

Toxoplasmosis may be congenital or may appear in adults, in whom the retinitis is a reactivation of the organisms that have been lying dormant in the retina since birth. These patients are systemically well. Histologically the protozoon is found free in pseudocysts or in true cysts in an area of coagulative necrosis of the retina (Fig. 21-16), which usually is sharply demarcated from contiguous normal retina.

Toxocara canis infection is found principally in children between 3 and 14 years of age who presumably contract the disease from puppies. These children do not have clinical evidence of systemic visceral larva migrans. Typically a single migrating larva reaches the eye hematogenously and comes to rest in the vitreous or inner surface of the retina. Severe endophthalmitis may result, and the retina may become detached. Such eyes are often enucleated. A less severe reaction produces only a white fibrotic mass in the retina, often with fibrous strands in the overlying vitreous. Histologically there is a granulomatous inflammatory reaction with an intense eosinophilia (Fig. 21-17). The worm is often not seen because it has totally disintegrated.

Presumed ocular histoplasmosis syndrome occurs in healthy young adults who have decreased vision as a result of a small hemorrhagic or serous detachment of the macula. These patients may have positive histoplasmin skin test results but no evidence of systemic histoplasmosis. Controversy still exists as to whether or not there has been unequivocal demonstration of *Histoplasma capsulatum* organisms in the eyes of such patients.

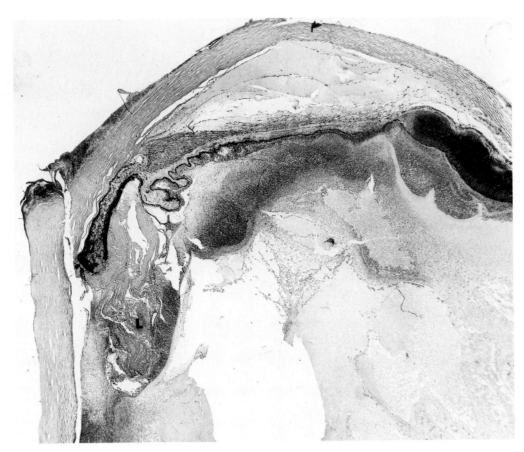

Fig. 21-15. Endophthalmitis showing infiltration of all intraocular structures by acute inflammatory cells. Lens, *L,* is necrotic. Organism presumably gained entrance through corneal wound. (15×; WU 67-4233; from Rosai, J.: Ackerman's surgical pathology, ed. 6, St. Louis, 1981, The C.V. Mosby Co.)

Cytomegalic inclusion disease may be a congenital infection, or it may occur in adults as an opportunistic infection. A typical example is the patient with acquired immunodeficiency syndrome. The disease characteristically produces massive hemorrhage and necrosis of the retina. Histologically the typical "owl's eye" cells with large intranuclear inclusion bodies surrounded by a clear halo are found within the necrotic retina.

Subacute sclerosing panencephalitis may produce a hemorrhagic macular lesion along with progressive central nervous system findings. Histologically the retina is necrotic, is infiltrated by lymphocytes, and often shows intranuclear inclusion bodies. A similar picture can be seen in herpes simplex retinitis and encephalitis.

Common ocular findings in congenital rubella syndrome include cataract, glaucoma, iritis, and a pigmentary retinopathy manifested opthalmologically as a pigmentary stippling of the retina referred to as a salt-and-pepper fundus. This is caused by alternating areas of retinal pigment epithelial atrophy and hypertrophy.

The cataract characteristically shows retention of lens cell nuclei in the embryonic lens nucleus.

Ocular complications occur in about 50% of cases of herpes zoster ophthalmicus. The most common problems are keratitis and iritis. The keratitis often leads to ulceration and eventual fibrosis and vascularization of the cornea. The iritis produces a patchy necrosis. There may also be involvement of the remaining uveal tract (ciliary body and choroid) as well as scleritis, retinitis, or papillitis. The characteristic histologic findings are perineural infiltration by lymphocytes, especially involving the long posterior ciliary nerves, and diffuse or patchy necrosis of the iris and pars plicata of the ciliary body.

Tuberculosis of the eye is now rare. It produces a chronic granulomatous inflammation of the uveal tract. Leprosy may involve the ocular adnexa and cornea, but intraocular involvement is rare. Syphilis may produce a nongranulomatous choroiditis, but the usual ocular manifestation is optic nerve atrophy. Congenital syphilis is the usual cause for intestinal keratitis.

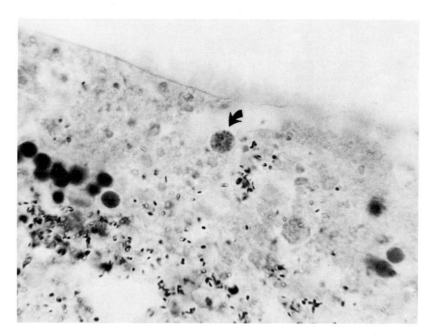

Fig. 21-16. Encysting proliferative forms *(arrow)* of *Toxoplasma gondii* found in necrotic retina. Small particles are pigment granules from necrotic retinal pigment epithelium, whereas larger round structures represent pyknotic retinal nuclei. (1000×; AFIP 754058; from Rosai, J.: Ackerman's surgical pathology, ed. 6, St. Louis, 1981, The C.V. Mosby Co.)

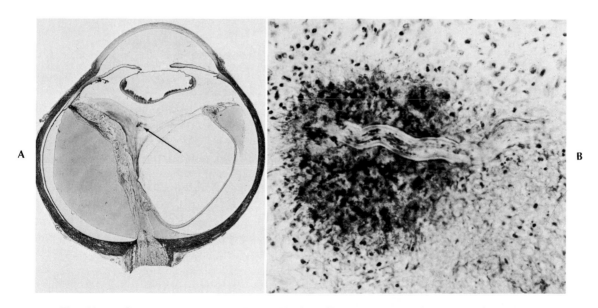

Fig. 21-17. Granulomatous endophthalmitis from *Toxocara canis.* **A,** Arrow indicates site of granuloma containing larva shown in **B.** Preretinal inflammatory membrane has led to total detachment of retina. **B,** Nematode larva in granuloma in vitreous. (**A,** 3×; **B,** 400×; **A** and **B** from Wilder, H.C.: Trans. Am. Acad. Ophthalmol. Otolaryngol. **55:**99, 1950; AFIP 198761.)

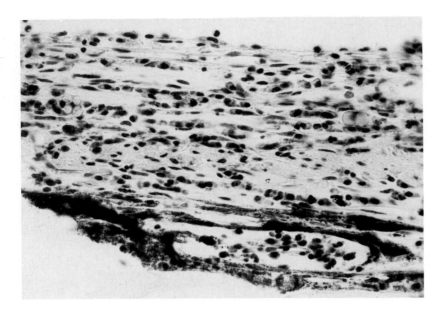

Fig. 21-18. Nongranulomatous iritis in which atrophic iris is diffusely infiltrated by plasma cells and several Russell bodies are present. Irregular degenerative and proliferative changes may be observed in pigment epithelium. (360×; AFIP 698722; from Rosai, J.: Ackerman's surgical pathology, ed. 6, St. Louis, 1981, The C.V. Mosby Co.)

Fig. 21-19. Nongranulomatous iritis with posterior synechiae. Iris is firmly attached to lens, which reveals widespread degeneration of its cortex and fibrous metaplasia of its subcapsular epithelium. (25×; AFIP 184111; from Rosai, J.: Ackerman's surgical pathology, ed. 6, St. Louis, 1981, The C.V. Mosby Co.)

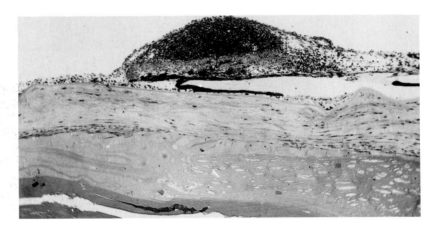

Inflammations

Most cases of nongranulomatous inflammation of the uveal tract (iritis, iridocyclitis, choroiditis) are not infectious in origin and are not associated with systemic disease. An important exception is the frequent association of chronic nongranulomatous iritis in girls with juvenile rheumatoid arthritis or in young men with ankylosing spondylitis. It is rare to obtain histologic specimens of such entities, but the few that have been reported show nonspecific changes, including a diffuse nongranulomatous chronic inflammation throughout the uveal tract (Fig. 21-18). Secondary sequelae include adhesions of the iris to lens (posterior synechia) (Fig. 21-19) or to the cornea (anterior synechia). Often a cataract is present, and there is usually some degree of chorioretinal scarring.

Sympathetic uveitis (also referred to as sympathetic ophthalmia) is a diffuse granulomatous uveitis in which a penetrating injury to one eye gives rise to a granulomatous inflammation in both eyes. Fortunately, it is rare, considering the number of injuries to which eyes are subjected (50% of all enucleations are the sequelae of accidental or surgical trauma). It is believed to be caused by an autoimmunity, with uveal pigment or retinal antigen or both acting as the inciting factor.

The histology of sympathetic uveitis is characterized by a diffuse infiltration of the uvea by lymphocytes, patchy aggregations of epithelioid cells, and eosinophils (Fig. 21-20). Plasma cells are usually sparse.

Although no systemic manifestations exist in sympathetic ophthalmia, there is a closely related disease in which there are systemic manifestations. Vogt-Koyanagi-Harada disease (uveomeningoencephalitis syndrome) has similar ocular findings, but there is no history of penetrating ocular injury; these patients also have fluctuating meningeal symptoms, vitiligo, poliosis, alopecia, and dysacusis.

Phacoanaphylaxis is another granulomatous inflammation that is concentrated around a ruptured lens and therefore usually follows penetrating ocular trauma.

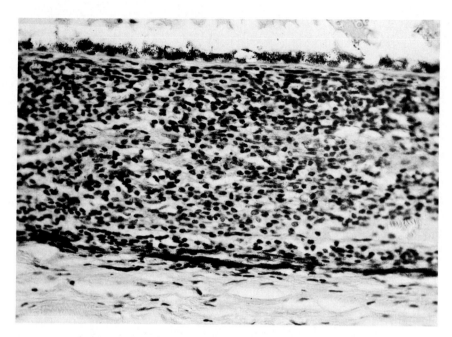

Fig. 21-20. Sympathetic uveitis. Uveal tissues are diffusely infiltrated by lymphocytes, and there are small, irregular collections of pale-staining epithelioid cells (300×; AFIP 731769; from Rosai, J.: Ackerman's surgical pathology, ed. 6, St. Louis, 1981, The C.V. Mosby Co.)

Clinically there is an intense inflammatory reaction in the anterior chamber that resembles an acute bacterial enophthalmitis. Histologically, in the area in which the lens capsule is broken, there is a massive invasion of the lens by inflammatory cells. Centrally and immediately surrounding individual lens fibers are polymorphonuclear leukocytes. Peripheral to this is a wall of epithelioid and giant cells about which is a broader zone of granulation tissue and round cell infiltration (Fig. 21-21). This disease is also believed to be autoimmune, with antilens antibodies being formed as a response to the sudden release of lens protein. No systemic manifestations are present.

About one third of patients with sarcoidosis have ocular manifestations, the most common of which is anterior uveitis. Other findings include eyelid nodules, nodular infiltrates in the palpebral conjunctiva, interstitial keratitis, retinochoroidal granulomas, optic neuritis, papilledema, retinal periphlebitis, and tumors in the orbit or lacrimal gland. Histologically the typical noncaseating granulomatous tubercle is seen (Fig. 21-22). A biopsy of the nodular infiltrates in the conjunctiva can easily be done to establish the diagnosis (Fig. 21-23).

Granulomatous scleritis is manifested clinically by intense inflammation and pain. It is associated with rheumatoid arthritis or collagen-vascular disease in less than 25% of cases. Histologically a zonal type of granulomatous inflammatory infiltrate surrounds a nidus of necrotic scleral collagen. The lesions, which may be focal or diffuse, resemble subcutaneous rheumatoid nodules.

Retinal vascular disease
Diabetes

Ocular diabetes is one of the leading causes of blindness in industrialized societies and is the leading cause of blindness in persons between 25 and 65 years of age. At present the most important factor influencing the occurrence of clinical retinopathy is the duration of the disease. Adequacy of control is probably just as important, but supportive data are only now accumulating. Retinopathy develops in many diabetics (65% or more) 15 years after the onset of the disease. There is a positive correlation between the presence of diabetic retinopathy and Kimmelstiel-Wilson nephropathy. Diabetes can cause a variety of pathologic conditions in the eye, often leading to blindness with pain, thus necessitating enucleation.

The selective retinal capillary microangiopathy appears to begin with a degeneration of the intramural pericytes and some loss of endothelial cells. Adjacent to these ischemic foci are saclike aneursymal dilatations of the capillaries (Fig. 21-24). Diapedesis of erythrocytes occurs, producing the so-called dot hemorrhages in the deeper layers of the retina. Also developing in the deeper layers of the retina as a result of this loss of

Text continued on p. 1062.

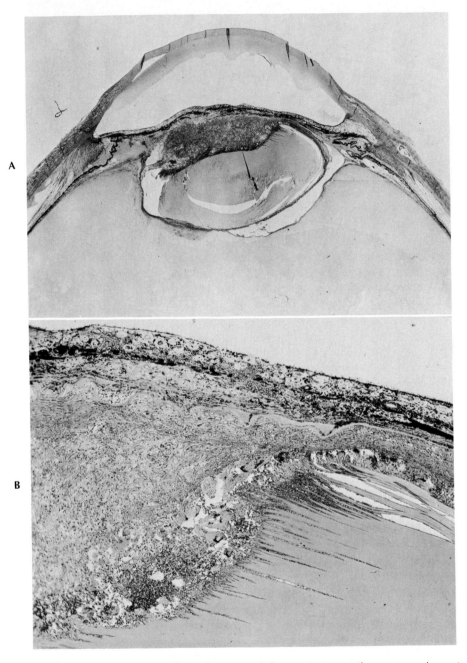

Fig. 21-21. Phacoanaphylaxis. Granulomatous inflammatory reaction surrounds ruptured lens. (**A,** 10×; AFIP 55-22260; **B,** 53×; AFIP 55-22261; from Zimmerman, L.E.: In Ackerman, L.V. [in collaboration with Butcher, H.R., Jr.]: Surgical pathology, ed. 2, St. Louis, 1959, The C.V. Mosby Co.)

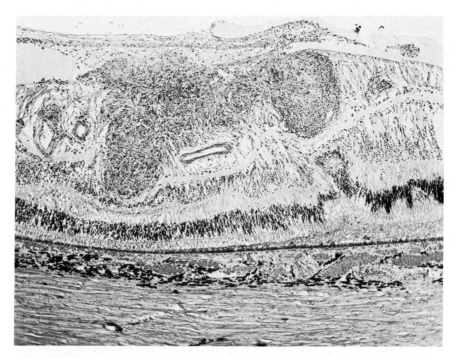

Fig. 21-22. Granulomatous tubercle within the retina in a patient with sarcoidosis. (50×; AFIP 63-1450.)

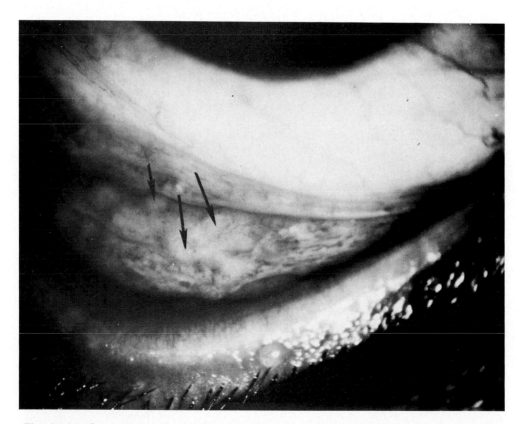

Fig. 21-23. Conjunctival granulomas in sarcoidosis. (WU 79-1632; from Rosai, J.: Ackerman's surgical pathology, ed. 6, St. Louis, 1981, The C.V. Mosby Co.)

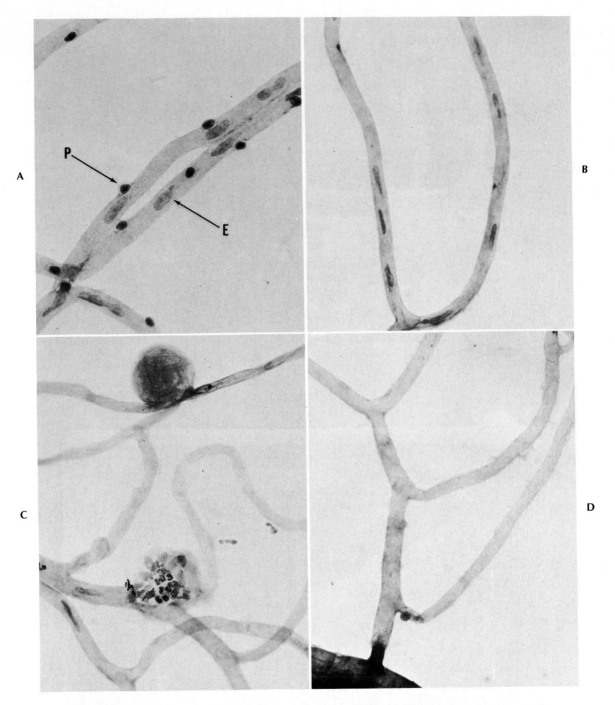

Fig. 21-24. Diabetic retinopathy. Whole mounts of retinal capillaries after digestion with trypsin. **A,** Nuclei of endothelial cells, *E,* and of pericytes or mural cells, *P,* are normally observed in about 1:1 ratio. **B,** Selective loss of mural pericytes, one of earliest changes in diabetes. **C,** Saccular microaneurysms characteristic of diabetic retinopathy. One in upper part of field is hyalinized, whereas one in lower part shows endothelial proliferation and adherent leukocytes. **D,** Many of ischemic vessels showing loss of all nuclei in advanced diabetic retinopathy. (**A,** AFIP 64-7004; **B,** AFIP 64-7010; **C,** AFIP 64-7009; **D,** AFIP 64-7008.)

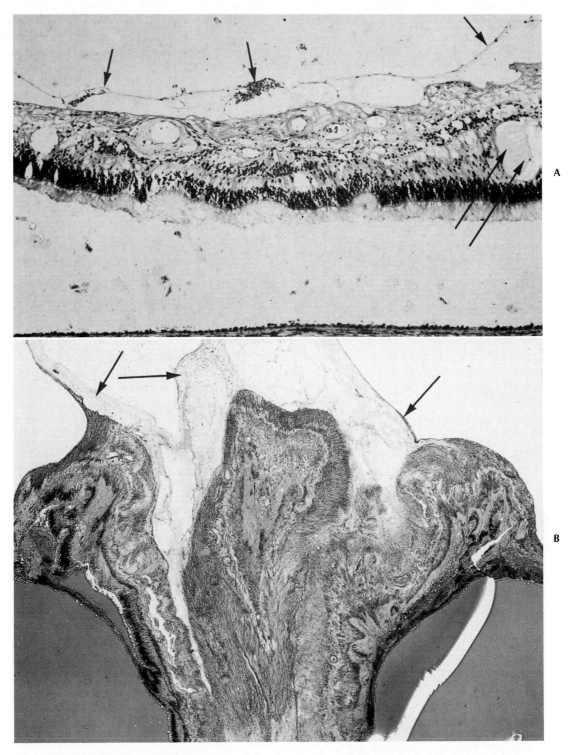

Fig. 21-25. A, Diabetic retinopathy with scattered exudates in deep retinal layers *(double arrows)* and early neovascularization extending from inner surface of retina into vitreous *(single arrows)*. **B,** Diabetic proliferative retinopathy *(arrows)* has caused complete retinal detachment. (**A,** 90×; WU 72-3170; **B,** 34×; WU 72-3171; **A** and **B** from Rosai, J.: Ackerman's surgical pathology, ed. 6, St. Louis, 1981, The C.V. Mosby Co.)

permeability of the capillaries are pockets of lipoproteinaceous material, referred to clinically as hard, waxy exudates. Soft "cotton-wool" spots may also appear, which are microinfarcts in the nerve fiber layer and are similar to those seen in hypertensive retinopathy.

All the aforementioned changes are referred to clinically as background retinopathy. In some cases the retinopathy eventually becomes proliferative. Under the influence of an angiogenesis factor, new capillaries proliferate, often at the optic disc or along one of the retinal veins, and eventually erupt through the internal limiting membrane of the retina. Bleeding into the vitreous may then occur; this blood organizes and contracts, producing traction on the retina with consequent retinal detachment (Fig. 21-25).

In many cases the diffuse ischemia of the retina is responsible for the development of a neovascular membrane on the anterior surface of the iris. This neovascular membrane on the anterior surface of the iris (clinically referred to as rubeosis iridis) contracts, pulling the root of the iris up against the trabecular meshwork (peripheral anterior synechia), thus occluding the outflow channels of the eye and producing an intractable glaucoma (Fig. 21-26). The contraction of the neovascular membrane also pulls the pigment epithelium of the iris forward around the pupil and onto the anterior surface of the iris (ectropion uveae).

Another characteristic histologic finding in ocular di-

abetes is the glycogen vacuolization of the pigment epithelium layer of the iris (see Fig. 21-25). This finding is analogous to Armanni-Ebstein nephropathy and is a reflection of a high serum glucose level in the 72-hour period before the specimen is obtained (either by enucleation in the living patient or at autopsy).

Hypertensive retinopathy

In hypertensive retinopathy there is generalized attenuation of retinal arterioles, often leading to retinal ischemia. Flame-shaped hemorrhages and soft cotton-wool spots are the characteristic ophthalmoscopic findings. Histologically both the hemorrhages and the cotton-wool spots are located in the inner layers of the retina, that is, in nerve fiber and ganglion cell layers. The cotton-wool spots are focal areas of ischemic infarction, producing the characteristic cytoid bodies that represent swollen axons or focal areas of axoplasmic stagnation (Fig. 21-27).

Central retinal artery or vein occlusion

Patients with generalized vascular disease, such as hypertension, arteriosclerotic cardiovascular disease, carotid artery disease, and diabetes, are prone to occlusions of the central retinal artery or vein. These patients typically complain of sudden, painless loss of vision in one eye. Sudden total occlusion of the central retinal artery is caused either by arthrosclerotic throm-

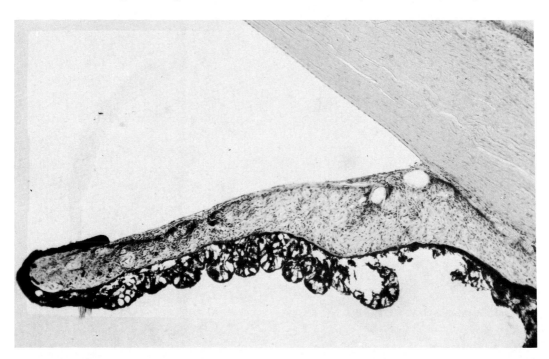

Fig. 21-26. Rubeosis iridis in diabetes. Angle of anterior chamber is occluded by peripheral anterior synechia, and fibrovascular membrane (rubeosis iridis) covers anterior surface of iris. Contraction of this membrane has pulled pigment epithelium anteriorly to produce "ectropion uvea." There is pronounced diabetic vacuolization of pigment epithelial cells. (90×; WU 67-4225; from Rosai, J.: Ackerman's surgical pathology, ed. 6, St. Louis, 1981, The C.V. Mosby Co.)

bosis of the artery within the lamina cribrosa portion of the optic nerve or by an embolism, usually from the carotid artery or heart valves. This vascular accident produces complete ischemic infarction of the inner layers of the retina, which are dependent for blood supply on the central retinal artery.

Histologically the retinal infarct is characterized by an early edematous thickening of the inner two-thirds of the retina with dissolution of nuclei in the ganglion cell and inner nuclear layers (Fig. 21-28). As the edema subsides, there is thinning of the inner retinal layers from which the nerve fibers, ganglion cells, and almost all the cells of the inner nuclear layer have disappeared.

Occlusion of the central retinal vein produces a hemorrhagic infarction of the retina. In most of these cases the vein is narrowed and eventually closed off by a thickened arteriosclerotic artery lying adjacent to the vein within the lamina cribrosa of the optic nerve. Histologically the inner layers of the retina are involved, as in the case of central artery occlusion. However, massive hemorrhage within these layers, rather than ischemia, is present. Later, as all the blood is resorbed, the histologic picture is similar to central artery occlusion in that thinning and loss of nuclei in the ganglion cell and inner nuclear layers occur. However, a stain for iron usually reveals the presence of the hemosiderin deposition.

Eyes in which central vein occlusion has developed may go on to develop neovascularization of the anterior surface of the iris ("rubeosis iridis") similar to that described earlier in the discussion of diabetes.

Branch retinal artery and vein occlusion, of course, cause only segmental infarctions to the retina.

Sickle cell retinopathy

Sickle cell retinopathy is most severe with sickle cell hemoglobin C disease but may also occur in other sickle hemoglobinopathies including sickle thalassemia and

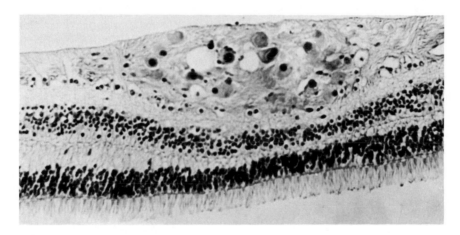

Fig. 21-27. Microinfarct of retina. "Cytoid bodies" are axonal enlargements in infarcted nerve fiber layer. (210×; AFIP 69808; from Friedenwald, J.S., et al.: Ophthalmic pathology, Philadelphia, 1952, W.B. Saunders Co.)

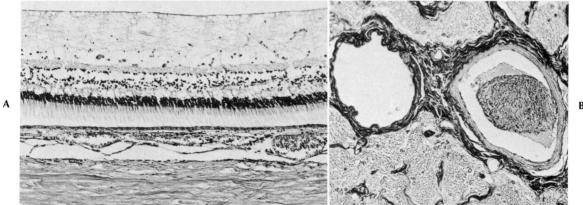

Fig. 21-28. Acute ischemic infarction of retina, **A,** produced by embolus in central retinal artery, **B,** from mural thrombus in left ventricle of patient who had sustained myocardial infarction. (AFIP 951983; **B,** from Zimmerman, L.E.: Arch. Ophthalmol. **73:**822, 1965.)

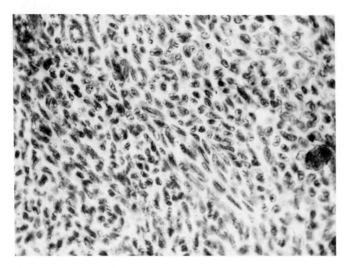

Fig. 21-29. Spindle A type of melanoma cells. (510×; AFIP 49801; from Rosai, J.: Ackerman's surgical pathology, ed. 6, St. Louis, 1981, The C.V. Mosby Co.)

sickle cell disease and even in occasional cases of sickle cell trait. First, there is arteriolar occlusion in the periphery of the retina, followed by the formation of arteriolovenular anastomoses. Neovascularization then occurs, which may lead to vitreous hemorrhage, fibrous proliferations, and eventual retinal detachment.

Primary intraocular neoplasms

The two important primary intraocular malignancies considered here are melanoma and retinoblastoma.

Malignant melanoma of the uvea typically occurs in white adults. It is slow growing and metastasizes very late. Clinically it is a painless mass recognized as an incidental finding or because it has caused some visual problem.

This neoplasm arises from the pigmented or potentially pigment-producing cells of the uvea, with the choroid and ciliary body being more frequently involved than the iris.

The cytologic characteristics of uveal melanomas have been classified and are used as one criterion to determine prognostic significance. Spindle cell melanomas are a mixture of spindle A cells and spindle B cells or

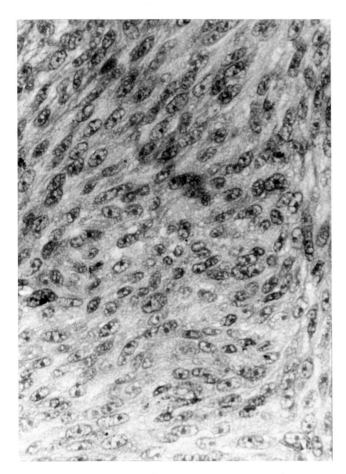

Fig. 21-30. Spindle B cells demonstrating moderate pleomorphism and ovoid nuclei with nucleoli. (600×.)

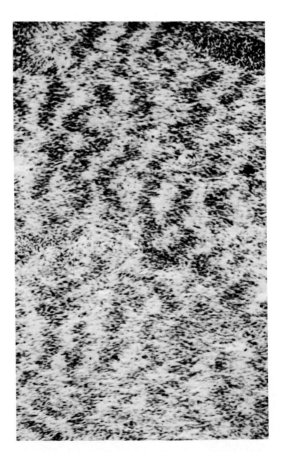

Fig. 21-31. Spindle B cells with fascicular pattern. (From del Regato, J.A., and Spjut, H.J.: Ackerman and del Regato's cancer, ed. 5, St. Louis, 1977, The C.V. Mosby Co.)

often only B cells. Spindle A cells are slender, spindle-shaped cells with fusiform nuclei and no or small nucleoli. Frequently the chromatin is arranged in a linear fashion along the central axis of the nucleus (Fig. 21-29). Spindle B cells are larger with ovoid nuclei containing a prominent nucleolus (Fig. 21-30). These spindle cell melanomas are cohesive and often have a fascicular pattern when viewed microscopically at low magnification (Fig. 21-31).

Epithelioid cell melanomas have cells that are larger, are irregular, and possess abundant cytoplasm. The nuclei are large, with strikingly prominent nucleoli. These cells are not cohesive (Fig. 21-32).

Most melanomas have a mixture of all these cell types and actually represent a continuum rather than distinct groups. However, general predictions concerning prognosis can be made. Roughly two thirds to three fourths of patients with spindle cell melanomas will still be alive in 5 years, whereas roughly two thirds to three fourths of patients with epithelioid melanomas will die of their tumors within 5 years. A patient with a mixed cell melanoma, such as spindle plus epithelioid, has roughly a 50% chance of surviving for 5 years.

Besides cell type, the other important criteria for predicting prognosis are extraocular extension and size of the tumor; larger tumors naturally have a worse prognosis than smaller ones (Figs. 21-33 and 21-34).

Another important fact concerning the prognosis of uveal tumors is the very benign behavior of almost all melanomas of the iris. Most of these are recognized early when they are quite small, and most are spindle cell. Distant metastasis from an iris melanoma is rare.

Choroidal melanoma tends to grow inward from the choroid toward the vitreous as a discoid, globular, or mushroom-shaped mass, first elevating and then detaching the retina (Fig. 21-35). Less commonly, choroidal melanomas spread diffusely and flatly along the choroid and may extend out along scleral canals into the orbit. Rarely a patient may not seek medical attention until the tumor has grown sufficiently to become necrotic and produce such complications as endophthalmitis, massive intraocular hemorrhage, and glaucoma. Metastasis is blood borne and can occur anywhere in the body, with a particular affinity for the liver.

All the preceding data are based on eyes that have been enucleated. A recent reappraisal of survival data on patients with uveal melanomas has led to the impression that the mortality is low before enucleation

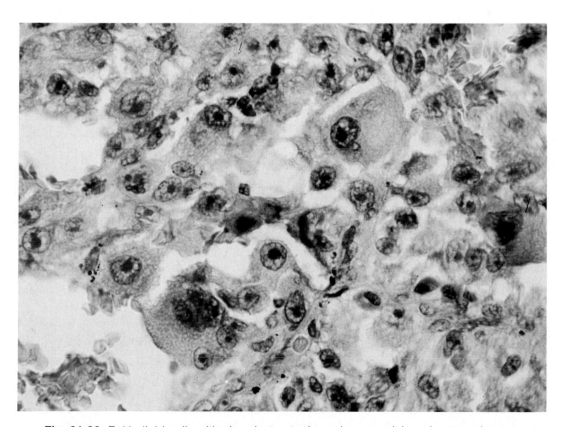

Fig. 21-32. Epithelioid cells with abundant cytoplasm, large nuclei, and extremely prominent nucleoli. (600×; WU 69-7517; from del Regato, J.A., and Spjut, H.J.: Ackerman and del Regato's cancer, ed. 5, St. Louis, 1977, The C.V. Mosby Co.)

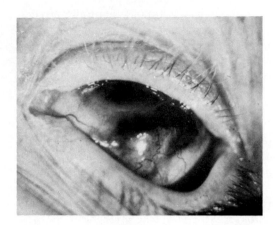

Fig. 21-33. Malignant melanoma of choroid breaking through sclera and appearing under conjunctiva. (WU 69-2213; from del Regato, J.A., and Spjut, H.J.: Ackerman and del Regato's cancer, ed. 5, St. Louis, 1977, The C.V. Mosby Co.; courtesy Registry of Ophthalmic Pathology, Armed Forces Institute of Pathology, Washington, D.C.)

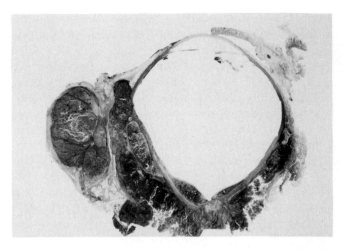

Fig. 21-34. Massive orbital extension from small choroidal melanoma that has occurred as result of diffuse spread along natural passages through sclera and optic nerve. (2×; AFIP 159090; from Friedenwald, J.S., et al.: Ophthalmic pathology: an atlas and textbook, Philadelphia, 1952, W.B. Saunders Co.)

but rises abruptly after enucleation. Many ophthalmologists now do not resort to immediate enucleation of eyes with small melanomas that remain relatively stationary in growth. Furthermore, a nationwide collaborative study is now being conducted to compare survival rates among various treatment modalities: observation versus irradiation versus enucleation.

Retinoblastoma, in contrast to melanoma, occurs almost exclusively in young children; no racial group is spared. Believed to be congenital and derived from incompletely differentiated retinal cells, tumors are nevertheless seldom recognized until these children are between 6 months and 2 years of age.

Although most cases arise sporadically, the influence of heredity is well established. Bilaterality is present in over 90% of the familial cases; survivors of bilateral retinoblastoma have a 50% chance of transmitting the disease to each of their progeny. In 80% of cases in which the retinoblastoma is sporadic and unilateral, the mutation is considered to be somatic. It has recently been shown that the defect is an antioncogene located at Re 14 locus of the q arm of chromosome 13.

These tumors characteristically appear as a leukokoria (white pupillary reflex) (Fig. 21-36), or less often as a strabismus when the tumor is in the macula. They may protrude into the vitreous (endophytic type), often with vitreous seeding, or they may grow between the retina and the pigment epithelium (exophytic type) (Fig. 21-37).

Histologically these tumors are composed of densely packed masses of round and angulated cells with hyperchromatic nuclei and scanty cytoplasm. In the more dif-

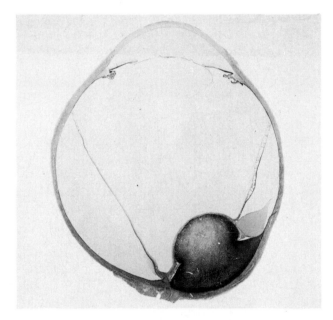

Fig. 21-35. Malignant melanoma of choroid that, by erupting through Bruch's membrane, has formed mushroom-shaped subretinal mass. (3×; AFIP 289600; from Rosai, J.: Ackerman's surgical pathology, ed. 6, St. Louis, 1981, The C.V. Mosby Co.)

ferentiated tumors the cells are often arranged in rosettes (Fig. 21-38). There are areas of necrosis and scattered foci of calcification (Fig. 21-39). Prognosis is most influenced by the extent of the tumor and is poorest in tumors that have invaded the optic nerve, especially if the tumor is present at the surgical plane of transection (Fig. 21-40). These tumors are likely to ex-

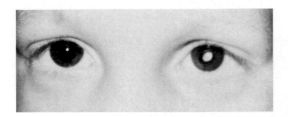

Fig. 21-36. Prominent white reflex present in dilated pupil of left eye attributable to retinoblastoma. (From Rosai, J.: Ackerman's surgical pathology, ed. 6, St. Louis, 1981, The C.V. Mosby Co.)

Fig. 21-37. Bilateral retinoblastoma showing presence of white mass consisting of detached retina and neoplastic tissue immediately behind lens in each eye. (AFIP 635460; from Rosai, J.: Ackerman's surgical pathology, ed. 6, St. Louis, 1981, The C.V. Mosby Co.)

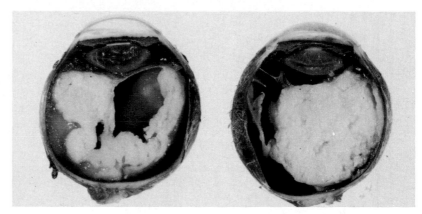

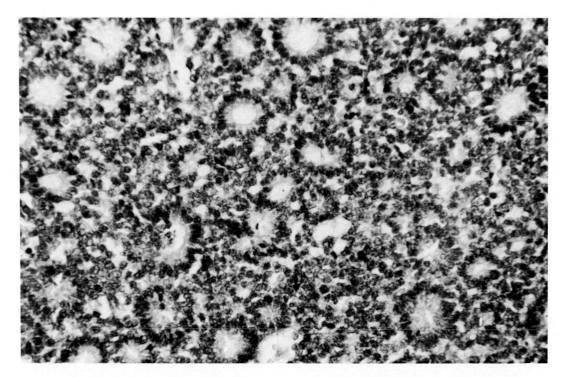

Fig. 21-38. Retinoblastoma with typical rosettes. (600×; WU 69-7513; from del Regato, J.A., and Spjut, H.J.: Ackerman and del Regato's cancer, ed. 5, St. Louis, 1977, The C.V. Mosby Co.)

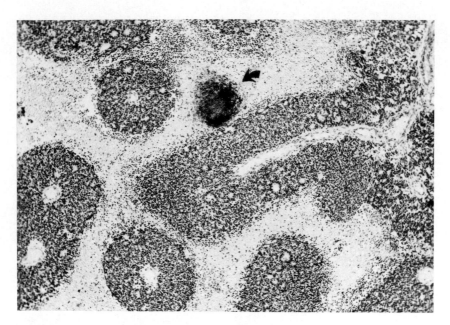

Fig. 21-39. Retinoblastoma showing typical pattern of collar of viable cells about nutrient vessels. Foci of calcification *(arrow)* occur within areas of coagulation necrosis. (80×; AFIP 147292; from Rosai, J.: Ackerman's surgical pathology, ed. 6, St. Louis, 1981, The C.V. Mosby Co.)

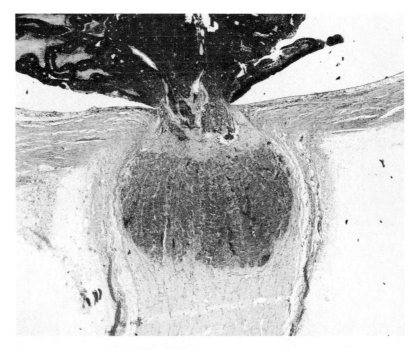

Fig. 21-40. Retinoblastomas exhibit definite tendency to spread out of globe by way of optic nerve. It is therefore of utmost importance for surgical pathologist to determine whether such optic nerve extension has occurred and, if it has, to what extent. (14×; AFIP 57-344; from Rosai, J.: Ackerman's surgical pathology, ed. 6, St. Louis, 1981, The C.V. Mosby Co.)

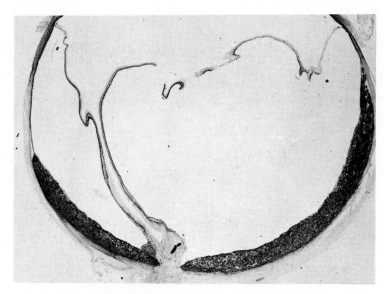

Fig. 21-41. Metastatic carcinoma from breast producing diffuse thickening of choroid posteriorly. (6×; AFIP 638509; from Rosai, J.: Ackerman's surgical pathology, ed. 6, St. Louis, 1981, The C.V. Mosby Co.)

tend along the nerve to the brain or to be carried there by the subarachnoid fluid. Another histologic finding that carries a grave prognosis is massive invasion of the uvea, in which there is a tendency for hematogenous dissemination. Survival is better than 90% in patients with unilateral retinoblastoma treated with immediate enucleation and in cases in which histologic study shows no optic nerve or uveal invasion.

Metastatic cancer

Metastatic neoplasms are the second most common intraocular neoplasms; they are second only to primary uveal melanomas. (If one were to review serial sections of autopsied eyes, the incidence of metastatic cancer would actually exceed that of melanoma.) Most metastatic neoplasms lodge in the choroid. The lids, orbit, and iris are less frequently involved. The breast is the most common primary site in women, and the lung is the most common in men. All other primary sites are relatively uncommon. Histologically these neoplasms tend to grow in a flat, diffuse manner within the choroid (Fig. 21-41).

Leukemic infiltration of the choroid or retinal hemorrhages or both are present in over 50% of patients who die of leukemia or allied disorders. Malignant lymphomas rarely involve the intraocular structures but often involve the orbit. An important exception is histiocytic lymphoma, which may involve the retina and choroid and often demonstrates characteristic vitreous cells. The diagnosis can be established by surgical vitrectomy and examination of the cells after processing through a Millipore filter.

Cysts of the pars plana filled with immunoglobulin

are present in multiple myeloma and other paraprotein disorders.

Cataracts

The term *cataract* merely refers to opacification of the lens. This process has a variety of causes: congenital (rubella, galactosemia, familial, chromosomal defects), toxic (long-term use of systemic steroids or dinitrophenol), traumatic (contusion, penetrating wounds, or electrical injury), metabolic (diabetics are prone to senile cataracts at an earlier age), or secondary (complication of chronic intraocular inflammation). The most common cause of cataracts is aging, whereby lens fibers formed constantly throughout life become compressed into the center of the lens.

The histologic characteristics of cataracts are similar regardless of the cause. The lens fibers degenerate and become fragmented and liquefied (Fig. 21-42). The nucleus often remains intact, since it is very sclerotic. Lens epithelial nuclei have migrated posteriorly beyond the equator to lie adjacent to the posterior lens capsule. A fibrous plaque on the anterior surface of the lens is sometimes seen, especially in cases of trauma or inflammation. This plaque, referred to as anterior polar cataract, represents fibrous metaplasia of the anterior epithelial cells. Cataract extraction with replacement by an intraocular lens implant is one of the most successful surgical procedures performed today.

Glaucoma

The essential feature of the glaucomas is a nonphysiologic state of increased intraocular pressure, which in almost all cases is caused by an impaired outflow of

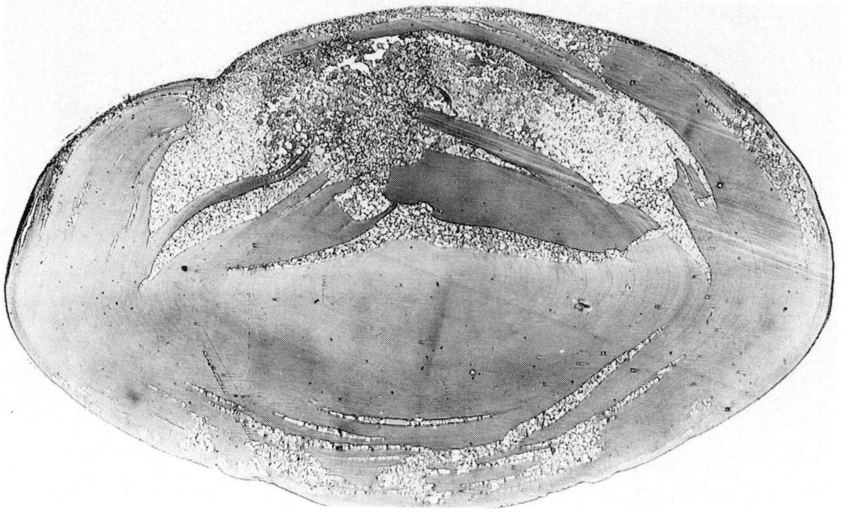

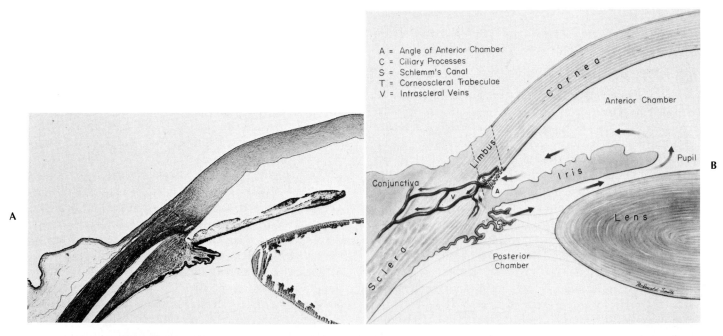

Fig. 21-42. Mature cortical and nuclear cataract. There is advanced degeneration of lens fibers, which are considerably fragmented. (27×; AFIP 66872; from DeCoursey, E., and Ash, J.E.: Atlas of ophthalmic pathology, Rochester, Minn., 1942, American Academy of Ophthalmology and Otolaryngology.)

A
A = Angle of Anterior Chamber
C = Ciliary Processes
S = Schlemm's Canal
T = Corneoscleral Trabeculae
V = Intrascleral Veins
Cornea
Anterior Chamber
Limbus
Pupil
Iris
Conjunctiva
Lens
Sclera
Posterior Chamber
B

Fig. 21-43. Normal eye. **A,** Actual section. **B,** Artist's drawing. (**A,** 11×; AFIP 56-11490; **B,** AFIP 57-18073; from Zimmerman, L.E.: In Saphir, O., editor: A text on systemic pathology, New York, 1958-1959, Grune & Stratton, Inc.; by permission.)

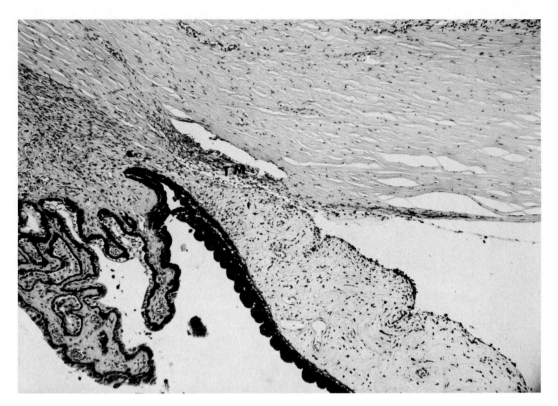

Fig. 21-44. Peripheral aspect of iris lying against trabecular meshwork, *TM,* producing peripheral anterior synechia and blocking outflow of aqueous humor. (90×; WU 67-4224; from Rosai, J.: Ackerman's surgical pathology, ed. 6, St. Louis, 1981, The C.V. Mosby Co.)

aqueous humor. Aqueous humor is produced by the ciliary processes and is discharged into the posterior chamber. It flows forward between the lens and the iris, through the pupil, and into the anterior chamber. It then leaves the anterior chamber through the trabecular meshwork that is present in the deep layers of the peripheral cornea, passes into Schlemm's canal, and leaves the eye through the plexus of the intrascleral and episcleral veins (Fig. 21-43).

The glaucomas are categorized according to the reason for the impairment of the aqueous humor: congenital, primary open-angle (synonomous with chronic simple glaucoma), primary angle-closure, and secondary. In congential glaucoma there is a malformation of the tissues in the region of the anterior chamber angle. The precise nature of this malformation is not clear, but there seems to be an incomplete separation of the iris root from the trabecular meshwork or the retention of an embryonic membrane or both.

Primary open-angle glaucoma, the most common type, appears to be a genetically determined disease that becomes evident with aging. It is characterized by an insidious onset and a slowly progressive rise in intraocular pressure resulting from an increased resistance to aqueous outflow of undetermined cause at an unde-

termined site. Untreated cases eventually go on to painless, progressive loss of vision.

Primary angle-closure glaucoma occurs most often in persons who have shallow anterior chambers and narrow anterior chamber angles (the angle formed by the peripheral cornea and the iris root). These peculiar anatomic features predispose to blockage of the ouflow channels by this root. During an attack of angle-closure glaucoma, the iris root actually apposes the trabecular meshwork. Chronic attacks may lead to adhesions of the iris root to the trabecular meshwork (peripheral anterior synechia), and the condition becomes permanent.

Secondary glaucoma is a complication of numerous primary processes, including trauma, inflammation, and neoplasia. The glaucoma in these secondary cases results from one or more of four main types of obstruction of the outflow of aqueous humor:

1. Adhesions of iris to lens (posterior synechiae)
2. Adhesions of iris to cornea (anterior synechiae) (Fig. 21-44)
3. Accumulation of cells or cellular debris in the anterior chamber angle (Fig. 21-45)
4. Direct damage to the outflow channels in the trabecular meshwork, canal of Schlemm, and so on

Regardless of the type and cause of glaucoma, certain

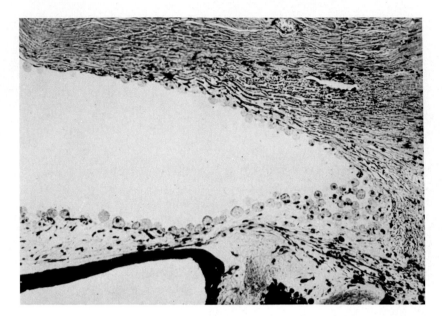

Fig. 21-45. Outflow channels blocked by macrophages in anterior chamber in phacolytic glaucoma (glaucoma resulting from lysis and escape of lens protein into aqueous humor). (75×; AFIP 609920; from Flocks, M., Littwin, C.S., and Zimmerman, L.E.: Phacolytic glaucoma: clinicopathologic study of 138 cases of glaucoma associated with hypermature cataract, Arch. Ophthalmol. **54:**37, 1955. Copyright 1955, American Medical Association.)

degenerative changes are typically produced after periods of variable duration. When glaucoma begins in childhood, the tissues tend to stretch and the globe may become enlarged (buphthalmos). When the glaucoma occurs in adult life, the effects are mostly in the retina and optic nerve and are easily recognized microscopically. There is virtually a total loss of retinal ganglion cells and thinning and gliosis of the nerve fiber layer while the outer nuclear layer and rods and cones remain intact (Fig. 21-46). The optic nerve shows pronounced excavation, posterior bowing of the lamina cribrosa, and generalized atrophy of nerve tissue (Fig. 21-47).

Retinal degenerative diseases
Retinal detachment

Retinal detachment is a separation of the sensory retina from its normally tenuous juxtaposition to the retinal pigment epithelium. The tips of the rods and cones are normally interdigitated with villous projections from the retinal pigment epithelium, but they are not attached by any specialized structures such as desmosomes. Thus these two structures separate readily as a result of many pathologic processes.

Retinal detachment can be expected to occur as a consequence of one of three main pathogenic mechanisms: (1) traction on the retina, resulting from pathologic processes developing in the vitreous or anterior segment of the eye, (2) exudation of fluid from the choroid, opening up the potential subretinal space, for example, from inflammation or tumor in the choroid, or (3) passage of liquefied vitreous through a hole or tear in the retina (Fig. 21-48).

Because the outer layers of the retina are dependent on the choroidal circulation for nutrition and oxygenation, retinal detachment leads to a spatial separation of the retina from the choroid and a consequent ischemic loss of function. The aim of surgical reattachment of the retina is to get it back in place before irreparable damage has occurred and to prevent the detachment from spreading to the macula.

Age-related macular degeneration

Age-related macular degeneration accounts for most cases of central visual loss in the elderly population. It is a bilateral, painless, progressive affliction of the macula. In the earliest stages of the disease degenerative changes are seen in Bruch's membrane, the basement membrane that separates the retinal pigment epithelial layer from the choroid. These changes consist of irregular thickening and calcium deposition.

The thickened Bruch's membrane may extend into the choriocapillaris, the innermost level of blood vessels of the choroid. Portions of the choriocapillaris may be obliterated. Secondary changes in the retinal pigment epithelium then may occur, including atrophy with de-

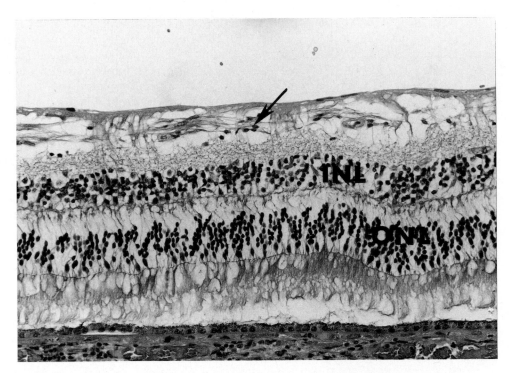

Fig. 21-46. Retina in glaucoma demonstrates loss of ganglion cells and gliosis of nerve fiber layer *(arrow)* but intact inner nuclear layer *(INL)* and outer nuclear layer *(ONL).* (260×.)

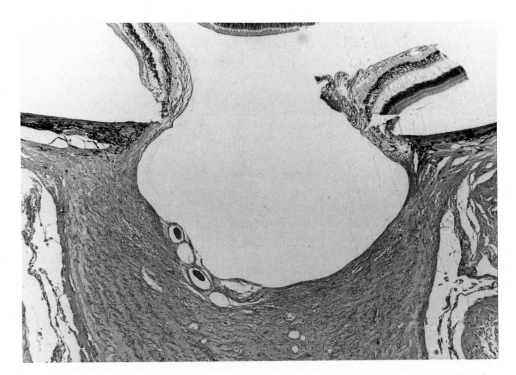

Fig. 21-47. Deep excavation (cupping) of optic disc secondary to glaucoma. (100×.)

pigmentation or hyperplasia. Consequently there is altered function of the rods and cones, as well as development of microcystoid changes in the sensory retina.

At times the early degenerative changes of Bruch's membrane may lead to actual cracks through which small capillaries grow from the choriocapillaris. This may progress to a subretinal pigment epithelial network of neovascularization, which then may leak serous fluid or even bleed, producing a subretinal hematoma that later organizes into a fibrous mass (Fig. 21-49). Naturally there is extensive damage to the overlying sensory retina and consequent loss of central vision.

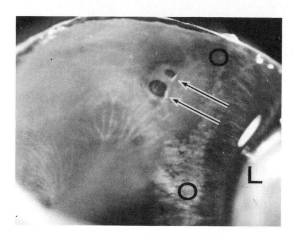

Fig. 21-48. Two holes are present in peripheral retina. Dense white retinal tissue at anterior border of each hole *(arrows)* is retracted operculum torn away in formation of holes. *O—O,* Ora serrata; *L,* posterior surface of lens. (AFIP 65-3203-1.)

Phthisis bulbi and atrophia bulbi

The clinical term *phthisis bulbi* represents the final stages of ocular degeneration and disorganization, in which the production of aqueous humor is so reduced that the intraocular pressure is decreased (hypotony) and the globe shrinks. Histologically there is pronounced atrophy of all ocular structures, and often there is intraocular ossification (atrophia bulbi).

OCULAR MANIFESTATIONS OF OTHER SYSTEMIC DISEASES

In Wilson's hepatolenticular degeneration, copper is deposited in Descemet's membrane of the peripheral cornea. This is recogized clinically as a greenish brown ring in the peripheral cornea and is referred to as a Kayser-Fleischer ring (Fig. 21-50).

In cystinosis, fine scintillating polychromatic cystine crystals are deposited in the subepithelial conjunctiva and in the corneal stroma.

A brownish discoloration in the sclera occurs in ochronosis (Fig. 21-51).

In hypercalcemia calcium salts may be deposited in Bowman's membrane of the cornea. This produces the clinical picture referred to as band keratopathy.

In familial hypercholesterolemia and in certain other forms of disturbed lipid metabolism, arcus senilis becomes prominent at an early age. Clinically it is a milky opacification of the peripheral cornea resulting from the accumulation of lipid in the corneal stroma.

In the mucopolysaccharidosis group of diseases, clouding of the cornea results from the accumulation of abnormal mucopolysaccharides throughout the central

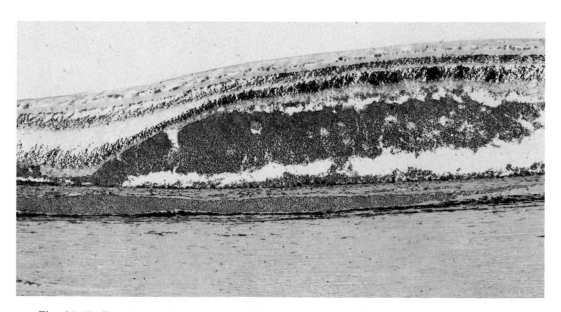

Fig. 21-49. Focal hemorrhage under retina was mistaken clinically for melanoma. (90×; WU 72-3167; from Rosai, J.: Ackerman's surgical pathology, ed. 6, St. Louis, 1981, The C.V. Mosby Co.)

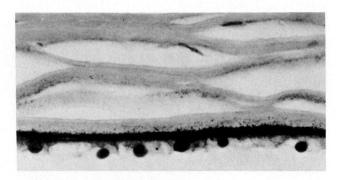

Fig. 21-50. Kayser-Fleischer ring. Dark band is copper compound that has been deposited in Descemet's membrane close to endothelium. (600×; AFIP 264768; from Hogan, M.J., and Zimmerman, L.E.: Ophthalmic pathology, ed. 2, Philadelphia, 1962, W.B. Saunders Co.)

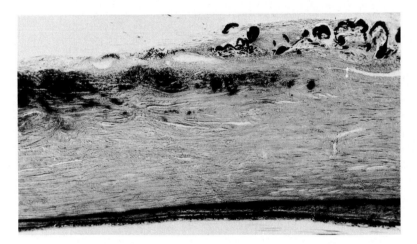

Fig. 21-51. Ochronosis. Pigmentation in degenerated elastic and collagenous tissues of sclera and episclera. (70×; AFIP 59-699; from Rones, B.: Am. J. Ophthalmol. **49**:440, 1960.)

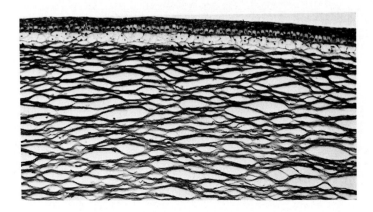

Fig. 21-52. Cells in superficial layers of corneal stroma are swollen with acid mucopolysaccharide. (90×; AFIP 68-4418.)

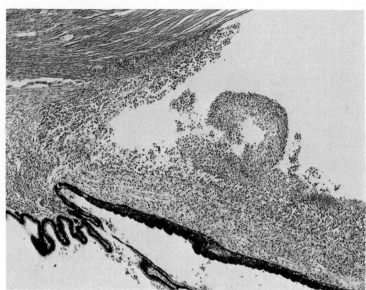

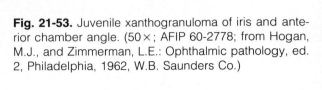

Fig. 21-53. Juvenile xanthogranuloma of iris and anterior chamber angle. (50×; AFIP 60-2778; from Hogan, M.J., and Zimmerman, L.E.: Ophthalmic pathology, ed. 2, Philadelphia, 1962, W.B. Saunders Co.)

stroma and endothelium (Fig. 21-52). Haziness of the cornea also occurs in Fabry's disease.

In juvenile xanthogranuloma, along with characteristic skin lesions, there may be tumors of the conjunctiva, orbit, or uveal tract (Fig. 21-53).

Although localized amyloid tumors may occur on the lids or conjunctiva, systemic amyloidosis usually has no ocular manifestations, with the important exception of primary familial amyloidosis, in which there are dense opacities in the vitreous.

REFERENCES

1. Apple, D.J., and Rabb, J.F.: Ocular pathology: clinical applications and self-assessment, ed. 3, St. Louis, 1985, The C.V. Mosby Co.
2. Spencer, W.H., editor: Ophthalmic pathology: an atlas and textbook, ed. 3, Philadelphia, 1985, W.B. Saunders Co.
3. Rosai, J., editor: Ackerman's surgical pathology, ed. 6, St. Louis, 1981, The C.V. Mosby Co.
4. Yanoff, M., and Fine, B.S.: Ocular pathology: a color atlas, Hagerstown, Md., 1987, J.B. Lippincott Co.

Index

A

A band, 2106
A-cells
  pancreatic tumors and, 1368
  type II diabetes and, 1360
Abdominal aorta, inflammatory aneurysm of, 779
Abdominal disease, suppurative, 1258-1259
Abdominal trauma, pancreatitis and, 1353
Abdominal wall desmoids, 1845
abl, 587t
Abnormalities
  congenital; *see* Congenital abnormalities
  fetal irradiation and, 269
ABO blood group, 149
ABO hemolytic disease, 1262
Abortion, spontaneous, 1700-1701
Abrasion, 112, *113*, 114
Abruptio placentae, *1703*
Abscess, 85, 87, 302
  alveolar, 1099
  Bartholin gland, 1628
  brain, 2158
    herniation and, *2129*
  endocarditis and, 657
  epidural, 2153-2154
  ischiorectal, 1169
  liver, 1252, 1258-1260
    amebic, *1259, 1260*
    laboratory examination of, 1259
    solitary, 1259
  lung aspirational, 939
  myocarditis and, 659
  perianal, 1169
  splenic, 1419
  urethral, 898
Absidia, 395t, 425
Absorption, impaired intestinal, 1171
Acalculous primary bacterial cholecystitis, 1327-1330
Acanthamoeba, 437
  meningitis and, 2154
Acantholysis, 1757
Acanthoma, clear cell or Degos, 1795
Acanthosis, 897, 1757
  oral mucosa and, 1109
Acanthosis nigricans, 1759-1760, *1760*
  tumors and, 605
Acarus scabiei, 1769
Accelerator, linear, 248
Accessory pulmonary lobes, 923
Accessory spleen, 1413
Accidental poisoning, chemicals and drugs in, 193-194t
ACE; *see* Angiotensin-converting enzyme
Acetabulum, defective development of, 2067

Acetaldehyde, ethanol and, 19-20
Acetaminophen, 150
  necrosis and, 1234t, 1236
  poisoning from, 193t
  submassive hepatic necrosis and, 1205
  toxicity of, 160-162
Acetoacetate accumulation, 37
Acetone poisoning, 193t
Acetophenetidin; *see* Phenacetin
Acetylcholine, 8, 964
Acetylcholine receptors, 506t, 508, 1496, 1503
  myasthenia gravis and, 2118
Acetylhydrazine toxicity, 169
Achalasia of esophagus, 1154
Achlorhydria, 31
Achondroplasia, 1946-1949, *1947, 1948*
AChR; *see* Acetylcholine receptors
Achromia, 1786
Achylia, pancreatic, 1173
Acid emissions, 230
Acid-fast bacilli
  leprosy and, 339, 341
  tuberculosis and, 1284
Acid maltase deficiency, 55, 2114-2115
Acidophilic adenoma, salivary gland, 1135, *1135*
Acidophilic bodies, hepatitis and, 1205, *1205*, 1218-1219
Acidophilic necrosis, hepatic, 1205
Acidophils
  adenohypophysis and, 1519
  myocardial infarction and, 636
Acidosis, chronic renal, 807
Acini
  liver and, 1199
  pancreatic
    cystic fibrosis and, 1350
    obstruction and, *1353*
Acinic cell carcinoma, salivary gland, 1139, *1139*
Acinous lesions in tuberculosis, 945
Acne, 302
Acne rosacea, 1077
Acoustic insult, 136
Acoustic schwannomas, 2175
Acquired immunodeficiency syndrome, 1471-1474, 1500t
  adrenal cortex and, 1607
  alimentary tract and, 1167
  central nervous system and, 2162, *2163*, 2163-2164
  Kaposi's sarcoma and, 797, 1821-1822
  liver and, 1286-1287
  lungs and, 947, 968-969, 1036-1037
  mycobacterial infections in, 947, *947*
  oral lesions and, 1104
  pneumocystosis and, 450
  pneumonia and, 948
  as primary immune deficiency, 499, 1502
  retroviruses and, 376

Acquired immunodeficiency syndrome— cont'd
  skin and, 1822-1823
  toxoplasmosis and, 449
Acral melanomas, 1818
Acrochordons, 1796
Acromegaly, 690, 1972
  osteoarthrosis and, 2074
Acrosclerosis, 1779
Acrospiroma, 1832
ACTH; *see* Adrenocorticotropic hormone
Actin, 6
Actinium, 284
Actinobacillus mallei, 321
Actinomadura madurae, 392t
Actinomadura pelletieri, 392t
Actinomyces bovis, 393t
Actinomyces israelii, 393t, *406, 407*, 1105
Actinomyces naeslundii, 393t
Actinomyces odontolyticus, 393t
Actinomyces viscosus, 393t
Actinomycetes, 396, 421; *see also* Actinomycosis; specific organism
Actinomycin D, 26, 606
Actinomycosis, 391-397, 393t, 406-407, *407*; *see also* Mycotic infections
  bladder and, 857
  cervicofacial, *406*
  gastrointestinal tract and, *406*, 1166
  granulomatous inflammation and, 91
  liver abscess and, 1260
  in oral soft tissue, 1105
Action potential, 8
Active junctional nevus, 1816
Activity per unit mass of radioactive substances, 249
Adamantinoma, 2053, *2054*
ADCC; *see* Antibody-dependent cell-mediated cytotoxicity
Addison's disease, 30, 1586-1588
  oral mucosa and, 1106
  pituitary gland and, 1525
  secondary, 1588
  skin and, 1786
Adenitis, submandibular, 1128
Adenoacanthoma, endometrium and, *1661*
Adenocarcinoma, 575, 576, 610
  of breast, 281
  bronchogenic, 582, 1007-1010, *1008, 1009*
    adrenal metastasis from, *1602*
  of cervix, 1649-1650, *1650, 1651*
  of colon, *1181*
  of endometrium, 1659-1661, *1660*
  of fallopian tubes, *1670*, 1670-1671, *1671*
  of gallbladder and biliary ducts, 1337, *1337, 1338, 1338, 1339, 1339*, 1342
  of kidney, 847-848, *848*
  of larynx, 1087
  of nasal mucosa, 1082
  nonbacterial thrombotic endocarditis and, 652, 653

Adenocarcinoma—cont'd
  ovarian, *1682*
    clear cell, *1683*
    metastatic, 1691, *1691*
  pancreatic, 1357, *1357, 1358*
  of periampullary region, *1359*
  of prostate gland, 915
  of salivary glands, 1140
  of stomach, 257*t*
  tracheal adenoid cystic, *1017*
  of vagina, 1641-1642, *1642*
  of vulva, 1637
Adenofibroma, endometrial, 1663
Adenohypophysis, 1517, 1519-1523, *1520, 1521, 1522*
  hormones and cells of, 1521*t*, 1525
  tumors of, 1530*t*
Adenoid cystic carcinoma
  breast and, 1746
  prostate gland and, 915
  salivary glands and, *1138*, 1138-1139
  skin and, 1833
  trachea and, *1017*
Adenoid squamous cell carcinoma in oral soft tissue, 1112
Adenolymphoma, salivary gland, 1134
Adenoma, 575, 577, 610
  adrenal glands and, 1588, 1595-1599, *1597, 1598, 1598t*
    Cushing's syndrome and, *1595*
  alimentary tract, *1175*, 1175-1179
  bile duct, 1291
  gallbladder and common duct, 1334
  hepatic, oral contraceptives and, 166-167
  hepatocellular, 1289, *1290*
  hyperparathyroidism and, 1573-1574, *1574*
  middle ear, 1088
  nephrogenic, 865, *865*
  of nipple, 1732
  pituitary gland, 1530-1535, *1532*
    alpha subunit, 1535
    chromophobe, 1530, *1531*
    corticotroph cell, 1534
    gonadotroph cell, 1534-1535
    mammosomatotrophic, 1534
    null cell, 1535
    oncocytic, 1535
    prolactin cell, 1533
    somatomammotrophic, 1534
    somatotroph cell, 1533
    thyrotroph cell, 1525, 1534
  salivary gland
    acidophilic, 1135, *1135*
    basal cell, 1135-1136
    canalicular, 1135-1136, *1136*
    monomorphic, 1134
    pleomorphic, 1132*t*, 1132-1134, *1133*
  thyroid gland, follicular, 1554-1556, *1555*
  tubular
    alimentary tract, 1179
    colonic, 1175, *1175*
    renal cortical, 847
Adenomatoid malformation in lung, congenital, 923, *924*
Adenomatoid tumors
  of epididymis, 891, *891*
  of fallopian tube, 1670
  of jaw, odontogenic, 1121
Adenomatosis
  multiple endocrine, 609, 1563
    pituitary gland and, 1535
    thymus gland and, 1508
  multiple hepatocellular, 1289-1290, *1291*

Adenomatous hyperplasia
  endometrium and, 1657-1659, *1658*
  liver and, 1291, *1291*
    alcoholic cirrhotic, 1246-1247
Adenomatous polyps
  alimentary tract and, 1175-1179
  gallbladder and common duct and, 1334, *1334*
Adenomyoma
  endometrium and, 1659
  gallbladder and, 1335, *1336*
  myometrium and, 1663-1664, *1664*
Adenosine-3,5-cyclic monophosphate, 300
Adenosine deaminase deficiency, 503, 1500*t*
  severe combined immune deficiency disease with, 501*t*
Adenosine diphosphate, 1-2
  aspirin and, 160
Adenosine triphosphate
  cellular injury and, 11
  energy and, 1, 2
  glucose oxidation and, 2
  ischemia and, 631
  skin and, 1754
Adenosis
  breast and, 1729-1730
  prostate gland and, 912
  vagina and, 1639-1640, *1640*
Adenosquamous carcinoma
  bronchogenic, 1011
  pancreatic, *1358*
Adenoviruses, *364*, 377-378, *378*
ADH; *see* Alcohol dehydrogenase; Antidiuretic hormone
Adhesions, 666-667, *667*, 1156, 1189
  chronic inflammation and, 90
Adiaspiromycosis, 393*t*, 407, *408*
Adipose tissue, fat necrosis and, 16
Adipose tissue tumors, 1873-1886
  bone and, 2054
  hibernoma in, 1885-1886
  lipoblastoma in, 1884-1885
  lipoma in, 1879-1884
  liposarcoma in, 1873-1879
ADL; *see* Adrenal leukodystrophy
Adnexal structures, 1047-1051
  microcystic carcinoma and, 1833
ADP; *see* Adenosine diphosphate
ADR; *see* Adverse drug reaction
Adrenal cytomegaly in newborn, 1583
Adrenal glands, 1580-1619
  Addison's syndrome and, 1586-1588
  alarm reaction and, 1607
  blood pressure regulation and, 1607
  calcification of, 1606
  chronic mucocutaneous candidiasis and, 412
  congenital hyperplasia of, 1584
    female genitalia and, 1627
  cortex of
    acquired immunodeficiency syndrome and, 1607
    adenoma in, 1595-1599, *1596*
    carcinoma of, 1599-1605, *1602, 1603*
    eosinophils and, 82
    hyperplasia of, 568, 1589-1592
    nodule of, 1588, *1589*
  Cushing's syndrome and, 1592-1593
  cysts of, 1606
  DDT toxicity and, 226, *228*
  development of, 1580-1581
  diffuse and nodular, 1591
  function of, 1581-1583

Adrenal glands—cont'd
  hemorrhage of, 1606-1607
  hyperaldosteronism and, 1593-1594
  hypocortisolism and, 1586-1588
  hypoplasia of, 1583
  infant and child disorders of, 1583-1586
  irradiation of, 1607
  lesion frequency in, 1593
  medulla of, 1607-1613
    neoplasms of, 1608-1613
    vascular lesions and hyperplasias of, 1608
  metastases to, 1605
  microadenomatous, with hypercortisolism, 1592
  multinodular, 1588-1589
  multinodular hyperplasia and hypercortisolism of, 1591-1592
  myelolipoma and, 1605-1606
  neoplasms of, 1595-1606, 1608-1613
    adenoma in, 1595-1599
    histologic assessment of, 1603*t*
    medullary, 1608-1613
    metastatic, 1605
    myelolipoma in, 1605-1606
    primary adrenocortical carcinoma in, 1599-1605
    unusual, 1606
  nodules of, 1588-1589, 1591-1592
  radiosensitivity of epithelium of, 257*t*
  structure of, 1580
  virilization and feminization and, 1594-1595
Adrenal insufficiency, 1586-1588
  chronic, oral pigmentation and, 1106
Adrenal leukodystrophy, 1583-1584, *1584*, 2180
Adrenal medullary hyperplasia, 1608
Adrenalitis, allergic, 536*t*
Adrenocorticotropic hormone
  adrenal glands and, 1581, 1589, *1590*
    ectopic, *1595*
    tumors with, 1593*t*
  lung cancer and, 1013
  melanogenesis and, 30
  necrosis from, 163
  pituitary gland and, 1517, 1525, 1534
  thyroid carcinoma and, 1563
Adrenogenital syndrome, 873, *1590*, 1625*t*
Adriamycin; *see* Doxorubicin
Adventitia, 753, 762
Adverse drug reaction, 146-168
  analgesic and antipyretic, 158-162
  androgenic-anabolic steroids in, 165
  antibiotics in, 150-158
  antihypertensive drugs in, 168
  causative components of, 146-149
  corticosteroids in, 162-165, 1164
  estrogens in, 167
  incidence of, 146
  morphologic aspects of, 150
  oral contraceptives in, 165-167
  tranquilizers in, 167-168
  unwarranted, 146
Adynamic ileus, 1157
Aedes, 370, 470
Aero–otitis media, 134-135
Aerosinusitis, 134-135
Aerosols, 277
  harmful, 232-239
Aflatoxin, 596, 597*t*, 599, 601
  liver cell carcinoma and, 1294
  liver injury and, 1232

AFP; *see* Alpha-fetoprotein
African histoplasmosis, 419-420
African trypanosomiasis, 439
Agammaglobulinemia, 501*t*
Aganglionic megacolon, 1154
Age
　of articular cartilage, 2070-2071
　pharmacogenetics and, 150
　thymus gland and, 1499
　vision loss and, 1072-1074
Agenesis
　of corpus callosum, 2139
　gonadal, 1625*t*, 1626
　pituitary gland and, 1526
　renal, 844
　thyroid, 1546
Aggregation factor, 531*t*
Aggretope, 494
Aglossia, 1096
Agonadism, 873
Agranulocytosis, 499
　in oral soft tissue, 1104
AIDS; *see* Acquired immunodeficiency
　syndrome
AIDS-dementia complex, 376, 2163-2164
AIDS-related complex, 376, 968, 1104
Air blast, 135
Air embolism, 953
Air pollution, 230-232, 989, 993
Airflow limitation, 987-996, 1040-1041; *see*
　also Lung, chronic airflow limitation
　and
Alagille syndrome, 922, 1267
Alanine aminotransferase, 1215, 1216*t*
Albinism, 31, 51-52, 1053
Albright's syndrome, 1898
　oral pigmentation and, 1106
Albuminuria, 516
Alcian blue stain, 396*t*
Alcohol, 18-20, 599
　amphetamines and methamphetamines
　　and, 169
　atherosclerosis and, 620
　barbiturates and, 193*t*, 218
　deaths attributed to, 192
　hemosiderosis and, 32
　hepatic oxidation of, 1238, *1239*
　metabolism of, 1238-1240
　methanol and, 198
　smooth endoplasmic reticulum and, 1240
　toxicity of, 191-198, 193*t*
Alcohol dehydrogenase, 1238-1239
　isoenzymes and enzyme polymorphisms
　　and, 1240
Alcoholic cardiomyopathy, *685*, 685-686
Alcoholic cerebellar degeneration, 2185
Alcoholic cirrhosis, 1202, 1238; *see also*
　　Alcoholic liver disease
　advanced stage of, 1246, *1247*
　atrophic stage of, *1246*, 1246-1247
　hepatocellular carcinoma and, 1294
　Mallory bodies and, 1203
　portacaval anastomosis and, 1247
　reversibility of, 1247
　salivary glands and, 1128
Alcoholic fibrosis, 1240, *1241*, 1244
　progressive perivenular, 1207
Alcoholic hepatitis, 1243, *1243*
Alcoholic hyaline body, 1203, 1203*t*, *1243*
Alcoholic liver disease, 16-18, 1202, 1238-
　　1247; *see also* Alcoholic cirrhosis
　acute, 1242-1244
　chronic, 1244-1247

Alcoholic liver disease—cont'd
　classification of, 1240-1241
　early asymptomatic, 1241
　ethanol metabolism and, 1238-1240
　fatty liver and, 1244, 1245
　Mallory bodies and, 1203, 1203-1204
　osteoporosis and, 1974
　pathology of, 1240-1241
Alcoholic myopathy, 194
Alcoholic pancreatitis, 1253
　hemorrhagic, 1353
Alcoholism, 1086
　liver and, 16-18; *see also* Alcoholic
　　cirrhosis
Aldomet; *see* Methyldopa
Aldosterone, 1581, *1582*, *1596*
　cirrhosis and, 1251
Aldosteronism, *1596*
Aldosteronoma, *1596*
Algal infections, 391-432; *see also* Mycotic
　　infections
Alimentary tract, 1153-1198
　acquired malformations of, 1155-1156
　anorectal lesions in, 1168-1169
　congenital anomalies in, 1153-1155
　flagellates of, 438-439
　functional states in, 1169-1172
　inflammations of, 1159-1168
　mechanical disturbances of, 1156-1158
　mesenteric disease in, 1189-1191
　nematodes of, 462-469
　neoplasms of, 1175-1188
　　adenomatous polyps in, 1175-1179
　　anal region carcinoma in, 1184
　　carcinoid tumor in, 1184-1186
　　colorectal carcinoma in, 1180
　　esophageal carcinoma in, 1183
　　gastric carcinoma in, 1180-1183
　　gastric polyps in, 1179
　　lymphoma in, 1186-1188
　　malignant melanoma in, 1184
　　papillary adenomas in, 1175-1179
　　rare tumors in, 1188
　　small intestinal carcinoma in, 1183
　　smooth muscle, 1186
　　tubular and papillary adenomas
　　　compared to colon carcinoma in, 1179
　omentum in, 1189-1191
　peritoneal disease in, 1189-1191
　radiation injury and, 278
　retroperitoneal disease in, 1189-1191
　systemic disease and, 1172-1175
　vascular disturbances of, 1158-1159
Alkaline phosphatase, 1932-1933, *1933*
　Paget's disease and, 2006
Alkaptonuria, 31
Alkylating agents, 606
　oxygen toxicity and, 180-182
ALL; *see* Leukemia, acute lymphoblastic
Allantoin, 36
Allele, 610
Allergens, atopic, 526
Allergic alveolitis, extrinsic, 965-967
Allergic angiitis, 772
　lungs and, 976
Allergic asthma, 962
Allergic bronchopulmonary mycosis, 964-965
Allergic encephalomyelitis, experimental,
　　535
Allergic granulomatosis, 538
　lungs and, 976
Allergic interstitial nephritis, 838
Allergic polyps, 1078

Allergy, 88, 487
　drug, 538
　　rifampin and, 170
　food, 525-526
　insect, 526
　larynx and, 1084
　nasal cavity and paranasal sinuses and,
　　1078-1080
Allescheria boydii, 423
Alloantigens, tissue, 493
Allograft rejection, 531
Allopurinol
　granulomas and, 1285
　liver necrosis and, 1236
Allosteric regulation, 10
Alloxan, 1359
Alobar holoprosencephaly, 2138
Alopecia, thallium toxicity and, 214-216
Alopecia areata, 539*t*
Alopecia mucinosa, 1787
Alpha₁-antichymotrypsin
　epithelioid sarcoma and, 1901
　malignant fibrous histiocytoma and, 1858-
　　1859
Alpha₁-antitrypsin
　epithelioid sarcoma and, 1901
　immunoperoxidase or
　　immunofluorescence and, 1264
　liver disease and, 1264
　malignant fibrous histiocytoma and, 1858
Alpha₁-antitrypsin deficiency, 1264-1265,
　　1788
　juvenile cirrhosis in, 1264, *1264*
　liver and, 1204
　neonatal and childhood cholestasis and,
　　1261*t*, 1262
Alpha emission, 248
Alpha-fetoprotein, 604, 880-881
　neural tube defects and, 2136
Alpha heavy-chain disease, 1470
Alpha-methyldopa
　chronic active hepatitis and, 1235*t*, 1237
　necrosis and, 1234*t*, 1236
Alpha particles, 23, 23*t*, 248
Alpha-thalassemia, 1381
Alpha-1-protease inhibitor, 993-994
Alphaviruses, 371
Alport's syndrome, 823
ALS; *see* Amyotrophic lateral sclerosis
ALT; *see* Alanine aminotransferase
Altitude
　exposure to increasing, 134
　pulmonary edema and, 960
Aluminum
　neurofibrillary degeneration and, 2133
　osteomalacia and, 1997, *1998*
Aluminum oxide in pneumoconiosis, 233
Alveolar abscess, periodontal, 1099
Alveolar capillary dysplasia, congenital, 921
Alveolar clearance mechanism, 233
Alveolar damage
　capillary endothelial, 960
　causes of, 961-962
　oxygen toxicity and, 176, *177-179*
Alveolar macrophages, 931
Alveolar microlithiasis, 982
　milk-alkali syndrome and, 189, *189*
Alveolar proteinosis, *981*, 981-982
Alveolar rhabdomyosarcomas, 1865, 1867-
　　1870, *1869*
　diagnostic molecular biology and, 603
Alveolar soft part sarcoma, 1903-1906, *1905*

Alveoli
lung development and, 920
pulmonary edema and, 958
radiation injury and, 276
sclerosing angiogenic tumor and, *1020*
Alveolitis
extrinsic allergic, 965-967
herbicide toxicity and, 230
methotrexate and, 185
Alymphoplasia, thymic, 501*t*, *1501*
Alzheimer type II astrocytes, 2134
Alzheimer's disease, *2181*, 2181-2182
Amanita toxin, 224, 1233
Amastigotes, 443
Ambisexual, 872
Amblyomma cajennense, 350
Amebas, 433-437
Amebiasis, 433-437, 1166-1167, *1167*
colitis and, 434, *434*, *435*
hepatic, 434
abscesses and, *1259*, *1259-1260*, *1260*
meningoencephalitis and, 437
Ameboma, 436
Amelanotic melanoma, 31
Ameloblastic fibroma, odontogenic, 1125, *1125*
Ameloblastic fibrosarcoma, odontogenic, 1126-1127
Ameloblastoma, odontogenic, 1121, *1122*, *1123*
Amenorrhea, hypopituitarism and, 1526
American trypanosomiasis, 440-441
Amethopterin; *see* Methotrexate
Amino acids
deficiencies of, 562
encephalopathy and, 1248
ethanol and, 18
peptides and, 2
Aminoaciduria, pancreatitis and, 1353
Aminoglycoside toxicity, 156-158
Aminophenol toxicity, 160-162
Aminopterine, 59
Aminorex, 957
Amiodarone toxicity, 176, 1238, 1546
Amitriptyline poisoning, 193*t*
Ammonia
bronchitis and, 238
liver disease and, 1248
pulmonary edema and, 237
Amnion, 1693, 1698
Amniotic fluid
emboli and, 953
infection and, 929
Amobarbital poisoning, 193*t*
Amosite, 235
Amphetamine toxicity, 168-169, 193*t*, 708
Amphotericin B, 410, 415
myocarditis and, 708
toxicity of, 153
Ampicillin, colitis and, 155
Ampulla of Vater, gallstone in, 1353
Amputation neuroma, 1335
Amylo-1,6-glucosidase deficiency, 57
Amylo-1,4→1,6-transglucosidase deficiency, 57
Amyloid, 38-41, *39*; *see also* Amyloidosis
arthropathy and, 2068
globular, 1204
in larynx, 1085
in prostate gland, 902
Amyloidosis, 695-696, 821-823, *822*
hemodialysis and, 2000
hepatic, 1286

Amyloidosis—cont'd
hypocortisolism and, 1587-1588
of islets of Langerhans, 1363, *1364*
leprosy and, 338
lung, 983
nitrogen mustard and, 182
pituitary gland and, 1529, *1529*
plasma cell proliferative disorders and, 1403
skin and, 1781, *1781*
spleen and, 1413
systemic, 821-823
thyroid gland and, 1554, *1554*
Amyotrophic lateral sclerosis, 2119, 2120, 2183
Anabolic steroids, 1234*t*, 1235
adverse reactions to, 165
hepatocellular adenoma and, 1289
hepatocellular carcinoma and, 1295
hypertrophy and, 568
Anaerobic bacteria
lung lesions and, 938-939
periodontal disease and, 1099
Anal ducts, 1168, *1169*
carcinoma of, 1184
Anal fissures, 1169
Analgesic toxicity, 158-162, 832
Anaphylactic reactions, 88, 148, 151*t*, 487, 516-527, 519, 523-524, 524, 526-527, 539*t*
cutaneous, 518, 523
passive, 519
mechanism of, 504*t*
pharmacologic control of, 528
symptoms of, 523*t*
Anaphylactoid purpura, 816
Anaplasia, 570-571, *572*, 610
endometrium and, 1659
Anaplastic astrocytoma, 2167-2168, *2168*
Anaplastic carcinoma
of bladder, 863, *863*
thyroid gland and, 1562
Anaplastic rhabdomyosarcoma tumor, 1866
Ancient neurilemomas, 1892
Ancylostoma braziliense, 467
Ancylostoma caninum, 464, 467
Ancylostoma duodenale, 463
Ancylostomiasis, 463-464
Androblastoma, 889
ovary and, 1685-1686
Androgen-insensitivity syndromes, 1624, 1626-1627
Androgenic anabolic steroids; *see* Anabolic steroids
Androgens, 902, 911
excess of, 873
prostate carcinoma and, 907
prostatic hyperplasia and, 567
Androstenedione, *1582*
Anemia, 31
amphotericin B and, 153
aplastic, 1375-1376, *1376*
chloramphenicol and, 155-156
benzene and, 222
blood-loss, 1379
bone marrow and megaloblastic, 1377-1378
bothriocephalus, 460
cirrhosis and, 1252
congestive cardiomyopathy and, 692-693
Fanconi's, 609, 1385
folic acid deficiency and, 557
hematopoietic syndrome and, 273

Anemia—cont'd
hemolytic, 1379-1382, *1380*
autoallergic, *511*
iron-deficiency, 1378-1379
myelophthisic, 1379
osteoporosis and, 1972
pernicious, 506*t*, 1169, 1378
vitamin B_{12} and, 560
pyridoxine deficiency and, 559
renal failure and, 807
sickle cell, 1380-1381, *1414*, *1417*
sideroblastic, 1379
tumors and, 605
Anencephaly, 2136, *2137*
hypoplasia of pituitary and, 1526
Anesthetic toxicity, 171
Aneuploidy, 46-47
Aneurysm, 778-785
aortic, 779, *780*, 782, 783, 784
dissecting, 780-784, *782*, *783*
rupture of, *664*
arteriovenous, 794
atherosclerotic, 778-780, *779*, *780*, *781*, *782*, *783*, *784*
cerebral hemorrhage and, 2151-2153, *2152*
Charcot-Bouchard, 2151
coronary artery disease and, 624
degenerative, 780
Dieulafoy's, 1159
false, 778
hemangiomas and, 1819
mycotic, 767
myocardial infarction and ventricular, 638
syphilitic, 780
true, 778
Aneurysmal bone cyst, 2022*t*, 2056-2057, *2058*
in jaws, 1120
Angiitis, 766-778; *see also* Arteritis
allergic, 772, 976
Angina, intestinal, 1158
Angina pectoris, 625-626, 675
Angiodysplasia, 1159
Angioedema, 524, *524*, 539*t*
Angioendotheliomatosis, malignant, 1465
Angiofibroma in nasopharynx, 1083
Angiofollicular lymph node hyperplasia, 1437, *1438*
Angiogenesis, 102, 581
Angiography, hemobilia and mesenteric, 1258
Angioimmunoblastic lymphadenopathy with dysproteinemia, 1439, *1441*
Angiokeratoma, 1820
Angiokeratoma corporis diffusum, 1780
Angioleiomyoma, 1860
Angiolipoma, 1792, 1883-1884, *1884*, 1888
Angiolymphoid hyperplasia with eosinophilia, 795, 1790, *1791*
Angioma
capillary, 1819
sclerosing, *1820*
Angiomatoid malignant fibrous histiocytoma, 1856, 1859
Angiomatoids, intra-arterial, 457
Angiomatosis, 795
encephalofacial, 1109
retinal, 1051
Angiomyolipomas in kidney, 847
Angiomyoma, 1824
Angiomyxoma, aggressive, 1632, 1898

Angionecrosis, thrombocytopenic verrucal, 1790-1791
Angiosarcoma, 797
  of bone, 2051
  of breast, *1748*, 1748-1749
  of skin, 1821
  of spleen, 1427, *1427*
Angiostrongyliasis, 468-469
Angiotensin-converting enzyme, 980
Angular cheilitis, 1105
Animal tumors, 292*t*
Anisakiasis, 462-463
Anitschkow cells, 659
Ankylosing spondylitis, 536, 650, 776, 2097-2098
  radiation injury and, 258-259, 279
ANLL; *see* Leukemia, acute nonlymphoblastic
Ann Arbor staging classification of Hodgkin's disease, 1450, 1452
Anodontia, 1096
Anogenital warts, 1794-1795
Anomalies
  congenital; *see* Congenital abnormalities of placenta, 1698
Anomalous pulmonary venous drainage, 737-738, *738*
Anopheles, 445, 470
Anorchia, bilateral, 873
Anorchidism, 871
Anorectal lesions, 1168-1169
Anorexia nervosa, 1981
Anovulatory bleeding pattern, 1657, *1657*
Anoxia
  encephalopathy and, 2146-2147
  intrauterine, 698
  liver necrosis and, 1278, *1278*, 1279
Antacids, osteomalacia and, 1994-1995
Anterior uveitis, 1057
Anthophyllite, 235
Anthracosis, 35, *35*
Anthracycline antibiotic toxicity, 183, 708
Anthralin, 598
Anthrax, 292*t*, 296-297, *298*
Antiarrhythmics, toxicity of, 175-176
Anti-*bcl*-2, 604
Antibiotics, 150-158; *see also* individual drug
  colitis and, 146, 155
  endocarditis and, 654
Antibody, 487, 488
  anti-idiotypic, 489, *489*, 498
  blocking, 498, 534
  cytophyllic, 531*t*
  fluorescent, 810, *810*, *811*
  to hepatitis B core antigen, 1213-1214
  homocytotropic, 519
  humoral, 499
  immune deficiency disease and defects in, 501*t*
  mitochondrial, primary biliary cirrhosis and, 1256
  monoclonal, 494
  oncogene products and, 604
  primary reaction of, 490
  reaginic, 519
  thyroid-stimulating, 1549
Antibody-antigen reactions, 490
  soluble antigen, *513*
Antibody-dependent cell-mediated cytotoxicity, 493, 507*t*
Antibody-mediated disease, 505, 511, *511*
Anticancer drug toxicity, 180-186, 606
Anticarcinogens, 597

Anticholinergics, children and, 150
Anticholinesterase agents in myasthenia gravis, 2118
Anticoagulants, hemopericardium and, 665
Anticonvulsants
  25-hydroxylation and, 1993
  osteoporosis and, 1972
  toxicity of, 171-174
Antidiabetic drug toxicity, 169
Antidiuretic hormone, 1523
Antiestrogens, 606
Antifreeze, 832
Antigen, 487
  B-lymphocyte and, *1456*
  carcinoembryonic, 1563
  cell surface, 507*t*
  colloid, 507*t*
  drug as, 148-149
  Epstein-Barr nuclear, 383
  incomplete, 488
  lymphoid cell and, 1454*t*, *1456*, 1496*t*
  microsomal, 507*t*
  neurofilament, as nervous system tumor marker, 2166*t*
  sex-specific histocompatibility, 1623
  T-lymphocyte, *1457*, 1496*t*
Antigen-antibody complex, 490
Antigen processing, 498
Antigenic drift, influenza and, 365
Antiglobulin test, 512
Anti-glomerular basement membrane disease, 515-516, 810
Anti-hepatitis B core antigen, 1213-1214
Anti-hepatitis B surface antigen, 1214
Antihypertensive drug toxicity, 168, 708
Anti-idiotypes, 489, *489*, 498
Antimetabolites, 606
  toxicity of, 183-186, *184*, *185*
Antimitochondrial antibody, 148
Antimony, 708
Antineoplastic toxicity, 180-186, 606
Antinuclear factor, 148
Antioncogenes, 589, 609
  radiation injury and, 265
Antipyretics, toxicity of, 158-162
Antistreptolysin O, 812
Antithyroid drug toxicity, 169
Antitrypsin, deficiency of; *see* Alpha$_1$-antitrypsin deficiency
Antitubercular drug toxicity, 169-171
Antivitamins, 551
Antoni A and B regions
  neurilemoma and, 1891, *1891*, 1891-1892
  in schwannoma, 2171
Antrochoanal polyps, 1078
Anuria, 809
Anus, 1153
  carcinoma of, 1184
  fissures of, 1169
Aorta
  aneurysm of, 778-784, *779*, *780*, *782*, *783*
    inflammatory abdominal, 779
    rupture of, *664*
  atheroma of, 760, *761*
  atheromatous plaques in, 623
  coarctation of, 740-743, *742*, *743*
  double-barreled, 782
  stenosis of, *674*, 674-675, *675*
    isolated, 739-740, *740*, *741*
    rheumatic fever and, 645, *646*
Aortic insufficiency, 675-676
  ankylosing spondylitis and, 650
  syphilis and, 650, *651*

Aortic regurgitation, syphilitic heart disease and, 650
Aortic sinus aneurysm, 784
Aortic tract, hypoplasia of, 748-749, *750*
Aortic valve
  rheumatic endocarditis and, 645, *646*
  syphilis and, 650
Aorticopulmonary septal defect, 737, *737*
Aortitis
  ankylosing spondylitis and, 650
  rheumatoid, 775-776
  syphilitic, 621, 767, *768*
  Takayasu's, 768
Aortocoronary vein bypass grafts, 791, 792-793
Apatite arthropathy, 2090
Aphthae, recurrent, 1104
Apical thrombosis, 442
Aplasia, 610
  bone marrow, 1375
  pure red blood cell, 1377
Aplastic anemia, 1375-1376, *1376*
  chloramphenicol and, 155-156
Aplysiatoxin, *598*
Apocrine glands, 1756
  cystadenomas of, 1832
Apoferritin, 31
Aponeuroses, clear cell sarcoma of, 2096
Aponeurotic fibroma, 1848-1849
Apophysomyces, 395*t*, 425
Apoplexy
  adrenal, 1585
  pituitary, 1527
Apoprotein of alveolar surfactant, 1009
Appendages
  diseases of, 1786-1787
  tumors of, 1830-1835
Appendicitis, 1165-1166
  diffuse type of, *88*
  necrosis and, *86*
Appendix
  balantidiasis of, *438*
  carcinoid tumors in, 1185
  inflammation of; *see* Appendicitis
  mucocele of, 1188
Apresoline; *see* Hydralazine
Arachidonic acid metabolism, 522, 635
Arachnia propionica, 393*t*
ARC; *see* AIDS-related complex
Arcus senilis, 1074
ARDS; *see* Respiratory distress syndrome, adult
Arenaviruses, 372-373
  encephalitis and, 2158
arg, 587*t*
Argentaffin tumors, 1184
  gastric polyps and, *1185*
Argentine fever, 373
Arginine, 562
Argyll Robertson pupils, 2158
Argyria, 36, 1785
Argyrophil cells, 1015, 1184
Ariboflavinosis, 558, *559*
Armanni-Ebstein lesion of kidney, 1062, 1366
Arnold-Chiari malformation, 2137
  hydrocephalus and, 2139, 2140, *2140*
Aromatics, poisoning from, 193*t*
Arrectores pilorum, 1756
Arrhenoblastoma, ovary and, 1685-1686
Arrhinencephaly, 2138, *2138*
Arrhythmias
  nonpenetrating cardiac injury and, 699

Arrhythmias—cont'd
  sudden cardiac death and, 627
Arsenic, 193t, 209-210, 599, 708
  keratosis and, 570
  liver and, 1232, 1237
Arterial air embolism in divers, 134
Arterial trunks, transposition of, 745-746,
    747
Arteries, 752-786
  aneurysms of, 778-785
  arteriopathy and, 785-786
  arteriosclerosis and, 754-766; see also
    Arteriosclerosis
  arteritis and, 766-778; see also Arteritis
  normal structure and age changes in, 752-
    754, 753-755
  primary tumors of large, 799
  radiation and, 276
Arteriohepatic dysplasia, 1267
Arteriole, 753, 754
  in bone marrow, 1406, 1407
  inflammatory response and, 68, 68
  inflammatory response of
    glomerular disease and, 826
    leukocytoclastic, in upper dermis, 1790
  nephrosclerosis and, 823
  radiation and, 274, 276
  repair of, 98
Arteriolitis, skin and, 1789
Arteriolosclerosis, 754
Arterionephrosclerosis, 842-843
Arteriopathy, 785-786
Arteriosclerosis, 754-766
  arteriolosclerosis and, 754-756
  atherosclerosis and, 757-766, 759, 760,
    761, 762, 763
  diabetes and, 1366
  hypertensive, 756, 756-757
  Mönckeberg's medial calcific sclerosis
    and, 757, 757
  senile, 753
Arteriosclerotic cardiovascular disease, 616
Arteriovenous aneurysm, 778
Arteriovenous fistula, 794
  chronic liver disease and, 1251
  hereditary hemorrhagic telangiectasia and,
    795
  liver injury and, 1275
Arteriovenous malformation, hemorrhage
    from, 2153, 2153
Arteritis, 766-778
  endarteritis obliterans in, 766
  Heubner's, 768
  infective, 766-768
  narcotic toxicity and, 219
  noninfective vasculitides in, 768-778
  nonsyphilitic, 766-767
  rheumatic, 623
  rheumatic fever and, 648
  rheumatoid, 623
  rheumatoid arthritis and, 649
  syphilitic, 767, 767-768
  Takayasu, 623
Arthritis, 516
  connective tissue diseases and, 2087
  enteropathic, 2086
  familial Mediterranean fever and, 2087
  gouty, 2089
  psoriasis and, 2086
  rheumatoid; see Rheumatoid arthritis
  sarcoidosis and, 2087
  Sjögren's syndrome and, 974
  skin and, 1792

Arthritis—cont'd
  traumatic, 2067
  tuberculous, 2006
  viral hepatitis and, 2087
Arthroconidium, 397
Arthropathy
  apatite, 2090
  diabetes mellitus and, 2091-2092
  with hemochromatosis, 2068-2069
  with hemophilia, 2069
  with ochronosis, 2068
  pyrophosphate, 2090
  sickle cell disease and, 2070
Arthropods, cutaneous reactions to, 1829
Arthus reaction, 88, 89, 148, 499, 512, 513,
    967
Articular cartilage, 2066
  aging of, 2070, 2070-2071
  calcinosis of, 2090
  inflammatory joint diseases and, 2075
Arylam; see Carbaryl
Arylsulfatase A, 2180
Asbestos, 594, 597, 599
  diseases related to, 235-236, 238, 1002-
    1005, 1003, 1004
Ascariasis, 462, 462, 1254
Ascaris, 462, 967, 1157
Aschoff bodies, 92, 623, 641-643, 642, 2077
Ascites, 1189
  ovary and, 1682, 1692
Ascorbic acid, 560-561
ASCVD; see Atherosclerotic cardiovascular
    disease
Aseptic inflammation, 129
Aseptic meningitis, 2158
ASH; see Asymmetric septal hypertrophy
ASHD; see Atherosclerotic heart disease
Asian influenza, 365
Asiatic cholera, 299
Askanazy cells, 1552
Askin tumor, 1611
ASO; see Antistreptolysin O
Aspergillosis, 393t, 407-410, 409
  cytomegalovirus pneumonia and, 382
  eye and, 1053
  heart and, 654, 655
  paranasal sinuses and, 1079
  pulmonary, 408-409, 410
Aspermia, 872
Asphyxia, perinatal, 2143
Aspiration
  bone marrow, 1375
  of food bolus, 192
  lipid, 985
  lung abscess and, 939
Aspiration pneumonia, 985
  botulism and, 293
Aspirin
  intolerance to, 526
  oral soft-tissue burns and, 1110
  papillitis necroticans and, 160-161
  Reye's syndrome and, 1269, 2185
  toxicity of, 158-160
    liver, 1237
Asplenism, 1411-1413
Asteroid bodies, 979
Asthma, 525, 962-964, 963
  chronic, 506t
  lung in, 525
Astrocytes, 2133-2134; see also Astrocytosis
  fusiform fibrillary, 2167, 2167
  hypertrophied, 2134
  mercury poisoning and, 203, 205

Astrocytoma
  with atypical or anaplastic foci, 2167-2168,
    2168
  juvenile pilocytic, 2167, 2167
  radiosensitivity of, 257t
  well-differentiated, 2167, 2167
Astrocytosis, 2133-2134; see also Astrocytes
  perinatal brain injury and, 2145
  subacute combined degeneration of spinal
    cord and, 2186
Astrogliosis, 2133
Asymmetric septal hypertrophy, 682-683
Ataxia, Friedreich, 694
Ataxia telangiectasia, 501t, 609, 1500t
  of eye, 1051
  leukemia and, 1385
Atelectasis, 986
Atherogenesis, 764
Atheroma, 758
  aortic, 623, 760, 761
Atherosclerosis, 617-621, 754, 762
  aneurysm and, 778-780, 779, 780
  angiogenesis and, 104
  placental lesions and, 1703-1704
  radiation-induced heart disease and, 699-
    700
Atherosclerotic cardiovascular disease, 616
Atherosclerotic heart disease, 616
Atherosclerotic plaque; see Plaque
Atmospheric pressure, injuries from, 133-
    136
Atomic bomb, injuries from, 136, 138, 260
  survivors of, 261t, 262, 263
Atopic reactions, 516-527, 518
  pharmacologic control of, 528
ATP; see Adenosine triphosphate
Atrabiliary capsules, 1580
Atresia
  alimentary tract and, 1153
  biliary, 1262-1263
    neonatal and childhood cholestasis and,
      1261t, 1262
  of fallopian tubes, 1627
Atresia complexes, 746-748
Atrial fibrillation, thrombi and, 623
Atrial infarcts, 629
Atrial septal defect, 731
Atrio-ventricular node, 705
Atrioventricular orifice, 735-736, 736, 737
Atrophia bulbi, 1074
Atrophic cirrhosis, 1247
Atrophic polychondritis, chronic, 2090
Atrophic rhinitis, 313
Atrophic thyroiditis, 1553
Atrophy, 42-43, 568-569, 610
  cardiac, 677
  epidermis and, 1805
  of fat, 1788
  gastric, 1169, 1170
  of hepatocytes, 1203
  muscle, 2108-2109, 2109
    childhood dermatomyositis and
      perifascicular, 2118, 2118
    infantile spinal, 2120-2121, 2121
    neurogenic, 2119, 2119-2121, 2120
  neuronal, 2132
  ovarian, 1674
  perinatal brain injury and, 2145
  of spleen, 1413, 1414
  of testicle, 876, 876
  vulvar, 1629-1630
Atypical bile ductules, 1207
Atypical carcinoids of bronchi, 1017

Atypical endometrial hyperplasia, *1658*, 1659
Atypical fibroxanthoma, 1792-1793
Atypical follicular adenoma, 1556
Atypical lipoma, 1881-1883
Atypical lymphocytes, 1419
Atypical lymphoid hyperplasia, 1443
Atypical mycobacteria, 946
Auerbach's plexus, 1154
Aural polyp, 1088
Auricular lesions, 1088-1089
Autoallergic diseases, *511*, 534-536; *see also* Autoimmune diseases
Autoantibodies, 535
    silicosis and, 998
    to thyroid antigens, 507t
Autocrine growth factors, 9, 591
Autograft, 531
Autoimmune diseases, 497, 498, 535-536, 536t
    adrenal glands and, 1586-1587
    hepatitis and, 1230
    major histocompatibility complex and, 536
    markers in, 148
    myopathies and, 2117-2119
    rheumatoid arthritis and, 2085
    thyroiditis and, 1545, 1551-1553
Autoinfection, 468
Autolysis, 13, *13*
    postmortem, 1205
Autophagy, 28, *29*, 43
Autosomal inheritance, *50*, 50-58
    agammaglobulinemia and, 501t
    hemochromatosis and, 32
    polycystic kidney and, 845-846, *846*
Autosomes, numeric abnormalities of, 46-48
Autosplenectomy, 1413, 1414
Axillary lymph nodes, 1741
Axon, 97
    myelinated, 2135
Axoneme, 950
Axonopathies, 2189-2190, *2190*
5-Azacytidine, 569
Azathioprine toxicity, 183, *185*, 185-186
Azoospermia, 875, 876
Azotemia, 516
Azotorrhea, 1172
Azygous vein, 921

B

B-cell tumors, 588, 1367
B-cells, 490-493, 495
    antigens and, *1456*
    diabetes and, 1359, 1360, *1361*
    differentiation of, *491*
    emiocytosis and, *1362*
    portal tracts and, 1206
    properties of, 490t
    thymus gland and, 1502
    thyroid gland and, 1565
    transformation of, *1429*
B-immunoblasts, 1430
B-K nevus, 1803
B-lymphocytes; *see* B-cells
Babesiosis, 451-452
Bacillary dysentery, 292t, 300, *301*
Bacillus anthracis, 297
Bacillus Calmette-Guérin, 999
Bacillus coli, 311
Bacillus megaterium, 83, *84*
Bacillus pyocyaneus, 311
Bacteremia; *see* Septicemia

Bacteria; *see also* Bacterial diseases
    aerobic, 936
    anaerobic, 938-939
    filamentous, 396
    phagocytosis of, 933
    pyogenic, 301
        lymphangitis and, 792
Bacterial cholecystitis, 1327-1330
Bacterial diseases, 289-331, 498t
    body surface, 294-301
        anthrax and, 296-297
        diphtheria and, 294-295
        gas gangrene and, 295-296
        pertussis and, 297-299
        Shigella and, 300-301
        vibrio and, 299-300
    disease versus lesion and, 290
    endocarditis as, 654
    exotoxicoses in, 292-294
        botulism in, 292-293
        staphylococcal, 293-294
        tetanus in, 294
    extracellular infections and, 301-314
        Enterobacter aerogenes and, 312
        Erysipelothrix and, 313
        Escherichia coli and, 311-312
        gonococci and, 309-310
        Haemophilus and, 310-311
        Klebsiella and, 312-313
        Legionella and, 311
        Listeria and, 313
        meningococci and, 307-309
        Mycoplasma and, 313-314
        pneumococci and, 306-307
        Proteus and, 311
        Pseudomonas aeruginosa and, 311
        staphylococci and, 301-303
        streptococci and, 303-306
    infection versus disease and, 289
    intracellular, 314-329
        brucellosis and, 317-318
        glanders and, 321-322
        granuloma inguinale and, 324
        melioidosis and, 322-324
        Pasteurella and, 321
        Salmonella and, 314-317
        spirochetes and, 324-329
        tularemia and, 318-320
        Yersinia and, 320-321
    of lung, 932-947; *see also* Lung, bacterial infections of
    myocarditis as, 659-660, *660*
    osteomyelitis as, 2004-2005
    pathogenesis of, 290-292
    pericarditis as, 668
    placenta and, 1704-1705
    pneumonia as, 928
    pseudomycosis as, 410-411
    vitamin A deficiency and, 553
Bacterial disseases, pneumonia as, 932-939
Bacterial toxins, 291, 1232
Bacterium; *see* Bacteria
Bacteroides, 938, 1189, 1657, 1667-1668, 1704
Bagassosis, 966t
Baker's cysts, 2092
Balanitis xerotica obliterans, 1776-1777, *1777*
Balantidiasis, 437-438, *438*
Balkan nephritis, 838
Balloon cells, 18, 195
    nevi and, 1804

Ballooned hepatocytes, hepatitis and, 1226, *1226*
Ballooning degeneration, skin and, 1757
Ballooning mitral valve, 676
Balo's concentric sclerosis, 2177
Bancroftian filariasis, 470
Bands of Büngner, 2190
Banti's syndrome, 1417
Bantu siderosis, 1273
Barbital poisoning, 193t
Barbiturate blister, 218, *218*
Barbiturates
    enzyme inducers and, 1232
    toxicity of, 193t, 217-219, *218*
Bare lymphocyte syndrome, 501t
Barium sulfate, 233
Barometric pressure, 133
Barr body, 59
Barrett's esophagus, 1159
Bartholin's gland
    carcinoma of, 1637
    cyst and abscess of, 1628
    inflammation of, 357
Basal cell adenomas, salivary gland, 1135-1136
Basal cell carcinoma, 1798-1799, *1800*
    multiple nevoid, 2166
Basal cell nevus syndrome, 1799-1800
Basal cells, 1753-1754
    prostate gland and hyperplasia of, 912, *913*
    tissue regeneration and, 96
Basal ganglia, carbon monoxide poisoning and, 222
Basaloid tumors, anal, 1184
Basedow's disease, 1549
Basement membrane
    diabetes and, *1365*
    glomerular, 804, *805*
    skin and, 1755
    tissue regeneration and, 96
    vascular permeability and, 73, 78
Basidiobolus ranarum, 393t, 426
Basilar crackles, 1003
Basophilia
    lead poisoning and, 205, *206*
    myeloproliferative disorders and, 1383
Basophilic degeneration, 465
    of myocardium, 687-688, *688*
Basophils, 516
    chemotaxis and, 80
    cutaneous hypersensitivity and, 530
    inflammation and, 82
    pituitary gland and, 1519, 1522
Basosquamous cell carcinoma, 1799
Bathing trunk nevi, 1816, *1817*
bcl-1, 587t
bcl-2, 587t, 603
bcr, 593
bcr/c-abl gene fusion, 593
Beau's lines, 1787
Beechey ground squirrel virus, 1211
Beef tapeworm, 458
Beer drinkers' heart disease, 212
Behçet's syndrome, 1104, 2086
Bence Jones protein, 839, 1402
    amyloidosis and, 40
    plasma cell myeloma and, 2048
Bends, 134
Benign cholestatic jaundice, 167
Benign eosinophilic leukemia, 467
Benign intraductal papilloma, 1731-1732
Benign jaundice of pregnancy, 1235

Benign lesions, 610; *see also* Benign tumors
  endometrial polypoid, 1659
  epidermal, 1794-1796
  fibro-osseous, of jaws, 1114
  of nasal cavity, 1081, *1081*
  neck lipomatosis and, 1142
  salivary gland lymphoepithelial, 1129
Benign mucous membrane pemphigoid, 1102
Benign nephrosclerosis, 842-843
Benign tumors, 573-575, *575*; *see also* Benign lesions
  bone
    chondroblastic, 2034-2040
    osteoblastic, 2025-2028
  of breast; *see* Breast, benign disease of
  of cervix, 1645
  characteristics of, 575*t*
  of fallopian tube, 1669-1670
  gallbladder and biliary duct, 1334-1335
  of penis, 896-897
  of prostate gland, 906-907
  pulmonary metastasizing leiomyomas and, 1020
  renal, 847
  of thyroid gland, 1554-1556
  of urethra, 899
  of vagina, 1640-1641
  of vulva, 1630-1633
Bentonite flocculation test, 466
Benzene, 193*t*, 222, 1385
Benzo*a*pyrene, 5, 239, 596, 597*t*
Benzoyl peroxide, 598
Berger's disease, 517*t*, 816, *816*
Bergonié and Tribondeau law, 264
Beriberi, 555-556, 692
Berry aneurysms, 2151-2153, *2152*
Bertin, columns of, 826
Beryllium
  inhalation of, 236-237, 1005
  neoplasia and, 599
  skin and, 1785
Beta emission, 248
Beta-endorphin, 1522
Beta-hemolytic streptococci, 303, 792, 935
  rheumatic fever and, 639, 640-641
Beta-lipoprotein deficiency, congenital, 1173
Beta-lipotropin, 1522, 1534
Beta$_2$-microglobulin amyloid bone disease, 2000
Beta particles, 23, 23*t*, 248
Beta-thalassemia, 1381
Bielschowsky stain, 1809, 2126*t*
Bile, 1189
  ethanol and, 192
  hepatocellular pigment and, 1204
Bile ducts
  benign tumors of, 1291-1292
  carcinoma of, liver fluke and, 1337
  extrahepatic
    cholangiocarcinoma and, 1293
    obstruction of, 1252-1253, 1255
    transhepatic cholangiogram of, 1253, *1253*
  intrahepatic
    congenital cystic dilatation of, 1257-1258
    obstruction of, 1252
    transhepatic cholangiogram of, 1253, *1253*
  liver abscess and, 1252
  obstruction of, 1252-1254
  primary disease of, 1255-1258

Bile stasis, 192, 1262, *1263*
Bilharziasis, 454-458, *455*
  prostate gland and, 901
  urinary, 458, 857
Biliary ascariasis, 462
Biliary atresia, 1262-1263
  neonatal and childhood cholestasis and, 1261*t*, 1262
Biliary canaliculi, 1200
Biliary cirrhosis, 165, 1254-1255, *1255*
  focal, 1351
  periportal connective tissue and, 1262, *1263*
  primary, 1255-1257, *1257*, 1294
    granulomas and, 1284
Biliary ducts; *see* Bile ducts
Biliary dysgenesis with protease inhibitor ZZ, 1264, *1264*
Biliary pleural fistula, 1275
Bilirubin, 33
  inborn errors in, 1275, 1276*t*
  perinatal brain injury and, 2145-2146
Bilirubinate calculi, 1323, *1324*
Billroth, cords of, 1408
Biologic agent–virus, 25-28
Biologic response modifiers, 607
Biologically active molecules, 504*t*, *505*
Biopsy
  biliary atresia and, 1262
  bone, 2024
    iliac crest, 1957-1958, 1965, *1966-1967*
  endomyocardial, 706-708
  excisional
    biliary atresia and, 1262
    soft-tissue tumors and, 1841
  infertility, unsuspected malignancy in, 875-876
  muscle, 2107-2108
  shave, 1814
  skin, 1751
  soft-tissue tumors and, 1841
  testicular, 881
Biotin, 559-560
Bipolaris, 395*t*, 402
Birbeck granules, 978, 1423, 1754
Bird-fancier's lung, 966*t*
Bird nests in syphilitic heart disease, 652
Bis ether, 596, 597*t*
Bishydroxycoumarin, 555
Bisphenol toxicity, 224
Bitot spots, 552
Bizarre leiomyoma, 1665, 1860
BK virus, 384
Black adenoma, *1598*, 1599
Black death, 320
Black fly, 472
Black piedra, 392*t*, 397
Black vomit, 372
Blackwater fever, 447-448
Bladder, urinary, 852-866; *see also* Urinary bladder
Blade-of-grass lesion, 2009, *2010*
Blandin-Nuhn cyst, 1128
Blaschko's ridges, 1752
Blast cells, 495
Blast crisis, 602, 1392
Blast injuries, 135, 136
Blastemas, gonadal, 1623
Blastoconidia, 397, 422, *422*
Blastoma, pulmonary, 1019, *1019*
Blastomycosis, 393*t*, 410, *411*
  endocarditis and, 654
  South American, 421-422

Bleb, 1757
Bleeding
  anemia and, 1379
  into gastrointestinal tract, 1158-1159
  from pulmonary capillaries, 985
  vitamin C deficiency and, 561
Bleomycin, 984
  toxicity of, 180
Blepharoplasts, 2169
Blindness, 1072
  diabetes and, 1057
  granulomatous arteritis and, 774
  onchocerciasis and, 472
  river, 473
  trachoma and, 357
Blister, 85
Blocking antibody, 498, 534
Blood
  and bone marrow, 1373-1408; *see also* Bone marrow and blood
  flagellates of, 439-445
  hepatocyte and, 1200
  inflammatory response and, 69
  in pericardial cavity, *664*, 664-665
  tumors and, 605
Blood cells; *see* Bone marrow and blood
Blood clot
  granulation tissue and, 98
  mechanical injury and, 132
Blood cysts of cardiac valves, 700
Blood donors, hepatitis and, 1215
Blood flow
  inflammation and, 70
  uteroplacental, 1703
Blood flukes, 454
Blood-loss anemia, 1379
Blood pressure, adrenal glands and, 1607
Blood vessels, 752-803
  arteries in, 752-786; *see also* Arteries
  burns and, 137
  inflammation and caliber of, *70*
  lymphatics and, 791-793
  radiation and wall of, 274
  repair of, 98, *99*
  of skin, 1756
  tumors and tumorlike conditions of, 794-799, 1818-1823
  veins in, 786-791
Blood volume, mechanical injury and, 131
Bloom's syndrome, 609, 1385
Blowout laceration, *115*
Blue nevi, 1810-1811
Blue rubber-bleb nevus, 795, 1820
Blue valve syndrome, 676
Blue velvet, 219
Blunt trauma
  of head, 2188
  of liver, 1275
Bochdalek hernia, 921, *922*
Bodian stain, 2126*t*
Boeck's sarcoid, 1287, 1784-1785
Boil, 85
Bolivian hemorrhagic fever, 373, 1205
Bomb survivors, 261*t*, 262, 263
Bombesin, 1012
Bone, 1929*t*, 1929-2017, 2023
  achondroplasia of, 1946-1949
  biopsy of, 2024
    iliac crest, 1957-1958, 1965, *1966-1967*
  chondrodystrophia calcificans congenita and, 1953-1956
  degenerative diseases of, 2010-2013, *2012*, *2013*

Bone—cont'd
extraosseous formation of, 107-108
formation of, 569
growth and development of, 1936-1941
  disorders of, 1946
hemangiomas of, in jaws, 1116
homeostasis and, 1944
in hyperparathyroidism, 1576
inflammatory skeletal disorders and, 2002-
  2010
mass of, 1944
metastases to, 911
mineralization of, 1944
  disorders of, 1957-2000; see also
    Metabolic bone diseases
  regulation of, 1945-1946
modeling of, 1941-1943
  cortical, 1943
  fractures and, 2001
multiple epiphyseal dysplasia and, 1957
osteogenesis imperfecta and, 1951-1953
osteopetrosis of, 1949-1951
radiation injury to, 280-281
radiosensitivity of, 257t
remodeling of, 1943-1944
  disorders of, 1957-2000; see also
    Metabolic bone diseases
  histomorphometric correlates of, 1959t
  osteoporosis and, 1971-1972
  regulation of, 1944t
structure of, 1929-1936, 1941-1943
tetracycline as in vivo marker of, 1945
trauma to, 2000-2002
tumors and tumorlike conditions of; see
    Bone tumors and tumorlike
    conditions
turnover of, 1960-1961
vitamin D deficiency and, 554
Bone cells, 1932-1936
Bone collagen, 1936
Bone cyst
aneurysmal, 2056-2057
in jaws, 1120
solitary, 2056
Bone-forming tumors, 2025-2034
Bone GLA protein, 1936
Bone marrow and blood, 1373-1408
aplastic marrow in, 1375-1376, 1376
arterioles and, 1406, 1407
benzene and, 222
blood cells and, 1374
cellularity in, 1375
development, structure, and function of,
  1373-1374
erythrocyte disorders in, 1375-1382
fibrosis in, 1405
  radiation injury and, 279
hyperplasia and, 1375
hypoplasia and, 1375
lymphocytes and, 495
marrow transplantation in; see Bone
    marrow transplantation
marrow tumors in, 2045-2050
mast cell proliferations in, 1403-1404,
  1404
megaloblastic dyspoiesis in, 1377
miliary tuberculosis and, 1406
necrosis in, 1405
plasma cell proliferative disorders in,
  1399-1403
primary evaluation of disorders of, 1374-
  1375
radiation injury and, 259, 261, 271, 279

Bone marrow and blood—cont'd
radium and, 259
sarcoid granuloma in, 1407
serous atrophy of adipose tissue and,
  1404, 1405
stromal reactions and lesions in, 1404-
  1408
white blood cell disorders of, 1382-1399
  leukocytosis and, 1382-1384
  leukopenia and, 1382-1384
  lymphoid cell proliferative disorders
    and, 1394-1399
  myeloid cell proliferative disorders and,
    1390-1394
  proliferative, 1384-1390
Bone marrow transplantation, 534
obliterative bronchiolitis after, 968, 968
veno-occlusive disease and, 1283
Bone mass, 1944
Bone matrix, 1932-1936
Bone mineralization, 1944
disorders of, 1957-2000; see also
    Metabolic bone diseases
regulation of, 1945-1946
Bone pain, 807
Bone tumors and tumorlike conditions,
  2018-2064
adamantinoma of long bones in, 2053
adipose tissue tumors and, 2054
of alleged histiocytic origin, 2054-2055
aneurysmal bone cyst in, 2056-2057
characteristics of, 2021-2022t
chondroblastic, 2034-2043
  benign, 2034-2040
  malignant, 2040-2043
chordoma in, 2052-2053
classification and distribution of, 2020-
  2023
diagnosis, treatment, and prognosis in,
  2023-2025
etiology and predisposing factors in, 2018-
  2020
fibrous tissue, 2051-2052
ganglion bone cyst in, 2057-2059
giant cell, 2043-2045
marrow tumors in, 2045-2050
metaphyseal fibrous defect in, 2059-2060
metastatic, 2055-2056
osteoblastic, 2025-2034
  benign, 2025-2028
  malignant, 2028-2034
peripheral nerve tumors and, 2053-2054
smooth muscle, 2055
solitary bone cyst in, 2056
vascular, 2050-2051
Bordetella pertussis, 297
Borellia vincentii, 329
Boric acid toxicity, 222-224
Boron poisoning, 193t
Borrelia, 324, 328-329, 1105
Bothriocephalus anemia, 460
Botryoid rhabdomyosarcoma, 1865, 1867,
  1869
Botryoid sarcoma in upper respiratory tract
    and ear, 1089
Botryomycosis, 410-411, 1768
Botulism, 292t, 292-293
Bourneville's disease, 1051, 1053
Boutonneuse fever, 349t, 353
Bovine tuberculosis, 941
Bowel, 1153
inflammatory disease of, 1161-1165
  liver abnormalities and, 1287

Bowel—cont'd
ischemic disease of, 1158
obstruction of, 1156
Bowenoid papulosis
of penis, 897, 1797, 1798
of vulva, 1633, 1635, 1636
Bowman's capsule, 806, 814, 846
Bowman's membrane of cornea, 1074
Bracht-Wachter bodies, 657
Bradykinin, 73
Brain
abscess of, 2158
  herniation and, 2129
boric acid toxicity and, 224
carbon monoxide intoxication and, 220
cysticercosis and, 459
edema of, 2125-2128, 2127, 2128
encephalopathy and energy metabolism
    in, 1248
herniation of, 2128-2130
heterotopic tissue and, 1077
injuries to; see Central nervous system
    pathology, injury in
lead toxicity and, 206, 208
malnutrition and, 563
mercury poisoning and, 203
of normal full-term infant, 2135-2136
parenchyma of; see Parenchyma, brain
perinatal injury to, 2141-2146
radiation injury and, 281
respirator, 1527
Brainstem
ischemic encephalopathy and, 2147
transtentorial herniation of, 2129
Branchial cyst, 1143
Bread-and-butter exudate, 647-648
Breakbone fever, 371
Breast, 1726-1750
angiosarcoma of, 1748-1749
benign disease of, 1727-1734
  cystic, 1728-1729
  epithelial proliferative lesions as, 1732-
    1734
  fibroadenoma as, 1730-1731
  granular cell tumor as, 1734
  gynecomastia as, 1734
  intraductal papilloma as, 1731-1732
  juvenile mammary hypertrophy as,
    1734
  mammary duct ectasia as, 1731
  sclerosing adenosis as, 1729-1730
carcinoma of, 1734-1748
  bone marrow and, 1408, 1408
  death rates for, 1735
  factors influencing risk of, 1734-1735
  favorable histologic types of infiltrating,
    1744-1746
  follow-up in, 1739
  histologic types of, 1741-1746
  hypophysectomy and, 1525
  in situ, 1735-1739
  invasive, 1739-1747
  invasive lobular, 1742, 1742
  metastatic, to eyes, 1069, 1069
  molecular biology and, 603
  pituitary gland and, 1520, 1525
  prognosis in, 1739-1741
  radiation injury and, 281
  radiosensitivity of, 257t
  risk of contralateral, 1745
  in situ lobular, 1736-1738
  tumor cell from, 581

Breast—cont'd
  carcinoma of—cont'd
    unusual clinical presentation of, 1746-1747
    unusual hosts of, 1747-1748
    epithelial radiosensitivity of, 257*t*
    gynecomastia and, 889
    lymphangiosarcoma and, 1823
    malignant mesenchymal tumors of, 1748
    radiation injury to, 281
    structure and function of, 1726-1727
Breast carcinoma; *see* Breast, carcinoma of
Breast lobule, *1727*
Brenner tumor, *1683*, 1683-1684
Breus mole, 1702
Brill-Zinsser disease, 349*t*, 354
Bromide poisoning, 193*t*
Brompheniramine poisoning, 193*t*
Bronchi
  carcinoids of, 1015-1017, *1016*
  infections of, 930-948, 1031-1033; *see also* Lung, infections of
  mucoepidermoid tumors of, 1017
Bronchial cartilage ossification, 983
Bronchial constriction, occupational, 238
Bronchiectasis, 948-951, *949*, 1033-1034
Bronchiolitis
  obliterative, 968, *968*, 971, 972
    interstitial pneumonia and, 971
    pediatric, 930
    silo-filler disease and, 232
  pediatric, 930
  viral, 931
Bronchioloalveolar carcinoma, 1009, *1009*, *1010*
Bronchioloalveolitis, ozone and, 231
Bronchitis
  asthmatic, 962
  chronic, 987-989
    small airways obstruction and, 996
  occupationally induced, 238
Bronchocentric granulomatosis, 965
Bronchogenic carcinoma; *see* Lung carcinomas
Bronchogenic cyst, 700, 923, 1024
Bronchopneumonia, 304, 306, 934
  staphylococcal, 935-936
  vitamin A deficiency and, 553
Bronchopulmonary dysplasia, 926-928, 927
Bronchopulmonary mycosis, allergic, 964-965
Bronchopulmonary sequestration, 922-923
Bronchus, carcinoma of, *594*
  epidermoid, *1007*
  melanocarcinoma in, *1818*
Bronze diabetes, 1272, 1786
Brood capsules, 461
Brown and Brenn stain, 396*t*
Brown atrophy
  of heart, 677
  inanition or starvation and, 692
Brown fat, 1885
Brown-Hopps stain, 396*t*
Brown tumor, *1976*, 1977
Brucellosis, 292*t*, 317-318, *318*
  arthritis and, 2076
  endocarditis and, 674
  granuloma in, 91
  myocarditis and, 660
  skin and, 1785
Brucellosis infection, granuloma in, 1284
Bruch's membrane, 1072
Brugia malayi, 471

Bruise, 114, *116*, *117*
Bruton's X-linked agammaglobulinemia, 501*t*
Bubonic plague, 320
Buccal mucosal carcinoma, 1111-1112
Buck's fascia, 895
Bud, 397
Budd-Chiari syndrome, 788, 790-791, 1282
  etiologic factors of, 1282
  hepatocellular carcinoma and, 1297
  oral contraceptives and, 165, *166*
Buerger's disease, 623, 777, *777*
Bulla, 1757
Bullets, *118*, 119-120
  firing of, 127-128
  heart and, 698
  retrieving, 126-127
  track of, 124, *125*, *126*
Bullous cystitis, 855
Bullous pemphigoid, 1763
Bundle of His, 705
Bungaro toxin, radiolabeled, 508
Bunina bodies, 2133
Bunyaviridae, 370
Buphthalmos, 1072
Burkitt's lymphoma, 588, 593*t*, 601, 1455, 1460, 1467
  malaria and, 446
Burns, 96
  cutaneous, 137-140, *138*, *139*
  electrical, 141-143, *142*, *143*
  radiation, 260, 261, 274
Bursa of Fabricius, 499
Bursae, 2065
  cysts of, 2092
  diseases of, 2090-2091
  tumors and tumorlike conditions of, 2092-2096
Bursitis, 2090-2091, *2091*
  olecranon, 403
Buschke-Löwenstein tumor, 385, 896
Buschke's disease, 1780
Bush tea, 224, *225*, 1283
Busulfan toxicity, 180-182, *181-182*, 984
  veno-occlusive disease and, 1283
Butabarbital poisoning, 193*t*
Butanol poisoning, 193*t*
Butchers' warts, 1794
Byler disease, 1268
Bypass grafts, aortocoronary vein, 791, 792-793
Byssinosis, 238, 996
Bystander effect, 27

C

c-*abl*, 588, 592-593
C-cells, 1544
  hyperplasia of, 1563
c-*erb*-a, 588
c-*erb*-b, 588
C-*erb* B oncogene, 1015
c-*fms*, 588, 591
c-*fos*, 587, 588
c-H-*ras*, 597, 603
c-Ha-*ras*, 587
c-*jun*, 588
c-*myb*, 588
c-*myc*, 588, 589, 603, 1457
c-*onc*, 586
C-peptide, 1360
c-*ras*, 588
c-*sis*, 588
c-*src*, 588
Cachectin, 569

Cachexia, 569, 605, 610
  endocarditis and, 652
CAD; *see* Coronary artery disease
Cadmium toxicity, 212-213, *213*, 237, 563, 907
Café-au-lait spots, 1825, 2175
Café coronary, 192
Caffeine poisoning, 193*t*
Caffey's disease, 1113
Cajal gold chloride sublimate stain, 2126*t*
Calabar swellings, 473
Calcification
  of adrenals, 1607
  aortic stenosis and, 674, *674*
  of arterial muscular media, 757, *757*
  dystrophic, 36, 693
  epiphyseal growth plate and, 1941
  of fibrous plaques, 761
  metastatic, 36, 37, 693
  of mitral valve anulus, 676-677
  of myocardium, 693
  pancreatitic, 1253
  parathyroid glands and, 1571, 1577
  of pericardium, 667, *668*
  periosteal, *1982*
  renal, 839-840
  of trichinas, 466
Calcifying epithelial odontogenic tumor, 1121, *1124*
Calcifying epithelioma, 1835
Calcifying odontogenic cyst, 1119, *1119*
Calcinosis; *see* Calcification
Calciphylaxis, 1571
Calcitonin, 1571
Calcitonin gene-related peptide, 964
Calcium, 36, *37*, 554, 562, 807
  accumulation of, 36, *36*
    gallbladder and, 1323, *1324*, *1329*, 1330
  bladder stones and, 854
  cell movement and, 6
  coagulation necrosis and, 22
  dystrophic calcification and, 693
  hormones regulating, 1944, *1945*
  metastatic calcification and, 693
  osteoporosis and, 1967
  parathyroid glands and, 1571
  renal stones and, 840
Calcium bilirubinate calculi, 1323, *1324*
Calcium carbonate calculi, 1323, *1325*
Calcium channels, 8
Calcium fluoride, 229
Calcium oxylate crystals, 198, *199*
Calcospheritis, 982
Calculi
  calcium, 840
  cystine, 854
  endemic, 854
  gallbladder; *see* Gallstones
  magnesium ammonium phosphate, 840
  phosphate, 840
  prostatic, 901-902
  renal; *see* Renal calculi
  ureteral, 851
  urinary bladder, 854
Calculus on tooth surfaces, 1100
Call-Exner bodies, 1672, 1684
Callus, fracture repair and, 2000-2001
Calmette-Guérin vaccine, 999
Calomel, 203
Calyces, 850-852
  dilatation of, 837
  diverticulum of, 850
Calymmatobacterium granulomatis, 324

cAMP-dependent kinase, 57-58
Campylobacter, 300, 1161
Canalicular adenoma, salivary gland, 1135-1136, *1136*
Cancer, 575, 610; *see also* Neoplasia
  chromosomal aberrations and, 593*t*
  death rates from, *598, 599*
  genetic analysis and, 60
  radiation and risk for, 267
  secondary immune deficiency and, 503
Cancrum oris, 1105
Candida, 382, 393*t*, 410, 411, *412; see also* Candidiasis
  alimentary tract and, 1166, 1167
  endocarditis and, 654, 655
  glossitis and, 1096
  granulomas and, 412
  lung and mediastinum and, 964
  myocarditis and, 660
  parathyroid glands and, 1572
  placenta and, 1705
  thrush and, 1105
  vagina and, 1638
Candidiasis, 393*t*, 411-413, *412; see also Candida*
  cerebral, 412
  chronic mucocutaneous, 503
  pulmonary, 412
  thrush and, 1105
  urinary bladder and, 857
  vulvovaginal, 412, 1638
Candle gutterings, 2175
Canker sores, 1104
Capillariasis, 466-467
Capillaries
  bleeding from pulmonary, 985
  burns and, 137
  granulation tissue and, 98
  hypothermal injury and, 137
  inflammatory response and, *68*
  pulmonary edema and, 960-961
  radiation and, 274, *276*
  sheathed, in spleen, 1409
Capillary angioma, 1819
Capillary hemangioma, 794, *794, 1886,* 1887
Capillary lymphangioma, 799
Caplan's syndrome, 1002
Carbamate toxicity, 229
Carbamazepine, *663*
Carbaryl, 229
Carbohydrate, 28-30
  corticosteroids and, 163
  metabolism disturbances and, 686-689, *687*
  thiamine deficiency and, 556
Carbon monoxide toxicity, 193*t*, 220-222, *221,* 694
Carbon tetrachloride toxicity, 16-18, *19,* 222, *223*
  flow sheet and, *19*
  liver and, 1209, 1232, 1233
Carboxyhemoglobin, 220
Carboxylase, 556
Carbuncle, 302
Carcinoembryonic antigen, 881, 1563, 1679
Carcinogenesis, 596, 596*t*, 597, 610
  arsenic and, 210
  benzene and, 222
  cigarette smoke and, 277, 1014
  cobalt toxicity and, 212
  dose-response curves for radiation and, *268*
  gallbladder cancer and, 1337

Carcinogenesis—cont'd
  radiation and, 257, 265, 274
  viral, 600*t*, 600-602
Carcinoids, 1184, 1185
  alimentary tract and, 1184-1186, *1185*
  heart and, 690-691
  lung and, 1015-1017
  prostate and, 915
  thymus gland and, 1508, *1509*
Carcinoma, 575, 610
  acinic cell, salivary gland, 1139, *1139*
  adenoid cystic, 1833
    prostate gland, 915
    salivary gland, *1138,* 1138-1139
  adrenocortical, 1599-1605, 1600*t, 1601, 1602, 1603*
  of anal region, 1184
  basal cell, 1798-1799
  bile duct, liver fluke and, 1337
  bladder, 860-863, *862, 863*
    radiosensitivity of, 257*t*
    schistosomiasis and, 458
  breast; *see* Breast, carcinoma of
  bronchioloalveolar, 1009, *1009, 1010*
  bronchogenic; *see* Lung carcinomas
  of cervix; *see* Cervix, carcinoma of
  cholangiolocellular, 1293
  colloid, of cecum, *1181*
  colonic, 1179, 1180, *1181*
    schistosomiasis japonica and, 458
  embryonal testicular, 884-885, *887*
  of esophagus, 1183
  in fibroadenoma of breast, 1730
  gallbladder, 1335-1343
  gastric, 1169
  of hand, 274
  in situ, 570, 581-582, *583,* 610
    cervical, *1646, 1648, 1649*
    conjunctival and corneal, *1050, 1051*
    endometrial, 1659
    gallbladder and, 1339-1342, *1341*
    laryngeal, 1086
    oral soft tissue, 1110-1111
    prostate, 915
    testicles and, *875, 876, 882*
    urinary tract, 864
    vulvar, 1632-1633, *1635, 1636*
  of limbus, *1051*
  liver, 601, 1293, 1294-1298
    B viral cirrhosis and, 1227
    clonorchiasis and, 453
    hepatocellular adenoma and, 1289
    intrasinusoidal growth of metastatic, 1299
    primary, 1293-1294
    radiation injury and, 279
    schistosomiasis and, 456
    trabecular cell, 1297, *1298*
  lung; *see* Lung carcinomas
  metastatic
    eyes and, 1069
    pituitary gland and, 1535
  mucoepidermoid, salivary gland, *1137,* 1137-1138
  nasal cavity, 1082
  nasopharyngeal, *1083,* 1083-1084
  neuroendocrine, 1339, *1340*
  nickel toxicity and, 214
  nutrition and, 563
  ovarian, *1681*
    stages of, 1692
  of pancreas, 1253, *1253,* 1354-1357, *1356, 1357, 1358*

Carcinoma—cont'd
  paranasal sinus, 1082
  parathyroid glands and, 1575
  of periampullary region, 1357-1358, *1359*
  pituitary gland and, 1535
  pleomorphic adenoma and salivary gland, 1139
  of rectum, 1180
  of sebaceous glands, 1833-1834
  of seminal vesicles, *916*
  of small intestine, 1183
  spindle cell
    laryngeal, 1086-1087
    oral soft tissue, 1112
  squamous
    bladder, 861, *862*
    bronchogenic, 1006-1007
    ear canal, 1088
    gallbladder and biliary duct, 1339, *1340*
    laryngeal, 1086
    oral soft tissue, 1110, 1111-1112
    penile, 898
    prostate gland, 915
    salivary gland, 1140
    scrotal, 894
    skin, 1800-1801
  stomach, 1180-1183, *1182*
    peptic ulcers and, 1161
  thymic, 1507
  thyroid, 1556-1563, *1558*
    natural history of, 1557*t*
    radiation injury and, 281
  undifferentiated
    prostate gland and, 915
    salivary gland, 1140
    sinonasal, 1082
  vaginal clear cell, 1639-1640
  vascular spread of, *584,* 584-585
  verrucous
    laryngeal, 1087
    oral soft tissue, 1112
    skin, 1801
  of vulva, *1634*
Carcinomatosis, meningeal, 2175
Carcinosarcoma, 610
  endometrial, 1662-1663
  esophageal, 1188
  pulmonary, 1019
  salivary gland, 1140
  soft tissue, 1898
Cardiac allograft rejection, 707
Cardiac arrhythmias, sudden death and, 627
Cardiac atrophy, 677
Cardiac biopsies, 706-708
Cardiac cirrhosis, 667, *1279,* 1279-1280
Cardiac damage
  alkylating agents and, 180
  endocarditis and, 657
Cardiac death, sudden, 627
Cardiac failure; *see* Heart failure
Cardiac fungal infection, 413
Cardiac growth disturbances, 677-681
Cardiac hypertrophy, 41, 677-681
Cardiac muscle
  cells of, 7
  coagulation necrosis of, *14*
Cardiac rupture, 638-639
Cardiac tamponade, 698
Cardiac valves
  blood cysts of, 700
  papillary tumors of, 703
  prosthetic, candidal infection of, 413
Cardiogenic shock, 637, 638

Cardiomegaly, acromegaly and, 690
Cardiomyopathies and myocardial disorders, 681-700
  alcoholic; 194, *685*, 685-686
  congestive, 684-695
    anemia and, 692-693
    drugs and toxic agents in, 693-694
    electrolyte disturbances and, 693
    endocrine disorders and, 689-692
    metabolic abnormalities in, 686-689
    nutritional deficiencies and, 692
    systemic diseases in, 694-695
  definition and classification of, 681-682
  diabetic, 691
  hypertrophic, 681, 682-684
  hypovolemic shock in, 698-700
  ionizing radiation in, 698-700
  ischemic, 638
  mechanical causes in, 698-700
  primary or secondary, 681
  restrictive, 695-698
Cardioplegia, 20
Cardiopulmonary schistosomiasis, 457-458
Cardiovascular radiation injury, 274
Cardiovascular surgery, endocarditis and, 654
Cardiovascular syphilis, 767
Caries, dental, 1098, *1098*
  fluoridation and, 229
Carnitine deficiency, 2115-2116
Carnitine palmityltransferase deficiency, 2116
Caroli's disease, 1257-1258, 1337
Carotenes, 551
Carotid artery occlusion, 2148
Carotid body tumor, 1141-1142, *1142*
  adrenal glands and, 1613
Carrier, 289, 487
  of hepatitis B virus, 1223
Cartilage, 1929
  articular, 2066
    inflammatory joint diseases and, 2075
  in embryo, 1937, *1937*
  extraosseous formation of, 107-108
  laryngeal tumors and, 1087
  neoplastic, 2041
  osteoarthrosis and, *2072*
  radiation injury to, 280-281
  radiosensitivity of, 257*t*
Cartilage extracts, angiogenesis and, 102-104
Caruncles, 899
Caseation necrosis, 13, *14*, 91
Caseous granulomas, 999
Castleman's disease, 1025
Cat liver fluke, 452
Cat-scratch disease, 313, 1442, *1443*
Cataracts, 281, 1069, *1070*
Catecholamines
  adrenal glands and overproduction of, 1609
  toxicity of, 216-217, 708
    cardiac, 693-694
Cathepsin, 433
Catheterization of bladder, 834
Caudate nucleus atrophy, 2182
Cavernous hemangioma, 794-795, 1819, 1886, *1887*
  liver and, 1292, *1292*
Cavernous lymphangioma, 799
Cavitary prostatitis, 901
Cavitary tuberculosis, *945*, 945-946
Cavum septi pellucidi, 2136
CD4 antigen, 1472

Cecum, colloid carcinoma of, *1181*
Celiac sprue, 1171-1172
Cell; *see also* specific cell
  blood; *see* Bone marrow and blood
  conversion of type of, 569-570
  daughter, 1624
  metabolic activity of, 12
  neoplastic transformation of, 587
  normal function of, 1-9
  progenitor, 495
  radiosensitivity of, 257*t*
  steady state of, *11*
Cell-cell interaction, 7, 8, 9
Cell communication, 7-8
Cell control mechanisms and homeostasis, 10-44; *see also* Cell injury, cell control mechanisms and homeostasis in
Cell cycle, 9
  blocks in postsynthetic gap and, *41*
  radiation and, 24-25, 254
Cell death, 11-16
  irradiation and, 250
  ischemic, 629-630, *630*
Cell excitation, 7-8
Cell fusion, 60
Cell growth
  interrelatedness of patterns of, 568
  neoplasia and, 567-743; *see also* Neoplasia
Cell injury, 1-65
  cell control mechanisms and homeostasis in, 10-44
    biologic agents and, 25-28
    cell injury and death and, 11-16
    chemical agents and, 16-20
    physical agents and, 20-25
    sustained sublethal injury and, 28-44; *see also* Cell injury, sustained sublethal
  genetic disorders and, 44-62
    autosomal inheritance in, 50-58
    cytogenetic disorders and, 45-49
    historical aspects in, 45
    maternal effects on, 61
    pedigree analysis in, 49-50
    sex-linked conditions in, 58-60
    somatic cell, 60-61
    therapeutic approaches to, 61-62
  irreversible, 633
  normal cell function and, 1-9
    cell movement in, 6-7
    cell recognition, communication, and excitation in, 7-8
    digestion and detoxication in, 4-6
    energy production in, 1-2
    intracellular storage in, 6
    protein and macromolecule synthesis in, 2-3
    reproduction in, 8-9
    transport, endocytosis, and exocytosis in, 3-4
  sustained sublethal, 28-44
    amyloid in, 38-41
    atrophy in, 42-43
    cellular accumulations in, 28-41
    glycogen, complex lipids, and carbohydrates in, 28-30
    hyperplasia in, 43-44
    hypertrophy and, 41-42
    pigments in, 30-36
    urate in, 36-38
Cell junctions, 7
Cell markers; *see* Tumor markers

Cell-mediated immunity, 490
Cell movement, 6-7
Cell proliferation, 85
Cell recognition, 7-8
Cell surface antigen, 507*t*
Cell volume, *10*, 11
Celloidin method, 2125
Cellular accumulations, 28-41
  amyloid in, 38-41, *39*
  calcium in, 36, 37
  glycogen, complex lipids, and carbohydrates in, 28-30
  pigments in, 30-36
  urate in, 36-38, *38*
Cellular atypia, 585
Cellular blue nevus, 1810, *1811*
Cellular fibroadenoma, 1731
Cellular hypersensitivity, 527, *529*
Cellular interstitial pneumonia, 516
Cellular leiomyoma of myometrium, 1665
Cellular oncogenes, 586-587
Cellular radiation biology, 250-255
Cellular reactions to stress, 11, *11*
Cellular schwannoma, 1892
Cellularity
  bone marrow, 1375
  tumor, 1842
Cellule claire, 1753, 1806
Cellulitis, 87, *88*, *304*
Cement, emphysema and, 238
Cemental dysplasia, periapical, 1115
Cemental tumors, 1125
Cementifying fibroma in jaws, 1114
Cemento-ossifying fibroma in jaws, 1114-1115
Cementoma, periapical, 1115
Central chromatolysis, 2132
Central core disease, 2112-2113, *2113*
Central nervous system depressants in elderly, 150
Central nervous system oxygen toxicity, 180
Central nervous system pathology, 2125-2189
  circulatory and vascular disorders in, 2146-2153
  degenerative diseases and, 2181-2183
  demyelinating diseases and, 2176-2180
  embryology and, 2135
  fetal irradiation and, 269
  hexachlorophene and, 224
  infections and, 2153-2164
    brain abscess in, 2158
    encephalitis in, 2158-2164
    meningitis in, 2154-2158
  injury in, 2125-2135
    brain edema and, 2125-2128
    brain herniation and, 2128-2130
    hydrocephalus and, 2130-2131
    intracranial pressure and, 2128-2130
    neurocellular reactions and, 2131-2135
  malformations and, 2135-2146
    congenital, 2136-2141
    embryology and development and, 2135
    normal full-term brain and, 2135-2136
    perinatal injury in, 2141-2146
  mercury poisoning and, 203
  metabolic diseases and, 2184-2185
  nutritional diseases and, 2185-2186
  radiation injury and, 265, 271, 271*t*, 281
  regenerative capacities in, 2124
  rheumatic fever and, 648
  toxoplasmosis, 449
  trauma and, 2186-2189

Central nervous system pathology—cont'd
  trichiniasis and, 466
  tumors and, 2165-2176
    frequency of different types of, 2165
    genetically determined disorders and, 2166
    hereditary neoplastic, 2175-2176
    immunohistochemical markers for, 2166t
    location of, 2165
    metastatic, 2165-2166, 2174-2175
    primary, 2165-2166, 2166-2174
  virus-like agents and, 387-388
Central papillary atrophy of tongue, 1096
Central pontine myelinolysis, 2179
Central retinal artery occlusion, 1062-1063
Centriacinar emphysema, 989-990, 990, 993
Centrilobular emphysema, 989
Centrilobular fibrosis, 1279, 1279
Centrilobular necrosis, anoxic, 1278, 1279
Centronuclear myopathy, 2113-2114
Cephalosporin toxicity, 156
Cephalothin toxicity, 150, 156
Cercariae, 452
Cerebellar herniation, ventral, 2129, 2129, 2130
Cerebellar herniation in foramen magnum, T9, 2130
Cerebellar roof nuclei bilirubin staining, 2146
Cerebellar sarcomas, 2171
Cerebellar vermis atrophy, 2185
Cerebral candidiasis, 412
Cerebral contusion, 2188-2189
Cerebral cortical lesions in perinatal injury, 2145
Cerebral cysticercosis, 459, 460
Cerebral edema, high-altitude, 133
Cerebral malaria, 447
Cerebral vasculature in newborn brain, 2136
Cerebrohepatorenal syndrome, 1267, 1268
Cerebromeningeal cryptococcosis, 415, 415
Cerebroside sulfatase deficiency, 2180
Cerebrospinal fluid
  cryptococcosis and, 415
  hydrocephalus and, 2130-2131
Cerebrovascular accidents, 15, 16
Ceroid, 554
Ceroid granuloma of gallbladder, 1332, 1332
Cerumen gland tumors, 1088
Cervical cyst, lateral, 1143
Cervical dysplasia, 1645-1650
  papillomaviruses and, 385
Cervical intraepithelial neoplasia, 1645-1650
Cervical thymic cyst, 1143-1144
Cervical thymus, 1142
Cervicitis, 1644-1645
Cervicofacial actinomycosis, 406
Cervix, 1643-1652
  anatomy and physiology of, 1643
  carcinoma of
    epidermoid, 257t, 1645-1650
    invasive, 1650-1652
    papillomaviruses and, 385
    in situ, 1645-1650
  hypoplasia of, 1627
  inflammation of, 1644-1645
  neoplasms of, 1645-1652
  polyps and papillomas of, 1645
  vestigial and heterotopic structures of, 1644-1645
Cestodes, 458-462

Chagas' disease, 440-442, 441, 442, 661, 661-662
Chalazia of eyelid, 1047, 1048
Chancre, 539t
  trypanosomal, 439
Chancroid, 310, 310, 895
Chandipura virus, 27
Charcot-Bouchard aneurysm, 2151
Charcot intermittent hepatic fever, 1254
Charcot joints, 2068, 2158
Charcot-Leyden crystals, 408, 963
Chastek paralysis, 551
Chediak-Higashi anomaly, 1384
Cheek-biting, habitual, 1110
Cheilitis, angular, 1105
Cheilosis, 555, 559, 559
Chemical pneumonia, 237, 928
Chemical signals, 7
Chemicals
  allergic response to, 531
  carcinogenesis and, 594-600, 1337
  in injury
    of cell, 16-20
    of liver, 1232-1238
  leukemia and, 1385
Chemodectoma, 1023, 1141-1142, 1142
Chemotaxis, 7, 79-81
Chemotherapy, 606
  bone tumors and, 2024, 2048
  malignant lymphoma and, 2048
  massive hepatic necrosis and, 1227
  in nonseminomatous germ cell tumors, 888
  pleomorphic rhabdomyosarcoma and, 1871
Chernobyl, 286
Cherubism, 1116
Chest fluoroscopy in radiation injury, 281
Chest pain, 625-626
Chiari malformations, 2137
  hydrocephalus and, 2139, 2140, 2140
  syringomyelia and, 2140
Chicken wire appearance of oligodendrogliomas, 2169
Chiclero ulcer, 444
Chief cell, 1570, 1573
Child
  adrenal glands and, 1583-1586
  amebiasis of vulva in, 436
  benign chronic bullous dermatosis in, 1762
  bladder tumor and, 866, 866
  Chagas' disease in, 441
  cholecystitis and, 1328
  cholelithiasis in, 1323, 1327t
  cholestasis in, 1261t
  Cushing's syndrome in, 1585
  of diabetic mother, 1262
  dwarfism and, 1577
  embryonal rhabdomyosarcoma and, 1867
  Ewing's sarcoma in, 1907
  exanthematous oral soft-tissue disease and, 1105-1106
  giant cell fibroblastoma in, 1909
  hepatocellular carcinoma and, 1298
  hyperaldosteronism in, 1586
  hypophosphatasia and, 1997
  idiopathic juvenile osteoporosis and, 1971
  liver diseases in, 1260-1269
  melanomas in, 1804
  mucocutaneous lymph node syndrome and, 774-775, 776, 1830

Child—cont'd
  non-Hodgkin's lymphoma staging and, 1471, 1471t
  osteomyelitis and, 2004
  rhabdomyosarcoma and, 1864
  rheumatoid arthritis and, 2086-2087
  scleredema and, 1780
  tuberculosis and, 944
  urinary tract obstruction in, 836
Childbed fever, 305
Chimerism, 534
Chimney-sweep's cancer, 894
Chimpanzee coryza agent, 367
Chinese liver fluke, 452
Chlamydial diseases, 356t, 356-357
  cervical infection and, 1645
  lymphogranuloma venereum and, 357, 1442
  pneumonitis and, 930
  premature labor and, 1704
  psittacosis and, 356-357
  salpingitis and, 1667
  skin and, 1774
  trachoma and, 357
  urethritis and, 898
Chlamydoconidium, 397
Chloracne, 229
Chloral hydrate poisoning, 193t
Chlorambucil, 180-182
Chloramphenicol, 155-156, 324, 1376, 1376
Chlordiazepoxide poisoning, 193t
Chlorella, 402, 404
Chlorinated biphenol toxicity, 224
Chlorinated hydrocarbons, organic, 226, 227, 228
Chlorinated naphthalenes, 1233
Chlorine
  bronchitis and, 238
  pulmonary edema and, 237
Chloroform, 193t, 599, 1232
Chloromas, 1389
Chloromethyl ether, 596, 597t
p-Chlorophenyl; see 1,1,1-Trichloro-2,2-bis ethane
Chlorothiazide toxicity, 169
Chlorpromazine, 167
  biliary cirrhosis–like disease and, 1237
  poisoning from, 193t
Chlorpropamide
  granulomas and, 1285
  toxicity of, 169
Choanal atresia, 1077
Choanal stenosis, 1077
Choke of gun muzzle, 128
Chokes, 134
Cholangiocarcinoma, 453, 1202
  etiology of, 1298
  extrahepatic, 1293
  hilar, 1293, 1298
  peripheral, 1293
  radiation injury and, 279
Cholangiography
  bile duct or pancreatic carcinoma and, 1253, 1253
  percutaneous transhepatic, 1323
Cholangiohepatitis, 1202
  recurrent pyogenic, 1254
Cholangiolocellular carcinoma, 1293
Cholangiopancreatography, endoscopic retrograde, 1323
Cholangiopathy, infantile obstructive, 1323
Cholangitis, 312
  acute, 1258

Cholangitis—cont'd
  diabetes and fatal, 1254
  primary sclerosing, 1257, 1333
  suppurative, multiple liver abscesses and,
    1254
Cholecystitis, 312
  acute
    clinical symptoms and signs of, 1328
    episodes of, 1331-1332
    hemorrhagic and fibrinopurulent
      deposits and, 1331, 1331
    primary bacterial, 1327-1330
  chronic, 1323, 1326t
    follicular, 1331
  Cryptosporidium, 1328, 1328t
  cytomegalovirus, 1328, 1328t
  mixed gallstones and, 1330, 1330
  mucosal attenuation and, 130, 1330
  xanthogranulomatous, 1332
Cholecystography, 1322
Cholecystokinin, 1322
Cholecystostomy, cancer and, 1337
Choledochal cyst, 1257-1258, 1261t
Choledocholithiasis, 1253, 1254
Cholelithiasis, 1323-1327
  in child, 1323, 1327t
Cholera, 292t, 299
Cholestasis, 1204, 1252-1260
  childhood, 1261t
  drug toxicity and, 1233, 1234t, 1235
    chlorpromazine in, 167
    oral contraceptives in, 166, 167
  familial, 1261t, 1266-1267, 1268
  fatty liver with, 1242
  herbicide toxicity and, 230
  neonatal, 1261t
  osteoporosis and, 1974-1975
  perivenular canalicular, 1218
Cholestatic hepatitis, 165
Cholesteatoma, 1087
Cholesterol, 3, 619, 1582
  neomycin and, 157
  nickel toxicity and, 214, 214, 215
Cholesterol crystal embolization, 1790
Cholesterol granuloma of paranasal sinuses,
  1078-1079
Cholesterol polyp, 1334-1335, 1335
Cholesterol stones in gallbladder, 1323,
  1324, 1333, 1334
Cholesterol sulfatase deficiency, 59-60
Cholesteryl esters, 758, 764
Choline, 560
Cholinergic urticaria, 527
Chondroblastic tumors, 2034-2043
  benign, 2034-2040
  malignant, 2040-2043
Chondroblastoma, 2021t, 2036-2039, 2038
Chondrocalcinosis, 2068
Chondrocytes, 1937, 2072
Chondrodermatitis nodularis chronica
  helicis, 1784
Chondrodystrophia calcificans congenita,
  1953-1956, 1956
Chondrodystrophies, 1946, 1953-1956, 1956
Chondroma, 2021t, 2034-2036
  in oral soft tissue, 1109
Chondromyxoid fibroma, 2021t, 2039, 2039-
  2040
Chondrosarcoma, 2021t, 2040, 2040-2043,
  2041, 2042, 2043
  dedifferentiated, 2043, 2043
  extraskeletal myxoid, 1909
  in jaws, 1117

Chondrosarcoma—cont'd
  of joint, 2096
  radiosensitivity of, 257t
Chordoma, 2022t, 2052-2053, 2053
Chorea minor, 648
Chorioamnionitis, 1704
Choriocarcinoma
  ovary and, 1688
  placenta and, 1708, 1709-1710
  testicular tumors and, 881, 885, 885-886
Chorionic gonadotropin, 1546
Chorionic somatomammotropin, 1696
Chorionic villi, 1696, 1696-1698
Choristoma, 573
  oral soft tissue and, 1109
  pituitary gland and, 1537
Choroid
  hemangioma of, 1051, 1052
  inflammation of, 1056
  malignant melanoma of, 1065, 1066
Choroid plexus
  papillomas of, 2169, 2169
  perinatal brain injury and, 2143
Choroiditis, 1056
Chromates, 239
Chromatid lesions, 24
Chromatolysis, 2132, 2190
Chromium, 239, 563, 599
Chromoblastomycosis, 392t, 399-400, 400
Chromophobe adenoma, 1530, 1531
Chromophobes, 1523
Chromosomal aberrations
  in cancers, 591, 593t
  of eye, 1051-1052
  female genitalia and, 874, 1624, 1627
  leukemia and, 1393
  origins of, 591-594
  radiation injury and, 261, 262
Chromosome
  double minute, 1387
  indentification of, 46
  intersex states and, 874, 1624, 1627
  Klinefelter's syndrome and, 874
  normal human, 591-592, 592
  radiation injury and, 24-25
  structure of, 591-594
    abnormalities of, 48-49, 49
  X and Y, 1623
Chromosome aberrations, 45-49, 49
  leukemia and, 1385, 1386t
Chromosome mapping, 60
Chromosome sites, fragile, 49
Chronic hepatitis; see Hepatitis, chronic
Chronic obstructive pulmonary disease, 987;
  see also Lung, chronic airflow
  limitation and
Chrysiasis, 1785
Chrysops, 319, 473
Chrysosporium parvum, 393t, 407, 408
Chrysotile, 235
Churg-Strauss syndrome, 538, 772, 976
Chwalla's membrane, 850
Chylangioma, 799
Chylomicrons, 764
Ci; see Curie
Cigarette smoking, 35, 990, 993, 1014
  asbestosis and, 236
  atherosclerotic coronary artery disease
    and, 759
  cadmium toxicity and, 213
  emphysema and, 238
  radiation and, 277
  thromboangiitis obliterans and, 777

Cilia, regeneration of, 96
Ciliary motility, pancreas and, 1349
Ciliated columnar cells, squamous
  metaplasia of pseudostratified, 107,
  107
Ciliated cysts, 700
Cimetidine toxicity, 169
Cingulate gyrus herniation, 2129, 4129,
  4130
Circulatory collapse, 131
  hypothermia and, 137
Circulatory disorders
  central nervous system, 2146-2153
  heart conducting system and, 705
  hepatic, 1278-1283
  spleen and, 1415-1417
Circumcision, 898
Circumoval precipitin test, 454
Circumscribed cerebellar sarcomas, 2171
Circumscribed glycogen disease of heart,
  687
Circumscribed myxedema, 1781-1782
Circumscribed scleroderma, 1779
Circumvallate placenta, 1699, 1699
Cirrhosis, 1238
  acidic glycosaminoglycans and, 1208
  alcoholic, 1202, 1238, 1244-1247, 1246
    Mallory bodies and, 1203
    salivary gland enlargement and, 1128
  atrophic, 1247
  biliary, 1254-1255, 1255
    focal, 1351
    granulomas and, 1284
    primary, 1255-1257, 1257
  cardiac, 667, 1279, 1279-1280
  chronic active hepatitis and, 1209, 1227
  clonorchiasis and, 453
  collagen and, 1207
  cryptogenic, 1202, 1209, 1212
    nodular, 1227, 1228
  fatty change and obliteration of veins in,
    1245, 1246
  hepatic, 1208-1210, 1209t
    choline deficiency and, 560
    IgA nephritis and, 516
    lymphocytes and, 82
    palpable splenomegaly and, 1415
    tests in, 1210t
  hepatitis and, 1225-1228, 1230
  histogenesis of, 1246
  idiopathic hemochromatosis with
    pigmentary, 1272, 1272
  immunologic defects and, 1252
  Indian childhood, 1268
  iron and, 1272
  juvenile, 1268
    alpha₁-antitrypsin deficiency and, 1264,
    1264
  Laënnec's, 192, 456, 1238
  morphologic pattern of, 1245-1246
  non-A, non-B viral, hepatocellular
    carcinoma and, 1295
  parasitic, 1286
  of portal vein, 1280, 1280
  radiation injury and, 279
  Sickle cell anemia and, 1287
Cirsoid aneurysm, 778
cis-Dichlorodiamine-platinum (II), 216, 606
Cisplatin; see cis-Dichlorodiamine-platinum
  (II)
Cisternae, 3
Citric acid cycle, 2
Civatte's bodies, 1774

Cladosporium carrionii, 392t, 399
Clara cells, 993, 1009
Clear cell acanthoma, 1795
Clear cell adenoma, of thyroid gland, 1555
Clear cell carcinoma of vagina, 1639-1640,
    1641, *1642; see also* Clear cell tumors
Clear cell chondrosarcoma, *2042*
Clear cell leiomyoma, 1665
Clear cell leiomyosarcoma, 1863, *1863*
Clear cell melanocytes, 1753
Clear cell sarcoma, 1902-1903
    of tendon sheaths and aponeuroses, 2096
Clear cell tumors; *see also* Clear cell
        carcinoma of vagina
    of kidney, 849
    of lung, 1021
    of ovary, 1683, *1683*
    of salivary glands, 1140-1141
Cleavage vesicles, 1761
Clefts, facial, 1095
Clindamycin toxicity, 153-155
Clonal elimination, 497
Clonorchiasis, 452-453
Clostridial cellulitis, 296
Clostridium, peritonitis and, 1189
Clostridium botulinum, 292-293
Clostridium difficile, 155, 1166
Clostridium novyi (oedematiens), 295
Clostridium perfringens, 155
Clostridium septicum, 295
Clostridium tetani, 130, 294
Clostridium welchii, 130, 295, *296*
Clotting; *see* Coagulation
Clubbing of fingers and toes, 2070
    alcoholic cirrhosis and, 1251
    asbestosis and, 1003
    interstitial pneumonia and, 969
Clubfoot, 2067
Clumping factor, 291
Cluster designation, lymphocytes and, 491,
        492t
Clutton's joint, 2076
Coagulase, 291, 302
Coagulation
    deficiencies in, 506t
    disseminated intravascular, adrenal glands
        and, 1585
Coagulation necrosis, 13, *14*, 1205
    electrical burns and, 141
    mercury poisoning and, 201, *201, 202*
Coal workers, 1000-1002
    emphysema and, 238
    pneumoconiosis and, 35, 233, *1000*, 1000-
        1001, *1001*
    tuberculosis and, *999*
Coarctation of aorta, 740-743
    adult, 741-743, *742, 743*
Cobalamin deficiency, 2185-2186, *2186*
Cobalt toxicity, 212, 562
    cardiac, 685
Cobblestone pattern of liver cords, 1203
Cocaine toxicity, 220
Coccidia, 445
Coccidioidomycosis, 393t, 404, 408, 413,
        413-415, 414, *414*
    endocarditis and, 654
    phagocytosis and, 93
    pulmonary, 414
Codeine poisoning, 193t
Coenzyme A, 1
    myocardial ischemia and, 631
Coin lesion, 473
Coke-oven emissions, 239

Colchicine, 38
Cold
    injuries from, 136-140
    parainfluenza and, 366
Cold sore, 1104
Colitis
    amebic, 434, *434, 435*, 1166-1167, *1167*
    antibiotic-associated, 146, 153, *154-155*,
        1166
        ulcerative colitis compared to, 155
    collagenous, 1168, *1168*
    infectious, 300
    ulcerative, 146, 1161, 1162, *1162*
        antibiotic-associated colitis compared to,
        155
Colitis cystica profunda, 1168
Collagen, 7, 754
    alcoholic and density of, 1202
    amyloidosis and, *1781*
    articular cartilage and, 2065
    aspirin and, 160
    bone and, 1934, 1936, *1936*
    cell of origin of, 1207-1208
    contraction of, 104
    iron and, 1273
    Ito cells and, 1207
    liver and, 1207
    neovascularization and, 102
    ovary and, 1673
    pleomorphic lipoma and, 1882
    rheumatic fever and, 641
    vitamin C and, 560-561
Collagen diseases, 516
    of dermis, 1776-1782
    pulmonary involvement in, 972-977, 1037-
        1038
Collagenase, 291, 433
Collagenous colitis, 1168, *1168*
Collagenous fibroconnective tissue in
        onchocerciasis, 472
Collateral circulation, coronary, 630
Colles' fracture, 1966
Colloid antigen, 507t
Colloid carcinoma
    of breast, 1743, *1743*
    of cecum, *1181*
Colloid goiter, 1547
Colloid milium, 1781, *1781*
Colloidal thorium dioxide, 259
Colon
    adenoma and, 1175, *1175*
    carcinoma of, 1179, 1180, *1181*
        radiosensitivity of, 257t
        schistosomiasis and, 458
    diverticulum of sigmoid, *1155*
    hyperplastic polyp of, *1177*
    melanosis of, 1156
    pellagra and, 557, *558*
    radiation injury and, 278
Colonization, 585
Colony forming unit–granulocyte, 1374
Colony forming unit–spleen, 1374
Colorado tick fever virus, 376
Columnar cells
    epithelial regeneration of, 96
    squamous metaplasia of, 107, *107*
Combined immune deficiency, 501t
Comedomastitis, 1731
Common bile duct, 1321
    strictures of, 1332-1333
Communicating hydrocephalus, 2131, 2139-
        2140

Complement, *510*, 511
    deficiencies of, 503t
    transfer of, 512t
Complement fixation test, 443
Complement-mediated injury, 811-812
Compound nevus, 1804, *1804*
Compression injury
    explosions and, 135
    of heart, 698-699
Concato disease, 667
Conchoid bodies, 979, 1005
Conducting system of heart, disturbances of,
        705-706
Conduction system of heart, ankylosing
        spondylitis and, 650
Condyloma acuminatum, 385, 1794-1795
    in cervix, 1645
    in oral soft tissue, 1106
    of penis, 896
    of vulva, *1631*, 1631-1632, *1632*
Confluent necrosis, 1205
Congenital abnormalities, 108
    of alimentary tract, 1153-1155
    in calyces, pelves, and ureters, 850-851
    of central nervous system, 2136-2141
    coronary artery disease and, 624
    of dental pigmentation, 1097
    of epididymis, 891
    of eye, 1051-1053
    of face and lips, 1095
    of female genital tract, 1627-1628
    of heart, 731
    infective endocarditis and, 655
    of jaws, 1113
    of joints, 2066-2067
    of kidneys, 844-847
    of larynx, 1084
    of liver, 1201-1202
    of lung, 921-925
    of mitral valve, 672-673
    of nose, 1077
    in offspring of atomic bomb survivors, 263
    of penis, 895
    phenytoin and, 174
    pituitary gland and, 1526-1527
    radiation injury and, 268
    of salivary gland, 1127
    of scrotum, 893
    of spermatic cord, 892
    of spleen, 1413
    of teeth, 1096-1098
    of testes, 871-872
    of thymus gland, 1499
    of thyroid gland, 1546
    of tongue, 1096
    of urinary bladder, 852-853
    vitamin deficiencies and, 561
Congenital adenomatoid malformation in
        lung, 923, *924*
Congenital adrenal hyperplasia, 1584, 1627
Congenital alveolar capillary dysplasia, 921
Congenital beta-lipoprotein deficiency, 1173
Congenital cervical erosion, 1643
Congenital cysts
    of bile duct, 1257-1258
    of liver, *1297*
Congenital encephalitis, 2160-2162, *2161*
Congenital epulis, 1108
Congenital fiber type disproportion, 2114
Congenital generalized fibromatosis, 1849-
        1850
Congenital glomerular diseases, 823

Congenital heart disease, 730-751
　cause of death in, 749-750
　conducting system and, 705
　isolated obstructions in, 739-743
　isolated shunts in, 731-738
　obstructions combined with shunts in,
　　743-749
　treatment of, 750-751
Congenital hepatic fibrosis, 1268, 1293
Congenital hydrocephalus, 2139-2140
Congenital jaundice of Crigler-Najjar type,
　　33
Congenital lip pits, 1095, 1096
Congenital lymphedema, 792
Congenital myopathies, 2112-2114
Congenital pneumonia, 929
Congenital pulmonary lymphangiectasis, 923
Congenital pulmonary overinflation, 923-925
Congenital spherocytosis, 1409, 1410
Congenital stenotic arteriopathy with medial
　　dysplasia, 786
Congenital syphilis, 1265
Congenital teratoma of neck, 1142-1143
Congenital thymic hypoplasia, 1500t
Congenital toxoplasmosis, 449, 1265
Congenital ureteral valves, 850
Congestive cardiomyopathy, 682, 684-695
　drugs and toxic agents and, 693-694
　electrolyte disturbances and, 693
　endocrine disorders and, 689-692
　metabolic abnormalities and, 686-689
　myocardial involvement in systemic
　　diseases and, 694-695
　nutritional deficiencies and, 692
　severe anemia and, 692-693
Congestive heart failure, 616
　cobalt toxicity and, 212
　diphtheria and, 295
　palpable splenomegaly and, 1415
Congestive splenomegaly, 1415, 1416
Congo Red stain, 39, 696, 1432
Conidiobolus coronatus, 393t, 426
Conidiophore, 397
Conidium, 397
Conjunctiva, 1051
　carcinoma in situ in, 1050, 1051
　loaiasis and, 473
　trachoma and, 357
Conjunctivitis in infant, 930
Connective tissue
　metaplasia in, 107-108
　radiosensitivity of, 257t
　regeneration and, 97
Connective tissue disease, 516, 1772
　pericarditis with, 670
Conn's syndrome, 1590
Constrictive cardiomyopathies, 682
Constrictive pericarditis, 667, 668
Contact dermatitis, 531, 532, 539t
Contact guidance, 8
Contraception
　hormonal, 1638
　　gallstones and, 1326
　　long-term use of, 1655
　hysterectomy and, 1656
　male, 893
Contraction-band necrosis, 632, 632-633,
　　636
Contraction of wound, 104, 106
Contractures, Dupuytren's, 2091
Contrast nephropathy, 832
Contrecoup contusions, 2188

Contusions, 114, 116, 117, 2188
　cerebral, 2188-2189
　chronologic changes in, 129
　myocardial, 699
Convalescent carrier, 289
Coombs' test, 148, 512
Copper, 562
Copper toxicity
　granulomas and, 1285
　liver and, 1232, 1233, 1269-1271
Cor bovinum, 678
Cor pulmonale, 679-680, 951
Cor villosum, 647
Cord factor, 940
Cords of Billroth, 1408
Corium of skin, 1823
Cornea
　carcinoma in situ in, 1050, 1051
　onchocerciasis and, 472
　riboflavin deficiency and, 558, 558
　vitamin A deficiency and, 552
Corneal, neovascularization of, 101, 102,
　　448, 558
Coronary artery
　angina pectoris and, 625-626
　anomalous origin of, 624
　atherosclerosis and, 617-621, 618, 758
　cocaine toxicity and, 220
　collateral circulation for, 630
　myocardial ischemia and, 627, 628
　radiation-induced heart disease and, 699-
　　700
Coronary artery aneurysms, 784-785
Coronary artery disease, 616-639
　atherosclerotic, 617-621, 618, 758
　consequences of, 624-639
　　angina pectoris in, 625-626
　　myocardial infarction in, 627-639; see
　　　also Myocardial infarction
　　sudden cardiac death in, 627
　diabetes and, 620
　etiology of, 617-624
　　aneurysms in, 624
　　atherosclerosis in, 617-621
　　congenital anomalies in, 624
　　embolism and, 623-624
　　inflammatory disorders in, 621-623
　　medial calcification in infancy in, 624
　　neoplasms in, 624
　　thrombotic diseases in, 624
　　trauma in, 624
　hypertension and, 619
　incidence of, 616-617
　physical activity and, 620
Coronary plaques, 617-618
Coronary thrombosis, 624
Coronaviridae, 369
Corpora amylacea, 901-902, 982
Corpus callosum, agenesis of, 2139
Corpus luteum, 1672, 1672
　cysts of, 1674
Corpus striatum
　hemorrhage in, 2150
　ischemic encephalopathy and, 2147
Corpuscles
　Hassall's, 1495, 1496, 1502, 1503
　Meissner, 1756
　Merkel-Ranvier, 1757
　pacinian, 1756, 1757
　Ruffini, 1757
Corrigan pulse, 676
Cortical bone
　modeling of, 1943

Cortical bone—cont'd
　osteoporosis and, 1975
Corticosteroids; see also Steroids
　polymyositis and dermatomyositis complex
　　and, 2117
　toxicity of, 162-165, 164
Corticosterone, 1582
Corticotrophs, 1522
　adenoma and, 1534
Corticotropin-releasing factor, 1581
Cortisol, 1582
Cortisone, 162-163, 164, 1581
　adrenal glands and, 1588
　amyloidosis and, 1781
　eosinophils and, 82
　gastric ulcers and, 1161
Corynebacterium, 294, 313
　eye and, 1084
　skin and, 1765
　wound infection and, 130
Cosmic radiation, 249-250
Cotton-mill workers
　byssinosis and, 996
　occupational bronchial constriction and,
　　238
Councilman bodies, 372, 1218-1219
Counterimmunoelectrophoresis, 466
Coup contusion, 2188
Cowden's syndrome, 1835
Cowdry type A inclusion bodies, 379, 1585
Cowper's gland, malignant tumors of, 899
Cowpox, 28, 386
Coxiella burnetii, 348, 349t, 354
Coxsackieviruses, 374
　encephalitis and, 2158
　group A, 1104
　jaundice and, 1265
　myocarditis and, 661
　pericarditis and, 668
Crackles, basilar, 1003
Cranial arteritis, 772-774, 773
Cranial nerve nuclei bilirubin staining, 2146
Craniopharyngioma, 1535-1537, 1536, 1537,
　　2173, 2173
Craniorachischises, 2136
Craniotabes, 1984
Creatine kinase in muscle diseases, 2108
Creeping eruption, 467
Crescent lesion, 814
Crescent sign, osteonecrosis and, 2013, 2013
Crescents, 85
　glomerular, 809
CREST syndrome, 974; see also CRST
　syndrome
Cretinism, 285, 1545
Creutzfeldt-Jakob disease, 387-388, 2163,
　　2164, 2164
Cri-du-chat syndrome, 48
Cribriform hyperplasia, 912
Cribriform tumor, 1833
Crigler-Najjar syndrome, 33, 1275-1277,
　　1276t
Crocidolite, 235
Crohn's disease, 1161, 1163, 1163, 1164
　arthritis and, 2086
　gallstones and, 1328
　liver and, 1287
　oral soft tissue and, 1104
Cronkhite-Canada syndrome, 1178
Crooke's hyaline change, 1524, 1525
Crotolaria fulva, 1283
Croup, 1084

CRST syndrome, 1780; *see also* CREST syndrome
Crush syndrome, 448
Crushing head injuries, 2188
Crust, 1757
Cruveilhier-Baumgarten syndrome, 1250
Cryoglobulinemia, mixed, 769
Cryoimmunoglobulinemia, 826
Crypt cells of intestinal epithelium, 257*t*
Cryptococcal meningitis, 415, *415*, 2155-2156, *2156*
Cryptococcosis, 394*t*, 415-416, *416*
    acquired immunodeficiency syndrome and, *1822*
    cerebromeningeal, 415, *415*, 2155-2156, *2156*
    pulmonary, 415
Cryptococcus, 1053
Cryptococcus neoformans, 394*t*, 410, 415, *415*
    acquired immunodeficiency syndrome and, 1287
    infective endocarditis and, 654
    meningitis and, 2154, 2155-2156
Cryptogenic chronic active hepatitis, 1230-1231
Cryptogenic cirrhosis, 1202, 1209
    hepatitis B virus and, 1212
    hepatocellular carcinoma and, 1295
    nodular, 1227, *1228*
Cryptogenic organizing pneumonitis, 971, *971*
Cryptorchidism, 871, *872*
Cryptosporidiosis, 445, 968, 1167
    cholecystitis and, 1328, 1328*t*
Crypts
    of Lieberkühn, 557, 1163, 1184
        and irradiation, 272
    of Morgagni, 1168
Crystal-deposition diseases, 2087-2091
Crystalline cholesterol stones, 1323, *1324*
Crystalloids of Reinke, 1687
CSF-1 and CSF-2, 590*t*
Ctenodactylus gundi, 448
Cuff cells, *1464*, 1464-1465
Culex, 470
Culicoides furans, 1777
Cuneate nuclei bilirubin staining, 2146
Cunninghamella, 395*t*, 425
Curie, 248, 249
Curling's ulcers, 1160, *1160*
Current, electrical, 140-141
Curvularia geniculata, 392*t*
Cushing's disease, 1534, 1589, 1592*t*
Cushing's syndrome, 163, 873, *1590*, 1592*t*, 1592-1593
    in child, 1585
    hyperadrenocorticism and, *1524*, 1525, *1594*, 1975
    pathophysiologic classification of, 1592*t*
Cusps, congenital heart disease and, 739
Cut, 114
Cutaneous anaphylaxis, 518, 539*t*; *see also* Skin
Cutaneous appendages, 1755
Cutaneous larva migrans, 467
Cutaneous reactions, 523
Cutaneous vasculitis, 539*t*
Cutaneous-visceral disease, 1758-1759
Cutis hyperelastica, 1782-1783
Cutis laxa, 1784
Cyanide poisoning, 193*t*
Cyanocobalamins, 560

Cyanotic tetralogy in newborn, 743, *744*
Cycasin, 596, *597*
Cyclic AMP, 8
Cyclists, injuries to, 118
Cyclophosphamide, 708, 825, 856
    oxygen toxicity and, 180-182
Cyclopia, agenesis of pituitary and, 1526
Cyclops, 473
Cyclosporin
    cholestasis and gallstones and, 1326
    lung transplantation and, 967
    orthotopic liver transplant and, 1300
    toxicity of, 182-183
Cyclotron, 248
Cylindrical cell papilloma in nasal cavity, 1081, *1081*
Cylindroid aneurysm, 778
Cylindroma, 1832
Cyst, 87
    adrenal glands and, 1606
    Baker's, 2092
    Bartholin's gland, 1628
    of Blandin-Nuhn, 1128
    bone, 2056-2057
        ganglionic, 2057-2059
    bronchogenic, 923, 1024
    bursal, 2092
    daughter, 461
    dermoid, 1077, 1835
    of echinococcosis, 461
    of *Entamoeba histolytica*, 433
    enteric, 1024, 1153-1154
    of epididymis, 892
    of fallopian tube, 1669-1670
    fissural, 1077
    Gartner's duct, 1639
    of heart, 700
    hydatid, 662
    intrasellar, 1537
    of jaws, 1117-1120
    of joints and para-articular tissues, 2092
    laryngeal, 1085
    liver, 1293
        congenital, *1297*
    mediastinal, 1024-1025, 1025*t*
    mesentery and, 1191
    mesonephric, 1669
    mother, 461
    Müllerian, *1626*
    myxoid, 1782
    neck, 1143-1144
    of nose, 1077
    ovarian
        follicular, oral contraceptives and, 165
        nonneoplastic, 1674-1677
        theca-lutein, 1674
    parathyroid, 1577
    of pars plana, 1069
    pericardial, 1024
    pilary, 1835
    pilosebaceous, 1835
    of prostate gland, 902
    salivary gland, 1127-1128
    sebaceous, 1835
    splenic, 1426
    sweat gland, *1764*
    synovial, 1782
    of thymus gland, 1502
    thyroglossal, 1546
    Toxoplasma, *449*
    trichilemmal, 1834
    urachal, 867
    of urethra, 899
    of vagina, 1639

Cystadenocarcinoma of pancreas, 1354
Cystadenofibromas of ovary, 1684
Cystadenoma, 610
    bile duct, 1291-1292
    eccrine, 1832
    of epididymis, 892
    of ovary, *1681*
    pancreatic, 1354, *1354*
    of salivary glands, 1134-1135, *1135*
Cystamine, 254, 1233
Cystectomy, *860*
Cysteine, 254
Cystic adventitial disease of popliteal artery, 785-786, *787*
Cystic bile duct, congenital, 1257-1258
Cystic breast disease, *1728*, 1728-1729
Cystic chondroblastoma, 2039
Cystic endometrial hyperplasia, 1657
Cystic fibrosis, 950-951
    gastrointestinal manifestations of, 1172-1173
    liver disease and, 1268
    pancreas and, 1348-1351, *1349*, *1350*
Cystic hygroma
    in mediastinum, 1024
    in neck, 1144
Cystic lung, herbicide toxicity and, 230
Cystic lymphangioma, 799, *799*
Cystic medial necrosis, 783, *784*
Cystic syringadenoma, 1832-1833
Cystic teratoma, 1689, *1689*
Cysticercosis, 459
    cerebral, *459*, *460*
    meningitis and, 2154
    of myocardium, *460*
Cystine stones, 854
Cystinosis, cornea and, 1074
Cystitis, 311, 834, 855, 855-857
    bullous, 855
    candidiasis and, 412
    emphysematous, 855
    encrusted, 856
    gangrenous, 856
    interstitial, 856
    irradiation, 856
    polypoid, 857
    tuberculous, 857
Cystitis cystica, 857, *858*
Cystitis glandularis, 458, 857
Cystoprostatectomy, *861*
Cystosarcoma, malignant breast, 1748
Cystosarcoma phyllodes, 1730-1731
Cystothionuria, 559
Cytochrome oxidase, 2, 558
Cytochrome P-450, 5, 16
    drug metabolism and, 1232
Cytogenetics, 45-49, 603, 1624-1627
Cytokeratin, 1012
    leiomyosarcomas and, 1863
    malignant fibrous histiocytomas and, 1859
    soft-tissue tumors and, 1840
Cytokines, 93
Cytology, 12, 610
    neoplastic cells and, 580-581
    in urothelial tumors, 866
    vaginal pathology and, 1638-1639
Cytolysis, 12, 504*t*, 509, *509*
Cytomegalic inclusion disease; *see* Cytomegalovirus
Cytomegalovirus, 379, *381*
    acquired immunodeficiency syndrome and, 1167, 1286
    alimentary tract and, 1054

Cytomegalovirus—cont'd
  cholecystitis and, 1328, 1328t
  cholestasis and liver cell necrosis and,
      1265, 1265
  Kaposi's sarcoma and, 1473
  liver and, 1231
      childhood cholestasis and, 1261t
      newborn and, 382, 1261t
          encephalitis in, 2160, 2161, 2161
      pneumonitis and, 382
      salivary gland and, 1130
Cytomegaly of adrenals in newborn, 1583
Cytopenia
  hypoplastic acute nonlymphoblastic
      leukemia and, 1388
  myelodysplastic syndromes and, 1390
Cytophilic antibody, 531t
Cytoplasm, radiation and, 24, 255
Cytoplasmic inclusion, 1825
Cytosine toxicity, 8, 185
Cytotoxic suppressor lymphocytes, 1219
Cytotoxicity, 88, 504t, 509, 509, 539t
  brain edema and, 2127, 2128
Cytotrophoblast, 885, 1709
Cytoxan; see Cyclophosphamide

D

2,4-D; see 2,4-Dichlorophenoxyacetic acid
D-cells
  diabetes and, 1360
  tumors of, 1368
Dallas criteria, 707
Dandy-Walker malformation, 2139, 2140
Dane particle, 387, 1212
Darier-Pautrier microabscesses, 1826, 1826
Darier-Roussy sarcoid, 1785
Darier's disease, 1103, 1759, 1759
Dartos, smooth muscle layer of, 871
Darvon; see Propoxyphene
Daughter cells, 1624
Daughter cysts, 461
Daunomycin; see Daunorubicin
Daunorubicin, 183
DDT, 226, 230
de Quervain's thyroiditis, 1550, 1550
Deaf-mutism, hypothyroidism and, 1545
Death
  alcohol and, 192
  alcohol-barbiturate intake and, 218-219
  arsenic and, 209
  from cancer, 607, 608t, 609t
  of cells from ionizing radiation, 250-251
  from coronary heart disease, 617
  ferrous sulfate toxicity and, 210
  by gunfire, 124-12
  herbicide toxicity and, 230
  isopropanol poisoning and, 198
  radiation injury and, 264-265
  sudden cardiac, 627
Decay of substance, radioactive, 248-249
Deceleration, protracted, 112
Decidual cells, 1190
Decomposition, 23
  of glycine, 23-24
Decompression sickness, 134
Deferentitis, 892
Deficiency diseases, 546-565; see also
    Malnutrition
Degenerative aneurysm, 780
Degenerative diseases
  of bone, 2010-2013, 2012, 2013
  central nervous system, 2181-2183
  of joints, 2071

Degos acanthoma, 1795
Degranulation, 520
  mast cell, 521, 522
Dehydroepiandrosterone, 1672
Dehydroisoandrosterone, 1581, 1582
Del Castillo syndrome, 873
Delayed hypersensitivity, 88-89, 490, 504t,
    505, 527, 529
  evolution of, 530
  lesions of, 539t
Delayed responses to cell injury, 76
Delayed skin reaction; see Delayed
    hypersensitivity
Deletions, 48
Delta hepatitis, 1210, 1215-1216
  chronic active hepatitis and, 1227
  fulminant hepatitis and, 1223
Dematiaceous granule, 396, 397
Demodex folliculorum, 1769
Demyelinating diseases, 2176-2180
Demyelination, 2176
  hexachlorophene and, 224
  organophosphates and, 226
  peripheral neuropathies and, 2190, 2190-
      2191
  radiation injury and, 281
Dendrites, junctional nevus and, 1802
Dendritic histiocytes, 492t
Dendritic macrophages, 494
Denervating diseases, 2119, 2119-2121, 2120
Denervation atrophy, 43
Dengue, 371
Dens in dente, 1097
Dens invaginatus, 1097
Dense-deposit disease, 517t, 811
Densely ionizing particles, 254
Dental caries, 1098, 1098
Dental granuloma, 1099, 1099
Dental pigmentation anomalies, 1097
Dentate nucleus, ischemic encephalopathy
    and, 2147
Dentigerous cyst, 1119
Dentin defects, 1097
Denture-injury tumor, 1107
Deoxycorticosterone, 217, 1582
Deoxycortisol, 1582
Deoxyribonucleic acid, 2, 9, 44
  cardiac hypertrophy and, 41
  genital neoplasms and, 1645
  hepatitis B virus and, 1212
  hyperplasia and, 43
  liver and, 1206
  non-Hodgkin's lymphomas and, 1455-
      1456, 1458
  radiation injury and, 254-255
  replication of, 8-9
  tumor-cell, 586-587
  viral, 26
  xeroderma pigmentosum and, 61
Dermacentor, 319, 350
Dermal appendages
  diseases of, 1786-1787
  tumors of, 1830-1835
Dermatan sulfate, 52
Dermatitis
  contact, 531, 532, 539t
  nickel toxicity and, 214
  pellagrous, 557
  radiation, 265
Dermatitis herpetiformis, 539t, 1761, 1761
Dermatitis medicamentosa, 218
Dermatitis venenata, 531
Dermatofibrosarcoma protuberans, 1819

Dermatographia, 526
Dermatolysis, 1784
Dermatomyositis, 1772, 2117-2118, 2118
  childhood, 2118, 2118
  and polymyositis complex, 2110, 2111,
      2117, 2118
  pulmonary involvement in, 974
  tumors and, 605
Dermatopathic lymphadenopathy, 1438,
    1438, 1439, 1827
Dermatopathology, 1751-1752
Dermatophytosis, 392t, 397-399
Dermatoses, 1759-1785
  dermal, 1775-1785; see also Dermis,
      diseases of
  epidermal, 1759-1769
    hyperplasia in, 1759-1767
    scabies in, 1769
    superficial mycoses in, 1768-1769
  intradermal neutrophilic, 1765
  shave biopsy and, 1759
  subcorneal pustular, 1765
  transient acantholytic, 1765
Dermis, 1755-1757
  burns and, 96, 138
  diseases of, 1775-1785
    berylliosis in, 1785
    brucellosis in, 1785
    chondrodermatitis nodularis chronica
        helicis in, 1784
    collagen, 1776-1782
    elastic tissue, 1782-1784
    erysipelas in, 85, 304, 304-305
    granulomas in, 1784-1785
    mucinous cysts in, 1782
    sarcoidosis, 1784-1785
    tuberculosis cutis in, 1784
    urticaria pigmentosa in, 1775-1776
    urticarial vasculitis in, 1776
  diseases of epidermis, 1769-1775
    dermatomyositis in, 1772
    keratoderma blennorrhagica in, 1774-
        1775
    lichen planus in, 1773-1774
    lupus erythematosus in, 1769-1772
    mixed connective tissue disease in,
        1772
    parapsoriasis in, 1773
    psoriasis in, 1772-1773
Dermoid cysts, 1835
  of nose, 1077
  oral, 1120
  of ovary, 1689, 1689
Desacetylrifampicin toxicity, 170
Descemet's membrane, 1074
Desensitization, 498
Desipramine poisoning, 193t
Desmin as marker in rhabdomyosarcoma,
    1866
Desmoid fibromatosis, 1845-1847, 1847
Desmoplasia, 568, 569, 610
  gastric carcinoma and, 1183
Desmoplastic fibroma, 2021t, 2051, 2051-
    2052
  in jaws, 1116
Desmosomes, 1755, 1802
Desquamative interstitial pneumonia, 970,
    970
Desquamative radiation injury, 273
Determinant, 488
Detoxification
  cells and, 4-6
  drug toxicity and, 147

Deuterons, 248
Developmental anomalies; *see* Congenital
  abnormalities
Developmental cysts
  of mediastinum, 1024-1025
  odontogenic, 1118-1119
Developmental rests, 571
Devic's disease, 2177
Dexamethasone, 163
Dextran, 655
Diabetes
  bronze, 1272
  steroid, 163
Diabetes insipidus, 1523, 1526
Diabetes mellitus, 1358-1367
  articular changes and, 2091-2092
  atherosclerosis and, 759
  candidiasis and, 412
  cardiac complications of, 620, 686-687,
    691-692
  etiology and pathogenesis of, 1359-1362
  glycogen deposits and, 30
  islet pathology and, 1362-1364
  liver disease and, 1287
  male infertility and, 873
  microangiopathy and, 1364-1367
  neoplasms and, 1367-1369
  nephropathy and, 822, 823
  neutralization reactions and, 506t
  placental lesions and, 1703-1704
  pregnancy and, 61, 1262, *1364*
  retinopathy and, 1057-1062, *1060*, *1061*,
    1364
  rubeosis iridis in, *1062*
  type I, 1359-1360, 1362
  type II, 1360, 1362-1363
Diabetic ketoacidosis, 37
Diabinese; *see* Chlorpropamide
Dialysis, 807
  arthropathy and, 2070
  beta$_2$-microglobulin amyloid bone disease
    in, 2000
  staphylococcal pneumonia and, 935
Diamond-Blackfan syndrome, 1377
Diapedesis, 78, 1057
Diaphragmatic hernia, 921-922
Diaphysis, 2022, *2022*
Diarrhea
  hepatic amebic abscess and, 1259
  tumors and, 1368
  watery, 1168
Diarthrodial joints, 2065-2066
Diastematomyelia, 2136
Diathrodial joints, 2065
Diatomaceous-earth pneumoconiosis, 234
Diazepam, 150, 193t
2,4-Dichlorophenoxyacetic acid, 193t
Dichorionic diamnionic twin placentas, 1699
Dicumarol; *see* Bishydroxycoumarin
Dieldrin poisoning, 194t
Dieterle's silver stain, 938
Diethyl *N*-substituted iminodiacetic acid,
  1262
Diethylene glycol toxicity, 198
Diethylstilbestrol, 1639-1640, 1642, *1642*
Dieulafoy's aneurysm, 1159
Differentiation, 610
  bladder transitional cell carcinoma and,
    862, *862*
  change in usual line of, 107
  of new epithelium, 96
  signals important in, 7

Diffuse alveolar damage, 961-962
  oxygen toxicity and, 176, *177-179*
Diffuse cerebral impact injury, 2189
Diffuse cirrhosis, 1238
Diffuse fibromuscular intimal thickening of
  arteries, 759
Diffuse fibrosis in cirrhosis, 1208
Diffuse glomerulonephritis, 812-815
Diffuse hyperplasia
  of adrenal glands, 568, 1589-1592, *1591*
  of lymph nodes, 1438-1440
Diffuse interstitial fibrosis, *174*, 175
  of myocardium, 699
Diffuse large-cell lymphomas, 1459, 1465-
  1467
Diffuse lymphocytic thyroiditis, 1551
Diffuse myocarditis, *661*, 663
Diffuse nontoxic goiter, 1546-1549
Diffuse pleural mesotheliomas, 1018, *1018*,
  1019
Diffuse proliferative glomerulonephritis, 825
Diffuse scleroderma, 1779-1780
Diffuse sclerosing thyroid papillary
  carcinoma, 1559
Diffuse septal amyloidosis, 983
Diffuse syringoma, 1832
Diffuse toxic goiter, 1549-1550, *1550*
DiGeorge syndrome, 501t
DiGeorge's syndrome, 1500t, 1978
Digestion and detoxication in cells, 4-6
Digestive tract; *see* Alimentary tract
Digital fibrous tumors of childhood, 1825
Digitalis
  gynecomastia and, 168
  toxicity of, 175
Dihydrotestosterone, 567, 1624
Dihydroxycholesterol, *1582*
1,25-Dihydroxyvitamin D, 1972
Diiodotyrosine, 1544
Diisocyanates, 238
Dilantin; *see* Phenytoin
Dilatation
  bile duct, 1257-1258
  cardiomyopathies and, 682
  congenital heart disease and, 730
  ureteral, 851
  urinary bladder, 853-854
Dimethyl busulfan; *see* Busulfan toxicity
7,12-Dimethylbenz*a*anthracene, 596
Dimorphic, definition of, 397
Dioxane toxicity, 200
Diphtheria, 292t, 294-295, *295*
  pseudomembranous inflammation and, 86
Diphtheroids, 1765
Diphyllobothriasis, 291, 460
Diplegia, spastic, 1545
Diplococcus pneumoniae, 306, *306*, 1087
Diploid female human karotype, *46*
Dipyridamole, 621
Diquat dibromide toxicity, 230
Direct agglutination test, 443
Direct fluorescent antibody stain, 396-397
Dirofilariasis, 473
Dirt-eating habits, 466
Disc disease, 2096
Discoid lupus erythematosus, 1769-1770,
  1770, 1785
Disease; *see also* Syndrome
  Addison's; *see* Addison's disease
  Alzheimer's, *2181*, 2181-2182
  Bowen's; *see also* Bowenoid papulosis
  Buerger's, 623
  Byler's, 1268

Disease—cont'd
  Caroli's, 1257-1258, 1337
  Chagas', 661, 661-662
  Concato's, 667
  Crohn's; *see* Crohn's disease
  Devic's, 2177
  Fabry's, 53, 55, 1173, 1780
  Gaucher's, 53, 1267
  Gilbert's, 33, 1275, 1276t, 1277
  Gorham's, 2051
  Graves'; *see* Graves' disease
  Grover's, 1765
  Hailey-Hailey, 1762
  Hippel's, 1820
  Hodgkin's; *see* Hodgkin's disease
  Hunter's, 53, 55, 59
  Huntington's, 2182, *2182*
  Hurler-Scheie, 52-55, *53*
  Hurler's, 53, 686, 1173, 1267, 1529
  Kawasaki's, 774-775, 776, 1433
    skin and, 1830
  Kikuchi's, 1434
  Kimmelstiel-Wilson, 823, 1057, 1364
  Kimura's, 1790, *1791*
  Krabbe's, 53, 2180, *2180*
  Kyrle's, 1784
  Lenègre's, 706
  Letterer-Siwe, 977, 1423
  Lev's, 706
  Libman-Sacks, 672-673, 1770
  Madelung's, 1142
  Majocchi's, 397, 1786
  Marie-Strümpell's, 650, 2097-2098
  Marion's, 853
  McArdle's, 2115, *2115*
  Ménétrier's, 1171
  Mikulicz's, 1129
  Milroy's, 792
  Mondor's, 1790
  Mseleni, 2075
  Niemann-Pick; *see* Niemann-Pick disease
  Osler-Weber-Rendu; *see* Osler-Weber-
    Rendu disease
  Paget's; *see* Paget's disease
  Parkinson's, 2182-2183, *2183*
  Peyronie's, 895-896, *896*, 1845
  Pick's, 667
  Plummer's, 1547
  Pompe's, 53, 55, 687
  Potter type I renal, 845-846
  Potter type IV renal, *845*, 845-846
  Pott's, 2006
  Reiter's; *see* Reiter's syndrome
  Scheie's, 53
  Schilder's, 2177
  silo-filler's, 231-232
  Still's, 2086-2087
  Takayasu's, 623, 768, 774, *775*
  Tay-Sachs', 52, 53, 1173
  Vincent's, 1105
  Vogt-Koyanagi-Harada, 1056
  von Gierke's, 687
  von Hippel-Lindau; *see* von Hippel-
    Lindau disease
  von Recklinghausen's; *see* von
    Recklinghausen's disease
  Weber-Christian, 1190, 1788, *1788*
  Weil's, 1232
  Werdnig-Hoffmann, 2119, 2120-2121,
    2121, 2183
  Wernicke's, 555, 556, 2185, *2185*
  Whipple's, 1173, *1174*, 2086
  Whitmore's, 322

Disease—cont'd
  Wilson's, 1074, 1269-1271, 1786
  Wolman's, 1173
  Woringer-Kolopp, 1827
Disse, space of, 1200
Dissecting aneurysm, 778, 780-784, 782, 783
Disseminated cutaneous leishmaniasis, 445
Disseminated gonococcal infection, 309
Disseminated herpetic infection of newborn, 379
Disseminated intravascular coagulation, 321
  adrenal glands and, 1585
  herpesviruses and, 379
  skin and, 1791
Disseminated spiked hyperkeratosis, 1795
Distal acinar emphysema, 990
Distal myopathy, 2112
Distal splenorenal shunt, 1250-1251
Distomiases, 452-454
Disuse osteoporosis, 1972
Diuretics
  thiazide; see Thiazides
  toxicity of, 169, 203
Divers, 134
Diverticular prostatitis, 901
Diverticulum
  bladder, 853
  bronchitis and, 988
  caliceal, 850
  gallbladder and mucosal, 1331, 1331
  gastrointestinal tract, acquired, 1155
  Meckel's, 1154, 1154
  urethral, 898
  Zenker's, 1155
DMF teeth, 1098
DNA; see Deoxyribonucleic acid
DNA genome, hepatitis B virus and, 387
DNA viruses, 377-387
  adenoviruses and, 377-378
  hepatitis B virus, 387
  herpesviruses and, 378-384
  papovaviruses and, 384-386
  poxviridae and, 386-387
Doca; see Deoxycorticosterone
Docking proteins, 3
Dog heartworm, 473
Dohm staging systems, 603
Doll-face appearance, 57
Donovanosis, 324
Dopamine, 30, 1248, 2183
Dorfman-Chanarin syndrome, 1793
Doriden; see Glutethimide
Dormia basket, 851
Double-barreled aorta, 782
Double minute chromosomes, 1387
Double-outlet right ventricle, 743
  with subaortic ventricular septal defect
    and pulmonary stenosis, 743-745, 745
  with subpulmonic ventricular septal
    defect, 744-745, 746
Double vulva, 1628
Doubling dose, mutations and, 262
Doubling times for cell, 580, 580
Down's syndrome, 47, 2141, 2141
  leukemia and, 1385
Doxorubicin, 183, 681, 708
DPI; see Phenformin
Dracontiasis, 473-474
Dracunculiasis, 473-474
Drechslera, 402
Dressler syndrome, 672
Droplet nuclei, 940
Drosophila, 261

Drug abuse
  foreign-body embolism and, 953, 953
  infective endocarditis and, 654
  viral hepatitis and, 1214, 1219, 1223, 1229
Drug allergy, 538
Drug injury and iatrogenic diseases, 146-226, 239-243
  amphetamines in, 168-169
  analgesics and antipyretics in, 158-162
  androgenic-anabolic steroids in, 165
  anesthetics in, 171
  anti-infective agents in, 174-175
  antiarrhythmics in, 175-176
  anticonvulsants in, 171-174
  antidiabetics drugs in, 169
  antihypertensives in, 168
  antineoplastic and immunosuppressive
    agents in, 180-186
  antithyroid drugs in, 169
  antitubercular drugs in, 169-171
  causative components of adverse reactions
    in, 146-149
  corticosteroids in, 162-165
  diuretics in, 169
  estrogens in, 167
  genetically related, 149-168; see also
    Pharmacogenetics
  H_2 receptor antagonists in, 169
  hemolytic reactions in, 511, 511-512, 512t
  hepatotoxicity in, 1232-1239, 1234-1235t
  incidence of, 146
  jaundice and, 1233
  lung and, 984-985
  methysergide in, 186
  milk and milk alkali in, 189-191
  mineral oil in, 191
  oral contraceptives in, 165-167
  oxygen in, 176-180
  potassium chloride in, 186-189
  sympathomimetic amines in, 168-191; see
    also Sympathomimetic amines
  thorotrast in, 186
  toxicologic aspects of forensic pathology
    in, 191-226
    alcohols and, 191-198
    arsenic and, 209-210
    barbiturates and, 217-219
    benzene and, 222
    boric acid and, 222-224
    cadmium and, 212-213
    carbon monoxide and, 220-222
    carbon tetrachloride and, 222
    catecholamines and, 216-217
    cobalt and, 212
    cocaine and, 220
    elemental phosphorus and, 224
    ferrous sulfate and, 210-212
    glycols and, 198-200
    hexachlorophene and, 224
    lead in, 205-209
    mercury in, 200-205
    metals and metallic salts in, 200-216
    narcotics and, 219-220
    nickel and, 214
    plant poisons and, 224-226
    platinum and, 216
    thallium and, 214-216
    uranium and, 216
  tranquilizers in, 167-168
Drug metabolism, liver and, 1232
Drug-oxidizing enzyme system, microsomal, 5, 5

Drugs
  as antigens, 148-149
  metabolism of, 5, 5-6
  as toxins, 146-147; see also Toxicity
Drummart-Ebstein lesion, 821
Dubin-Johnson pigment, 1204
Dubin-Johnson syndrome, 1275, 1276t, 1277, 1277
Duchenne muscular dystrophy, 60, 2110, 2111
Duct
  of Hering, 1200
  of Santorini, 1347
  of Wirsung, 1347
Ductus arteriosus, 734
Duffy blood group determinant, 446
Duhring's disease, 1761
Dukes system for colon cancer, 603
Duodenum
  strongyloidiasis and, 468
  ulcers of, 87, 1159-1161
Duplication
  alimentary tract, 1153-1154
  of fallopian tubes, 1627
  of ureter, 850, 850
Dupuytren's contracture, 895, 2091
Dupuytren's exostosis, 2036
Dupuytren's type of fibromatoses, 1845
Dural sinuses, septic thrombophlebitis of, 2153-2154
Dürck's glial nodes, 447
Duret hemorrhages, 2130
Durozier sign, 676
Dust particles
  emphysema and, 238
  fibrogenic, 233-236
  hypersensitivity pneumonitis and, 236
  lung deposition and clearance of, 996
  nonfibrogenic, 233
  in normal lung, 996-997
  tracheobronchial tree and, 232
Dutcher bodies, 1400
Duval endodermal sinuses, 1688
Dwarfism
  achondroplastic, 1947
  parathyroid glands and, 1577
  short-limbed, 1500t
Dynein, 950, 950
Dysbaric caisson disease, 134
Dyschondroplasia, 795
Dyscrasias; see also Bone marrow and blood
  plasma cell, 1400
  radium and, 259
Dysentery, bacillary, 292t, 300, 301
Dysfunctional uterine bleeding, 1656-1657
Dysgenesis, gonadal, 880, 1625t, 1626
Dysgerminoma, 1687, 1687-1688
  radiosensitivity of, 257t
Dyshormonogenic goiters, 1547
Dyskeratosis, 1757-1758
Dyskeratosis congenita, 1795
Dysplasia, 570, 585, 610
  cervical, 1645-1650, 1646, 1649
  epiphyseal, 1957
  fibromuscular, 786, 787
  renal, 845, 845-846
  thymic, 1499, 1501
  vulva and, 1632-1633
Dysplastic nevi, 1803, 1816
Dyspoiesis in bone marrow, 1377
Dysproteinemia with angioimmunoblastic
  lymphadenopathy, 1439, 1441
Dysrhythmias, 637

Dysthyroid ophthalmopathy, 1047
Dystopia of hypophysis, 1526
Dystrophic calcification, 36, 693, 1571
Dystrophies
  muscular, *2109*, 2110, 2111-2112
  vulvar, 1629-1630
Dystrophin, 60

E

Ear; *see also* Upper respiratory tract and ear
  external, 1088-1089
  middle, 1087-1088
Early viral antigens, 383
Eastern equine encephalitis, 371
Eaton-Lambert syndrome, 1013
Ebola viruses, 376, 1231
Eccrine adenoma, 1832
Eccrine cystadenomas, 1832
Eccrine glands, 1755
  pancreas and secretions of, 1348
Eccrine poroepithelioma, 1832
Eccrine poroma, 1831
Eccrine spiradenoma, 1832
Echinococcal cyst
  of liver, 1293, *1293*
  of prostate gland, 901
Echinococcosis, 460-462, 700, 857, 1426
  myocarditis and, 662
Echoviruses, 374
  encephalitis and, 2158
  jaundice and, 1265
  myocarditis and, 661
Eck fistula, 2184
Eclampsia, 827-828, *828*, 1701-1702
  liver and, *1274*, 1274-1275
Ectasia
  juvenile melanoma and, 1808-1809
  mammary duct, 1731
  vascular, 1159
Ecthyma gangrenosum, 311
Ecto-5'-nucleotidase deficiency, 503
Ectodermal placodes, 2135
Ectomesenchyme, 1095
Ectomesenchymomas, malignant, 1896
Ectopic adrenal carcinoma, 1605
Ectopic adrenocorticotropic hormone, 1592-1593, *1595*
  tumors with, 1593*t*
Ectopic granulomatous schistosomiasis, 458
Ectopic pancreas, 1348
Ectopic pinealoma, 2174
Ectopic pregnancy, 1669, 1700
Ectopic sebaceous glands, 1756
Ectopic testis, 871
Ectopic thyroid, 573, *573*, 1546
Ectromelia, 386
Ectropion uveae, 1062
Eczema, 526, 531, 1761
Edema
  accumulation of, 69
  brain, 2125-2128, *2127*, *2128*
  in heart failure, 616
  hydropericardium and, 664
  inflammation and, 84
  juvenile melanoma and, 1808
  mechanisms of, 958-959
  onchocerciasis and, 472
  ovarian, 1676
  pregnancy and, 827
  pulmonary, 958-962, 1035-1036
  radiation and, 271
  secondary, 129
  subintimal, radiation and, 274
  villous, of placenta, 1703

Edrophonium, 2118
Edward's syndrome, 47-48
Effector lymphocyte populations, 492, 492*t*
EGF; *see* Epithelial growth factor
Ehlers-Danlos syndrome, 986, 1782-1783, 2067
Ehrlichia, 349*t*, 357-358
Ehrlichial diseases, 357-358
Ehrlichiosis, canine, 358
El Tor organism, 299
Elastic arteries, 752
Elastic lamellae, 951
Elastic pulmonary arteries, 951
Elastic tissue diseases, 1782-1784
Elastica Van Gieson stain, 1809
Elasticity, force and, 112
Elastin, 754, 992
Elastofibroma dorsi, 1783-1784
Elastosis perforans serpiginosa, 1784
Elavil; *see* Amitriptyline
Electrical injury, 140-144, *142*, *143*
Electrical signals, 8
Electrolyte-concentrating mechanism, 1349
Electrolytes
  disturbances of, 693
    congestive cardiomyopathy and, 693
  transport of, 806
Electromagnetic radiation, *247*, 247-248
Electromyography, 2108
Electron capture, 248
Electron microscopy, 517*t*
  liposarcoma and, 1879
  neurofibroma and, 1893
  rhabdomyosarcoma and, 1866
  soft-tissue tumors and, 1839
  synovial sarcoma and, 1900
Electron volts, particulate radiation and, 248
Electrothermal injuries, 141-143, *142*, *143*
Elemental mercury, 200
Elemental phosphorus, toxicity of, 224
Elements, essential, 562-563
Elephantiasis
  bancroftian filariasis and, 471
  of scrotum, 893-894
Embden-Meyerhof glycolytic pathway, 30
Embolism
  air, 953
  amniotic fluid, 953
  cardiac tumors and, 704
  central nervous system infarct and, 2148, *2148*
  coronary artery disease and, 623-624
  coronary occlusion and, 627
  foreign-body, 953, 953-954
  infective endocarditis and, 657
  mechanical injury and, 132
  pulmonary, 952
  pulmonary candidiasis and, 413
  rheumatic fever and, 649
Embryo, *1695*
  exogenous deoxyribonucleic acid and, 62
  female genitalia in, *1620*, 1620-1628
  liver and, 1199-1201
  radiation of, 259
  skeleton and, 1937, *1937*
  splenic fusions and, 1413
Embryonal carcinoma
  of ovary, 1688
  of testes, 884-885, *887*
Embryonal rhabdomyosarcoma, 603, 1865, 1867, *1868*
  of biliary tract, 1343, *1343*
  of vagina, 1642, *1643*

Embryonal sarcoma
  bladder and, 866, *866*
  liver and, 1299
Emetine, 708
Emmonsia, 393*t*, 407
Emphysema, 987, 989-995
  bullae and, 992
  cadmium toxicity and, 212
  centriacinar, 989-990, *990*, *993*
  centrilobular, 989
  classification of, 989-992
  congenital lobar or segmental, 923-925
  distal acinar, 990
  etiology of, 993-994
  focal, 1000
  irregular, 990
  morphogenesis of lesions in, 992
  natural history of chronic airflow limitation in, 995
  occupational, 238
  panacinar, 990, *991*
  paraseptal, 990
  pathogenesis of, 994-995
  pathophysiology of, 992-993
  pertussis and, 299
  pulmonary interstitial, 928, *928*
  silo-filler disease and, 232
  small airways obstruction in absence of, 996
Emphysematous cystitis, 855
Empty sella syndrome, 1527
Empyema, 935, 937, 939
  subdural, 2153-2154
Enamel
  fluoridation and, 229
  hereditary defects of, 1097
  mottled, 1098
Encapsulated tumors, 581
Encephalitis, 2158-2164
  California, 370
  Eastern equine, 371
  herpes simplex virus and, 379, *381*
  Japanese B, 371-372
  lymphocytes and, 82, *82*
  microglia and, 2135
  mumps, *366*, 367
  Russian spring-summer, 372
  St. Louis, 371-372
  tick-borne, 371-372
  Toxoplasma, 449, 450
  Venezuelan equine, 371
  Western equine, 371
Encephalocele, 2136
Encephalofacial angiomatosis, 1109
Encephalomalacia, multicystic, 2139
Encephalomyelitis, 2158
  acute disseminated, 2177-2178, *2178*
  allergic, 536*t*
    experimental, *535*
Encephalopathy, 1248
  acute toxic, 2184-2185
  aliphatic amino acids and, 1248
  hepatic, 2184
  ischemic, 2146-2147, *2148*
  perinatal injury and bilirubin, 2145-2146
  portal-systemic, 2184
  spongiform, 387-388
  transmissible mink, 387
  Wernicke's, 556, 2185, *2185*
Encephalotrigeminal angiomatosis, 1051
Enchondroma, 2034, *2034*, *2035*
Enchondromatosis, multiple, 2034
Encrustation theory, 621, *623*, 762

Encrusted cystitis, 856
End bulbs of Krause, 1757
End-capillary loops, 629
Endarteritis
   schistosomal, 457
   syphilis and, 650, 2157
Endarteritis obliterans, 766, *766*, 842
Endocardial fibroelastosis
   endocardial thickening in, *697*, 697-698
   mitral stenosis and, 672-673
   mumps and, 366
   restrictive cardiomyopathy and, 695
Endocardial hypertrophy, 730
Endocardial pockets in syphilitic heart
      disease, 652
Endocardial sclerosis, 730
Endocarditis, 306, 652-658, *653*, *655-656*,
      657
   infective arteritis and, 767
   Libman-Sacks, 672-673
   Q fever, 356
   rheumatic fever and, 643-645, *644*, *645*
Endochondral ossification, 1937, *1938*, 1947
Endocrine disorders
   cholestasis and, 1261*t*
   congestive cardiomyopathy and, 689-692
   multiple adenomatosis in, 1535, 1563
      thymus gland and, 1508
   pituitary in, 1523-1525
   testicular tumors and, 880
   tumors and, 606
   vaginal cytology and, 1638
Endocrine glands, 7; *see also* Endocrine
      disorders
   reproduction and hormones of, 9
Endocrine pancreas, 1358-1369
Endocytosis, 3-4, 508
Endocytotic vesicles, 4
Endodermal sinus tumor
   ovary and, 1688, *1688*
   testes and, 885, *885*
   vagina and, 1642
Endogenous autoinfection, 468
Endolymphangitis, polypoid, 470
Endolymphatic stromal myosis, 1661, *1662*
Endometrial stromal neoplasms, 1661-1662
Endometrioid tumors of ovary, 1682, *1682*
Endometriosis, 1669
   alimentary tract and, 1156, 1190
   ovarian, 1676-1677, *1677*
   in vulva, 1632
Endometritis, 1657
   puerperal, 306
Endometrium, 1652-1663
   anovulatory, *1655*
   benign polypoid lesions of, 1659
   dysfunctional uterine bleeding and, 1656-
      1657
   hormonal effects on, 1654-1656
   hyperplasia of, 1657-1659
   hysterectomy and, 1656
   inflammation of, 1657
   neoplasms of, 1659-1663
   normal cyclic changes in, 1652-1654
Endomyocardial biopsy, 706-708
Endomyocardial fibrosis, 696-697
   methysergide and, 186
Endophthalmitis, 1053, *1054*
   phacoanaphylactic, 536*t*
Endoplasmic reticulum, 1200-1201
   DDT toxicity and, 226, *227*
Endosalpingiosis, 1190

Endoscopic retrograde
      cholangiopancreatography, 452, 1323
Endospore, 397
Endothelium
   atherosclerosis and, 764
   capillary, injury to
      alveolar, 960
      hypothermia and, 137
      granulation tissue and, 98
   intravascular papillary hyperplasia of, 796
   neutrophil adherent to, 79
   oral contraceptives and, 165
   radiation and, 257*t*, 274
   vascular permeability and, 73, 78
Endotoxins, 291
   adrenal glands and, 1585
Endovasculitis, placental hemorrhagic, 1705-
      1706
Energy
   cells and production of, 1
   joule of, 249
   mechanical trauma and transfer of, 111-
      112
   of spinning object, 111
Energy metabolism
   encephalopathy and cerebral, 1248
   myocardial ischemia and, 630-631
Entactin, 805
Entamoeba coli, 436
Entamoeba histolytica, 433, 1166
   liver abscess and, 1259
   pericarditis and, 670
Enteric cysts, 1024, 1153-1154
Enteric fevers, 314-315
Enteric organisms
   meningitis and, 2154
   as opportunists, 292*t*
Enteritis of terminal ileum, 1164
Enterobacter, 312, 936, 1585
Enterobiasis, 464-465, *465*, 1165
Enterococcus, 834, 1189
Enterocolitis, 1166
   antibiotic-associated, 146, 153, *154-155*,
      155, 1166
Enteropathic arthritis, 2086
Enteropathy, protein-losing, 1172
Enterotoxin, staphylococcal, 293
Entomophthoromycosis, 393*t*, 426-427
Environmental pathology, 226-239
   air pollutants in, 230-232
   carbamates in, 229
   fluorine compounds in, 229
   herbicides in, 230, *231*
   insecticides and pesticides in, 226
   occupational chest diseases in, 232-239
   polychlorinated biphenyls in, 226-229
Environmental radiation, 249-250
Enzootic zoonoses, 314
Enzymatic activation unit, 511
Enzyme-linked immunosorbent assay, 440,
      450
Enzyme polymorphisms, 1240
Enzymes
   adaptive synthesis of, 487
   adrenal glands and, 1581, *1582*
   barbiturates and, 218
   cell death and hydrolytic, 12
   detoxification, 147
   in eccrine glands, 1756
   fluorine compound toxicity and, 229
   lead poisoning and, 205
   lysosomal, leukotrienes and, 75
   muscle fibers and, 2107

Enzymes—cont'd
   oxygen and, 176
   proteolytic, 73, 291
   vascular permeability and, 73
   vitamins and, 550
   yellow respiratory, 558
Eosinophil chemotactic factor A, 519*t*
Eosinophil phospholipase, 963
Eosinophilia
   angiolymphoid hyperplasia with, 795,
      1790
   echinococcosis and, 461
   myocardial infarction and, 636
   parasitic infestation and, 82
   pulmonary infiltration and, 967
      nitrofurantoin in, 174
   tropical, 467, 471
Eosinophilic fasciitis, 1780
Eosinophilic gastroenteritis, 1159
Eosinophilic granulocytes, chemotaxis and,
      80
Eosinophilic granuloma, 537
   bone tumors and, 2022*t*
   common duct and, 1334
   spleen and, 1422
Eosinophilic granulomas, skin and, 1829
Eosinophilic meningoencephalitis, 468, *469*
Eosinophilic neuronal necrosis, 2132
Eosinophilic pneumonia, 978
Eosinophilic pustular folliculitis, 1787
Eosinophilic ulcer of soft tissues, 1104-1105
Eosinophils
   bladder wall and, 856
   chemotaxis and, 80
   drug reaction and, 149
   inflammation and, 81-82
      chronic, 93-94
   onchocerciasis and, 472
   oral contraceptives and, 166
   schistosomiasis and, 454
Ependymal granulations in neurosyphilis,
      2157
Ependymoma, 2168-2169, *2169*
Ephedrine toxicity, 216-217
Epidemic parotitis, 1130
Epidemic typhus, 349*t*, 660
Epidermal cleavage, 1806-1808
Epidermal epithelium, radiosensitivity of,
      257*t*
Epidermal growth factor, 568
Epidermal necrolysis, toxic, 1765
Epidermis, 1753-1755
   abrasion and, 112, *113*
   basal cell layer of, 1753-1754
   basement membrane of, 1753, 1755
   benign neoplasms of, 1794-1796
   burns of, 96
      electrical, 141
   diseases of, 1759-1769
      dermal diseases and, 1769-1775
      hyperplasia in, 1759-1767
      scabies in, 1769
      superficial mycoses in, 1768-1769
   diseases of dermis and, 1769-1775
      dermatomyositis in, 1772
      keratoderma blennorrhagica in, 1774-
         1775
      lichen planus in, 1773-1774
      lupus erythematosus in, 1769-1772
      mixed connective tissue disease in,
         1772
      parapsoriasis in, 1773
      psoriasis in, 1772-1773

Epidermis—cont'd
electrical burns and, 141
gun wounds and, 123
healing by first intention and, 104-105
precancerous lesions of, 1796-1798
prickle cell layer of, 1754
stratum corneum of, 1755
stratum granulosum of, 1754-1755
Epidermoid carcinoma, 575, 610
of cervix, 1645-1650, *1651*
of conjunctiva, *1050*
of hand, radiation injury and, 274
of lung, *1006-1008*
of vagina, 1641
of vulva, 1633-1635, *1634*
Epidermoid cysts, splenic, 1426
Epidermoid metaplasia, 107
Epidermolysis bullosa, 1764, *1764*
in oral soft tissue, 1103
Epidermophyton, 392*t*, 397, 1768
Epididymis, 871, 891-892
absence of, 876
cysts of, 892
inflammation of, 357
tuberculosis of, 878
Epididymitis, 357
Epididymo-orchitis, 877, 891
Epidural abscesses, 2153-2154
Epidural hematoma, *2187*, 2187-2188
Epiglottis, 1084
Epinephrine, 519, 526
aspirin and, 160
bacteria in skin and, 89
myocardial injury and, 693
toxicity of, 216-217
Epiphyseal center, 1939
Epiphyseal dysplasia, multiple, 1957, *1957, 1958*
Epiphyses, *1940*, 2022, *2022*
Epispadias, 895
Epithelial cysts
of heart, 700
of vagina, 1639
Epithelial growth factor, 9, 590*t*, 591
Epithelial proliferation
breast and, 1731-1734
liver and, 1252
Epithelial tumors, 575
of ovary, 1678-1684
of salivary gland origin, 1131-1137
in urinary bladder, 858-866, *859, 860*
Epithelioid cells, 92, 505, 536
melanomas of eye and, 1065, *1065*
Epithelioid hemangioendothelioma, 796, *1296, 1299*
liver and, 1299
Epithelioid hemangioma, 795
Epithelioid leiomyoma, 1860
Epithelioid leiomyosarcoma, 1863, *1863*
Epithelioid sarcoma, 1900-1902, *1902*
Epithelioma
calcifying, 1835
superficial, 1799
Epithelium
alveolar capillary, 960
asthma and, 964
breast, hyperplasia of, *1733*
differentiation of, 96
gallbladder and biliary ducts and, 1321, *1322*
glomerular, 805, *805*
metaplasia in, 107
in nasal cavity, 1081

Epithelium—cont'd
of optic lens, 257*t*
pancreatic malignancy and, 1356-1357
regeneration of, *94*, 95, *95*, 96
of small intestine, *272*
sutures and, 105-106
of testes, 280
tumor origin in, 574*t*
vitamin A deficiency and, 552
Epitopes, 488
Epitype, 488
Epstein-Barr virus, 382-383, 601, 1500*t*
liver and, 1231
non-Hodgkin's lymphoma and, 1460, 1467
rheumatoid arthritis and, 2084
Epulis of newborn, 1108
erb A, 587, 587*t*, 591
erb B, 587, 587*t*, 591
erb B2, 587*t*
Erdheim pregnancy cells, 1521
Erosion, 1757
congenital cervical, 1643
Errors of metabolism, 51-58; *see also* Cell injury
Eruption cyst, 1119
Eruption of teeth, anomalies of, 1097
Erysipelas, 85, *304*, 304-305
Erysipelothrix, 313
Erythema
boric acid toxicity and, 224
radiation injury and, 273
Erythema induratum, 1787-1788
Erythema marginatum, 539*t*
Erythema multiforme, 539*t*
in oral soft tissue, 1103
phenytoin and, 172
Erythema nodosum, 539*t*, 1788-1789
Erythema nodosum leprosum, 337-338, 341-342
Erythema pernio, 1789
Erythroblastosis fetalis, *511*, 1262, 1706
Erythrocytes
burns and, 139
cratered, 1412
disorders of, 1375-1382
granulation tissue and, 98
Erythrocytosis, 1382
Erythroid cells, myeloid cell ratio to, 1373
Erythroid hyperplasia, osteoporosis and, 1972, *1973*
Erythroleukemia, 222
Erythrophagocytosis, 353, 1425
Erythroplakia, 1109-1110
Erythroplasia of Queyrat, 897, 1797-1798
Erythropoiesis
decreased, 1379
disorders with increased, 1379-1382
methotrexate and, 183
Erythropoietin, 807
Escherichia coli, 311-312, 411
alimentary tract and, 1189
jaundice and, 1265
lung and mediastinum and, 936-937
meningitis and, 2154
placenta and, 1704
pyogenic abscesses and, 1259
urinary system and, 834, 855
wound infection and, 130
Eserine; *see* Physostigmine
Esophageal varices, 788, 1158, 1249, *1251*
Esophageal web, congenital, *1153*
Esophagitis, 1159

Esophagus, 1153, *1153*, 1159
achalasia of, 1154
carcinoma of, 1183
pseudodiverticulosis of, 1159
radiation and, 257*t*, 278
Espundia, 445
Esthesioneuroblastoma, 1082
Estradiol, *1582*
Estrogen receptors, gallbladder and, 1323
Estrogens, 597, 599, 902
adverse reactions to, 167
breast carcinoma and, 1747
endometrium and, 1654, 1654-1656, 1660
excess of, 872
gynecomastia and, 168
hepatocellular adenoma and, 1289
jaundice and, 1235
obstetric cholestasis and, 1274
osteoporosis and, 1967
ovary and, 1672
Estrone; *see* Estrogens
Ethanol; *see* Alcohol
Ethchlorvynol poisoning, 194*t*
Ethylene dibromide, 599
Ethylene glycol toxicity, 194*t*, 198, 832
ets and *ets* 1, 587*t*
Eumycete, 396
mycetoma and, 392*t*
Eunuchoidism, 1526
Ewald's node, 1183
Ewing's sarcoma, 579, 2045-2047
adrenal glands and, 1612
bone tumors and, 2021*t*, 2023, *2046*
cytogenetics and, 603
extraskeletal, 1907-1909
in jaws, 1117
Exanthema, viral, 539*t*
Exanthematous disease in oral soft tissue, 1105-1106
Excision biopsy
biliary atresia and, 1262
soft-tissue tumors and, 1841
Excoriation, 1757
Exercise, hypertrophy and, 568
Exocytosis, 3-4
Exogenous autoinfection, 468
Exogenous molecules, 506
Exogenous photosynthesizer, 286
Exophiala jeanselmei, 392*t*, 393*t*, 402
Exophthalmos, 1047, 1549
Exostoses
in jaws, 1113
osteochondroma and, 2036
Exotoxins, 292-294
Explosions, injuries from, 135-136
Exposure to radiation, 258-261, 263
whole-body, 264
Exstrophy of bladder, 852
External ear, 1088-1089
Extracellular matrix, 7
reproduction and, 9
Extrachorial implantation, 1699, *1699*
Extragonadal germ cell tumors, 888, 1026
Extrahepatic biliary tract
cholangiocarcinoma of, 1293
obstruction of, 1252-1253, 1255
transhepatic cholangiogram of, 1253, *1253*
Extrahepatic effects of hepatic diseases, 1287
Extramammary Paget's disease
skin and, 1798, 1830
vulva and, 1635-1636, *1636*
Extraskeletal Ewing's sarcoma, 1907-1909
Extraskeletal myxoid chondrosarcoma, 1909

Extraskeletal osteosarcoma, 1909
Extrauterine life, pulmonary adaptation to, 925-929
Extravascular accumulation of blood, 129
Extrinsic allergic alveolitis, 965-967
Extrinsic asthma, 962
Exudate, pericarditis and, 666, 670, *671*
Exudation, 85
  of plasma, 69, 71-76
  tuberculosis and, 943
Exudative glomerulonephritis, 813
Eye; *see* Ophthalmic pathology
Eye worm, 473
Eyelids, 1047
  xanthomas of, 1257, *1792*

F
F-cells, 1360
Fab radioimmunoassay of procollagen III, 1207
Fabricius bursa, 499
Fabry angiokeratoma, 1820
Fabry's disease, *53*, 55, 1780
  gastrointestinal manifestations of, 1173
Face and lips, 1095
Facial bones, radiation injury to, 280
Facial clefts, 1095
Facial dysmorphism, 2113
Facial erysipelas, *304*
Facioscapulohumeral dystrophy, 2111-2112
Factitious panniculitis, 1788
FAD; *see* Flavin adenine dinucleotide
FADH₂; *see* Flavin adenine dinucleotide, reduced form of
Falciparum malaria, *448*
Fallopian tube, 1667-1671
  developmental anomalies of, 1627
  Walthard cell rests and, 1190
Fallot tetralogy, 743, *744*
Fallout, radioactive, 281, 286
False aneurysm, 778
False lumen, 781, 782, *783*
Familial cholestasis, 1261*t*, 1266-1267, 1268
Familial fibrous dysplasia of jaws, 1116
Familial hemophagocytic lymphohistiocytosis, 1424
Familial histiocytic proliferative syndromes, 1424, 1424*t*
Familial hypercholesterolemia, 50, 61
Familial hypophosphatemia, 1993
Familial Mediterranean fever, 1189, 2087
Familial recurring polyserositis, 1189
Fanconi's anemia, 206, 609, 1385
Farcy, 321
Farmer's lung, 965, 966*t*
Fasciae, diseases of, 2090-2091
Fasciculata, 1580
Fasciitis
  eosinophilic, 1780
  nodular, 1850-1852, *1851*
  proliferative, 1852
Fasciola hepatica, 452, *452*
Fasciolopsis buski, 453
Fat
  brown, 1885
  Wucher atrophy of, 1788
Fat cells, 6
Fat embolism, 132
Fat infiltration of heart, 688, *689*
Fat necrosis, *15*, 16
  of pancreas, *1351*, *1352*
  subcutaneous, in newborn, 1789
Fatal fulminant hepatitis, 1220

Fatal infectious mononucleosis, 1502
Fatal submassive hepatic necrosis, 1230
Fatal viral hepatitis, 1219-1223
Fatty acids
  adrenoleukodystrophy and, 2180
  deficiencies of, 562
  ethanol and, 19, 1239
  free plasma, 132
  myocardial ischemia and, 631
Fatty change, 12
Fatty degeneration
  of heart, 688-689, *689*
  of liver; *see* Fatty liver
Fatty liver, 17, *17*, 1203, 1241, *1242*, 1244
  alcoholic, 192, 1245; *see also* Alcoholic liver disease
  cholestasis and, 1242
  lipid metabolism in, *17*, 17-18
  precirrhotic changes in, 1244-1245
  pregnancy and, 1274
  tetracycline and, 151, *152*
Fatty streaks in atherosclerosis, *759*, 759-760
Fatty tumors, 1881
Fecalith, 1165
Felon, 302
Felton's immunologic paralysis, 498
Felty's syndrome, 1383, 2083
Female genitalia, 1620-1725
  cervix and, 1643-1652; *see also* Cervix
  embryology of, 1620-1628, *1622*, 1622*t*
  endometrium and, 1652-1663; *see also* Endometrium
  fallopian tube and, 1667-1671
  myometrium and, 1663-1667
  ovary and, 1671-1692; *see also* Ovary
  placenta and, 1692-1710; *see also* Placenta
  radiation injury to, 279-280
  vagina and, 1637-1642
  vulva and, 1628-1637; *see also* Vulva
Female karotype, normal diploid, *46*
Female prostate, 900
Female pseudohermaphroditism, 1627
Female sex differentiation, 1623-1624
Feminization, adrenal glands and, 1594-1595, 1598*t*
Femur
  avascular necrosis of, *2012*, *2013*
  chondrosarcoma and, *2040*
  osteoarthrosis and, *2073*
  osteosarcoma of, *2030*
  rheumatoid arthritis and, *2079*
Fenestrations, 804
Fernandez reaction, 337
Ferric ferrocyanide, 31
Ferritin, 31
  liver and, 1271, 1273
Ferrous sulfate
  hepatotoxins and, 1233
  toxicity of, 210-212, *211*
Ferruginous bodies, 235, 1003
fes, 587*t*
Fetal adrenal cortex, 1581
Fetal alcohol syndrome, 2141
Fetal circulation, persistent, 929
Fetal coarctation, 741, *742*
Fetal hemoglobin, 1373
Fetal irradiation, abnormalities and, 269
Fetal membranes, rupture of, 1704
Fetal rhabdomyomas, 1872
α-Fetoprotein, 604, 880-881, 2136
Fetus
  radiation injury and, 269
  radiation of, 259

Fetus—cont'd
  rubella virus and, 370-371
  toxoplasmosis and, 449
Fever, Lassa, 1231
Fever blister, 26, 1104
FGF, 590*t*, 591
fgr, 587*t*
Fiber, muscle; *see* Muscle fiber
Fibrillary astrocytosis, 2134, 2167, *2167*, 2186
Fibrillation, electrical injury and, 140
Fibrin
  clotting and, 94, 95, *95*
  in crescentic glomerulonephritis, 814
  granulation tissue and, 98
  inflammation and, 89
  oxygen toxicity and, 176, *177-179*
Fibrinoid necrosis, *513*
  cholecystitis and, 1328
  pulmonary hypertension and, 955
  rheumatic fever and, 641, 648, *648*
  systemic lupus erythematosus and, 824
Fibrinolysin, 582
Fibrinopurulent pericarditis, 666
Fibrinous exudate, 85, *85*
  pericarditis and, 665, 665-666
  tuberculous, 670, *671*
Fibro-osseous lesions of jaws, 1114
Fibroadenoma
  breast and, *1730*, 1730-1731
  prostate gland and, 903, *904*
  vulva and, 1630-1631
Fibroblast growth factor, 568
Fibroblastoma, giant cell, 1909
Fibroblasts, 93, 97
  healing by second intention and, 106
  pancreas and, 1349
  radiosensitivity of, 257*t*
  repair and, 99
  silicosis and, 36
  spindle-shaped, *1855*
  wound contraction and, 104
Fibrocongestive splenomegaly, 1415, *1416*
Fibroconnective tissue, onchocerciasis and, 472
Fibrocystic disease of breast, 1728-1729
Fibroelastosis in heart
  congenital disease and, 743
  endocardial
    mumps and, 366
    restrictive cardiomyopathy and, 695
Fibroepithelial polyp of vagina, 1640
Fibrofatty plaque, 758
Fibrogenic dusts, 233-236
Fibrohistiocytic tumors, 1850-1860
Fibrolamellar hepatocellular carcinoma, *1296*, 1298
Fibroleiomyoma, myometrium and, 1666
Fibroma, 1292
  aponeurotic, 1848-1849
  chondromyxoid, 2039-2040
  cutaneous, 1825
  desmoplastic, 2051-2052
  in oral soft tissue, 1107
  ovary and, 1685
  of tendon sheath, 1909
Fibromatoses, 1844-1850
  aponeurotic, 1848-1849
  desmoid, 1845-1847
  fibrous hamartoma of infancy and, 1847-1848
  myofibromatosis in, 1849-1850
  neck and, 1142, *1142*

Fibromatoses—cont'd
  oral soft tissue and, 1106, 1107
  palmar and plantar, 1845
  subcutaneous pseudosarcomatous, 1850
Fibromuscular dysplasia, 785, 786, 787
Fibromyxoid sarcoma, 1909
Fibronectin, 805, 1208
Fibronectin receptors, 582
Fibrosarcoma, 1842-1844, 1843
  bone and, 2022t, 2052
  grading systems of, 1844
  in jaws, 1117, 1126-1127
  odontogenic ameloblastic, 1126-1127
  of spermatic cord, 893
Fibrosis, 191, 191
  chronic inflammation and, 90
  endomyocardial, 696-697
    methysergide and, 186
  hepatic, 1207-1208
    alcoholic, 1207, 1240, 1241, 1244
    centrilobular, 1279, 1279
    cirrhosis and diffuse, 1208
    congenital, 1293
    diffuse interstitial, 174, 175
    mushroom toxicity and, 226
  medial, in blood vessels, 754
  myocarditis and, 660
  pleural, 238
  pulmonary
    asbestosis and, 235
    cadmium toxicity and, 212, 213, 213
    herbicide toxicity and, 230
    ozone and, 231
  valvular, methysergide and, 186
Fibrous ankylosis, rheumatoid arthritis and,
    2080
Fibrous bands in chronic inflammation, 90
Fibrous defect, metaphyseal, 2059-2060
Fibrous dysplasia
  bone tumors and, 2019, 2022t
  jaws and, 1114
Fibrous hamartoma of infancy, 1847-1848,
    1848
Fibrous histiocytoma
  benign, 1853
  malignant, 1853-1860, 1855
Fibrous pericarditis, radiation and, 274
Fibrous plaque
  in atherosclerosis, 760-762
  carcinoid heart lesions and, 691
Fibrous pseudotumor in tunica vaginalis,
    894
Fibrous-tissue lesions, 1842-1852
  bone tumors and, 2051-2052
  fibromatoses in, 1844-1850
  fibrosarcoma in, 1842-1844
  pseudosarcomatous fibrous lesions in,
    1850-1852
  repair and, 98
Fibrous union in fracture healing, 2001-2002
Fibrous variant of Hashimoto's thyroiditis,
    1552
Fibroxanthomas, 1853
  atypical, 1792-1793
  in lung, 1021
Fibroxanthosarcoma, 1855, 1856
Fibula, aneurysmal bone cyst and, 2058
FIGO system, 603
Filamentous bacterium, 396
Filariasis, 470, 470-474, 894
Fillers, drugs and, 953
Filtration-slit membrane, 805

Finger clubbing; see Clubbing of fingers and
    toes
Fingernails, arsenic clippings of, 209
Firearm injuries, 118, 119-128
  cutaneous entrance wounds in, 120, 120-
    123, 121, 122, 123, 124
  cutaneous exit wounds in, 123-124, 124
  disability after, 128
  guns and bullets in, 118, 119-120
    direction of fire of, 127
    number and sequence of, 127-128
  liver and, 1275, 1275
  medicolegal evidence in, 124-128
  retrieving bullets or fragments in, 126-127
  rifle wounds in, 123, 124
  shotgun wounds in, 128
First degree burns, 96
First-set rejection, 532
Fish
  irradiation of, 267
  raw, 462
Fish tapeworm, 460, 2185
Fissural cysts, 1077
Fissure, 1757
Fissured tongue, 1096
Fistula
  arteriovenous, 794
    liver injury and, 1275
    pulmonary, 795, 922
    skin, 1251
  biliary pleural, hepatic trauma and, 1275
  gastrojejunocolic, 1161
  in urinary bladder, 854
  vesicointestinal, 854, 854
  vesicovaginal, 854
Fite-Faraco stain, 345, 396t
  granulomas and, 1284
Flagellate protozoa, 438-445
  of blood and tissues, 439-445
  of digestive tract and genital organs, 438-
    439
Flagellated promastigotes, 443
Flare, 67-68, 518, 520, 523
Flash burns, 138
  radiation injury and, 260, 261
Flattened gyri, 2147
Flavin adenine dinucleotide, 1
  reduced form of, 1
Flaviviruses, 371-372
Flax, 996
Flea, plague and, 320
Flea-bitten kidney, 844
Floating spleen, 1418
Floppy baby syndrome, 150, 293, 2112,
    2120
Floppy mitral valve, 676
Floret cells, 1882, 1883
Flow cytometry, 604
  adrenal glands and, 1604
Flukes, 452-458
Fluorescent antibodies, 810, 810, 811
  mycetomas and, 396-397
Fluoride
  dental caries and, 229, 1098
  poisoning from, 194t
Fluorine toxicity, 229, 563
5-Fluorocytosine, 415
Fluorodeoxyuridine
  sclerosing cholangitis and, 1333
  toxicity of, 185
Fluoroscopy, 263
  radiation injury and, 281
5-Fluorouracil, 606, 708

Fluorspar miners, 276
Fly
  black, 472
  Chrysops, 473
  sand, 444
  tsetse, 439
Flying missile, 111
Flying squirrel typhus, 349t
fms, 587t
Foam cells, 2093
Foamy degeneration in liver, 1242, 1243
Focal autophagy, 43
Focal biliary cirrhosis, 1351
Focal embolic glomerulonephritis, 815
Focal emphysema, 1000
Focal epithelial hyperplasia in oral soft
    tissue, 1107, 1107
Focal glomerulonephritis, 815, 815
  nodular, infective endocarditis and, 658
  proliferative, 825
Focal lymphocytic thyroiditis, 1553, 1553
Focal nodular hyperplasia, 1290-1291
  oral contraceptives and, 166-167
Focal segmental glomerulosclerosis, 820-
    821, 821
Folic acid, 555, 560
  deficiency of, 1378
    alcoholic liver disease and, 1252
Folic acid antagonists, toxicity of, 183, 185
Follicle
  lymphoid, 495, 1430
  thyroid, 1544
Follicle-stimulating hormone, 872, 881,
    1522, 1676
Follicular adenoma of thyroid, 1554-1556,
    1555
Follicular carcinoma of thyroid, 602, 1559-
    1561, 1560
  clear cell type, 1562
  histologic differential diagnosis of, 1559t
  minimally invasive, 1561
  oxyphil cell type, 1562
  widely invasive, 1561
Follicular cells
  in lymph nodes, 1431
  in lymphoma, 1461-1462
Follicular cholecystitis, 1331
Follicular cysts
  oral contraceptives and, 165
  ovarian, 1674
Follicular hyperkeratosis, 553, 553
Follicular hyperplasias of lymph nodes,
    1435-1438, 1437
Follicular lymphomas, 603, 1459
Follicular mucinosis, 1787, 1787
Follicular salpingitis, 1668
Follicular urinary cystitis, 855
Folliculitis, eosinophilic pustular, 1787
Fonsecaea, 392t, 399
Fontana-Masson stain, 396t, 1903
Food allergy, 525-526
Food poisoning, 292t, 293
Force
  functional disturbances and, 112
  mechanical trauma and, 111
Fordyce's granules, 1095
Fordyce's spots, 1644
Fordyce's type of angiokeratoma, 1820
Forebrain, 2135
Foreign body
  as embolus, 953, 953-954
  penetrating wounds of heart and, 698
  reactions to, 92, 93

Foreign-body giant cells, 979
Foreign-body granulomas of fallopian tubes, 1668
Foreskin, 898
Formaldehyde, 599
    methanol and, 197
Formic acid, 197
fos, 587*t*
Foshay intradermal test, 320
Fouling, *119*, 120
4P-syndrome, 1095
Fox-Fordyce disease, 1787
Fractionization, *283*
Fracture, 114-115
    complications of, 2001-2002
    hypercortisolism and, 1975
    nonunion of humeral, *2002*
    pathologic, 115
    repair of, *2000*, 2000-2001
Fracture contusions, 2188
Fragile chromosome sites, 49
Francisella tularensis, 318
Franklin's disease, 1470
Freckle, Hutchinson, 1802
Free bilirubin, 34-35
Free energy of adenosine triphosphate hydrolysis, 2
Free radicals
    drug toxicity and, 147
    myocardial ischemia and, 631
    oxygen and, 176
    radiation-induced formation of, 253
French-American-British classification
    of acute leukemias, 1386*t*, 1388
    of myelodysplastic syndromes, 1388*t*
Friedländer's bacillus, 312
Friedreich ataxia, 694
Frozen-section of soft-tissue tumors, 1841
Fructosemia, 1261*t*, 1262, 1266
FSH; *see* Follicle-stimulating hormone
FSH dystrophy; *see* Facioscapulohumeral dystrophy
FUDR; *see* Fluorodeoxyuridine
Fugitive swellings, 473
Full-thickness burns, 96
Fulminant hepatitis, 1219-1222, *1220*
    delta, 1215
    pregnancy and, 1273
Fulminant meningococcemia, 308, *308*
Fulminant tuberculosis, 561
Fulvine toxicity, 224
Fungi, 391, 498*t*; *see also* Mycotic infections
    alimentary tract and, 1166
    arthritis and, 2076-2077
    endocarditis and, 654, 657
    epidermis and, 1768-1769
    myocarditis and, 659-660, *660*
    osteomyelitis and, 2005
    pericarditis and, 666
    phagocytosis and, 93, *93*
    placenta and, 1705
    true, 396
Fungiform papilloma of nasal septum, *1080*
Fungus ball, 408-409
Funiculitis, 892
    filarial, *470*
Furadantin; *see* Nitrofurantoin
Furosemide toxicity, 169
Furuncle, 302
Fusariosis, 394*t*, 410, 416-417, *417*, 2075
Fusiform aneurysm, 778
    ruptured, 2151

Fusiform fibrillary astrocytes, 2134, 2167, *2167*, 2186
Fusobacterium nucleatum, 938
Fusospirochetosis, 895, 1105
    synergistic, 329

G

G-cells
    pancreatic tumors and, 1368
    type II diabetes and, 1360
GABA; *see* Gamma-aminobutyric acid
Gait disorder in hydrocephalus, 2131
Galactocerebroside accumulation, 2180
Galactorrhea, 168, 1533
Galactosemia, 1266, *1266*
    neonatal and childhood cholestasis and, 1261*t*, 1262
α-Galactosidase, 55
β-Galactosidase, 52
Galactosyl ceramide–beta-galactosidase, absence of, 2180
Gallbladder and biliary ducts, 1321-1346
    absorptive rate of, 1321
    acute hydrops of, 1333
    acute inflammation of, 1327-1330
    anatomy and, 1321
    carcinoma of, 1335-1337
    cholesterosis of, 1333
    chronic inflammation of, 1330-1333
    morphology and, 1321
    physiology of, 1321-1327
    spontaneous perforation of, 1333
    trabeculated surface of, 1330, *1330*
    tumors of, 1334-1343
        benign, 1334-1335
        malignant, 1335-1343
    ulcerated mucosa in cholesterol granuloma and, 1332, *1332*
Gallbladder carcinoma, 1342
Gallstones, 1323-1327
    biliary obstruction and, 1253, 1254
    combined, 1323, 1325*t*, 1330
    gallbladder carcinoma and, 1335-1337
    mixed, 1323, *1324*, 1325*t*, 1330
        cholecystitis and, 1330, *1330*
    pure, 1323, 1325*t*
    paired, 1323, *1324*
Gambian trypanosomiasis, 439
Gametocytes, 445
Gamma-aminobutyric acid
    encephalopathy and, 1248
    Huntington's disease and, 2182
Gamma globulin, rheumatoid arthritis and, 2085
Gamma heavy-chain disease, 1470
Gamma-interferon, 81
Gamma rays, 23, 23*t*, 247, 283
Gammopathy, benign monoclonal, 1403
Gamna-Gandy bodies, 456, *1416*, 1417
Ganglion cells, radiosensitivity of, 257*t*
Ganglion cyst of bone, 2057-2059
Ganglioneuroma
    adrenal glands and, 1613
    benign, 602
    radiosensitivity of, 257*t*
Gangliosides, 52
Gangliosidosis, 1267, 1419, 1419*t*
Gangrene
    cholecystitis and, 1328
    cystitis and, 856
    gas, 292*t*, 295-296, *296*
    protracted nonfreezing hypothermia and, 137

Gangrene—cont'd
    of scrotum, 893
    stomatitis and, 1105
Gap junction, 7
Gardnerella vaginalis, 1638
Gardner's syndrome, 1334
    desmoids and, 1846
    polyposis of colon and, 1178
Gargoylism, 686, 1529
Garré's osteomyelitis, chronic sclerosing, 1113, 2004
Gartner's duct cysts, 1639
Gas
    harmful, 232-239
    inhalation of toxic, 139-140
    physical properties of, 133
    in portal vein, 1281
    trapped in body cavities, 133
Gas exchange, pulmonary edema and, 958
Gas gangrene, 292*t*, 295-296, *296*
Gastrectomy, osteoporosis and, 1981
Gastric anisakiasis, 463
Gastric atrophy, 1169, *1170*
Gastric carcinoma, 1169, 1182
Gastric epithelium-lined cysts, 1120
Gastric mucosa, radiosensitivity of, 257*t*
Gastric polyps, 1179
Gastric rugal hypertrophy, 1169, *1171*
Gastric ulcers, 1160-1161
Gastrinomas, 1368
Gastritis, 1159
    alcoholics and, 197
    allergic, 536*t*
Gastroenteritis, 1159
    eosinophilic, 1159
    mushroom toxicity and, 224
    Salmonella, 317
Gastrointestinal anthrax, 297
Gastrointestinal cytomegalovirus disease, 382
Gastrointestinal hemorrhage, 1158-1159
    herbicide toxicity and, 230
Gastrointestinal inflammation, 1168
Gastrointestinal lesions, 1166
    malignant lymphoma and, 1186
Gastrointestinal lymphoid tissue, 495
Gastrointestinal lymphoma, 1187
Gastrointestinal manifestations of systemic disease, 1172-1175
Gastrointestinal muscle tumors, 1186
Gastrointestinal radiation injury, 265, 277-278
Gastrointestinal syndrome, 271, 271*t*
Gastrointestinal tube; *see* Alimentary tract
Gastrojejunocolic fistula, 1161
Gastropathy, 1170
    hypertrophic, 1169-1171
Gaucher's disease, 53
    gastrointestinal manifestations of, 1173
    hepatosplenomegaly and, 1419, 1419*t*, *1420*, *1421*
    osteonecrosis and, 2010
    postneonatal disease and, 1267
Gay bowel syndrome, 433
Gel diffusion test, 437, 466
Gel-sol transition, 6-7
Gemistocytes, 2134
Gene mapping, 47, 50
Gene mutations, 262
Gene rearrangements, 1386*t*, 1387
Gene replacement therapy, 62
General adaptation syndrome, 131-132, 1607
Genetic analysis, 60-61

Genetic disorders, 44-62; *see also* Cell injury, genetic disorders in
Genetic factors
    atherosclerosis and, 618
    cancer and, 607-609
    dentin or enamel defects and, 1097
    drug hepatotoxicity and, 1233
    neoplastic disorders, 2175-2176
    radiation carcinogenesis and, 267
    radiation injury and, 261-263
    rheumatoid arthritis and, 2085
Genetically conditioned deficiencies, 559
Genital anomalies, embryology and, 1624-1628
Genital infections, 309, 357; *see also* specific organ
Genital ridges, 1620-1621
Genital warts, 1794
Genitalia, female; *see* Female genitalia
Genome
    cellular injury and, 12
    hepatitis B virus and DNA, 387
    virus, 362
        influenza, 365
Genotoxic carcinogens, 596, 597
Genotype, 1624-1626
Gentamicin toxicity, 150, 156-157
Genu valgum, 1986
Genu varum, 1986
Geotrichosis, 394*t*, *417*, 417-418
Germ cell tumors, 1687-1691
    central nervous system, 2174, *2174*
    histopathologic classification of, 882-888
    mediastinal, 1026
    ovarian, 1687*t*
    testicular, 879-891
    thymus gland and, 1508-1509, *1510*
Germ cells, 871
    absence of, 873-874
    female genitalia and, 1621
    intratubular malignant, 875, *875*
    of ovary, 1671
Germ tube, 397
German measles, 370
Germinal center cells, 496, *496*
    reactive lymphoid hyperplasia and, 1436, *1437*
Germinal epithelium
    ovarian, *1679*
    testicular, radiation injury and, 280
Germinal tumors of pituitary gland, 1538
Germinoma, pineal, 2174, *2174*
Gerstmann-Sträussler syndrome, 2164
Gestation
    multiple, 1698-1699
    prolonged, 1703
    radiation and, 269
Gestational choriocarcinoma, 1710
GFAP; *see* Glial fibrillary acidic protein
GGT; *see* Glutamyl transpeptidase
GH; *see* Growth hormone
GH cells; *see* Somatotroph cell
Ghon's focus, 943
Giant aneurysm, ruptured, 2151
Giant bathing trunk nevus, *1817*
Giant cell arteries, 772-774, *773*
Giant cell bone tumor, 2021*t*, 2043-2045, *2044*
Giant cell carcinoma, 602
    bronchogenic, 1010, *1011*
Giant cell fibroblastoma, 1909
Giant cell granuloma, 1108, *1115*, 1115-1116
Giant cell hepatitis, 1263

Giant cell myocarditis, 663, 694
Giant cell pneumonia of infants, 369
Giant cell soft-tissue tumor, 1906-1907, *1907*
Giant cell thyroiditis, 1550
Giant cells
    foreign body, 979
    infective endocarditis and, 657
    juvenile melanoma and, 1808
    Langhans', 979
    multinucleated, 91, *91*, 92, *92*, *93*
        radiation injury and, 250
        viruses and, 28
    radiation-induced, 25, *25*
    rheumatic fever and, 641-643, *642*
Giant condyloma of penis, 896
Giant fibroadenoma of breast, 1731
Giant keratoacanthomas, 1796
Giant mitochondria in alcoholic liver disease, 1204
Giant urticaria, 539*t*
Giardiasis, 438
Giemsa stain, 451, 948
Gilbert's disease, 33, 1275, 1276*t*, 1277
Ginger Jake paralysis, 226
Gingiva
    cyst of, 1119
    enlargement of, 1106
    fibromatosis of, 1106
    hyperplasia of, *1101*
        phenytoin and, *173*, 173-174
    lung lesions and, 938
    pregnancy tumor on, 1108
    squamous cell carcinoma of, 1111
Gingivitis, 1100
    acute necrotizing ulcerative, 1105
Gingivostomatitis, herpetic, 1103-1104
Glabrous skin, 1752
Gland/wall ratio, 987, *988*
Glanders, 292*t*, 321-322
Glands of von Ebner, 1127
Glaucoma, 1069-1072, *1071-1073*
    onchocerciasis and, 473
Gleeson staging systems, 603
Glia, myelination of, 2135
Glial cells, 27
    radiosensitivity of, 257*t*
Glial fibrillary acidic protein, 1523, 2133, 2166*t*
    tuberous sclerosis and, 2176
Glial heterotopia in lung parenchyma, 921
Gliding contusions, 2189
Glioblastoma multiforme, 2168, *2168*
Gliomas, 2166-2170, *2167*, *2168*, *2169*, *2170*
    nasal, 1077
    peritoneal, 1191
Gliosis, 2133
Glisson capsule, 1199, 1202
Globin gene transfection, 62
Globoid cell leukodystrophy, 2180, *2181*
Globular amyloidosis, 1204, 1286
Globulomaxillary cysts, 1077, 1120
Globus pallidus
    bilirubin staining of, 2146
    necrosis of, *221*, 222
Glomangioma, 795-796, *796*
Glomerular basement membrane, 804, *805*
    foot processes of, 805, *805*
Glomerular disease, 808, 810-829
    chronic injury and, 808*t*, *828*, 828-829, *829*
    congenital glomerular diseases in, 823
    diabetic nephropathy and, *822*, 823
    diffuse glomerulonephritis and, 812-815

Glomerula disease—cont'd
    focal glomerulonephritis and, 815, *815*
    focal segmental glomerulosclerosis and, 820-821, *821*
    immune injury and, 810-812
    membranoproliferative glomerulonephritis and, 816-818, *817-819*
    membranous nephropathy and, 819-820, *820*, *821*
    mesangioproliferative glomerulonephritis and, 815-816
    minimal change disease and, 818-819, *819*
    secondary, 826
    systemic disease in, 824-827
        amyloidosis and, 821-823
        toxemia of pregnancy and, 827-828, *828*
Glomerular ischemic obsolescence, 843
Glomerular vasculitides, 824
Glomerulitis, 815
Glomerulonephritis, 515-516, 517*t*
    acute, 808-809
        exudative, 813
        necrotizing, 813
        nonstreptococcal, 814
        poststreptococcal, *812*, 812-813, *813*
        proliferative, 813
    alternative-pathway, 516
    anti–glomerular basement membrane, 515-516
    diffuse, 812-815
        proliferative, 825
    focal, 815, *815*
        infective endocarditis and, 658
        proliferative, 825
        systemic bacterial infection and, 815, *815*
    hypocomplementemic, 516, 817
    idiopathic membranous, 819
    immunologic reaction to drugs and, 148
    membranoproliferative, 457, 517*t*, 816-818, *817-819*
    membranous, *514*, 516
        heavy metals and, 203
        lupus, 825
        mesangial, 825
        ibuprofen toxicity and, 162
    mesangiocapillary, 817
    mesangioproliferative, 815-816
    postinfectious, 517*t*
    rapidly progressive, 810, *813*, *814*, 814-815
Glomerulopathy, schistosomal, 457
Glomerulosa, 1580
Glomerulosclerosis, 823
    focal segmental, 820-821, *821*
Glomus, 1756
Glomus tumor, 795-796, *796*, 1088
    skin and, 1823
Glossina, 439
Glossitis, syphilitic, 1105
Glossoptosis, 1095
Glottis, laryngeal carcinoma in, 1086
Glucagonomas, 1368
Glucocerebroside in Gaucher's disease, 1419
Glucocorticoids, 163, 1581
    excess of, 873
Gluconeogenesis, activation of, 10
Glucose
    adenosine triphosphate from oxidation of, 2
    diabetes and, 1360
Glucose-6-phosphatase, defects in, 57

Glucose-6-phosphate dehydrogenase, 765
  leukemia and, 1384
Glucose-6-phosphate dehydrogenase
    deficiency, 149, 446, 1381
α-Glucosidase, 57
Glucuronyl transferase, 34
  Gilbert's disease and, 1277
Glutamine, encephalopathy and, 1248
Glutamyl transpeptidase, 1262
Gluten-sensitive enteropathy, 1171
Glutethimide poisoning, 193t
Glycine, decomposition of, 23-24
Glycogen, 28-30
  infiltration of, in heart, 686-687
  pathways of, 56
  quantitative analysis of, 30
  storage of, 6
Glycogen nuclei, 1204
Glycogen-rich cystadenoma, 1354
Glycogen storage diseases, 30, 53, 55-57,
    2114-2115
  heart and, 687, 687
  hepatocellular adenoma and, 1289
  therapy of, 62
  type I, 37
Glycogenosis, 55, 1267
  of B-cells, 1362, 1363
Glycol toxicity, 198-200
Glycolipids, 3
Glycolysis, 2, 10
Glycoprotein
  healing and, 102
  Tamm-Horsfall, 808
  thyroglobulin, 1544
Glycosaminoglycans, 52-55, 764
Glycoside toxicity, 175-176
Glycosylation, 3
  diabetes and, 1365
Goblet cells, 96
Goiter, 1546-1549
  amyloid, 1554
  diffuse toxic, 1549-1550, 1550
Goitrogens, 1547
Goitrous autoimmune thyroiditis, 1551
Gold, 36, 150
Golden pneumonia, 215
Golgi apparatus, 3, 4, 1201
Golgi complex, 1360
  enlargement of, 1525
Golgi zone, 1347
Gomori methenamine-silver stain, 334, 396t,
    407, 948, 1084
Gonad, 871
  streak, 1626
Gonadal agenesis, 1625t, 1626
Gonadal blastemas, 1623
Gonadal dysgenesis, 880, 1625t, 1626, 1626
Gonadal hormones, 1525
Gonadal-splenic fusion, 892
Gonadal stromal tumors, 888-890, 890
Gonadoblastoma
  of ovary, 1690, 1690-1691
  of testis, 890
Gonadotrophs, 1522
  adenoma and, 1534-1535
Gonadotropin, 1546
  genetic defects and, 872
Gonococci, 309, 309-310
  oral soft tissue and, 309, 1105
  pharyngitis and, 309
  urethritis and, 898, 1774
  vulvovaginitis and, 310
Gonorrhea; see Gonococci

Goodpasture's syndrome, 516, 517t, 810,
    814
  nonpulmonary, 815
  pulmonary involvement in, 976-977
Gorham's disease, 2051
Gorlin cyst, 1119, 1119
Gout, 37-38, 38, 2087-2090, 2088
  arthritis and, 2089
  nephropathy in, 839
  with sodium monourate crystals in
    dermis, 1782
Gracile nuclei, bilirubin staining of, 2146
Grading of neoplasia, 602, 602-603, 610
  fibrosarcoma and, 1844
  soft-tissue sarcomas and, 1842
Graft facilitation, 534
Graft rejection, 531-534, 533
  corticosteroids and, 162
Graft-versus-host disease, 534, 968, 1502
  skin and, 1828, 1829
Gram-negative organisms
  meningitis and, 2154
  pericarditis and, 666
  pneumonia and, 936
Gram's stain, 938, 948
Granular cell tumor
  of biliary tract, 1334
  of breast, 1734
  of larynx, 1087
  of oral soft tissue, 1108
  of pituitary gland, 1537
  of vulva, 1630
Granular ependymitis, 2157
Granulation tissue, 98-102, 100-102, 104
  myocardial infarction and, 635, 637
Granule, 397
  mycetomas and, 396
Granulocyte macrophage–colony-stimulating
    factor, 590t, 1386t
Granulocytes, 80
Granulocytic sarcoma of ovary, 1691
Granuloma, 90-91
  arteritis and, 772-774, 773
  colitis and, 1163, 1163
  common duct and, 1334
  dental, 1099, 1099
  dermal, 1784-1785
  giant cell, 1108, 1115, 1115-1116
  liver and, 1283-1285, 1284
    antihypertensives in, 168
  mastocytosis and, 1980
  methotrexate and, 185
  in oral soft tissue, 1104, 1108
  of paranasal sinuses, 1078-1079
  pituitary gland and, 1527-1528
  pulmonary involvement in noninfectious,
    975-981
  reticulohistiocytic, 1792
  rheumatoid, 649-650
  spermatic, 878-879
  tuberculosis and, 942, 943, 943, 1284
Granuloma annulare, 1777-1778, 1778
Granuloma inguinale, 324, 895
  in oral soft tissue, 1105
Granuloma pyogenicum, 1819
Granulomatosis, 772
  allergic, 505, 536-538, 537
    pulmonary involvement in, 976
  bronchocentric, 965
  necrotizing sarcoid, 981
  skin and lymphomatoid, 1827
  Wegener's, 769-772, 771, 826
    pulmonary involvement in, 975-976,
    976

Granulomatosis infantiseptica, 313
Granulomatous disease, 91-92
  of blood vessels, 772-774, 773
    in Wegener's granulomatosis, 976
  chronic, 1258
  of eyes, 1057
  of fallopian tubes, 1668
  hypocortisolism and, 1587-1588
  immune reactions and, 504t, 539t
  of lymph nodes, 1434, 1435t
  of mediastinum, 1024
  of myocardium, 660, 662, 663
  of oral soft tissues, 1105-1106
  of pericardium, 666
  of prostate, 901
  rheumatic fever and, 641
  schistosomiasis and, 458
  of spleen, 1418, 1419
  of testes, 877
  of thyroid, 1550-1551
Granulomatous hypersensitivity, 505, 536-
    538, 537
Granulomatous orchitis, 877
Granulosa cells, 1672
Granulosa-theca cell tumors, 1684-1685,
    1685
  radiosensitivity of, 257t
Graves' disease, 1047, 1549-1550, 1550
  hyperthyroidism and, 1546
  myxedema and exophthalmic, 1781
Grawitz tumor, 579
Gray hepatization, 933, 934
Gray matter necrosis
  mercury poisoning and, 203, 204
  perinatal brain injury and, 2145
Gray tubercles, 670
Gray unit, 249
Green herring, 462
Grey-Turner spots, 1351
Gridley fungus stain, 396t
Ground glass cells, 1204, 1225, 1225
Ground substance, 2065
  of media of arteries, 754
  repair and, 98
Grover's disease, 1765
Growth
  failure of, 549
  neoplastic cells and, 579-580
  radiation injury and, 268
  signals important in, 7
Growth factors, 9, 568, 588, 589-591, 590t;
    see also Growth hormone
Growth hormone, 1520, 1521, 1521, 1521t;
    see also Growth factors
  acromegaly and, 1972
Growth plate disorders, 1947t
  rickets and, 1986
Guarnieri bodies, 386, 1767
Guillain-Barré syndrome, 2132
Guinea worm infection, 473-474
Gummas, 92
  myocardium and, 650
Guns; see Firearm injuries
Gy unit; see Gray unit
Gynandroblastoma, 1686
Gynecomastia, 880, 885, 889, 1734
  phenothiazines and, 168
Gyri
  flattening of, 2129, 2130, 2147
  in normal newborn brain, 2135

H

H-ras, 587t, 589, 600
H2 receptor antagonist toxicity, 169

H-Y antigen, 1623
Hadziyannis cells, 1204, 1225, *1225*
Haemaphysalis leporis palustris, 319
Haemophilus aegyptius, 310
Haemophilus ducreyi, 310, 895
Haemophilus influenzae, 306, 310-311
    epiglottitis and, 1084
    immune deficiency diseases and, 499
    meningitis and, 2154
    otitis media and, 1087
    pulmonary infection and, 932, 936, 937, 988
    in superinfection in viral influenza, 365
    wound infection and, 130
Haemophilus vaginalis, 310
Hageman factor, 37, 2090
Hailey-Hailey disease, 1762
Hair, 1756
    arsenic clippings of, 209
    diseases of, 1787
Hair follicles
    radiation injury and, 257t, 274
    tumors of, 1834-1835
Hairy cell leukemia, 375, 1397-1398, *1398*
    liver and, *1428*, 1429
Hairy leukoplakia, 1104
Hairy tongue, 1103
Half-life of isotopes, 249
Halo nevi, 1812
Halogenated hydrocarbon toxicity, 222
Halogenated pyrimidines, 254
Halothane toxicity, 171, 1205, 1234t, 1236
Hamartoma, 571, *573*, 610, 1880
    fibrous, in infant, 1847-1848
    in lung, 1021
    mesenchymal, 1293
    mixed, 1291
    myxoid, 1878, 1909
    splenic, 1426
    ventricular, 2175
Hamman-Rich syndrome, 969
Hand, epidermoid carcinoma of, 274
Hand-foot-and-mouth disease, 1104
Hand-Schüller-Christian disease, 1422, 1529
Handgun wounds, 119-120, 123, *125*
Haptens, 487-488, 512t
Harelip, 1095
Harrison's groove, 1984
Hartmann pouch, 1321
Hashimoto's thyroiditis, 1549, 1551-1553, *1551-1553*
Hassall's corpuscles, 1025, 1144, *1495*, 1496, 1502, *1503*
Hay fever, 525, 526
Head
    injuries to
        penetrating, 2189
        traffic, 116, *117*
        irradiation and, 281
Healing, 94-108
    chemical estimations of constituents of, 102
    inflammation and, 67; *see also* Inflammation
    metaplasia and, 106-108
    regeneration in, 94-98
    repair in, 98-106
        contraction of wounds and, 104
        granulation tissue and, 98-102
        healing by first intention and, 104-106
        healing by second intention and, 106
        organization and, 102-104
Hearing loss from noise exposure, 136

Heart, 615-729
    cardiac failure in, 615-616
    cardiomyopathies and myocardial disorders in, 681-700; *see also* Cardiomyopathies and myocardial disorders
    Chagas' disease and, 441, 442
    conducting system disturbances of, 705-706
    congenital disease of, 730-751; *see also* Congenital heart disease
    coronary artery disease and, 616-639; *see also* Coronary artery disease
    endomyocardial biopsy of, 706-708
    growth disturbances of, 677-681
    infective endocarditis and, 655
    inflammatory diseases of, 639-672; *see also* Inflammatory heart diseases
    ischemic injury to, 20-21, *21*
    radiation-induced disease of, 274
    tumors of, 700-705
    valvular and hypertensive heart diseases in, 672-681; *see also* Valvular and hypertensive heart diseases
Heart block, 706
Heart failure, 615-616
    amyloidosis and, 696
    aortic insufficiency and, 675
    Chagas' disease and, 442
    congestive, 616
        diphtheria and, 295
        palpable splenomegaly and, 1415
    edema in, 616
    forward, 616
    high-output, 616
    left-sided, 615, 959-960
    potassium deficiency and, 693
    Rh incompatibility and, 692
    rheumatic fever and, 649
    right-sided, 615
    schistosomiasis and, 457
    sickle cell anemia and, 692
Heart failure cells, 32
Heart-lung transplantation, alveolar wall fibrosis and, 968
Heart septum, asymmetric hypertrophy of, 682-683
Heart valves; *see* Cardiac valves
Heartworm, 473
Heat
    inflammation and, 84
    injuries from, 136-140
Heath-Edwards grading scheme in pulmonary hypertension, 954-955
Heatstroke, 140
Heavy-chain diseases, 1470
Heavy metals, 214-216
    myocardial changes and, 694
    pigmentation and, 36
    transmembranous glomerulonephritis and, 203
Heavy-particle irradiation, 284
Heberden's nodes, 2074
Heerfordt's syndrome, 1130-1131, *1131*
Heidenhain, sulci of, 1752
Heinz bodies, 1382
Heister, valves of, 1321
Helicase, 9
Heliotropium, 1283
Helminthic diseases, 452-474
    cestodes in, 458-462
    nematodes in, 462-474
        digestive tract, 462-469

Helminthic diseases—cont'd
    nematodes in—cont'd
        filarial, 470-474
    trematodes in, 452-458
Helminthosporium, 964
Hemagglutinin, influenza and, 365
Hemangioblastoma, central nervous system, *2173*, 2173-2174
Hemangioendothelioma, 796, 797, *797*, 1820-1821
    benign, 797
    bone and, 2051
    epithelioid, *1296*, 1299
    infantile, 1292
    radiation injury and, 279
    vegetant intravascular, 1820
Hemangioma, *794*, 794-795
    bone, 1116, 2021t
    capillary, 794, *794*
    cavernous, 794-795, 1292, *1292*
    of choroid, 1051, *1052*
    cutaneous, 1819-1821
    epithelioid, 795
    intramuscular, 1884, 1886-1888, *1887*
    of larynx, 1087
    in oral soft tissue, 1108
    sclerosing, in lung, 1021
    of spleen, 1427, *1427*
Hemangiopericytoma, 796-797, 1888-1890, *1889*
Hemangiosarcoma, 797
Hematemesis, 1159, 1186
Hematin, 33
Hematocele, 894
Hematogenous pneumonia, 935
Hematoma
    cerebral, 2150, 2151
    epidural, *2187*, 2187-2188
    fracture repair and, 2001
    intraplacental, 1702
    of scrotum, 893
    subcapsular, in newborn, 1275
    subdural, *2187*, 2188
        alcoholics and, 192
    subretinal, 1074, *1074*
Hematomyelia, 2189
Hematopoietic syndrome, 271t, 273
Hematopoietic system; *see also* Bone marrow and blood; Lymph nodes; Spleen
    maturation phases in, *500*
    neoplasms and, 1428-1429
    radiation injury and, 257t, 264-265
Hematoxylin and eosin stain, 396t, 2126t
Hematoxylin bodies of Gross, 652
Hematoxylin–basic fuchsin–picric acid staining, 634
Hematuria, 516, 808, 823
    prostate gland and, 906
Hemobilia, 1258, 1275
Hemochromatosis, 212, 686, *686*, 1786
    arthropathy with, 2068-2069
    hepatocellular carcinoma and, 1295
    idiopathic, 1271-1273
    neonatal, 1273
    oral mucosa pigmentation and, 1106
    osteoporosis and, 1972-1974
    primary, 32-33
    secondary, 32, 1273
Hemodialysis; *see* Dialysis
Hemoglobin
    fetal, 1373
    glycosylation of, 1365

Hemoglobin—cont'd
  osteoporosis and, 1972
Hemoglobin Barts, 1381
Hemoglobin H disease, 1381, 1409, *1410*
Hemoglobinopathy, 1380; *see also* specific
      disease
Hemoglobinuria, 1380, 1382
Hemoglobinuric fever, 447-448
Hemolysins, 291
Hemolysis
  bacteria and, 303; *see also* Hemolytic
      streptococci
  burns and, 139
  immune, 510*t*
  pharmacogenetics and, 149
Hemolytic anemia, 1379-1382, *1380*; *see also*
      Hemolytic disease
  autoallergic, *511*
  cardiac tumors and, 704
  spur cell, 1252
Hemolytic disease
  antibody-induced, 511, *511*
  of newborn, 1261-1262
Hemolytic drug reactions, *511*, 511-512,
      512*t*
Hemolytic jaundice, 33
Hemolytic streptococci
  acute diffuse glomerulonephritis and, 812
  diffuse inflammatory lesions and, 87
  meningitis and, 2154
Hemolytic uremic syndrome, 826, 827
Hemopericardium, *664*, 664-665, 698
Hemophagocytic syndrome, 1424, 1425,
      1425
Hemophilia, 59
  arthropathy with, 2069
Hemoproteins, pigments from, 31
Hemoptysis, 453, 977
Hemorrhage
  adrenal, 1585, 1606-1607
  atherosclerotic plaques and, 762, *763*
  central nervous system, 2150-2153, *2152*,
      2188
    boric acid toxicity and, 224
    brain herniation and, *2129*, 2130
    carbon monoxide poisoning and, 222
    herpes simplex encephalitis and, 2160,
      2160
    perinatal brain injury and, 2141-2143,
      2142
  gallbladder and, 1328
  gastrointestinal, 1158-1159
  healing by first intention and, 104
  hepatic disease and, 1252
  inflammation and, 69-70
  mechanical injury and, 128-129, 131
  methotrexate and, 183
  pancreatitis and, 1351-1353
  pituitary gland and, 1527
  placenta and, 1705-1706
  pulmonary, 985
    neonatal, 928-929
    systemic lupus erythematosus and, *973*
  retinal, leukemia and, 1069
  in tunica vaginalis, 894
  vitamin K deficiency and, 555
Hemorrhagic bone cyst in jaw, 1120
Hemorrhagic diathesis, hemopericardium
      and, 665
Hemorrhagic fever, Bolivian, 1205
Hemorrhagic inflammation, 85
Hemorrhagic leukoencephalitis, 2178, *2178*
Hemorrhagic pericarditis, 666

Hemorrhagic telangiectasia; *see*
      Telangiectasia
Hemorrhoids, 788, 1158
Hemosiderin, 32
  liver and, 1271, 1272, 1273
  macrophages and, 985
  malignant fibrous histiocytoma and, 1857
Hemosiderosis, 32, *32*, 212, 1271, 1272,
      1273
Hemp dust, 996
Henle's loop, 806, 846, 1575
Henoch-Schönlein purpura, 516, 769, 816,
      1789, 1790
Hepadnaviruses, 1211
Hepar lobatum, 1202
Hepar lobatum syphiliticum, *1285*, 1285-
      1286
Heparan sulfate, 39, 52
Heparin, 104
Hepatic amebiasis, 434
Hepatic artery diseases, 1280
Hepatic carcinoma; *see* Hepatocellular
      carcinoma
Hepatic distomiasis, 452
Hepatic encephalopathy, 2184
Hepatic fibrosis
  congenital, 1268, 1293
  mushroom toxicity and, 226
  schistosomiasis and, 456, *456*
Hepatic necrosis
  bridging, 1205
  carbon tetrachloride and, 222, *223*
  ferrous sulfate toxicity and, 210
  massive or submassive, 1205
    immunosuppressant therapy and, 1230
Hepatic osteodystrophy, 1974-1975
Hepatic portoenterostomy, 1262
Hepatic sinusoid lining cells, 1199
Hepatic tumors, 1288*t*, 1288-1289
Hepatic veins, 1282-1283
  thrombosis of, 790-791, 1282
  oral contraceptives and, 165, *166*
Hepatic venule, terminal, 1199
Hepaticola hepatica, 466
Hepatis peliosis, 1292
Hepatitis
  alcoholic, 192, 195, 1243
  amiodarone and, 176
  chronic, 1223-1231
    chronic active hepatitis and delta
      hepatitis in, 1228
    chronic active hepatitis B and B viral
      cirrhosis in, 1225-1228
    definition of, 1223
    hepatitis non-A, non-B, 1228-1231
    lobular, 1228
    persistent viral hepatitis type B, 1224-
      1225
  chronic active, 1223
    autoimmune, 1230
    cryptogenic, 1230-1231
    delta hepatitis and, 1227
    drug hepatotoxicity and, 1235*t*, 1237
    non-A, non-B, 1230
    portal fibrosis in, 1207
  chronic persistent, 1223
    survival in, 1227
  giant cell, 1263
  granulomatous
    antihypertensives and, 168
    chronic, 1283-1285
  halothane and, 171
  isoniazid and, 170, *170*

Hepatitis—cont'd
  Lábrea, 1223
  methoxyflurane and, 171
  neonatal, 1263, *1263*, 1264
  pregnancy and fulminant, 1273
  quinidine and, 176
  radiation, 278
  rifampin and, 171
  Santa Marta, 1223
  viral; *see* Viral hepatitis
Hepatitis A, 377, 1210-1211
  neonatal and childhood cholestasis and,
      1261*t*
Hepatitis-associated antigen, 2087
Hepatitis B, 1211-1215; *see also* Hepatitis B
      virus
  chronic active, 1225-1228, *1226*
  cirrhosis and, 1225-1228
  hepatocellular carcinoma and, 1294-1295
  neonatal and childhood cholestasis and,
      1261*t*
  persistent, 1224-1225
Hepatitis B core antigen, 1213
Hepatitis B surface antigen
  hepatocellular carcinoma and, 1294
  screening blood donors for, 1215
  vaccine from plasma-derived, 1215
Hepatitis B virus, 27, 387, 601, 1210; *see*
      also Hepatitis B
  carriers of, 1223
  clinical and immunologic aspects of, 1212
  deoxyribonucleic acid replication and,
      1212
  nucleotide base sequence of genome of,
      1211-1212
  structure of, 1211, *1212*
  transmission of, 1224
  vaccine for, 1215
Hepatitis delta antigen, 1215
Hepatitis non-A, non-B, 1216-1217
Hepatoadrenal necrosis, 379, 1585
Hepatobiliary ascariasis, 1254
Hepatoblastoma, 579
Hepatocanalicular injury, 1235
Hepatocellular adenoma, 1289-1290, *1291*
Hepatocellular carcinoma, 601, 1249, 1293-
      1298
  B viral cirrhosis and, 1227
  radiation injury and, 279
Hepatocellular jaundice, 34
Hepatocellular lysosomes, 1204
Hepatocellular necrosis, 1204-1205
  ethanol and, 192
  halothane and, 1236, *1237*
Hepatocellular tumors, benign, 1289-1291
  hepatoma and, 575
Hepatocyte, 1200-1201
  atrophy of, 1203
  ballooned, 1226, *1226*
  carbon tetrachloride and, 18, *18*
  Wilson disease and, 1270, *1270*
Hepatocytolysis, 1204-1205
Hepatography, Budd-Chiari syndrome and
      percutaneous, 1282
Hepatolenticular degeneration, 1269-1271,
      1786
Hepatomegaly, 1269
  asymptomatic alcoholism and, 1241
  leukemia and, 1388
Hepatopoietin, 9
Hepatosplenic schistosomiasis, 455-457
Hepatotoxicity, 1232
  acetaminophen, 160, *161*

Hepatotoxicity—cont'd
  amiodarone, 1238
  chlorpromazine and, 168
  genetic factors and, 1233
  phosphorus and, 224
  pregnancy and tetracycline, 1274
Herbicides, 230, *231*
Hereditary; *see* Genetic factors
Hereditary hemorrhagic telangiectasia, 795, 1109
Hereditary hyperbilirubinemias, 1275-1278, *1276t*
Hereditary spherocytosis, 1380
Hering duct, 1200
Hermaphroditism, 872, 1624, *1625t*
  true, 1626
Hernia
  alimentary tract, 1156
  Bochdalek, 921, *922*
  brain, 2128-2130
  diaphragmatic, 921-922
Herniation contusions, 2188-2189
Heroin toxicity, 219
Herpangina, 1767
Herpes, recurrent, 1104
Herpes gestationis, 539t, 1766
Herpes labialis, 26
Herpes neonatorum, *380*
Herpes progenitalis, 895
Herpes simplex, 379, 1103, 1167, *1768*
  cholestasis and, 1261t
  encephalitis and, 379, *381*, 2158, 2159-2160, *2160*
  hepatic necrosis and, 1231
  neonate and, 379, 1260, 1261t, 1265
  of vagina, *1638*
  of vulva, *1628*, 1628-1629
Herpes zoster, 382
Herpes zoster ophthalmicus, 1054
Herpesviruses, 28, 378-384
  encephalitis and, 2158, 2159-2150, *2160*
  gingivostomatitis and, 1103-1104
Herringbone pattern of fibrosarcoma, 1843, *1843*
Heterotopia, 108
  alimentary tract and, 1153
  of brain tissue, 921, 1077
  cervical, 1644
  in lung parenchyma, 921
  ovarian tissue, 1677
HETEs; *see* Hydroxyeicosatetraenoic acids
Heubner's arteritis, 768
Hexachlorophene toxicity, 224
Hexosamine, 102
HGPRT deficiency, 60
HHF-35, 1867
Hibernoma, 1885-1886, *1886*
Hidradenoma papilliferum, 1832
  in vulva, 1630, *1631*
Hidrocystoma, *1831*
High-altitude cerebral edema, 133
High-altitude pulmonary edema, 133
High-density lipoproteins, 619, 764
High-output heart failure, 616
Hilar cholangiocarcinoma, 1293, 1298
Hilum cells of ovary, 1673
Hilum of lymph node, 495
Hindbrain, 2135
Hip articular cartilage, *2070*
Hip dysplasia, 2067
Hippel-Lindau disease, 1051
Hippel's disease, 1820
Hirano bodies, 2133, 2182

Hiroshima, *260, 262*
Hirsch-Peiffer acidified cresyl violet stain, 2180, *2180*
Hirschsprung's disease, 1154
His bundle, 705
Histamine, 519t, 962
  release of, 499, 519
  triple response and, 70
  vascular permeability and, 71-72, *72*
Histidine, 546, 562
Histiocyte, 492t
  atherosclerosis and, 765
  sea-blue, 1420
Histiocytic hyperplasia of spleen, 1418
Histiocytic necrotizing lymphadenitis, 1434
Histiocytoma
  of bone, 2054-2055, *2055*
  malignant, 1856
    fibrous, 1853, 1853-1860, 1856, *1858*
Histiocytosis, *1422*, 1422-1426, *1423, 1424, 1426*
  in jaws, 1114, *1114*
  pulmonary, 977-978
  skin and, 1754
Histocompatibility complex, 1496
Histogenesis, 7
Histoplasmosis, 394t, 410, 418-420, *419, 420*, 1084, *1406*
  endocarditis and, 654
  hepatic granulomas and, 1285
  intestinal, 1166
  in oral soft tissue, 1105
History of neuropathology, 2123
HIV; *see* Human immunodeficiency virus
HLA (human lymphocyte antigens)
  ankylosing spondylitis and, 2098
  disease associations with, 536t
  Goodpasture's syndrome and, 977
  Hashimoto's thyroiditis and, 1551
  pharmacogenetics and, 150
HMB45, 604
HMG CoA; *see* 3-Hydroxy-3-methylglutamyl coenzyme A
Hobnail cirrhosis, 1238
Hodgkin's disease, 579
  actuarial survival and, *1451*
  bone tumors and, 2047
  Lukes-Butler-Hicks classification of, 1446
  lymph nodes and, *1444-1449*, 1444-1452
  lymphocytic depletion type, 1449, *1449*
  lymphocytic predominance type, 1447, *1448*
  mediastinal, 1025
  nodular sclerosis type, *1447*
  phenytoin and, 173
  radiation-induced heart disease and, 699
  Rye classification of, 1446
  skin and, 1827
  staging classification for, 1450
  therapeutic radiation for, 274
  thymus and, 1509, *1511*
    cysts of, 1502
Holandric inheritance patterns, 58
Holiday heart syndrome, 194
Holocrania, 2136
Holocrine glands, 1756
Holoprosencephalies, 2138
Holzer stain, 2126t
Homeostasis
  bone and mineral, 1944
  cell, 10-44; *see also* Cell injury, cell control mechanisms and homeostasis in
  intracellular ion, 21-22

Homer Wright rosettes, 1611-1612
  medulloblastoma and, *2170*, 2170-2171
Homicidal poisoning, 193-194t
Homocystinurea, 559, 1053
Homocytotropic antibody, 519
Homogentisic acid, 51
Homograft rejection, 531
Homosexuals, 1214, 1219, 1223
Homovanillic acid, 1612
Homozygosity, 58
  hemochromatosis and, 1271
  Wilson's disease and, 1270
Honeycombing in lung, 965, *969*
Hookworm disease, 463-464
Hormone receptors, 508-509
Hormones, 7; *see also* specific hormone
  calcium-regulating, 1944, *1945*
  cells of adenohypophysis and, 1521t
  chemotaxis and, 8
  endometrium and, 1654-1656
  reproduction and, 9, 1525
Horror autotoxicus, 497
Horse serum, 515, 708
Hortega silver carbonate stain, 2126t
Host immune response, 27
Host of organism, 289, 290
Hot spots, 280
Housemaid's knee, 2090
Howell-Jolly bodies, 1412
Howship's lacunae, 1934, *1935*, 1943
5 HT; *see* 5-Hydroxytryptamine
HTLV; *see* Human T-cell leukemia virus
Human chorionic gonadotropin, 880-881
  ovary and, 1688
  placenta and, 1696
Human immunodeficiency virus, 375-376, 1104, 1471-1472
  central nervous system infection and, 2162
  classification of, 1472t
Human papillomavirus, 601
  Bowenoid papulosis of penis and, 1798
  cervix and, 1647
  vulva and, 1632, *1632*
Human placental lactogen, 881, 1696, 1709
Human T-cell leukemia virus, 375-376, 602, 1385, 1460
Humberstone stain, 396t
Humerus, 2022, *2022*
  chondroblastoma of, *2058*
  chondrosarcoma of, *2040*
  nonunion of fracture of, *2002*
Humoral antibody, 499
Hunter's disease, 53, 55, 59
Huntington's disease, 2182, *2182*
Hurler-Hunter syndrome, 1267
Hurler-Scheie disease, 52-55, *53*
Hurler's disease, 52, *53*, 686, 1267, 1529
  gastrointestinal manifestations of, 1173
Hürthle cells, 1552
  adenoma and, 1555, *1556*
  carcinoma and, 1562
Hutchinson's freckle, 1802, 1811-1812
Hutchinson's syndrome, 1612
Hutchinson's teeth, 327, 1105
Hx cells, 977-978
Hyaline arteriolosclerosis, 755, *756*, 823, 842
Hyaline bodies, alcoholic, 192, 195, 1203, 1203t, *1243*
Hyaline degeneration of splenic arteries, 1413-1414
Hyaline granules, mycetomas and, 396

Hyaline membrane in alveolar duct, *961*
Hyaline membrane disease, 925-926, *926*
  oxygen toxicity and, 176-180
Hyaline necrosis
  acute liver disease and, 1243
  Wilson disease and, 1270, *1270*
Hyaline nodule in silicosis, 998
Hyaline thrombi, 624, *624*
Hyalinization of islets of Langerhans, 1363
Hyalinizing trabecular adenoma of thyroid
      gland, 1556
Hyalinosis cutis et mucosae, 1103, 1780-
      1781
Hyaluronidase-sensitive acid
      mucopolysaccharide myxoid material,
      1897
Hyaluronidases, 87, 291, *291*, 302
Hybrid cells, 60
Hybridoma cells, 494-495
Hydatid of Morgagni, 892
Hydatid disease, 460-462
Hydatid diseases, myocarditis and, 662
Hydatidiform mole, *1706*, 1706-1709, *1707*,
      1708
Hydralazine
  adverse reactions to, 168
  granulomas and, 1285
  lupus erythematosus and, 149
Hydranencephaly, 2139
Hydrocarbons, toxicity of, 226, *227*, *228*
Hydrocele, 471, 894, *894*
Hydrocephalus, 2130-2131, *2131*
  congenital, 2139-2140
  edema of, 2127, 2128
  neural tube defects and, 2136, 2137
Hydrogen peroxide, 84
Hydrolysis of adenosine triphosphate, 2
Hydrolytic enzymes, 12
Hydromyelia, 2137, 2140
Hydronephrosis, 836, 906
  with renal stones, 840, *840*
Hydropericardium, 664
Hydropic change, 12
  hepatocyte and, 1202-1203
Hydrops, gallbladder and, 1333
Hydrops fetalis, erythroblastosis fetalis and,
      511, 1262, 1706
Hydrostatic effect, 112
Hydroureter, 836, 906
3-Hydroxy-3-methylglutamyl coenzyme A,
      51
Hydroxyapatite accumulation, 36, *36*
β-Hydroxybutyrate accumulation, 37
Hydroxychloroquine poisoning, 194*t*
Hydroxycholesterol, *1582*
Hydroxycorticosterone, *1582*
Hydroxyeicosatetraenoic acids, 635
5-Hydroxyindoleacetic acid, 690-691
Hydroxyl radicals, 631
Hydroxylation
  anticonvulsants and, 1993
  bone and, 1944
  hepatic disease and, 1993
Hydroxylysine, 561
Hydroxypregnenolone, *1582*
Hydroxyprogesterone, *1582*
Hydroxyproline, 102, 560, 1572
2-Hydroxystilbamidine, 410
5-Hydroxytryptamine, 1184, 1563
  carcinoid tumors and, 690
  vascular permeability and, 72-73
25-Hydroxyvitamin D, 807

Hygroma, 799, *799*, 1819
  in mediastinum, 1024
  in neck, 799, 1144
Hyper-alpha-2-globulinemia, 1797
Hyperacidity, 1161
Hyperadrenocorticism, 1525
Hyperaldosteronism, 1593-1594, 1598*t*
  child and, 1586
  substrata of, 1593*t*
Hyperbilirubinemia
  direct-acting, 1262-1265
  exchange transfusions and, 1261
  hereditary, 1275-1278, 1276*t*
  indirect-acting, 1260, 1261-1262
  physiologic neonatal, 1260-1262
Hypercalcemia, 839-840
  cornea and, 1074
  milk-alkali syndrome and, 189, *189*
Hypercalciuria, 839
Hypercholesterolemia, 619, 1074
  familial, 50, 61
Hyperchromatic nuclei, 570
Hypercortisolism, 1591-1592, 1598*t*
  osteoporosis and, 1975
Hyperdiploidy, 1387
Hyperelastosis cutis, *1783*
Hyperemia, hepatic passive, 1279-1280
Hypereosinophilia, 697
Hypergammaglobulinemia, 443
Hyperglobulinemia
  sarcoidosis and, 980
  silicosis and, 998
  Sjögren's syndrome and, 974
  of Waldenström, 1789
Hyperglycemia, 1362
Hyperimmune gamma globulin, 1211
Hyperinfection, 468
Hyperkalemia, 693, 807, 831
Hyperkeratosis, 1757
  cervical, 1643
  disseminated spiked, 1795
  follicular, 553, *553*
  oral mucosa and, 1109
  vulvar, 1629, *1629*
Hyperlipidemia, atherosclerosis and, 766
Hyperlipoproteinemia
  atherosclerotic, 758
  spleen and, *1422*
Hypermature placenta, 1703
Hypernephroma, 847, 1565
Hyperosteoidosis, *1992*
Hyperostosis, infantile cortical, 1113
Hyperoxia, pulmonary edema and, 962
Hyperparathyroidism, 1572-1577
  osteitis fibrosa and, *1975*
  osteoporosis and, 1975-1977, *1976*, *1977*
  renal osteodystrophy and, 1577
  skeletal disease and, *1974*
  tertiary, 1574
Hyperpigmentation, radiation and, 273
Hyperplasia, 567, 567-568, 610
  adenomatous, 1291, *1291*
    alcoholic cirrhosis and, 1246-1247
  adrenal
    congenital, 1584
    cortical, 1589-1590, 1591, *1591*
    diffuse, 1590, *1591*
    medullary, 1608
    microadenomatous, 1592
    multinodular, 1591-1592
  angiolymphoid, with eosinophilia, 1790
  bone marrow and, 1375
  cells and, 43-44

Hyperplasia—cont'd
  cervical microglandular, 1643-1644
  compensatory, 568
  endometrial, 1657-1659
  epidermal, 1759-1767
  erythroid, osteoporosis and, 1972
  hepatic
    focal nodular, 1290-1291
    Kupffer cell, 1206
    nodular regenerative, 1249
    portal lymphoid, 1206
  neoplasia and, 44
  ovarian, 1674-1677
  parathyroid glands and, *1573*, 1573-1574
  peritoneum and, 1190
  pituitary gland and, 1529
  prostate gland, 902-906, *903*, *906*
    malignant change and, 915
  thymic, 1502-1504, *1503*
  thyroid gland and, 1549
    adenoma of, 1563
  trophoblastic, 1706-1710
Hyperplastic arteriolosclerosis, 755-756, *756*
Hyperplastic dystrophy of vulva, 1629
Hyperplastic nodules in cirrhosis, 1208
Hyperplastic polyp of colon, 1177
Hyperprolactinemia, 1534
Hypersensitivity, 487-545; *see also*
      Immunopathology
  barbiturates and, 218
  chronicity and, 94
  cutaneous basophil, 530
  delayed, 490, 504*t*, 505, 527, 529
    evolution of, *530*
  granulomatous, 505, 536-538, *537*
  immediate type of, 88
  inflammation in, 87-89
  methyldopa and, 168
  phenytoin and, 172
  tubercle bacilli and, 941-942
  tuberculin type of, 527
Hypersensitivity angiitis, 976
Hypersensitivity myocarditis, *663*, 664
  biopsy and, 707
Hypersensitivity pneumonitis, 236-237, 965-
      967, *966*
  dust-related, 236
Hypersensitivity vasculitis, 769, *771*, 976
Hypersideritis anemia, 559
Hyperspermatogenesis, 873
Hypersplenism, 1411-1413
Hypertension
  accelerated, 843
  adrenal glands and, 1607
  atherosclerosis and, 619, 754, 756, 759
  cardiac hypertrophy and, 677-678, *678*,
      680-681, *681*
  cerebral hemorrhage and, 2150-2151
  coronary heart disease and, 619, 759
  diabetic nephropathy and, 823
  dissecting aneurysm and, 782
  inferior vena cava, 1251
  paroxysmal, 1609, *1609*
  placental lesions and, 1703-1704
  polyarteritis nodosa and, 825
  portal, 1248-1251
    idiopathic, *1281*, 1281-1282
    intrahepatic, 1248
    liver and, 1202
    posthepatic, 1249
    prehepatic, 1249
    spleen and, 1415
  pregnancy and, 827

Hypertension—cont'd
pulmonary, 735, *736*
renal, 841-842
retinopathy and, 1062
vascular disease and, 841-842
Hyperthecosis, ovarian, 1676
Hyperthermia
injuries from local, 137-140
malignant, 149
systemic, 140
Hyperthyroidism, 506, 506*t*, 1546
heart disease and, 689-690
pituitary gland and, 1525
Hypertransaminasemia, 1237
Hypertrophic cardiomyopathy, 682-684
Hypertrophic gastropathy, 1169-1171
Hypertrophic osteoarthropathy, 2070
Hypertrophy, 568, 610
cardiac, 677-681
acromegaly and, 690
cells and, 41-42
chronic airflow limitation and, 995
in cirrhosis with jaundice, 1255
congenital heart disease and, 730
muscle, 2109
Hyperuricemia, 37, 2089
Hypervitaminosis, 36, 547
Hypervitaminosis A, 553
bone metabolism and, 1982, *1982*
Hypervitaminosis D, 554
Hypha, 397
Hypoalbuminemia, 443, 1251
Hypocalcemia
neonatal, 1572
osteopetrosis and, 1951
Hypocomplementemic glomerulonephritis, 516, 817
Hypocortisolism, 1586-1588
Hypodontia, 1096
Hypoglossia-hypodactylia syndrome, 1096
Hypoglycemia, 57, 1269
central nervous system disorders and, 2185
Hypoglycemic agent toxicity, 169
Hypogonadism, 874
osteoporosis and, 1977
Hypogonadotrophic eunuchoidism, 1526
Hypokalemia, 693
Hypokalemic nephropathy, 834, *834*
Hypoparathyroidism, 1571-1572
chronic mucocutaneous candidiasis and, 412
osteoporosis and, 1978
Hypophosphatasia, 1997-2000
Hypophosphatemia
osteomalacia and, 1993-1995
X-linked, 1993-1994
Hypophysectomy, 1525-1526
Hypophysis
dystopia of, 1526
pharyngeal, 1525-1526
Hypophysitis, lymphocytic, 1528-1529
Hypopituitarism, 872, 1526
Hypoplasia
adrenal, 1583
of aortic tract complexes, 748-749, *750*
bone marrow and, 1375
cervical, 1627
lung, 921*t*, 921-922
pituitary gland and, 1526
renal, 844
splenic, 1413
Hypoproteinemia, 516

Hypospadias, 895
Hypospermatogenesis, 873, *874*
Hypospermia, 872
Hyposplenism, 1411-1413
Hypotension, ischemic necrosis of central nervous system and, 2146
Hypothalamic corticotropin-releasing factor, 1581
Hypothalamohypophyseal nerve tract, 1519
Hypothalamus, 1519
Hypothermia, 20
elderly and, 137, *138*
injuries from local, 136-137
injuries from systemic, 137
protracted nonfreezing, 137
Hypothyroidism, 506*t*, 1545
cardiovascular disturbances and, 690
causes of, 1545
male infertility and, 873
neonatal and childhood cholestasis and, 1261*t*
pituitary gland and, 1523-1525
Hypovolemic shock, 700
Hypoxanthine-guanine phosphoribosyl transferase, 59, 2089
deficiency of, 503
Hypoxemia, 961
Hypoxic encephalopathy, 2146-2147
Hypoxic necrosis
hepatic, 1278-1279, 1278-12279
perinatal injury and, 2143-2145
Hypoxic vasoconstriction, 956, 995
Hysterectomy, 1649, 1656

I
I-cell disease, 55, *56*
Ibuprofen toxicity, 162
Ichthyosis, 59-60
ICSH; *see* Interstitial cell–stimulating hormone
Icterus
intravenous drugs and hepatitis, 1219
neonatal, 1262
Idiopathic adrenocortical atrophy, 1586, *1587*
Idiopathic calcification
of adrenals, 1607
arterial, of infancy, 757
Idiopathic fatty liver of pregnancy, 1274
Idiopathic hemochromatosis, 1271-1273
Idiopathic hypertrophic subaortic stenosis, 682, 739
Idiopathic hypoparathyroidism, 1572
Idiopathic hypoplasia of adrenals, 1583
Idiopathic inflammatory disease of bone, 2006
Idiopathic juvenile osteoporosis, 1971
Idiopathic lymphedema, 792-793
Idiopathic membranous glomerulonephritis, 819
Idiopathic midline destructive disease, 1079
Idiopathic multiple pigmented sarcoma, 797
Idiopathic osteoporosis, 1971
Idiopathic Parkinson's disease, 2183
Idiopathic portal hypertension, *1281*, 1281-1282
Idiopathic retroperitoneal fibrosis, 1190
Idiosyncrasy, drug, 150
Idiotypes, 488-489, 508-509
Iduronidase deficiency, 52
L-Iduronosulfate sulfatase, 55
Ig; *see* Immunoglobulins
IGF-I or IGF-II, 590*t*

IL-1, 81
IL-2, 590*t*, 591
IL-3, 590*t*
Ileocecal intussusception, *1157*
Ileum
enteritis of terminal, 1164
polyp of, *1179*
potassium chloride and ulcer of, 186-189, *189*
small noncleaved cell lymphoma in, *1468*
Ileus, adynamic, 1157
Iliac crest bone biopsy, 1957-1958
osteoporosis and, 1965, *1966-1967*
Imipramine poisoning, 194*t*
Immature sinus histiocytosis, 1442
Immature teratoma of ovary, 1689
Immature testes, 874-875, *875*
Immediate responses to cell injury, 75-76
Immediate type of hypersensitivity, 88, 151*t*; *see also* Anaphylactic reactions
Immersion blast, 135
Immersion foot, 137
Immotile cilia syndrome, 950, *950*
Immune activation mechanism, 504*t*, *505*
Immune complex, 512*t*
damage by, 88
Immune complex disease, 148, 515-516, 811
infective endocarditis and, 657
penicillin and, 156
Immune deficiency diseases, 499, 501-502*t*, 534
malignant lymphomas in, 1471-1474
primary, 499-503
secondary, 503
thymus gland and, 1499-1502, 1500*t*
Immune glomerular injury, 810-812
Immune hemolysis, 510*t*
Immune inactivation mechanism, 504*t*, *505*
Immune mechanisms, 498-499, 504*t*
in skin diseases, 539*t*
in viral diseases, 363
Immune-mediated myopathies, 2117-2119
Immune-mediated skin diseases, 538
Immune paralysis, 498
Immune reactions; *see also* Immunologic reactions
classification of, 151*t*
experimental, 538-540
methotrexate and, 185
rheumatoid arthritis and, 2085
viruses and, 27
Immune response region, 536
Immune tolerance, 26, 497-498
Immunity, 487
cell-mediated, 490, 591*t*
Immunoblasts
cardiac biopsy and, 707
lymphadenopathy and, 1439
lymphoma and, *1466*
Immunocyte dyscrasia with amyloidosis, 1286
Immunodeficiency, severe combined, 1499, *1501*; *see also* Immune deficiency diseases
Immunogen, 487
Immunoglobulins, 488
A, 489*t*
deficiency of, 502*t*
dermatitis herpetiformis and, 1762
dermatosis and, 1765
giardiasis and, 439
nephropathy and, 516, 517*t*, 810, 816, *816*

Immunoglobulins—cont'd
  D, 489t
  E, 489t, 519
    allergen reactions with, 518
  G, 489t
    bullous pemphigoid and, 1763
    deficiency of, with increased IgM, 501t
    dermatitis herpetiformis and, 1762
    hypoalbuminemia and, 443
    increased, 443
    molecular structure of, 488
    multiple sclerosis and, 2176
    viral hepatitis and, 1211
  leprosy and, 344-345
  lupus erythematosus and, 1770
  M, 489t
    nephropathy and, 816
    viral hepatitis and, 1211
  plasma cell myeloma and, 2048
  properties of, 489t
Immunohematologic diseases, 509
Immunohistochemical markers for nervous
      system tumors, 2166t
Immunohistochemistry in lymphomas, 604
Immunologic lung disease, 962-964
Immunologic reactions; see also Immune
      reactions
  cirrhosis and, 1252
  Felton's paralysis of, 498
  pharmacogenetics and, 149, 150, 151t
  rheumatic fever and, 641
  toxic drug reactions compared to, 147t
Immunology, 487-490; see also
      Immunopathology
Immunopathology, 487-545; see also
      Lymphocyte
  antibody-induced hemolytic diseases and,
      511, 511
  antibody-mediated disease and, 505
  antiglobulin test and, 512
  Arthus' reaction and, 512, 513
  atopic and anaphylactic reactions and,
      516-527
  autoallergic diseases and, 534-536
  autoimmunity and, 498
    tolerance and, 497
  B- and T-cells and, 490-493
  basic immunology in, 487-490
  cell-mediated disease and, 505
  cellular interactions and antibody
      formation and, 494-495
  cellular or delayed hypersensitivity and,
      527
  clinical findings related to, 516
  complement and, 511
  control of immune response and, 495
  cytotoxic or cytolytic reactions and, 509
  deficiencies in inflammatory mechanisms
      and, 503-505
  delayed skin reaction and, 527, 529
  drug allergy and, 538
  drug-induced hemolytic reactions and,
      511, 511-512
  granulomatous hypersensitivity and, 536-
      538, 537
  idiotype networks, internal images, and
      hormone receptors and, 508-509
  immune complex disease and, 515-516
  immune deficiency diseases and, 499
    primary, 499-503
    secondary, 503
  immune effector mechanisms and, 498-
      499

Immunopathology—cont'd
  immune-mediated skin diseases and, 538
  immune paralysis and, 498
  immune tolerance and, 497-498
  insulin resistance and, 506
  lymphocyte mediators and, 527-534
  lymphocytes in, 490-538
  lymphoid organs and, 495
  lymphoid tissue and, 495-497
  major histocompatibility complex and, 493
    autoimmune diseases and, 536
    tissue transplantation and, 493
  myasthenia gravis and, 508
  neutralization of biologically active
      molecules and, 505-506
  serum sickness and, 512-515, 514
  thyroid disease and, 506-508
  toxic complex reactions and, 512
Immunoperoxidase
  alpha₁-antitrypsin and, 1264
  hepatitis B surface antigen and, 1225,
      1225
Immunoproliferative small intestinal disease,
      1470
Immunosuppressives, 162
  autoimmune hepatitis and, 1230
  toxicity of, 180-186
Impact injury, cerebral, 2189
Impetigo, 302, 303, 303, 1765
Imuran; see Azathioprine
In situ carcinoma
  of breast, 1735-1739, 1736, 1737, 1738
  of cervix, 1645-1650
In situ hybridization, 604
In vivo antibody-antigen reaction, 490
Inborn errors of metabolism, 51
Incision, 114
Incisional biopsy, 1841
Inclusion bodies, 27, 27
  neuronal, 2133
  viral diseases and, 362
Incomplete antigen, 488
Incubation period, 289
Indian childhood cirrhosis, 1268
Indirect-acting hyperbilirubinemia, 1260-
      1262
Indirect-effects theory of radiation damage,
      252-253
Industrial bronchitis, 238
Inertia, 112
Infant
  adrenal glands and, 1581, 1583-1586
    neuroblastoma and, 1611
  arterial calcification and, 624, 757
  beriberi and, 556
  bladder tumor and, 866
  botulism and, 293
  candidiasis and, 412
  cortical hyperostosis in jaws of, 1113
  cytomegalic inclusion disease of, 382
  embryonal carcinoma of testes of, 885,
      885
  fibrous hamartoma of, 1847-1848
  giant cell pneumonia of, 369
  gingival cysts of, 1119
  hemangioendothelioma of, 1292
  hemorrhagic disease in, 555
  hepatoadrenal necrosis and, 379
  hepatocellular carcinoma and, 1298
  hypophosphatasia in, 1997
  liver disease in, 1260-1269
  malignant osteopetrosis of, 1949-1951,
      1950, 1952

Infant—cont'd
  melanotic neuroectodermal jaw tumor in,
      1116
  myofibromatosis in, 1849-1850
  obstructive cholangiopathy in, 1323
  osteomyelitis in, 2004
    jaw and, 1113
  polyarteritis nodosa in, 775
  polycystic kidney in, 845-846, 846
  spinal muscular atrophy in, 2120-2121,
      2121
  subcutaneous fat necrosis of, 1789
  subdermal fibromatous tumors in, 1847
  teratoma and, 1556
  thymus gland in, 1495
  vaginal adenocarcinoma in, 1642
Infarction
  bone, 2010
  central nervous system, 2147-2150, 2148,
      2149, 2150
    septic, 2153-2154
  gallbladder hemorrhagic, 1328
  hepatic, 1280-1281
  infective arteritis and, 767
  placental, 1702
  prostate gland and, 902, 906
  repair in, 102
  retinal, 1063, 1063
  splenic, 1417-1418, 1418
  testicular, 876
Infection; see also Sepsis
  adrenal glands and, 1585
  arteritis and, 766-768, 767, 768
  arthritis and, 2075-2077
  bone, 2002-2010
  central nervous system, 2153-2164
    brain abscess and, 2158
    encephalitis and, 2158-2164
    meningitis in, 2154-2158
  cytocidal, 362
  disease versus, 289
  endocarditis and, 658, 658t
  extracellular, 301-314
  of eye, 1053-1055
  healing by second intention and, 106
  hepatic, 1210-1232; see also Liver,
      infections of
  intracellular, 314-329
  larynx and, 1084
  local, 130
  lung, 930-948, 1031-1033; see also Lung,
      infections of
  nasal cavity and paranasal sinus, 1078-
      1080
  oral soft tissue, 1103-1105
    granulomatous, 1105-1106
  parasitism and, 292t
  pathogenesis of, 290-292
  penetrating wounds of heart and, 698
  placenta and, 1704-1706
  spleen and systemic, 1418-1419
  steady state, 363
  of surfaces of body, 294-301
  thyroiditis and, 1550
Infectious inoculum, 290
Infectious mononucleosis, 383, 1104
  fatal, 1502
  lymph nodes and, 1439, 1440
  splenic rupture and, 1418
Infective agents, immune defense reactions
      to, 498t
Inferior olives, bilirubin staining of, 2146

Inferior vena cava
  hypertension and, 1251
  obstruction of
    Budd-Chiari syndrome and, 1282
    hepatic outflow, 791
Inferior vena caval syndrome, 790, *791*
Infertility, male, 872-877
Infiltrating angioma, 1820
Infiltrating lipoma, 1880-1881
Infiltrations, pituitary gland and, 1529
Inflammation, 67-94, 95, 108-109
  abscess formation and, 87
  acute, 84-87
  alimentary tract and, 1159-1168
  aseptic, 129
  atherogenesis and, 765
  bone marrow and, 1405
  cardinal signs of, 84
  cellulitis and, 87
  cervical, 1644-1645
  chronic, 84, 89-94
  corticosteroids and, 162, 165
  definition of, 67
  endometrial, 1657
  of eye, 1056-1057
  factors in variation of, 84-86
  of fallopian tube, 1667-1668
  functions of, 89
  gallbladder and biliary ducts and, 1327-
      1330
  granulomatous
    lymph nodes and, 1434, 1435*t*
    spleen and, *1418*, 1419
  healing and, 67, 94-108; *see also* Healing
  heart conducting system and, 705
  historical perspective on, 67
  hypersensitivity and, 87-89
  of jaws, 1113-1116
  juvenile melanoma and, 1809
  leukocytes in, 81-84
  of liver, 1206
  lymph flow in, 84
  of male urethra, 898-899
  of nasal cavity and paranasal sinuses,
      1078-1080
  neck, 1144
  odontogenic cysts and, 1118
  of penis, 895-896
  of peritoneum, 1189
  permeability responses in, 71, *71*
  pituitary gland and, 1527-1529
  polyarteritis nodosa and, 769
  of prostate gland, 901
  pseudomembranous, 86-87
  salivary gland enlargement and, 1128-1131
  scrotal, 891
  of seminal vesicles, 916
  sequential accumulation of cells in, 78-79
  signs of, 67
  of spermatic cord, 892
  systemic effects of, 89
  of tendons, 2091
  testicular, 877-879
  ulceration and, 87
  of ureter, 851-852
  of urinary bladder, 854-857
  of uveal tract, 516, 1056
  vaginal, 1638-1639
  of vas deferens, 892
  vascular reaction in, 67-84
    exudation and, 71-76
    leukocytes and, 81-84
    lymph flow and, 84

Inflammation—cont'd
  vascular reaction in—cont'd
    microscopy and, 68-70
    neutrophil emigration and, 76-81
    vasodilatation and, 70-71
  vulvar, 1628-1629
Inflammatory aneurysm, 779, *781*
Inflammatory bowel disease, 1161-1165
  liver abnormalities and, 1287
Inflammatory carcinoma of breast, 1746-
    1747, *1747*
Inflammatory disorders of skeleton, 2002-
    2010
Inflammatory fibroid polyp, 1159, *1160*
Inflammatory fibrous histiocytoma, 1854,
    1857
Inflammatory heart diseases, 639-672
  ankylosing spondylitis and, 650
  coronary artery disease and, 621-623
  endocarditis in, 652-658
  hemopericardium in, 664-665
  hydropericardium in, 664
  myocarditis in, 659-664
  pericarditis in, 665-672
  rheumatic fever and rheumatic heart
      disease in, 639-649; *see also*
      Rheumatic fever and rheumatic heart
      disease
  rheumatoid arthritis and, 649-650
  syphilitic, 650-652
Inflammatory histiocytomas, 1856
Inflammatory infiltrates, interstitial, 2111
Inflammatory joint diseases, 2075-2086
  arthritis with rheumatic fever in, 2077
  brucellosis and, 2076
  fungal disease and, 2076-2077
  infectious agents in, 2075-2077
  rheumatoid arthritis in, 2077-2086; *see
      also* Rheumatoid arthritis
  syphilitic, 2076
  toxic arthritis in, 2077
  tuberculous, 2075-2076
  viral, 2075
Inflammatory myofibroblastic tumor, 1292-
    1293
Inflammatory myopathies, 2117-2119
Inflammatory papillary hyperplasia in oral
    soft tissue, 1106
Inflammatory pseudotumor, 1292-1293
  in lung, 1021, *1022*
Inflammatory response, 67, *510*
  deficiencies in, 503-505
  functions of, 89
  lymph nodes and, 1433-1443
  myocardial infarction and, 635-637
  variation of, 84-87
Influenza, 363-365, 935
  Asian, *365*
Infrared rays, 285*t*
Infundibular process, 1518
Infundibular proliferation, hair follicle
    tumors and, 1834
Infundibular stem, 1518
Infundibulum, 1518
INH; *see* Isoniazid
Inhalation injury, 139-140
Inhalation, 274
Iniencephaly, 2136
Injury
  bone, 2000-2002
  cell; *see* Cell injury
  central nervous system, 2186-2189
    general reactions to, 2125-2135

Injury—cont'd
  central nervous system—cont'd
    neurocellular reactions to, 2131-2135
  coronary artery disease and, 624
  extrathoracic, 962
  head
    blunt, 2188
    crushing, 2188
    penetrating, 2189
  heart conducting system and, 705
  hemorrhagic pancreatitis and, 1353
  hepatic, 1275
    radiation, 1283
  joint disorders and, 2067-2068
  muscle, 2108-2111
  myocardium and, 698-699
  perinatal brain, 2141-2146
  radiation, 247-288; *see also* Radiation
      injury
  spinal cord, 2189
  spleen and, 1414
  ureteral, 850-851
  to urinary bladder, 853
Inoculum, infectious, 290
Inoperable tumor, 284
Insect allergy, 526
Insect bites, 1829
Insecticide toxicity, 226
Insulin, 506*t*
  binding of, 4
  glycolysis and, 10
  synthesis of, 1360
Insulin-like growth factor, 568
Insulin resistance, 506
Insulinoma, 578, 1367
Insulitis, lymphocytic, 1362
int 2, 587*t*
Interdigitating reticulum cells, 492*t*
Interferon, 531*t*
Interferon-gamma, 433
Intergroup Rhabdomyosarcoma Study
    Group, 1865, 1866, 1871
Interleukin-1, 81
Interleukin-2, 590*t*, 591
Interleukin-3, 590*t*
Intermediate filaments, 1203
Intermittent hepatic fever of Charcot, 1254
Intersex states, 872, 1624-1627, 1625*t*
Interstitial brain edema, 2127, 2128
Interstitial cell–stimulating hormone, 1522
Interstitial cells of Leydig, 1526
Interstitial cystitis, 856
Interstitial emphysema
  of lung, 928, *928*
  of mediastinium, 1024
Interstitial nephritis, 837-839
  rifampin and, 171
Interstitial pneumonia, 969-972, *970*, 1037
  acquired immunodeficiency syndrome
      and, 968
  cellular, 516
  desquamative, 970, *970*
  lymphoid, 1022, *1022*
  plasma cell, 948
  usual, 971
Interstitial pulmonary fibrosis
  cadmium toxicity and, 212, 213, *213*
  diffuse, *174*, 175
  hydralazine and, 168
  ozone and, 231
  silo-filler's disease and, 232
Interstitial pulmonary inflammatory
    infiltrates, 2111

Interstitial reactions in skeletal muscle diseases, 2111
Interstitial sclerosis of testes, 875
Intestinal absorption, 1171
Intestinal angina, 1158
Intestinal disorders, dermatoses and, 1786
Intestinal distomiasis, 453
Intestinal epithelial crypt cells, 257t
Intestinal epithelium-lined cysts, 1120
Intestinal histoplasmosis, 1166
Intestinal lipodystrophy, 1173, *1174*
Intestinal lumen, 7
Intestinal mucosa hyperinfection, 468
Intestinal obstruction, 1157-1158
Intestinal schistosomiasis, 455
Intestine; *see also* Alimentary tract
    cystic fibrosis and, 1350
    digitalis and venous engorgement of, *175,* 175-176
    pneumatosis cystoides of, 1155-1156, *1156*
    radiation injury to, *272, 278*
    schistosomiasis japonica in, 458
Intimal thickening, 753-754, *755*
Intra-arterial angiomatoids, 457
Intracellular ion homeostasis, 21-22
Intracellular milieu, 12
Intracellular storage, 6
Intracranial pressure, increased, 2128-2130
Intracytoplasmic brown pigment, 1277, *1277*
Intradermal neutrophilic dermatosis, 1765
Intradermal nevus, *1803,* 1803-1804
Intraductal carcinoma of breast, 1737-1739
Intraductal papilloma of breast, 1731-1732
Intraepithelial neoplasia
    of cervix, 1645-1650
    of prostatic ducts, 915
    of vulva, 1632-1633, *1633*
Intrahepatic bile duct
    congenital cystic dilatation of, 1257-1258
    obstruction of, 1252
    transhepatic cholangiogram of, 1253, *1253*
Intrahepatic cholestasis
    chlorpromazine and, 167
    familial, 1261t, 1266-1267
    herbicide toxicity and, 230
Intrahepatic portal hypertension, 1248
Intramuscular hemangioma, 1884, 1886-1888, *1887*
Intramuscular myxoma, *1897*
Intranuclear inclusions
    Cowdry type A, 1585
    lead-containing, 206, *207*
    of virus, 27, *27*
Intraocular lesions, 1051-1074; *see also* Ophthalmic pathology, intraocular lesions in
Intraocular neoplasms, primary, 1064-1069
Intraperitoneal adhesions, 1189
Intraplacental hematoma, 1702
Intrascrotal inflammation, 891
Intrasellar cyst, 1537
Intrasinusoidal growth, 1299
Intratubular malignant germ cells, 875, *875*
Intrauterine anoxia, 698
Intrauterine contraceptive devices, 1657
Intravascular bronchoalveolar tumor, 1020
Intravascular hemolysis, burns and, 139
Intravascular malignant lymphomatosis, 1465
Intravascular papillary endothelial hyperplasia, 796
Intravascular stasis, 130
Intravenous drug users; *see* Drug abuse
Intravenous leiomyomatosis, 1666

Intraventricular hemorrhage, perinatal, *2142,* 2142-2143
Intrinsic asthma, 962
Intrinsic factor, 506t
Intubation granuloma in larynx, 1085
Intussusception, 1157, *1157*
Invasion, 581, 610
    breast carcinoma, 1739-1747, *1742*
    cervical carcinoma, 1650-1652
    fibrous thyroiditis and, 1553-1554
Inversions, 48
Inverted papilloma of bladder, 864, *865*
Involution
    of fetal adrenal cortex, precocious, 1583
    of thymus, *1498,* 1499
Involutional osteoporosis, 1967-1971
Iodine, 563
    radioactive, 270, 281, 285
    toxicity of, 169
Iodopsin, 553
Ion homeostasis, intracellular, 21-22
Ionizing particles, 254
Ionizing radiation; *see* Radiation
Ions, 247
    transport of, 3
Iridocyclitis, 1056
Iris, juvenile xanthogranuloma of, 1076, *1076*
Iritis, 1054, 1056, *1056*
Iron
    cirrhosis and, 1272
    collagen and, 1273
    hepatocellular pigment and, 1204
    idiopathic hemochromatosis and, 1271-1272
    liver disease and metabolism of, 1271-1273
    poisoning from, 194t
    storage of, 31
        liver and, 1271
    tissue, 31-33
Iron-deficiency anemia, 1378-1379
Iron deposition in bone tissue, 1974
Iron ore miners, 276
Iron overload, 1271-1273
    multiple transfusions and, 1273
Iron oxide, 233
Iron salts, liver injury and, 1232
Irradiation; *see* Radiation
Irritant gases, 86, 237
Ischemia, 13
    cryptorchidism and, 872
    hemorrhagic pancreatitis and, 1353
    hypothermia and, 137
    myocardial, 624-625, *626*; *see also* Coronary artery disease
    pituitary gland and, 1527
Ischemic acute tubular necrosis, 832-833, *833*
Ischemic bowel disease, 1158
Ischemic cardiomyopathy, 681
    myocardial infarction and, 638
Ischemic cell death, 629-630, *630*
Ischemic cell injury, irreversible, 633
Ischemic encephalopathy, 2146-2147, *2148*
Ischemic forearm test, 2114
Ischemic heart disease, 616; *see also* Coronary artery disease
Ischemic injury, 20-22, *22*
Ischemic necrosis
    central nervous system and, 2146-2150
    infective arteritis and, 767
    neuronal, 2132

Ischemic necrosis—cont'd
    perinatal injury and, 2143-2145
    secondary, 130
        electrical injury and, 142
Ischiorectal abscess, 1169
Islet cell adenoma, 578
Islet cell tumor, *575*
Islet cells, 492t, 506t
    aurophilic, 1754
    diabetes and transplantation of, 1366
    granulomatosis of, spleen and, 1422-1423, *1423, 1424*
Islets of Langerhans, 1348, 1359
    hyalinization of, 1363
Isoenzymes, 10
    alcohol dehydrogenase and, 1240
    leukemia and mosaicism of, 1384
Isoleucine, 546, 562
Isoniazid, 559
    gynecomastia and, 168
    myocarditis and, 708
    necrosis and, 1232, 1234t, 1236
    pharmacogenetics and, 150
    toxicity of, 169-170, *170*
Isonicotinic acid, 149
Isopropanol toxicity, 198
Isoproterenol
    aortic outflow obstruction and, 684
    myocardial injury and, 693-694
    toxicity of, 216-217, *217*
Isosporiasis, 445, 1167
Isotopes, 284-285
    radioactive, 263
        half-life of, 249
Ito cells, 1199, 1200
    collagen and, 1207
    wound contraction and, 104
Ixodes dammini tick, 451

J

Jaccoud's arthritis, 2077
Jadassohn nevus, 1810, 1833
Janeway lesions, 657-658
Japanese B encephalitis, 371-372
Jaundice, 33-34
    bacterial infections and, 1231-1232
    drug-induced, 149, 1233
    hypertropic cirrhosis with, 1255
    oral contraceptives and, 166, 167
    pediatric
        less common causes of, 1265-1267
        neonatal, 1260-1262
    of pregnancy, 1235
Jaws, 1113-1127
    cysts of, 1117-1120
    developmental lesions of, 1113
    inflammations and metabolic lesions of, 1113-1116
    malignant tumors of, 1116-1117
    odontogenic tumors of, 1121-1127
    radium, 280
    uncommon benign tumors of, 1116
JC virus, 384, 2178, 2179
Jejunum, *1172*
    lipoma of, *1188*
    peptic ulcers and, 1161
        potassium chloride and, 186-189, *189*
    strongyloidiasis and, 468
Jerne's hypothesis of idiotype networks, 508
Jessner's lymphocytosis of skin, 1829
Jodbasedow hyperthyroidism, 1546
Joint
    diarthrodial, 2065-2066

Joint—cont'd
  vertebral, 2067
Joint diseases, 2065-2104
  congenital malformations in, 2066-2067
  crystal-deposition diseases in, 2087-2091
  cysts in, 2092
  developmental defects in, 2066-2067
  diabetes mellitus and, 2091-2092
  inflammatory, 2075-2086
    brucellosis and, 2076
    fungal arthritis in, 2076-2077
    infectious agents in, 2075-2077
    rheumatic fever and, 2077
    rheumatoid arthritis and, 2077-2086
    syphilitic, 2076
    toxic arthritis in, 2077
    tuberculous, 2075-2076
    viral, 2075
  noninflammatory, 2067-2075
  normal joint structure and function and, 2065-2066
  seronegative spondyloarthropathies in, 2086-2087
  tumors and tumorlike conditions in, 2092-2096
  vertebral column and, 2096-2098
Joint mice, 2067, 2069, *2069*
Joule of energy, 249
Jugular paraganglioma, 1088
jun, 587*t*
Junctional alteration of epidermis, 1805-1806
Junctional nevus, 1802-1803
  active, 1816
  malignant melanomas and, 1815-1816
Junín virus, 372-373
Juvenile cirrhosis, 1264, *1264*, 1268
Juvenile mammary hypertrophy, 1734
Juvenile melanoma, 1804-1810, *1806*, *1807*
Juvenile osteoporosis, idiopathic, 1971
Juvenile papillomatosis, 1084-1085
Juvenile periodontitis, 1100
Juvenile pilocytic astrocytoma, 2167, *2167*
Juvenile polyp of rectum, *1177*, *1178*
Juvenile rheumatoid arthritis, 2086-2087
Juvenile thyroiditis, 1552, *1552*
Juvenile xanthogranuloma of iris, 1076, *1076*
Juxtacortical chondroma, 2034, *2035*
Juxtacortical chondrosarcoma, 2040
Juxtacortical osteosarcoma, 2021*t*
Juxtaductal coarctation, 741-743, *742*, *743*

K

K-*ras* gene, 587*t*, 589, 1015
Kala-azar, 443, *444*
Kallidin, 73
Kallikreins, 37, 73
Kallman's syndrome, 874, *875*
Kanamycin toxicity, 157-158, *158*
Kangri cancers, 1800
Kaolin, 233
Kaolinite, 997
Kaposi's sarcoma, 797-799, *798*
  acquired immunodeficiency syndrome and, 1113, 1286, *1473*
    gastrointestinal tract symptoms in, 1167
    oral symptoms in, 1113
    pulmonary symptoms in, 968
  idiopathic hemorrhagic, 1821-1822
Kaposi's varicelliform eruption, 1767
Kappa Ig gene, *1458*
Kappa light chains, 491

Kartagener's triad of sinusitis, bronchiectasis, and situs inversus, 950
Karyolysis, 12
  myocardial infarction and, 636
Karyorrhexis, 255, 824
Karyotype
  normal human, *46*, *592*
  pure gonadal dysgenesis and, 1625*t*
  true hermaphroditism and, 1626
Kasabach-Merritt syndrome, 795
Kasai operation, 1262, 1263
Kashin-Beck disease, 2074-2075
Katayama fever syndrome, 455
Kawasaki's disease, 774-775, *776*, 1433
  skin and, 1830
Kayser-Fleischer ring, 1074, *1075*, 1270
Kearns-Sayre syndrome, 2116
Keloid, 568, 1776
Kemerovo virus, 376
Keratin, 1007, 1755
  disorder of, 1795
  warts and, 1794
Keratinizing cyst, 1119, *1119*
Keratinocytes, 1754
Keratitis, 1054
  onchocerciasis and, 472
Keratoacanthoma, 1796, *1796*
  in oral soft tissue, 1107
Keratocyst, odontogenic, 1119, 1799
Keratoderma, 1752
Keratoderma blennorrhagica, 1774-1775
Keratoma, 1087
Keratomalacia, 552
Keratosis, 1085-1086
  seborrheic, 1795, *1795*
  senile, 1796-1797
  vulvar, 1629-1630
Keratosis arsenica, *570*
Keratosis follicularis, 1103, 1759
Kerley-A or -B lines, 957, 960
Kernicterus, 34, 2145-2146
  neonatal hyperbilirubinemia and, 1260-1261
  parenchymal necrosis and, 2143
Kernohan's notch, 2130
Ketoacidosis, diabetic, 37
Kidneys, 804-849, 867-869
  adenocarcinoma radiosensitivity and, 257*t*
  anatomy of renal failure and, 807-809
  calcification in, 36, 37
  classification of disease of, 809-810
  congenital anomalies of, 844-847
  cytomegalovirus infection of, *381*
  diabetes and, 1365-1366
  flea-bitten, 844
  flow abnormalities and, 836-839
  glomerular disease of, 810-829
    anti–glomerular basement membrane disease in, 810
    chronic injury and, 828-829
    complement-mediated injury and, 811-812
    congenital, 823
    diabetic nephropathy and, 823
    diffuse glomerulonephritis and, 812-815
    focal glomerulonephritis and, 815
    focal segmental sclerosis and, 820-821
    immune complex, 811
    membranoproliferative glomerulonephritis and, 816-818
    membranous nephropathy and, 819-820

Kidneys—cont'd
  glomerular disease of—cont'd
    mesangioproliferative glomerulonephritis and, 815-816
    minimal change disease and, 818-819
    systemic amyloidosis and, 38-39, *39*, 821-823
    systemic disease and, 824-827
    toxemia of pregnancy and, 827-828
  graft rejection and, 533
  hypertrophy of, 41, *42*
  ischemic injury to, 20
  lithiasis and, 840
  mercury bichloride poisoning in, 831
  metabolic tubulointerstitial toxicity and, 839-840
  myeloma and, 839, 1402
  neoplasms of, 847-849
  parathyroid adenoma and, *1576*
  pathophysiology and, 806-807
  pelvic ectopic, 844
  pressure abnormalities and, 836-839
  pressure and flow abnormalities of, 836-839
  pyelonephritis and, 834-836
  radiation injury and, 273, 279
  shock, 131
  structure and function of, 804-806
  tubulointerstitial disease and, 829-834
  vascular renal disease and, 841-844
Kiel classification of non-Hodgkin's lymphomas, 1452-1453
Kikuchi's disease, 1434
Kimmelstiel-Wilson disease, 823
  diabetes and, 1364
  nephropathy in, 1057
Kimura's disease, 1790, *1791*
Kinetic energy, 111
Kininogens, 73
Kinins, 70, 73
Kinyoun's stain, 396*t*
Klatskin tumor, 1337, *1337*, 1342
Klebsiella, 312-313, *313*, 834, 936, 1079
  pyogenic abscesses and, 1259
  wound infection and, 130
Klinefelter's syndrome, 48, 874, *874*
  leukemia and, 1385
  male breast carcinoma and, 1747
Klippel-Trenaunay syndrome, 795
Knee joint, arthritis and, *2081*
Knuckle pads, 1845
Koch's postulates, 362
Koch-Weeks bacillus, 310
Kohn, pores of, 933, 992
Koilocytes, 385, *385*, 1104
Koilocytosis, 1631, 1633, *1633*
Koilonychia, 1787
Koplik spots, 367
Korsakoff's psychosis, 556, 2185
Krabbe's disease, *53*, 2180, *2180*
Kraurosis, 1629
Krause end bulbs, 1757
Krebs cycle, 1239
Krükenberg's tumor, 1183, 1691
Kulchitsky cell, 1184
Kupffer cells, 1199-1200
  hyperplasia of, 1206
  radiation injury and, 279
Kuru, 387-388, 2164
Kveim test, 980, 1785
Kwashiorkor, 549, *549*, 692
  experimental models of, 550
  fatty change in hepatocytes and, 1203

Kyphoscoliosis, 956
Kyphosis, 2096
Kyrle's disease, 1784

L

L-*myc*, 587*t*
La Crosse virus, 370
Labial glands, 1127
Labial papillomatosis, 1103
Labile cells, 94-96
Lábrea hepatitis, 1223
Laceration, 112, *113*, 114, *115*
Lacrimal glands in Sjögren's syndrome, 974
Lactational adenomas, 1730
Lactic acidemia, 37
  glycogen storage diseases and, 2114
Lactotrophs, 1521, 1521*t*, 1523
Lacunar cells, 1446, *1447*
Lacunar infarct, 2150, *2150, 2151*
Laënnec's cirrhosis, 456, 1238
Lafora bodies, 2133
Lambda light chains, 491
Lamellar bone, 2023
Lamellar necrosis of gray matter, 222
Lamellar unit, 752
Lamina densa, 804-805
Lamina rara externa, 805
Lamina rara interna, 804
Laminar necrosis, 2147
Laminin, 582, 805
  neovascularization and, 102
  neurofibroma and, 1893
Lancefield group A streptococci, 935
Langerhans' cells, 492*t*, 506*t*
  aurophilic, 1754
  spleen and granulomatosis of, 1422-1423,
    1423, 1424
  transplantation of, 1366
Langerhans' islets, 1348, 1359
  hyalinization of, 1363
Langhans' giant cells, 91, *91*, 324, 467, 942,
  979, 1528, 1778
Lanugo, 1756
Laplace equation, 958
Large cell lymphomas
  mediastinum and, 1511
  thyroid
    diffuse, 1465-1467
    follicular, 1461
Large cell undifferentiated carcinoma of
  lung, 1010-1011
Large intestine; *see* Intestine
Larva migrans, 467-469, *468*
Laryngeal atresia, 1084
Laryngeal cysts, 1085
Laryngeal papillomas, 385-386, 1020, 1084-
  1085
Laryngopyocele, 1085
Laryngotracheal sulcus, 920
Laryngotracheobronchitis, 1084
Larynx, 1084-1087
Laser radiation, 285
Lassa fever, 372-373, 1231
LATS; *see* Long-acting thyroid stimulator
LATSP; *see* Long-acting thyroid stimulator
  protector
Launois-Bensaude syndrome, 1142
Law of Bergonié and Tribondeau, 264
LDL; *see* Low-density lipoprotein
Lead
  as carcinogen, 239, 277
  toxicity of, 36, 194*t*, 205-209, *206, 207*
    nephropathy and, 832

Lead sulfite deposition in gums, 206
Leaking aneurysm, 779
Leather-bottle stomach, Plate 2 *F*, 1183
Lecithin, 560
Lecithinase, 296
Left-sided heart failure, 615, 959-960
Left-to-right shunt
  at atrial level, 731, *732-734*
  at ductus level, 734-735, *735*
  at ventricular level, 731-734, *734*
Legionella, 311, 937-938
Legs
  lymphedema praecox and, 792-793
  varicose veins of, 786-788
  white, painful, 789
Leiomyoblastoma, myometrial, 1665
Leiomyoma, 1838, 1860-1861, *1861*
  aggressive, 1864
  of cervix, 1645
  of epididymis, 892
  in lung, 1020
  myometrial, 1664-1665, *1665*
  in oral soft tissue, 1108
  of skin, 1823-1824
  of stomach, 1186, *1186*
  of vagina, 1640
Leiomyomatosis peritonealis disseminata,
  1190
Leiomyosarcoma, 799, 1838, 1861-1864,
  1862
  deep-seated, 1862
  myometrial, 1666, *1666*
  radiosensitivity of, 257*t*
Leishman-Donovan bodies, 443
Leishmaniasis, 419, 442, 443-445, *444*
Lenègre disease, 706
Lennert's lymphoma, 1466
Lens
  nonionizing radiation and, 285
  opacification of, 1069
Lentiginosis, generalized, 1786
Lentigo, senile, 1811
Leonine facies, *473*
Leopard syndrome, 1786
Lepra cells, 339
Lepromatous leprosy, 335, *338*, 338-339,
  503
  histoid variety of, 342
Lepromin test, 337
Leprosy, 333-347, 538
  borderline, 335, 339, 341
  classification of, 335-337
  clinical features of, 337
  control of, 345
  definition, history, and prevalence of,
    333-334
  diagnosis of, 345
    differential, 345
  granulomatous inflammation and, 91
  histopathology of, 338-342
  immunology and, 344-345
  indeterminate, 335, 337, 341, *342*
  lepromatous, 335, *338*, 338-339, 503
    histoid variety of, 342
  leprosy bacillus and, 334
  lymph node involvement in, 344
  nerve involvement in, 342-343
  reactions in, 337-338
  temperature selectivity and pathology of,
    344
  transmission of, 334
  tuberculoid, 335, *336*, 339-341, 539*t*
  as zoonosis, 334-335

Leprosy bacillus, 334
Leptomeningitis, 2154-2158
Leptospiral infections, 324, 325, 328, 392*t*
Lesch-Nyhan syndrome, 37, 51, 59, 503
Leser-Trélat sign, 1795
Lesion versus disease, 290
Lethal dose of radiation, 264
Lethal factor, 297
Lethal granuloma
  midline, 1079
  in oral soft tissue, 1104
Letterer-Siwe disease, 977, 1423
Leucine, 546
Leucine aminopeptidase, 1754
Leucine threonine, 562
Leukemia, 1384-1399
  acute lymphoblastic, 1384, 1386*t*, 1388,
    1395-1396, 1469
    morphologic, immunologic, and
      cytogenetic correlations in, 1389*t*
  acute nonlymphoblastic, 1384, 1386*t*,
    1388, 1390-1391
    morphologic, immunologic, and
      cytogenetic correlations in, 1389*t*
  acute nonlymphocytic, 593*t*
  acute promyelocytic, 1391
  acute undifferentiated, 1386*t*
  benign eosinophilic, 467
  benzene and, 222
  chronic lymphocytic, 1384, 1388, 1396,
    1396, 1397
  chronic myelocytic, 1384, 1386*t*, 1388,
    1391-1393, *1392, 1393*
  chronic myelogenous, 588, 592-593, 602,
    1384
  cytogenetics and, 603
  eyes and, 1069
  fetal irradiation and, 269
  French-American-British classification of,
    1386*t*, 1388
  hairy-cell, 375, 1397-1398, *1398*
    liver and, *1428*, 1429
  hemopericardium and, 665
  kidney and, 849
  pathophysiology of, 1388-1390
  prolymphocytic, 1397
  radiation injury and, *266*, 279
  radiosensitivity of, 257*t*
  radium and, 259
  skin and, 1827
  viral carcinogenesis and, 601
Leukemia-lymphoma syndrome, 1460, 1469
Leukins, 84
Leukocidins, 291, 302
Leukocyte-inhibitory factor, 531*t*
Leukocytes
  adherence of, 76, *77*
  chemotaxis and, 79-81
  granulation tissue and, 98
  inflammation and, 76, 76-81, *78*, 81-84
  polymorphonuclear, 499
Leukocytoclasis, 1776, 1789, 1790
Leukocytosis, 935, 1382-1384
  chronic myelocytic leukemia and, 1392
Leukoderma acquisitum centrifugum, 1812
Leukodystrophies, 2179, 2179-2180
  adrenal, 1583-1584, *1584*
Leukoencephalitis
  acute hemorrhagic, 2178, *2178*
  progressive multifocal, 2162
Leukoencephalopathy
  metachromatic, 1173
  progressive multifocal, *2178*, 2178-2179

Leukoerythroblastic reaction, 1379
Leukokeratosis nicotina palati, 1110
Leukokoria, 1066, *1067*
Leukomalacia, periventricular, 2143-2145, *2144*
Leukonychia, 1787
Leukopenia, 316, 935, 1382-1384
    radiation and, 264, 284
Leukoplakia, 1797
    bladder and, 857
    hairy, 1104
    larynx and, 1086
    oral mucosa and, 1109, 1110, *1110*
    schistosomiasis, 458
    vulva and, 1629
Leukotrienes, 519*t*, 964
    vascular permeability and, 73-75
Lev disease, 706
Lever action, 112
Levodopa, 30, 1248, 2183
Lewy bodies, 2133, 2183, *2183*
Leydig cells, 871, 1526
    ovarian tumor and, 1673
    testicular tumor and, 888-889
LFA-1, 80
LH; *see* Luteinizing hormone
Libman-Sacks disease, 672-673, 1770
Librium; *see* Chlordiazepoxide
Lichen amyloidosis, 1781
Lichen planus, 1100-1102, *1102*, 1773-1774, *1774*
    white oral lesions of, 1110
Lichen sclerosus, 1629-1630, *1630*, 1777
Lichen simplex chronica, 1629
Lichenification, 526, 1757
Lichtheim plaques, 2186
Lids of eye, 1047
    xanthomas and, 1257, *1792*
Lieberkühn crypts, 557, 1163, 1184
    irradiation and, 272
Liesegang rings, 943
Ligands, 508
Light-chain disease, 826
Light-chain excretion, 839
Lightning, 144, *144*
    cutaneous hyperemia and, 144, *144*
Limb bud development, 1936-1937
Limb-girdle dystrophy, 2112
Limbus, carcinoma of, *1051*
Lime, 234
Limiting plate, 1200, 1202
Lindau's disease, 892
Lindau's tumor, 795
Linear accelerator, 248, 284
Linear energy transfer, 23, 253-254, 265
Linear laceration, 114, *114*
Lines of Zahn, 952
Lingual thyroid gland, 1096
Linitis plastica, 1183
Linoleic acid deficiency, 562
Lip, 1095
    cleft, 1095
    squamous cell carcinoma of, 1111
Lip pits, congenital, 1095, *1096*
Lipid cell tumors of ovary, 1686-1687
Lipid-infiltration theory, 620-621
Lipid-laden foamy cells, 1333, *1334*
Lipid peroxides, 176
Lipid pneumonia, 985-986, *986*
Lipid proteinosis, 1780-1781
Lipid-storage diseases, 686, 2115-2116, *2116*
Lipids
    atherosclerosis and, 765

Lipids—cont'd
    complex, 28-30
    fatty liver and, *17*, 17-18
    myocardial ischemia and, 631
    storage of neutral, 6
    Whipple's disease and, 1173
Lipoatrophy, 1789
Lipoblastoma, 1884-1885, *1885*
Lipocaic, 560
Lipochrome pigment, 1277, *1277*
Lipodystrophy, 1173, *1174*, 1190
Lipofuscin, *34*, 35, 43
    central nervous system neurons and, 2132
    hibernoma and, 1886
    liver and, 1201, 1204
Lipogranuloma
    of eyelid, 1047, *1048*
    mineral oil and, *190*, 191
    retroperitoneum and mesentery and, 1190
    sclerosing, 896, *897*
Lipolysis, pancreatitis and, 1351
Lipoma, 1292, 1838
    cardiac, 703
    gastrointestinal tract, 1188, *1188*
    infiltrating intramuscular, 1881
    myometrium and, 1667
    neural tube defects and, 2136
    soft tissue, 1879-1884
        infiltrating, 1880-1881
        oral, 1109
        pleomorphic, *1883*
        spindle cell, *1882*
    of spermatic cord, 893
    subcutaneous, 575
Lipoma-like liposarcoma, 1874-1875, *1876*
Lipomatosis, benign symmetric neck, 1142
Lipophagic phagocytosis, 1440
Lipophilic chemical transformation, 147
Lipoprotein-tetracycline complexes, 153
Lipoproteins, atherosclerosis and, 764
Liposarcoma, 578, *578*, 1838, *1874*
    dedifferentiated, 1856, 1877
    radiosensitivity of, 257*t*
    soft tissue, 1873-1879
Lipping, osteoarthrosis and, 2073, *2073*
Lipschütz bodies, 1760, 1767
Liquefaction necrosis, 13-16, *15*
    skin and, 1758, 1771
Lisch nodules, 2175
Lissencephaly, 2139
Listeria, 313, 1657, 1704
    meningitis and, 313, 2154
    neonatal encephalitis and, 2160, 2162
Lithiasis, 1323, *1326*
    complications of, 1327
    pancreatic, 197
    renal, 840
Lithium, 276, 708
Liver, 1199-1320
    abnormalities of, 1201-1202
    abscesses of, 1252, 1258-1260
        amebic, *435*, *1259*, *1260*
        cholangitis and, 1254
    alcoholic disease of; *see* Alcoholic liver disease
    alpha$_1$-antitrypsin and, 1264
    biliary cirrhosis and, 1254-1255
    biopsy of, 1217, 1219, 1222
    capillariasis and, 466
    carcinoma of, 1293-1298
        choline deficiency and, 560
        clonorchiasis and, 453
        metastatic, from stomach, 1183

Liver—cont'd
    carcinoma of—cont'd
        radiosensitivity of, 257*t*
        trabecular, 1297, *1298*
    chemical and drug injury of, 1232-1238
    cholestatic disorders of, 1252-1260
        osteoporosis and, 1974-1975
    chronic disease of, 1283-1287
        complications of, 1248
        pathophysiology of, 1247-1252
    circulatory disturbances and, 1278-1283
    cirrhosis of; *see* Cirrhosis
    copper in, 1270-1271
    cystic fibrosis and, 1351
    cysts of, 1293
        echinococcal, 461
        hydatid, 461
    disease of, in nonhepatic disorders, 1287
    drug-induced disease of, 1233
    embryology of, 1199-1201
    emphysema and, 994
    ethanol oxidation and, 1238, *1239*
    extrahepatic effects of disease of, 1287
    fatty; *see* Fatty liver
    hairy cell leukemia and, *1428*, 1429
    hemosiderosis of, 1273
    hereditary hyperbilirubinemia and, 1275-1278
    histopathology of, 1202-1210
        cirrhosis and, 1208-1210
        fibrosis and, 1207-1208
        hepatocellular changes in, 1202-1204
        hepatocellular necrosis in, 1204-1205
        portal and lobular inflammation in, 1206
        regeneration and, 1206-1207
    25-hydroxylation and, 1993
    hyperplasia and, 43-44
    infant and child diseases of, 1260-1269
    infections of, 1210-1232
        bacterial, 1231-1232
        chronic, 1283-1287
        chronic hepatitis and, 1223-1231
        cytomegalovirus and, 1231
        Epstein-Barr virus and, 1231
        herpes simplex viruses and, 1231
        viral hepatitis and, 1210-1223; *see also* Viral hepatitis
    injuries of, 1275
    iron metabolism and, 1271-1273
    kwashiorkor and, 549
    methotrexate and, 183-185, *184*
    microscopic anatomy of, 1199
    necrosis of; *see* Necrosis, liver
    oral contraceptives and adenomas of, 166-167
    polychlorinated biphenyls and, 229
    pregnancy and disease of, 1273-1275
    radiation injury to, 278-279
    radiosensitivity of epithelium of, 257*t*
    regeneration of, 97
    secondary hemochromatosis and siderosis and, 1273
    stages of disease of, 1270
    Swiss-cheese appearance of, 52
    syphilis of, 1285-1286
    tetracycline and vacuolization of, 1237, *1237*
    transplantation of, 1300
    tumors and tumorlike lesions of, 1287-1300
        benign bile duct, 1291-1292
        benign hepatocellular, 1289-1291
        benign mesodermal, 1292

Liver—cont'd
  tumors and tumorlike lesions of—cont'd
    benign tumorlike lesions in, 1292-1293
    cholangiocarcinoma in, 1298
    hepatocellular carcinoma in, 1294-1298;
      see also Liver, carcinoma of
    mesodermal tumors in, 1298-1299
    metastatic, 1299-1300
    primary hepatic carcinoma in, 1293-
      1294
  vascular and biliary supply of, 1199
  weight of, 1208
  Wilson's disease and, 1269-1271
  yellow atrophy of, 1221
    pregnancy and, 1274
Liver biopsy, 1217, 1219, 1222
Liver fluke, 1337
Liver rot, 452
Liver scan, Budd-Chiari syndrome and,
  1282
Lobar emphysema, congenital, 923-925
Lobar pneumonia, 935
  interstitial, 191, *191*
Lobomycosis, 392*t*, 400
Lobular capillary hemangioma in nasal
  cavity, 1081, *1081*
Lobular carcinoma of breast, 1735-1737
Lobular hepatitis, 1228
Lobular inflammation of liver, 1206
Lobular syringoma, 1832, *1832*
Local hyperthermia injuries, 137-140
Local hypothermia injuries, 136
Local infection, 130
Local invasion, neoplastic cells and, 581-
  584, *582*
Lochia, 306
Lockjaw, 294
Löffler's syndrome, 156, 467, 537
  nitrofurantoin and, 174
Löfgren's syndrome, 980
Loiasis, 473
Long-acting thyroid stimulator, 506, 506*t*
  myxedema and, 1781
Long-acting thyroid stimulator protector,
  506, 506*t*
Long bone, 2022, *2022*
Long-chain fatty acids, 2180
Long QT syndrome, 627
Loop
  of Henle, 806, 846, 1575
  of vasa recta, 806
Looser's zones, 1986
Lordosis, 2096
Louis-Bar syndrome, 1051
Low-density lipoprotein, 50-51, 619-620,
  764
  binding of, 4
Low-grade fibromyxoid sarcoma, 1909
Lower urinary tract infection, 834
Lowe's syndrome, 1053
Loyez stain, 2126*t*
LSD; *see* Lysergic acid diethylamide
Lucio, 337
Ludwig's angina, 303, 1144
Luetic aneurysm, 780
Luetic heart disease, 650-652
Lukes-Butler-Hicks classification of
  Hodgkin's disease, 1446
Lukes-Collins classification of non-Hodgkin's
  lymphomas, 1452-1453
Lumbosacral anomalies, 2136
Lung, 920-1046
  acquired immunodeficiency syndrome
    and, 947, 968-969, 1036-1037

Lung—cont'd
  adrenal metastasis from, *1602*
  alveolar microlithiasis and, 982
  alveolar proteinosis and, 981-982
  amyloidosis of, 983
  aspiration pneumonia and, 985
  in asthma, 525
  bacterial infections of, 932-947
    acquired immunodeficiency syndrome
      and, 947
    acute tracheobronchitis in, 932
    anaerobic, 938-939
    mycobacterial, 939-947
    pneumonia and, 932-939
  blast injury and, 135
  bronchiectasis and, 948-951, 1033-1034
  carcinoids of, 1015-1017
  carcinoma of; *see* Lung carcinomas
  chronic airflow limitation and, 987-996,
    1040-1041
    chronic bronchitis in, 987-989
    definitions in, 987
    emphysema in, 989-995
    incidence of, 987
    natural history of, 995
    small airways obstruction in absence of
      atypical chronic bronchitis and
      emphysema in, 996
  collagen-vascular disease and, 972-977,
    1037-1038
  collapse of, 986-987
  congenital anomalies of, 921-925
  development of, 920
  drug- and radiation-induced disease of,
    984-985
  dusts in, 996-997
  extrathoracic injuries and damage to, 962
  herbicide toxicity and, 230
  histiocytosis X and, 977-978
  hypoplasia of, 921-922
  immunologic disease of, 962-967, 1036
  infections of, 930-948, 1031-1033
    bacterial, 932-947; *see also* Lung,
      bacterial infections of
    infant and, 929-930
    mycoplasmal pneumonia in, 932
    Pneumocystis carinii pneumonia and,
      948
    pulmonary defenses in, 931
    routes of, 930-931
    viral, 931-932
  interstitial pneumonia and, 969-972, 1037
  lipid pneumonia and, 985-986
  lymphangiomyomatosis of, 983-984
  mediastinum and, 1023-1026
  metastatic calcification and ossification of,
    982-983
  necrotizing sarcoid granulomatosis and,
    981
  ossification of, 982-983
  osteosarcoma and, *2030*
  parathyroid adenoma and, *1576*
  pediatric disease of, 920-930, 1026-1031
    bronchiolitis and bronchiolitis obliterans
      in, 930
    congenital anomalies in, 921-925
    extrauterine life adaptation and, 925-
      929
    infectious, 929-930
    lung development and, 920
  pneumoconiosis in, 996-1005, 1051-1052;
    see also Pneumoconiosis
  pneumothorax and, 986-987

Lung—cont'd
  pulmonary edema and, 958-962, 1035-
    1036
  pulmonary hemorrhage and, 985
  pulmonary vascular disease of, 951-958,
    1034-1035
  radiation injury to, 274-277
  rheumatic fever and, 648
  sarcoidosis in, 978-981
  sclerosis of skin and, 1780
  shock, 131
  transplantation of, 967-968, 1036-1037
  tumorlike proliferations of, 1023
  tumors of, 1005-1023, 1042-1045
    benign, 1020-1021
    carcinoids in, 1015-1017
    carcinoma in; *see* Lung carcinomas
    carcinosarcoma and pulmonary blastoma
      in, 1019
    lymphoproliferative diseases and, 1021-
      1023
    mesothelial, 1018-1019
    metastatic, 1020
    mucous glands and, 1017
    sarcomas in, 1020
Lung carcinomas, 578, 1004, 1005-1015
  adenocarcinoma in, 582
  adenosquamous, 1011
  asbestosis and, 236
  beryllium compounds and, 237
  bronchogenic, 1006-1013
  classification of, 1006
  clinical manifestations of, 1013
  epidermoid, *1006*, *1007*, *1008*
  etiology of, 1014-1015
  giant cell, 1010, *1011*
  incidence of, 1005-1006
  large cell undifferentiated, 1010-1011
  molecular biology of, 1015
  mortality from, *1005*
  occupational, 238, 1015
  silicosis and, 235
  small cell, 593*t*, *594*, 1011-1012, *1012*
    radiosensitivity of, 257*t*
  undifferentiated, radiation injury and,
    277
  staging and prognosis of, 1013-1014
  superior vena caval syndrome and, 790
Lupoid hepatitis, 1230
Lupus erythematosus, 1769-1772, *1770*
  acute, 1770-1772, *1771*
  cutaneous, 539*t*
  hydralazine and, 168
  pharmacogenetics and, 149
  systemic, 149
    cardiac manifestation of, 652, *653*
    liver disease and, 1287
    pulmonary involvement in, 973-974
    renal manifestations of, 175, 515
Lupus erythematosus cell phenomenon, 148
Lupus erythematosus preparations, 1230
Lupus erythematosus profundus, 1769
Luschka ducts, 1321
Luteal phase defect, 1656
Luteinization, 1672
Luteinizing hormone, 872, 1522
Luteoma of pregnancy, 1674-1675
Lutzomya, 442, 444
Luxol fast blue stain, 2126*t*
Lycopodium, 1189
Lyell's disease, 1765, *1766*
Lyme disease, 451
Lymph flow in inflammation, 84

Lymph nodes, 1429-1474
  abnormalities of structure in, 1431-1433
  axillary, breast carcinoma and, 1741
  cortical sinus of, 1430
  enlargement of, 357
    trypanosomiasis and, 439
  of germ-free and normal animals, 497
  inflammatory-immune reactions of, 1433-
    1443
    reactive lymphoid hyperplasia and,
      1434-1443; see also Lymphoid
      hyperplasia, reactive
  leprosy and, 344
  malignant lymphoma and, 1443-1474; see
    also Lymphoma, malignant
  schema of, 1430
  structure and function of, 1429-1431
    abnormalities of, 1431-1433
  tissue of, clonal analysis of, 1459
  tuberculosis and, 943
Lymphadenitis
  acute necrotizing, 1434
  onchocerciasis, 473
  Toxoplasma, 449
Lymphadenopathies, 1434
  angioimmunoblastic, with dysproteinemia,
    1439, 1441
  dermatopathic, 1438, 1438, 1439
  immunoblastic, 1439
  leukemia and, 1389
  phenytoin, 172, 172, 1439
  proteinaceous, 1432, 1433
  sinus histiocytosis with massive, 1440,
    1441, 1442
Lymphangiectasia
  congenital pulmonary, 923
  of jejunum, 1172, 1172
Lymphangioendothelioma of heart, 700
Lymphangioma, 799, 799
  cutaneous, 1818-1819
  mediastinum and, 1024
  in oral soft tissue, 1109
  salivary glands and, 1141
  of spleen, 1427, 1427
Lymphangioma cavernosum, 1818
Lymphangioma cutis circumscriptum, 1818
Lymphangioma cysticum coli, 1819
Lymphangioma simplex, 799, 1818
Lymphangiomyoma, 799
  pulmonary, 983-984
Lymphangiosarcoma, 797
  postmastectomy, 1823
Lymphangitis, 791
  ascending, 471
  spermatic cord and, 892
Lymphatic leukemia; see Leukemia
Lymphatics, 791-793
  absolute alcohol and, 195-197, 196
  metastasis and, 584
    prostatic carcinoma, 911
  repair and, 98
  of skin, 1756
  urothelial tumors and, 866
Lymphedema, 792-793
  angiosarcoma and, 797
  congenital, 792
Lymphoblastic lymphoma, 1468, 1469
Lymphocyte, 490-538; see also
    Immunopathology
  atypical, 1419
  B-lymphocyte; see B-cells
  chemotaxis and, 80-81
  chronic inflammation and, 93

Lymphocyte—cont'd
  drugs and, 508
  inflammation and, 82
  lymphomas and small, 1462-1464, 1463
  perivascular accumulation and, 527
  radiosensitivity of, 257t
Lymphocyte-permeability factor, 531t
Lymphocyte-stimulating factor, 531t
Lymphocytic choriomeningitis virus, 372-
  373
Lymphocytic cuff, 1430-1431
Lymphocytic depletion type of Hodgkin's
  disease, 1449, 1449
Lymphocytic hypophysitis, 1528-1529
Lymphocytic insulitis, 1362
Lymphocytic leukemia, 849
Lymphocytic predominance type of
  Hodgkin's disease, 1447, 1448
Lymphocytic thyroiditis, 1551-1553, 1553
Lymphocytosis, 1469
  thymic hyperplasia and, 1502
Lymphoepithelial carcinoma in oral soft
  tissue, 1112
Lymphoepithelial cyst
  in neck, 1143, 1143
  in oral cavity, 1120
Lymphoepithelial lesion of salivary glands,
  1129
Lymphoepithelioma, nasopharyngeal, 1083
Lymphogranuloma venereum, 356t, 357
Lymphohistiocytosis, familial
  hemophagocytic, 1424
Lymphoid cell surface receptors, 493
Lymphoid cells, proliferative disorders of,
  1394-1399
Lymphoid follicles, 1430
Lymphoid follicular hyperplasia, 1503
Lymphoid hyperplasia, 534, 1398-1399
  atypical, 1443
  portal, 1202, 1206
  reactive, 1433-1443, 1436
    diffuse, 1438-1440
    follicular, 1435-1438, 1437
    mixed, 1442-1443
    paracortical, 1438-1440
    sinus, 1440-1442
  thymic gland and, 1503
Lymphoid interstitial pneumonia, 1022,
  1022
Lymphoid nodules in Crohn's disease, 1164,
  1164
Lymphoid rosette, 491
Lymphoid system, 487, 495
Lymphoid tissue, 495
  antigenic stimulation and, 496
  central, 499
  gastrointestinal, 495
  testicular tumor metastasis and, 888
Lymphoid tumors initially manifested as
  testicular tumors, 890
Lymphokine-activated killer cells, 493
Lymphokines, 93, 530, 531t
Lymphoma, 578, 610
  acquired immunodeficiency syndrome
    and, 968
  alimentary tract and, 1186-1188
  Burkitt's, 588, 593t, 601, 1455, 1460, 1467
    malaria and, 446
  composite, 1462
  of cuff cells, 1464, 1464-1465
  cutaneous, 1825-1829
  diagnostic and ancillary studies for, 1461
  diffuse
    large cell, 1465-1467

Lymphoma—cont'd
  diffuse—cont'd
    small cleaved cell, 1474
  of follicular cells, 1461-1462
  immunoblastic, 1466
  large cell, 1465-1467
    mediastinum and, 1511
  Lennert's, 1466
  lymphoblastic, 1468, 1469
  malignant, 1443-1474
    bone tumors and, 2021t, 2047, 2047-
      2048
    breast, 1748
    Hodgkin's disease and, 1444, 1444-
      1452, 1445, 1446, 1447, 1448, 1449
    immunodeficiency states and, 1471-1474
    jaws and, 1117
    metastatic neoplasms and, 1474
    non-Hodgkin's, 1452-1474
    oral soft tissue, 1112-1113
    ovarian, 1691
    radiation therapy and, 284
    sinonasal, 1082
    thymus gland and, 1509-1511
    thyroid gland and, 1563-1565, 1565
  of mantle zone cells, 1464, 1464-1465
  Mediterranean type of, 1470
  microgliomas and, 2134
  molecular biology and, 603
  non-Hodgkin's, 1398-1399, 1399
  peripheral T-cell, 1466
  primary central nervous system, 2174
  radiosensitivity of, 257t
  Sjögren's syndrome and, 974
  small cell, 1396-1397, 1462-1464, 1463
    noncleaved, 1467-1469, 1474
  spleen and, 1428-1429
  thymic, radiation and, 266
Lymphomatoid granulomatosis
  in lung, 1022, 1023
  sinonasal, 1082, 1083
  skin and, 1827
Lymphomatoid papulosis, 1827-1829
Lymphomatosis, intravascular malignant,
  1465
Lymphopathia venereum, 895
Lymphopenia, hematopoietic syndrome and,
  273
Lymphopoiesis, 1499
Lymphoproliferative disease, of
  mediastinum, 1025-1026
Lymphoproliferative diseases, of lung, 1021-
  1023
Lymphosarcoma, skin and, 1827
Lymphotoxin, 531t
Lyon hypothesis, 59
Lysergic acid diethylamide, 880
Lysine, 546, 562
Lysis, 12
Lysosomal membrane receptors, 5
Lysosomal overloading, 28
Lysosomal storage diseases, 52-57, 53
Lysosome-phagosome fusion, 942
Lysosomes, 28, 29
  arthritis and, 2075
  leukotrienes and, 75
  liver and, 1201, 1204
  phagocytosis and, 84
Lytic necrosis of hepatocytes, 1242-1243

M
MAC-1, 80
MacCallum patch, 644

Machupo virus, 372-373
Macrocytic anemia, 557
Macrodantin; *see* Nitrofurantoin
Macrodontia, 1097
Macrodystrophia lipomatosa, 1880
Macrofollicular adenoma, 1555
Macroglobulinemia of Waldenström, 1402-
    1403, *1403*, 1470
Macroglossia, 1096
Macromolecules
    radiation and, 254-255
    synthesis of protein, 2-3
Macronodular cirrhosis, 1208
Macrophage, 4
    alveolar, 931
    atherosclerosis and, 764-765
    chronic inflammation and, 92-93
    cordal, 1418
    dendritic, 494
    emphysema and, 995
    granulation tissue and, 98
    hemosiderin-filled, 985
    lung and, 934
    nickel toxicity and, 214, *214, 215*
    starry-sky, 1431
    subpopulation and, 492*t*
    T-B cell cooperation and, *494*
    of tubercle, *90*
Macrophage-activating factor, 531*t*
Macrophage-chemotactic factor, 531*t*
Macrophage-derived growth factors, 765
Macrophage–colony-stimulating factor, 1386*t*
Macroregenerative nodule, 1291, *1291*
Macrovesicular fatty change, 1203
Macula densa, 806
Macular degeneration, age-related, 1072-
    1074
Macule, 1757
Madelung's disease, 1142
Madura foot, 400-402
Maduromycosis, 392*t*, 400-402
Maffucci's syndrome, 795, 1820, 2034, *2035*
Magnesium
    endomyocardial fibrosis and, 697
    lithiasis and, 840
Mahon stain, 2126*t*
Majocchi's disease, 397, 1786
Major histocompatibility complex, 493, 536,
    1496, 1500*t*
Malabsorption syndrome, 467, 1171
Malakoplakia, 856, *857*, 877-878
    alimentary tract and, 1167
    with Michaelis-Gutmann bodies, *1331,
        1332, 1333*
Malaria, 445-448, *448*
    hemolytic anemia and, 1382
Malassez rests, 1099
Malasseziasis, 392*t*, 420, *421*
Malate-asparate shuttle, 1239
Malathion toxicity, 226
Male
    breast carcinoma and, 1747-1748
    infertility and, 872-877
    pseudohermaphroditism and, 1626-1627
    sex differentiation and, 1623-1624
Male reproductive system, 871-919
    epididymis in, 891-892
    penis in, 895-898
    prostate gland and, 899-915, 919; *see also*
        Prostate gland
    radiation injury to, 279-280
    rete testis in, 892
    scrotum in, 893-894

Male reproduction system—cont'd
    seminal vesicles in, 916-917
    spermatic cord in, 892-893
    testes in, 871-891; *see also* Testes
    tunica vaginalis in, 894-895
    urethra in, 898-899
Male XX syndrome, 1625*t*
Malformations, congenital; *see* Congenital
    abnormalities
Malignant angioendotheliomatosis, 1465
Malignant ectomesenchymomas, 1896
Malignant external otitis, 1088
Malignant fibrous histiocytoma, 1853-1860,
    1858
Malignant hemangioendothelioma, 797
    epithelioid, 1299
Malignant histiocytoma, 1856
Malignant histiocytosis, 1425, *1426*
Malignant hyperthermia, 149
Malignant lymphoma, 1443-1474; *see also*
    Lymphoma, malignant
Malignant melanoma, 31, 575, *582*, 594,
    595, 1812-1818
    gastrointestinal, 1184
    histology and histogenesis of, 1814
    melanocarcinomas and, 1817-1818
        pediatric, 1816-1817
    minimal deviation, 1814-1815
    nevi and, 1815-1816
    nodular, *1813*
    in oral soft tissue, 1113
    of soft parts, 1903
    of uvea, 1064
    in vulva, 1637
Malignant mesenchymal tumors of breast,
    1748
Malignant mixed tumor
    müllerian, 1662-1663
    salivary glands and, 1139-1140
Malignant nephrosclerosis, *843*, 843-844,
    844
Malignant nerve sheath tumor, 1894-1896,
    1895
Malignant odontogenic tumor, 1126
Malignant rhabdoid soft-tissue tumor, 1909
Malignant schwannoma, 1894-1896, 2173
Malignant teratoma of ovary, 1689, *1690*
Malignant thymoma, 1507
Malignant tissue, 610; *see also* Neoplasia
Malignant tumors, 575, 575*t*
Malleomyces, 321, 322
Mallory bodies, 192, 195, 1203, 1203*t*, 1270
Mallory Weiss syndrome, 1158
Malnutrition, 546-565
    amino acid deficiencies in, 562
    brain function and, 563
    essential elements and, 562-563
    fatty acid deficiencies in, 562
    heart disease and, 692
    melanosis of Riehl and, 1786
    nutrition and cancer and, 563
    pathogenesis of, 547
    primary and secondary nutritional
        inadequacy in, 547-548
    protein-calorie, 548-550
    salivary gland enlargement and, 1128
    starvation and, 548
    vitamin deficiencies in, 550-561
Malt-worker's lung, 966*t*
Malta fever, 317-318
Mamillary body atrophy, 2185, *2185*
Mammary carcinoma; *see* Breast, carcinoma
    of

Mammary duct ectasia, 1731
Mammary gland involution after weaning,
    42, 43
Mammary hypertrophy, juvenile, 1734
Mammography, 281
Mammoplasty, 1779
Mammosomatotrophic adenoma, 1534
Mammosomatotrophic cells, 1521
Mandible, radiation injury to, 280
Manganese, 562, 563
    chemical pneumonia and, 237
Mannitol, 216
Mannose-6-phosphate, 5
Manson's schistosomiasis, *455*
Mantle zone lymphoma, *1464*, 1464-1465
MAO inhibitor; *see* Monoamine oxidase
    inhibitor
Maple bark stripper's disease, 966*t*
Marasmus, 549
Marbling, perinatal injury and, 2145
Marburg viruses, 376, 1231
March hemoglobinuria, 1382
Marchi stain, 2126*t*
Marfan's syndrome, 50, 780, 783, *784*
    eyes and, 1053
    lung collapse and, 986
Marginal sinus tear of placenta, 1698
Marie-Strümpell disease, 650, 2097-2098
Marinesco bodies, 2133
Marion's disease, 853
Marjolin ulcer, 1801
Markers
    of autoimmunity, 148
    tumor; *see* Tumor markers
Marrow; *see* Bone marrow and blood
Marschalko plasma cells, 1826
Masson bodies, 971
Mast cell, 516, 520
    proliferative disorders of, 1403-1404, *1404*
Mast cell degranulation, *521, 522*
Mast cell mediators, 519*t*
Mastectomy, 1726-1727
    lymphangiosarcoma and, 1823
    survival rate and radical, 1740*t*
Mastocytosis, *1979*
    osteoporosis and, 1979-1981
    systemic, 1404
Mastoid air cells, 1087
Masugi nephritis, 810
Maternal effects on pregnancy, 61
Maternal floor infarcts, 1702
Matrix, repair and, 98
Maturation arrest, male infertility and, 873,
    873
Maxilla, radiation injury to, 280
Maximum tolerated dose, 239
May-Grunwald stain, 396*t*
Mayer's mucicarmine stain, 396*t*
McArdle's disease, 2115, *2115*
McCune-Albright syndrome, 1114
Measles, 367-368
    giant cell pneumonia and, *368*, 368-369
Measles virus, 28
Mebutamate poisoning, 194*t*
Mechanical trauma, 111-133
    amount of force in, 111
    local effects of, 112-130
        firearm injuries and, 119-128
        sequelae of, 128-130
        traffic injuries in, 115-119
        wounds and, 112-115
    myocardial, 698-700
    physical principles in, 111-112

Mechanical trauma—cont'd
  rate of energy transfer and, 111-112
  surface area and, 112
  systemic effects of, 130-133
  target area and, 112
Meckel's diverticulum, 1154, *1154*
Meconium aspiration syndrome, 928
Meconium ileus, 1349, 1350
Meconium peritonitis, 1173
Media, atherosclerosis and, 762, *763*
Medial calcification in infancy, 624
Medial fibrosis, 754
Median rhomboid glossitis, 1096
Mediastinal cysts, 1024-1025, 1025*t*
Mediastinal tumors, 1025*t*, 1025-1026
Mediastinitis, 163, 1024
Mediastinopericarditis, 667
Mediastinum, 1023-1026, 1511
  anatomic division of, 1023-1024
  developmental cysts of, 1024-1025, 1025*t*
  mediastinitis and, 163, 1024
  pneumomediastinum and, 1024
  therapeutic radiation to, 274
  thoracic thyroid and parathyroids and, 1026
  tumors of, 1025*t*, 1025-1026
Medicolegal evidence in death by gunfire, 124-125
Medicolegal problems with traffic injuries, 118-119
Medina worm infection, 473-474
Mediterranean fever, 317-318, 1189
Mediterranean type of lymphoma, 1470
Medulla
  adrenal, 1580, 1607-1613
  bone and, 2022
  lymph node, 495
Medullary carcinoma
  of breast, 1743, *1743*
  of thyroid gland, 1562-1563, *1564*
Medullary cystic diseases, 846-847, *847*
Medullary sinuses, 1430
Medullary tumor, 610
Medulloblastoma, 579, *2170*, 2170-2171
Megacolon, aganglionic, 1154
Megakaryocytes, 1373
Megaloblastic anemia, *1377*, 1377-1378
Megalonodular B-viral cirrhosis, 1227, *1227*
Megamitochondria in hepatocytes, 1241, *1242*
Meigs' syndrome, 1685
Meissner's corpuscles, 1756
Meissner's plexus, 1154
Melanin, 30-31
Melanin-stimulating hormone, 30
Melanocarcinoma, *1815*
  of bronchus, *1818*
  of mucous membranes, 1817-1818
  pediatric, 1816-1817
  in situ, 1815-1816
Melanocyte-stimulating hormone, 1522, 1534
Melanocytes, 1753
Melanoma
  juvenile, 1804-1810, *1806*, *1807*
  malignant; *see* Malignant melanoma
  thin, 1813
Melanophores, 1803
Melanosis
  of colon, 1156
  of Riehl, 1786
Melanotic freckle of Hutchinson, 1811-1812

Melanotic neuroectodermal tumor of infancy, 1116
Melanotic pigmentation in oral soft tissue, 1106
Melasmic staining, 1106
Melena, 1186
Melioidosis, 292*t*, 322-324
Melkersson-Rosenthal syndrome, 1103
Membrane potential, 8
Membranoproliferative glomerulonephritis, 457, 517*t*, 816-818, *817*, *818*, *819*
Membranous glomerulonephritis, *514*, 516
  lupus, 825
Membranous nephropathy, 517*t*, 819-820, *820*, *821*
Membranous obstruction of vena cava
  Budd-Chiari syndrome and, 1282
  hepatocellular carcinoma and, 1295-1296
Membranous ossification, *1940*, 1941
Ménétrier's disease, 1171
Meninges
  carcinomatosis and, 2175
  cysticercosis and, 459
Meningioma, 2171, *2171*
  cutaneous, 1821
Meningitis, 290, 306, 2154-2158
  acute purulent, *2154*, 2154-2155, *2155*
  aseptic, 2158
  chronic, 2155-2158
  complications of, 2155
  cryptococcal, 2155-2156, *2156*
  meningococcal, 307
  mumps and, 366
  tuberculous, 2155, *2156*
Meningocele, 2137
Meningococcemia, fulminant, 308, *308*
Meningococci, 307-309
  wound infection and, 130
Meningoencephalitis, 370, 2158
  amebic, 437
  eosinophilic, 468, *469*
Meningoencephalocele, 1077
Meningomyelocele, 2136, 2137, *2137*
  mediastinum and, 1024
  syringomyelia and, 2140
Menkes' syndrome, 2116
Menopause, 1674
  hyperparathyroidism and, 1572
Menstrual cycle, corpus luteum in, *1672*
Mental retardation
  fetal irradiation and, 269
  X chromosome–linked, 49
Meperidine poisoning, 194*t*
Meprobamate poisoning, 193*t*
Mercaptopurine
  cholestasis with necrosis and, 1234*t*, 1235
  toxicity of, 183, 185
Mercurial diuretic toxicity, 203
Mercuric chloride, 200
Mercuric oxide, 203
Mercuric sulfide, 1785
Mercury toxicity, 194*t*, 200-205, *201*, *202*, *204-205*, 831
Merkel cell tumor, 1801-1802
Merkel-Ranvier corpuscles, 1757
Merocrania, 2136
Mesangial glomerulonephritis, 825
  ibuprofen toxicity and, 162
Mesangiocapillary glomerulonephritis, 817
Mesangioproliferative glomerulonephritis, 815-816
Mesangium, 805, *805*
Mesencephalon, 2135

Mesenchymal breast tumors, 1748
Mesenchymal chondrosarcoma, 2021*t*, *2042*
Mesenchymal hamartoma, 1293
Mesenchymal malignant fibrous histiocytoma, 1858
Mesenchymal neoplasms, 574*t*, 847
Mesenchymal odontogenic tumors, 1123-1125
Mesenchymal sarcoma of liver, 1299
Mesenchyme-sex cord tumors, 1684-1686
Mesenteric angiography, hemobilia and, 1258
Mesentery, 1190-1191
  neoplasms of, 1191
    leiomyosarcoma of, 1864
    metastatic, 1191
  panniculitis and, 1190
Mesodermal tumor
  endometrial, 1662-1663
  hepatic, 1292, 1298-1299
Mesonephric cysts, 1669
Mesonephroma, 1652, 1683
Mesorchium, 871
Mesothelial cells, 599
Mesothelial lesions of tunica vaginalis, 895
Mesothelial tumors of lung, 1018-1019
Mesothelioma, 578
  asbestos exposure and, 236, 1004
  of heart, 700
  occupational, 238
  peritoneum and, 236, 1191
Mesotheliomas, of pleura, 236
Mesothelium of ovary, 1673
Mesothorium toxicity, 186
Messenger ribonucleic acid, 2, 3
met, 587*t*
Metabolic activity of cell, 12
Metabolic bone diseases, 1957-2000
  beta$_2$-microglobulin amyloidosis in hemodialysis and, 2000
  definition of, 1957
  morphologic diagnosis of, 1957-1958
  osteomalacia and rickets in, 1983-2000
    classification of, 1983-1984
    clinical manifestations of, 1984-1986
    histologic features of, 1986, 1988-1990
    25-hydroxylation and, 1993
    hypophosphatasia and, 1997-2000
    hypophosphatemic, 1993-1995
    radiography of, 1986-1988
    renal osteodystrophy and, 1995-1997
    vitamin D deficiency and, 1990-1993
    vitamin D–dependent rickets in, 1993
  osteoporosis in, 1958-1982
    general features of, 1958-1959
    histopathology of, 1959-1965
    primary, 1965-1971
    secondary, 1971-1982; *see also*
      Osteoporosis, secondary
  vitamin A and, 1982
  vitamin C and, 1982-1983
Metabolic control, 10-11
Metabolic disorders
  of bone; *see* Metabolic bone diseases
  central nervous system, 2184-2185
  congestive cardiomyopathy and, 686-689
  jaundice and, 1266-1267
  jaws and, 1113-1116
  liver diseases of postneonatal infancy and, 1261*t*, 1267
  pituitary gland and, 1529
  skeletal muscle, 2114-2117
Metabolic pools of molecules, 6

Metabolic transformation of lipophilic
    chemical, 147
Metabolic tubulointerstitial toxicity, 839-840
Metabolism
    arachidonic acid, 522
    errors of, 51-58
        cell injury and; see Cell injury
    ethanol, 1238-1240
    liver disease and iron, 1271-1273
    myocardial ischemia and, 630-631
    purine, 499
    tumors and, 605
Metabolites
    accumulation of, 57, 631
    gastrointestinal inflammation and, 1168
    reactive, 147-148
Metacercariae, 452
Metachromasia, pancreas and, 1349
Metachromatic leukodystrophy, 2180, 2180
Metachromatic leukoencephalopathy, 1173
Metallic abnormalities of cutaneous
    pigmentation, 1785
Metallic conductor, 143
Metallic salts; see Metals and metallic salts
Metallothioneine
    cadmium toxicity and, 213
    renal concentration of, 200
Metals and metallic salts, 200-216
    arsenic in, 209-210
    cadmium in, 212-213, 213
    cobalt in, 212
    ferrous sulfate in, 210-212, 211
    lead in, 205-209, 206, 207
    mercury in, 200-205, 201, 202, 204-205
    nickel in, 214, 214, 215, 216
    platinum in, 216
    thallium in, 214-216
    uranium in, 216
Metanephric kidney, 850
Metaphyseal fibrous defect, 2022t, 2059,
    2059-2060
Metaphyses, 2022, 2022
Metaplasia, 106-108, 569-570, 610
    in bladder, 857-858
    in connective tissues, 107-108
    endometrium and, 1656
    in epithelium, 107
    fallopian tube papillary tumor and, 1670
    peritoneum and, 1190
    squamous; see Squamous metaplasia
    transitional cell prostate, 912, 914
Metarteriole, 796
Metastases, 575, 576, 581, 583, 584-585, 610
    to adrenal, 1605
    from adrenal gland neuroblastomas, 1612
    from adrenocortical carcinoma, 1604-1605
    angiogenesis and, 102
    assay for potential, 585
    bone, 2055-2056
    bone marrow and, 1406-1408
    to brain, 2174-2175
    breast carcinoma, 1069, 1069
    cervical adenocarcinoma, 1652
    endometrial carcinoma, 1663
    to eyes, 1069, 1069
    fallopian tube carcinoma, 1671
    to heart, 704, 704t, 704-705
    hepatic, 1299-1300
    liver carcinoma, 1299
    lung, calcification in, 982-983
    lymph node, 1474
        testicular tumor in, 888
    myometrial leiomyoma, 1665-1666

Metastases—cont'd
    ovarian, 1691
    pituitary gland carcinoma, 1535
    prostatic carcinoma, 911
    pulmonary, 1020
    salivary gland pleomorphic adenoma, 1140
    skin and, 1830
    spleen and, 1427
    testicular, 888
    to thyroid gland, 1565
    vaginal carcinoma, 1641
    vulvar carcinoma, 1637
Metastatic calcification, 36, 37, 693
    parathyroid glands and, 1575
Methacholine, 962
Methamphetamine poisoning, 194t
Methanol toxicity, 193t, 197-198
Methapyrilene poisoning, 194t
Methaqualone poisoning, 194t
Methionine, 546, 562
Methotrexate toxicity, 183, 984, 1235t, 1238
Methoxyflurane toxicity, 171, 1236
Methoxypsoralin, 286
Methyl alcohol toxicity, 197-198
Methyl mercury, 200
Methyl salicylate toxicity, 158-160
Methyldopa
    adverse reactions to, 168
    granulomas and, 1285
Methylmercaptan, 1248
2-Methyl-1,4-naphthoquinone, 555
Methyltestosterone
    adverse reactions to, 165
    hepatocellular adenoma and, 1289
Methyprylon poisoning, 194t
Methysergide toxicity, 186
Metronidazole, colitis and, 155
MHC; see Major histocompatibility complex
Mibelli angiokeratoma, 1820
Michaelis-Gutmann bodies, 856, 857, 878
    malakoplakia and, 1331, 1332, 1333
Microadenoma
    adrenal, with hypercortisolism, 1592
    pituitary gland and, 1530
Microangiopathy, diabetic, 1364-1367
Microatelectasis, 932
Micrococcus, 293, 301, 302
Microcystic adnexal carcinoma, 1833
Microcystic liver disease, 1293
Microdontia, 1097
Microfilaments, neurofibrillary degeneration
    and, 2133
Microfilariae, 470
Microfollicular adenoma, 1555
Microglandular hyperplasia of cervix, 1643-
    1644, 1644
Microglia, 2134-2135
Microgliomas, 2134
Microglossia, 1095, 1096
Micrognathia, 1095
Microinvasive carcinoma of cervix, 1645-
    1650, 1646
Microlithiasis, alveolar, 189, 189, 982
Micronodular cirrhosis, 1208
    sickle cell anemia and, 1287
Microsomal antigen, 507t
Microsomal ethanol-oxidizing system, 1240
Microsporum, 392t, 397, 398, 399
Microtubules, neurofibrillary degeneration
    and, 2132-2133
Microvilli of hepatocyte, 1200
Microwaves, 285, 285t
    testicular germ cell tumors and, 880

Midbrain, 2135
Middle ear, 1087-1088
Midline destruction in nasal cavity, 1079-
    1080
Midline lethal granuloma, 1104
Midline malignant reticulosis, 1082, 1083
Migrating cells, 95, 96
Migration disorders, congenital central
    nervous system, 2138-2139
Migration-inhibitory factor, 527, 531t
Mikulicz cells, 1079
Mikulicz's disease, 1129
Miliary tuberculosis, 944, 944-945
    of spleen, 1418, 1419
Milieu, cellular, 12
Milk-alkali syndrome, 189, 189-191, 982
Milk spots, 667
Milkman's syndrome, 1986
Millirem, 249
Milroy's disease, 792
Mine dust, 997
Mineral dusts, 35
Mineral homeostasis, 1944
Mineral oil toxicity, 190, 191
Mineralization, bone, 1959
    disorders of, 1957-2000; see also
        Metabolic bone diseases
    regulation of, 1945-1946
Mineralocorticoids, 1581
Miners
    dust and, 997
    lung carcinoma and, 276-277
    terrestrial radiation and, 250
Minimal change disease, 517t, 818-819, 819
    ibuprofen toxicity and, 162
Minimal deviation melanoma, 1814-1815
Minor histocompatibility antigens, 493
Minute chemodectoma, 1023
Miscarriage, 1700-1701
Missed abortion, 1700
Mitochondria, 292t
    cobalt toxicity and, 212
    ethanol toxicity and, 195, 195, 1204
    ferrous sulfate toxicity and, 212
    lead toxicity and, 206, 207
    liver and, 1201, 1204
    radiation injury and, 255
Mitochondrial antibody test, 1256
Mitochondrial myopathies, 2116-2117, 2117
Mitomycin C toxicity, 180-182, 596, 597t
Mitoses
    ionizing radiation and, 24-25
    leiomyosarcomas and, 1863-1864
    lymphoblastic lymphomas and, 1469
    radiosensitivity and, 256
Mitral insufficiency, 673-674
    rheumatic fever and, 645
Mitral regurgitation, myocardial infarction
    and, 638
Mitral stenosis, 672-673, 673
    rheumatic endocarditis and, 645, 645, 647
Mitral valve, rheumatic endocarditis and,
    645, 645, 646, 647
Mitral valve calcification, 676-677
Mitral valve prolapse, 676
Mitsuda reaction, 337
Mixed connective tissue disease, 1772
Mixed-function oxidase system, 1232
Mixed gallstones, 1323, 1324, 1325t, 1330
    cholecystitis and, 1330, 1330
Mixed gliomas, 2170
Mixed gonadal dysgenesis, 1626

Mixed hamartoma, 1291
Mixed medullary-follicular carcinoma, 1563
Mixed mesodermal tumor of endometrium, 1662-1663
Mixed odontogenic tumors, 1125-1127
Mixed osteomalacia–osteitis fibrosa, 1995-1997
Mixed rhabdomyosarcoma tumor, 1866
Mixed salivary gland tumor, 1132t, 1132-1134
    malignant, 1139-1140
Mixed tumor, 610
Modeling of bone, 1941, 1941, 1943
    fractures and, 2001
Molar trophoblast, 1708
Mole, 1813
    hydatidiform, 1706, 1706-1709, 1707, 1708
Molecular abnormalities, 47
Molecular biology, diagnostic, 603
Molecular radiation biology, 250-255
Molecules
    biologically active, 505, 505-506
    exogenous, 506
Molluscum contagiosum, 386, 387, 1760
Molybdenum, 563
Mönckeberg's medial calcific sclerosis, 754, 757
Mondor's disease, 1790
Mongolian spot, 1810
Monkeypox, 386
Monoamine oxidase inhibitor, 168
Monochorionic twin placentas, 1699
Monoclonal antibody, 494
Monoclonal gammopathies, 1403, 1469-1470
Monoclonal hypothesis, 621
Monocytes, 492t, 934
    atherosclerosis and, 764-765
    chemotaxis and, 80
    inflammation and, 82-83
    perivascular accumulation of, 527
Monocytoid B-cells, 1442
Monoiodotyrosine, 1544
Monokines, 93
Monomorphic salivary gland adenoma, 1134
Monomorphous rhabdomyosarcoma tumor, 1866
Mononucleosis, infectious; see Infectious mononucleosis
Monorchidism, 871
Monosodium urate, 2087
Monosomy, 46
Monosporium apiospermum, 423
Morfamquat dichloride toxicity, 230
Morgagni
    crypts of, 1168
    hydatid of, 892
Morphea, subcutaneous, 1780
Morphea guttata, 1779
Morphine
    oxygen toxicity and, 219
    toxicity of, 193t, 219
Morsicatio buccarum, 1110
Morton's neuroma, 1890
Morula, 403
mos, 587t
Mosaic cells, 422
    leukemia and isoenzyme, 1384
Mosquito, 445, 470, 529
Mothballs, 198
Mother cysts, 461
Motor end plate, 2118
Motor neuron disease, 2120, 2183
Mottled enamel, 1098

Mouth
    radiosensitivity of, 257t
    squamous cell carcinoma of, 1111
    trench, 1105
mRNA; see Messenger ribonucleic acid
Mseleni disease, 2075
MSH; see Melanin-stimulating hormone; Melanocyte- stimulating hormone
Mu heavy-chain disease, 1470
Mucin, 1180
Mucin-producing cells, 1556
Mucinous adenocarcinoma of prostate gland, 915
Mucinous ascites, 1682
Mucinous cysts of dermis, 1782
Mucinous tumors of ovary, 1680-1683, 1681
Mucocele
    of appendix, 1188
    in orbit of eye, 1047, 1050
    of paranasal sinuses, 1078-1079
    of salivary glands, 1127-1128, 1128
Mucocutaneous diseases of oral soft tissues, 1100-1103
Mucocutaneous lymph node syndrome, 774-775, 776
    skin and, 1830
Mucoepidermoid tumors
    of bronchi, 1017
    of salivary glands, 1137, 1137-1138
Mucoid degeneration
    of mitral valve, 676
    of myocardium, 687-688, 688
Mucolipidoses, 53, 55-57
Mucophages, 1078
Mucopolysaccharidoses, 52-55, 53, 686
    cornea and, 1074, 1075
Mucormycosis, 395t, 425-426
    infective endocarditis and, 654
    upper airway and, 426, 1079
Mucosa
    gallbladder
        diverticula of, 1331, 1331
        ulcerated, 1332, 1332
    herpetic infection of, 379
    squamous cell carcinoma of buccal, 1111-1112
Mucous glands
    pancreas and, 1348
    tumors of pulmonary, 1017
Mucous membranes
    melanocarcinomas of, 1817-1818
    pemphigoid and, 1102
    radiosensitivity of, 257t
Mucoviscidosis, 1348
Mucus plugs, 993
Mucus retention phenomenon, 1127-1128, 1128
Muir-Torre syndrome, 1833
Mulberry molars, 1105
Müllerian ducts
    cysts of, 902, 1626
    embryology and, 1620-1623
Müllerian elements, 873
Müllerian endometrial tumor, 1662-1663, 1663
Müllerian inhibiting substance, 569, 582, 1624, 1625t
Müllerian system, 1627
    secondary, 1684
Müller's tubercle, 1623
Multi-CSF, 590t
Multicentric angiofollicular lymph node hyperplasia, 1437

Multicystic encephalomalacia, 2139
Multidrug resistance, 606
Multifocal leukoencephalopathy, progressive, 2162, 2178, 2178-2179
Multinodular adrenals, 1588-1589, 1591-1592
Multinucleated giant cells, 91, 91, 92, 92, 93
    neonatal hepatitis and, 1263, 1263
    radiation injury and, 250
    viruses and, 28
Multiple deficiency states, 546
Multiple endocrine adenomatosis, 609, 1563
    pituitary gland and, 1535
Multiple epiphyseal dysplasia, 1957, 1957, 1958
Multiple gestation, 1698-1699
Multiple hepatocellular adenomatosis, 1289-1290, 1291
Multiple mucosal neuromas of thyroid gland, 1563
Multiple myeloma
    jaws and, 1117
    kidneys and, 839, 839
Multiple neurofibromatosis, 50
Multiple nevoid basal cell carcinoma syndrome, 2166
Multiple pulmonary fibroleiomyoma, 1666
Multiple sclerosis, 2176-2177
Multiplication of new cells, 96
Mumps, 366, 366, 1130
Mumps orchitis, 876, 877
Mural endocardial lesions of rheumatic fever, 644
Mural thrombi, 701, 703t, 778
Murine typhus, 349t, 354
Murphy staging system for childhood non-Hodgkin's lymphoma, 1471, 1471t
Muscle
    atrophy of, 42-43, 2108-2109, 2109
        chilhood dermatomyositis and perifascicular, 2118, 2118
        infantile spinal, 2120-2121, 2121
        neurogenic, 2119, 2119-2121, 2120
    biopsy of, 2107-2108
    gas gangrene and, 296
    hypertrophy of, 2109
    injury to, 2108-2111
    regeneration of, 97-98
    skeletal; see Skeletal muscle diseases
    smooth; see Smooth muscle
    striated, 2105
    tumors of, 1823-1825
    ultrastructure of, 58, 2105
Muscle cell
    radiosensitivity of, 257t
    ultrastructure of, 58, 2105
Muscle clamp, 2108
Muscle fiber, 2105, 2106
    atrophy of; see Muscle, atrophy of
    parasitized, 465
    ragged-red, 2116, 2117
    skeletal; see Skeletal muscle fiber
    target, 2119-2120, 2120
    vacuolization of, 2110, 2110
Muscle spindle, 2105
Muscular arteries, 752, 753
Muscular dystrophies, 2109, 2111-2112
    fiber necrosis and, 2110
    myocardial involvement and, 694
Muscular subaortic stenosis, 682
Musculoaponeurotic fibromatoses, 1846
Mushrooms, 224, 966t, 1233

Mutagen, radiation as, 261
Myasthenia gravis, 506t, 2118-2119
    experimental allergic or naturally
        occurring, 507
    lymphocytes and, 508
    myocardial degeneration and necrosis and,
        694
    thymic hyperplasia and, 1504
    thymomas and, 1506, 1508
myb, 587t
myc, 587, 587t, 600
Mycelium, 397
Mycetoma, 392t, 400-402, 401
Mycobacterial infection, 498t
    in acquired immunodeficiency syndrome,
        947
    of lung, 939-947
    nontuberculous, 946-947
Mycobacterium avium-intracellulare, 946,
        947, 1167, 1473
    acquired immunodeficiency syndrome
        and, 1286
Mycobacterium bovis, 940
Mycobacterium chelonei, 946
Mycobacterium fortuitum, 946
Mycobacterium kansasii, 946
Mycobacterium leprae, 333, 939; see also
        Leprosy
Mycobacterium marinum, 946
Mycobacterium scrofulaceum, 946
Mycobacterium tuberculosis, 314, 382, 939,
        1084, 1668
    bone and, 2006
    caseation necrosis and, 13
    initial response to, 90
    meningitis and, 2154, 2155
Mycoplasma, 313-314, 1657, 1705
    placenta and, 1705
    pneumonia and, 314, 932, 988
Mycosis fungoides, 1469, 1825-1827
    with Pautrier-Darier abscesses, 1826
Mycosis fungoides d'emblée, 1826
Mycotic infections, 391-432; see also Fungi
    allergic bronchopulmonary, 964-965
    aneurysm and, 767, 778
        hemorrhage from ruptured, 2151
    cutaneous and subcutaneous, 399-406
        chromoblastomycosis in, 399-400
        lobomycosis in, 400
        mycetoma in, 400-402
        mycosis fungoides and, 1826, 1826
        phaeohyphomycosis in, 402
        prototheceosis in, 402-404
        rhinosporidiosis in, 404
        sporotrichosis in, 404-406
    superficial, 397-399
    systemic, 406-427
        actinomycosis in, 406-407
        adiaspiromycosis in, 407
        aspergillosis in, 407-410
        blastomycosis in, 410
        botryomycosis in, 410-411
        candidiasis in, 411-413
        coccidioidomycosis in, 413-415
        cryptococcosis in, 415-416
        fusariosis in, 416-417
        geotrichosis in, 417-418
        histoplasmosis capsulati in, 418-419
        histoplasmosis duboisii in, 419-420
        malasseziasis in, 420
        nocardiosis in, 420-421
        paracoccidioidomycosis in, 421-422
        penicilliosis marneffei in, 422-423

Mycotic infections—cont'd
    systemic—cont'd
        pseudallescheriasis in, 423
        torulopsosis in, 423-424
        trichosporonosis in, 424-425
        zygomycosis in, 425-427
Myelin, 97
    loss of, 2176-2180
        beriberi and, 556
Myelinated axons, 2135
Myelination glia, 2135
Myelinolysis, central pontine, 2179
Myeloblastic leukemia, 602
Myelodysplastic syndromes, 1386t, 1390
    colony-stimulating factors and, 1390
    French-American-British classification of,
        1388t
Myelofibrosis, primary, 1394, 1394, 1395
Myelogenous leukemias, radiation and, 279
Myeloid cells
    erythroid cell ratio to, 1373
    proliferative disorders of, 1390-1394
    stem cell and, 1374
Myeloid metaplasia, spleen and, 1411
Myelolipoma, adrenal gland, 1605-1606,
        1606
Myeloma
    amyloidosis and, 695
    multiple
        jaws and, 1117
        kidneys and, 839, 839
        plasma cell, 1399-1401, 1400-1402
            bone and, 2048-2050
        radiation injury and, 279
Myeloma kidney, 1402
Myelophthisic anemia, 1379
Myeloproliferative disorders, chronic, 1393-
        1394
Myelotoxins, 1385
Myleran; see Busulfan
Myoblastoma, 1824-1825
    biliary tract and, 1334
    in oral soft tissue, 1108
    skin and, 1824
Myoblasts, rhabdomyosarcoma and, 1865
Myocardial contusion, 699
Myocardial fibrosis
    Chagas' disease and, 442
    radiation and, 699
Myocardial hypertrophy, 690
Myocardial infarction, 627-639
    cellular consequences of ischemia in, 630-
        633
    early and late cardiac complications of,
        637-639
    early diagnosis of, 633-635
    expansion of, 638
    hemopericardium and, 664
    inflammatory response and reparative
        phase of, 635-637
    location of, 628, 628-629
    organization of, 637
    pericarditis in, 672
    sudden cardiac death and, 627
    sudden onset of ischemia in, 627-628
    transmural extent and course of, 629-630
Myocardial ischemia, 20-21, 21, 627; see
        also Myocardial infarction
    aortic stenosis and, 675
    causes and consequences of, 624-625, 626
    cellular consequences of, 630-633
Myocardial reperfusion, 629, 632-633
Myocardial scars, 636

Myocarditis, 659-664, 660, 661, 662, 663
    cellular infiltrate in, 659
    Chagas' disease and, 442, 442
    endomyocardial biopsy and, 707-708
    infective endocarditis and, 657
    methyldopa and, 168
    rheumatic fever and, 645
    specific and nonspecific, 659
    in typhus fever, 353
Myocardium
    abscess of, 87
    alcoholics and, 194
    alkylating agents and, 180
    calcification of, 693
    carbon monoxide poisoning and, 222
    catecholamine toxicity and, 217, 217
    cocaine toxicity and, 220
    cysticercosis of, 460
    diphtheria toxin and, 295
    disorders of, 681-700; see also
        Cardiomyopathies and myocardial
        disorders; Myocardial infarction
    ischemia of; see Myocardial ischemia
    lacework appearance of, 687
    trichiniasis and, 466
Myocyte
    hypertrophy of, 679
    hypovolemic shock and, 700
Myoepithelioma, salivary gland, 1136
Myofiber disarray, 683-684
Myofibril, 2105-2106
Myofibrillar change
    catecholamines and, 217
    cocaine and, 220
Myofibroblastic tumor, inflammatory, 1292-
        1293
Myofibroblasts, 1844, 1858
    healing by second intention and, 106
    wound contraction and, 104
Myofibromatosis, 1849-1850
Myogenesis of rhabdomyosarcoma, 1865
Myoglobin
    electrical burns and urinary, 143
    rhabdomyosarcoma and, 1866
Myoid cells, 1494
Myometrium, 1661, 1663-1667
Myopathies
    alcoholic, 194
    centronuclear, 2113-2114
    congenital, 2112-2114
    distal, 2112
    immune-mediated, 2117-2119
    inflammatory, 2117-2119
    mitochondrial, 2116-2117, 2117
    nemaline, 2113, 2114
Myophosphorylase deficiency, 2115
Myosin, cell movement and, 6
Myosin-ribosome complex, 1866
Myositis, proliferative, 1852, 1852
Myositis ossificans, 107
Myospherulosis, 1079
Myotonic muscular dystrophy, 2112
Myotubular myopathy, 2114
Myxedema, 1523, 1524, 1545
    cardiovascular disturbances and, 690
    circumscribed, 1781-1782
    pericarditis and, 666
Myxoid cysts, dermal, 1782
Myxoid hamartoma, 1878, 1909
Myxoid leiomyosarcoma, 1863
Myxoid liposarcoma, 1874, 1875
Myxoid malignant fibrous histiocytoma, 1856
Myxoid tumors, 1854

Myxoma, 1896-1898
  of heart, 701-703, *702*
  intramuscular, *1897*
  odontogenic, 1123, *1125*

N

N-*myc*, 587*t*, 588, 589
N-*ras*, 587*t*, 589
NAD; *see* Nicotinamide adenine
    dinucleotide
NADH; *see* Reduced nicotinamide adenine
    dinucleotide
NADPH; *see* Reduced nicotinamide adenine
    dinucleotide phosphate
Naegleria, 437
  meningitis and, 2154
Nail diseases, 1787
Naphthalene, 198
Narcotics
  children and, 150
  toxicity of, 219-220
Nasal cavity, 1078-1083
  carcinoma of, 1082
  destructive midline processes in, 1079-
      1080
Nasal glioma, 1077
Nasal polyps, 525, 1078, *1078*
  asthma and, 964
Nasal septum, fungiform papilloma of, *1080*
Nasoalveolar cyst, 1120
Nasolabial cyst, 1077, 1120
Nasopalatine duct cyst, 1120
Nasopharyngitis, 303
Nasopharynx, 1083-1084
  carcinoma of, *1083*, 1083-1084
Natural killer cells, 492
Natural tolerance, 497
Nebenkerns, 1521
Necator americanus, 463
Neck, 1141-1144
  cysts of, 1120
  irradiation and, 281
  traffic injuries and, 116, *117*
Necrobiosis lipoidica diabeticorum, *1778*,
    1778-1779
Necrosis, 13, 85-86, *86*
  acidophilic, 1205
  caseation, 91
  central nervous system and, 2146-2150
  cholecystitis and, 1328
  chronic inflammation and, 90
  coagulation, 1205
    electrical burns and, 141
  confluent, 1205
  electrical injury and, 142
  fibrinoid, *513*
    rheumatic fever and, 648, *648*
  of globus pallidus, *221*, 222
  hepatoadrenal, 379
  liver, 379, 1202, 1204-1205, 1220, *1220*
    anoxic, 1278, *1278*, *1279*
    bridging, 1205
    carbon tetrachloride and, 222, *223*
    drug toxicity and, 1234*t*, 1235-1236
    halothane and, 1236, *1237*
    hypoxic, 1278-1279
    immunosuppressants and, 1230
    ischemic neuronal, 2132
    lead poisoning and, 206, *209*
    massive, 1205, 1220, *1220*, 1221, 1227
    perivenular, 1278
    sclerosing hyaline, 1243
    submassive, 1205, *1220*, 1220-1221

Necrosis—cont'd
  liver—cont'd
    viral hepatitis and, 1218, 1226
    Wilson disease and, 1270, *1270*
    zonal, 1204
  mercury poisoning and, 203, *204*
  myocardial, *632*, 632-633; *see also*
      Myocardial infarction
  perinatal injury and, 2143-2145
  renal tubular, 830-832, 1252
    ischemic acute, 832-833, *833*
  rheumatic fever and, 641
  types of, 13-16
Necrotizing angiitis, 172
Necrotizing enterocolitis, 1166
Necrotizing glomerulonephritis, 813
Necrotizing lymphadenitis, 1434
Necrotizing panarteritis, 623
Necrotizing pancreatitis, 137, *138*
Necrotizing pneumonia, 939
Necrotizing renal papillitis, 837
Necrotizing sarcoid granulomatosis of lung,
    981
Necrotizing sialometaplasia, 1131, *1131*
Necrotoxin, 302
Needle biopsy
  biliary atresia and, 1262
  bone tumors and, 2024
Negri bodies, 370, *370*, 2133
Neisseria, 292*t*
Neisseria gonorrhoeae, 309, 1105, 1638,
    1667
Neisseria meningitidis, 307, *308*, 2154
Nelson's syndrome, 1534
Nemaline myopathy, 2113, *2114*
Nematodes, 462-474
  digestive tract, 462-469
    capillariasis in, 466-467
    larva migrans in, 467-469
  filarial, 470-474
Neo-Silvol, 1785
Neoantigen, 512*t*
Neocholangioles, 1207
Neomycin toxicity, 157
Neonate; *see* Newborn
Neoplasia, 566-614; *see also* Tumor; specific
      organ
  adrenal
    adrenocortical, 1599-1605, *1602*, *1603*,
      1603*t*
    child and, 1586
    histologic assessment of, 1603*t*
    medullary, 1608-1613
  alimentary tract, 1156-1157, 1175-1188
    carcinoid and, 1184-1186, *1185*
    smooth muscle, 1186
  azathioprine toxicity and, 185-186
  bone
    characteristics of, 2021-2022*t*
    chondroblastic, 2040-2043
    giant cell, 2043-2045
    osteoblastic, 2028-2034
    vascular, *2050*
  cartilage and, 2041
  cell characteristics in, 579-586; *see also*
      Neoplastic cells
  cell growth variations and, 567-573
  cervical, 1645-1652
  coronary artery disease and, 624
  course and treatment of, 606-607
  definition of, 566-567
  demographic and familial aspects of, 607-
      610

Neoplasia—cont'd
  diagnostic approaches to, 603-605
  endometrial, 1659-1663
  etiology and pathogenesis of, 586-602
    carcinogens in, 594-602
    chromosomal changes in, 591-594
    growth factors in, 589-594
    oncogenes in, 586-589
  of exocrine pancreas, 1354-1357
  of fallopian tube, 1670-1671
  fibrosis and, 1207
  future prospects for diagnosis and
      treatment of, 589
  gallbladder and biliary ducts and, 1335-
      1343
  genetic analysis of, 60-61
  grading and staging in, 602-603
  of heart, 700-705
  heart conducting system and, 705-706
  hyperplasia and, 44
  interrelationship of tumor and host in,
      605-606
  liver and; *see* Liver, tumors and tumorlike
      lesions of
  myometrial, 1664-1667
  nasal cavity, 1081-1083
  nomenclature and taxonomy of, 573-579
  nonbacterial thrombotic endocarditis and,
      652, 653
  ovarian; *see* Ovary, neoplasms of
  pericarditis and, 670
  radiation injury and, 269, 274
  renal, 847-849
  in seminal vesicles, 916-917
  skin, 1793-1802; *see also* Skin, neoplasms
      of
  Thorotrast toxicity and, 186, *187-188*
  thymus gland and, 1504-1512
  thyroid gland and, 1556-1565
  trophoblastic, 1706-1710
  of urethra, 899
  of vagina, 1640-1642
  of vulva, 1630-1637
Neoplastic cells, 579-586
  angiogenesis and stromal support of, 581
  characteristics of, 579-586
  cytologic features of, 580-581
  growth rate and differentiation of, 579-580
  local growth of, 581-582
  local invasion of, 582-584
  metastasis of, 584-585
  progression of, 585-586
  regional extension and, 584
  transformation of, 587
Neostigmine, 229
Neovascularization, *101*, 102
  in atherosclerotic plaque, *103*, 104
Nephrectomy, 41, *42*
Nephritic factor, 818
Nephritic syndrome, 808*t*
Nephritis
  allergic, 838
    experimental, 536*t*
  Balkan, 838
  IgA, 516
  interstitial, 837-839
    cyclosporin A and, 183
    diphtheria and, 295
    vasculitis and, 838
  Masugi, 810
  radiation, 279, 832
Nephroblastoma, 579, 848-849, *849*
Nephrocalcinosis, 153, 1575

Nephrogenic adenoma, 865, *865*
Nephrolithiasis, 553
Nephron, 804
Nephropathy
  analgesic abuse, 832
  contrast, 832
  diabetic, *822*, 823
  gout, 839
  hypokalemic, 834, *834*
  IgA, 517t, 810, 816, *816*
  IgM, 816
  lead, 832
  light-chain, 826
  membranous, 517t, 819-820, *820*, *821*
  mercury, 831, *831*
  phenacetin, 832
  reflux, 836
  sclerosing, 825
  sickle cell, 837
Nephrosclerosis, 808
  benign, 842-843
  malignant, *843*, 843-844, *844*
Nephrosis
  osmotic, 833, *833*
  platinum toxicity and, 216
  tubular
    boric acid toxicity and, 224
    carbon tetrachloride poisoning and, 222
Nephrotic syndrome, 808t, 818
  hydropericardium and, 664
Nephrotoxic serum, 810
Nerve gas toxicity, 226
Nerve sheath tumors, 2171-2173, *2172*
  malignant, 1894-1896, *1895*
Nerves of skin, 1756
Nervous system
  pathology of; *see* Nervous system
    pathology
  regenerative capacities of, 2124
  selective vulnerability and, 2124-2125
Nervous system pathology, 2123-2196
  central, 2125-2189; *see also* Central
    nervous system pathology
  diagnosis and classification of, 2124
  evolution of study of, 2123
  fixatives and, 2125
  ground rules of study of, 2123-2125
  morphologic techniques in, 2125
  peripheral, 2189-2191
  specimen selection and, 2124
Nesidioblastosis, 1369
neu, 587t, 589, 603
Neural tube defects, 2136-2138
Neuraminidase, 365
Neurilemoma, 1890-1892, *1891*, 2053
  in oral soft tissue, 1107
  vagina and, 1640
Neuritis, allergic, 536t
Neuroblastoma, 579, 588, 589, 602
  adrenal glands and, 1611, *1612*
  olfactory, 1082
  radiation and, 267
Neuroendocrine system
  carcinoma of, 1339, *1340*
  dispersed, 1613
  tumor of, 1184
    skin and, 1801
    thymus gland and, 1508, *1509*
Neurofibrillary degeneration, 2132-2133
Neurofibrillary tangles, *2181*, 2182
Neurofibroma, 1825, 1892-1894, *1893*, 2171-
  2173, *2172*
  in oral soft tissue, 1107

Neurofibroma—cont'd
  vagina and, 1640
Neurofibromatosis, 50, 609, 2175
  of eye, 1051
  von Recklinghausen's, 2166
Neurofibrosarcomas, 1894
Neurofilament antigen, 2166t
Neurofilaments, 2133
Neurogenic atrophy, *2119*, 2119-2121, *2120*
Neurogenic tumors
  mediastinal, 1026
  soft-tissue, 1890-1896
Neurohypophysis, 1517, 1518, 1523, 1526
Neurokinin A, 964
Neurologic defects, fetal irradiation and, 269
Neurologic signs and symptoms, 2124
Neuromas, *1890*
  amputation, 1335
  Morton's, 1890
  multiple mucosal, 1563
  in oral soft tissue, 1107
Neuromelanin, 2132
Neuromyelitis optica, 2177
Neuron-specific enolase, 1012, 1017, 2166t
Neuronal atrophy, 2132
Neuronal injury, 2132-2133
Neuronal storage, metabolic diseases and,
  2133
Neurons, injury of, 2131-2133
Neuropathic joint disease, 2068
Neuropathies, demyelinative, *2190*, 2190-
  2191
Neuropathology; *see* Nervous system
  pathology
Neurophysins, 1523
Neurosarcoma, 1894-1896
Neurosyphilis, 2156-2158, *2157*
  microglia and, 2134
Neurotransmitter receptors, 508
Neurotransmitters, 8
  Huntington's disease and, 2182
Neurulation defects, 2136
Neutralization, 149, 506t
Neutrino, 248
Neutrons, 23, 23t, 248
  in therapy, 284
Neutropenia, 273, 1383
Neutrophil chemotactic factor, 519t
Neutrophils
  adherent to endothelium, 79
  ameba-mediated lysis of, 436
  emigration of, 69, *70*
    inflammation and, 76, 76-81, *78*
  escape of, 78
  inflammation and, 81
  polymorphonuclear, *510*
    myocardial infarction and, 637, *637*
  pseudopod of, 77
  sticking of, 77, 78
Nevoid basal cell carcinoma syndrome, 2166
Nevus, 31
  balloon cell, 1804
  bathing trunk, 1816
  blue, 1810-1811, *1811*
  blue rubber-bleb, 1820
  compound, 1804, *1804*
  dysplastic, 1803, 1816
  halo, 1812
  intradermal, *1803*, 1803-1804
  Jadassohn, 1810, 1833
  junctional, 1802-1803, 1816
    malignant melanomas and, 1815-1816
  in oral soft tissue, 1109

Nevus—cont'd
  of Ota, 1810
  pigmented, 1802-1804
  Spitz, *1806*, *1807*
Nevus flammeus, 794
New cells, multiplication of, 96
Newborn
  adrenals of, *1581*
    cytomegaly in, 1583
    hyperplasia in, 1584-1585
  candidiasis and, 412
  cholestasis and, 1261t, 1262
  congenital epulis of, 1108
  cystic fibrosis and, 1350
  cytomegalic inclusion disease of, 382
  disseminated herpetic infection of, 379
  encephalitis and, 2160-2162
  gingival cysts of, 1119
  hemochromatosis and, 1273
  hemorrhagic disease in, 555
  hepatitis and, 1215, 1261t, 1262, 1263,
    1264
    multinucleated giant cells in, 1263,
    1263
  hypocalcemia and, 1572
  infections in, 356t, 357
  jaundice in, 1260-1262
  massive pulmonary hemorrhage in, 928-
    929
  meningitis and, 2155, *2155*
  osteomyelitis of jaw of, 1113
  pancreas of, 1363-1364
  subcutaneous fat necrosis of, 1789
  thyroid teratoma and, 1556
  toxoplasmosis in, 449
  transient tachypnea of, 925
  wet lung and, 925
Newcastle disease virus, 366
Nezelof's syndrome, 1500t
β-NGF, 590t
Niacin, 555, 556-558
Nickel, 214, *214*, *215*, 238, 599
Nicotinamide adenine dinucleotide, 1
  ethanol and, 197, 1239
  infarction and, 635
  ischemia and, 631
Nicotine
  poisoning from, 193t
  stomatitis and, 1110
Niemann-Pick disease, 53, 1267
  gastrointestinal manifestations of, 1173
  hepatosplenomegaly and, 1419t, 1419-
    1420
Night blindness, 552
Nikolsky's sign, 1764
Nipple, 1726
  adenomas of, 1732
Nissl stain, 2126t
Nissl substance, 2132
Nitrates as air pollutants, 232
Nitric oxide as air pollutant, 231
p-Nitroblue tetrazolium, 634
Nitrofurantoin toxicity, 174-175, 1235t, 1237
Nitrogen dioxide, 231-232, 989
  emphysema and, 238
  pulmonary edema and, 237
Nitrogen mustard toxicity, 180-182, 596,
  597t
NK cells; *see* Natural killer cells
No-reflow phenomenon, 633
Nocardiosis, 382, 392t, 394t, 420-421, *421*,
  1053
Nocturnal hemoglobinuria, paroxysmal, 1380

Nodular, suppurative, febrile, relapsing panniculitis, 1788
Nodular cryptogenic cirrhosis, 1227, *1228*
Nodular fasciitis, 1850-1852, *1851*
Nodular goiter, 1546-1549, *1547*, *1548*
Nodular hyperplasia
  of adrenal cortex, 1591, *1591*
  hepatic
    focal, 1290-1291
    portal hypertension and regenerative, 1249
  of prostate gland, 903, 904-906
Nodular periorchitis, 894
Nodular sclerosis, 1446, *1447*, 1451
Nodular vasculitis, 1789
Nodules, 1757
  adrenal glands and, 1588
  prostatic hyperplasia and, 903, 904-906
  vocal, 385-386, 1020, 1084-1085
Noise, injuries from, 136
Noludar; *see* Methyprylon
Noma, 1105
Non-A, non-B viral hepatitis, 1210, 1295
Noncommunicating hydrocephalus, 2139-2140
Non–epithelium lined jaw cysts, 1120
Non-Hodgkin's lymphomas, 1398-1399, *1399*, 1452-1474
  classification of
    Kiel, 1452-1453
    Lukes-Collins, 1452-1453
    Rappaport, 1452-1453
  of cuff or mantle zone cells, 1464-1465
  diffuse, of large cells, 1465-1467
  of follicular cells, 1461-1462
  heavy-chain disease and, 1470
  histopathology of, 1460-1461
  in immunodeficiency states, 1471-1474
  of lymphoblasts, 1469
  lymphocytosis and, 1469
  monoclonal gammopathies and, 1469-1470
  Murphy staging system for, 1471, 1471t
  in oral soft tissue, 1112
  pathogenesis of, 1453-1460
  of small lymphocytes, 1462-1464
  of small noncleaved cells, 1467-1469
  spleen and, *1428*, 1429
  staging of, 1470-1471
Non–collagen matrix components, 1208
Noncommunicating hydrocephalus, 2131
Nonepithelial salivary gland tumors, 1141
Nonfibrogenic dusts, 233
Nongonococcal urethritis, 357
Noninfective vasculitides, 768-778, *770*, *771*, *773*, *775*, *776*, *777*
Nonionizing radiation, 285t, 285-286
Nonkeratinizing carcinoma in oral soft tissue, 1112
Nonmelanotic pigmentation in oral soft tissue, 1106
Nonodontogenic cysts, 1119-1120
Nonparasitic cyst, 1293
Nonpenetrating injuries, 698-699
Nonportal hepatotrophic factors, 1206
Nonsteroidal anti-inflammatory agent toxicity, 158-162
Nonstochastic radiation injury, 257
Nontropical sprue, 1171-1172
Nontuberculous mycobacteria, 946-947
Nonunion of fractures, 2001, *2002*
Norepinephrine toxicity, 216-217
  encephalopathy and, 1248
  myocardium and, 632, 664, 693

Normal-pressure hydrocephalus, 2131
Normofollicular thyroid adenoma, 1555
North Asian tick typhus, 349t, 353
Nortriptyline poisoning, 194t
Norwalk-like agents, 377
Nose, 1077; *see also* Nasal cavity
Novobiocin toxicity, 1235t, 1238
NSE; *see* Neuron-specific enolase
Nuclear antigen, Epstein-Barr, 383
Nuclear-cytoplasmic asynchrony, 1377
Nuclear fallout, 281
Nuclear glycogen, 1200
Nuclear hyperchromicity, 581
Nuclear inclusions, 1265; *see also* Inclusion bodies
Nuclear karyolysis, 636
Nuclear karyorrhexis, 824
Nuclear streaming, 141
Nuclear weapons testing, 260, 286
Nucleus
  pyknotic, 255
  radiation and, 24, 255
Nuclides, 248
Null cell adenoma, 1535
Nurse cell–parasite unit, 465
Nutrition
  carcinoma and, 563
  congestive cardiomyopathy and, 692
  dietary components of, 546
  imbalances in, 546-547
  inadequacy of, 547-548; *see also* Nutritional diseases
Nutritional diseases
  central nervous system, 2185-2186
  factors in, 548
  scheme of pathogenesis of, *547*

O

Oat cell carcinoma, *594*, 1082
Obesity
  atherosclerosis and, 620
  diabetes and, 1360
  lipomas and, 1879
  osteoarthrosis and, 2074
Obliterative bronchiolitis, 968, *968*
Obliterative lymphangitis, 892
Obliterative pericarditis, 666-667, *667*
Obstetric cholestasis, 1274
Obstetric shock, 1527
Obstruction
  biliary, 1252-1254
  congenital heart disease and, 739-743
    shunts in, 743-749
  intestinal, 1156-1158
  prognosis in, 1254
  prostatic, 854
  urinary tract, 836-837
    ureteral, 851
    urethral, 898, 906
Obstructive cholangiopathy, infantile, 1323
Obstructive jaundice, 33-34
Obstructive lymphedema, 793
Obstructive renal dysplasia, *845*, 845-846
Obturation obstruction, 1157
Occipital lobe infarction, *2129*, 2130
Occlusion of portal vein, 1280
Occult carcinoma of thyroid, 1559
Occult spina bifida, 2136, 2137
Occupational bladder tumors, 860
Occupational chest diseases, 232-239
Occupational lung carcinomas, 1015
Ochronosis, 1074, *1075*, 2097
  arthropathy with, 2068

Ocular disorders; *see* Ophthalmic pathology
Oculocraniosomatic neuromuscular disease with ragged-red fibers, 2116
Oculocutaneous albinism, 51
Oculoglandular listeriosis, 313
Oddi, sphincter of, 1353
Odontogenesis, 1121
Odontogenic adenomatoid tumor, 1121
Odontogenic cysts, 1118-1119, *1119*
Odontogenic fibroma, 1123-1125
Odontogenic keratocyst, 1119, 1799
Odontogenic tumors, 1121-1127
  malignant, 1126
Odontoma, 1126, *1126*
Odoriferous glands, 1756
Old tuberculin, 940
Olecranon bursitis, 403
Olfactory-genital syndrome, 874
Olfactory neuroblastoma, 1082
Oligodendrocytes, 384
Oligodendrogliomas, 2169, *2170*
Oligodontia, 1096
Oligohydramnios, 844
Oligomeganephrony, 844
Oliguria, 809, 830-831
Ollier's disease, 2034
Omentum, 1191
  neoplasms of, 1191
Omphalomesenteric veins, 1199
Onchocerciasis, 471-473, *472*, *473*
Onchocercoma, 472, *472*
Onchocercosis, 471-473, *472*, *473*
Oncocytic adenoma, 1535
Oncocytoma, salivary gland, 1135, *1135*
Oncogenes, *571-572*, 586-589, 610
  antibodies to, 604
  bioassays for, 239
  chemical carcinogens and, 597
  diagnosis of neoplasia and, 588
  functions and intracellular locations of, 588
  leukemia and, 1387
  occupational disease and, 238-239
  radiation injury and, 265, 266
Oncogenic osteomalacia, 1994
Oncogenic viruses, 600t, 600-602
Oncology, 610
Onion-bulb neuropathy, *2190*, 2191
Onion-skin lesion, *756*
  pulmonary hypertension and, 954, *954*
Onycholysis, 1787
Onychomycosis, 397
Onychorrhexis, 1787
Oocyst, *Toxoplasma*, 448-449
Oocytes, 1671, 1674
Oogonia, 1621
Oophorectomy, 1676
Opacities, radiation injury and, 281
Open-circulation theory, spleen and, 1409
Ophthalmia, sympathetic, 1056, *1057*
Ophthalmic pathology, 1047-1076
  adnexal structures in, 1047-1051
  diabetes and, 1366
  intraocular lesions in, 1051-1074
    cataracts and, 1069
    congenital and developmental, 1051-1053
    glaucoma and, 1069-1072
    infections and inflammations in, 1053-1057
    primary neoplasms and, 1064-1069
    retinal degenerative diseases and, 1072-1074

Ophthalmic pathology—cont'd
  intraocular lesions in—cont'd
    retinal vascular disease and, 1057-1064
  lightning and, 144
  nonionizing radiation and, 285
  normal eye and, *1070*
  onchocerciasis and, 472
  radiation and, 281
  systemic disease manifestations and, 1074-1076
  systemic diseases and, 1074-1076
Opisthorchiasis, 452, 453
Opisthorchis, 452
Opportunism, 301
  fungal, 391
Opsonins, 83
Optic lens, radiation and, 257t, 281
Oral cavity infection, 412
Oral contraceptives
  adverse reactions to, 165-167, *166*
  breast carcinoma and, 1747
  and cholestatic action, 1234t, 1235
  gallstones and, 1326
  hepatocellular tumors and, 1289
  pharmacogenetics and, 149
Oral floor cysts, 1120
Oral hypoglycemic agent toxicity, 169
Oral soft tissues, 1100-1113
  infections of, 1103-1105
    granulomatous, 1105-1106
  mucocutaneous diseases of, 1100-1103
  pigmentation disturbances of, 1106
  tumors and tumorlike lesions of, 1106-1113
  white lesions of, 1109-1110
Orbit of eye, 1047-1051
Orbiviruses, 376
Orchiectomy, 881
Orchitis, 367, 536t, 877-879
  mumps, 876, 877
Organ
  of contraction, 104
  of Corti, 136
Organic arsenical drugs, 1237
Organic chlorinated hydrocarbon toxicity, 226, *227*, *228*
Organization
  of myocardial infarct, 637
  wound healing and, 102-104, *105*
Organizing mural thrombi, cardiac myxomas and, 701, 703t
Organogenesis, radiation and, 269
Organophosphate toxicity, 226
Oriental sore, 444
Orinase; *see* Tolbutamide
Oroanal sexual practices, 433
Oropharynx, epidermoid carcinoma of, 257t; *see also* Pharynx
Orthomyxoviruses, 363-365
Orthotopic liver transplant, 1300
Orungo virus, 376
Osler nodes, 657
Osler-Weber-Rendu disease, 795, 922, 1109, 1292
  gastrointestinal tract and, 1188
Osmotic nephrosis, 833, *833*
Osseous metaplasia, 107-108
  in heart, 693
Osseous metastases of prostatic carcinoma, 911
Ossification, 107, 1937-1941, *1939*
  in lung, 982-983
  membranous, *1940*, 1941

Ossifying fibroma in jaws, 1114
Osteitis deformans, 2006-2010
  in jaws, 1114
Osteitis fibrosa, *1963*, 1977
  hyperparathyroidism and, *1975*
  osteomalacia and, *1991*, *1995*, 1995-1997
  pure, 1997
Osteitis fibrosa cystica
  parathyroid glands and, 1575
  of ulna, *1976*
Osteoarthropathy, hypertrophic, 2070
  bronchogenic carcinoma and, 1013
Osteoarthrosis, 2071-2075, *2072*, *2073*
  acromegaly and, 2074
  etiology and pathogenesis of, 2073-2074, *2074*
  histogenesis of, 2071-2073
  Kashin-Beck disease and, 2074-2075
  prevalence and distribution of, 2071
Osteoblastic tumors, 2025-2034
Osteoblastomas, 2021t, 2025-2028, *2027*
  in jaws, 1116
Osteoblasts, 1932, *1932*
Osteocalcin, 1936
Osteocartilaginous exostosis, 2036
Osteochondrodystrophies, 1946
Osteochondroma, 2021t, 2036, *2037*
Osteochondromatosis, 2093-2094, *2094*
  multiple, *2036*
Osteochondroses, 2069-2071
Osteochondrosis dissecans, 2069
Osteoclast-activating factor, 531t, 1400
Osteoclastoma, 2043-2045
Osteoclasts, 1934-1936, *1935*
  soft-tissue tumors and, 1906
Osteocytes, 1932-1934, *1934*
Osteodystrophy
  hepatic, 1974-1975
  renal, 1995-1997, *1996*
    osteosclerosis of, 1997, *1999*
    parathyroid glands and, 1577
Osteogenesis imperfecta, 1951-1953, *1952*, *1953*, *1954*, *1955*
  osteosarcoma and, 2019
Osteogenic sarcoma
  in jaws, 1116-1117
  radiosensitivity of, 257t
Osteoid, 569, 1944, 1958, 2022
Osteoid osteoma, 2021t, 2025-2028, *2026*
Osteoid seam, 1944
Osteolysis, massive, 2051
Osteoma, 1825, 2025
  osteoid, 2021t, 2025-2028, *2026*
  soft-tissue, 1109
Osteoma cutis, 1780
Osteomalacia and rickets, 807, 1983-2000, *1987*, *1989*
  antacid-induced, 1994-1995
  classification of, 1983-1984, 1985t
  clinical manifestations of, 1984-1986
  histology of, 1986, 1988t, 1988-1990
  25-hydroxylation in, 1993
  hypophosphatasia in, 1997-2000
  hypophosphatemic, 1993-1995
  oncogenic, 1994
  polymorphic mesenchymal tumors and, 1909
  pure, 1997
  radiographic features of, 1986-1988
  renal osteodystrophy in, 1995-1997
  risk factors for, 1988t
  vitamin D deficiency and, 554, 1990-1993
  vitamin D–dependent rickets in, 1993

Osteomatosis in jaws, 1113
Osteomyelitis, *2003*, *2004*
  Garré's, 1113, 2004
  hematogenous, 2004
  in jaws, 1113
  plasma cell, 2050
Osteonecroses, 2010-2013, *2012*, *2013*
Osteons, 1931, *1931*, 1941-1943
  secondary, *1942*
Osteopathy, drug-induced, 1972
Osteopenia, *1968*
  disuse, 1972
  secondary osteoporosis and, 1971
Osteopetrosis, *1949*, 1949-1951
Osteophytes, 2097
Osteoporosis, 1958-1982
  active, *1960*, *1962*, *1963*, *1973*
    histology of, 1961t
  disuse, 1972
  general features of, 1958-1959
  histopathology of, 1959-1965, 1961t, *1964*, *1965*
  inactive, 1961, 1961t, *1964*, *1965*
  involutional, 1967-1971
  primary, 1965-1971
  risk factors for, 1965-1966
  secondary, 1971-1982
    acromegaly and, 1972
    anticonvulsant drug-induced, 1972
    chronic anemias with erythroid hyperplasia and, 1972
    disuse, 1972
    hemochromatosis and, 1972-1974
    hepatic osteodystrophy and, 1974-1975
    hypercortisolism and, 1975
    hyperparathyroidism and, 1975-1977
    hypogonadism and, 1977
    hypoparathyroidism and, 1978-1979
    mastocytosis and, 1979-1981
    partial gastrectomy and, 1981
    primary hyperparathyroidism and, 1975-1977
    secondary hyperparathyroidism and, 1975-1977
    starvation and, 1981
    thyrotoxicosis and, 1981-1982
  type I, 1966-1967
  type II, 1967
Osteoradionecrosis, 113-114, 280
Osteosarcoma, 2021t, *2028*, 2028-2034, *2029*, *2030*, *2031*, *2032*, *2033*
  extraskeletal, 1909
  in jaws, 1116-1117
  therapeutic irradiation and, 281
Osteosarcomas, 2018-2020
Osteosclerosis, 1949
  of renal osteodystrophy, 1997, *1999*
OT; *see* Old tuberculin
Ota, nevus of, 1810
Otic polyp, 1088
Otitis, malignant external, 1088
Otitis media, 1087
  chronic, 1079
Otosclerosis, 1088
Ototoxicity, cisplatin and, 216
Ovarian stroma, 1673
Ovary, 1671-1692
  anatomy and physiology of, 1671-1674
  cells of, 1671-1674
  cystic teratoma of, *578*
  developmental anomalies of, 1627
    agenesis in, 1977
  in embryo, 1621, *1621*

Ovary—cont'd
  embryology and, 1621
  heterotopic tissue of, 1677
  neoplasms of, 1677-1692
    carcinoma of stomach and, 1183
    classification of, 1677-1678, 1678t
    germ cell, 1687-1691
    lipid cell, 1686-1687
    malignant lymphoma, 1691
    metastatic, 1691
    prognosis in, 1691-1692
    sex cord stromal, 1684-1686
    stages of, 1692
    surface epithelial, 1678-1684
  nonneoplastic cysts and hyperplasia of,
    1674-1677
  polycystic, 1675-1676
  postmenopausal, 1674
  radiation and, 257t, 280
  senescence, failure, and atrophy of, 1674
Ovulation, 1653
Ovum, superficially implanted, 1694
Oxalate crystals, 198, 199
Oxidative drug-induced hemolysis, 1382
Oxidative enzyme reactions, 2
  muscle fibers and, 2107
11-Oxy steroids, 163
Oxygen effect, 254
Oxygen toxicity, 176-180
  concentrations and, 962
  morphine and, 219
Oxymetholone, 1289
Oxyphenisatin, 1237
Oxyphil adenoma
  salivary gland, 1135, 1135
  thyroid gland, 1555, 1556
Oxyphil cell
  parathyroid glands and, 1570
  thyroid adenoma and, 1555, 1556
  thyroid carcinoma and, 1562
Oxytocin, 1523
Oxyuriasis, 464-465
Ozone, 230-231, 989

P

P component, 39
Pacemaker, cardiac, 654, 705
Pachygyria, 2138, 2139
Pacinian corpuscles, 1757
PAF; see Platelet-activating factor
Pagetoid reticulosis, 1827
Paget's disease
  of bone, 1114, 2006-2010, 2007, 2008,
    2009, 2010, 2011, 2018-2019
    and osteosarcoma, 2028
  of breast, 1746, 1746
  extramammary
    skin and, 1798, 1830
    vulva and, 1635-1636, 1636
Pain
  bone, 807
  inflammation and, 84
Painless thyroiditis, 1554
Paint, radium-containing, 259
Paired pure gallstones, 1323, 1324
Palate
  cleft, 1095
  squamous cell carcinoma of, 1112
Palliation, 606
Palmar fibromatoses, 1845
Palpation thyroiditis, 1551
Panacinar emphysema, 990, 991
Panarteritis, necrotizing, 775

Pancarditis, trypanosomiasis and, 440
Pancreas, 1347-1372
  ectopic, 1348
  endocrine, 1358-1369
    diabetes mellitus and, 1358-1367; see
      also Diabetes mellitus
    neoplasms of pancreatic islets and,
      1367-1369
  fat necrosis of, 15, 16
  form and development of
    abnormalities of, 1348-1351
    normal, 1347-1348
  neoplasms of exocrine, 1253, 1253, 1354-
    1357
  pancreatitis and, 1351-1353
  periampullary tumors and, 1357-1358
  radiation and, 257t, 278
  systemic disease and, 1354
Pancreatic achylia, 1173
Pancreaticoduodenectomy, 1355
Pancreatitis, 1351, 1351-1353, 1352
  acute hemorrhagic, 1351-1353
  alcoholics and, 197, 1253
  chronic, 1253, 1353
  hypothermia and necrotizing, 137, 138
Pancreatoblastoma, 1355, 1355
Pancytopenia, 1376
Panencephalitis, subacute sclerosing, 369,
    369, 1054
Panhypopituitarism, 1261t, 1526
Panhypoplasia of bone marrow, 279
Panniculitis, 1787-1789, 1788-1789
  lupus erythematosus, 1769
  mesenteric, 1190
Panophthalmitis, 1053
Pantothenic acid, 559
PAP; see Prostatic acid phosphatase
Papanicolaou smear, 580
Papillary adenocarcinoma
  pancreatic, 1358
  of periampullary region, 1359
  prostatic, 915
Papillary adenomas, 1175-1179
Papillary carcinoma
  of breast, 1743
  thyroid gland, 1556, 1558, 1559, 1561
    histologic differential diagnosis of, 1559t
Papillary cystadenoma
  of epididymis, 892
  of salivary gland, 1134, 1134
Papillary hyperplasia
  oral soft tissue, 1106
  prostatic, 904, 905
Papillary necrosis, 837
  candidiasis and, 412
Papillary tumors
  alimentary tract and, 1191
  bladder and, 861-862
  of cardiac valve, 703
Papillitis necroticans, 837
  aminophenols and, 160
  aspirin and, 160-161
Papilloma, 292t, 575, 610
  bladder and, 864, 865
  breast and, 1731-1732, 1732, 1733
  cervical, 1645
  laryngeal, 385-386, 1020, 1084-1085
  of nasal cavity, 1080, 1080-1081
  oral soft tissue and, 1103, 1106
Papillomaviruses, 384, 2178
Papillon-Lefèvre syndrome, 1097
Papovaviruses, 384-386, 2178
Papule, 1757

Papulosis
  bowenoid
    penile, 1798
    vulva and, 1633, 1635
  lymphomatoid, skin and, 1827-1829
Para-articular tissues cyst, 2092
Paracicatricial emphysema, 990
Paracoccidioidomycosis, 394t, 421-422, 422
Paracortical hyperplasia, 1438-1440
Paracrine growth factors, 9
Paradental cyst, 1118
Paraductal coarctation, 741-743, 742, 743
Paraffin method, 2125
Paraffinoma, 191, 191, 896, 897, 986
Parafollicular cells, 1544
Paraganglioma
  of adrenal glands, 1613
  of gallbladder, 1334
  of mediastinum, 1026
Paragonimiasis, 453-454
Parainfluenza virus, 28, 366
Parakeratosis, 896, 1757
Paraldehyde poisoning, 194t
Paralysis, 2134, 2157
  Chastek, 551
  immune, 498
Paralytic ileus, 1157
Paramyxoviruses, 365-369, 2010
  encephalitis and, 2158
Paranasal sinus, 1078-1083
  carcinoma of, 1082
Paraphimosis, 895
Paraplegia, radiation injury and, 281
Paraproteinemia, 826
Paraproteins, interstitial disease and, 838-
    839
Parapsoriasis, 1773
Paraquat toxicity, 230, 708
Paraseptal emphysema, 990
Parasitism, 292t
  alimentary tract and, 1166-1167
  cirrhosis and, 1286
  eosinophilia with, 82
  muscle fibers and, 465
  prostate gland and, 901
Parathion toxicity, 226
Parathyroid glands, 1570-1579
  adenoma of, 1563
  calcium metabolism regulation and, 1571
  cysts of, 1143, 1577
  development of, 1570
  ectopic, 1026
  hyperparathyroidism and, 1572-1577
  hypoparathyroidism of, 1571-1572
  inflammatory processes of, 1577
  parathyroid hormone and; see Parathyroid
    hormone
  pathologic calcification of, 1571
  pseudohypoparathyroidism and, 1572
  structure of, 1570
Parathyroid hormone, 1570-1571
  bone and, 1944, 1944t, 1945
  osteoporosis and deficiency of, 1978
Paratopes, 488
Paratubal cyst, fallopian, 1669
Paratyphoid fever, 314-315
Paravaginal hematoma, 893
Paregoric and tripelennamine hydrochloride
    toxicity, 219
Parenchyma
  brain
    astrocytic reactions to injuries of, 2134
    hemorrhage of, 2142, 2150-2153

Parenchyma—cont'd
  brain—cont'd
    inflammation of, 2158-2164
      perinatal injury and, 2142, 2143
    pulmonary
      asthma and, 964
      radiation injury to, 277
    radiation injury and, 256, 277
Parenteral nutrition, cholestasis and, 1261t,
    1267
Paresis; see Paralysis
Parietal cells, 506t
Parkinsonism, 2183
Parkinson's disease, 2182-2183, 2183
Paronychia, 302
Parotid gland, 1127
Parotitis
  acute, 1128
  epidemic, 1130
  mumps and, 366
Parovarian cysts, fallopian, 1669
Paroxysmal hypertension, 1609, 1609
Paroxysmal nocturnal hemoglobinuria, 1380
Pars distalis, 1518, 1519
Pars intermedia, 1518
Pars nervosa, 1518, 1523
Pars plana cyst, 1069
Pars tuberalis, 1518
Partial-thickness burns, 138, 138, 139
Particulate radiation, 248
Passive cutaneous anaphylaxis, 519
Passive hyperemia, hepatic, 1279-1280
Passive leukocyte-sensitizing activity of
    serum, 519
Passive smoking, 1015
Pasteurella, 318, 321
Patent ductus arteriosus, 734-735, 735
Pathogenicity, 289
Pathologic fracture, 115
Paul-Bunnell test, 450
Pautrier-Darier abscesses, 1826
Pearls, 610
Pedestrians, injuries to, 116-118
  hit and run, 118-119
Pediatric lung disease, 920-930, 1026-1031
Pedigree analysis, 49-50
Pedunculated vesicles, 461
Peking duck hepatitis virus, 1211
Peliosis hepatis, 165, 1292
  azathioprine and, 183, 185
Pellagra, 555, 556-557, 557, 558
Pelves, renal, 850-852
Pelvic ectopic kidneys, 844
Pelvic endometriosis, 1669
Pelvic inflammatory disease, 309, 1667-1668
Pelvis
  chondrosarcoma and, 2041
  osteomalacia and, 1987
  Paget's disease and, 2009
Pemphigoid, 539t, 1764
  benign mucosal, 1102, 1763
Pemphigus, 539t, 1102, 1102, 1103, 1762,
    1762-1764
Penetrating injury, 114
  of brain, 2189
  of heart, 698
Penetration-enhancing factor, 449
Penicillamine
  hepatocellular carcinoma and, 1294
  lupus erythematosus and, 149
  pharmacogenetics and, 150
  Wilson disease and, 1270

Penicillins, 655
  actinomycosis and, 407
  hypersensitivity and, 148, 168, 538, 708
  myocarditis and, 168, 708
  pharmacogenetics and, 150
  toxicity of, 156, 157
Penicillium marneffei, 395t, 422-423, 423
Penis, 895-898
  bowenoid papulosis of, 1798
Pentachlorophenol poisoning, 194t
Pentobarbital
  alcohol and, 195
  poisoning from, 193t
Pentrane; see Methoxyflurane
Peptic ulcer, 1160-1161
Peptides
  amino acids and, 2
  phagocytosis and, 84
  vasoactive intestinal, 519t
Peptostreptococcus, 1704
Percutaneous hepatography, 1282
Percutaneous transhepatic cholangiography,
    1323
Periampullary tumors, 1357-1358
Perianal abscess, 1169
Periapical cemental dysplasia, 1115
Periapical cementoma, 1115
Periapical periodontal disease, 1098, 1099-
    1100, 1100, 1101
Periappendicitis, 1165
Periarteriolar lymphoid sheath, 1409
Pericardial cysts, 700, 1024
Pericardial plaques, 667-668
Pericarditis, 665, 665-672, 667, 668, 669,
    671, 672
  acute nonspecific, 668
  ankylosing spondylitis and, 650
  chronic
    adhesive, 666-667, 667
    constrictive, 667, 668
  purulent, 302
  radiation-induced, 699
  rheumatic fever and, 647-648
  rheumatoid, 649
Pericardium
  cysts of, 700, 1024
  hemorrhage and, 129
  inflammation of; see Pericarditis
Pericyte, 796, 1889
Perifascicular atrophy, 2118, 2118
Periglandular basement membrane, 1756
Perikaryon, neuronal, 2132
Perimenopausal exogenous estrogen, 1747
Perinatal brain injury, 2141-2146
Perinatal lung disease, 925-929
Perinatal telencephalic
    leukoencephalopathy, 2145
Perinatal transmission of hepatitis virus,
    1214-1215
Perineum, embryology of, 1622
Perineurial cell, 1892
Periodic disease, 1189
Periodontal cyst, 1119
Periodontal disease, 1099-1100, 1100, 1101
Periodontitis, 1099-1100, 1100, 1101
Periorchitis, 878
Periosteal chondroma, 2034
Periosteitis, proliferative, 1113
Periosteum, 2022
  blood beneath, 129
  inflammation of, 1113
  syphilis and, 2005
Peripheral anterior synechia, 1062

Peripheral cholangiocarcinoma, 1293
Peripheral nerves
  diabetes and, 1366
  diseases of, 2189-2191
  injury to, 2189-2191
  morphology of, 2189
  regeneration of, 97, 2124
  tumors of, 2053-2054
Peripheral odontogenic fibroma, 1125
Peripheral ossifying fibromas in oral soft
    tissue, 1107
Peripheral T-cell lymphomas, 1466
Peritoneal leiomyomatosis, 1665
Peritoneal splenic implants, 1414
Peritoneal stromal cell mutation, 1190
Peritoneum, 1189-1190
  inflammation of; see Peritonitis
  neoplasms of, 1191
    asbestos mesotheliomas in, 236
    metastatic, 1191
Peritonitis, 1189
  meconium, 1173
  salmonella, 317
  sclerosing, 1189
    propranolol and, 168
  tuberculous, 1189
Perivascular edema in lead poisoning, 206,
    209
Perivenous demyelination, 2177, 2178
Perivenous mononuclear inflammatory cell
    infiltration, 2177, 2178
Periventricular-intraventricular hemorrhage,
    2142, 2142-2143
Periventricular leukomalacia, 2143-2145,
    2144
Perivenular canalicular cholestasis, 1218
Perivenular necrosis, 1278
Periwinkle alkaloid toxicity, 185
Perlèche, 1105
Permanent cells, 94
  regeneration of, 97-98
Permeability factors, 71, 71-75
Pernicious anemia, 506t, 1169, 1378
  vitamin B_{12} and, 560
Pernio, 1789
Peroxisomes, liver, 1201
Persistent fetal circulation, 929
Persistent viral hepatitis, 1223, 1224-1225
  cobblestone pattern in, 1224, 1225
  morphologic pattern in, 1225
  pathologic changes of, 1229
Pertussis, 292t, 297-299, 299
Pest, 320
Pesticides
  air pollutants and, 230
  toxicity of, 226
Petechiae, endocarditis and, 657
Petriellidium boydii, 423
Peutz-Jeghers syndrome, 1786
  oral mucosal pigmentation and, 1106
  polyps and, 1178
Peyer's patches, 316
Peyronie's disease, 895-896, 896, 1845
Pfeiffer's bacillus, 310
Phacoanaphylaxis, 536t, 1056, 1058
Phacomatoses of eye, 1051
Phaeoannellomyces werneckii, 392t
Phaeohyphomycosis, 393t, 395t, 402, 403
Phagocytes
  disorders of, 503t
  emphysema and, 995
  tuberculosis and, 942
Phagocytic pouch, 83

Phagocytin, 84
Phagocytosis, 4, 83-84, 498, *509*
  of bacteria, 933
  macrophages and, 92, *93*
Phagosome, 83
Pharmacogenetics, 149-168
  hazards of therapy and, 150-168
    analgesics and antipyretics in, 158-162
    androgenic-anabolic steroids in, 165
    antibiotics and, 150-158
    antihypertensives in, 168
    corticosteroids in, 162-165
    estrogens in, 167
    oral contraceptives in, 165-167
    tranquilizers in, 167-168
  morphology and, 150
Pharyngeal hypophysis, 1517, *1518*, 1525-
    1526
Pharynx
  inflammation of, 303
    gonococcal, 309
  radiosensitivity of, 257*t*
Phenacetin toxicity, 160-162
  nephropathy and, 832
Phenformin toxicity, 169
Phenobarbital
  bilirubin and, 33
  Crigler-Najjar syndrome, 1277
  cytochrome P-450 and, 5
  Dubin-Johnson syndrome and, 1277
  hyperbilirubinemia and, 1261
  osteopathy and, 1972
  poisoning from, 193*t*
Phenomenona, no-reflow, 633
Phenothiazines, 708
  adverse reactions to, 167-168
  cholestasis with necrosis and, 1234*t*, 1235
Phenotype, 1626
Phenylalanine, 546, 562
  ochronosis and, 2068
Phenylbutazone
  granulomas and, 1285
  myocarditis and, 708
  necrosis and, 1234*t*, 1237
Phenylketonuria, 61
Phenytoin, 1100, *1101*, 1106
  enzyme inducers and, 1232
  lymphadenopathy and, 1439
  myocarditis and, *663*, 708
  necrosis and, 1234*t*, 1236
  osteopathy and, 1972
  pharmacogenetics and, 150
  toxicity of, 171-174, *172*, *173*, 194*t*
Pheochromocytoma, 1563, 1607, 1608, *1609*,
    1610
Pheochromocytoma cells, 588
Phialophora, 392*t*, 393*t*, 399, 402
Philadelphia chromosome, 588, 591, 1384
Phimosis, 895
Phlebothrombosis, 788-791, *789*
Phlebotomus, 442, 444
Phlegmasia alba dolens, 789
Phlegmasia cerulea dolens, 790
Phlegmon, 302
Phorbol esters, 599
Phosgene, 237
Phosphate
  bone and, 1944
  ionized, 982
  lithiasis and, 840
Phosphaturic mesenchymal tumors, 1909
Phosphofructokinase deficiency, 57, 2115
Phospholipases, 11

Phospholipids, 3
Phosphorus
  liver injury and, 1232, 1233
  metabolism of, 1570
  radioactive, 270
Phosphorylase
  congenital absence of, 57
  myocardial infarction and, 634
Phosphorylase kinase deficiency, 57
Phosphotungstic acid–hematoxylin stain,
    2126*t*
Photosynthesizer, exogenous, 286
Phototherapy, 1261
Phthisis bulbi, 473, 1074
Phycomycosis; *see* Mucormycosis
Physical agents in cell injury, 20-25
Physical carcinogens, 594-600
Physical injuries, 111-145
  atmospheric pressure changes and, 133-
    136
  electrical, 140-144
  heat and cold in, 136-140
  joint disorders and, 2067-2068
  mechanical trauma in, 111-133; *see also*
    Mechanical trauma
  sound waves and, 136
Physiologic death, instantaneous, 112
Physiologic neonatal hyperbilirubinemia,
    1260-1262
Physiology
  of cervix, 1643-1644
  of fallopian tube, 1667
  of ovary, 1671-1674
  of placenta, 1693-1698
  of vagina, 1637-1638
Physostigmine toxicity, 229
Pian bois, 444
Pica, 205
Pick bodies, 2133
Pick disease, 667
Pickwickian syndrome, 956
Picornaviruses, 374-375
  encephalitis and, 2158
Piecemeal necrosis of liver, 1202
  acute viral hepatitis and, 1218
  chronic active viral hepatitis and, 1226
Piedraia hortae, 392*t*
Pig-bel, 295
Pig roundworm, 462
Pigment, 30-36
  changes in, 129
  dental anomalies of, 1097
  Dubin-Johnson, 1204
  endogenous, 30
  exogenous, 30-31
  lipofuscin, 34, *35*, 1886
  oral soft tissue, 1106
  radiation injury and increased, 273-274
  skin disorders of, 1785-1786
Pigmentary cirrhosis, 1272, *1272*
Pigmented moles, 31
Pigmented nevi, 1802-1804
Pigmented papilloma, 1795
Pilary cysts, 1835
Piloid or pilocytic astrocytes, 2167
Pilomatricoma, 1835
Pilosebaceous cysts, 1835
pim, 587*t*
Pinealomas, 2174, *2174*
Pinta, 328
Pinworm, 464
Pipestem hepatic fibrosis, 456, *456*
Piriform sinus carcinomas, 1086

Piroplasmosis, 451-452
Pit of lower lip, 1095, *1096*
Pit cells, 1199, 1200, 1206
Pittsburgh pneumonia agent, 938
Pituicytes, 1523
Pituitary apoplexy, 1527
Pituitary follicle-stimulating hormone, 1676
Pituitary gland, 1517-1543
  anatomy of, 1518-1519
  anomalies of, 1526-1527
  in disorders of other endocrine glands,
    1523-1525
  embryology of, 1517-1518
  empty sella syndrome and, 1527
  hemorrhage and, 1527
  histology and function of, 1519-1523
  hypophysectomy and, 1525-1526
  hypopituitarism and, 1526
  infiltrations and metabolic disorders and,
    1529
  inflammation of
    acute, 1527
    chronic, 1527-1529
  ischemia and, 1527
  malposition of, 1526-1527
  midsagittal section of, *1517*
  pharyngeal, 1517, *1518*
  pituitary apoplexy and, 1527
  postpartum necrosis of, *1528*
  pregnancy and, 1523
  secondary Addison's disease and, 1588
  tumors of, 1529-1538
    adenomas in, 1530-1535, *1532*
    carcinoma in, 1535
    craniopharyngioma in, 1535-1537
    germinal, 1538
    granular cell, 1537
    intrasellar cyst in, 1537
    irradiated, 267
    multiple endocrine adenomatosis and,
      1535
Pituitary snuff user's lung, 966*t*
Pityrosporon furfur, 1768
Placenta, 1692-1710
  abnormal implantation of, *1699*, 1699-1700
  anatomy and physiology of, 1693-1698
  anomalies of, 1698
  circulatory lesions of, *1702*, 1702-1704
    accelerated maturation and, 1703
  erythroblastosis fetalis and, 1706
  examination of, 1692-1693
  hypermature, 1703
  infectious diseases and, 1704-1706
  multiple gestation and, *1698*, 1698-1699
  spontaneous abortion and, 1700-1701
  toxemia of pregnancy and, 1701-1702
  trophoblastic hyperplasia and neoplasia
    and, 1706-1710
Placenta accreta, 1699-1700
Placenta membranacea, 1698
Placenta previa, 1700
Placental circulation, disturbances of, 1702-
    1704
Placidyl; *see* Ethchlorvynol
Placodes, ectodermal, 2135
Plague, 292*t*, 320, *321*
Plant poison toxicity, 224-226
Plant pollens, 525
Plantar fibromatoses, 1845
Plaque, 668
  in aorta, 623
    atherosclerotic, *763*
      myocardial infarcts and, 627

Plaque—cont'd
dental, 1098, *1099*
Lichtheim, 2186
multiple sclerosis and, 2176-2177, *2177*
neovascularization in, *103*, *104*
Plaquenil; *see* Hydroxychloroquine
Plasma
burns and loss of, 139
chemotactic factors in, 80
exudation of, 69
Plasma cell dyscrasias, 1400
Plasma cell granulomas in lung, 1021, *1022*
Plasma cell inflammation, 93, *93*
Plasma cell myeloma, *1399*, *1400*, 1400-
1402, *1401*, *2049*
amyloidosis and, 40
bone and, 2021t, 2048-2050
Plasma cell osteomyelitis, 2050
Plasma cell proliferative disorders, 1399-
1403
Plasma free fatty acids, 132
Plasma kallikrein, 73
Plasma lipoproteins, 764
Plasma membrane, 3
Plasmacytoma
solitary, 1113
in upper respiratory tract and ear, 1089
Plasmalemma, 2105
Plasmodium(a), 445, 446, 1381, 1460
Plastic films, 597, 599
Plastic induration, 895-896
Plasticity, 112
Platelet-activating factor, 519t, 765, 964
Platelet aggregation, aspirin and, 160
Platelet-derived growth factor, 568, 590t,
591, 621, 764
Platelet factor IV, 160
Platinum toxicity, 216
Pleomorphic adenoma, salivary gland, 1132t,
1132-1134, *1133*
Pleomorphic carcinoma, pancreatic, *1358*
Pleomorphic fibrosarcoma, 1853
Pleomorphic lipoma, 1881-1883, *1883*
Pleomorphic liposarcoma, 1873, 1877, *1877*
Pleomorphic rhabdomyosarcoma, 1865,
1870-1871, *1871*
Pleomorphism, 570, 581, 610
Pleura
asbestos and, 236, 1004
mesotheliomas of, 1018-1019
asbestosis and, 236
occupational fibrosis of, 238
rheumatic fever and, 648
Pleural-biliary fistula, 1275
Pleural cavity, 935
Pleurisy, 973
Plexiform lesion
endometrium and, 1661
in muscular pulmonary artery, *955*, 955-
956
Plummer's disease, 1547
Plummer-Vinson syndrome, 1153, 1787
Plutonium, 260, 270
Pneumatoceles, 936
Pneumatosis cystoides intestinalis, 1155-
1156, *1156*
Pneumobilia, 1258
Pneumococci, 292t, 306-307
pericarditis and, 666
pneumonia and, 932-935, *933*
wound infection and, 130
Pneumoconiosis, 233-236, 996-1005, 1041-
1042
asbestos and, 1002-1005

Pneumoconiosis—cont'd
beryllium disease and, 1005
coal workers and, 35, *1000*, 1000-1002,
1001
dust and, 996-1000
pathogenesis of, 998
silicosis and, 997-998
tuberculosis and, 999
Pneumocystis carinii, 382, 450-451, *451*,
948, 968, 1405
Pneumomediastinum, 1024
Pneumonia, 312, *313*; *see also* Pneumonitis
adenovirus, 377, *378*
aspiration, 985
botulism and, 293
bacterial, 928, 932-939
beta-hemolytic streptococcal, 935
cadmium toxicity and, 212
chronic destructive, 939
eosinophilic, 978
gram-negative, 936
Haemophilus, 932, 936, 937, 988
hematogenous, 935
interstitial; *see* Interstitial pneumonia
Klebsiella, 936
lipid, 985-986, *986*
lobar, 306, *306*, 935
measles giant cell, *368*, 368-369
mycoplasmal, 932
necrotizing, 939
neonatal pulmonary infection and, 929
pneumococcal, 932-935, *933*
Pneumocystis, 450, 948
Pseudomonas, 937, *937*
psittacosis and, 356
Rocky Mountain spotted fever and, 352
staphylococcal, 935
transplacental, 930
uremic, 807
varicella, *383*
viral, 931
Pneumonitis; *see also* Pneumonia
chemical, 928
chlamydial, 930
cryptogenic organizing, 971, *971*
cytomegalovirus, 382
hypersensitivity, 965-967, *966*
causes of, 966t
dust-related, 236
occupationally induced, 236-237
radiation, 276, 984
Pneumothorax, 986-987
radiation injury and, 281
Podocytes, 805, *805*
POEMS syndrome, 1791
Point mutations, 261, 262
Poiseuille's law, 993
Poison ivy, 531
Poisoning, 193-194t
food, 292t, 293
gastrointestinal inflammation and, 1168
mercury bichloride, 831
uremia and, 807
Poliomyelitis, 374, *375*
encephalitis and, 2158
Pollen, 525
Pollutants, air, 230-232, 993
Polonium 210, 277
Polyarteritis nodosa, *537*, 623, 768-769, *770*,
825-826, *877*, 976
barbiturates and, 218
myocarditis in, 663
subcapsular infarct and, 1280, *1280*

Polyarthritis, 648
Polychlorinated biphenyls, 226-229, 599
cytochrome P-450 drug-metabolizing
enzyme system and, 5
toxicity of, 226-229
Polychondritis
chronic atrophic, 2090
relapsing, 776, 1089, 2090
Polycyclic hydrocarbons, 596
Polycyclic organic matter in oncogenesis,
239
Polycystic disease, 1268
hepatic, 461, 1293
ovarian, 1675-1676, *1676*
renal, 845-846, *846*
Polycythemia
bone marrow and, 1375, 1382
chronic myeloproliferative disorders and,
1393
cobalt toxicity and, 212
Polyembryoma, 885
ovary and, 1688
Polygonal cells, 1506
histiocyte-like, 1856
Polyhistiomas, 2043
Polykaryocytes, 28
Polymerase chain reaction, 1648
Polymicrogyria, 2139, *2139*
Polymorphic reticulosis, *1082*, 1083
Polymorphisms, enzyme, 1240
Polymorphonuclear leukocytes, 4, 499, *510*
myocardial infarction and, 636, 637, *637*
Rocky Mountain spotted fever and, 350
Polymyalgia rheumatica, 772
Polymyositis
and dermatomyositis complex, 2110, 2111,
2117, *2118*
pulmonary involvement in, 974
Polymyxin toxicity, 156-157
Polyomaviruses, 384, 2178
Polyorchidism, 871
Polyostotic fibrous dysplasia of oral mucosa,
1106
Polyp, 610
alimentary tract, 1175-1179, *1177*, *1178*
aural, 1088
cervical, 1645
endometrial, 1659
nasal, 525, 1078, *1078*
vaginal stromal, 1640
vocal, 1085
vulvar stromal, 1631
Polypeptides, pancreatic, 1368
Polypoid cystitis, 857
Polypoid endolymphangitis, 470
Polypoid gastric carcinoma, 1182
Polysaccharide capsules, 291
Polyserositis, 667
familial recurring, 1189
Polysplenia, 1413
Pompe's disease, 53, 55, 687, 1096
Pontiac fever, 311, 938
Pontine myelinolysis, *2179*
Popliteal artery adventitial disease, 785-786,
787
Porcelain gallbladder, *1329*, 1330
Porencephaly, 2139
Pores of Kohn, 933, 992
Pork tapeworm, 458
Poroepithelioma, eccrine, 1832
Porphyria, 149, 1771
Port-wine stain on face, 1819
Portacaval shunt
esophageal varices and, 1250

Portacaval shunt—cont'd
    portal hypertension and, 1249
Portal of entry for infectious diseases, 290
Portal amyloidosis, 1286
Portal area of liver, 1202
Portal cirrhosis, 1238
Portal fibrosis, alcoholism and, 1244
Portal hepatotrophic factors, 1206
Portal hypertension, 1248-1251
    idiopathic, 1281, 1281-1282
    intrahepatic, 1248
    liver and, 1202
    posthepatic, 1249
    prehepatic, 1249
    spleen and, 1415
Portal inflammation of liver, 1206
Portal lymphoid hyperplasia, 1202, 1206
Portal pressure, 1249
Portal-systemic encephalopathy, 2184
Portal-systemic shunt
    esophageal varices and, 1250
    portal hypertension and, 1249
Portal vein, 1249
    cirrhosis and thrombosis of, 1280, 1280
    collateral circulation and, 1249, 1250
    gas in, 1281
    obstruction of, 791
    occlusion of, 1280
Portoenterostomy, hepatic, 1262
Postcollapse cirrhosis, 1208
Posthepatic portal hypertension, 1249
Postinfectious glomerulonephritis, 812, 812-
        813, 813
Postintubation granulation tissue in larynx,
        1085
Post–kala-azar dermal leishmaniasis, 443
Postmastectomy lymphangiosarcoma, 1823
Postmortem autolysis, 1205
Postmortem change, 13
Postnatal hydranencephaly, 2139
Postnatal period, radiation and, 269
Postnecrotic cirrhosis, 1208
Postpartum cardiomyopathy, 684
Postprimary tuberculosis, 945-946
Postsinusoidal block, 1251
Poststeroid atrophy of adrenal glands, 1588
Postsynaptic receptor protein, 2118
Posttransfusion hepatitis, 1219, 1229
Postulates of Rivers, 362
Potassium, 807
    deficiency of
        heart failure and, 693
        hypokalemic nephropathy of, 834, 834
    sodium ratio to, 634
    transport of, 3-4
Potassium chloride toxicity, 186-189
Potassium ferrocyanide, 31
Potassium-sparing diuretic toxicity, 169
Potbelly, rachitic, 1986
Potter type I renal disease, 845-846
Potter type IV renal disease, 845, 845-846
Pott's disease, 2006
Poxviridae, 386-387
Prausnitz-Küstner test, 519
Preacher's node, 1085
Precancerous lesions of epidermis, 1796-
        1798
Precarcinogens, 596
Precirrhosis, 1244-1247
Precocious involution of fetal adrenal cortex,
        1583
Precocious puberty, 1106
Prednisone, 825
    adverse reactions to, 165

Prednisone—cont'd
    hepatic hepatitis B and, 1227
Preeclampsia, 827-828, 828, 1701-1702
Pregnancy, 42
    benign jaundice of, 1235
    choriocarcinoma and, 1710
    dissecting aneurysm and, 780
    ectopic, 1669
        placenta and, 1700
    fibroadenoma of breast in, 1730-1731
    hyperthyroidism and, 506
    liver diseases in, 1273-1275
    luteoma of, 1674-1675
    pituitary in, 1523
    placenta and, 1697
    radioactive isotopes and, 285
    termination of, 1700
    toxemia of, 827-828, 828, 1701-1702
    toxoplasmosis and, 449
Pregnancy cells, 1523
    of Erdheim, 1521
Pregnancy luteoma, 1675
Pregnancy-specific antigen 1, 881
Pregnancy tumor, 1819
    on gingiva, 1108
Pregnenolone, 1581, 1582
Prehepatic portal hypertension, 1249
Preinfarction angina, 626
Preleukemia, 1385, 1390
Premature loss of teeth, 1097
Premature separation of placenta, 1702-1703
Prenatal syphilis, 1105
Prepro-opiomelanocortin, 1522
Pressure hypertrophy in congenital heart
        disease, 730
Pretracheal fascia, 1024
Prickle cells, 1754, 1802
Primary biliary cirrhosis, 1255-1257, 1257,
        1294
    granulomas and, 1284
Primary complex in tuberculosis, 943
Primary hemochromatosis, 32-33
Primary ossification center, 1937-1939
Primary sclerosing cholangitis, 1257, 1333
Primary union in healing, 104
Primitive mesenchymal cells, 1858
Prinzmetal angina, 626
Procainamide, 149, 150
Procollagen III, 1207
Profile burns, 260, 261
Progenitor cells, 495
Progesterone, 1582
    endometrium and, 1654-1656
    obstetric cholestasis and, 1274
Progesterone receptors, 1323
Progestogens; see Progesterone
Progression in cell neoplasia, 585-586, 599
Progressive multifocal leukoencephalopathy,
        27, 384, 2178, 2178-2179
    as slow virus infection, 2162
Progressive muscular dystrophy, 694
Progressive perivenular alcoholic fibrosis,
        1207, 1244, 1245
Progressive primary tuberculosis, 944-945
Progressive systemic sclerosis, 826, 974
    gastrointestinal manifestations of, 1173
    pulmonary involvement in, 974
Prolactin, 1521, 1521t
Prolactin cell adenoma, 1533
Prolapse
    of spine, 2096-2097
    of urethra, 898

Proliferation, 85; see also Proliferative
        disorders
    in lung, tumorlike, 1023
Proliferation-inhibitory factor, 531t
Proliferative arteriolosclerosis, 755-756, 756
Proliferative disorders
    of lymphoid cells, 1394-1399
    of mast cells, 1403-1404, 1404
    of myeloid cells, 1390-1394
    of plasma cells, 1399-1403
    of white blood cells, 1384-1390
Proliferative fasciitis, 1852
Proliferative glomerulonephritis, 813
Proliferative mucosal lesions
    in ureter, 852
    in urinary bladder, 857-858
Proliferative myositis, 1852, 1852
Proliferative periorchitis, 878
Proliferative periosteitis, 1113
Prolonged gestation, 1703
Prolymphocytic leukemia, 1397
Promastigotes, flagellated, 443
Promoter, 602, 610
Proofreading, 8
Propagation of thrombus, 130
Propanol poisoning, 193t
Properdin, 511
Prophylactic antibiotics in endocarditis, 654
Propoxyphene poisoning, 193t
Propranolol, adverse reactions to, 168
Propylene glycol toxicity, 198
Prosencephalon, 2135
Prosoplasia, cervical squamous, 1643
Prostacyclin, 764
Prostaglandins, 519t
    ibuprofen toxicity and, 162
Prostate gland, 899-915, 919
    carcinoma in, 907-912
        ductal, 915
        lesions that simulate, 912, 913
        transitional cell, 915
        undifferentiated, 915
    distribution of glandular tissue in, 900
    female, 900
    hyperplasia of, 567, 567, 900
    malignant tumors of, 907-915
    nontumorous conditions of, 900-902
    obstruction of, 854
    tumorlike lesions of, 902-907
Prostate-specific antigen, 908, 915
Prostatectomy, 911
Prostatic acid phosphatase, 908, 915
Prostatic ductal dysplasia, 915
Prostatitis, 357, 900-901
Prosthetic valve infection, 413, 654
Prostigmin; see Neostigmine
Protamine, angiogenesis and, 102-104
Protease inhibitor system, 1264
Proteases, 994
Protection standards, radiation, 286
Protein, 546
    altered, 44
    amyloid, 40-41
    cobalt toxicity and, 212
    irradiation of, 23-24
    serum, 487
    synthesis of, 2-3
    Tamm-Horsfall, 851
    in urine; see Proteinuria
Protein-calorie malnutrition, 548-550
Protein catabolism, 631
Protein II, 309
Protein-losing enteropathy, 467, 1172

Proteinaceous infectious particle, 2164
Proteinaceous lymphadenopathy, 1432, *1433*
Proteinosis, alveolar, 981-982
Proteinuria, 516, 805, 820, 823
    Bence Jones, 839
    pregnancy and, 827
    radiation injury and, 279
Proteoglycans, 2, 752, 754
Proteolytic enzymes, 73, 291
Proteus, 311, 411
    alimentary tract and, 1189
    pulmonary infection and, 936
    urinary system and, 834, 851, 855
    vagina and, 1704
    wound infection and, 130
Prothrombin, 555
Proto-oncogene, 610
Protons, 23, 23*t*, 248
Protothecosis, 391, 392*t*, 402-404, *404*
Protozoal diseases, 433-452, 498*t*
    amebiasis in, 433-437
    amebic meningoencephalitis in, 437
    balantidiasis in, 437-438
    flagellates in
        blood and tissue, 439-445
        digestive tract and genital organ, 438-
            439
    myocarditis and, 661, 661-662
    placenta and, 1705
    sporozoans in, 445-452
        babesiosis and, 451-452
        isoporiasis and, 445
        malaria and, 445-448
        pneumocystosis and, 450-451, *451*
        toxoplasmosis and, 448-450, *449*
Protracted nonfreezing hypothermia, 137
Protracted viral hepatitis, 1222
Proximal convoluted tubules
    coagulative necrosis of, 201, *201*, 202
    epithelial proliferation of, 1252
    platinum toxicity and, 216
Pruritus
    atopic eczema and, 526
    enterobiasis and anal, 465
    primary biliary cirrhosis and, 1255-1256
Prussian blue reaction, 31
Psammoma bodies, 1559, 1571, 1679
Pseudallescheriasis, 392*t*, 395*t*, 402, 408,
    410, 423, *424*
Pseudarthrosis, 2002
Pseudobuboes, 310
Pseudocholangioles, 1207
Pseudocholinesterase, 149
Pseudocysts
    myocarditis and, 661
    splenic, 1426
Pseudodiverticulosis, 1159
Pseudoectasia of vessels, 1808-1809
Pseudoepitheliomatous hyperplasia, 1758
    in oral soft tissue, 1108
    skin and, 1796, 1805
Pseudofibromatous periorchitis, 878, *879*
Pseudofractures, 1986, *1988*
Pseudogout, 2090
Pseudohermaphroditism, 872, 1624, 1625*t*
    female, 1627
    male, 1626-1627
Pseudohypha, 397
Pseudohypoparathyroidism, 1572
    osteoporosis and, *1978*, 1978-1979, *1979*
Pseudolaminar necrosis, 2147
Pseudolobules, hepatic
    cirrhosis and, 1246, *1247*
    hypoxic necrosis and, 1278-1279

Pseudolymphomas, pulmonary, 1022
Pseudomembranous enterocolitis, 153, *154-
    155*, 155, 1166
Pseudomembranous inflammation, 86-87
Pseudomonas, 311, 322, 410-411
    adrenal glands and, 1585
    pregnancy and, 1704
    pulmonary infection and, 930, 936, 937,
        937, 951
    upper respiratory tract and, 1088
    urinary system and, 834, 855
    wound infection and, 130
Pseudomyxoma peritonei, 1191, 1682
Pseudopalisades, 2168
Pseudopod of neutrophils, 77
Pseudopolyps of colon, 1163
Pseudosarcoma of gallbladder, *1342*, 1343
Pseudosarcomatous fibrous lesions, 1850-
    1852
Pseudostratified ciliated columnar cell
    metaplasia, 107, *107*
Pseudotubercles, bilharzial, 455, *455*
Pseudotumor
    gallbladder and biliary ducts and, 1334-
        1335
    inflammatory, 1292-1293
    in tunica vaginalis, 894
Pseudoxanthoma elasticum, 757, 1783
Psittacosis, 356*t*, 356-357
Psoriasis, 539*t*, 1772-1773
    arthritis and, 2086
Psorospermosis, 1759
Psychosis, Korsakoff's, 556
Pteroylglutamates, 560
Ptyalism, 1127
Puberty, 871
    precocious, 1106
Puerperal sepsis, 305-306
Pulex irritans, 320
Pulmonary agenesis, 921
Pulmonary alveolar microlithiasis, 189, *189*
Pulmonary amyloidosis, *983*
Pulmonary arteriovenous fistula, 795, 922
Pulmonary artery aneurysms, 785
Pulmonary artery sling, 922
Pulmonary aspergillosis, 408-409, *410*
Pulmonary atresia with intact ventricular
    septum, 747-748, *749*
Pulmonary blastoma, 1019, *1019*
Pulmonary candidiasis, 412
Pulmonary coccidioidomycosis, 414
Pulmonary cryptococcosis, 415
Pulmonary defenses against infection, 931
Pulmonary distomiasis, 453-454
Pulmonary edema, 958-962, 1035-1036
    capillary permeability and, 960-961
    extrathoracic injuries and, 962
    hemodynamics and, 960
    high-altitude, 133
    hyperoxia and, 962
    left-sided heart failure and, 959-960
    mechanisms of, 958-959
    occupationally induced, 237
Pulmonary eosinophilia, 967
    and granuloma, 977
    nitrofurantoin and, 174
    penicillin therapy and, 156
Pulmonary epithelial radiosensitivity, 257*t*
Pulmonary fibroleiomyoma, 1666
Pulmonary fibrosis
    asbestosis and, 235
    hemorrhage and, 985
Pulmonary heart disease, 679-680

Pulmonary hemorrhage, 985
    in newborn, 928-929
    systemic lupus erythematosus and, *973*
Pulmonary hemosiderosis, 985
Pulmonary histiocytosis X, 977-978, *978*
Pulmonary hypertension, 954-958
    shunts and, 735, *736*
Pulmonary hypoplasia, 921
    etiology of, 921*t*
Pulmonary infiltrates with eosinophilia; *see*
    Pulmonary eosinophilia
Pulmonary insufficiency, 676
Pulmonary interstitial emphysema, 928, *928*
Pulmonary isomerism, 921
Pulmonary lymphangiectasia, congenital,
    923
Pulmonary mechanical injury, 131
Pulmonary metastasis of prostatic carcinoma,
    911
Pulmonary mucormycosis, 426
Pulmonary nocardiosis, *421*
Pulmonary overinflation, congenital, 923-925
Pulmonary paracoccidioidomycosis, 422
Pulmonary parenchyma
    asthma and, 964
    radiation injury to, 277
Pulmonary stenosis, 676
    carcinoid tumors and, 691
    isolated, 739, *739*
Pulmonary tuberculosis; *see* Tuberculosis
Pulmonary vascular anomalies, 922
Pulmonary vascular disease, 951-958, 1034-
    1035
    emboli and
        air, 953
        amniotic fluid, 953
        fat, 953
        foreign-body, 953-954
    histology of normal vasculature and, 951-
        952
    hypertension in, 954-958
    infarcts and, 953
    thromboembolism and, 952
Pulmonary veno-occlusive disease, 957
Pulmonary venous drainage, total
    anomalous, 737-738, *738*
Pulmonary venous obstruction, 738
Pulmonary venous thrombi, 623, 738, 952,
    957
Pulmonary wedge pressure, 954
Pulmonic infections, chronic, 312
Pulp disease, dental, 1098
Pulpitis, 1098
Pulsion diverticula, 1155
Pump failure in myocardial infarction, 638
Pure gallstones, 1323, *1324*, 1325*t*
Pure gonadal dysgenesis, 1625*t*
Pure neural leprosy, 343
Pure osteitis fibrosis, 1997
Pure osteomalacia, 1997
Pure red blood cell aplasia, 1377
Purified protein derivative, 999
Purine antagonist toxicity, 183
Purine metabolism, 36-37, 499
Purine nucleoside phosphorylase deficiency,
    501*t*, 503, 1500*t*
Purpura
    cutaneous, 1786
    Henoch-Schönlein, 816, 1789, 1790
    hyperglobulinemia of Waldenström and,
        1789
    thrombotic thrombocytopenic, 827
Purulent meningitis, *2154*, 2154-2155, *2155*

Purulent pericarditis, 666
Pus, 85, 87
Pustular dermatosis, subcorneal, 1765
Pustular folliculitis, eosinophilic, 1787
Pustule, 1757
Pyelonephritis, 823, 834-836, 835
   candidiasis and, 412
   chronic, 835, 836, 836
   lymphocytes and, 82
   parathyroid glands and, 1577
   tuberculous, 835-836
Pyelophlebitis, 1202
Pyknosis, 12
   myocardial infarction and, 636
   radiation injury and, 255
Pylephlebitis, 791, 1258
Pyloric obstruction, 1161
Pyloric stenosis, 1154
Pyocyanine, 311
Pyocystis, 860
Pyoderma, 302
Pyoderma gangrenosum, 1766
Pyogenic abscesses of liver, 1258-1259
Pyogenic bacteria, 301
   lymphangitis and, 792
Pyogenic cholangiohepatitis, recurrent, 1254
Pyogenic granuloma
   in larynx, 1085
   in nasal cavity, 1081, 1081
Pyonephrosis, 837
Pyorrhea, 938
β-Pyridine carboxylic acid, 556
Pyridoxal 5′-phosphate, 559
Pyridoxine, 556, 558-559
Pyrimidines, halogenated, radiosensitivity of
   cells and, 254
Pyrophosphate arthropathy, 2090
Pyrrolizidine toxicity, 224
   liver and, 1232
   veno-occlusive disease and, 1282
Pyruvate kinase, 10
Pyuria, 808

Q

Q fever, 349t, 354-356, 1232
   granulomas and, 1284-1285
   infective endocarditis and, 654
Queensland tick typhus, 349t, 353
Queyrat, erythroplasia of, 897
Quinidine, 708
   granulomas and, 1285
   hypersensitivity reaction, 1236
   sensitization and, 148
   toxicity of, 176
Quinine
   hypersensitivity reaction to, 219
   poisoning from, 194t
   sensitization and, 148
Quinsy, 303

R

R-ras, 589
Rabbit fever, 318-320
Rabies, 369-370, 370
   encephalitis and, 2158, 2159
Racemose aneurysm, 778
Rachitic potbelly, 1986
Raccoon parasite, 473
Rad, 249
Radar devices, 285
Radiation, 22-25, 23t, 249; see also Radiation
   injury; Radiation oncogenesis
   cosmic, 249-250, 250t

Radiation—cont'd
   electromagnetic, 247, 247-248
   environmental, 249-250
   exposure to, 250t
   factors in response to, 253-254
   gastrointestinal inflammation and, 1168
   generator types and, 283-284
   heavy-particle, 284
   human populations and, 258t
   laser, 285
   lethal dose of, 264
   macromolecules and, 254-255
   man-made, 250, 250t
   microwave, 880
   mutations and, 261, 262
   nonionizing, 285t, 285-286
   particulate, 248
   skin and, 1801
   terrestrial, 250
   tumor response to, 268
   ultraviolet, 30, 286
   whole-body, 264, 270
Radiation biology, cellular and molecular,
   250-255, 251
   tumor and, 282-283
Radiation hits, 251
Radiation injury, 247-288; see also Radiation
   oncogenesis
   acute radiation syndrome in, 270-273
   to bone marrow, 279
   to breast, 281
   to cardiovascular system, 274
   to cartilage and bone, 280-281
   cellular and molecular radiation biology
     in, 250-255, 251
   to central nervous system, 281
   cystitis and, 856
   dose and, 251, 251t, 252, 253
   early lethality of, 264-265
   environmental radiation and, 249-250
   exposed populations and, 258-261
   to eyes, 281
   factors affecting degree of, 253-254
   to gastrointestinal tract, 277-278
   general effects of, 256-258
   genetic effects of, 261-263
   to genitourinary system, 279-280
   to liver, 278-279, 1283
   to lung, 274-277, 984-985
   morphologic features of, 255-256
   to myocardium, 699-700
   nephritis and, 279, 832
   nonionizing radiation in, 285t, 285-286
   nonstochastic, 257
   protection and concept of relative risk
     and, 286
   radiation spectrum and, 247-248
   radiation units and, 249
   radioactive substances and, 248-249
   radiotherapy and, 282-285
   repair of sublethal, 254
   of skin, 273-274
   somatic effects of, 263-264
     late, 265-270
   stochastic, 257
   testicular, 876, 880
   thymic, 259
   to thyroid, 281, 1554
Radiation oncogenesis, 239, 257, 594, 595;
   see also Radiation injury
   bone tumors and, 2018, 2019
   dose and, 268, 268
   leukemia and, 1385

Radiation oncogenesis—cont'd
   linear energy transfer and, 265
   of skin, 274
Radiation spectrum, 247-248
Radiation therapy; see Radiation;
   Radiotherapy
Radiation units, 249
Radical mastectomy, survival rate and, 1740t
Radicular cyst in jaws, 1118
Radicular dentin dysplasia, 1097
Radio waves, 285t
Radioactive fallout, 281, 286
Radioactive isotopes, 248, 263, 284-285; see
   also Radionuclides
Radioactive substances, 248-249
   oncogensis and; see Radiation oncogenesis
Radioallergosorbent test, 520
Radiodermatitis, 273-274
Radioimmunoassay, 448
Radioisotopes, 248, 263, 284-285; see also
   Radionuclides
Radiolabeled bungaro toxin, 508
Radiology, diagnostic, 263
Radiology personnel, 262
Radiomimetic drugs, 255
Radionuclide angiography, 2, 26, 51
Radionuclides; see also Radioisotopes
   bone-seeking, 280
   internally deposited, 259
Radiosensitivity, 256, 257t
Radiotherapy, 263, 282-285, 606
   bone tumors and, 2024
   prostate gland and, 911
Radiothorium toxicity, 186
Radium, 249, 284
   in paint, 259
Radium jaw, 280
Radium water, 280
Radon 222, 277, 594
raf 1, 587t
Ragged-red fibers, 2116, 2117
Ranula, 1127
Ranvier, ring of, 1937, 1941, 1941
Rapidly progressive glomerulonephritis, 813,
   814, 814-815
Rappaport classification of non-Hodgkin's
   lymphomas, 1452-1453
Rappaport zone of hepatocytes, 1200
ras, 585, 587, 587t, 588, 589
Rat fibroblasts, 599
Rat urothelium, 599
Rathke's pouch, 1517
   craniopharyngioma and, 2173
Raynaud's phenomenon, 777-778
   pulmonary hypertension and, 957
Reactive lymphoid hyperplasia, 1433-1443,
   1436
Reactive perforating collagenosis, 1784
Reactive systemic amyloidosis, 1286
Reaginic antibody, 519
Recognition unit, complement, 511
Recombinant-deoxyribonucleic acid therapy,
   62
Rectal shelf, 1180
Rectal tonsil, 1186
Rectum
   carcinoid tumors in, 1185
   carcinoma of, 1180
   hyperinfection in, 468
   juvenile polyp of, 1177, 1178
   lymphoma of, 1186
   papillary adenoma of, 1176
Recurrent aphthae, 1104

Recurrent herpes, 1104
Recurrent pyogenic cholangiohepatitis, 1254
Recurring polyserositis, 1189
Red blood cell aplasia, 1377
Red blood cell production, decreased, 807,
    1375-1379
Red devil, 219
Red flare, 67
Red pulp in spleen, 1408
Redness of skin, 84
    scarlatina and, 305
Reduced nicotinamide adenine dinucleotide,
    1
    ethanol and, 19, 197, 1239
    oxidation of, 2
Reduced nicotinamide adenine dinucleotide
        phosphate, 5
    ethanol and, 19
Reduplications, 1024
Reed-Sternberg cells, *1444*, 1444-1447,
    1445, 1466, 1509
Reed-Sternberg-like cells, 1856
Reflux, vesicoureteral, 851
Reflux nephropathy, 836
Regeneration, 94-98
    of labile cells, 94-96
    of liver, 1206-1207
        and cirrhosis, 1208
    of stable cells, 97
Regional extension of tumors, 584
Regional vascular spasm, 129-130
Regurgitation, aortic, 650
Reid index, 951, 987
Reifenstein's syndrome, 1627
Reinke's crystals, 889, 1687
Reinke's space, 1085
Reiter's syndrome, 776, 2086
    keratoderma blennorrhagica and, 1774
    urinary system disorders and, 855, 898-
        899
Reither's syndrome, 1104
Rejection, graft, 531-534, *533*
Relapsing polychondritis, 776, 1089, 2090
Relative biologic effectiveness, 253
Rem, 249
Remodeling of bone, 1943-1944, *1944*
    disorders of, 1957-2000; *see also*
        Metabolic bone diseases
    histomorphometric correlates of, 1959*t*
    osteoporosis and, 1971-1972
    regulation of, 1944*t*
Renal acidosis, chronic, 807
Renal adenocarcinoma, 847
Renal agenesis, 844
Renal azotemia, 808
Renal calculi, 839-840, *840*
    parathyroid glands and, 1575
    shock waves and, 136
    staghorn, 840
    vitamin A deficiency and, 553
Renal cell carcinoma metastasis, *2056*
Renal cortex, tubular adenomas of, 847
Renal differentiation, defective, 845, *845*
Renal disease
    classification of, 809-810
    metastatic calcification and ossification
        and, 982
    myeloma and, 1402
    parathyroid glands and, 1575-1577
    pharmacogenetics and, 150
    polycystic, 845-846, *846*
    thrombotic, 826-827
    vascular, 841-844

Renal dysplasia, 845, *845*
    obstructive, *845*, 845-846
Renal epithelial radiosensitivity, 257*t*
Renal failure
    anatomy of, 807-809
    chronic, 807
    cirrhosis and, 1252
    mercury and, 201
    pulmonary edema and, 960
Renal function, cirrhosis and, 1251
Renal glomerular insufficiency, parathyroid
        glands and, 1573
Renal graft rejection, 532-533, *533*
Renal hypertension, 841-842
Renal hypoplasia, 844
Renal infarction, 841
Renal injury, irreversible, 131
Renal insufficiency, acute, 806-807
Renal lithiasis; *see* Renal calculi
Renal medullary necrosis, 837
Renal neoplasms, 847-849, *849*
Renal osteodystrophy, 1995-1997, *1996*
    osteitis fibrosa and osteomalacia and, *1995*
    osteosclerosis of, 1997, *1999*
    parathyroid glands and, 1577
    pure form of osteomalacia of, 1997, *1998*
Renal papillary necrosis, 837
Renal pathophysiology, 806-807
Renal pelvis, tumors of, 849, *849*
Renal stones; *see* Renal calculi
    parathyroid glands and, 1577
Renal transplantation, 533-534
Renal tubular hyperplasia, 43
Renal tubular injury; *see* Tubular injury
Renal tubular loss; *see* Tubular loss
Rendu-Osler-Weber disease, 1159, 1820
Renin, 841
Reoviridae, 370
Repair, 94, 98-106
    myocardial infarction and, 635-637
    with organization, 102-104
    of sublethal radiation injury, 254
Reperfusion, myocardial, 629, 632-633
    injury in, 21, 633
Replication of deoxyribonucleic acid, 8-9
Reproduction, cells and, 8-9
Reproductive system; *see also* Female
        genitalia; Male reproductive system
    cystic fibrosis and, 1351
    ionizing radiation and, 250-251
Reserpine
    adverse reactions to, 168
    gynecomastia and galactorrhea and, 168
Reserve cells, 569
Residency training programs in
        neuropathology, 2123
Residual bodies, 4
Resistance, electrical injury and, 141
Resistance syndromes, female genitalia and,
        1624, 1626-1627
Respirator brain, 1527, 2147
Respiratory distress syndrome
    adult, 961
    oxygen toxicity and, 176-180
Respiratory oxidative metabolism, 1
Respiratory syncytial virus, 367, 931
Respiratory tract; *see also* Pulmonary entries
    cystic fibrosis and, 1349, 1350
    parainfluenza viral disease of, 366
    upper; *see* Upper respiratory tract and ear
Response-to-injury hypothesis, 621, 622
Restriction point, 9
Restrictive cardiomyopathies, 682, 695-698

Rests of Malassez, 1099
Rete malpighii, 1764, 1796
    spongiosis in, 1761
Rete ridges, 1755
Rete testis, 892
Reticular colliquation, 1757
Reticular dysgenesis, 501*t*, 1500*t*
Reticularis zone of adrenal glands, 1580
Reticulin, healing and, 105
Reticulin stain, 1533, *1533*
Reticulocytosis, 1379
Reticuloendothelial system, 52, 515
    phagocytosis and, *509*
Reticulohistiocytic granuloma, 1792
Reticulohistiocytoma, 1792, *1793*
Reticulosis, 1826
    midline malignant, *1082*, 1083
    pagetoid, 1827
Reticulum cells, interdigitating, 492*t*
Retina
    degenerative diseases of, 1072-1074
    detachment of, 1072, *1074*
    hemorrhage of, *1074*
        leukemia and, 1069
    infarct of, 1063, *1063*
    nonionizing radiation and, 285
    vascular disease of, 1057-1064
Retinal vessels, oxygen toxicity and, 180,
        1052
Retinitis pigmentosa, 1052
Retinoblastoma, 579, 593*t*, 1064, 1066,
        1067, *1068*
    chromosomal alterations and, 593-594
    radiosensitivity of, 257*t*
Retinopathy
    diabetic, *1060*, *1061*, 1364
    hypertensive, 1062
    of prematurity, 1052
    sickle cell, 1063-1064
Retinyl palmitate, 551
Retrolental fibroplasia, 1052
Retroperitoneum, 1190-1191
    idiopathic fibrosis of, 1190
    leiomyosarcoma of, 1864
    liposarcoma of, 1879
    lymph node dissection and, 884
Retroperitonitis, sclerosing, 163
Retroviruses, 375-376, 586
Reverse smoking, 1112
Reverse transfusion reaction, *511*
Reversible ischemic neurologic deficit, 2149
Reversible tubular lesions, 833-834
Reye's syndrome, 1268-1269, 2184-2185
    carnitine deficiency and, 2115
    phosphorus poisoning and, 224
Rhabditiform larvae, 463, 468
Rhabdoid tumor
    of kidney, 849
    of soft tissue, 1909
Rhabdomyoblasts, 866
Rhabdomyoma, 1871-1873
    adult, 1872, *1872*
    of myocardium, 703
    in oral soft tissue, 1108
    in upper respiratory tract and ear, 1089
Rhabdomyosarcoma, 603, 1864-1871
    alveolar, 1867-1870
    differentiation of, 1866
    embryonal, 1867
        biliary tract and, 1343, *1343*
        vaginal, 1642, *1643*
    of head, 1089
    in nasal cavity, 1083
    pleomorphic, 1870-1871

Rhabdomyosarcoma—cont'd
  radiosensitivity of, 257*t*
  sites of, 1867
  in upper respiratory tract and ear, 1089
Rhabdoviridae, 369-370
Rhagades, 1757
Rhagocytes, 2085
Rheumatic fever and rheumatic heart
          disease, 639-649
  aortic stenosis and, 674
  arteritis in, 623, 775
  arthritis and, 2077
  Aschoff nodule in, 92
  cardiac manifestations of, 641-648
    valvulitis healing and, 644-645
  causes of death in, 649
  etiology and pathogenesis of, 640-641
  extracardiac lesions in, 648
  immunologic mechanism and, 641
  incidence of, 639-640
  postmortem diagnosis of old, 648-649
  pulmonary involvement in, 972
  vasculitis in, 623, 775
Rheumatic heart disease; *see* Rheumatic
          fever and rheumatic heart disease
Rheumatoid aortitis, 775-776
Rheumatoid arteritis, 623, 775
Rheumatoid arthritis, 649-650, 768, 2077-
          2086, *2080*, *2081*
  distribution and prevalence of, 2078
  etiology and pathogenesis of, 2084-2086
  lesion in, 2079
  pathologic anatomy of, 2078-2084
  pericarditis with, 670
  synovial fluid and, *2077*
Rheumatoid diseases, 516, *973*
  granuloma and, *2084*
  pulmonary involvement in, 972-973
Rheumatoid factor, 148
Rheumatoid nodule, 92, 648, *648*, 1777-
          1778, 2079, *2082*, *2083*
Rheumatoid pannus, *2081*
Rheumatoid synovitis, *2078*
Rhinitis
  acute, 1078
  atrophic, 313
  seasonal allergic, 525
Rhinocerebral mucormycosis, 426, *426*
Rhinocladiella aquaspersa, 392*t*, 399
Rhinofacial zygomycosis, 426-427
Rhinophyma, 1077
Rhinoscleroma, 313, 1079
Rhinosporidiosis, 393*t*, 404, *404*, 1079
Rhinoviruses, 375
Rhipicephalus sanguineus, 350, 358
Rhizomucor, 395*t*, 425
Rhizopus, 395*t*, 425, 426
Rhodesian trypanosomiasis, 439
Rhodopsin, 552
Rhombencephalon, 2135
Rhomboid glossitis, 1096
Rhoptries, 449
Rib markings, 135
Riboflavin, 555, 558
Ribosomes, 2-3
  mercury poisoning and, 205
Rickets, 554, 1983-2000, *1985*, *1986*, *1987*;
          see also Osteomalacia and rickets
  dentin and, 1097-1098
  growth plate and, *1986*
  polymorphic mesenchymal tumors and,
          1909

Rickettsial diseases, 348-356, 349*t*, *350*
  murine typhus and, 354
  myocarditis and, 660-661
  neonatal encephalitis and, 2162
  Q fever and, 354-356
  Rocky Mountain spotted fever and, 350-
          353
  scrub typhus group and, 354
  typhus and, 354
Rickettsialpox, 349*t*, 353
Riedel lobe, 1201
Riedel's thyroiditis, 1553-1554
Rifadin; *see* Rifampin
Rifampin, 155, 170
Rifle wounds, 123, *124*
Rifles, 119-120
Right-sided heart failure, 615
Rimactane; *see* Rifampin
Rimifon; *see* Isoniazid
Rimmed vacuoles, 2112
RIND; *see* Reversible ischemic neurologic
          deficit
Ring of Ranvier, 1937, 1941, *1941*
Ringworm, 1768-1769
Risus sardonicus, 294
River blindness, 473
Rivers' postulates, 362
RNA
  cervical tumors and, 1647
  radiation injury and, 254-255
RNA polymerase, rifampin and, 171
RNA viruses, 363-377, 586, 600
  alphaviruses and, 371
  Arenaviridae and, 372-373
  Bunyaviridae and, 370
  Coronaviridae and, 369
  flaviviruses and, 371-372
  human retroviruses and, 375-376
  orthomyxoviruses and, 363-365
  paramyxoviruses and, 365-369
  Picornaviridae and, 374-375
  Rhabdoviridae and, 369-370
  rhinoviruses and, 375
  Togaviridae and, 370-371
Rocky Mountain spotted fever, 349*t*, 350-
          353, *351*, *352*
  myocarditis and, 660
Rod myopathy, 2113, *2114*
Roentgen, 249
Romaña's sign, *441*
Romanowsky stain, 1374, 1390
Romberg sign, 2158
Rosenthal fibers, 2134
Rotavirus group, 376-377
Rothia dentocariosa, 393*t*
Rotor syndrome, 1275, 1276*t*, 1277-1278
Rough endoplasmic reticulum, 3, 1244
Round cell liposarcoma, 1877, *1878*
Rounded atelectasis, 986
Roundworm, pig, 462
Rous sarcoma virus, 586, 587*t*
RSV; *see* Respiratory syncytial virus
Rubella, 370
  cholestasis and, 1261*t*
  encephalitis and, 2160, 2162
  jaundice and, 1265
  rheumatoid arthritis and, 2084
Rubeola, 367-368
Rubeosis iridis, 1062, *1062*, *1063*
Rubiviruses, 370
Ruffini corpuscles, 1757
Ruffled border of osteoclasts, 1936
Runting, 534

Rupture
  of bladder, 853
  cardiac, 638-639
  of ovarian carcinoma, 1692
  of spleen, 1414
Russell's bodies, 440, 1021, 1400, 2050
Russian spring-summer encephalitis, 372
Rye classification of Hodgkin's disease, 1446

S

S-100 protein
  as nervous system tumor marker, 2166*t*
  neurilemoma and, 1892
S phase of cell cycle, 9
Saber shins, 2006
Sabin-Feldman dye test, 449
Sabouraud's agar, 1768
Saccharin, 597, 599
Saccular aneurysms, 778
  hemorrhage from ruptured, 2151-2153,
          2152
Saccules, 920
Safety belt injuries, 116, *117*
Safrole, 596, 597*t*
St. Louis encephalitis, 371-372
St. Vitus's dance, 648
Saksenaea, 395*t*, 425, *425*
Salicylates, 158-160
  children and, 150
  Reye's syndrome and, 2184-2185
Salivary glands, 1127-1141
  adenoid cystic carcinoma and, 1833
  cysts of, 1120, 1127-1128
  development of, 1127
  enlargements of, 1127, 1128
  inflammatory diseases of, 1128-1131
  radiation injury and, 277-278
  salivary flow and, 1127
  Sjögren's syndrome and, 974
  squamous metaplasia of, 107, *107*
  structure and types of, 1127
  tumors of, 1131-1141
Salmonella, 294, 314-317, 1419
  food poisoning and, 294
  osteomyelitis and, 2005
Salpingitis, 1165, 1667-1668
Salpingitis isthmica nodosa, 1669
Sand, inflammatory lesions from, 90
Sand fly, 444
Sansert; *see* Methysergide
Santa Marta hepatitis, 1223
Santorini duct, 1347
Saphenous vein, 787
Saponification, 16
Saprophytes, 391
Sarcocystis, 445
Sarcoid granuloma
  of bone marrow, *1407*
  of liver, 1284, *1284*
  pulmonary necrotizing, 981
Sarcoidosis, 539*t*
  arthritis and, 2087
  Boeck, 1287
  bone and, 2006
  eyes and, 1057, *1059*
  frequency of organ involvement in, 980*t*
  granulomatous inflammation and, 91, *91*
  liver and, 1287, 1299
  lymph nodes and, *1436*
  myocarditis and, 660
  pulmonary, 978-981, *979*
  skin and, 1784-1785
  urinary system and, 838

Sarcolemmal damage, 633, *634*, 2109-2110
Sarcoma, 578, 610, 1838, 1841
　alveolar soft part, 1903-1906, *1905*
　botryoid, 1089, 1642, *1643*
　of breast, 1748
　chordoid, 1909
　circumscribed cerebellar, 2171
　clear cell, 1902-1903, 2096
　embryonal
　　bladder and, 866, *866*
　　liver and, 1299
　endometrium and, *1662*
　epithelioid, 1900-1902, *1902*
　Ewing's, 579, 2045-2047
　　cytogenetics and, 603
　　extraskeletal, 1907-1909
　fibromyxoid low-grade, 1909
　grading systems for, 1842
　idiopathic multiple pigmented, 797
　Kaposi's; *see* Kaposi's sarcoma
　mesenchymal, 1299
　osteogenic
　　jaws and, 1116-1117
　　radiosensitivity of, 257*t*
　of ovary, 1684
　of penis, 898
　of prostate gland, 915
　pulmonary, 1020
　soft-tissue, 1113
　synovial, 1898-1900, *1899*, 2094-2096
　of undetermined histogenesis, 1865
Sarcomatoid carcinoma in oral soft tissue,
　1112
Sarcomeres, 2105-2106
Sarcoplasm, abnormalities of, 2110
Sarcoplasmic reticulum, 2106
Sarcotubular complex, 2106
Sashimi, 462
Scabies, 1769
Scale, 1757
Scaling skin syndrome, 1766
Scar
　chronic inflammation and, 90
　glomerular tuft, 809
　myocardial, 636
　　endomyocardial fibrosis and, 696
Scarlatina, 305
Scarlet fever, 305
Scedosporium apiospermum, 423
Schaumann bodies, 979, 1005
Scheie's disease, 53
Schilder's disease, 2177
Schistosomiasis, 454-458, *456*, *457*, 1167
　bladder carcinoma and, 860
　cardiopulmonary, 457-458
　granulomas and, 458, 1284
　hepatosplenic, 455-457, 1286
　intestinal, 455
Schizogony, 446
Schizonts, 445
Schlemm's canal, *1070*, 1071
Schmidt's syndrome, 1525, 1587
Schmorl's nodules, 2096
Schönlein-Henoch purpura, 516, 769, 816,
　1789, 1790
Schultz-Charlton phenomenon, 305
Schultz-Dale test, 519
Schwann cells, 97, 1366, 1537, 1890
　concentric proliferation around, *2190*,
　2191
Schwannoma, 1890, 2053, 2171-2173, *2172*
　malignant, 1894-1896
　in mediastinum, 1026

Schwannoma—cont'd
　skin and, 1825
　von Recklinghausen's neurofibromatosis
　　and acoustic, 2175
SCIDS; *see* Severe combined immune
　deficiency diseases
Scimitar syndrome, 922
Scirrhous carcinoma, 610
　of breast, *1742*, 1742-1743
Scleredema, 1780
Sclerema neonatorum, 1780, 1789
Sclerodactylia, 1779
Scleroderma, 826, *1779*, 1779-1780
　alimentary tract and, 1173
　myocarditis and, 663
Sclerosing adenosis of breast, *1729*, 1729-
　1730
Sclerosing angiogenic tumor of alveoli, *1020*
Sclerosing angioma, 1820
Sclerosing cholangitis, 1257, 1333
Sclerosing hemangioma, 1819
　in lung, 1021
Sclerosing hyaline necrosis, 1243
Sclerosing lipogranuloma, 896, *897*
Sclerosing mediastinitis, 163, 1024
Sclerosing nephropathy, 825
Sclerosing peritonitis, 163, 1189
　propranolol and, 168
Sclerosing retroperitonitis, 163
Sclerosing well-differentiated liposarcoma,
　1874-1875
Sclerosis
　amyotrophic lateral, 2119, 2120
　tuberous, *2175*, 2175-2176
Scoliosis, 2096
Scrapes, 112
Scrapie, 387
Scratch, 112
Screamer's node, 1085
Scrotum, 871, 893-894
　tumors of, 879-891
Scrub typhus, 349*t*, 354
　myocarditis and, 660
Scuba divers, 134
Scurvy, 560-561, 1982, *1983*, *1984*
　heart disease and, 692
　hemopericardium and, 665
Sea-blue histiocyte, 1420
Seasonal allergic rhinitis, 525
Sebaceous cyst, 1835
Sebaceous glands, 1077, 1756
　diseases of, 1787
　radiosensitivity of, 257*t*
　tumors of, 1833-1834
　　eyelid and, *1047*, *1049*
　　salivary glands and, 1136-1137, *1137*
Seborrheic keratosis, 1795, *1795*
Secobarbital poisoning, 193*t*
Seconal toxicity, 219
Second-degree burns, 96, 138, *138*
Second-set rejection, 532
Secondary ossification center, 1939-1941
Secondary osteons, *1942*
Secondary shock
　burns and, 139
　mechanical injury and, 130-131
Secondary spongiosa, 1941
Secondary vitamin D deficiency, 1990-1993
Secretory carcinoma of breast, 1746
Segmental emphysema, congenital, 923-925
Selective vulnerability, 2124-2125
Selenium, 563
Self-eating, 28, *29*

Self-tolerance, mechanisms breaking, 498
Semilunar cartilage cyst, 2092
Seminal vesicles, 916-917
Seminiferous tubules, 871
Seminoma, 882-883, *883*, 1538
　cryptorchidism and, 872
　radiosensitivity of, 257*t*
Sendai virus, 28
Senear-Usher syndrome, 1762
Senecio, 1283
Senile arteriosclerosis, 753
Senile cardiac amyloidosis, 695
Senile elastosis, 1783, *1783*
Senile keratosis, 1796-1797
Senile kyphosis, 2096
Senile lentigo, 1811
Senile osteoporosis, 1967
Sennetsu rickettsiosis, 349*t*
Sepsis; *see also* Infection; Septicemia
　hypophyseal inflammation and, 1527
　neonatal and childhood cholestasis and,
　　1261*t*
　puerperal, 305-306
Septal cirrhosis, 1238
Septal hypertrophy, asymmetric, 682-683
Septate, 397
Septic infarcts in central nervous system,
　2153-2154
Septic splenitis, 1418
Septic thrombophlebitis of dural sinuses,
　2153-2154
Septicemia, 826, 1258; *see also* Sepsis
　liver abscesses and, 1259
　　Pseudomonas, 937
　　Salmonella, 317
　typhoid fever and, 315
Sequestration, bronchopulmonary, 922-923
Sequoiosis, 966*t*
Serofibrinous pericarditis, 665-666
Seronegative spondyloarthropathies, 2086-
　2087
Serotonin, 433, 519*t*, 1184
　aspirin and, 160
　carcinoid tumors and, 690
　encephalopathy and, 1248
　vascular permeability and, 72-73
Serous exudate, 85
Serous pericarditis, 665-666
Serous tumors of ovary, 1679-1680, *1680*
Serpentine aneurysm, 778
Serpentine rock, 235
Serpiginous lesion, 1182
Serratia, 930
Sertoli cell—only syndrome, 873-874
Sertoli cells, 871, 875
　testicular tumor and, 888-889
Sertoli-Leydig cell tumors of ovary, 1685-
　1686, *1686*
Serum
　horse, 515
　passive leukocyte-sensitizing activity of,
　　519
Serum globulin, *497*
Serum protein alpha$_1$-antitrypsin, 993
Serum proteins, 487
Serum sickness, 512-515, *514*, 769
Severe combined immune deficiency
　diseases, 501*t*, 1499, 1500*t*
　thymic dysplasia and, *1501*
Sevier-Munger stain, 2126*t*
Sevin; *see* Carbaryl
Sex chromosomal abnormalities, 48
Sex cord stromal tumors, 1684-1686

Sex hormones, 902
Sex-linked conditions, 58-60
Sex-specific histocompatibility antigen, 1623
Sex steroids, 1581
Sexual differentiation, 1623-1624
Sexual practices, oroanal, 433
Sexually transmitted infections, 356t
Sézary's syndrome, 375, 1469, 1826
Shaggy heart, 647
Sharpey's fibers, 2003
Shave biopsy, 1814
Sheath
    periarteriolar lymphoid, 1409
    splenic capillaries in, 1409
Sheehan's syndrome, 1527
Sheep liver fluke, 452
Shigella, 300-301, *301*
Shin spots, 1778
Shingles, 382
Shock
    adrenal glands and, 1585
    anaphylactic, 519, 523-524
    burns and, 139
    cardiogenic, 637, 638
    ferrous sulfate toxicity and, 210
    hypovolemic, 700
    obstetric, 1527
Shock kidney, 131
Shock lung, 131
Shock waves, 135, 136
Shope papillomavirus, 600
Short-chain fatty acids, 1248
Short-limbed dwarfism, 1500t
Shotgun wounds, 128
Shunts, 730
    combined with obstructions, 743-749
    isolated, 731-738
Shwartzman phenomenon, 89, 311, 487
SI units, 249
Sialadenitis, allergic, 536t
Sialadenoma papilliferum, 1137
Sialolithiasis, 1129-1130
Sialometaplasia, necrotizing, 1131, *1131*
Sialorrhea, 1127
Sialosis, *1129*
Sicca complex, 838
Sickle cell anemia, 446
    arthropathy with, 2070
    atrophy of spleen in, *1414*
    bone marrow and, 1380-1381
    cardiac failure and, 692
    central nervous system infarct and, 2148
    micronodular cirrhosis and, 1287
    nephropathy in, 837
    retinopathy in, 1063-1064
    spleen and, *1417*
Sickle thalassemia, 1063
Sideroblastic anemias, 1379
Siderophages, 985
Siderosis, 1273
Siderosomes, liver and, 1201
SIDS; see Sudden infant death syndrome
Sieve plate, 1200
Sievert, 249
Sigma toxin, 296
Sigmoid colon
    diverticulum of, *1155*
    hyperinfection in, 468
Signet-ring cells, 1180, 1556
Signet-ring lipoblasts, 1877
Signs
    Durozier, 676
    Leser-Trélat, 1795
    Romberg, 2158

Silica, 35-36, 999
    augmentation mammoplasty and, 1779
    emphysema and, 238
    granulomas and, 1285
    inflammatory lesions from, 90
Silicosis, 35-36, 233-235, *234*, 997-998
    nodule in, 234, *234*, *998*
    pathogenesis of, 998
    tuberculosis and, 999
Silicotuberculosis, 999
Silo-filler's disease, 231-232, *232*
Silver, 36
Silver nitrate, 310
Silver stain, 1809
Simian vacuolating virus, 2178
Simmonds' disease, 1526
Simon's focus, 944
Simple bone cyst, in jaws, 1120
Simulium, 472
Single deficiency states, 546
Single-strand deoxyribonucleic acid–binding
    protein, 9
Sinoatrial node, 705
Sinus
    dural, septic thrombophlebitis of, 2153-
        2154
    endodermal
        ovarian tumor and, 1688, *1688*
        vaginal tumor and, 1642
    lymph node, 1430
    medullary, 1430
    paranasal, 1078-1083
    piriform, 1086
    subcapsular, 1430
    of Valsalva, 740, 776
Sinus barotrauma, 134-135
Sinus histiocytosis with massive
    lymphadenopathy, 1440, *1441*, *1442*
Sinus hyperplasia, 1440-1442
Sinusitis, 1078
    chronic, 1079
    in Kartagener's triad, 950
Sinusoid lining cells of liver, 1199
sis, 587t
Situs inversus, 950
Sjögren's syndrome, 830t, 838, 1127, 1129,
    1129
    biliary cirrhosis and, 1256
    pulmonary involvement in, 974
    rheumatoid arthritis and, 2083
    skin and, 1790
Skeletal dysplasias, 1946
Skeletal failure, 1967
Skeletal muscle, staining pattern of normal,
    2107
Skeletal muscle diseases, 2105-2122
    congenital myopathies and, 2112-2114
    denervating diseases and, *2119*, 2119-
        2121, *2120*
    disfigurative changes in injury and, 2110
    dysvoluminal changes in injury and, 2108-
        2109
    fiber necrosis and, 2110, *2110*
    fiber regeneration and, 2110-2111
    inflammatory and immune-mediated
        myopathies in, 2117-2119
    internal nuclei and, 2109-2110
    interstitial reactions and, 2111
    lipid storage diseases and, 2115-2116,
        2116
    metabolic diseases and, 2114-2115
    muscle biopsy and, 2107-2108
    muscle reactions to injury in, 2108-2111

Skeletal muscle diseases—cont'd
    muscular dystrophies and, 2111-2112
    normal structure and, 2102-2107
    sarcolemmal nuclei reactions to injury in,
        2109-2110
Skeletal muscle fiber
    necrosis of, 2110, *2110*
    regeneration of, 2110-2111
Skeletal muscle tumors, 1864-1873
Skeleton, 1929, *1930*
    in embryo, 1937, *1937*
    inflammatory disorders of, 2002-2010
    radium in, 280
    vitamin C deficiency and, 561
ski, 587t
Skin, 1751-1837
    amebiasis of vulvar, *436*
    angiolipoma and, 1792
    angiosarcoma in, 797
    appendage diseases and, 1786-1787
    arteriovenous fistulas of, 1251
    arthropods and, 1829
    atypical fibroxanthoma and, 1792-1793
    basophil hypersensitivity and, 530
    biopsy of, 1751
    blue nevus and, 1810-1811
    burns of, 137-140, *138*, *139*; see Burns
    capillary hemangioma of, *794*
    cutaneous fibroma and, 1825
    cutaneous-visceral disease and, 1758-1759
    definitions and, 1757-1758
    dermatoses and, 1759-1769
        hyperplasia of epidermis in, 1759-1767
        scabies in, 1769
        shave biopsy and, 1759
        superficial mycoses and, 1768-1769
    dermis in; see Dermis
    digital fibrous tumors of childhood and,
        1825
    elasticity of, 1782-1784
    Entamoeba histolytica and ulcers of, 436
    epidermis in; see Epidermis
    fibroma of, 1825
    halo nevus and, 1812
    herpetic infection of, 379
    immune mechanism and, 538, 539t
    immunologic reaction to drugs and, 148
    juvenile melanomas and, 1804-1810
    Kawasaki disease and, 1830
    leishmaniasis and, 443
    lupus and, 539t
    lymphomas and allied diseases and, 1825-
        1829
    malignant melanomas and, 1812-1818
    melanotic freckle of Hutchinson and,
        1811-1812
    meningioma of, 1821
    muscle tumors and, 1823-1825
    mycoses and, 391, 392t, 399-406
    neoplasms of, 30, 1793-1802
        benign epidermal lesions in, 1794-1796
        classification of, 1793-1794
        dermal appendage, 1830-1835
        ionizing radiation and, 1801
        malignant epidermal, 1798-1801
        Merkel cell tumor and, 1801-1802
        metastatic, 1830
        mineral oil and, 191
        precancerous epidermal, 1796-1798
        radiosensitivity of, 257t
        ultraviolet radiation and, 286
    neurofibroma and, 1825
    normal, 1752, *1753*

Skin—cont'd
  of nose, 1077
  onchocerciasis and, 472
  osteoma and, 1825
  panniculitis and, 1787-1789
  of penis, 897
  pigmentations of, 1785-1786
    metallic, 1785
    nonmetallic, 1785-1786
  pigmented nevi and, 1802-1804
  POEMS syndrome and, 1791
  radiation and, 257t, 273-274
  reticulohistiocytoma and, 1792
  of scrotum, 893
  senile lentigo and, 1811
  vascular disorders and, 1789-1791
  vessel tumors and, 1818-1823
  warts of, 385
  xanthoses and, 1791-1792
Skin neoplasms; see Skin, neoplasms of
Skin reaction, 531t
  Arthus, 513
  delayed, 527, 529
Skin tags, 1796
Skin testing, 519
Skin warts, 385
Skip lesions, 774, 2029
Skull, pagetic, 2009
Sleeping sickness, 439, 440
Sliding hernia, 1156
Sloughing of epithelium in asthma, 964
Slow virus infections, 2162-2163
Slugs, 468
Small cell lung carcinoma, 593t, 594, 1011-
    1012, 1012
  radiation and, 257t, 277
Small cleaved-cell type of follicular
    lymphoma, 1461, 1462
Small intestine, 1153
  carcinoma of, 1183
  digitalis and venous engorgement of, 175,
    175-176
  epithelial radiation injury in, 272
  immunoproliferative disease of, 1470
  schistosomiasis and, 458
  Whipple's disease and, 1174
Small lymphocytic lymphoma, 1396-1397,
    1462-1464, 1463
Small noncleaved-cell lymphoma, 1467-1469
Smallpox, 28, 386, 386, 1766-1767, 1767
Smoking, 1086
  atherosclerotic coronary artery disease
    and, 759
  cigarette, 990, 993, 1014
    passive, 1015
  in pregnancy, 61
  radiation and, 277
  reverse, 1112
  thromboangiitis obliterans and, 777
Smooth endoplasmic reticulum, 5, 1232
Smooth muscle
  anaphylactic reaction and, 527
  arterial atherosclerosis and, 762-764
  cigar-shaped nuclei of cells in, 1860, 1861
  tumors of, 1860-1864
    bone and, 2055
    gastrointestinal tract and, 1186
    myometrial, 1664-1667
Smudging, 119, 120, 378
Snails, 468
Sodium channels, 8
Sodium fluoride toxicity, 229
Sodium potassium pump, 3

Sodium retention, 806-807
Sodium transport, 3-4
Soft tissue
  eosinophilic ulcer of, 1104-1105
  oral; see Oral soft tissues
Soft-tissue tumors and tumorlike conditions,
    1838-1928
  adipose tissue tumors in, 1873-1886
    hibernoma and, 1885-1886
    lipoblastoma and, 1884-1885
    lipoma and, 1879-1884
    liposarcoma and, 1873-1879
  calcification in, 1577
  deep, 1887
  fibrohistiocytic tumors in, 1852-1860
  fibrous-tissue lesions in, 1842-1852
    fibromatoses and, 1844-1850
    fibrosarcoma and, 1842-1844
    pseudosarcomatous fibrous lesions and,
      1850-1852
  giant cell tumor in, 1906-1907
  myxoma in, 1896-1898
  neurogenous tumors and, 1890-1896
  osteoma, 1109
  sarcomas in, 1113
    alveolar soft part, 1903-1906
    clear cell, 1902-1903
    epithelioid, 1900-1902
    extraskeletal Ewing's, 1907-1909
    synovial, 1898-1900
  skeletal muscle tumors in, 1864-1873
  smooth muscle tumors in, 1860-1864
  vascular tumors in, 1886-1890
Solar radiation, 594
Soldier spots, 668
Solid blast, 135
Solid cell nests
  adrenal glands and, 1609
  thyroid gland and, 1544, 1545
Solitary abscesses of liver, 1259
Solitary bone cyst, 2022t, 2056, 2057
Solitary mesotheliomas, pleural, 1018, 1018
Solitary plasmacytoma in oral soft tissue,
    1113
Solitary squamous papilloma of larynx, 1085
Somatomammotrophic adenoma, 1534
Somatomammotrophic cells, 1521
Somatostatin, 2182
Somatostatinomas, 1368
Somatotroph cell, 1521, 1521t
  adenomas of, 1533
Somatotroph-prolactin adenomas, 1534
Somatotropin, 9
S-100 protein
  fibrous hamartoma and, 1848
  liposarcoma and, 1877
  neurofibroma and, 1893
  spindle cell lipoma and, 1881
Soot, 233
Sore throat, 303
Sound waves, injuries from, 136
South American blastomycosis, 421-422
Southgate's mucicarmine stain, 396t
Space of Disse, 1200
Sparsely ionizing particles, 254
Spastic diplegia, hypothyroidism and, 1545
Speckled erythroplakia, 1109
Spermatic cord, 892-893
Spermatic granuloma, 878-879
Spermatocele, 892
Spermatocytic seminoma, 883, 883-884
Spermatogenesis, 871
Spermatogonia, radiation and, 257t, 280

Spermatozoa, 871, 875
Spherocytosis, congenital, 1380, 1409, 1410
Spherule, 397
Sphincter of Oddi, 1353
Sphingolipidoses, 52, 53, 1419t, 1419-1422
Spider angiomas, 1820
Spider cells, 1021
Spiegler-Fendt sarcoid, 1827
Spina bifida, 2068
Spinal bifida occulta, 2136, 2137
Spinal cord
  injury of, 2189
  irradiation of, 281
  subacute combined degeneration of, 1377-
    1378, 2185-2186
Spinal muscular atrophy, 2183
  infantile, 2120-2121, 2121
Spindle cell carcinoma
  in larynx, 1086-1087
  in oral soft tissue, 1112
Spindle cell fibroblast, 1844, 1855
Spindle cell lipoma, 1881, 1882
Spindle cell sarcomas, 1863
Spindle cell thymoma, 1506
Spindle cells, 1562
  measles and, 368
  sarcoma and, 1863, 1899-1900
Spindle melanoma cells in eyes, 1064, 1064-
    1065
Spine
  bone loss in, 1968
  deformities of, 2096
  osteomalacia and, 1987
  radiation injury to, 258, 258t
Spirillum minor, 329
Spirochetes, 324-329, 878
Spironolactone bodies, 1599, 1599
Spironolactone toxicity, 168, 169
Spitz's nevus, 1806, 1807
Spleen, 1408-1429
  abnormalities of structure in, 1413
  asplenism and, 1411-1413
  autotransplantation and, 1414
  circulatory disorders of, 1415-1417
  cysts of, 1426
  degenerative changes of, 1413-1414
  hairy cell leukemia and, 1398
  histiocytoses and, 1422, 1422-1426
  Hodgkin's disease and, 1450
  hypersplenism and, 534, 1411-1413
  hyposplenism and, 1411-1413
  infarction of, 1417-1418, 1418
  leishmaniasis and, 443
  mass lesions and, 1426-1429
  mononucleosis and, 383
  peritoneal implants and, 1414
  rupture of, 1414
  sphingolipidoses and, 1419t, 1419-1422
  splenomegaly and, 1411, 1412t
  structure and functions of, 1408-1411,
    1411t
    abnormalities of, 1413
  systemic infection and, 1418-1419
  tumors and mass lesions of, 1426-1429
  vascular system of, 1409
Splendore-Hoeppli material, 397, 426
Splenectomy, 1426
Splenitis, septic, 1418
Splenomegaly, 1411, 1412t
  acute reactive hyperplasia and, 1418
  congestive, 1415, 1416
  fibrocongestive, 1415, 1416
  leukemia and, 1388
  schistosomiasis and, 456

Splenosis, 1189-1190, 1414
Split papule of mouth, 1105
Split tolerance, 503
Spondylitis, ankylosing, 650, 2097-2098
Spondyloarthropathies, seronegative, 2086-2087
Spondylosis, 2097
  hyperostotic, 2097
Spongiform encephalopathies, 387-388
Spongiosa, secondary, 1941
Spongiosis, 531, 1757
  in rete Malpighii, 1761
Spontaneous abortion, 1700-1701
Spontaneous hypothyroidism, 1553
Spontaneous perforation of biliary tract, 1333
Spontaneous reactivation of hepatitis B, 1227
Spontaneous rupture of spleen, 1414
Sporadic goiter, 1547
Sporogony, 446
Sporotrichosis, 393t, 404-406, 405
Sporozoa, 445-452
  babesiosis in, 451-452
  cryptosporidiosis in, 445
  isoporiasis in, 445
  malaria in, 445-448
  pneumocystosis in, 450-451, 451
  toxoplasmosis in, 448-450, 449
Spotted fever, 307, 349t, 350-354
Spotted leprosy, 337
Spreading factor, 87
Sprue, celiac, 1171-1172
Spur cell hemolytic anemia, 1252
Squamous cell carcinoma, 575, 577, 610, 1339, 1340
  of bladder, 861, 862
  of buccal mucosa, 1111-1112
  of ear canal, 1088
  of floor of mouth, 1111
  of gingiva, 1111
  of larynx, 1086
  of lip, 1111
  of lung, 1006-1007
  in oral soft tissue, 1110
  of palate, 1112
  of penis, 898
  of prostate gland, 915
  of salivary glands, 1140
  of scrotum, 894
  of skin, 1800-1801
  of tongue, 1111
Squamous cell epithelium, regeneration of, 96
Squamous hyperplasia in vulva, 1629, 1629
Squamous metaplasia, 107, 107
  of bladder, 857
  of cervix, 1643, 1644
  cigarette smoke–induced, 569
  of endometrium, 1656
  vitamin A deficiency and, 553
src, 586, 587t
Stab wounds, 114
  heart and, 698
Stable cells, 94
  regeneration of, 97
Stafne cyst, 1120
Staggers, 134
Staghorn calculi, 840
Staging in neoplasia, 602, 602-603, 610
Stannic oxide, 233
Staphylococci, 292t, 301-303, 792, 930
  abscesses and, 87, 1259
    splenic, 1419

Staphylococci—cont'd
  cystic fibrosis and, 951
  endocarditis and, 654
  exotoxicoses and, 293-294
  focal necrotizing, 658
  leukocidins and, 291
  osteomyelitis and, 2005
  pericarditis and, 666
  pneumonia and, 935-936
  skin and, 1765, 1766, 1768
  urinary system and, 834
  wound infection and, 130
Staphylococcus aureus, 302, 411
  arthritis and, 2075
  lymph nodes and, 1434
  myocarditis and, 660
  osteomyelitis and, 1113, 2003
  parotitis and, 1128
  pericarditis and, 666
  pulmonary infection and, 932, 935
  skin and, 1762, 1765
  toxic shock syndrome and, 1639
  urinary system and, 855
Staphylococcus pyogenes, 293
Staphylokinase, 291
Starch, 219
Starling equation, 958
Starry-sky macrophage, 1431
Starvation, 548
  balanced, 549
  osteoporosis and, 1981
Stasis, intravascular, 130
Status marmoratus, 2145
Status thymolymphaticus, 1502
  radiation injury and, 281
  x-rays for, 259
Steady state of cell, 11
Steady state infection, 363
Steatorrhea, 1172
Stein-Leventhal syndrome, 1638, 1654, 1675-1676, 1676
  oral contraceptives and, 165
Stem cells, 492t, 1373
  radiation and, 273
Stenella araguata, 392t
Stenosing tenovaginitis, 2091
Stensen's duct, 366, 1127
Stensen's papilla, 1095
Stercoraceous ulcers, 1168
Sterile fluid collection, 87
Steroid diabetes, 163
Steroids
  adrenal, 1582
  anabolic, 1581
    adverse reactions to, 165
    hepatocellular adenoma and, 1289
    hepatocellular carcinoma and, 1295
  angiogenesis and, 104
  fatty liver and, 1203
  polymyositis and dermatomyositis complex and, 2117
  secondary immune deficiencies and, 503
  toxicity of, 162-165, 164
  zona fasciculata cells and, 1588
Stevens-Johnson syndrome, 1103, 1763
Stillbirths in offspring of Japanese atomic bomb survivors, 263
Still's disease, 2086-2087
Stippling, 120, 120, 1953, 1956
Stochastic radiation injury, 257
Stomach, 1170
  adenocarcinoma radiosensitivity and, 257t
  hyperplastic polyp of, 1179, 1179

Stomach—cont'd
  inflammatory fibroid polyp of, 1160
  leather-bottle, Plate 2F, 1183
  leiomyoma of, 1186, 1186
  malignant lymphoma of, 1187
  radiation injury and, 278
  ulcers of, 86, 87, 1159-1161
  watermelon, 1159
Stomatitis
  nicotine, 1110
  vesicular viral, 27
Stones; see Calculi
Storage cell, 104
Storage diseases, 30, 53
  gastrointestinal manifestations of, 1173-1175
Storage iron, 1271
Storiform pattern of histiocytoma, 1855, 2055, 2055
Strange reaction, 516
Stratum corneum, 1755
Stratum granulosum, 1754-1755
Stratum lucidum, 1755
Streak gonad, 1624, 1626
Streptobacillus moniliformis, 329
Streptococci, 292t, 303-306, 411
  abscesses and, 1419
  endocarditis and, 654
  focal necrotizing, 658
  hemolytic
    diffuse inflammatory lesions and, 87
    glomerulonephritis and, 812
    meningitis and, 2154
    pneumonia and, 935
  incidence of infections from, 640-641
  infective endocarditis and, 654
  leukocidins and, 291
  osteoporosis and, 2005
  pericarditis and, 666
  pyogenic abscesses and, 1259
  rheumatic fever and, 639
  vagina and, 1704
  wound infection and, 130
Streptococcus faecalis, 312, 855
Streptococcus mutans, 1098
Streptococcus pneumoniae, 932, 988, 1412
  meningitis and, 2154
Streptococcus pyogenes, 303
Streptococcus viridans, 306
  focal necrotizing, 658
Streptokinase, 291
Streptomyces somaliensis, 392t
Streptomycin toxicity, 158, 159
  myocarditis and, 708
Streptozotocin, 1359
Striate pons, hemorrhage in, 2150
Striated muscle, 2105
Strictures
  intestinal, 1157
  urethral, 898
Stroke, 2146, 2153
Stromal breast sarcoma, 1748
Stromal cell
  bone tumors and, 2045
  hemangioblastoma and, 2173
Stromal endometrial neoplasms, 1661-1662
Stromal ovarian hyperplasia, 1676
Stromal ovarian luteoma, 1675
Stromal polyp
  vagina and, 1640
  vulva and, 1631
Stromal pulmonary fibrosarcoma, 1019
Stromal sex cord tumors, 1684-1686

Stromal support, 581
Stromolysin, 582
Strongyloidiasis, 467-468, *469*, 857, 967
Strongyloidosis, 467-468
Strontium, radioactive, 270
Strychnine poisoning, 194t, 219
Sturge-Weber syndrome, 795, 1051, *1052*, 1109, 1820
Subacute combined degeneration of spinal cord, 1377-1378, 2185-2186
Subacute hepatic necrosis, 1222
Subacute nodular migratory panniculitis, 1788
Subacute sclerosing panencephalitis, 369, *369*, *2162*, 2162-2163
  microglia and, 2135
Subacute yellow atrophy, 1221
Subarachnoid hemorrhage, 2150-2153, 2188
  perinatal injury and, 2142
Subcapsular hematoma of newborn, 1275
Subcapsular infarct, polyarteritis nodosa and, 1280, *1280*
Subcapsular sinus, 1430
Subcorneal pustular dermatosis, 1765
Subcutaneous fat necrosis of newborn, 1789
Subcutaneous morphea, 1780
Subcutaneous mycoses, 391, 392t, 399-406
Subcutaneous nodules of rheumatic fever, 92, 648, *648*, 1777-1778, *2082*, *2083*
Subcutaneous phaeohyphomycosis, 393t
Subcutaneous pseudosarcomatous fibromatosis, 1850
Subcutaneous zygomycosis, 393t, 426-427
Subdermal fibromatous tumors of infancy, 1847
Subdural empyema, 2153-2154
Subdural hematoma, *2187*, 2188
  alcoholics and, 192
  perinatal injury and, 2141-2142
Subepithelial cysts of vagina, 1639
Subfalcial herniation of cingulate gyrus, 2129
Sublingual gland, 1127
Submandibular adenitis, 1128
Submandibular gland, 1127
Submassive hepatic necrosis, 1205, *1220*, 1220-1221
  immunosuppressant therapy and, 1230
Subretinal hematoma, 1074, *1074*
Substance P, 964
Substrate specificity, 10
Succinic dehydrogenase, 634
Succinylcholine, 149
Sucquet-Hoyer canal, 1756, 1823
Sucrose nephrosis, 833, *833*
Sudan Red dyes, 2126t
Sudan stain, 986
Sudden cardiac death, 627
Sudden infant death syndrome
  adrenal medulla and, 1608
  botulism and, 293
  larynx and, 1084
  maternal effects and, 61
Sugar tumor, 1021
Suicidal poisoning, 193-194t
Sulci
  of Heidenhain, 1752
  in normal newborn brain, 2135
Sulfasalazine, 150
Sulfhydryl amines, 254
Sulfinpyrazone, 621
Sulfonamides
  cholestasis with necrosis and, 1234t, 1235
  chronic active hepatitis and, 1237

Sulfonamides—cont'd
  granulomas and, 1285
  myocarditis and, 168, 708
  pharmacogenetics and, 150
Sulfonated toluidine blue stain, 948
Sulfonylurea toxicity, 169
  cholestasis and, 1234t, 1235
Sulfur, 562
Sulfur dioxide, 989
  bronchitis and, 238
  pulmonary edema and, 237
Sulfur granules, 1105
Sunlight
  exposure to, 286
  pellagra and, 557
Sunomono, 462
Superficial epitheliomatosis, 1799
Superficial mycoses, 391, 392t, 397-399, 1768-1769
Superficial proteins, 3
Superinfection, hepatitis and, 1223, 1228
Superior vena caval syndrome, 790, 1504
Superoxide, 631, 1269
Supervoltage machine, 284
Suppressor cells, 497
Suppressor gene, 609
Suppuration, 85, 87
  abdominal disease and, 1258-1259
  cholangitis and, 1254
Suprarenal capsules, 1580
Surface inclusion cysts of ovary, 1674
Surface phagocytosis, 83
Surgery
  bone tumors and, 2024
  cancer therapy and, 606
  soft-tissue tumors and, 1841
Sushi, 462
Sutton's disease, 1104
Sutton's nevus, 1812
Sutures, response to, *105*, 105-106
Sweat, pancreas and, 1349
Sweat glands
  adenomas of, 1833
  cystic fibrosis and, 1351
  cysts in, *1764*
  diseases of, 1786-1787
  hemochromatosis and, 1786
  tumors of, 1830-1833
Swelling, inflammation and, 84; *see also* Edema
Swiss-cheese appearance of liver, 52
Swiss agammaglobulinemia, 501t
Swyer's syndrome, 930, 1625t
Syburn-Mason syndrome, 1051
Sydenham chorea, 648
Symbiotic relationship, 289
Sympathetic ophthalmia, 1056, *1057*
Sympathomimetic amines, 168-191
  amphetamines in, 168-169
  anesthetics in, 171
  anti-infective agents in, 174-175
  antiarrhythmics in, 175-176
  anticonvulsants in, 171-174
  antidiabetics in, 169
  antineoplastic and immunosuppressive agents in, 180-186
  antithyroid drugs in, 169
  antitubercular drugs in, 169-171
  diuretics in, 169
  H_2 receptor antagonists in, 169
  methysergide in, 186
  milk and milk alkali and, 189-191
  mineral oil and, 191

Sympathomimetic amines—cont'd
  oral hypoglycemic agents in, 169
  oxygen and, 176-180
  potassium chloride and, 186-189
  Thorotrast in, 186, *187-188*
Synaptic cleft, 8
Synaptic junctions, 8
Synaptophysin, 1012
Syncytial variant, 1447
Syncytiotrophoblasts, 881, 885-886, *1696*, 1696-1697
Syndrome; *see also* Disease
  Alagille's, 922
  Albright's, 1106, 1898
  Alport's, 823
  Banti's, 1417
  Behçet's, 1104, 2086
  Bloom's, 609, 1385
  Budd-Chiari; *see* Budd-Chiari syndrome
  Caplan's, 1002
  Churg-Strauss, 538, 772, 976
  Conn's, *1590*
  Cowden's, 1835
  Crigler-Najjar, 1275-1277, 1276t
  Cronkhite-Canada, 1178
  Cruveilhier-Baumgarten, 1250
  Cushing's; *see* Cushing's syndrome
  Dandy-Walker, 2139, 2140
  Del Castillo's, 873
  Diamond-Blackfan, 1377
  DiGeorge's, 501t, 1500t, 1978
  Dorfman-Chanarin, 1793
  Down's, 47, 1385, 2141, *2141*
  Dressler's, 672
  Dubin-Johnson, 1275, 1276t, 1277, *1277*
  Eaton-Lambert, 1013
  Edward's, 47-48
  Ehlers-Danlos, 986, 1782-1783, 2067
  Fanconi's, 206, 609, 1385
  Felty's, 2083
  Gardner's, 1178, 1846
  Gerstmann-Sträussler, 2164
  Goodpasture's; *see* Goodpasture's syndrome
  Guillain-Barré, 2132
  Hamman-Rich, 969
  Heerfordt's, 1130-1131, *1131*
  Hunter's, *53*, 55, 59
  Hurler-Hunter, 1267
  Hurler's, *52*, *53*, 686, 1173, 1267, 1529
  Hutchinson's, 1612
  Kallman's, 874, *875*
  Kasabach-Merritt, 795
  Katayama fever, 455
  Kearns-Sayre, 2116
  Kimmelstiel-Wilson, 823, 1057, 1364
  Klinefelter's; *see* Klinefelter's syndrome
  Klippel-Trenaunay, 795
  Launois-Bensaude, 1142
  Lesch-Nyhan, 37, 51, 59, 503
  Löffler's, 156, 174, 467, *537*
  Löfgren's, 980
  Louis-Bar, 1051
  Lowe's, 1053
  Maffucci's, 795, 1820, 2034, *2035*
  Mallory-Weiss, 1158
  Marfan's; *see* Marfan's syndrome
  McCune-Albright, 1114
  Meigs', 1685
  Melkersson-Rosenthal, 1103
  Menkes', 2116
  Milkman's, 1986
  Muir-Torre, 1833

Syndrome—cont'd
Nelson's, 1534
Nezelof's, 1500t
Osler-Weber-Rendu; see Osler-Weber-Rendu disease
Papillon-Lefèvre, 1097
Peutz-Jeghers, 1106, 1178, 1786
Plummer-Vinson, 1153, 1787
POEMS, 1791
Reifenstein's, 1627
Reiter's; see Reiter's syndrome
Reither's, 1104
Reye's; see Reye's syndrome
Rotor's, 1275, 1276t, 1277-1278
Schmidt's, 1525, 1587
Senear-Usher, 1762
Sertoli cell–only, 873-874
Sézary's, 375, 1469, 1826
Sheehan's, 1527
Sjögren's, 830t, 838, 1127, 1129, 1129
    biliary cirrhosis and, 1256
    pulmonary involvement in, 974
    rheumatoid arthritis and, 2083
    skin and, 1790
Stein-Leventhal, 1638, 1654, 1675-1676, 1676
    oral contraceptives and, 165
Stevens-Johnson, 1103, 1763
Sturge-Weber, 795, 1051, 1052, 1109, 1820
Swyer's, 930, 1625t
Syburn-Mason, 1051
Torre's, 1833
Turcot's, 1178, 2166
Turner's, 48, 1625t, 1626
    osteoporosis and, 1977
Urbach-Wiethe, 1103
von Hippel-Lindau; see von Hippel-Lindau disease
Waterhouse-Friderichsen, 309, 1585
Weber's, 1820
Weil-Marchesani, 1053
Wermer's, 1535
Wernicke-Korsakoff, 556
Wilson-Mikity, 926
Wiskott-Aldrich, 384, 501t, 1500t
Zellweger's, 1267, 1268, 2116
Zieve, 197
Zinsser-Engman-Cole, 1110
Zollinger-Ellison, 1170, 1680
Synechia, peripheral anterior, 1062
Synergistic fusospirochetosis, 329
Syngraft, 531
Synorchidism, 871
Synovial cysts, dermal, 1782
Synovial fluid in rheumatoid arthritis, 2077
Synovial joints, 2065
Synovial sarcoma, 1898-1900, 1899, 2094-2096, 2095
Synoviocytes, 2066
Synovioma, 2094-2096
Synovitis, villinodular, 2093
Syphilis, 92, 325-328, 539t, 621-623, 895
    aneurysm in, 780
    aortitis in, 767, 768
    arteritis in, 767, 767-768
    arthritis and, 2076
    benign late, 327
    of bone, 2005, 2005-2006
    congenital, 327, 1105
        jaundice and, 1265
    glossitis in, 1105
    granulomatous inflammation and, 91

Syphilis—cont'd
    gummatous stage of, 1286, 1286
    heart disease in, 650-652
    of liver, 1285-1286
    lymphocytes and, 82
    neonatal and childhood cholestasis and, 1261t
    neonatal encephalitis and, 2160, 2162
    nonvenereal, 328
    oral soft tissue and, 1105
    secondary, 326
    testes and, 878
Syringadenoma, 1830, 1831
Syringobulbia, 2141
Syringocarcinoma, 1833
Syringocystadenoma papilliferum, 1832
Syringomyelia, 2140-2141
Système Internationale units, 249
Systemic amyloidosis, 821-823
    reactive, 1286
Systemic disease
    gastrointestinal manifestations of, 1172-1175
    glomerular injury and, 824-827
    ocular manifestations of, 1074-1076
    thymomas in, 1508
Systemic lupus erythematosus, 149, 768, 824, 824-825, 825, 838
    cardiac manifestation of, 652, 653
    liver disease and, 1287
    pulmonary involvement in, 973-974
    spleen in, 1414, 1415
Systemic mastocytosis, 1404
Systemic mycoses, 391, 393-395t, 406-427
    actinomycosis in, 406-407
    adiaspiromycosis in, 407
    aspergillosis in, 407-410
    blastomycosis in, 410
    botryomycosis in, 410-411
    candidiasis in, 411-413
    coccidioidomycosis in, 413-415
    cryptococcosis in, 415-416
    fusariosis in, 416-417
    geotrichosis in, 417-418
    histoplasmosis capsulati in, 418-419
    histoplasmosis duboisii in, 419-420
    malasseziasis in, 420
    nocardiosis in, 420-421
    paracoccidioidomycosis in, 421-422
    penicilliosis marneffei in, 422-423
    pseudallescheriasis in, 423
    torulopsosis in, 423-424
    trichosporonosis in, 424-425
    zygomycosis in, 425-427
Systemic reactions, 523-524
Systemic sclerosis, 974, 1779
Systolic anterior motion, 683

T

T-cell leukemia-lymphoma, 1460, 1469
T-helper lymphocytes, leprosy and, 344-345
T-lymphocyte cell surface marker antigens, 1496t
T-lymphocyte subsets, 492t
T-lymphocytes, 490-493, 495, 527
    antigens and, 1457
    defects of, 501t
    lymphomatoid papulosis and, 1828
    portal tracts and, 1206
    properties of, 490t
    splenic transformation of, 1429
    thymus gland and, 1496, 1507
    tuberculosis and, 941-942

T-suppressors, 495, 1773
Tabby-cat pattern, 692
Tabes dorsalis, 2157-2158
Tachypnea of newborn, transient, 925
Tachyzoites, Toxoplasma, 449
Taenia, 458-460
Tagamet; see Cimetidine
Takayasu's arteritis, 623, 768, 774, 775
Talc
    granulomas and, 1285
    inflammatory lesions and, 90, 236
    narcotic abuse and, 219
Tamm-Horsfall protein, 808, 851
Tamoxifen; see Antiestrogens
Tamponade, cardiac, 698
Tampons, vaginal, 293-294, 1638-1639
Tangier disease, 1173
Tapeworms, 458-462
Target cells, 527
Target fibers, 2119-2120, 2120
Target theory, radiation damage and, 251-252
Target-tissue specificity, 148
Tatlockia, 938
Tattoo, 120, 120, 1785, 1785
Tay-Sachs disease, 52, 53
    gastrointestinal manifestations of, 1173
Teeth, 1096-1100
    developmental anomalies of, 1096-1098
    diseases of, 1098-1100
    premature loss of, 1097
    vitamin A deficiency and, 553
    vitamin C deficiency and, 561
Teething, 1127
Telangiectasia, 794-795
    hepatosplenic schistosomiasis and, 456
    hereditary hemorrhagic, 1109
    osteosarcoma and, 2031, 2032
    wart and, 1820
Telencephalic leukoencephalopathy, 2145
TEM; see Triethylenethiophosphoramide
Temperature
    cryptorchidism and, 872
    injury and, 136-140
Temporal arteritis, 772-774, 773
Temporal bone, 1089
Temporal lobe transtentorial herniation, 2129
Tendinitis, 2091
Tendon sheaths
    clear cell sarcoma of, 2096
    fibroma of, 1909
    tumors and tumorlike conditions of, 2092-2096
Tendons
    diseases of, 2090-2091
    tumors and tumorlike conditions of, 2092-2096
"1080" [Ten-eighty], toxicity of, 229
Tenovaginitis, 2091
Teratocarcinoma, 887
Teratology, 610
Teratoma, 578, 578, 579, 610
    congenital neck, 1142-1143
    fallopian tube, 1670
    gonadal, 1538
    ovarian, 1688-1690, 1689, 1689, 1690
    of testes, 886-888, 887
    thyroid gland and, 1556
Terminal deoxynucleotidyl transferase, 1395
Terminal hepatic venule, 1199
Terminal ileum, enteritis of, 1164

Testes, 871-891
    anomalies of, 871-872
    atrophy of, 876, *876*, 1251-1252
    biopsy of, 881
    ectopic, 871
    female genitalia and, 1624
    immature, 874-875, *875*
    infarction of, 876, *877*
    inflammation of, 877-879
    interstitial sclerosis of, 875
    in male infertility, 872-877
    radiation damage to, 280, 876
    syphilis and, 878
    thrombosis of, 876
    torsion of, 876-877
    tuberculosis of, 878
    tubular sclerosis of, 875
    tumors of, 879-891, *882*
        burned-out, 888
        diagnosis of, 880-881
        etiology of, 879-880
        germ cell and gonadal stromal elements
            combined in, 890
        histogenesis of, 881-882
        histopathologic classification of germ
            cell, 882-888
        incidence and prevalence of, 879
        lymphoid tumors and, 890
        metastasis of, 888
        more than one histologic type in, 886-
            888
        secondary, 890-891
        specialized gonadal stroma derivation
            of, 888-890
        symptoms of, 880
        teratoma in, *579*
Testicular adnexa, 871
Testicular feminization syndrome, 1625*t*
Testosterone, *1582*
    female genitalia and, 1624, 1625*t*, 1676
Tetanus, 292*t*, 294
2,3,7,8-Tetrachlorodibenzo-*p*-dioxin, 598
Tetracycline
    antibiotic-associated colitis and, 155
    myocardial infarction and, 634
    myocarditis and, 708
    toxicity of, 150-153, 1235*t*, 1237-1238
        fatty liver and, 1203
        pregnancy and, 1274
    as in vivo bone marker, 1945, *1946*
        in bone remodeling, 1959*t*, 1961
        in mixed osteomalacia–osteitis fibrosa,
            1995, *1996*
        in osteomalacia, 1990, *1991*
Tetradeconylphorbol acetate, 597, 598
Tetraiodothyronine, 1544
Tetralogy of Fallot, 743, *744*
Textile workers, 996
TGF-α and TGF-β, 582, 590*t*, 591
Thalamus
    bilirubin staining of, 2146
    hemorrhage in, 2150
    ischemic encephalopathy and, 2147
Thalassemia, 1381
    osteoporosis and, 1972
    therapy in, 62
Thallium toxicity, 214-216
Theca cells, ovary and, 1672
Theca granulosa cell, 871
Theca-lutein cysts, 1674
Thecomas, 1685
Theiler virus, 27
Theophylline, 708

Thermal edema, 137
Thermal injury, 136-140
Thiaminase, 551
Thiamine, 555-556
    cobalt toxicity and deficiencies of, 212
Thiazides, 37
    cholecystitis and, 1327
    secondary gout and, 37
    toxicity of, 169
Thioridazine poisoning, 194*t*
Thiouracil
    cholestasis with necrosis and, 1234*t*, 1235
    toxicity of, 169
Third-degree burns, 96, 139
Thoracic irradiation, 276
Thoracic kyphosis, 1986
Thoracic thyroid and parathyroids, 1026
Thorazine; *see* Chlorpromazine
Thorium, 259, 279, 284
    cholangiocarcinoma and, 1298
    endomyocardial fibrosis and, 697
    hepatocytes and, 1204
    mesodermal tumors and, 1298
    osteosarcoma and, 2018
    toxicity of, 186, *187-188*
Thorotrast; *see* Thorium
Threadworm, 464
Threonine, 546
Threshold for safe radiation dose, 268
Throat, sore, 303
Thrombin, 764
Thromboangiitis obliterans, 623, 777, *777*
Thrombocythemia, primary, 1393-1394
Thrombocytopenia
    hematopoietic syndrome and, 273
    methotrexate and, 183
    radiation therapy and, 284
Thrombocytopenic verrucal angionecrosis,
    1790-1791
Thromboembolism
    oral contraceptives and, 165
    pharmacogenetics and, 149
Thrombophlebitis, 788-791, *790*
    of dural sinuses, 2153-2154
    subcutaneous, 1790
    superficial, 789
Thrombophlebitis migrans, 789
Thrombosis, 95
    atherosclerosis and, 762
    cardiac myxomas and, 701, 703*t*
    central nervous system infarct and, 2148,
        2148-2149, *2149*
    Chagas' disease and, 442
    coronary artery disease and, 624
    coronary occlusion and, 627-628
    fibrous plaques and, 761-762
    narcotic toxicity and, 219
    oral contraceptives and, 165
    prostate gland and, 902
    renal disease and, 826-827
    repair and, 102
    testicular, 876
    types of, 789-791
    venous, 789-791
        hepatic, 790-791, 1282
        portal, 1280, *1280*
        varicose, 788
Thrombospondin, 447
Thrombotic thrombocytopenic purpura, 624,
    624, 827
Thromboxane, 519*t*, 764
Thrombus; *see also* Thrombosis
    mural, 778
    propagation of, 130

Thrush, 412, 1105
Thymic nurse cells, 1495
Thymic primordium, 1499
Thymidine, 59
Thymocyte differentiation, 1497*t*
Thymolipomas, 1511-1512
Thymomas, 1500*t*, 1504-1508, *1505*, *1506*
    clinical staging classification for, 1507*t*
    immune deficiency with, 502*t*
    malignant, 1507
    spindle cell, 1506
Thymus, 495, 1142, 1493-1516
    alymphoplasia of, 501*t*, *1501*
    congenital anomalies of, 1499, 1500*t*
    cortex of, 1496
    cysts of, 1143-1144, 1502
    development of, 1493-1494
    dysplasia of, *1501*
    function of, 1496-1499
    hyperplasia of, 1502-1504
    immunodeficiency disorders and, 1499-
        1502, 1500*t*
    involution of, *1498*, 1499
    irradiation of, 259
    neoplasms of, 1504-1512
        carcinomas in, 1507
        germ cell tumors in, 1508-1509
        malignant lymphomas and, 266, 1509-
            1511
        neuroendocrine tumors in, 1508
        thymolipomas and, 1511-1512
        thymomas in, 1504-1508
    structure of, 1494-1496, *1495*
    weight of, 1494*t*
Thymus-derived lymphocytes, 495; *see also*
    T-lymphocytes
Thyroglobulin, 507*t*
Thyroglossal cyst, 1143, 1546
Thyroid antigens, autoantibodies to, 507*t*
Thyroid gland, 1544-1569
    benign tumors of, 1554-1556
    development of, 1544-1545
        anomalies in, 1546
    ectopic, 573, *573*, 1026
    functional disorders of, 1545-1546
    goiter and, 1546-1549
    Graves' disease and, 1549-1550
    hyperplasia of, 568
    lingual, 1096
    lymphocytes and, 506-508
    malignant tumors of, 1556-1565
        carcinoma in, 602, 1556-1563, 1557*t*
        malignant lymphoma in, 1563-1565
        radiation injury and, 281
    radiation injury to, 260, 281
    radiosensitivity of, 257*t*, 1554
    structure and function of, 1544-1545
    thyroiditis and, 1550-1554
Thyroid hormone synthesis, 1544
Thyroid-stimulating antibody, 1549
Thyroid-stimulating autoantibodies, 506
Thyroid-stimulating hormone, 507*t*, 1517,
    1522, 1525, 1544, 1547
Thyroiditis, 1550-1554
    allergic, 536*t*
    anti-immune, 506
    autoimmune, 1545
Thyroid-stimulating hormone receptor, 506,
    506*t*, 507*t*
Thyrotoxicosis, 1546
    heart disease and, 689-690
    osteoporosis and, *1981*, 1981-1982
    radiation injury and, 281

Thyrotrophs, 1522, 1525
  adenomas and, 1525, 1534
Thyrotropin-releasing hormone, 1546
Thyroxine, 9, 507t, 1544
Tibial adamantinoma, 2054
Ticks, 319, 451
  encephalitis and, 371-372
  pseudoepitheliomatous hyperplasia and,
    1829
Tight contact wound, 120, 121
Tigroid pattern, 692
Tinea, 392t, 397, 398
  radiation injury and, 281
Tissue alloantigens, 493
Tissue disruption in lacerations, 112, 113
Tissue injury
  reactive metabolites in, 147
  regeneration and repair in, 567
Tissue iron, 31-33
Tissue kallikreins, 73
Tissue placement, inappropriate, 571-573
Tissue reaction in delayed-type
    hypersensitivity, 89
TNM system; see Tumor, node, metastasis
    system of staging
Toad skin, 552, 553
Tobacco leaf, 277
Tobacco smoke, 993
Tocopherols, 554-555
Toe, clubbing of, 2070
Toenails, arsenic clippings of, 209
Tofranil; see Imipramine
Togaviruses, 370-371, 2158
Tolbutamide toxicity, 169, 195, 1237
Tolerance, 497
  split, 503
Toluene 2,4-diisocyanate, 238
Tongue, 1096
  fissured, 1096
  hairy, 1103
  pellagra and, 557
  squamous cell carcinoma of, 1111
Tonofilaments, 1755
  skin and, 1802
Tonsil, rectal, 1186
Tonsillar crypts, 938
Tonsillar herniation, 2130
Tophi, gouty, 38, 38
TORCH syndrome, 2160
Tori in jaws, 1113
Torre's syndrome, 1833
Torsion
  omental, 1191
  testicular, 876-877
Torticollis, 1142, 1142
Torulopsosis, 395t, 423-424, 424
Total anomalous pulmonary venous
    drainage, 737-738, 738
Total parenteral nutrition
  cholecystitis and, 1323, 1327t
  hepatic fibrosis and fatal liver failure and,
    1267
Tourniquet test, 2114
Toxemia of pregnancy, 827-828, 828, 1701-
    1702
Toxic arthritis, 2077
Toxic complex reactions, 504t, 512, 535
Toxic encephalopathy, 2184-2185
Toxic epidermal necrolysis, 172, 1765
Toxic gas inhalation, 139-140
Toxic metabolites in hepatic
    encephalopathy, 1248
Toxic nephropathy, 831

Toxic nodular goiter, 1547
Toxic reactions, 150, 151t
  immunologic drug reactions compared to,
    147t
Toxic-shock syndrome, 293-294, 1639
Toxins
  alpha, 296
  bacterial, 291
    liver injury and, 1232
  botulinus, 293
  congestive cardiomyopathy and, 693-694
  diphtheria, 295
  drugs as, 146-147
  erythrogenic, 305
  gas-forming clostridial, 296
  healing by second intention and, 106
  inflammation and, 89
  radiolabeled bungaro, 508
  sigma, 296
  staphylococcal, 302
  tetanus, 294
Toxocara, 467, 967, 1053, 1055
  granulomas and, 1285
Toxoplasmosis, 419, 448-450, 449, 1053,
    1055
  central nervous system, 449, 450
  congenital, 449, 1261t, 1265, 2160, 2161
  encephalitis and, 449, 450
    neonatal, 2160, 2161
  eye and, 1053
  hepatic granuloma-like lesion in, 1285
  lymphadenitis and, 449
  lymphoid hyperplasia and, 1442
  myocarditis and, 661
  neonatal and childhood cholestasis and,
    1261t
  pulmonary infection and, 968
  in TORCH syndrome, 2160
TPA; see Tetradeconylphorbol acetate
Trabecula
  primary, 1941
  prostate gland and, 906
Trabecular adenoma of thyroid gland, 1555
Trabecular bone, 1931, 1931-1932
Trabecular carcinoma
  liver cell, 1297, 1298
  of skin, 1801
Trace-element deficiencies, 693
Tracheal adenoid cystic adenocarcinoma,
    1017
Tracheobronchial amyloidosis, 983
Tracheobronchitis, 932
Tracheobronchopathia osteoplastica, 983
Trachoma, 356t, 357
Traffic injuries, 115-119, 117
Tranquilizers, adverse reactions to, 167-168
Transaminase, 1278
Transcobalamin 2 deficiency, 502t
Transcription, 2, 610
Transcytose, 764
Transfection of globin gene, 62
Transfer factor, 531t
Transfer ribonucleic acid, 2
Transferrin, 31, 1271
Transformation, 106-108
  viral diseases and, 363
Transforming growth factor B, 568
Transfusion reaction, 511
Transfusions
  hepatitis and, 1229
  iron overload after, 1273
Transient acantholytic dermatosis, 1765
Transient eosinophilic pulmonary infiltrates,
    156

Transient ischemic attack, 2149
Transient tachypnea of newborn, 925
Transition energy, 248
Transition zone, 1643
Transitional cell carcinoma
  bladder, 862, 863
  nasopharyngeal, 1083
  prostatic, 915
Transitional cell metaplasia of prostate
    gland, 912, 914
Transitional coarctation, 741
Transitional epithelium in nasal cavity, 1081
Translocation, 48
Transmembranous glomerulonephritis, 203;
    see also Glomerulonephritis,
    membranous
Transmural extent and course of myocardial
    infarction, 629-630
Transplacental pneumonia, 930
Transplantation
  bone marrow, 534
    obliterative bronchiolitis after, 968, 968
    veno-occlusive disease and, 1283
  islet cell, 1366
  liver, 1300
  lung, 967-968, 1036-1037
  major histocompatibility complex and, 493
  renal, 533-534
Transport, cellular, 3-4
Transposition of arterial trunks, 745-746, 747
Transtentorial herniation of temporal lobe
    and brainstem, 2129
Transudate, 69
Transurethral biopsy, 865
Transverse myelitis, 281
Transverse tubules, 2106
Trauma; see Injury
Traumatic arthritis, 2067
Traumatic bone cyst in jaw, 1120
Traumatic bursitis, 2090
Traumatic neuroma in oral soft tissue, 1107
Traumatic pericarditis, 672
Trehalose 6,6'-dimycolate, 940
Trematodes, 452-458
Trench foot, 137
Trench mouth, 1105
Trendelenburg gait, 1986
Treponema pallidum, 324, 1232, 1704, 2005
  meningitis and, 2154, 2156-2158
  neonatal encephalitis and, 2160, 2162
Treponematoses, 324, 329; see also
    Treponema pallidum
  features of, 327t
  nonvenereal, 327-328
TRH; see Thyrotropin-releasing hormone
Triatoma, 440
Trichilemmal cysts, 1834
Trichilemmoma, 1834-1835
Trichinella, 465-466, 466
  myocarditis and, 662
Trichinosis, 465-466
1,1,1-Trichloro-2,2-bis ethane, toxicity of,
    226
Trichloroethane poisoning, 194t
Trichloroethanol; see Chloral hydrate
Trichloroethylene poisoning, 194t
Trichocephaliasis, 463
Trichoepithelioma, 1834
Trichomatricoma, 1835
Trichomonas, 439, 901, 1638, 1638, 1639,
    1667
Trichophyton, 392t, 397, 398, 1768
Trichosporon, 392t, 395t, 424, 424-425

Trichuriasis, 463
Tricuspid atresia without transposition, 747, 748
Tricuspid insufficiency, 676
   carcinoid tumors and, 691
Tricuspid stenosis, 676, 746-748
   with severe pulmonary stenosis or atresia, 747-748, 749
Triethylenethiophosphoramide toxicity, 180-182
Triglycerides
   carbon tetrachloride and, 17
   ethanol and, 19
Triiodothyronine, 507t, 1544
Tripelennamine hydrochloride toxicity, 219
Triphenyltetrazolium chloride, 634-635
Triple-barreled aorta, 782
Triple response, 68
   exudation of plasma and, 71-76
   neutrophilic leukocyte emigration and, 76-81
   vasodilatation and, 70-71
Triploidy, 1700
Trisomies, 46, 47-48
   eyes and, 1051
   facial clefts and, 1095
   leukemia and, 1385
   tongue and, 1096
Tritium, radioactive, 270
Triton tumors, 1865, 1895, 1896
tRNA; see Transfer ribonucleic acid
Trophic factors, 588
Trophoblast, 1697, 1697
   hyperplasia and neoplasia of, 1706-1710, 1708
   invagination of, 1701
Trophozoites, 433
Tropical eosinophilia, 467, 471
True aneurysm, 778
True cysts, 1127
   splenic, 1426
True fungus, 396
True hermaphroditism, 1626
Trypanosomiasis, 419, 439, 440-441, 442, 661-662
Tryptophan, 546, 556, 557, 562
Tsetse fly, 439
TSH; see Thyroid-stimulating hormone
TTC; see Triphenyltetrazolium chloride
Tubal ectopic pregnancy, 1700
Tubercle, macrophages of, 90
Tubercle bacillus, 940, 942
   response to, 90, 91, 92
Tuberculin, 89
   old, 940
Tuberculin test, 539t, 940, 943
Tuberculin type of hypersensitivity, 527
Tuberculoid leprosy, 335, 336, 339-341, 538, 539t
Tuberculosis, 292t, 537-538, 939-947
   alimentary tract and, 1166
   arthritis and, 2006, 2075-2076
   bone and, 2006
   caseation necrosis in, 14
   caseation necrosis in pulmonary, 14
   cavitary, 945, 945-946
   cystitis and, 857
   endometritis and, 1657
   of eye, 1054
   granulomatous inflammation and, 91
   hemopericardium and, 665
   hepatic granuloma and, 1284
   hypocortisolism and, 1587, 1587

Tuberculosis—cont'd
   meningitis and, 2155, 2156
   miliary, 944, 944-945
      spleen and, 1418, 1419
   Mycobacterium tuberculosis and, 314
   myocarditis and, 660
   in oral soft tissue, 1105
   pericarditis and, 666, 667, 669, 670, 671
   peritonitis and, 1189
   postprimary, 945-946
   progressive primary, 944-945
   pyelonephritis and, 835-836
   pyridoxine deficiency and, 559
   skin and, 1784
   of spermatic cord, 892
   of testicle and epididymis, 878, 891
   ureteral inflammation and, 852
   vitamin C deficiency and, 561
Tuberculum impar, 1096
Tuberous sclerosis, 2175, 2175-2176
   central nervous system neoplasia and, 2166
   of eye, 1051, 1053
Tubular adenomas
   alimentary tract and, 1175, 1175, 1179
   renal cortical, 847
Tubular carcinoma of breast, 1744, 1745
Tubular injury
   acute, 809, 830-832
      renal failure and, 1252
   boric acid and, 224
   cadmium and, 213
   carbon tetrachloride and, 222
   glycol and, 198, 199
   isopropanol and, 198
   mercury and, 201
   methoxyflurane and, 171
   platinum and, 216
   secondary to therapeutic agents, 832-833
   uranium and, 216
Tubular interstitial sclerosis, 875
Tubular loss
   acute, 809, 830-832, 833
      renal failure and, 1252
   chronic, 809
   reversible, 833-834
Tubular sclerosis of testes, 875
Tubulointerstitial disease, 829-834, 830t
   cyclosporin A and, 183
   metabolic toxicity and, 839-840
Tubulorrhexis, 833
   mercury and, 201
Tularemia, 292t, 318-320, 1443
Tumor, 610; see also Neoplasia
   alveolar, sclerosing angiogenic, 1020
   Askin, 1611
   bladder, 857-866, 859, 860
   blood vessels and lymphatic, 794-799, 1818-1823
   breast carcinoma and size of, 1740, 1740
   brown, 1976, 1977
   Burkitt's; see Burkitt's lymphoma
   Buschke-Lowenstein, 896
   carotid body, 1141-1142, 1142
   central nervous system, 2165-2176
      hereditary neoplastic, 2175-2176
      metastatic, 2174-2175
      primary, 2166-2174
   cerumen gland, 1088
   denture-injury, 1107
   of epididymis, 891-892
   of gallbladder and biliary ducts, 1334-1343
   germ cell, 1687-1691

Tumor—cont'd
   germ cell—cont'd
      thymus gland and, 1508-1509, 1510
   giant cell
      bone, 2021t, 2043-2045, 2044
      soft-tissue, 1906-1907, 1907
   glomus, 795-796, 796, 1088
      skin and, 1823
   of hair follicle, 1834-1835
   of heart, 700-705
   inoperable, radiation therapy and, 284
   irradiation and, 265, 274, 280
   of jaws, 1116-1117
   of kidney, 847-849
   Klatskin, 1337, 1337, 1342
   Krükenberg's, 1183, 1691
   of larynx, 385-386, 1020, 1084-1085
   Lindau's, 795
   liver, 1287-1300; see also Liver, tumors and tumorlike conditions of
   of lymph nodes; see Lymphomas
   of lymphatics and blood vessels, 794-799
   lymphedema and, 793
   malignant Triton, 1865, 1895, 1896
   mediastinal, 1025t, 1025-1026
   metastases of; see Metastases
   of muscle, 1823-1825
   neck, 1141-1143
   neuroendocrine, 1184
      thymus gland and, 1508, 1509
   odontogenic, 1121-1127, 1124
   of oral soft tissues, 1106-1113
   oxygen effect and, 254
   of pancreatic islets, 1367-1369
   of parathyroid glands, 1563
   of penis, 896-898
   periampullary, 1357-1358
   pituitary gland, 1528-1538
      irradiated, 267
   pregnancy, 1819
   progression from benign to malignant, 585-586
   of prostate; see Prostate gland
   radiosensitivity of, 257t
   of renal pelvis, 849, 849
   rhabdoid, 849
   salivary glands and, 1131-1141, 1132t, 1833
   of scrotum, 894
   of sebaceous glands, 1136-1137, 1137
   in seminal vesicles, 916
   of skeletal muscles, 1864-1873
   smooth muscle; see Smooth muscle, tumors of
   soft-tissue; see Soft-tissue tumors and tumorlike conditions
   of spermatic cord, 893
   of spleen, 1426-1429
   sugar, 1021
   testicular; see Testes, tumors of
   of thymus, 1504-1512
   of thyroid gland, 1554-1565
      and radiation injury, 281
   Triton, 1865, 1895, 1896
   in tunica vaginalis, 894-895
   turban, 1832
   in ureter, 852
   of urethra, 899
   vaginal, 1639-1642
      botryoid, 1869
   of vessels, 794-799, 1818-1823
   von Hippel's, 795
   Warthin's, 579, 1134
   Wilms', 579, 593t, 594, 848-849, 849

Tumor, node, metastasis system of staging, 603
Tumor-cell DNA, 586-587
Tumor cells
    cytoskeleton and, 582-584
    of hepatocellular carcinoma, 1297-1298
    radiotherapy and, 282, 284
Tumor doublings, 580, 580
Tumor enhancement, 534
Tumor-host system, radiation dose and, 283
Tumor markers, 604t, 604-605
    carcinoembryonic antigen and, 1563
    fibrohistiocytic, 1858
    nervous system, 2166t
    non-Hodgkin's lymphomas and, 1454, 1455t
    prostate gland and, 908
    rhabdomyosarcoma and, 1866
    soft-tissue tumors and, 1840
    thymus and, 1496t
Tumor matrix, bone and, 2024
Tumor necrosis factor, 81, 569
Tumor promoters, 597, 598, 610
Tumorigenic virus, 266
Tumorlet, 1023
Tungsten miners, 276
Tunica adventitia, 752
Tunica albuginea, 877
    mesothelial lesions of, 895
Tunica intima, 752
Tunica media, dissecting aneurysm and, 783
Tunica propria, 871
Tunica vaginalis, 878, 894-895
    hydrocele of, 471
Turban tumor, 1832
Turcot's syndrome, 1178, 2166
Turner's syndrome, 48, 1625t, 1626
    osteoporosis and, 1977
Twin placentas, 1698, 1698-1699
Tylenol; see Acetaminophen
Tympanic membrane, 1088
Tympanosclerosis, 1088
Type A behavior pattern, 620
Typhoid fever, 292t, 314-315, 315, 316
    inflammatory process in, 85
    Salmonella typhosa and, 314
Typhus, 349t, 351, 353, 354
Tyrosine, 1266
    hepatocellular adenoma and, 1289
    inborn errors of metabolism and, 51, 52
    neonatal and childhood cholestasis and, 1261t, 1262
    ochronosis and, 2068
    oxidation of, 30
Tzanck cells, 1762

U
Ulcer, 86, 87
    alcoholics and, 197
    burns and, 139
    chiclero, 444
    in fibrous plaques, 761-762
    gallbladder mucosal, 1332, 1332
    Marjolin, 1801
    osteoarthrotic, 2072
    peptic, 1159-1161
        potassium chloride and, 186-189, 189
    radiation injury and, 273, 278
    skin, 1757
        Entamoeba histolytica and, 436
    stercoraceous, 1168
Ulcer carcinoma, 1182

Ulcerative colitis, 146, 1161, 1162, 1162
    antibiotic-associated colitis and, 155
    liver abnormalities and, 1287
Ulegyria, 2145
Ulex europaeus I marker, 1900, 1901
Ulna, osteitis fibrosa cystica of, 1976
Ultrasound
    gallbladder and common duct and, 1323
    hepatic amebic abscess and, 1259
    injuries from, 136
Ultraviolet radiation, 30, 285t, 286, 594
    warts and, 1794
Umbilical artery, single, 1698
Umbilical cord formation, 1693-1696
Uncal herniation, 2129, 2129-2130
Uncinariasis, 463-464
Unconventional viruses, 387
Undifferentiated carcinoma
    of oral soft tissue, 1112
    of ovary, 1684
    of prostate gland, 915
    of salivary glands, 1140
    sinonasal, 1082
    of thyroid gland, 1562
Undifferentiated intratubular malignant
        germ cells, 882
Undulant fever, 317-318
Unstable angina, 626
Upper respiratory tract and ear, 1077-1094
    external ear and, 1088-1089
    larynx in, 1084-1087
    middle ear in, 1087-1088
    nasal cavity and paranasal sinuses in, 1078-1083
    nasopharynx in, 1083-1084
    nose in, 1077
    plasmacytoma and, 1089
    relapsing polychondritis and, 1089
    rhabdomyoma and, 1089
    rhabdomyosarcoma and, 1089
    temporal bone and, 1089
Urachus, 853, 866-867
Uranium, 216, 260, 276
Urate, 36-38, 38
    gout and, 2089
Urbach-Wiethe syndrome, 1103
Uremia
    hemolytic syndromes and, 826, 827
    medullary cystic disease and, 847
    myocarditis and, 664
    pericarditis and, 666, 670-671, 671
    pneumonia and, 807
    poisons in, 807
Ureter, 850-852
    calculi in, 851
    duplication of, 850, 850
    inflammation of, 851-852
Ureteral valves, congenital, 850
Ureteritis cystica lesions, 852
Ureteritis follicularis, 852
Ureterocele, 850
Ureteropelvic stenosis, 850
Urethan, 606
Urethra
    lithiasis and, 899
    male, 898-899
    obstruction of, 906
Urethritis, nongonococcal, 357
Uricase, 36
Urinary bilharziasis, 458
Urinary bladder, 852-866
    calculous disease in, 854
    carcinoma of, 860

Urinary bladder—cont'd
    carcinoma of—cont'd
        schistosomiasis and, 458
    catheterization of, 834
    congenital malformations in, 852-853
    connective tissue tumors of, 866
    dilatation of, 853-854
    diverticulum of, 853
    embryonal sarcoma and, 866
    epithelial tumors in, 858-866, 859, 860
    exstrophy of, 852
    fistulas in, 854
    inflammation of, 854-857
    metaplastic mucosal lesions in, 857-858
    proliferative and metaplastic mucosal
            lesions of, 857-858
    radiation injury and, 279
    radiosensitivity of epithelium of, 257t
    rupture of, 853
    trauma to, 853
Urinary collecting system, 850-867, 869-870
    calices, pelves, and ureters in, 850-852
    infection of, 834, 855
        candidiasis and, 412
    obstruction of, 836-837
    urachus in, 866-867
    urinary bladder in; see Urinary bladder
Urinary shutdown, 906
Urinary system, 804-870
    alkylating agents and atypias of, 180
    collecting system in, 850-867, 869-870; see
        also Urinary collecting system
    kidneys in, 804-849, 867-869; see also
        Kidneys
Urine, failure of formation of, 809
Urogastrone–eosinophil chemotactic factor,
        1206
Urogenital organs, female; see Female
        genitalia
Urothelial tumors in urinary bladder, 858-
        866, 859, 860
Urovaginal septum, caudad growth of, 1622
Urticaria
    cholinergic, 527
    giant, 539t
Urticaria pigmentosa, 1775, 1775-1776
    systemic mastocytosis and, 1404
Urticaria solaris, 1776
Urticarial vasculitis, 1776
Ussing chambers, 433
Usual interstitial pneumonia, 971
Uteroplacental blood flow, reduced, 1703
Uterus
    developmental anomalies of, 1627-1628
    in embryo, 1620, 1621
    granulosa-theca cell tumors and bleeding
            from, 1685
    hemangiopericytoma of, 1667
    hypertrophy of, 42
    involution of, 42
Uveitis, 516, 1056
    allergic, 536t
    anterior, 1057
    sympathetic, 1056, 1057
Uveomeningoencephalitis syndrome, 1056
Uveoparotid fever, 1130-1131, 1131
Uveoparotitis, 1127

V
Vaccinia, 26, 27, 28, 386
Vacuolar nephropathy, 834, 834
Vacuoles
    disfigurative changes and muscle fiber,
            2110, 2110

Vacuoles—cont'd
distal myopathy and rimmed, 2112
tetracycline and hepatic, 1237, *1237*
Vagina, 1637-1642
adenosis of, 1639-1640
anatomy and physiology of, 1637-1638
botryoid rhabdomyosarcoma of, *1869*
clear cell carcinoma and, 1639-1640
cysts and nonneoplastic growths of, 1639
cytology in pathology of, 1638-1639
developmental anomalies of, 1627-1628
inflammation of, 1638-1639
neoplasms of, 1640-1642
in utero diethylstilbestrol exposure and,
1639-1640
Vaginitis, 1638
chronic, 878
nodular, 879
Vaginitis emphysematosa, 1639, *1639*
Valine, 546, 562
Valium; *see* Diazepam
Valsalva, sinuses of, 740, 776
Valves
cardiac
blood cysts of, 700
disorders of, 672-681
endocarditis and, 652
papillary tumors of, 703
rheumatic fever and, 639, 643-645, *644,
645*
of Heister, 1321
Valvular and hypertensive heart diseases,
672-681
acquired, 672-677
cardiac growth disturbances and, 677-681
Valvular fibrosis, methysergide and, 186
Van de Graaff generator, 284
Van Gieson stain, 1809
Vanillylmandelic acid, 1612
Vanishing testis syndrome, 873
Variant angina, 626
Variant follicular bronchiectasis, 949
Varicella pneumonia, 383
Varicella-zoster virus, 382
Varicoceles, 788, 892-893
Varicosities, 786-788
Variola, 28, 386
Vas deferens
absence of, 876
inflammation of, 892
Vasa recta loops, 806
Vasa vasorum, 767
Vascular disorders
alimentary tract and, 1158-1159
central nervous system, 2146-2153
hepatic, 1280-1281
peripheral neuropathies and, 2191
pulmonary, 922
pulmonary hypertension and, 954
radiation and, 256, 274
skin, 1789-1791
Vascular ectasia, 1159
Vascular lesions, 539*t*
adrenal medulla and, 1608
bone marrow and, 1405-1406
Vascular malformation, cerebral hemorrhage
from ruptured, 2151-2153, *2152*
Vascular permeability, 71-75
increased, *75*, 75-76
Vascular renal disease, 841-844
Vascular shunt, *68*
Vascular spiders, 1251
Vascular spread of carcinomas, *584*, 584-585

Vascular sprouts, 98, *99*, 106
Vascular tumors
of bone, *2050*, 2050-2051
gastrointestinal tract and, 1188
soft tissue, 1886-1890
Vasculitis, 766
antithyroid drugs and, 169
central nervous system infarct and, 2148
cholecystitis and, 1328
cutaneous, 539*t*
glomerular, 824, 826
hypersensitivity, 769, *771*
infective endocarditis and, 657
interstitial nephritis and, 838
nasal cavity and, 1079
nodular, 1789
noninfective, 768-778, *770, 771, 773, 775,
776, 777*
rheumatic, *775*
rheumatoid arthritis and, 649
trichiniasis and, 466
urticarial, 1776
Wegener's granulomatosis and, 975
Vasectomy, 893
Vasitis, 892, *893*
Vasoactive intestinal peptide, 519*t*, 1368-
1369
gallbladder and, 1322
Vasoconstriction
mechanical injury and, 131
pulmonary hypertension and, 956
Vasodilatation
inflammation and, 70
local, *68*
Vasogenic brain edema, 2125-2127, *2127,
2128*
Vasomotor nerve repair, 98
Vasopressin, 1523
Vasopressor amine toxicity, 216
Vater ampulla
atresias and, 1153
gallstone in, 1353
Vater-Pacini corpuscles, 1756
Vegetant intravascular
hemangioendothelioma, 796, 1820
Vegetations, 654, *655*, 655-656, *656, 657*
Veins, 786-791
aortocoronary bypass grafts of, 791, *792,
793*
digitalis and engorgement of intestinal,
175, 175-176
normal structure and age changes in, 786,
787
phlebothrombosis and thrombophlebitis
in, 788-791
primary tumors of large, 799
retinal, 1062-1063
of Retzius, 1250
saphenous, 787
of Sappey, 1250
varicosities of, 786-788, 1250
Vena cava
hypertension of, 1251
syndrome of, 790, 1504
Venezuelan equine encephalitis, 371
Veno-occlusive disease, hepatic, 1282-1283,
1283
Venous sinuses in spleen, 1408
Venous stasis, 952
Venous thrombosis; *see* Thrombosis
Ventral cerebellar herniation, 2129, *2129,
2130*

Ventricles
endomyocardial fibrosis and, 696
infarcts of, 629
Ventricular aneurysm, 638
Ventricular fibrillation, 140, 143, 144
Ventricular hamartomas, 2175
Ventricular septal defects, 731, 743
muscular artery necrosis in, *956*
Ventricular tachycardia, 637
Ventriculitis, 2157
Ventromedial occipital lobe infarction, *2129*,
2130
Venules
inflammatory response and, *68*
interendothelial gaps in, *74, 75*
terminal hepatic, 1199
Venulitis, 1790
Vermis, atrophy of cerebellar, 2185
Verocay bodies, 1892, 2171, *2172*
Verruca, 292*t*, 1794-1795
cutaneous, 385
endocarditis and, 652
of penis, 897
telangiectatic, 1820
thrombocytopenic angionecrosis, 1790-
1791
Verruca senilis, 1795
Verruca vulgaris, 385, 1794
in larynx, 1087
in oral soft tissue, 1106
Verrucae, endocarditis and, 653, 654
Verruciform xanthoma in oral soft tissue,
1107
Verrucous carcinoma
of cervix, 1652
of larynx, 1087
of oral soft tissue, 1112
of penis, 896
of skin, 1801
of vulva, 1635
Verrucous endocarditis, 643-644, *644*
Vertebral artery occlusion, 2148
Vertebral column diseases, 2096-2098
Vertebral joints, 2067
Vertebral osteoporosis, 1969, *1969, 1970*
Very-low-density lipoproteins, 619, 764
Vesicles, 85, 1757
endocytotic, 4
skin, 1760-1761
viral, 1766-1767, *1767*
Vesicointestinal fistula, 854, *854*
Vesicoureteral reflux, 851
Vesicovaginal fistula, 854
Vesicular stomatitis virus, 27
Vessels; *see* Blood vessels
Vestigial structures
cervical, 1644
ovarian, 1674
Vibrio, 299-300
Vietnamese time bomb, 324
Villinodular synovitis, 2093
Villitis, chronic, 1704-1705
Villous adenomas of gallbladder and
common duct, 1334
Villous edema of placenta, 1703
Vimentin, 1863, 1893, 2166*t*
Vimentin intermediate filament protein,
1863
Vinblastine toxicity, 185
Vinca alkaloids, neurofibrillary degeneration
and, 2133
Vincent's disease, 1105
Vincent's organisms, 557

Vincristine toxicity, 185
Vinyl chloride, 1298-1299
Viral antigens
  capsid, 383
  early, 383
Viral deoxyribonucleic acid, 26
Viral diseases, 362-390
  DNA, 377-387
    adenoviruses and, 377-378
    hepatitis B virus and, 387
    herpesviruses and, 378-384
    papovaviruses and, 384-386
    Poxviridae and, 386-387
  RNA, 363-377
    alphaviruses and, 371
    Arenaviridae and, 372-373
    Bunyaviridae and, 370
    Coronaviridae and, 369
    flaviviruses and, 371-372
    hepatitis A virus and, 377
    human retroviruses and, 375-376
    orthomyxoviruses and, 363-365
    paramyxoviruses and, 365-369
    Picornaviridae and, 374-375
    Rhabdoviridae and, 369-370
    rhinoviruses and, 375
    Togaviridae and, 370-371
  unconventional, 387
  virus-like agents and, 387-388
Viral exanthema, 539t
Viral factories, 386
Viral hepatitis, 1210-1223
  acute
    electron microscopy of, 1218
    histologic changes in, 1217, 1218
    needle biopsy of, 1217
    neonate and, 1265
    pathogenesis of, 1219
    recovery of, 1220
  arthritis and, 2087
  chronic active, 1225-1228, 1226
  delta, 1215-1216
    acute viral hepatitis B and, 1215, 1215t
    course of, 1225, 1228
    fulminant, 1223
  fatal, 1219-1223
  fulminant, 1219-1222, 1220
  in homosexuals, 1219
  impaired regeneration syndrome and,
    1222
  infectivity of, 1222
  Marburg, 1231
  morphologic changes in, 1217
  pathology of, 1217-1219
  persistent, 1223
  protracted, 1222
  relapse of, 1223
  type A, 1210-1211
    neonatal and childhood cholestasis and,
      1261t
  type B, 1211-1215
    acute delta hepatitis with, 1215, 1215t
    clinical, serologic, and biochemical
      course of, 1213
    course of, 1213, 1213
    epidemiology of, 1214
    neonatal and childhood cholestasis and,
      126t
  type non-A, non-B, 1216-1217
Viral oncogenes, 586, 589
Viral vesicles, 1766-1767, 1767
Virchow's lepra cells, 339
Virchow's node, 1183

Virchow's triad, 788
Virchow-Robin spaces, 440
Virilization, 1594-1595, 1598t
Virion, 1215
Virulence, 289
Virus-associated hemophagocytic syndrome,
    1425, 1425
Virus-host cell interaction, 362
Virus-like agents, 387-388
Virus-specific receptors, 26
Viruses, 498t
  arthritis and, 2075
  bronchiolitis and, 931
  carcinogenesis and, 600t, 600-602
  Chandipura, 27
  Ebola, 1231
  encephalitis and, 82, 82
  intranuclear inclusions and, 2133
  leukemia and, 1385
  lung and, 931-932
  Marburg, 376, 1231
  myocarditis and, 661, 661
  oncogenic, 266
  pericarditis and, 666, 668
  placenta and, 1705
  radiation and tumorigenic, 266
  Theiler, 27
  uncoating phenomenon and, 26
Visceral larva migrans, 467, 468, 1285
Visceral leishmaniasis, 443
Visceral tide, 447
Visible light, 285t
Vision loss, 1072; see also Blindness
Visual purple, 552
Vitamin D–dependent rickets, type I and
    type II, 1993
Vitamin deficiencies, 550-561
  A, 551-554, 552
    bone metabolism and, 1982
  B₁₂, 2185-2186, 2186
    bone marrow and, 1377-1378
  B group, 555-560
  C, 560-561
    heart disease and, 692
  congenital abnormalities and, 561
  D, 554
    diagnosis of, 1993
    osteomalacia and, 1984
    osteoporosis and, 1978
    primary, 1990
    secondary, 1990-1993
  E, 554-555, 2186
    axonopathy and, 2190
    central nervous system disorders and,
      2186
    heart disease and, 692
  K, 555
Vitamin D–resistant osteomalacia, 1994
Vitamin D–resistant rickets, 1097-1098
Vitamins
  A
    bone metabolism and, 1982
    metabolic bone diseases and, 1982
    smokers and, 1015
  B₁₂, diphyllobothriasis and, 460
  C
    bone metabolism and, 1982-1983
    metabolic bone diseases and, 1982
  D
    osteomalacia and, 1987
    osteopathy and, 1972
    osteoporosis and malabsorption of, 1981
    parathyroid glands and, 1571, 1573
  deficiencies of; see Vitamin deficiencies

Vitiligo, 539t
VLDL; see Very-low-density lipoproteins
Vocal cord papillomas, 385-386, 1020, 1084-
    1085
Vocal nodule, 1085
Vogt-Koyanagi-Harada disease, 1056
Volkmann's canals, 1931
Voltage
  electrical injury and, 141
  particulate radiation and, 248
Volume hypertrophy congenital heart
    disease, 730
Volvulus, 1157
Vomit, black, 372
von Brunn's nests, 852, 857
von Ebner glands, 1127
von Gierke's disease, 687
von Hansemann cells, 856
von Hippel-Lindau disease, 795
  central nervous system tumors and, 2166,
    2176
  eye and, 1051
  hemangioblastoma and, 2174
von Recklinghausen's disease, 50, 609, 866,
    1051, 1053
  malignant nerve sheath tumors and, 1894
  neurofibromas and, 1026, 1892-1893,
    2166, 2172, 2172-2173, 2175
  parathyroid glands and, 1575
  skin and, 1825
Vulva, 1628-1637
  amebiasis of, 436
  anatomy of, 1628
  developmental anomalies of, 1627-1628
  double, 1628
  dysplasia subclassifications and, 1633
  dystrophies, keratoses, and atrophy of,
    1629-1630
  embryology and, 1623
  herpes simplex of, 1628
  inflammation of, 1628-1629
  neoplasms of, 1630-1637
Vulvovaginal candidiasis, 412
Vulvovaginitis, gonococcal, 310

W

Waldenström's macroglobulinemia, 1402-
    1403, 1403, 1470, 1789
Waldeyer's throat ring, 1465
Wallerian degeneration, 2176, 2189
Walthard cell rests, 1190, 1667
Wandering spleen, 1418
Wangiella dermatitidis, 393t
Wart; see Verruca
Warthin-Finkeldey cells, 368, 1087, 1106,
    1106
Warthin-Starry stain, 1903
Warthin's tumor, 579, 1134
Wasting, 569
Watanabe hereditary hyperlipoproteinemic
    strain, 764
Water
  radiation and, 253
  radiochemistry of, 23, 24t
  radium, 280
  retention of, 806-807
Water-clear cell hyperplasia, 1570, 1574
Waterhammer pulse, 676
Waterhouse-Friderichsen syndrome, 309,
    1585
Watermelon stomach, 1159
Watery diarrhea, 1168
Wavelengths, radiation, 283

Weaning, mammary gland involution after, 42, 43
Wear-and-tear disease, 2073-2074
Web in pulmonary artery, 952, *952*
Weber-Christian disease, 1190, 1788, *1788*
Weber's syndrome, 1820
Weber's glands, 1127
Wegener's granulomatosis, 769-772, *771*, 826
   limited, 975
   in nasal cavity, 1079-1080
   in oral soft tissue, 1104
   in orbit of eye, 1047, *1049*
   pulmonary involvement in, 975-976
Weibel-Palade bodies, 1819, 1884
Weigert's stain for elastic tissue, 1782, *1783*
Weil disease, 1232
Weil-Marchesani syndrome, 1053
Weil stain, 2126*t*
Werdnig-Hoffmann disease, 2119, 2120-2121, *2121*, 2183
Wermer's syndrome, 1535
Wernicke-Korsakoff syndrome, 556
Wernicke's disease, 556
Wernicke's encephalopathy, 555, 556, 2185, *2185*
Western equine encephalitis, 371
Wet desquamation, 273
Wet lung, neonatal, 925
Wheal, 68, 518
Wheal-and-flare reaction, *520, 523*
Whipple's disease
   arthritis and, 2086
   gastrointestinal manifestations of, 1173, *1174*
Whipworm, 463
White, painful leg, 789
White arsenic, 210
White blood cell disorders, 1382-1399
   leukocytosis and, 1382-1384
   leukopenia and, 1382-1384
     radiation sickness and, 261
   proliferative, 1384-1390
     lymphoid cells and, 1394-1399
     myeloid cells and, 1390-1394
White graft reaction, 532
White oral mucosa lesions, 1109-1110
White piedra, 392*t*, 397
White pulp in spleen, 1408
White pupillary reflex, 1066, *1067*
White-spot disease, 1779
Whitmore's disease, 322
Whole-body irradiation, 264
Whooping cough, 297-299
Wickham's striae, 1102, 1110, 1774
Wilms' tumor, 579, 593*t*, *594*, 848-849, *849*
Wilson-Mikity syndrome, 926
Wilson's disease, 1074, 1269-1271, 1786
Winterbottom's sign, 439
Wintergreen oil toxicity, 158-160
Wire-loop lesion, 824
Wirsung duct, 1347
Wiskott-Aldrich syndrome, 384, 501*t*, 1500*t*
Wolbach's stain, 396*t*

Wolffian structures, 873
Wolff's law, 2001
Wolman's disease, gastrointestinal manifestations of, 1173
Wood alcohol poisoning, 197-198
Woodchuck hepatitis virus, 1211
Wool-sorter's disease, 297
Woringer-Kolopp disease, 1827
Work load, hypertrophy and, 568
World Health Organization, 548
Worms
   infection from, 498*t*
   lung disease and, 967
Wound track, 124, *125, 126*
Wounds, 112-115
   abrasion, 112, *113*
   contraction of, 104
   contusion, 114, *116*
   cutaneous entrance, 120-123, *121, 122, 123*
   cutaneous exit, 123-124, *124*
   fracture, 114-115
   handgun, 123, *125*
   incision, 114
   laceration, 112-114, *113, 114, 115*
   mechanical trauma and, 111
   penetrating injury, 114
   rifle, 123, *124*
   vitamin C and repair of, 560
Woven bone, 2023
Wright's stain, 1374, *1406*
Wryneck, 1142
Wucher atrophy of fat, 1788
Wuchereria bancrofti, 470, 893

X

X chromosome
   abnormalities in, 48
   disorders of, 58
   fragile chromosome sites and, 49
   mental retardation and, 49
   sexual differentiation and, 1623
X granules, 1423
X-linked enzyme glucose-6-phosphate dehydrogenase, 1384
X-linked hypophosphatemia, 1993-1994, *1994*
X rays, 23, 23*t*, 247, 283
Xanthelasma of eyelid, *1792*
Xanthofibroma, 2092-2093
   of tendon sheath, *2093*
Xanthogranuloma, 1856, *1857*
   cholecystitis and, 1332
   of iris, 1076, *1076*
   of joints, 2092
Xanthoma
   bone and, 2054
   of eyelid, biliary cirrhosis and, 1257
   pulmonary fibrous, 1021
   skin and, *1791*
Xanthoses, 1791-1792
Xanthurenic aciduria, 559
Xenobiotic compound biotransformation, 5

Xenograft, 531
Xenopsylla cheopsis, 320
Xeroderma pigmentosum, 61, 597, 609, 1797
Xerophthalmia, 552, 838
Xerostomia, 838, 1127
   radiation injury and, 277
Xylohypha bantiana, 395*t*, 402

Y

Y chromosome, 59
   sexual differentiation and, 1623
Yaws, 328, *328*
Yeast, 397
Yellow atrophy of liver, 1221
   pregnancy and, 1274
Yellow fever, 371-372, *373*
Yellow nail syndrome, 1787
Yellow-phosphorus toxicity, 224
Yellow respiratory enzyme, 558
Yersinia, 320-321, 1434
   arthritis and, 2086
yes 1, 587*t*
Yolk sac endoderm, 1621
Yolk-sac hematopoiesis, 1373
Yolk sac tumors of testes, 885, *885*

Z

Z band, 2106
   rhabdomyoma and, 1872
   rhabdomyosarcoma and, 1865, 1866
Z protein, 994
Zahn lines, 952
Zebra bodies, 52, 1529
Zeis glands, 1047
Zellballen, 1610
Zellweger's syndrome, 1267, 1268, 2116
Zenker's degeneration, 316
Zenker's diverticulum, 1155
Ziehl-Neelsen stain, 396*t*, 940, 1287
Zieve syndrome, 197
Zinc, 562
   oncogensis and, 239
Zinsser-Engman-Cole syndrome, 1110
Zirconium, 539*t*, 1785
Zollinger-Ellison syndrome, 1170, 1680
Zona fascicularis, *1590*
Zona fasciculata
   nodular hyperplasia of, *1594*
   poststeroid atrophy of, *1588*
Zona glomerulosa, *1590*
Zona reticularis, *1590*
   DDT toxicity and, 226, *228*
Zonal necrosis, 1204
Zonulae occludentes, 958
Zoonoses, 314, 348, 451-474
   leprosy as, 334-335
Zoster bodies of Lipschütz, 1767
Zoster cutaneous lesion, 382
Zygomycosis, 393*t*, 395*t*, *425*, 425-427, *426*
Zygote, 1624, 1699
Zygotic gene replacement therapy, 62
Zymogen granules, 1347